THE JOURNAL OF PEDIATRICS

MOSBY–YEAR BOOK, INC. JANUARY-JUNE 1995 VOLUME 126

THE JOURNAL OF PEDIATRICS
VOLUME 126

Mosby

THE JOURNAL OF PEDIATRICS

Contents

JANUARY 1995

Medical progress

Cancer in children with primary or secondary immunodeficiencies 1
Brigitta U. Mueller, MD, and Philip A. Pizzo, MD, Bethesda, Maryland

Original articles

Progression of premature thelarche to central precocious puberty 11
Anna Maria Pasquino, MD, Ida Pucarelli, MD, Franca Passeri, MD, Maria Segni, MD, Maria Antonietta Mancini, MD, and Giovanna Municchi, MD, Rome, Italy

One hundred girls thought to have premature thelarche were followed for several years, and 14 eventually progressed into precocious puberty. No clinical or laboratory studies at the time of onset differentiated the minority of girls who progressed into puberty from those with isolated thelarche.

Increased fat oxidation in prepubertal obese children: A metabolic defense against further weight gain? 15
C. Maffeis, MD, L. Pinelli, MD, and Y. Schutz, PhD, Verona, Italy, and Lausanne, Switzerland

Obese children were found to have a higher postabsorptive rate of fat oxidation than nonobese children. Thus a reduction of fat intake plus increased physical activity should favor fat loss by achieving a negative fat balance.

Measured versus predicted resting energy expenditure in infants: A need for reappraisal 21
M. A. Thomson, MRCP(UK), S. Bucolo, GDID, P. Quirk, BSc(Hons), and R. W. Shepherd, MD, FRACP, Brisbane, Australia

Measurements of resting energy expenditure in well infants and in those with cystic fibrosis showed that the formulas used to predict REE were often inaccurate. These data call into question many recommendations for caloric and fluid intake for infants, at least for the individual infant.

Vol. 126, No. 1, January 1995. The Journal of Pediatrics (ISSN 0022-3476) is published monthly (six issues per volume, two volumes per year) by Mosby–Year Book, Inc., 11830 Westline Industrial Dr., St. Louis, MO 63146-3318. Second-class postage paid at St. Louis, Mo., and additional mailing offices. POSTMASTER: Send changes of address to The Journal of Pediatrics, Mosby–Year Book, Inc., 11830 Westline Industrial Dr., St. Louis, MO 63146-3318, (800)453-4351. Annual subscription rates: domestic, $102.00 for individuals and $211.00 for institutions. Printed in U.S.A.

CONTENTS *continued*

Normal energy expenditure in the infant with presymptomatic cystic fibrosis 28

Michele N. Bronstein, PhD, Peter S. W. Davies, PhD, K. Michael Hambidge, FRCP(Ed), ScD, and Frank J. Accurso, MD, Denver, Colorado, and Cambridge, United Kingdom

Infants with cystic fibrosis who had no symptoms of the disease had normal energy expenditure when body composition was taken into account. However, such infants may need an increased caloric intake to maintain normal fat tissue stores.

Chronic constipation as a symptom of cow milk allergy 34

G. Iacono, MD, A. Carroccio, MD, F. Cavataio, MD, G. Montalto, MD, M. D. Cantarero, MD, and A. Notarbartolo, MD, Palermo, Italy

Infants and young children referred because of constipation often responded well to introduction of a diet free of cow milk, especially if they had a history of colic or other symptoms possibly related to cow milk allergy, or laboratory evidence of atopy.

Spectrum of disease associated with anti-neutrophil cytoplasmic autoantibodies in pediatric patients 40

Eileen N. Ellis, MD, Ellen G. Wood, MD, and Phillip Berry, MD, Little Rock, Arkansas, and St. Louis, Missouri

Five children with anti-neutrophil cytoplasmic antibodies and a spectrum of disease, including glomerulonephritis with or without respiratory disease, are described. Progression to end-stage renal disease was common. Measurement of ANCA seems appropriate in children with glomerulonephritis and systemic vasculitis.

Somatosensory evoked potentials for prediction of outcome in acute severe brain injury 44

J. Beca, MBChB, FRACP, P. N. Cox, MBChB, FFARCS, FRCPC, M. J. Taylor, PhD, D. Bohn, MBBCh, FRCPC, W. Butt, MBBS, FRACP, W. J. Logan, MD, FRCPC, J. T. Rutka, MD, FRCSC, and G. Barker, MBBS, FFARACS, Toronto, Ontario, Canada, and Melbourne, Victoria, Australia

In children with brain injury of various types, the absence of somatosensory evoked potentials was found to predict an unfavorable outcome with high accuracy. Such studies may be helpful in determining whether withdrawal of treatment should be considered.

Catheter-related thrombosis in critically ill children: Comparison of catheters with and without heparin bonding 50

Brian Krafte-Jacobs, MD, Carlos J. Sivit, MD, Rodrigo Mejia, MD, and Murray M. Pollack, MD, FCCM, Washington, D.C.

The use of heparin-bonded catheters in an intensive care unit was associated with a lower incidence of thromboses and of catheter-related infections than in children with standard femoral venous catheters. The absence of clinical signs did not rule out the presence of thromboses.

CONTENTS *continued*

Clinical and laboratory observations

Fisher syndrome after *Campylobacter jejuni* enteritis: Human leukocyte antigen and the bacterial serotype 55
Nobuhiro Yuki, MD, PhD, Hiroo Ichikawa, MD, and Ayumi Doi, MD, Tokyo, Fukuyama City, and Hiroshima, Japan

Acute pancreatitis associated with acute hepatitis A in a young child 57
Lydia A. Shrier, MD, Saul J. Karpen, MD, PhD, and Colston McElvoy, MD, Boston, Massachusetts, and New Haven, Connecticut

Methemoglobinemia associated with acidosis of probable renal origin 59
Susanne Sager, PhD, MD, Guy H. Grayson, MD, and Stephen A. Feig, MD, Los Angeles, California

Intact survival with transfusion-associated graft-versus-host disease proved by human leukocyte antigen typing of lymphocytes in skin biopsy specimens 61
R. Hentschel, MD, E. B. Broecker, MD, G. Kolde, MD, M. Frosch, MD, W. Friedrich, MD, W. Holzgreve, MS, MD, E. Westphal, MD, and E. Harms, MD, Münster, Würzburg, Ulm, and Kiel, Germany

Neonatal onset of medium-chain acyl–coenzyme A dehydrogenase deficiency with confusing biochemical features 65
John Christodoulou, MBBS, PhD, FRACP, Julie Hoare, BSc, Judith Hammond, MAppSc, Wai Ching Ip, BSc, and Bridget Wilcken, MBChB, FRACP, Sydney and Camperdown, Australia

Transient organic aciduria and persistent lacticacidemia in a patient with short-chain acyl–coenzyme A dehydrogenase deficiency 69
D. Brian Dawson, PhD, Lewis Waber, MD, PhD, Daniel E. Hale, MD, and Michael J. Bennett, PhD, MRCPath, Dallas, Texas, and Philadelphia, Pennsylvania

Congenital lacticacidemia caused by lipoamide dehydrogenase deficiency with favorable outcome 72
O. N. Elpeleg, MD, W. Ruitenbeek, PhD, C. Jakobs, PhD, V. Barash, PhD, D. C. De Vivo, MD, and N. Amir, MD, Jerusalem, Israel; Nijmegen and Amsterdam, The Netherlands; and New York, New York

Fetal and neonatal medicine

Secular changes in the outcomes to eighteen to twenty-four months of age of extremely low birth weight infants, with adjustment for changes in risk factors and severity of illness 75
Max Perlman, MB, Olivier Claris, MD, Yong Hao, MD, PhD, Paresh Pandit, MB, Hilary Whyte, MB, Mary Chipman, MSc, and Peter Liu, MD, Toronto, Ontario, Canada

An analysis of changes in rates of death and of major impairment during the 1980s was conducted in a regional neonatal intensive care unit for outborn infants. Despite increasing referrals of less mature and more severely ill infants, and more aggressive care, the rate of major impairment fell significantly.

CONTENTS *continued*

Acuity scores as predictors of cost-related outcomes of neonatal intensive care 88

Uma R. Kotagal, MBBS, Paul H. Perlstein, MD, Harry D. Atherton, MSEE, and Edward F. Donovan, MD, Cincinnati, Ohio

Two proprietary scoring systems for stratifying patients so as to compare the care they received were evaluated in a neonatal intensive care unit. One correlated well with lengths of stay, use of ancillary resources, and hospital discharges; the other was no better than birth weight. Better instruments are needed to compare cost-related elements of medical care.

Synthetic surfactant for rescue treatment of respiratory distress syndrome in premature infants weighing from 700 to 1350 grams: Impact on hospital resource use and charges 94

Josephine A. Mauskopf, PhD, Martin E. Backhouse, MSc, David Jones, MS, Diane E. Wold, PhD, Mark C. Mammel, MD, Martha Mullett, MD, Robert Guthrie, MD, and Walker A. Long, MD, Research Triangle Park and Chapel Hill, North Carolina; St. Paul, Minnesota; Morgantown, West Virginia; and Pittsburgh, Pennsylvania

A cost analysis of data from a controlled study of the use of synthetic surfactant in preterm infants indicated that long-term charges for infants treated with surfactant were not likely to be higher, at least through the first year after birth, even though more treated infants survived. Rescue therapy with surfactant can improve survival without increasing hospital charges.

Glucose-6-phosphate dehydrogenase deficiency and carboxyhemoglobin concentrations associated with bilirubin-related morbidity and death in Nigerian infants 102

Tina M. Slusher, MD, Hendrik J. Vreman, PhD, Donald W. McLaren, MD, Laura J. Lewison, BA, Audrey K. Brown, MD, and David K. Stevenson, MD, Dallas, Texas; Stanford, California; Brooklyn, New York; and Eku, Nigeria

In jaundiced Nigerian neonates, carboxyhemoglobin concentrations correlated well with serum bilirubin values and, when G6PD deficiency was present, with bilirubin-related morbidity and death. Earlier recognition of increased bilirubin production might allow effective intervention and fewer serious sequelae.

Internal potassium shift in premature infants: Cause of nonoliguric hyperkalemia 109

Kazuo Sato, MD, Tsutomu Kondo, MD, Hatsuo Iwao, MD, Sunao Honda, MD, and Kohji Ueda, MD, Fukuoka City, Japan

Studies of potassium balance in preterm infants during the first 3 days of life indicated that nonoliguric hyperkalemia is due to a shift of K from the intracellular to the extracellular space, which is greatest in the smallest infants.

CONTENTS *continued*

Use of the urine-to-blood carbon dioxide tension gradient as a measurement of impaired distal tubular hydrogen ion secretion among neonates 114
Jin-Yao Lin, MD, Jin-Shoei Lin, MD, and Chang-Hai Tsai, MD, Taiwan, Republic of China

The urine-to-blood partial pressure of the CO_2 gradient was found to have a linear relation to urinary bicarbonate concentrations in neonates, as in older infants and children, and is a useful indicator of distal urinary acidification in evaluating whether renal tubular acidosis is present.

Newborn screening for congenital adrenal hyperplasia in New Zealand 118
W. S. Cutfield, MBChB, and D. Webster, PhD, Auckland, New Zealand

Experience in neonatal screening for congenital adrenal hyperplasia in New Zealand indicates that it is a cost-effective and sensitive way to identify affected boys and some unrecognized affected girls. Early notification of results and prompt treatment are necessary to achieve maximal benefit from screening.

Reference ranges for newer thyroid function tests in premature infants 122
Linda M. Adams, MD, Janet R. Emery, MD, Susan J. Clark, MD, Esther I. Carlton, MT, and Jerald C. Nelson, MD, Loma Linda and San Juan Capistrano, California

Reference ranges for thyroid function were determined for preterm infants. Free thyroxine concentration correlated positively with gestational age, as did the logarithm of thyrotropin values.

Clinical and laboratory observations

Vitamin A and E status in very low birth weight infants: Development of an improved parenteral delivery system 128
T. E. Inder, MBChB, A. C. Carr, BScHons, C. C. Winterbourn, PhD, N. C. Austin, MBChB, FRACP, and B. A. Darlow, MD, FRACP, Christchurch, New Zealand

Possible fetal effects of cervical dilation and uterine curettage during the first trimester of pregnancy 131
Lewis B. Holmes, MD, Boston, Massachusetts

Pediatric pharmacology and therapeutics

Use of a visual panel detection method for drugs of abuse: Clinical and laboratory experience with children and adolescents 135
Jimmie L. Valentine, PhD, and Eva M. Komoroski, MD, Little Rock, Arkansas

A device that rapidly identifies seven classes of drugs in urine was evaluated in a hospital setting. Reasonable specificity and positive predictive values were found when confirmation was attempted by gas chromatography–mass spectrometry. The primary advantages were the ease of use and rapid availability of results, which were helpful in differential diagnosis.

CONTENTS *continued*

Clinical and laboratory observations

Successful treatment of Finnish congenital nephrotic syndrome with captopril and indomethacin 140
A. Pomeranz, MD, B. Wolach, MD, J. Bernheim, MD, Z. Korzets, MBBS, and J. Bernheim, MD, Kfar Saba and Tel Aviv, Israel

Treatment of intractable gastrointestinal manifestations of chronic granulomatous disease with cyclosporine 143
Joel R. Rosh, MD, Hope B. Tang, MD, Lloyd Mayer, MD, Gabriel Groisman, MD, Sheeja K. Abraham, MD, and Alice Prince, MD, New York, New York

Healing of rickets during vitamin D therapy despite defective vitamin D receptors in two siblings with vitamin D–dependent rickets type II 145
Klaus Kruse, MD, and Evemarie Feldmann, MD, Luebeck and Neunkirchen, Germany

Current literature and clinical issues

Abstracts from the literature 149

Profiles in pediatrics II

C. Henry Kempe 152
Vincent A. Fulginiti, MD, Denver, Colorado

Editorial correspondence

Incidence of liver disease in patients with cystic fibrosis and meconium ileus 155
Anders Lindblad, MD, Birgitta Strandvik, MD, PhD, and Lena Hjelte, MD, PhD, Göteborg and Stockholm, Sweden

Reply 155
Carla Colombo, MD, Annamaria Giunta, MD, and Pier Maria Battezzati, MD, Milan, Italy

Short-term, high-dose corticosteroid therapy in childhood acute immune thrombocytopenic purpura 156
Haluk Yavûz, MD, Ahmet Özel, MD, and İbrahim Erkul, MD, Konya, Turkey

Reply 156
Victor S. Blanchette, MRCP(UK), FRCP(C), Toronto, Ontario, Canada

Diagnostic accuracy of urinary tract infection and subsequent development of renal scars 157
Olli Koskimies, MD, Helsinki, Finland

Reply 158
Alejandro Hoberman, MD, and Ellen R. Wald, MD, Pittsburgh, Pennsylvania

Local reactions to luteinizing hormone releasing hormone analog therapy 159
Giorgio Tonini, MD, Stefano Marinoni, MD, Vincenzo Forleo, MD, and Mariangela Rustico, MD, Trieste, Italy

Reply 159
E. Kirk Neely, MD, and Darrel M. Wilson, MD, Stanford, California

CONTENTS *continued*

Hypotension in preterm infants 160
Jay M. Milstein, MD, Davis, California

Reply 160
Roger G. Faix, MD, Ann Arbor, Michigan

Terbutaline powder for acute asthma 161
P. Rufin, MD, M. R. Benoist, MD, J. de Blic, MD, and P. Scheinmann, MD, Paris, France

Familial Guillain-Barré syndrome subsequent to *Campylobacter jejuni* enteritis 162
Nobuhiro Yuki, MD, PhD, and Yoshihiro Tsujino, Tokyo and Osaka, Japan

Reader services

Instructions to authors 14A

Information for readers 17A

Scheduled meetings 19A

News and notes 21A

Annual listing of fellowships 25A

Professional opportunities 78A

Index to advertisers 86A

THE JOURNAL OF PEDIATRICS

Contents

FEBRUARY 1995

Medical progress

Allergic colitis in infants 163
Robert D. Odze, MD, FRCP(C), Barry K. Wershil, MD, Alan M. Leichtner, MD, and Donald A. Antonioli, MD, Boston, Massachusetts

Original articles

Enhanced adrenomedullary response and increased susceptibility to neuroglycopenia: Mechanisms underlying the adverse effects of sugar ingestion in healthy children 171
Timothy W. Jones, MD, Walter P. Borg, MD, Susan D. Boulware, MD, Gregory McCarthy, PhD, Robert S. Sherwin, MD, and William V. Tamborlane, MD, New Haven, Connecticut

Metabolic studies of the responses to ingestion of sugar showed that children, in comparison with adults, had higher adrenomedullary responses to modest reductions in plasma glucose concentrations and more hypoglycemic symptoms at similar plasma glucose values. These data may explain the symptoms attributed to glucose ingestion in some children. *See* related article on page 178.

Effects of acute hyperglycemia on mental efficiency and counterregulatory hormones in adolescents with insulin-dependent diabetes mellitus 178
Sylvia Gschwend, MD, Christopher Ryan, PhD, Joy Atchison, MD, Silva Arslanian, MD, and Dorothy Becker, MBBCh, Pittsburgh, Pennsylvania

In adolescents with diabetes mellitus, studies during an insulin-glucose clamp showed that mild hypoglycemia caused transient decreases in cognitive function. Neither hyperglycemia nor a rapid change from hyperglycemia to euglycemia affected cognitive function or other symptoms. *See* related article on page 171.

Vol. 126, No. 2, February 1995. The Journal of Pediatrics (ISSN 0022-3476) is published monthly (six issues per volume, two volumes per year) by Mosby–Year Book, Inc., 11830 Westline Industrial Dr., St. Louis, MO 63146-3318. Second-class postage paid at St. Louis, Mo., and additional mailing offices. POSTMASTER: Send changes of address to The Journal of Pediatrics, Mosby–Year Book, Inc., 11830 Westline Industrial Dr., St. Louis, MO 63146-3318, (800)453-4351. Annual subscription rates: domestic, $102.00 for individuals and $211.00 for institutions. Printed in U.S.A.

CONTENTS *continued*

Subsequent insect stings in children with hypersensitivity to Hymenoptera 185

Pia Hauk, MD, Katrin Friedl, Klaus Kaufmehl, MD, Radvan Urbanek, MD, and Johannes Forster, MD, Freiburg, Germany, and Vienna, Austria

Children who had allergic reactions to Hymenoptera stings were challenged with a sting by the relevant insect under controlled conditions. The subsequent reactions were better predictors of the need for venom immunotherapy than were results of skin-prick tests or serologic evidence of sensitization.

Relation between infant feeding and infections during the first six months of life 191

Micheline Beaudry, PDt, MNS, PhD, Renée Dufour, MSc, and Sylvie Marcoux, MD, PhD, Sainte-Foy, Quebec, Canada

A retrospective cohort study of infants of primiparous women showed a protective effect of breast-feeding on both respiratory and gastrointestinal illnesses during the first 6 months of life, even when socioeconomic status, maternal smoking, and other risk factors were taken into account.

Effect of neonatal immunization with diphtheria and tetanus toxoids on antibody responses to *Haemophilus influenzae* type b conjugate vaccines 198

Jay M. Lieberman, MD, David P. Greenberg, MD, Victor K. Wong, MD, Susan Partridge, RN, Swei-Ju Chang, MS, Chung-Yin Chiu, MS, and Joel I. Ward, MD, Los Angeles and Torrance, California

Neonatal immunization with *Haemophilus* conjugate vaccine did not increase the antibody response to subsequent doses of vaccine given at the usual time. Neonatal administration of diphtheria–tetanus toxoid may have led to suppression of responses to subsequent doses of *Haemophilus* conjugate vaccine with DT antigens.

Enhanced antibody responses in infants given different sequences of heterogeneous *Haemophilus influenzae* type b conjugate vaccines 206

David P. Greenberg, MD, Jay M. Lieberman, MD, S. Michael Marcy, MD, Victor K. Wong, MD, Susan Partridge, RN, Swei-Ju Chang, MS, Chung-Yin Chiu, MS, and Joel I. Ward, MD, Los Angeles, Torrance, Panorama City, and Downey, California

Heterogeneous schedules of different *Haemophilus* conjugate vaccines given in infancy were as immunogenic as schedules of single conjugate vaccines. Some schedules may provide protection earlier in infancy and may be especially useful in populations at high risk.

CONTENTS *continued*

Pediatric Investigators Collaborative Network on Infections in Canada (PICNIC) prospective study of risk factors and outcomes in patients hospitalized with respiratory syncytial viral lower respiratory tract infection 212
Elaine E. L. Wang, MDCM, Barbara J. Law, MD, Derek Stephens, MS, and other members of PICNIC, Toronto, Ontario, Canada

A prospective study of infants with lower respiratory tract infections caused by respiratory syncytial virus was carried out in seven Canadian tertiary care hospitals. Hypoxia on admission, a history of apnea, and the presence of pneumonia increased the need for intensive care and prolonged hospitalization, as did aboriginal race and the presence of underlying heart or lung disease.

Hospitalization for lower respiratory tract illness in infants: Variation in rates among counties in New York State and areas within Monroe County 220
Kenneth M. McConnochie, MD, MPH, Klaus J. Roghmann, PhD, and Gregory S. Liptak, MD, MPH, Rochester, New York

Hospitalization rates for infants with lower respiratory tract illness varied substantially within small geographic areas, and were related more closely to socioeconomic than to identifiable medical factors, although physician discretion is probably a major determinant. Substantial cost savings and better service to families may be possible by using less expensive alternatives to hospitalization.

Binding of *Pseudomonas aeruginosa* to respiratory epithelial cells from patients with various mutations in the cystic fibrosis transmembrane regulator 230
Heather Zar, MBBCh, Lisa Saiman, MD, Lynne Quittell, MD, and Alice Prince, MD, New York, New York

Pseudomonas aeruginosa bound significantly better to epithelial cells of patients with cystic fibrosis than to cells from carriers of a CF mutation or from normal subjects. However, no correlation between quantity of binding and clinical status could be demonstrated.

Expanded spectrum of herpes simplex encephalitis in childhood 234
Yechiel Schlesinger, MD, Richard S. Buller, PhD, Janice E. Brunstrom, MD, Christopher J. Moran, MD, and Gregory A. Storch, MD, St. Louis, Missouri

Three young children eventually shown to have herpes simplex encephalitis had atypical findings, including multifocal or diffuse involvement of the brain, shown by MRI. Polymerase chain reaction for detection of HSV DNA in spinal fluid was helpful in diagnosis.

Lipid abnormalities in Turner syndrome 242
Judith L. Ross, MD, Penelope Feuillan, MD, Lauren L. Long, RN, Karen Kowal, PA, Harvey Kushner, PhD, and Gordon B. Cutler, Jr., MD, Bethesda, Maryland, and Philadelphia, Pennsylvania

Serum cholesterol values in girls with Turner syndrome were higher than in a control group, and the increase preceded any treatment with estrogen or growth hormone. This constitutes another cardiovascular risk factor in Turner syndrome.

CONTENTS *continued*

Lysinuric protein intolerance characterized by bone marrow abnormalities and severe clinical course 246
Giancarlo Parenti, MD, Gianfranco Sebastio, MD, Pietro Strisciuglio, MD, Barbara Incerti, MD, Carmine Pecoraro, MD, Luigi Terracciano, MD, and Generoso Andria, MD, Naples and Catanzaro, Italy

Nine patients with lysinuric protein intolerance from southern Italy are described. Unusual clinical features in some patients (erythroblastophagocytosis, pancreatitis, kidney failure) indicate that genetic heterogeneity may be present. Pulmonary disease is the most severe complication.

Long-term reduction in bone mass after severe burn injury in children 252
Gordon L. Klein, MD, David N. Herndon, MD, Craig B. Langman, MD, Thomas C. Rutan, MSN, William E. Young, MS, Gregory Pembleton, CNMT, Martin Nusynowitz, MD, Joseph L. Barnett, BSN, Lyle D. Broemeling, PhD, Dawn E. Sailer, MS, and Robert L. McCauley, MD, Galveston, Texas, and Chicago, Illinois

Children with severe burns were found to have persistently reduced bone density compared with values in matched children with moderate burns. The changes may contribute to an increased risk of fractures and to osteoporosis later in life.

Editor's column

Venom immunotherapy: Who should receive it? 257
C. Warren Bierman, MD, Seattle, Washington

Clinical and laboratory observations

Critical illness neuromuscular disease in children manifested as ventilatory dependence 259
Raj D. Sheth, MD, William E. M. Pryse-Phillips, MD, Jack E. Riggs, MD, and John B. Bodensteiner, MD, Morgantown, West Virginia, and St. John's, Canada

Transient elevation of sweat chloride concentration in a malnourished girl with the Mauriac syndrome 261
Fernando P. Polack, MD, David J. Transue, MD, William M. Belknap, MD, Bishara J. Freij, MD, and David J. Aughton, MD, Royal Oak, Michigan

Transformation of congenital neutropenia into monosomy 7 and acute nonlymphoblastic leukemia in a child treated with granulocyte colony-stimulating factor 263
Mark E. Weinblatt, MD, Philip Scimeca, MD, Anne James-Herry, MD, Indira Sahdev, MD, and Joseph Kochen, MD, PhD, Manhasset, New York

CONTENTS *continued*

Painful keratoderma and photophobia: Hallmarks of tyrosinemia type II 266
Linda G. Rabinowitz, MD, Lynn R. Williams, MD, MPH, Carol E. Anderson, MD, Alice Mazur, RN, MS, and Paige Kaplan, MB,BCh, Milwaukee, Wisconsin; Cleveland, Ohio; and Philadelphia, Pennsylvania

Loss of detectable antibody to hepatitis B surface antigen in immunized patients with hemophilia but without human immunodeficiency virus infection 269
John M. Maris, MD, Regina B. Butler, RN, and Alan R. Cohen, MD, Philadelphia, Pennsylvania

Fetal and neonatal medicine

Effect of maternal glucocorticoid exposure on risk of severe intraventricular hemorrhage in surfactant-treated preterm infants 272
Jeffery S. Garland, MD, SM, Rosanne Buck, MSN, CNNP, and Alan Leviton, MD, SM, Boston, Massachusetts

A retrospective study confirmed that antenatal administration of corticosteroids to mothers reduced the risk of severe intraventricular hemorrhage in their preterm infants. Steroid therapy was associated with a reduced risk of hypotension and its consequences, but not with pulmonary function improvement after surfactant therapy.

Reducing blood donor exposures in low birth weight infants by the use of older, unwashed packed red blood cells 280
David A. Lee, MD, Terri A. Slagle, MD, Thomas M. Jackson, MD, and Cherie S. Evans, MD, San Francisco and Oakland, California

The use of dedicated eight-packs of erythrocytes reduced donor exposures in preterm infants needing transfusions, and was technically simple and logistically feasible. The data indicate that washing erythrocytes and using only younger cells are not necessary.

Effects of parenteral L-carnitine supplementation on fat metabolism and nutrition in premature neonates 287
Cynthia M. Bonner, MD, Karan L. DeBrie, RD, George Hug, MD, Evelyn Landrigan, BS, and Bonnie J. Taylor, MD, Little Rock, Arkansas, and Cincinnati, Ohio

Intravenous administration of carnitine in parenterally fed preterm infants increased plasma carnitine concentrations and enhanced ketogenesis, probably because of an increase in carnitine stores. Amount of lipid tolerated and weight gain also were improved in infants weighing more than 1000 gm.

Clinical and laboratory observations

Congenital cytomegalovirus infection as a result of nonprimary cytomegalovirus disease in a mother with acquired immunodeficiency syndrome 293
Kay Schwebke, MD, Keith Henry, MD, Henry H. Balfour, Jr., MD, Douglas Olson, MD, R. Thomas Crane, MS, and M. Colin Jordan, MD, St. Paul and Minneapolis, Minnesota

The book shelf

Book reviews 296

CONTENTS *continued*

Pediatric pharmacology and therapeutics

Growth and the growth hormone axis in prepubertal children with asthma 297
Suzanne Crowley, MRCP, Peter C. Hindmarsh, MD, David R. Matthews, MD, and Charles G. D. Brook, MD, London and Oxford, United Kingdom

Studies of the growth hormone axis in children with asthma showed that slow growth was common in those treated with corticosteroids, whether given orally or by inhalation, but there were no significant changes in growth hormone secretion or insulin-like growth factor I.

Corticosteroid therapy for ventricular tachycardia in children with silent lymphocytic myocarditis 304
Toshihiro Ino, MD, Mataichi Okubo, MD, Katsumi Akimoto, MD, Kei Nishimoto, MD, Keijiro Yabuta, MD, Sachio Kawai, MD, and Ryozo Okada, MD, Tokyo, Japan

Four patients with unexplained ventricular tachycardia were found to have lymphocytic myocarditis on endomyocardial biopsy. Corticosteroid therapy was followed by remission of the tachycardia, whereas antiarrhythmic therapy was ineffective in three patients.

A randomized comparison of intravenously administered granisetron versus chlorpromazine plus dexamethasone in the prevention of ifosfamide-induced emesis in children 309
Karel Hählen, MD, PhD, Erica Quintana, MD, C. Ross Pinkerton, MD, DCH, FRCPI, and Eve Cedar, MSc, Rotterdam, The Netherlands; Paris, France; and Sutton and Harlow, United Kingdom

Intravenously administered granisetron was superior to a combination of chlorpromazine and dexamethasone in preventing ifosfamide-induced emesis, and undesirable side effects were less common with granisetron.

Clinical and laboratory observations

Short-term use of amoxicillin-clavulanate during upper respiratory tract infection for prevention of acute otitis media 313
Terho Heikkinen, MD, Olli Ruuskanen, MD, Thedi Ziegler, PhD, Matti Waris, PhD, and Heikki Puhakka, MD, Turku, Finland

Current literature and clinical issues

Antenatal corticosteroid therapy to prevent respiratory distress syndrome 317
C. Anthony Ryan, MB, FRCPC, and Neil N. Finer, MD, FRCPC, Cork, Ireland, and Edmonton, Alberta, Canada

The book shelf

Book reviews 320

Editorial correspondence

Usefulness of cerebrospinal fluid bacterial antigen tests 321
C. R. Warren, DO, and W. R. Kiser, MD, MA, Jacksonville, Florida

Reply 321
M. Suzanne Maxson, MD, Mary Jo Lewno, BS, and Gordon E. Schutze, MD, Little Rock, Arkansas

CONTENTS *continued*

Infectious hazards of immune globulin 321
Leslie L. Barton, MD, Tucson, Arizona

Reply 322
Padmani Karna, MD, Dennis L. Murray, MD, and John W. Dyke, PhD, Lansing, Michigan

Differences in clinical significance of maternal-infant blood group incompatibility in mothers with blood type O, A, or B 322
Harold Perl, MD, Hackensack, New Jersey

Reply 322
John A. Ozolek, MD, Jon F. Watchko, MD, and Francis B. Mimouni, MD, Pittsburgh, Pennsylvania, and Brooklyn, New York

Screening neonates for intrauterine cocaine exposure 323
Daniel R. Neuspiel, MD, MPH, Bronx, New York

Reply 324
Rita M. Ryan, MD, and Dale L. Phelps, MD, Rochester, New York

Accuracy of aural infrared temperature device 324
Naja E. McKenzie, RN, MN, Carlsbad, California

Reply 324
Robert Yetman, MD, Houston, Texas

The book shelf — **New books received** 326

Reviewers — **Acknowledgment of reviewers** 327

Reader services — **Instructions to authors** 13A

Information for readers 16A

Scheduled meetings 17A

Professional opportunities 26A

Index to advertisers C3

THE JOURNAL OF PEDIATRICS

Mosby

THE JOURNAL OF PEDIATRICS

Contents

MARCH 1995

Medical progress

Cardiovascular, renal, and endocrine actions of dopamine in neonates and children 333
Istvan Seri, MD, PhD, Philadelphia, Pennsylvania

Original articles

Definition and application of the discretionary screening indicators according to the National Cholesterol Education Program for Children and Adolescents 345
Philip M. Diller, MD, PhD, Gertrude A. Huster, MHS, Alan D. Leach, MS, Peter M. Laskarzewski, PhD, and Dennis L. Sprecher, MD, Cincinnati, Ohio

The addition of secondary screening indicators, such as high fat intake, to the current guidelines for cholesterol screening in childhood increased the number of children identified as having high serum low-density lipoprotein values. The absence of any indicators was associated with a very low risk of having high cholesterol values.

Relation of activity levels to body fat in infants 6 to 12 months of age 353
Ruowei Li, MD, PhD, Lisa O'Connor, MEd, Donna Buckley, BA, and Bonny Specker, PhD, Cincinnati, Ohio

A study of healthy infants found that body fatness was related more to activity levels than to energy intake; babies with higher body fatness tended to become less active later in infancy. Perhaps physical activity should be encouraged in fat infants.

A cross-sectional study of catheter-related thrombosis in children receiving total parenteral nutrition at home 358
Maureen Andrew, MD, Velma Marzinotto, RN, Paul Pencharz, MD, Stanley Zlotkin, MD, PhD, Patricia Burrows, MD, Joanne Ingram, RN, Margaret Adams, and Robert Filler, MD, Toronto, Ontario, Canada

In children receiving total parenteral nutrition at home, the risk of extensive deep venous thrombosis of the upper limbs and superior vena cava was found to be high. Prevention of this potentially serious complication (best demonstrated by venography) with low doses of warfarin deserves further study.

Continued on page 5A

Vol. 126, No. 3, March 1995. The Journal of Pediatrics (ISSN 0022-3476) is published monthly (six issues per volume, two volumes per year) by Mosby–Year Book, Inc., 11830 Westline Industrial Dr., St. Louis, MO 63146-3318. Second-class postage paid at St. Louis, Mo., and additional mailing offices. POSTMASTER: Send changes of address to The Journal of Pediatrics, Mosby–Year Book, Inc., 11830 Westline Industrial Dr., St. Louis, MO 63146-3318, (800)453-4351. Annual subscription rates: domestic, $102.00 for individuals and $211.00 for institutions. Printed in U.S.A.

CONTENTS *continued*

Precocious puberty in children with neurofibromatosis type 1 364
Reema Habiby, MD, Bernard Silverman, MD, Robert Listernick, MD, and Joel Charrow, MD, Chicago, Illinois

Studies of a large cohort of children with neurofibromatosis type 1 showed that 3% had precocious puberty, and that precocious puberty develops in more than a third of those with tumors of the optic chiasma. Biochemical evidence of puberty can be found before clinical signs are apparent.

Immunologic characterization of children vertically infected with human immunodeficiency virus, with slow or rapid disease progression 368
Alessandra Viganò, MD, Nicola Principi, MD, Maria Luisa Villa, MD, Chiara Riva, PharmD, Lina Crupi, MD, Daria Trabattoni, BS, Gene M. Shearer, PhD, and Mario Clerici, MD, Milan, Italy, and Bethesda, Maryland

Children with vertically acquired human immunodeficiency virus infection had decreased production of type 1 cytokines and increased production of type 2 cytokines; the latter was associated with high IgE concentrations and with progressive symptoms of HIV infection. Therapy to counteract type 2 cytokines might result in immunologic benefit. *See* related article on page 375.

Cognitive assessment of school-age children infected with maternally transmitted human immunodeficiency virus type 1 375
Marc Tardieu, MD, Marie-Jeanne Mayaux, BA, Nathalie Seibel, PsyD, Isabelle Funck-Brentano, PsyD, Elisabeth Straub, PsyD, Jean-Paul Teglas, PhD, and Stéphane Blanche, MD, Paris, France

Schoolchildren who had been vertically infected with human immunodeficiency virus were examined after 6 years of age. Two thirds had normal school achievement, but almost half had neuropsychologic abnormalities when tested. The percentage of circulating $CD4^+$ lymphocytes early in life correlated to some extent with good school performance. *See* related article on page 368.

Long-term effects of L-thyroxine therapy for congenital hypothyroidism 380
Joanne F. Rovet, PhD, and Robert M. Ehrlich, MD, FRCP(C), Toronto, Ontario, Canada

In children with congenital hypothyroidism, a higher initial dose of L-thyroxine was associated with better intellectual outcome but more behavior problems. A prospective study of different doses seems justified. *See* related article on page 389.

Editor's column

Adolescent medicine 1995 387
S. Jean Emans, MD, Boston, Massachusetts

CONTENTS *continued*

Clinical and laboratory observations

Brain metabolite changes on in vivo proton magnetic resonance spectroscopy in children with congenital hypothyroidism 389
Rakesh K. Gupta, MD, Vijayalakshmi Bhatia, MD, Harish Poptani, MSc, and Ratni B. Gujral, MD, Lucknow, India

Lead poisoning: Low rates of screening and high prevalence among children seen in inner-city emergency departments 392
James F. Wiley II, MD, Louis M. Bell, MD, Lisa S. Rosenblum, MD, MPH, Jayne Nussbaum, MPA, Richard Tobin, MS, and Fred M. Henretig, MD, Philadelphia, Pennsylvania, and Atlanta, Georgia

Resolution of breath-holding spells with treatment of concomitant anemia 395
Kenneth F. Colina, MD, and Herbert T. Abelson, MD, Seattle, Washington

Overinterpretation of gastroduodenal motility studies: Two cases involving Munchausen syndrome by proxy 397
Howard I. Baron, MD, David C. Beck, MD, Jorge H. Vargas, MD, and Marvin E. Ament, MD, Los Angeles, California

A missense mutation in a patient with guanosine triphosphate cyclohydrolase I deficiency missed in the newborn screening program 401
N. Blau, PhD, H. Ichinose, PhD, T. Nagatsu, PhD, MD, C. W. Heizmann, PhD, F. Zacchello, MD, and A. B. Burlina, MD, Zurich, Switzerland; Toyoake, Japan; and Padua, Italy

The book shelf

New books received 406

Fetal and neonatal medicine

Improved oxygenation during synchronized intermittent mandatory ventilation in neonates with respiratory distress syndrome: A randomized, crossover study 407
John P. Cleary, MD, Graham Bernstein, MD, Frank L. Mannino, MD, and Gregory P. Heldt, MD, San Diego, California

Synchronized intermittent mandatory ventilation improved oxygenation in spontaneously breathing preterm neonates with an endotracheal tube in place, compared with that during conventional ventilation. This might allow reduction of ventilator pressure or oxygen exposure.

Partial liquid ventilation in premature lambs with respiratory distress syndrome: Efficacy and compatibility with exogenous surfactant 412
Corinne Lowe Leach, MD, PhD, Bruce Holm, PhD, Frederick C. Morin III, MD, Bradley P. Fuhrman, MD, Michele C. Papo, MD, David Steinhorn, MD, and Lynn J. Hernan, MD, Buffalo, New York

Partial liquid ventilation with perflubron improved gas exchange and lung mechanics in preterm lambs with respiratory distress syndrome, was compatible with the preliminary use of surfactant, and was superior to surfactant alone in this model.

CONTENTS *continued*

Efficacy and cost analysis of treating very low birth weight infants with erythropoietin during their first two weeks of life: A randomized, placebo-controlled trial 421
Robin K. Ohls, MD, Karen A. Osborne, RN, and Robert D. Christensen, MD, Gainesville, Florida, and Salt Lake City, Utah

Very low birth weight infants given erythropoietin daily required fewer blood transfusions than were needed by a matched group given placebo. The charges associated with erythropoietin therapy were less than those associated with transfusions. No significant side effects were noted.

Neonatal mortality rate: Is further improvement possible? 427
Alistair G. S. Philip, MD, FRCPE, Portland, Maine

Neonatal mortality rates in a regional NICU were evaluated for a period of 10 years. The number of possibly preventable deaths is now very small. For a reduction in mortality rates, it will be necessary to lower the rates of preterm births.

Twenty-month outcome in ventilator-dependent, very low birth weight infants born during the early years of dexamethasone therapy 434
L. Furman, MD, M. Hack, MB,ChB, C. Watts, MD, E. Borawski-Clark, PhD, J. Baley, MD, S. Amini, PhD, and B. Hook, MD, Cleveland, Ohio

Outcome at 20 months of corrected age was compared in a nonrandomized manner, in very low birth weight infants who were not treated with dexamethasone for chronic lung disease. No differences in pulmonary status, growth, or neurodevelopmental outcome were identified. Large prospective and controlled studies are needed.

Postnatal attainment of intrauterine macromineral accretion rates in low birth weight infants fed fortified human milk 441
Richard J. Schanler, MD, and Steven A. Abrams, MD, Houston, Texas

Mineral balance and bone mineral content were compared in two groups of preterm infants given different fortifiers in feedings of their mothers' milk. Intrauterine accretion rates of calcium and phosphorus were achieved with both formulations; the amount ingested was more important than the source. Factors such as fecal fat excretion and total fluid intake need further evaluation.

Clinical and laboratory observations

Diagnosis of neonatal enterovirus infection by polymerase chain reaction 447
Mark J. Abzug, MD, Michael Loeffelholz, PhD, and Harley A. Rotbart, MD, Denver, Colorado, and Branchburg, New Jersey

CONTENTS *continued*

Inhaled nitric oxide for premature infants after prolonged rupture of the membranes 450
Abraham Peliowski, MD, Neil N. Finer, MD, Philip C. Etches, MB, Anne J. Tierney, MB, and C. Anthony Ryan, MB, Edmonton, Alberta, Canada

Administration of granulocyte colony-stimulating factor to neutropenic low birth weight infants of mothers with preeclampsia 454
Rita A. Makhlouf, MD, Mia W. Doron, MD, Carl L. Bose, MD, Wayne A. Price, MD, and Alan D. Stiles, MD, Chapel Hill, North Carolina

Effect of granulocyte colony-stimulating factor on preeclampsia-associated neonatal neutropenia 457
Edmund F. La Gamma, MD, Oral Alpan, MD, and Prabhakar Kocherlakota, MD, Stony Brook, New York

The book shelf

Book reviews 460

Pediatric pharmacology and therapeutics

Intravenous morphine pharmacokinetics in pediatric patients with sickle cell disease 461
Carlton D. Dampier, MD, B. N. Y. Setty, PhD, Joann Logan, BS, Jacqueline G. Ioli, MS, and Roger Dean, PharmD, Philadelphia, Pennsylvania, and Chicago, Illinois

Pharmacokinetic studies of morphine in the treatment of patients with painful crises of sickle cell disease showed wide variation in plasma clearance values. Individualization of morphine dosing is needed for optimal analgesia and minimal adverse effects.

Combination treatment with growth hormone and gonadotropin-releasing hormone analogs in short normal girls 468
Giuseppe Saggese, MD, Graziano Cesaretti, MD, Stefania Barsanti, MD, and Anna Rossi, MD, Pisa, Italy

Combination treatment with growth hormone and gonadotropin-releasing hormone improved predicted height in a small group of otherwise normal short girls. The GnRH-induced block of pubertal maturation may permit the growth-promoting effect of growth hormone without a rapid increase of bone age.

Response to growth hormone therapy in patients with growth hormone deficiency who at birth were small or appropriate in size for gestational age 474
Antonio Balsamo, MD, Paola Tassoni, MD, Alessandra Cassio, MD, Cristina Colli, MD, Davide Tassinari, MD, Alessandro Cicognani, MD, and Emanuele Cacciari, MD, Bologna, Italy

Children with growth hormone deficiency had smaller growth responses to growth hormone therapy if they had been small for gestational age at birth than if their birth size had been appropriate. Longer follow-up will be needed to determine whether GH therapy improves eventual height in children who were SGA at birth.

CONTENTS *continued*

Clinical and laboratory observations

Effect of growth hormone therapy on final versus predicted height in short twelve- to sixteen-year-old boys without growth hormone deficiency 478
Paul B. Kaplowitz, MD, Richmond, Virginia

Neurodevelopmental disabilities

Otitis media, hearing sensitivity, and maternal responsiveness in relation to language during infancy 481
Joanne Erwick Roberts, PhD, Margaret R. Burchinal, PhD, Lynn P. Medley, MS, Susan A. Zeisel, EdD, Martha Mundy, MS, Jackson Roush, PhD, Stephen Hooper, PhD, Donna Bryant, PhD, and Frederick W. Henderson, MD, Chapel Hill, North Carolina

A prospective study of infants in day care showed that the presence of otitis media with effusion and hearing loss was indirectly associated with language and cognitive development at 1 year of age; the effect was mediated by child-rearing factors such as interaction style of the mother and the home environment.

Bacteriuria in children with neurogenic bladder treated with intermittent catheterization: Natural history 490
Theresa A. Schlager, MD, Susan Dilks, MD, Julie Trudell, RN, Thomas S. Whittam, PhD, and J. Owen Hendley, MD, Charlottesville, Virginia, and University Park, Pennsylvania

Children with neurogenic bladder and on a regimen of clean intermittent catheterization had frequent cultures of urine for 6 months. Bacteriuria and pyuria were present in three fourths of specimens, but symptomatic infections were uncommon. The benefit of attempting to eradicate the bacteria is questionable if urinary tract anatomy and function are normal.

Clinical and laboratory observations

Neurodevelopmental outcome of infants with hypoplastic left heart syndrome 496
B. T. Rogers, MD, M. E. Msall, MD, G. M. Buck, PhD, N. R. Lyon, PNP, M. K. Norris, NP, J.-M. A. Roland, MD, R. L. Gingell, MD, D. C. Cleveland, MD, and D. R. Pieroni, MD, Buffalo, New York

Current literature and clinical issues

Abstracts from the literature 499

Editorial correspondence

Isolation of *Ureaplasma urealyticum* from low birth weight infants
Ken B. Waites, MD, Gail H. Cassell, PhD, Lynn B. Duffy, MT(ASCP), and Karen B. Searcey, MSPH, Birmingham, Alabama 502

Dennis T. Crouse, MD, PhD, and Judith M. Reese, Memphis, Tennessee 502

CONTENTS *continued*

Reply 503
Alfred D. Heggie, MD, Michael R. Jacobs, MD, PhD, Verleria T. Butler, BA, MASCP, Jill E. Baley, MD, and Bernard Boxerbaum, MD, Cleveland, Ohio

Band neutrophil counts in neonates 504
Charles R. Rosenfeld, MD, Dallas, Texas

Reply 505
Robert L. Schelonka, MD, Bradley A. Yoder, MD, and Robert B. Hall, MD, Lackland Air Force Base, Texas

Electrocardiographic findings in Rett syndrome 506
Manuel Fuster-Siebert, PhD, and Manuel Castro-Gago, PhD, Santiago de Compostela, Spain

Reader services

Instructions to authors 12A

Information for readers 15A

Scheduled meetings 16A

News and notes 18A

Professional opportunities 37A

Index to advertisers 37A

Mosby

THE JOURNAL OF PEDIATRICS

Contents

APRIL 1995

Special article

Impact of attitudes on maternal decisions regarding infant feeding 507

Mary Losch, PhD, Claibourne I. Dungy, MD, MPH, Daniel Russell, PhD, and Lois B. Dusdieker, MD, MS, Iowa City and Ames, Iowa

Original articles

A multicenter study of alternate-day prednisone therapy in patients with cystic fibrosis 515

Howard Eigen, MD, Beryl J. Rosenstein, MD, Stacey FitzSimmons, PhD, Daniel V. Schidlow, MD, and the Cystic Fibrosis Foundation Prednisone Trial Group, Indianapolis, Indiana; Baltimore and Bethesda, Maryland; and Philadelphia, Pennsylvania

Alternate-day therapy with prednisone produced significant improvement in pulmonary function in patients with cystic fibrosis who were colonized with *Pseudomonas aeruginosa*. Larger doses were not more effective and were associated with more severe side effects.

Kawasaki disease in infants less than one year of age 524

Elaine A. Rosenfeld, MD, Kathleen E. Corydon, RN, and Stanford T. Shulman, MD, Chicago, Illinois

Infants with Kawasaki disease were more likely to have coronary artery aneurysms if they were less than 6 months of age when affected. Intravenous immune globulin therapy reduced the risk of coronary lesions if given within 10 days of onset.

Cell-mediated immune status of children with recurrent infection 530

Henry G. Herrod, MD, Michael S. Blaiss, MD, William R. Valenski, BS, and Sharon Gross, BS, Memphis, Tennessee

Cell-mediated immune function was evaluated in children referred because of frequent infections. These studies were of little benefit in explaining susceptibility to infection, but many patients had evidence of immunoglobulin deficiencies.

Vol. 126, No. 4, April 1995. The Journal of Pediatrics (ISSN 0022-3476) is published monthly (six issues per volume, two volumes per year) by Mosby–Year Book, Inc., 11830 Westline Industrial Dr., St. Louis, MO 63146-3318. Second-class postage paid at St. Louis, Mo., and additional mailing offices. POSTMASTER: Send changes of address to The Journal of Pediatrics, Mosby–Year Book, Inc., 11830 Westline Industrial Dr., St. Louis, MO 63146-3318, (800)453-4351. Annual subscription rates: domestic, $102.00 for individuals and $211.00 for institutions. Printed in U.S.A.

Supplementary sensorimotor area seizures in children and adolescents 537
Nancy Bass, MD, Elaine Wyllie, MD, Youssef Comair, MD, Prakash Kotagal, MD, Paul Ruggieri, MD, and Hans Holthausen, MD, Cleveland, Ohio

Supplemental sensorimotor area seizures characterized by brevity, nocturnal timing, gross limb movements, and preserved consciousness were recognized after prolonged video-EEG monitoring. The standard EEG was often normal. Most patients responded poorly to antiepileptic medications; surgery was often required to achieve control of seizures.

Predictive factors in the determination of final height in boys with constitutional delay of growth and puberty 545
A. Albanese, MD, and R. Stanhope, MD, FRCP, London, England

A study of boys with constitutional delay of growth and puberty showed that one of the main features was a relatively short upper body segment. Neither testosterone nor oxandrolone therapy modified final height attainment or body disproportion. Absence of these anthropometric features indicates that another diagnosis should be considered.

Effects of dairy products on bone and body composition in pubertal girls 551
Gary M. Chan, MD, Karen Hoffman, and Martha McMurry, MS, Salt Lake City, Utah

Adolescent girls who increased the amounts of dairy products in their diets had improved calcium, vitamin D, and protein intakes, and for a period of a year had gains in total body mineral content and lumbar bone density without excess weight gain or increased body fat. This might help prevent osteoporosis in later life.

Mineral homeostasis and bone mass at diagnosis in children with acute lymphoblastic leukemia 557
Jacqueline M. Halton, MD, Stephanie A. Atkinson, PhD, Laurence Fraher, PhD, Colin E. Webber, PhD, W. Peter Cockshott, MB,ChB, MD, Cherk Tam, MD, and Ronald D. Barr, MB,ChB, MD, Hamilton, London, and Toronto, Ontario, Canada

Most children with acute lymphoblastic leukemia were found to have alterations in bone mass and bone metabolism at the time of initial diagnosis and before treatment. These abnormalities may indicate which patients will develop clinically important bone disease during therapy.

CONTENTS *continued*

Pulmonary function abnormalities in Prader-Willi syndrome 565
Hákon Hákonarson, MD, Jay Moskovitz, MS, Karen L. Daigle, MD, Suzanne B. Cassidy, MD, and Michelle M. Cloutier, MD, Farmington, Connecticut, and Cleveland, Ohio

Children and adults with Prader-Willi syndrome had evidence of restrictive ventilatory impairment primarily as a result of thoracic muscle weakness. This could predispose patients to pulmonary infections, hypoxemia, and cor pulmonale, which are causes of morbidity and death in patients with this syndrome.

Pulmonary arteriovenous shunting in children with liver disease 571
Thierry Barbé, MD, Jean Losay, MD, Gilles Grimon, MD, Denis Devictor, MD, Anne Sardet, MD, Frédéric Gauthier, MD, Didier Houssin, MD, and Olivier Bernard, MD, Paris, France

Pulmonary arteriovenous shunting was demonstrated in 25 children with cirrhosis of various causes, and in one with portal vein obstruction. Early recognition of shunting is important so that liver transplantation can be done; shunting usually then regresses in those who survive transplantation.

The book shelf

Book review 580

Clinical and laboratory observations

Life-threatening infection in two children with hemoglobin S–beta-thalassemia 581
Amy Lynch, MD, and Joseph D. Tobias, MD, Nashville, Tennessee

Development of a vaccine tracking system to improve the rate of age-appropriate primary immunization in children of lower socioeconomic status 583
Jon S. Abramson, MD, T. Michael O'Shea, MD, MPH, D. Lee Ratledge, BS, Michael R. Lawless, MD, and Laurence B. Givner, MD, Winston-Salem, North Carolina

Portal vein thrombosis caused by protein C and protein S deficiency associated with cytomegalovirus infection 586
Ravit Arav-Boger, MD, Shimon Reif, MD, and Yoram Bujanover, MD, Tel Aviv, Israel

Absence of infection in breast-fed infants born to hepatitis C virus–infected mothers 589
Ho-Hsiung Lin, MD, PhD, Jia-Horng Kao, MD, Hong-Yuan Hsu, MD, PhD, Yen-Hsuan Ni, MD, Mei-Hwei Chang, MD, Su-Cheng Huang, MD, Lih-Hwa Hwang, PhD, Pei-Jer Chen, MD, PhD, and Dong-Shinn Chen, MD, Taipei, Taiwan, Republic of China

Viral measurement by polymerase chain reaction–based assays in human immunodeficiency virus–infected infants 592
Paul E. Palumbo, MD, Shirley Kwok, BA, Sharon Waters, BS, Yvonne Wesley, RN, Dan Lewis, MS, Nancy McKinney, MS, Arlene Bardeguez, MD, Edward M. Connor, MD, and James M. Oleske, MD, MPH, Newark, New Jersey, and Alameda, California

CONTENTS *continued*

Outcome of partial splenectomy for type I Gaucher disease 596
A. Zimran, MD, D. Elstein, PhD, R. Schifmann, MD, A. Abrahamov, MD, M. Goldberg, MD, J. A. Bar-Maor, MD, R. O. Brady, MD, P. C. Guzzetta, MD, and N. W. Barton, MD, PhD, Jerusalem and Haifa, Israel; Bethesda, Maryland; and Dallas, Texas

Deletion of mitochondrial DNA in patient with chronic tubulointerstitial nephritis 597
Agnès Rötig, PhD, Françoise Goutières, MD, Patrick Niaudet, MD, Pierre Rustin, PhD, Dominique Chretien, PhD, Geneviève Guest, MD, Jacqueline Mikol, MD, Marie-Claire Gubler, MD, and Arnold Munnich, MD, PhD

Plasma erythropoietin reference ranges in children 601
Brian Krafte-Jacobs, MD, Jacqueline Williams, MD, and Steven J. Soldin, PhD, Washington, D.C.

The book shelf

Book review 604

Fetal and neonatal medicine

Changing trends in the epidemiology and pathogenesis of neonatal chronic lung disease 605
Mario A. Rojas, MD, Alvaro Gonzalez, MD, Eduardo Bancalari, MD, Nelson Claure, MS, Catherine Poole, MD, and Galdino Silva-Neto, MD, Miami, Florida

Most very low birth weight infants with chronic lung disease were found not to have had severe respiratory distress syndrome. The presence of a symptomatic patent ductus arteriosus, especially in conjunction with sepsis, was strongly associated with subsequent development of CLD.

Long-chain polyunsaturated fatty acids in preterm infants: Status at birth and its influence on postnatal levels 611
Magritha M. H. P. Foreman–van Drongelen, MD, Adriana C. van Houwelingen, MD, PhD, Arnold D. M. Kester, PhD, Tom H. M. Hasaart, MD, PhD, Carlos E. Blanco, MD, PhD, and Gerard Hornstra, PhD, Maastricht, The Netherlands

The long-chain polyunsaturated fatty acid status of preterm infants was studied at birth and at term postconceptional age. The LCP status at birth and the diet (human milk vs formula) significantly affected the later values. Further study of the effect of maternal diet is needed because of the importance of these fatty acids in neural development.

Influence of energy substrates on respiratory gas exchange during conventional mechanical ventilation of preterm infants 619
Philippe Chessex, MD, Sylvie Bélanger, MD, Bruno Piedboeuf, MD, and Marjolain Pineault, PhD, Montreal, Quebec, Canada

Ventilator-dependent preterm infants fed parenterally with glucose-based energy intake compensated for the enhanced carbon dioxide production by increasing their respiratory drive. The net effect on oxygenation was beneficial compared with that when energy was derived largely from lipids.

CONTENTS *continued*

Birth order, delivery route, and concordance in the transmission of human immunodeficiency virus type 1 from mothers to twins 625
Anne-Marie Duliège, MD, MS, Christopher I. Amos, PhD, Susanne Felton, MA, Robert J. Biggar, MD, the International Registry of HIV-Exposed Twins, and James J. Goedert, MD, Emeryville, California; Houston, Texas; Washington, D.C.; and Rockville, Maryland

A study of twins born to mothers infected with human immunodeficiency virus showed that A twins were more likely to be infected than B twins, and vaginally delivered infants more likely to be infected than those delivered by cesarean section. Reducing intrapartum exposure to the virus may reduce transmission from mother to infant.

Clinical and laboratory observations

Placement of umbilical venous catheters with use of bedside real-time ultrasonography 633
Mark Greenberg, MD, Hamid Movahed, MD, Beverly Peterson, and Raul Bejar, MD, San Diego, California

Relation between meconium concentration of the cocaine metabolite benzoylecgonine and fetal growth 636
Mark Mirochnick, MD, Deborah A. Frank, MD, Howard Cabral, MPH, Adrian Turner, BSc, and Barry Zuckerman, MD, Boston, Massachusetts

Pediatric pharmacology and therapeutics

Effiacy of frequent nebulized ipratropium bromide added to frequent high-dose albuterol therapy in severe childhood asthma 639
Suzanne Schuh, MD, David W. Johnson, MD, Sheilagh Callahan, RN, Gerald Canny, MD, and Henry Levison, MD, Toronto, Ontario, Canada

Addition of one or three inhalations of ipratropium to repeated nebulized doses of albuterol increased the effectiveness of therapy for acute asthma in children, particularly if symptoms were severe. Some hospitalizations may be averted by the use of combination therapy.

Treatment of purpura fulminans in meningococcemia with protein C concentrate 646
George E. Rivard, MD, Michèle David, MD, Catherine Farrell, MD, and Hans Peter Schwarz, MD, Montreal, Quebec, Canada, and Vienna, Austria

Protein C concentrate was given to patients with meningococcemia, purpura fulminans, and diffuse intravascular coagulation. The coagulation values were improved, as were evidences of organ dysfunction. A controlled clinical trial seems justified.

Control of severe pain in children with terminal malignancy 653
John J. Collins, MBBS, FRACP, Holcombe E. Grier, MD, Hannah C. Kinney, MD, and Charles B. Berde, MD, PhD, Boston, Massachusetts

Some children with terminal malignancy were found to require massive doses of opioids or other extraordinary measures to achieve adequate relief of pain. Those with solid tumors that spread to nerves or spinal cord were particularly difficult to treat. Guidelines for controlling pain in these patients are provided.

CONTENTS *continued*

Clinical and laboratory observations

Diarrhea associated with enteral benzodiazepine solutions 657
J. D. Marshall, MD, H. C. Farrar, MD, and G. L. Kearns, PharmD, Little Rock, Arkansas

Prepubertal gynecomastia during growth hormone therapy 659
Saul Malozowski, MD, PhD, and Bruce V. Stadel, MD, MPH, Rockville, Maryland

The book shelf

New books received 662

Clinical conference

A three-month-old girl with fever and hepatomegaly 663
V. Faye Jones, MD, and John J. Buchino, MD, Louisville, Kentucky

Profiles in pediatrics II

Josef Warkany 669
Robert W. Miller, MD, Bethesda, Maryland

Editorial correspondence

Motor and cognitive development in children with congenital hypothyroidism 673
Marvin L. Mitchell, MD, and Robert Z. Klein, MD, Jamaica Plain, Massachusetts, and Lebanon, New Hampshire

Reply 673
Thomas Vulsma, MD, PhD, and Libbe Kooistra, MSc, Amsterdam and Groningen, The Netherlands

Opsoclonus-myoclonus, ataxia, and coincident neuroblastoma 675
Marc C. Chamberlain, MD, La Jolla, California

Blood flow velocities and neonatal asphyxia 675
Stephen J. Elliott, MD, Houston, Texas

Reply 676
H. Akinbi, MD, V. Bhutani, MD, and S. Abbasi, MD, Philadelphia, Pennsylvania

A new defect in vitamin D metabolism 676
Walter Nützenadel, MD, Otto Mehls, MD, and Günter Klaus, MD, Heidelberg, Germany

Reply 677
Samuel J. Casella, MD, and Laurence Finberg, MD, Baltimore, Maryland, and Brooklyn, New York

Criteria for studies of antibiotic therapy for acute otitis media 677
Richard H. Schwartz, MD, and William J. Rodriguez, MD, Washington, D.C.

Adult respiratory distress syndrome in children, associated with miliary tuberculosis 678
Amelia Martinez-Azagra, MD, Ana Serrano, MD, and Juan Casado-Flores, MD, Madrid, Spain

Reply 678
Susan L. Davis, MD, Houston, Texas

CONTENTS *continued*

Techniques for measurement of resting energy expenditure in children 679
Dale A. Schoeller, PhD, and Amy Luke, PhD, Chicago and Maywood, Illinois

Reply 679
Michael I. Goran, PhD, and Rachel Johnson, RD, PhD, Birmingham, Alabama, and Burlington, Vermont

Placebo-controlled versus comparative studies of drug effects 680
Miles M. Weinberger, MD, Iowa City, Iowa

Reply 681
Stanley P. Galant, MD, Orange, California

Reply 681
Joseph M. Garfunkel, MD, Chapel Hill, North Carolina

Standards for home care of sick children 681
Mark S. McConnell, MD, and Ronald M. Perkin, MD, Stanford and Loma Linda, California

Reply 682
Allen I. Goldberg, MD, M. Harry Gardner, MD, and Lewis E. Gibson, MD, Maywood, Illinois

Correction

Fellowships (J Pediatr 1995;126:25A-70A) 682

Reader services

Instructions to authors 13A

Information for readers 16A

Scheduled meetings 17A

News and notes 19A

Professional opportunities 30A

Index to advertisers 36A

THE JOURNAL OF PEDIATRICS

Mosby

THE JOURNAL OF PEDIATRICS

Contents

MAY 1995, PART 1

Medical progress

Bone mineralization, hypothalamic amenorrhea, and sex steroid therapy in female adolescents and young adults 683
Albert C. Hergenroeder, MD, Houston, Texas

Original articles

Relationship between insulin resistance and abnormal lipid profile in obese adolescents 690
Julia Steinberger, MD, Catherene Moorehead, MS, Victor Katch, EdD, and Albert P. Rocchini, MD, Minneapolis, Minnesota, and Ann Arbor, Michigan

Obese adolescents were found to have serum lipid abnormalities, and these correlated with their degree of insulin resistance as evaluated during a euglycemic clamp procedure. Weight reduction probably would improve both metabolic abnormalities.

Differences in morbidity between breast-fed and formula-fed infants 696
Kathryn G. Dewey, PhD, M. Jane Heinig, PhD, and Laurie A. Nommsen-Rivers, MS, RD, Davis, California

In a relatively affluent population, breast-feeding for a year was associated with fewer diarrheal illnesses, and fewer or less-prolonged episodes of otitis media during the first 2 years of life. Common upper respiratory tract infections were not less frequent than in a formula-fed control group.

Use of polymerase chain reaction for improved diagnosis of tuberculosis in children 703
Christophe Delacourt, MD, Jean-Dominique Poveda, MD, Corinne Chureau, Nicole Beydon, MD, Bruno Mahut, MD, Jacques de Blic, MD, Pierre Scheinmann, MD, and Guy Garrigue, MD, Paris, France

The polymerase chain reaction was used to detect *Mycobacterium tuberculosis* infection in children. Most children with active disease and some with no evidence of clinical disease had at least one positive PCR result with repeated testing. The technique seems applicable when a rapid diagnosis is needed.

Vol. 126, No. 5, Part 1, May 1995. The Journal of Pediatrics (ISSN 0022-3476) is published monthly (six issues per volume, two volumes per year) by Mosby–Year Book, Inc., 11830 Westline Industrial Dr., St. Louis, MO 63146-3318. Second-class postage paid at St. Louis, Mo., and additional mailing offices. POSTMASTER: Send changes of address to The Journal of Pediatrics, Mosby–Year Book, Inc., 11830 Westline Industrial Dr., St. Louis, MO 63146-3318, (800)453-4351. Annual subscription prices effective through September 30, 1995: domestic, $102.00 for individuals and $211.00 for institutions. Printed in U.S.A.

CONTENTS *continued*

Encephalopathy in children with perinatally acquired human immunodeficiency virus infection 710
Mark N. Lobato, MD, M. Blake Caldwell, MD, MPH, Paulus Ng, MPH, Margaret J. Oxtoby, MD, and the Pediatric Spectrum of Disease Clinical Consortium, Atlanta, Georgia

Encephalopathy was found to be a common complication of perinatally acquired human immunodeficiency virus infection in children, and to be associated with other AIDS-defining conditions and lower $CD4^+$ T-lymphocyte counts. Median time of survival after diagnosis was 22 months.

Long-term efficacy of recombinant hepatitis B vaccine and risk of natural infection in infants born to mothers with hepatitis B e antigen 716
Ping-Ing Lee, MD, Chin-Yun Lee, MD, Li-Min Huang, MD, PhD, and Mei-Hwei Chang, MD, Taipei, Taiwan, Republic of China

Children born to mothers who were carriers of hepatitis B were vaccinated after birth and followed for 5 years; 4% became carriers and 12% had serologic evidence of natural infection. A booster dose of HB vaccine seems unnecessary before 5 years of age.

Cerebral vein thrombosis in childhood systemic lupus erythematosus 722
Yosef Uziel, MD, MSc, Ronald M. Laxer, MD, FRCPC, Susan Blaser, MD, FRCPC, Maureen Andrew, MD, FRCPC, Rayfel Schneider, MBBCh, FRCPC, and Earl D. Silverman, MD, FRCPC, Toronto and Hamilton, Canada

Cerebral venous thrombosis occurred in three girls with systemic lupus erythematosus. Severe headache was the initial diagnostic clue, and should lead to appropriate radiologic investigations. Long-term anticoagulation therapy is recommended.

Low-density lipoprotein apheresis as long-term treatment for children with homozygous familial hypercholesterolemia 728
R. Jeff Zwiener, MD, Ricardo Uauy, MD, PhD, Mary L. Petruska, RN, and Beverley A. Huet, MS, Dallas, Texas

Weekly low-density lipoprotein apheresis was used for several years to treat two children with receptor-negative homozygous familial hypercholesterolemia. Blood cholesterol values decreased by about two thirds, and xanthomas regressed. The procedures were well tolerated.

Pathophysiology of calcium metabolism in children with vitamin D–deficiency rickets 736
Klaus Kruse, MD, Luebeck, Germany

Biochemical studies related to bone metabolism were carried out in children with various stages of rickets and during the healing phase after vitamin D therapy. The data help to clarify the pathophysiologic events associated with vitamin D deficiency.

Use of peritoneal dialysis, continuous arteriovenous hemofiltration, and continuous arteriovenous hemodiafiltration for removal of ammonium chloride and glutamine in rabbits 742
Denis S. Semama, MD, Frédéric Huet, MD, Jean-Bernard Gouyon, MD, Christian Lallemant, MD, and Jean Desgres, PhD, Dijon, France

Continuous hemodiafiltration was more effective than peritoneal dialysis or continuous arteriovenous hemofiltration for removing ammonium in rabbits with artificially induced hyperammonemia.

Editor's column

Use of intravenous lipids in neonates 747
Harold J. Helbock, MD, and Bruce N. Ames, PhD, Berkeley, California

Clinical and laboratory observations

Disseminated intravascular coagulation associated with granulocyte colony-stimulating factor therapy in a child with human immunodeficiency virus infection 749
Brigitta U. Mueller, MD, Richard Burt, MD, Leslie Gulick, MD, Freda Jacobsen, RN, Philip A. Pizzo, MD, and McDonald Horne, MD, Bethesda, Maryland; and Brooklyn, New York

Association of symptoms with *Helicobacter pylori* infection in children 753
Siobhan M. Gormally, MD, Nan Prakash, MRCP, Marie T. Durnin, SRN, Leslie E. Daly, PhD, Marguerite Clyne, PhD, Barry M. Kierce, MB, and Brendan Drumm, MD, Dublin, Ireland

Use of the gonadotropin-releasing hormone agonist triptorelin in the diagnosis of delayed puberty in boys 756
Giorgio Zamboni, MD, Franco Antoniazzi, MD, and Luciano Tató, MD, Verona, Italy

Relationship of growth hormone deficiency and leukemia 759
Robert Rapaport, MD, Sharon E. Oberfield, MD, Leslie Robison, PhD, Sonia Salisbury, MD, Raphael David, MD, Jayashree Rao, MD, and Geoffrey P. Redmond, MD, Newark, New Jersey; New York, New York; Minneapolis, Minnesota; Halifax, Nova Scotia, Canada; New Orleans, Louisiana; and Beachwood, Ohio

Permanent heterotopic ossification at the injection site after diphtheria-tetanus-pertussis immunizations in children who have fibrodysplasia ossificans progressiva 762
Thomas F. Lanchoney, BS, Randolph B. Cohen, MD, David M. Rocke, PhD, Michael A. Zasloff, MD, PhD, and Frederick S. Kaplan, MD, Philadelphia, Pennsylvania, and Davis, California

CONTENTS *continued*

Dysmorphic features in patients with complex glycerol kinase deficiency 764
Angela Scheuerle, MD, Frank Greenberg, MD, and Edward R. B. McCabe, MD, PhD, Houston, Texas

The book shelf

Book review 768

Fetal and neonatal medicine

Effect of pulse dexamethasone therapy on the incidence and severity of chronic lung disease in the very low birth weight infant 769
Beverly S. Brozanski, MD, Judith G. Jones, BSN, RNC, Carol H. Gilmour, MD, Michael J. Balsan, MD, Roger L. Vazquez, MD, Barbara A. Israel, MD, Beverley Newman, MD, Francis B. Mimouni, MD, and Robert D. Guthrie, MD, Pittsburgh, Pennsylvania

Pulse dexamethasone therapy led to improved pulmonary outcome in preterm infants at risk of the development of chronic lung disease; the survival rate without the need for supplemental oxygen was also improved. Pulse therapy may be associated with fewer side effects than continuous steroid therapy.

Effect of the arterial oxygenation level on cardiac output, oxygen extraction, and oxygen consumption in low birth weight infants receiving mechanical ventilation 777
Andreas Schulze, MD, Robin K. Whyte, MBBS, R. Clifton Way, MD, and John C. Sinclair, MD, Hamilton, Ontario, and Halifax, Nova Scotia, Canada

A comparison of the effects on oxygenation of targeting lower rather than higher recommended pulse oximetry measurements was conducted in preterm infants. The lower target range allowed for less oxygen exposure without requiring an increase in cardiac output and without reducing oxygen consumption, at least during the short duration of the study.

Oxidation of parenteral lipid emulsion by ambient and phototherapy lights: Potential toxicity of routine parenteral feeding 785
Jiři Neužil, PhD, Brian A. Darlow, MD, Terrie E. Inder, MBChB, Karl B. Sluis, BSc, Christine C. Winterbourn, PhD, and Roland Stocker, PhD, Sydney, Australia, and Christchurch, New Zealand

Laboratory studies of a lipid emulsion used for parenteral nutrition of preterm infants showed that exposure to phototherapy and other light resulted in the formation of relatively high levels of oxidized lipids. This may represent a source of morbidity and is easily preventable by minimizing the exposure to light. *See* commentary *on page 747.*

Plasma mineral concentrations in preterm infants fed a nutrient-enriched formula after hospital discharge 791
Sujatha Rajaram, PhD, Susan E. Carlson, PhD, Winston W. K. Koo, MBBS, and W. Emmett Braselton, PhD, Memphis, Tennessee, and East Lansing, Michigan

Preterm infants fed a preterm formula for 2 months after discharge from the hospital achieved plasma zinc concentrations comparable to those of term infants, without adverse effects on other measures of mineral homeostasis.

Clinical and laboratory observations

Evidence of increased intrauterine bone resorption in term infants of mothers with insulin-dependent diabetes 796
Sergio Demarini, MD, Bonny L. Specker, PhD, Rosa I. Sierra, MS, Menachem Miodovnik, MD, and Reginald C. Tsang, MBBS, Cincinnati, Ohio

Pediatric pharmacology and therapeutics

Bacteriologic failure of amoxicillin-clavulanate in treatment of acute otitis media caused by nontypeable *Haemophilus influenzae* 799
Janak A. Patel, MD, Barbara Reisner, PhD, Negar Vizirinia, MD, Mary Owen, MD, Tasnee Chonmaitree, MD, and Virgil Howie, MD, Galveston, Texas

Bacteriologic treatment failure rates were higher in children treated with amoxicillin-clavulanate for acute otitis media caused by nontypeable *Haemophilus influenzae* than for that caused by other bacteria, and higher than during a preceding study. Contributing factors were nonwhite race, male gender, recurrent otitis, and associated viral infections.

Clinical trial of vitamin A as adjuvant treatment for lower respiratory tract infections 807
Chris L. Kjolhede, MD, MPH, Francisco J. Chew, MD, Anne M. Gadomski, MD, MPH, and Diana P. Marroquin, MD, Baltimore, Maryland, and Guatemala City, Guatemala

In a controlled trial, administration of vitamin A, 100,000 IU in oil, had no measurable clinical effect on young children hospitalized for acute lower respiratory tract infection. Studies of larger doses and in populations deficient in vitamin A may still be justified.

Clinical and laboratory observations

Fatal hemolysis induced by ceftriaxone in a child with sickle cell anemia 813
Juan C. Bernini, MD, Mahmoud M. Mustafa, MD, Laurie J. Sutor, MD, and George R. Buchanan, MD, Dallas, Texas

Fatal hemolysis caused by ceftriaxone 816
André D. Lascari, MD, and Kristina Amyot, MD, Albany, New York

Furosemide-associated fever 817
Herbert W. Clegg, MD, and Donald A. Riopel, MD, Charlotte, North Carolina

CONTENTS *continued*

Rebound severe methemoglobinemia from ingestion of a nitroethane artificial-fingernail remover 819
Kevin C. Osterhoudt, MD, Catherine C. Wiley, MD, Robert Dudley, MD, Sandra Sheen, BSN, and Fred M. Henretig, MD, Philadelphia, Pennsylvania

Effect of corticosteroids on survival of children with acquired immunodeficiency syndrome and *Pneumocystis carinii*–related respiratory failure 821
Gwenn E. McLaughlin, MD, Satranjan S. Virdee, MBBS, Charles L. Schleien, MD, Bernard H. Holzman, MD, and Gwendolyn B. Scott, MD, Miami, Florida

Human synthetic calcitonin therapy for hypercalcemia of immobilization 825
Sushma Kaul, MD, and Joseph J. Sockalosky, MD, Minneapolis and St. Paul, Minnesota

Neurodevelopmental disabilities

Estimation of energy requirements in persons with severe central nervous system impairment 828
Linda G. Bandini, RD, PhD, Heidi Puelzl-Quinn, MS, RD, Julie A. Morelli, BS, and Naomi K. Fukagawa, MD, PhD, Boston and Cambridge, Massachusetts, and New York, New York

The energy balance technique, in which energy intakes are adjusted for weight changes, was found to be a valid method of determining energy requirements in individuals with central nervous system disorders. Standardized equations based on height and weight overestimate energy needs in these patients.

Body composition in children with spastic quadriplegic cerebral palsy 833
Virginia A. Stallings, MD, Christine E. Cronk, ScD, Babette S. Zemel, PhD, and Edward B. Charney, MD, Philadelphia, Pennsylvania, and Carbondale, Illinois

Prepubertal children with spastic quadriplegia were found to have a high incidence of growth failure and abnormal body composition, easily recognized by appropriate anthropometric measurements. Prevention of malnutrition or effective nutritional rehabilitation should improve growth and may improve function in these patients.

The book shelf

Book review 840

Current literature and clinical issues

Abstracts from the literature 841

Profiles in pediatrics II

Edith Potter 845
Enid Gilbert-Barness, MD, Tampa, Florida

Editorial correspondence

Cost of ribavirin therapy for respiratory syncytial virus infection 847
Eric D. Marquardt, PharmD, Sacramento, California

CONTENTS *continued*

Reply 847
Janet A. Englund, MD, Pedro A. Piedra, MD, and Brian E. Gilbert, PhD, Houston, Texas

Opsoclonus-myoclonus and recurrent neuroblastoma 847
William T. Basco, Jr., MD, Miguel Abboud, MD, and Kenton R. Holden, MD, Charleston, South Carolina

Cystic fibrosis and episodic arthritis 848
G. Taccetti, MD, S. Campana, MB, L. Marianelli, MD, and S. Turchini, MD, Florence, Italy

Reply 849
N. M. Wulffraat, MD, PhD, E. R. de Graeff-Meeder, MD, PhD, G. T. Rijkers, PhD, H. van der Laag, MD, and W. Kuis, MD, PhD, Utrecht, The Netherlands

***Helicobacter pylori* infection in neurologically impaired children** 849
Joyce Elizabeth Mauk, MD, Philadelphia, Pennsylvania

Reply 850
Roy Proujansky, MD, Stephen Shaffer, MD, Nancy Vinton, MD, and Steven Bachrach, MD, Wilmington, Delaware

Promotion of healthy eating habits in children 850
Sherry R. Crump, MD, Atlanta, Georgia

Reply 850
Robert C. Whitaker, MD, MPH, Jeffrey A. Wright, MD, Thomas D. Koepsell, MD, MPH, Bruce M. Psaty, MD, PhD, and Anita J. Finch, MS, RD, Seattle and Bellevue, Washington

Congenital nephrotic syndrome in neonatal lupus syndrome 851
P. J. Westenend, MD, Nijmegen, The Netherlands

Pancreatitis and organic acidemias 852
A. Fiumara, R. Barone, F. Nigro, A. Ribes, and L. Pavone, Catania, Italy, and Barcelona, Spain

Reader services

Instructions to authors 13A

Information for readers 16A

Scheduled meetings 17A

News and notes 18A

Professional opportunities 28A

Index to advertisers 34A

THE JOURNAL OF PEDIATRICS

Mosby

THE JOURNAL OF PEDIATRICS

COPYRIGHT© 1995 BY MOSBY–YEAR BOOK, INC.

Contents

JUNE 1995

Medical progress

Recent developments in the pathophysiology and treatment of persistent pulmonary hypertension of the newborn 853
John P. Kinsella, MD, and Steven H. Abman, MD, Denver, Colorado

Original articles

Vertical transmission of human immunodeficiency virus type 1: Autologous neutralizing antibody, virus load, and virus phenotype 865
Robert N. Husson, MD, Yan Lan, MD, Eiji Kojima, MS, David Venzon, PhD, Hiroaki Mitsuya, MD, PhD, and Kenneth McIntosh, MD, Boston, Massachusetts, and Bethesda, Maryland

In human immunodeficiency virus–infected women matched for $CD4^+$ cell percentage, low titers of autologous neutralizing antibody, high virus load, and syncytium-inducing virus phenotype were not associated with increased risk of transmission of HIV-1 to their infants. Other variables apparently determine whether vertical transmission will occur.

Cytokine elevations in infants with bacterial and aseptic meningitis 872
Susan J. Dulkerian, MD, Laurie Kilpatrick, PhD, Andrew T. Costarino, Jr., MD, Lisa McCawley, BS, Joel Fein, MD, Linda Corcoran, BSN, Sharon Zirin, BSN, and Mary Catherine Harris, MD, Philadelphia, Pennsylvania

Measurements of the cytokines interleukin-6 and tumor necrosis factor were helpful in differentiating aseptic from bacterial meningitis in infants; the presence of IL-6 was uniformly sensitive in the prediction of bacterial meningitis.

Vol. 126, No. 6, June 1995. The Journal of Pediatrics (ISSN 0022-3476) is published monthly (six issues per volume, two volumes per year) by Mosby–Year Book, Inc., 11830 Westline Industrial Dr., St. Louis, MO 63146-3318. Second-class postage paid at St. Louis, Mo., and additional mailing offices. POSTMASTER: Send changes of address to The Journal of Pediatrics, Mosby–Year Book, Inc., 11830 Westline Industrial Dr., St. Louis, MO 63146-3318, (800)453-4351. Annual subscription prices effective through September 30, 1995: domestic, $102.00 for individuals and $211.00 for institutions. Printed in U.S.A.

Efficacy of an observation scale in detecting bacteremia in febrile children three to thirty-six months of age, treated as outpatients 877
Stephen J. Teach, MD, MPH, Gary R. Fleisher, MD, and the Occult Bacteremia Study Group, Buffalo, New York, and Boston, Massachusetts

In a large multicenter study of young febrile children with no apparent focal infection, the Yale Observation Scale scores were higher in those with bacteremia, but the difference was too small to be clinically reliable in detecting occult bacteremia in this population.

Clinical characteristics and risk factors for *Vibrio cholerae* infection in children 882
Juan M. Fukuda, MD, Augusto Yi, MD, Luis Chaparro, MD, Miguel Campos, MD, PhD, and Elsa Chea, MD, Lima, Peru

During an epidemic of cholera, children 2 to 14 years of age were more likely to be affected than infants. Diarrhea and vomiting were more severe and dehydration was more likely to require hospitalization than in children with non-cholera-associated diarrhea. With a simple, rapid rehydration regimen the case-fatality rate was very low.

A reexamination of the risk factors for the sudden infant death syndrome 887
James A. Taylor, MD, and Maureen Sanderson, MPH, RD, Seattle, Washington

Analysis of information about infant deaths in a national data set indicated that maternal smoking during pregnancy was significantly more common among infants who died of sudden infant death syndrome than among infants who died of other causes. If pregnant women did not smoke, up to 30% of SIDS might be prevented.

Economic comparison of a tissue adhesive and suturing in the repair of pediatric facial lacerations 892
Martin H. Osmond, MD, CM, Terry P. Klassen, MD, and Jim V. Quinn, MD, Ottawa, Ontario, Canada

An economic analysis showed that a tissue adhesive, rather than a suture method, is the preferred method for closing facial lacerations because it makes the most efficient use of resources and is preferred by most parents.

Risk of recurrent stroke in patients with sickle cell disease treated with erythrocyte transfusions 896
Charles H. Pegelow, MD, Robert J. Adams, MD, Virgil McKie, MD, Miguel Abboud, MD, Brian Berman, MD, Scott T. Miller, MD, Nancy Olivieri, MD, Elliott Vichinsky, MD, Winfred Wang, MD, and Donald Brambilla, PhD, Miami, Florida; Augusta, Georgia; Charleston, South Carolina; Cleveland, Ohio; Brooklyn, New York; Toronto, Ontario, Canada; Oakland, California; Memphis, Tennessee; and Watertown, Massachusetts

A retrospective, multiinstitutional review of patients with sickle cell disease who were receiving long-term transfusion therapy showed that maintaining hemoglobin level at 30% or lower reduces the rate of recurrent stroke but does not prevent transient neurologic events.

Coagulation factor deficiencies during initiation of extracorporeal membrane oxygenation 900
Michael L. McManus, MD, Sherwin V. Kevy, MD, Lynne K. Bower, RRT, and Paul R. Hickey, MD, Boston, Massachusetts

Infants and young children were found to have a high incidence of coagulation abnormalities before and after the initiation of ECMO. These deficiencies may increase the risk of hemorrhage during the procedure. The practice of using factor-deficient priming solutions may need to be reevaluated.

Prediction of the outcome of growth hormone therapy in children with idiopathic short stature: A multivariate discriminant analysis 905
Anna Spagnoli, MD, Gian Luigi Spadoni, MD, Stefano Cianfarani, MD, Anna Maria Pasquino, MD, Simonetta Troiani, MD, and Brunetto Boscherini, MD, Rome, Italy

A mathematical model was derived to identify factors that might predict response to growth hormone therapy in short children without hormone deficiency. A formula including pretreatment growth velocity and bone age was found to have good predictive ability and may be helpful in selecting patients for therapy.

Clinical and biochemical characterization of short-chain acyl–coenzyme A dehydrogenase deficiency 910
Ajay Bhala, BS, Steven M. Willi, MD, Piero Rinaldo, MD, Michael J. Bennett, PhD, MRCPath, Eberhard Schmidt-Sommerfeld, MD, and Daniel E. Hale, MD, Philadelphia, Pennsylvania; Charleston, South Carolina; New Haven, Connecticut; Dallas, Texas; and New Orleans, Louisiana

Clinical and biochemical findings in six patients (four previously reported) with SCAD deficiency are described. All the patients had neurologic abnormalities; four had neonatal onset of metabolic acidosis, but none had hypoglycemia. It may be necessary to study several urine or plasma specimens to confirm the diagnosis.

Neonatal-onset propionic acidemia: Neurologic and developmental profiles, and implications for management 916
Kathryn N. North, MD, Mark S. Korson, MD, Yasodha R. Gopal, MD, Frances J. Rohr, MS, RD, T. Berry Brazelton, MD, Susan E. Waisbren, PhD, and Matthew L. Warman, MD, Boston, Massachusetts

Follow-up studies in six children with neonatal-onset propionic acidemia showed that dietary management and early gastrostomy have improved survival rates and nutritional status, but hypotonia and neurodevelopmental delay are universal, even in the absence of significant metabolic decompensation.

Prolonged dysphagia caused by congenital pharyngeal dysfunction 923
Elie Mbonda, MD, Dominique Claus, MD, C. Bonnier, MD, P. Evrard, MD, J. F. Gadisseux, MD, and G. Lyon, MD, Brussels, Belgium

A severe, congenital disorder of swallowing is described in four infants, two of whom died after tracheal aspiration. The paralysis gradually resolved in the other two children. A dysfunction of the central nervous system seems to be the most likely cause.

The book shelf

Book review 928

Editor's column

Prevention of recurrent febrile seizures 929
Peter R. Camfield, MD, FRCP(C), Carol S. Camfield, MD, FRCP(C), Kevin Gordon, MD, FRCP(C), and Joseph M. Dooley, MB, FRCP(C), Halifax, Nova Scotia, Canada

Clinical and laboratory observations

Comparison of an optical immunoassay technique with two culture methods for the detection of group A streptococci in a pediatric office 931
Oliver F. Roddey, Jr., MD, Herbert W. Clegg, MD, Edward S. Martin, MD, Raymond L. Swetenburg, MD, and Elizabeth W. Koonce, MD, Charlotte, North Carolina

Diagnosis of group A streptococcal pharyngitis in a private clinic: Comparative evaluation of an optical immunoassay method and culture 933
Stephen M. Fries, MD, Boulder, Colorado

Relationship between parental occupation and children's oropharyngeal colonization with *Neisseria meningitidis* 937
W. James King, MD, FRCP(C), Noni E. MacDonald, MD, FRCP(C), George Wells, PhD, Doug Manion, MD, FRCP(C), Frank Chan, MSc, and Upton D. Allen, MD, FRCP(C), Ottawa, Ontario, Canada

CONTENTS *continued*

Consumption of soft drinks with phosphoric acid as a risk factor for the development of hypocalcemia in children: A case-control study 940
Efraín Mazariegos-Ramos, MD, Fernando Guerrero-Romero, MD, Martha Rodríguez-Morán, MD, Gloria Lazcano-Burciaga, MD, Ramón Paniagua, MD, and Dante Amato, MD, DSc, Mexico City, Mexico

Cerebral artery stenoses in Williams syndrome cause strokes in childhood 943
Paige Kaplan, MBBCh, Martin Levinson, MD, and Bernard S. Kaplan, MBBCh, Philadelphia, Pennsylvania, and Detroit, Michigan

Ischemic stroke and intracranial multifocal cerebral arteriopathy in Williams syndrome 945
Robert Soper, MD, John C. Chaloupka, MD, Pierre B. Fayad, MD, John M. Greally, MB,BCh, BAO, Bennett A. Shaywitz, MD, Issam A. Awad, MD, and Barbara R. Pober, MD, New Haven, Connecticut

Pancreatic glucagon levels in infants and children with hyperinsulinemia 948
Ewa Pronicka, Beata Gruszczyńska, Bogdan Woźniewicz, Andrzej Cedro, Wojciech Kamiński, and Anna Leśniewska, Warsaw, Poland

Chronic pancreatitis in a patient with cystic fibrosis and clinical pancreatic insufficiency 951
J. Fernando del Rosario, MD, Philip E. Putnam, MD, and David M. Orenstein, MD, Pittsburgh, Pennsylvania

Beneficial effect of growth hormone on atherogenic risk in children with growth hormone deficiency 953
Hitoshi Kohno, MD, Nami Ueyama, MD, Shinji Yanai, MD, Koutaro Ukaji, MD, and Sunao Honda, MD, Fukuoka, Japan

Bayley-Pinneau method of height prediction in girls with central precocious puberty: Correlation with adult height 955
A. Bar, MD, B. Linder, MD, E. H. Sobel, MD, P. Saenger, MD, and J. DiMartino-Nardi, MD, Bronx, New York

Acquired platelet dysfunction with eosinophilia in white children 959
Man-Chiu Poon, MD, FRCP(C), Soo Chin Ng, MBBS, FRCPA(A), and Max J. Coppes, MD, PhD, Calgary, Alberta, Canada, and Petaling Jaya, Selangor, Malaysia

Effect of airway pressure on inferior vena cava pressure as a measure of central venous pressure in children 961
Zacharia Reda, MD, Sion Houri, MD, Alan L. Davis, MD, and Victor C. Baum, MD, Los Angeles and Long Beach, California

Peutz-Jeghers syndrome in a neonate 965
M. J. Fernandez Seara, MD, M. I. Martinez Soto, MD, J. R. Fernandez Lorenzo, MD, S. Trabazo, MD, E. Gamborino, MD, and J. Forteza Vila, MD, Santiago de Compostela, Spain

CONTENTS *continued*

The book shelf

New books received 968

Fetal and neonatal medicine

Double-blind, randomized trial of one versus three prophylactic doses of synthetic surfactant in 826 neonates weighing 700 to 1100 grams: Effects on mortality rate 969
Anthony Corbet, MB, FRACP, Jeffrey Gerdes, MD, Walker Long, MD, Emilio Avila, MD, Asha Puri, MD, Adam Rosenberg, MD, Kathleen Edwards, MSc, Larry Cook, MD, and American Exosurf Neonatal Study Groups I and II, Atlanta, Georgia; Philadelphia, Pennsylvania; Chapel Hill, North Carolina; Los Angeles, California; Denver, Colorado; Anchorage, Alaska; Research Triangle Park, North Carolina; and Louisville, Kentucky

A large clinical trial showed that three prophylactic doses of synthetic surfactant, given at 12-hour intervals starting soon after birth, were associated with significant reductions in the severity of respiratory distress syndrome and reduced morbidity and mortality rates for small preterm infants in comparison with treatment with only one dose.

Clinical and laboratory observations

Effects of central apnea on cerebral blood flow velocity in healthy term infants 979
Virender K. Rehan, MD, MRCP, MRCPI, Ruben E. Alvaro, MD, Jaques Belik, MD, FRCPC, Doug W. Allen, RRT, Kim Kwiatkowski, RN, and Carlos A. Fajardo, MD, Winnipeg, Manitoba, Canada

Soluble interleukin-2 receptor as a predictor of neonatal sepsis 982
Michael L. Spear, MD, John L. Stefano, MD, Paul Fawcett, PhD, and Roy Proujansky, MD, Newark and Wilmington, Delaware, and Philadelphia, Pennsylvania

Reference ranges for serum cortisol and 17-hydroxyprogesterone levels in preterm infants 985
Saad Al Saedi, MD, FRCPC, Heather Dean, MD, FRCPC, William Dent, MSc, and Catherine Cronin, MD, MRCPI, FRCPC, Winnipeg, Manitoba, Canada

Conjugated hyperbilirubinemia in a newborn infant after maternal (transplacental) treatment with flecainide acetate for fetal tachycardia and fetal hydrops 988
Andre L. Vanderhal, MD, Jose Cocjin, MD, Thomas V. Santulli, Jr., MD, Dru E. Carlson, MD, and Philip Rosenthal, MD, Los Angeles, California

Pediatric pharmacology and therapeutics

Effect of acetaminophen and of low intermittent doses of diazepam on prevention of recurrences of febrile seizures 991
M. Uhari, MD, H. Rantala, MD, L. Vainionpää, MD, and R. Kurttila, BM, Oulu, Finland

In a placebo-controlled, double-masked trial, low doses of acetaminophen or diazepam or both, given at the time of fever, had no significant effect on the recurrence of febrile seizures in children who had one febrile seizure. *See* commentary on page 929.

CONTENTS *continued*

Benign intracranial hypertension in children with growth hormone deficiency treated with growth hormone 996
Saul Malozowski, MD, PhD, L. Ann Tanner, RPh, MPH, Diane K. Wysowski, PhD, G. Alexander Fleming, MD, and Bruce V. Stadel, MD, MPH, Rockville, Maryland

Benign intracranial hypertension developed in 13 children being treated with growth hormone for GH deficiency, and resolved with time, usually after administration of GH was discontinued. The recent use of higher doses may be responsible for this complication of treatment.

Comparative safety and efficacy of two immune globulin products in Kawasaki disease 1000
Elaine A. Rosenfeld, MD, Stanford T. Shulman, MD, Kathleen E. Corydon, RN, William Mason, MD, Masato Takahashi, MD, and Chieko Kuroda, BS, Chicago, Illinois, and Los Angeles, California

The safety and efficacy of two commercially available preparations of immune globulin for intravenous use were compared in patients with Kawasaki disease. Efficacy was similar, but rigors and other reactions were more common after administration of one of the products.

Clinical and laboratory observations

A randomized trial comparing the efficacy of epinephrine with salbutamol in the treatment of acute bronchiolitis 1004
Kusum Menon, MD, Teresa Sutcliffe, RN, and Terry P. Klassen, MD, Ottawa, Ontario, Canada

Antibiotic-associated hemorrhagic colitis without *Clostridium difficile* toxin in children 1008
Seiichi Kato, MD, Kyoko Ebina, MD, Akira Ozawa, MD, Hiroshi Naganuma, MD, and Hiroshi Nakagawa, MD, Sendai, Japan

Neurodevelopmental disabilities

Abnormalities in control of ventilation in newborn infants with myelomeningocele 1011
Mario C. Petersen, MD, Mark Wolraich, MD, Andrea Sherbondy, MD, and Jeff Wagener, MD, Iowa City, Iowa; Nashville, Tennessee; and Denver, Colorado

Ventilatory control studies in neonates with myelomeningocele frequently showed abnormal patterns including an abnormal response to CO_2. However, these abnormalities did not predict the later development of symptoms related to Arnold-Chiari deformity.

The book shelf

New books received 1016

CONTENTS *continued*

Editorial correspondence

Discordance for hyperinsulinemic hypoglycemia in monozygotic twins 1017
René Santer, MD, Heike Hoffmann, MD, Meinolf Suttorp, MD, Eva Simeoni, MD, and Jürgen Schaub, MD, Kiel, Germany

Reply 1017
Paul S. Thornton, MBBCh, MRCPI, Lester Baker, MD, and Charles A. Stanley, MD, Philadelphia, Pennsylvania

Comparison of fiberoptic and conventional phototherapy for neonatal hyperbilirubinemia 1018
Jakob Larsen, MD, and Andrew Whitelaw, MD, FRCP, Oslo, Norway

Reply 1018
K. L. Tan, MBBS, FRCPE, FRACP, DCH, Singapore, Republic of Singapore

Single-day therapy for rickets 1019
F. Mimouni, MD, Brooklyn, New York

Reply 1019
Binita R. Shah, MD, and Laurence Finberg, MD, Brooklyn, New York

Hemoglobin A_{1c} levels in young patients with diabetes beyond the "honeymoon" period 1020
Harry Dorchy, MD, PhD, Brussels, Belgium

Reply 1021
William V. Tamborlane, MD, and David M. Nathan, MD, Bethesda, Maryland

Lactic acidosis in a patient with acute lymphoblastic leukemia 1021
William Lane M. Robson, MD, FRCP(C), FRSH, MRCP(Glasg), and Alexander K. C. Leung, MBBS, FRCP(C), FRCP(Edin), Greenville, South Carolina, and Calgary, Alberta, Canada

True hermaphroditism with 46,XY karyotype and a point mutation in the *SRY* gene 1022
Olaf Hiort, MD, Britta Gramss, and George T. Klauber, MD, Lübeck, Germany, and Boston, Massachusetts

Supplement: Perspectives on infant feeding

Guest Editor's note S103
Steven Shelov, MD, Bronx, New York

Introduction S104
Allen Erenberg, MD, Kansas City, Kansas

Abnormal tympanography after supine bottle feeding S105
Susan B. Tully, MD, Yehuda Bar-Haim, MD, and Richard L. Bradley, PA-C, Los Angeles, California, and Rehovot, Israel

CONTENTS *continued*

The clinician's role in teaching proper infant feeding techniques S112
Ruth Lawrence, MD, Rochester, New York

Quantitative and qualitative video analysis of infants feeding: Angled- and straight-bottle feeding systems S118
Shereen D. Farber, PhD, OTR, FAOTA, Rory L. Van Fossen, MS, and Stephen W. Koontz, PhD, Indianapolis, Indiana, and Skillman, New Jersey

Nipple confusion: Toward a formal definition S125
Marianne Neifert, MD, Ruth Lawrence, MD, and Joy Seacat, RN, CHA, MS, Denver, Colorado, and Rochester, New York

Imaging evaluation of breast-feeding and bottle-feeding systems S130
Arthur J. Nowak, DMD, Wilbur L. Smith, MD, and Allen Erenberg, MD, Iowa City, Iowa, and Kansas City, Kansas

Reader services

Instructions to authors 13A

Information for readers 16A

Scheduled meetings 17A

News and notes 18A

Professional opportunities 25A

Index to advertisers 32A

Indexes

Author index 1025

Subject index 1039

THE JOURNAL OF PEDIATRICS

THE JOURNAL OF PEDIATRICS

JANUARY 1995 *Volume 126* *Number 1*

MEDICAL PROGRESS

Cancer in children with primary or secondary immunodeficiencies

Brigitta U. Mueller, MD, and Philip A. Pizzo, MD

From the Pediatric Branch, National Cancer Institute, Bethesda, Maryland

With improvements in supportive care and other therapeutic advances, children with congenital or acquired immunodeficiencies are surviving longer. Unfortunately, with a more prolonged life span, they also become vulnerable to malignancies. In this review, we will concentrate on the malignancies that occur in children with congenital and acquired immunodeficiencies and highlight new insights in epidemiology, pathogenesis, and treatment.

In the United States, about 7220 new cases of cancer are diagnosed each year in children less than 15 years of age. Leukemias represent 30% of all childhood malignancies; these are mainly of the lymphoblastic type (75%) and of B-cell origin.[1] Lymphomas and brain tumors each account for 12% of pediatric neoplasms. Most of the lymphomas (55%) are of the non-Hodgkin type; the incidence of Hodgkin disease does not increase until adolescence.[2]

The overall risk for children with a congenital immunodeficiency to develop a malignancy has been calculated to be 4%, nearly 10,000 times higher than expected in healthy control groups of similar age.[3] In 1992 the Immunodeficiency Cancer Registry in Minneapolis, Minn., contained more than 500 case records of patients with primary immunodeficiencies in whom a malignancy had developed. The largest numbers of cases were found in patients with either ataxia-telangiectasia or common variable immunodeficiency, representing 30% and 24%, respectively, of all cases registered.[4, 5] After infections, malignancies are the second leading cause of death in children and adults with congenital immunodeficiency disorders.

Autoimmune disorders are also associated with an increased risk of acquiring neoplastic diseases. In one series, 11.4% of the patients with systemic lupus erythematosus-acquired a malignancy.[6] Survivors of childhood cancer have a 10 to 20 times higher risk of having a second cancer than age-matched control subjects. Organ allograft recipients have a 100 times higher risk of having a malignancy than the general population.[3] Through July 1993 the Cincinnati (Ohio) Transplant Tumor Registry had received data on 7070 patients in whom 7539 different cancers developed after transplantation, including 346 children with 354 tumors.[7] Children had a higher proportion of lymphomas (52% vs 15% of all neoplasms) and sarcomas (4% vs 1% of all tumors) than adults.

Children with the acquired immunodeficiency syndrome are at a higher risk of having a malignancy, although an exact incidence rate is currently not available. Neoplastic

AIDS	Acquired immunodeficiency syndrome
AT	Ataxia-telangiectasia
EBV	Epstein-Barr virus
HIV	Human immunodeficiency virus
HPV	Human papillomavirus
WAS	Wiskott-Aldrich syndrome

Reprint requests: Brigitta U. Mueller, MD, Visiting Scientist, Pediatric Branch, National Cancer Institute, Building 10, Room 13N240, Bethesda, MD 20892-1928.

THE JOURNAL OF PEDIATRICS 1995;126:1-10
9/18/61122

Table I. Incidence of malignancies in immunodeficiency disorders

Syndrome	Tumor	Risk (%)	Latency period (yr)
X-linked agammaglobulinemia	Leukemia, NHL	6	10
Wiskott-Aldrich syndrome	NHL, leukemia, Hodgkin disease	>10	6
Bloom syndrome	Leukemia, NHL, Hodgkin disease, adenocarcinomas	25	During first four decades
Ataxia-telangiectasia	Leukemia, NHL, Hodgkin disease, miscellaneous tumors	>12	9
Common variable immunodeficiency syndrome	NHL, stomach cancer	8-10	16
Severe combined immunodeficiency syndrome	NHL	5	0.9
X-linked lymphoproliferative syndrome	NHL	24	After EBV infection
Selective IgA deficiency	NHL, gastric carcinoma, thymoma	?	?
Autoimmune diseases	Hodgkin disease, multiple myeloma, cervical carcinoma, skin cancer	11	37
Chemotherapy/radiotherapy	Leukemia, NHL	3-12	Within 20 yr after treatment
Transplantation (renal, cardiac, or bone marrow)	NHL, skin cancer, anogenital cancer	6	Depends on kind of transplant, preparative regimen and posttransplant immunosuppression
AIDS	NHL, Kaposi sarcoma, cervival and anal neoplasia, soft tissue tumors in children	5-10	Kaposi sarcoma often early, NHL often during end stages of disease but can occur at any time

NHL, Non-Hodgkin lymphoma.

disease was the AIDS-defining illness in 99 (1.9%) of the 5228 children less than 13 years of age reported to the Centers for Disease Control and Prevention (CDC) as of December 1993.[8] Twenty-five had Kaposi sarcoma and 64 had non-Hodgkin lymphoma. It is not clear how many children infected with the human immunodeficiency virus will acquire a neoplastic disease during the course of their illness, but it currently appears to be less common than in the adult population. However, HIV-infected children can acquire a malignancy even before they reach an advanced stage of disease (e.g., when their CD4-positive cell counts are only moderately decreased).

Although the overexpression of cancer in children and adults with congenital and acquired immunodeficiency states underscores the important association of the immune system with neoplasia, it is notable that a relatively limited repertoire of cancers has been observed (Table I). Non-Hodgkin lymphomas and Kaposi sarcomas are the most common tumors, followed by carcinomas of the skin, Hodgkin lymphomas, and leukemias.[5]

PATHOPHYSIOLOGY OF ONCOGENESIS

Virtually all parts of the immune system have the potential to contribute to the eradication of tumor cells. The most important immunologic host response is provided by T cells, which are able to kill directly or to activate other components of the immune system to destroy tumor cells. In animal models, neonatal thymectomy or treatment with antilymphocytic serum results in increased tumor occurrence. Lysis of tumor cells can occur through the action of CD8-positive cytotoxic T cells that are capable of directly recognizing and killing tumor targets by disrupting their cell membrane and nucleus. CD4-positive (helper) T cells are major histocompatibility complex class II restricted, and because most tumors do not express these class II antigens, they do not recognize the tumor cells directly. However, through the interaction with antigen-presenting macrophages, CD4-positive cells are activated and begin to secrete lymphokines that stimulate other effector cells, including cytotoxic T cells and antibody-producing B cells. Other cells also are capable of direct cytotoxic activity, including the natural killer cells, the function of which is augmented by interleukin-2, interferon, possibly interleukin-12, and macrophages that can become cytolytic if activated by certain T-cell lymphokines.[9] This complex network of interactions can be disturbed at various levels, and in immunodeficiency disorders may culminate in a defective response to the proliferation of a malignant cell clone.

The transformation of a normal into a malignant cell is a multistep process. It can be induced by a variety of factors, including chemical or physical carcinogens, or spontaneously occurring random mutations and gene rearrangements.[9] Inherited defects can cause damage in the DNA itself or in its repair mechanisms, and can render the cell more susceptible to neoplastic transformation.[10] Oncogenic DNA viruses, which include papovaviruses, herpesviruses, and adenoviruses, can lead to the development of highly immunogenic tumors despite the absence of any significant viral replication. Several cancers have a strong correlation with certain DNA viruses, including the link of Epstein-Barr virus infection with Burkitt lymphoma and nasopharyngeal carcinoma, and of herpes simplex infection with cervical carcinoma. The hepatitis B virus also has a strong association with primary liver cancer. Oncogenic RNA viruses belong to the family of retroviruses because they contain the gene for reverse transcriptase, a polymerase that allows the transcription of single-stranded RNA into double-stranded DNA. Infection with the oncogenic tumor virus leads to the uptake (transduction) of copies of cellular genes into the viral genome, followed by the activation and subsequent malignant transformation of the infected cell.[11] The mechanisms leading to this transformation may include the introduction or activation of proto-oncogenes, inactivation of tumor suppressor genes, stimulation of growth factors, and suppression of "immune surveillance."[12] Perhaps one of the best known of the human retroviruses, HIV-1, has been closely associated with cancer in adults and increasingly so in children with AIDS. Although generally not considered to be oncogenic per se, HIV contributes to oncogenesis by transactivating a coinfecting oncogenic virus such as EBV or cytomegalovirus, or it may act as a stimulatory factor for already transformed cells.[13] By destroying the immune system, HIV indirectly contributes to the heightened risk of cancer.

MALIGNANCIES IN CHILDREN WITH CONGENITAL IMMUNODEFICIENCIES

Non-Hodgkin lymphomas account for more than 60% of the tumors found in children with congenital immunodeficiency disorders.[10] This prevalence of the non-Hodgkin lymphomas over the leukemias (65% vs 8%) is markedly different from the general distribution of childhood tumors.[14] The risk for the development of a cancer is dependent on the kind of underlying immunodeficiency, the age of the patient, and possibly the presence of cofactors, such as viral infections.

Wiskott-Aldrich syndrome. The risk of malignancy is 100 times higher in patients with Wiskott-Aldrich syndrome than in the general pediatric population.[15] Non-Hodgkin lymphomas account for the majority of these malignancies (Table II).[16] Most of the children have diffuse, high-grade disease, frequently with extranodular involvement. In a group of eight patients with WAS and non-Hodgkin lymphoma, the brain was involved in seven patients, the skin in two, and small bowel and mediastinum in one each.[15] Histologically, the large cell type is predominant, 47% being histiocytic and 38% diffuse immunoblastic, and more than one third appear to have B-cell features.[5, 14, 15] The appearance of a non-Hodgkin lymphoma in a patient with WAS can be preceded by a long period of persistent, indolent lymphadenopathy. As in non-Hodgkin lymphomas encountered in patients after transplantation or in patients with AIDS, infection with EBV appears to play an important role in lymphomagenesis (Table III).[17]

Hodgkin disease is about 10 times less frequent than non-Hodgkin lymphoma and appears to be mostly of the nodular sclerosing type in patients with WAS.[14, 15] These patients also may have a variety of other malignancies, including myelogenous leukemia, cerebellar astrocytoma, or, rarely, smooth muscle tumors.

Ataxia telangiectasia. Patients with AT represent the largest single cohort (approximately 33% of cases) in the Immunodeficiency Cancer Registry.[5] The risk of malignancy appears to be especially high in black patients with AT, in whom a 750-fold excess for lymphomas and a 500-fold excess for leukemias has been described.[18] White patients have an excess of 252-fold for lymphomas and 71-fold for leukemias. It is assumed that the increased chromosome breakages typical of AT, especially those occurring in chromosome regions 11q22 to 11q23, combined with a deficient DNA repair mechanism, predispose persons to these cancers.[19, 20] About 1% of the population carry the AT gene, and carriers have been reported to have a twofold to sixfold increased risk of having cancer. They might be predisposed to the development of breast cancer and cancers of the

Table II. Frequency of different types of neoplasm in immunodeficient children with cancer

	Non-Hodgkin lymphoma (%)	Hodgkin disease (%)	Leukemia (%)	Other tumors
General pediatric population	6.7	5.6	30	Brain tumors, 11.7%
Wiskott-Aldrich syndrome	59-75	4	9	
Ataxia-telangiectasia	41-66	7-10	17-27	Adenocarcinoma, 9.4%
Common variable immunodeficiency syndrome	45-62	4-8	7-19	Adenocarcinoma, 16.4%
Severe combined immunodeficiency syndrome	31-76	7-20	12-20	Adenocarcinoma, 2.4%
Other primary immunodeficiences	16-33	8-14	7-33	Cervical carcinoma, multiple myeloma, Bowen carcinoma
Iatrogenic immunodeficiency	27	3		Kaposi sarcoma, 3.2%; carcinoma of skin, 38%
Acquired immunodeficiency syndrome (AIDS)	66* 9-31†	1.5-12	1-2	Children: Kaposi sarcoma, 16%; leiomyoma or leiomyosarcoma (?%) Adults: Kaposi sarcoma, 59% to 70%; cervical and anal cancer

*In children.
†In adults.

Table III. Non-Hodgkin lymphoma in the immunocompetent and the immunocompromised host

Immunodeficiency	Pathology	Phenotype	Site	Comment
None	Small non-cleaved-cell tumors, 50%; lymphoblastic, 33%; large cell, 15%	B and T cell	Abdominal lymph nodes, bone marrow, nasopharynx, other lymph nodes	14;18 translocation; associated with EBV infection in African (endemic) Burkitt lymphoma
Congenital	Large cell, 52%	Mostly B cell, except for AT, where T-cell tumors are more common	Extranodal sites: primary CNS tumors in WAS and SCID; gastrointestinal tract in common variable immunodeficiency	Association with EBV infection in X-linked lymphoproliferative syndrome
Iatrogenic	Large cell, 70%; immunoblastic, 20%	T cell, 12%; rarely polyclonal	Primary CNS tumors in 33%; allograft can be affected	Association with EBV in transplant patients
AIDS	Small non-cleaved-cell tumors, 80% to 90% (Burkitt and non-Burkitt type)	Mostly B cell	Primary CNS tumors, 17% to 42%; bone marrow, 30%	8;14 translocation; in CNS tumors, association with EBV infection

CNS, Central nervous system; *SCID*, severe combined immunodeficiency.

stomach, pancreas, bladder, and ovary, as well as leukemia.[21]

Sixty percent of the malignancies in patients with AT are lymphomas, often with a 14q+ chromosomal abnormality.[14, 18, 22] The ratio of T-cell to B-cell lymphoid malignancy (leukemias and lymphomas) is 6:1, which is different from that in the general population.[21] Hodgkin disease occurs in patients with AT at a significantly younger age than in the general pediatric population (mean age 7.8 years vs. 11.5 years).[23] A large proportion of these patients also have tumors with mixed cellularity (42%) or lymphocyte depletion (33% vs 3% in the general population), whereas the nodular sclerosing type prevails in the general pediatric population.[14, 23] Among 119 patients with cancer and AT, 31 had solid tumors (brain tumors, gastric carcinomas, ovarian or uterine tumors).[20]

Severe combined immunodeficiency syndrome. Severe combined immunodeficiency syndrome is the most severe of the congenital immunodeficiencies. Despite improved antibiotic therapy, affected children rarely survive beyond the first 2 years of life unless a successful bone marrow transplant is performed, or, in the case of adenosine deaminase deficiency syndrome, enzyme substitution or gene therapy or both are used. Because the number of children who survive for a prolonged period is small, the accurate incidence rate for malignancies is difficult to assess but is estimated to be about 1.5%. In 1987 the Immunodeficiency Cancer Registry listed 31 patients with non-Hodgkin lymphoma, 4 with Hodgkin disease, and 5 with leukemia.[16] This represents an estimated 30-fold increase in lymphomas compared with that in the general population.[24] These tumors occurred in infants or very young children with a median age of 0.9 year.[3, 25]

Common variable immunodeficiency syndrome, selective IgA deficiency, X-linked agammaglobulinemia and Bloom syndrome. Common variable immunodeficiency syndrome is the most common form of immunodeficiency and has a broad spectrum of disease manifestations, including late-onset hypogammaglobulinemia, recurrent sinopulmonary infections, and autoimmune disorders. If the immunodeficiency has its onset before the age of 16 years, the incidence of cancer has been estimated to be about 2.5%; if the onset is later, the incidence rises to 8.5%.[25] Non-Hodgkin lymphomas account for about half of the neoplasms, a 30-fold excess over the normal population. Epithelial tumors are seen in 39%, including carcinomas of the stomach (with a 47-fold excess), breast, bladder, and cervix.[4, 5, 14, 25] As in other immunodeficiency disorders, lymphoproliferative lesions ranging from chronic lymphomatous inflammation to malignant lymphomas have been described.[26]

Disorders involving immunoglobulin production are also associated with an increased number of malignancies, mostly of lymphoreticular origin. Selective IgA deficiency, in contrast, is associated with a high incidence of epithelial tumors (comprising 75% of all tumors), mostly gastric carcinomas.[16] The IgA system is primarily involved in the local defense of the mucosa against pathogens, especially in the respiratory and gastrointestinal tract. The development of pulmonary and gastric carcinomas has been attributed to a defect in local immune surveillance, but definitive proof is lacking.

Children with sex-linked agammaglobulinemia (Bruton type) appear to have a risk of 6% for the development of a malignancy.[25] The neoplasms observed are mostly of lymphoreticular origin, and the children have a median age of 4 years at the time of diagnosis of the malignancy.[14]

Bloom syndrome is a rare disorder characterized by an increased frequency of chromosomal breaks, rearrangements, and abnormalities in DNA repair. As of 1987, a total of 130 persons were registered in the Bloom Syndrome Registry, and 57 malignant neoplasms had been detected among them.[27] Several different malignancies have been reported, including acute leukemias, non-Hodgkin lymphomas, and Hodgkin disease. The majority of patients have solid tumors of skin, breast, or gastrointestinal tract, which occur during the second or third decade of life.

X-linked lymphoproliferative syndrome (Duncan disease). In 1975 Purtilo et al.[28] described a kindred with 18 boys, of whom 6 died of a lymphoproliferative disorder. This syndrome has since been linked to infection with the EBV. The affected boys have a T-cell regulatory defect that makes them extremely vulnerable to EBV infection, which often is fatal.[24, 29] The immune defect allows an explosive proliferation of B-cells after exposure to EBV. Of the patients who survive the initial infection with EBV, 24% will acquire a malignant lymphoproliferative disorder, at a median age of 4.9 years. All neoplasms have a B-cell phenotype; 45% are of the small and noncleaved type. The majority of the non-Hodgkin lymphomas occur in the intestinal region, especially the ileocecal area. The overall risk of having a lymphoma has been estimated to be 200 times higher than for the general population.[24] This disease bridges the gap between benign proliferation and malignant lymphoma. A similar phenomenon is observed in patients receiving immunosuppressive therapy after an allograft transplant, or in patients with AIDS.

MALIGNANCIES IN CHILDREN WITH ACQUIRED IMMUNODEFICIENCIES

Autoimmune disease. There are numerous case reports that associate autoimmune disorders with malignancies, but a true incidence rate is difficult to establish because of the protracted course and variable degree of immunosuppression. Cancers usually occur several years after the onset of the autoimmune disease and are therefore rarely seen during childhood. There is an increased incidence of lymphoid proliferation, mostly of B-cell origin, in patients with Sjögren syndrome, and the incidence of malignant lymphomas has been calculated to be 44 times greater than in the general population. Patients with celiac disease, who also have an increased cancer risk, have a tendency to acquire either lymphomas or carcinomas of the gastrointestinal tract.[4] In addition, there have been several reports of patients in whom cancers develop during therapy with immunosuppressive agents given for diseases such as psoriasis, ulcerative colitis, and other autoimmune states.

Chemotherapy- and radiotherapy-associated immunodeficiency. Within the first 20 years after the initial diagnosis and treatment of a neoplastic disease, the incidence of second malignancies is between 3% and 12%.[30] A major etiologic factor is presumably the carcinogenicity of the cancer therapy per se. Exceptions are patients who have been treated for Hodgkin disease, in whom the risk of having a second cancer during the first 10 years after diagnosis is between 1.3% for non-Hodgkin lymphomas and 6.7% for solid tumors. It has been suggested that the development of a non-Hodgkin lymphoma is related to the immunocompromised state of the patient as a result of the Hodgkin disease, and that the risk of having solid tumors is a sequel of the toxic effects of chemotherapy or radiotherapy.

Transplant-associated immunodeficiency. The type and intensity of the immunosuppressive regimen appear to influence both the rate and the time of occurrence of a neoplastic disease after organ transplantation. The average time from transplantation to the appearance of cancer is between 33 and 61 months,[31, 32] but lymphoproliferative disorders may occur as early as 10 months afterward.[33] Most of the experience comes from the observation of patients after renal allograft transplantation, but malignancies have been seen after cardiac, lung, and bone marrow transplantation as well.

The most prevalent malignancies are non-Hodgkin lymphomas (98% in children), mostly of B-cell origin.[7] Extranodal involvement is seen in two thirds of all cases, and more than 25% have a primary central nervous system tumor (Table III). The allograft itself is affected in 18% of renal transplants and in 86% of liver transplants, and this rate has also been described for cardiac transplant patients with non-Hodgkin lymphoma.[32, 34] In addition, an increasing number of patients have a lymphoproliferative disorder.[33-35] Several studies have documented the association between EBV infection and posttransplantation lymphoproliferative disorder.[36] Continued B-cell activation after the initial infection may promote a polyclonal proliferation, which, with time, can develop into a monoclonal malignancy.[26] The lymphoproliferative disorder is reversible after discontinuation or reduction of the immunosuppressive regimen. The addition of the monoclonal antibody OKT3, which is T-cell specific, has shortened the time to the appearance of lymphoproliferative disease and has increased the incidence.[35] Combination regimens using OKT3 together with one to three additional immunosuppressive agents seem to have enhanced this problem even further.[33]

Although uncommon in children, carcinomas of the skin account for 38% of the neoplastic diseases in adult patients after an allograft transplantation, a 4- to 21-fold increase compared with the general population.[22] In patients who have received a bone marrow transplant, this is thought, at least in part, to be due to chronic graft-versus-host disease. Malignant melanomas have also been described, and they arise from a dysplastic precursor nevus. Kaposi sarcoma is seen with a 400-fold excess in organ transplant recipients, with a male/female ratio of 2.3:1, an unusually high incidence for women.

Children with the acquired immunodeficiency syndrome. About 10% to 15% of HIV-infected adult patients have a malignancy (i.e., non-Hodgkin lymphoma or Kaposi sarcoma) as their AIDS-indicator disease.[8] Further, between 15% and 40% of HIV-infected adults may have a malignancy during the course of their illness.[37] A multicenter study from Italy reported only seven malignancies (4 non-Hodgkin lymphomas, 1 Kaposi sarcoma, 1 hepatoblastoma, 1 B-cell leukemia) among 1321 children with HIV infection.[38] In our group of more than 400 affected children we have observed 10 with a non-Hodgkin lymphoma, one adolescent with a localized Kaposi sarcoma, and four children with leiomyomas or leiomyosarcomas. The most common cancer in children and adults with HIV infection is non-Hodgkin lymphoma, occurring either as a systemic disease or as a primary CNS tumor.[38, 39] One study found a 360-fold excess of non-Hodgkin lymphomas in HIV-infected children less than the age of 19 years.[40] Most of the non-Hodgkin lymphomas in adults and children with HIV infection are high-grade malignancies, consisting of small non-cleaved-cell, B-cell immunoblastic, or diffuse large–cell lymphomas.

Patients with HIV infection have profound cellular and humoral immune suppression and dysfunction, and they tend to be infected with other, potentially oncogenic viruses such as cytomegalovirus, EBV, human papillomavirus, and hepatitis B virus. It is also possible that increased levels of growth factors such as interleukin-1, interleukin-6, and tumor necrosis factor sustain uncontrolled proliferation of malignant cells.[41]

Epstein-Barr virus DNA can be demonstrated in only 30% to 50% of the systemic non-Hodgkin lymphomas, although it is found in the majority of CNS lymphomas. There appear to be geographic areas that have a higher frequency of EBV positivity in non-Hodgkin lymphomas, and some have described a distinct EBV-positive polyclonal type of non-Hodgkin lymphoma. High-grade non-Hodgkin lymphomas, specifically the small, non-cleaved-cell type occurring in association with HIV disease, have frequent chromosomal translocations, including 8;14, 8;22, and 2;8 translocations. This results in alterations of the regulatory region of c-*myc*, which, through inappropriate expression of the c-*myc* protein, leads to uncontrolled growth. Although the majority of the non-Hodgkin lymphomas are of B-cell origin, there have been several reports of T-cell lymphomas, including Ki-1+ anaplastic lymphomas and cutaneous T-cell malignancies.[42, 43]

Involvement of extranodal sites occurs in up to 87% of HIV-infected patients. Primary CNS disease accounts for 4% to 40% of the non-Hodgkin lymphomas in HIV-infected adults.[40] Patients often have confusion, lethargy, memory loss, and sometimes seizures or other neurologic findings. A computed tomogram of the brain usually shows isodense or hypodense single lesions that are enhanced with contrast medium. Histopathologic evaluation reveals multicentric tumors with an angiocentric distribution. The brain stem and spinal cord can be involved, with focal leptomeningeal and perivascular lymphomatous infiltrates. Other extranodal sites commonly involved are the gastrointestinal tract, bone marrow, heart, kidneys, liver, and bone.

As in patients receiving immunosuppressive therapy after an allograft transplantation, a polyclonal, polymorphic B-cell lymphoproliferative disorder that is strongly associated with EBV has been observed in patients with HIV infection, in children often in conjunction with lymphocytic interstitial pneumonitis.[44, 45]

Because the incidence of Hodgkin disease peaks among young adults (when HIV disease is most prevalent), it has been difficult to demonstrate an excess incidence in HIV-infected adults. However, recent data from San Francisco indicate an excess risk of Hodgkin disease of 19.3 cases per 100,000 person-years.[46] There are no data yet to indicate an increased incidence of Hodgkin disease in HIV-infected children.

KAPOSI SARCOMA

More than 29,000 cases of Kaposi sarcoma in HIV-infected adults have been reported to the Centers for Disease Control and Prevention as of 1993. However, it is uncommon in HIV-infected children, only 25 pediatric cases having been reported as an AIDS-defining illness.[8] Published reports include the case of a child with transfusion-acquired HIV infection several years after a kidney transplantation and the cases of six children with perinatally acquired HIV infection.[47] Most children had the lymphadenopathic form, sometimes with diffuse nodular skin lesions.

Kaposi sarcoma has a spindle cell component, and recently published data indicate a relationship of cultured Kaposi sarcoma cells to leiomyoblasts. Histopathologic findings range from a granulation-like lesion in early stages to one in later stages that is reminiscent of angiosarcoma or fibrosarcoma. The pathogenesis of AIDS-associated Kaposi sarcoma is not completely understood, and it is even questionable whether Kaposi sarcoma is a "true" neoplasm. This includes the observation that Kaposi sarcoma often arises with a multifocal origin rather than as primary tumor with metastases, that cytogenetic abnormalities are rare, and that spontaneous tumor regression can occur in some patients.

OTHER TUMORS

Fewer than 10% of malignancies in HIV-infected adults are neither Kaposi sarcomas nor non-Hodgkin lymphomas. They include seminomas, lung cancer, brain tumors, and epithelial and mucosal malignancies, as well as germ cell tumors.[48] Estimates of incidence rely heavily on case reports because these tumors are not diagnostic of AIDS and are therefore not registered in a systematic way. In children it is even more difficult to discern trends because of the relatively small number of HIV-infected children. In addition, pediatric HIV disease is often rapidly progressive, and the overall incidence of cancer in childhood is much lower than in adults.

The incidence of soft tissue tumors in the general pediatric population is 8.4 cases per million, and smooth muscle tumors account for fewer than 2% of these.[49] Several reports of soft tissue tumors in pediatric patients with AIDS have been published, including eight cases of leiomyomas or leiomyosarcomas, one fibrosarcoma, and one rhabdomyosarcoma. We are also aware of five additional children with leiomyomatous tumors.[50]

Cervical and anal neoplasms have also been seen with increased frequency in HIV-infected adults. In one study the incidence of squamous intraepithelial cervical lesions was 40% in HIV-infected women versus 9% in uninfected women, and the cervical neoplasias progress more rapidly and are associated with early and widespread metastatic disease.[51] Anal epithelial abnormalities were found in 14% of homosexual HIV-infected men and were strongly associated with certain HPV genotypes.[52] Cervical and anal neoplasias may also occur in the child with HIV infection. One of the published cases of invasive cervical carcinoma occurred in a 16-year-old girl.[53] Children with HIV infection have been described with either widespread cutaneous flat warts, or severe and extensive perineal condylomata acuminata caused by HPV infection.

PRINCIPLES OF MANAGEMENT

Progress in the treatment of cancer has been made in large part through the systematic study of pediatric malignancies. As new syndromes or diseases evolve, it is important to collect surveillance and prevalence data. A nationwide registry to assess incidence, risk factors, biologic features, and outcome of neoplastic diseases in immunosuppressed patients is therefore of great value.[16] A registry of HIV-infected children and adolescents with malignancies has recently been initiated in collaboration with the AIDS Clinical Trial Groups and the Pediatric Oncology Group.

Comparison with the treatment of cancer in nonimmunosuppressed hosts. A detailed review of therapeutic regimens for the different cancers observed in immunosuppressed patients is beyond the scope of this review. Treatment is similar to strategies used in the general population, with the exception that in the patient receiving immunosuppressive drugs, a regression of the neoplastic lesion can often be induced by a reduction or interruption of the iatrogenic immune suppression. If possible, radiation therapy should not be used in patients with AT or Bloom syndrome because of their impaired DNA repair mechanisms. The decision to treat a malignancy in the immunosuppressed child, and especially the child with HIV infection, must be guided by the stage of the cancer as well as the overall performance status of the patient. If treatment is initiated, it should be with the intention to cure the malignancy. Aggressive supportive care combined with antiinfective prophylaxis during chemotherapy is of great importance, because many children will be at risk of having opportunistic infections such as *Pneumocystis carinii* pneumonia or fungal infections. Granulocyte colony-stimulating factor can shorten the duration and diminish the severity of neutropenia. Its use in HIV-infected children may allow the delivery of the dose of chemotherapy that is necessary for cure. In the patient with HIV infection it is also important to deliver concomitant antiretroviral therapy, because therapy for cancer will be of benefit only if disease progression during times of added iatrogenic immunosuppression is avoided and the clinical manifestations of HIV infection can be controlled. Our recent experience with six immunosuppressed patients treated for non-Hodgkin lymphoma with a dose-intensive chemotherapeutic regimen of short duration has been encouraging. After three courses of the combination of cyclophosphamide and methotrexate administered systemically and methotrexate and cytarabine administered intrathecally, four of the children reached a complete remission and two a partial remission, and all patients tolerated chemotherapy well. The five patients with HIV infection received concomitant antiretroviral therapy.

PREVENTION, AND RESEARCH TOPICS FOR THE FUTURE

The number of successful allograft transplants is increasing and patients are surviving longer. Although the immunosuppressive regimens used are becoming more selective, some of them also appear to have a higher oncogenic potential.[35] The knowledge accumulated through the care of these patients provides a unique opportunity to gain insight into the pathophysiologic mechanisms that lead to primary and secondary immunodeficiencies. This is particularly important because an estimated 14 million adults and 500,000 children are infected with HIV.

In several of the neoplastic diseases that occur in patients with immunodeficiency disorders, there is strong evidence of an interaction between, and perhaps a causative role for, viruses. The influences of EBV on non-Hodgkin lymphoma, of HPV on the development of cervical neoplasias, and of cytomegalovirus on Kaposi sarcoma are being studied. Leiomyomas and leiomyosarcomas appear to occur more frequently in children with HIV infection and have occasionally been seen in other immunodeficiency states. Insulin-like growth factor genes have recently been shown to be important in the pathogenesis of smooth muscle tumors; insulin-like growth factor I is expressed at high levels in leiomyomas, whereas growth factor II is seen predominantly in leiomyosarcomas and other sarcomas.[54] Both growth factors are markedly influenced by nutritional status and caloric intake, which are often suboptimal in chronically ill children with an immunodeficiency. Although malignancies occurring in immunodeficiency states represent only a small percentage of all cancers, they help us understand many immunopathogenic mechanisms important not only for this group but also for tumor immunology and oncogenesis in general.

REFERENCES

1. Poplack DG. Acute lymphoblastic leukemia. In: Pizzo PA, Poplack DG, eds. Principles and practice of pediatric oncology. 2nd ed. Philadelphia: JB Lippincott, 1993:431-81.
2. Magrath IT. Malignant non-Hodgkin's lymphomas in children. In: Pizzo PA, Poplack DG, eds. Principles and practice of pediatric oncology. 2nd ed. Philadelphia: JB Lippincott, 1993:537-75.
3. Ioachim HL. The opportunistic tumors of immune deficiency. Adv Cancer Res 1990;54:301-17.
4. Penn I. Lymphoproliferative diseases in disorders of the immune system. Cancer Detect Prev 1990;14:415-22.
5. Filipovich AH, Mathur A, Kamat D, Kersey JH, Shapiro RS. Lymphoproliferative disorders and other tumors complicating immunodeficiencies. Immunodeficiency 1994;5:91-112.
6. Canoso JJ, Cohen AS. Malignancy in a series of 70 patients with systemic lupus erythematosus. Arthritis Rheum 1974; 17:383-90.
7. Penn I. De novo tumors in pediatric organ transplant recipients. Transplant Proc 1994;26:1-2.
8. Centers for Disease Control and Prevention. HIV/AIDS Surveillance Report [year-end edition] 1994;5:1-33.
9. Greenberg PD. Mechanisms of tumor immunology. In: Stites DP, Terr AI, ed. Basic and clinical immunology. 7th ed. Norwalk, Connecticut: Appleton & Lange, 1991:580-7.
10. Müller H. Recessively inherited deficiencies predisposing to cancer. Anticancer Res 1990;10:513-8.
11. Israel MA. Cancer cell biology. In: Pizzo PA, Poplack DG, ed. Principles and practice of pediatric oncology. 2nd ed. Philadelphia: JB Lippincott, 1993:57-80.

12. Cremer KJ, Spring SB, Gruber J. Role of human immunodeficiency virus type 1 and other viruses in malignancies associated with acquired immunodeficiency disease syndrome. J Natl Cancer Inst 1990;82:1016-24.
13. Shiramizu B, Herndier BG, McGrath MS. Identification of a common clonal human immunodeficiency virus integration site in human immunodeficiency virus–associated lymphomas. Cancer Res 1994;54:2069-72.
14. Frizzera G, Rosai J, Dehner LP, Spector BD, Kersey JH. Lymphoreticular disorders in primary immunodeficiencies: new findings based on an up-to-date histologic classification of 35 cases. Cancer 1980;46:692-9.
15. Cotelingam JD, Witebsky FG, Hsu SM, Blaese RM, Jaffe ES. Malignant lymphoma in patients with the Wiskott-Aldrich syndrome. Cancer Invest 1985;3:515-22.
16. Filipovich AH, Heinitz KJ, Robison LL, Frizzera G. The immunodeficiency cancer registry: a research resource. Am J Pediatr Hematol Oncol 1987;9:183-4.
17. Gatti RA, Good RA. Occurrence of malignancy in immunodeficiency diseases: a literature review. Cancer 1971;28:89-98.
18. Morrell D, Cromartie E, Swift M. Mortality and cancer incidence in 263 patients with ataxia telangiectasia. J Natl Cancer Inst 1986;77:89-92.
19. Hecht F, Kaiser-McCaw Hecht B. Chromosome changes connect immunodeficiency and cancer in ataxia-telangiectasia. Am J Pediatr Hematol Oncol 1987;9:185-8.
20. Hecht F, Hecht BK. Cancer in ataxia-telangiectasia patients. Cancer Genet Cytogenet 1990;46:9-19.
21. Taylor AMR. Ataxia telangiectasia genes and predisposition to leukaemia, lymphoma and breast cancer. Br J Cancer 1992; 66:5-9.
22. Ziegler JL. Cancer in the immunocompromised host. In: Stites DP, Terr AI, eds. Basic and clinical immunology. 7th ed. Norwalk, Connecticut: Appleton & Lange, 1991:588-98.
23. Robison LL, Stoker V, Frizzera G, Heinitz K, Meadows AT, Filipovich AH. Hodgkin's disease in pediatric patients with naturally occurring immunodeficiency. Am J Pediatr Hematol Oncol 1987;9:189-92.
24. Seibel NL, Cossman J, Magrath IT. Lymphoproliferative disorders. In: Pizzo PA, Poplack DG, eds. Principles and practice of pediatric oncology. 2nd ed. Philadelphia: JB Lippincott, 1993:595-616.
25. Groopman JE, Broder S. Cancers in AIDS and other immunodeficiency states. In: DeVita VT, Hellman S, Rosenberg SA, eds. Cancer: principles and practice of oncology. 3rd ed. Philadelphia: JB Lippincott, 1989:1953-70.
26. Sander CA, Medeiros J, Weiss LM, Yano T, Sneller MC, Jaffe ES. Lymphoproliferative lesions in patients with common variable immunodeficiency syndrome. Am J Surg Pathol 1992;16:1170-82.
27. German J, Passarge E. Bloom's syndrome. XII. Report from the Registry for 1987. Clin Genet 1989;35:57-69.
28. Purtilo DT, Yang JPS, Cassel CK, et al. X-linked recessive progressive combined variable immunodeficiency (Duncan's disease). Lancet 1975;1:935-41.
29. Weinberg KI, Parkman R. Interface between immunodeficiency and pediatric cancer. In: Pizzo PA, Poplack DG, eds. Principles and practice of pediatric oncology. Philadelphia: JB Lippincott, 1989:65-79.
30. Blatt J, Copeland DR, Bleyer WA. Late effects of childhood cancer and its treatment. In: Pizzo PA, Poplack DG, eds. Principles and practice of pediatric oncology. 2nd ed. Philadelphia: JB Lippincott, 1993:1091-114.
31. Vogt P, Frei U, Repp H, Bunzendahl H, Oldhafer K, Pichlmayr R. Malignant tumours in renal transplant recipients receiving cyclosporine: survey of 598 first-kidney transplantations. Nephrol Dial Transplant 1990;5:282-8.
32. Penn I. Cancers complicating organ transplantation. N Engl J Med 1990;323:1767-9.
33. Cockfield SM, Preisaitis J, Harvey E, et al. Is sequential use of ALG and OKT3 in renal transplants associated with an increased incidence of fulminant posttransplant lymphoproliferative disorder? Transplant Proceed 1991;23: 1106-7.
34. Abu-Farsakh H, Cagle PT, Buffone GJ, Bruner JM, Weilbaecher D, Greenberg SD. Heart allograft involvement with Epstein-Barr virus–associated posttransplant lymphoproliferative disorder. Arch Pathol Lab Med 1992;116:93-5.
35. Swinnen LJ, Costanza-Nordin MR, Fisher SG, et al. Increased incidence of lymphoproliferative disorder after immunosuppression with the monoclonal antibody OKT3 in cardiac-transplant recipients. N Engl J Med 1990;323:1723-8.
36. Sokal EM, Caragiozoglou T, Lamy M, Reding R, Otte JB. Epstein-Barr virus serology and Epstein-Barr virus–associated lymphoproliferative disorders in pediatric liver transplant recipients. Transplantation 1993;56:1394-8.
37. Monfardini S, Vaccher E, Lazzarin A, et al. Characterization of AIDS-associated tumors in Italy: report of 435 cases of an IVDA-based series. Cancer Detect Prev 1990;14:391-3.
38. Arico M, Caselli D, D'Argenio P, et al. Malignancies in children with human immunodeficiency virus type 1 infection. Cancer 1991;68:2473-7.
39. DiCarlo FJ, Joshi VV, Oleske JM, Connor EM. Neoplastic diseases in children with acquired immunodeficiency syndrome. Prog AIDS Pathol 1990;2:163-85.
40. Beral V, Peterman T, Berkelman R, Jaffe H. AIDS-associated non-Hodgkin lymphoma. Lancet 1991;337:805-9.
41. Matsuyama T, Kobayashi N, Yamamoto N. Cytokines and HIV infection: is AIDS a tumor necrosis factor disease? AIDS 1991;5:1405-17.
42. Ruff P, Bagg A, Papadopoulos K. Precursor T-cell lymphoma associated with human immunodeficiency virus type 1 (HIV-1) infection. Cancer 1989;64:39-42.
43. Gold JE, Ghali V, Gold S, Brown JC, Zalusky R. Angiocentric immunoproliferative lesion/T-cell non-Hodgkin's lymphoma and the acquired immune deficiency syndrome: a case report and review of the literature. Cancer 1990;66:2407-13.
44. Joshi VV, Kauffman S, Oleske JM, et al. Polyclonal polymorphic B-cell lymphoproliferative disorder with prominent pulmonary involvement in children with acquired immune deficiency syndrome. Cancer 1987;59:1455-62.
45. Katz BZ, Berkman AB, Shapiro ED. Serologic evidence of active Epstein-Barr virus infection in Epstein-Barr virus–associated lymphoproliferative disorders of children with acquired immunodeficiency syndrome. J PEDIATR 1992;120:228-32.
46. Hessol NA, Katz MH, Liu JY, Buchbinder SP, Rubino CJ, Holmberg SD. Increased incidence of Hodgkin disease in homosexual men with HIV infection. Ann Intern Med 1992; 117:309-11.
47. Connor E, Boccon-Gibod L, Joshi V, et al. Cutaneous acquired immunodeficiency syndrome–associated Kaposi's sarcoma in pediatric patients. Arch Dermatol 1990;126:791-3.

48. Monfardini S, Vaccher E, Pizzocaro G, et al. Unusual malignant tumours in 49 patients with HIV infection. AIDS 1989; 3:449-52.
49. Miser JS, Triche TJ, Pritchard DJ, Kinsella TJ. The other soft tissue sarcomas of childhood. In: Pizzo PA, Poplack DG, eds. Principles and practice of pediatric oncology. 2nd ed. Philadelphia: JB Lippincott, 1993:823-40.
50. Mueller BU, Shad AT, Magrath IT, Horowitz ME. Malignancies in children with HIV infection. In: Pizzo PA, Wilfert CM, eds. Pediatric AIDS: the challenge of HIV infection in infants, children, and adolescents. 2nd ed. Baltimore: Williams & Wilkins, 1994:603-22.
51. Rellihan MA, Dooley DP, Burke TW, Berkland ME, Longfield RN. Rapidly progressing cervical cancer in a patient with human immunodeficiency virus infection. Gynecol Oncol 1990;36:435-8.
52. Palefsky JM. Anal human papillomavirus infection and anal cancer in HIV-positive individuals: an emerging problem. AIDS 1994;8:283-95.
53. Maiman M, Fruchter RG, Serur E, Remy JC, Feuer G, Boyce J. Human immunodeficiency virus infection and cervical neoplasia. Gynecol Oncol 1990;38:377-82.
54. Gloudemans T, Prinsen I, Van Unnik JAM, Lips CJM, Otter WD, Sussenbach JS. Insulin-like growth factor gene expression in human smooth muscle tumors. Cancer Res 1990; 50:6689-95.

FELLOWSHIPS

Fellowships available in pediatric subspecialties and those for general academic pediatric training are listed once a year, in **January,** in THE JOURNAL OF PEDIATRICS. Each **June,** forms for listing fellowships available for the academic year beginning 18 months after publication are sent to the Chairman of the Department of Pediatrics at major hospitals in the United States and Canada. In addition, **a copy of the application form appears in the July, August, and September issues** of THE JOURNAL (please use the current form). Should you desire to list fellowships, a separate application must be made *each* year for *each* position. All applications must be returned to Mosby–Year Book, Inc., by **October 15** preceding the listing year to ensure publication. Additional forms will be supplied on request from the Journal Editing Department, Mosby–Year Book, Inc., 11830 Westline Industrial Drive, St. Louis, MO 63146-3318/800-325-4177, ext. 4317, or 314-453-4317.

Progression of premature thelarche to central precocious puberty

Anna Maria Pasquino, MD, Ida Pucarelli, MD, Franca Passeri, MD, Maria Segni, MD, Maria Antonietta Mancini, MD, and Giovanna Municchi, MD

From the Pediatric Endocrinology Unit, Pediatric Department, University "La Sapienza," Rome, Italy

To evaluate whether girls with premature thelarche progress to central precocious puberty (CPP) and to analyze their clinical and hormonal characteristics, we retrospectively examined 100 girls with premature thelarche who were followed for several years. Fourteen of the patients with characteristics diagnostic of premature thelarche (isolated breast development before age 8 years, bone age advancement within 2 SD of normal, normal growth velocity, follicle-stimulating hormone–predominant response to luteinizing hormone–releasing hormone) progressed during follow-up to precocious or early central puberty (progressive breast size increase, bone age acceleration, and significant decrease in predicted adult height). The chronologic age of this group of 14 girls was 5.1 ± 2.0 years at the onset of premature thelarche and 7.8 ± 0.6 years (mean ± SD) after progression to central early or precocious puberty. Pelvic ultrasonography showed significant differences in measurements between the time of diagnosis of premature thelarche and progression to CPP. Nine of these patients required treatment, three with cyproterone acetate and six with luteinizing hormone–releasing hormone analogs, and all responded as expected for classic CPP. At baseline evaluation, no clinical or hormonal characteristics could be established that separated the 14 children who progressed to precocious or early puberty from the 86 girls who did not. We conclude that premature thelarche is not always a self-limited condition and may sometimes accelerate the timing of puberty. (J Pediatr 1995;126:11-4)

Premature thelarche is characterized by isolated breast development without any other clinical signs of sexual maturation in girls before age 8 years; the highest prevalence is during the first 2 years of life.[1] The relationship between premature thelarche and central precocious puberty has been discussed in several reports; the current concept is that premature thelarche is a benign self-limited condition that only rarely progresses to CPP.[2, 3] We reexamined the clinical and hormonal characteristics of 100 girls with premature thelarche to determine how many of this large cohort had progressed into CPP.

Submitted for publication Aug. 9, 1993; accepted Aug. 11, 1994.

Reprint requests: Anna Maria Pasquino, MD, Pediatric Endocrinology Unit, Pediatric Department, University "La Sapienza," Viale Regina Elena 324, 00161 Rome, Italy.

0022-3476/95/$3.00 + 0 **9/20/59782**

CPP	Central precocious puberty
FSH	Follicle-stimulating hormone
LH	Luteinizing hormone
LH-RH	Luteinizing hormone–releasing hormone
PAH	Predicted adult height

METHODS

Subjects. One hundred girls with premature thelarche were examined in our pediatric endocrine unit between 1975 and 1990. After other causes of breast development (estrogen intake, CPP, estrogen-secreting tumors) were ruled out, premature thelarche was diagnosed according to the classic criteria: breast development without other signs of puberty

Table. Clinical and hormonal characteristics of 14 girls with premature thelarche who progressed to CPP, compared with 86 girls with premature thelarche who did not progress to CPP

Characteristics	Nonprogressive (n = 86)	Progressive (n = 14)	After progression (n = 14)
Chronologic age (yr)	4.7 ± 2.7	5.1 ± 2.0	7.8 ± 0.6
Bone age (yr)	5.6 ± 2.8	5.9 ± 2.3	10.3 ± 0.4
Breast regression	No (n = 48); yes (n = 48)	No (n = 7); yes (n = 7)	
Peak FSH (IU/L)	31.7 ± 15.9	24.2 ± 8.6	20.9 ± 6.0
Peak LH (IU/L)	10.5 ± 4.2	13.2 ± 5.0	21.4 ± 19.2
Breast stage	2.2 ± 0.3	2.3 ± 0.5	3.1 ± 0.8*
Uterine length (cm)	3.2 ± 0.6 (n = 52)	3.4 ± 0.7	4.5 ± 0.7†
Ovarian volume (cm^3)	1.4 ± 0.7 (n = 52)	1.4 ± 0.7	2.4 ± 0.9†
PAH		161.7 ± 6.6 (n = 10)	154.9 ± 5.3 (n = 10)†

Values are mean ± SD.
*p <0.005 versus time of original diagnosis of premature thelarche.
†p <0.05 versus time of original diagnosis of premature thelarche.

before age 8 years (we restricted the limit to age 7 years), bone age within 2 SD of normal, normal growth velocity, and luteinizing hormone–releasing hormone stimulation test characterized by a follicle-stimulating hormone–predominant response.[4, 5] The degree of breast development was assessed according to the stages given by Marshall and Tanner.[6] Bone age was determined according to the method of Greulich and Pyle.[7] Growth velocity was determined from the height increment during a 6- to 12-month period. The predicted adult height was calculated by the Bayley-Pinneau method.[8] Before 1980, diagnostic evaluation included vaginal smears according to Papanicolaou, and afterward included ultrasound examination of the uterus and ovaries.[9] The LH-RH stimulation test (dose 100 μg) was performed between 8 and 9 AM, and plasma gonadotropin concentrations were determined at time zero and then at 15, 30, 60, 90, and 120 minutes after LH-RH. In several cases the initial screening visit was later than the age at onset reliably reported by the parents and the referring physician; all patients were followed by us to monitor clinical progression of sexual development. The girls were examined at least at yearly intervals: physical examination, with pubertal staging and height measurement, was performed at each visit; at yearly intervals and when either growth velocity or bone age or breast development was progressing more than expected, the follow-up examination included bone age assessment, pelvic ultrasonography, and, at least once during the follow-up period, an LH-RH stimulation test.

Computed tomography scan or magnetic resonance imaging of the brain and pituitary gland was performed in all the girls who had progression to CPP.

Plasma LH and FSH were measured in duplicate by polyclonal radioimmunoassay (Serono Biodata, Milan, Italy).

Statistical analysis. Results are expressed as mean ± SD unless otherwise stated. Statistical significance of mean differences was assessed by paired *t* test. A p value of <0.05 was considered significant.

RESULTS

After a follow-up period that varied from 2 to 6 years, 14 of these girls with the initial diagnosis of premature thelarche had an increase in breast size from 2.3 ± 0.5 to 3.1 ± 0.8, in pubic hair development from Tanner stage 1.0 ± 0.0 to 1.7 ± 0.6 (p <0.05), and in bone age advancement from 0.8 ± 0.3 to 2.4 ± 0.4 years (p <0.005). The mean chronologic age of this group of 14 girls was 5.1 ± 2.0 years (range, 1.1 to 7 years) at the time of clinical and laboratory diagnosis of premature thelarche, whereas the age at onset had been birth to 5 years, and the girls were 7.8 ± 0.6 years of age (range, 6.6 to 8.5 years) when identified as having progressed to CPP (Table). The PAH significantly decreased from 161.7 ± 6.6 to 154.9 ± 5.3 cm (p <0.05). Pelvic ultrasound examination showed significant differences in measurements between the time of diagnosis of premature thelarche and progression to CPP: uterine length had increased from 3.4 ± 0.7 to 4.5 ± 0.7 cm; ovarian volume had increased from 1.4 ± 0.7 to 2.4 ± 0.9 cm^3 (both p <0.05). In retrospect, the 14 girls who progressed to CPP had an initially FSH-predominant response to LH-RH and an LH/FSH ratio <1, but a more dominant LH response then developed: peak FSH level was 24.2 ± 8.6 IU/L at observation during premature thelarche and 20.9 ± 6.0 IU/L after progression to CPP, and peak LH was 13.2 ± 5.0 IU/L at observation during premature thelarche and 21.4 ± 19.2 IU/L after progression to CPP (both p values not significant) (Table). Computed tomography scan or magnetic resonance imaging of the brain and pituitary gland showed normal findings for all patients. On the basis of development of precocious or early puberty (breast size increase, pubic hair appearance, uterine and ovarian volume increase, growth velocity increment, bone age acceleration, decreased PAH, low mid-parental height, and/or psychologic problems), nine of these patients were treated, three with cyproterone acetate (150 mg/m^2 body surface area per day by mouth) and six with LH-RH analog (depot preparation of triptorelin, 120 μg/kg given intramuscularly every 21 days). All girls responded to treatment; they had arrest or regression of breast development, reduction of uterine and ovarian volume, complete gonadotropin suppression in the patients treated with LH-RH analogs, and deceleration of bone maturation. Five patients were not treated: one, who refused treatment, had menarche at age 9 years, 3 years after pubertal progression, and reached a final height of 144 cm (below the 3rd percentile and the mid-parental height); the other patients have not yet reached final height but are progressing in pubertal development and are showing progressive reduction of PAH.

The remaining 86 patients had clinical and hormonal characteristics comparable to those of the 14 patients at the time of the diagnosis of premature thelarche (Table). Pelvic ultrasonography, performed after 1980 in 52 patients, showed prepubertal values (uterine length, 3.2 ± 0.6 cm; ovarian volume, 1.4 ± 0.7 cm^3) comparable to those of the 14 girls who progressed to CPP (Table).

DISCUSSION

The pathophysiologic mechanism of premature thelarche is still unknown; it has been postulated to result from increased breast sensitivity to estrogen,[10] transient estrogen secretion by follicular cysts of the ovary,[11] increased production of estrogens from precursors of adrenal origin,[12] increased dietary estrogen as a result of exogenous contamination of food,[13] and transient partial activation of the hypothalamic-pituitary-gonadal axis with excessive secretion of FSH.[4, 14-17] Our data have not resolved these questions. There are few studies of the natural history of premature thelarche, and their conclusions remain controversial. In a retrospective study of 46 girls with premature thelarche, Mills et al.[2] reported that none of them had any other problems of sexual development or function during a period of 7 years, and concluded that premature thelarche is a benign condition and that referral to an endocrinologist is not necessary. A more recent retrospective study[3] showed that in the majority of girls there was regression of breast volume during a period of 6 months to 6 years after diagnosis; in about 10%, breast development persisted until puberty, with no untoward effects on later health, growth, or fertility. Ilicki et al.,[10] in a long-term follow-up of 68 girls, reported regression of thelarche in 44% after approximately 3 years and an overall progression into normal puberty at the appropriate time. Pescovitz et al.[5] stated that girls with isolated premature thelarche had an FSH-predominant response to LH-RH, and girls with complete sexual development had an LH-predominant response; girls with early or intermediate manifestations of CPP had LH and FSH responses to LH-RH indistinguishable from the FSH-predominant responses of girls with isolated thelarche. On the basis of these data, the authors hypothesized that premature thelarche and CPP may represent different positions along a continuum of hypothalamic LH-RH neuron activation; the authors, however, did not report longitudinal follow-up of their patients.

Our data indicate that in a number of cases (14 in our cohort of 100 girls), simple premature thelarche may develop into precocious or early puberty. The patients with pubertal progression are not to be confused with the "thelarche variant" described by Stanhope and Brook[18] and the "exaggerated thelarche" described by Garibaldi et al.[19]; their patients failed to respond to LH-RH analog treatment altogether, whereas our patients responded clinically and hormonally just as patients with classic CPP would.

On the basis of our experience, the clinician should keep in mind that premature thelarche may not always be a self-limited condition with no impact on the timing of puberty. We strongly recommend that all girls with this condition be monitored clinically for accelerated pubertal progression. Currently there are no predictive clinical or laboratory tests that can identify at time of onset which patients are at risk of having early or precocious puberty. This should not dissuade the pediatrician caring for these children from offering sympathetic reassurance, because in most instances the condition does not progress or may turn out to be fully reversible.

We thank Dr. Paul Saenger for reviewing the manuscript.

REFERENCES

1. Wilkins L. Diagnosis and treatment of endocrine disorders of childhood and adolescence. 3rd ed. Springfield, Illinois: Charles C Thomas, 1965:206.
2. Mills JL, Stolley PD, Davies J, Moshang T Jr. Premature thelarche: natural history and etiologic investigation. Am J Dis Child 1981;135:743-5.
3. Van Winter JT, Noller KL, Zimmerman D, Melton LJ III. Natural history of premature thelarche in Olmsted County, Minnesota, 1940 to 1984. J PEDIATR 1990;116:278-80.
4. Pasquino AM, Piccolo F, Scalamandré A, Malvaso M, Ortolani R, Boscherini B. Hypothalamic-pituitary-gonadotropic function in girls with premature thelarche. Arch Dis Child 1980;55:941-4.
5. Pescovitz OH, Hench KD, Barnes KM, Loriaux DL, Cutler GB Jr. Premature thelarche and central precocious puberty: the relationship between clinical presentation and the gonadotropin response to luteinizing hormone–releasing hormone. J Clin Endocrinol Metab 1988;67:474-9.
6. Marshall WA, Tanner JM. Variations in pattern of pubertal changes in girls. Arch Dis Child 1969;44:291-303.

7. Greulich WW, Pyle SI. Radiographic atlas of skeletal development of the hand and wrist. 2nd ed. Stanford: Stanford University Press, 1959.
8. Zachmann M, Sobradillo B, Frank M, Frisch H, Prader A. Bayley-Pinneau, Roche-Wainer-Thissen, and Tanner height predictions in normal children and in patients with various pathologic conditions. J PEDIATR 1978;93:749-55.
9. Salardi S, Orsini LF, Cacciari E, et al. Pelvic ultrasonography in girls with precocious puberty, congenital adrenal hyperplasia, obesity, or hirsutism. J PEDIATR 1988;112:880-7.
10. Ilicki A, Prager Lewin R, Kauli R, Kaufman H, Schachter A, Laron Z. Premature thelarche: natural history and sex hormone secretion in 68 girls. Acta Paediatr Scand 1984;73:756-62.
11. Sizonenko PC. Preadolescent and adolescent endocrinology: physiology and physiopathology. II. Hormonal changes during abnormal pubertal development. Am J Dis Child 1978;132:797-805.
12. Dumic M, Tajic M, Mardesic D, Kalafatic Z. Premature thelarche: a possible adrenal disorder. Arch Dis Child 1982; 57:200-3.
13. Saenz de Rodriguez CA, Bongiovanni AM, Conde de Borrego L. An epidemic of precocious development in Puerto Rican children. J PEDIATR 1985;107:393-6.
14. Job JC, Guilhaume B, Chaussain JL, Garnier PE. Le developement premature isole des seins chez les fillettes. Arch Fr Pediatr 1975;32:39-48.
15. Reiter EO, Kaplan SL, Conte FA, Grumbach MM. Responsivity of pituitary gonadotropins to luteinizing hormone–releasing factor in idiopathic precocious puberty, precocious thelarche, precocious adrenarche and in patients treated with medroxyprogestrone acetate. Pediatr Res 1975;9:111-5.
16. Beck W, Stubbe P. Pulsatile secretion of luteinizing hormone and sleep-related gonadotropin rhythms in girls with premature thelarche. Eur J Pediatr 1984;141:168-70.
17. Pasquino AM, Tebaldi L, Cioschi L, et al. Premature thelarche: a follow-up study of 40 girls. Arch Dis Child 1985;60:1180-2.
18. Stanhope R, Brook CGD. Thelarche variant: a new syndrome of precocious sexual maturation? Acta Endocrinol (Copenh) 1990;123:481-6.
19. Garibaldi LR, Aceto T Jr, Weber C. The pattern of gonadotropin and estradiol secretion in exaggerated thelarche. Acta Endocrinol 1993;128:345-50.

Increased fat oxidation in prepubertal obese children: A metabolic defense against further weight gain?

C. Maffeis, MD, L. Pinelli, MD, and Y. Schutz, PhD

From the Department of Pediatrics, Regional Center for Juvenile Diabetes, University of Verona, Verona, Italy, and the Institute of Physiology, University of Lausanne, Lausanne, Switzerland

The purpose of this study was to measure postabsorptive fat oxidation at rest and to assess the association between fat mass and fat oxidation rate in prepubertal children, who were assigned to two groups: 35 obese children (weight, 44.5 ± 9.7 kg; fat mass; 31.7 ± 5.4%) and 37 nonobese children (weight, 30.8 ± 6.8 kg; fat mass, 17.5 ± 6.7%). Postabsorptive fat oxidation expressed in absolute value was significantly higher in obese than in nonobese children (31.4 ± 9.7 mg/min vs 21.9 ± 10.2 mg/min; p <0.001) but not when adjusted for fat-free mass by analysis of covariance with fat-free mass as the covariate (28.2 ± 10.6 mg/min vs 24.9 ± 10.5 mg/min). In obese children and in the total group, fat mass and fat oxidation were significantly correlated (r = 0.65; p <0.001). The slope of the relationship indicated that for each 10 kg additional fat mass, resting fat oxidation increased by 18 gm/day. We conclude that obese prepubertal children have a higher postabsorptive rate of fat oxidation than nonobese children. This metabolic process may favor the achievement of a new equilibrium in fat balance, opposing further adipose tissue gain. (J Pediatr 1995;126:15-20)

Fat balance, calculated from the ratio between dietary fat and fat oxidation, may play a critical role in the regulation of body weight.[1] Fat intake does not promote fat oxidation[2]; the latter, which includes the proportion of energy expenditure that is not included by protein and carbohydrate oxidation, does not affect fat intake per se.[3] Therefore if the lipid content of the diet is higher than the overall fuel mix oxidized, a positive fat balance will produce fat storage. The maintenance of this process leads to a progressive increase in body fat mass. It has been hypothesized that increased fat stores, induced by a high proportion of fat in the diet, might promote fat oxidation,[1] favoring lipid balance readjustment and the maintenance of a new weight equilibrium at a higher level.

This study was undertaken to determine the relationship between fat mass and postabsorptive fat and carbohydrate oxidation rates in obese and nonobese prepubertal children studied in the same experimental conditions.

ANCOVA	Analysis of covariance
BMI	Body mass index
FFM	Fat-free mass
FM	Fat mass
PMR	Postabsorptive metabolic rate
RQ	Respiratory quotient
$\dot{V}CO_2$	Carbon dioxide output
$\dot{V}O_2$	Oxygen uptake

Supported by the National Research Council Target Project "Prevention and Control Disease Factors," project No. 7, contract No. 93.00.164PF41.

Submitted for publication Jan. 31, 1994; accepted Aug. 9, 1994.

Reprint requests: Claudio Maffeis, MD, Department of Pediatrics, Polyclinic, 37134 Verona, Italy.

0022-3476/95/$3.00 + 0 **9/20/59696**

METHODS

Subjects. We studied 80 prepubertal white children aged 7 to 10 years who formed two groups: 40 obese children and 40 nonobese children. Some of the children participated in previous studies exploring the validity of energy intake reported by obese and nonobese children[4] or of energy expenditure during walking and running.[5] Obesity was defined as body mass index >97th percentile of the reference values for age and sex. Control children were selected based on BMI ≤97th percentile of the reference values for age and sex.[6] Physical examination and routine laboratory tests excluded health problems other than obesity. Pubertal stage was assessed according to Tanner.[7] None of the subjects reported significant changes in body weight during the month preceding the study. No child was taking any drugs. Informed consent was obtained from the parents of all subjects. The protocol was approved by the ethics committee of the University Hospital of Verona.

Physical characteristics. Anthropometric measurements (weight, height, and skin-fold thicknesses) were performed by the same investigator. Height was measured to the nearest 0.5 cm on a standardized, wall-mounted height board. Weight was determined to the nearest 0.1 kg by standard physician's beam scale with the child dressed only in light underwear and without shoes. Body mass index was calculated as weight (in kilograms) divided by height squared (in square meters). Skin-fold thicknesses were measured in triplicate to the nearest millimeter at the triceps and subscapular sites by means of an Harpenden skin-fold caliper (CMS Weighing Equipment Ltd., London, United Kingdom). The Lohman formulas were used to calculate the percentage of body fat from the sum of the two skin folds.[8] Fat mass was obtained by multiplying the percentage of body fat by body weight. Fat-free mass was obtained by subtracting body fat from body weight.

The expected error of predicting body fat from triceps and subscapular measurements in the age-specific group of 8- to 9-year-old children is ≅5% of body fat predicted by densitometry. The prediction error is slightly higher than the prediction error of percentage body fat from more skin folds, and is comparable with that reported in adults.[9, 10] Although the use of skin-fold thickness to assess FM is not completely satisfactory, particularly in obese subjects, other more valid techniques such as underwater weighing may lead to practical problems when applied to prepubertal children because of fear of the water or incomplete immersion. In addition, because the density of FFM changes during childhood,[8] further uncertainty is involved unless body density and total body water are measured simultaneously.

Experimental design. Before the postabsorptive metabolic rate measurement, children consumed an unrestricted diet. The day before the test they did not perform any intense physical exercise. The children arrived by car at the Department of Pediatrics at 7:30 AM in fasting condition; the last meal had been eaten at 8 PM the day before. After 30 minutes of rest on a hospital bed in a comfortable, temperature-controlled environment, continuous respiratory exchange was initiated by indirect calorimetry. During the 30-minute measurement period, children rested quietly watching cartoons. Throughout the PMR measurement, a technician observed the child to verify that he or she was motionless and relaxed during the respiratory exchange measurement. Special attention was given to prevent extra body movements or hyperventilation because the former increase PMR and the latter increases the respiratory quotient. Data from eight children (five obese and three nonobese) were not included in the statistical analysis because hyperventilation induced RQs greater than 1.0.

In a subsample of 23 obese and 11 nonobese children, a blood sample was taken from an antecubital vein immediately after the PMR measurements, to measure plasma immunoreactive insulin, glucose, and free fatty acids concentrations. Blood could not be drawn from the other children because either the children or parent refused. Plasma glucose[9] and free fatty acids[10] were measured enzymatically, whereas the plasma immunoreactive insulin level was assayed by radioimmunoassay.[11]

Postabsorptive metabolic rate. Postabsorptive metabolic rate was measured by respiratory gas exchange for 30 minutes as previously described.[12] An open-circuit computerized indirect calorimeter (Deltatrac, Datex Division, Instrumentarium OY, Helsinki, Finland) connected to a transparent hood system was used. The instrument was calibrated before each test with a gas mixture (95.2% oxygen and 4.8% carbon dioxide). Records of oxygen consumption and carbon dioxide production were printed out at 1-minute intervals. The mean of the last 20 minutes was used to evaluate PMR. The energy expenditure was derived from oxygen uptake and carbon dioxide output according to the formula by Lusk.[13]

Macronutrient oxidation rate. The macronutrient oxidation rate was calculated from $\dot{V}O_2$, $\dot{V}CO_2$, and RQ by means of the following formulas[14]:

$$F_{ox}\ (\text{gm/min}) = 1.67\ \dot{V}O_2\ (\text{L/min}) - 1.67\ \dot{V}CO_2\ (\text{L/min}) - 0.307\ P_{ox}$$

$$G_{ox}\ (\text{gm/min}) = 4.55\ \dot{V}CO_2\ (\text{L/min}) - 3.21\ \dot{V}O_2\ (\text{L/min}) - 0.459\ P_{ox}$$

where F_{ox} = fat oxidation; G_{ox} = glucose oxidation, and P_{ox} = protein oxidation. The protein oxidation was estimated as follows:

$$P_{ox}\ (\text{gm/min}) = \frac{\text{PMR (kJ/min)} \cdot 0.15}{16.74\ \text{kJ}}$$

We assumed that protein oxidation covered 15% of PMR in both obese and nonobese children. This assumption does not affect the relative partition between carbohydrate and fat oxidation determined by indirect calorimetry; 16.74 kJ is the energy produced by the oxidation of 1 gm of protein.

Table I. Physical characteristics of obese and nonobese children

	Obese (n = 35)	Nonobese (n = 37)	p
Gender (M/F)	18/17	19/18	
Age (yr)	8.7 ± 1.5	8.8 ± 1.0	NS
Weight (kg)	44.5 ± 9.7	30.8 ± 6.8	<0.001
Height (cm)	134 ± 9	133 ± 7	NS
BMI (kg/m²)	24.5 ± 2.9	17.0 ± 2.1	<0.001
FM (%)	31.7 ± 5.4	17.5 ± 6.7	<0.001
FM (kg)	14.5 ± 5.2	5.7 ± 3.8	<0.001
FFM (kg)	30.0 ± 5.7	24.1 ± 3.9	<0.001
Skin-fold thickness			
Triceps (mm)	22.6 ± 6.4	11.8 ± 4.2	<0.001
Suscapular (mm)	25.3 ± 9.2	8.4 ± 4.8	<0.001

Data reported as mean ± SD.
NS, Not significant.

Statistical analysis. The results are expressed as mean ± SD. An unpaired *t* test was used to compare obese and nonobese children. The degree of association between two variables was quantified by using the Pearson product-moment linear correlation coefficient. Analysis of covariance, with FFM as the covariate, was used to calculate PMR and macronutrient oxidation rates adjusted for FFM (i.e., the metabolic active tissue). To assess the relationship between fat oxidation as the dependent variable and body weight, FFM, and FM as the independent variables, a stepwise regression procedure was used. The Statistical Analysis Systems/STAT statistical package, version 6.0 (SAS Institute Inc., Cary, N.C.) was used to analyze the data.

RESULTS

Age and height were comparable in the two groups; weight, BMI, percentage of FM, FM, and FFM were significantly higher in the obese group (Table I). The measurement of skin-fold thickness confirmed the diagnosis of obesity estimated by means of the BMI. In each of the obese children the triceps skin fold was greater than the reference value (85th percentile for age and sex, assessed on the tables devised by Tanner and Whitehouse[15]), frequently used as a cutoff point to define obesity in children.[16] In addition triceps and subscapular thicknesses were both significantly correlated to BMI ($r = 0.92$ and $r = 0.91$; $p < 0.001$, respectively).

Postabsorptive metabolic rate was significantly higher in obese than in nonobese children (Table II). Postabsorptive metabolic rate adjusted for FFM by means of ANCOVA, with FFM as the covariate, was comparable in the two groups. The postabsorptive RQ was slightly lower in obese than in nonobese children (Table II).

The postabsorptive fat oxidation rate was significantly higher in obese than in nonobese children. When expressed as a percentage of PMR (32.3 ± 7.5% vs 25.5 ± 12.1%) or of PMR adjusted for FFM (32.7 ± 9.6% vs 25.9 ± 12.5%), it was significantly ($p < 0.01$) higher in obese than in nonobese children. In obese children, FFM explained 48.6% of the variance of fat oxidation ($r = 0.697$), versus 14.6% ($r = 0.382$) in nonobese children. In the whole group, a significant positive correlation was found between postabsorptive fat oxidation rate and FM expressed both in absolute values and as a percentage of body weight (Table III). The degree of correlation was higher in the obese group and not significant in the nonobese group. The narrow range of body fat in the nonobese group may explain these results. When the postabsorptive fat oxidation was adjusted for FFM by

Table II. Postabsorptive metabolic rate, respiratory quotient, fat and glucose postabsorptive oxidation rates in obese and nonobese children

	Obese (n = 35)	Nonobese (n = 37)	p
PMR (kJ/day)	5218 ± 718	4559 ± 499	<0.001
PMR adjusted for FFM (kJ/day)	4953 ± 421	4810 ± 421	NS
RQ	0.862 ± 0.024	0.882 ± 0.039	<0.01
F_{ox} (mg/min)	31.4 ± 9.7	21.9 ± 10.2	<0.001
F_{ox} adjusted for FFM (mg/min)	28.2 ± 10.6	24.9 ± 10.5	NS
G_{ox} (mg/min)	110.9 ± 19.1	110.4 ± 25.8	NS
G_{ox} adjusted for FFM (mg/min)	109.1 ± 26.5	112.0 ± 26.5	NS

Data are reported as mean ± SD.
F_{ox}, Fat oxidation; G_{ox}, glucose oxidation; *NS*, not significant; see text for other abbreviations.

Table III. Correlation coefficients between body weight, fat-free mass, body fat, and fat and carbohydrate postabsorptive oxidation rates in obese, nonobese, and obese and nonobese children combined

	Obese (n = 35)	Nonobese (n = 37)	Total (n = 72)
Body weight (kg) vs:			
F_{ox} (mg/min)	0.746*	0.300†	0.635*
G_{ox} (mg/min)	0.135	0.164	0.127
Fat-free mass (kg) vs:			
F_{ox} (mg/min)	0.697*	0.382	0.627*
G_{ox} (mg/min)	0.143	0.151	0.108
Fat mass (kg) vs:			
F_{ox} (mg/min)	0.651*	0.103	0.555*
G_{ox} (mg/min)	0.103	0.140	0.008
Fat mass (%) vs:			
F_{ox} (mg/min)	0.326†	−0.007	0.414*
G_{ox} (mg/min)	0.006	0.122	0.052

F_{ox}, Fat oxidation; G_{ox}, glucose oxidation; see text for abbreviations.
*$p < 0.001$.
†$p < 0.05$.

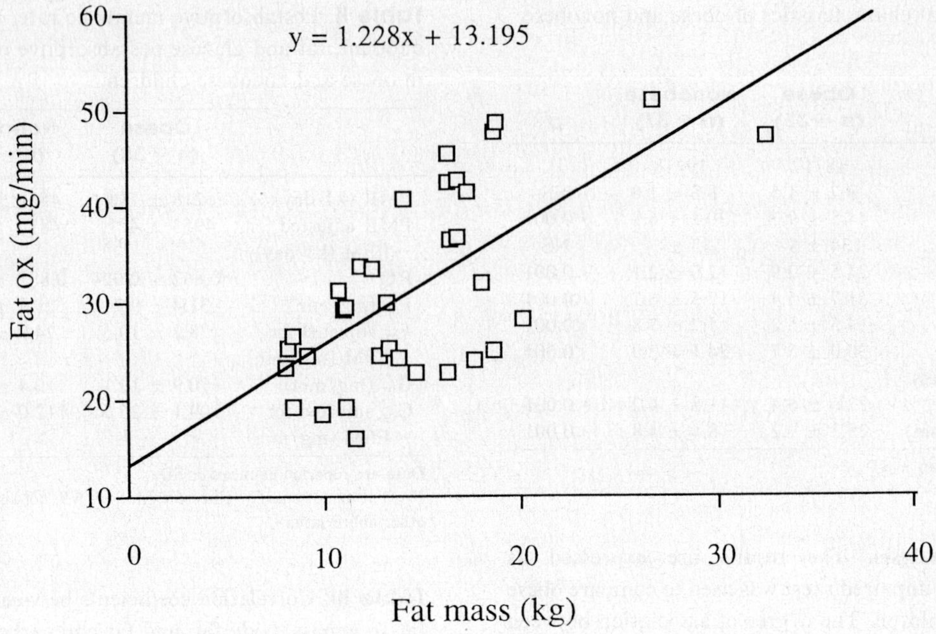

Fig. 1. Regression line between absolute fat mass (in kilograms) and postabsorptive fat oxidation *(fat ox)* rate in 35 obese children. The regression equation is as follows: Postabsorptive fat oxidation rate (mg/min) = 1.228 · Fat mass (kg) + 13.195 ($r = 0.651$; $p < 0.001$).

ANCOVA, it was comparable in both the obese and nonobese children. In the obese group only, when a stepwise regression analysis was performed, addition of FM in the model increased by 8.1% ($r^2 = 0.567$), the proportion of the variance of postabsorptive fat oxidation already explained by FFM. As expected, postabsorptive fat oxidation was positively correlated to PMR in obese children ($r = 0.726$; $p < 0.001$), in nonobese children ($r = 0.454$; $p < 0.01$), and in the total group of children ($r = 0.663$; $p < 0.001$).

No significant difference in postabsorptive glucose oxidation rate was found in the two groups of children, and glucose oxidation was not correlated to FM (Table II). In the subgroup studied (n = 34), fasting insulin plasma levels were significantly higher in obese than in nonobese children (104 ± 32 pmol/L vs 73 ± 21 pmol/L, respectively; $p < 0.05$), whereas blood glucose (4.42 ± 0.22 mmol/L vs 4.35 ± 0.48 mmol/L; *p* not significant) and free fatty acid (591 ± 75 μmol/L vs 668 ± 227 μmol/L; *p* not significant) concentrations were comparable in the two groups of children. Plasma insulin concentration was significantly ($p < 0.05$) correlated to FM expressed both as an absolute value ($r = 0.551$) and as a percentage of body weight ($r = 0.546$). No significant association was found between insulin levels and postabsorptive fat oxidation rate ($r = 0.107$; *p* not significant) or postabsorptive glucose oxidation rate ($r = 0.367$; *p* not significant).

DISCUSSION

The results of this study show that moderately obese children had a greater fat oxidation rate than that in nonobese children. Obese children had a significant association between postabsorptive fat oxidation rate and FM. Postabsorptive fat oxidation rate adjusted for FFM by ANCOVA was comparable in the obese and in the nonobese groups. This relationship is expected because FFM is the only tissue in which fat oxidation occurs. However, after taking FFM into account, FM explained an additional 8.1% of the residual variance in postabsorptive fat oxidation. Therefore the expansion of FM seems directly involved in the mechanisms leading to an increased fat oxidation rate. Other factors, which were not evaluated in our study, might affect residual variance in fat oxidation (e.g., the degree of insulin resistance). Fasting insulin plasma levels, available for only a subgroup of children, were higher with increasing FM, confirming previous results.[17] In a previous study in children and adolescents, basal insulin levels were not associated with fat oxidation at rest.[18] Because in normal adults the sensitivity of lipid oxidation to hyperinsulinemia was about half the sensitivity of lipolysis to hyperinsulinemia,[19, 20] it might be argued that only a sufficient degree of hyperinsulinemia may reduce lipid oxidation, by stimulating glucose oxidation. Therefore it might be assumed that in the study by

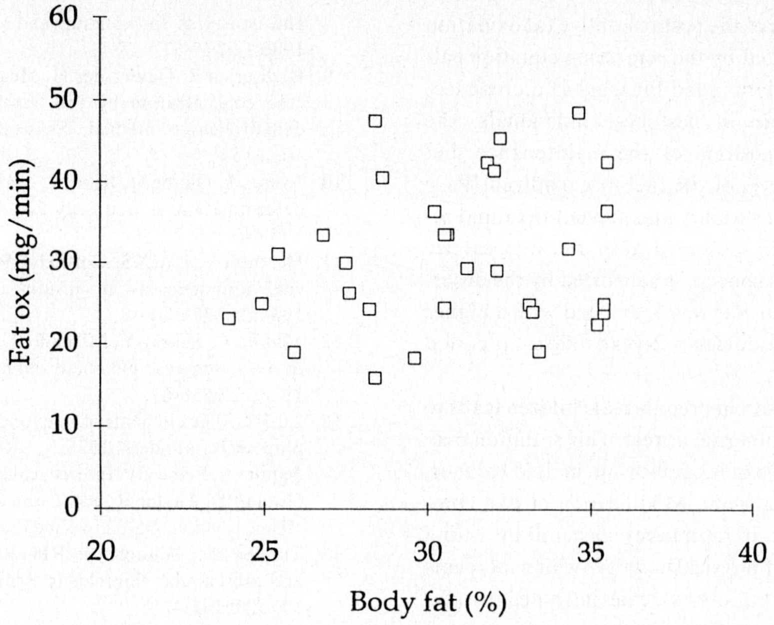

Fig. 2. Regression between relative fat mass (percentage) and postabsorptive fat oxidation *(Fat ox)* rate in 35 obese children. The regression equation is as follows: Postabsorptive fat oxidation rate (mg/min) = 0.599 · Fat mass (%) + 12.11 ($r = 0.336$; $p < 0.05$).

Le Stunff and Bougneres,[18] hyperinsulinemia did not reach a sufficient level to stimulate glucose oxidation and reduce fat oxidation in children and adolescents. An improvement in insulin sensitivity, leading to an increase in carbohydrate oxidation and a reduction of the fat oxidation rate, has been shown to increase the risk for further weight gain, as suggested by the results of a large study on insulin sensitivity and obesity in adult Pima Indians.[21] No association between postabsorptive fat oxidation rate and age, pubertal status, and duration of obesity was found in obese children.[18]

Increased postabsorptive fat oxidation in obese prepubertal children is important for two reasons: first, it shows that obese children must eat more fat than their lean counterparts to maintain fat balance. Second, the rise in fat oxidation in the obese children can be considered as a buffer mechanism to offset the excess fat intake, the possible initial defect in fat oxidation, or both, that must have occurred in their preobese state, by favoring a new lipid equilibrium. With the regression equation between FM (independent variable) and fat oxidation (dependent variable), it is possible to predict an increase of 18 gm/day in fat oxidation for each 10 kg increase in FM. This result is comparable to that previously reported for obese adult women.[22] The increased fat oxidation accompanying fat gain might explain why, after a dynamic phase of body weight gain, apparent FM stability might be reached, despite the fact that lipid continues to account for a relatively high proportion of energy intake.[23]

Although our results are not necessarily extensible to the postprandial state (a period when the contribution of fat oxidation to energy expenditure is lower than in the postabsorptive state), and the estimates of body composition by means of skin-fold thickness have a margin of error, the clinical implications of these results are evident: a modification in the proportion of the macronutrients in the diet by selectively reducing lipid intake is essential, and should be combined with the avoidance of a sedentary lifestyle (e.g., reduced TV viewing, using stairs instead of elevators) and with increased physical activity (programmed exercise and sports) so that the fat oxidation rate and thus fat loss will be enhanced. Reduced energy (fat) intake and increased activity are necessary to produce the negative energy (fat) balance, without which fat loss is impossible. Physical exercise of low intensity and of long duration (e.g., walking at various paces) appears to be realistic in practice and induces the utilization of fat as the major substrate for covering energy expenditure, and favors the maintenance of a negative fat balance.[1] In addition, the choice of a mixed diet with a low-lipid content favors the maintenance of a high rate of fat oxidation. This is particularly useful because the enhanced postabsorptive fat oxidation in obese individuals seems to be counteracted with fat loss. Data obtained in adults show that a weight loss of 12.7 kg, 77% of which was fat, produced a reduction of the postabsorptive fat oxidation rate equal to that predicted by the regression equation calculated between fat oxidation and fat mass in a cross-sectional study.[22] Therefore in postobese individuals, the adjustment of the composition of the maintenance diet (food quotient) to the level of the fuel mix oxidized (RQ) should favor body weight stability and prevent the rapid relapse of obesity generally observed after the hypocaloric diet is discontinued. This concept is supported by the observation that a high 24-hour RQ was associated with a higher risk of body weight gain during a 2-year follow-up period in adult Pima Indians.[24]

We conclude that obesity in prepubertal children leads to an increased lipid oxidation rate at rest. This situation may favor the achievement of a new equilibrium in lipid balance, opposing further body fat gain. Modification of diet composition (i.e., a reduction in fat intake) concomitant with a stimulation of the level of physical activity (which increases fat oxidation) will favor fat loss by achieving a negative fat balance.

We thank Ray E. Gleason of the Clinical Research Center, at Massachusetts Institute of Technology, Cambridge, for his invaluable help with the statistical analysis of the data.

REFERENCES

1. Flatt JP. Dietary fat, carbohydrate balance and weight maintenance: effects of exercise. Am J Clin Nutr 1987;45:296-306.
2. Schutz Y, Flatt JP, Jequier E. Failure of dietary fat to promote fat oxidation: a factor favoring the development of obesity. Am J Clin Nutr 1989;50:307-14.
3. Flatt JP. Opposite effects of variations in food intake on carbohydrate and fat oxidation in ad libitum fed mice. J Nutr Biochem 1991;2:186-192.
4. Maffeis C, Schutz Y, Zaffanello M, Piccoli R, Pinelli L. Elevated energy expenditure and reduced energy intake in obese prepubertal children: Paradox of poor dietary reliability in obesity? J PEDIATR 1994;124:348-54.
5. Maffeis C, Schutz Y, Schena F, Zaffanello M, Pinelli L. Energy expenditure during walking and running in obese and nonobese prepubertal children. J PEDIATR 1993;123:193-9.
6. Rolland-Cacherà MF, Sempà M, Guillaud-Bataille M, et al. Adiposity indices in children. Am J Clin Nutr 1982;36:178-84.
7. Tanner JM. Growth at adolescence, 2nd ed. Oxford: Blackwell, 1962.
8. Lohman TG. Applicability of body composition techniques and constants for children and youth. Exerc Sport Sci Rev 1986;14:325-57.
9. Richterich R, Dauwalder H. Measurement of the plasma glucose concentration by the hexokinase-glucose-6-phosphate-dehydrogenase method. Schweiz Med Wochenschr 1971; 101:615-8.
10. Noma A, Okabe H, Kita M, et al. A new colorimetric microdetermination of free fatty acids in serum. Clin Chim Acta 1973;43:317-20.
11. Hertbert V, Lau KS, Gottlieb CW, Bleicher SJ. Coated charcoal immunoassay of insulin. J Clin Endocrinol Metab 1965;25:1375-84.
12. Maffeis C, Schutz Y, Micciolo R, et al. Resting metabolic rate in six- to ten-year-old obese and nonobese children. J PEDIATR 1993;122:556-62.
13. Lusk G. The elements of science of nutrition, 4th ed. Philadelphia: WB Saunders, 1928.
14. Jequier E, Felber JP. Indirect calorimetry. In: Alberti KGMM, Home PD, Taylor R, eds. Clinical endocrinology and metabolism. London: Bailliere Tindall, 1987:911-35.
15. Tanner JM, Whitehouse RH. Revised standards for triceps and subscapular skinfolds in British children. Arch Dis Child 1975;50:142-4.
16. Must A, Dallal GE, Dietz WH. Reference data for obesity: 85th and 95th percentiles of body mass index (wt/ht^2) and triceps skinfold thickness. Am J Clin Nutr 1991;53:839-46.
17. Deschamps I, Guron BJ, Lestradet H. Blood glucose, insulin, and free fatty acid levels during oral glucose tolerance test in 158 obese children. Diabetes 1977;26:89-93.
18. Le Stunff C, Bougneres PF. Time course of increased lipid and decreased glucose oxidation during early phase of childhood obesity. Diabetes 1993;42:1010-6.
19. Thiebaud D, Jacot E, De Fronzo R, Maeder E, Jequier E, Felber J. The effect of graded doses of insulin on total glucose uptake, glucose oxidation, and glucose storage in man. Diabetes 1982;31:957-63.
20. Golay A, Chen Y-D, Reaven G. Effect of differences in glucose tolerance on insulin's ability to regulate carbohydrate and free fatty acid metabolism in obese individuals. J Clin Endocrinol Metab 1986;62:1081-8.
21. Swinburn BA, Nyomba BL, Saad MF, et al. Insulin resistance associated with lower rates of weight gain in Pima Indians. J Clin Invest 1991;88:168-73.
22. Schutz Y, Tremblay A, Weinsier RL, Nelson KM. Role of fat oxidation in the long-term stabilization of body weight in obese women. Am J Clin Nutr 1992;55:670-4.
23. Sims EAH, Danforth E Jr, Horton ES, Bray GA, Glennon JA, Salans LB. Endocrine and metabolic effects of experimental obesity in man. Recent Prog Horm Res 1973;29:457-64.
24. Zurlo F, Lillioja S, Esposito-Del Puente A, et al. Low ratio of fat to carbohydrate oxidation as predictor of weight gain: study of 24-h RQ. Am J Physiol 1990;E650-E657.

Measured versus predicted resting energy expenditure in infants: A need for reappraisal

M. A. Thomson, MRCP(UK), S. Bucolo, GDID, P. Quirk, BSc(Hons), and R. W. Shepherd, MD, FRACP

From the Department of Child Health, Children's Nutrition Research Center, Royal Children's Hospital, and the Queensland Institute of Medical Research, Brisbane, Australia

The reliability of commonly used predictive equations for estimating energy expenditure in infants in both health and disease was assessed by comparing resting energy expenditure (REE, measured by indirect calorimetry) in relation to weight, height, and body cell mass (by total body potassium analysis) with predictive equations (Harris-Benedict, Food and Agriculture Organization/World Health Organization/United Nations University (FAO/WHO/UNU), Schofield weight-only, and Schofield weight-and-height equations) in 36 healthy infants (age 0.43 ± 0.27 years; 19 male) and in 9 infants with cystic fibrosis (age 0.41 ± 0.30 years; 4 male). Mean ± SD REE for healthy boys was 0.205 ± 0.019 MJ $kg^{-1}day^{-1}$ and for healthy girls 0.217 ± 0.026 MJ kg^{-1} day^{-1}. Infants with cystic fibrosis had a significantly higher REE (0.258 ± 0.034 vs 0.210 ± 0.024 MJ kg^{-1} day^{-1}; $p<0.005$). Compared with measured values, predicted REE values varied markedly among equations, overestimating REE in healthy infants (Harris-Benedict equation, 182% ± 63% (SD) of measured values; FAO/WHO/UNU equation, 104% ± 14%; Schofield weight-only equation, 107.5% ± 14%; and Schofield weight-and-height equation, 106% ± 11%) and underestimating REE in those with cystic fibrosis (84% to 88% for the FAO/WHO/UNU, Schofield weight-only, and Schofield weight-and-height equations) except the Harris-Benedict equation (152%). On regression analysis both weight and body cell mass were related significantly to REE ($r^2 = 0.87$ and $r^2 = 0.61$, respectively) for normal infants and ($r^2 = 0.92$ and $r^2 = 0.94$) for those with cystic fibrosis. Using a generalized linear model of variance, we saw a significant ($p<0.001$) variability among all REE measures. Thus we could rely on none of the predictive equations to give an accurate estimate of REE, and hence energy and fluid requirements, in individual infants. We suggest that when accurate estimates are needed, measurement of REE in individual infants should be attempted, especially in disease states, and that the continued use of current formulas should be reexamined. (J PEDIATR 1995;126:21-7)

For many years the determination of nutritional and fluid requirements in infants has been based on equations used to predict values of basal metabolic rate derived from studies using indirect calorimetry. Forster[1] measured the gaseous metabolism of infants in 1877, and a number of metabolic studies using indirect calorimetry were performed in the first half of this century.[2-4] Harris and Benedict,[5] in 1919, formulated their predictive equations based on weight, height, and age to the nearest whole year. The data of Talbot et al.[2] formed the basis for the 1973 Food and Agriculture Organization/World Health Organization/United Nations University recommendations for energy requirements in childhood[6, 7] but their reliability was questioned by

Submitted for publication March 3, 1994; accepted July 26, 1994.

Reprint requests: R.W. Shepherd, MD, FRACP, Department of Child Health, Royal Children's Hospital, Brisbane, Queensland 4029, Australia.

0022-3476/95/$3.00 + 0 **9/20/59481**

BCM	Body cell mass
CF	Cystic fibrosis
FAO/WHO/UNU	Food and Agriculture Organization/World Health Organization/United Nations University [equation]
H-B	Harris-Benedict [equation]
REE	Resting energy expenditure
TBK	Total body potassium
$\dot{V}O_2$	Volume of oxygen consumption
$\dot{V}CO_2$	Volume of carbon dioxide production

Schofield,[7] who presented new equations derived from pooled measurements of resting energy expenditure from a number of studies divided into gender and limited age categories (e.g., infants were in the birth to 3-year age group) and based on height and weight or weight alone. In addition, the data collected by Talbot[8] have provided the theoretical cornerstone for prediction of infant caloric and, hence, maintenance fluid requirements in infants developed by Holliday and Segar.[9] These formulas are widely quoted today in standard pediatric texts.[10] These equations have also been used by some groups to evaluate changes in energy expenditure in various disease states,[11, 12] but their validity in disease states might be questioned partly because of the alterations in body composition, particularly of the body cell mass, which represents the oxygen-exchanging, work-performing body compartment. Studies in healthy individuals who have altered body composition (such as obesity) have highlighted their unreliability in these situations.[13, 14]

Review of the derivation of these equations calls into question the validity of using them in the infant age group at all, particularly in predicting an individual infant's energy expenditure, or if a disease state with altered body composition is present. All current equations have been either extrapolated down from older age groups, or have been developed by calorimetric techniques of limited accuracy for infants. We therefore measured REE using a dedicated infant indirect calorimeter in relation to weight, height, and BCM (by total body potassium). The BCM appears to be the most appropriate frame of reference against which energy expenditure should be studied.[15]

METHODS

Subjects. Thirty-six healthy infants (age 0.43 ± 0.27 years; 19 male) and nine infants with cystic fibrosis homozygous for the δF508 mutation (age 0.41 ± 0.30 years; 4 male) were studied. Sixteen of the healthy infants received more than 90% of their daily caloric intake as human milk, and neither the infants nor any of the breast-feeding mothers were taking medications, or had intercurrent infections or pyrexia. Infants were volunteered for this noninvasive study by their parents, and written informed consent was obtained. The study was approved by the ethics committee of the Royal Children's Hospital, Brisbane.

Table I. Equations used for estimation of basal energy expenditure in infants

1. Harris-Benedict (kcal/day)*
   - Boys: REE = 66.473 + 5.003 × Height (cm) + 13.752 × Weight (kg) − 6.755 × age (yr)
   - Girls: REE = 655.096 + 1.850 × Height (cm) + 9.563 × Weight (kg) − 4.676 × Age (yr)
2. Schofield, weight only (MJ/day)
   - Children less 3 years of age
     - Boys: REE = 0.249 × Weight (kg) − 0.127
     - Girls: REE = 0.244 × Weight (kg) − 0.130
3. Schofield, weight and height (MJ/day)
   - Children less than 3 years of age
     - Boys: REE = 0.0007 × Weight (kg) + 6.349 × Height (m) − 2.584
     - Girls: REE = 0.068 × Weight (kg) + 4.281 × Height (m) − 1.730
4. FAO/WHO/UNU (kcal/day)*
   - Children less than 3 years of age
     - Boys: REE = 60.9 × Weight (kg) − 54
     - Girls: REE = 61.0 × Weight (kg) − 51

*1 kcal = 4.186 kJ.

Resting energy expenditure

Predicted REE. Details of the equations used in prediction of the REE are set out in Table I.

Measured REE. The REE was measured with a portable indirect calorimeter designed primarily for use with spontaneously breathing children and infants. The system is based on the open-circuit principle[16] and uses a small canopy to collect expired respiratory gases. Gas flow is measured with a mass flow meter (Bronkhorst F-103D-HB; Anri Instruments, Melbourne, Australia), which has an accuracy of ±1% over the flow range of 0 to 100 L/min. Carbon dioxide is measured by a single-beam infrared analyzer (ADC, type RF; Analytical Development Co., Hoddeston, England), which has a response time of <4 seconds, a resolution of 0.001%, and a nonlinearity error of 0.05% for carbon dioxide concentrations up to 10%. Oxygen is measured by a differential paramagnetic analyzer (Datex OM-11; Instrumentarium OY, Helsinki, Finland), which has a response time of 130 msec, resolution of 0.01%, and a nonlinearity error of <1% for oxygen concentrations up to 100%. The associated software was designed to enable calculations of the volumes of oxygen consumption and carbon dioxide production to be displayed continuously, to define steady state concentrations, and to enable later editing for noise from episodes of agitation and so forth.

Validation of the system was based on the combustion of methanol to simulate infant values of $\dot{V}O_2$, $\dot{V}CO_2$, and respiratory quotient.[17] Thirty studies of 15 minutes were performed, with a flame and chimney substituted for the canopy used in patient studies. The amount of methanol con-

Table II. Characteristics of infants

	Healthy infants: Total (n = 36)	Healthy infants: Male (n = 19)	Healthy infants: Female (n = 17)	CF infants (total) (n = 9)
Age (yr)	0.43 ± 0.27	0.43 ± 0.29	0.43 ± 0.26	0.41 ± 0.30
Weight (kg)	6.75 ± 2.07	7.24 ± 2.40	6.20 ± 1.44	5.75 ± 2.25
Height (cm)	64.8 ± 7.6	65.5 ± 8.2	63.9 ± 6.7	61.5 ± 9.1
%Predicted weight/height	97.5 ± 10.6	99.5 ± 8.9	95.9 ± 7.8	96 ± 9.5
%Predicted weight/age	102.0 ± 10.9	107.6 ± 10.3	95.9 ± 11.2	91 ± 11.3
TBK* (gm)	10.1 ± 3.4	10.9 ± 3.9	9.1 ± 2.6	9.1 ± 3.8
%Expected TBK*/age	98.8 ± 17.2	99.4 ± 18	97.9 ± 16.4	89.3 ± 10.4
%Expected TBK*/weight	98.9 ± 16	98.1 ± 14	99.2 ± 17	94.1 ± 7.8

Values expressed as mean ± SD.
*TBK, total body potassium from ^{40}K analysis.

sumed was controlled by adding an additional flame inside the chimney; this allowed varying values of $\dot{V}O_2$ and $\dot{V}CO_2$ to be simulated within a range expected of the study population (approximately 20 to 250 ml/min). This validation study showed that the system has an accuracy of 0.59% ± 2.21% (mean ± SD) for $\dot{V}O_2$, 1.053% ± 1.45% (mean ± SD) for $\dot{V}CO_2$, and 1.01% ± 1.93% (mean ± SD) for respiratory quotient.

Measurement protocol. Weight and height of each naked infant were obtained by a single observer before each measurement. The *z* scores for weight and height, and the weight-for-height and weight-for-age percentages were calculated with the Anthro software program,[18] and standard definitions of underweight and overweight were adopted[19] with the use of Australian reference standards.[20]

Two measurements of REE were obtained in the mid morning, 2 to 3 hours after a feeding, and separated by a 30-minute rest period, and the average was taken. The infants were quiet and awake during the 3-minute stabilization period, followed by a 20-minute period of sampling, which was performed while the infant was enclosed in a humidity- and temperature-controlled environment within a canopy system. Measurement started only after a steady state in $\dot{V}O_2$ and $\dot{V}CO_2$ was obtained as defined by variance of <5% for a 30-second period. Thereafter, $\dot{V}O_2$ and $\dot{V}CO_2$ were calculated every 20 seconds, and any episodes of crying, agitation, coughing, and so forth could be edited out later.

Body composition analysis. The BCM, which is the actively metabolising, the work performing, and in children the actively growing body compartment, was measured by TBK analysis.[21-23] Potassium is the major intracellular cation and is maintained within strict concentration limits within each cell; 98% of body potassium is located within the BCM[21] and contains a small, fixed proportion of the natural isotope ^{40}K. The TBK was measured with a body-counter facility adapted for use in infants, as previously described.[22, 23] Calculation of the percentage of expected TBK for age, height, and weight was performed by comparing with pooled normal data as described previously.[22-24]

Statistical methods. Analysis of variance was performed to determine whether there were any differences between measured REE and that predicted by the four different equations for each individual. This was performed for all healthy subjects (and within the following subsets: male; female; those from birth to 6 months of age; those from 6 to 12 months of age; those with ideal body weight; and those with less than ideal body weight) and subjects with CF. Multiple regression analysis was performed to determine the influence of patient age, weight, height, and TBK on measured REE. Analysis of covariance was performed in the healthy group to determine whether there were any differences between (1) breast-fed and formula-fed infants and (2) boys and girls in REE after adjustment for the covariates age, weight, length, and TBK. All analyses were performed with the SAS statistical package (SAS Institute Inc., Cary, N.C.).

RESULTS

The age, weight, height, weight/height percentage, BCM represented by the TBK in grams, and the TBK expected for age and weight are represented in Table II. The CF group had a lower-than-expected BCM for age but also a lower BCM per unit of weight than normal infants, indicating altered body composition. The measured REE expressed in terms of weight and TBK are represented in Figs. 1 and 2 for the healthy group (also divided into subsets of male, female, birth to 6 months of age, and 6 to 12 months of age) and for the CF group. The infants with CF had a significantly higher mean REE than the healthy group expressed both per unit of weight (0.258 ± 0.036 vs 0.21 ± 0.024 MJ/kg per 24 hours) and per unit of TBK (0.163 ± 0.027 vs 0.142 ± 0.027 MJ/gm K per 24 hours). Infants' mean REEs for weight, for male versus female infants, were 0.217 ± 0.027 versus 0.205 ± 0.019 MJ/kg per 24 hours and for TBK were 0.15 ± 0.03 versus

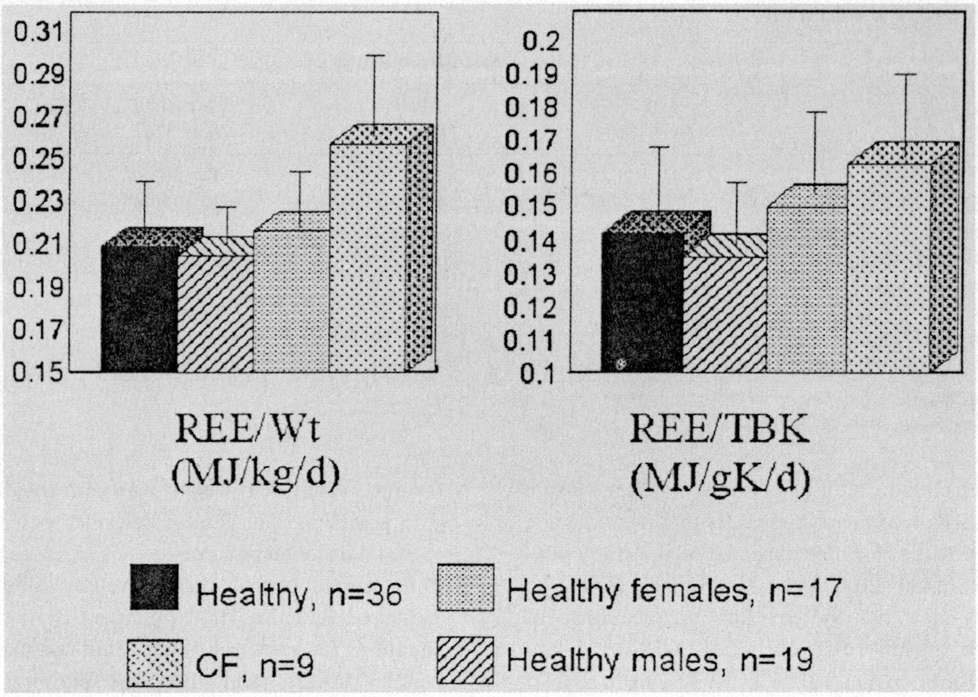

Fig. 1. Measured REE (expressed in terms of weight and TBK). It was significantly greater in infants with CF than in healthy infants (p <0.005). *gK*, Grams of potassium.

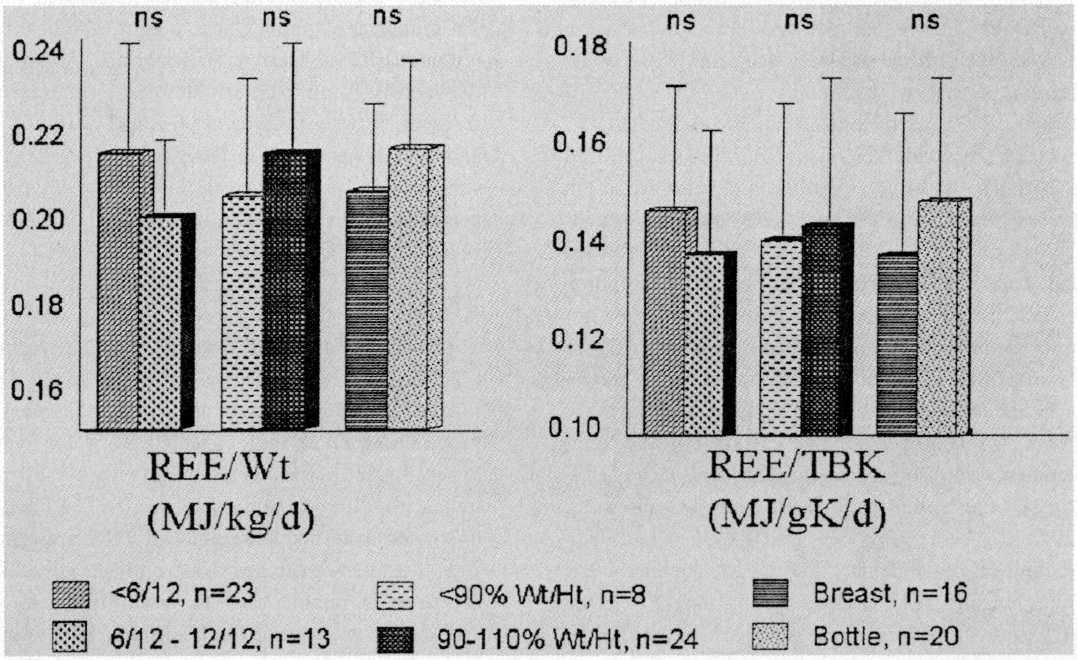

Fig. 2. Measured REE (expressed in terms of weight and TBK), analyzed for age, source of energy intake, and state of nutrition. No statistically significant differences emerged. *gK*, Grams of potassium.

0.135 ± 0.021 MJ/gm K per 24 hours; these differences were not statistically significant. Similarly, no significant differences were noted between mean REE for weight when the groups less than versus more than 6 months of age, less than versus more than the 90th percentile weight-for-length, or bottle versus breast fed were compared.

Using a generalized linear model of variance, we saw a significant (p <0.001) variability in the variance of the five

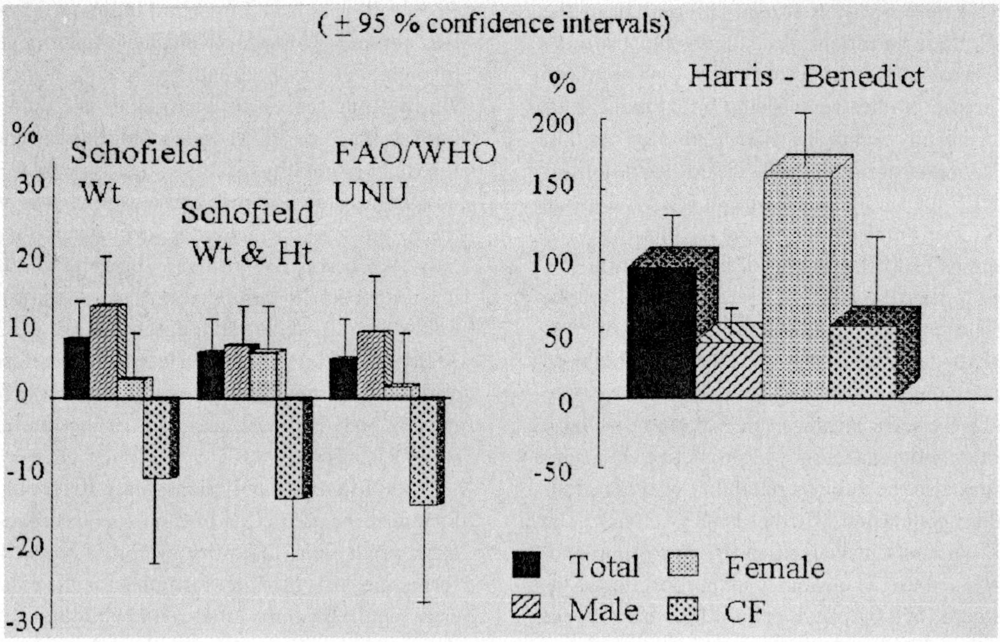

Fig. 3. Predicted/measured REE for the four equations examined. On multiple-range test analysis, the H-B equation was significantly worse than the other equations (p 0.05), but all four overestimated REE in healthy infants and (except H-B) underestimated REE in infants with CF. When a generalized linear model of variance was used, all five equations were at significant variance ($p < 0.001$) for all subjects, as well as for subsets in Fig. 2. (Age, breast vs bottle, weight/height percentile data not shown.)

different values for REE (measured and four predicted), for all subjects combined as well as for the subsets analyzed (i.e., male/female; birth to 6 months/6 to 12 months of age; and those with ideal body weight/those below ideal body weight). Subsequent use of the studentized Newman-Keuls multiple range test showed a significant difference between the mean predicted energy expenditure from the Harris-Benedict equation and the other three predicted REEs, as well as the measured REE ($p < 0.05$) in both the healthy and the CF groups, and in all subsets of healthy subjects (Fig. 3). There was a consistent overestimation of REE, by up to 16% in one subset (Schofield weight-only equation in the 6- to 12-month age group) in healthy infants, and a consistent underestimation in infants with CF (excepting the H-B equation). The 95% confidence limits of up to 12% for predicted/measured REE with the Schofield weight-only, Schofield weight-and-height, and FAO/WHO/UNU equations (and up to 48% if one uses the H-B equation) were unacceptably large and, if added to the aforementioned overestimation, could result in a variation of up to 23% of measured REE. For example, the measured REE for a 7 kg male infant in this study was 1.43 MJ/day; by FAO/WHO/UNU equation the REE would be 1.56 MJ/day, but the 95% confidence limits would be 1.45 to 1.67 MJ/day. In the healthy infants <90% ideal body weight, the 95% confidence limits were wider: 1.37 to 1.75 MJ/day. The infants with CF who have altered body composition had wider prediction confidence limits (for a 7 kg infant with CF, REE measured 1.81 [1.63 to 1.99] MJ/day, and the predicted value was 1.56 MJ/day [1.36 to 1.76]). In the healthy group, by linear regression, subject weight and TBK were significantly related to REE ($r^2 = 0.87$, $p < 0.0001$ and $r^2 = 0.61$, $p < 0.0001$, respectively); however, subject age and sex were not ($p > 0.4$ and $p > 0.7$, respectively). In the CF group, similar relationships were found with REE for weight ($r^2 = 0.92$, $p < 0.0001$) and for TBK ($r^2 = 0.94$, $p < 0.0001$). When the relation of TBK to REE was compared between the healthy group and the CF group by analysis of covariance, the difference was not significant ($p = 0.08$).

DISCUSSION

Estimation of nutritional and fluid requirements based on determination of energy expenditure by the use of predictive formulas is, on the basis of this study, prone to inaccuracy in individual infants, consistently overestimating energy and fluid requirements in healthy infants, and sometimes significantly underestimating them in disease states.

Schofield[7] emphasised the wide coefficient of variation when these formulae are used to predict REE in healthy subjects, as opposed to group estimates (n >100), for which their accuracy was not disputed. The 95% confidence limits of up to 12% for predicted versus measured REE (and up to 48% if one uses the H-B equation) are unacceptably large and, if added to the aforementioned overestimation, could result in a variation of up to 23% of measured REE. Although by multiple range test the calculated REEs (other than by H-B) were not statistically different from the measured REE, these variations nevertheless illustrate the magnitude of error that may occur when one employs equations to predict values for specific individuals. This point was underlined by Schofield[7] when he pointed out that in the group <3 years of age a coefficient of variation for prediction of REE for an individual was 19.4%, for a group of ten 6.3%, for one hundred 2.5%, and for one thousand 1.6%. This demonstrates the danger of using pro rata formulas on which to base estimates of energy expenditure for individual cases, especially in this age group. In our relatively small population group, no differences between male and female infants or between those being breast fed or formula fed were seen. However, in this study we have highlighted not only the inaccuracy of predictive equations in individuals but also the dubious reliability of these equations in the infant population, whether healthy or sick. The H-B equation[5] is grossly inaccurate in this age group and, despite its continued use, is obviously inappropriate for infants: the intercept (655.096 kcal, or 2.74 MJ) is too great for a female infant. This is also obvious from the fact that the H-B predicted mean value for girls is 1.69 that for males. Nevertheless, when the newer equations are used, there remains a consistent overestimation of REE in healthy infants. The FAO/WHO/UNU equation particularly overestimates REE in males and in infants 6 to 12 months of age. Recent work from the Dunn Nutrition Unit on total energy expenditure in infants and young children suggests that a decline in energy intake in recent years may be one reason for the apparent gradual decrease in TEE through the years,[25, 26] and this may be a contributing factor in the overestimation of REE in our study, given that the predictive equations are largely based on infant studies from the first half of this century.

In contrast, however, in the group with CF the predictive equations markedly underestimated the actual REE, indicating that CF infants have a higher energy requirement than realized.[27] Schofield[7] noted that many of the studies on which these predictive equations are based were carried out with a single measurement only, which may also bias the data.[28] We took the average of two measurements under strictly controlled conditions and were able to edit out "noise," a practical problem when studying infants.

These data also highlight the fact that body composition is important in the context of energy expenditure. Differences in body composition occur in obese but healthy children, in whom these equations have a large predictive error.[13, 14] Previous studies of infants with CF had mean REE values for weight which were significantly different from those predicted by these equations[29, 30] but body composition was not measured. Because all the equations cited are based on standard anthropometric variables, they fail to take into account possible alterations in body composition. Body cell mass is an important indicator of nutritional status, comprising the actively metabolizing, the work-performing, and, in children, the growing-body compartment. On multiple regression analysis of the data in our study, both weight and BCM were predictors of energy expenditure in both healthy infants and those with CF, but age was not. In healthy infants, body composition was comparatively uniform (coefficient of variation of TBK/weight was only 19%, compared with 33% for weight). We suggest that it is important to compare energy expenditure and intake data on a unit-weight and, if possible, on a BCM basis. The BCM should be the appropriate term of reference in an examination of metabolic processes, especially in states of abnormal body composition in which the relation of BCM to weight is altered.

In addition to predictions for nutritional requirement, formulas for prediction of fluid requirements are based on REE prediction. The work of Holliday and Segar,[9] which forms the basis of many formulas for the calculation of energy requirements in infancy and childhood quoted in modern textbooks,[10] is founded on the dubious assumption of the energy expenditure of what was termed "an average hospital patient." Their assumption that 100 to 115 ml of water is lost as insensible loss by the skin, lungs, and kidneys for each 100 calories expended led to formulas that constitute the cornerstone of our present-day fluid management in infants. However, their assumptions were based on REE data from as far back as 1914, the validity of which is highly questionable (measurements on ill children tested in the outpatient department of the Massachusetts General Hospital, Boston, were included[30-32]). The inapplicability of such formulas to the energy and fluid requirements of the present-day infant cannot be too strongly emphasized, especially in disease states in which fluid and energy requirements are known to differ markedly from those in well infants, and are also prone to wide and rapid fluctuations.

We advocate the wider use of actual measurement of energy expenditure in the infant population, especially in disease states, and we suggest caution in relying solely on equations for estimating energy expenditure and fluid requirements in individual infants.

REFERENCES

1. Forster E, Amtl Ber d50. Versammlung deutsch Naturfarscher u Aezte in München, Munich, 1877.
2. Talbot F, Wilson E, Worcester J. Basal metabolism of girls: physiological background and application of standards. Am J Dis Child 1937;53:274-7.
3. Boothby W, Berkson J, Halbert D. Studies of the energy of metabolism of normal individuals: a standard for basal metabolism with nomogram for clinical application. Am J Physiol 1936;116:468-83.
4. Robertson J, Reid D. Standard for the basal metabolism of normal people in Britain. Lancet 1952;1:940-3.
5. Harris J, Benedict F. A biometric study of basal metabolism

in man [publication No. 279]. Washington, D.C.: Carnegie Institute of Washington, 1919.
6. World Health Organisation. Energy and protein requirements: report of a joint FAO/WHO/UNU expert consultation [WHO Technical Report Series No. 724]. Geneva: World Health Organization, 1985.
7. Schofield C. Predicting basal metabolic rate, new standards and review of previous work. Hum Nutr Clin Nutr 1985; 39c(suppl 1):5-42.
8. Talbot FB. Basal metabolism in children. In: Brennemann's practice of paediatrics. Hagerstown, Maryland: Prior, 1949.
9. Holliday MA, Segar WE. The maintenance need for water in parenteral fluid therapy. Paediatrics 1957;19:823-32.
10. Robson AM. Parenteral fluid therapy. In: Behrman RE, Vaughan VC, eds. Nelson's textbook of paediatrics. 13th ed. 191-4.
11. Tilden S, Watkins S, Tong T, Jeevanandam M. Measured energy expenditure in pediatric intensive care patients. Am J Dis Child 1989;143:490-2.
12. Vaisman N, Pencharz P, Corey M, Canny G, Hahn E. Energy expenditure of patients with cystic fibrosis. J PEDIATR 1987; 111:496-500.
13. Maffeis C, Schutz Y, Micciolo R, Zoccante L, Pinelli L. Resting metabolic rate in six- to ten-year-old obese and nonobese children. J PEDIATR 1993;122:556-62.
14. Dietz WH, Bandini LG, Schoeller DA. Estimates of metabolic rate in obese and nonobese adolescents. J PEDIATR 1991; 18:146-9.
15. Kinney JM, Lister J, Moore FD. Relationship of energy expenditure to total exchangeable potassium. Ann NY Acad Sci 1963;110:711-22.
16. Branson R. The measurement of energy expenditure: instrumentation, practical considerations and clinical applications. Respir Care 1990;35:640-59.
17. Marks KH, Coen P, Kerrigan JR, Francalancia NA, Nardis EE, Snider MT. The accuracy and precision of an open circuit system to measure oxygen consumption and carbon dioxide production in neonates. Pediatr Res 1986;21:58-65.
18. Anthro software program; version 1.01. Geneva: Division of Nutrition, Center for Disease Control, World Health Organization.
19. Dixon NJ, Massey FJ. Introduction to statistical analysis. 2nd ed. New York: McGraw-Hill, 1967:61.
20. National Health and Medical Research Council. Heights and masses of Australian infants and children. Sydney: Australian Government Publishing, 1973.
21. Coward WA, Parkinson SA, Murgatroyd PR. Body composition measurements for nutrition research. Nutrition Research Reviews 1988;1:115-24.
22. Shepherd RW, Holt TL, Greer R, Cleghorn GJ, Thomas BJ. Total body potassium in cystic fibrosis. J Pediatr Gastroenterol Nutr 1989;9:200-5.
23. Shepherd RW, Oxborough D, Holt TL, Thomas BJ, Thong YH. Longitudinal study of the body composition of weight gain in exclusively breast-fed and intake-measured whey-based formula-fed infants to age 3 months. J Pediatr Gastroenterol Nutr 1988;7:732-9.
24. Pierson RN, Lind DH, Phillips RA. Total body potassium in health: effects of age, sex, height and fat. Am J Physiol 1974;226:206-12.
25. Prentice AM, Lucas A, Vasquez-Velasquez L, Davies PS, Whitehead RG. Are current dietary guidelines for young children a prescription for overfeeding? Lancet 1988;2:1066-9.
26. Davies PS, Ewing G, Lucas A. Energy expenditure in early infancy. Br J Nutr 1989;62:621-9.
27. Shepherd RW, Holt TL, Vasques-Velasquez L, Coward WA, Prentice A, Lucas A. Increased energy expenditure in young children with cystic fibrosis. Lancet 1988;1:1300-3.
28. Robertson JD. The determination of basal metabolism from outpatients. BMJ 1944;1:617-27.
29. O'Rawe A, McIntosh I, Dodge JA, et al. Increased energy expenditure in cystic fibrosis is associated with specific mutations. Clin Sci (Colch) 1992;82:71-6.
30. Fried MD, Durie PR, Tsui LC, Corey M, Levison H, Pencharz PB. The cystic fibrosis gene and resting energy expenditure. J PEDIATR 1991;119:913-6.
31. Talbot FB. Basal metabolism standards for children. Am J Dis Child 1938;55:455-9.
32. Benedict FG, Talbot FB. The gaseous metabolism of infants with special reference to its relation to pulse rate and muscular activity. Washington, D.C.: Carnegie Institute, 1914:1-168. (Publication No. 201.)

Normal energy expenditure in the infant with presymptomatic cystic fibrosis

Michele N. Bronstein, PhD, Peter S. W. Davies, PhD,
K. Michael Hambidge, FRCP(Ed), ScD, and Frank J. Accurso, MD

From the Department of Pediatrics, University of Colorado School of Medicine and Children's Hospital, Denver, and the Infant and Child Nutrition Group, M. R. C. Dunn Nutrition Unit, Cambridge, United Kingdom

To investigate whether a fundamental lesion in energy metabolism is a feature of cystic fibrosis, we measured total energy expenditure using the doubly labeled water technique in 19 infants with presymptomatic cystic fibrosis (0.8 to 6.6 months of age) identified through newborn screening. Total energy expenditure data collected in a cohort of healthy infants by the same method were used for comparison. Energy balance studies were additionally performed in 10 of the infants with cystic fibrosis. Total energy expenditure levels in infants with cystic fibrosis, expressed as either kilocalories per day or kilocalories per kilogram of fat free mass per day, did not differ from control levels. When expressed on the basis of body weight (in kilocalories per kilogram per day), expenditure levels in infants with cystic fibrosis were greater ($p < 0.05$) than control levels. No differences in expenditure were observed between those infants who were homozygous ($n = 10$) for the ΔF508 mutation and the heterozygous infants ($n = 7$), regardless of how expenditure was expressed. Assessment of energy balance indicated that infants with cystic fibrosis grow at a normal rate for metabolizable energy intakes similar to those reported for healthy infants. We conclude that there are no differences in energy expenditure between infants with presymptomatic cystic fibrosis and healthy infants, once differences in body composition are taken into account. This finding indicates that the primary cystic fibrosis defect is not an energy-requiring one. (J Pediatr 1995;126:28-33)

A dietary energy intake of 120% to 150% of the recommended dietary allowance has been recommended as an appropriate intake for either the infant or child with cystic fibrosis, to cover the additional energy costs associated with nutrient malabsorption and increased energy expenditure.[1, 2] The need for promoting such a high energy intake has been questioned, however, in the absence of steatorrhea and significant progression of disease. Nutritional guidelines published in a 1990 consensus report generated by the Cystic Fibrosis Foundation state that if growth is normal and steatorrhea is minimal, the daily energy requirement for the child with cystic fibrosis is the same as that of the healthy, normal child.[3]

The assumption made in formulating these new dietary guidelines is that the cystic fibrosis patient in good pulmonary status does not have an augmented metabolism. This conclusion remains controversial; some evidence suggests that the primary cystic fibrosis defect is an energy-requiring one. Oxygen consumption studies performed with cultured fibroblasts from patients with cystic fibrosis have indicated that the mitochondrial electron transport system is unusually active, suggesting increased energy expenditure.[4] More recently, it was proposed that the basic cystic fibrosis defect may be characterized by impaired hydrolysis of adenosine triphosphate, because the primary cystic fibrosis

Supported by grant No. M01 RR00069 from the General Clinical Research Centers Program, National Center for Research Resources, National Institutes of Health; and the Cystic Fibrosis Foundation.

Submitted for publication Jan. 3, 1994; accepted Aug. 5, 1994.

Reprint requests: Frank J. Accurso, MD, Children's Hospital, B395, 1056 E. 19th St., Denver, CO 80218.

0022-3476/95/$3.00 + 0 **9/20/59592**

mutation is located in a nucleotide-binding domain in the cystic fibrosis gene product.[5] It has been further suggested that variability in energy expenditure levels may be related to genotype. O'Rawe et al.[6,7] found the resting energy expenditure of patients homozygous for the ΔF508 mutation to be greater than that of other genotypes, even after adjustment for differences in pulmonary function.

Efforts to assess energy expenditure in patients with cystic fibrosis have yielded conflicting results. Some researchers have observed elevated energy expenditure levels in patients with minimal pulmonary disease[8-10]; others have not found energy expenditure to be notably elevated in the absence of significant pulmonary disease.[11] One explanation for the lack of agreement among studies has been the difficulty in ensuring that other aspects of the disease, such as infection, pulmonary disease, medication, or altered body composition, are not influencing energy metabolism.[12,13] With this concern in mind, we studied total energy expenditure, body composition, and energy balance in a "presymptomatic" cystic fibrosis population, the young (1 to 6½ months of age) infants identified by newborn screening. Study of these infants offered the opportunity to assess energy expenditure when the influence of confounding factors on energy metabolism would be minimal. Furthermore, because energy expenditure has not been assessed in the infant with cystic fibrosis, these data should provide a scientific basis from which an energy requirement can be devised.

METHODS

Study population. Ten infants (3½ to 8 weeks of age) identified as having cystic fibrosis through a Colorado statewide newborn screening program[14] participated in a study of energy balance and expenditure. An additional nine infants with cystic fibrosis (15 to 29 weeks of age) identified through an East Anglia (United Kingdom) newborn screening program[15] were recruited for study of energy expenditure only. At the time of study, none of the 19 infants was receiving medications or had clinically apparent pulmonary disease or infection. One of the ten Colorado infants (subject 10) and five of the nine East Anglia infants were receiving pancreatic enzyme replacement therapy. Energy expenditure data for normal, healthy infants were obtained from recent work in using the doubly labeled water technique.[16,17] The Colorado study protocol was approved by the University of Colorado Health Sciences Center, and the East Anglia study protocol was approved by the East Anglia Area Health Authority. Informed parental consent was obtained before infant participation.

Study design. Colorado infants were admitted to the inpatient Clinical Research Center for clinical assessment, anthropometric measurements, and evaluation of nutrient balance. Evaluation of total energy expenditure took place during both the inpatient stay and for the 3-day period after discharge. The total energy expenditure of East Anglia infants was measured during a 7-day period at home. Physical examination and anthropometric measurements were also performed at home.

Clinical assessment

Evaluation and pulmonary status. Pulmonary status was evaluated in the Colorado infants only. To obtain viral culture specimens, we washed nasal passages by injecting 2 ml of saline solution into the nose and recovering the fluid with a DeLee trap. Throat culture specimens were obtained in the standardized manner[18] and were assessed for the presence of *Haemophilus influenzae*, *Staphylococcus aureus*, and *Pseudomonas aeruginosa*. A blood sample was drawn for total leukocyte count; the range of 5.0 to 15.0 cells $\times 10^6$/L was defined as normal.[19] Chest radiographs were scored in a blinded fashion by three independent observers using the standard Brasfield scoring system, the maximal possible score being 25.[20]

Genotype. For all infants, the presence of the ΔF508 mutation, the most common mutation associated with cystic fibrosis, was determined by the method of Rommens et al.[21] Subjects were categorized into two groups on the basis of their genotype, homozygous for the ΔF508 mutation and heterozygous for the Δ508 mutation.

Anthropometric measurements. For both Colorado and East Anglia infants, weight was measured on a daily basis to the nearest gram with a pediatric scale (Sartorius; Brinkmann Instruments, Inc., Westbury, N.Y.). For all infants, length (measured in millimeters) was assessed with a stadiometer while the infant was supine. We standardized weight and length data for age and sex by expressing these measurements as *z* scores (number of standard deviations above or below the 50th percentile value for age and sex), employing the National Center for Health Statistics database for reference values.[22] Total body water was assessed by isotope dilution.[16] Fat free body mass was estimated from total body water by applying published values for the hydration of lean tissue.[23] The percentage of fat mass was determined from the following formula: [(Body weight − Fat free mass)/Body weight]100.

Nutrient Balance. Nutrient balance studies were performed in the Colorado infants only. Milk intake was assessed during a 72-hour period by weighing the breast-fed infant before and after feeding and by weighing the bottle before and after feeding of the bottle-fed infants. Use of these weighing techniques introduces an uncertainty of up to 4% in the estimation of milk intake. Stool and urine were collected continuously between brilliant blue markers given at the beginning and end of the 72-hour period of milk intake measurement. To collect stools, we kept the infants on a metabolic bed for the majority of the balance study; an adhesive polyethylene bag was used for the separate collection of urine. Energy content of stools was measured by bomb calorimetry; energy content of urine was estimated by assuming that 72% of urinary nitrogen was derived from urea and that each gram of urea nitrogen represented an energy loss of 5.4 kcal.[24] Urinary nitrogen was measured by Kjeldahl analysis.[25] Fecal fat was analyzed by the method of Van der Kamer et al.[26] No infant was fed a formula containing medium-chain triglycerides. The coefficient of excretion for fat was calculated from [(fecal loss of fat)(100)/(intake of fat)]. Infants with a coefficient of fat excretion $\geq$15% were considered to have pancreatic insufficiency.[27] Literature values were used for gross human milk composition (4.1 gm fat, 1.1 gm protein, 7.2 gm carbohydrate per 100 gm milk),[28, 29] and manufacturers' reported values were used for gross formula composition. Gross calorie intake was computed from calculated macronutrient intake and published gross energy conversion factors (9.25 kcal/gm fat, 5.65 kcal/gm protein, 3.95 kcal/gm carbohydrate).[30] Metabolizable energy intake was calculated from the difference between gross energy intake and the sum of energy in feces and urine. The recommendations of the Food and Agriculture Organization/World Health Organization/United Nations University (FAO/WHO/UNU) were employed as reference values for dietary energy intake.[31] For the infant from birth to 3 months of age, the metabolizable energy recommendation is 116 kcal/kg per day, which assumes, a priori, that approximately 5% of milk calories are lost by excretion. Consequently the gross energy requirement was estimated by applying a factor of 1.05 (122 kcal/kg per day).

Total energy expenditure. Total energy expenditure was assessed by the doubly labeled water technique ($H_2{}^{18}O$; ${}^2H_2O$).[16] For the Colorado infants, water labeled with ^2H (99.96 atom%; MSD Isotopes, Los Angeles, Calif.) and ^{18}O (92.8 to 99.4 atom%; Isotec Inc., Miamisburg, Ohio) was administered orally with a sterile syringe in doses of 0.15 gm/kg body weight and 0.45 gm/kg body weight, respectively. The syringe was capped and reweighed immediately after dose administration; the amount of dose water given was calculated to the nearest 0.1 mg. The dose was not administered until at least 2½ hours after feeding, and the infant was closely monitored for 45 minutes after dosing to ensure no regurgitation of the labeled waters. Urine samples were obtained from the infants immediately before isotope administration for determination of naturally occurring levels of ${}^2H_2O$ and $H_2{}^{18}O$. After dosing, a urine sample was collected daily for the next 6 days in conjunction with the infant's first feeding of the morning. Urine samples were collected in adhesive polyethylene bags. Nurses and parents were instructed to monitor the infants carefully so that the time of void could be accurately recorded.

For the East Anglia infants, details regarding the doubly labeled water protocol are published elsewhere.[16] The East Anglia infants received 0.10 gm ${}^2H_2$ O/kg body and 0.28 gm $H_2{}^{18}$ O/kg body weight.

The calculation of ^2H and ^{18}O dilution spaces (N_dN_o) and of ^2H and ^{18}O elimination rate constants (k_d, k_o), and the subsequent determination of carbon dioxide production from the difference between ^2H and ^{18}O turnover, were performed as previously described.[16] Total energy expenditure was determined from carbon dioxide production by estimation of the mean respiratory quotient for the metabolic period and application of the formula of Weir.[32] For Colorado infants, the dietary quotient computed from the nutrient balance studies was used as an estimate of the mean respiratory quotient.[33] This estimate of respiratory quotient was adjusted for growth, as recommended by Black et al.[33] for 1- to 4-month-old infants. The mean ($\pm$SD) computed respiratory quotient for the 10 Colorado infants was 0.87 $\pm$ 0.02. For the East Anglia infants, a mean respiratory quotient of 0.85 was assumed.

To compare the normality of cystic fibrosis energy expenditure with that of the healthy infant, we expressed the total energy expenditure level of each affected infant as a *z* score (number of standard deviations above or below the 50th percentile value for age), employing the East Anglia infant database as reference values for healthy infant energy expenditure.[16, 17]

Statistical analysis. Unpaired *t* tests were used to compare intake and balance data collected for pancreatic sufficient and insufficient infants, and to compare total energy expenditure *z* scores for cystic fibrosis genotypes. Paired *t* tests were used to compare the percentage of fat mass in the infant with cystic fibrosis with age- and sex-matched reference values obtained from healthy East Anglia infants.[34] One-sample *t* tests were used to evaluate mean anthropometric *z* scores and mean total energy expenditure *z* scores obtained for infants with cystic fibrosis relative to reference values. The level of significance was defined as $p < 0.05$. Results are expressed as means $\pm$ SD.

RESULTS

Evaluation of pulmonary status. Specimens for viral and bacterial cultures were obtained from nine of the Colorado infants. All subjects had negative results except for subject 4, whose bacterial culture was positive for *S. aureus*. Total leukocyte counts were within the normal range for all Colorado infants except for one who had a total leukocyte count of 18.6×10^6/L. Chest x-ray scores for 9 of the 10 infants fell within the normal range[23-25]; the one remaining infant had a score of 22. On reevaluation at 6 months of age, the chest x-ray score of this subject had become normal.

Genotype. Eleven infants were homozygous and seven in-

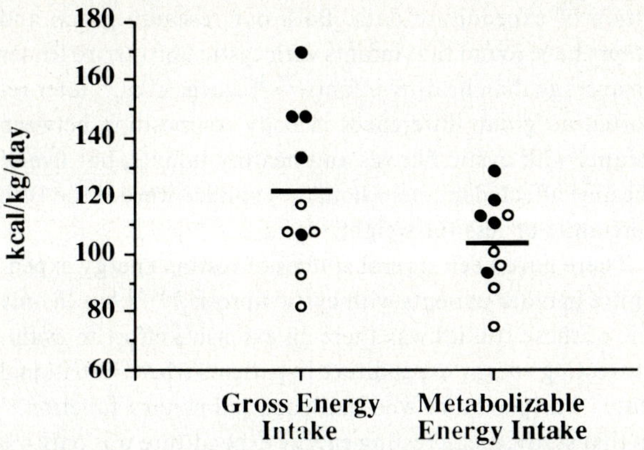

Figure 1. Gross energy intake and metabolizable energy intake in Colorado infants with cystic fibrosis. *Clear circles* represent pancreatic-sufficient infants; *darkened circles* represent pancreatic-insufficient infants. *Bars* represent mean energy intakes for the 10 infants examined for energy balance.

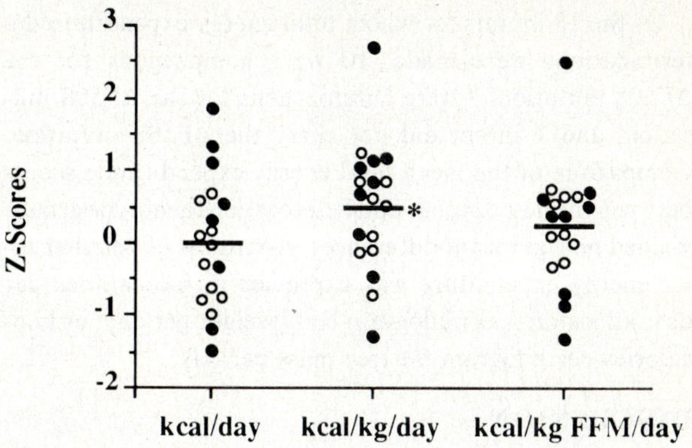

Figure 2. Total energy expenditure z scores for the Colorado and East Anglia infants with cystic fibrosis combined (n = 18). *Clear circles* represent the Colorado infants; *darkened circles* represent the East Anglia infants. *Bars* represent the mean z scores. Mean total energy expenditure z scores did not differ from the reference value of zero, when total energy expenditure was expressed either as kilocalories per day or as kilocalories per kilogram of fat free mass *(FFM)* per day. When total energy expenditure was expressed as kilocalories per kilogram per day, the mean total energy expenditure z score *(asterisk)* was greater ($p < 0.05$) than the reference value of zero.

fants were heterozygous for the ΔF508 deletion. One infant did not carry the ΔF508 deletion.

Anthropometric assessment. The mean age of the infants was 2.56 ± 0.55 months. The mean weight was 4.88 ± 1.19 kg, and the mean weight-for-age z score was −0.49 ± 0.75. Mean length was 56.8 ± 4.6 cm, and the mean length-for-age z score was −0.66 ± 0.76. Thus the mean z scores for weight and length of the 19 infants fell below the normal reference value ($p = 0.01$). The percentage of fat mass (15.8% ± 6.9%) of the infants was significantly ($p = 0.01$) less than age- and sex-matched reference values.[34]

Nutrient balance. Results from the nutrient balance studies in the Colorado infants are shown in Fig. 1. Mean gross energy intake (122 ± 28 kcal/kg per day) mirrored the FAO/WHO/UNU recommended level of 122 kcal/kg per day, whereas mean metabolizable energy intake (104 ± 16 kcal/kg per day) was less ($p < 0.05$) than the recommended level of 116 kcal/kg per day. Mean weight gain for the Colorado infants, computed during the 3-day balance study (27.8 ± 11.2 gm/day) and the 7-day energy expenditure study (28.3 ± 16.5 gm/day), was similar to that of the National Center for Health Statistics 50th percentile for infants (both male and female) from birth to 3 months of age (26.8 gm/day).[22] Mean weight gain for the East Anglia infants (31.9 ± 20.5 gm/day) for the 7-day energy expenditure study was also similar to the reference standard. The mean coefficient of fat excretion for the 10 infants who underwent balance studies was 17% ± 13%. Comparison of pancreatic-insufficient (≥15% coefficient of fat excretion; n = 5) and pancreatic-sufficient (n = 5) infants revealed different gross energy intakes (141 ± 23 vs 102 ± 14 kcal/kg per day; $p = 0.01$), but similar metabolizable energy intakes and rates of weight gain (Fig. 1).

Total energy expenditure. Total energy expenditure determinations were made for 18 of the 19 infants; data from subject 6 was excluded because of inability to obtain good duplication of urinary isotope analysis. Mean ^2H and ^{18}O elimination rate constants (k_d, k_o) were 0.238 ± 0.040 day^{-1} and 0.281 ± 0.043 day^{-1}, respectively. Mean ^2H and ^{18}O dilution space (N_d, N_o) values were 3415 ± 730 ml and 3319 ± 707 ml, respectively. The mean ratio of N_d and N_o was 1.029 ± 0.01, varying from 1.013 to 1.049.

Mean total energy expenditure for the 18 infants, expressed as kilocalories per day, kilocalories per kilogram per day, and kilocalories per kilogram fat free mass per day was 401 ± 157, 79.0 ± 15.7, and 94.3 ± 18.3, respectively. Expressions of total energy expenditure were converted into z scores to evaluate the normality of energy expenditure in infants with cystic fibrosis relative to that of healthy infants. In comparison with the z score for a normal population (i.e., z score = 0), total energy expenditure, expressed as either kilocalories per day (mean z score = 0.01 ± 0.91) or kilocalories per kilogram fat free mass per day (mean z score = 0.25 ± 0.82) did not differ significantly (Fig. 2). Expressed as kilocalories per kilogram per day, the mean total energy expenditure z score of 0.51 ± 0.90, differed significantly ($p < 0.05$) from zero. One infant had a much higher level of expenditure than the other infants; he was the eldest child studied (6.58 months). Exclusion of this infant's data did not change our findings. The mean total energy expenditure z scores of the Colorado and East Anglia infants with cystic fibrosis did not differ.

Of the 18 infants for whom total energy expenditure determinations were made, 10 were homozygous for the ΔF508 mutation, 7 were heterozygous for the ΔF508 mutation, and 1 infant did not carry the ΔF508 mutation. Comparison of the mean total energy expenditure *z* scores between the homozygous and heterozygous genotype groups yielded no significant differences, regardless of whether total energy expenditure was expressed as kilocalories per day, kilocalories per kilogram body weight per day, or kilocalories per kilogram fat free mass per day.

DISCUSSION

We observed no differences in energy expenditure between infants with cystic fibrosis and healthy infants once differences in body composition were taken into account. The results of energy balance studies substantiated our expenditure data. On average, infants with cystic fibrosis had a metabolizable energy intake of 104 ± 16 kcal/kg per day, which is similar to the most recent estimates of energy intake for 1-month-old normal, healthy infants: 110 kcal/kg per day.[35] For this similar metabolizable energy intake, infants with cystic fibrosis grew at a rate equivalent to that of the healthy, normal infant. Thus neither energy expenditure nor energy balance data were supportive of a differential rate of energy use in the infant with cystic fibrosis.

To achieve a similar metabolizable energy intake, pancreatic-insufficient infants needed to consume 40% more calories than pancreatic-sufficient infants. This high energy intake was achieved in the circumstances of an inpatient nutrition study; it is doubtful that pancreatic-insufficient infants consume adequate calories before diagnosis and initiation of pancreatic enzyme replacement therapy. Previously we reported significant growth failure in the pancreatic-insufficient infant at diagnosis, but not in the pancreatic-sufficient infant.[27] This observation supports the notion that dietary energy is not a special concern in the absence of steatorrhea in the infant with cystic fibrosis.

These conclusions contrast with those of the one previous investigation of total energy expenditure by the doubly labeled water technique in older infants with cystic fibrosis (0.7 to 2.0 years of age)[10]; Shepherd et al.[10] reported that nine clinically well infants had a 25% greater level of expenditure than either age- or weight-matched normal infants. Energy expenditure in that study was expressed, however, on the basis of body weight, rather than fat free mass. We also found differences in energy expenditure when the data are reported on the basis of body weight. Because lean tissue, rather than fat tissue, is the major energy-consuming component of the body mass, it is generally agreed that it is preferable to express energy data relative to the lean tissue.[16] In this way, adjustment can be made for differences in body composition that may confound interpretation of expenditure data. Both our research group and others have found that infants with cystic fibrosis are leaner on average than healthy infants.[27, 36] Lucas et al.[37] later reported no group differences in body composition between infants with cystic fibrosis and healthy infants, but five of the nine affected infants whom they studied were at the 10th percentile or less for weight.

There have been several studies of resting energy expenditure in older patients with cystic fibrosis,[6-9, 11] but in only one of these studies was there an extensive effort to evaluate resting energy expenditure in patients whose nutritional status was good and who had good pulmonary function.[11] In that study, mean resting energy expenditure was only 4% higher than the predicted normal value. Although the authors acknowledged that the slight elevation in resting energy expenditure may have been due to the primary defect, it seemed equally feasible that mild pulmonary disease may also have been responsible. Similar to our findings, no significant differences in resting energy expenditure were observed between different cystic fibrosis genotypes. It seems likely that previous reports[6, 7] of augmented energy expenditure in patients homozygous for the ΔF508 mutation may reflect genotype-related differences in disease severity, rather than intrinsic differences in energy metabolism.

We conclude that energy expenditure is normal in patients with cystic fibrosis before the development of significant disease progression. Thus, when malabsorption is under control and growth is normal, the infant's need for energy is comparable to that of a healthy infant. However, at diagnosis of cystic fibrosis, energy needs may be high initially because of growth failure resulting from prolonged malabsorption. In addition, the infant with cystic fibrosis is likely to require increased caloric intake to achieve and maintain normal adipose tissues stores.

Readers interested in having data on individual patients can obtain such data from the authors.

REFERENCES

1. Hubbard VS, Mangrum PJ. Energy intake and nutrition counseling in cystic fibrosis. J Am Diet Assoc 1982;80:127-31.
2. Michel SH, Mueller DH. Practical approaches to nutrition care of patients with cystic fibrosis. Topics in Clinical Nutrition 1987;2:10-20.
3. Ramsey BW, Farrell PM, Pencharz P, Consensus Committee. Nutritional assessment and management in cystic fibrosis: a consensus report. Am J Clin Nutr 1992;55:108-16.
4. Feigal RJ, Shapiro BL. Mitochondrial calcium uptake and oxygen consumption in cystic fibrosis. Nature 1979;278:276-7.
5. Thomas PJ, Shenbagamurthi P, Ysern X, Pedersen PL. Cystic fibrosis transmembrane conductance regulator: nucleotide binding to a synthetic peptide. Science 1991;251:555-7.
6. O'Rawe A, Dodge JA, Redmond AOB, McIntosh I, Brock DJH. Gene/energy interaction in cystic fibrosis. Lancet 1990;1:552-3.

7. O'Rawe A, McIntosh I, Dodge JA, et al. Increased energy expenditure in cystic fibrosis is associated with specific mutations. Clin Sci (Colch) 1992;82:71-6.
8. Vaisman N, Pencharz PB, Corey M, Canny GJ, Hahn E. Energy expenditure of patients with cystic fibrosis. J PEDIATR 1987;111:496-500.
9. Buchdahl RM, Cox M, Fulleylove C, et al. Increased resting energy expenditure in cystic fibrosis. J Appl Physiol 1988; 64:1810-6.
10. Shepherd RW, Vasques-Velasquez L, Prentice A, Holt TL, Coward WA, Lucas A. Increased energy expenditure in young children with cystic fibrosis. Lancet 1988;1:1300-3.
11. Fried MD, Durie PR, Tsui L-C, Corey M, Levison H, Pencharz PB. The cystic fibrosis gene and resting energy expenditure. J PEDIATR 1991;119:913-6.
12. Pencharz PB, Durie PR. Nutritional management of cystic fibrosis. Ann Rev Nutr 1993;13:111-36.
13. Pencharz PB, Berall G, Vaisman N, Corey M, Canny G. Energy expenditure in children with cystic fibrosis [Letter]. Lancet 1988;2:513-4.
14. Hammond KB, Abman SH, Sokol RJ, Accurso FJ. Efficacy of statewide neonatal screening for cystic fibrosis by assay for persistent elevation of trypsinogen concentrations. N Engl J Med 1991;325:769-74.
15. Heeley AF, Heeley ME. Biochemical screening of the neonatal population for the early detection of cystic fibrosis in East Anglia, 1980–1986. In: Kuzemko JA, Joint GS, eds. Insights into paediatrics. Macclesfield, United Kingdom: Gardiner-Caldwell Communications, 1987;1:49-59.
16. Davies PSW, Ewing G, Lucas A. Energy expenditure in infancy. Br J Nutr 1989;62:621-9.
17. Davies PSW, Cameron JE, Lucas A. Reference data for total energy expenditure in early infancy. In: Schurch B, Scrimshaw NS, eds. Activity, energy expenditure and energy requirements of infants and children. Vienna, Austria: IDECG Publication, 1990:103-16.
18. Abman SH, Ogle JW, Butler-Simon N, Rumack CM, Accurso FJ. Role of respiratory syncytial virus in early hospitalizations for respiratory distress of young infants with cystic fibrosis. J PEDIATR 1988;113:826-30.
19. Silver HK, Kempe CH, Bruyn H, eds. Handbook of pediatrics. Los Altos, California: Lange, 1977:674.
20. Brasfield D, Hicks G, Soong S-J, Tiller R. The chest roentgenogram in cystic fibrosis: a new scoring system. Pediatrics 1979;63:24-9.
21. Rommens JM, Iannuzzi MC, Kerem B, et al. Identification of the cystic fibrosis gene: chromosome walking and jumping. Science 1989;245:1059-65.
22. Hamill PVV, Drizd TA, Johnson CL, Reed RB, Roche AF, Moore WM. Physical growth: National Center for Health Statistics percentiles. Am J Clin Nutr 1979;32:607-29.
23. Fomon SJ, Haschke F, Ziegler EE, Nelson SE. Body composition of reference children from birth to age 10 years. Am J Clin Nutr 1982;35:1169-75.
24. Reichman BL, Chessex P, Putet G, et al. Partition of energy metabolism and energy cost of growth in the very low-birth-weight infant. Pediatrics 1982;69:446-51.
25. Horwitz N, ed. Official methods of analysis. 12th ed. Washington, D.C.: Association of Official Analytical Chemists, 1975.
26. Van der Kamer JG, ten Bokkel Huinink H, Weger HA. Rapid method for determination of fat in feces. J Biol Chem 1949;177:347-55.
27. Bronstein MN, Sokol RJ, Abman SH, et al. Pancreatic insufficiency, growth and nutrition in infants identified by newborn screening as having cystic fibrosis. J PEDIATR 1992;120:533-40.
28. Fomon SJ. Protein requirements of term infants. In: Fomon SJ, Heird WC, eds. Energy and protein needs during infancy. Orlando, Florida: Academic Press, 1985:55-68.
29. Paul AA, Southgate DAT. McCance and Widdowson's the composition of foods. 4th ed. New York: Elsevier/North Holland Biomedical Press, 1978:70-1.
30. Watt BK, Merrill AL. Composition of foods. Agricultural Handbook No. 8. Washington, D.C.: Agricultural Research Services, U.S. Department of Agriculture, 1963.
31. Food and Agriculture Organization/World Health Organization/United Nations University Expert Consultation. Energy and protein requirements. Technical Report Series 724. Geneva: World Health Organization, 1985.
32. Weir JB de V. New methods for calculating metabolic rate with special reference to protein metabolism. J Physiol 1949; 109:1-9.
33. Black AE, Prentice AM, Coward WA. Use of food quotients to predict respiratory quotients for the doubly-labeled water method of measuring energy expenditure. Hum Nutr: Clin Nutr 1986;40C:381-91.
34. Davies PSW. Estimates of body fatness in infancy and childhood. Am J Human Biol 1992;4:621-4.
35. Prentice AM, Lucas A, Vasquez-Velasquez L, Davies PSW, Whitehead RG. Are current dietary guidelines for young children a prescription for overfeeding? Lancet 1988;2:1066-9.
36. Greer R, Shepherd R, Cleghorn G, Bowling FG, Holt T. Evaluation of growth and changes in body composition following neonatal diagnosis of cystic fibrosis. J Pediatr Gastroenterol Nutr 1991;13:52-8.
37. Lucas A, Prentice AM, Shepherd RW. Energy expenditure and cystic fibrosis [Letter]. Lancet 1988;2:737.

Chronic constipation as a symptom of cow milk allergy

G. Iacono, MD, A. Carroccio, MD, F. Cavataio, MD, G. Montalto, MD, M. D. Cantarero, MD, and A. Notarbartolo, MD

From the Cattedra di Patologia Medica II, Universitá di Palermo Ospedale Pediatrico G. Di Cristina, Palermo, Italy

Twenty-seven consecutive infants (mean age, 20.6 months) with chronic "idiopathic" constipation were studied to investigate the possible relation between constipation and cow milk protein allergy (CMPA). The infants were initially observed on an unrestricted diet, and the number of stools per day was recorded. Subsequently the infants were put on a diet free of cow milk protein (CMP) for two periods of 1 month each, separated by two challenges with CMP. During the CMP-free diet, there was a resolution of symptoms in 21 patients; during the two consecutive challenges, constipation reappeared within 48 to 72 hours. In another six patients the CMP-free diet did not lead to improvement of constipation. Only four of the patients who improved on the CMP-free diet had concomitant symptoms of suspected CMPA, but a medical history of CMPA was found in 15 of the 21 patients cured and in only one of the six patients whose condition had not improved (*p* <0.05); in addition, in 15 of the 21 cured patients, results of one or more laboratory tests (specific IgE, IgG, anti-β-lactoglobulin, circulating eosinophils) were positive at the time of diagnosis, indicating hypersensitivity, compared with one of the six patients whose condition did not improve (*p* <0.05). The endoscopic and histologic findings at the time of diagnosis showed proctitis with monocytic infiltration in two patients cured with the CMP-free diet; after 1 month on this diet, they were completely normal. We conclude that constipation in infants may have an allergic pathogenesis. (J Pediatr 1995;126:34-9)

Most chronic constipation in infants and young children is thought to have a psychogenic cause[1, 2] or to be related to an intestinal motility disorder.[3-7] Our experience in dealing with chronic constipation, however, has led us to suspect that the illness in the first 2 to 3 years after birth may be a manifestation of cow milk protein allergy. However, there have been no studies evaluating the relation between CMPA and constipation, although there have been two sporadic reports of patients in the same age group that we considered.[8, 9]

The aim of our prospective study was to ascertain whether there is a relation between chronic constipation and CMPA.

Submitted for publication April 21, 1994; accepted Aug. 5, 1994.

Reprint requests: Antonio Carroccio, MD, via Coffaro No. 25, 90124 Palermo, Italy.

0022-3476/95/$3.00 + 0 **9/20/59591**

METHODS

The study group included all the patients with chronic constipation, aged <3 years, referred to our pediatric gastroenterology clinic during the preceding 12 months. Two patients with mental retardation and one with Hirschsprung disease were excluded. Anorectal manometry and biopsy of

CMP	Cow milk protein
CMPA	CMP allergy

the intestinal mucosa were also performed in two cases of suspected megacolon and megarectum (patients with marked abdominal distention and clinical signs of malnutrition). Twenty-seven infants (15 boys) were considered to have chronic idiopathic constipation and were included in the study. Their mean age ($\pm$SD) was 20.6 $\pm$ 13.4 months (range, 5 to 36 months). The diagnosis of constipation was made on the basis of a history of reduced frequency of stools—one evacuation every 3 to 7 days—and of pain in the passage of hard stools. Furthermore, in all the patients included in the study, the frequency of stools per day was lower than the 3rd percentile of the values observed in a large population of healthy subjects participating in an Italian multicenter study.[10] At the time of diagnosis, a detailed chart was compiled; it contained the clinical data obtained at physical examination, plus historical information such as previous illnesses and a family history of atopic disease. A record was made of soiling, encopresis, abdominal pain, anal fissures, and perianal erythema or edema. In addition, on first observation and after 4 weeks of a CMP-free diet, a blood sample was taken to determine serum levels of IgG anti-β-lactoglobulin (by enzyme-linked immunosorbent assay: Beta-lactotest, Eurospital, Trieste, Italy), total serum IgE (Phadebas IgE paper radioimmunosorbent test kit, Pharmacia Diagnostics, Uppsala, Sweden), and peripheral eosinophil counts. The following values were considered elevated: β-lactoglobulin, >36% above a standard control; IgE, >60 kallikrein units per liter (mean value ± 2 SD, observed in our laboratory in healthy infants of the same age range); and eosinophils, >400/mm^3. In patients with elevated levels of total IgE, specific IgE was also measured (Phadebas radioallergosorbent test kit); a score >1 was regarded as positive (>4 sorbent units per milliliter). Moreover, three patients whose parents had given informed consent underwent sigmoidoscopy at the time of diagnosis, and in two of them mucosal biopsy specimens were taken both then and after 1 month of a CMP-free diet. Biopsy specimens were fixed in 10% neutral buffered formalin, embedded in paraffin wax, and stained with hematoxylin and eosin. The parents of the other children in the study had not given their consent to endoscopy.

At the time of diagnosis, all the patients were being fed either various forms of commercial formula derived from cow milk or whole cow milk and its derivatives. This diet was not modified during the first 7 days of the study, and then all patients started a CMP-free diet: three patients aged <12 months were fed a formula containing soy protein, and in the others whole cow milk was replaced with soy milk or ass milk (eight cases) and all milk derivatives were excluded. After 1 month of this exclusion diet, the patients whose symptoms had abated underwent a cow milk challenge, with cow milk being given for a maximum of 10 days; these patients again started an exclusion diet for 1 month, and then a second cow milk challenge was performed. In contrast, the patients with no abatement in symptoms during the first CMP-free diet period were permanently given an unrestricted diet, except for one infant who had episodes of recurrent bronchospasm related to ingestion of cow milk.

The parents of the infants were given a diary in which they noted the number of stools of the patients during the

Table I. Clinical characteristics at time of diagnosis

	Patients on CMP-free diet	
	Cured	**Unimproved**
Age (mo)	24.4 ± 14.0	31.4 ± 11.6
Sex	13 M; 8 F	2 M; 4 F
Duration of illness (mo)	3.4 ± 4.8	3.6 ± 4.2
History of CMPA	4/21	0/6
Associated symptoms of CMPA	4/21	1/6
History of infantile colic	8/21	0/6
Soiling or encopresis	1/21	1/6
Abdominal pain	12/21	3/6
Anal fissures and perianal erythema and edema	19/21	4/6
Family history of CMPA	5/21	0/6

Values for age and duration of illness are expressed as mean ± SD.

various study periods; they also included a description of the stools and the difficulty in passing them. A score was established: 3 = hard feces, difficulty and pain in passing stools; 2 = soft feces, no pain; and 1 = mushy or liquid stool. The parents were also requested to note any eventual changes in feeding habits during the various phases of the study.

On the basis of the clinical response to the periods of CMP-free diet and the successive challenges, the patients were divided into two groups: cured with a CMP-free diet, and not improved (Table I). At the time of diagnosis, there was no difference between the two groups in mean age or in mean duration of the illness. Four of the patients whose condition improved with a CMP-free diet had previously been identified as having CMPA, by a double-blind, controlled food challenge performed twice; in three patients there had been enteropathy with diarrhea and malabsorption during the first 3 months of life, and in the fourth, atopic dermatitis. These four infants, after a period of a CMP-free diet varying between 6 and 10 months, had resumed feeding with cow milk without any similar disturbances, and growth rate was satisfactory. In addition, a further eight patients in this group had colic during the first few months of life, whereas none of the six infants with constipation that did not respond to the dietary treatment had a history of severe infantile colic. Furthermore, four of the infants cured with the CMP-free diet had symptoms at diagnosis compatible with overt CMPA: two had atopic dermatitis and two had recurrent episodes of bronchospasm. None of the six patients whose condition was unimproved with the CMP-free diet had a clinical history of CMPA, although one at diagnosis had suspected CMPA and associated episodes of recurrent bronchospasm. In summary, a history of symptoms of CMPA or current symptoms of CMPA were recorded in 15 of the 21 patients who were cured with the CMP-free diet, and in only 1 of the 6 patients whose con-

Table II. Mean number (±SD) of stools per day during unrestricted diet and during CMP-free diet

	Stools from patients on CMP-free diet	
	Cured (n = 21)	Unimproved (n = 6)
Control	0.24 ± 0.10[a]	0.18 ± 0.12
CMP-free diet	1.04 ± 0.12[b]	0.20 ± 0.13
CMP challenge	0.31 ± 0.14[c]	—
CMP-free diet	1.05 ± 0.11[d]	—

Significance: b and d versus a and c, $p < 0.0005$ (Wilcoxon rank sum test).

dition did not improve with this diet (chi-square statistic = 3.75; $p < 0.05$). Among the other symptoms present at diagnosis, soiling or encopresis was observed in only two patients of the 27 studied; more frequent symptoms included abdominal pain, which was equally distributed in the two groups, and anal fissures. There was a family history of atopic disease in the parents and or siblings of patients in 24% (5/21) of the infants cured and no family history in any of the infants whose condition showed no improvement with the CMP-free diet (chi-square statistic, 0.530; not significant).

Follow-up procedures. The study patients were then followed monthly for a mean period of 18 months (range, 10 to 30 months); a complete physical examination was performed and a case history was elicited on each occasion. For the patients with abnormal laboratory data at diagnosis, tests were repeated every 6 to 8 months.

The parents of the patients had given their informed consent to the study, and it was approved by the ethics committee of the Institute of Internal Medicine Faculty of Medicine.

Challenge method. All the challenges were performed in the hospital, and the reactions were evaluated by physicians and by members of the nursing staff. In all cases during the challenge, the infants received an infusion of 0.9% sodium chloride solution to facilitate immediate intervention in the event of anaphylactic shock. Before the challenge a prick test was performed with CMP. In the patients with a negative test result, the challenge was performed by giving whole cow milk in a single feeding; if there were no clinical reactions, the same food was given on the following days. In patients with a positive prick test result, the challenge was performed by giving a formula containing CMP, beginning with an initial quantity of 10 ml and gradually increasing the amount to reach the dose equivalent to a full feeding after 48 hours. No other change in diet was made.

Statistical analysis. The analysis of frequency was performed with the chi-square test. The Wilcoxon rank sum test was employed to compare the number of evacuations per day and the qualitative score of the stools during the various study periods. The Student *t* test was used to compare the mean values of the laboratory results.

RESULTS

During the first month of the CMP-free diet there was a significant improvement in symptoms in 21 patients: the frequency of stools significantly increased, feces were soft, and none of the infants had any discomfort when passing stools. These improvements were rapid; in all patients the bowel frequency became normal within the first 3 days of the CMP-free diet. In the remaining six study patients, the CMP-free diet did not lead to any changes, either in the number of stools or in the symptoms associated with constipation (Table II).

In the 21 patients who were cured during the CMP-free diet, there was also a resolution of the episodes of abdominal pain, the perianal fissures, and the edema and erythema of the anus and perianal area accompanying the constipation. During the first challenge the perianal erythema and edema reappeared, and constipation then returned within 48 hours after the reintroduction of cow milk, passing stools became painful, and seven patients had renewed abdominal pain; in these seven patients, ingestion of cow milk was discontinued on day 4. During the second period of CMP-free diet, the stools became normal once again in the 21 patients and the symptoms accompanying constipation disappeared. During the second challenge, symptoms reappeared within 24 to 48 hours: all 21 patients had painful passage of stools, and for this reason the challenge was suspended on the third day. In six patients the CMP-free diet did not lead to any improvement in symptoms; there was no change in the frequency of stools between periods 1 and 2 of the study (Table II). There was also no improvement in the qualitative score of the feces in these patients during the second study period; as in all patients the score for each stool was still 3. In the other 21 patients, however, the qualitative score was 2.85 ± 0.05 and 2.75 ± 0.11 during cow milk protein feeding, and fell to 1.90 ± 0.08 and 1.85 ± 0.10 during the CMP-free diet ($p < 0.001$, Wilcoxon rank sum test).

Analysis of the patients' dietary diaries did not show any significant variations in daily fiber and liquid intake during the various study periods.

The IgG anti-β-lactoglobulin values were elevated in 8 of 21 patients whose condition improved with the CMP-free diet; these subjects did not include any of the four infants with previous CMPA but did include three infants who had atopic dermatitis (two cases) or bronchospasm (one case) at the time of diagnosis. In the group of patients without lessening of constipation when a CMP-free diet was used, one infant who had recurrent episodes of bronchospasm also had elevated beta-lactoglobulin values; the frequency of positive

Table III. Laboratory results

	Cured (n = 21)		Unimproved (n = 6)	
	Diagnosis	No CMP	Diagnosis	No CMP
Subjects with positive assay				
β-Lactoglobulin	8/21	4/21	1/6	0/6
Serum IgE	7/21	7/21	0/6	0/6
Circulating eosinophils	6/21	2/6	0/6	0/6
Laboratory values*				
β-Lactoglobulin	64 + 30[a]	42.5 + 15[a]		
Serum IgE	126 + 63	111 + 75		
Circulating eosinophils	766 + 222[b]	371 + 71[b]		

Mean comparison: a = p <0.005; b = p <0.0001 (Student t test).
No CMP, Diet free of CMP.
*Values are expressed as mean ± SD. To calculate the mean ± SD, we considered only patients who had elevated values at diagnosis.

test results in the two groups was not significantly different (Table III).

Values for circulating IgE were greater than normal in 7 of the 21 patients cured with the CMP-free diet; among them were two patients with previous CMPA and three infants with symptoms probably associated with current CMPA (two atopic dermatitis, one bronchospasm). In all seven patients, specific IgE to CMPs were demonstrated. In the group of patients with no abatement in constipation with a CMP-free diet, no infants had elevated IgE values; the frequency of elevated IgE in the two groups of patients was not significantly different.

An increase in the number of circulating eosinophils was observed in six patients cured with the CMP-free diet; all of them also had contemporaneous elevated IgE values. In the patients with no improvement after the CMP-free diet was started, there was no increase in the number of circulating eosinophils. The frequency of the increase in eosinophils in the two groups was not significantly different.

In summary, we observed alterations in one or more laboratory results at the time of diagnosis in 15 of 21 patients cured and in 1 of 6 not cured with the CMP-free diet: this different frequency was significant (chi-square statistic, 3.75; p <0.05). There was no difference in sex and age between the subjects with positive and those with negative immunologic data.

After the CMP-free diet, the β-lactoglobulin values were almost halved in all the patients, and in four they returned within normal limits. A similar change occurred in the circulating eosinophil values, which in four of six cases were below the maximum reference limits after the diet. In contrast, in the patients with elevated total IgE levels there was no significant reduction in values between the first study phase and the following CMP-free diet phase (Table III). Rectosigmoidoscopy performed at diagnosis in three infants, two of whom showed improvement after a CMP-free diet was used, showed signs of proctitis with hyperemia of the mucosa, but without erosions or ulcerations; histologic examination of the mucosa showed moderate edema and monocytic infiltration, without the presence of eosinophils (Figure); after 1 month of the CMP-free diet, the two patients in whom constipation had disappeared again underwent endoscopy and biopsy of the rectal mucosa. Both the endoscopic and histologic findings were completely normal.

The monthly follow-up of the patients cured with the CMP-free diet confirmed the resolution of constipation in all of them; the patients with associated atopic dermatitis or recurrent bronchospasm were all free of symptoms; all manifestations associated with constipation—soiling, anal edema, erythema and fissures, recurrent abdominal pain—had disappeared. The patients with positive laboratory findings at diagnosis no longer had increased eosinophil or IgG anti-lactoglobulin values. Height-weight growth was completely satisfactory in all cases. Reintroduction of cow milk into the diet was cautiously attempted in 16 infants, 6 to 9 months after the diagnosis of CMPA-dependent constipation. In eight children CMP did not cause the onset of any problems, and it was reintroduced on a permanent basis; in eight patients CMP led to the reappearance of constipation within 2 to 3 days after reintroduction, and these infants are still following a CMP-free diet. The six infants whose condition did not improve on the CMP-free diet were treated with lactulose, and only a partial regression in symptoms was observed during follow-up; these also included the infant with recurrent bronchospasm who followed a CMP-free diet for approximately 7 months and whose constipation did not improve, although no further episodes of bronchospasm were recorded.

DISCUSSION

These data indicate that some cases of "idiopathic" constipation were due to CMPA; 21 of 27 of the patients showed rapid improvement. Symptoms completely regressed when a CMP-free diet was used, and there was a

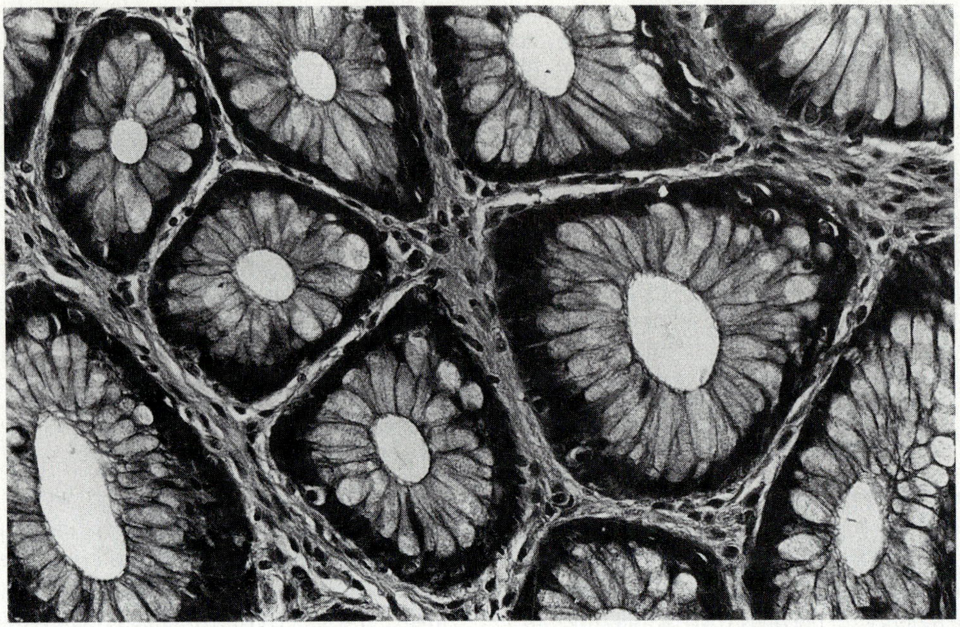

Figure. Histologic study of the rectal mucosa in a patient with a CMPA-related proctitis, showing monocytic infiltration.

clinical relapse during two subsequent cow milk challenges. The possibility that CMPA might be manifested only by the presence of constipation has rarely been reported[8, 9]; apart from single case reports, the presence of constipation as a symptom of CMPA has been reported only in association with other, more typical symptoms of food allergy.[11] Only a few of our patients with CMPA-dependent constipation had other symptoms attributable to CMPA; all the others had constipation accompanied by abdominal pain or anal fissures or both, as reported in cases of chronic idiopathic constipation.[1, 12] However, a detailed history revealed previous disturbances, such as infantile colic, attributable to CMPA[13, 14] in more patients. There had been reports of a frequent history of infantile colic in infants with idiopathic constipation when the hypothesis of a colic-CMPA relationship had not been advanced[15]; furthermore, Davidson et al.[16] reported that patients with constipation showed considerable improvement when treatment included the exclusion of cow milk and its derivatives from the diet.

Apart from the clinical evidence of the reactions to the challenges, the laboratory data also support the hypothesis of constipation as a symptom of CMPA; in most of the infants cured with a CMP-free diet, we recorded an increase in either IgG anti-lactoglobulin, total IgE, or circulating eosinophil values. Furthermore, there was a consistent drop in values of β-lactoglobulin values and circulating eosinophils after the diet was started. Only the total IgE values were not significantly lower in the CMP-free period, but it is probable that the amount of anti-CMP IgE in the total serum IgE pool was so small that the differences in total IgE were not apparent. We believe that an abnormal finding in one of these laboratory studies in an infant with constipation should lead to a possible diagnosis of CMPA. However, some patients cured with the CMP-free diet had no abnormal laboratory values. It would be useful to investigate the immune mechanisms involved in causing constipation.

Rectoscopy, performed in our study on only two patients who were cured with the CMP-free diet, showed nonspecific proctitis with considerable monocytic infiltration but without the eosinophils that usually characterize allergic proctitis[17, 18]; however, neither of the two patients who underwent biopsy had an increase in circulating IgE, a finding usually associated with eosinophilic proctitis.[18, 19] Consequently, it is possible that the histologic pattern may differ depending on the immune mechanisms that cause the CMPA-dependent proctitis.

The follow-up of the patients confirmed the good tolerability of ass milk, which we had already used in patients with multiple food allergy[20]; this milk has also proved to be acceptable from a nutritional point of view, as witnessed by the excellent weight-height growth that we observed in our patients.

We conclude that many cases of chronic constipation in young children are due to CMPA. A clinical history of previous CMPA or of symptoms associated with CMPA increases the probability that the constipation may be an allergic manifestation; this probability also increases if serum data point to abnormalities of immune mechanisms.

However, this was open, preliminary research, and other studies, possibly on a double-blind basis, will be necessary to confirm these data and to clarify the immune mechanisms underlying this association.

REFERENCES

1. Abrahamian FP, Lloyd-Still JD. Chronic constipation in childhood: a longitudinal study of 186 patients. J Pediatr Gastroenterol Nutr 1984;3:460-7.
2. Olatawura MO. Encopresis: a review of thirty-two cases. Acta Pediatr Scand 1973;62:358-64.
3. Meunier P, Marechal JM, De Beaujeu MJ. Rectoanal pressures and rectal sensitivity studies in chronic childhood constipation. Gastroenterology 1979;77:330-6.
4. Emery Y, Descos L, Meunier P, Louis D, Valancogne G, Weil G. Constipation terminale par asychronisme abdomino-pelvien: analyse des donnees etiologiques, cliniques, manometriques, et des resultats therapeutiques apres rééducation par biofeedback. Gastroenterol Clin Biol 1988;12:6-11.
5. Loening-Baucke V, Cruikshank BM. Abnormal defecation dynamics in chronically constipated children. J PEDIATR 1986;108:562-6.
6. Corazziari E, Cucchiara S, Staiano AM. Gastrointestinal transit time, frequency of defecation and ano-rectal manometry in healthy and constipated children. J PEDIATR 1985; 103:379-82.
7. Staiano AM, Cucchiara S, Andreotti MR, Minella R, Manzi G. Effect of Cisapride on chronic idiopathic constipation in children. Dig Dis Sci 1991;36:733-6.
8. Chin KC, Tarlow MJ, Allfree AJ. Allergy to cow's milk presenting as a chronic constipation. BMJ 1983;287:1593.
9. McGrath J. Allergy to cow's milk presenting as a chronic constipation. BMJ 1984;288:236.
10. Fontana M, Bianchi C, Cataldo F, et al. Bowel frequency in healthy children. Acta Paediatr Scand 1989;78:682-4.
11. Buisseret PD. Common manifestations of cow's milk allergy in children. Lancet 1978;1:304-5.
12. Levine MD. Children with encopresis: a descriptive analysis. Pediatrics 1975;56:412-6.
13. Iacono G, Carroccio A, Montalto G, et al. Severe infantile colic and food intolerance: a long-term prospective study. J PEDIATR Gastroenterol Nutr 1991;12:332-5.
14. Lothe L, Lindberg T. Cow's milk whey protein elicits symptoms of infantile colic in colicky formula-fed infants: a double-blind, crossover study. Pediatrics 1989;83:262-6.
15. Jorup S. Colonic hyperperistalsis in neurolabile infants: studies in so-called dyspepsia in breast-fed infants. Acta Paediatr 1952(suppl 85):41-5.
16. Davidson M, Kugler MM, Baue CH. Diagnosis and management in children with severe and protracted constipation and obstipation. J PEDIATR 1963;62:261-75.
17. Jenkins HR, Pincott JR, Soothill JF, Milla PJ, Harries JT. Food allergy: the major cause of infantile colitis. Arch Dis Child 1984;59:326-9.
18. Rosekrans PCM, Meijer CJLM, Van der Wal AM, Lindeman J. Allergic proctitis, a clinical and immunopathological entity. Gut 1980;21:1017-23.
19. Pittschieler K. Cow's milk protein-induced colitis in the breast-fed infants. J Pediatr Gastroenterol Nutr 1990; 10:548-9.
20. Iacono G, Carroccio A, Cavataio F, Montalto G, Soresi M, Balsamo V. Use of ass's milk in multiple food allergy. J Pediatr Gastroenterol Nutr 1992;14:177-81.

Spectrum of disease associated with anti-neutrophil cytoplasmic autoantibodies in pediatric patients

Eileen N. Ellis, MD, Ellen G. Wood, MD, and Phillip Berry, MD

From the Department of Pediatrics, Arkansas Children's Hospital and University of Arkansas for Medical Sciences, Little Rock, and Department of Pediatrics, Cardinal Glennon Children's Hospital and St. Louis University Health Sciences Center, St. Louis, Missouri

Anti-neutrophil cytoplasmic autoantibodies (ANCA) are usually determined during the diagnostic evaluation of systemic vasculitis and glomerulonephritis syndromes in adult patients, but few pediatric patients with ANCA have been reported. We describe five pediatric patients with ANCA and glomerulonephritis, with and without upper or lower respiratory tract disease. We compared these five patients and six previously described patients to affected adults; the spectrum of ANCA-associated disease appears to be similar in adults and children, but a female predominance may exist in the pediatric patients. Pediatric patients often had end-stage renal disease within 1 year after onset. We conclude that ANCA is a useful diagnostic tool in both pediatric and adult patients with systemic vasculitis and glomerulonephritis. (J PEDIATR 1995;126:40-3)

Anti-neutrophil cytoplasmic autoantibodies are associated with various syndromes of systemic arteritis, glomerulonephritis, and pulmonary vasculitis syndromes in adult patients.[1] Thus the testing for ANCA has become an important tool in such diseases as Wegener granulomatosis, polyarteritis nodosa, and idiopathic crescentic glomerulonephritis. Several types of ANCA autoantibodies have been described: C-ANCA, with cytoplasmic staining of alcohol-fixed neutrophils on indirect immunofluorescence microscopy; P-ANCA, with artifactual perinuclear staining of alcohol-fixed neutrophils; and an atypical pattern.[2] The C- and P-ANCA types can be found in the various associated clinical syndromes, but C-ANCA is more frequently present in patients with renal, lung, and sinus diseases and P-ANCA in patients with renal-limited disease.[1] The atypical pattern has not been associated with a specific disease entity.[2] The renal biopsy lesion most often seen with ANCA-associated disease is pauci-immune crescentic glomerulonephritis.[1]

Submitted for publication May 16, 1994; accepted Aug. 4, 1994.

Reprint requests: Eileen N. Ellis, MD, Pediatric Nephrology, Arkansas Children's Hospital, 800 Marshall, Little Rock, AR 72202.

0022-3476/95/$3.00 + 0 **9/20/59590**

The ANCA-associated diseases have rarely been reported in children and adolescents.[3-5] We report five cases of ANCA-associated disease in pediatric patients and compare the spectrum of ANCA-associated disease in adults with that in children.

CASE REPORTS

The clinical characteristics of our five patients are listed in Table I.

ANA	Antinuclear antibody
ANCA	Anti-neutrophil cytoplasmic autoantibodies
BUN	Blood urea nitrogen
C3	Third component of complement
C4	Fourth component of complement
C-ANCA	ANCA with cytoplasmic staining of neutrophils
CCPD	Continuous-cycling peritoneal dialysis
ELISA	Enzyme-linked immunosorbent assay
IIF	Indirect immunofluorescence [microscopy]
P-ANCA	ANCA with artifactual perinuclear staining of neutrophils

Patient 1. Patient 1, a white boy 4 years 11 months of age, had a history of intermittent abdominal pain, fever, gross hematuria, and proteinuria persisting for several months. At that time he was

Table I. Patient characteristics

Characteristic	Patient No. 1	2	3	4	5
Age at onset (yr)	4	14	13	14	13
Prodrome	Fever Abdominal pain	Fever Cough	Weight loss Malaise Headache	Weight loss Joint pain	Fever Malaise Abdominal pain
Laboratory values at onset					
Hematuria	Many RBC/hpf	Many RBC/hpf	25-35 RBC/hpf	12-15 RBC/hpf	12-15 RBC/hpf
Proteinuria	>1000 mg/dl	300 mg/dl	300 mg/dl	30 mg/dl	100 mg/dl
BUN (mmol/L)	22.5	60.6	50.3	3.6	52.8
Serum creatinine (μmol/L)	159	1644	1220	44	1574
C3, C4	Normal	Normal	Normal	Normal	Normal
ANA	1:80	1:640	Negative	Negative	Negative
Anti-GBM antibodies	Negative results	Negative	Negative	Negative	Negative
ANCA	Not done (see text)	C-ANCA$^+$	P-ANCA$^+$	C-ANCA$^+$	P-ANCA$^+$
Renal biopsy results	Crescentic GN with immune complexes	ESRD only	Crescentic pauci-immune GN	Focal necrotizing GN (Wegener)	Crescentic pauci-immune GN
Other organ involvement					
Lung	Immune-complex vasculitis with hemorrhage	Granulomatous inflammation (Wegener)	None	None	None
Sinus	None	None	None	Necrotizing vasculitis	None
Skin	Raynaud phenomenon	None	Rash	None	None
Joint	None	None	None	Arthalgias	None
Renal outcome	ESRD	ESRD	ESRD	Normal	Normal

RBC/hpf, Red blood cells per high-power field; *GBM*, glomerular basement membrane; *GN*, glomerulonephritis; *ESRD*, end-stage renal disease.

pale and chronically ill in appearance but had normal blood pressure and physical examination findings. The laboratory evaluation showed hematuria; proteinuria; blood urea nitrogen concentration, 22.5 mmol/L (63 mg/dl); serum creatinine concentration, 159 μmol/L (1.8 mg/dl); erythrocyte sedimentation rate, 69 mm/hr; normal values for the third and fourth components of complement; antinuclear antibody titer, 1:80 in a homogeneous pattern; no antistreptolysin O antibodies; no anti-DNA antibodies; no anti-glomerular basement membrane antibodies; and no cryoglobulins. A renal biopsy revealed crescentic glomerulonephritis; 9 of 11 glomeruli had crescents and IgM, IgG, and C3 deposition in a mesangiocapillary pattern. The patient received intravenous methylprednisolone therapy, but 1 month later his blood urea nitrogen and serum creatinine levels had risen to 75.0 mmol/L (210 mg/dl) and 451 μmol/L (5.1 mg/dl), respectively, and continuous cycling peritoneal dialysis was begun.

The patient did well on the CCPD regimen until 2 years later, when he underwent one-antigen-match cadaveric renal transplantation, with immunosuppression consisting of prednisone, azathioprine, and cyclosporine. He had a smooth posttransplantation course for 14 months and then was noted to have hematuria and proteinuria. A renal allograft biopsy specimen showed recurrent crescentic glomerulonephritis with subendothelial, intramembranous, and mesangial deposits by electron microscopy. On review and comparison with the original native kidney biopsy specimen, both showed idiopathic crescentic glomerulonephritis of immune complex origin, the allograft showing a recurrence of the original disease. Laboratory evaluation at this time showed an ANA titer of 1:320, no anti-DNA antibodies, normal C3 and C4 values, no anti-glomerular basement membrane antibodies, no cryoglobulins, the presence of P-ANCA with anti-myeloperoxidase antibodies, and repeated positive results on IIF microscopy to detect P-ANCA, with an enzyme-linked immunosorbent assay value of 77.1 (normal, <40). After the child's parents refused treatment with cyclophosphamide, monthly intravenous infusions of immune globulin were added to the usual immunosuppression. The boy had continued hematuria and proteinuria and worsening renal function; CCPD was restarted.

During CCPD 1 year later, Raynaud phenomena developed. The boy's P-ANCA remained detectable by IIF and ELISA at 6-month intervals. The patient subsequently had malaise, worsening anemia despite erythopoeitin therapy, and weight loss; he refused to attend school. He was hospitalized for evaluation of these problems in February 1994 (sixth year of illness) and was noted to have bilateral interstitial infiltrates on a chest radiograph, maxillary mucosal thickening on sinus x-ray study, and hypoxemia. An open lung biopsy showed alveolar hemorrhage with hemosiderin and hemosiderin-laden macrophages, and results of immunofluorescence for

Table II. Disease characteristics of reported children

	All patients (n = 11)	Patients with C-ANCA (n = 7)	Patients with P-ANCA (n = 4)
Hematuria, proteinuria	11	7	4
Acute renal failure	7	4	3
End-stage renal disease	5	3	2
Upper respiratory tract disease*	2	2	0
Lower respiratory tract disease*	2	1	1
Pulmonary hemorrhage	1	0	1
Arthritis	4	3	1
Rash	3	1	2
Raynaud phenomena	1	0	1

*Represents biopsy-proved upper or lower respiratory tract disease (see Results section).

IgG, IgM, Clq, and fibrin were consistent with immune complex–associated vasculitis. Treatment with prednisone was restarted and resulted in a gradual improvement in the patient's exercise tolerance and resolution of supplemental oxygen requirement after 1 month. The P-ANCA test result remains positive.

Patient 2. Patient 2, a 14-year-old white girl, was referred to our hospital after a 2-week history of sore throat, fever, and cough. On initial evaluation, she had oliguria; microscopic hematuria; proteinuria; BUN concentration, 60.6 mmol/L (168 mg/dl); and serum creatinine concentration, 1644 μmol/L (18.6 mg/dl). Dialysis was begun, and after stabilization the patient underwent a renal biopsy that showed end-stage renal disease of uncertain origin. Further laboratory evaluation showed an ANA titer of 1:640 in a homogeneous pattern; no anti-DNA antibodies; normal C3 and C4 values; normal serum concentrations of IgG, IgM, and IgA; and the presence of C-ANCA by IIF, with an ELISA finding of 77.6.

One month after CCPD was started, the patient was noted on chest x-ray study to have an enlarging cavitary lesion in her right lung base that had not been present previously. She underwent a right lower lobe resection, which showed nodular liquefactive necrosis with a rim of granulomatous inflammation and multinucleated giant cells consistent with Wegener granulomatosis. She received oral prednisone and cyclophosphamide therapy for several months, after which her pulmonary lesion resolved and no other symptoms of vasculitis developed.

One year later, the patient underwent two-antigen-match cadaveric renal transplantation; the kidney continues to function well after 4 years. Her immunosuppression regimen has consisted of prednisone and cyclosporine; oral cyclophosphamide therapy was tried on several occasions after transplantation but was discontinued quickly because of leukopenia. Complications after transplantation have included several steroid-responsive rejection episodes, a perforated gastric ulcer, and gallstones requiring cholecystectomy. The ANCA are measured at 6-month intervals, and the patient intermittently has C-ANCA detected but no symptoms of vasculitis.

METHODS

In all patients except No. 3, ANCA were detected by IIF microscopy and by ELISA in the nephropathology laboratory at the University of North Carolina (J. Charles Jennette, director, Chapel Hill, N.C.); normal values on the ELISA are <40. In patient 3, ANCA determinations were done by flow cytometry and IIF antibody microscopy at Specialty Laboratories Inc. (Santa Monica, Calif.); the normal value for flow cytometry is <22. The pattern of ANCA (C- or P-ANCA) was determined by IIF microscopy.

We retrospectively reviewed the charts of all five patients. We also compared the characteristics of our patients with those of the six previously described pediatric patients with positive ANCA determinations.[3-5]

RESULTS

All pediatric patients in our study had a prodrome lasting several weeks to months, which often consisted of abdominal pain, fever, or weight loss. Of the 11 patients, 9 were female; the age at onset averaged 11.5 ± 2.5 years and was most often the early adolescent years. Although race is not listed in the previously reported cases, all five of our patients were white, a disproportionate number in view of the racial makeup of our population base. Seven of the pediatric patients had C-ANCA detected and four had P-ANCA detected.

All patients had evidence of renal disease; seven had acute renal failure and five eventually had end-stage renal disease (Table II). Upper or lower respiratory tract disease was noted in four patients; granulomatous inflammation was seen on sinus biopsy in two and on lung biopsy in one patient, and immune complex vasculitis with hemorrhage was seen on the lung biopsy in one. Polyarthritis was also an early complaint in four.

DISCUSSION

Our five patients have a spectrum of ANCA-associated disease from renal-limited disease to renal disease with other systemic symptoms or pulmonary vasculitis. In addition, one of our patients had recurrent crescentic glomerulonephritis in a cadaveric renal allograft, which resulted in loss of transplant function; this same patient had onset of pulmonary symptoms with pulmonary vasculitis and hemorrhage 6 years after the onset of renal disease.

Of adult patients in several reported series,[6-8] 113 were male and 100 were female, whereas 9 of 11 pediatric cases were female. The reason for this marked sex difference is unclear, although in one adult series a female predominance was noted in patients with P-ANCA.[8] A seasonal variation with a preponderance of adult patients having onset of symptoms in winter has been reported.[6, 8] Although the season of the year in which symptoms started is not noted in the previously reported pediatric cases, four of our five patients had onset of symptoms in December or January.

Acute renal failure at onset and end-stage renal disease are apparently more common in pediatric patients with ANCA, whereas pulmonary disease is more common in adults. Patient and kidney survival has been about 75% at 2 years in adult patients[6, 7]; most of the deaths have been associated with pulmonary hemorrhage. There has been only one death thus far in the reported pediatric patients, and this death was associated with fungal sepsis during peritoneal dialysis.[3] End-stage renal disease has been present in less than one fourth of adult patients but in half of the pediatric patients. In one of the adult series,[6] the only significant predictor of renal outcome was the elevation of the serum creatinine concentration at onset; the serum creatinine level was inversely correlated with kidney survival time. Four of the five pediatric patients with end-stage renal disease had marked elevations of serum creatinine levels at onset, and only one patient with a similar elevation in the serum creatinine concentration at onset had resolution of her renal failure. Immunosuppressive therapy did not prevent development of end-stage renal disease. Whether the apparently worse outcome in pediatric patients is a result of some confounding factor, such as delay in diagnosis, cannot be determined from this study.

Although only 11 pediatric patients with detectable ANCA have been reported, and thus only limited conclusions can be drawn, it appears that the clinical disease spectrum is similar in pediatric and adult patients but that there is a trend for pediatric patients to be female and to have rapid progression to end-stage renal disease. We conclude that the ANCA test is an important tool in the evaluation of both pediatric and adult patients with various vasculitis and glomerulonephritis syndromes, and should be performed for any patient with rapidly progressive renal failure or with combined renal and upper or lower respiratory tract disease.

REFERENCES

1. Jennette JC, Falk RJ. Anti-neutrophil cytoplasmic autoantibodies and associated diseases: a review. Am J Kidney Dis 1990;15:517-29.
2. Kallenberg CGM, Brouwer E, Weening JJ, Tervaert JWC. Anti-neutrophil cytoplasmic antibodies: current diagnostic and pathophysiological potential. Kidney Int 1994;46:1-15.
3. Walters MDS, Savage COS, Dillon MJ, Lockwood CM. Antineutrophil cytoplasm antibody in crescentic glomerulonephritis. Arch Dis Child 1988;63:814-7.
4. Baldree LA, Gaber LW, McKay CP. Anti-neutrophil cytoplasmic autoantibodies in a child with pauci-immune necrotizing and crescentic glomerulonephritis. Pediatr Nephrol 1991;5:296-9.
5. Nash MC, Jones CL, Walker RG, Powell HR. Anti-neutrophil cytoplasmic antibody–associated glomerulonephritis in children. Pediatr Nephrol 1993;7:11-4.
6. Falk RJ, Hogan S, Carey TS, Jennette JC. Clinical course of anti-neutrophil cytoplasmic autoantibody–associated glomerulonephritis and systemic vasculitis. Ann Intern Med 1990; 113:656-63.
7. Gans ROB, Kuizinga MC, Goldschmeding R, et al. Clinical features and outcome in patients with glomerulonephritis and antineutrophil cytoplasmic autoantibodies. Nephron 1992;64: 182-8.
8. Geffriaud-Ricouard C, Noel LH, Chauveau D, Houhou S, Grunfeld JP, Lesavre P. Clinical spectrum associated with ANCA of defined antigen specificities in 98 selected patients. Clin Nephrol 1993;39:125-36.

Somatosensory evoked potentials for prediction of outcome in acute severe brain injury

J. Beca, MBChB, FRACP, P. N. Cox, MBChB, FFARCS, FRCPC, M. J. Taylor, PhD, D. Bohn, MBBCh, FRCPC, W. Butt, MBBS, FRACP, W. J. Logan, MD, FRCPC, J. T. Rutka, MD, FRCSC, and G. Barker, MBBS, FFARACS

From the Departments of Critical Care, Neurology, and Neurosurgery, Hospital for Sick Children, Toronto, Canada, and the Department of Critical Care, Royal Children's Hospital, Melbourne, Victoria, Australia

The purpose of this study was to evaluate prospectively short-latency somatosensory evoked potentials (SEPs) as a predictor of outcome in acute, severe brain injury, and to compare this with the predictive power of the motor component of the Glasgow Coma Scale score and computed tomographic scan. Outcome was measured with the Glasgow Outcome Scale at a minimum of 6 months after injury. We studied 109 patients (aged 0.1 to 16.8 years) with SEPs within 4 days of the onset of coma. Four patients had absent SEPs and a favorable outcome by the Glasgow Outcome Scale (full recovery or moderate disability); two of these patients had meningitis with bilateral subdural effusions, one had a midbrain hemorrhage, and one had a decompressive craniectomy for uncontrolled intracranial hypertension. Normal SEPs had a positive predictive value for favorable outcome of 93% (95% confidence interval (CI), 77% to 99%), and absent SEPs had a positive predictive value for unfavorable outcome by the Glasgow Outcome Scale (severe disability, survival in a persistent vegetative state, or death) of 92% (95% CI, 80% to 98%). If the above identifiable clinical situations in which a physical barrier existed to impede cutaneous reception of the electrical impulse were excluded, the positive predictive value of absent SEPs for poor outcome reached 100% (95% CI, 92% to 100%). An absent motor response to painful stimulus also had 100% positive predictive value (95% CI, 84% to 100%) for unfavorable outcome; however, 23% of patients could not be evaluated because of the effects of muscle relaxants or sedatives. In patients with traumatic brain injury, results of computed tomography did not reliably predict outcome. Of the 59 patients with unfavorable outcome, 76% could be identified with SEPs compared with 36% with examination of motor function. We suggest that SEPs be performed in children with acute severe brain injury because they add an important tool to the physician's prognostic armamentarium. We conclude that in the absence of the above mentioned identifiable clinical situations, absent SEPs predict 100% unfavorable outcome, and this finding may warrant consideration of withdrawal of treatment in children with brain injuries. (J Pediatr 1995;126:44-9)

Reliable and early prediction of neurologic outcome in patients with acute brain injury remains a challenge for the intensivist; early identification of patients with a poor neurologic prognosis would enable physicians to counsel families to agree to stop futile and costly treatment. Short-latency somatosensory evoked potentials have been shown to

Submitted for publication May 9, 1994; accepted July 28, 1994.

Reprint requests: P. N. Cox, MBChB, FFARCS, FRCPC, Department of Critical Care, Hospital for Sick Children, 555 University Ave., Toronto, Ontario M5G 1X8, Canada.

0022-3476/95/$3.00 + 0 **9/20/59569**

CI	Confidence interval
CT	Computed tomographic
SEPs	Somatosensory evoked potentials

provide accurate prognostic information in both adults and children with an acute brain injury.[1-8] In particular, bilateral absence of SEPs appears to be uniformly associated with a poor outcome. SEPs can be obtained relatively easily; they are noninvasive and require 30 to 40 minutes to perform. Short-latency SEPs reflect the subcortical and primary cortical aspects of the somatosensory pathways. They are not affected by the sedative and analgesic drugs used in intensive care[9-11] and can be used in patients receiving muscle relaxants, in whom clinical assessment is impossible. Studies have been done on auditory and visual evoked potentials as predictors of outcome, but these indicators do not add further prognostic information; both may be unaffected by brain injury so that, although loss of either is associated with poor outcome, neither is reported to be as sensitive as SEPs.[1, 2, 7, 12]

It has been proposed that evoked potentials be used as an adjunct in planning therapy[13]; Judson et al.[5] have incorporated SEPs into the management of head injury in adults. There are only a few studies of SEPs in children with brain injuries,[2, 6, 7, 14] and no studies, of either pediatric or adult patients, provide details of confidence limits. The aims of this study were to evaluate SEPs prospectively as a predictor of neurologic outcome in a large number of children with acute, severe brain injury. Our hypothesis was that no child would have a good recovery if SEPs were absent bilaterally at any time. If this generalization was not true, we wished to determine whether exceptions could be defined—in particular, whether focal intracranial abnormalities could lead to loss of SEPs but the child could still make a good recovery. We also compared the predictive power of SEPs with clinical assessment and, in patients with traumatic brain injury, with computed tomographic scan.

METHODS

Patients. Children eligible for this study were those older than 1 month of age with severe brain injury who were admitted to the intensive care unit at the Hospital for Sick Children (HSC), Toronto, Canada, from July 1990 to February 1992, and at the Royal Children's Hospital (RCH), Melbourne, Australia, from February 1991 to February 1992. Severe brain injury was defined as (1) a Glasgow Coma Scale score <8, (2) the inability to localize painful stimuli if a full Glasgow Coma Scale was not performed (i.e., motor score <4), or (3) a history suggestive of severe brain injury in a patient who could not be examined neurologically. All patients had endotracheal tubes in place and were supported by mechanical ventilation. Intracranial pressure was monitored in children with traumatic brain injury. Patients were excluded if they were known to have neurological deficits before the acute event, or if they subsequently died from nonneurologic causes, or if a diagnosis of brain death was made before SEPs were performed.

We performed SEPs in 120 patients with acute traumatic and nontraumatic brain injury. Of these, 11 were excluded from further analysis either because they died from nonneurologic causes (n = 8) or had neurodevelopmental disabilities before the injury (n = 3). The median age of the remaining 109 patients was 4.8 years (range, 2 months to 16.8 yrs). Infants younger then 1 month of age were not included because of the requirement of some history of normal neurologic development before injury (for our criteria), and we did not wish to include the range of possible perinatal injuries. The application of evoked potentials in both term and preterm infants warrants separate studies. Somatosensory evoked potentials can be reliably recorded in all normal infants if measurements used for older children are modified for those younger than 4 months[15, 16]; if these modifications are not made, this is not the case.[17, 18] In our study there were only two children younger than 4 months of age (both were 2 months of age).

The mechanisms of brain injury were trauma in 53 (48.6%) patients, hypoxic ischemic encephalopathy in 33 (30.3%), and other in 23 (21.1%). The latter group included meningitis (n = 6), hemorrhage (n = 3), tumor (n = 3), cardiopulmonary bypass (n = 3), hemolytic uremic syndrome (n = 2), insulin overdose (n = 1), hepatic encephalopathy (n = 1), and encephalopathy of unknown cause (n = 4). Children with acute brain dysfunction after cardiopulmonary bypass were classified as "other" because of the several possible mechanisms of injury.

The Glasgow Coma Scale score or the motor score alone was recorded at the time of admission. If the patient was unable to be examined clinically because of the effects of muscle relaxants, the most recent assessment before admission was used (for example, by the referring hospital or an ambulance attendant). All patients had CT scans as part of their diagnostic evaluation. The first CT scan after admission was classified according to the Traumatic Coma Data Bank scale for patients with traumatic brain injury.[19]

The outcome was assessed with the Glasgow Outcome Scale[20] at a minimum of 6 months after injury. This scale consists of five categories of patient outcomes: good (normal or mild disability), moderate (disabled but independent), severe (conscious but severely disabled and dependent), persistent vegetative state, and death. For analysis these groups were further simplified into favorable outcome (including good or moderate disability) and unfavorable outcome (including severe disability, vegetative state, or death). Outcome assessment was performed by pediatric neurologists with no knowledge of the results of the SEPs.

Table I. Result and outcome of SEPs

	Outcome	
	Favorable* (No.)	Unfavorable† (No.)
Initial SEPs		
Normal	31	3
Unilateral delay	4	0
Bilateral delay	5	5
Unilateral absent	9	10
Bilateral absent	1	41
Worst SEPs		
Normal	26	2
Unilateral delay	5	0
Bilateral delay	4	4
Unilateral absent	11	8
Bilateral absent	4	45

*Normal or moderate disability.
†Severe disability, vegetative state, or death.

Somatosensory evoked potentials. The SEPs were recorded with a model 2000 measuring unit (Nicolet Instruments, Madison, Wis.) (HSC) or a Medilec Maestro measuring unit (Medilec, Old Woking, Surrey, England) (RCH). The right and left median nerves were stimulated at the wrist, and SEPs were recorded over the cervical spine (C_7) and contralateral somatosensory cortex (C_3' and C_4') with a frontal reference electrode (Fpz). If the wrist was inaccessible, stimulation was performed at the antecubital fossa. If the cervical spine was inaccessible, peripheral SEPs were recorded at the Erb point (over the brachial plexus). At least two averages of 256 artifact-free responses were recorded per arm. The bandpass was 30 to 3000 Hz (HSC) and 20 to 2000 Hz (RCH), the sweep interval was 50 ms, and the stimulation rate was 4.1 Hz. In infants younger than 4 months of age, 64 trials were averaged; the bandpass was 30 to 3000 Hz and 5 to 1500 Hz (HSC), or 20 to 2000 Hz and 3 to 1000 Hz (RCH), with a sweep of 200 ms, and a stimulation rate of 1.1 Hz.[19] The SEPs were classified into five categories: (1) normal, (2) unilateral increased latency, (3) bilateral increased latency, (4) unilateral absence, and (5) bilateral absence. Latency was considered prolonged if it was greater than 2.5 SD above normal for the child's age.[15, 21] The first three categories were further subdivided into normal and low amplitude; category 4 was subdivided according to whether the unilateral response was normal or delayed. If there was uncertainty about classification, SEPs were recorded as the better alternative. When possible, SEPs were recorded within 48 hours of admission, and in all cases they were recorded within 4 days of the onset of coma. They were repeated within the first week in 67 of the 109 patients.

The positive and negative predictive values, and the sensitivity and specificity[22] were calculated for the first SEPs and the worst SEPs recorded for each child. Confidence intervals were derived with the binomial distribution.[23]

RESULTS

For 80% of the patients, initial SEPs were performed within 48 hours, and for 91% within 72 hours; 54% of patients had SEPs repeated one to three times during the first week. The overall outcome was good in 34 (31.2%) of the 109 children, and there was moderate disability in 16 (14.7%), severe disability in 13 (11.9%), persistent vegetative state in 9 (8.3%), and death in 37 (33.9%), yielding an overall favorable outcome of 44.9%. Reduced SEP amplitude did not appear to be predictive of outcome, but numbers within these subgroups were too small for meaningful analysis. Favorable outcome was associated with normal (category 1) SEPs at initial testing in 31 of 34 children (91% positive predictive power) (Table I). If the worst SEP recording was considered, the positive predictive power increased to 93% (95% CI, 77% to 99%). Of 42 children with bilaterally absent SEPs (category 5) at initial SEP testing, 41 had an unfavorable outcome (98% positive predictive power). This included a single child in whom SEPs were bilaterally absent for anatomic reasons (subdural effusions). In 49 children, SEPs were absent in the worst recording. Of these, 45 had an unfavorable outcome (92% positive predictive power; 95% CI, 80% to 98%); 4 of these 45 children had an evoked response (categories 1 to 4) present on the initial recording that became absent on later testing. The sensitivity, specificity, and predictive value of later versus initial SEPs were compared; minimal differences were found (Table II). An additional four patients had bilaterally absent SEPs (category 5) at either initial or after additional testing and a favorable outcome (normal or moderate disability) (Table I). Two of these four children had meningitis with subdural effusions; one had a favorable outcome and one had moderate disability at follow-up. Of the remaining two children, one had traumatic brain injury with hemorrhage in the tegmentum of the mesencephalon and the right cerebral peduncle and contusion to the posterior limb of the left internal capsule; she had a favorable outcome with moderate disability. The fourth patient also had traumatic brain injury and grade 1 SEPs on the first recording; the SEPs became absent after decompressive craniectomy for uncontrolled intracranial hypertension, and then returned by day 7; she also had moderate disability. Each of these four children had identifiable clinical features known to interfere technically with the recording of SEPs. If these four patients are excluded, the positive predictive value for absent SEPs is 100% (95% CI, 92% to 100%). Of the 45 children with bilaterally absent SEPs (category 5) on either initial or subsequent testing and poor outcome, 27% were alive at 6 months, but were either

Table II. Predictive value, sensitivity, and specificity for SEPs and motor score

	Positive predictive value	Negative predictive value	Sensitivity	Specificity
Worst SEPs				
Absent (category 5)/unfavorable	45/49 (92)	46/60 (77)	45/59 (76)	46/50 (92)
Normal (category 1)/favorable	26/28 (93)	57/81 (70)	26/50 (52)	57/59 (97)
Initial SEPs				
Absent (category 5)/unfavorable	41/42 (98)	49/67 (73)	41/59 (69)	49/50 (98)
Normal (category 1)/favorable	31/34 (91)	56/75 (75)	31/50 (62)	56/59 (95)
Motor score				
Flaccid/unfavorable	21/21 (100)	38/63 (60)	21/46 (46)	38/38 (100)

Data are presented as number with test result/number with outcome. Numbers in parentheses indicate percentages.

severely disabled or in a persistent vegetative state. Of the 32 patients with abnormal but present SEPs (categories 2 to 4), 20 (63%) had favorable outcomes.

All the patients with no response to pain had an unfavorable outcome (Table III). Of the 32 patients with flexor or extensor posturing responses, 14 (44%) had a favorable outcome, and 24 (77%) of 31 with withdrawal or a localizing response had a favorable outcome. The motor score could not be recorded in 25 (22.9%) of the patients, usually because muscle relaxants or large doses of sedative drugs were used, but some motor assessments were either incorrectly performed or not recorded by the admitting physicians. An absent motor response to painful stimulus had a positive predictive power of 100% (95% CI, 84% to 100%) for unfavorable outcome. However, sensitivity was 46% in those who could be clinically assessed and only 36% in all patients, compared with sensitivity of 69% for initial SEPs.

No specific CT scan appearance in patients with traumatic brain injury was invariably associated with either a good or bad outcome (Table IV); 38 (72%) of the 53 patients had diffuse injury II or III (Traumatic Coma Data Bank scale), and in these groups CT scan had poor predictive power. Numbers in other categories were very small.

DISCUSSION

This study shows that bilaterally absent SEPs accurately predict unfavorable outcome in the setting of both traumatic and nontraumatic coma. In any test of neurologic function that attempts to predict neurologic outcome, the positive predictive power and the specificity are of much greater importance than the sensitivity. It would be highly undesirable for treatment to be withdrawn because a test incorrectly predicted a poor outcome, but less unacceptable if treatment were continued because a test incorrectly predicted a good outcome. Knowledge of the CIs is essential, to proper test use, but in published studies on SEPs these have not been provided. For a test to be clinically useful, it is necessary to know the outcome for a large number of patients with the poor prognostic sign.[24, 25] The clinician needs

Table III. Motor score related to outcome: Number of children (percent)

	Outcome			
	Favorable		Unfavorable	
	No.	%	No.	%
Motor score				
Localizes	6	75	2	25
Withdrawal	18	78	5	22
Flexor	7	41	10	59
Extensor	7	47	8	53
Flaccid	0	0	21	100
Inaccessible	12	48	13	52

Table IV. Computed tomographic scan related to outcome of traumatic brain injury

	Outcome			
	Favorable		Unfavorable	
	No.	%	No.	%
Diffuse injury				
I (normal)	1	50	1	50
II (minor abnormality)	9	60	6	40
III (edema)	12	52	11	48
IV (shift)	1	25	3	75
Evacuated mass	5	83	1	17
Nonevacuated mass	1	33	2	67

to know what proportion of children with absent SEPs will have a poor outcome.

In this study initial SEPs were only slightly different than additional SEPs performed later. Although many children had SEPs that showed some improvement or deterioration in latency and amplitude, only a few children had additional SEPs that crossed the present/absent boundaries. A larger series is needed to determine the significance of the changes, such as from abnormal to normal latencies. Normal SEPs, regardless of when recorded, predicted good outcome in 91% to 93% of children; abnormal but present responses predicted good outcome in 63%. Absent SEPs predicted unfavorable outcome in 92% of children. Absent SEPs on later studies in patients with no identifiable anatomic cause for their absence always predicted poor outcome (95% CI, 92% to 100%). If the lower limit of the 95% CI is used, this study shows that up to 8% of children with absent SEPs could still have a favorable outcome. However, given the very high predictive power shown in many adult and a few pediatric studies,[13] the risk must be much lower than this. With Bayesian methods, the actual risk is likely to be 2% for this sample size.[25] Huge numbers would be required to reduce the lower limit of the 95% CI to less than 1%, and ultimately the decision about how to use this information will depend on the individual doctor, hospital, and country.

Although we have shown that absent SEPs have high sensitivity and specificity, in certain instances they cannot be relied on to predict outcome accurately; these include extraaxial collections, brain stem hemorrhage, and after cranial decompression. Extraaxial collections, such as subdural effusions in meningitis, increase the physical distance between the brain and recording electrodes, which can be sufficient to prevent the recording of responses. However, because CT scanning is part of the management of such conditions, the presence of these collections will be known at the time. Likewise, CT scanning will reveal brain stem hemorrhage, which can interfere with conduction in the subcortical somatosensory pathways. Deep cerebral hemorrhages in traumatic brain injury, especially if in the brain stem, are in themselves associated with poor outcome. Midbrain hemorrhage in adults has been shown to lead to loss of SEPs and has been uniformly associated with poor outcome.[26, 27] However, because the child with brain stem hemorrhage in this study survived with moderate disability, we suggest that absent SEPs should not be used to predict outcome in cases with brain stem hemorrhage. The final exception, of cranial decompression for intracranial hypertension, has been previously reported in children with Reye syndrome.[2] Taylor and Farrell[7] also identified a child with brain injury as a result of a lightning strike who had transient loss of SEPs and good outcome. Both these clinical situations are encountered so rarely that it will be difficult to get further information, but in the former, SEPs recorded before decompression accurately predicted the outcome. If these conditions are considered, we have shown that absent SEPs are relatively specific in predicting poor outcome.

It is essential that technically satisfactory SEPs be obtained, and recordings in which the components are obscured by artifact should not be used clinically. We have found that electrical interference is rarely a problem, even in an intensive care setting. The most common source of artifact is from muscle activity in nonparalyzed patients. Clear cervical or brachial plexus potentials, demonstrating the integrity of the peripheral nervous system, must be obtained before absent cortical potentials are regarded as significant.

Absence of motor response to painful stimuli was as specific as bilaterally absent SEPs for predicting unfavorable outcome but considerably less sensitive. In evaluating clinical assessment in this study, motor response was used for two reasons. First, it is likely that most, if not all, the predictive power of the Glasgow Coma Scale is derived from the motor score.[28] Moreover, patients with nontraumatic coma commonly had only the motor score rather than the full Glasgow Coma Scale score recorded. Muscle relaxants and sedative and analgesic agents are frequently used in neurointensive care; thus it is often difficult to obtain additional clinical assessments of patients with acute brain injury, but SEPs can be used in these patients. No CT scan appearance had absolute specificity, although assessment was limited by the small number of patients in the several subgroups.

The distinction between moderate and severe disability at clinical follow-up is difficult in children, and becomes more difficult with younger age; this distinction is critical because we used it to separate favorable from unfavorable outcome in this study. However, all our patients with severe disabilities had profound developmental delay (functioning at less than half the appropriate level for age) and severe motor disabilities (preventing independent mobility).

We suggest that SEPs be performed in all children with acute, severe brain injury, because they are the best predictor of outcome in this group. The SEPs should be performed within 24 to 48 hours of admission and be repeated within 24 to 48 hours to increase positive predictive power. If a CT scan excludes the presence of extraaxial fluid collections or brain stem hemorrhage, the presence of normal SEPs suggests a 93% chance of a favorable outcome, whereas the absence of SEPs predicts a 92% chance of an unfavorable outcome. In patients who had no physical barrier impeding the recording of the cortical response, absent SEPs predicted a 100% chance of unfavorable outcome. If SEPs are absent and clinical assessment is compatible with an unfavorable outcome, we believe that consideration should be given to withdrawal of treatment.

We thank L. J. MacMillan, N. K. Keenan, and B. G. Carter for their excellent technical support.

REFERENCES

1. De Meirleir DJ, Taylor MJ. Evoked potentials in comatose children: auditory brainstem responses. Pediatr Neurol 1986; 2:31-4.
2. De Meirleir LJ, Taylor MJ. Prognostic utility of SEPs in comatose children. Pediatr Neurol 1987;3:78-82.
3. Greenberg RP, Newlon PG, Becker DP. The somatosensory

evoked potential in patients with severe head injury: outcome prediction and monitoring of brain function. Ann N Y Acad Sci 1982;388:683-8.
4. Hume AL, Cant BR. Central somatosensory conduction after head injury. Ann Neurol 1981;10:411-9.
5. Judson JA, Cant BR, Shaw NA. Early prediction of outcome from cerebral trauma by somatosensory evoked potentials. Crit Care Med 1990;18:363-8.
6. Lutschg J, Pfenninger J, Ludin HP, Vassella F. Brain-stem auditory evoked potentials and early somatosensory evoked potentials in neurointensively treated comatose children. Am J Dis Child 1983;137:421-6.
7. Taylor MJ, Farrell EJ. Comparison of the prognostic utility of VEPs and SEPs in comatose children. Pediatr Neurol 1989; 5:145-50.
8. Taylor MJ, Murphy WJ, Whyte HE. Prognostic reliability of somatosensory and visual evoked potentials of asphyxiated term infants. Dev Med Child Neurol 1992;34:507-15.
9. Ganes T, Lundar T. The effect of thiopentone on somatosensory evoked responses and EEGs in comatose patients. J Neurol Neurosurg Psychiatry 1983;46:509-14.
10. Newlon PG, Greenberg RP, Hyatt MS, Enas GG, Becker DP. The dynamics of neuronal dysfunction and recovery following severe head injury assessed with serial multimodality evoked potentials. J Neurosurg 1982;57:168-77.
11. Sutton LN, Frewen T, Marsh R, Jaggi J, Bruce DA. The effects of deep barbiturate coma on multimodality evoked potentials. J Neurosurg 1982;57:178-85.
12. Cant BR, Hume AL, Judson JA, Shaw NA. The assessment of severe head injury by short-latency somatosensory and brain-stem auditory evoked potentials. Electroencephalogr Clin Neurophysiol 1986;65:188-95.
13. Goodwin SR, Friedman WA, Bellefleur M. Is it time to use evoked potentials to predict outcome in comatose children and adults? Crit Care Med 1991;19:518-24.
14. Frank LM, Furgiuele TL, Etheridge JE Jr. Prediction of chronic vegetative state in children using evoked potentials. Neurology 1985;35:931-4.
15. George SR, Taylor MJ. Somatosensory evoked potentials in neonates and infants: developmental and normative data. Electroencephalogr Clin Neurophysiol 1991;80:94-102.
16. Bongers-Schokking CJ, Colon EJ, Hoogland RA, Van den Brande JL, De Groot CJ. The somatosensory evoked potentials of normal infants: influence of filter bandpass, arousal state and number of stimuli. Brain Dev 1989;11:33-9.
17. Willis J, Seales D, Frazier B. Short latency somatosensory evoked potentials in infants. Electroencephalogr Clin Neurophysiol 1984;59:366-73.
18. Laureau E, Majnemer A, Rosenblatt B, Riley P. A longitudinal study of short latency somatosensory evoked responses in healthy newborns and infants. Electroencephalogr Clin Neurophysiol 1988;71:100-8.
19. Marshall LF, Marshall SB, Klauber MR, et al. A new classification of head injury based on computerised tomography. J Neurosurg 1991;75:S14-20.
20. Jennett B, Bond M. Assessment of outcome after severe brain damage. Lancet 1975;1:480-4.
21. Taylor MJ, Fagan ER. SEPs to median nerve stimulation: normative data for paediatrics. Electroencephalogr Clin Neurophysiol 1988;71:323-30.
22. Altman DG. Practical statistics for medical research. 1st ed. London: Chapman and Hall, 1990:409-16.
23. Lentner C. Geigy scientific tables. basel: Ciba Geigy, 1982:89-102.
24. Bates D. Defining prognosis in medical coma. J Neurol Neurosurg Psychiatry 1991;54:569-71.
25. Shewmon DA, De Giorgio CM. Early prognosis in anoxic coma: reliability and rationale. Neurol Clin 1989;7:823-43.
26. Rosenblum WI, Greenberg RP, Seelig JM, Becker DP. Midbrain lesions: frequent and significant prognostic feature in closed heart injurt. Neurosurgery 1981;9:613-20.
27. Marshall LF, Gautille T, Klauber MR, et al. The outcome of severe closed head injury. J Neurosurg 1991;75:S28-36.
28. Jagger J, Jane JA, Rimel R. The Glasgow Coma Scale: To sum or not to sum? Lancet 1983;2:97.

Catheter-related thrombosis in critically ill children: Comparison of catheters with and without heparin bonding

Brian Krafte-Jacobs, MD, Carlos J. Sivit, MD, Rodrigo Mejia, MD, and Murray M. Pollack, MD, FCCM

From the Departments of Critical Care and Diagnostic Imaging, Children's National Medical Center, Washington, D.C., and the Departments of Anesthesiology and Pediatrics, George Washington University School of Medicine, Washington, D.C.

Objective: To compare the incidence of and factors associated with vascular thrombosis after placement of heparin-bonded and standard femoral venous catheters.
Design: Prospective, masked, clinical study.
Setting: Multidisciplinary, tertiary, pediatric intensive care unit.
Patients: Consecutive cases (n = 50) of critically ill children admitted to a pediatric intensive care unit in whom either a heparin-bonded (n = 25) or a standard (n = 25) femoral venous catheter was placed.
Measurements and main results: Patients were examined by ultrasonography within 3 days of catheter insertion, weekly while the catheter was in place, and after catheter removal for evidence of vascular thrombosis. Data were collected prospectively regarding clinical evidence of catheter thrombosis, infusate composition, and positive blood culture results. Of 50 patients, 13 (26%) had thrombotic complications, 11 (44%) of the 25 patients in the standard-catheter group, in comparison with 2 (8%) of the 25 patients in the heparin-bonded catheter group ($p = 0.004$). In addition, there was a significantly higher incidence of positive blood culture results among patients in the standard-catheter group (24% vs 0%; $p = 0.009$). Positive catheter blood culture results were obtained in 38% of patients with thrombosis versus 3% without thrombosis ($p = 0.001$). Clinical evidence of thrombosis was found in 69% of patients with, versus 27% of patients without, ultrasound-proved thrombosis ($p = 0.007$).
Conclusion: Heparin bonding of catheters is associated with significantly fewer thrombotic complications. A reduced incidence of positive catheter-related blood culture results may be associated with the absence of thrombosis. (J PEDIATR 1995;126:50-4)

Vascular thrombosis is a major complication associated with the use of deep venous catheters. Factors associated with the initiation and propagation of thrombosis include endothelial damage during catheter placement, blood vessel occlusion and low flow states, turbulent flow, patient and infusate characteristics, and catheter composition.[1-4] Successful inhibition of thrombosis would be a substantial clinical advantage. Although heparin-bonded catheters have been available for many years, there is limited clinical information regarding the effect of heparin bonding on vascular thrombosis. Short-term placement of standard pulmonary artery catheters in adult patients results in the formation of surface thrombi, a complication that is eliminated by the use of heparin-bonded catheters.[5] In addition, both catheter material and specific catheter coatings (such as

Supported in part by a research grant from Cook Incorporated.

Presented at the Society of Critical Care Medicine 1994 Educational and Scientific Symposium.

Submitted for publication May 3, 1994; accepted Aug. 16, 1994.

Reprint requests: Brian Krafte-Jacobs, MD, Division of Critical Care Medicine, Children's Hospital Medical Center, 3333 Burnet Ave., Cincinnati, OH 45229.

0022-3476/95/$3.00 + 0 **9/20/59943**

heparin) are important in the prevention of initiation and propagation of vascular thrombosis.[6, 7] Because the femoral and iliac veins and the inferior vena cava are much smaller in children than in adults, thrombosis may be more likely in children.

There have been no prospective studies addressing either the incidence and factors associated with thrombus formation, or the protective effect of heparin bonding on thrombosis after venous catheter placement in infants and children. The purpose of this study was to investigate by ultrasonography the incidence of and factors associated with vascular thrombosis after placement of heparin-bonded and standard femoral venous catheters in critically ill infants and children. We hypothesized that the use of heparin-bonded catheters would be associated with a lower incidence of thrombosis.

METHODS

Patients. The study took place prospectively between March and December 1993 in our 16-bed, multidisciplinary unit with more than 1000 admissions each year. Deep venous catheters are used in approximately 20% of the patients admitted to this unit. All patients between birth and the age of 8 years who had 8 to 15 cm femoral venous catheters placed were eligible for entry into the study. Patients were excluded from the study if there was a history of vascular thrombosis, previous femoral venous catheterization, or thrombolytic therapy, or if they had an ongoing coagulopathy (prothrombin or partial thromboplastin times >95th percentile for age, thrombocytopenia $<150 \times 10^9$/L [150,000/mm^3], or thrombocytosis $>1000 \times 10^9$/L [1,000,000/mm^3]). The study was approved by the Children's Hospital Institutional Review Board, and consent was obtained from the patient's parent(s) or guardian(s).

Femoral venous catheters. The catheters used in this study were size 3F, 4F, and 5F in diameter, 8 to 15 cm in length, and of polyurethane or polyethylene composition (Cook Inc., Bloomington, Ind.). The study was limited to patients with 8 to 15 cm catheters to permit ultrasonographic visualization of the inferior vena cava while minimizing catheter distortion of the image. Patients were sequentially enrolled during periods when only standard catheters were available, when both standard and heparin-bonded catheters were available, and when only heparin-bonded catheters were available. These changes corresponded to a change in practice in the intensive care unit.

Data. Data consisting of patient demographics, diagnoses, history, and physical and laboratory examination findings (platelets, prothrombin and partial thromboplastin times), catheter characteristics, date of placement, number of placement attempts, placement by cutdown, and composition of the infusate (parenteral nutrition, lipid, and heparin) were recorded on entry to and throughout the study as indicated. Clinical evidence of venous thrombosis, including leg swelling, leg discoloration, loss of pulses, changes in perfusion, and inability to flush or draw back from the catheter, were recorded daily. Blood culture specimens were obtained from the catheter with aseptic technique when clinically indicated (fever or hemodynamic instability). Positive blood culture results were noted on the data collection sheet.

Ultrasonography. All studies were performed with a 3.5, 5.0, or 7.5 MHz transducer (Acuson, Inc., Mountain View, Calif.). Scanning was begun at the level of the groin and extended as far cephalad and caudad as possible. Color Doppler flow imaging was used in all cases. Venous thrombosis was diagnosed if there was an absence of a Doppler signal or gray-scale visualization of a thrombus. All ultrasonographic studies were analyzed by one of us (C.J.S.), who was masked to the catheter composition. Examinations were performed within 3 days of catheter insertion and then weekly until the catheter was removed. After catheter removal, ultrasonographic evaluation was performed before hospital discharge.

Statistical analysis. Fifty patients were enrolled on the basis of an estimated 25% difference in the incidence of thrombosis in standard and heparin-bonded catheters, a chance of 0.8 of detecting such a difference, and a significance level of 0.05. Demographic data were analyzed by descriptive statistics. The differences between the heparin-bonded and standard-catheter groups, as well as between the thrombosis and no-thrombosis groups, were analyzed by chi-square tests for categorical data, and by the Mann-Whitney U test for continuous variables.

Table. Patient characteristics with heparin-bonded and standard catheters

	Heparin-bonded catheters (n = 25)	Standard catheters (n = 25)	p
Age (mo)*	6 (0.5-88)	7 (0.75-84)	0.45
Attempts (No.)*	1 (1-5)	2 (1-10)	0.25
Duration (days)*	5 (2-29)	5 (1-40)	0.21
Heparin	6 (24%)	4 (16%)	0.48
Cutdown	1 (4%)	2 (8%)	0.53
TPN/lipid	6 (24%)	5 (20%)	0.73
Clinical evidence†	8 (32%)	11 (44%)	0.38
Positive culture result	0 (0%)	6 (24%)	0.009
Thrombosis	2 (8%)	11 (44%)	0.004

TPN, Total parenteral nutrition.
*Median (range). Statistical analysis by Mann-Whitney U test or chi-square.
†Clinical evidence of thrombosis, including leg swelling, leg discoloration, loss of pulses, changes in perfusion, and inability to flush or draw back from the catheter.

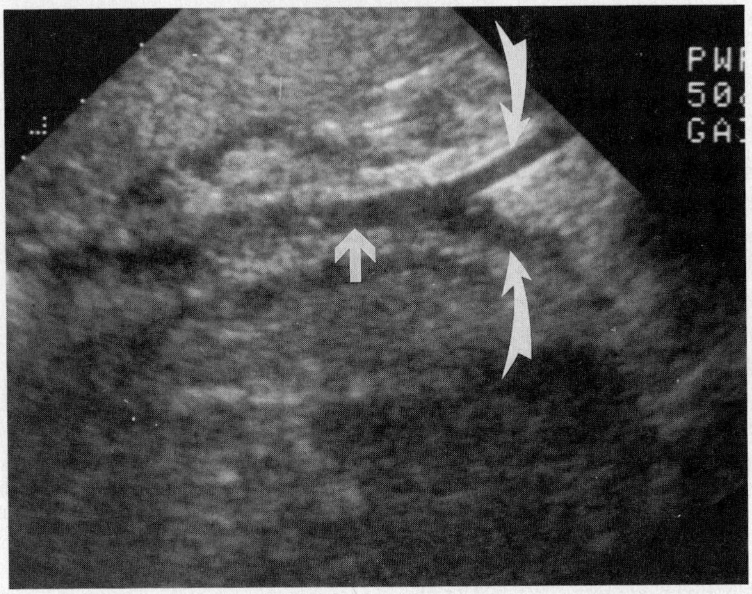

Fig. 1. Normal iliac bifurcation. Coronal sonogram at the level of the iliac bifurcation demonstrates a normal inferior vena cava *(straight arrow)* and iliac veins *(curved arrows)*.

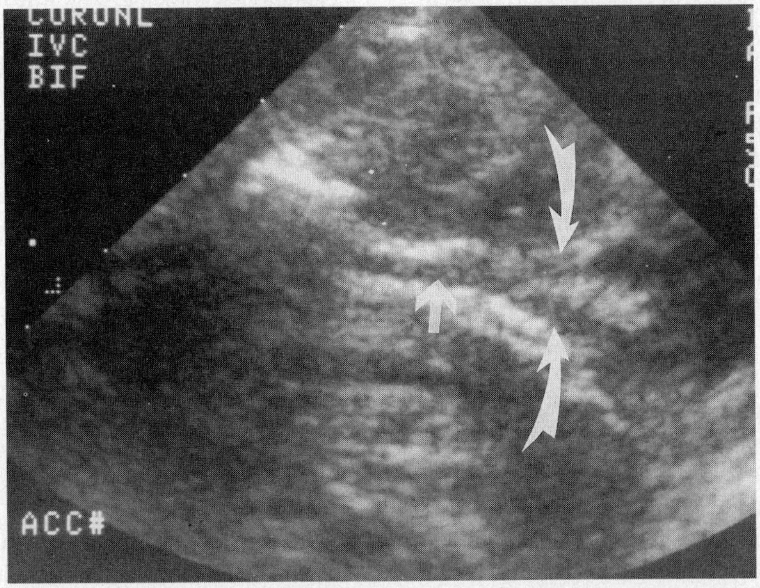

Fig. 2. Thrombosis at iliac bifurcation. Coronal sonogram at the level of the iliac bifurcation demonstrates intraluminal low-level echoes in the lower inferior vena cava *(straight arrow)* and iliac veins *(curved arrows)*.

RESULTS

Fifty patients were enrolled at a median age of 6.5 months (range, 0.5 to 88 months); 25 were enrolled in the heparin-bonded and 25 in the standard-catheter groups (Table). Patient, infusate, and catheter data did not differ with the exception that one group had heparin-bonded catheters placed and the other group had standard catheters placed. Vascular thrombosis developed in 13 (26%) of 50 patients overall, 11 (44%) of 25 patients in the standard-catheter group and 2 (8%) of 25 patients in the group using heparin-bonded catheters ($p = 0.004$). In addition, there was a significantly higher incidence of positive blood culture results among the patients in the standard-catheter group (6/25, 24%) than among the patients in the group using heparin-bonded catheters (0/25; $p = 0.009$). Positive blood culture results were also significantly more frequent among children with thrombosis (5/13, 38%) than among those without thrombosis (1/37, 3%; $p = 0.001$).

Clinical evidence of thrombosis was noted significantly more frequently in patients with ultrasound-proved thrombosis (9/13, 69%) than in those without ultrasound-proved thrombosis (10/37, 27%; $p = 0.007$). There was no clinical evidence of pulmonary embolism or any other serious thrombosis-related complication in any patient in the study.

The most common locations for thrombus formation were the iliac vein in 11 (85%) of 13 patients, the femoral vein in 5 (38%) of 13 patients, and the inferior vena cava in 3 (23%) of 13 patients. Typical ultrasound findings in normal and thrombosed vessels are shown in Figs. 1 and 2.

DISCUSSION

Heparin prevents thrombosis and thrombus extension[8-10] and is therefore a logical coating in attempts to decrease catheter-related thrombosis. Heparin-bonded catheters have been associated with diminished adherent thrombi and fibrin sheath formation around the catheter in adults[5, 11] and with decreased vascular thrombosis in an animal model.[12] The effect of heparin-bonded catheters on the formation of mural thrombosis has not been studied in human subjects.

Our patients with heparin-bonded catheters had a significantly lower incidence of vascular thrombosis, compared with those with standard catheters. Heparin-bonded catheters were also associated with a significantly lower incidence of positive catheter blood culture results, presumably related to the lower incidence of thrombosis. The association of vascular thrombosis and infection has been noted previously in catheter-related thrombosis.[13-15] By decreasing the incidence of thrombosis, heparin-bonded catheters may indirectly reduce the incidence of infection.

We did not observe any complications from the heparin-bonded catheters, but their use has been linked with heparin-associated thrombocytopenia.[16] Therefore patients with heparin-associated antiplatelet antibodies should not undergo placement of heparin-bonded catheters. Patients in whom thrombocytopenia develops should be examined for heparin-associated anti-platelet antibodies and have heparin-bonded catheters removed or replaced with standard catheters if these antibodies are present.

The overall incidence of catheter-related thrombosis in the standard-catheter group was consistent with reported catheter-related thrombosis in prospective studies using venography or ultrasonography in adults or on autopsy.[8, 13, 17-23] Almost one third of children with ultrasound-proved thrombosis had no clinical evidence of vessel obstruction, findings similar to those of previous studies of adults.[19, 20, 22, 24, 25] The lack of clinical evidence of thrombosis is likely related to residual flow within the partially occluded vessel or to the development of collateral flow, or both. These findings were noted on sonograms of several study patients with thrombosis.

Duration of catheter placement and the use of total parenteral nutrition and lipid have been noted by previous investigators to be associated with an increased incidence of thrombosis.[2, 3, 8, 23] In our study there was an equivalent duration of catheter placement as well as a similar percentage of patients receiving total parenteral nutrition and lipid in the heparin and standard groups. Moreover, neither the duration of catheter placement nor the use of total parenteral nutrition or lipid was associated with an increased incidence of thrombosis in the standard catheter group.

We conclude that the use of heparin-bonded femoral venous catheters is associated with significantly lower thrombotic and infectious complications. Furthermore, the absence of clinical evidence of thrombosis does not rule out the presence of a thrombotic process.

We thank Linda Rebolo, RDMS, and Cathy Brown-Jones, RDMS, for assistance with the study.

REFERENCES

1. McDonough JJ, Altemeier WA. Subclavian venous thrombosis secondary to indwelling catheters. Surg Gynecol Obstet 1971;133:397-400.
2. Wakefield A, Cohen Z, Craig M, et al. Thrombogenicity of total parenteral nutrition solutions. I. Effect on induction of monocyte/macrophage procoagulant activity. Gastroenterology 1989;97:1210-9.
3. Montemurro P, Lattanzio A, Chetta G, et al. Increased in vitro and in vivo generation of procoagulant activity (tissue factor) by mononuclear phagocytes after Intralipid infusion in rabbits. Blood 1985;65:1391-5.
4. Pottecher T, Forrler M, Picardat D, Krause JP, Bellocq JP, Otteni JC. Thrombogenicity of central venous catheters: prospective study of polyethylene, silicone, and polyurethane catheters with phlebography or postmortem examination. Eur J Anaesthesiol 1984;1:361-5.
5. Hoar PF, Wilson RM, Mangano DT, Avery GJ, Szarnicki RJ, Hill D. Heparin bonding reduces thrombogenicity of pulmonary-artery catheters. N Engl J Med 1981;305:993-5.
6. Welch GW, McKeel DW, Silverstein P, Walker HL. The role of catheter composition in the development of thrombophlebitis. Surg Gynecol Obstet 1974;138:421-4.
7. Borow B, Crowley JG. Evaluation of central venous catheter thrombogenicity. Acta Anaesthesiol Scand 1985;81:59-64.
8. Brismar B, Hardstedt C, Jacobson S, Kager L, Malmborg AS. Reduction of catheter-associated thrombosis in parenteral nutrition by intravenous heparin therapy. Arch Surg 1982; 117:1196-9.
9. Pini M, Pattacini C, Quintavalla R, et al. Subcutaneous vs intravenous heparin in the treatment of deep venous thrombosis: a randomized clinical trial. Thromb Haemost 1990;64:222-6.
10. Fabri PJ, Mirtallo JM, Ruberg RL, et al. Incidence and pre-

vention of thrombosis of the subclavian vein during total parenteral nutrition. Surg Gynecol Obstet 1982;155:238-40.
11. Peters WR, Bush WH, McIntyre RD, Hill LD. The development of fibrin sheath on indwelling venous catheters. Surg Gynecol Obstet 1973;137:43-7.
12. DiConstanzo J, Sastre B, Choux R, et al. Experimental approach to prevention of catheter-related central venous thrombosis. JPEN J Parenter Enteral Nutr 1984;8:293-7.
13. Warden GD, Wilmore DW, Pruitt BA. Central venous thrombosis: a hazard of medical progress. J Trauma 1973;13:620-5.
14. Rupar DG, Herzog KD, Fisher MC, Long SS. Prolonged bacteremia with catheter-related central venous catheters. Am J Dis Child 1990;144:879-82.
15. Raad II, Luna M, Khalil SM, Costerton JW, Lam C, Bodey GP. The relationship between the thrombotic and infectious complications of central venous catheters. JAMA 1994; 271:1014-6.
16. Laster JL, Nichols WK, Silver D. Thrombocytopenia associated with heparin-coated catheters in patients with heparin-associated antiplatelet antibodies. Arch Intern Med 1989; 149:2285-7.
17. Ahmed N, Payne RF. Thrombosis after central venous cannulation. Med J Aust 1976;1:217-20.
18. Moncrief JA. Femoral catheters. Ann Surg 1958;147:166-72.
19. Valerio D, Hussey JK, Smith FW. Central vein thrombosis associated with intravenous feeding: a prospective study. JPEN J Parenter Enteral Nutr 1981;5:240-2.
20. Bozzeti F, Scarpa D, Terno G, et al. Subclavian vein thrombosis due to indwelling catheters: a prospective study on 52 patients. JPEN J Parenter Enteral Nutr 1983;7:560-2.
21. Karnik R, Valentin A, Winkler WB, Donath P, Slany J. Duplex sonographic detection of internal jugular venous thrombosis after removal of central venous catheters. Clin Cardiol 1993;16:26-9.
22. Wanscher M, Frifelt JJ, Smith-Sivertsen C, et al. Thrombosis caused by polyurethane double-lumen subclavian superior vena cava catheter and hemodialysis. Crit Care Med 1988; 16:624-8.
23. Chastre J, Cornud F, Bouchama A, Viau F, Benacerraf R, Gilbert C. Thrombosis as a complication of pulmonary-artery catheterization via the internal jugular vein. N Engl J Med 1982;306:278-81.
24. Moore RA, McNicholas KW, Naidech H, Flicker S, Gallagher JD. Clinically silent venous thrombosis following internal and external jugular central venous cannulation in pediatric cardiac patients. Anesthesiology 1985;62:640-3.
25. Berman W, Fripp RR, Yabek SM, Wernly J, Corlew S. Great vein and right atrial thrombosis in critically ill infants and children with central venous lines. Chest 1991;99:963-7.

CLINICAL AND LABORATORY OBSERVATIONS

Fisher syndrome after *Campylobacter jejuni* enteritis: Human leukocyte antigen and the bacterial serotype

Nobuhiro Yuki, MD, PhD, Hiroo Ichikawa, MD, and Ayumi Doi, MD

From the Department of Biochemistry, Faculty of Medicine, Tokyo Medical and Dental University, Tokyo, the Department of Neurology, Faculty of Medicine, Showa University, Tokyo, and the Department of Pediatrics, National Fukuyama Hospital, Fukuyama City, Hiroshima, Japan

We describe two children who had Fisher syndrome subsequent to *Campylobacter jejuni* enteritis. The *C. jejuni* isolates from both patients, who lived in different areas, belonged to PEN 2: LIO 4. One patient had the following human leukocyte antigens (HLAs): HLA-A24, 33; B44, 52; DQ1; and DR2, 6 antigens. Another had the HLA-A24, 33; B44, 54; Cw1; DQ1, 4; and DR4, 6. An effort should be made to isolate *C. jejuni* from patients with Fisher syndrome and to perform HLA typing so that the pathogenesis of this syndrome can be clarified. (J PEDIATR 1995;126:55-7)

Fisher syndrome is defined as a monophasic illness of acute onset, characterized by external ophthalmoplegia, cerebellar ataxia, and the absence of tendon reflexes. It is generally considered a variant form of Guillain-Barré syndrome, which is characterized by the acute onset of symmetric limb weakness and areflexia. Serologic studies suggest the possibility that *Campylobacter jejuni*, a gram-negative bacterium that frequently causes acute enteritis, is the most common infection preceding GB syndrome.[1] In contrast, there are only a few reports of FS subsequent to *C. jejuni* enteritis,[2-5] and no children were included. We earlier found a significant association between HLA-B35 antigen and GB syndrome occurring after *C. jejuni* infection,[6] but HLA antigens of patients with FS were not studied. The specific serotype PEN 19, of *C. jejuni*, is frequently isolated from patients with GB syndrome,[7, 8] whereas no isolates from patients with FS subsequent to *C. jejuni* enteritis have been serotyped. We describe two children who had FS after *C. jejuni* infection, the patients' HLA typing, and the bacterial serotype.

Supported in part by Uehara Memorial Foundation.

Submitted for publication May 9, 1994; accepted July 28, 1994.

Reprint requests: Nobuhiro Yuki, MD, PhD, Department of Biochemistry, Faculty of Medicine, Tokyo Medical and Dental University, 1-5-45 Yushima, Bunkyo-ku, Tokyo 113, Japan.

0022-3476/95/$3.00 + 0 **9/22/59570**

METHODS

Serotyping of *C. jejuni* was performed by the method of Penner and Hennessy,[9] which is based on heat-stable antigens. The isolates also were serotyped by the method of Lior et al.,[10] which is based on heat-labile antigens.

CASE REPORTS

Patient 1. A 13-year-old boy with bronchial asthma had watery diarrhea accompanied by headache, cough, and fever, which resolved within 3 days. Six days after resolution, headache, nausea, diplopia, and difficulty in walking developed, and he was admitted to Showa University Hospital, Tokyo, on the same day. On examination, he was afebrile and fully conscious and had normal visual acuity. The fundi were normal, but there was left blepharoptosis.

FS	Fisher syndrome
GB	Guillain-Barré [syndrome]
HLA	Human leukocyte antigen

The pupils were dilated and responded sluggishly to light. Accommodation was normal. Limitation of ocular movement was detected in the lateral gaze of both eyes and in the vertical gaze of the left eye. The oculocephalic reflex was absent. Nystagmus was noted on lateral and downward gaze. The patient's muscle bulk, tone, and power were normal. Deep tendon reflexes were absent. Pathologic reflexes were not present. Formal tests of limb coordination showed mild decomposition. There was considerable ataxia of stance and gait; the Romberg test result was negative. There was no sensory dysfunction.

The erythrocyte sedimentation rate, C-reactive protein determination, blood cell count, and serum biochemistry study results were normal. Serum values for IgG, IgA, and IgM, respectively, were

1.82, 0.132, and 0.296 gm/L on day 2, and 1.69, 0.123, and, 0.346 on day 88; cerebrospinal fluid protein was 0.009 gm/L on day 3 and 0.029 gm/L on day 22, with normal cellularity on both days. He had the following HLA antigens: HLA-A24, 33; B44, 52; DQ1; and DR2, 6. A computed tomographic scan of the brain on day 2 with and without enhancement was normal; magnetic resonance imaging on days 12 and 44 with and without enhancement showed no abnormalities in the brain stem. An electroencephalogram on days 4 and 22 showed bilateral delta activity. Nerve conduction study results on day 20 were normal. The stool culture grew *C. jejuni* on days 5 and 8; the isolate belonged to PEN 2: LIO 4.

The patient was given prednisolone, 50 mg/day. Cerebellar ataxia reached a peak on day 2, his gait being unstable and tandem gait impossible. The left eyeball became completely fixed and right ocular movement was limited in all directions on day 8, but ocular movement began to improve on day 9. The boy had no ataxia of tandem gait on day 13. Three months after the onset of these conditions, left blepharoptosis, bilateral abducens nerve palsy, and areflexia remained.

Patient 2. A 9-year-old girl had a 1-day bout of fever, headache, and diarrhea, and then headache and diplopia 12 days later. The next day she had nausea, vomiting, and difficulty in walking, and was admitted to National Fukuyama Hospital (Hiroshima). She was afebrile and fully conscious and had normal visual acuity. The fundi and pupils were normal, and her light reflexes were prompt. Accommodation was normal. Lateral gaze of the left eye was limited. There was no Bell phenomenon. The oculocephalic reflex was absent. There were no other cranial nerve abnormalities. Muscle bulk, tone, and power were normal. Deep tendon reflexes were diminished. Pathologic reflexes were absent. Abdominal reflexes were retained. Finger-to-nose and heel-to-knee tests showed dysmetria and decomposition. There was ataxia of tandem gait. The result of a Romberg test was negative. The patient complained of dysesthesia in her left hand. Senses of touch, pain, proprioception, and vibration were normal. There were no meningeal signs.

The patient's leukocyte count was 11.3×10^6/L (11,300/μl). The erythrocyte sedimentation rate was 40 mm (1 hour). Results of serum C-reactive protein and biochemistry determinations were normal; IgG, IgA, and IgM values, respectively, were 1.23, 0.131, and 0.443 gm/L on day 6 and 1.21, 0.141, and 0.417 gm/L on day 77. The cerebrospinal fluid protein was 0.035 gm/L on day 7, 0.049 gm/L on day 10, 0.064 gm/L on day 22, and 0.023 gm/L on day 45. Cellularity was increased (8 mononuclear cells per microliter) on day 10 but was normal on the other days. The girl had the following HLA antigens: HLA-A24, 33; B44, 54; Cwl; DQ1, 4; and DR4, 6. With and without enhancement, computed tomography on day 3 and magnetic resonance imaging on days 5 and 22 showed no abnormalities in the brain stem. The results of electroencephalography, electromyography, and nerve conduction studies were normal, as was the auditory brain-stem response. *C. jejuni* was grown from a stool culture taken on day 6; the isolate belonged to PEN 2: LIO 4. Treatment with erythromycin for 14 days cleared the patient's stools of the organism.

The girl could not walk on day 8. Limitation and nystagmus in lateral and upward gaze reached a peak on day 8. Accommodation was absent. Deep tendon reflexes were absent in the legs. Headache lessened on day 11. Upward-gaze palsy disappeared on day 13. The patient could walk, but tandem gait was unstable on day 16. The tendon reflexes in the legs returned to normal on day 19. Tandem gait became stable on day 34. Left abducens nerve palsy worsened again on day 51 and reached a peak on day 71; 3 months after the onset of symptoms, left abducens nerve palsy remained.

DISCUSSION

These two patients had typical FS. The isolation of *C. jejuni* demonstrated the antecedent infection. Although a Penner serotype may correspond to a different Lior serotype, the isolates from our patients, who live in different areas, belonged to PEN 2: LIO 4. The PEN 19 serotype of *C. jejuni* is often isolated from patients with GB syndrome but is isolated from fewer than 2% of patients with *C. jejuni* enteritis in Japan.[7, 8] In contrast, PEN 2 and LIO 4 are common serotype isolates in cases of *C. jejuni* enteritis in Japan, PEN 2 being isolated from 15%[8] and LIO 4 from 12% of the patients with this condition.[11] It is necessary to determine whether there is an epidemiologic association between FS and *C. jejuni* (PEN 2: LIO 4).

The dependence of postinfection neurologic disorders on "molecular mimicry" between infectious agents and surface components of neural tissue has been postulated. Very frequently, FS is associated with autoantibody to GQ1b ganglioside.[12, 13] Using monoclonal anti-GQ1b antibodies, we have found that lipopolysaccharides of *C. jejuni* (PEN 2: LIO 4) isolated from the patients with FS bear the GQ1b epitope.[14] In contrast, *C. jejuni* (PEN 2: LIO 4) isolated from a patient with enteritis who had no neurologic disorder also had a lipopolysaccharide that bears the GQ1b epitope; serum from the patient had no anti-GQ1b antibody. A particular immunogenetic background in the host, therefore, may be necessary for FS to develop in addition to the antigenic components of the infectious agent.

Although previous studies did not show a clear association between HLA typing and GB syndrome, a significant association has been shown between the presence of HLA-B35 antigen and GB syndrome subsequent to *C. jejuni* enteritis.[6] In contrast, there is a significant association between HLA-B39 antigen and FS,[15] which suggests that the antecedent infections of FS are relatively homogeneous in comparison with those of GB syndrome. The previously described patient with *C. jejuni* (PEN 2: LIO 4) enteritis had the following HLA antigens: HLA-A26, 31; B39, 48; and Cw4, 7 (we did not investigate the patient's class II antigens [reported in part in reference 7]). These differed from the HLA antigens in our patients. For clarification of the pathogenesis of FS, it is necessary to determine whether there is an association between a specific HLA antigen and FS subsequent to *C. jejuni* infection.

We assume that infection by agents that bear the GQ1b epitope induces a high rate of production of anti-GQ1b antibody in patients with particular immunogenetic backgrounds, leading to loss of tolerance, and that anti-GQ1b antibody has a role in the development of FS. Approximately 5% of patients acquire FS after gastrointestinal infection,[16] and we speculate that some episodes are preceded by *C. jejuni* infection. An effort should be made to isolate *C. jejuni* from patients' stool cultures and to perform HLA typing to clarify the pathogenesis of this syndrome.

We thank Drs. Kahiko Saito and Masaki Takahashi (Department of Microbiology, Tokyo Metropolitan Research Laboratory of Public Health) for serotyping *C. jejuni*.

REFERENCES

1. Rees JH, Gregson NA, Griffiths PL, Hughes RAC. *Campylobacter jejuni* and Guillain-Barré syndrome. Q J Med 1993; 86:623-34.
2. Wroe SJ, Blumhardt LD. Acute polyneuritis with cranial nerve involvement following *Campylobacter jejuni* infection [Letter]. J Neurol Neurosurg Psychiatry 1985;48:593.
3. Roberts T, Shah A, Graham JG, McQueen I. The Miller Fisher syndrome following *Campylobacter* enteritis: a report of two cases. J Neurol Neurosurg Psychiatry 1987;50:1557-8.
4. Fross RD, Daube JR. Neuropathy in the Miller Fisher syndrome: clinical and electrophysiologic findings. Neurology 1987;37:1493-8.
5. Köhler A, de Torrente A, Inderwildi B. Fisher's syndrome associated with *Campylobacter jejuni* infection. Eur Neurol 1988;28:150-1.
6. Yuki N, Sato S, Itoh T, Miyatake T. HLA-B35 and acute axonal polyneuropathy following *Campylobacter* infection. Neurology 1991;41:1561-3.
7. Yuki N, Sato S, Fujimoto S, et al. Serotype of *Campylobacter jejuni*, HLA, and the Guillain-Barré syndrome. Muscle Nerve 1992;15:968-9.
8. Kuroki S, Saida T, Nukina M, et al. *Campylobacter jejuni* strains from patients with Guillain-Barré syndrome belong mostly to Penner serogroup 19 and contain *β-N*-acetylglucosamine residues. Ann Neurol 1993;33:243-7.
9. Penner JL, Hennessey JN. Passive hemagglutination technique for serotyping *Campylobacter fetus* subsp. *jejuni* on the basis of soluble heat-stable antigens. J Clin Microbiol 1980; 12:732-7.
10. Lior H, Woodward DL, Edgar JA, Laroche LJ, Gill P. Serotyping of *Campylobacter jejuni* by slide agglutination based on heat-labile antigenic factors. J Clin Microbiol 1982;15:761-8.
11. Saito K, Shingaki M, Takahashi M, et al. Serological studies on *Campylobacter jejuni/coli:* establishment of national reference system for serological typing in Japan [in Japanese with English abstract]. Kansenshogaku zassi 1992;66:340-8.
12. Chiba A, Kusunoki S, Shimizu T, Kanazawa I. Serum IgG antibody to ganglioside GQ1b is a possible marker of Miller Fisher syndrome. Ann Neurol 1992;31:677-9.
13. Yuki N, Sato S, Tsuji S, Ohsawa T, Miyatake T. Frequent presence of anti-GQ1b antibody in Fisher's syndrome. Neurology 1993;43:414-7.
14. Yuki N, Taki T, Takahashi M, et al. Molecular mimicry between GQ1b ganglioside and lipopolysaccharides of *Campylobacter jejuni* isolated from patients with Fisher's syndrome. Ann Neurol (in press).
15. Yuki N, Sato S, Tsuji S, Ogawa K, Miyatake T. Human leukocyte antigens in Fisher's syndrome. Ann Neurol 1993; 33:655-7.
16. Berlit P, Rakicky J. The Miller Fisher syndrome: review of the literature. J Clin Neuro-ophthalmol 1992;12:57-63.

Acute pancreatitis associated with acute hepatitis A in a young child

Lydia A. Shrier, MD,[a] Saul J. Karpen, MD, PhD, and Colston McEvoy, MD

From the Division of Adolescent/Young Adult Medicine, Children's Hospital, Boston, Massachusetts, and the Division of Gastroenterology/Hepatology, Department of Pediatrics, Yale–New Haven Hospital, New Haven, Connecticut

Acute hepatitis A infection is an unusual cause of pancreatitis in adults and has not been reported previously in young children. We describe a 4-year-old girl with acute pancreatitis associated with hepatitis A infection. (J PEDIATR 1995; 126:57-9)

Supported in part by Project No. MCJ-MA259195 from the Maternal-Child Health Bureau (Title V, Social Security Act), Health Resources and Services Administration, U.S. Department of Health and Human Resources.

Submitted for publication Aug. 3, 1994; accepted Aug. 22, 1994.

Reprint requests: Lydia A. Shrier, MD, Division of Adolescent/ Young Adult Medicine, Children's Hospital, 300 Longwood Ave., Boston, MA 02115.

[a]Formerly a resident in the Yale–New Haven Hospital Department of Pediatrics.

0022-3476/95/$3.00 + 0 **9/22/60148**

Acute pancreatitis is a relatively uncommon disease in children; trauma, biliary tract disease, and systemic diseases are the most frequent causes. Less often, viral infections may be associated with acute pancreatitis. The viruses most commonly identified include mumps,[1] rubella,[2] coxsackievirus B,[3, 4] and Epstein-Barr virus.[5] Pancreatitis complicating infection with influenza A[6] and varicella[7] also has been observed. Acute pancreatitis as a complication of acute hepatitis A infection has been noted rarely in older individuals,[8, 9] but this association has not been reported in a young child.

CASE REPORT

A 4-year-old Korean girl had a 1-day history of intermittent, severe, supraumbilical pain that migrated to the periumbilical region. She was vomiting all oral intake and had decreased appetite. She had no fever, diarrhea, upper respiratory tract symptoms, dysuria, or urinary frequency. There was no history of abdominal trauma. She had a normal bowel movement 1 day before being examined. Medical history was noncontributory and immunizations were current. She was not taking any medications. There was no family history of hepatitis, parasitic infections, gallstones, or hemolytic anemias.

On physical examination the patient had jaundice, mild periumbilical tenderness, and a tender liver palpable 2 cm below the right costal margin. There were no stigmata of chronic liver disease. Initial laboratory evaluation showed the following values: leukocyte count $6.2 \times 10^6/L$, hemoglobin 125 gm/L, serum bicarbonate 17 mmol/L, total bilirubin 85 μmol/L (4.97 mg/dl), direct bilirubin 48 μmol/L (2.80 mg/dl), aspartate aminotransferase 1110 U/L (normal, 0 to 35 U/L), alanine aminotransferase 379 U/L (normal, 0 to 35 U/L), and alkaline phosphatase 695 U/L (normal, 100-300 U/L for ages 2 to 10 years). The patient was hospitalized. Further laboratory findings included serum amylase 2130 U/dl (normal, 40 to 150 U/dl), serum lipase 84.0 U/ml (normal, <1.5 U/ml), random total cholesterol 5.25 mmol/L (203 mg/dl), triglycerides 2.34 mmol/L (207 mg/dl), and normal serum calcium concentration. Ultrasound examination of the abdomen showed increased echogenicity and thickening of the entire pancreas and a prominent pancreatic duct. There was no evidence of a mass, abnormal calcifications, or pancreatic cysts. The liver parenchyma and vasculature, the spleen, and the kidneys appeared normal. Moderate ascites was noted. A computed tomography scan with and without intravenous contrast medium showed a diffusely swollen pancreas without focal abnormality; no mass or evidence of trauma was seen.

Hepatitis A IgM and IgG antibodies were present; hepatitis B surface antibody was detectable, but hepatitis B surface antigen and hepatitis B core antibody were not. Results of tests for hepatitis C antibody and heterophile antibody were also negative.

The patient's abdominal pain and tenderness dissipated by the fourth day of hospitalization, after standard supportive therapy. Attempts at oral intake were associated initially with recurrence of abdominal pain, but by the tenth hospital day the patient was advanced to a regular diet. Serum amylase and lipase values gradually decreased to 203 U/dl and 14.0 U/ml, respectively, 1 day before discharge. The serum total bilirubin level had decreased to 17 μmol/L (0.97 mg/dl), aspartate aminotransferase to 89 U/L, alanine aminotransferase to 171 U/L, and alkaline phosphatase to 378 U/L.

The pancreas appeared normal on an ultrasound examination 1 month after discharge. By 11 weeks after onset, all of the patient's liver function and pancreatic enzyme findings were within normal limits. She continued to complain of occasional abdominal discomfort, usually after meals, sometimes with vomiting. However, she was gaining weight and physical examination findings were unremarkable.

DISCUSSION

In adults, acute pancreatitis has been associated only rarely with nonfulminant acute viral hepatitis; hepatitis A,[8, 9] hepatitis B,[10] and non-A, non-B hepatitis[11] all have been implicated. To our knowledge, no cases of acute pancreatitis complicating acute hepatitis A infection have been reported in young children. Recent reviews of cases of pancreatitis in the pediatric population have not included hepatitis A among the causes.[6, 12-14]

The mechanism by which viral hepatitis may cause pancreatitis is unknown. Shimoda et al.[10] detected hepatitis B surface and core antigens in the cytoplasm of pancreatic acinar cells, which suggests that direct infection of the pancreas may occur in patients with hepatitis B. Animal studies of other viral infections and pancreatitis have suggested either direct inflammation and acinar cell destruction.[4, 15] or edema of the ampulla of Vater causing obstruction of pancreatic outflow.[3] Autodigestion may play a role in potentiating pancreatic damage.[16] No direct evidence of hepatitis A infection of the pancreas has been described.

In our patient no coincidental causes of acute pancreatitis, such as alcohol abuse, gallstone disease, drug- or toxin-induced pancreatic injury, trauma, or anomalies of the pancreaticobiliary tree, were evident. Hyperlipidemia was mild and likely not responsible for the clinical and laboratory severity of the pancreatitis. We conclude that acute hepatitis A infection should be considered as another possible cause of acute pancreatitis in children.

REFERENCES

1. Naficy K, Nategh R, Ghadimi H. Mumps pancreatitis without parotitis. BMJ 1973;1:529.
2. Bunnell CE, Monif GRG. Interstitial pancreatitis in the congenital rubella syndrome. J PEDIATR 1972;80:465-6.
3. Tsui CH, Burch GE, Harb JM. Pancreatitis in mice infected with Coxsackie virus B1. Arch Pathol 1972;93:379-89.
4. Ursing B. Acute pancreatitis in Coxsackie B infection. BMJ 1973;3:524-5.
5. Wislocki LC. Acute pancreatitis in infectious mononucleosis. N Engl J Med 1966;275:322-3.
6. Jordan SC, Ament ME. Pancreatitis in children and adolescents. J PEDIATR 1977;91:211-6.
7. Kirschner S, Raufman JP. Varicella pancreatitis complicated by pancreatic pseudocyst and duodenal obstruction. Dig Dis Sci 1988;33:1192-5.
8. Davis TV, Keeffe EB. Acute pancreatitis associated with acute hepatitis A. Am J Gastroenterol 1992;87:1648-50.
9. Lopez Morante A, Rodriguez de Lope C, San Miguel G, Pons Romero F. Acute pancreatitis in hepatitis A infection. Postgrad Med J 1986;62:407-8.
10. Shimoda T, Shikata T, Karasawa T, Tsukakoshi S, Yoshimu S, Sakurai I. Light microscopic localizations of hepatitis B virus antigens in the human pancreas: possibility of multiplica-

tion of hepatitis B virus in the human pancreas. Gastroenterology 1981;81:998-1005.
11. Eugene C, Cadranel JF, Bergue A, Anciaux ML. Acute pancreatitis associated with non-A, non-B hepatitis. J Clin Gastroenterol 1990;12:195-7.
12. Vane DW, Grosfeld JL, West KW, Rescorla FJ. Pancreatic disorders in infancy and childhood: experience with 92 cases. J Pediatr Surg 1989;24:771-6.
13. Weizman A, Duire PR. Acute pancreatitis in childhood. J PEDIATR 1988;113:24-9.
14. Ziegler DW, Long JA, Philippart AI, et al. Pancreatitis in childhood. Ann Surg 1988;207:257-61.
15. Burch GE, Harb JM. Electron microscopic studies of viral pancreatitis in coxsackie B4 virus infected mice. Exp Mol Pathol 1979;31:23-35.
16. Vuorinen T, Kallajoki M, Hyypia T, et al. Coxsackievirus B3–induced acute pancreatitis: analysis of histopathological and viral parameters in a mouse model. British Journal of Experimental Pathology 1989;70:395-403.

Methemoglobinemia associated with acidosis of probable renal origin

Susanne Sager, PhD, MD, Guy H. Grayson, MD, and Stephen A. Feig, MD
From the Divisions of Nephrology and Hematology/Oncology, Gwynne Hazen Cherry Memorial Laboratory, Department of Pediatrics, University of California at Los Angeles School of Medicine

We describe an infant who had methemoglobinemia related to acidosis, probably on the basis of renal tubular acidosis. Methemoglobinemia may indicate the presence of a clinically significant underlying disorder. (J PEDIATR 1995; 126:59-61)

Neonatal methemoglobinemia and renal tubular acidosis are both infrequent, and there are no reports describing these two abnormalities in the same infant. Here we describe an infant with methemoglobinemia as a result of acidosis, probably because of RTA.

CASE REPORT

A 1-month-old infant, the term product of a healthy 19-year-old Hispanic woman (gravida 2, para 1, aborta 1), was born by normal, spontaneous vaginal delivery. His birth weight was 3.345 kg, and Apgar scores were normal. The mother had good prenatal care and had no prenatal complications. The mother took only prenatal vitamins during the pregnancy and did not smoke or use drugs or alcohol. Mother and child were discharged after 24 hours. There was no consanguinity, nor any family history of renal or hematologic disease.

The infant was seen at 1 month of age with a 5-day history of intermittent nonprojectile vomiting with normal urine and stool pattern. He also had not fed well since he was discharged from the nursery, and had not gained weight. The infant was being fed a standard commercial formula, and there were no errors in preparation. He was taking no medications, although the family had given him a small amount of mint tea to try to relieve his vomiting. He had not consumed any well water, and had not been exposed to any dyes or other toxic substances.

Physical examination revealed a thin, pale, cyanotic, lethargic infant. Weight was 3.232 kg, temperature 36.4° C, pulse 140 beats/min, respirations 40/min, and blood pressure 82/46 mm Hg. There was a right preauricular skin tag. The lungs were clear, and there were no chest retractions. The heart rate was regular, and no murmurs were present. The abdomen was soft and nontender and had no masses. The extremities had acrocyanosis and no edema. The infant was easily arousable and had no focal neurologic deficits. The skin had no lesions, but there was minimal subcutaneous fat.

Laboratory evaluation revealed a leukocyte count of 21×10^6/L (21,000/μL), hemoglobin level 108 gm/L, hematocrit 0.30 (30%), and methemoglobin value 0.43 (43%). Arterial blood gas values in room air were as follows: pH, 7.25; P_{CO_2}, 17 mm Hg; P_{O_2}, 84 mm Hg; and base deficit, 17.3 mmol/L. In 100% oxygen his P_{O_2} was 294 mm Hg. Serum electrolyte concentrations were as follows: sodium, 135 mmol/L; potassium, 2.5 mmol/L; chloride, 117 mmol/L; and bicarbonate, 5 mmol/L. The blood urea nitrogen was 3.9 mmol/L (11 mg/dl) and arterial ammonia 28 μmol/L (48 mg/dl). Urinalysis showed a specific gravity of 1.005 and pH 6.0. Results of chest and abdominal x-ray studies were normal.

Submitted for publication April 11, 1994; accepted Aug. 2, 1994.
Reprint requests: Stephen A. Feig, MD, Department of Pediatrics, Division of Hematology/Oncology, University of California at Los Angeles School of Medicine, 10833 Le Conte Ave., Los Angeles, CA 90024.

0022-3476/95/$3.00 + 0 **9/22/59562**

NADH	Nicotinamide adenine dinculeotide, reduced form
P_{CO_2}	Partial pressure of carbon dioxide
P_{O_2}	Partial pressure of oxygen
RTA	Renal tubular acidosis

The infant was given a blood transfusion and subsequently treated with intravenously administered methylene blue (2 mg/kg), with a prompt fall in the methemoglobin value to 0.019 (1.9%). Acidosis was treated with intravenous administration of fluids and bicarbonate. During the ensuing hospitalization, he tolerated an oral electrolyte solution and then a commercial soy formula without further vomiting. Methemoglobin levels remained less than 0.1 (10%), and serum bicarbonate concentrations ranged between 14 and 16 mmol/L. Because the patient had received a transfusion, methemoglobin reductase (NADH–ferricyanide reductase) levels were not measured. Pretransfusion hemoglobin electrophoresis showed a normal electrophoretic pattern for age. The evaluation for metabolic acidosis revealed normal concentrations of serum organic acids, carnitine, and urinary amino and organic acids. After discharge home, the patient tolerated soy formula without cyanosis.

The patient was readmitted to the hospital 5 days later with a 4-day history of frequent emesis and watery green stools with progressive cyanosis and lethargy. Laboratory evaluation showed the following: leukocyte count, 17.7×10^6/L (17,700/μl); hemoglobin level, 108 gm/L; hematocrit, 0.30 (30%); and methemoglobin level, 0.21 (21%). The arterial blood gas values were pH, 7.29; P_{CO_2}, 15 mm Hg; P_{O_2}, 126 mm Hg; bicarbonate, 7.1 mmol/L; and base deficit, 16.3 mmol/L. Serum electrolyte values were sodium, 136 mmol/L; potassium, 4.0 mmol/L; chloride, 118 mmol/L; and bicarbonate, 8 mmol/L (anion gap = 14). Urinalysis revealed a specific gravity of 1.014 and pH 6.0 by dipstick. Urinary electrolytes yielded a urine anion gap of 20 (urinary sodium, 59 mmol/L; potassium, 20 mmol/L; chloride, 59 mmol/L). Because a positive urine anion gap in a phase of nonanion gap metabolic acidosis might indicate distal RTA, fractional excretion of bicarbonate was measured in the following manner: the patient was treated with intravenously administered sodium bicarbonate, and then orally administered sodium citrate and citric acid up to 7 mEq/kg per day to increase the serum bicarbonate level to 26 mmol/L. At that time the patient was euvolemic and stable with the use of oral feedings and medications. Urine pH by meter was 7.66. Arterial blood gas values were, pH 7.36; P_{CO_2}, 47 mm Hg; and bicarbonate, 26 mmol/L. Urine collected in a syringe was immediately processed in the laboratory and had a sodium concentration of 21 mmol/L; potassium, 23 mmol/L; chloride, 15 mmol/L; bicarbonate, 20 mmol/L; and creatinine, 0.539 μmol/L (6.1 mg/dl). From these data the fractional excretion of bicarbonate was 0.05 (5%), consistent with a distal RTA (type I).

Maintenance of a serum bicarbonate level between 23 and 26 mmol/L has required an intake of sodium citrate and citric acid, 7 to 9 mEq/kg daily, with frequent monitoring of serum electrolytes. On this medical regimen the patient has thrived; his height and weight were at the 50th percentile at 42 months of age. Renal ultrasound studies have revealed no evidence of nephrocalcinosis. No further episodes of methemoglobinemia have occurred. At routine follow-up, when the patient was 6 months of age, NADH–ferricyanide reductase levels in the patient and his parents were normal (Table).

Table. NADH–ferricyanide reductase

Subject	Value (IU/gm hemoglobin)
Patient	24.22
Father	26.21
Mother	21.22
Control	22.79
(Normal)	(11.51-26.91)

Assays were kindly performed by Ernest Beutler, MD, Scripps Clinic, San Diego, Calif.

DISCUSSION

Methemoglobin is hemoglobin in which the heme iron is in the ferric state. Methemoglobin does not bind O_2; this diminishes the oxygen-carrying capacity of blood and diminishes oxygen delivery to the tissues. Methemoglobin, even at low concentrations, causes cyanosis because of the color of the compound.

Methemoglobin normally makes up only 1% of total erythrocyte hemoglobin because several pathways exist to reduce methemoglobin to hemoglobin. Primary methemoglobinemia can result from partial or complete deficiencies in the methemoglobin reductase or, rarely, from the presence of unstable hemoglobins that are readily oxidized (M hemoglobins).[1] Enzyme assays of this patient at 6 months of age and of his parents effectively eliminated the possibility that a hereditary heterozygous or homozygous methemoglobin reductase deficiency was present. Hemoglobin electrophoresis revealed normally migrating hemoglobin.

Acquired methemoglobinemia has been reported to occur in infants after exposure to aniline dyes, dietary nitrates, and many oxidizing medications.[1-3] In addition, secondary methemoglobinemia has been described in infants with metabolic acidosis on the basis of severe diarrhea.[4, 5] No renal abnormalities were demonstrated in these infants. The proposed mechanism for methemoglobinemia was an immature erythrocyte enzyme system in the presence of increased oxidant stress caused by unidentified oxidants and diarrhea-induced acidosis. Others have postulated that an increased synthesis of intestinal nitrates by colonic bacteria during diarrheal illnesses oxidized the hemoglobin to methemoglobin.[6] Newborn infants are thought to be particularly sensitive to the development of secondary methemoglobinemia because neonatal red cells are relatively deficient in methemoglobin reductase activity.[7] The apparent oxidant stress in this infant was the severe metabolic acidosis, probably caused by uncorrected RTA.

This report demonstrates the development of clinically significant methemoglobinemia in an infant whom we believe had untreated renal tubular acidosis. Although the diarrhea may have contributed to acidosis during the second episode of methemoglobinemia, the acidosis was out of proportion to the severity of diarrhea and dehydration. Furthermore, the first episode of methemoglobinemia was associated with vomiting, but not with diarrhea. Nevertheless, the patient was severely acidotic, probably as a result of RTA.

This case stresses the need for a thorough search for an underlying cause of methemoglobinemia as a means of identifying other clinically important conditions.

REFERENCES

1. Curry S. Methemobloginemia. Ann Emerg Med 1982;11:214-21.
2. Dolan MA, Luban NCL. Methemoglobinemia in two children: disparate etiology and treatment. Pediatr Emerg Care 1987;3:171-5.
3. Keating JP, Lell ME, Strauss AW, Zarkowsky H, Smith GE. Infantile methemoglobinemia caused by carrot juice. N Engl J Med 1973;288:824-6.
4. Yano SS, Danish EH, Hsia YE. Transient methemoglobinemia with acidosis in infants. J PEDIATR 1982;100:415-8.
5. Lanir A, Borochowitz Z, Kaplan T. Transient methemoglobinemia with acidosis and hyperchloremia in infants. Am J Pediatr Hematol Oncol 1986;8:353-5.
6. Murray KF, Christie DL. Dietary protein intolerance in infants with transient methemoglobinemia and diarrhea. J PEDIATR 1993;122:90-2.
7. Ross JD. Deficient activity of DPNH-dependent methmoglobin diaphorase in cord blood erythrocytes. Blood 1963;21:51-62.

Intact survival with transfusion-associated graft-versus-host disease proved by human leukocyte antigen typing of lymphocytes in skin biopsy specimens

R. Hentschel, MD, E. B. Broecker, MD, G. Kolde, MD, M. Frosch, MD, W. Friedrich, MD, W. Holzgreve, MS, MD, E. Westphal, MD, and E. Harms, MD

From the Departments of Pediatrics, Dermatology, and Obstetrics and Gynecology, University Hospital, Münster, Germany; the Department of Dermatology, University Hospital, Würzburg, Germany; the Department of Pediatrics, University Hospital, Ulm, Germany; and the Institute of Immunology, University of Kiel, Kiel, Germany

A transient transfusion-associated graft-versus-host disease occurred in a premature infant of 30 weeks of gestation. We demonstrated donor lymphocytes in a skin biopsy specimen with a two-step immunoperoxidase technique using monoclonal antibodies against human leukocyte antigen determinants specific for the donor. The girl survived and is immunocompetent. (J PEDIATR 1995;126: 61-4)

Submitted for publication Nov. 22, 1993; accepted Aug. 8, 1994.

Reprint requests: R. Hentschel, MD, Department of Pediatrics, University of Munster, Albert-Schweitzer-Str. 33, 48129 Munster, Germany.

0022-3476/95/$3.00 + 0 **9/22/59700**

Transfusion-associated graft-versus-host disease has been reported in immunocompromised patients[1, 2] and in subjects after mass transfusion,[3, 4] exchange transfusion, multiple intrauterine transfusions, or transfusion in premature infants.[5-7] The disease is usually lethal.[2] Diagnosis may be suggested by the history, typical clinical symptoms, and the

GVHD	Graft-versus-host disease
HLA	Human leukocyte antigen
TGVHD	Transfusion-associated graft-versus-host disease

latency time; however, the disease often is unrecognized because symptoms are not specific.[1, 3, 4, 7]

CASE REPORT

After 30 weeks of gestation a female premature infant was delivered by cesarean section to healthy parents. The mother was Rh negative and the father was Rh positive. It was the mother's fifth pregnancy; the first had no complications, and anti-D prophylaxis was not administered. The second child and the third child had hemolytic disease of the newborn and required postnatal transfusions or exchange transfusion. A fourth pregnancy ended in abortion. During the fifth pregnancy the mother's anti-D antibody titers rose from 1:128 in the third week of gestation to 1:1024 in the twenty-second week. The fetus had pericardial and abdominal effusions from the twenty-fourth week until delivery. Because of a low hemoglobin level, the fetus received four intrauterine transfusions with nonirradiated type O, Rh-negative packed erythrocytes between weeks 25 and 29. The infant's birth weight was 1520 gm, and the Apgar scores were 8 and 9 at 5 and 10 minutes. There were no signs of hydrops and the liver was not markedly enlarged. After an exchange transfusion with 180 ml of type O, Rh-negative, nonirradiated fresh whole blood, the infant's hemoglobin level increased from 90 gm/L after birth to 141 gm/L. She received three additional transfusions of 15 to 20 ml of nonirradiated packed erythrocytes on days 3 and 12. On day 7 a scattered pale exanthem developed on the infant's face and thighs. The rash was follicular but not confluent, remained discrete, and seemed to regress. However, on the twelfth day of life, the rash became more intense and spread centrifugally with a maximum intensity in the groin area. The final stage was erythroderma with palmar and plantar edema. On day 16 histologic examination of a skin biopsy specimen and immunofluorescence staining confirmed the clinical diagnosis of acute graft-versus-host disease.

Because some of the blood donors were men, we attempted to identify blood leukocyte chimerism by karyotyping of the circulating cells on day 18. A normal female genotype was found in 100 cells examined. We performed human leukocyte antigen typing of the child, her parents, and siblings on the same day. No blood chimerism was found in the child's blood; T cells and non-T cells (DR-positive B cells and monocytes) were of patient origin. A total of 40% of the cells were identified as T cells (38% $CD4^+$; 11% $CD8^+$), 3% were B cells, 40% of the cells were contaminating monocytes (37% DR-positive). We also tested the HLA antigens of all four blood donors. These tests enabled us to prove that the infant had TGVHD by use of an immunohistologic technique on a frozen skin section.

With a rapid regression of the exanthem beginning on day 18, temporary desquamation of the entire integument began on the thighs and on interdigital skin surfaces, and was complete by day 27. Skin manifestations had totally disappeared on day 32. When the exanthem first appeared, the patient's leukocyte count was $9.0 \times 10^9/L$, the platelet count was $142 \times 10^9/L$, and the hemoglobin level was 153 gm/L. Between day 16 and day 30 a marked eosinophilia was present, with a maximum of 39% of eosinophils in a total of 24×10^9 leukocytes per liter. A diagnosis of hepatitis was excluded by serum studies; all other laboratory values were within the normal range.

Unexpectedly, the child survived without specific therapy. At the age of 48 months she has no clinical abnormalities, her growth is adequate, and there are no indications of a primary or secondary immunodeficiency. She has received vaccine against tuberculosis without side effects; vaccination against *Haemophilus influenzae*, diphtheria, tetanus, and poliomyelitis yielded normal antibody titers, and quantitative determination of IgG classes and subclasses verified normal serum levels. Intracutaneous tests of delayed-type hypersensitivity showed normal reactivity. Subpopulations of lymphocytes are normal, and T cells show adequate proliferation on stimulation in vitro.

RESULTS

Immunohistologic studies of frozen sections. We used a two-step immunoperoxidase technique to incubate monoclonal antibodies against supertypic HLA epitopes (class I and class II), Langerhans cells (CD1), T lymphocytes (CD3, CD4, CD8, and CD25), and against subtypic HLA-A and B-alleles[8, 9] on acetone-fixed sections of fresh-frozen skin. We found a complete absence of $CD1^+$ dendritic cells, a homogeneous HLA-DR expression of epidermal keratinocytes, and predominance of $CD8^+$ T cells in the epidermotropic infiltrate. Anti–HLA-A1 antibody 108A6 reacted preferentially with the epidermis but expressed only a weak reaction with infiltrating lymphocytes, which in contrast were stained by anti–HLA-BW6 antibody 2BC4 (Figure). Antibody 48C1, which is directed against HLA-A2 or HLA-A28, did not react with lymphocytes or epidermal structures. Because HLA-BW6 is associated with B7, B8, B14, B35, B60, and B65, this antibody could not discriminate between the lymphocytes of the mother and those of all four blood donors (Table). However, blood donors 1, 2, and 3 could be excluded because the third monoclonal antibody, 48C1, did not detect HLA-A2 or HLA-A28 on the infiltrating lymphocytes.

DISCUSSION

In addition to marked eosinophilia, the leading clinical criterion for the diagnosis of GVHD in this infant was the skin manifestation.[2, 5, 6] However, toxic drug reactions, viral infections (especially cytomegalovirus), and septicemia may produce similar rashes.[6] Even histologic and routine immunohistologic examination of a skin biopsy specimen, though quite typical, is not specific for TGVHD; similar alterations can be found in toxic drug reactions and after chemotherapy or radiation treatment.[2] The proof of TGVHD requires the demonstration of infiltrating lymphocytes of donor origin in affected organs[10] that are not part of the reticulohistiocytic system, because it can be assumed that circulating viable or decaying lymphocytes should undergo phagocytosis in this compartment. Change of HLA

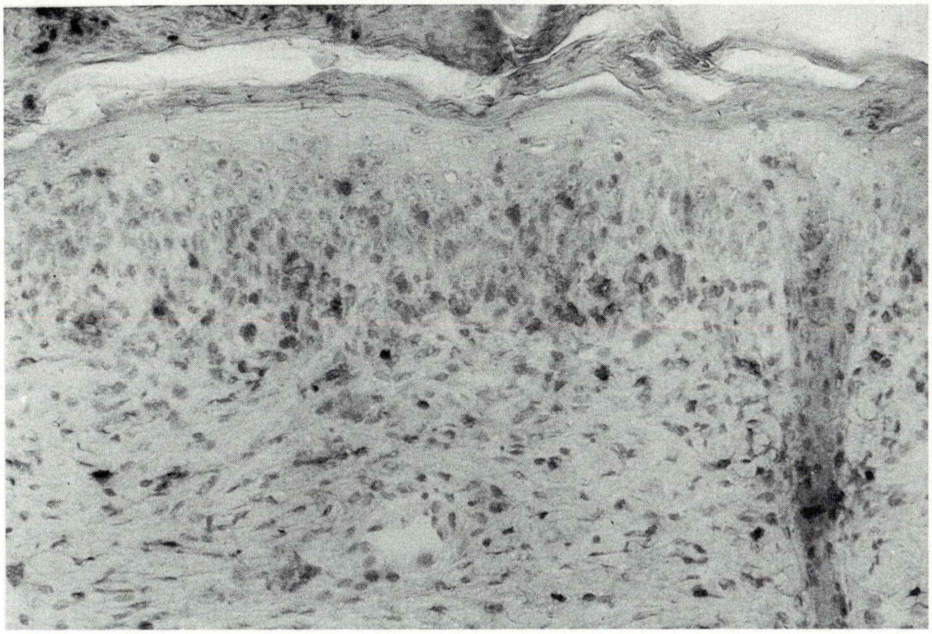

Figure. Immunohistologic findings of frozen sections of the skin on day 16. Monoclonal antibody 2BC4 was used to identify infiltrating lymphocytes presenting HLA-BW6 or associated antigens.

Table. HLA types of the patient, her parents, and blood donors for intrauterine transfusions and for exchange transfusion

	Histocompatibility antigens				
	HLA-A	HLA-B	HLA-C	HLA-DR	HLA-DQ
Family member					
Patient	1, 29	57, 58	w6 w7	2, 4	6, 8
Mother	26, 29	14*, 58	w7 w8	1, 2	5, 6
Father	1, 68	7*, 57	w6 w7	2, 4	6, 8
Blood donor					
1	2, 29	35*, 44	w4	3, 4	2, 3
2	2, 11	35*, 38	w4 w7	1, 9	1, 3
3	28, 33	44, 65*	w5 w8	1, 11	1, 3
4†	1, 24	8*, 60*	w3 w7	3, 13	1, 2

Blood donors are indicated in chronologic order.
*HLA-B locus antigens associated with HLA-Bw6.
†Exchange transfusion.

type within 2 days[11] and demonstration of two different haplotypes on circulating lymphocytes,[5] of donor HLA in lymph nodes,[12] or of donor DNA from peripheral blood[13] is not sufficient to diagnose TGVHD, because cells may survive for a period of time before they are successfully eradicated by the host defense.

We believe that GVHD and TGVHD are seldom proved without doubt; in 1990 Decoste et al.[2] stated after a review of the medical literature that "many cases of TGVHD lack absolute confirmation." We suggest that only the detection of lymphocytes with an HLA type that is not that of the patient, in an organ that is affected by TGVHD (for example, the skin), provides definitive proof of the disease. However, this type of proof has not been previously reported.

We believe that infiltrating lymphocytes were not of the patient's origin, because they also reacted with HLA-BW6–associated antigens and these were not expressed by the patient. The numbers of $CD8^+$ T cells and HLA-BW6–positive cells in skin biopsy specimens were identical; thus a host-versus-graft reaction was unlikely. By exclusion, the only possible source of lymphocytes that could have caused TGVHD was the blood for exchange transfusion (donor 4). The potential risk of exchange transfusion with nonirradiated whole fresh blood, in contrast to intrauterine transfusions, can be attributed to three circumstances: transfusion of a larger amount of blood, use of whole blood components, and use of blood that was not older than 2 days. In contrast, the probability of induction of TGVHD by one of the three postnatal transfusions of packed erythrocytes, is low, but cannot be excluded absolutely, because the donors could not be identified.

In posttransfusion GVHD the risk depends on the number of viable lymphocytes that survive and proliferate in the host so that the host defense is overrun.[1] On the other hand, transfusion of only a few viable or decaying lymphocytes might induce tolerance so that a subsequent challenge with lymphocytes of an identical haplotype cannot be rejected. This hypothesis may explain the risk of neonates and premature infants for TGVHD after intrauterine transfusion(s) with or without postnatal exchange transfusion, even if the relative immunoincompetence incumbent with prematurity is not considered. Parkman et al.[5] provided evidence that TGVHD after exchange transfusion has been observed only after intrauterine transfusions had been introduced as therapy for hemolytic disease. The younger a fetus, the more probable that tolerance will occur. Conversely, cellular immunity is suppressed in newborn infants after exchange transfusion (and without a former intrauterine transfusion), which leads to tolerance to skin allografts.

Our patient shares two HLA antigens with the incriminated blood donor (HLA-A1 and Cw7), and thus a primary immune tolerance related to the mechanism of self-recognition may have been a factor in addition to the mechanisms discussed above. It has been assumed that coincidence of HLA haplotype(s) between blood donor(s) and the patient might be causally relevant in TGVHD.[3, 4, 14] In a case of TGVHD after transfusion of fresh blood pooled from three donors, the lymphocytes from the donor who shared the most determinants with the host survived.[11] Thus four immunologic mechanisms may have been important in our patient: primary immunoincompetence caused by immaturity, tolerance induced by former transfusion(s), immunosuppression as a result of antigenic overloading, or partial self-recognition.

In our patient lymphocytes with HLA-BW6 antigenic structures could unequivocally be demonstrated in a cryopreserved skin biopsy specimen. Therefore after detection of engrafted lymphocytes we reassessed blood samples that had been taken at the time of skin biopsy. However, HLA-BW6–positive lymphocytes could not be detected. Perhaps engrafted lymphocytes circulate only in an early stage of disease, when clinical signs may not yet be evident. In a later stage engrafted lymphocytes may have become sessile and thus were protected from attacks of circulating recipient cells. Our case shows that lack of blood chimerism does not exclude TGVHD.

We believe that of all reported cases of TGVHD in patients without immunodeficiency, this is the first patient who survived.[3] Maturation of the immune system may have led to rejection of engrafted lymphocytes, and therefore the TGVHD was only transient. This experience demonstrates that TGVHD can affect "healthy" premature infants without any detectable immune deficiency, and that the patient can survive even when there is no doubt about the diagnosis of this disease. Prophylactic irradiation of blood products should be used to bypass the potential hazards of transfusion in populations at risk.

We thank Gabriele Walther-Wenke, Deutches Rotes Krenz Münster, for identification of the blood donors; H. Grosse-Wilde, University of Essen, for HLA typing; P. Bartmann, University of Ulm, for all other immunologic tests and techniques; and the four blood donors for their readiness to help us clarify this case.

REFERENCES

1. Brubaker DB. Human posttransfusion graft-versus-host disease. Vox Sang 1983;45:401-20.
2. Decoste SD, Boudreaux C, Dover JS. Transfusion-associated graft-vs-host disease in patients with malignancies. Report of two cases and review of the literature. Arch Dermatol 1990; 126:1324-9.
3. Greenbaum BH. Transfusion-associated graft-versus-host disease: historical perspectives, incidence, and current use of irradiated blood products. J Clin Oncol 1991;9:1889-902.
4. Holland PV. Prevention of transfusion-associated graft-vs-host disease. Arch Pathol Lab Med 1989;113:285-91.
5. Parkman R, Mosier D, Umansky I, Cochran W, Carpenter CB, Rosen FS. Graft-versus-host disease after intrauterine and exchange transfusions for hemolytic disease of the newborn. N Engl J Med 1974;290:359-63.
6. Berger RS, Dixon SL. Fulminant transfusion-associated graft-versus-host disease in a premature infant. J AM ACAD DERMATOL 1989;20:945-50.
7. Sanders MR, Graeber JE. Posttransfusion graft-versus-host disease in infancy. J PEDIATR 1990;117:159-63.
8. Harpprecht J, Westphal E, Mueller-Ruchholtz W. Production and applications of new monoclonal antibodies against human lymphocyte antigen-A and -B antigens. Diagn Clin Immunol 1988;5:388-92.
9. Kandzia J, Anderson MJD, Mueller-Ruchholtz W. Cell separation by antibody-coupled magnetic microspheres and their application in conjunction with monoclonal HLA-antibodies. J Cancer Res Clin Oncol 1981;101:165-70.
10. Ferrara JLM, Deeg HJ. Graft-versus-host disease. N Engl J Med 1991;324:667-74.
11. Ito K, Yoshida H, Yanagibashi K, et al. Change of HLA phenotype in postoperative erythroderma [Letter]. Lancet 1988;1:413-4.
12. Dinsmore RE, Straus DJ, Pollack MS, et al. Fatal graft-versus-host disease following blood transfusion in Hodgkin's disease documented by HLA typing. Blood 1980;55:831-4.
13. Funkhouser AW, Vogelsang G, Zehnbauer B, et al. Graft versus host disease after blood transfusions in a premature infant. Pediatrics 1991;87:247-50.
14. Shivdasani R, Haluska FG, Dock NL, et al. Graft-versus-host disease associated with transfusion of blood from unrelated HLA-homozygous donors. N Engl J Med 1993;328:766-70.

Neonatal onset of medium-chain acyl–coenzyme A dehydrogenase deficiency with confusing biochemical features

John Christodoulou, MBBS, PhD, FRACP, Julie Hoare, BSc, Judith Hammond, MAppSc, Wai Ching Ip, BSc, and Bridget Wilcken, MBChB, FRACP

From the Department of Paediatrics and Child Health, University of Sydney, Sydney, Australia, and the Oliver Latham Laboratory, Royal Alexandra Children's Hospital, Camperdown, Australia

A female neonate was seen because of shock, ketosis, and undetectable blood glucose. Initial urinary findings indicated the possibility of a defect of fatty acid β-oxidation; subsequent studies showed that she had medium-chain acyl–coenzyme A dehydrogenase deficiency. This case highlights the fact that the initial symptoms may occur in the first few days of life, and that the presence of ketosis does not exclude the possibility of a fatty acid oxidation defect; the profiles of urinary organic acids and acylglycines may not be characteristic at that time. (J PEDIATR 1995;126:65-8)

Medium-chain acyl–coenzyme A dehydrogenase deficiency (McKusick 22274) is the most common of the inborn errors of fatty acid β-oxidation.[1] Typically, the initial manifestations occur between 2 months and 4 years of age, when hypoketotic hypoglycemia is provoked by the catabolic stress of an acute infection or prolonged fasting.[2, 3] However, in up to a third of cases of MCAD deficiency, suggestive symptoms may first develop in the neonatal period.[4] We describe a 10-month-old girl with MCAD deficiency, who had her first near-fatal episode on day 2 of life. The correct diagnosis was not initially made because of an atypical urinary biochemical profile.

CASE REPORT

The infant, the second child of unrelated Australian parents, was born by spontaneous vaginal delivery at term after an uncomplicated pregnancy. Apgar scores were 9 and 10 at 1 and 5 minutes, respectively. Birth weight was 3020 gm. She breast fed well for the first day of life and was discharged home at 36 hours of age. However, she then fed poorly and became progressively irritable and lethargic. She was examined at home the next morning by a community nurse, having slept through the night without being fed, and was extremely lethargic and cold and had extreme bradycardia.

Submitted for publication May 20, 1994; accepted Aug. 9, 1994.
Reprint requests: John Christodoulou, MBBS, PhD, University Teaching Unit, Royal Alexandra Children's Hospital, Pyrmont Bridge Rd., Camperdown, New South Wales 2050 Australia.

0022-3476/95/$3.00 + 0 **9/22/59697**

Physical examination at a local hospital revealed hypothermia (axillary temperature, 33.7° C), poor peripheral perfusion, and lethargy. Heart rate was 40 beats/min, and respirations were 50 breaths/min. Blood glucose concentration was undetectable; resuscitation included intravenous administration of dextrose, bicarbonate, and ampicillin and gentamicin. Arterial blood gas values indicated a compensated metabolic acidosis. The blood lactate concentration was 8.1 mmol/L (normal, <2.1) (73 mg/dl [normal, <18.9]), and the ammonium concentration was 136 μmol/L (normal, <100) (245 μg/dl, [normal <180]). Serum concentrations of

See related article, p. 69.

HGL	Hexanoylglycine
MCAD	Medium-chain acyl–coenzyme A dehydrogenase

potassium (6.5 mmol/L [normal, 3.8 to 5.5]), urea (22.9 mmol/L [normal, 1 to 13] [63 mg/dl; [normal, 2.8 to 36]), and creatinine (160 μmol/L [normal range, 1 to 100] [1.8 mg/dl; normal range, 0.011 to 1.1]) were elevated. Plasma liver enzyme values were normal except for aspartate aminotransferase, which was 154 U/L (normal, up to 90). Urine contained a moderate amount of ketones.

The patient was transferred to the Royal Alexandra Children's Hospital for diagnostic evaluation and further management. She was now active, was well perfused, and had a strong cry. She had tachypnea (rate, 60 breaths/min) and mild intercostal retractions; findings of cardiovascular and respiratory examinations were otherwise unremarkable. The liver was palpable 1 cm below the costal margin. By day 3 the serum electrolyte, aspartate aminotransferase, lactate, and ammonium values had returned to normal, and treatment consisted of intravenous administration of fluids (glucose intake, 8 mg/kg per minute) and antibiotics. Urinary organic acid analysis, performed on a urine sample collected on admission to our center, indicated the possibility of a fatty acid oxidation disorder but did not suggest MCAD deficiency (see Results section, below). On day 4, seizures began; they were brief but recurred every 2 to 3 hours and were eventually brought under control during the next 48 hours with phenobarbital. An electroencephalogram showed severe abnormalities with frequent multifocal discharges; cranial ultrasonography showed possible cerebral edema. An electrocardiogram and echocardiogram were normal. Frequent oral feedings begun on day 6 consisted of 40% Nan 1 (Nestlé Vevey, Switzerland), 9.5% Poly-Joule (Sharpe Laboratories, Ermington, NSW, Australia), Combined Amino Acid Mix (Scientific Hospital Supplies, Ermington), and modified Seravit vitamin and mineral mix (Scientific Hospital Supplies), giving fat, carbohydrate, and protein intakes of 20%, 74%, and 6%, respectively, of total caloric intake. Skin fibroblasts were cultured for later enzyme assay. The patient was discharged home, apparently well, on day 13.

The patient was followed regularly on an outpatient basis. Phenobarbital therapy was discontinued at 1 month of age. Growth was normal except for the head. She remained well, with normal early developmental progress and no clinical evidence of a cardiomyopathy or hepatopathy. When she was 4 months of age, the cultured skin fibroblast fatty acid oxidation results became available and suggested a defect involving medium-chain rather than long-chain fatty acid oxidation. Deficiency of MCAD was quickly confirmed by molecular analysis, which showed her to be homozygous for the common A985G MCAD mutation (Dr. S. Forrest, Murdoch Research Institute, Melbourne, Australia). A normal diet was recommended. Because of low plasma carnitine levels, glycine therapy (200 mg/kg per day) was commenced. A urine sample obtained subsequently for urinary organic acid analysis was then consistent with MCAD deficiency.

At 6 months of age the patient had a focal seizure, which was not associated with fever, alteration of feedings, or an acute illness. Blood chemistry values were normal, and no cause of the seizure was found. When the patient was last seen at 11 months of age, developmental progress was normal and weight and length were between the 50th and 75th percentiles, but head circumference had decreased from the 75th to the 2nd percentile. Physical examination findings, including neuromuscular assessment, were otherwise unremarkable. A skull x-ray study showed no abnormalities; a computed tomographic scan of the head showed mild cerebral atrophy. The patient has had no further episodes of hypoglycemia or encephalopathy.

The patient's sister, now aged 4 years, has enjoyed good health. Both she and her parents are heterozygous for the A985G MCAD mutation.

METHODS

Urinary organic acids and acylglycines. Trimethylsilyl derivatives of urinary organic acids were analyzed by capillary gas chromatography–mass spectrometry on a Hewlett-Packard MSD system using an HP1 column. Derivatized urine was applied to the column according to the creatinine value. Hexanoylglycine was estimated with postscan data acquired from the analysis of the urinary organic acid profile. The combined areas of three characteristic ions of the two trimethylsilyl derivatives, and the area of the characteristic ion for the internal standard, were obtained. The amount of HGL present was calculated by comparison with areas obtained in an HGL control sample.

Plasma carnitine. Total and free carnitines in plasma were estimated by using [1-^{14}C]acetyl–coenzyme A and carnitine acetyltransferase.[5]

Cultured fibroblast fatty acid oxidation assay. Fibroblast culture and the assay conditions for determination of ^3H_2O release from [9,10-^{3}H]myristic and [9,10-^{3}H]palmitic acids in intact cells were substantially those of Manning et al.[6] The enhanced protocol of the Pierce bicinchoninic acid (BCA) protein assay (Pierce Chemical Co., Rockford, Ill.) was performed on the fibroblasts from each microtiter well.[7] The cells had been digested with sodium hydroxide, 2 mol/L, and neutralized before protein analysis.

RESULTS

Urinary organic acids and acylglycines. Initial urinary organic acid analysis on day 2 (Figure) showed large amounts of hexanedioate (adipate), moderate amounts of lactate, 3-hydroxybutyrate, acetoacetate, octanedioate (suberate), decanedioate (sebacate), octenedioate, decenedioate, and 3-hydroxydecanedioate. The octanedioylglycine (suberylglycine) concentration was slightly elevated. The hexanoylglycine concentration, though estimated at 6 μmol/mmol creatinine, was thought not to be significantly elevated in the presence of a moderate ketosis; five other neonates with symptoms of MCAD deficiency, previously investigated by us, had urinary HGL values from 13 to 124 μmol/mmol creatinine. Phenylpropionylglycine was not detectable in this sample. Further urinalysis at 5 months of age, when the patient had no symptoms, showed the HGL level to be 74 μmol/mmol creatinine. The octanedioylglycine (suberylglycine) concentration was slightly increased. Phenylpropionylglycine was still not detected, and there were no other abnormalities.

Plasma carnitine. The initial plasma total carnitine level on day 3 was 108 μmol/L (normal range, 35 to 60), and free carnitine was 15 μmol/L (normal range, 30 to 60). Two days later, total and free plasma carnitine values were 10 and 6 μmol/L, respectively. At 1 month of age, total and free plasma carnitine levels had returned to 29 and 24 μmol/L, respectively, without supplementation, but at 8 months were 15 and 11 μmol/L, respectively. Three months after glycine therapy was begun, total and free plasma carnitine values recovered to 27 and 17 μmol/L, respectively.

Cultured skin fibroblast fatty acid oxidation studies. Intact fibroblasts were assayed for patency of the fatty acid

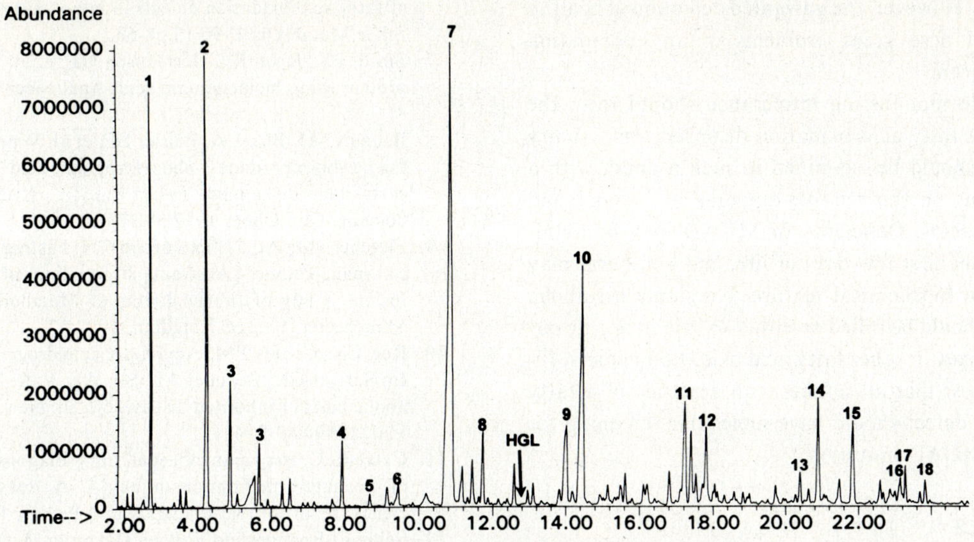

Figure. Urinary organic acid profile of our patient from a sample collected during the neonatal episode and separated on HP1 capillary column. The peaks are the trimethylsilyl derivatives of the following: *1*, lactate; *2*, 3-hydroxybutyrate; *3*, acetoacetate; *4*, 5-hydroxyhexanoate; *5*, glutarate; *6*, 3-hydroxyhexanedioate lactone; *7*, hexanedioate (adipate); *8*, 7-hydroxyoctanoate; *9*, octenedioate (unsaturated suberate); *10*, octanedioate (suberate); *11*, decenedioate (unsaturated sebacate); *12*, decanedioate (sebacate); *13*, 3-hydroxydecenedioate; *14*, 3-hydroxydecanedioate; *15*, internal standard (heptadecanoate); *16*, octanedioylglycine (suberylglycine); *17*, 3-hydroxydodecenedioate; and *18*, 3-hydroxydodecanedioate.

oxidation pathway on three occasions. Tritium release from both 9,10-labeled palmitate and 9,10-labeled myristate was greatly reduced. Release from palmitate was a mean of 19% of three intrabatch controls; release from myristate was a mean of only 3% of the controls. These results suggested mild electron transport flavoprotein deficiency or MCAD deficiency, although the activities found, especially for palmitate, were lower than those which we and others have found in MCAD-deficient patients.

DISCUSSION

The initial urinary findings in our patient were confusing, with prominent ketosis (unusual in the neonatal period and unusual in MCAD deficiency) in association with a pattern suggestive of a defect of long-chain fatty acid β-oxidation. Characteristic metabolites seen in the urine of patients with MCAD deficiency include hexanedioate (adipate), octanedioate (suberate), and decanedioate (sebacate), as well as hexanoylglycine and octanedioylglycine (suberylglycine).[3] Phenylpropionylglycine is not usually found before 4 months of age.[8] Hypoketosis is usual, though total ketone-body production can be nearly normal in unstressed MCAD-deficient patients.[9] In our patient the concentrations of dicarboxylic acids were elevated, and HGL was present but not elevated; in addition, there were a few longer-chain 3-hydroxy derivatives (including 3-hydroxydecanedioate, 3-hydroxydecenedioate, 3-hydroxydodecanedioate, and 3-hydroxydodecenedioate), which are more commonly seen in defects of long-chain fatty acid β-oxidation than in MCAD deficiency. Patients with long-chain fatty acid β-oxidation defects usually have severe liver dysfunction, skeletal myopathy, and cardiomyopathy during acute episodes,[10] which were not evident in our patient at any stage. Cultured skin fibroblast fatty acid oxidation studies in our patient, however, showed much lower activities, but the ratio of palmitate to myristate oxidation was typical of a medium-chain defect; MCAD deficiency was confirmed by mutation analysis.

The development of symptoms in the neonatal period has been described infrequently,[11] but Wilcken et al.[4] recently reported that 6 of 16 infants with MCAD deficiency had significant symptoms within the first 3 days of life. One of these infants died during the first episode; the other five have remained well, apart from one subsequent acute episode in each of four. The unpredictability of the onset and the high mortality rate during the first episode,[10] coupled with its relatively high prevalence,[1] have led some to recommend newborn screening for MCAD deficiency.[12] With the recognition that more than 97% of MCAD-deficient individuals are either heterozygous or homozygous for a common point mutation, a guanosine-to-adenine transversion at position 985 of the MCAD coding sequence,[13] has come the capability to use a simple and sensitive method, based on the polymerase chain reaction, to screen infants for MCAD deficiency.[14, 15] However, the unwanted detection of healthy carriers would pose great problems in any population screening program.

We conclude that fasting intolerance should raise the possibility of a fatty acid oxidation disorder, and urinary organic acids should be examined in such a child, with a particular focus on the relative amounts of ketones and other organic acids. Deficiency of MCAD may be manifested within the first few days of life, and ketonuria may be a prominent biochemical feature. No single metabolic intermediate should be relied on either to rule in or rule out MCAD deficiency or other fatty acid oxidation defects. Finally, we suggest that all infants with evidence of a fatty acid oxidation defect should have molecular screening for the common MCAD mutation.

REFERENCES

1. Matsubara Y, Narisawa K, Tada K. Medium-chain acyl-CoA dehydrogenase deficiency: molecular aspects. Eur J Pediatr 1992;151:154-9.
2. Touma EH, Charpentier C. Medium-chain acyl-CoA dehydrogenase deficiency. Arch Dis Child 1992;67:142-5.
3. Hale DE, Bennett MJ. Fatty acid oxidation disorders: a new class of metabolic diseases. J PEDIATR 1992;121:1-11.
4. Wilcken B, Carpenter KH, Hammond J. Neonatal symptoms in medium-chain acyl coenzyme A dehydrogenase deficiency. Arch Dis Child 1993;69:292-4.
5. de Sousa C, English NR, Stacey TE, Chalmers RA. Measurement of L-carnitine and acylcarnitines in body fluids and tissues in children and adults. Clin Chim Acta 1990;187:317-28.
6. Manning NJ, Olpin SE, Pollitt RJ, Webley J. Comparison of [9,10-^{3}H]palmitic and [9,10-^{3}H] myristic acids for detection of fatty acid oxidation defects in intact cultured fibroblasts. J Inher Metab Dis 1990;13:58-68.
7. Smith PK, Krhn RI, Hermanson GT, et al. Measurement of protein using bicinchoninic acid. Anal Biochem 1985;150:76-85.
8. Bennett MJ, Bhala A, Poirier SF, et al. When do gut flora in the newborn produce 3-phenylpropionic acid? implications for early diagnosis of medium-chain acyl-CoA dehydrogenase deficiency. Clin Chem 1992;38:278-81.
9. Fletcher JM, Pitt JJ, Thompson GN. Fasting MCAD patients can make ketones [Abstract]. Proceedings of the 31st Society for the Study of Inborn Errors of Metabolism Symposium, Manchester, United Kingdom, 1993:57.
10. Roe CR, Coates PM. Acyl-CoA dehydrogenase deficiencies. In: Scriver CR, Beaudet AL, Sly WS, Valle D, eds. The metabolic basis of inherited disease. 6th ed. New York: McGraw-Hill, 1989:889-914.
11. Catzeflis C, Bachmann C, et al. Early diagnosis and treatment of neonatal medium-chain acyl-CoA dehydrogenase deficiency: report of two siblings. Eur J Pediatr 1990;149:577-81.
12. Schmidt-Sommerfeld E, Penn D, Duran M, et al. Detection of inborn errors of fatty acid oxidation from acylcarnitine analysis of plasma and blood spots with the radioisotopic exchange–high-performance liquid chromotographic method. J PEDIATR 1993;122:708-14.
13. Workshop on Molecular Aspects of MCAD Deficiency. Mutations causing medium-chain acyl-CoA dehydrogenase deficiency: a collaborative compilation of the data from 172 patients. In: Coates PM, Tanaka K, eds. New developments in fatty acid oxidation. New York: Wiley-Liss, 1992:499-506.
14. Matsubara Y, Narisawa K, Tada K, et al. Prevalence of K329E mutation in medium-chain acyl-CoA dehydrogenase gene determined from Guthrie cards. Lancet 1991;338:552-3.
15. Christodoulou J, Clarke JTR, Rupar CA, Gordon BA, Kelly DP. Retrospective diagnosis of medium-chain acyl-CoA dehydrogenase deficiency. J Paediatr Child Health 1993;29:237-8.

Transient organic aciduria and persistent lacticacidemia in a patient with short-chain acyl–coenzyme A dehydrogenase deficiency

D. Brian Dawson, PhD, Lewis Waber, MD, PhD, Daniel E. Hale, MD, and Michael J. Bennett, PhD, MRCPath

From the Departments of Pathology and Pediatrics, University of Texas Southwestern Medical Center, Dallas, and the Department of Pediatrics, Children's Hospital of Philadelphia, Pennsylvania

A neonate with signs of neurologic dysfunction was noted to have elevated blood lactic acid levels. Organic acid analysis revealed transient elevations in ethylmalonate, methylsuccinate, butyrylglycine, and butyrylcarnitine. Enzyme assay in cultured skin fibroblasts confirmed short-chain acyl coenzyme A dehydrogenase deficiency. The intermittent nature of the characteristic metabolic markers for this deficiency make diagnosis difficult. The apparent rarity of the disorder may be the result of underdiagnosis. (J Pediatr 1995;126:69-71)

Under prolonged fasting conditions, oxidation of fatty acids provides the primary source of energy for maintaining metabolic homeostasis. Enzymatic and transport protein defects within the fatty acid oxidation pathway are associated with high mortality and morbidity rates. Signs and symptoms noted during fasting include muscle weakness, organ fat deposition, and lethargy. The biochemical abnormalities frequently include hypoketotic hypoglycemia, changes in plasma or tissue carnitine and acylcarnitine values, hyperammonemia, acidosis, and dicarboxylic aciduria.[1] This acute metabolic decompensation enhances excretion of abnormal urinary metabolites. Therefore organic acid analysis of urine samples collected while the patient has symptoms provides a transient opportunity to make a diagnosis.[2]

Short-chain acyl coenzyme A dehydrogenase deficiency is a deficiency of the last cycle of fatty acid oxidation, and is specific for fatty acids of chain length 4 to 6.[3] Only four cases of confirmed systemic SCAD deficiency have been reported[4-6]; thus either the defect is very uncommon or the diagnosis is difficult to establish. The metabolic markers in the urine of patients with SCAD deficiency include elevated ethylmalonate, methylsuccinate, butyrylcarnitine, and butyrylglycine.[4-5, 7] We describe the intermittent elevation of all of these markers in a child with SCAD deficiency in whom the only consistent biochemical finding was an elevated blood lactate concentration.

CASE REPORT

A black male infant with a birth weight of 3.55 kg was delivered without complications. On day 1 of life hypertonicity, staring spells, and jitteriness were noted. Results of studies to detect sepsis were negative, as was the result of a drug screen performed on a meconium sample. An initial electroencephalogram was interpreted as abnormal, but subsequent electroencephalograms and results of a magnetic resonance image study were normal. A plasma lactic acid level was 4.7 mmol/L (reference range, 0.3 to 1.3 mmol/L). Lactic acid levels ranged from 1.5 to 7.3 mmol/L during the first week. Organic acid analysis of urine collected on day 2 of life revealed elevated concentrations of ethylmalonate, methylsuccinate, and butyrylglycine (Table). The infant was fed a standard formula with added corn oil and was discharged home on day 7. Lactic acid values continued to be elevated.

On day 14 the infant was referred to Children's Medical Center of Dallas for further evaluation. Slight hypertonia and hyperreflexia were noted. Blood gas, β-hydroxybutyrate, and ammonia

See related article, p. 65.

CoA	Coenzyme A
ETF	Electron transfer flavoprotein
SCAD	Short-chain acyl-CoA dehydrogenase

Submitted for publication May 10, 1994; accepted July 19, 1994.

Reprint requests: D. Brian Dawson, PhD, Department of Pathology, University of Texas Southwestern Medical Center, 5323 Harry Hines Blvd., Dallas, TX 75235-9072.

0022-3476/95/$3.00 + 0 **9/22/59278**

Table. Quantitative urinary organic acid and blood lactic acid values in our patient

Compound	Values at specified ages: 6 days (symptoms)	15 days (symptoms)	6 mo (no symptoms)	7 mo (no symptoms)	30 mo (no symptoms)	Reference values*
Ethylmalonate	3900	1460	25	16	175	0-18
Methylsuccinate	630	180	10	<10	215	0-8
Glutarate	<10	130	<10	<10	<10	0-10
Adipate	640	150	<10	<10	<10	0-46
Suberate	600	<10	<10	<10	<10	0-34
Unsaturated suberate	530	<10	<10	<10	<10	ND
Sebacate	160	<10	<10	<10	<10	0-22
Butyrylglycine	0.44	1.09	ND	ND	ND	ND
Lactate (mmol/L; nonfasting state)	4.1 (9 day) (reference range, 0.3-1.3)	9.9 (12 days)	5.2	2.7	2.1	0.7-2.3 (fasting)

ND, Not detected.
Units are expressed as millimoles per mole creatinine measured by selected ion monitoring. Limits of detection (five times the baseline value) = 10 mmol/mol creatinine, except butyryl glycine = 0.1 mmol/mol creatinine.
*Sweetman L (personal communication, June 1994).

values were normal; the plasma lactate concentration was 4.1 mmol/L. Organic acid analysis revealed elevated ethylmalonate, methylsuccinate, and glutarate concentrations, consistent with either SCAD deficiency or a multiple acyl-CoA dehydrogenation defect (glutaric aciduria type II). The absence of elevated hexanoylglycine and suberylglycine would rule out glutaric aciduria type II. The patient was given riboflavin therapy (200 mg/day) in the hope that large doses of the vitamin might enhance residual enzyme activity. Carnitine therapy, 50 mg/kg per day, was initiated to correct any intramitochondrial free CoA deficiency and to enhance butyrylcarnitine excretion. The medications were tolerated well except for the riboflavin, which the infant often spit out because of its bitter taste. Follow-up plasma lactate values were 7.3 and 9.9 mmol/L. To minimize the production of butyryl-CoA, we planned for the patient a low-fat diet (calculated to provide 20% of total calories), with essential fatty acids, the recommended daily allowance for protein, and the remainder of the dietary calories as carbohydrate. The parents were instructed to feed the child every 3 to 4 hours to minimize fatty acid oxidation from fasting. The total plasma carnitine concentration was within normal limits, but an acylcarnitine profile revealed an elevated butyrylcarnitine concentration consistent with SCAD deficiency (Dr. D. Millington, Duke University Medical Center Durham, N.C.). Enzyme assay in cultured fibroblasts using butyryl-CoA as substrate indicated a decreased value of 0.98 nmol ETF reduced per minute per milligram protein for the patient, compared with 2.10 nmol ETF reduced per minute per milligram protein for the control cell line (reference values, 2.20 ± 0.24 nmol ETF reduced per minute per milligram protein; n = 126). The SCAD deficiency was confirmed by the addition of anti–medium-chain acyl-CoA dehydrogenase antibody (courtesy Dr. A. W. Strauss, Washington University, St. Louis, Mo.) to the assay, which resulted in values of 0.07 and 0.77 nmol ETF reduced per minute per milligram protein for the patient and for the control cell line, respectively.

A pruritic, excoriated papular rash of unknown origin subsequently developed and covered the patient's face, cheeks, arms, and trunk. The rash was managed with application of a gentle skin cleanser every other day, no use of soap, applications of 1% hydrocortisone cream to the face only, triamcinolone 0.025% ointment to the extremities twice a day, and a dry skin care ointment applied twice a day after the application of hydrocortisone and triamcinolone. The fatty acid content and composition of the patient's diet were modified without noticeable effects on the rash. The patient continued to receive L-carnitine, riboflavin, and a low-fat diet until he was 12 months of age; he had no serious illnesses but did have a few recurrences of staring spells. When he was 1 year of age, his parents changed medical providers and discontinued the riboflavin and carnitine supplements and the special diet. When he was 18 months old, the skin rash disappeared. Contact was reestablished when the child was 30 months of age. No serious illnesses or hospitalizations had been recorded. Several colds and other minor infections were noted. Physical examination findings were noncontributory. The patient was walking and beginning to talk in sentences. Laboratory values were as follows: total serum carnitine, 30 μmol/L (47 ± 11 μmol/L); free carnitine, 18 μmol/L (38 ± 11 μmol/L); and short-chain acylcarnitines, 12 μmol/ml (9 ± 5 μmol/L). Analysis of urinary organic acids showed elevated concentrations of ethylmalonate and methylsuccinate and no detectable butyrylglycine by selected ion monitoring (Table). A nonfasting lactic acid level (2.1 mmol/L) was near the upper end of the reference range for normal, fasting individuals.

RESULTS

The Table summarizes the quantitative urinary organic acids and blood lactic acid values. Lactate concentration was consistently elevated during the first 7 months. However, the urinary excretion of ethylmalonate, methylsuccinate, and butyrylglycine was not persistently excessive. The diagnosis of SCAD deficiency would not have been made on the basis of analysis of the urine specimens collected at 6 and 7 months of age. A recently obtained urinary organic acid analysis revealed elevated ethylmalonate and methylsuccinate values; the lactate level was again near the upper end of the normal range.

DISCUSSION

We report the fifth case of SCAD deficiency in the neonatal period. The clinical features were primarily neurologic and were not related to those of fasting intolerance. Neurologic signs appear to be a consistent feature of SCAD deficiency, perhaps because of an intracellular accumulation of short-chain volatile intermediates. Although the first urine specimens collected from our patient contained the metabolites predicted for SCAD deficiency, with abnormal elevations of medium-chain dicarboxylic acids consistent with the newborn period,[8] on a number of occasions we could not detect the presence of excess metabolites in the urine. These results emphasize the need for collection of urine samples when the patient has symptoms so that the proper diagnosis can be made, as noted by Sewell et al.[6] The presence of persistent lactic acidemia in our patient indicates that an incorrect diagnosis of a primary lactic acidemia may be made in many cases and that such patients should be reexamined by enzymatic assay for SCAD. Our patient had initial symptoms that differed from those of other patients with SCAD deficiency. A review of published cases led us to expect a poor prognosis and prompted what we regarded as maximal therapy for his disorder. When the patient responded to therapy, all treatment modalities were continued. Disappearance of the biochemical markers consistent with the disorder provided confidence in the prescribed therapy and a reluctance to discontinue any part of that regimen. Now that the child has had no therapy for 18 months without demonstrable sequelae, whether treatment had any positive effect on the clinical course is uncertain. This case may indicate that therapeutic intervention may not drastically influence the outcome of SCAD deficiency. Whether the clinical course in patients with a more severe phenotype could be altered is unknown. However, in a maturing central nervous system, a decrease in sensitivity to short-chain fatty acids as the blood-brain barrier develops and increases in efficiency cannot be ruled out. For rare disorders of unknown variability, reliable evaluation of therapeutic efficacy must rely on proper clinical trials and not on individual case reports.

The gene for SCAD is located on chromosome 12[9] and codes for a tetrameric mitochondrial flavoprotein.[10, 11] Defects within the gene appear to be heterogeneous, which makes development of a simple DNA-based screening assay unlikely.[1] This emphasizes the need to obtain proper functional, enzymatic assessment to establish the diagnosis. The perception that SCAD deficiency is a rare condition may be a result of underdiagnosis because of the intermittent nature of metabolite excretion plus the presence of neurologic abnormalities, rather than because of the fasting hypoglycemia that is encountered in other fatty acid oxidation disorders.

This case illustrates the utility of performing repeated testing of patients in whom the clinical course suggests an underlying metabolic defect. The yield may be small, but when children have unusual symptoms that are not explained well by more common diagnoses, appropriate metabolic investigation is indicated.

REFERENCES

1. Hale DE, Bennett MJ. Fatty acid oxidation disorders: a new class of metabolic diseases. J PEDIATR 1992;121:1-11.
2. Bennett MJ. The laboratory diagnosis of inborn errors of fatty acid oxidation. Ann Clin Biochem 1990;27:519-31.
3. Furuta S, Miyazawa S, Hashimoto T. Purification and properties of rat liver acyl-CoA dehydrogenases and electron transfer flavoprotein. J Biochem 1981;90:1739-50.
4. Amendt BA, Greene C, Sweetman L, et al. Short-chain acyl-CoA dehydrogenase deficiency. J Clin Invest 1987;79:1303-9.
5. Coates PM, Hale DE, Finocchiaro G, Tanaka K, Winter SC. Genetic deficiency of short-chain acyl-coenzyme A dehydrogenase in cultured fibroblasts from a patient with muscle carnitine deficiency and severe muscular weakness. J Clin Invest 1988;81:171-5.
6. Sewell AC, Herwig J, Bohles H, Rinaldo P, Bhala A, Hale DE. A new case of short-chain acyl-CoA dehydrogenase deficiency with isolated ethylmalonic aciduria. Eur J Pediatr 1993; 152:922-4.
7. Turnbull DM, Bartlett K, Stevens DL, et al. Short-chain acyl-CoA dehydrogenase deficiency associated with a lipid storage myopathy and secondary carnitine deficiency. N Engl J Med 1984;311:1233-6.
8. Downing M, Rose P, Bennett MJ, Pollitt RJ. Generalised dicarboxylic aciduria as a common finding in neonates. J Inherit Metab Dis 1989;12(suppl 2):321-4.
9. Barton DE, Yang-Feng TL, Finocchiaro G, Ozasa H, Tanaka K, Francke U. Short-chain acyl-CoA dehydrogenase (ACADS) maps to chromosome 12 (q22-qter) and electron transfer flavoprotein (ETFA) to 15 (q23-q25). Cytogenet Cell Genet 1987;46:577.
10. Ikeda Y, Okamura-Ikeda K, Tanaka K. Purification and characterization of short-chain, medium-chain, and long-chain acyl-CoA dehydrogenases from rat liver mitochondria. J Biol Chem 1985;260:1311-25.
11. Finocchiaro G, Ito M, Tanaka K. Purification and properties of short chain acyl-CoA, medium chain acyl-CoA, and isovaleryl-CoA dehydrogenases from human liver. J Biol Chem 1987;262:7982-9.
12. Naito E, Indo Y, Tanaka K. Identification of two variant short chain acyl-coenzyme A dehydrogenase alleles, each containing a different point mutation in a patient with short chain acyl-coenzyme A dehydrogenase deficiency. J Clin Invest 1990; 85:1575-82.

Congenital lacticacidemia caused by lipoamide dehydrogenase deficiency with favorable outcome

O. N. Elpeleg, MD, W. Ruitenbeek, PhD, C. Jakobs, PhD, V. Barash, PhD, D. C. De Vivo, MD, and N. Amir, MD

From the Metabolic and Neuropediatric Units, Shaare-Zedek Medical Center, Jerusalem, Israel, the Department of Pediatrics, University Hospital, Nijmegen, The Netherlands, the Department of Pediatrics, Free University Hospital, Amsterdam, The Netherlands, the Department of Clinical Biochemistry, Hadassah Medical Center, Jerusalem, Israel, and the Department of Neurology, Columbia Presbyterian Medical Center, New York, New York

A 5-year-old boy had recurrent vomiting and lethargy with lacticacidemia and ketoacidemia since birth. Lipoamide dehydrogenase deficiency was found in muscle and fibroblasts. Therapy with sodium dichloroacetate, thiamine, and carnitine was associated with reduction of the severity and frequency of the decompensation episodes and near normal plasma lactate levels. At 5 years of age, the patient has normal cognitive function and moderate motor impairment. (J Pediatr 1995;126:72-4)

Inborn errors of metabolism associated with combined lacticacidemia and ketoacidemia usually cause life-threatening metabolic decompensation in infancy. In many cases the primary enzymatic defect can be localized to the pyruvate dehydrogenase complex or to the mitochondrial respiratory chain. The most common defect in the PDHC resides in its E1 subunit; deficiency of the E3 subunit (lipoamide dehydrogenase) has been reported in only a few patients,[1-5] whose clinical course was characterized by progressive neurologic deterioration; most died during early childhood.

We describe a 5-year-old boy with LAD deficiency who has been treated for the past 3 years with sodium dichloroacetate, thiamine, and carnitine. His cognitive functions were age appropriate, but his motor development was moderately impaired.

CASE REPORT

A 7-month-old boy was admitted because of refusal to eat and recurrent vomiting for 24 hours. He was the third child of nonconsanguineous Ashkenazi-Jewish parents. Two older sisters were healthy. He was born in another hospital after an uneventful pregnancy and delivery; birth weight was 4000 gm. He had an episode of tachypnea and vomiting 12 hours after birth, with a plasma lactate concentration of 7.0 mmol/L (normal, <2.4 mmol/L) and total ketone bodies of 1.27 mmol/L (normal, <0.24 mmol/L). Thereafter he was hospitalized every 6 to 8 weeks for loss of appetite, recurrent vomiting, and hyperlactatemia (Figure). Thiamine, riboflavin, coenzyme Q, and biotin were given for a suspected mitochondrial disorder. None of these agents had reduced the frequency of the attacks.

Physical examination revealed tachycardia, tachypnea, pallor, hepatomegaly, and muscle hypotonia. Blood pH was 7.15, partial pressure of carbon dioxide 19 mm Hg, plasma lactate concentration 9.8 mmol/L, and total ketone bodies 6.61 mmol/L. Plasma carnitine concentration was 21.8 μmol/L (normal, ≥ 30 μmol/L). Serum aspartate aminotransferase activity was 10,000 IU/L (normal, < 50 IU/L), alanine aminotransferase 12,000 IU/L (normal, < 56 IU/L), and prothrombin time 40% of the control value. Creatine kinase activity was normal. Plasma amino acid values were normal except for an increased alanine concentration. Cerebrospinal fluid lactate concentration was 1.4 mmol/L. Abdominal ultrasonography revealed liver and kidneys of normal size. Findings of echocardiography and cranial computed tomography were normal. The patient gradually improved after intravenous administration of glucose and Na bicarbonate solution. However, when he was clinically well, plasma lactate concentration and ketone bodies remained elevated. Open muscle biopsy was performed with the patient under general anesthesia, and muscle tissue was obtained from the right quadriceps. Electron microscopic findings, including mitochondrial size and shape, were normal. The main portion was immediately frozen at −70° C for enzymatic analysis.

Similar episodes during the following 2 months were accompa-

DCA	Sodium dichloroacetate
LAD	Lipoamide dehydrogenase
NADH	Nicotinamide adenine dinucleotide (reduced form)
PDHC	Pyruvate dehydrogenase complex

Submitted for publication March 17, 1994; accepted Aug. 24, 1994.

Reprint requests: Orly N. Elpeleg, MD, Metabolic Unit, Shaare-Zedek Medical Center, Jerusalem 91031, Israel.

0022-3476/95/$3.00 + 0 **9/22/60180**

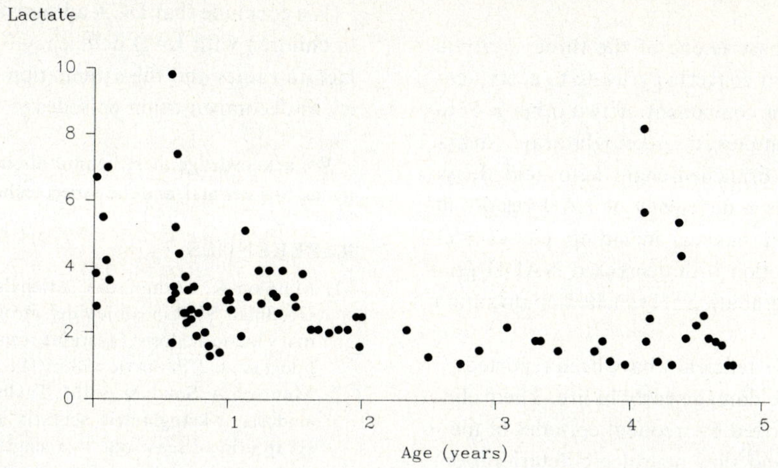

Figure. Lactate concentration (in millimoles per liter) as a function of year of life. Therapy was started at 9 months of age. The increased lactate concentrations after 4 years of age were associated with the discontinuation of DCA administration.

nied by moderate neurologic deterioration with severe generalized hypotonia and inability to sit unsupported. A therapeutic trial with DCA, carnitine, thiamine, lipoic acid, Na succinate, and restriction of branched-chain amino acids was initiated. This regimen was associated with normalization of plasma lactate values, but plasma ketones remained elevated.

Since 2 years of age the patient had been treated with DCA, thiamine, and carnitine. In addition to his regular oral intake, supplementary nasogastric feeding was maintained because of periods of anorexia. During the second year he had only four episodes of recurrent vomiting in association with elevated liver transaminase values, moderate hyperketonemia, and nearly normal plasma lactate levels. No such episodes were noted thereafter. Repeated attempts since 4 years of age to reduce DCA dosage to less than 25 to 30 mg/kg every 12 hours resulted in hyperlactatemia (Figure). At 5 years, the patient's weight was at the 50th percentile, length at the 75th percentile, and head circumference at the 50th percentile. The patient had hepatomegaly and general muscular hypotonia. He walked freely on a broad base, comprehension was age appropriate, and he spoke fluently. Cranial computed tomography, electroencephalography, electromyography, nerve conduction velocity, visual evoked potentials, electroretinography, electrocardiography, echocardiography, and abdominal ultrasonography, performed every year, showed results within the normal range.

METHODS

Plasma lactate levels were determined in 15 samples before therapy was started and in 66 samples during therapy. Urinary organic acids were identified with a Hewlett-Packard 5970 mass selective detector as previously described.[6]

In muscle homogenate, the activities of rotenone-sensitive NADH:ubiquinone oxidoreductase, antimycine-sensitive succinate:cytochrome *c* oxidoreductase, cytochrome *c* oxidase, citrate synthase, PDHC, the E1 subunit, LAD, and α-ketoglutarate dehydrogenase complex were determined according to previously described methods.[7, 8] In sonicated fibroblasts, the activities of PDHC, LAD, and α-ketoglutarate dehydrogenase complex were determined as previously described.[9, 10]

Dichloroacetic acid, succinic acid (Sigma Chemical Co., St. Louis, Mo.), and lipoic acid (Astra Pharma, Frankfurt, Germany) were converted to their sodium salt (pH 5.0 to 7.0) with sodium hydroxide. These drugs were administered orally after Ministry of Health approval and informed parental consent.

RESULTS

Mean plasma lactate concentrations were significantly lower after therapy (2.4 ± 0.9 mmol/L) than before (4.8 ± 2.1 mmol/L) (Figure).

On admission, urinary organic acid analysis revealed elevated lactic, β-hydroxybutyric, α-ketoglutaric, and α-ketoadipic acid levels (11.63, 1.47, 4.14, and 0.27 mol/mol creatinine, respectively). After introduction of therapy, only mild organic aciduria was found (0.18, 0.04, 0.94, and 0.15 mol/mol creatinine, respectively).

In muscle, PDHC activity was 0.51 mU/gm wet weight, LAD 11.0 mU/gm, and α-ketoglutarate dehydrogenase complex 0.54 mU/gm (control values, 5.0 ± 1.8, 101 ± 26, and 3.8 ± 1.2 mU/gm, respectively). The activities of the other enzymes were within the normal range. In fibroblasts, the activity of PDHC was 14.1 nmol/hr per milligram of protein, LAD 235 nmol/hr per milligram, and α-ketoglutarate dehydrogenase complex 14.4 nmo/hr per milligram (control values, 23.4 ± 3.0, 2334 ± 288, and 22.2 ± 4.8 nmol/hr per milligram of protein, respectively).

DISCUSSION

Lipoamide dehydrogenase is one of the three catalytic proteins of the PDHC that converts pyruvate to acetyl–coenzyme A. LAD is also a component of two other α-keto acid dehydrogenase complexes: α-ketoglutarate dehydrogenase complex and branched-chain keto acid dehydrogenase complex. Thus a deficiency of LAD results in extensive metabolic disturbances, including lacticacidemia, Krebs cycle dysfunction with decreased NADH production, and impaired degradation of branched-chain amino acids.

Five patients with LAD deficiency have been reported.[1-5] All had severe neurologic damage early in life. Their clinical course was characterized by frequent episodes of metabolic decompensation and slow neurologic deterioration. Therapy with thiamine, glutamine, biotin, lipoic acid, restriction of branched-chain amino acids, and a low-carbohydrate, high-fat diet did not seem to influence their neurologic course; only lipoic acid was reported to be of some biochemical benefit. Three patients died at 7 to 21 months of age, and two remained severely retarded.

For the past 3 years our patient has been treated with DCA, thiamine, and carnitine. During this period the frequency and severity of his decompensation episodes decreased markedly, and his plasma lactate concentration was maintained at nearly normal levels. No adverse effects of this therapy have been observed, and at 5 years of age his cognitive functions were age appropriate, whereas his motor development was moderately impaired. The reason for this favorable outcome is unclear. DCA is effective in lowering plasma lactate levels, but its administration has not been associated with improvement of preexisting neurologic damage.[11] Our patient had only mild neurologic impairment when therapy was initiated. In view of the normal level of cerebrospinal fluid lactate and the normal results on neuroimaging and neurophysiologic studies, the possibility of a high residual LAD activity in the central nervous system cannot be excluded. We speculate that the main contribution of this therapy was preventive, by reducing the frequency and severity of the decompensation episodes. In previously described patients with LAD deficiency, such events worsened preexisting neurologic damage.[4, 5]

We conclude that DCA administration may be of benefit in children with LAD deficiency for the control of plasma lactate values and the attenuation of frequency and severity of decompensation episodes.

We acknowledge most helpful discussions with Prof. C. Bachmann, Switzerland, and the expert technical assistance of E. Chen.

REFERENCES

1. Matalon R, Stumpf DA, Michals K, Hart RD, Parks JK, Goodman SI. Lipoamide dehydrogenase deficiency with primary lactic acidosis: favorable response to treatment with oral lipoic acid. J PEDIATR 1983;104:65-9.
2. Munnich A, Saudubray JM, Taylor J, et al. Congenital lactic acidosis, α-ketoglutaric aciduria and variant form of maple syrup urine disease due to a single enzyme defect: dihydrolipoyl dehydrogenase deficiency. Acta Paediatr Scand 1982; 71:167-71.
3. Robinson BH, Taylor J, Sherwood WG. Deficiency of dihydrolipoyl dehydrogenase (a component of the pyruvate and α-ketoglutarate dehydrogenase complexes): a cause of congenital chronic lactic acidosis in infancy. Pediatr Res 1977; 11:1198-202.
4. Robinson BH, Taylor J, Kahler SG, Kirkman HN. Lactic acidemia, neurological deterioration and carbohydrate dependence in a girl with dihydrolipoyl dehydrogenase deficiency. Eur J Pediatr 1981;136:35-9.
5. Sakaguchi Y, Yoshino M, Aramaki S, et al. Dihydrolipoyl dehydrogenase deficiency: a therapeutic trial with branched-chain amino acid restriction. Eur J Pediatr 1986;145:271-4.
6. Elpeleg ON, Havkin S, Barash V, Jakobs C, Glick B, Shalev RS. Familial benign hypotonia of childhood due to isolated 3-methylcrotonyl-CoA carboxylase deficiency. J PEDIATR 1992;121:407-10.
7. Fischer JC, Ruitenbeek W, Gabreels FJM, et al. A mitochondrial myopathy: the first case with an established defect at the level of coenzyme Q. Eur J Pediatr 1986;144:441-4.
8. Sperl W, Ruitenbeek W, Kerkhof CMC, et al. Deficiency of the α and β subunits of pyruvate dehydrogenase in a patient with lactic acidosis and unexpected sudden death. Eur J Pediatr 1990;149:487-92.
9. Robinson BH, Taylor J, Sherwood WG. The genetic heterogeneity of lactic acidosis: occurrence of recognizable inborn errors of metabolism in a pediatric population with lactic acidosis. Pediatr Res 1980;14:956-62.
10. Taylor SI, Mukherjee C, Jungas RL. Studies on the mechanism of activation of adipose tissue pyruvate dehydrogenase by insulin. J Biol Chem 1973;248:73-81.
11. Stacpoole PW. The pharmacology of dichloroacetate. Metabolism 1989;38:1124-44.

Secular changes in the outcomes to eighteen to twenty-four months of age of extremely low birth weight infants, with adjustment for changes in risk factors and severity of illness

Max Perlman, MB, Olivier Claris, MD, Yong Hao, MD, PhD, Paresh Pandit, MB, Hilary Whyte, MB, Mary Chipman, MSc, and Peter Liu, MD

From the Departments of Pediatrics, Preventive Medicine and Biostatistics, and Radiology, University of Toronto and the Hospital for Sick Children, Toronto, Ontario, Canada.

Objectives: **To analyze secular changes in the rates of death and of major impaired outcome in surviving outborn infants who weighed ≤800 gm at birth and were admitted in 1980 to 1989, with adjustment for changes in risk factors and severity of illness around the time of birth; and to identify changes in these factors that might explain changes in outcomes.**
Design: **Retrospective cohort study with follow-up to a minimum of 18 months of postterm age. After preliminary screening, multivariate models of association between risk/severity of illness factors and outcomes were constructed, validated, and used to adjust outcomes (death and major impairment to 18 to 24 months of age).**
Setting: **Regional neonatal intensive care unit for referral of "outborn" infants.**
Patients: **Two hundred eighty-seven consecutively admitted infants who weighed ≤800 gm at birth (97% follow-up).**
Results: **The death rate during the 1980s did not fall significantly (*p* adjusted for risk factors = 0.115). The major impairment rate fell (odds ratio, 0.24 (95% confidence interval, 0.10, 0.60); *p* = 0.002, adjusted for delivery route and respiratory failure measures), mainly because of a reduced rate of blindness, not attributable to cryotherapy. The risk factors that improved and were possibly related to the reduced impairment rate were blood pH and glucose concentration, and serum sodium concentration in the first 48 hours of life.**
Conclusions: **Despite an increasing selection for referral of less mature and more severely ill outborn babies near the "limit of viability," and despite more aggressive care, the rate of major impairment fell significantly during the 1980s. This trend was enhanced by adjustment for severity of illness. The fall was attributable to a reduced rate of blindness, and was associated with evidence of improved control of physiologic balance after birth. (J PEDIATR 1995;126:75-87)**

Submitted for publication March 11, 1994; accepted Aug. 4, 1994.

Reprint requests: Max Perlman, MB, Department of Pediatrics, University of Toronto, Hospital for Sick Children, 555 University Ave., Toronto, Ontario M5G 1X8, Canada.

0022-3476/95/$3.00 + 0 **9/23/59589**

Historically, the survival of premature infants has steadily increased and the perceived "limit of viability" has fallen. During the 1980s, the expectation that this trend would continue, together with increased regionalization of perinatal care, was associated with important changes in referral patterns. Threatened delivery in the late second trimester in level I and II centers was increasingly a reason for re-

AGA	Appropriate size for gestational age
BW	Birth weight
ELBW	Extremely low birth weight
GA	Gestational age
IVH	Intraventricular hemorrhage
NICU	Neonatal intensive care unit
Pa_{O_2}	Partial pressure of arterial oxygen
P_{CO_2}	Partial pressure of carbon dioxide
P_{O_2}	Partial pressure of oxygen
SGA	Small for gestational age

ferral to level III centers.[1, 2] At the same time, extremely low birth weight infants (birth weight ≤800 gm) born in level I and II ("outborn" infants), as well as level III centers, received more aggressive but inconsistent resuscitation and referral.[3, 4]

For medical and logistic reasons, only about 60% to 85% of mothers of ELBW infants can be transported to tertiary care centers.[5-7] This leaves a proportion of obligatory outborn infants, with whom we deal. Because of the changes noted above in the perception of viability and in referral patterns, we would expect a selection of outborn ELBW infants with increasingly borderline viability and at high risk of having adverse outcomes. The pertinence of concerns raised about the provision of neonatal intensive care to premature infants near the perceived limit of viability[8, 9] is heightened for outborn infants because of their observed disadvantages compared with inborn infants.[10-13] Thus the secular trends in the outcomes of recently born outborn ELBW infants deserve rigorous evaluation.

Evaluations of these trends usually employ BW or gestational age to define, stratify, and make adjustment for population differences. There is recent evidence in neonates in general and in infants of ≤800 and ≤1500 gm BW that, for avoidance of confounding factors, comparisons of mortality rates should make adjustments for risk factors and measures of severity of illness, as well as for BW.[7, 14-17] To allow adjusted outcome comparisons, models specific to ELBW infants were desirable.

The overall purpose of this study was to determine whether the outcomes of outborn ELBW infants weighing ≤800 gms improved, stabilized, or worsened during the 1980s, a period in which no striking therapeutic innovations were introduced to our neonatal intensive care unit. Specific goals were (1) to describe, analyze, and interpret the changes in the rates of death by 2 years of age, and major impairment at 18 to 24 months postterm age, with adjustment for changes in pertinent risk and severity of illness factors, and (2) to identify the changes in associated risk and severity of illness factors that might explain the observed changes in outcomes during the period of study.

METHODS

Setting. The NICU at the Hospital for Sick Children is a referral center for infants derived from more than 60,000 annual births from about 50 regionalized hospitals. About 90% of deliveries occur within 35 miles of this hospital, and others at distances up to 550 miles. The neonatal transport team, funded by the Province of Ontario since 1977, transports by ambulance, helicopter, or fixed-wing aircraft.

Referral patterns changed during the period of study because of several changes in regionalization and in attitudes to resuscitation of tiny infants. A second perinatal center, including a newly established NICU, began to accept maternal referrals for extreme prematurity in 1982. The resuscitation of tiny infants and their referral to our NICU became more active in 1982, fostered by the recommendation of a coroner's inquest to hospitals in our region to consult immediately with the tertiary care center about the birth of premature infants.[18] In addition, the number of pediatricians with at least 1 year of additional training in our neonatology program serving in our regional hospitals increased by about 15 in the 1980s, compared with less than 5 in the 1970s. In 1985 to 1989 there was an approximate 2.5-fold increase in the numbers of maternal referrals resulting in the birth of ELBW infants in the two regional level III perinatal centers ("inborn" infants), compared with 1980 to 1984. At the same time, the number of referrals to our level III regional outborn NICU fell by 22%. There was an overall approximate 1.75-fold increase in the total number of referrals of inborn and outborn infants combined.

There were no striking therapeutic advances during the period of study. Preterm infant feeding formulas were introduced to our NICU in 1983, a manual of guidelines for neonatal care created by staff consensus in 1985, surfactant therapy in October 1989, and cryotherapy for severe retinopathy of prematurity in 1988. Refinements occurred in noninvasive monitoring of blood gases and in the ultrasound diagnosis of patent ductus arteriosus and intracranial lesions.

Study population. The sample consisted of 287 infants admitted between 1980 and 1989. Inclusion criteria were BW ≤800 gm and arrival at our NICU or establishment of care by our transport team before 8 hours of age. Exclusion criteria were multiple congenital anomalies, major single anomalies, death before 8 hours of age, and moribund condition or withholding or withdrawal of respiratory support before or at 8 hours of age. Patients were excluded from analyses after support was withheld or withdrawn.

Withholding or withdrawal of life support. The following criteria were used to define withholding or withdrawal of support (henceforth termed "withdrawal of support") up to 168 hours of age: (1) a progress note written by the respon-

Table I. Comparison of clinical characteristics (categorical) in the three subgroups defined by outcome (N = 287; 9 cases lost to follow-up)

Risk factor	Total cohort (N = 287): No. (% of total)	Deaths (n = 142; 49% of total): No. (% of 142 cases)	Deaths: OR (CI); p	Survivors with major impairment (n = 36; 13% of total): No. (% of 36 cases)	Survivors with major impairment: OR (CI); p	Survivors without major impairment (n = 100; 36% of total): No. (% of 100 cases)	Survivors without major impairment: OR (CI); p
Spontaneous abortion ≥1	99 *(34.5)*	42 *(30)*	0.58 (0.34, 0.97); 0.027	15 *(42)*	0.53 (0.08, 2.78); 0.972	42 *(42)*	1.54 (0.90, 2.63); 0.095
Delivery			0.98 (0.53, 1.83)*		0.18 (0.03, 0.84)*		1.64 (0.87, 3.12)*
Vaginal vertex	149 *(53.6)*	76 *(54)*		21 *(58)*		52 *(52)*	
Vaginal breech	74 *(26.6)*	38 *(27)*	0.994	13 *(36)*	0.031	23 *(23)*	0.224
Cesarean section	55 *(19.8)*	28 *(20)*		2 *(6)*		25 *(25)*	
Bruising	131 *(45.6)*	82 *(58)*	2.44 (1.48, 4.05); 0.000	14 *(39)*	1.18 (0.50, 2.78); 0.677	35 *(35)*	0.46 (0.27, 0.79); 0.002
Air leak (<48 hr)	81 *(40.3)*	41 *(69)*	3.40 (1.57, 7.37); 0.001	7 *(19)*	1.77 (0.57, 5.45); 0.269	12 *(12)*	0.34 (0.15, 0.76); 0.004
Glucose							
Maximal ≥11.1 mmol/L†	54 *(26.9)*	30 *(51)*	3.64 (1.76, 7.57); 0.000	6 *(17)*	0.91 (0.29, 2.75); 0.857	18 *(18)*	0.42 (0.21, 0.87); 0.011
Minimal ≤2.1 mmol/L†	79 *(39.3)*	43 *(73)*	0.76 (0.34, 1.68); 0.462	4 *(11)*	0.27 (0.17, 0.88); 0.015	32 *(32)*	2.21 (1.06, 4.63); 0.022
IVH (≥120 hr)‡ (n = 191)			1.87 (0.81, 4.33); 0.108§		5.09 (1.18, 14.54); 0.000§		6.25 (0.10, 0.59); 0.000§
Absent	79 *(40.9)*	12 *(24)*	0.003‖ (Absent to Grade 4)	15 *(42)*	0.002‖ (Absent to Grade 4)	47 *(47)*	0.004‖ (Absent to Grade 4)
Grade 1-2	77 *(39.9)*	23 *(45)*		8 *(22)*		43 *(43)*	
Grade 3	21 *(10.9)*	4 *(8)*		10 *(28)*		6 *(6)*	
Grade 4	16 *(8.3)*	9 *(18)*		3 *(8)*		4 *(4)*	

Patients who died (n = 142) were compared with survivors to hospital discharge (n = 145), survivors without major impairment (n = 100) were compared with patients who died or survived with major impairment (n = 178), and survivors with major impairment (n = 36) were compared with survivors without major impairment (n = 100). Univariate analyses were by chi-square or Fisher Exact tests.

Italicized numbers in parentheses represent the percentage of infants with the risk or severity of illness factor (denominator is the group or subgroup indicated at the head of the column). Results are expressed as odds ratios (confidence intervals) and *p* values.

OR, Odds ratio; *CI*, confidence interval.

*Compares cesarean section with vaginal delivery.

†Defined as hyperglycemia and hypoglycemia, respectively.

‡Of the nine survivors to hospital discharge who were lost to follow-up, five had no IVH, three had grade 1 to 2 IVH, and one had grade 3 IVH.

§Compares grades 3 and 4 IVH with absent and grades 1 and 2 IVH.

‖Comparison of all four categories in 2 × 4 contingency table.

sible physician indicating intent to withhold or withdraw active treatment or, after the introduction of the hospital's "Do not resuscitate" policy, a signed order in the patient record; (2) failure to respond to documented hypoxia (Po_2 <50 mm Hg) by increasing fraction of inspired oxygen or ventilation pressures or rates, or to documented hypercapnia (Pco_2 >60 mm Hg) by increasing ventilator rate, or to acidosis (pH <7.25) by increasing ventilator rate or by administration of sodium bicarbonate; and (3) any respiratory death of a patient receiving mechanical ventilation at the time of death in whom the peak inspiratory pressure was <30 cm H_2O (the 99th percentile for peak inspiratory pressure in surviving patients was 30 cm H_2O). Data collected before withdrawal of intensive care were included in all analyses, and data collected after withdrawal were excluded from all subsequent analyses.

Risk and severity of illness data. Risk data and data on deaths and early complications of prematurity during the initial hospitalization were collected retrospectively from patient records in the health records department. The data collector was masked to the outcome of survivors but not to deaths. Maternal, obstetric, and neonatal resuscitation and initial stabilization data, and histories taken directly from parents at the time of transfer, were recorded routinely by our neonatal transport team from referring hospital records and staff. Routine NICU nursing records were made hourly. Routine cranial ultrasonography of very low birth weight infants was initiated in 1979. Follow-up data were obtained later from records in the neonatal follow-up clinic.

More than 40 variables were selected for their recognized relevance to outcomes, definability, and availability. Demographic factors included maternal race (white, black, or

Table II. Comparison of clinical characteristics (continuous) of infants of birth weight ≤800 gm in the three subgroups defined by outcome (N = 278; 9 cases lost to follow-up)

Risk factor	Total (N = 287) (n of observations)	Deaths (n = 142) No. (%)*	p	Survivors with major impairment (n = 36) No. (%)†	p	Survivors without major impairment (n = 100) No. (%)‡	p
Gestational age (wk)	282	24.1 (1.7)	0.000	24.4 (1.2)	0.060	24.9 (1.5)	0.000
Apgar score	268	4.8 (2.1)	0.002	5.4 (2.1)	0.406	5.7 (2.0)	0.005
Birth weight (gm)	287	696.6 (75.6)	0.000	680.0 (86.1)	0.120	702.8 (70.6)	0.000
Hemoglobin concentration (gm/dl)	284	13.2 (2.5)	0.001	13.9 (2.3)	0.359	14.4 (2.4)	0.001
Leukocyte count (per mm^3)	283	14.8 (10.4)	0.001	19.9 (19.4)	0.892	19.5 (13.3)	0.029
Platelet count (per mm^3)	269	200 (77)	0.000	250 (115)	0.460	234 (80)	0.032

Patients who died were compared with survivors to hospital discharge, survivors without major impairment were compared with patients who died or survived with major impairment, and survivors with major impairment were compared with survivors without major impairment. Analyses were by the Student t test. Results are expressed as means (SD) and p values.
*Proportion of total 49%.
†Proportion of total 13%.
‡Proportion of total 36%.

other) and maternal age. Reproductive and obstetric risk factors included the number of prior abortions, gravidity, parity, hypertension in pregnancy, rupture of membranes for >12 hours, multiple gestation, maternal fever, foul amniotic fluid, cesarean versus vaginal delivery, and antepartum hemorrhage (defined as any bleeding more than spotting within 7 days of birth, of any cause). Variables reflecting maturity and growth at birth were as follows: GA in completed weeks based on dates and ultrasound study; BW reported by the referring hospital or, when admission weight was outside this weight ±50 gm, defined by the admission weight; fused eye(s); and growth as defined in the Appendix. Condition soon after birth was characterized by 5-minute Apgar score, endotracheal intubation within 5 minutes of birth, and bruising documented as extensive or marked, or at two separate body sites. Severity of illness at 8, 16, 24, and 48 hours was measured by axillary temperature, systolic blood pressure measured by limb cuff and Doppler or by strain gauge connected to an arterial catheter, blood gas values (pH, Pa_{O_2}, Pc_{O_2}) at designated times ±2 hours, and respiratory variables (see Appendix). Hematologic variables included the first hemoglobin concentration and total leukocyte and platelet counts. Blood chemistry variables included maximal serum sodium and potassium concentrations and blood glucose concentrations during the first 48 hours (based on the 75th percentiles derived from our own data, respectively ≥152, ≥7.2, and ≥11.1 mmol/L, defining hypernatremia, hyperkalemia, and hyperglycemia), and the minimal serum sodium and blood glucose concentrations (based on 25th percentiles, respectively ≤135 and ≤2.1 mmol/L, defining hyponatremia and hypoglycemia). Early complications included air leaks in the first 48 hours, defined as interstitial emphysema or free air in chest or abdomen, neonatal seizures in the first 48 hours, and intraventricular hemorrhage (see Appendix).

Outcomes. Follow-up methods and definitions of impairment have been described previously.[19] The Hospital for Sick Children Neonatal Follow-up Clinic has been using standardized procedures with intent to perform outcome studies resulting in a high percentage of follow-up since 1975.[20] Scores on the Bayley Scales of Infant Development were obtained at 18 months of corrected age, with a few exceptions for logistic reasons or in children unable to cooperate, who were tested at 24 months. Death was defined as death before 24 months of chronologic age. Deaths occurring after 3 months of age were described as postponed neonatal deaths. Unannounced late deaths were ascertained by the neonatal follow-up clinic when patients failed to attend. All postponed neonatal deaths were attributable to bronchopulmonary dysplasia (sudden infant death syndrome did not occur in this cohort). Death rates, expressed as percentages, are the number of known deaths by age 24 months divided by the number of admitted patients. Major impairment was defined as including any one of the following: Bayley corrected Mental Development Index ≤68, spastic cerebral palsy of any limb(s) sufficient to delay walking beyond 18 months of corrected age, any degree of athetoid cerebral palsy, severe unilateral or bilateral hearing loss partially corrected with hearing aids, blindness, or hydrocephalus treated with shunt surgery.

Statistical analysis. Comparisons were made between (1) deaths and survivors, (2) survivors with major impairment and survivors without major impairment, (3) survival with-

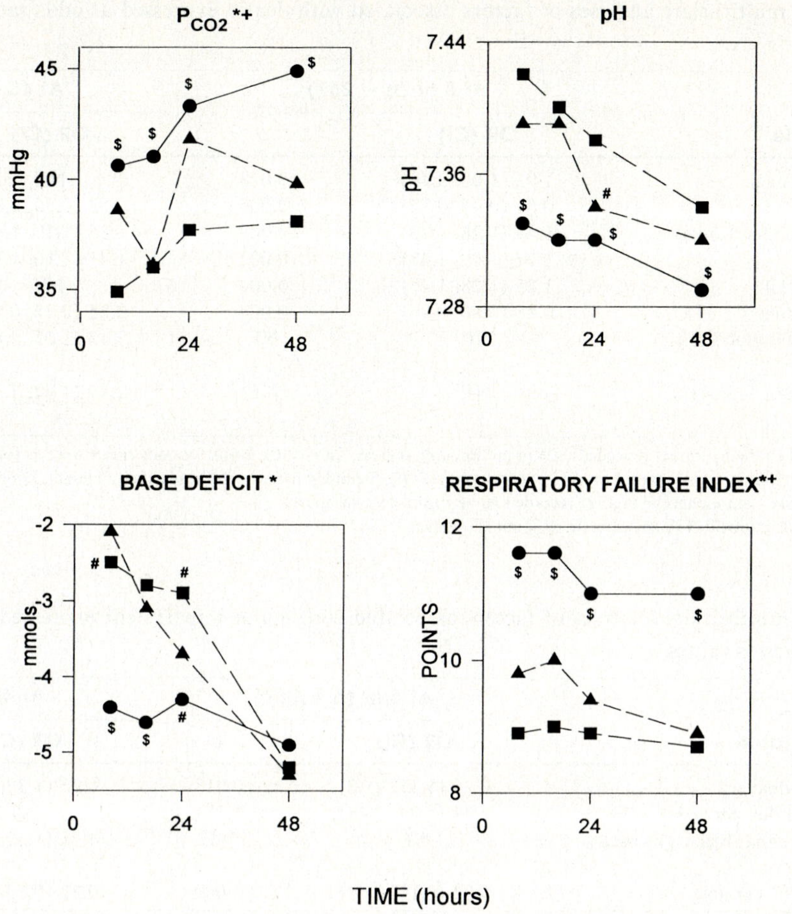

Figure. Mean values of blood gas variables (P_{CO_2}, pH, base deficit) and a respiratory failure index incorporating ventilatory variables, at 8, 16, 24, and 48 hours of age. *Circles* represent patients who died, *triangles* those who had major impairment at 18 or 24 months of corrected age, and *squares* those who survived without major impairment. The symbols beside data points for patients who died or had major impairment represent *p* values of *t* tests comparing the marked measurements with parallel measures of those with good outcome (*dollar sign, p* <0.001; *number sign, p* <0.05 >0.001). The symbols beside the names of severity of illness factors indicate those which were entered into multivariate analyses of death *(asterisk)* and major impairment *(plus sign)*.

out major impairment and death or major impairment, (4) admissions from 1980 to 1984 (period 1) and from 1985 to 1989 (period 2), and (5) small for GA or large for GA infants, and infants whose size was appropriate for GA. Analyses were performed at 8 hours for secular comparisons of outcome rates, and at 48 hours to identify factors that might explain the observed changes in outcomes.

To identify associations between the various factors and each outcome, we performed preliminary univariate analyses (chi-square statistic, odds ratio with 95% confidence intervals, and the two-tailed Student *t* test) at each time point. Variables with *p* values <0.15 in univariate analyses were entered into multivariate logistic regression analyses. A backward elimination procedure was used. Variables staying in final logistic models with *p* <0.05 were regarded as exhibiting independent associations.

Preliminary multivariate analyses for the development of models for adjustment of outcomes. In addition to the univariate analyses described above, the numbers of variables were further reduced by performing preliminary comparative multivariate analyses on the whole cohort to determine the measures that contributed most to multivariate models. Analyses were done with and without BW or GA or both; with and without ventilator rate, arterial/alveolar P_{O_2} ratio (a/A ratio), and/or respiratory failure measures aggregated in a respiratory failure index (Appendix); with and without P_{CO_2}, base deficit, and/or pH; and with and without SGA infants.

Table IIIA. Results of multivariate analyses of factors associated with death, expressed as odds ratios (confidence intervals) and *p* values

Variable	At 8 hr (n = 267)		At 48 hr (n = 190)	
	OR (CI)	*p*	OR (CI)	*p*
Antepartum hemorrhage	1.93 (1.07, 3.48)	0.028	NE	NE
Birth weight (gm)	0.51 (0.37, 0.72)	0.000	0.53 (0.33, 0.85)	0.001
Respiratory failure index (units)	1.49 (1.28, 1.73)	0.000	1.35 (1.10, 1.66)	0.005
P_{CO_2} (mm Hg)	1.27 (1.09, 1.48)	0.003	1.41 (1.16, 1.73)	0.001
Base deficit (mmol/L)	1.25 (1.08, 1.45)	0.004	NS	NS
Platelet count (per mm^3)	0.88 (0.80, 0.96)	0.004	0.85 (0.74, 0.96)	0.011
Hyperglycemia: blood $glucose_{max}$ ≥11.1 mmol/L	NE	NE	3.43 (1.05, 5.87)	0.003
Hypernatremia: serum $sodium_{max}$ ≥152 mmol/L	NE	NE	2.49 (1.52, 7.74)	0.038

Variables were not entered when their *p* values exceeded 0.05 in preliminary analyses (n = 136). Units for odds ratios were as follows: BW, 100 gm increments; respiratory failure index, 1-unit increments (range, 3 to 15; 15 most severe), P_{CO_2}, 5 mm Hg increments; base deficit, 2 mmol/L increments; platelet count, 25,000 increments. The subscript "max" represents the highest recorded value in the first 48 hours.
OR, Odds ratio; *CI*, confidence interval; *NE*, not entered; *NS*, not significant.

Table IIIB. Results of multivariate analyses of factors associated with major impairment expressed as odds ratios (confidence intervals) and *p* values

Variable	At 8 hr (n = 284)		At 48 hr (n = 190)	
	OR (CI)	*p*	OR (CI)	*p*
Vaginal vs cesarean delivery	6.25 (1.37, 25.0)	0.018	6.25 (1.37, 25.0)	0.018
Respiratory failure index per unit	1.24 (1.04, 1.48)	0.016	NS	NS
Absence of hypoglycemia: blood $glucose_{min}$ ≥2.2 mmol/L	NE	NE	4.16 (1.35, 12.5)	0.016
"Period 2 vs period 1" variable	0.24 (0.10, 0.60)	0.002	0.32 (0.13, 0.74)	0.008

Variables were not entered when their *p* values exceeded 0.05 in preliminary analyses (N = 136). Units for odds ratios were as follows: respiratory failure index, 1-unit increments (range, 3 to 15, with 15 most severe), and blood $glucose_{min}$, 1 mmol/L increments. The subscript "min" represents the lowest recorded value in the first 48 hours.
OR, Odds ratio; *CI*, 95% confidence interval; *NS*, not significant; *NE*, not entered.

Multivariate outcome models. Multivariate models were constructed, entering variables determined from the above analyses (see Results section, below). Details of validation procedures by the "split sample" method, with comparison of two groups of subjects randomly selected by computer after stratification into 100 gm BW subgroups, will be provided in a future publication.

Secular comparisons and associations. In addition to univariate comparisons, period comparisons of risk and severity-of-illness factors, as well as outcomes, were performed by multivariate analyses of subcohorts born from 1980 to 1984 and from 1985 to 1989. Because of sample size constraints for major impairment, a "period indicator" variable was added to the whole cohort for analysis of this outcome.

RESULTS

Among 287 infants admitted before 8 hours of age in viable condition, 142 deaths were ascertained by 2 years of age. Twenty-five infants were considered to be nonviable on admission, 10 died by 8 hours of age, and the other 15 were moribund or had withdrawal of support before that age and died between 9 and 41 hours of age. The mean BW and GA of these 25 infants were 619 gm and 23.5 weeks, respectively. Of 9 postponed neonatal deaths, 2 infants died after discharge to their homes and 7 remained in our hospital until their deaths.

Major impairment was present in 36 infants at 18 to 24 months of corrected age, 100 survived without major impairment, and nine were lost to follow-up. One lost patient was later found at 6 years of age, two were last seen at 15 months, and two at 9 months of adjusted age; development was appropriate for age in all areas in all five patients. The only infant in this cohort who received cryotherapy is now legally blind. Of 135 patients followed to at least 18 months of adjusted age, 106 had Bayley scores measured at 18 or 24 months of adjusted age, 19 were ineligible for testing because of blindness or severe cerebral palsy, and 10 eligible patients were not tested for logistic reasons.

Data on race were missing in 10 cases, together with data on intraventricular hemorrhage in 63 of the 92 subjects who died before 120 hours of age. The median age of arrival at our NICU was 5 hours, and all but nine infants were admitted to the NICU by 8 hours of age. The remaining nine infants were in the care of our transport team between 3 and 8 hours of age and were admitted to the NICU at 9 to 13 hours of age. Withdrawal of support was implemented in 66 patients who died, in 59 between 8 and 48 hours, and in 7 between 48 and 168 hours of age. There were 161 eligible cases from 1980 to 1984 and 126 from 1985 to 1989 (periods 1 and 2, respectively).

Preliminary analyses to nominate risk and severity of illness factors

Univariate analyses. The risk characteristics associated with outcomes that had p values <0.05 for at least one of the comparisons are shown in Tables I and II and in the Figure. The results of other variables with p values between 0.15 and 0.05 that were also entered into multivariable analyses are given in the text below.

The following variables were associated with death, with p values ≤ 0.001: at 8 hours of age, marked bruising (Table I), low temperature, low BW, low GA (Table II), low blood pressure, and high base deficit (Figure); at each time point, high measures of severity of respiratory failure, high P_{CO_2}, and low pH (Figure); and at 48 hours, air leak syndrome, high maximal blood sugar concentrations ≥ 2.2 mmol/L (vs blood sugar concentrations <2.2 mmol/L) (Table I), and low platelet count (Table II). Variables associated with death, with p values between 0.15 and 0.05, were male gender ($p = 0.113$), a history of therapeutic abortion(s) ($p = 0.091$), the occurrence of antepartum hemorrhage ($p = 0.088$), absence of foul liquor ($p = 0.109$), presence of fused eye(s) ($p = 0.087$), a maximal serum sodium concentration during the first 48 hours of ≥ 152 mmol/L ($p = 0.058$), a minimal serum sodium concentration during the first 48 hours of <143 mmol/L ($p = 0.071$), and the occurrence of seizures ($p = 0.118$).

None of the variables associated with major impairment had p values <0.001. Those variables with p values ≤ 0.05 at 8 hours of age were vaginal delivery (Table I), high P_{CO_2}, low pH, and high respiratory failure index (Figure), and, at 48 hours, high minimal blood sugar concentrations ≥ 2.2 mmol/L (vs <2.2 mmol/L) (Table I). Birth weight, GA, marked bruising, air leak syndrome, and first platelet count were not associated with major impairment. For infants still alive at 120 hours of age, IVH was strongly associated with both death ($p = 0.003$) and major impairment ($p = 0.002$) (Table I). Variables associated with major impairment with p values between 0.15 and 0.05 were no endotracheal intubation at birth ($p = 0.097$), presence of fused eye(s) ($p = 0.073$), and a maximal serum sodium concentration during the first 48 hours of ≥ 152 mmol/L ($p = 0.139$).

Table IVA. Univariate period comparisons for risk and severity of illness factors: Continuous variables

	1980–1984 Mean (SD)	1985–1989 Mean (SD)	p
GA (wk)	24.7 (1.8)	24.1 (1.6)	0.008
BW (gm)	682 (88)	664 (85)	0.080
Temperature (C)			
At 8 hr	35.5° (1.2°)	35.8° (1.3°)	0.030
At 48 hr	36.4° (0.6°)	36.7° (0.4°)	0.000
Ventilator rate (breaths/min)			
At 8 hr	41 (31)	58 (24)	0.000
At 48 hr	25 (28)	41 (27)	0.000
PIP (cm H_2O)			
At 8 hr	15.5 (8.3)	21.8 (6.8)	0.000
At 48 hr	13.6 (8.6)	19.2 (8.6)	0.000
F_{IO_2}			
At 8 hr	0.53 (0.28)	0.56 (0.29)	0.473
At 48 hr	0.36 (0.20)	0.42 (0.25)	0.057
P_{O_2} (mm Hg)			
At 8 hr	63 (29)	65 (33)	0.543
At 48 hr	63 (22)	67 (31)	0.282
P_{CO_2} (mm Hg)			
At 8 hr	39 (12)	37 (12)	0.189
At 48 hr	41 (11)	39 (9)	0.256
pH (units)			
At 8 hr	7.36 (0.13)	7.39 (0.11)	0.019
At 48 hr	7.31 (0.09)	7.33 (0.07)	0.097

Values are means (SD).
PIP, Peak inspiratory pressure; *F_{IO_2}*, fraction of inspired oxygen.

The SGA infants (n = 22) and AGA infants had similar death and major impairment rates. The SGA condition was associated with birth from 1980 to 1984 (17 SGA and 145 AGA infants vs 5 SGA and 114 infants born from 1985 to 1989, $p = 0.035$), maternal hypertension ($p = 0.000$), birth by cesarean section (68% vs 16%, $p = 0.000$), and absence of fused eyes ($p = 0.002$). The SGA infants had lower axillary temperature but less severe respiratory failure at 8 hours of age, lower leukocyte and platelet counts, and less hypernatremia during the first 48 hours. The SGA infants also had lower rates of patent ductus arteriosus ($p = 0.014$) and bronchopulmonary dysplasia ($p = 0.000$). The infants who were large for gestational age (n = 22) resembled AGA infants with respect to both outcomes and risk and severity of illness factors, except for lower 8-hour temperature, blood pressures, and hemoglobin concentration. They had a high rate of withdrawal of life support.

Preliminary multivariate analyses. In multivariate analyses of both outcomes, the performance of the respiratory failure index was marginally but consistently superior to that of all or any of the respiratory measures included in its

Table IVB. Period comparisons of risk and severity of illness factors: Categorical variables

	1980-1984 (n = 161)		1985-1989 (n = 126)			
	No.	(%)	No.	(%)	OR (CI)	*p*
Maternal hypertension	16	(10)	7	(6)	0.53 [0.19, 1.44]	0.175
Multiple gestation	19	(12)	25	(20)	0.54 [0.27, 1.08]	0.061
PROM	43	(27)	24	(19)	0.65 [0.35, 1.18]	0.128
Cesarean section	35	(22)	22	(18)	0.76 [0.40, 1.43]	0.283
Intubation at birth	71	(44)	80	(63)	2.20 [1.33, 3.66]	0.001
Fused eye(s)	76	(47)	69	(55)	1.35 [0.83, 2.22]	0.204
SGA	17	(11)	5	(4)	0.35 [0.11, 1.04]	0.035
Air leak	12	(7)	28	(22)	3.40 [1.50, 7.65]	0.001
Hyperglycemia	20	(12)	32	(25)	2.10 [1.05, 4.22]	0.020
Hypernatremia	32	(20)	24	(19)	0.95 [0.50, 1.78]	0.387
Hyperkalemia	32	(20)	20	(16)	0.60 [0.30, 1.20]	0.119
Withdrawal of support	55	(34)	11	(9)	0.18 [0.09, 0.39]	0.000

Percentage of patients shown in parentheses.
OR, Odds ratio; *CI*, 95% confidence interval; *PROM*, premature rupture of membranes.

Table VA. Comparisons of outcomes in periods 1 and 2

	1980-1984 (n = 161)		1985-1989 (n = 126)			
Outcome variable	No.	(%)	No.	(%)	OR (CI)	*p*
Death	82	(51)	60	(48)	0.88 [0.53, 1.43]	0.578
Postponed neonatal death	7	(4)	9	(7)	1.89 [0.60, 6.09]	0.229
Lost to follow-up	6	(4)	3	(2)	0.58 [0.11, 2.76]	0.449
Major impairment	25	(16)	11	(9)	0.41 [0.17, 0.98]	0.027
*Risk adjusted**	—		—		0.24 [0.10, 0.60]	0.002
Blindness	14	(9)	2	(2)	0.14 [0.02, 0.68]	0.004
Other major impairment	15	(9)	10	(8)	0.73 [0.28, 1.91]	0.483
CMDI scores ≤68	7	(4)	5	(4)	0.81 [0.21, 3.06]	0.735
Severe neurodeficit	4†	(2)	4‡	(3)		
Deafness	4§	(2)	1	(1)		

Percentage of period total shown in parentheses.
OR, Odds ratio; *CI*, 95% confidence interval; *CMDI*, corrected Mental Development Index (Bayley).
**Risk adjusted* refers to the period comparison for major impairment rates, adjusted for risk and severity of illness factors at 8 hours of age.
†One was also blind and deaf.
‡One was also blind.
§Three were also blind, and one also had spastic quadriplegia.

formulation. In subsequent analyses the index was entered in place of those measures.

Birth weight and GA were mutually exclusive in most multivariate analyses of both outcomes. Comparative analyses, alternatively excluding GA or BW, showed that the contribution of each to the models was similar, and that inclusion of both neither changed the variables associated with outcomes nor improved model performance. Entry of an SGA variable did not influence the performance of models. Because of the missing values for GA (n = 5) and the definition of the cohort by BW, the GA was excluded from final analyses. There was no advantage substituting pH for P_{CO_2} and base deficit for either outcome.

Multivariate outcome models. Detailed results of validation analyses will be reported in a second article on prognostic models. The multivariable models were validated for death. It was not possible to validate the models for major impairment because of sample size limitations (n = 36). Subsequent analyses (excluding period comparisons) were performed on the whole cohort (n = 287).

Variables that consistently contributed to the models for death were the respiratory failure index and the maximal blood glucose concentration ≥2.2 mmol/L (vs <2.2 mmol/L) (absence of hypoglycemia) during the first 48 hours (Table IIIA). Between 8 and 48 hours the importance of BW and base deficit for models of death diminished, as did the importance of the respiratory failure index for models of major impaired outcome.

Variables contributing to the final multivariable models for major impairment (with the addition of the "period in-

Table VB. Univariate period comparisons of intermediate outcomes

Variable (age at entry for denominator)	1980-1984 (n = 161) No.	(%)	1985-1989 (n = 126) No.	(%)	OR (CI)	p
IVH* (5 days)	18	(18)	19	(20)	1.17 [0.5, 2.54]	0.668
PDA (28 days)	56	(65)	62	(83)	2.55 [1.15, 5.76]	0.012
BPD (28 days)	72	(84)	73	(97)	7.10 [1.46, 46.97]	0.004
NEC (28 days)	12	(14)	6	(8)	0.54 [0.17, 1.65]	0.232
Retinopathy†	11	(14)	3	(5)	0.29 [0.06, 1.21]	0.057

Age at entry and denominators shown with each variable.
Percentage of period total shown in parentheses.
OR, Odds ratio; *CI*, confidence interval; *PDA*, patent ductus arteriosus; *BPD*, bronchopulmonary dysplasia; *NEC*, necrotizing enterocolitis.
*Grades 3 and 4 IVH.
†Grades 4 and 5 retinopathy at hospital discharge.

dicator" variable) at 8 and 48 hours of age are reported in Table IIIB. Of 57 babies born by cesarean section, 29 survived and two had major impairment: one visual and the other a low Bayley Mental Development Index. Both vaginal delivery route and absence of hypoglycemia ($\geq$2.2 mmol/L) were independently associated with major impairment during the first 48 hours, but BW and GA were not associated with this outcome.

Because of the strong association between SGA and both cesarean section and maternal hypertension, additional multivariate analyses were performed in a subcohort that excluded the 22 SGA infants. The results were similar to those of the whole cohort with respect to both the identity of independent variables and the predictive accuracy. Thus no adjustment of outcomes was made for the SGA condition.

Secular comparisons and associations

Risk and severity of illness factors. Period comparisons analyzed by univariate methods are shown in Tables IVA and IVB. Period 2 was characterized by biases toward admission of fewer infants whose mothers could be transferred to the regional perinatal centers (fewer SGA infants, less maternal hypertension, and premature rupture of membranes), less mature infants (lower GA, lower BW), more severe illness (high respiratory failure index, more air leaks), and more aggressive neonatal resuscitation and provision of respiratory support (but not obstetric intervention) (Tables IVA and IVB). Some treatment-dependent factors (temperature, pH, electrolytes) showed a trend toward normalization. Hematologic values (not shown) were 5% to 13% lower. Intermediate outcomes showed varied secular trends: IVH (grades 3 and 4) showed no change, patent ductus arteriosus and bronchopulmonary dysplasia occurred more frequently, and severe retinopathy of prematurity (grades 4 and 5) was diagnosed less frequently.

Multivariate analyses revealed that the respiratory failure index was the most important association of death in both periods. Other trends in the associations of death were, for period 1, antepartum hemorrhage, low pH, hypernatremia, and hyperglycemia during the first 48 hours, and, for period 2, BW and gender. Separate multivariate period analyses for major impairment were not possible because of limited sample sizes.

Crude and adjusted secular outcome comparisons. The results of univariate analyses indicated that infants born in period 2 had a similar death rate but a lower major impairment rate at 18 to 24 months of age, attributable to the reduced proportion of blind survivors (Tables VA and VB). Of the intermediate outcomes, the incidence of patent ductus arteriosus and bronchopulmonary dysplasia was significantly higher in period 2, whereas that of retinopathy of prematurity tended to fall (Table VB). Bowel perforation occurred in five and two survivors in periods 1 and 2, and subglottic stenosis in six and three survivors, respectively. The mean corrected Bayley Mental Development Index was 90 for both periods; the mean corrected Bayley Psychomotor Development Index was 84 for period 1 and 91 for period 2.

After statistical control for changes in risk factors and severity of illness (BW, respiratory failure index, P_{CO_2}, and base deficit at 8 hours of age), the death rate in infants born in period 2 was not significantly lower than that in infants born in period 1 ($p = 0.115$). The reduction in the major impairment rate at 18 to 24 months of age in period 2 was enhanced by control for the delivery route and the respiratory failure index at 8 hours of age (odds ratio, 0.24 [0.10, 0.60]; $p = 0.002$).

DISCUSSION

Secular trends in death and major impairment rates, and in risk and severity of illness factors. For our outborn infants, the 1980s were characterized by increasing immaturity and severity of illness, and increasingly aggressive postnatal care, evidenced by an increasing rate of endotracheal intubation at birth and a diminishing rate of withdrawal of respiratory support. The number of admissions to this outborn NICU declined, with a corresponding fall in the percentage of infants of mothers with obstetric risks that permitted transfer. The frequency of intermediate outcomes associated with immaturity that provide clear evidence of impending irreversible impairment (severe IVH and retinopathy of prematurity) showed no tendency to increase with time. The significant reduction in the proportion of survivors with major impairment was reinforced with statistical control for the changes in risk and severity of illness.

The reduced incidence of severity of retinopathy of prematurity and of blindness accounted for the observed reduction in the major impairment rate. Certainly this trend cannot be explained by greater maturity of the infants admitted from 1985 to 1989, nor were these infants treated less aggressively, two possible explanations for a reduced rate of impairment. The improvement may be attributable to more precise control of PaO_2 levels because of the increased use of noninvasive monitoring of transcutaneous PO_2 and oxygen saturation and/or because of changes in other, unrecognized cofactors that may increase or decrease the susceptibility of the retinal vessels to severe damage by oxygen.[21] The blood PO_2 data of our patients in the first 48 hours do not indicate any advantage for infants admitted in the 1985–1989 period, but in another study the PO_2 effect was more important during weeks 2 to 4 of life, for which we did not collect data.[21] Other factors suggested by our study that may have reduced the susceptibility of the retina to severe damage by oxygen in the 1985–1989 group include improved acid-base and serum electrolyte balance.

Although there was a reduction in the incidence of severe visual loss, there were no apparent changes in the rates of other types of major impairment (Table VA). The numbers of patients with major nonvisual impairment were too small to permit adjustment for risk and severity of illness for each specific impairment. However, the increased risk in the 1985–1989 group, together with the reduced rate of withdrawal of support, led us to expect an increased rate for all types of impairment. That this was not demonstrated is encouraging.

The clues to more precise external control of the neonatal internal environment during the first 48 hours include maintenance of more physiologic levels and tighter control of ranges of temperature and blood gas values from as early as 8 hours of age, together with determination of blood glucose and serum electrolyte values from 48 hours of age. We speculate that lower serum potassium and sodium concentrations and hematologic values in the 1985–1989 period indicate that there was less hemoconcentration or "extracellular fluid contraction"[22] in that period. That these variables remained in models for death in the 1980–1984 but not in the 1985–1989 multivariate analyses reinforces the idea that control of these variables may have implications for outcome. Outside the context of a controlled trial, we cannot comment on whether these associations are causative or attributable to unidentified surrogate effects.

Recent reports of nonadjusted secular trends of the major impairment rate in infants of BW ≤800 gm and 501 to 750 gm have shown either improvement or no change.[2, 23-28] These discrepancies may represent, among other factors, maternal or neonatal referral biases, differences in resuscitation and ventilation, delay in diffusion of technical advances to outborn compared with inborn infants, or failure to account for increased severity of illness in analyses of outcome. The increase in the number of trained neonatologists serving our referral hospitals during the 1980s, as well as our increasing experience in the treatment of these patients, may have contributed to the observed improvement in outcomes for outborn infants from our region.

Factors associated with death. The independent associations with death in our present study were measures of respiratory failure, acidosis (both respiratory and metabolic), BW (or GA), and high maximal blood glucose and serum sodium concentrations during the first 48 hours (Table IIIA). These findings are similar to those of our previous report on ELBW infants (≤800 gm BW) at 8, 16, and 24 hours of age,[29] and to other published multivariate models for infants of BW <1500 gm at 1 minute to 12 hours of age.[7, 15, 16] The absence of spontaneous breathing in our previous report was probably analogous to high ventilator rate in the present report. Temperature, an independent variable at 16 and 24 hours in our previous study, was not important in either the present 1980–1989 cohort or the 1985–1989 subcohort, a difference than can be explained by the secular trend for admission temperature to increase. Temperature may be a proxy for quality of resuscitation and medical care in the first hour or two after birth, before the arrival of the transport team, or it may directly influence outcome.

Disagreement exists about the relative importance and utility of BW and GA as associations of death, and about the Apgar score.[7, 15, 16, 28, 30-33] The Apgar score may be confounded by the strong association between low values and immaturity,[34] other measures of which remained in the multivariate models. The association between respiratory distress (or measures of its severity) with death is well recognized.[7, 16, 30, 33]

Race, associated with outcomes in other studies of infants of BW <1000 gm,[32] did not remain in our multivariate models, probably because of sampling differences. Male gender, also variably associated with death and impairment,[10, 15, 16, 26, 30-33] was associated with death in the 1985–1989 group but not in the 1980–1984 group or in the whole cohort. Other reported risk factors based on univariate analyses, such as fused eyes, bruising, air leak syndrome, and hyperkalemia,[35-38] were eliminated in our multivariate analyses, which suggests that they were not independent variables.

Inclusion of IVH diagnosed before each of the ages of study as a risk factor might contribute to the models, but its presence or absence at frequent intervals was not (and, for logistic reasons, is at present not potentially) detectable on a routine basis. Severe IVH is obviously a cause of death when its detection leads to the withdrawal of respiratory support.[39] Patients who died with severe IVH often had poor predictions of outcome based on other risk and severity of illness factors (to be published).

Factors associated with major impairment. Vaginal delivery versus cesarean section consistently stayed in models of major impairment, not unique to the present cohort.[26, 40] This delivery mode appeared to be associated with reductions in both central nervous system and retinal impairments. Sample sizes were inadequate for more precise statistical analysis. Associations between delivery mode and outcomes in infants of BW <1500 gm or ≤1000 gm have been attributed to correlation with other factors such as maternal hypertension and the SGA condition. The construction of models after exclusion of SGA infants (which included 10 of 22 of the mothers with hypertension) produced similar results. Controlling for the above conditions by multivariate analyses, we were unable to detect an alternative explanation for the consistency of delivery route in models for major impairment. It was not dependent on a secular change, as indicated by the similar proportion of cesarean deliveries in the 1985–1989 and 1980–1984 periods (Table IVB).

Other associations of major impairment (respiratory and metabolic acidosis and measures of respiratory failure) might prove to be more consistent with longer "exposures"[41] or in larger samples of patients. The association of minimal blood glucose values ≥2.2 mmol/L in the first 48 hours after birth with major impairment was unexpected in light of the finding that hypoglycemia was associated with impairment in preterm infants but with a broader spectrum of that outcome.[41] High blood glucose values in the present study may represent homeostatic immaturity.

Several investigators have pointed to differences between the cause of death and the cause of impairment.[33, 42] Birth weight and GA were relatively unimportant associations of major impairment,[30, 33] as in our study. The 5-minute Apgar score, not associated with major impairment in this study, has had variable associations with this outcome.[26, 30, 31, 33] The association between cerebral palsy and prematurity may be partly explained by common antecedents, rather than indicating that prematurity per se causes cerebral palsy.[43]

Methodologic considerations. A full discussion of the methods of secular outcome studies is beyond the scope of this article, but a number of features related to risk and severity of illness factors, the timing of adjustments, and outcome variables call for comment.

We used risk and severity of illness measures that were recorded routinely for clinical purposes. Prospective biochemical and radiographic testing at predetermined postnatal ages would require additional blood sampling and irradiation, not feasible for either ethical or logistic reasons. Some limitations of retrospective data collections, such as those subject to detection or documentation biases, may be insurmountable in outborn infants. We selected risk and severity of illness factors on the basis of their definability and availability.

The 8-hour period was the shortest time in which severity of illness data were available for virtually all patients of ≤800 gm BW admitted to our NICU from 1980 to 1989, and therefore represented "zero time" for this cohort. The 8-hour variables would already reflect the effects of treatment after birth, to some extent inseparable from the basic risk factors for outborn infants. Even at birth the infant's condition may reflect obstetric treatment, especially in situations proximal to the limit of viability. Measures of severity of illness for the period up to 48 hours of age reflected the effects of interactions among maturity, severity of illness, and therapy.

The choice of outcome variable may bias the interpretation of secular trends. Death and major impairment are competing events, but a comprehensive outcome variable that accounts for all possible adverse outcomes would be preferable. Descriptions of prognostic models for this cohort and the results of analyses that deal with this issue, as well as the justification of our strategy of dealing with patients who had withdrawal of support, will be published separately.

Conclusions. Despite an increasing selection for referral of less mature and more severely ill outborn babies near the "limit of viability," and despite a marked reduction in the rate of withdrawal of respiratory support, the rate of major impairment fell significantly during the 1980s. This trend was enhanced by adjustment for severity of illness. The fall was attributable to a reduced rate of blindness, and was associated with evidence of improved control of physiologic balance in the first 48 hours after birth. The observed secular association between less aberrant physiologic measures and a reduced rate of major impairment suggests that fine-tuning of the external control of the ELBW infant's internal environment may be important for the prevention of impairment. Further research should be conducted on the role of failures of homeostasis as possible contributors to specific impairments. The consistent association between delivery route and major impaired outcome in this cohort of infants of BW ≤800 gm, not changed by adjustment for some of the factors associated with cesarean section, suggests that this subject deserves further study in larger samples.

We thank Drs. Jill Boulton and Andrew Shennan for providing details of admissions to the Mount Sinai and Women's College Hospitals, respectively.

REFERENCES

1. Victorian Infant Collaborative Study Group. Improvement of outcome of infants of birth weight under 1000 grams. Arch Dis Child 1991;66:765-9.
2. Saigal S, Rosenbaum P, Hattersley B, Milner R. Decreased disability rate among 3-year-old survivors weighing 501 to 1000 grams at birth and born to residents of a geographically defined region from 1981 to 1984 compared with 1977 to 1980. J PEDIATR 1989;114:839-46.
3. Hack M, Fanaroff AA. Changes in the delivery room care of the extremely small infant (<750 g). N Engl J Med 1986; 314:660-4.
4. Day C, Primhak RA. Current practices in neonatal intensive care in the United Kingdom. BMJ 1993;307:362.
5. Campbell MK, Chance GW, Natale R, Dodman N, Halinda E, Turner L. Is perinatal care in southwestern Ontario regionalised? Can Med Assoc J 1991;144:305-12.
6. Erkkola RU, Kero PO. Impact of prematurity on perinatal mortality and morbidity. Ann Med 1991;23:663-9.
7. Patterson CC, Halliday HL. Prediction of outcome after delivery for the very low birth weight (≤1500 g) infant. Paediatr Perinat Epidemiol 1988;2:221-28.
8. McCormick MC. The contribution of low birth weight to infant mortality and childhood morbidity. N Engl J Med 1985;312:82-90.
9. Avery GB. Ethical dilemmas. Clin Perinatol 1987;14:361-5.
10. Paneth N, Kiely JL, Wallenstein S, Markus M, Pakter J, Susser M. Newborn intensive care and neonatal mortality in low-birth-weight infants. N Engl J Med 1982;307:149-55.
11. Verloove-Vanhorick SP, Verwey RA, Ebeling MCA, Brand R, Ruys JH. Mortality in very preterm and very low birth weight infants according to place of birth and level of care: results of a national collaborative survey of preterm and very low birth weight infants in the Netherlands. Pediatrics 1988;81: 404-11.
12. Powell TG, Pharoah POD. Regional neonatal intensive care: bias and benefit. BMJ 1987;295:690-2.
13. Field D, Hodges S, Mason E, Burton P. Survival and place of treatment after premature delivery. Arch Dis Child 1991; 66:408-11.
14. Richardson DK, Tarnow-Mordi WO. Measuring illness severity in newborn intensive care. Journal of Intensive Care Medicine 1994;9:20-33.
15. Horbar JD, Onstad L, Wright E, et al. Predicting mortality risk for infants weighing 501 to 1500 grams at birth: a National Institutes of Health Neonatal Research Network report. Crit Care Med 1993;21:12-8.
16. Tarnow-Mordi W, Ogston S, Wilkinson AR, et al. Predicting death from initial disease severity in very low birth weight infants: a method for comparing the performance of neonatal units. BMJ 1990;300:1611-4.
17. International Neonatal Network. The CRIB (clinical risk index for babies) score: a tool for assessing initial neonatal risk and comparing performance of neonatal intensive care units. Lancet 1993;342:193-8.
18. Verdict of Coroner's Jury. Baby girl J. January 20, 1982. Office of the Chief Coroner, 26 Grenville St., Toronto, Ontario M7A 2G9, Canada.
19. Wojtulewicz J, Alam A, Brasher P, et al. Changing survival and impairment rates at 18-24 months in outborn very low-birth-weight infants: 1984-87 versus 1980-83. Acta Paediatr 1993;82:666-71.
20. Fitzhardinge PM. Follow-up studies of the high-risk newborn. In: Avery GB, ed. Neonatology: pathophysiology and management of the newborn. Philadelphia: JB Lippincott, 1987: 400-17.
21. Flynn JT, Bancalari E, Snyder E, et al. A cohort study of transcutaneous oxygen tension and the incidence and severity of retinopathy of prematurity. N Engl J Med 1992;326:1050-4.
22. Stefano JL, Norman ME. Nitrogen balance in extremely low birth weight infants with nonoliguric hyperkalemia. J PEDIATR 1993;123:632-5.
23. Hack M, Fanaroff AA. Outcomes of extremely-low-birth weight infants between 1982 and 1988. N Engl J Med 1989; 321:1642-7.
24. Kilbride HW, Daily DK, Calfin K, Hall RT, Maulik D, Grundy H. Improved survival and neurodevelopmental outcome for infants less than 801 grams birth weight. Am J Perinatol 1990;7:160-5.
25. Kitchen WH, Doyle LW, Ford GW, et al. Changing two-year outcome of infants weighing 500 to 999 grams at birth: a hospital study. J PEDIATR 1991;118:938-43.
26. Hoffman EL, Bennett FC. Birth weight less than 800 grams: changing outcomes and influences of gender and gestation number. Pediatrics 1990;86:27-34.
27. Grogaard JB, Lindstrom DP, Parker RA, Culley B, Stahlman MT. Increased survival rate in very low birth weight infants (1500 grams or less): no association with incidence of handicaps. J PEDIATR 1990;117:139-46.
28. Lipper EG, Ross GS, Auld PAM, Glassman MB. Survival and outcome of infants weighing <800 grams at birth. Am J Obstet Gynecol 1990;163:146-50.
29. Zarfin J, Van Aerde J, Perlman M, Pape K, Chipman M. Predicting survival of infants of birth weight less than 801 grams. Crit Care Med 1986;14:768-72.
30. Yu VYH, Downe L, Astbury J, Bajuk B. Perinatal factors and adverse outcome in extremely low birth weight infants. Arch Dis Child 1986;61:554-8.
31. Skouteli HN, Dubowitz LMS, Levene MI, Miller G. Predictors associated with survival and normal neurodevelopmental outcome in infants weighing less than 1001 grams at birth. Dev Med Child Neurol 1985;27:588-95.
32. Amon E, Sibai BM, Anderson GD, Mabie WC. Obstetric variables predicting survival of the immature newborn (≤1000 gm): a five-year experience at a single perinatal center. Am J Obstet Gynecol 1987;156:1380-9.
33. Shennan AT, Milligan JE, Hoskins EM. Perinatal factors as-

sociated with death or handicap in very preterm infants. Am J Obstet Gynecol 1985;151:231-8.
34. Schmidt B, Kirpalani H, Rosenbaum P, Cadman D. Strengths and limitations of the Apgar score: a critical appraisal. J Clin Epidemiol 1988;41:843-50.
35. Cross G, Becker M, Congdon P. Prognosis for babies born with fused eyelids. Arch Dis Child 1985;60:479-80.
36. Powers WF, Clemens JD. Prognostic implications of age at detection of air leak in very low birth weight infants requiring ventilatory support. J PEDIATR 1993;123:611-7.
37. Andrew M, Castle V, Saigal S, Carter C, Kelton JG. Clinical impact of neonatal thrombocytopenia. J PEDIATR 1987;110:457-64.
38. Shortland D, Trounce JQ, Levene MI. Hyperkalaemia, cardiac arrhythmias and cerebral lesions in high risk neonates. Arch Dis Child 1987;62:1139-43.
39. van de Bor M, Ens-Dokkum M, Schreuder AM, Veen S, Brand R, Verloove-Vanhorick SP. Outcome of periventricular-intraventricular haemorrhage at five years of age. Dev Med Child Neurol 1993;35:33-41.
40. Malloy MH, Onstad L, Wright E, National Institute of Child Health and Human Development Neonatal Research Network. The effect of cesarean delivery on birth outcome in very low birth weight infants. Obstet Gynecol 1991;77:498-503.
41. Brazy JE, Eckerman CO, Oehler JM, Goldstein RF, O'Rand AM. Nursery Neurobiologic Risk Score: Important factors in predicting outcome in very low birth weight infants. J PEDIATR 1991;118:783-92.
42. Marlow N, Hunt LP, Chiswick ML. Clinical factors associated with adverse outcome for babies weighing 2000 g or less at birth. Arch Dis Child 1988;63:1131-6.
43. Pharoah POD, Cooke T, Cooke RWI, Rosenbloom L. Birthweight specific trends in cerebral palsy. Arch Dis Child 1990;62:602-6.
44. Papile L-A, Burstein J, Burstein R, Koffler H. Incidence and evolution of subependymal and intraventricular hemorrhage: a study of infants with birth weights less than 1500 gm. J PEDIATR 1978;92:529-34.

APPENDIX

Infants small and large for gestational age. Infants who were small and those who were large for gestational age were at <10th percentile and >90th percentile, respectively, based on our own database with rounding off, with the exclusion of infants whose mothers had hypertension in pregnancy. The weights above the 90th percentile for 22, 23, and 24 weeks of gestation were, respectively, >540, >670, and >780 gm. The weights below the 10th percentile for 25, 26, 27, and 28 or more weeks of gestation were, respectively, ≤550, ≤630, ≤720, and ≤800 gm.

Respiratory variables. The respiratory variables were based on routine hourly records of fraction of inspired oxygen (FIO_2), ventilator rate, and peak inspiratory pressure (PIP) in centimeters of H_2O. For patients who received continuous positive airway pressure (CPAP), PIP was taken to equal the CPAP pressure and the ventilator rate was zero. The arterial/alveolar (a/A) ratio was calculated by the standard "short" formula $[PO_2/(FIO_2 \times 713) - (PCO_2 \times 1.25)]$. The "respiratory failure index" was based on a points system employing the three variables a/A ratio, ventilator rate, and PIP, as follows: One point if <10th percentile, 2 points between the 10th and 25th percentiles, 3 points between the 26 and 75th percentiles, 4 points between the 76th and 90th percentile, and 5 points >90th percentile. The index was determined at each postnatal age (8, 16, 24, and 48 hours), excluding infants who died. Thus minimal and maximal scores were 3 and 15 points, respectively. The scoring criteria for 8 hours are given in the Appendix Table. The following 90th percentiles were defined at 16, 24, and 48 hours of age: for a/A ratio 0.125, 0.095, and 0.099, respectively; for ventilator rate 60, 56, and 70 breaths/min, respectively; and for PIP 22, 22, and 24 cm H_2O, respectively.

Definition of intraventricular hemorrhage at 120 hours. Intraventricular hemorrhage was graded by the Papile classification,[44] derived from the radiologic reports in patient health records, up to 1 week of age. The reliability of the findings was tested by comparing the findings in a random sample of 40 cranial ultrasound examinations done during the first 5 days with the findings of one of us (P.L.), who was masked to the reports and to the clinical variables. The mean (±SD) kappa statistic was 0.87 ± 0.08 (z value, 10.32; $p < 0.000$). Cranial ultrasonography was performed in all patients by 5 days of age and, between 2 and 5 days of age, in all patients who died.

Appendix Table. Scoring criteria for "respiratory failure index" 8 hours of age

Percentile	Points	a/A ratio	Ventilator rate	PIP
<10th	1	>0.735	<1	<1
10th-25th	2	0.529-0.735	1-14	1-12
26th-75th	3	0.181-0.528	15-59	13-19
76th-90th	4	0.107-0.181	60-71	20-23
>90th	5	<0.107	>71	>23

Acuity scores as predictors of cost-related outcomes of neonatal intensive care

Uma R. Kotagal, MBBS, Paul H. Perlstein, MD, Harry D. Atherton, MSEE, and Edward F. Donovan, MD

From the Pediatrics Clinical Outcomes Research Evaluation Group and the Center for Clinical Effectiveness, Institute for Health Policy and Health Services Research, University of Cincinnati, University Hospital and Children's Hospital Medical Center, Cincinnati, Ohio

***Objective*: The Medicus Patient Classification System (PCS) and the Iameter Acuity Index Method (AIM) are two proprietary scoring systems in common use for stratifying patient populations before making comparisons of the medical care they receive. In this study the validities of these scores were tested when the scores were used to evaluate cost-related elements of high-risk neonatal intensive care.**

***Methods*: A total of 687 surviving inborn infants cared for in a university hospital newborn intensive care unit provided data for these analyses. The infants were stratified into the five diagnosis-related groups (DRGs) for surviving neonates (386, 387, 388, 389, and 390), as determined from their discharge diagnoses. Each infant's summed total of daily PCS scores, a single AIM score, and birth weight were extracted from the hospital's decision-support data files and used as independent variables in regression analyses to determine correlations with lengths of hospital stay, ancillary resource utilizations, and hospital charges.**

***Results*: The Medicus scores, which are computed prospectively on a daily basis, when summed retrospectively, correlated highly with lengths of stay, ancillary resource utilization, and associated hospital charges. The Iameter scores, which are assigned retrospectively, were far less predictive of these outcome variables and generally worse than birth weight in explaining outcome variances.**

***Conclusions*: Although in common use, the Iameter AIM could not be validated as an appropriate method for assessing cost-related outcomes after newborn intensive care. The Medicus PCS produced daily scores that, when summed after patient discharge, correlated highly with the same outcome variables. There is a need to test further these and other proprietary methods now used to compare the cost-related elements of care provided by different hospitals and physicians. (J PEDIATR 1995;126:88-93)**

Supported by the Cincinnati Children's Hospital Research Foundation.

Submitted for publication May 31, 1994; accepted Aug. 4, 1994.

Reprint requests: Uma R. Kotagal, MBBS, Medical Science Building, University of Cincinnati Medical Center, Cincinnati, OH 45216-0541.

0022-3476/95/$3.00 + 0 **9/23/59587**

Various acuity scores have been proposed for normalizing patient populations so that valid conclusions about effectiveness, patient outcomes, and costs can be made when methods of delivery of services by different hospitals and

AIM	Acuity Index Method (Iameter)
DRG	Diagnosis-related group
NICU	Neonatal intensive care unit
PCS	Patient Classification System (Medicus)

Table I. Data elements contributing to each acuity score

Iameter AIM score: Uniform Hospital Discharge Data Set	Medicus PCS score
• DRG • Hospital number • Age • Sex • Length of stay • Principal diagnosis code (ICD-9-CM) • Secondary diagnosis codes (ICD-9-CM) • Procedure codes (ICD-9-CM) • Discharge status • Total charges	• Admit or transfer onto service • Discharge or transfer from service • Altered mental status • Communication barrier • Self, partial, or complete assisted care • Fluid balance assessment or management • Incontinence management • Preventive skin care • Wound management and complexity • Pulmonary management and complexity • Vital signs frequency • Noninvasive monitoring and risk • Invasive monitoring and risk • Learning needs and intensity • Emotional needs and intensity • Medication management and frequency • Specimen collection and complexity • Patient in isolation • Use of drainage devices • Preparation for test or procedure • One-to-one care required

ICD-9-CM, International Classification of Diseases (ninth revision), Clinical Modification.

physicians are compared. These scores have been better tested and standardized as predictors of morbidity and death than of cost-related features of care, and better standardized for adult than for older pediatric patients in intensive care.[1, 2] Only a few scoring systems have been introduced and subjected to preliminary testing for applicability to assessment of the outcomes of care delivered to neonatal intensive care populations.[3] The current rapidly changing market forces in health care have resulted in pressures to contain health care costs without including any requirement for validation of methods. As a result, proprietary acuity scores are being marketed without peer review; without convincing proof of efficacy, they are being used to generate "report cards" of performance by hospitals and physicians, including neonatal intensive care unit providers.[4] We attempted to produce the missing validation of two proprietary acuity measurement scoring methods now employed to evaluate and characterize health care delivery by hospitals and physicians. In this study, the validities of these scores were tested when the scores were used for evaluating high-risk newborn care, with lengths of hospital stay, ancillary resource utilization, and hospital charges as outcome variables.

Table II. DRG categories

DRG	Definition	Population No.
386	Extreme immaturity or RDS	101
387	Premature infants with major problems	140
388	Premature infants without major problems	104
389	Term infants with major problems	228
390	Neonates with other significant problems	114
	TOTAL	687

RDS, Respiratory distress syndrome.

METHODS

Subjects. Six hundred eighty-seven inborn infants of all weights and gestations provided the data used for the study. Each infant was selected from a sequential population of 717 infants born at the University Hospital in Cincinnati and admitted to that hospital's NICU. Each of the infants selected was discharged home alive from the NICU between July 1, 1992, and May 1, 1993. Of the 717 infants, 30 (4.2%) died or were transferred to other hospitals before discharge home; data on these infants were not included in analyses. The exclusion of nonsurviving and transferred infants was elected because of the inconsistent and large variances in the outcome variables used in the analyses. The results are not affected by the exclusion because of the manner in which the study population was subsequently stratified to reflect the manner by which acuity scores are used to make interhospital comparisons.

Data sources. The hospital's decision support unit provided all information relating to the studied score values assigned to each infant. They also provided for each infant the daily charges generated from the utilization of all ancillary resources, and the daily charges for room and bed use. Data for population characterization, including birth weights, were obtained from a second computerized file (Southwest Ohio Alcyon Regional Database) of information maintained on every patient served by the university

Table III. Correlations between "scores" and cost-related variables

	Total daily Medicus scores								Iameter AIM scores			
	Total resource units		Total ancillary charges		Total hospital charges		Length of stay		Total resource units		Total ancillary charges	
DRG	r	r^2	r	r^2	r	r^2	r	r^2	r	r^2	r	r^2
386	0.849	0.721	0.742	0.551	0.932	0.869	0.986	0.972	0.487	0.237	0.409	0.167
387	0.914	0.835	0.662	0.438	0.996	0.992	0.996	0.992	0.475	0.226	0.432	0.187
388	0.949	0.901	0.789	0.623	0.996	0.992	0.997	0.994	0.429	0.184	0.351	0.123
389	0.479	0.229	0.471	0.222	0.487	0.237	0.995	0.990	0.125*	0.016	0.118*	0.014
390	0.685	0.469	0.471	0.222	0.918	0.843	0.961	0.924	0.298	0.089	0.265	0.070

All r values significant at $p < 0.01$ except if marked by asterisk.
*Not significant.

neonatology staff since 1974. The data files were merged, with the infant's hospital numbers used as key fields.

Data definition. Two scoring systems were tested: the proprietary Acuity Index Method, or AIM score, developed by Iameter Corp., San Mateo, Calif., and the proprietary Patient Classification System, or PCS score, marketed by Medicus Systems Corp., Evanston, Ill.

The AIM score is generated by Iameter on the basis of information submitted from the hospital. An unpublished algorithm is used to stratify patient populations on the basis of data routinely collected on each patient by means of the Uniform Hospital Discharge Data Set (Table I). The AIM score is derived with the ninth revision of the Clinical Modification of the International Classification of Diseases diagnostic codes and ranges between 1, for patients considered to have the lowest illness severity, to 5, for those with the highest. In the Iameter assessment method, after the scores are adjusted for severity, infants in common diagnosis-related groups are separated by hospital. Comparative statistics are then performed to determine interhospital variations in care efficiencies as reflected in differences in average length of stay and average charges when hospitals provide care for apparently similar patients.

Unlike the Iameter AIM score, which is produced retrospectively, the Medicus PCS score is generated daily on each patient. The method employs a format that allows NICU nurses to create profiles of the population to be served (Table I). The profile elements are then used in algorithms that anticipate nursing workloads, providing a basis for prospectively scheduling and locating personnel throughout the hospital. The daily PCS score ranges from 1, describing the patient with the least complex nursing care needs, to 6, for the most complex.

For purposes of this study, the AIM score, the Medicus score, and the number, type, and charges for each ancillary resource unit used on each day of care by each member of the study population were extracted from the decision support records. The ancillary units included all patient services that generated a hospital charge not included in the daily charge for bed space utilization. Thus a single resource unit was defined as any single use of a service such as a laboratory test, x-ray study, equipment, or device, or as the utilization of selected supply items.

Data analysis. The AIM score, which was assigned independently for each patient by Iameter, was tabulated without modification along with each infant's total ancillary resource utilization units and the charges incurred for those units only. In addition, the total hospital charges combining the ancillary charges and the charges for daily bed utilization were tabulated, as were the infants' lengths of hospital stay.

The Medicus scores generated daily throughout each infant's stay were added together to produce a summed score, providing a value that was weighted to reflect each infant's unique and cumulative demand on the hospital's system resources. These score assignments are generated before the actual delivery of each day's care, and thus reflect a measure of acuity as perceived prospectively by those delivering the care.

The tabulated data were sorted according to the DRG assigned to each of the 687 infants at discharge. For each of the five DRGs used for more complex illnesses (386-390), the dependencies of total ancillary resource units used, total charges for the ancillary resource units, total hospital charges, and lengths of stay were tested by means of regression analyses, with either the AIM scores, the summed Medicus scores, or the infants' birth weights as independent variables. The five DRG categories are defined in Table II. Nonsurviving and transferred infants were excluded from analyses; thus DRG 385, used to classify these infants, was not applicable for the study population.

Because the analysis was intended as a test of the utility of these methods for predicting cost-related outcomes, none of the data provided by the decision support group was re-

Iameter AIM scores—cont'd				Birth weight							
Total hospital charges		Length of stay		Total resource units		Total ancillary charges		Total hospital charges		Length of stay	
r	r^2	r	r^2	r	r^2	r	r^2	r	r^2	r	r^2
0.583	0.340	0.599	0.359	0.619	0.383	0.495	0.245	0.736	0.542	0.763	0.582
0.437	0.191	0.411	0.169	0.626	0.392	0.346	0.120	0.747	0.558	0.766	0.587
0.422	0.178	0.414	0.171	0.579	0.335	0.484	0.234	0.626	0.392	0.617	0.381
0.117*	0.014	0.374	0.140	0.008*	0.000	0.064*	0.004	0.004*	0.000	0.023*	0.001
0.164*	0.027	0.079*	0.006	0.132*	0.017	0.142*	0.020	0.029*	0.001	0.004*	0.000

fined or corrected in any way. For example, for the Iameter score analysis, the data presented are the same as those reported to and received from Iameter without modification or adjustments for any errors in clinical facts, DRG coding, or possible errors in the transcription of information. The only necessary compromise in analysis was the elimination of some individual data sets when information on a variable required for computation was missing from the infant's computer file, disallowing meaningful use for correlation purposes. Therefore, in the reported results, the number of subjects tabulated is the total population available for each DRG stratification subset. Because of missing data, the number contributing to each of the specific correlations varied slightly from the total but never by more than 5%. Missing data appeared to be randomly distributed in the data sets, and no population characteristics were altered significantly by the individual patient data exclusions.

RESULTS

For each of the five DRG populations, all outcome measures were characterized by frequency distribution curves skewed to the right. The skewing was accentuated by outlier data at the very extremes of the dependent variable ranges. We display in Fig. 1 the frequency histogram for the lengths of stay of infants in DRG 389, and in Fig. 2 the histogram of the total charges incurred by these same infants.

The correlation coefficients (r) and the corresponding r^2 values resulting from the regression analyses are listed in Table III. The summed total of the daily Medicus scores in all DRG groups provided near unity correlation coefficient values with lengths of stay, as expected from the method of summation, because length of stay determines the number of values contributing to the total scores. The Medicus score sums also correlated highly with total resource units utilized, the total ancillary charges, and the total hospital charges for DRGs 386, 387, 388, and 390. The correlations for these relationships in DRG 389, although significant ($p < 0.001$), were less useful as indicated by the r^2 values signaling that less than 25% of the population variance was enveloped by the resulting equations.

The low r^2 values document that the Iameter AIM scores also were poor predictors of cost-associated outcomes. Although Iameter publishes interhospital comparison charts displaying hospital variance from group mean length of stay and mean total hospital charge, for this population of study infants the r^2 values for these two elements exceeded 0.33 only for infants in DRG 386; the relation between the AIM score and the length of stay generated the very modest peak r^2 of 0.359.

When birth weight was used as an independent variable, it produced higher correlation coefficients than the AIM score for DRGs 386, 387, and 388. Only for total ancillary charges in DRG 387 did the AIM score ($r = 0.432$) exceed the birth weight ($r = 0.346$) as a predictor of the outcome values. For total hospital charges and length of stay in DRGs 386, 387, and 388, birth weights produced far better r^2 values than the AIM score. However, even birth weight, when used as an independent variable, did not explain more than 58% of the variance in results, and this value was achieved only for length of stay analyses for the DRG 386 and 387 populations.

For DRG 389, none of the scores, including birth weight, proved useful except for the previously noted near unity relation between the total Medicus score and the length of stay. The Medicus score predicted the outcomes better for infants in DRG 390 than for those in DRG 389.

DISCUSSION

The utilization of hospital resources to provide patient care is highly variable among countries, regions, hospitals, and physicians.[5-7] The explanations for variations are numerous, and include differences in the severity of illnesses treated in different medical centers, the additional costs incurred by providing programs in medical education, and differences in medical practice and expertise. Between the extremes are complex confounding influences on care deci-

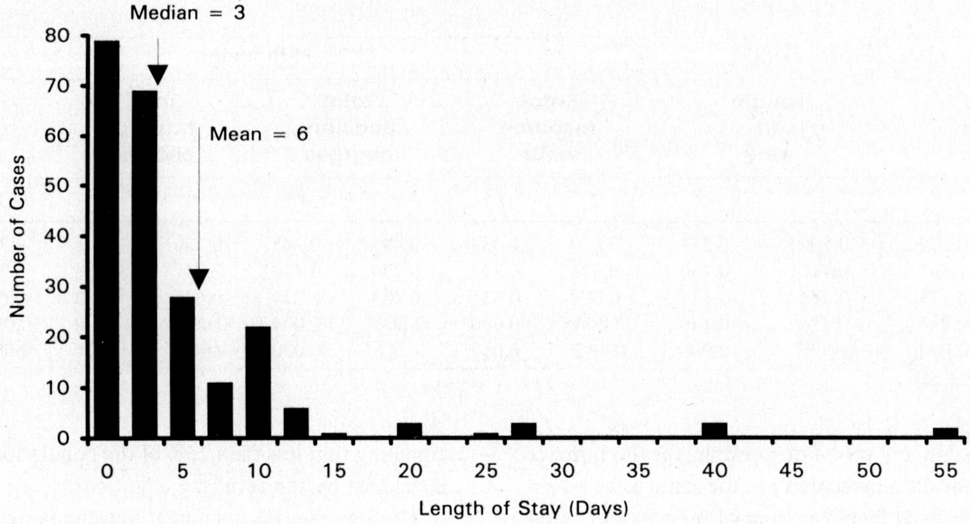

Fig. 1. Frequency histogram of length of stay for infants discharged with a DRG assignment of 389, illustrating the skewing of the distribution accentuated by outlier data.

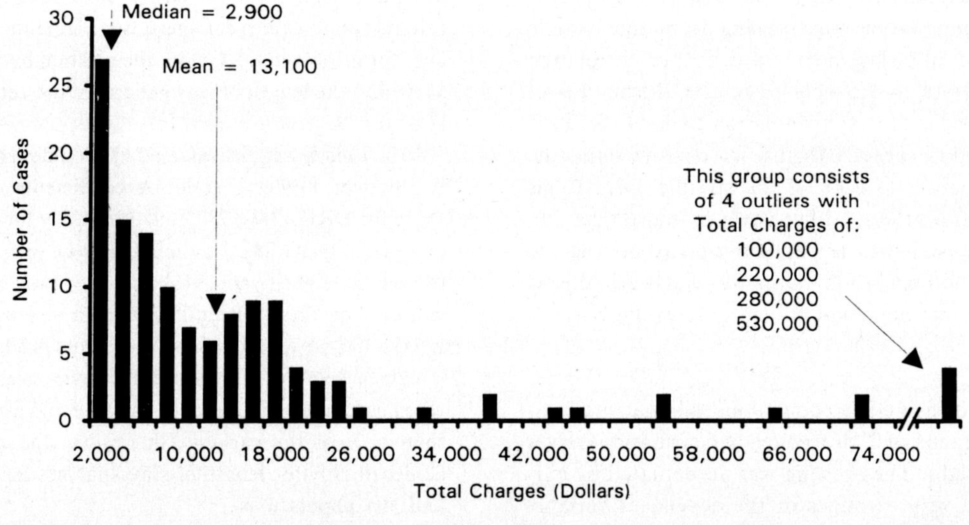

Fig. 2. Frequency histogram of total hospital charges billed for the care of infants in DRG 389, illustrating that the skewing to the right is increased by outlier patients who accumulated extraordinary charges.

sions, including regional differences in pressures from insurance and peer review organizations, and variability in the nature of rules and incentives that modify hospital and physician income. Although the characteristics and elucidation of all the variable factors influencing variations in care remain elusive and under study, the pressure to reduce health care costs has produced a demand for standardization of care and associated costs. A question remains as to whether existing methods of care assessment meet the requirements of this demand.

We have demonstrated that the Medicus PCS score is well correlated and may be a good predictor of resource utilization, hospital charges, and length of stay for surviving newborn infants cared for in a level III NICU in the inner city. The demonstration is tempered by the score's limitation in retrospectively assessing length of stay, which itself influences the score value. In addition, it would be premature to recommend the use of a total Medicus score, even as a predictor of any outcome variables, until there is proof that the daily Medicus score generation does not predestine resource utilization, because it is also used to distribute hospital personnel who ultimately implement the use of ancillary services and supplies.

Unlike the Medicus score, the Iameter AIM score was

developed specifically as a method for stratifying patient populations retrospectively. The method attempts to take into account the fact that patients with similar disease problems, as defined by DRG assignment, may have varying disease severities and, most important, may also have coincident problems identified through the discharge diagnoses coding of comorbidities. Although there is some evidence that the AIM algorithm stratifies and groups adult patients in a useful manner, our study indicates that AIM scores have little predictive value when applied to a neonatal population and, in fact, are less effective than birth weights, which also are a mediocre basis for assessing cost-related outcomes.

Some of the reasons for the failure of the application of AIM scoring to a neonatal population are evident. For example, when used for purposes of comparing hospitals or physicians by means of a regional, local, or other basis for establishing a norm or standard, the Iameter method expresses that norm or standard as an average value. As illustrated in this report, resource utilization, lengths of stay, and charges billed for care are not distributed normally when newborn populations are analyzed. The skewing of data precludes the valid use of averages to characterize cost-related population data. The results also illustrate a likelihood that accurate stratification by severity of disease is not achieved by using the secret AIM algorithm for incorporating comorbidities in the grouping equation. As well articulated by others, the seven DRG groups used to classify infants for reimbursement purposes are too simplistic and bear little relationship to actual care costs or patient outcomes.[8, 9] The DRGs need to be expanded if they are to be useful. Unfortunately, our results indicate that the augmentation of the DRG classification using the AIM score does not take into account the profound effect of outlier patients and other influences that create demands for hospital services, and apparently in other ways is not able to produce description or separation of submembership groups within the broad and heterogeneous populations identified by simple DRG assignments.

The current results were derived with the use of data from patients cared for in only one hospital, but there is no reason to doubt that the results are generalizable to other hospitals. Only a multicenter study could certify this as a fact, and our study confirms that there is a need for additional research that can provide hard data on which to construct clinical care outcome assessment tools applicable to newborn care. Because hospital charges are used for making interhospital comparisons, our study was limited only to examination of cost-related elements as reflected in billed charges. There is great variation in the way hospitals relate costs to charges; further analysis of these variations is needed to better understand how the differing balances between costs and reimbursement for care in different regions contribute to apparent discrepancies in hospital efficiencies. The need for additional research applies also to outcome studies that address changes in the quality of care as cost containment efforts are introduced.

Planning for health care programs is rapidly progressing. Without an equally rapid generation of additional data, the medical provider system will continue to be scrutinized and patient care uncritically modified because of the use of methods shaped more by competition than by scientific study and validation.

We thank Mark Sattler, Jerry Volker, and other Cincinnati University Hospital Decision Support Systems staff members for assistance in obtaining access to data used in this study.

REFERENCES

1. Knaus WA, Draper EA, Wagner DP, Zimmerman JE. APACHE II: a severity of disease classification system. Crit Care Med 1988;13:818-29.
2. Pollack MM, Ruttimann UE, Getson PR. Pediatric Risk of Mortality (PRISM) score. Crit Care Med 1988;16:1110-6.
3. Richardson DK, Phibbs CS, Gray JE, et al. Birthweight and illness severity: independent predictors of neonatal mortality. Pediatrics 1993;91:969-75.
4. Kassirer JP. The use and abuse of practice profiles [Editorial]. N Engl J Med 1994;330:634-5.
5. Pfaff M. Differences in health care spending across countries: statistical evidence. J Health Polit Policy Law 1990;15:1-24.
6. Wennberg JE. Outcomes research: the evaluative clinical sciences. Dartmouth: Hitchcock Medical Center Research, 1991;3(2):106.
7. Greenfield S, Nelson EC, Zubkoff M, et al. Variations in resource utilization among medical specialties and systems of care. JAMA 1992;267:1624-30.
8. Poland RL, Bollinger RO, Bedard MP, Cohen SN. Analysis of the effect of applying federal diagnosis-related grouping (CDRG) guidelines to a population of high-risk newborn infants. Pediatrics 1985;76:104-9.
9. Schwartz RM, Michelman T, Pezzullo J, Phibbs CS. Explaining resource consumption among non-normal neonates. Health Care Financing Review 1991;13:21-8.

Synthetic surfactant for rescue treatment of respiratory distress syndrome in premature infants weighing from 700 to 1350 grams: Impact on hospital resource use and charges

Josephine A. Mauskopf, PhD, Martin E. Backhouse, MSc, David Jones, MS, Diane E. Wold, PhD, Mark C. Mammel, MD, Martha Mullett, MD, Robert Guthrie, MD, and Walker A. Long, MD

From Burroughs Wellcome Co., Wellcome Research Labs, Research Triangle Park, North Carolina; the Department of Neonatal Medicine, Children's Hospital of St. Paul, St. Paul, Minnesota; the Department of Pediatrics, West Virginia School of Medicine, Morgantown; the Department of Pediatrics, Magee-Women's Hospital, Pittsburgh, Pennsylvania; the Department of Pediatrics, University of North Carolina at Chapel Hill; and the American Exosurf Neonatal Study Group I[a]

To determine the impact of the use of synthetic surfactant on hospital resource use and charges, we analyzed the economic data from a multicenter, randomized, placebo-controlled clinical trial of synthetic surfactant in infants with neonatal respiratory distress syndrome and birth weights between 700 and 1350 gm. Two 5 ml/kg doses of a synthetic surfactant (Exosurf Neonatal) or air placebo were administered to 419 infants who were receiving mechanical ventilation and had an arterial/alveolar oxygen tension ratio <0.22. In addition to the clinical endpoints for safety and efficacy, data were collected on length of hospital stay, days in the neonatal intensive care unit, days of mechanical ventilation, days of oxygen supplementation, and hospital charges until the infant reached 1 year adjusted age. Growth and development of infants who received synthetic surfactant therapy in the study and survived to 1 year adjusted age were equivalent to those of the survivors in the air placebo group. For 1-year survivors, synthetic surfactant reduced the average length of stay at the different levels of care needed during the hospitalization such as neonatal intensive care unit days, days of mechanical ventilation, and days of oxygen supplementation. For nonsurvivors, synthetic surfactant increased the average length of stay, especially at more intense levels of care. Total hospital charges for the initial hospitalization and through 1 year adjusted age for a hypothetic cohort of 100 infants treated with synthetic surfactant were, on average, the same as those for a comparable cohort of infants in the air placebo group. These results indicate that rescue therapy with synthetic surfactant in infants with respiratory distress syndrome and birth weights from 700 to 1350 gm can result in significantly improved survival without significant increases in hospital charges. (J Pediatr 1995;126:94-101)

Supported by Burroughs Wellcome Co.

Submitted for publication Jan. 31, 1994; accepted July 27, 1994.

Reprint requests: Josephine Mauskopf, PhD, Burroughs Wellcome Co., 3030 Cornwallis Rd., Research Triangle Park, NC 27709.

[a]Members of the American Exosurf Neonatal Study Group I are listed between the text and the reference list.

0022-3476/95/$3.00 + 0 **9/23/59568**

In the past few years, several clinical trials have shown that the use of surfactants is effective for treatment or prevention of neonatal respiratory distress syndrome. In a review of many of these studies, Jobe[1] showed that the use of surfactants is associated with an improvement in survival with no significant effect on the incidence of bronchopulmonary dysplasia or intraventricular hemorrhage, and with a reduction in the incidence of other complications from RDS, such as pneumothorax. In addition, when long-term follow-up of the infants has been included in the clinical trials, there has been no difference between the treatment and control groups in developmental disabilities.[2, 3]

CI	Confidence interval
NICU	Neonatal intensive care unit
RDS	Respiratory distress syndrome

A recent retrospective study[4] has demonstrated overall cost savings in several U.S. hospitals with the introduction of surfactant therapy for treatment of RDS in premature infants. Several studies have prospectively estimated the costs associated with the use of surfactants in premature infants with different birth weights[5-10] and demonstrated that preventive or rescue therapy is cost effective relative to other types of treatment for a range of drug prices. Most of these studies estimate an increase in total costs for the initial hospitalization, primarily because of the increased number of infants who survive and require prolonged stays in the neonatal intensive care unit. The estimates in all the prospective studies have been based on small numbers of infants.

In this article, we present the results of an economic evaluation using data from a large, placebo-controlled clinical trial of synthetic surfactant in premature infants with RDS and birth weights between 700 and 1350 gm. In addition to the clinical endpoints, data were collected on hospital resource use and hospital charges until the baby reached 1 year adjusted age. These data allow us to obtain a more complete picture of the impact of synthetic surfactant therapy on the clinical and economic outcomes for premature infants of this size range. The results are presented from the perspective of third-party payers and from that of the hospital.

METHODS

Data collection

Trial design. Two 5 ml/kg doses of a synthetic surfactant (Exosurf Neonatal, Burroughs Wellcome Co., Research Triangle Park, N.C.) were administered to 419 infants weighing 700 to 1350 gm at birth who had RDS with an arterial/alveolar oxygen tension ratio <0.22 in a multicenter, double-blind, placebo-controlled rescue trial conducted at 21 U.S. hospitals. The first dose was given between 2 and 24 hours of age; the second dose was given 12 hours later to those infants who still required mechanical ventilation. Infants were stratified at entry by birth weight and gender.

Clinical outcome measures. Clinical outcomes that were measured during the trial included survival at 28 days and 1 year adjusted age, and incidence rates of complications of RDS and prematurity, such as bronchopulmonary dysplasia, pulmonary interstitial emphysema, pneumothorax, nosocomial infections, and intraventricular hemorrhage. These data have been reported elsewhere.[11] In addition, follow-up at 1 year adjusted age included measurement of mental and physical development and an overall classification of level of impairment.[2]

Resource use measures. In addition to these clinical outcomes, the duration and intensity of hospital care were measured for two periods, from birth to 28 days, and from 29 days to 1 year of adjusted age. Measurements during hospitalization included days in hospital, days in the NICU, days of oxygen supplementation, and days of mechanical ventilation. Of all the infants in the trial, for approximately 7% resource use data were missing, and 10% of those with some resource use data had incomplete data capture during the 1-year follow-up period.

Charge measures. Hospital charge data for room, laboratory, medications, physician, and total charge categories for both the first 28 days and the remaining period through 1 year adjusted age were collected by persons masked to the treatment group. Investigators were instructed to include in the room charges category all other charges not included in the laboratory, medications, or physician categories. When physician charge data were not available or were incomplete, total charges were considered to be incomplete and were not computed. Investigators were also instructed to collect charge and resource use data from hospitalizations at sites other than the study site. If they suspected that the infant had had a non-study-site hospital stay but could not obtain the resource use and charge data, they were instructed not to complete the resource use and charge case report forms for that period, indicating incomplete data capture. The database was not finalized until approximately 18 months after the end of the trial to allow for more complete capture of the charge data. Of all the infants in the trial, for approximately 35% charges data were missing, and 9% of those had some incomplete charges data capture during the 1-year follow-up period. Rates of missing data (39% vs 31%) and losses to follow-up (11% vs 7%) were higher in the group treated with synthetic surfactant than in the air placebo group.

Statistical methods

Clinical effectiveness. The findings on clinical effectiveness, reported by Long et al.,[11] were used in the analysis of the economic outcomes as follows. The differential survival rates at 1 year of age were used in conjunction with survival data from the U.S. life tables[12] to calculate the additional years of life saved with synthetic surfactant treatment. The female/male ratio in the trial was approximately 38:62. Discounted years of life saved for each additional 1-year survivor were calculated from the survival data using a discount rate of 5%, a rate commonly used in cost-effectiveness studies.[13] Discounting adjusts the benefits to account for the greater value generally assigned to immediate gains compared with those further in the future.

Resource utilization and charges. Conventional methods were used to compute the means and SD of the resource utilization and charges data for all variables for patients with complete 1-year follow-up, and subdivided by survivors at 1 year and nonsurvivors. Differences in mean resource utilization and total charges between the two groups were also computed. The 95% confidence intervals were calculated for differences in the mean resource utilization or charges based on a standard normal statistic to define plausible ranges for the resource use and charge variables.

Ratio of incremental charges to effectiveness. The key purpose of this analysis was to report the outcomes of the economic variables observed in the trial; we also used the results to assess the ratio of incremental charges to effectiveness of surfactant treatment, which involves weighing the survival benefits of therapy against the charges associated with achieving them. The effectiveness and total charges data were therefore combined in two ways. First, total charges for a cohort of 100 infants were divided by the number of expected survivors in that cohort to calculate a "charge per survivor" for each group. This calculation is in keeping with the reporting of results from other studies in neonatal care.[9] Second, and more appropriately for decision making, incremental analysis was performed whereby the differences in charges were compared with the differences in survival outcomes, measured in terms of incremental 1-year survivors and number of life years gained (additional number of survivors multiplied by life expectancy per survivor). Results reported in this way permit comparisons with findings from other health care evaluations.

Sensitivity analysis. It is standard practice in economic evaluations to examine the extent to which the results are sensitive to changes in the values of key variables, assumptions made, or both.[14] Hospital resource utilization and charges data for the complete 1-year time period were censored because of loss to follow-up or incomplete reporting for some patients. Thus Kaplan-Meier product limit estimation, a method commonly used to estimate survival when the observed data are censored,[15] was used to estimate the means and SD for total hospital days, NICU days, and charges from birth to 1 year adjusted age. The differences in the means between the two groups were also computed. The 95% CIs were calculated for differences in the mean resource utilization and charges based on a standard normal statistic.

The Kaplan-Meier estimation was used in the sensitivity analysis, and the results were compared with the estimates from data for infants with complete follow-up, because it allows for inclusion of incomplete data in the analysis. For example, for a patient who never returned for follow-up assessments after initial hospital discharge, Kaplan-Meier estimation makes use of the data for that patient on hospital days and total charges up to the point at which the patient records were discontinued. The ability to make use of incomplete data seemed particularly important for the 1-year total charges data, for which a significant portion of the data was missing.

In addition, the total charge data were converted to cost estimates using each hospital's total cost/charge ratio where available (19 of the 21 study hospitals). The missing cost/charge ratios were imputed using the median known rates by type of hospital (children's hospital, state university hospital, and private university hospital). Cost/charge ratios for non-study-site hospitals were assumed to be the same as those for the study site where the patient was enrolled.

RESULTS

Clinical effectiveness. The mortality rate at 1 year of age was lower for the group treated with synthetic surfactant than for the air placebo group (0.16 vs 0.29, respectively). Thus it is estimated that 13 additional lives would be saved for every 100 infants treated with synthetic surfactant. On the basis of the 95% CIs on the differences between the survival rates (0.05, 0.21), the plausible range of outcomes is between 5 and 21 additional survivors per 100 infants treated.

When the U.S. life table for 1984 is used, the actuarial life expectancy weighted by the female/male ratio for infants aged 1 year is 74 years. Clinical follow-up data for this trial show that, although there were more total survivors in the synthetic surfactant group than in the air placebo group, there were no more infants with developmental disabilities.[2] This finding supports the assumption that the life expectancy of the additional survivors is equal to that of all infants. This life expectancy, discounted at 5%, gives 19 discounted life years:

$$\left(\sum_{i-1}^{90} 1/[1.05]^{i-1} \times \text{Probability [Alive at age i]} \right)$$

where i−1 is age minus 1 year. Multiplying the number of survivors by the undiscounted and discounted life expectancy yields an expected gain of 962 undiscounted and 247 discounted life years attributable to the use of synthetic surfactant treatment for every 100 infants treated (with 95% CIs of [370, 1,554], undiscounted, and [95, 399], discounted).

Medical care resource utilization. Tables I and II show the mean levels of medical care resource utilization ob-

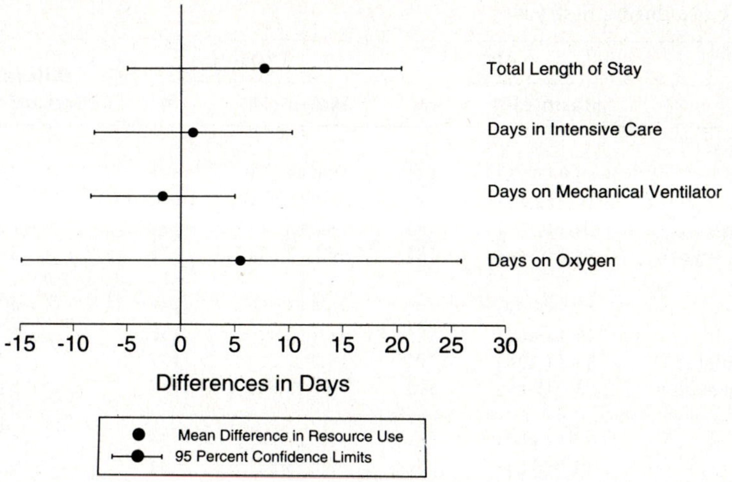

Fig. 1. Difference in 1-year resource use (synthetic surfactant vs air placebo) for all infants.

Table I. Hospital resource use—initial hospitalization only

	Air		Exosurf			
	Mean (SE)	n	Mean (SE)	n	Difference (Exosurf vs air)	95% CI
All infants*						
Total days in hospital	55.7 (4.13)	181	64.1 (3.74)	171	8.4	−2.5, 19.3
Days in intensive care	36.2 (3.57)	181	38.5 (2.74)	170	2.3	−6.5, 11.1
Survivors at 1 yr						
Total days in hospital	72.7 (4.78)	120	71.0 (3.69)	137	−1.7	−13.8, 10.4
Days in intensive care	44.2 (4.20)	121	40.7 (2.61)	136	−3.5	−13.8, 6.8
Nonsurvivors at 1 yr						
Total days in hospital	22.3 (5.89)	61	36.4 (10.32)	34	14.1	−9.7, 37.9
Days in intensive care	20.2 (5.51)	60	29.8 (8.82)	34	9.6	−11.2, 30.4

*Excluding infants lost to follow-up.

served in the trial for each treatment group as well as the 95% CIs for the initial hospitalization and first year, respectively. During the initial hospitalization stay, the use of synthetic surfactant resulted in an average increase of 8.4 hospital days overall and 2.3 days in intensive care for all infants (Table I). Rehospitalization rates were slightly higher for the synthetic surfactant group than the air placebo group (34% vs 28%), but total rehospitalization days and NICU days were lower for the synthetic surfactant group. Thus during the first year, the overall increase in hospital stay was less than for the initial hospitalization, 7.7 days with an overall increase of 1.1 days in intensive care (Table II; Fig. 1). Also during the first year, the synthetic surfactant group had 1.7 fewer days of mechanical ventilation and 5.5 more days of oxygen supplementation (Table II; Fig. 1). Use of most medical care resources measured in the trial was significantly less for nonsurvivors than for survivors (Tables I and II). Survivors treated with synthetic surfactant had reductions in each component of resource use; however, the trend was reversed for nonsurvivors.

Hospital charges. Use of synthetic surfactant resulted in no change in mean hospital charges for the initial hospitalization or the first year (Table III). Total charges for all infants in the synthetic surfactant and air placebo groups for the initial hospitalization were both approximately $97,500 and for the first year $100,500, equal charges despite the large number of extra survivors who required prolonged care in the NICU. The equal charges are in contrast to the increased resource utilization for the synthetic surfactant group (Tables I and II), indicating that the overall resource use might be less intensive with synthetic surfactant. When analyzed separately, charges were lower for survivors in the synthetic surfactant group, but for those infants who died, charges were higher for those treated with synthetic surfactant than for the air placebo group. These findings reflect the trends in medical care resource utilization. Laboratory charges, other medication charges (excluding the synthetic surfactant), and physician charges were reduced in infants treated with surfactant; total charges (including the synthetic surfactant) and room charges were not (Fig. 2). The higher room charges reflect the longer length of stay for the cohort of treated infants because of the additional survivors;

Table II. Hospital resource use during first year

	Air		Exosurf		Difference (Exosurf vs air)	95% CI
	Mean (SE)	n	Mean (SE)	n		
All infants*						
Total days in hospital	60.9 (4.78)	181	68.6 (4.37)	171	7.7	−5.0, 20.4
Days in intensive care	37.7 (3.81)	181	38.8 (2.75)	170	1.1	−8.1, 10.3
Days of mechanical ventilation	20.3 (2.77)	183	18.6 (2.01)	171	−1.7	−8.4, 5.0
Days of oxygen supplementation	56.7 (7.14)	182	62.2 (7.57)	171	5.5	−14.9, 25.9
Survivors at 1 yr						
Total days in hospital	80.5 (5.79)	120	76.4 (4.58)	137	−4.1	−18.9, 10.7
Days in intensive care	46.4 (4.82)	121	41.1 (2.63)	136	−5.3	−16.3, 5.7
Days of mechanical ventilation	23.3 (3.74)	122	18.2 (2.20)	137	−5.1	−13.8, 3.6
Days of oxygen supplementation	75.6 (9.89)	121	70.0 (8.98)	137	−5.6	−32.3, 21.1
Nonsurvivors at 1 yr						
Total days in hospital	22.3 (5.89)	61	37.5 (10.49)	34	15.2	−8.9, 39.3
Days in intensive care	20.2 (5.51)	60	29.8 (8.82)	34	9.6	(−11.2, 30.4)
Days of mechanical ventilation	14.4 (3.51)	61	20.2 (4.96)	34	5.8	−6.4, 18.0
Days of oxygen supplementation	19.2 (6.00)	61	30.7 (10.25)	34	11.5	−12.3, 35.3

*Excluding infants lost to follow-up.

Table III. Charges for initial hospitalization and first year

	Air		Exosurf		Difference (Exosurf vs air)	95% CI
	Mean (SE)	n	Mean (SE)	n		
All infants*						
Initial hospitalization	$ 97,452 (11,959)	135	$ 97,642 (6,586)	113	$ 190	−26,569, 26,949
First year	100,531 (12,224)	135	$100,732 (7,043)	113	206	−27,445, 27,857
Survivors at 1 yr						
Initial hospitalization	132,857 (17,550)	80	$111,927 (7,021)	82	−20,930	−58,735, 16,875
First year	137,978 (17,936)	80	$115,464 (7,609)	82	−22,514	−61,481, 16,452
Nonsurvivors at 1 yr						
Initial hospitalization	45,955 (11,522)	55	$59,855 (13,137)	31	13,901	−21,048, 48,849
First year	46,065 (11,529)	55	$61,784 (13,849)	31	15,719	−20,320, 51,758

*Excluding infants lost to follow-up.

the lower ancillary and physician charges indicate that the care needed while in the hospital was less intensive.

Ratio of incremental charges to effectiveness. The ratio of incremental charges to effectiveness may be assessed either by comparing charge per survivor for the two patient groups, or by comparing the ratio of the incremental charges with the incremental benefits, measured in lives saved and life years gained for the two patient groups (Table IV). The charge per survivor (total charges for a cohort of 100 infants divided by expected number of survivors in the cohort) was lower for the synthetic surfactant group, $119,919, than for the air placebo group, $141,593. The incremental charges per additional 1-year survivor were $1585. The incremental charges per life year gained were only $21 per undiscounted life year gained, and $82 per discounted life year gained. Even in the worst possible case, the upper 95% CI for incremental charges and lower 95% CI for life years gained, the cost-effectiveness ratio was only $28,720 per life year gained (Fig. 3).

Sensitivity analysis. Although the numeric estimates for infants with both complete and incomplete follow-up differed, the direction of the effects was generally similar (Table V). The product limit method estimates mean charge savings and reduced days in the NICU, but the 95% CI limits are wide. The differences in costs, obtained by multiplying the patients' total charges by the hospital cost/charge ratio, were similar in magnitude to the estimated differences in charges (Table V).

DISCUSSION

These data indicate that the total hospital charges through 1 year adjusted age for a cohort of infants treated with synthetic surfactant are similar to those for a comparable cohort of infants receiving air placebo treatment, despite the fact that more babies in the synthetic surfactant cohort survive and thus require prolonged hospital care during their first year of life. Rates of missing charges data were slightly higher in the synthetic surfactant group than in the air group, as were losses to follow-up for those with some charge data, most likely because data were more likely

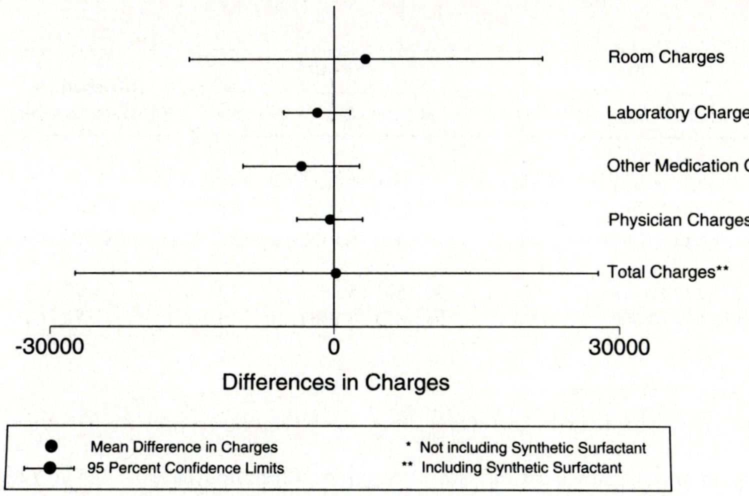

Fig. 2. Differences in disaggregated 1-year charges (synthetic surfactant vs air placebo) for all infants.

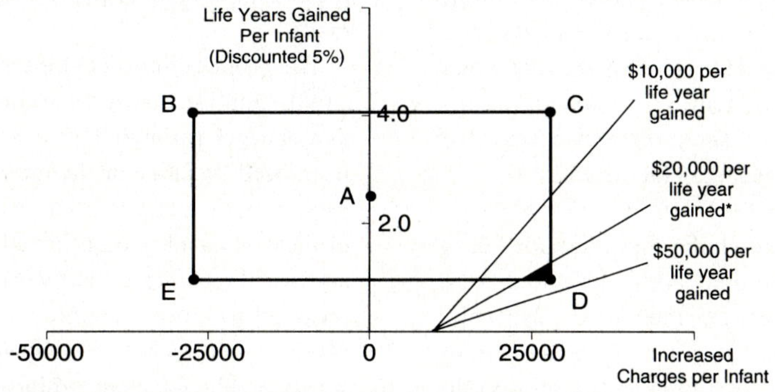

Fig. 3. Value of synthetic surfactant rescue therapy for RDS for infants weighing between 700 and 1350 gm. *Asterisk:* Commonly used benchmark of very good value for money; any new product above this line is generally considered very good value for money. *A*, Mean increased charges and life years gained per infant; *BC*, 95% confidence limits for charges; *CD*, 95% confidence limits for life years gained; *D*, worst-case increased charges and life years gained per infant.

to be complete for infants who died and there were more deaths in the air placebo group.

The lack of difference in total charges is in contrast to the increased total number of hospital days for the synthetic surfactant cohort. The increase in hospital days is attributable both to the extra survivors and some prolongation of life in nonsurvivors. The number of hospital days in surviving babies of this size is primarily determined by their birth weight and gestational age. However, as has been shown in other studies,[5-7] the level of care required is very dependent on the need for mechanical ventilation, which in turn is related to the incidence and severity of RDS.

Discounting of the life years gained, assigning a lower value to years gained further in the future than to the current year, is generally recommended for economic analyses of new treatments[14] and has been used in previous economic analyses of neonatal intensive care. For example, Boyle et al.[17] justify their use of discounting for life years gained-

Table IV. Economic value analysis

	Difference (Exosurf vs air)	95% CI
Charges per infant	$206	−27,445, 27,857
Additional 1 yr survival probability	0.13	0.05, 0.21
Life years gained (undiscounted) per infant	9.62	3.70, 15.54
Life years gained (5% discount) per infant	2.47	0.95, 3.99
Charges per survivor*	$−21,674	
Charges per extra survivor	$1,585	
Charges per life year gained (undiscounted)	$21	
Charges per life year gained (discounted)	$82	

*Total charges for a cohort of 100 infants divided by the expected number of survivors at 1 year.

Table V. Sensitivity analysis

	Air		Exosurf		Difference	
	Mean (SE)	n	Mean (SE)	n	(Exosurf vs air)	95% CI
Product limit estimates*						
Total days in hospital	68.1 (5.46)	198	75.5 (5.06)	192	7.4	−7.5, 22.3
Days in intensive care	45.3 (4.96)	199	42.7 (2.99)	191	−2.6	−14.2, 9.0
Charges	$132,543 (19,824)	145	$115,440 (8,157)	127	$−17,108	−59,976, 25,770
Cost estimates†						
Initial hospitalization	$77,232 (9,579)	135	$79,545 (5,857)	113	$2,313	−19,693, 24,319
First year	$79,670 (9,803)	135	$81,833 (6,106)	113	$2,163	−20,473, 24,799

*All infants with resource use data.
†Excluding infants lost to follow-up.

from neonatal care with the argument that new treatments in the NICU require the early expenditures of large sums of money to achieve later gains in numbers of life years or productivity. Because it is assumed that people prefer to receive money and health benefits sooner rather than later, this difference in timing of the costs and the benefits of treatment in the NICU should be taken into account when the impacts of the new treatment are analyzed. Thus discounted survival benefits are the most appropriate for economic evaluation of new neonatal therapies.

We estimated total charges for the time period through 1 year of adjusted age. Previous studies have included data for only the initial hospitalization. Although there were small increases in rehospitalization rates for the synthetic surfactant group, probably because of the higher number of survivors in this group, small reductions in the total number of hospital days and NICU days were observed in the subsequent hospitalizations for the group treated with synthetic surfactant, thereby further controlling their total charges.

For the baseline analysis, differences in total charges and not total costs were estimated. The financial data collected during the trial were hospital charges (the amounts that appear on the patient bill). These data are relevant for third-party payers who reimburse the hospital based on charges and for the hospital in terms of revenue estimation for charged-based patients. Charges are generally higher than costs because the hospital attempts to generate funds for new programs, equipment, and building replacement, as well as to cover bad debts and costs disallowed by third-party payers. Economic costs (the prices paid by the hospital for the resources consumed) are more relevant from a societal perspective, and accounting costs (economic costs allocated to each unit of service) are more relevant for those who reimburse providers on the basis of costs.[18] As part of the sensitivity analysis, we adjusted the total charge data by the hospital accounting cost/charge ratios. This adjustment was only approximate because total cost/charge ratios were obtained for only a subset of the study sites and for none of the hospitals that were not listed as study sites. The missing values were imputed from the available data. The results of the sensitivity analysis illustrate that the cost differences are slightly larger than the charge differences in absolute magnitude, but in the same direction. Thus our conclusions from the charge estimates do not change when this adjustment is made.

The product limit techniques[15] that were used in the sensitivity analysis to estimate the level of resource utilization and charges through 1 year are similar to those that have been used recently in the analyses of the costs of treating persons with acquired immunodeficiency syndrome.[19-21] All of these research groups have recognized the value of using statistical techniques that were developed for obtaining the most information possible from incomplete data. Use of product limit techniques allowed us to use all the data that we were able to collect, while adjusting for incompleteness. The results were sensitive to the analysis method chosen. In particular, the differences in 1-year charges were close to zero when only infants with complete follow-up data were used, but negative when using the product limit data. No systematic differences in infants with complete and incomplete data were identified except that infants who died were more likely to have complete data.

Eidelman[22] has suggested, based on several published studies, that in the United States the total cost of surfactant use for infants in the 700 to 1350 gm birth weight range might be between $280 million and $350 million per year. In contrast to Eidelman's assumed incremental cost per survivor of $100,000, the incremental cost per survivor estimated in this study is $1585. With Eidelman's computation, this would imply an increase in annual costs of $5 million to $6 million for infants in this size range. This increase in costs would likely be offset by decreased charges for larger infants treated with surfactants, as implied by the study by Schwartz et al.[4]

The economic value of a new drug depends both on its impact on health care expenditures and on the quality of life during the patient's lifetime. Our estimates focus on the infants with birth weights between 700 and 1350 gm, and suggest equivalent total hospital charges during the first year of life for infants in this size range with RDS who are treated with synthetic surfactant compared with those treated with an air placebo. Clinical follow-up data for this trial show that although there are more total survivors in the synthetic surfactant group than in the air placebo group, there are no more infants with developmental disabilities.[2] This finding suggests that the long-term charges for care for babies treated with synthetic surfactant are likely to be no higher than those for an untreated cohort. The study results therefore suggest that rescue therapy with synthetic surfactant in infants with RDS and birth weights between 700 and 1350 gm can result in improved survival without significant increases in hospital charges.

Members of the American Exosurf Neonatal Study Group I were as follows: David Stevenson, MD, Stanford University Medical Center, Palo Alto, Calif; Steven Goldman, MD, Children's Hospital of San Francisco, San Francisco, Calif; Frans Walther, MD, Women's Hospital, University of Southern California, Los Angeles, Calif; Stephen Boros, MD, and Mark Mammel, MD, Children's Hospital of St. Paul, St. Paul, Minn; Theodore Thompson, MD, University of Minnesota, Minneapolis; Richard Bucciarelli, MD, and David Burchfield, MD, University of Florida, Gainesville; Anthony Corbet, MB, FRACP, Baylor College of Medicine, Houston, Texas; Martha Mullett, MD, West Virginia University Medical Center, Morgantown; Robert Cotton, MD, and Hakan Sundell, MD, Vanderbilt University Medical Center, Nashville, Tenn; Ross Vaughn, MD, Wake Area Health Education Center, Raleigh, N.C.; Michael LeBlanc, MD, University of Mississippi Medical Center, Jackson; Carl Bose, MD, University of North Carolina at Chapel Hill; Donnal Walter, MD, Arkansas Children's Hospital, Little Rock; Thomas Pauley, MD, Albert Chandler Medical Center, University of Kentucky, Lexington; Robert Schumacher, MD, C. S. Mott Women's Hospital, University of Michigan, Ann Arbor; Alice Gong, MD, Santa Rosa Hospital, University of Texas Health Sciences Center, San Antonio; Matthew Sell, MD, St. Luke's Regional Medical Center, Boise, Idaho; Sherry Courtney, MD, Children's Medical Center, Wright State University, Dayton, Ohio; Jeffrey Gerdes, MD, Pennsylvania Hospital, University of Pennsylvania, Philadelphia; Douglas Derleth, MD, Mayo Medical Center, Rochester, Minn; Endla Anday, MD, Hospital of the University of Pennsylvania, Philadelphia; Frank Volberg, MD, Bowman Gray School of Medicine, Wake Forest University, Winston Salem, N.C.

REFERENCES

1. Jobe A. Pulmonary surfactant therapy. N Engl J Med 1993; 328:861-8.
2. Gong AK, Phillips L, Gold R, et al. One-year outcome of 419 700 to 1350 gram infants with respiratory distress syndrome randomized to two rescue doses of synthetic surfactant or air. Am J Perinatol 1992;9:5-6.
3. Ware J, Taeusch HW, Soll RF, McCormick MC. Health and developmental outcomes of a surfactant controlled trial: follow-up at 2 years. Pediatrics 1990;85:1103-7.
4. Schwartz R, Luby A, Scanlon J, Kellogg R. Effect of surfactant on morbidity, mortality, and resource use in newborn infants weighing 500 to 1500 grams. N Engl J Med 1994; 330: 1476-80.
5. Maniscalco WM, Kendig JW, Shapiro DL. Surfactant replacement therapy: impact on hospital charges for premature infants with respiratory distress syndrome. Pediatrics 1989; 83:1-6.
6. Tubman TRJ, Halliday HL, Normand C. Cost of surfactant replacement treatment for severe neonatal respiratory distress syndrome: a randomised controlled trial. Br Med J 1990;301: 842-5.
7. Mugford M, Piercy J, Chalmers L. Cost implications of different approaches to the prevention of respiratory distress syndrome. Arch Dis Child 1991;68:757-64.
8. Merritt TA, Hallman M, Vaucher Y, McFeeley E, Tubman TRJ. Impact of surfactant treatment on cost of neonatal intensive care: a cost-benefit analysis. J Perinatol 1991; 10: 416-9.
9. Mugford M, Howard S. Cost-effectiveness of surfactant replacement in preterm babies. PharmacoEconomics 1993; 3:362-73.
10. Phibbs CS, Phibbs RH, Wakely A, Schlueter MA, Sniderman S, Tooley WH. Cost effects of surfactant therapy for neonatal respiratory distress syndrome. J PEDIATR 1993;123:953-62.
11. Long W, Thompson T, Sundell H, et al. Effects of two rescue doses of a synthetic surfactant on mortality rate and survival without bronchopulmonary dysplasia in 700- to 1350-gram infants with respiratory distress syndrome. J PEDIATR 1991; 118:595-605.
12. National Center for Health Statistics 1987. Vital statistics of the United States, 1984 volume II, section 6, life tables. Washington, D.C.: U.S. Public Health Service, DHHS publication no. (PHS) 87-1104.
13. Goldman L, Weinstein MW, Goldman PA, Williams LW. Cost-effectiveness of HMG-CoA reductase inhibition for primary and secondary prevention of coronary heart disease: projection of coronary heart disease model. JAMA 1991;265:1145-51.
14. Drummond M, Brandt A, Luce B, Rovira J. Standardizing methodologies for economic evaluations in health care: practice, problems, and potential. Int J Technol Assess Health Care 1993;9:26-36.
15. Yamaguchi K. Event history analysis. Newbury Park, California: Sage Publications, 1991.
16. Laupacis A, Feeny D, Detsky A, Tugwell P. How attractive does a new technology have to be to warrant adoption and utilization? Tentative guidelines for using clinical and economic evaluations. Can Med Assoc 1992;146:473-81.
17. Boyle M, Torrance G, Sinclair J, Horwood S. Economic evaluation of neonatal intensive care of very low birth weight infants. N Engl J Med 1983;308:1330-7.
18. Finkler S. The distinction between costs and charges. Ann Intern Med 1982;96:102-9.
19. Crystal S, Sambamoorthi U, Merzal C. Estimating the per-case cost of AIDS care [Abstract]. Annual meeting of the American Health Planning Association, Washington, DC, November 8-12, 1992.
20. Markson L, McKee L, Mauskopf J, Fanning T, Turner B. Medicaid expenditures for AIDS diagnosis, mid-illness, and death. Presented at the annual meeting of the American Health Planning Association, Washington, DC, November 8-12, 1992.
21. Drummond M, Vella S, Backhouse M, et al. Cost-effectiveness of zidovudine therapy for people with AIDS: results from long-term follow-up. Presented at the Seventh International AIDS Conference, Florence, Italy, June 16-21, 1991.
22. Eidelman A. Economic consequences of surfactant therapy. J Perinatol 1993;13:137-9.

Glucose-6-phosphate dehydrogenase deficiency and carboxyhemoglobin concentrations associated with bilirubin-related morbidity and death in Nigerian infants

Tina M. Slusher, MD, Hendrik J. Vreman, PhD, Donald W. McLaren, MD, Laura J. Lewison, BA, Audrey K. Brown, MD, and David K. Stevenson, MD

From the Departments of Pediatrics, University of Texas Southwestern Medial Center at Dallas, Stanford University School of Medicine, Stanford, California, State University of New York Health Science Center at Brooklyn, Eku Baptist Hospital, Eku, Nigeria, and Children's Medical Center of Dallas, Dallas, Texas

Our objective was to determine whether glucose-6-phosphate dehydrogenase (G6PD) deficiency and elevated carboxyhemoglobin (COHb) levels correlated with bilirubin-related morbidity and mortality rates. For this purpose, we studied 55 clinically jaundiced infants admitted to a rural mission hospital in southern Nigeria. Total serum bilirubin levels (range, 80 to 1016 μmol/L (4.7 to 59.4 mg/dl)) correlated with the percentage COHb concentrations (COHb = 0.45 + 0.08* Total serum bilirubin; *r* = 0.72). Infants were divided into two groups of equal size around the median COHb concentration (COHb range, 0.43% to 5.93% (median = 1.40%), with ambient carbon monoxide of 0.65 ± 0.03 μL/L). The COHb levels ≥1.40% were associated with the need for exchange transfusion (15/28, or 54%, vs 5/27, or 19%; *p* <0.01) and with an increased incidence of clinical findings compatible with kernicterus (9/28, or 32%, vs 0/27, or 0%; *p* <0.01). Mortality rate was 29% (8/29) among infants with higher COHb levels, and 7% (2/28) in those with lower levels (*p* = 0.08). Thirty-one percent (14/45) of the clinically jaundiced infants tested had G6PD deficiency. Thirty-six percent of the infants with G6PD deficiency died with presumed kernicterus, compared with only 3% (1/31) of the infants with a normal G6PD screening test result (*p* <0.01). These data suggest that G6PD deficiency and increased bilirubin production, as indexed by COHb, are associated with jaundice-related morbidity and death in Nigerian infants. (J Pediatr 1995;126:102-8)

Neonatal jaundice is a significant cause of morbidity and death in Nigerian infants[1-7] and an important contributing cause of cerebral palsy in that country.[2, 3, 6, 8] A major cause of neonatal jaundice is increased bilirubin production, which may be particularly important if hemolysis occurs in infants deficient in glucose-6-phosphate dehydrogenase.

COHb	Carboxyhemoglobin
G6PD	Glucose-6-phosphate dehydrogenase
TSB	Total serum bilirubin [concentration]

The catabolism of heme results in the equimolar production of bilirubin and carbon monoxide, which is firmly bound to hemoglobin to form carboxyhemoglobin. The latter disso-

Supported in part by National Institute of Child Health and Development grants HD14426 and RR00070, by the Mary L. Johnson Research Fund, and by designated gifts from individuals of Pike County Methodist and Baptist churches.

Submitted for publication May 16, 1994; accepted Aug. 4, 1994.

Reprint requests: David K. Stevenson, MD, Department of Pediatrics, Stanford University School of Medicine, Stanford, CA 94305-5119.

0022-3476/95/$3.00 + 0 **9/23/59586**

Table I. Individual data for infants with kernicterus

Patient No.	Age (days)	Sex	Weight (kg)	Birth-place*	Hematocrit (%)	Bilirubin maximum (mg/dl)†	G6PD	COHb (%)‡	Death	Notes
1	4	M	2.5	0	30	38	+	2.0	Yes	Moribund, fever, possible sepsis
2	5	M	3.5	0	28	31	+	2.2	Yes	Fever, possible sepsis, cephalhematoma
3	5	M	3.1	0	50	59	−	2.8	No	Fever, possible sepsis, mild asphyxia
4	6	F	3.0	0	53	36	−	3.2	Yes	Fever, possible sepsis, hepatomegaly
5	4	M	2.8	Unknown§	26	39	+	3.7	Yes	Moribund, early death, possible sepsis
6	5	M	2.7	0	Unknown§	40	Unknown§	4.1	Yes	Early death, chart lost
7	4	M	3.6	0	27	59	+	5.0	Yes	Fever, possible sepsis
8	4	M	2.5	Eku	29	38	+	5.8	Yes	Fever, possible sepsis
9	6	M	2.7	0	33	55	+	5.9	No	Fever, possible sepsis

This table lists characteristics of all infants with kernicterus and probable kernicterus as defined in the Methods section.
*0 = Other (village or other hospital).
†Numbers rounded to nearest whole number for clarity.
‡Numbers rounded to nearest 0.1 for clarity.
§Data not recorded.

ciates in the lungs, resulting in the excretion of CO from the body. Therefore the production of bilirubin can be estimated by measuring CO in breath or the COHb concentration in blood.[9]

To ascertain whether COHb measurements were associated with hyperbilirubinemia-related morbidity and death in Nigerian infants, we studied jaundiced infants at Eku Baptist Hospital in the former Bendel State (now Delta State), Nigeria. Our objective was to determine whether G6PD deficiency and elevated COHb levels correlated with jaundice-related morbidity and mortality rates.

METHODS

Patients. The study protocol was approved by the institutional review board at the University of Texas Southwestern Medical Center at Dallas, as well as by the hospital administrator at Eku Baptist Hospital, Eku, Nigeria, and included informed consent from the parents or guardians of the infants who served as subjects of this investigation. Fifty-five clinically jaundiced infants, ≤10 days of age, admitted to Eku Baptist Hospital were enrolled from June to October 1991 and during June and July of 1992, regardless of place of birth, gestational age, or health status.

Data collection. At enrollment, all patients had blood samples drawn for total serum bilirubin concentration, hematocrit, total hemoglobin level, and COHb concentration. Blood typing and a G6PD screen were performed for most patients enrolled in the study. Additional blood samples were drawn for bilirubin levels as clinically necessary. Data obtained included physical examination, age, sex, and weight. Medical history included place of birth (hospital/clinic or village) and age at onset of disease. Therapy, outcome, and condition at discharge were also recorded. COHb levels were not available or considered in therapeutic decisions. The diagnosis of kernicterus (Table I) was based on clinical signs and symptoms and made by two of us (T.M.S. or D.W.M.) or the house staff. These signs and symptoms included lethargy, poor feeding, respiratory distress, opisthotonos, twitching of the face or limbs, shrill high-pitched cry, seizures, and spasms.[10] Although we did not attempt to stage the kernicterus, most infants had a combination of the signs noted above, and all had progressed beyond simple lethargy and poor feeding. Infants who died with significant hyperbilirubinemia and presumed sepsis were classified as having probable kernicterus and were included in our analysis. No autopsies were performed.

Exchange transfusions were performed on sick term infants with a TSB concentration of >342 μmol/L (20.0 mg/dl); a modification of the University of Texas Southwestern Medical School criteria for exchange transfusion was used as a guideline.[11] Although this guideline generally held true, the need for exchange transfusions was determined by the physician on a clinical basis. For the purpose of analysis, patients who met the criteria for exchange transfusions, but who died before treatment was administered, were grouped together with patients who had exchange transfusions.

Laboratory analysis. The TSB concentration was measured by the van den Bergh reaction.[12] G6PD deficiency was detected with a colorimetric screening assay (kit No. 400K; Sigma Diagnostics, St. Louis, Mo.). In accordance with the guidelines accompanying the kit, 60 minutes was selected as the end point for a normal G6PD screening test result, although this value was derived from blood sample data on adults. All laboratory investigations, with the exception of COHb and total hemoglobin concentration were carried out in the clinical laboratory at Eku. Results of blood cultures, reticulocyte counts, and Coombs tests were not reliable in this setting. Consequently the diagnoses of sepsis and ABO incompatibility could not be confirmed.

Blood samples for COHb measurement, collected in custom-made tubes,[13] were refrigerated and shipped on ice to Stanford University, Stanford, Calif. The COHb concentrations in blood samples (120 to 140 μl) were determined with a sensitive gas chromatographic method within 1 month of storage at 4° C.[13, 14] Briefly, 2 μl of blood was injected in triplicate into 2 ml septum-sealed, CO-free gas chromatography vials with 20 μl of 10% (wt/vol) potassium ferricyanide in potassium phosphate buffer (0.1 mol/L), pH 6.0, containing 1% (wt/vol) saponin. The vials were incubated at 0° C for at least 30 minutes, but no longer than 1 hour. The CO liberated into the vial headspace was then injected into the gas chromatograph with a reduction gas detector (model RGA2; Trace Analytical, Inc., Menlo Park, Calif.). The CO was separated from other compounds on a 68 × 0.53 cm (inner diameter) molecular sieve column at 125° C with a carrier gas flow rate of 50 ml of CO-free air per minute. The analyzer was standardized before and after each run with volumes of standard gas containing 25.0 μl CO per liter of N_2 (Airco Air and Specialty Gases, Santa Clara, Calif.). The within- and between-day coefficient of variation for reference blood samples when this method is used are 3% and 8%, respectively.[15] The minimal detectable concentration is 0.005% COHb.[15] COHb concentrations are expressed as a percentage of the total hemoglobin concentration.

The COHb levels were not corrected for CO in inhaled air.[9] Information regarding exposure of subjects to passive cigarette smoking or cooking fires within the home environment was not obtained. Cigarette smoking is extremely rare in rural Nigeria. Representative environmental levels of CO in the hospital area were obtained by periodically collecting room air samples in bistable gas samplers (model V-12; Chemical Projects Ltd., Rexdale, Ontario, Canada) followed by subsequent gas chromatographic analysis at Stanford University.

Concentrations of total hemoglobin (measured in grams per deciliter), used for the calculation of COHb concentrations, were measured with a manual cyanmethemoglobin method (kit No. 525, from Sigma). Four microliters of blood, pipetted with a gas-tight syringe (Hamilton Co., Reno, Nev.) in a Hamilton repeating dispenser, was allowed to react with 2.0 ml of modified Drabkin reagent (Sigma) for a minimum of 2 hours at room temperature. The absorbance of the resultant cyanmethemoglobin was determined at 540 nm with a spectrophotometer (model UV-160; Shimadzu Scientific Instruments, Columbia, Md.). The within- and between-day coefficient of variation for reference blood samples when this method is used are 2.2% and 3.0%, respectively.[15]

Data analysis. Data are presented either as mean ± SD or as median (25th to 75th percentiles). Continuous variables (COHb, TSB) were analyzed with either the Student *t* test, Mann-Whitney Rank Sum test, or Kruskal-Wallis one-way analysis of variance on ranks where applicable. Dichotomous variables (death, kernicterus, exchange transfusion) were analyzed with the chi-square or Fisher Exact tests when appropriate. In the latter case, groups were divided around the median COHb, which left 27 subjects in the group with COHb <1.40% and 28 subjects in the group with COHb ≥1.40%. Results were considered significant if $p < 0.05$. Continuous data were analyzed with the Pearson correlation coefficient and regression analysis. All statistical analysis was performed with SigmaStat Statistical Software (Jandel Scientific, San Rafael, Calif.).

RESULTS

Infants ranged in age from 1 to 10 days, with a mean of 3.9 ± 1.6 days, (n = 55). Average weight was 2.7 ± 0.8 kg, with a range of 1.1 to 4.2 (n = 54; one not recorded). Twenty-one infants (39%) were ≤2.5 kg. There were 39 boys and 15 girls (one not recorded); all infants were black. Twenty-two infants were born in the hospital at Eku and admitted directly from the obstetrics department. Twenty were born in outlying hospitals or clinics and subsequently came to Eku without a documented stay at home; 12 were admitted from home (one not recorded). All infants were breast fed. Mean TSB concentration at the time of enrollment into the study was 338 ± 226 μmol/L (19.8 ± 13.2 mg/dl) (n = 54), with a range of 80 to 1016 μmol/L (4.7 to 59.4 mg/dl). Mean maximal TSB concentration was 383 ± 227 μmol/L (22.4 ± 13.3 mg/dl) (n = 54), range

Table II. Comparison of patients with and without kernicterus

	Kernicterus		
	No (n = 46)	Yes (n = 9)	p
Age (days)*	4.0 (3.0-5.0)	5.0 (4.0-5.3)	0.021
Weight ≤2500 gm	19/45 (42.2%)	2/9 (22.2%)	0.46
Male	31/45 (68.9%)	8/9 (88.9%)	0.42
Born at Eku	21/45 (46.7%)	1/9 (11.1%)	0.07
COHb (%)*	1.3 (0.43-5.44)	3.72 (2.13-5.93)	<0.001
TSB (μmol/L)*	224 (183-287)	672 (643-942)	<0.001
TSB (mg/dl)*	13.1 (10.7-16.8)	393 (376-558)	<0.001
Hematocrit (%)*	48.0 (38-58)	29.5 (27-50)	0.001
G6PD deficiency	8/37 (22%)	6/8 (75%)	0.007

Data in parentheses denote a fraction or the range of values recorded, where appropriate.
*Data are presented as median (interquartile range).

Table III. Comparison of G6PD-deficient and normal patients

	G6PD status		
	Normal (n = 31)	Deficient (n = 14)	p
Age (days)*	4.0 (3.0-5.0)	4.0 (3.0-4.0)	0.830
Weight ≤2500 gm	15/30 (50%)	2/14 (14.3%)	0.023
Male	21/30 (70%)	13/14 (93%)	0.130
Born at Eku	14/30 (47%)	5/19 (26%)	0.500
COHb (%)*	1.2 (1.0-1.7)	2.3 (1.3-4.2)	0.005
TSB (μmol/L)*	224 (183-301)	518 (250-657)	0.004
TSB (mg/dl)*	13.1 (10.7-17.6)	303 (146-384)	0.004
Hematocrit (%)*	49.0 (43.0-53.0)	37.5 (28.0-49.0)	0.014

Data in parentheses denote a fraction or the range of recorded values, where appropriate.
*Data are presented as median (interquartile range).

94 to 1074 mol/L (55.0 to 62.8 mg/dl). Twenty-four infants (44%) had a maximal TSB concentration >342 μmol/L (20.0 mg/dl). Mean COHb concentration at or near the time of initial bilirubin determination was 1.97% ± 1.40% (n = 55), range 0.43% to 5.93%; the median COHb was 1.40%. All infants with TSB ≥513 μmol/L (30.0 mg/dl) had a COHb <2.00%. Random samples of room air contained 0.65 μl/L of CO; therefore, for correction of our COHb values for room air, 0.11% needed to be subtracted from the stated values.[9] Exchange transfusions were indicated in 20 of the 55 infants. Ten infants died; of these, seven had kernicterus and were considered to have had jaundice-related deaths, and three with TSB <256 μmol/L (15.0 mg/dl) were judged to have died of other factors. Nine patients had presumed kernicterus (Table I); the lowest TSB concentration at the time of enrollment in this group was 535 μmol/L (31.3 mg/dl); the TSB value at the onset of symptoms of kernicterus was unknown. All infants with kernicterus had COHb levels >2.00%. Infants with kernicterus had a mean TSB level that was significantly higher than in the group without kernicterus (Table II). Additionally, the infants with kernicterus were older and had lower hematocrits and a higher rate of G6PD deficiency than the nonkernicteric group. Thirty-one infants (56%) had a normal G6PD screening test result, and 14 infants (25%) had G6PD deficiency (10 [18%] not identified). Four of the "normal" infants (all boys) had a prolonged G6PD test decolorization time that was intermediate between those for normal and G6PD-deficient infants.

Figure 1 shows that TSB levels at the time of enrollment were correlated with COHb concentrations, with $r = 0.72$ (Pearson Product Moment Correlation). The COHb regression equation was COHb = 0.45 + 0.08*TSB (p <0.001).

For analysis, infant data were divided into two groups on either side of the median blood COHb concentration. Twenty-seven infants (49%) had a COHb range of 0.43% to 1.39%, and 28 (51%) had a COHb range of 1.40% to 5.93%. There was no difference in either age or weight between the groups. However, elevated COHb levels (≥1.40%) were positively associated with morbidity and death (Fig. 2).

We examined the relation of G6PD deficiency to COHb and outcome (n = 45). There was no difference in age between the normal (n = 31) and the G6PD-deficient (n = 14) groups. G6PD-deficient babies had significantly higher COHb levels than G6PD-normal babies, 2.26% (1.30% to 4.24%) versus 1.23% (0.98% to 1.74%) (p <0.01). As noted in Table III, the infants with G6PD deficiency also varied significantly from their G6PD-normal colleagues with respect to body weight ≤2500 gm, TSB and COHb levels, and hematocrit. Infants in our study with a normal G6PD screen result had better outcome than infants with G6PD deficiency with regard to jaundice-related death, kernicterus, and the number who met the criteria for exchange transfusion (Fig. 3).

On entry into the study, children born at Eku (n = 22) were slightly younger, 3.0 (2.0 to 4.0) days, than children admitted from home (n = 12), 4.0 (4.0 to 5.5) days, and than those from other hospitals/clinics (n = 20), 4.0 (3.5 to 5.0) days (p <0.001); there was no difference in their weights.

In the mothers tested (n = 45), none were Rh negative; Rh incompatibility was therefore unlikely. Coombs testing was not reliable, but ABO heterospecificity between mother and infant was found in only 7 of the 48 infants tested; of

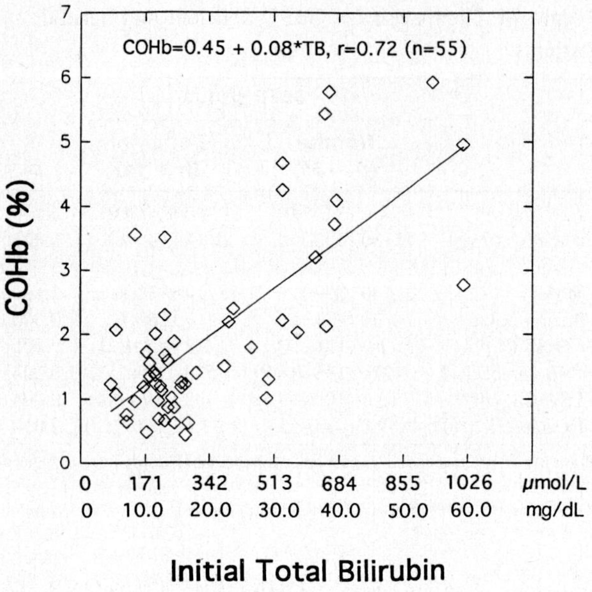

Fig. 1. COHb correlated with total bilirubin. The COHb levels are plotted against initial indirect serum bilirubin concentrations (n = 55).

these, it may have played a role in only one infant who required an exchange transfusion. Most of the infants were treated with intravenously administered ampicillin and gentamicin for possible sepsis. However, in at least two of the nine infants with kernicterus, there was strong supportive evidence for concurrent sepsis, and in most of the others, sepsis was also a possibility.

DISCUSSION

The COHb level is an accepted index of total bilirubin production in neonatal subjects under various clinical conditions.[16, 17] Although COHb concentrations in this study correlated with bilirubin levels, half of the variability cannot be explained by this relationship, most likely because of individual differences in bilirubin elimination from the body during the first several days of life. Except when bilirubin production is extremely high and associated consequently with extremely high bilirubin levels, such a relationship would not be expected, reflecting the importance of bilirubin elimination in determining the pattern of transitional jaundice. COHb levels also were associated with bilirubin-related morbidity and death in this patient sample.

We showed that infants with G6PD deficiency had increased COHb levels compared with those whose G6PD screen results were normal at the time of presentation with jaundice. However, no information about total bilirubin production was available before the onset of jaundice, and thus it is impossible to know whether earlier measurement of the COHb concentration would be predictive of jaundice in this population.

Infants with G6PD deficiency also had increased morbidity and mortality rates, consistent with findings in other studies.[1, 6, 18-20] G6PD deficiency is the most common enzymatic disorder of human beings, with prevalence as high as 35% in parts of Africa.[21] It has been identified as a major cause of neonatal jaundice in Nigerian infants[1, 4, 6, 8, 22-25] and in other groups.[21, 26-28] In a large study done in Ibadan, Nigeria,[6] 53 of 741 jaundiced babies required exchange transfusion. In the infants requiring exchange transfusion, 62% of the boys and 19% of the girls had G6PD deficiency.

The incidence of G6PD deficiency among jaundiced infants had not been determined at Eku before our study. Previous authors have raised doubts concerning the role of hemolysis in the production of neonatal jaundice in G6PD-deficient infants,[29, 30] and researchers cited by Luzzatto[30] had speculated that the jaundice may be of hepatic rather than hemolytic origin. Our data, however, indicate that increased bilirubin production plays a major role in hyperbilirubinemia in G6PD-deficient neonates with jaundice. The majority of our patients with G6PD deficiency had COHb levels greater than the median of 1.40%, indicating that, in our population, hemolysis was an important contributing cause of hyperbilirubinemia in G6PD-deficient infants readmitted for jaundice.

As expected, infants admitted from home had a higher incidence of exchange transfusion, clinical evidence of kernicterus, and death. Poorer outcome in outborn infants with neonatal jaundice has been documented previously in Nigeria[6, 18]; the possible reasons include later identification and treatment of jaundice.[7, 22, 25] Owa[20] and others have reported that increased morbidity in outborn versus inborn infants may be due to increased exposure to tribal medicines and agents associated with neonatal jaundice in patients with G6PD deficiency.[23, 25, 30] These include agents such as mentholated dusting powder, naphthalene, and herbs,[20, 31] and perhaps others yet to be identified. Although a history of exposure to such agents was sought, many of the medical histories were too incomplete for meaningful analysis.

Although ABO incompatibility was a potential cause of jaundice in only 15% of the infants tested, the low incidence may be attributed to missing blood type information. In other studies, such as reported by Azubuike,[18] it accounted for 17% of outborn and 26% of inborn cases of jaundice. In some studies, such as that by Owa et al.,[22] ABO incompatibility alone accounted for only 2% of the kernicterus but increased to 18% when multifactorial causes were included. Rh incompatibility is rare because of a very low incidence of Rh negativity in Nigeria. Consistent with other studies,[5, 6, 20] it was not a significant cause of jaundice in our study.

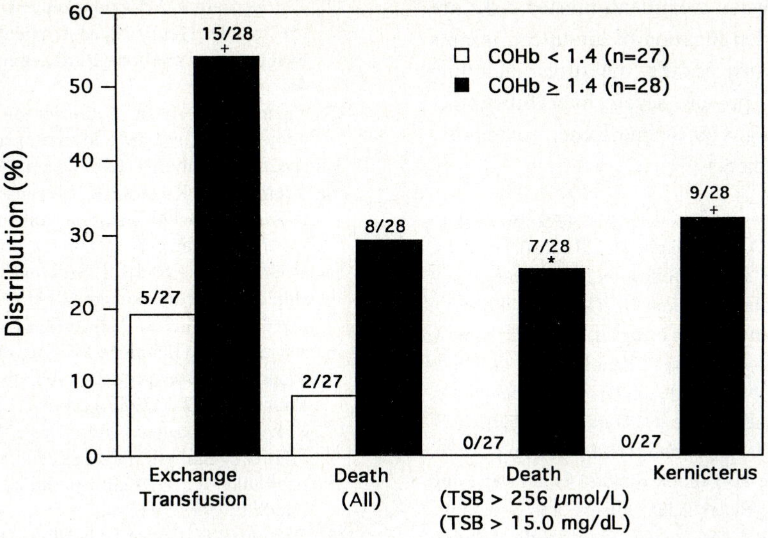

Fig. 2. COHb levels were positively associated with morbidity and death. The percentages of infants who met the criteria for exchange transfusion, those who died, and those in whom kernicterus developed was greater in the group of infants with COHb levels ≥1.40%. $^{*}p<0.05$; $^{+}p<0.01$. The numbers shown above each *bar* are expressed as ratios of subjects for each group.

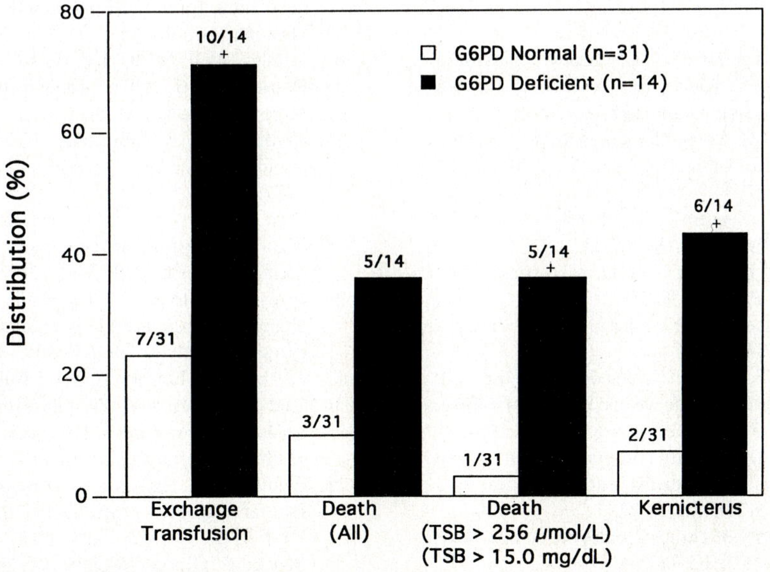

Fig. 3. G6PD deficiency was a major determining factor of outcome. The percentages of infants who met the criteria for exchange transfusion, those who died, and those in whom kernicterus developed was greater in the group of infants with G6PD deficiency. $^{+}p<0.01$. The numbers shown above each bar are expressed as ratios of subjects for each group.

Sepsis may also be an important cause of kernicterus[5, 6, 22-24, 28] and can be very difficult to distinguish from both the early and very late stages of kernicterus.[32] We were unable to obtain reliable blood culture results, and it was not possible to diagnose sepsis definitively as either a primary or a contributing etiologic factor.

We conclude that COHb levels correlated well with bilirubin levels in Nigerian infants admitted to the hospital for jaundice. Elevated COHb levels and G6PD deficiency were associated with bilirubin-related morbidity and death in these infants. In developing countries such as Nigeria, much of the blood supply is not screened for blood-borne disease and exchange transfusions are often performed under less than ideal conditions with minimal monitoring. Consequently, exchange transfusion treatment–related risks are extremely high. Earlier identification of jaundiced infants might allow for phototherapy or other measures, including exchange transfusions, to prevent severe hyperbilirubinemia and kernicterus among infants predisposed to hemolysis because of G6PD deficiency.

This research was made possible by the hard work of many both here and abroad, including Dr. Jedi Agbowu, Medical Director, Eku Baptist Hospital (EBH), and the following house staff, whom we thank for their help in data collection: Dr. O. Olanubi, Dr. O. Chukwu, Dr. O. P. Oyakhilome, Dr. B. Nzegwu, Dr. B. E. Aimua, Dr. I. Ofotokun, Dr. R. Agbowu, Dr. G. Ologidi, Dr. E. O. Chidume, Dr. H. A. Ladibile, Dr. N. M. Ashaka, Dr. O. P. Dienye, Dr. E. B. Akpochafo, Dr. E. Ofoegbu, Dr. O. Oaikhinam, Dr. O. S. Nonju, Dr. G. W. Nsirim, Dr. A. Oiowu, Dr. P. U. Agu, Dr. O. Omoruyi, Dr. J. Ojiabo. We also thank Sunday Ishiekwene and Laboratory personnel, EBH; Sister Edah, nurses, and assistants, EBH; fellow missionaries, EBH; Dr. Daniel Levin, Medical Director, and Dr. Brett Giroir, Co-Fellow, Children's Medical Center at Dallas Pediatric Intensive Care Unit; Svetlana A. Alshvang, of Stanford University School of Medicine, for total hemoglobin and COHb analysis of samples; and Sigma Chemical Co., St. Louis, Mo., for the gift of G6PD screening kits.

REFERENCES

1. Bienzle U, Effiong C, Luzzatto L. Erythrocyte glucose-6-phosphate dehydrogenase deficiency (G6PD type A) and neonatal jaundice. Acta Paediatr Scand 1976;65:701-3.
2. Ike Izuora G, Okoro ABO. Some clinical aspects of cerebral palsy among Nigerian Igbo children. Cent Afr J Med 1981; 27(8):155-9.
3. Duggan MB, Ogala W. Cerebral palsy in Nigeria: a report from Zaria. Ann Trop Paediatr 1982;2:7-11.
4. Ransome-Kuti O. Child health in Nigeria: past, present, and future. Arch Dis Child 1986;61:198-204.
5. Mee J, Scott D. Phototherapy for neonatal jaundice in rural Africa. Trop Doct 1977;7:33-4.
6. Effiong CE, Aimaku VE, Bienzle U, Ohedeji GA, Ikpe DE. Neonatal jaundice in Ibadan: incidence and etiologic factors in babies born in hospital. J Natl Med Assoc 1975;67:208-13.
7. Oyebola DDO. Care of the neonate and management of neonatal jaundice as practised by Yoruba traditional healers of Nigeria. J Trop Paediatr 1983;29:18-22.
8. Animashuan A. Aetiology of cerebral palsy in African children. Afr J Med Sci 1971;2:165-71.
9. Ostrander CR, Cohen RS, Hopper AO, Cowan BE, Stevens GB, Stevenson DK. Paired determinations of blood carboxyhemoglobin concentration and CO excretion rate in term and preterm infants. J Lab Clin Med 1992;100:745-55.
10. Behrman RE, Kleigman RM, Nelson WE, Vaughan VC. Nelson textbook of pediatrics. Philadelphia: WB Saunders, 1992.
11. Perlman JM, Rosenfeld CR. House staff nursery manual. Dallas: Division of Neonatal-Perinatal Medicine, Department of Pediatrics, University of Texas Southwestern Medical School, 1992.
12. Zimmerman HJ. Evaluation of the function and integrity of the liver. In: Henry JB, ed. Clinical diagnosis and management by laboratory methods. Philadelphia: WB Saunders, 1979;305-46.
13. Vreman HJ, Zwart A, Stevenson DK. Analysis for carboxyhemoglobin by gas chromatography and multicomponent spectrophotometry. Clin Chem 1987;33:694-6.
14. Vreman HJ, Kwong LK, Stevenson DK. CO in blood: an improved micro–blood sample collection system with rapid analysis by gas chromatography. Clin Chem 1984;30:1382-6.
15. Widness JA, Lowe LS, Stevenson DK, et al. Direct relationship of fetal carboxyhemoglobin with hemolysis in alloimmunized pregnancies. Pediatr Res 1994;35:713-9.
16. Ferguson JE II, Schutz TE, Stevenson DK. Neonatal bilirubin production after preterm labor tocolysis with nifedipine. Dev Pharmacol Ther 1989;12:113-7.
17. Peevy KJ, Landaw SA, Gross SJ. Hyperbilirubinemia in infants of diabetic mothers. Pediatrics 1980;66:417-9.
18. Azubuike JC. Neonatal jaundice in eastern Nigeria. J Trop Paediatr 1985;31:82-4.
19. Dowodu AH, Owa JA, Familusi JB. A prospective study of the role of bacterial infection and G6PD deficiency in severe neonatal jaundice in Nigeria. Trop Geogr Med 1984;36:127-32.
20. Owa JA. Relationship between exposure to icterogenic agents, glucose-6-phosphate dehydrogenase deficiency and neonatal jaundice in Nigeria. Acta Paediatr Scand 1989;78:848-52.
21. WHO Working Group. Glucose-6-phosphate dehydrogenase deficiency. Bull World Health Organ 1989;67:601-11.
22. Owa JA, Dowdu AH, Familusi JB. Kernicterus in Nigerian infants. West Afr J Med 1987;6:11-20.
23. Ransome-Kuti O. The problems of paediatric emergencies in Nigeria. Nigerian Medical Journal 1972;2:62-70.
24. Coulter JBS, Akpabio MA, Jikeme SON, Kay T. Neonatal jaundice in northern Nigeria. Nigerian Journal of Paediatrics 1977;5:12-5.
25. Owa JA, Durosinmi MA, Alabi AO. Determinants of severity of neonatal hyperbilirubinemia in ABO incompatibility in Nigeria. Trop Doct 1991;21:19-22.
26. Brown WR, Boon WH. Hyperbilirubinemia and kernicterus in glucose-6-phosphate dehydrogenase–deficient infants in Singapore. Pediatrics 1968;41:1055-62.
27. Kaplan M, Abramov A. Neonatal hyperbilirubinemia associated with glucose-6-phosphate dehydrogenase deficiency in Sephardic-Jewish neonates: incidence, severity, and the effects of phototherapy. Pediatrics 1992;90:401-5.
28. Fleming AF. Hematologic diseases. In: Strickland GT, ed. Hunter's tropical medicine. Philadelphia: WB Saunders, 1991:36-64.
29. Beutler E. Glucose-6-phosphate dehydrogenase deficiency. N Engl J Med 1991;324:169-74.
30. Luzzatto L. G6PD deficiency and hemolytic anemia. In: Nathan DG, Oski F, eds. Hematology of infancy and childhood. Philadelphia: WB Saunders, 1993:674-95.
31. Olowe SA, Ransome-Kuti O. The risk of jaundice in glucose-6-phosphate dehydrogenase–deficient babies exposed to menthol. Acta Paediatr Scand 1980;69:341-5.
32. Maisels MJ, Newman TB, Von Stockhausen H-B. Neonatal jaundice. In: Eichenwald HF, Ströder J, eds. Pediatric therapy. 3rd ed. St. Louis: Mosby–Year Books, 1993.

Internal potassium shift in premature infants: Cause of nonoliguric hyperkalemia

Kazuo Sato, MD, Tsutomu Kondo, MD, Hatsuo Iwao, MD, Sunao Honda, MD, and Kohji Ueda, MD

From the Department of Neonatology, Fukuoka Children's Hospital and Medical Center for Infectious Diseases, and the Department of Pediatrics, Faculty of Medicine, Kyushu University, Fukuoka, Japan

To study the pathophysiology of nonoliguric hyperkalemia, we measured serum potassium concentration and external K balance (intake and excretion), and estimated internal K balance (a shift from intracellular space to extracellular space) in 24 nonoliguric premature infants during the first 72 hours after birth. Data were analyzed from two aspects: gestational age (group 1, 24 to 28 weeks, n = 9; group 2, 29 to 32 weeks, n = 9; group 3, 33 to 36 weeks, n = 6) and postnatal age (0 to 72 hours). Serum K concentration rose from baseline (0 hour) to 24 hours in groups 1 and 2 (p <0.01) but did not rise in group 3. The external K balance was negative in all groups during the study period, and was more negative in the more premature infants (group 1 > group 2 > group 3) during the second 24 hours. There was a significant difference (p <0.01) between the internal K balance of the three groups during the first 24 hours (group 1 > group 2 > group 3), and the K shift decreased significantly (p <0.05) during the study period in groups 1 and 2. The more premature the infants, the larger the K shift and the larger the rise in serum K concentration during the first 24 hours, and the more negative the external K balance after 24 hours. These data indicate that K loading caused by the K shift associated with prematurity produces a rapid rise in serum K concentration, resulting in an increase in urinary K excretion. We conclude that an internal K shift inversely proportional to gestational and postnatal age is the primary cause of nonoliguric hyperkalemia in very premature infants. (J Pediatr 1995;126:109-13)

In very premature infants during the first 48 hours after birth, hyperkalemia develops even though oliguria is not observed.[1-5] If K intake is negligible, hyperkalemia could be produced only by decreased K excretion or K shift or both. Two mechanisms have been considered as causes of this nonoliguric hyperkalemia. One mechanism is decreased urinary K excretion as a result of distal tubular dysfunction[2-4, 6, 7]; the other is an internal K shift from the intracellular to the extracellular space.[8-10] In either case, nonoliguric hyperkalemia is associated strongly with prematurity and postnatal age, because it does not occur in mature infants or after 72 hours of age.

ATPase	Adenosinetriphosphatase
BW	Body weight
ECS	Extracellular space
ECV	Extracellular volume
ICS	Intracellular space

The purpose of this study was to determine the changes in serum K concentration, the K external balance (urinary

Submitted for publication March 1, 1994; accepted July 13, 1994.

Reprint requests: Kazuo Sato, MD, Department of Neonatology, Fukuoka Children's Hospital and Medical Center for Infectious Diseases, 2-5-1, Tohjin-machi, Chuo-ku, Fukuoka City 810, Japan.

0022-3476/95/$3.00 + 0 **9/23/59057**

K excretion), and the internal K balance (K shift) with gestational and postnatal age in premature infants without oliguria.

METHODS

Twenty-four male premature infants of appropriate size for gestational age (gestational age <37 weeks) who were admitted soon after birth to the neonatal intensive care unit of Fukuoka Children's Hospital, Fukuoka, Japan, were studied during the first 72 hours after birth. The gestational age of the patients was determined from the last menstrual period or prenatal ultrasound estimates or both. Female infants (because of difficulty in urine collection) and infants with severe asphyxia (Apgar score <3 at 1 minute), intracranial hemorrhage, acidosis (pH <7.25), or oliguria (urine output <1.0 ml/kg per hour of more than 24 hours' duration) were excluded. Informed consent was obtained from the parents.

Infants were divided into three groups according to gestational age: group 1, 24 to 28 weeks (n = 9); group 2, 29 to 32 weeks (n = 9); group 3, 33 to 36 weeks (n = 6). The average gestational age and birth weight of the three groups were 26.2 ± 1.5, 30.4 ± 1.3, and 34.8 ± 1.3 weeks and 963 ± 235, 1752 ± 339, and 2013 ± 315 gm, respectively. Differences in the serum K concentration, the external balance (urinary K extretion), and the internal balance (K shift) were compared among the three groups and among the time periods for each group.

Serum K concentration in nonhemolyzed blood samples obtained from a radial artery were determined every 24 hours (0, 24, 48, 72 hours). Body weight was also measured every 24 hours; BW changes in the three groups were within the normal range (group 1, 958 ± 230, 928 ± 220, 865 ± 228, and 820 ± 211 gm; group 2, 1752 ± 338, 1720 ± 344, 1635 ± 336, and 1578 ± 318 gm; and group 3, 2001 ± 323, 1931 ± 329, 1990 ± 318, and 1867 ± 313 gm).

Urine was collected continuously with a test tube or a finger portion of a latex glove for each 24-hour interval up to 72 hours (0 to 24, 24 to 48, 48 to 72 hours). The urine was immediately evacuated and placed in a capped refrigerated container to prevent evaporative losses. Urine volume and potassium concentration were determined for each 24-hour interval. Total urinary K excretion was equal to the negative external K balance because parenteral fluids did not include K.

Calculation of K shift. The internal K balance was calculated as follows:

The amount of K in ECS is extracellular volume (in liters per kilogram) × serum K (in millimoles per liter).

The amount of K after 24 hours is ECV' × serum K'.

The K shift (in millimoles per kilogram per 24 hours) is added, and urinary K excretion (in millimoles per kilogram per 24 hours) is subtracted for each 24-hour period.

$$(\text{ECV} \times \text{Serum K}) + \text{K shift} - (\text{Urine volume} \times \text{Urine K}) = (\text{ECV}' \times \text{Serum K}')$$

$$\therefore \text{K shift} = (\text{ECV}' \times \text{Serum K}') - (\text{ECV} \times \text{Serum K}) + (\text{UV} \times \text{Urine K})$$

It is assumed that ECV at birth = {0.57 − 0.06BW}, in liters per kilogram,[11] BW loss after birth = ECV loss, and ECV' = ECV − BW loss. These assumptions are based on the changes in body fluid composition during intrauterine growth and postnatal contraction of ECV.

Statistical analysis. All data are presented as mean ± SD. Differences among the three groups were tested with the Kruskal-Wallis test. After confirmation, the Mann-Whitney test was performed to detect differences between two groups. Differences between times or periods within each group were tested with the Friedman test (all study periods) and Wilcoxon signed rank test (two periods). The correlation between the K shift and gestational age was tested with linear regression analysis. A probability of <0.05 was considered significant.

RESULTS

There were significant differences among the serum K concentrations of the three groups at baseline (group 1 < group 2 < group 3; $p < 0.05$) and at 24 hours (group 1 > group 2 > group 3; $p < 0.01$). At baseline the serum K concentration of group 1 was significantly lower than that of group 3 (<0.05). At 24 hours the serum K values of group 1 and group 2 were higher than that of group 3 ($p < 0.01$ and $p < 0.05$, respectively). The serum K concentration of group 1 rose rapidly from baseline (3.97 ± 0.42 mmol/L) to 24 hours (6.00 ± 0.97 mmol/L) and fell from 24 hours to 72 hours (4.62 ± 0.67 mmol/L) ($p < 0.01$) (Fig. 1). Group 2 had a significant change in serum K similar to that in group 1, but group 3 had no significant change during the study period.

The external K balance was negative in the three groups during all three 24-hour intervals (Fig. 1). Urinary flow for the three intervals was 46.4 ± 30.0, 94.5 ± 23.6, and 88.6 ± 16.8 ml/kg per 24 hours in group 1, 38.3 ± 16.8, 70.9 ± 26.5, and 56.1 ± 21.0 ml/kg per 24 hours in group 2, 45.9 ± 15.4, 46.6 ± 23.7, and 49.1 ± 9.1 ml/kg per 24 hours in group 3, respectively. There was a significant difference in the degree of negative external balance of the three groups during the second 24 hours (group 1 > group 2 > group 3; $p < 0.01$). During the second 24 hours, the degree of negative external K balance in group 1 was larger than that of the other two groups ($p < 0.05$). The degree of negative balance in group 1 increased from the first 24 hours

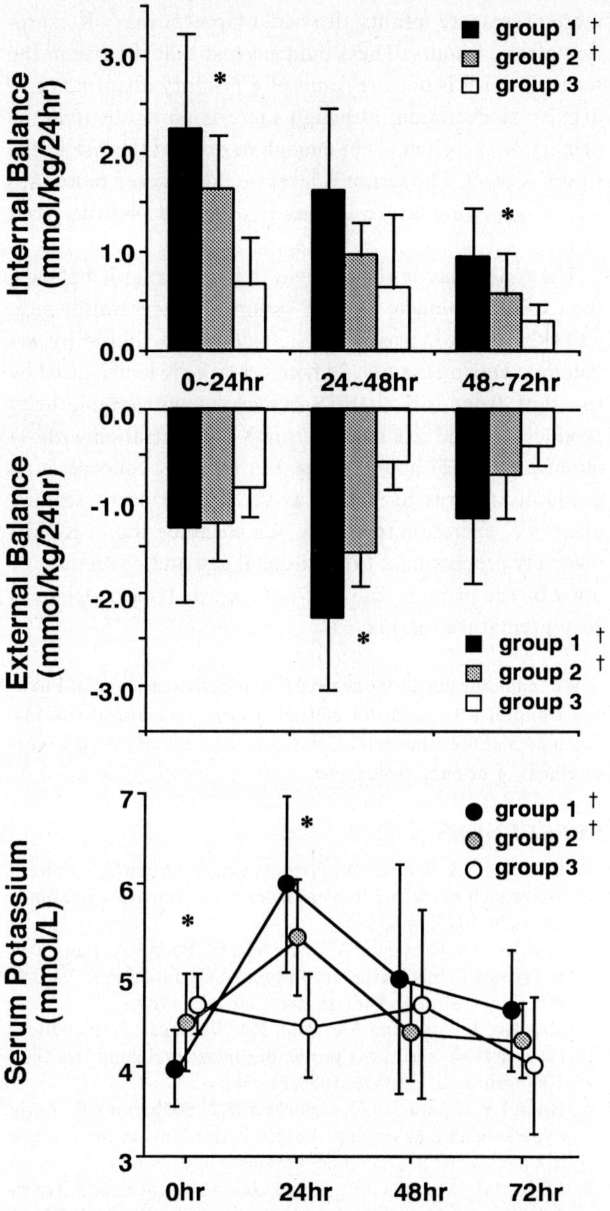

Fig. 1. Internal potassium balance, external potassium balance, and serum potassium concentration. Group 1, 24 to 28 weeks, n = 9; group 2, 29 to 32 weeks, n = 9; group 3, 33 to 36 weeks, n = 6. *Asterisk* indicates significant differences between groups (p <0.05). *Dagger* indicates significant differences between times or periods (p <0.05).

(1.30 ± 0.81 mmol/kg per 24 hours) to the second 24 hours (2.29 ± 0.78 mmol/kg per 24 hours) and decreased from the second to the third 24-hour interval (1.20 ± 0.72 mmol/kg per 24 hours) (p <0.05). Group 2 had a change similar to that in group 1. Group 3 had no significant change in the external K balance.

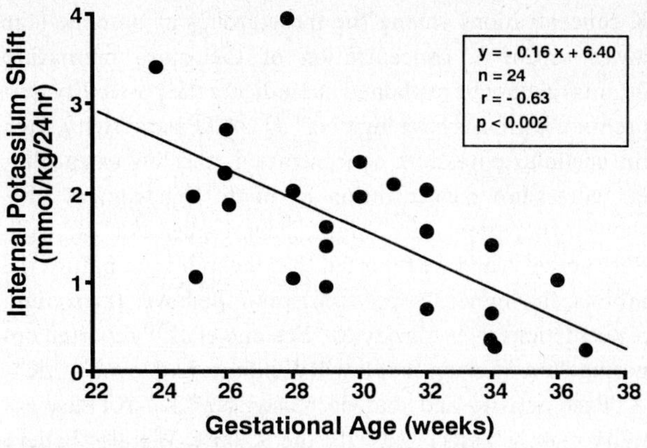

Fig. 2. Correlation between internal potassium shift from ICS to ECS during the first 24 hours and gestational age.

There was a significant difference between the internal K balance of the three groups during the first 24 hours (group 1 > group 2 > group 3; p <0.01) (Fig. 1). During the first 24 hours, the K shift (internal K balance) of group 1 was larger than that of group 3 (p <0.01), and the K shift of group 2 was also larger than that of group 3 (p <0.05). The K shift of the first 24 hours was inversely correlated with gestational age (r = −0.63; p <0.002) (Fig. 2). The K shift of group 1 decreased from the first 24 hours (2.25 ± 0.98 mmol/kg per 24 hours) to the third 24 hours (0.94 ± 0.50 mmol/kg per 24 hours) (p <0.01). Group 2 had a significant decrease, as in group 1 (p <0.05). Group 3 had no significant change in the K shift.

The time delay in the changes in the internal K balance, the external K balance, and the serum K concentration are also demonstrated in Fig. 1. In group 1 a large K shift occurred and serum K concentration rose rapidly during the first 24 hours, and then a large urinary K excretion was observed during the second 24 hours, after which the serum K level fell gradually with a decline of the K shift. Group 2 had similar but smaller changes than in group 1. Group 3 did not show any changes.

DISCUSSION

Nonoliguric hyperkalemia occurs in very premature infants during the first 48 hours after birth, but not in mature infants or after 72 hours of age. Previous studies have reported hyperkalemia in extremely low birth weight infants but not a rapid rise in serum K during the first 24 hours.[3, 7, 10, 12] Our data indicate that the serum K level is normal (not high) soon after birth but rises rapidly in very premature infants, and that the degree of rise is proportional to the degree of prematurity (moderately premature infants have a smaller rise in serum K). The differences of serum

K concentrations among the three groups at baseline (the lower serum K concentration of the more premature infants) cannot be explained but indicate the possibility that premature infants have high Na^+,K^+-ATPase activity, high intracellular potassium concentration, and low extracellular potassium concentration at birth. Sigström et al.[13] showed that premature infants have higher Na^+,K^+-ATPase activity, and we reported that the more premature the infants, the higher the potassium and the lower the sodium concentrtions in erythrocytes.[9] Stefano et al.[10] reported opposing data showing that low BW infants had low Na^+,K^+-ATPase activity and that decreased Na^+,K^+-ATPase activity may be associated with the K shift. We also believe that Na^+,K^+ pump failure after birth might be associated with cellular K loss. The serum K level is normal, not high, soon after birth and then rises rapidly, but the serum K on day 1 (first measurement) in their article had already increased and was higher than at any time during the first 3 days of life. Therefore we assume that Stefano et al. failed to demonstrate a normal serum K level before it rose and high Na^+,K^+-ATPase activity before it decreased, because their measurements were not taken soon after birth.

The internal potassium balance was deduced, rather than measured, from the serum K concentration and the external potassium balance measurements, but the calculations and assumptions are considered to be reasonable. The differences in the internal K balance among the three groups (the more premature infants had a larger K shift) could be the reason that nonoliguric hyperkalemia occurs in very premature infants and not in mature infants. Hyperkalemia probably does not develop in mature infants because the K shift is very small. The decline in the internal K balance with postnatal age could be the reason that nonoliguric hyperkalemia occurs during first the 48 hours and not after 72 hours. Hyperkalemia does not develop after 72 hours because the K shift is very small. The cause of the K shift has not been elucidated. Stefano et al.[10] reported that Na^+,K^+-ATPase activity was lower in hyperkalemic extremely low birth weight infants than in a normokalemic group, and concluded that the K shift from ICS to ECS associated with decreased erythrocyte Na^+,K^+-ATPase activity was probably the cause of nonoliguric hyperkalemia. The Na^+, K^+-ATPase activity may be disturbed by stress caused by preterm birth. The other possible causes of the K shift from ICS to ECS are increased cell K production,[14] insulin insufficiency,[15] and relative hypoaldosteronism.[8, 16]

There were no differences in the degree of negative balance (urinary K excretion) among the three groups during the first 24 hours, although the more premature infants had a larger rise in serum K levels during the same period. The more premature infants also had a larger urinary K excretion after 24 hours. These data suggest that the rise in the serum K level is not the result of a primary disturbance of urinary K excretion, although there is no doubt that the urinary K excretion is not enough to prevent the rise in the serum K level. The serum K level would rise even more rapidly in very premature infants if they had oliguric renal failure.

The time delay in the changes in the internal K balance, the external balance, and the serum K concentration suggests the following pathophysiology of nonoliguric hyperkalemia: During the first 24 hours, a large K load caused by the shift from ICS to ECS associated with prematurity produces a rapid rise in the serum K concentration without oliguria; after 24 hours of age, the serum K concentration gradually returns to normal as the K shift decreases and urinary K excretion increases. We conclude that a K shift inversely proportional to gestational age and postnatal age must be the primary cause of nonoliguric hyperkalemia in very premature infants.

We thank the nurses in the neonatal intensive care unit at Fukuoka Children's Hospital for collecting urine. We also thank Ms. Iwamoto and the other staff of the clinical laboratory for the measurement of urinary electrolytes.

REFERENCES

1. Herscher ES, Berman W, Friedman Z, Whitman V. Left bundle-branch block due to hyperkalemia in premature infants. J Pediatr 1979;94:654-6.
2. Gruskay JA, Costarino AT, McNelis W, Polin RA, Baumgart S. Hyperkalemia secondary to tubular dysfunction in VLBW infants [Abstract]. Pediatr Res 1986;20:349A.
3. Gruskay J, Costarino AT, Polin RA, Baumgart S. Nonoliguric hyperkalemia in the premature infant weighing less than 1000 grams. J Pediatr 1988;113:381-6.
4. Brion LP, Schwartz GJ, Campbell D, Fleischman AR. Early hyperkalaemia in very low birthweight infants in the absence of oliguria. Arch Dis Child 1989;64:270-2.
5. Leslie GI, Carman G, Arnold JD. Early neonatal hyperkalaemia in the extremely premature newborn infant. J Paediatr Child Health 1990;26:58-61.
6. Fukuda Y, Kojima T, Ono A, Matsuzaki S, Iwase S, Kobayashi Y. Factors causing hyperkalemia in premature infants. Am J Perinatol 1989;6:76-9.
7. Shaffer SG, Kilbride HW, Hayen LK, Meade VM, Warady BA. Hyperkalemia in very low birth weight infants. J Pediatr 1992;121:275-9.
8. Lorenz JM, Kleinman LI. Nonoliguric hyperkalemia in preterm neonates [Letter]. J Pediatr 1989;114:507-8.
9. Sato K, Kondo T, Iwao H, Honda S, Ueda K. Sodium and potassium in red blood cells of premature infants during the first few days: risk of hyperkalaemia. Acta Paediatr Scand 1991; 80:899-904.
10. Stefano JL, Norman ME, Morales MC, Goplerud JM, Mishra OP, Delivoria PM. Decreased erythrocyte Na^+, K^+-ATPase

activity associated with cellular potassium loss in extremely low birth weight infants with nonoliguric hyperkalemia. J PEDIATR 1993;122:276-84.
11. Brans YW. Fetal and neonatal body fluid composition with reference to growth and development. In: Polin RA, Fox WW, eds. Fetal and neonatal physiology. Philadelphia: WB Saunders, 1992:1299-313.
12. Stefano JL, Norman ME. Nitrogen balance in extremely low birth weight infants with nonoliguric hyperkalemia. J PEDIATR 1993;123:632-5.
13. Sigström L, Waldenström J, Karlberg P. Characteristics of active sodium and potassium transport in erythrocyte of healthy infants and children. Acta Paediatr Scand 1981;70:347-52.
14. Aiken CG, Sherwood RA, Kenney IJ, Furnell M, Lenney W. Mineral balance studies in sick preterm intravenously fed infants during the first week after birth: a guide to fluid therapy. Acta Paediatr Scand Suppl 1989;355:1-59.
15. Goldman SL, Hirata T. Attenuated response to insulin in very low birthweight infants. Pediatr Res 1980;14:50-3.
16. Sulyok E, Nemeth M, Tenyi I, et al. Postnatal development of renin-angiotensin-aldosterone system, RAAS, in relation to electrolyte balance in premature infants. Pediatr Res 1979;13:15-27.

Use of the urine-to-blood carbon dioxide tension gradient as a measurement of impaired distal tubular hydrogen ion secretion among neonates

Jin-Yao Lin, MD, Jin-Shoei Lin, MD, and Chang-Hai Tsai, MD

From the Department of Pediatrics, China Medical College Hospital, Taichung, Taiwan, Republic of China

To evaluate the utility of the urinary-minus-blood partial pressure of carbon dioxide (U-B P_{CO_2}) gradient for the diagnosis of distal renal tubular acidosis in neonates, we measured the U-B P_{CO_2} gradient corresponding to different urinary bicarbonate concentrations in 40 neonates. The U-B P_{CO_2} gradient in these neonates had a significant linear relationship to the urinary bicarbonate concentration. When the urinary bicarbonate concentration was >10 mmol/L, in all the neonates the U-B P_{CO_2} could be increased above the 20 mm Hg level. We conclude that it is appropriate to determine the U-B P_{CO_2} gradient as an index of distal urinary acidification and that it is a necessary test for diagnosis of distal renal tubular acidosis in neonates. (J PEDIATR 1995;126:114-7)

The observation that urinary partial pressure of carbon dioxide increases considerably after alkalinization of the urine as a consequence of distal hydrogen ion secretion is not new.[1, 2] However, in recent years this phenomenon has been used increasingly as an index of distal acidification.[3-6]

In adults and children, measurement of the urinary-minus-blood P_{CO_2} gradient during maximal urine alkalinization has been considered the most sensitive method of detecting impairment of distal tubular H^+ secretion.[7-12] To our knowledge, no data are available for use of this measurement in neonates.

We measured the U-B P_{CO_2} gradient of 40 term neonates and plotted the value against urinary bicarbonate concentration. The specific aim was to determine whether the capacity of distal nephron H^+ secretion in term neonates is mature enough to validate the use of U-B P_{CO_2} gradient in evaluating the possible presence of distal renal tubular acidosis.

Submitted for publication Feb. 28, 1994; accepted July 18, 1994.

Reprint requests: Jin-Yao Lin, MD, Division of Pediatric Nephrology, Department of Pediatrics, China Medical College Hospital, No. 75 Yuh Der Rd., Taichung, Taiwan, Republic of China.

0022-3476/95/$3.00 + 0 **9/23/59062**

METHODS

During a period of 1 year, 63 term neonates admitted to China Medical College Hospital, Taichung, Taiwan, were considered for participation in this study. These neonates were hospitalized because of fever or jaundice. Of the 63 neonates, 40 infants without any type of renal or nonrenal disease that might affect water and electrolyte or acid-base metabolism were enrolled in the study. Their ages ranged from 1 to 29 days with a mean of 10.3 days; the sex ratio (female/male) was 21:19. The weights of all subjects were between the 10th and 75th percentiles for age.

dRTA	Distal renal tubular acidosis
P_{CO_2}	Partial pressure of carbon dioxide
U-B P_{CO_2}	Urinary-minus-blood P_{CO_2}
$UHCO_3^-$	Urinary bicarbonate concentration

Antibiotics, including ampicillin and gentamicin, were given intravenously in 20 subjects because of suspicion of infection pending the results of cultures. In addition, 15 icteric subjects were first treated with phototherapy.

The investigations were performed with institutional approval, and informed parental consent was obtained before study.

Urine collection. To avoid suprapubic aspiration or ure-

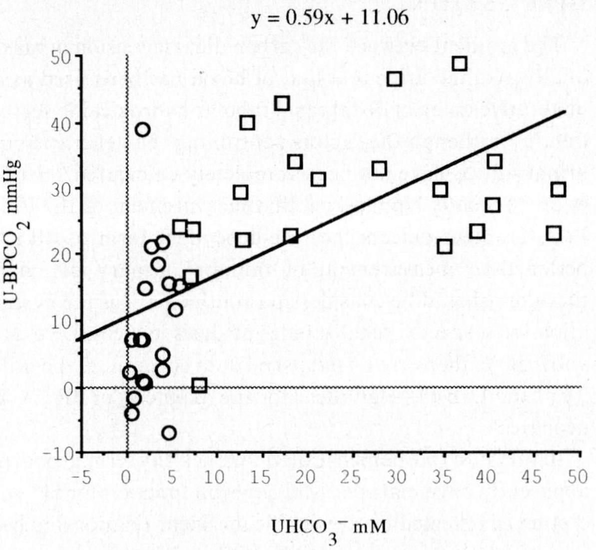

Fig. 1. Linear regression for urinary-minus-blood Pco_2 *(U-BP-CO_2)* gradient/urinary bicarbonate concentration *($UHCO_3^-$)* in healthy neonates with *(squares)* and without *(circles)* sodium bicarbonate loading; $p < 0.01$.

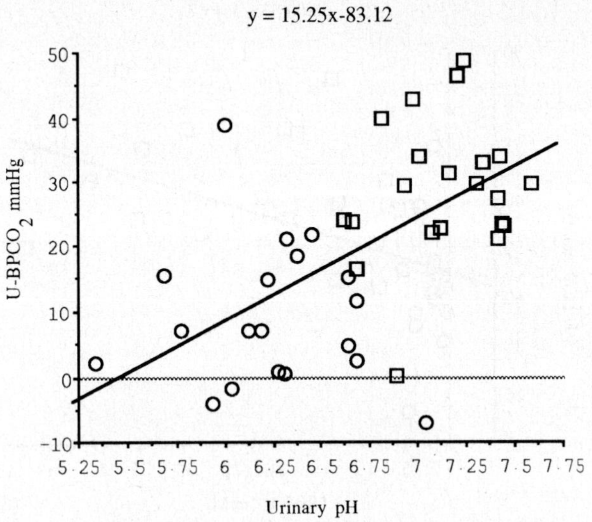

Fig. 2. Linear regression for urinary-minus-blood Pco_2 *(U-BP co_2)* gradient/urinary pH in normal neonates with *(squares)* and without *(circles)* sodium bicarbonate loading; $p < 0.01$.

thral catheterization, we collected urine by the following method. A full bladder was first confirmed by echographic study; thereafter we massaged the bladder gently and collected the urine in a test tube containing 0.5 ml mineral oil. When the urine was voided into the tube, it was covered by the oil spontaneously. We easily collected an adequate volume of urine for analysis in this manner.

Blood sampling. Arterial blood samples were obtained by anaerobic radial artery puncture after an aseptic procedure for measurement of Pco_2 and pH.

Study procedure. Urine sodium, potassium, and creatinine were measured with a standard chemistry automatic analyzer (model 763-15; Hitachi, Tokyo, Japan). Urinary pH was measured by a pH meter (model 6071 Microcomputer pH meter; Jenco, San Diego, Calif.). Urinary CO_2 and blood pH and CO_2 were measured with a standard blood gas analyzer (model 278 blood gas analyzer; Ciba Corning Diagnostics Corp., Medfield, Mass.). Urinary HCO_3^- content was calculated as described by Edelmann et al.,[13] with the negative logarithm of the ionization constant of the urine corrected for ionic strength.

To obtain different $UHCO_3^-$ values and the corresponding U-B Pco_2 gradient among the neonates with a minimum number of artery punctures, we developed the following procedures. First, the neonates were assigned to icteric (19 neonates) and nonicteric (21 neonates) groups. No $NaHCO_3$ was given to infants in the icteric group because of the possible adverse effect of metabolic alkalosis in icteric neonates. These icteric neonates received hydration fluids overnight; in the morning urine and blood samples were obtained simultaneously. Thus we obtained 19 sets of $UHCO_3^-$ data and the corresponding U-B Pco_2 gradient.

The nonicteric infants were studied after sodium bicarbonate loading. A solution of 5% dextrose containing 100 mmol $NaHCO_3$ per liter was given intravenously at a rate of 1500 ml/m^2 per day. We could not predict the individual response to $NaHCO_3$ loading in these subjects; therefore we performed the study case by case sequentially in the following manner. Urine and blood samples were collected from the first subject after $NaHCO_3$ loading for 1 hour. Thereafter we studied the remaining subjects sequentially by increasing the loading interval for at least 30 minutes. Urine was collected during 30-minute intervals. The $UHCO_3^-$ was calculated immediately, which required only 2 minutes. When the $UHCO_3^-$ for a particular infant was greater than that of the previous subject, the artery was punctured to measure the U-B Pco_2 gradient and the study was terminated. If the $UHCO_3^-$ was equal to or less than that of the previous subject, the $NaHCO_3$ infusion would be continued and urine was collected again after an interval of 30 minutes. When the $UHCO_3^-$ was satisfactory, the study was terminated after measurement of the U-B Pco_2 gradient. The $NaHCO_3$ loading was also terminated when the total amount infused was 40 mmol in a single subject, regardless of the $UHCO_3^-$. Therefore it was sometimes necessary to collect urine more than once in some subjects to obtain a satisfactory $UHCO_3^-$, but arterial puncture was done only once in all neonates. In this manner we obtained 21 different sets of $UHCO_3^-$ data and the corresponding U-B Pco_2 gradient.

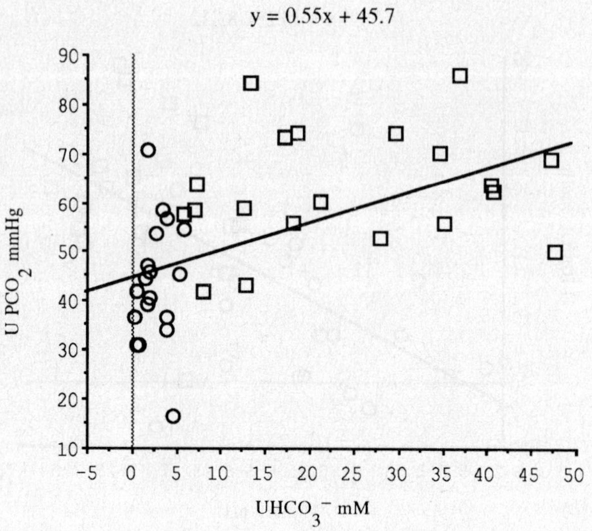

Fig. 3. Linear regression for urinary P_{CO_2} *(UPco₂)*/urinary bicarbonate concentration *($UHCO_3^-$)* in normal neonates with *(squares)* and without *(circles)* sodium bicarbonate loading; $p < 0.01$.

Statistical analysis of the data was performed with a standard bivariate correlation technique on an Apple computer (Macintosh IIvi, Cupertino, Calif.).

RESULTS

All the neonates were discharged home and no complications developed because of the study procedure. We followed these subjects for at least 6 months; none showed any evidence of renal tubular acidosis or other renal disease.

The U-B P_{CO_2} gradient in normal neonates varied widely when $UHCO_3^-$ was low; however, the value increased markedly when $UHCO_3^-$ increased after sodium bicarbonate loading (Fig. 1). All the subjects had a U-B P_{CO_2} gradient well in excess of 20 mm Hg when the $UHCO_3^-$ increased above 10 mmol/L. The regression equation for U-B P_{CO_2} gradient/$UHCO_3^-$ was U-B P_{CO_2} gradient = 0.59 $UHCO_3^-$ + 11.06 (Fig. 1). The correlation coefficient for the regression equation was 0.60 ($p < 0.01$). There was a significant linear correlation between the U-B P_{CO_2} gradient and the $UHCO_3^-$ at values of urinary bicarbonate between 0 and 50 mmol/L. We also found a linear relationship between U-B P_{CO_2} gradient and urinary pH ($p < 0.01$) (Fig. 2).

When urinary P_{CO_2} was plotted against U-B $UHCO_3^-$, there was also a significant linear relationship between urinary P_{CO_2} and $UHCO_3^-$, though the correlation was less than that of the U-B P_{CO_2} gradient and $UHCO_3^-$ ($p < 0.01$) (Fig. 3).

DISCUSSION

The gradient between the carbon dioxide tension in maximally alkaline urine and that of blood has been used as a qualitative index of distal renal tubular hydrogen ion secretion,[5, 12] although the factors controlling the generation of urinary P_{CO_2} have not been completely elucidated.[8] Strife et al.[14] recently emphasized that measurement of the U-B P_{CO_2} gradient detects the rate-dependent form of dRTA better than measurement of minimal urinary pH, and therefore should be considered a routine part of the evaluation for suspected renal tubular acidosis in a child. To our knowledge, there are no published data concerning the utility of the U-B P_{CO_2} gradient for the diagnosis of dRTA in neonates.

In this study we demonstrated that healthy term neonates apparently have mature distal nephron function for H^+ secretion as reflected by the significant linear relationship between U-B P_{CO_2} gradient and $UHCO_3^-$. It is thus necessary to measure the U-B P_{CO_2} gradient for diagnosis of dRTA in neonates. Batlle[5] stressed that the change in urine P_{CO_2} is a more accurate index of distal acidification than U-B P_{CO_2} gradient when urinary P_{CO_2} and blood P_{CO_2} vary widely. The linear changes of urinary P_{CO_2} against $UHCO_3^-$ in our study confirmed that the change in P_{CO_2} is also a good index of distal acidification in neonates. It would be convenient to need only urine samples at different intervals shortly after $NaHCO_3$ loading, rather than to require puncture of the vessel after maximal alkalization of urine to evaluate distal nephron H^+ secretion. Because the regression coefficient of urinary $P_{CO_2}/UHCO_3^-$ is less than that of U-B $P_{CO_2}/UHCO_3^-$, we might have to infuse more $NaHCO_3$ to obtain a significant gradient between each urinary P_{CO_2} measurement than would be needed for a significant U-B P_{CO_2} gradient. However, the change in P_{CO_2} is a good index of distal acidification in hypercapnic states and might obviate unnecessary blood sampling.[5]

Sodium bicarbonate loading may result in hypernatremia, metabolic alkalosis, volume overload, and cerebral spinal fluid acidosis.[15] Therefore it is safe to perform the study with moderate or minimal alkalization of the patient. In our study, in all the normal neonates the U-BP_{CO_2} gradient could be increased above 20 mm Hg when the $UHCO_3^-$ was >10 mmol/L. Therefore it may be appropriate to collect urine during approximately 30- to 60-minute intervals and to terminate the $NaHCO_3$ infusion if the U-B P_{CO_2} gradient is >20 mm Hg, because the majority of our subjects had $UHCO_3^-$ >10 mmol about 3 to 5 hours after infusion, and the urinary bladder would become full enough for urine collection by massage within 30 to 60 minutes. With this method we can rule out dRTA after moderate alkalization of neonates; furthermore, plotting the U-B P_{CO_2}

gradient or change in P_{CO_2} against $UHCO_3^-$ is also a good method in the study of distal tubular acidification, and makes unnecessary the maximal alkalization of urine, as described by Rodriguez-Soriano et al.[16] Conversely, in our study, in all neonates the U-B P_{CO_2} could be increased >20 mm Hg when the urinary pH was >7.0; therefore, checking the urinary pH rather than $UHCO_3^-$ might be used as an alternative for determining when to obtain blood samples.

We conclude that the U-B P_{CO_2} gradient is an appropriate index of distal urinary acidification and is a necessary test for diagnosis of dRTA in neonates.

REFERENCES

1. Kennedy TJ Jr, Orloff J, Berliner RW. Significance of carbon dioxide tension in urine. Am J Physiol 1952;169:596-608.
2. Ochwadt BK, Pitts RF. Effect of intravenous infusion of carbonic anhydrase on carbon dioxide tension of alkaline urine. Am J Physiol 1956;185;426-39.
3. Batlle DC. Hyperkalemic hyperchloremic metabolic acidosis associated with selective aldosterone deficiency and distal renal tubular acidosis. Semin Nephrol 1981;1:260-74.
4. Batlle DC, Sehy JT, Roseman MK, Arruda JAL, Kurtzman NA. Clinical and pathophysiologic spectrum of acquired distal renal tubular acidosis. Kidney Int 1981;20:389-96.
5. Batlle D. Delta urine PCO_2 rather than U-$BPCO_2$ as an index of distal acidification [Editorial]. Semin Nephrol 1982;2:189-90.
6. Batlle D, Kurtzman NA. Distal renal tubular acidosis: pathogenesis and classification. Am J Kidney Dis 1982;1:328-44.
7. Batlle DC, Grupp M, Gariria M, Kurtzman NA. Distal renal tubular acidosis with intact capacity to lower urinary pH. Am J Med 1982;72:751-8.
8. Kurtzman NA. Acquired distal renal tubular acidosis. Kidney Int 1983;24:807-19.
9. Stinebaugh BJ, Esquenazi R, Schloeder FX, Suki WN, Goldstein MB, Halperin ML. Control of the urine-blood PCO_2 gradient in alkaline urine. Kidney Int 1980;17:31-9.
10. Batlle DC, Arruda JAL. The renal tubular acidosis syndromes. Miner Electrolyte Metab 1981;5:83-99.
11. Arruda JAL, Nascimento L, Mehta PK, et al. The critical importance of urinary concentrating ability in the generation of urinary carbon dioxide tension. J Clin Invest 1977;60:922-35.
12. Halperin ML, Goldstein NB, Haig A, Johnson M, Stinebaugh B. Studies on the pathogenesis of type I (distal) renal tubular acidosis as revealed by the urinary PCO_2 tension. J Clin Invest 1974;53:669-77.
13. Edelmann CM, Rodriguez-Soriano J, Boichis H, Gruskin AB, Acosta M. Bicarbonate reabsorption and hydrogen ion excretion in normal infants. J Clin Invest 1967;46:1309-17.
14. Strife CF, Clardy CW, Varade WS, Prada AL, Waldo FB. Urine-to-blood carbon dioxide tension gradient and maximal depression of urinary pH to distinguish rate-dependent from classic distal renal tubular acidosis in children. J PEDIATR 1993;122:60-5.
15. Posner J, Plum F. Spinal-fluid pH and neurologic symptoms in systemic acidosis N Engl J Med 1967;277:605-13.
16. Rodriguez-Soriano J, Vallo A, Castillo G, Oliveros R. Pathophysiology of primary distal renal tubular acidosis. Int J Pediatr Nephrol 1985;6:71-8.

Newborn screening for congenital adrenal hyperplasia in New Zealand

W. S. Cutfield, MBChB, and D. Webster, PhD

From the Department of Pediatrics, University of Auckland, and the National Testing Centre, Greenlane Hospital, Auckland, New Zealand

Objective: **To evaluate the efficacy and efficiency of newborn screening for classic congenital adrenal hyperplasia (CAH) in New Zealand.**
Design: **All infants younger than 6 weeks of age identified by newborn screening between December 1984 and December 1993 were included.**
Results: **23 cases of classic CAH (20 salt-losers) were identified. The incidence of classic CAH was 1 in 23,344. Screening identified 3 of 9 virilized female infants whose disease had not been detected clinically. Screening alone identified all 11 male infants. Notification of cases occurred at 11 ± 3 days of age. There was a delay in treatment of the group identified by screening alone (n = 14) until 13 days of age (range, 4 to 35 days); at that time 11 infants had hyponatremia and 10 had hyperkalemia. Symptoms of vomiting, poor feeding, and shock were common after 10 days of age (2/10, <10 days, and 8/8, 11 to 16 days of age).**
Conclusions: **Newborn CAH screening is the only method of identifying male infants with classic CAH without a family history of CAH before symptoms develop, as well as a significant portion of overlooked virilized female infants. So that clinical or significant biochemical deterioration can be avoided, pediatrician notification of screening results and treatment should be started before 10 days of age. (J Pediatr 1995;126:118-21)**

Classic congenital adrenal hyperplasia as a result of 21-hydroxylase deficiency is divided into salt-wasting and simple virilizing forms. Salt-wasting CAH is a rapidly evolving, life-threatening disorder that typically is apparent within the first month.

The development of a 17α-hydroxyprogesterone assay from a filter paper–dried blood spot has allowed classic CAH to be added to newborn screening programs.[1] Although newborn screening for CAH began 14 years ago, there are only 23 CAH screening programs in 10 countries worldwide.[2] Such limited international acceptance of CAH screening is a reflection of skepticism of likely benefits gained for the cost entailed. Screening for CAH was added to the newborn screening program in New Zealand in December 1984 and continues to the present. The purpose of this study was to evaluate the efficacy and efficiency of newborn CAH screening in New Zealand.

Submitted for publication May 23, 1994; accepted August 10, 1994.

Reprint requests: W. S. Cutfield, MBChB, Department of Pediatrics, University of Auckland, Private Bag, Auckland, New Zealand.

0022-3476/95/$3.00 + 0 **9/23/59780**

METHODS

All children in whom CAH was diagnosed by neonatal screening, family history, or clinical evaluation within the first 6 weeks of life, from December 1984 to December 1993, were included in the study. Newborn screening is conducted by a single laboratory in New Zealand, the National Testing Centre located in Auckland. Whole blood 17-OHP was measured initially by a double-antibody radioimmunoassay. The samples with 17-OHP values that were ≥2 SDs above the assay mean were reassayed after diethyl ether extraction. These sequential assays were completed within 24 hours to provide a sense of timing. Extracted whole blood 17-OHP values of ≥23 nmol/L from infants who weighed >1500 gm, and of ≥32

CAH	Congenital adrenal hyperplasia
17-OHP	17-α-Hydroxyprogesterone

nmol/L (approximately 51 and 71 nmol/L of plasma, respectively) from infants who weighed <1500 gm, were set as the levels used to indicate a positive screening result for CAH (reference 3; M. Wallace, personal communication, 1994). The intraassay and interassay variabilities for a whole blood 17-OHP value of 23 nmol/L were 15%. Clinical and laboratory data from the initial hospital evaluation were collected for analysis of all subjects. Hyponatremia was defined as a serum sodium concentration <136 mmol/L, and hyperkalemia was defined as a serum potassium concentration ≥7.0 mmol/L. Values are expressed as means with either SD or range. Simple linear regression was used to compare serum sodium and potassium concentrations with treatment age.

RESULTS

A total of 536,915 newborn samples were screened for CAH by 17-OHP measurement. During this period 23 cases of CAH were identified within the first 6 weeks of life. The newborn screening 17-OHP sample was collected at 4.3 ± 1.0 (SD) days, similar to the collection time of 3 to 5 days for most centers performing CAH screening.[4] The incidence of CAH in New Zealand as identified by the newborn screening program was 1:23,344, an annual rate of 2.6 cases per year. The cost of each 17-OHP test performed as an additional test to an established newborn screening program was 30¢ (U.S.), which includes labor, reagents, and confirmatory testing. This equates to $8527 for each case of classic CAH identified and $12,181 for each case of classic CAH identified by the screening program alone. A total of 1180 samples were initially incorrectly identified as indicating CAH when the above criteria were used; 80% of false-positive results occurred in infants with a birth weight <2.7 kg. No known cases of classic CAH were incorrectly identified as normal. Therefore the sensitivity and specificity of screening for classic CAH were 100% and 99.78%, respectively.

Three infants (2 boys and 1 girl) with presumed late-onset, simple virilizing CAH were identified by screening. The cases were characterized by a lack of symptoms, absence of virilization, and no detectable biochemical abnormality (except the elevated 17-OHP level) at the time of markedly delayed treatment (42, 60, and 2190 days of age). These three subjects have been excluded from further analysis unless otherwise stated.

Although all cases were ultimately identified by screening, six were initially identified by clinical evaluation (i.e., family history or physical examination); the remaining 14 cases were identified by screening alone (Table I). The majority of infants identified by screening alone had no symptoms when treatment was initiated. Five infants had poor feeding, eight had vomiting, and three had hypotension with poor peripheral perfusion. When all cases identified by screening or clinical evaluation just before treatment were considered, symptoms occurred in only 2 of 10 infants ≤10 days of age; between 11 and 16 days of age, all 8 infants had symptoms. Two additional infants were treated at later ages (18 and 34 days).

Table. Characteristics of infants identified with classic CAH

Initial identification	Screening	Clinical evaluation
Number	14	6
Sex (M/F)	11:3	0:6
Age at diagnosis days ± SD)	10 (±8)	2 (±2)
Symptomatic pretreatment	10	1
Virilization (M/F)	10:3	0:6
Salt-wasting	14	6

The majority of infants identified by screening alone were boys (Table 1); however, three girls not initially recognized as virilized by their pediatricians were detected by screening. One girl had Prader type 2 virilization (clitoromegaly and posterior labial fusion), and the other two girls had severe Prader type 5 virilization with penile transformation of the clitoris and urethra, and complete fusion of the labial folds; sex assignment was incorrect until the screening result was known. Almost all (10 of 11) of the boys had subtle evidence of virilization or excess levels of corticotropin, including macrogenitosomia (stretched penile length ≥2 SD above the mean), scrotal hyperpigmentation, or both. All 20 infants had markedly elevated plasma renin levels for age.

Notification of the diagnosis of CAH by the National Testing Centre was made at 11 ± 3 (SD) days of age. Treatment was started in the screening group at 13 days of age (range, 4 to 35 days). From the time of screening diagnosis, there was a delay of 3 days (range, 0 to 26 days) before steroid therapy was initiated.

At the time treatment was initiated, 11 of the 13 infants identified by screening alone had hyponatremia (serum sodium, 124 ± 7.2 mmol/L). Hyperkalemia was present in 10 of the 13 infants (potassium, 7.8 ± 0.7 mmol/L). Furthermore, when those identified by clinical evaluation and screening were considered together, there was a strong correlation between age of treatment and severity of hyponatremia ($r = -0.77$; $p = 0.001$) or hyperkalemia ($r = 0.56$; $p = 0.015$) as shown in Figs. 1 and 2.

DISCUSSION

New Zealand has one of the lowest incidences of classic CAH in the world; the incidence from other screening programs is 1:14,199.[2, 4] Of the 23 patients identified, 20 had

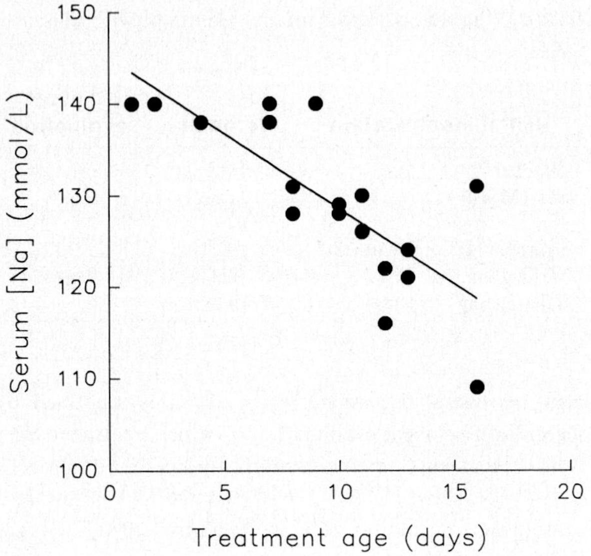

Fig. 1. The relationship between the serum sodium *(Na)* concentration in blood samples drawn just before treatment and the age at which treatment was started for infants with classic CAH identified by screening ($r = -0.77$; $p < 0.001$).

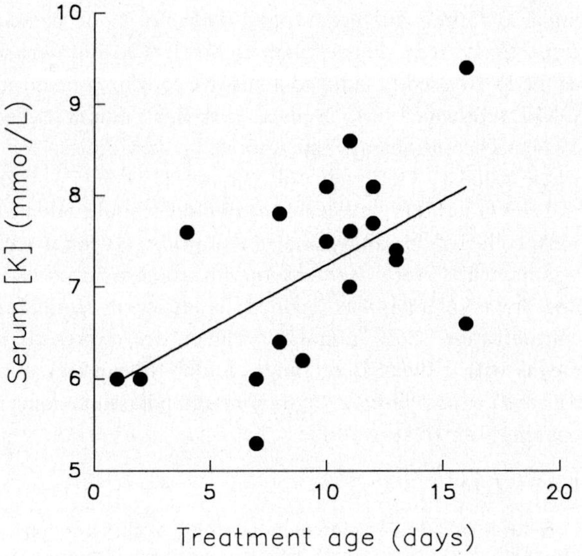

Fig. 2. The relationship between the serum potassium *(K)* concentration in blood samples drawn just before treatment and the age at which treatment was started for infants with classic CAH identified by screening ($r = 0.56$; $p = 0.015$).

mineralocorticoid deficiency. This is a much higher rate of the salt-losing form of classic CAH than previously reported (33% to 66% from case survey studies[5] and 77% from newborn screening programs worldwide[4]).

The cost of a CAH screening test in New Zealand is at least half the cost of a sample analyzed by other CAH programs (60¢ [U.S.] to $2).[4, 5] The cost of identifying an infant with classic CAH by newborn screening is also considerably cheaper in New Zealand ($8527 compared with an average of $10,495 in other countries[4, 5]), illustrating the benefit of achieving low assay costs with in-house rather than kit assays if such rare disorders are to be screened.

The rate of biochemical and clinical deterioration is extremely rapid in the salt-losing form of classic CAH. Until 10 days of age, symptoms are uncommon, but shortly afterward poor feeding and vomiting develop, together with marked hyponatremia and hyperkalemia. Salt-wasting episodes in infancy are associated with a reduced intelligence quotient in later childhood, reinforcing the importance of early screening.[6] Despite the genetic heterogeneity of salt-losing classic CAH, the majority of infants have a remarkably similar temporal course of biochemical deterioration. To avoid this precipitous deterioration, a newborn CAH screening program must consistently identify infants with positive test results and notify their pediatricians before 10 days of age. Effective CAH screening therefore places considerable pressure on a newborn screening program to strive for expeditiousness. To reduce delay, sample collection time in New Zealand has been shortened from 5 to 3 days of age, priority has been given to 17-OHP assay over thyroid-stimulating hormone or phenylalanine assays, and mailing of completed newborn screening cards in batches has been discouraged.[7] There is no evidence to suggest that a 1- to 2-day delay in diagnosis of congenital hypothyroidism or phenylketonuria alters the outcome in either disorder.

The effectiveness of any screening test depends on prompt and optimal treatment. The 3-day treatment delay was principally the result of the pediatrician awaiting formal laboratory confirmation of an elevated 17-OHP level before commencing treatment. To maximize the benefits achieved by early CAH screening, it is essential to evaluate the infant and obtain blood for measurement of serum electrolytes, 17-OHP, and plasma renin on the day of notification. Treatment with hydrocortisone, 20 to 25 mg/m^2 per day, 9-α-fludrocortisone, 0.2 mg/m^2 per day, and sodium chloride, 2.2 mmol/kg per day,[8] should then be undertaken immediately. If the plasma renin level is not elevated, 9-α-fludrocortisone therapy can be discontinued.

In girls, mild or even severe virilization is not reliably identified at delivery or during the neonatal period. International experience suggests that at least one third of virilized female infants with CAH are either overlooked or incorrectly identified as boys.[4, 9] Screening does not reduce the incidence of initial incorrect sex assignment in severely virilized females, but it considerably shortens the period of parental misconception about their child's sex from 40 to less than 10 days.[9] Almost all boys with classic CAH identified by screening had macrogenitosomia or scrotal hyperpigmentation. Such subtle signs invariably are not detected in the early neonatal period. It is in this group that CAH screening is most beneficial, because these patients would otherwise be recognized during extreme illness because of markedly disordered electrolyte levels. In Sweden there is a higher incidence of classic CAH in girls than boys at a ratio of 1.8:1.0[9]; because it is assumed that the sex incidence is equal, some boys with classic CAH apparently are dying during infancy without a diagnosis established.

Despite apparently high specificity (98.78%) of screening for classic CAH in New Zealand, the low incidence of the disease means that the positive predictive value of a positive 17-OHP screening result in identifying a child with CAH is only 1.9%. These false-positive results create two problems: the additional cost and inconvenience of repeated testing, and, more importantly, the distress to parents created by repeated testing for a serious disease. The 17-OHP values are considerably higher in preterm and sick neonates.[4, 10] Approximately half of the measured 17-OHP in the serum of preterm infants consists of 17-OHP–conjugated metabolites.[10] Illness results in elevation of the levels of cortisol and its precursors, including 17-OHP.

After analysis of false-positive results, the criteria for a positive 17-OHP screening result in the New Zealand program can be modified to improve the specificity substantially without compromising sensitivity. We propose graded cutoff criteria that accommodate prematurity and illness. An increase in whole blood concentrations of 17-OHP to >30 nmol/L for infants >2700 gm, >40 nmol/L for infants 1500 to 2700 gm, and >50 nmol/L for infants <1500 gm are recommended, which would further increase specificity 87%, 90%, and 60%, respectively. The lowest whole blood 17-OHP value for a term infant with classic CAH was 65 nmol/L. In addition, sick neonates with an identified illness should have newborn screening sampling delayed until the infant is either 2 weeks of age or is discharged from the neonatal unit, whichever occurs first. Collectively these amendments could improve the positive predictive value to 41% or more.

We conclude that newborn screening for classic CAH is the only means of identifying affected male infants without a family history of CAH, before the development of symptoms or significant biochemical deterioration. Screening also identifies a significant number of virilized female infants whose disease is not detected clinically. The rapid and very consistent rate of biochemical and clinical deterioration that occurs in the salt-losing form of this disease after 10 days of age demands both early pediatrician notification of positive results and prompt treatment to achieve maximal benefit from screening.

REFERENCES

1. Pang S, Hotchkiss J, Drash AL, et al. Microfilter paper method for 17-hydroxyprogesterone radioimmunoassay: its application for rapid screening for congenital adrenal hyperplasia. J Clin Endocrinol Metab 1977;45:1003-8.
2. Pang S, Clark A. Congenital adrenal hyperplasia due to 21-hydroxylase deficiency: newborn screening and its relationship to the diagnosis and treatment of the disorder. Screening 1993;2:105-39.
3. Cacciari E, Balsamo A, Cassio A, et al. Neonatal screening for congenital adrenal hyperplasia using a microfilter paper method for 17-α-hydroxyprogesterone radioimmunoassay. Horm Res 1982;16:4-9.
4. Pang S, Wallace MA, Hofman L, et al. Worldwide experience in newborn screening for classical congenital adrenal hyperplasia due to 21-hydroxylase deficiency. Pediatrics 1988; 81:866-74.
5. Cicognani A. The experience of neonatal screening for congenital adrenal hyperplasia. Horm Res 1992;37(suppl 3):34-48.
6. Nass R, Baker S. Learning disabilities in children with congenital adrenal hyperplasia. J Child Neurol 1991;6:306-12.
7. Farriaux JP, Dhont JL. Neonatal screening for congenital adrenal hyperplasia [Letter]. J PEDIATR 1989;115:1022.
8. Mullis PE, Hindmarsh PC, Brook CG. Sodium chloride supplement at diagnosis and during infancy in children with salt-losing 21-hydroxylase deficiency. Eur J Pediatr 1990; 150: 22-5.
9. Thilen A, Larsson A. Congenital adrenal hyperplasia in Sweden 1969–1986. Acta Paediatr Scand 1990;79:168-75.
10. Larsson A, Haganfeldt L, von Dobeln U, Curstedt T, Gustafsson J, Svensson E. Neonatal screening for congenital adrenal hyperplasia using 17-hydroxyprogesterone assay in filter paper blood spots. Horm Res 1988;30:235-40.

Reference ranges for newer thyroid function tests in premature infants

Linda M. Adams, MD,[a] Janet R. Emery, MD, Susan J. Clark, MD, Esther I. Carlton, MT, and Jerald C. Nelson, MD

From the Departments of Pediatrics, Medicine, and Pathology, Loma Linda University School of Medicine, Loma Linda, California, and Nichols Institute References Laboratories, San Juan Capistrano, California

***Objective*: To establish reference ranges for recently developed assays of thyroid function in premature infants.**
***Methods*: We measured serum free thyroxine (T_4) by direct equilibrium dialysis and serum thyrotropin by a sensitive immunometric method in 104 preterm infants (25 to 36 weeks of gestational age) during the first week of life.**
***Results*: The free T_4 level correlated positively with gestational age (p <0.0001; $r^2 = 0.09$) and differed significantly between adjacent gestational age groups (p <0.05). Free T_4 concentrations (mean ± SD) for the 25- to 27-, 28- to 30-, 31- to 33-, and 34- to 36-week groups were 18.0 ± 5.2, 25.7 ± 9.0, 30.9 ± 9.0, 36.0 ± 10.3 pmol/L (1.4 ± 0.4, 2.0 ± 0.7, 2.4 ± 0.7, and 2.8 ± 0.8 ng/dl), respectively. Two reference ranges for free T_4 were determined, one for 25 to 30 weeks (6.4 to 42.5 pmol/L (0.5 to 3.3 ng/dl)) and one for 31 to 36 weeks (16.7 to 60.5 pmol/L (1.3 to 4.7 ng/dl)). The logarithm of the value for thyrotropin correlated positively with gestational age (p < 0.001; $r^2 = 0.08$); one reference range of 0.5 to 29 mU/L was determined for thyrotropin.**
***Conclusion:* This study extends information on thyroid function of preterm infants and establishes reference ranges for this population. (J PEDIATR 1995;126:122-7)**

In newborn premature infants, interpretation of some standard thyroid function tests, such as total thyroxine or free T_4 index, is confounded by simultaneous changes in both hypothalamic-pituitary-thyroid function[1, 2] and serum T_4 binding proteins.[3-6] Previous studies used a variety of free T_4 methods that were often inaccurate and variably biased by changes in serum proteins and in protein-bound T_4.[7-15] Newer and more accurate free T_4 assays and improved thyrotropin assays are available. Direct equilibrium dialysis measurements of free T_4 are not biased by changes in serum proteins[13, 16, 17] or protein binding of T_4.[15] The increased sensitivity of immunometric thyrotropin assays allows definition of the lower limit of the normal range.[18-20] Age-specific normal ranges for these assays in premature infants have not been reported. We report a prospective study of the normal values for serum free T_4 by direct equilibrium dialysis and serum thyrotropin by sensitive immunometric assay during the first week of life for premature infants less than 37 weeks of gestational age who were healthy except for their prematurity. Normal values for infants 37 to 42 weeks of gestational age using these methods have been reported previously.[21]

T_4	Thyroxine

Submitted for publication May 2, 1994; accepted Aug. 2, 1994.

[a]Current address: Utah Valley Regional Medical Center, 1034 North 500 West, Provo, UT 84604.

Reprint requests: Janet R. Emery, MD, Loma Linda University Children's Hospital, Department of Pediatrics, 11262 Campus St., WH 135, Loma Linda, CA 92354.

0022-3476/95/$3.00 + 0 **9/23/59563**

METHODS

Subjects. Infants of 25 to 36 weeks of estimated gestational age who were born at or transported to Loma Linda University Medical Center between March 1990 and Octo-

Table I. Patient characteristics

	Gestational age			
	25-27 wk (n = 12)	28-30 wk (n = 33)	31-33 wk (n = 65)	34-36 wk (n = 64)
Age at sampling (days)	3.5 ± 2.5	3.4 ± 2.1	3.3 ± 1.5	3.5 ± 1.6
Weight (gm)	772 ± 233	1260 ± 238	1786 ± 255	2125 ± 376
Length (cm)	35 ± 2	39 ± 2	43 ± 3	45 ± 3
Head circumference (cm)	24 ± 0.7	27 ± 1.6	30 ± 1.6	32 ± 1.4
Systolic blood pressure (mm Hg)	49 ± 5	57 ± 11	63 ± 11	64 ± 9

Values presented as mean ± SD.

ber 1993 were considered candidates for study. Infants were excluded if they had clinical or laboratory evidence of infection, required more than 10 ml/kg of blood products in the first day of life, had congenital anomalies, had an intraventricular hemorrhage during the first week of life, or had a positive result of urine or meconium drug screening tests. Infants with respiratory distress syndrome were also excluded because previous reports suggested an effect of respiratory distress syndrome on thyroid hormones.[22] Patients who died within 2 weeks of blood sampling were excluded. Infants whose mothers had endocrine disease were also excluded.

Infants were stratified by gestational age at birth into four groups: 25 to 27 weeks, 28 to 30 weeks, 31 to 33 weeks, and 34 to 36 weeks of gestation. Gestational age was assigned by early obstetric ultrasound studies and maternal dates whenever those data were available. Otherwise, gestational age was assessed by the Ballard Maturational Score after examination performed within 24 hours of delivery.[23]

The following inclusion criteria were used. Infants 34 to 36 weeks of gestation were included when their height, weight, and head circumference at birth were appropriate for gestational age, they had an Apgar score of ≥ 7 by 5 minutes of life, were spontaneously breathing in room air, had normal blood pressure for gestational age,[24] and were free of intraventricular hemorrhage as assessed by cranial ultrasonography in the first week of life. Infants 31 to 33 weeks of gestation were included when they met the 34- to 36-week criteria; infants were also included if they had a 5-minute Apgar score of 6 and when mechanical ventilation or supplemental oxygen were required for 24 hours or less. Infants of 25 to 30 weeks of gestation were included when they met the 31- to 33-week criteria; infants were also included who required mechanical ventilation or supplemental oxygen for more than 24 hours.

This study was approved by our institutional review board. Blood samples were obtained from infants during the first week of life. Only infants older than 24 hours of age were included. If an umbilical arterial or venous catheter was already in place for clinical reasons, the blood sample was drawn from it. Otherwise, 1 ml samples were obtained by venipuncture when blood samples were drawn for other routine laboratory work. All assays were performed at Nichols Institute Reference Laboratories, San Juan Capistrano, Calif.

Assay methods. Free T_4 was measured by direct equilibrium dialysis[16] with an interassay coefficient of variation of 8.5% at 20 pmol/L (1.56 ng/dl). This method uses a semipermeable dialysis membrane to separate serum proteins and protein-bound T_4 from free T_4. Free T_4 is then directly measured by radioimmunoassay of the protein-free dialysate. The thyrotropin level was determined by a highly sensitive immunoradiometric assay (HS-TSH Allegro, Nichols Institute Diagnostics) with an interassay coefficient of variation of 20% at a thyrotropin concentration of 0.1 mU/L.[25] Some serum sample volumes were inadequate to perform both tests.

Data analysis. Statistical outliers were identified with the Grubbs test.[26, 27] Skewness and kurtosis were determined with a software program (Systat Inc., Evanston, Ill.). Differences between adjacent groups were analyzed by the Student t test. Differences were regarded as significant at values of $p \leq 0.05$. Differences among multiple groups were determined by analysis of variance. Relationships between variables were evaluated by linear regression.

RESULTS

Study group. Clinical characteristics of the study infants are summarized in Table I. There were 104 boys and 70 girls, a sex distribution consistent with the admission demographics of neonatal intensive care unit patients in general. There were no differences in free T_4 or thyrotropin levels related to gender as determined by analysis of variance. Differences among the four gestational age groups in the mode of delivery or the day of postnatal life on which the sample was drawn were insignificant ($p > 0.05$).

In all groups the mean weight, length, and head circumference were within the 40th to 60th percentile range for their respective gestational ages using standard curves for

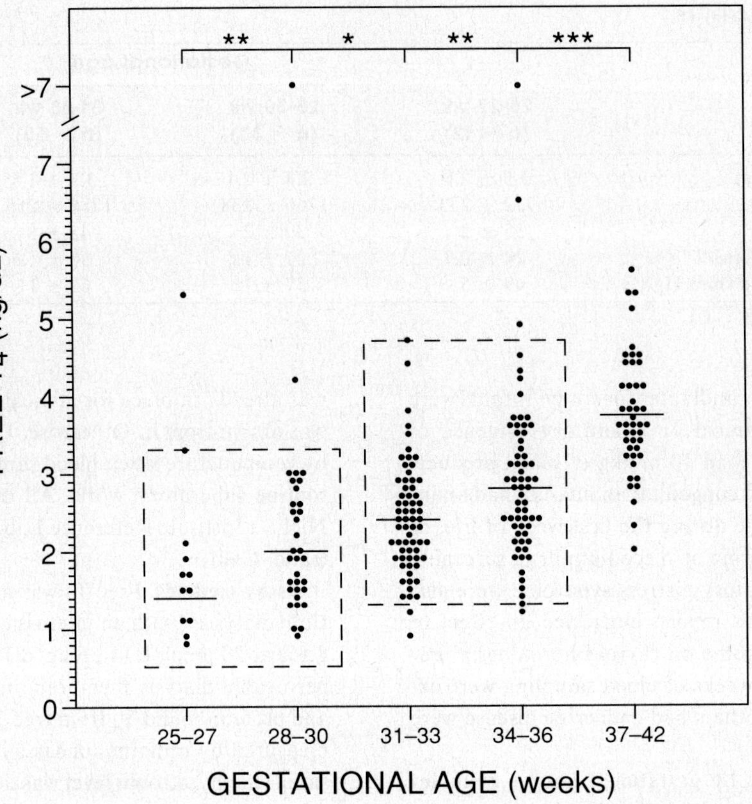

Fig. 1. Serum free T_4 concentrations (12.87 pmol/L = 1 ng/dl) by gestational age in all healthy preterm infants (including statistical outliers) during the first week of postnatal life. Horizontal *solid lines* represent the arithmetic means: $*p<0.05$; $**p<0.01$; $***p<0.001$. *Dashed lines* represent the arithmetic mean ± 2 SD reference ranges (after outlier deletion) for two gestational age ranges: 25 to 30 weeks and 31 to 36 weeks. The data for term infants (37 to 42 weeks) have been published previously[21] and are presented for comparison with data for preterm infants.

infants born at sea level.[28, 29] Blood pressures in all infants were within the normal range for the gestational age.[24]

In the 25- to 27-week group (n = 12), 7 infants required mechanical ventilation, 4 were receiving supplemental oxygen, and 1 was receiving enteral feedings. In the 28- to 30-week group (n = 33), 2 infants received mechanical ventilation, 4 received supplemental oxygen, and 14 were receiving enteral feedings. In the 31- to 33-week group (n = 65), 4 infants received mechanical ventilation, 9 received supplemental oxygen, and 45 were receiving enteral feedings. None of the infants in the 34- to 36-week group (n = 64) required mechanical ventilation, 6 received supplemental oxygen, and 57 were receiving enteral feedings. In no instance was there a significant difference (Student *t* test) between the free T_4 or thyrotropin concentrations in infants requiring supplemental oxygen or mechanical ventilation compared with infants of similar gestational age who did not require these treatments.

Free thyroxine. There was a weak correlation between free T_4 concentrations and gestational age ($r^2 = 0.09$; free $T_4 = 0.11$ gestational age in weeks − 0.97; $p < 0.001$). This correlation with age was stronger when previously reported data[21] from term infants were added ($r^2 = 0.26$; free $T_4 = 0.15$ gestational age − 2.32; $p < 0.001$). There was a slight but significant decline in free T_4 concentration during the first week of life ($r^2 = 0.03$; $p = 0.03$).

Free T_4 concentrations increased progressively with increasing gestational age (Fig. 1) and differed significantly ($p<0.05$) between adjacent groups (18.0 ± 5.2, 25.7 ± 9.0, 30.9 ± 9.0, 36.0 ± 10.3 pmol/L [1.4 ± 0.4, 2.0 ± 0.7, 2.4 ± 0.7, and 2.8 ± 0.8 ng/dl], respectively, mean ± SD). Statistical outliers were deleted before reference ranges were determined. Two outliers were deleted from the 25- to 27-week group, two from the 28- to 30-week group, one from the 31- to 33-week group, and two from the 34- to 36-week group. The remaining data satisfied the gaussian assumption based on skewness and kurtosis. Reference ranges were calculated as the arithmetic mean ± 2 SD range for each gestational age group (Table II). To simplify clinical reference range citations, data were com-

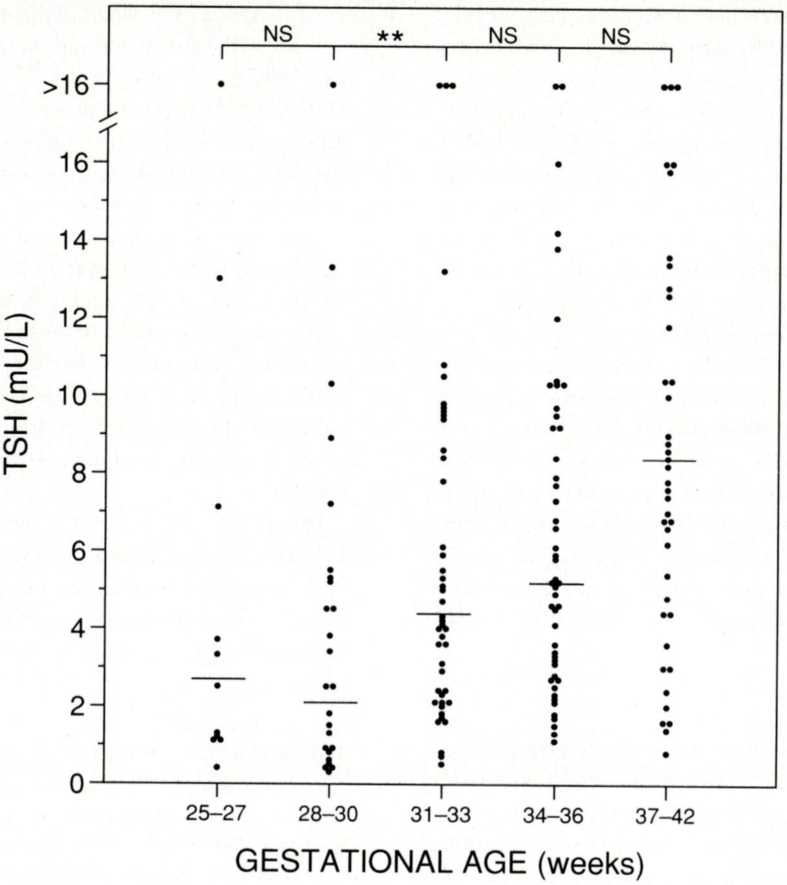

Fig. 2. Serum thyrotropin (*TSH*, thyroid-stimulating hormone) concentrations by gestational age in healthy preterm infants during the first week of postnatal life. Horizontal *solid lines* represent the geometric means for each group. The *asterisks* indicate a significant difference between means (** p <0.01); *NS* indicates no significant differences. The data for term infants (37 to 42 weeks) have been published previously[21] and are presented for comparison with data for preterm infants. The geometric mean ± 2 SD range for infants 25 to 36 weeks of gestational age was 0.5 to 29.0 mU/L. The reference range was not depicted because the upper limit was off scale.

Table II. Reference ranges for serum free T_4 and thyrotropin in premature infants during the first week of life

Age groups	Age (wk)	Free T_4 (pmol/L (ng/dl))	Thyrotropin (mU/L)
Premature infants	25-27	7.7-28.3 (0.6-2.2)	0.2-30.3
	28-30	7.7-43.8 (0.6-3.4)	0.2-20.6
	31-33	12.9-48.9 (1.0-3.8)	0.7-27.9
	34-36	15.4-56.6 (1.2-4.4)	1.2-21.6
Combined premature infants	25-30	6.4-42.5 (0.5-3.3)	
	31-36	16.7-60.5 (1.3-4.7)	
	25-36		0.5-29
Term infants[21]	37-42	25.7-68.2 (2.0-5.3)	1.0-39

bined into two gestational age ranges: 25 to 30 weeks and 31 to 36 weeks (Table II). These two ranges included 94.8% (164/173) of the data. The range for the 25- to 30-week group included 93.3% (42/45) of the data, and the range for the 31- to 36-week group included 95.3% (122/128) of the data. This is similar to the expectation that the mean ± 2 SD range will include the central 95.4% of the data.

Thyrotropin. The thyrotropin data were logarithmically distributed as determined by skewness and kurtosis. There was a weak correlation between the logarithm of thyrotropin concentrations and gestational age ($r^2 = 0.08$; log thyrotropin = 0.05 gestational age in weeks − 0.85; $p < 0.001$). This correlation with age was stronger when previous data from term infants[21] were added ($r^2 = 0.11$; log thyrotropin = 0.03 gestational age − 0.50; $p < 0.001$). There was also a decline in serum thyrotropin concentration during the first week of life ($r^2 = 0.13$; $p < 0.001$), as expected.

Because the data distribution was logarithmic, the geometric means were calculated for each gestational age group and compared between adjacent groups by Student *t* test; the only significant difference was between the 28- to 30-week and the 31- to 33-week age groups (Fig. 2). The value in the single statistical outlier, who was in the 28- to 30-week group, was deleted before reference range determination. Data from all age groups, 25 to 36 weeks, were used to determine a single reference range as the geometric mean ± 2 SD range (Table II) that included 95.4% (124/130) of the data.

DISCUSSION

Because the definition of a "healthy" preterm infant is problematic, we used prospective criteria with sufficient detail to identify the patient groups from which these reference ranges were determined. Comparison of previous studies of serum free T_4 in healthy preterm infants[4, 30-34] with the present data is confounded by different (or absent) patient selection criteria. Patients in previous studies were classified by birth weight; our patients were classified by gestational age. A variety of nondialysis free T_4 measurement methods that are not directly comparable to dialysis methods[2-20]; were used in these other studies; direct equilibrium dialysis differentiates central hypothyroidism from low T_4 states caused by reduced protein binding.[16] None of these former studies provided reference ranges. Two previous studies examined the relationship between serum free T_4 and gestational age[31, 34]; both reported a significant increase in free T_4 with gestational age, in agreement with our data.

The contribution of gestational age to normal serum free T_4 concentrations was small, warranting the evaluation of combined ranges for clinical use. In our judgment, the use of two reference ranges for the premature infants is superior to a single reference range because it provides a better definition of the lower end of the normal range in the youngest infants.

Serum thyrotropin levels in this study were as low as 0.3 mU/L. Two previous studies of thyrotropin in healthy preterm infants used assays capable of measuring thyrotropin at this level; neither of these studies provided reference ranges. Fuse et al.[33] reported a positive correlation of thyrotropin with gestational age in 26 infants weighing less than 2500 gm. Mantagos et al.[35] did not evaluate the correlation between serum thyrotropin and gestational age. Other studies of serum thyrotropin in premature infants used older, less sensitive thyrotropin assays and provided conflicting results.[5, 32, 36-40]

The thyrotropin values in our premature infants were significantly lower than in term infants.[21] Fuse et al.[33] also reported lower thyrotropin levels in premature than in term infants. Mantagos et al.[35] reported similar levels in preterm infants and term infants, but they did not include infants younger than 32 weeks of gestational age. Furthermore, wide variability in serum thyrotropin values among preterm infants of all ages confounds the detection of age-related changes.

This study confirms and extends previous data on the thyroidal status of healthy preterm infants during the first week of life and provides reference ranges not previously available. These reference ranges do not apply to other free T_4 measurement methods or to less sensitive thyrotropin assays.

REFERENCES

1. Fisher DA. Euthyroid low thyroxine (T_4) and triiodothyronine (T_3) states in prematures and sick neonates. Pediatr Clin North Am 1990;37:1297-1312.
2. Fisher DA. Thyroid physiology in the perinatal period and during childhood. In: Ingbar SH, Braverman LE, eds. The thyroid, 5th ed. Philadelphia: JB Lippincott, 1986:1387-95.
3. Jacobsen BB, Peitersen B, Andersen HJ, Hummer L. Serum concentrations of thyroxine-binding globulin, prealbumin and albumin in healthy full term, small-for-gestational age and preterm newborn infants. Acta Paediatr Scand 1979;68:49-55.
4. Hirano T, Singh J, Srinivasan G, Pildes R. Postnatal thyroid function in low birth weight infants: a cross-sectional assessment of free thyroxine and thyroid hormone binding globulin. Eur J Pediatr 1982;139:244-6.
5. Hirano T, Singh J, Srinivasan G, Pildes R. Postnatal thyroid function in low birth weight infants; a longitudinal assessment of free thyroxine and thyroid hormone binding globulin. Acta Endocrinol 1985;110:56-60.
6. Mercado M, Yu VYH, Francis I, Szymonowicz W, Gold H. Thyroid function in very preterm infants. Early Human Dev 1988;16:131-41.
7. Amino N, Niski K, Nakatani K, et al. Effect of albumin concentration on the assay of serum free thyroxin by equilibrium radioimmunoassay with labeled thyroxin analog (Amerlex free T_4). Clin Chem 1983;29:321-5.
8. Bayer MF. Free thyroxine results are affected by albumin concentration and nonthyroidal illness. Clin Chim Acta 1983; 130:391-96.
9. Helenius T, Liewendahl K. Improved dialysis method of free thyroxin in serum compared with five commercial radioimmunoassays in nonthyroidal illness and subjects with abnormal concentrations of thyroxin-binding globulin. Clin Chem 1983; 29:816-22.

10. Csako G, Zweig MH, Benson C, Ruddel M. On the albumin-dependence of measurements of free thyroxin. II. Patients with nonthyroidal illness. Clin Chem 1987;33:87-92.
11. Csako G, Zweig MH, Glickman J, Ruddel M, Kestner J. Direct and indirect techniques for free thyroxin compared in patients with nonthyroidal illness. II. Effect of prealbumin, albumin, and thyroxin-binding globulin. Clin Chem 1989;35:1655-62.
12. Nelson JC, Tomei RT. Dependence of the thyroxin/thyroxin-binding globulin (TBG) ratio and the free thyroxin index on TBG concentrations. Clin Chem 1989;35:541-4.
13. Nelson JC, Wilcox RB, Pandian MR. Dependence of free thyroxine estimates obtained with equilibrium tracer dialysis on the concentration of thyroxine-binding globulin. Clin Chem 1992;38:1294-300.
14. Wong TK, Pekary AE, Hoo GS, Bradley ME, Hershman JM. Comparison of methods for measuring free thyroxin in nonthyroidal illness. Clin Chem 1992;38:720-4.
15. Nelson JC, Weiss RM, Wilcox RB. Underestimates of serum free T_4 concentrations by free T_4 immunoassays. J Clin Endocrinol Metab 1994;79:76-9.
16. Nelson JC, Tomei RT. Direct determination of free thyroxin in undiluted serum by equilibrium dialysis/radioimmunoassay. Clin Chem 1988;34:1737-44.
17. Nelson JC, Wilcox RB. Further studies on thyroxin-binding globulin-dependence in equilibrium dialysis assays of free thyroxin. Clin Chem 1991;37:128-9.
18. Spencer CA. Clinical utility and cost-effectiveness of sensitive thyrotropin assays in ambulatory and hospitalized patients. Mayo Clin Proc 1988;63:1214-22.
19. Nicoloff JT, Spencer CA. Clinical review 12: the use and misuse of the sensitive thyrotropin assays. J Clin Endocrinol Metab 1990;71:553-8.
20. Kaptein EM. Clinical application of free thyroxine determinations. Clin Lab Med 1993;13:653-72.
21. Nelson JC, Clark SJ, Borut DL, Tomei RT, Carleton EI. Age-related change in serum free thyroxine during childhood and adolescence. J PEDIATR 1993;123:899-905.
22. Delange F, Bourdoux P, Ermans AM. Transient disorders of thyroid function and regulation in preterm infants. Pediatr Adolesc Endoc 1985;14:369-93.
23. Ballard JL, Novak KK, Driver MA. A simplified score for assessment of fetal maturation of newly born infants. J PEDIATR 1979;95:769-74.
24. Versmold HT, Kitterman JA, Phibbs RH, Gregory GA, Tooley WH. Aortic blood pressure during the first 12 hours of life in infants with birth weight 610-4220 grams. Pediatrics 1981;67:607-13.
25. Odell WD, Griffin J, Zahradnik R. Two-monoclonal-antibody sandwich-type assay for thyrotropin, with use of avidin-biotin separation technique. Clin Chem 1986;32:1873-8.
26. Conover WJ. Practical non-parametric statistics, 2nd ed. New York: John Wiley & Sons, 1980.
27. Grubbs FE, Green B. Extension of sample sizes and percentage points for significance tests of outlying observations. Technometrics 1972;14:847-54.
28. Usher R, McLean F. Intrauterine growth of live-born caucasian infants at sea level: standards obtained from measurements in 7 dimensions of infants born between 25 and 44 weeks of gesation. J PEDIATR 1969;74:901-10.
29. Babson SG, Benda GI. Growth graphs for the clinical assessment of infants of varying gestational age. J PEDIATR 1976; 89:814-20.
30. Hadeed AJ, Asay LD, Klein AH, Fisher DA. Significance of transient postnatal hypothyroxinemia in premature infants with and without respiratory distress syndrome. Pediatrics 1981;68:494-8.
31. Sakaguchi M, Suzuki S, Nagashima K, et al. Longitudinal study of free throxine in low-birth-weight infants by paper disk method. J PEDIATR 1983;103:793-6.
32. Franklin RC, Purdie GL, O'Grady CM. Neonatal thyroid function: prematurity, prenatal steroids, and respiratory distress syndrome. Arch Dis Child 1986;61:589-92.
33. Fuse F, Shimizu M, Uga N, et al. Maturation of feedback control of thyrotropin in premature infants. J Dev Physiol 1990;14:17-22.
34. Kodama S, Mori Y, Miyoshi M, et al. Thyroid function in premature infants. Kobe J Med Sci 1992;38:109-16.
35. Mantagos S, Koulouris A, Makri M, et al. Development of thyrotropin circadian rhythm, in infancy. J Clin Endocrinol Metab 1992;74:71-4.
36. Bongers-Schokking JJ, Schopman W. Thyroid function in healthy normal, low birthweight and preterm infants. Eur J Pediatr 1984;143:117-22.
37. Uhrmann S, Marks KH, Maisels MJ, et al. Thyroid Function in the preterm infants: a longitudinal assessment. J PEDIATR 1978;92:968-73.
38. Jacobsen BB, Andersen JH, Peitersen B, Dige-Petersen H, Hummer L. Serum levels of thyrotropin, thyroxine, and triiodithyronine in fullterm, small-for-gestational age and preterm newborn babies. Acta Paediatr Scand 1977;66:681-87.
39. Klein AH, Foley B, Kenny F, Fisher D. Thyroid hormone and thyrotropin responses of parturition in premature infants with and without the respiratory distress syndrome. Pediatrics 1979;63:380-5.
40. Desai M, Dabholkar C, Colaco MP. Thyroid function in fullterm and preterm newborns. Indian J Pediatr 1985;52:599-607.

Clinical and laboratory observations

Vitamin A and E status in very low birth weight infants: Development of an improved parenteral delivery system

T. E. Inder, MBChB, A. C. Carr, BScHons, C. C. Winterbourn, PhD,
N. C. Austin, MBChB, FRACP, and B. A. Darlow, MD, FRACP

From the Departments of Paediatrics, Christchurch and Dunedin Hospitals, and the Department of Pathology, Christchurch School of Medicine, University of Otago, Christchurch, New Zealand

Plasma vitamin A and E levels were inadequate in very low birth weight infants receiving a continuous infusion of a parenteral multivitamin preparation, 1.5 ml/kg per day, in dextrose–amino acid solution. A new delivery system using 2 ml/kg per day, infused for 6 hours from the first day of life, avoided loss during infusion and significantly improved plasma vitamin A and E levels during the first 28 days of life in very low birth weight infants. (J Pediatr 1995;126:128-31)

Premature infants usually receive vitamins A and E in a multivitamin preparation added to the dextrose–amino acid–electrolyte mixture of total parenteral nutrition. Current evidence favors maintaining plasma levels of vitamin A and vitamin E at greater than 200 μg/L and 10 mg/L, respectively.[1-6] This study aimed to examine whether the low serum levels of vitamin A and E measured in very low birth weight infants (<1500 gm) receiving a conventional multivitamin preparation delivered in parenteral nutrition fluids could be improved by using a new method of delivery.

METHODS

Conventional delivery of vitamins A and E in our NICU consists of MVI Paediatric (Rhône-Poulenc Rorer, Auckland, New Zealand), 1.5 ml/kg per day, added to a 24-hour dextrose–amino acid (Vaminolact; Kabi Pharmacia, Stockholm, Sweden) infusion solution with black bag shielding, commencing on a mean of day 3 (SD 0.6) and infused at a rate of up to 150 ml/kg per day. Vitadol C (Karitane Products Society; distributed by Douglas Pharmaceuticals, Auckland, New Zealand), containing vitamins A, D, and C, is administered at a dose of 780 μg retinol palmitate per day to all VLBW infants established on full oral feeding. No oral vitamin E supplementation is given in our NICU. Throughout the study period nutritional policy unrelated to parenteral multivitamin administration was unchanged.

This study consisted of three phases. All phases of the study protocol were approved by the Canterbury and Otago ethics committees of the Southern Regional Health Authority of New Zealand; informed parental consent was obtained.

Phase I. A prospective study of 95% (n = 68) of all eligible VLBW infants admitted to level III neonatal intensive care units in Christchurch or Dunedin, New Zealand, from February through October 1993 was undertaken to analyze plasma vitamin A and E levels. Their mean gestational age was 29.1 weeks (SD 3.0 weeks) and birth weight 1084 gm (SD 266 gm). Sixty-one of these infants (90%) received total parenteral nutrition from day 2 or 3 for a mean period of 14 days (SD 10 days). Plasma vitamin A and E levels

NICU	Neonatal intensive care unit
VLBW	Very low birth weight

Supported by the New Zealand Lottery Board, New Zealand Health Research Council, and the Grand Lodge of New Zealand Freemasons.

Submitted for publication May 18, 1994; accepted July 26, 1994.

Reprint requests: B.A. Darlow, MD, FRACP, Department of Paediatrics, Christchurch Hospital, Private Bag, Christchurch, New Zealand.

0022-3476/95/$3.00 + 0 **9/24/59439**

Table. Plasma concentrations of vitamins A and E in VLBW infants after use of conventional and new multivitamin delivery systems

	Vitamin A (μg/L)			Vitamin E (μg/L)		
	Conventional (n = 68)	New (n = 20)	*p*	Conventional (n = 68)	New (n = 20)	*p*
Mother's blood: mean (SD)	387 (131)	250 (105)	0.02	14.1 (4.6)	14.0 (3.3)	NS
Cord blood: mean (SD)	145 (59)	155 (64)	NS	3.5 (1.5)	4.2 (2.2)	NS
At 48 hr: mean (SD)	162 (64)	223 (60)	0.003	5.6 (3.4)	13.7 (4.4)	<0.0001
% Below recommended value	75	25		91	5	
At 1 wk: mean (SD)	191 (96)	224 (67)	NS	14.3 (5.6)	13.7 (4.4)	NS
% Below recommended value	50	30		25	15	
At 4 wk: mean (SD)	181 (67)	281 (181)	0.02	13.1 (5.9)	13.9 (6.6)	NS
% Below recommended value	70	20		30	30	

Recommended levels are as follows: vitamin A, >200 μg/L, and vitamin E, >10 mg/L.[7]
NS, Not significant.

were measured in cord blood; in maternal blood within 48 hours of parturition; and in infants' blood at 48 hours and at 1 and 4 weeks of age.

Phase II. To investigate the infants' inadequate plasma vitamin levels, we studied the efficacy of the conventional multivitamin delivery system. Vitamin concentrations in the solution bag and in the efflux of the intravenous line were measured from time zero every 2 hours for a 24-hour period in standard level III ambient lighting nursery conditions (n = 1). A new multivitamin delivery system infusing MVI-Paediatric, 2 ml/kg per day for 6 hours, by syringe pump (Graseby Medical, Watford, U.K.) placed in a black bag connected by minimal tubing to the lowest entry point into the intravenous line infusing parenteral nutrition, was then examined in the same nursery conditions (n = 1). The dose administered was increased to 2 ml/kg, consistent with recommendations of the American Society for Clinical Nutrition.[6] The length of tubing from syringe to intravenous line in the new system was 3.4 cm, compared with 38 cm in the conventional system.

Phase III. From November 1993, all VLBW infants admitted to a level III NICU in Christchurch or Dunedin received MVI-Paediatric, 2 ml/kg per day, by the new infusional method from the first day of life. Plasma vitamin A and E levels were monitored prospectively in the first 20 VLBW infants receiving the new delivery system between November 1993 through February 1994. Levels were monitored as in phase I with additional weekly levels until 4 weeks of age unless parenteral nutrition continued, in which case the levels continued to be monitored weekly until full oral feeding was established, to monitor plasma vitamin levels for possible toxicity. The mean gestational age of these 20 infants was 27.6 weeks (SD 2.8 weeks) and mean birth weight 1020 gms (SD 227 gm). Oral supplementation with Vitadol C was given as previously described.

Assay. Blood samples were taken from the infants outside the 6-hour multivitamin infusional period. A time series study of two infants' plasma vitamin A and E levels before, during (at midpoint), and immediately after a 6-hour multivitamin infusion on days 2 and 5 showed a 10% rise in plasma vitamin A levels and a 15% rise in plasma vitamin E levels during the infusion. Blood was stored in glass tubes in the dark at 4° C for no longer than 8 hours before separation of plasma to be stored at −80° C. Vitamin A and E levels in plasma, and vitamin A and α-tocopherol acetate levels in nutrient solution, were measured by high-performance liquid chromatography.[7] The total parenteral nutrition fluid was measured as for plasma; the MVI Paediatric multivitamin was diluted 40-fold with distilled water before analysis.

Statistics. Statistical analysis was carried out with the Epi Info data-entry program, version 5.01B (USD, Inc., Stone Mountain, Ga.), and Statistical Analysis Systems, version 6.07 (SAS Institute Inc., Cary, N.C.). Unpaired *t* tests were used except for the 4-week vitamin A levels, for which Wilcoxon rank-sum analysis was used because the data were not normally distributed. Values are represented as means (SD) unless stated otherwise.

RESULTS

Plasma vitamin A and E levels were low in our population of VLBW infants receiving multivitamins by a conventional parenteral delivery system (Table). Vitamin A levels declined in the solution bag from 73% to 25% of prescribed values during a 24-hour period (Figure). At the efflux of the intravenous line, vitamin A levels were only 4% to 21% of prescribed values. By measuring the area under the curve, we found that this corresponded to a 24-hour calculated delivery of 6% of the prescribed vitamin A (equivalent to 12 μg/kg per day). Efflux vitamin E levels were initially low but

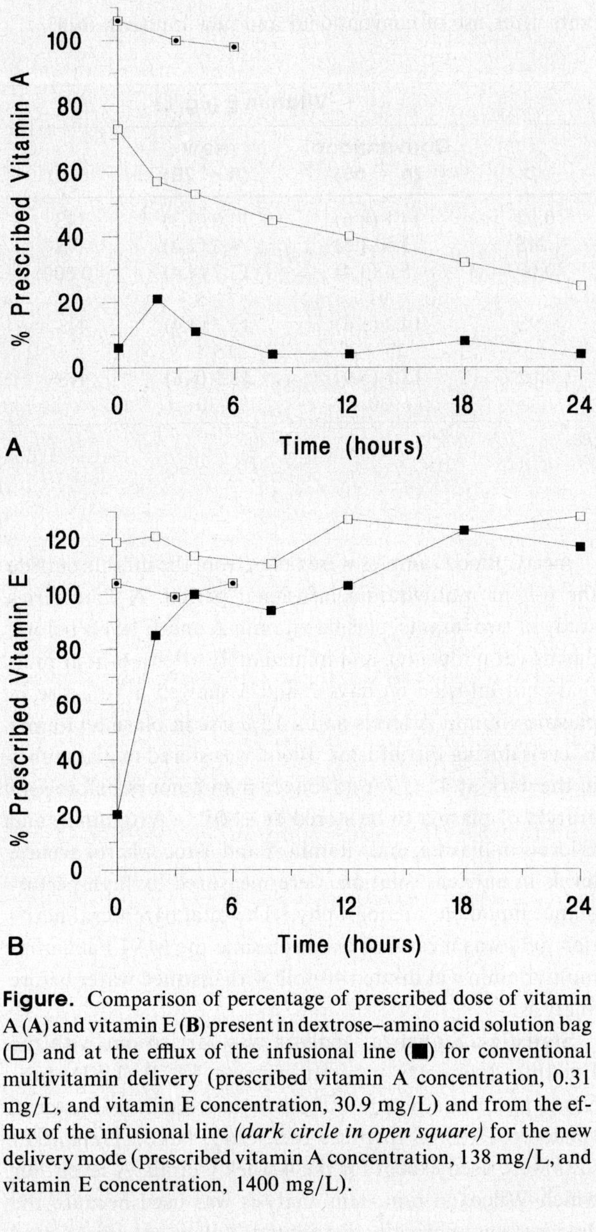

Figure. Comparison of percentage of prescribed dose of vitamin A (**A**) and vitamin E (**B**) present in dextrose–amino acid solution bag (□) and at the efflux of the infusional line (■) for conventional multivitamin delivery (prescribed vitamin A concentration, 0.31 mg/L, and vitamin E concentration, 30.9 mg/L) and from the efflux of the infusional line *(dark circle in open square)* for the new delivery mode (prescribed vitamin A concentration, 138 mg/L, and vitamin E concentration, 1400 mg/L).

rose to give a 24-hour calculated delivery of 88% of prescribed vitamin E (equivalent to 1.9 mg/kg per day).

With the new delivery system, however, there was no loss of vitamin E and only minimal loss of vitamin A during the 6-hour infusion period. This would result in delivery of all of the prescribed vitamin A (280 μg/kg per day) and vitamin E (2.8 mg/kg per day) to the infant. Compared with levels in infants receiving conventional vitamin delivery, mean plasma vitamin A and E levels were significantly elevated at 48 hours (Table). Vitamin A levels remained higher at 4 weeks. The initial rise in vitamin E was not sustained, however, and by 4 weeks there was no difference from conventional delivery values. These differences between the two populations were not due to their having different baseline values, because maternal vitamin A levels were significantly lower in infants receiving the new multivitamin delivery system, but maternal vitamin E levels and cord vitamin A and E levels did not differ significantly. No infants receiving the new delivery mode had vitamin A levels exceeding 800 μg/L or vitamin E levels exceeding 30 mg/L, which are regarded as the upper limits of vitamin A and E levels in healthy children and adults.

DISCUSSION

Our results show that many VLBW infants had plasma levels of vitamin A and E well below recommended minimal levels when a conventional multivitamin parenteral delivery mode was used. Investigation of the parenteral delivery system showed that the infants were receiving almost none of the vitamin A but most of the vitamin E prescribed. Previous studies have shown that this is caused by tubal adherence and photodegradation.[8-10] In our study, adherence to the tubing can account for the initial vitamin E loss in the efflux line. Photodegradation of vitamin A with time also appeared to be an important factor despite shielding of the solution bag. We devised a system to minimize surface contact and light exposure by delivering the multivitamin solution without prior dilution into the lowest entry point of the infusion line. Using this system, and increasing the dose of MVI-Paediatric from 1.5 to 2 ml/kg per day beginning on day 1 instead of day 3, we were able to increase plasma levels of vitamins A and E significantly. With vitamin A, there was a significant rise from the cord levels by 48 hours, and elevated values were sustained for 4 weeks. Early administration of vitamin E allowed an initial rise to acceptable levels; these were not maintained at 4 weeks, probably because of the switch to oral feeding without vitamin E supplementation.

Other alternative delivery strategies have been devised. The addition of MVI-Paediatric to a lipid emulsion reduces losses to 15%[8] but would result in delay of vitamin administration if lipid administration is not commenced until after the first week of life. Increasing evidence is mounting that early administration of lipids may be detrimental,[11] potentially exposing the infants to toxic endoperoxides.[12] Increased doses of multivitamins have been recommended to achieve adequate plasma levels of vitamin E,[13] but these will lead to excessive doses of riboflavin, ascorbic acid, and pyridoxine. Photodegradation of riboflavin occurs through the skin of neonates during phototherapy, and elevated levels could increase the formation of reactive oxygen species[14]; this risk should prompt caution in increasing the dose of multivitamins administered to premature infants. A dose of 2 ml/kg, as used in our multivitamin infusion, is associated with appropriate thiamine, riboflavin, folate, and vitamin B_{12} status in VLBW infants, whereas 3 ml/kg significantly elevates these levels.[15]

The specific needs of VLBW infants should be addressed by designing a multivitamin preparation for their use. However, until a more appropriate formulation is available, it would seem advisable to maximize the efficiency of delivery of available preparations. The method that we have described resulted in significant improvement in plasma vitamin A and E status, but individual infants still had low vitamin levels. Further improvements in parenteral delivery are therefore desirable.

We acknowledge the assistance of the medical and nursing staff of the Dunedin and Christchurch NICU and the work of V. Aebli and K. Sluis in the handling of samples.

REFERENCES

1. Frank L. Antioxidants, nutrition and bronchopulmonary dysplasia. Clin Perinatol 1992;19:541-61.
2. Shenai JP, Chytil F, Stahlman MT. Vitamin A status of neonates with bronchopulmonary dysplasia. Pediatr Res 1985; 19:185-7.
3. Law MR, Wijewardene K, Wald NJ. Is routine vitamin E administration justified in very low birthweight infants? Dev Med Child Neurol 1990;32:442-50.
4. Shenai JP, Kennedy KA, Chytil F, Stahlman MT. Clinical trial of vitamin A supplementation in infants susceptible to bronchopulmonary dysplasia. J PEDIATR 1987;111:269-77.
5. Pearson E, Bose C, Snidow T, et al. Trial of vitamin A supplementation in very low birthweight infants at risk of bronchopulmonary dysplasia. J PEDIATR 1992;121:420-7.
6. Subcommittee on Paediatric Parenteral Nutrient Requirements, Committee on Clinical Practice Issues, American Society for Clinical Nutrition. Greene HL, Hambridge KM, Schanler R, Tsang RC. Am J Clin Nutr 1988;48:1324-42.
7. Bieri J. Simultaneous determination of alpha-tocopherol and retinol in plasma or red cells by high-pressure liquid chromatography. Am J Clin Nutr 1979;32:2143-9.
8. Greene HL, Phillips BL, Franck L, et al. Persistently low blood retinol levels during and after parenteral feeding of very low birthweight infants: examination of losses into intravenous administration sets and a method of prevention by addition to a lipid emulsion. Pediatrics 1987;79:894-900.
9. Henton DB, Merritt RJ. Vitamin A sorption to polyvinyl and polyolefin intravenous tubing. JPEN J Parenter Enteral Nutr 1990;14:79-81.
10. Thomas DG, James SL, Fudge A, Odgers C, Teubner J, Simmer K. Delivery of vitamin A from parenteral nutrition solutions in neonates. J Paediatr Child Health 1991;27:180-3.
11. Sosenko IRS, Rodriguez-Pierce M, Bancalari E. Effect of early initiation of intravenous lipid administration on the incidence and severity of chronic lung disease in premature infants. J PEDIATR 1993;123:975-82.
12. Helbock HJ, Motchnik PA, Ames BN. Toxic hydroperoxides in intravenous lipid emulsions used in preterm infants. Pediatrics 1993;91:83-7.
13. Amorde-Spalding K, D'Harlingue AE, Phillips BL, et al. Tocopherol levels in infants <1000 grams receiving MVIP. Pediatrics 1992;84:992-4.
14. Ennever JT, Carr JHS, Speck WT. Potential for genetic damage from multivitamin solutions exposed to phototherapy illumination. Pediatr Res 1983;17:192-4.
15. Levy R, Herzberg GR, Andrews WL, Brajendra S, Friel JK. Thiamine, riboflavin, folate and vitamin B_{12} status of low birth weight infants receiving parenteral and enteral nutrition. JPEN J Parenter Enteral Nutr 1992;16:241-7.

Possible fetal effects of cervical dilation and uterine curettage during the first trimester of pregnancy

Lewis B. Holmes, MD

From the Department of Newborn Medicine, Brigham and Women's Hospital, and the Department of Pediatrics, Harvard Medical School, Boston, Massachusetts

We describe two malformed infants whose mothers had cervical dilation and uterine curettage. One mother had the procedure at 8 weeks and the other at 6 weeks of gestation. One infant had a facial cleft, hypertelorism, scalp defects, brain malformations, and absent fingernails and a constricting band on the fourth and fifth fingers. The other infant had an area of diminished scalp hair, vertebral anomalies, and a heart defect. (J PEDIATR 1995;126:131-4)

Submitted for publication May 29, 1994; accepted July 25, 1994.

Reprint requests: Lewis B. Holmes, MD, Genetics and Teratology Unit, Massachusetts General Hospital, Warren 801, Boston, MA 02114-2696.

0022-3476/95/$3.00 + 0 **9/24/59435**

Two procedures in the first trimester of pregnancy, chorionic villus sampling[1-3] and the selective reduction of multiple gestations by the infusion of saline solution,[4] have been

D&C	Cervical dilation and uterine curettage

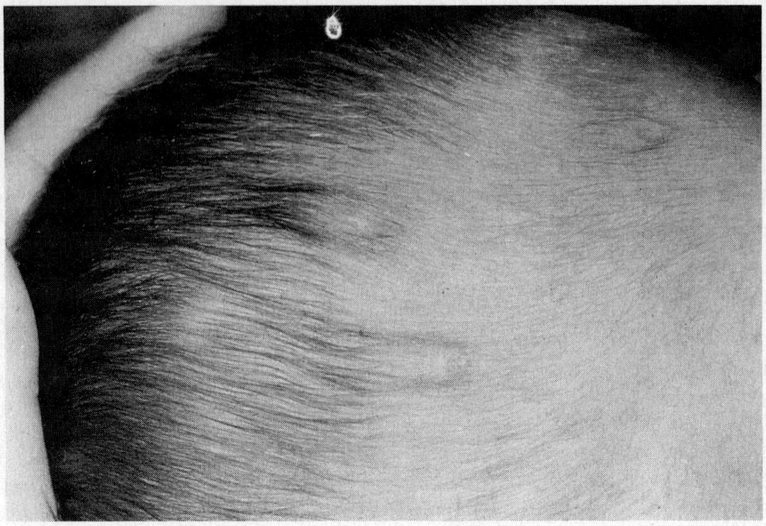

Fig. 1. Small parietal scalp defects in patient 1 are surrounded by a ring of hyperpigmentation.

associated with the occurrence of a higher frequency of malformations in the exposed infants. Exposure during the first trimester to the synthetic prostaglandin misoprostol also has been associated with the occurrence of terminal transverse limb defects[5] and scalp defects.[6] The postulated mechanisms of action of these exposures is a disruptive process caused by changes in the blood flow in the embryo, either by shock and hypoperfusion or vasoconstriction, followed by ischemia, hypoxia, hemorrhage, and tissue loss.

As part of an Active Malformations Surveillance Program,[7] a pregnancy history has been obtained to identify potential teratogenic exposures. Two infants were identified as having been exposed to a cervical dilation and uterine curettage during pregnancy among all of the malformed infants ascertained during a 19-year period (1972 to 1974, 1979 to present).

CASE REPORTS

Patient 1. A female infant was born to a primigravid 22-year-old white woman who had a D&C at approximately 8 weeks of gestation after a presumed spontaneous abortion. She had general anesthesia for the procedure and took doxycycline twice a day for 1 week thereafter. Subsequently she was found still to be pregnant. Ultrasonography at 18 weeks after the last menstrual period showed an intrauterine pregnancy and no fetal abnormalities. However, ultrasonography at 28 weeks identified several fetal abnormalities, including hydrocephalus, facial cleft deformity, and intrauterine growth retardation. At 37½ weeks of gestation, a cesarean section was performed because of the hydrocephalus. The infant weighed 3180 gm (25th percentile), was 50 cm long (50th percentile), had a head circumference of 38.8 cm (>97th percentile[8]), and had Apgar scores of 7 and 9 at 1 and 5 minutes, respectively. The cranium was large, with prominence of the forehead and both temporal areas; the sagittal suture was up to 3 cm in width. There were three 0.5 cm scalp defects with a surrounding halo of hyperpigmentation and increased hair growth over the temporal area (Fig. 1). The infant had marked hypertelorism (Fig. 2) with the inner canthal distance 4.2 cm (>97th percentile) and outer canthal distance 7.6 cm (>97th percentile). The palpebral fissures were shortened (right, 1.4 cm; left, 1.6 cm; <3rd percentile). The nose was broad and shortened markedly. There was a left lateral cleft of the lip that extended up through the lateral aspect of the left nostril into the maxilla; the right nostril was misshapen (Fig. 2). The soft palate and uvula were cleft; the premaxilla was present and the tongue was not hypoplastic. The right ear was low set; both ears were normal in size (3.5 cm and 3.2 cm in length). Neither hand had fingernails on the fourth and fifth fingers; the distal phalanx of the fifth finger was short. Bandlike threads encircled the left fourth finger at the level of the distal interphalangeal joint; a constriction-like ring was present at the same level of the fourth and fifth fingers. The toenails were considered smaller than normal.

The infant had recurrent apnea and died at 11 days of age. The brain had an abnormal gyral pattern, fused basal ganglia, and atresia of the aqueduct, hydrocephalus, and absence of the corpus callosum. The general autopsy identified no other internal malformations, although interstitial chronic pancreatitis was present.

The placenta was large and mature; it weighed 570 gm (normal). There was extensive squamous epithelial proliferation at the cord surface and extensive absence of amniotic epithelium from the extraplacental membrane and placental surface.

A review of the pregnancy history in the postpartum period identified no additional harmful exposures except cigarette smoking (one pack per day).

Patient 2. A male infant was born after an estimated 41-week pregnancy that had been complicated by lysis of intrauterine synechiae, a D&C, air insufflation, and hysterosalpingography at 6 weeks of gestation. It was difficult to date the procedure because the mother had had no menstrual period during the 2 years before conception. The infant was born 35 weeks after the procedure and was considered to be a term infant; thus the procedure probably occurred at about 6 weeks of gestation. Delivery was by cesarean section because of a prolapsed umbilical cord. The birth weight was 3495 gm (97th percentile), length was 50.5 cm (75th percentile), and head circumference was 35.5 cm (75th percentile). Initially, the infant was hypotonic and had a protrusion (5 × 6 cm) in the right parietal area and decreased scalp hair in this area, widely spaced eyes (inner canthal distance, 2.5 cm), right preauricular tag, a low-set and posteriorly rotated right ear, a heart murmur, and scoliosis. Cardiac catheterization at 2 weeks of age showed that he had a right-to-left transposition of the great arteries, ventricular septal defect, and infundibular pulmonary stenosis. Radiographs showed an extra parietal skull suture, several abnormalities of the vertebrae, and scoliosis. Chromosome analysis showed no abnormalities.

In childhood the boy's gross and fine motor functions were poor but improved with age. The boy had a severe conductive hearing loss in the left ear and a mild hearing loss in the right ear; the eardrums were normal in appearance. An angiogram showed normal kidneys. When we examined the child at age 8 years, he had an area of diminished hair growth in the right parietal region. An endocrine evaluation at 15 years of age showed normal thyroid function and insulin-like growth factor I levels, and prepubertal levels of luteinizing hormone, follicle-stimulating hormone, and testosterone. Radiographs at age 17 years showed fused hemivertebrae at T2 and T9, and fusion of the vertebral bodies L3 and L4. He had an extra rib on the left side.

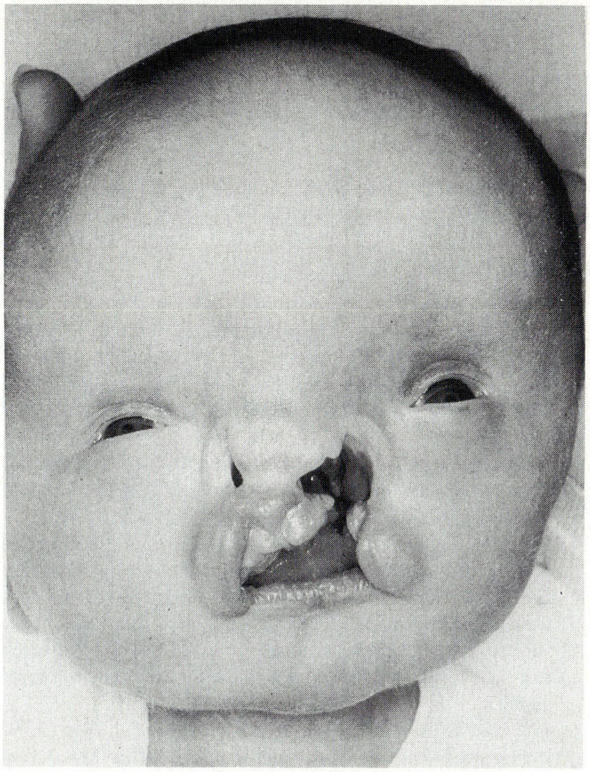

Fig. 2. Patient 1 had widely spaced eyes with lateral cleft extending up into maxilla on one side of the face, with a shortened, broad nose, and long, narrow right nostril.

DISCUSSION

We have not found any published descriptions of infants who had been exposed to D&C during the first 8 weeks of pregnancy. We cannot rule out the possibility of a coincidence between this exposure and the fetal abnormalities, but several fetal injuries or exposures have been associated with phenotypic features similar to those of patient 1, who had the features of the amniotic band syndrome. The loss of nails, the constriction bands, and the terminal transverse limb deficiencies have been associated with the following: (1) exposure to chorionic villus sampling between 8 and 10 menstrual weeks[1-3]; (2) selective reduction of multiple gestations by the infusion of saline solution at 10 weeks after the last menstruation[4]; (3) the ingestion of misoprostol, a synthetic prostaglandin, in the second month of pregnancy[5]; and (4) abdominal trauma.[9]

One important corollary of the clinical diagnosis of amniotic band syndrome is the absence of the amniotic epithelium in the extraplacental membrane.[10] This histologic change was observed in the placenta of patient 1; there was no description of this part of the placenta of patient 2.

Each of these teratogenic exposures has been postulated to cause abnormal vascular perfusion of the fetus, hypoxia, ischemia, and tissue loss. Several experimental models of this phenomenon have been developed. For example, a similar pattern of facial defects, constriction bands, and tissue loss in rat fetuses was observed after clamping the uterine artery for 45 minutes on days 14 to 16.[11] The authors postulated that the interruption of uterine blood supply produced hypoxia, hemorrhage, and subsequent tissue loss. Two common areas of tissue loss were the central mid-face area and the digits, which were the areas of tissue disruption in patient 1. Cocaine-induced hypoxia has been shown in vitro to produce terminal transverse limb defects, presumably as a consequence of vasoconstriction, which leads to ischemia, hemorrhage, and tissue loss.[12] Placental trauma produced at 8 and 10 menstrual weeks was observed by fetoscopy to be associated with numerous ecchymoses over the scalp, chest, and arms.[13] Perhaps similar scalp ecchymoses could have been precursors of the scalp defect in patient 1 or the scalp hair loss in patient 2.

A fetus exposed to the D&C procedure would be reacting, if the pregnancy continued, to marked and acute mechanical forces on the circulatory system, such as fluid shear stress. In vitro studies have shown that the exposure of cultured vascular endothelial cells to steady shear stress has a direct effect on the function of these cells, which in turn release vasoactive modulators such as endothelin-1, a potent vasoconstrictor.[14-16] This endothelial cell response could lead to vasoconstriction, hypoxia, and ischemia and, if sustained, to tissue loss.

These case histories raise the question of whether fetal exposure to the D&C procedure is teratogenic. Further experience is needed to determine the magnitude of the risk, if any, and the spectrum of phenotypic features in such infants.

I thank Drs. S. G. Driscoll, D. Genest, M. F. Greene, and B. R. Pober for discussions of the findings in patient 1.

REFERENCES

1. Firth HV, Boyd PA, Chamberlain P, et al. Severe limb abnormalities after chorionic villus sampling at 56-66 days' gestation. Lancet 1991;337:762-3.
2. Burton KB, Schulz CJ, Burd LI. Limb anomalies associated with chorionic villus sampling. Obstet Gynecol 1992;79:726-30.
3. Mastroiacovo P, Botto LD, Cavalcanti DP, et al. Limb anomalies following chorionic villus sampling: a registry based case-control study. Am J Med Genet 1992;44:856-64.
4. Roze JM, Tschupp MJ, Arvis P, et al. Interruption sélective de grossesses et malformations embryonnaires des extrémités. J Gynecol Obstet Biol Reprod (Paris) 1989;18:673-7.
5. Gonzalez CH, Vargas FR, Perez ABA, et al. Limb deficiency with or without Möbius sequence in seven Brazilian children associated with misoprostol use in the first trimester of pregnancy. Am J Med Genet 1993;47:59-64.
6. Fonseca W, Alencar AJC, Pereira RMM, et al. Congenital malformation of the scalp and cranium after failed first trimester abortion attempt with misoprostol. Clin Dysmorphol 1993;2:76-80.
7. Nelson K, Holmes LB. Malformations due to presumed spontaneous mutations in newborn infants. N Engl J Med 1989; 320:19-23.
8. Niklasson A, Ericson A, Fryer JG, et al. An update of the Swedish reference standards for weight, length and head circumference at birth for given gestational age (1977-1981). Acta Paediatr Scand 1991;80:756-62.
9. Ossipoff V, Hall BD. Etiologic factors in the amniotic band syndrome: a study of 24 patients. Birth Defects 1977;13 (3D):117-32.
10. Honoré LH, Sekhon PS, Curry CJR. The essential role of placental examination in the diagnosis of amniotic band syndrome: a study of 23 cases [Abstract]. Teratology 1993;47:421.
11. Webster WS, Lipson AH, Brown-Woodman PDC. Uterine trauma and limb defects. Teratology 1987;35:253-60.
12. Fantel AG, Barber CV, Carda MB, Tumbic RW, Machler B. Studies of the role of ischemia/reperfusion and superoxide anion radical production in the teratogenicity of cocaine. Teratology 1992;46:293-300.
13. Quintero RA, Romero R, Mahoney MJ, et al. Embryoscopic demonstration of hemorrhagic lesions on the human embryo after placental trauma. Am J Obstet Gynecol 1993;168:756-9.
14. Davies PF, Dewey CF Jr, Bussolari SR, Gordon EJ, Gimbrone MA Jr. Influence of hemodynamic forces on vascular endothelial function. J Clin Invest 1983;73:1121-9.
15. Malek A, Izumo S. Physiological fluid stress causes downregulation of endothelin-1 mRNA in bovine aortic endothelium. Am J Physiol 1992;32:C389-C396.
16. Davenport A, Maguire JJ. Is endothelin-induced vasoconstriction mediated only by ET_A receptors in humans? Trends Pharmacol Sci 1994;15:9-11.

Use of a visual panel detection method for drugs of abuse: Clinical and laboratory experience with children and adolescents

Jimmie L. Valentine, PhD, and Eva M. Komoroski, MD

From the Sections of Clinical Pediatric Pharmacology and Pediatric Emergency Medicine, Department of Pediatrics, University of Arkansas for Medical Sciences, Arkansas Children's Hospital, and Arkansas Children's Hospital Toxicology and Therapeutics Laboratory, Little Rock

We evaluated the Triage panel for drugs of abuse, a visual method that simultaneously detects seven distinct drug classes in a single aliquot of urine, by use of 1214 urine specimens obtained from children and adolescent patients whose clinical findings warranted a toxicology evaluation. A total of 295 positive results were confirmed by gas chromatography–mass spectrometry. Additional toxicology investigations were not performed on specimens with negative results unless the clinical findings did not correspond with the urine Triage results. The positive predictive value of the test was found to be >85% for detection of barbiturates, cannabinoid metabolite, cocaine metabolite, and opiates; for the benzodiazepines the positive predictive value was 77%. Positive predictive values were 53% for amphetamines and 40% for phencyclidine, although only five specimens were available for evaluation of the latter drug. Correlation between clinical findings of patients and results from the Triage test were good except for ingestion of sympathomimetic amines (because of selectivity of the antibodies used in the test for amphetamines) and in patients receiving either antianxiety or antidepressant drugs (some members of these classes of drugs or their metabolites appeared to cross-react with the benzodiazepine test). The primary advantages of the Triage test were the rapid turnaround time, the ease with which a specimen could be processed, and the ability to use rapidly provided information as part of a differential diagnosis. (J Pediatr 1995;126:135-40)

Children and adolescents are often seen for emergency treatment because of symptoms possibly resulting from accidental or intentional drug exposure. Rapid identification of the commonly abused drugs in such patients can be helpful in the differential diagnosis. Because of the potential importance of drug abuse in patients in the emergency department, physicians need a rapid, sensitive way to determine the presence of these substances in their patients. Such a need potentially could be met by the Triage panel for drugs of abuse, a clinical screening test that simultaneously detects seven distinct drug classes in a single urine specimen in less than 15 minutes.[1]

GC-MS	Gas chromatography–mass spectrometry
9-carboxy-THC	11-Nor-Δ^9-tetrahydrocannabinol-9-carboxylic acid

This study was conducted in patients seen at our institution in whom drug abuse was considered in the differential diagnosis. No previous information was available to suggest whether this technique had useful applications in children

Submitted for publication June 21, 1994; accepted Aug. 4, 1994.

Reprint requests: Jimmie L. Valentine, PhD, Arkansas Children's Hospital, 800 Marshall St., Little Rock, AR 72202.

0022-3476/95/$3.00 + 0 **9/25/59588**

Table I. Drugs identified in various drug classes by GC-MS analysis

Drug class	Drugs identified
Amphetamines	Amphetamine,* ephedrine, fenfluramine, methamphetamine,* phentermine, phenylephrine, phenylpropanolamine, pseudoephedrine
Barbiturates	Butalbital, butabarbital, pentobarbital, phenobarbital, secobarbital*
Benzodiazepines	Desmethylflurazepam, α-hydroxy-alprazolam, α-hydroxy-triazolam, lorazepam, nordiazepam, oxazepam,* temazepam
Opiates	Codeine,* hydrocodone, hydromorphone, morphine*
Cannabinoids	11-Nor-Δ^9-tetrahydrocannabinol-9-carboxylic acid*
Cocaine metabolite	Benzoylecgonine*
Phencyclidine	Phencyclidine*

*Analyte also quantitated.

and adolescent patients, although some information was available in an adult population.[2] Our study was designed to evaluate the clinical utility of the Triage device by addressing the following question: Do positive findings from urine tests for drugs of abuse performed with the Triage test in children and adolescents correlate with gas chromatography–mass spectrometry studies?

METHODS

Clinical information. Urine specimens from all children and adolescents in the study were collected during 4 months of 1992 and throughout the 1993 calendar year. Most children and adolescents were examined in the Arkansas Children's Hospital Emergency Department. Patients whose clinical findings warranted a toxicology investigation provided a freshly voided urine specimen. Some patients transported to our hospital bypassed the emergency department and were admitted directly to a patient care unit, where a urine drug screen was ordered as part of their evaluation. A total of 1214 urine specimens were available for evaluation. The evaluating physician made the decision to order the urine drug screen and we did not attempt to influence this decision. Required clinical information was obtained by chart review. This study was approved and judged exempt from the requirement for informed consent by the University of Arkansas for Medical Sciences Human Research Advisory Committee.

Principle of analysis with the Triage device. Tests were performed by dispensing an aliquot of urine into a well on the device containing three beads: one containing monoclonal antibodies directed against seven different classes of drugs of abuse or their metabolites, one containing gold particles conjugated to multiple drug derivatives, and one containing buffer. This solution was allowed to incubate for 10 minutes. During this time, seven distinct immunoassay reactions occurred to detect any drug present in the urine that had displaced free drug conjugate from antibody binding sites. Any free drug conjugate present after the initial competitive reaction was available to bind the solid phase (detection zone), which consisted of immobilized monoclonal antibodies in seven discrete drug zones, in addition to a positive and negative control zone. The solution from the well was pipetted onto the detection zone and at cutoff concentrations, different for most drugs, a color response was generated. Multiple drugs or drug classes were detected simultaneously.

Laboratory methods. All urine specimens were sent to the Arkansas Children's Hospital clinical laboratory where an on-duty medical technologist performed the Triage test and made the determination of a negative or positive finding. The Food and Drug Administration–approved Triage device was purchased from Biosite Diagnostics (San Diego, Calif.). We performed daily quality control tests with urine specimens that showed a positive and a negative result on two different devices from the same lot on days when urine drug of abuse tests were ordered. Negative results were reported by the technologist to the emergency department or other ordering unit. When a positive result was obtained, the technologist was required to contact one of us (J.L.V.), who reported the finding to the ordering physician; the toxicologist and the physician jointly made the decision whether additional toxicology testing was warranted. All specimens that yielded positive results were refrigerated and studied within 48 hours by GC-MS in the toxicology laboratory with a selective ion monitoring method. Limits of quantitation and detection for all analytes by GC-MS were as specified by the College of American Pathologists. The analytes in each drug class identified by GC-MS analyses are listed in Table I, with an indication of which analytes were quantitatively measured. All GC-MS confirmation results were made available to the ordering physician, and a comparison was made by us with the Triage findings to determine the correctness of the initial screen.

Analysis of data. If GC-MS analysis did not produce evidence of either the parent drug or a metabolite from the drug or drug class indicated by Triage testing, the result was considered to be a false positive. Extensive analysis of false-negative results was not possible because specimens producing a negative screening result with the Triage test were not evaluated with GC-MS. Additional toxicology testing was required in some instances when the amphet-

Table II. Positive predictive value and specificity of Triage device in children and adolescents

Drug class	Number of true positives	Number of false positives	Percent positive predictive value	Percent specificity
Amphetamines	16	14	53.3	98.8
Barbiturates	39	4	90.7	99.7
Benzodiazepines	72	21	77.4	98.1
Cannabinoids	46	2	95.8	99.8
Cocaine metabolite	40	6	87.0	99.5
Opiates	26	4	86.7	99.7
Phencyclidine*	2	3	40.0	99.8

*Insufficient data for reliable determinations.

amines test from the Triage device produced a negative result that did not appear to correlate with the clinical findings.

The percent positive predictive value for the Triage results were determined by the following formula:

$$\frac{\text{Total true positive results}}{\text{Total true positives + Total false positives}} \times 100$$

The percent specificity of the Triage test was determined by the following formula:

$$\frac{\text{Total true negative results}}{\text{Total true negatives + Total false positives}} \times 100$$

Examination of patient records for drugs that might have produced false-positive results. Four of the drug classes identified by the Triage device, which are commonly used therapeutically (amphetamines, barbiturates, benzodiazepines, and opiates) produced some false-positive results (Table II). Therefore medical records of patients whose urine specimens had yielded false-positive results for these drug classes were further evaluated to determine the following: (1) whether a drug available to the patient was in the class that had produced the positive result; (2) whether a drug available to the patient, but not in the class with the positive test result, had been identified in multiple patient specimens; and (3) whether an available drug had previously been described by the manufacturer of the Triage device to produce potential cross-reactions. Medical records were not evaluated if notations could not be found concerning drugs available to the patient. If, after medical chart review, it was found that the patient was in the first category, the test result was not considered to be a false-positive finding.

RESULTS

Assessment of the positive predictive value of the Triage device (Table II). Of the 1214 Triage devices utilized in the study, 295 (24.3%) showed positive results for a drug or drug group. This represented the number of positive test results, not the number of devices that were used, because one device might have had more than one positive result, as in the case of multiple ingestions. Only five urine specimens were available for confirmation as a result of a positive phencyclidine test; therefore the results given for this drug class were not further evaluated.

Table III. Correlation of medical records with false-positive results in children and adolescents

Drug class giving false-positive result	Drugs available to patient	No. patients with available drug
Amphetamines	Isometheptene*	1
	Nicotine	4
	Ranitidine*	3
	Terfenadine	1
Barbiturates	Diphenhydramine	1
	Phenytoin*	1
Benzodiazepines	Albuterol	2
	Amitriptyline	1
	Fluoxetine	3
	Hydroxyzine*	3
	Imipramine	2
	Sertraline*	4

*Listed by the manufacturer as cross-reacting with specified drug test antibody.

Examination of patient records for available drugs: adjustment of false-positive results. If a GC-MS confirmation revealed that a Triage result was falsely positive for amphetamines, barbiturates, benzodiazepines, or opiates, that patient's medical records were evaluated. If this review revealed that a drug was available to the patient in the class that produced the positive Triage result, the result was considered to be a true positive. This resulted in adjustments of apparent false positives for two specimens with barbiturates and five with benzodiazepines.

Assessment for potential cross-reacting drugs that produced false-positive results. Review of patient records revealed multiple instances in which a given drug was available to a patient whose urine specimen had given a false-positive result (Table III). This was an indication that the parent drug or its metabolites might cross-react with the antibody used in the device and produce a false-positive result. In some instances, the availability of a particular drug could be determined in only one specimen, but the drug was a structural analog or possessed similar pharmacologic action and therefore was included as a potential cross-reacting drug. For example, urine specimens from two patients receiving imipramine therapy produced false-positive results, whereas its structural analog, amitriptyline, produced only one false-positive result. Other drugs were listed if the manufacturer had reported a cross-reaction or if the drug was one frequently used in pediatric emergency medicine and might be found to be a cross-reacting drug if more specimens were studied. Examples of the latter are isometheptene, frequently used for adolescent migrainelike headaches, and terfenadine and diphenhydramine, drugs widely used to treat allergic disease.

DISCUSSION

The standard methods for toxicology analysis (gas chromatography, GC-MS, high-performance liquid chromatography, thin-layer chromatography) are not available to all institutions for use in emergency evaluations. A point-of-care device that permits a rapid and accurate screen for drugs of abuse and that could be performed by clinical unit personnel would therefore be a helpful adjunct for patient evaluations. This study investigated the utility of one such system, the Triage test, a visual method that can simultaneously identify seven different classes of drugs of abuse. Two similar methods, the ONTRAK system (Roche Diagnostic Systems, Somerville, N.J.), which is based on latex agglutination, and the accu-PINCH (Hycor Biomedical, Garden Grove, Calif.), which is based on enzyme immunoassay, analyze only one drug per device.[3, 4] A potential disadvantage of all these systems is that interpretation depends on visual inspection. This may lead to a false interpretation of results, either judging a result too marginal to be positive when the drug is actually present (false negative), or judging a faint test result as being positive when the drug is not present (false positive). Advantages to visual systems include point-of-care use and elimination of instrument calibration and maintenance. If the test is to have utility in point-of-contact care, the number of false-negative and false-positive results must be at a minimum, or be predictable based on knowledge of drugs or drug classes that will produce an inaccurate result.

False-negative results with the Triage device might arise from two causes: the workplace cutoff values established by the U.S. Department of Health and Human Services for the common drugs of abuse and the lack of reactivity of the antibody with other members of a drug class, including unidentified urinary metabolites. Five of the drug classes found in the Triage device (i.e., amphetamines, cannabinoid metabolite [9-carboxy-tetrahydrocannabinol], cocaine metabolite [benzoylecgonine], opiates, and phencyclidine) require a cutoff value of 1000, 50, 300, 300, and 25 ng/ml, respectively. Concentrations of these drugs in the workplace population may not correlate with clinical findings in children and adolescents; care must be exercised in using such cutoff concentrations to establish the presence or absence of a particular drug. The other two drugs detected with the Triage device, barbiturates and benzodiazepines, are not part of the U.S. Department of Health and Human Services guidelines for workplace drug testing and have been assigned a cutoff value of 300 ng/ml by the manufacturer, which is similar to cutoff concentrations for other immunoassay screening methods. Another consideration in using the Triage device is that the antibody used to discriminate members of a drug class may be so selective that a false-negative result may occur even though that drug might be important in a clinical setting. An example of this was found in an afebrile child with seizures of unknown origin. The Triage device had been designed to interact more selectively with the D-isomers of amphetamine and methamphetamine while requiring very high levels of ephedrine to produce a positive result, and gave a negative result. The inability of this screening test to reveal the presence of ingested ephedrine led to an extensive neurologic evaluation before confirmatory toxicology testing demonstrated the presence of ephedrine, a finding which prompted the parent's admission that the child had been given multiple doses of an over-the-counter preparation containing ephedrine.

Some false-positive results were observed in all drug classes. Comparison of the manufacturer's specificity tables with our results indicated that only a few of the drugs available to our patients should have cross-reacted with the test. Variance between our findings and those listed by the manufacturer could be related to differences in the metabolism of drugs in children and adolescents studied compared with previous studies that are presumed to have primarily involved adult populations.

The marijuana metabolite test had the greatest positive predictive value. The false-positive result found in one patient mostly likely occurred because of a cross-reaction of the antibody for 9-carboxy-THC with one of the other drugs being taken, or alternately, as a result of misreading of the device because cannabinoids and opiates are adjacent on the Triage device. This false-positive finding did not alter the course of short-term treatment for the patient but might have presented a problem for the physician confronting the patient concerning marijuana use. The cutoff values for marijuana metabolite used in the Triage device were decreased from 100 to 50 ng/ml during the course of the study. The majority of the study was conducted with the 100 ng/ml cutoff, and 41% of the confirmed cannabinoid-positive values were >100 ng/ml. Eight (13%) of the specimens were true positives that had levels of 9-carboxy-THC by GC-MS below the 50 ng/ml cutoff value; the lowest value was 22.5 ng/ml. That levels of 9-carboxy-THC were determined below the cutoff value was not surprising because the Triage test, as well as other immunoassay procedures, may react to varying degrees with a variety of cannabinoid metabolites that are not readily available and are required to determine the true cross-reactivity of the test. Additionally, this may account for the large difference in the screening cutoff concentration compared with the confirmatory concentration for the cannabinoids.

Cocaine testing with the Triage device appeared reliable in most patients and was found to be useful in neonatal drug screening. The positive predictive value with the cocaine test might permit a negative finding to be used in the differential diagnosis of cardiac arrhythmias. However, we observed apparent false-positive results with the Triage device for cocaine during the study; therefore caution should be used in relying on it alone to provide an accurate differential diagnosis of a patient with, for example, cardiac arrhythmias, or chest pain.

Positive predictive value with the opiate test was acceptable. Dihydrocodeine, which is known to react with the Triage test, was not measured in this study but has been confirmed by GC-MS in specimens that produced "apparent false positive results" (Dr. John F. Bruni, Biosite Diagnostics: personal communication, April 1994).

More patients had positive screening results in the benzodiazepine class than any other drug or drug class when the Triage device was used. Perhaps this was to be expected in a series of children and adolescent patients because short-lived benzodiazepines, such as lorazepam, oxazepam, or temazepam, are frequently used therapeutically. This conclusion was borne out in our GC-MS findings; almost 60% of all benzodiazepines confirmed were one of these drugs. Midazolam, which is frequently used in pediatric procedures, was not identified by GC/MS but its presence would be apparent from medical record reviews. Flurazepam is rarely used in children or adolescents, and its desmethyl metabolite was not identified in our study population. Positive results for benzodiazepines in urine specimens could not be adequately explained in one third of the cases, for a variety of reasons. Probably the most significant was the variety of benzodiazepines that are available and the lack of laboratory standards required for the confirmation and identification of various metabolites in urine. Our GC-MS procedure required a minimum of 3 ml urine and could determine only some of the potential metabolites. As a class, benzodiazepines initially undergo oxidative metabolism followed by glucuronidation, and are largely excreted in urine as the glucuronides.[5] Because the Triage product has been designed to detect the glucuronide conjugates of the hydroxylated metabolites, it could potentially cross-react with other drug metabolites also being excreted as glucuronides. Patients receiving some type of antidepressant, such as sertraline, may have accounted for some unconfirmed false-positive results. This drug class has the potential to undergo oxidative hydroxylation followed by glucuronide conjugation that might potentially cross-react with the Triage antibodies. Other immunoassays for benzodiazepines have antibodies designed to react with oxazepam; although not giving cross-reactions with glucuronidated metabolites, such assays will not be as sensitive to the benzodiazepines found in urine principally as the glucuronides. Other drugs available to patients that were found to produce apparent false-positive test results for benzodiazepines were hydroxyzine and albuterol. Finally, review of patient records demonstrated that three specimens with positive results for benzodiazepines by Triage were not confirmed by GC-MS but came from patients who had received diazepam or lorazepam. The failure to confirm the findings in these specimens may have been related to urine concentrations below the limit of quantitation.

The positive predictive value for the amphetamines test was lower than for the other immunoassays in the panel. Results from a test that gave a 50% probability of being correct when positive were less useful for patient management, even though the specificity was 98.8%. Some of the false-positive results may have been produced as a result of the presence of histamine H_1 and H_2 blockers in addition to the presence of other sympathomimetic amines. In young children (<3 years of age), central nervous system hyperactivity with or without seizures is, in our opinion, an indication for toxicology testing to determine whether a sympathomimetic-like drug is producing the symptoms. Although amphetamine or methamphetamine may be involved, it is more likely that common over-the-counter drugs such as ephedrine, pseudoephedrine, and phenylpropanolamine may have been ingested accidentally or may represent an iatrogenic overdose.

Apparent false-positive results with the barbiturates could be attributed to extensive metabolism of the barbiturates, which cannot be confirmed by GC-MS because of the lack of available standards for the metabolites, or to the presence of other unidentified cross-reacting substances. Some of the patients who had such false-positive test results were receiving drugs known to cross-react with the antibody for barbiturates in the Triage test. For example, one patient was receiving phenytoin, which is listed as cross-reacting by the manufacturer.

The primary advantages of the Triage panel for drugs of abuse were the rapid turnaround time, the ease with which a urine specimen could be processed, the ability to correlate clinical findings rapidly with a positive result for some drug classes, and the specificity in ruling out use of drugs of abuse. False-positive results were noted with all drug classes detected by the device and were believed to be caused by two factors: misinterpretation of the intensity of visual color band produced (which can be minimized through adequate training) and cross-reactivity of the antibody with drugs or their metabolites in classes other than those being tested. Positive results provided reasonable correlations with GC-MS confirmations for marijuana metabolite, cocaine metabolite, and opiates—and with barbiturates and benzodiazepines when potentially cross-reacting drugs were also considered. Less acceptable correlations were found with the amphetamines test as the consequence of potential cross-reactivity with commonly administered therapeutic drugs. Interpretation of a positive benzodiazepines test requires that the clinician know if the patient has received antidepressants. Results from the amphetamines test were of limited value given the cross-reactivity with some therapeutic drugs and the inability to detect the presence of other sympathomimetic amines that may lead to seizures and hyperactivity in children.

A definitive diagnosis should never be based solely on tests such as the Triage device. A chromatographic method, preferably GC-MS or liquid chromatography–mass spectrometry, should be used to confirm initial results and determine a final diagnosis when drugs are suspected to be the cause of poisoning in children.

We thank Vicki Jackson, Steve Rankin, Carolyn Sparks, and James Weddle, Jr., for technical assistance, Drs. John Bruni, Greg Kearns, and Henry Farrar III for review of the manuscript, and faculty members in the Pediatric Emergency Medicine Section for their contributions to this study.

REFERENCES

1. Buechler KF, Moi S, Noar B, et al. Simultaneous detection of seven drugs of abuse by the Triage panel for drugs of abuse. Clin Chem 1992;38:1678-84.
2. Wu AHB, Wong SS, Johnson KG, et al. Evaluation of the Triage system for emergency drugs-of-abuse testing in urine. J Anal Toxicol 1993;17:241-5.
3. Armbruster DA, Krolak JM. Screening for drugs of abuse with the Roche ONTRAK assay. J Anal Toxicol 1992;16:172-5.
4. Anderson G, Vekich AJ, Scott M. Evaluation of a rapid qualitative EIA test for drugs of abuse [Abstract]. Clin Chem 1990;36:1021.
5. Goodman LS, Gilman A. The pharmacological basis of therapeutics. New York: Macmillan, 1985:347-8.

Clinical and laboratory observations

Successful treatment of Finnish congenital nephrotic syndrome with captopril and indomethacin

A. Pomeranz, MD, B. Wolach, MD, J. Bernheim, MD, Z. Korzets, MBBS, and J. Bernheim, MD

From the Departments of Nephrology, Pediatrics, and Pathology, Meir General Hospital, Kfar Saba, and the Sackler School of Medicine, Tel Aviv University, Tel Aviv, Israel

Two infants with biopsy-proven microcystic Finnish congenital nephrotic syndrome (onset at birth) were treated with a combination of captopril and indomethacin for 2½ and 2 years, respectively; they had a marked reduction of urinary protein excretion without further need for albumin infusions. One infant has end-stage renal disease; the other infant's glomerular filtration rate has remained within normal limits. (J Pediatr 1995;126:140-2)

Submitted for publication April 18, 1994; accepted July 26, 1994.

Reprint requests: J. Bernheim, MD, Head, Department of Nephrology, Meir General Hospital, Kfar Saba, Israel.

0022-3476/95/$3.00 + 0 **9/26/59437**

Finnish congenital nephrotic syndrome is characterized by massive proteinuria beginning within the first 3 months of life, and is refractory to treatment with corticosteroids and immunosuppression. Without aggressive treatment, most children die within a year of severe protein malnutrition and

ACE	Angiotensin-converting enzyme
FCNS	Finnish congenital nephrotic syndrome
GFR	Glomerular filtration rate

sepsis.[1,2] In patients with intractable disease, bilateral nephrectomy and subsequent dialysis[2,3] or, recently, unilateral nephrectomy[4,5] has been advocated. Captopril, an angiotensin-converting enzyme inhibitor, and indomethacin, a prostaglandin synthetase inhibitor, have antiproteinuric effects.[6-9] We describe the successful treatment of two infants with microcystic FCNS treated with a combination of captopril and indomethacin.

CASE REPORTS

Patient 1. An Israeli Arab boy was born to nonconsanguineous parents at 38 weeks of gestation after an uneventful pregnancy. At delivery, a large placenta was noted. During the first 10 days after birth, edema developed. Laboratory evaluation revealed the following: proteinuria, 500 mg/dl; serum albumin, 7 gm/L; serum creatinine, 35.4 μmol/L (0.4 mg/dl); urea, 14.4 mmol/L (87 mg/dl); and cholesterol, 7.3 mmol/L (284 mg/dl). The family history was noncontributory; a 3-year-old sister is healthy. A renal biopsy specimen showed fetal glomeruli with microcystic changes of the tubules, compatible with FCNS. Initial treatment consisted of the infusion of albumin and plasma expanders, diuretics, and a high-calorie (140 calories/kg per day), high-protein (3 gm/kg per day), low-salt formula. At 2 months of age, combined therapy with captopril (gradually increasing dosage to a maximum of 5 mg/kg body weight) and indomethacin (maximum dosage 4 mg/kg) was begun.

During the next 4 months, the edema resolved, proteinuria decreased to 60 mg/dl, and the serum albumin concentration increased to between 28 and 32 gm/L. Albumin infusions were tapered and then stopped. The serum cholesterol value decreased to 4.4 mmol/L (170 mg/dl), and the serum urea level decreased to 2.2 mmol/L (13 mg/dl); the creatinine level remained at 26.5 μmol/L (0.3 mg/dl). After 2½ years, the child is developing normally; his weight is 12 kg and height is 92 cm. He has recurrent *Pseudomonas* ear infections despite maintenance infusions of intravenously administered immune globulin (serum IgG concentration, 0.66 gm/L).

Patient 2. A white infant of Yemenite-Iranian parentage was born at 38 weeks of gestation. The mother had glucose-6-phosphatase deficiency and had become pregnant after treatment of secondary infertility caused by endometriosis. The patient's 7-year-old brother is healthy. The parents are not related. Edema was noted soon after birth; within the first month of life the infant's weight increased from 3.2 to 6 kg. Results of laboratory investigations were as follows: proteinuria, 500 mg/dl; serum albumin, 15 gm/L; creatinine, 61.8 μmol/L (0.7 mg/dl); urea, 14.9 mmol/L (90 mg/dl), and cholesterol, 7.1 mmol/L (275 mg/dl); IgM was not detectable. Antibodies to Epstein-Barr virus, cytomegalovirus, toxoplasmosis, herpes simplex, and syphilis were not detectable.

A renal biopsy specimen showed 18 fetal-appearing glomeruli with mild mesangial proliferation. Cystic dilation of proximal tubules was seen. The interstitium showed a slight degree of fibrosis with round cell infiltration. These changes were interpreted as representative of FCNS.

Initial treatment was similar to that described for patient 1. Despite the daily infusions of albumin, the serum concentration did not increase above 20 gm/L. Indomethacin (4 mg/kg) and captopril (5 mg/kg) were then given. Within 2 months, proteinuria decreased to 60 mg/dl, and the serum albumin concentration increased to 32 gm/L. Albumin infusions were then stopped. At 21 months of age, the serum creatinine level increased to 194.5 μmol/L (2.2 mg/dl); the urea concentration was 21.6 mmol/L (130 mg/dl) and the albumin concentration was 37 gm/L.

The decrease in the glomerular filtration rate was partly attributed to the treatment with captopril and indomethacin and the drugs were withdrawn. Proteinuria promptly increased to 500 mg/dl with a reduction of the serum albumin concentration to 22 gm/L, and renal function did not improve. Captopril and indomethacin therapy was reinstituted and there was a resultant decrease of urinary protein excretion. However, the patient's renal function continued to deteriorate rapidly with elevation of blood pressure (140/95 mm Hg), and anuria developed. Continuous ambulatory peritoneal dialysis was commenced at 2 years of age. After 2 months of dialysis the patient's weight was 10.5 kg and his height was 89 cm. After having dialysis for a year, he underwent transplantation with a cadaver kidney.

DISCUSSION

These two infants had severe proteinuria within the first month of life. Renal biopsy specimens from both infants showed findings typical of FCNS (Prof. R. Habib, Hôpital des Enfants Malades, Necker Hôpital, Paris, corroborated our interpretation). The onset of the nephrotic syndrome within 3 months of birth, coupled with the biopsy findings, established the diagnosis of microcystic FCNS.

Accepted treatment regimens for FCNS have included a high-protein, high-calorie, low-salt diet; repeated (daily) infusions of albumin; use of diuretics; injections of immune globulin; antibiotic prophylaxis; thyroxine supplements; and low doses of aspirin and dipyridamole. Despite these conservative measures, most children fail to thrive and fewer than 2% survive to the age of 4 years. Renal transplantation has resulted in significant improvement in prognosis.[2]

Therefore the aim of early management is to allow the child to reach a sufficient age and size so that early transplantation can be performed. It is essential, however, that the infant reach the stage of transplantation with the least amount of developmental delay.

Because protein malnutrition, which leads to a negative nitrogen balance, is the prime factor affecting prognosis, a reduction of the urinary protein loss and subsequent protein catabolism is important. Bilateral nephrectomy followed by dialysis has therefore been a treatment option.[2,3] In a series of 17 patients described by Mahan et al.,[2] normal serum albumin levels were achieved within 4 to 6 weeks after nephrectomy. An average 6.2 years after transplantation, 14 of the children were alive with a functioning graft. Normal or accelerated growth was seen in those with good graft function, as was marked improvement in developmental skills. Similar results were noted by Holmberg et al.[3] in eight patients. However, bilateral nephrectomy induces a state of anuria with the need for severe fluid restriction and maintenance dialysis until the patient has a transplant. In an attempt to circumvent dialysis and its many inherent complications, unilateral nephrectomy has recently emerged as an alternative form of therapy[4, 5]; the rationale consists of a reduction in total protein excretion to a level tolerated by most patients while maintaining some degree of renal function and urine output.

Based on the antiproteinuric action of ACE inhibitors and nonsteroidal antiinflammatory drugs in various nephrotic states,[6-9] we decided to treat our two patients with this combined regimen. A reduction of proteinuria after ACE inhibition has been documented in animal models[10] and in adult patients with proteinuric renal diseases.[11, 12] Representative of this effect is the antiproteinuric action of captopril in diabetic nephropathy.[13] The decline of proteinuria by ACE inhibition is independent of the antihypertensive effect or a decrease in GFR; the effect is apparent after a week or more and persists for several weeks after discontinuation of the agent.[11] The nonsteroidal antiinflammatory drugs also lower urinary protein excretion; their mode of action is rapid and reaches a maximum effect within 1 to 3 days of onset and dissipates very quickly on cessation of therapy.[8, 9]

Although the antiproteinuric effect of both drugs is probably the result of a reduction of the glomerular capillary hydrostatic pressure, they achieve this reduction by different mechanisms. Captopril acts by preferential dilation of the efferent arteriole,[14] and indomethacin acts by selective vasoconstriction of the afferent arteriole.[15] The combination has been reported to have an additive antiproteinuric effect in nephrotic patients.[16] Our patients had a marked reduction in proteinuria with a parallel elevation of serum albumin to almost normal levels. Their body weight and height were maintained along the 10th growth percentile. In keeping with the predicted course of FCNS, in one infant end-stage renal disease developed at the age of 2 years.

Both captopril and indomethacin can produce a decrease of GFR, particularly in states of reduced effective plasma volume, but whether the combined therapy contributed to the rapid decline of this patient's GFR is impossible to determine. In contrast, the GFR in patient 1 has remained within normal limits. Mahan et al.[2] reported that the mean age at which creatinine clearance was less than 50% of normal was 23 months (range, 6 to 52 months). The balance between a decline of GFR or its protection may be hemodynamically finely poised.

On the basis of this limited experience, we suggest that a therapeutic trial with combined captopril and indomethacin treatment be considered in patients with FCNS before either unilateral or bilateral nephrectomy is performed.

REFERENCES

1. Huttunen NP. Congenital nephrotic syndrome of Finnish type: study of 75 patients. Arch Dis Child 1976;51:344-8.
2. Mahan JD, Mauer SM, Sibley RK, Vernier RL. Congenital nephrotic syndrome: evolution of medical management and results of renal transplantation. J PEDIATR 1984;105:549-57.
3. Holmberg C, Jalanko H, Leijala M, Salmeva K, Ahonen J, Koskimies O. Results of active treatment of 17 children with congenital nephrotic syndrome of the Finnish type (CNF). Pediatr Nephrol 1988;2:C124.
4. Coulthard MG. Management of Finnish congenital nephrotic syndrome by unilateral nephrectomy. Pediatr Nephrol 1989; 3:451-3.
5. Matoo TK, Al-Sowailem AM, Al-Harbi MS, Mahmoud MA, Katawee Y, Hassab MH. Nephrotic syndrome in 1st year of life and the role of unilateral nephrectomy. Pediatr Nephrol 1992;6:16-8.
6. Lagrue G, Robeva R, Laurent J. Antiproteinuric effect of captopril in primary glomerular disease. Nephron 1987;46:99-100.
7. Heeg JE, de Jong PE, van der HEM GK, de Zeeuw D. Reduction of proteinuria by angiotensin converting enzyme inhibition. Kidney Int 1987;32:78-83.
8. Donker AJM, Brentjens JRH, van der HEM GK, Arisz L. Treatment of the nephrotic syndrome with indomethacin. Nephron 1978;22:374-81.
9. Vriesendorp R, Donker AJM, de Zeeuw D, de Jong P, van der Hem GK, Brentjens JRH. Effects of non-steroidal anti-inflammatory drugs on proteinuria. Am J Med 1986;81:84-94.
10. Podjarny E, Rathaus M, Bernheim J, Shapira J, Kariv N, Pomeranz A, Bernheim J. Captopril but not diltiazem favorably affects the course of chronic renal disease in rats. Nephron 1990;55:196-202.
11. Glassock RJ. Focus on proteinuria. Am J Nephrol 1990;10(suppl 1):88-93.
12. Bernheim J. Effects of different converting enzyme inhibitors on the course of non-diabetic glomerulopathies. Nephrol Dial Transplant 1990;5:837-40.
13. Taguma Y, Kitamoto Y, Futaki G, Ueda H. Effect of captopril on heavy proteinuria in azotemic diabetics. N Engl J Med 1985;313:1617-20.
14. Hall JE, Coleman TG, Guyton AC, Kastner PR, Granger JP. Control of glomerular filtration rate by circulating angiotensin II. Am J Physiol 1981;241:R190-7.
15. Jensen PK, Steven K, Blaehr H, Christiansen JS, Parving HH. Effects of indomethacin on glomerular hemodynamics in experimental diabetes. Kidney Int 1986;29:490-5.
16. Heeg JE, de Jong PE, Vriesendorp R, de Zeeuw D. Additive antiproteinuric effect of the NSAID indomethacin and the ACE inhibitor lisinopril. Am J Nephrol 1990;10(suppl 1):94-7.

Treatment of intractable gastrointestinal manifestations of chronic granulomatous disease with cyclosporine

Joel R. Rosh, MD,[a] Hope B. Tang, MD, Lloyd Mayer, MD, Gabriel Groisman, MD, Sheeja K. Abraham, MD, and Alice Prince, MD

From the Departments of Pediatrics, Medicine, and Pathology, Mt. Sinai School of Medicine, New York, and the College of Physicians and Surgeons, Columbia University, New York, New York

Gastrointestinal manifestations of chronic granulomatous disease of childhood include granulomatous inflammatory bowel disease. Severe colitis and perirectal disease developed in a 12-year-old boy with chronic granulomatous disease while he was receiving interferon gamma therapy. The boy had a deficiency of the 22 kd light chain of the cytochrome *b* heterodimer. After conventional medical therapy proved to be ineffective, a rapid clinical response was obtained to cyclosporine. (J PEDIATR 1995;126:143-5)

Chronic granulomatous disease of childhood is a phagocytic disorder characterized by recurrent pyogenic infections caused by catalase-producing organisms; the phagocytes are unable to produce superoxide and other reactive oxygen intermediates because of the deficient production of reduced nicotinamide adenine dinucleotide phosphate oxidase.[1] Several different mutations are associated with this disorder.[2] In addition to pulmonary infections, these patients frequently have perirectal abscesses; inflammatory disease of the bowel is less common. The findings of luminal narrowing, the presence of granuloma, and the involvement of both the small and the large bowel can make this clinical entity indistinguishable from Crohn disease.[3] The general management of CGD has included prophylactic antimicrobial agents to attempt to prevent infection and immunomodulatory therapy with interferon gamma.[4] We describe the use of cyclosporine, a suppressor of T-cell function, in the short-term management of severe colitis in a child with CGD unresponsive to conventional therapy.

CASE REPORT

A 12-year-old boy was found at birth to have CGD caused by a deficiency in the 22 kd light chain component of the cytochrome *b* heterodimer.[2] Medical management from infancy included daily administration of trimethoprim-sulfamethoxasole. At the age of 9 years he had pneumonia caused by *Aspergillus fumigatus* that was treated initially with amphotericin B and then maintenance therapy with itraconazole. Injections of interferon-γ were also begun. Throughout this time, the patient intermittently had perirectal abscesses that resolved slowly after incision and drainage, and appropriate antibiotic therapy. In July 1992 the diagnosis of granulomatous colitis was made, and the patient's condition improved with a regimen consisting of metronidazole, ciprofloxacin, and orally administered prednisone; the doses were slowly tapered during the next 6 months.

The patient remained well until August 1993 when severe bloody diarrhea, extensive perirectal abscesses, and abdominal pain again developed. Flexible sigmoidoscopy revealed continuous mucosal involvement from the rectum to the splenic flexure. He was given nothing by mouth and treated with high doses of corticosteroids, parenteral alimentation, imipenem, and local care for the perirectal disease. Administration of interferon–γ was also stopped. However, his symptoms persisted and left knee pain and swelling, a presumed reactive arthritis, developed. Because of the refractory nature of this patient's disease, a cyclosporine infusion (4 mg/kg per day) was begun; the infusion was adjusted to maintain a blood level of approximately 300 ng/ml (monoclonal assay, Abbott Laboratories, Abbott Park, Ill.). By the third day of therapy the number of bowel movements decreased from six per day with gross blood to two or three per day without blood. Flexible sigmoidoscopy and biopsy after 5 days of cyclosporine treatment revealed the characteristic changes associated with CGD colitis, namely an inflammatory infiltrate that included macrophages containing granules in the cy-

CGD	Chronic granulomatous disease
IFN-γ	Interferon gamma

Submitted for publication Aug. 4, 1994; accepted Sept. 12, 1994.

Reprint requests: Alice Prince, MD, Division of Infectious Disease, College of Physicians and Surgeons, Columbia University, 650 W. 168th St., New York, NY 10031.

[a]Now at the Department of Pediatrics, Morristown Memorial Hospital, Morristown, N.J.

0022-3476/95/$3.00 + 0 **9/26/60555**

toplasm that stained with periodic acid–Schiff reagent, but with diminished inflammation in comparison with the biopsy specimens taken earlier in the course of this patient's disease. A contrast radiogram of the small bowel showed no evidence of disease. Oral preparations of metronidazole and mesalamine were given for long-term maintenance, and the patient was able to resume a regular diet without any increase in stool output. The dosage of corticosteroids was also successfully tapered and eventually discontinued.

On the seventh day of cyclosporine therapy, the patient's temperature increased to 39.4° C accompanied by pleuritic chest pain and decreased breath sounds on examination. Chest x-ray study demonstrated three new nodular densities. *Paecilomyces variotii*, a pathogen previously associated with infection in CGD,[5, 6] was recovered from specimens obtained by bronchoalveolar lavage; the patient was treated with amphotericin B for a total dose of 40 mg/kg administered during 2 months, and resumption of long-term itraconazole therapy. Follow-up studies demonstrated complete resolution of the pulmonary nodules. The bowel symptoms have been controlled for more than 9 months of follow-up with a regimen of metronidazole and mesalamine.

DISCUSSION

Gastrointestinal manifestations of CGD include involvement of the terminal ileum and colon, similar to that of Crohn disease,[7] and of the gastric antrum in children, producing symptoms of gastric outlet obstruction. Histopathologically, the finding of granules that stain with periodic acid–Schiff reagent within the histiocytes of the lamina propria is important in differentiating CGD from Crohn disease. As with Crohn disease, the management of patients with CGD has been directed at suppressing the amount of inflammation with 5-aminosalicylic acid and corticosteroids, along with antimicrobial agents, particularly metronidazole.[7] The only therapeutic alternative not explored in this case, colectomy, is not always successful in these patients, particularly because their disease may not be limited to the colon. In addition, with the prospects of gene therapy for this disorder within the conceivable future, we hoped to avoid such irreversible modalities.

In CGD it has been speculated that the chronic antigenic stimulation of the bowel flora, organisms that are not readily killed by the local phagocytes, results in granuloma formation and bowel wall thickening; the predilection for involvement of the terminal ileum and colon of both CGD and Crohn disease suggests similarities in their pathogenesis.[7] Although the biochemical defect(s) associated with CGD have been defined, it is not clear how deficient phagocytic capabilities eventually result in granulomatous colitis. Animal studies suggest a more complex defect of immunoregulation in the pathogenesis of Crohn disease and, by analogy, CGD colitis.[8]

The use of cyclosporine in the treatment of inflammatory bowel disease is controversial.[9-14] Although sulfasalazine, 5-aminosalicylic acid, and corticosteroids are the mainstays of conventional therapy, the indications for other immunosuppressive agents and their inherent risks are less clear. Cyclosporine blocks the activation of T cells by interfering with the expression of interleukin-2 and interferon-γ.[8] The rapid response to intravenous cyclosporine therapy in our patient was quite typical of that described in patients with Crohn disease who were treated similarly for perirectal disease.[10] However, the duration of maintenance of this remission and how cyclosporine might be administered for a more prolonged period remain unknown. When given orally, low doses of cyclosporine have not been reported to be efficacious in the long-term management of Crohn disease.[12] The long-term risks and benefits of the use of cyclosporine remain uncertain.[13, 14] The clinical response to an agent that suppresses T-cell function suggests that infection may initiate bowel inflammation in CGD, but dysregulation of the immune response may perpetuate and exacerbate this process. The contribution of pharmacologic doses of interferon-γ to the gastrointestinal abnormalities remains uncertain.[15]

Because patients with CGD are already at significant risk of a variety of bacterial and fungal infections, the use of potent immunosuppressive agents is not to be undertaken lightly. Both corticosteroids and cyclosporine, by diminishing T-cell function, further increase the spectrum of infectious agents to which these patients are susceptible. Our patient had a significant fungal pneumonia shortly after treatment with cyclosporine was initiated and still receives long-term oral antifungal therapy.

This case demonstrates both the advantages and disadvantages of cyclosporine therapy for granulomatous colitis in children with CGD. Our patient's clinical response was rapid but complicated by a potentially fatal pneumonia. For patients with CGD and intractable bowel disease, a very brief course of intravenous cyclosporine therapy may provide marked and rapid amelioration, both clinically and histopathologically. However, the risk/benefit ratio must be carefully weighed, and infectious complications should be anticipated.

We thank John Shullinger, MD, Janna Collins, MD, and Philip Kazlow, MD, at Columbia University for their help in the management of this patient and Charlotte Cunningham-Rundles, MD, PhD, Neal LeLeiko, MD, PhD, and Keith Benkov, MD, at Mt. Sinai for many useful discussions.

REFERENCES

1. Tauber, AI, Borregaard N, Simons E, Wright J. Chronic granulomatous disease: a syndrome of phagocyte oxidase deficiencies. Medicine (Baltimore) 1983;62:286-309.
2. Dinauer MC, Pierce EA, Bruns GAP, Curnutte JT, Orkin ST.

Human neutrophil cytochrome *b* light chain (p22-phox). J Clin Invest 1990;86:1729-37.
3. Isaacs D, Wright VM, Shaw DG, Raafat F, Walker-Smith JA. Chronic granulomatous disease mimicking Crohn's disease. J Pediatr Gastroenterol Nutr 1985;4:498-501.
4. International Chronic Granulomatous Disease Study Group. A controlled trial of interferon gamma to prevent infection in chronic granulomatous disease. N Engl J Med 1991;324:509-16.
5. Silliman CC, Lawellin DW, Lohr JA, Rodgers BM, Donowitz, LG. *Paecilomyces lilacinus* infection in a child with chronic granulomatous disease. J Infect 1992;24:191-5.
6. Williamson PR, Kwon-Chung KJ, Gallin JI. Successful treatment of *Paecilomyces variotii* infection in a patient with chronic granulomatous disease and a review of *Paecilomyces* species infections. Clin Infect Dis 1992;14:1023-6.
7. Werlin SL, Chusid MJ, Caya J, Oechler HW. Colitis in chronic granulomatous disease. Gastroenterology 1982;82:328-31.
8. Strober W, Ehrhardt RO. Chronic intestinal inflammation: an unexpected outcome in cytokine or T cell receptor mutant mice. Cell 1993;75:203-5.
9. Brynskov J, Freund L, Rasmussen SN. A placebo-controlled double-blind randomized trial of cyclosporine therapy in active chronic Crohn's disease. N Engl J Med 1989;321:845-50.
10. Present D, Lichtiger S. Efficacy of cyclosporine in treatment of fistula in Crohn's disease. Dig Dis Sci 1994;39:374-80.
11. Lichtiger S, Present DH, Kornbluth A, et al. Cyclosporine in severe ulcerative colitis refractory to steroid therapy. N Engl J Med 1994;330:1841-5.
12. Feagan BG, McDonald JWD, Rochon J, Laupacis A, Fedorak RN, et al. Low-dose cyclosporine for the treatment of Crohn's disease. N Engl J Med 1994;330:1846-51.
13. Treem WR, Davis PM, Hyams JS. Cyclosporine treatment of severe ulcerative colitis in children. J PEDIATR 1991;119:994-7.
14. Benkov KJ, Rosh JR, Schwersenz AH, Janowitz HD, LeLeiko NS. Cyclosporine as an alternative to surgery in children with inflammatory bowel disease. J Pediatr Gastroenterol Nutr 1994;19:290-4.
15. Sechler JMG, Malech HL, White CJ, Gallin JI. Recombinant human interferon-γ reconstitutes defective phagocyte function in patients with chronic granulomatous disease of childhood. Proc Natl Acad Sci U S A 1988;85:4874-8.

Healing of rickets during vitamin D therapy despite defective vitamin D receptors in two siblings with vitamin D–dependent rickets type II

Klaus Kruse, MD, and Evemarie Feldmann, MD

From the Departments of Pediatrics, University of Luebeck and Neunkirchen, Germany

We report the healing of severe rickets despite hypocalcemia in two siblings with absent vitamin D receptors; long periods of treatment with excessive doses of vitamin D led to relative hypoparathyroidism and a return to normal of calcium metabolism during calcitriol treatment. This finding suggests that some other regulating factor may substitute for the defective vitamin D receptor. (J PEDIATR 1995;126:145-8)

Vitamin D–dependent rickets type II is a rare disorder characterized by early-onset rickets, hypocalcemia, secondary hyperparathyroidism, and increased circulating levels of 1,25-dihydroxyvitamin D.[1] About half of the affected children have total alopecia, which does not improve with otherwise satisfactory therapy. Two main classes of defects have been identified, reflecting point mutations in the gene that codes for the vitamin D receptor–hormone-binding domain mutations and DNA-binding mutations.[2]

1,25-$(OH)_2D$	1,25-Dihydroxyvitamin D
1,25-$(OH)_2D_3$	1,25-Dihydroxyvitamin D_3 (calcitriol)
PTH	Parathyroid hormone
VDDR II	Vitamin D–dependent rickets type II
VDR	Vitamin D receptor

Presented in part at the Seventh Workshop on Vitamin D, Rancho Mirage, Calif., April 24-29, 1988.

Submitted for publication June 10, 1994; accept Aug. 16, 1994.

Reprint requests: Klaus Kruse, MD, Klinik fuer Paediatrie der Medizinischen Universitaet zu Luebeck, Kahlhorststrasse 31-35, D-23538 Luebeck, Germany.

0022-3476/95/$3.00 + 0 **9/22/59942**

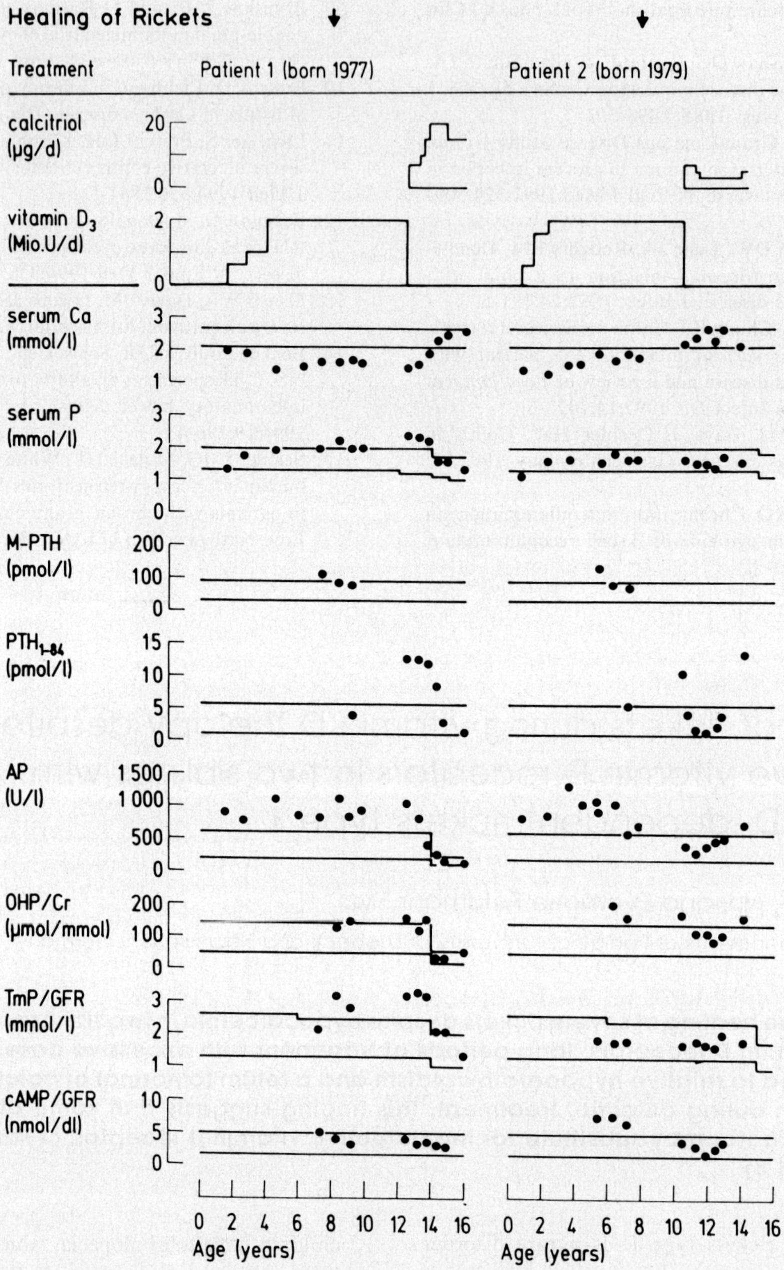

Figure. Treatment regimens, serum calcium *(Ca)*, phosphate *(P)*, mid-regional PTH *(M-PTH)*, intact PTH *(PTH$_{1-84}$)*, alkaline phosphatase activity *(AP)*, urinary hydroxyproline in relation to creatinine *(OHP/Cr)*, tubular maximal rate of phosphate reabsorption in relation to the glomerular filtration rate *(TmP/GFR)* and adenosine 3':5'-cyclic phosphate in relation to the glomerular filtration rate *(cAMP/GFR)* in patient 1 *(left panel)* and patient 2 *(right panel)*. The age-dependent normal ranges are indicated.

Some patients may be cured by high-dose vitamin D therapy, whereas those with receptor-negative mutations and truncated VDRs usually have no response to therapy with excessive doses of vitamin D or vitamin D metabolites. The absence of effective therapy may have severe consequences; death during the first years of life, mainly caused by pulmonary complications and hypocalcemic convulsions, has been reported.[1]

We report the healing of severe rickets in two siblings with absent VDRs after long periods of treatment with excessive doses of vitamin D in the presence of hypocalcemia, and a return to normal of calcium metabolism during calcitriol treatment.

CASE REPORTS

Patient 1. Patient 1, a girl, was born in 1977 after an uneventful gestation and labor. The Turkish parents were first cousins and were healthy, as were the patient's three elder siblings. Alopecia developed within the first 5 weeks of life. At the age of 19 months, she was unable to walk and was referred with clinically and radiologically severe rickets and total absence of body and scalp hair. Her initial serum calcium concentration was 2.0 mmol/L (normal, 2.1 to 2.6 mmol/L), phosphate 1.26 mmol/L (normal, 1.3 to 2.0 mmol/L), and alkaline phosphatase activity 990 U/L (normal, 200 to 600 U/L).

Patient 2. The brother, born in 1979, had convulsions because of hypocalcemia (1.4 mmol/L), complete alopecia, and rickets at the age of 10 months. His serum phosphate concentration, was 1.1 mmol/L, alkaline phosphatase activity 810 U/L, and the serum 1,25-$(OH)_2D$ concentration >360 pg/ml (normal, 20 to 60 pg/ml).

In vitro studies in fibroblasts of patient 1, kindly done by J. Barsony and S. Marx (National Institutes of Health, Bethesda, Md.[3]) showed no significant induction of 24-hydroxylase at the highest tested concentration of 1,25-$(OH)_2D_3$ (10^{-6} mol/L) and no detectable saturable binding of tritium-labeled 1,25-$(OH)_2D_3$ in soluble extracts from whole fibroblasts ("hormone-binding negative").

The mutational analysis (kindly done by K. Kristjansson, Houston, Tex.[4]) revealed a C → T transition at codon 149 (CAG to TAG), which replaced the normal glutamine codon with a termination codon and resulted in a truncated receptor missing the total hormone-binding domain.

RESULTS

During oral treatment with 2 million units (50 mg) of vitamin D daily and calcium, 1 to 2 gm, the serum levels of 1,25-$(OH)_2D$ were extremely elevated to >13440 pmol/L (normal, 48 to 144 pmol/L) without calcemic responses in both siblings (Figure). Despite chronic hypocalcemia the mid-regional parathyroid hormone concentrations in serum were suppressed to 75 to 86 pmol/L (normal, 30 to 90 pmol/L), and intact PTH values in serum were 4.8 and 5.5 pmol/L (normal, 1.1 to 5.8 pmol/L) at the age of 9 and 7 years, in patients 1 and 2, respectively. The relative hypoparathyroidism was associated with high-normal tubular maximum for phosphate reabsorption (in relation to the glomerular filtration rate) and serum phosphate levels, and normal or slightly elevated urinary excretion of cyclic adenosine monophosphate.

Both children had a decreased growth rate until the age of 7 years, when the rate returned to normal; the children had healing of rickets at the ages of 9 and 8 years, respectively.

High-dose oral vitamin D preparations were no longer available in Germany in 1989, and the treatment was changed to calcitriol (1,25-$[OH]_2D_3$) at the ages of 12 and 10 years, respectively. During the overlap phase, there was a slight transient increase of the serum concentration of PTH; during daily calcitriol doses of 15 to 20 μg and 3 to 7.5 μg, the PTH concentration returned to normal in patients 1 and 2, respectively, in association with serum levels of 1,25-$(OH)_2D$ between 2712 and 20280 pmol/L. During this treatment regimen, the calcium metabolism became normal in association with subsidence of bone pain and acceleration of growth in both patients. There was no improvement in hair growth. Probably because of a pubertal growth spurt with a greater calcium requirement of the skeleton, patient 1 acquired slight secondary hyperparathyroidism associated with a small increment of bone turnover, making an increase of the calcitriol dosage to 7.5 μg necessary (Figure).

DISCUSSION

These two siblings have the most severe form of VDDR II because of a premature stop mutation and truncation of the VDR, resulting in the absence of calcitriol binding and biologic activity.[4] Our two patients had total alopecia and lacked an in vitro response of 25-hydroxyvitamin D_3–24-hydroxylase, suggesting the highest degree of resistance to calcitriol in vivo.[1] Although both siblings at first had no calcemic response to excessive doses of vitamin D_3 that induced circulating 1,25-$(OH)_2D$ levels more than 100 times the mean normal range, they showed striking improvement, clinically and radiologically, at the ages of 9 and 8 years, respectively. The healing of rickets in the presence of low serum calcium concentrations has also been observed by Hochberg et al.[5] in a 6-year-old patient with a form of VDDR II that was as severe as in our siblings.

In our patients bone healing was associated with PTH suppression, which caused an increase in the extracellular calcium X phosphate product. The relative hypoparathyroidism may result from the supression of the parathyroid glands by the excessive circulating 1,25-$(OH)_2D$ levels, mediated by vitamin D receptors.[6] This possibility suggests that there may be selective differences in the resistance to calcitriol in VDDR II, or that these effects may be caused by nongenomic actions of vitamin D or its metabolites mediated by different receptors.[7] The return to normal of calcium metabolism was probably not due to the change from vitamin D to calcitriol, but it might also have occurred during continuation of the vitamin therapy. In other words, it was the induction of very high serum levels of 1,25$(OH)_2D$ for a long time during treatment with vitamin D or calcitriol that at first led to relative hypoparathyroidism, saturation of bone minerals, and healing of rickets, and then to a return to normal of calcium and bone metabolism. With further therapy, intermediate doses of calcitriol (or vitamin D) and orally administered calcium seem to be able to support continued remission of calcium and bone disturbances in our patients.

Bone healing between 7 and 8 years of age, accompanied by a return to normal of serum phosphate concentrations, but without a change in vitamin D treatment, has also been described in two other patients with VDDR II.[5, 8] Balsan et al.[9] observed spontaneous healing of rickets in a child with VDDR II at the age of 6 years, followed by a relapse despite continuous treatment with increasing doses of vitamin D derivates. This indicates that the degree of resistance to calcitriol may vary with time within a subject, and that in some patients with the severest type of VDDR II spontaneous improvement may occur; some other regulating factor may substitute for the defective VDR.

We thus recommend long-term therapy with high doses of vitamin D or its analogs even in patients with the most severe form of VDDR II. The healing process in the patients reported by us and others began in later years; we recommend high doses of intravenously or orally administered calcium (in addition to very large doses of vitamin D or its analogs) during the first years of life.[10]

REFERENCES

1. Marx SJ, Liberman KA, Eil C, Gamblin GT, DeGrange DA, Balsan S. Hereditary resistance to 1,25-dihydroxyvitamin D. Recent Prog Horm Res 1984;40:589-620.
2. Hughes MR, Malloy PJ, O'Malley BW, Pike JW. Genetic defects of the 1,25-dihydroxyvitamin D_3 receptor. J Recept Res 1991;11:699-716.
3. Barsony J, McKoy W, DeGrange DA, Liberman KA, Marx S. Selective expression of a normal action of 1,25-dihydroxyvitamin D_3 receptor in human skin fibroblasts with hereditary severe defects in multiple action of this receptor. J Clin Invest 1989;83:2093-101.
4. Kristjansson K, Rut AR, Hewison M, O'Riordan JLH, Hughes MR. Two mutations in the hormone binding domain of the vitamin D receptor cause tissue resistance to 1,25-dihydroxyvitamin D_3. J Clin Invest 1993;92:12-6.
5. Hochberg Z, Benderli Z, Levy J, Weisman Y, Chen T, Feldman D. 1,25-Dihydroxyvitamin D resistance, rickets, and alopecia. Am J Med 1984;77:805-11.
6. Silver J, Nareh-Many T, Mayer H, Schmelzer HJ, Popovtzer MM. Regulation by vitamin D metabolites of parathyroid hormone gene transcription in vivo in the rat. J Clin Invest 1986;78:1296-301.
7. Norman AW, Nemere J, Zhou L-X, et al. 1,25$(OH)_2$-Vitamin D_3, a steroid hormone that produces biologic effects via both genomic and nongenomic pathways. J Steroid Biochem Mol Biol 1992;41:231-40.
8. Tsuchiya Y, Matsao N, Cho H, et al. An unusual form of vitamin D–dependent rickets in a child: alopecia and marked end-organ hyporesponsivity to biological active vitamin D. J Clin Endocrinol Metab 1980;51:685-90.
9. Balsan A, Garabédian M, Liberman KA, et al. Rickets and alopecia with resistance to 1,25-dihydroxyvitamin D: two different clinical courses with two different cellular defects. J Clin Endocrinol Metab 1983;57:803-11.
10. Hochberg Z, Tiosano D, Even L. Calcium therapy for calcitriol-resistant rickets. J J PEDIATR 1992;121:803-8.

CURRENT LITERATURE AND CLINICAL ISSUES

The purpose of this section is to help readers keep up with the literature in pediatrics. We scan current journals and select clinically relevant articles according to explicit validity criteria, summarize these articles in structured abstracts, and provide brief commentary from clinical experts. For every issue, *Archives of Disease in Childhood, Journal of the American Medical Association, Lancet, The New England Journal of Medicine*, and *Pediatric Infectious Disease Journal* are reviewed. For this issue, the following additional journals were reviewed: *American Journal of Pediatric Hematology/Oncology, Biology of the Neonate, Blood*, and *Pediatric Pulmonology*.—*V. A. Moyer, MD, MPH*

We are grateful to Dr. Virginia Moyer for the development of this section, which we believe to be a service for our readers. Obviously, she has had excellent help from individuals who have made a commitment to review specific journals on a regular basis; we thank this core group of contributors, whose names are listed below. We are pleased that Dr. Moyer has succeeded in enlisting the help of additional individuals, including members of the Editorial Board; this will allow the regular review of 12 to 15 journals. Comments from readers would be welcome, and may be sent to Dr. Moyer or to me.—*J. M. Garfunkel, MD, Editor*

1993 AND 1994 REVIEWERS

Michelle S. Barratt, MD, MPH
University of Texas Medical School at Houston
Houston, Texas

Mark Farnie, MD
University of Texas Medical School at Houston
Houston, Texas

Lynnette J. Mazur, MD, MPH
University of Texas Medical School at Houston
Houston, Texas

Virginia A. Moyer, MD, MPH
University of Texas Medical School at Houston
Houston, Texas

Daniel R. Neuspiel, MD, MPH
Albert Einstein College of Medicine
Montefiore Medical Center
Bronx, New York

Kimberly Connelly Smith, MD, MPH
University of Texas Medical School at Houston
Houston, Texas

David C. Waagner, MD
Texas Tech Health Science Center
Lubbock, Texas

Robert Yetman, MD
University of Texas Medical School at Houston
Houston, Texas

Abstracts from the literature

Consequences of varicella and herpes zoster in pregnancy: Prospective study of 1739 cases

Enders G, Miller E, Cradock-Watson J, Bolley I, Ridehalgh M. Lancet 1994;343:1548-51.

Objective: To define the risk of congenital varicella syndrome after maternal varicella-zoster virus (VZV) infection in different stages of pregnancy, and to estimate the frequency of fetal infection in the absence of this syndrome.
Design: Prospective study.
Setting: Germany and the United Kingdom.
Patients: All patients with maternal varicella or zoster whose cases occurred during pregnancy and were reported to the Institut für Virologie, Infektiologie, und Epidemiologie e.V., Stuttgart, Germany, from 1980 to 1993, and to the Communicable Disease Surveillance Centre, London, United Kingdom, from 1980 to 1991.
Main outcome measures: Outcome of pregnancy, specifically evidence of congenital varicella syndrome. Blood from a subset of infants was tested for the presence of VZV IgM (by antibody-capture radioimmunoassay) shortly after birth and/or VZV IgG (by enzyme-linked immunosorbent assay) at age 10 to 12 months.
Results: In 1373 cases of maternal varicella, nine cases of congenital varicella syndrome were identified, all having occurred after maternal varicella during the first 20 weeks of gestation. The highest risk (7/351, or 2.0%) was observed after maternal varicella between 13 and 20 weeks of gestation. Zoster occurred in infancy or early childhood in 10 infants born to mothers who had maternal varicella. No cases of congenital varicella syndrome or zoster in infancy were

9/34/61125

reported in infants born to the 366 women with maternal zoster or to the 97 women with maternal varicella given anti-VZV immune globulin after exposure. VZV IgG was detected in 4 (25%) of 16 infants with congenital varicella syndrome and 76 (12%) of 615 symptom-free infants; VZV IgG persisted in 5 of 7 infants with symptoms and in 22 (7%) of 335 symptom-free infants tested.
Conclusions: The risk of congenital varicella syndrome after maternal varicella is small, peaking at 2.0% when varicella occurs between weeks 13 and 20 of gestation. Asymptomatic varicella infection of the fetus is not infrequent with maternal varicella.

Comment: This study is the largest reported prospective study to date of the outcome of varicella in pregnancy. Risk estimates of congenital varicella syndrome reported here, which are similar to results in two other recent studies,[1,2] provide a firm basis for counseling women with varicella (or zoster) in pregnancy. Despite continued research, reliable means of early prenatal detection of symptomatic infection or reactivation do not exist. Although the possible role of antiviral therapy was not addressed in this study, postexposure prophylaxis with VZV IgG was efficacious in decreasing the risk of congenital varicella syndrome. Because varicella exposures are often unidentified, future consideration should be given to the use of varicella vaccine in varicella-susceptible women of childbearing age.

Tom Belhorn, MD, PhD
University of Texas Medical School at Houston
Houston, TX 77030

REFERENCES

1. Jones K, Johnson KA, Chambers CD. Offspring of women infected with varicella during pregnancy: a prospective study. Teratology 1994;49:29-32.
2. Pastuszak AL, Levy M, Schick B, et al. Outcome after maternal varicella infection in the first 20 weeks of pregnancy. N Engl J Med 1994;330:901-5.

Intellectual, educational, and behavioral sequelae after cranial irradiation and chemotherapy

Anderson V, Smibert E, Ekert H, Godber T. Arch Dis Child 1994;70:476-83.

Objective: To investigate differences in cognitive and educational sequelae after cranial irradiation for acute lymphoblastic leukemia, with control for the effects of chemotherapy and psychosocial factors.
Design: Case comparison.
Setting: Regional cancer center in Australia.
Patients: Three groups were evaluated: 100 children with acute lymphoblastic leukemia treated with cranial irradiation and chemotherapy; 50 children with acute lymphoblastic leukemia or other cancers treated with chemotherapy alone; and a healthy control group of 100 children. Children in the clinical groups stopped treatment at least 2 years before evaluation and had no history of relapse. Children were aged between 7 and 16 years at the time of assessment.
Main outcome measures: Evaluation included cognitive, educational, and behavioral measures.
Results: Children receiving cranial irradiation and chemotherapy performed more poorly than nonirradiated groups on intellectual and educational tests, with verbal and attentional deficits most pronounced. Children receiving chemotherapy alone performed similarly to control subjects, which suggests that such treatment is not associated with adverse neurobehavioral sequelae.
Conclusions: Children with acute lymphoblastic leukemia treated with cranial irradiation do have problems in cognitive and educational abilities that cannot be explained by environmental or psychosocial factors.

Comment: The findings in this report are consistent with the axiom derived from prior studies that, within the age range studied (2 to 12 years at the time of irradiation), the majority of children with acute lymphoblastic leukemia eventually have mild to moderate central-nervous-system dysfunction after 24 Gy to the brain, and mild or no deficits after 18 Gy. What is relatively new in this study is the evaluation of social competence and behavioral effects of CNS therapy, which showed surprisingly few sequelae attributable to the radiotherapy. Also important and novel is the evidence that socioeconomic status cannot explain the observed CNS dysfunction. It is unfortunate that there are no comparisons among the irradiated patients of radiation dose (24 Gy vs 18 Gy), age, sex, or exposure to intrathecally administered methotrexate during the month before radiotherapy, all of which have been reported to be prognostic and could have been analyzed. Although the number of patients in subgroups is undoubtedly too small to test for statistically significant differences, these factors could have been assessed. In addition, the fact that one of the control groups comprised patients treated with systemic chemotherapy, a minority of whom also received intrathecal chemotherapy, does not eliminate some role of intrathecal or systemic chemotherapy in contributing to the adverse outcomes of radiotherapy.

W. Archie Bleyer, MD
University of Texas Medical School
M. D. Anderson Cancer Center
Houston, TX 77030

Effect of vitamin A supplementation on diarrhoea and acute lower-respiratory-tract infection in young children in Brazil

Barreto ML, Santos LMP, Assis AMO, et al. Lancet 1994;344:228-31.

Objective: To determine whether vitamin A supplementation, in a population of children with biochemical evidence of inadequate vitamin A nutriture, would reduce morbidity rates for diarrheal and respiratory disease.
Design: Randomized, placebo-controlled, double-blind intervention trial, which also controlled for duration of breast-feeding, anthropometric indexes, previous illnesses, immunization, and socioeconomic status. Children with clinical signs of vitamin A deficiency, recent measles, and severe growth failure, and who had previously received high doses of vitamin A supplements, were excluded. Each child was visited at home by field workers three times weekly for 1 year to quantify respiratory and diarrheal illnesses.
Setting: A low-income community in northeastern Brazil where suboptimal vitamin A nutriture was considered a public health problem (at least 7% of preschool children had low serum retinol levels).
Patients: 1240 children 6 to 48 months of age.
Intervention: Dietary supplements (either 100,000 to 200,000 IU vitamin A or placebo) were administered by investigators at 4-month intervals.
Main outcome measure: Frequency, severity, and duration of diarrheal and acute lower respiratory tract infections.
Results: The incidence of diarrheal disease in both study groups was less than expected (six or seven episodes per child per year), and there was no difference in reports of mild diarrhea. Both clinical and statistical differences were noted with increasing severity; the incidence and prevalence of severe diarrheal disease were 20% to 23% less in the vitamin A–supplemented group. There was no significant difference in acute lower respiratory tract infections.
Conclusions: Reduction in severity of diarrheal disease may be of major clinical importance in the reduced mortality rates that follow vitamin A supplementation in populations of children in developing societies.

Comment: Preschool children in developing societies are confronted by a wide range of sociologic and biologic inadequacies, including inadequate nutrition. It is assumed that a public health problem exists whenever 5% of preschool children have plasma vitamin A levels less than 10 μg/dl. There also is a consensus that, in geographic areas where children are at risk of having inadequate vitamin A nutriture, mortality rates for infectious diseases (especially measles and diarrheal and respiratory tract infections) may be reduced by vitamin A supplementation. Whether morbidity rates for these infections may also be reduced is less clear. This carefully designed study reports that vitamin A supplementation, in a population of children at risk of having inadequate vitamin A nutriture but without clinical evidence of deficiency, resulted in a significant reduction in morbidity rates for severe diarrhea. If there is any clinical evidence of inadequate vitamin A nutriture in a population of preschool children, all children should be considered as candidates for periodic prophylactic vitamin A supplementation.

George R. Kerr, MD
University of Texas School of Public Health
Houston, TX 77225

ALSO NOTED

A population-based study of the risk of recurrence of birth defects

Lie RT, Wilcox AJ, Skjaerven R. N Engl J Med 1994;331:1-4.

In this study in Norway, women whose first child had a birth defect were at increased risk of having another child with the same (7.6× risk) or different (1.5× risk) birth defects. The risk of recurrence of birth defects was found to be twice as high for women who had not changed municipalities between pregnancies as for those who had moved since the previous pregnancy. These data suggest a role for environmental as well as genetic factors in the recurrence of birth defects.

Effects of age of introduction of complementary foods on infant breast milk intake, total energy intake, and growth: A randomized intervention study in Honduras

Cohen RJ, Brown KH, Canahuati J, Rivera LL, Dewey KG. Lancet 1994;343:288-93.

This randomized trial indicates that breast-fed infants regulate their total energy intake by decreasing their milk intake when solids are introduced. Growth did not differ between groups. Delaying the introduction of complementary foods may be indicated when exposure to contaminated weaning foods is likely.

Factors predictive of maternal-fetal transmission of HIV-1

Boyer PJ, Dillon M, Naviae M, et al. JAMA 1994;271:1925-30.

In this prospective cohort study, the authors found increased risk of transmission with immune complex dissociated p24 antigenemia at term and with intrapartum events that increase fetal exposure to maternal blood.

C. Henry Kempe

There are few Renaissance men in pediatrics, but C. Henry Kempe (1922–1984) was one of them, in the view of his colleagues, students, and friends. He combined superb academic skills and interest with a keen appreciation for the humanities, the arts, and the quality of life in general. Not only did he forge this combination in his personal life, but he extended that philosophy to the institutions in which he worked and to the people he educated, influenced, and mentored. This profile details the career of a dynamic, influential, intellectual giant in our discipline.

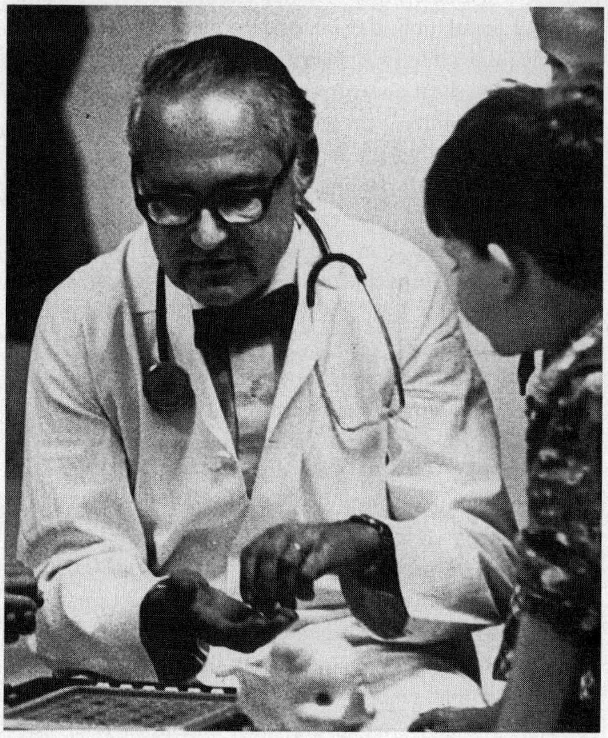

Dr. Kempe was born in Germany in 1922 and grew up under the cloud of Hitlerism, which caused his family to leave that country in 1937. He and his parents were separated by the force of circumstance. Henry went to England with Quaker sponsorship, and in 1938 he migrated to the United States, where he survived on his own with the help of an occasional friend. He was educated in the California system, receiving his medical degree in 1945 from the University of California School of Medicine in San Francisco. Like many others of German descent, he was at first an enemy resident and was then transformed into a citizen so that he could enter the U.S. Army on graduation from medical school. Physicians were badly needed by the services, and at that time entire classes of emerging physicians were recruited into the accelerated programs in U.S. medical schools.

Dr. Kempe's first interest in one of his ultimate fields, infectious diseases, was initiated in medical school under the influence of the pediatric department and by Dr. Edward Shaw, and was furthered by his career sequence after graduation. He was an intern in pediatrics for a portion of the first year after school, and then was assigned to the graduate school in Bethesda and then to the Virology Research Laboratory of the Army Medical Research Unit, where he served for the next 2 years. It was here that he was mentored by Dr. Joseph Smadel and was introduced to the poxviruses. He was told by some of his colleagues that this research was a "dead end" of no significance, but Dr. Smadel convinced him that the problems were interesting and the issues important—a prediction that turned out to be true, as his later activities with vaccinia and smallpox viruses demonstrate.

Dr. Kempe completed his pediatric training under the watchful eye and mentorship of Dr. Grover Powers at Yale University School of Medicine. He was part of a remarkable group of residents, many of whom became leaders of pediatrics in their own right, and one of whom, Ruth Svibergson, became his wife. Those years instilled in Henry a passion for improving the lot of children, which was reflected throughout his clinical career. He often spoke of the strong influence of Dr. Powers in helping him to shape his intellectual and emotional direction toward the improvement of children's health and welfare, the latter being echoed in his future activities in the identification and prevention of child abuse, among other interests in the well-being of children.

Dr. Kempe's affection for his earlier institutional affiliation led him to accept a position on the faculty at the University of California at San Francisco. Here, another powerful influence was Dr. Edward Shaw, a gentle but dedicated professional. Henry sharpened his critical focus under this mentor and learned much about the science and art of pediatrics. These years also furthered his interest in the breadth of pediatrics, as he also became expert in, and ac-

THE JOURNAL OF PEDIATRICS 1994;125:152-4

0022-3476/95/$3.00 + 0 **9/20/54238**

tive in, social welfare issues, lecturing on that subject during his time there.

In 1956 Henry took the position that established him ultimately as a leader in pediatrics. He was appointed by the dean, Robert Glaser, to be professor and chairman of the department of pediatrics at the University of Colorado School of Medicine in Denver, at the young age of 34 years. Dr. Glaser assembled a remarkable group of vigorous young persons, and the University of Colorado rose from relative oblivion to become one of the leading medical schools in the West and then in the nation. Persons such as Ted Puck, Arthur Robinson, Gordon Meikeljohn, David Talmage, Henry Silver, Tom Starzl, and others were the authors of this revival, and Henry Kempe was among the leaders. His department of pediatrics became a scientific core of top-notch investigators, each of whom was encouraged, cajoled, supported, and led to become a superb teacher as well. Henry also stressed compassionate, competent clinical care, and all the faculty members that he recruited were expected to be superb clinicians. One can safely say that in those days the faculty at the University of Colorado Department of Pediatrics were true triple-threat academicians. Henry went further, however, and insisted that there be only a single pediatric community in the city. All pediatricians were invited to join the volunteer faculty, to teach students in both the outpatient and inpatient settings, and to participate actively in the department. In exchange, Henry instituted superb, heavily attended conferences, grand rounds, and continuing education courses. Today this approach to building a pediatric community does not sound remarkable, but the time was the late 1950s and early 1960s, when town-gown problems abounded throughout the nation and in other disciplines in Denver. Henry, however, was at the forefront of change, and his pattern, now so common, was unique.

Dr. Kempe, during his tenure as chairman together with the faculty whom he recruited and nurtured, taught thousands of students and hundreds of residents, many of whom later became leaders in pediatrics. He brought to the faculty both experienced veterans, such as Henry Silver, Lula Lubchenco, Conrad Riley, Arthur Robinson, and Jack Githens, and young, promising professionals, such as Joseph Butterfield, Ray Helfer, Joseph Brazie, Joseph French, Ida Nakashima, Fred Battaglia, Donough O'Brien, Bill Hathaway, Henry Cooper, and many others. As a member of that faculty, I can attest to the spirit that prevailed. We were curious investigators, avid clinicians, and enthusiastic teachers—all traits fostered and inspired by Dr. Kempe. Although his personal accomplishments are considered by many people to be his most spectacular achievements, many of us believe that his mentoring of hundreds did as much for pediatrics, because we multiplied his effect by our own efforts, cultivated by his mentorship. His was a true contribution to the legacy that will persist beyond his individual accomplishments.

Consider the remarkable results that came from this group, a sampling of which include the following: (1) the discovery of new forms of immunodeficiency; (2) the first clinical descriptions of graft-versus-host disease in human beings; (3) the widely used Denver Developmental Screening Test; (4) a tremendous amount of definitive information about the newborn infant, particularly the premature infant, and about hyperbilirubinemia and respiratory physiology and disease; (5) the institution and development of nonphysician health care professions, such as that of pediatric nurse practitioner; (7) enhancements in microchemistry that saved thousands of children from needless large-volume blood sampling; (8) major advances in our understanding of bleeding disorders; (9) institution of community pediatric health centers, a concept novel for its time; (10) significant participation in the development of the nomenclature for chromosomes; (11) delineation of unique genetic and metabolic disorders; and (12) many innovations in medical education. Dr. Kempe's influence was felt in all these activities of his faculty and students; in many of these, he was either a collaborator or had stimulated the quest in the first place.

Not that the personal achievements of Dr. Kempe were minor; indeed, they were significant. His first interest, infectious diseases, led him to become a leading figure in the research of poxviruses, which eventually led to elimination of smallpox vaccination (a consequence of his pioneer work with complications of vaccinia infection) and to worldwide elimination of smallpox. I can vividly remember his presenting his case for elimination of smallpox vaccination at a Society for Pediatric Research/American Pediatric Society meeting in Philadelphia. After his presentation, a number of the leading figures of the day attacked his reasoning and declared him "misguided." Within several years national authorities and committees recommended that smallpox vaccination be discontinued, and within a decade and a half, smallpox was eradicated from the world. Dr. Kempe was a crusader, often recognizing facts before the rest of the world was ready to accept them, but that did not deter him from the crusade, and ultimately he was proved right.

The work with persons who had complications of smallpox vaccination led to other avenues pursued by Dr. Kempe and by his colleagues. These included (1) the delineation of various forms of immunodeficiency, many of which were pioneer observations (e.g., thymic dysplasia, graft=versus=host disease); (2) novel antiviral approaches, such as the use of thiosemicarbazone and anti-vaccinia γ-globulin for treatment of smallpox and for treatment of complications of vaccination, and the use of lymphoid tissue for transplantation to immunodeficient patients; (3) diagnostic meausres that ultimately were used in routine laboratory studies (immunodiffusion, fluorescent antibody techniques); (4) evaluation of a variety of vaccines now in routine use; (5) studies of adverse consequences of other vaccine viruses (e.g., atypical measles, enhanced respiratory syncytial virus infection after immunization); and (6) nascent studies of the association of viruses with chronic neurologic diseases, which, although unsuccessful, pointed the way toward delineation of this association. In addition to the research efforts, Dr. Kempe led a clinical team that cared for a large group of infants with severe infectious diseases. Children with puzzling infections were referred from all over the West, from the remainder of the United States, and, on occasion, from abroad, and such patients were often given correct diagnoses and received expert care, with return in health to their point of origin.

What came as a surprise to many in the infectious diseases community, but not to those who knew Dr. Kempe, was his seminal report on the "battered child syndrome" in the *Journal of the American Medical Association.* Who would envision that an eminent virologist would be the first to adequately inform the medical community of what he termed a "hidden epidemic" of major proportions? Today, we take for granted that there is child abuse, and society has developed the means for its identification and prevention. In the late 1950s and early 1960s, however, such a suggestion was met with disbelief, and many judges, law officers, physicians, and others refused to accept the fact that parents could beat and otherwise abuse their children. Dr. Kempe taught them that their beliefs were a myth and that all of us needed to wake up to reality. He often considered this to be his major contribution, with the greatest impact on children's welfare, notwithstanding his other accomplishments. His work with his colleagues, Ruth Kempe, Brandt Steele, Ray Helfer, Dick Krugman, and many others, has provided a legacy that will stretch far into the future.

Dr. Kempe also had a major impact nationally and internationally. Among his most significant contributions was the conception, implementation, development, and finalization of the Task Force on Pediatric Education, which mapped a direction for pediatric education that has helped to shape current styles and content. He assembled a group of expert educators, somehow found funding for an unpopular undertaking, set out the task for the group members, and then guided them in multiple meetings (at such exciting places as O'Hare Airport) to create a set of usable, practical, but important recommendations. They did so, and their document was used by many national organizations and local departments to determine educational policy and content.

Internationally, Dr. Kempe established a smallpox research laboratory in Madras, India, and together with Gordon Meikeljohn and others, and with the assistance of Leone St. Vincent, accomplished much of the research on the diagnosis and treatment of smallpox. In addition, he trained investigators in India, who remained there to continue their own work. Together, we trained Dr. Jacob John, of Christian Medical College in Vellore, India; he is now a major international virologist who is assisting the International Rotary in their Polio Plus campaign, an attempt to eradicate the disease by the year 2005. Many other students and faculty trained at the University of Colorado Health Sciences Center and now populate medical centers throughout the world.

Dr. Kempe's commitment to issues other than pediatric medicine and infectious diseases, and his activities with art, the humanities, and social concerns, demonstrate his breadth. He introduced art and music to the cloistered students and residents at the University of Colorado Health Sciences Center. He learned that there was radioactive contamination at home sites in Grand Junction, Colo., long before there was "environmental awareness," and embarked on a campaign to protect children who lived on the sites. The government resisted this effort, but eventually the danger was realized and appropriate steps were taken.

In sum, Henry Kempe—he never used his first name—was a consummate scientist, clinician, teacher, and humanist, in the broadest and best sense of these words. He inspired thousands during his illustrious career and his ideas carry on through these individuals. No greater tribute can be paid; no greater legacy can be given to the future of children's health.

Vincent A. Fulginiti, MD
Chancellor, Professor of Pediatrics
University of Colorado
Denver, CO 80262

Incidence of liver disease in patients with cystic fibrosis and meconium ileus

To the Editor:

Colombo et al.[1] reported prospective screening of all patients at the cystic fibrosis (CF) center of the University of Milan for overt liver disease (LD) and related this to genotype, sex, pancreatic insufficiency, and a past history of meconium ileus (MI) or distal intestinal obstruction syndrome (DIOS). They did not find any statistically significant risk related to sex, genotype, or pancreatic status, but there was an almost fourfold increased risk for patients with a history of MI, DIOS, or both to have LD. Because of this increased risk and a prevalence of 33% of overt LD at the age of 5 years in the MI group (results presented at the European Working Group for Cystic Fibrosis conference in Paris in June 1994), the authors suggest a prospective, randomized, and placebo-controlled multicenter study of this group of patients.

The outcome of such a study depends on whether other centers have the same prevalence of liver disease in the MI group. We investigated the prevalence of LD in patients older than 3 years of age at the CF centers of Stockholm and Gothenburg (median age 17 and 13 years, respectively), comprising approximately 70% of the CF population in Sweden. The patients have had yearly liver function tests since 15 years and yearly ultrasound study of the liver for the latest 4 years. The prevalence of MI/DIOS is similar in Milan and Stockholm/Gothenburg. The percentage of LD also corresponds fairly well; the MI/DIOS part of the group with LD is larger in Milan (Table).

The largest difference is seen in the group consisting of patients with MI; Stockholm and Gothenburg have had no cases of LD developing (0/23) at the age of 5 versus an incidence of 33% in Milan. In 3 of the 23 patients with a history of MI, LD developed at the age of 9, 9, and 15 years, respectively. This means that the prerequisite for a multicenter study of a high prevalence of LD in this group is not fulfilled in the Swedish centers. A study with the proposed design including centers like Stockholm and Gothenburg would therefore be neither ethical nor cost effective. Before a study starts, we recommend that other centers determine their prevalence of overt LD in this group of patients with CF. If the prevalence is lower also in other centers, another risk factor should be sought.

Anders Lindblad, MD
Birgitta Strandvik, MD, PhD
Göteborg University
Göteborg, Sweden

Lena Hjelte, MD, PhD
Huddinge Hospital
Karolinska Institutet
Stockholm, Sweden
9/35/59704

REFERENCE

1. Colombo C, Apostolo MG, Ferrari M, et al. Analysis of risk factors for the development of liver disease associated with cystic fibrosis. J PEDIATR 1994;24:393-9.

Reply

To the Editor:

Dr. Lindblad and colleagues report data on the association between liver disease and meconium ileus or its equivalent, distal intestinal obstruction syndrome, in Sweden. Indeed there is fairly good agreement between the prevalence of liver disease in the Swedish population with cystic fibrosis and the prevalence that we observed in Milan.[1] There is also good agreement (particularly for patients followed in Milan and Stockholm) in the prevalence of liver disease within the group who have a history of meconium ileus or meconium ileus equivalent. According to the data reported by Lindblad and colleagues, the risk (odds ratio) of development of liver disease in patients with cystic fibrosis who have a history of meconium ileus and meconium ileus equivalent, compared with patients unaffected by these complications, is 2.9 and 1.7 times higher in Stockholm and Gothenburg, respectively. The corresponding figure for the patients followed in Milan is 3.9.[1] These data support the hypothesis that patients with CF and with a history of meconium ileus or its equivalent are at risk for the development of liver disease and suggest that a study aimed at evaluat-

Table. Prevalence of MI/DIOS

	MI/DIOS of total (%)	Overt LD of total (%)	MI/DIOS of overt LD (%)	MI/DIOS with overt LD (%)
Milan	31/189 (16)	34/189 (18)	12/34 (35)	12/31 (38)
Stockholm	20/120 (17)	19/120 (16)	6/19 (32)	6/20 (30)
Gothenburg	11/88 (12)	11/88 (12)	2/11 (18)	2/11 (18)

ing the prophylactic efficacy of ursodeoxycholic acid treatment would be cost effective. Moreover, as far as ethical issues are concerned, it should be considered that ursodeoxycholic acid therapy is virtually free of serious side effects.

Data reported by Lindblad et al. indicate that there is apparently a more delayed onset of liver disease in the Swedish compared with the Italian patients. Several factors may have played a role, including genetic and environmental differences between the two populations or differences in the criteria used for the diagnosis of liver disease,[1] which in turn may have conditioned different diagnostic sensitivities. In their letter, Lindblad and colleagues do not specify which criteria they adopted for diagnosis of liver disease. Regardless of the cause, while supporting the need for a prophylactic treatment, the Swedish data suggest that enrollment of patients with CF at a later age than the first year of life, as we have recently proposed,[2] would be more appropriate.

We agree that a survey on the prevalence of liver disease in patients with meconium ileus and its equivalent is a prerequisite for a study of ursodeoxycholic acid therapy as a preventive measure for development of liver disease. This had been planned when the study was designed, and a questionnaire is being mailed to CF centers in Europe specifically to address this issue.

Carla Colombo, MD
Annamaria Giunta, MD
Department of Pediatrics, University of Milan
Pier Maria Battezzati, MD
Department of Internal Medicine, School of Medicine
San Paolo Hospital, University of Milan
Milan, Italy
9/35/59703

REFERENCES

1. Colombo C, Apostolo MG, Ferrari M, et al. Analysis of risk factors for the development of liver disease associated with cystic fibrosis. J PEDIATR 1994;124:393-9.
2. Colombo C, Battezzati PM, Genoni S, Giunta A. Prophylactic treatment with UDCA in infants with cystic fibrosis at high risk for the development of liver disease: is a multicenter European study feasible? Proceedings of the 19th European Cystic Fibrosis Conference, 1994. (Book of abstracts, No. 49.)

Short-term, high-dose corticosteroid therapy in childhood acute immune thrombocytopenic purpura

To the Editor:

We read with interest the article by Blanchette et al.[1] A therapeutic regimen that increases the platelet count above a safe level for preventing intracranial hemorrhage by use of orally administered corticosteroids in relatively low doses would be the preferred form of therapy, but we think that the continuation of this therapy for 3 weeks is disadvantageous because of the development of untoward effects and the prolongation of therapy. Side effects may occur with the continued daily use of corticosteroids, and the hypothalamus-pituitary-adrenal system would be suppressed if steroids were administered for periods longer than 15 days.[2] Moreover, effective treatment without any side effects have been reported in studies in which methylprednisolone was used in very high doses orally for 1 week.[3] We are still investigating the effect of orally administered methylprednisolone, 10 mg/kg per day, for 5 days in the treatment of acute immune thrombocytopenic purpura in children. The preliminary data for 10 patients revealed mild elevation of the blood glucose concentration in two patients on day 3 and in the occult blood in the stool in one patient on day 7, which were transient. The mean platelet count increased from 21×10^9/L, to 47×10^9/L on the third day of therapy. The platelet count decreased below 20×10^9/L in only one patient during follow-up.

We believe that short-term therapy with high doses of corticosteroids is as effective as long-term therapy and may decrease the side effects of steroid use. In addition, administration of intravenous immune globulin G, which is very expensive and also has adverse reactions, should be preserved for patients who are unresponsive to high doses of prednisolone or who have serious bleeding.

Halûk Yavûz, MD
Ahmet Özel, MD
İbrahim Erkul, MD
Department of Pediatrics
Selçuk University
Konya, Turkey
9/35/59786

REFERENCES

1. Blanchette VS, Luke B, Andrew M, et al. A prospective, randomized trial of high-dose intravenous immune globulin G therapy, oral prednisone therapy, and no therapy in childhood acute immune thrombocytopenic purpura. J PEDIATR 1993;123:989-95.
2. Del Principe D, Menichelli A. Methylprednisolone in childhood idiopathic thrombocytopenic purpura. Acta Haematol 1988;79:224-6.
3. Özsoylu Ş, Ertürk G. Oral megadose methylprednisolone for childhood acute idiopathic thrombocytopenic purpura. Blood 1991;77:1856-7.

Reply

The comments of Drs. Buchanan, Özsoylu (J PEDIATR 1994;125:503), and Yavûz and colleagues are important; they focus on the two most important issues concerning treatment of children with acute idiopathic thrombocytopenic purpura (ITP), namely whom to treat and what modality to select if a decision to treat is made.

Dr. Buchanan favors a "noninterventionist" approach with treatment of the child rather than the platelet count. He cites a very low incidence of intracranial hemorrhage (ICH), high cost of intravenous immune globulin therapy, and adverse effects of therapy as support for his opinion. Our approach is different. We believe that children with acute ITP and platelet counts $<20 \times 10^9$/L are the group "at risk" for ICH, and that such children should immediately be offered the minimum therapy necessary to a rapid increase in their platelet counts to a safe hemostatic level.[1] This opinion is based on a 0.9% (16 of 1802 cases) incidence of ICH in children with ITP,[1-8] and the fact that the treating physician cannot accurately identify the individual child with acute ITP who will have this rare but life-threatening complication.

Dr. Özsoylu favors intervention, and cites evidence from studies in favor of oral very high dose ("megadose") methylprednisolone therapy (30 mg/kg for 3 days, followed by 20 mg/kg for 4 days). Although Dr. Özsoylu reports no adverse effects with this protocol when administered once daily before 9 AM, others have reported significant adverse effects with much smaller doses of orally administered corticosteroids.[9] Our results with oral prednisone therapy at a starting dose of 4 mg/kg per day are similar to those reported by Dr. Özsoylu for the oral megadose methylprednisolone regimen, so we favor use of the lower dose of corticosteroids if this modality of therapy is selected.

Dr. Yavûz reports results for 10 children with acute ITP who received 10 mg/kg per day of methylprednisolone orally for 5 days. A case is made for short-term therapy to minimize corticosteroid-related adverse effects.

Although the cost of intravenous immune globulin therapy is much higher than that for oral corticosteroid therapy, the more predictable platelet response to intravenous immune globulin therapy and the recommendation, accepted by many pediatric hematologists, that a bone marrow aspiration be performed in children with acute ITP before the start of orally administered corticosteroids should be considered. We believe that the final choice should be made by the treating physician, and that this choice should involve discussion of both risks and benefits of management options with the parents or guardians of the child.

Victor S. Blanchette, MRCP(UK), FRCP(C)
Division of Hematology/Oncology
Hospital for Sick Children
Toronto, Ontario, Canada
9/35/59785

REFERENCES

1. Blanchette VS, Turner C. Treatment of acute idiopathic thrombocytopenic purpura. J PEDIATR 1985;108:326.
2. Benham ES, Taft LI. Idiopathic thrombocytopenic purpura in children: results of steroid therapy and splenectomy. Aust Pediatr J 1972;8:311-7.
3. Lammi AT, Lovric VA. Idiopathic thrombocytopenic purpura: an epidemiologic study. J PEDIATR 1973;83:31-6.
4. Simons SM, Main CA, Yaish HM, et al. Idiopathic thrombocytopenic purpura in children. J PEDIATR 1975;87:16-22.
5. McClure PD. Idiopathic thrombocytopenic purpura in children: diagnosis and management. Pediatrics 1975;55:68-74.
6. Ramos MEG, Newman AJ, Gross S. Chronic thrombocytopenia in childhood. J PEDIATR 1978;92:584-6.
7. Lusher JM, Emami A, Ravindranath Y, et al. Idiopathic thrombocytopenic purpura in children: the case for management without corticosteroids. Am J Pediatr Hematol Oncol 1984;6:149-57.
8. Imbach P, Wagner HP, Berchtold W, et al. Intravenous immunoglobulin versus oral corticosteroids in acute immune thrombocytopenic purpura in childhood. Lancet 1985;2:464-8.
9. Suarez CR, Rademaker DO, Hasson A, et al. High-dose steroids in childhood acute idiopathic thrombocytopenia purpura. Am J Pediatr Hematol Oncol 1986;8:111-5.

Diagnostic accuracy of urinary tract infection and subsequent development of renal scars

To the Editor:

My colleagues and I read with interest the article by Hoberman et al.[1] and the commentary by Hellerstein,[2] and I wish to discuss these articles in the light of our own experience.

The two important issues, as pointed out by Dr. Hellerstein, are the diagnosis of significant bacteriuria, and the criteria used for localizing the site of infection. We have performed a study in which we compared the results obtained with clean-voided urine specimens (CVUS) with those obtained with suprapubic aspiration of urine (SPA).[3] To our knowledge this is the only investigation in children in which the CVUS findings were critically evaluated in two patient populations by comparing those patients with true bacteriuria (positive SPA results) with those whose bladder urine was sterile.

Of 477 infants and children studied, 322 had bacteria in the SPA specimen. Numerous bacteria or > 200 leukocytes/mm^3 in the microscopic examination of uncentrifuged CVUSs, or 10^5 colony-forming units (CFU) per milliliter in quantitative bacterial culture, were found in 42%, 59%, and 81% of the patients with symptomatic infection. The diagnostic accuracies of these indexes were 94%, 88%, and 95%, respectively. When the quantitative bacterial culture results for 199 patients with symptoms and positive SPA results were further evaluated, 18 had 10^4 and 20 had 10^3 CFU/ml in the CVUSs, indicating reduced bladder incubation time. Therefore, if "significant bacteriuria" of 10^5 CFU/ml had been the sole criterion of infection, 19% of our patients would have been missed; these results are similar to those obtained in the study of adult women.[2]

To standardize the diagnostic criteria of CVUS and minimize undue delay in starting treatment, we developed a simple diagnostic procedure based on the scoring of the findings of two consecutive CVUSs.[4] The score was based on the number of bacteria and leukocytes in an uncentrifuged CVUS. The scoring allowed immediate start of treatment in 48 of 50 children with symptoms whose diagnosis was later proved by urine culture.

The second important issue is the localization of the site of infection to the kidney or to the lower urinary tract. Although I agree that the indirect methods of localization of the infection are sometimes unreliable, it would be clinically relevant to distinguish pyelonephritis from cystitis because treatment and eventual risk of scarring of the two conditions are different. We have followed 252 infants and children with a first urinary tract infection for 2 and later for 5 years.[5] The level of initial infection was determined with the aid of fever, C-reactive protein, sedimentation rate, and renal concentrating capacity. Renal scars developed in 12 subjects (5%) during the study. Among infants, the frequency of new scars was 10%. No renal injury was detected in those 88 infants and children who had lower urinary tract infection or asymptomatic bacteriuria. These data have been applied in our hospital when treatment, follow-up, and imaging studies are planned.

Olli Koskimies, MD
Children's Hospital, University of Helsinki
00290 Helsinki, Finland
9/35/60448

REFERENCES

1. Hoberman A, Wald ER, Reynolds EA, Penchansky L, Charron M. Pyuria and bacteriuria in urine specimens obtained by catheter from young children with fever. J PEDIATR 1994; 124:513-9.
2. Hellerstein S. Evolving concepts in the evaluation of the child with a urinary tract infection. J PEDIATR 1994;124:589-92.
3. Pylkkänen J, Vilska J, Koskimies O. Diagnostic value of symptoms and clean-voided urine specimen in childhood urinary tract infection Acta Paediatr Scand 1979;68:341-4.
4. Pylkkänen J, Vilska J, Koskimies O. Scoring of urinary findings as an aid in diagnosis for childhood urinary tract infection. Acta Paediatr Scand 1981;70:875-8.
5. Pylkkänen J, Vilska J, Koskimies O. The value of level diagnosis of childhood urinary tract infection in predicting renal injury. Acta Paediatr Scand 1981;70:879-83.

Reply

To the Editor:

We appreciate the comments of Dr. Koskimies, and are aware of the study comparing clean-voided specimens with suprapubic aspirations. Clean-voided specimens, more properly termed "best catch possible" urine,[1] are not obtained from infants and young children who were the subjects of our study. At our institution, suprapubic aspirations are rarely performed and use of catheterized specimens is standard. We reported that microscopic analysis of uncentrifuged urine, in which leukocytes were counted in a hemocytometer and bacteria were visualized on Gram-stained smears (Enhanced Urinalysis), resulted in high sensitivity and positive predictive value for identification of positive culture results.[2] On the basis of data from 2181 urine specimens obtained by catheter from infants and young children with fever, we concluded that urinary tract infection was best defined by both a leukocyte count $\geq 10/mm^3$ and growth of bacteria at a concentration of $\geq 50{,}000$ colony-forming units (CFU) per milliliter.[3] Dr. Koskimies points out that 19% of patients in their study had clean-voided specimens, with growth at a concentration less than 10^5 CFU/ml,[4] and expresses concern that these patients would have been missed if "significant bacteriuria" (10^5 CFU/ml) had been used as the sole criterion for defining infection. We agree, and accordingly defined urinary tract infection as the recovery of bacteria in a density of $\geq 50{,}000$ CFU/ml, rather than 100,000 CFU/ml, and we added the presence of ≥ 10 leukocytes/mm^3 as an indication of local inflammatory response. Although our report included 2181 urine specimens, our experience is currently based on 3257 specimens. Of the reported 110 specimens with growth of single pathogens at a concentration $\geq 10{,}000$ CFU/ml—a minimum standard used to define significant bacteriuria in catheterized specimens—8 (7.2%) had 10,000 to 49,000 CFU/ml and 10 (9%) had 50,000 to 99,000 CFU/ml. Thus our findings are also consistent with previous studies in children and with the study of adult women.[5] Specimens with bacterial counts between 1 and 49,000 CFU/ml were more likely to yield nonpathogens or mixed organisms than to yield single pathogens. Specimens with counts of 50,000 CFU/ml or more were most likely to yield single pathogens. Therefore the criteria that we used almost always discriminated true urinary tract infection from bacteriuria resulting from contamination of the urine specimen or colonization of the urinary tract (asymptomatic bacteriuria). In our report we also acknowledged that counts less than 50,000 CFU/ml are likely to represent contamination in the majority of instances, and that bacterial colony counts may fall below the range that is characteristic of infections when (1) a bacteriostatic agent is present in the urine; (2) there is a rapid rate of urine flow with reduced incubation time; (3) obstruction of the ureter interferes with discharge of bacteria into the bladder; or (4) infection is limited to areas of the kidney not directly accessible to renal tubules. We also recommended that when patients with bacterial colony counts between 10,000 and 49,000 CFU/ml have persistent symptoms, the urine culture should be repeated and management individualized.[3]

With regard to Dr. Koskimies' second concern—localization of the site of infection to the upper or lower urinary tract—our ongoing randomized clinical trial comparing oral and intravenous antimicrobial therapy in febrile children aged 1 to 24 months uses renal scarring as the outcome measure to determine the equivalence of the two treatment modalities. Renal scans are performed with technetium 99m–labeled dimercaptosuccinic acid (DMSA) at study entry and at 6 months. Of the 115 patients enrolled to date, approximately 80% have DMSA scan findings consistent with the presence of acute pyelonephritis at entry, and renal scarring developed in 45% of them 6 months later. Neither patients with febrile cystitis (pyuria, positive urine culture result, and normal initial scan), nor those with asymptomatic bacteriuria (no pyuria, positive urine culture result, and normal initial scan) have had renal scarring 6 months later.[6] Our finding of a significantly higher incidence of renal scarring (overall, 35% vs 5%) than previously reported by Pylkkanen et al.[7] is probably related to our use of more sensitive imaging procedures—DMSA scans—rather than intravenous pyelograms, as was the case in 1974 to 1977, when that study was conducted.

Alejandro Hoberman, MD
Ellen R. Wald, MD
Department of Pediatrics
Children's Hospital
Pittsburgh, PA 15213
9/35/60447

REFERENCES

1. Todd JK. Diagnosis of urinary tract infections. Pediatr Infect Dis J 1982;1:126-31.
2. Hoberman A, Wald ER, Penchansky L, Reynolds EA, Young S. An enhanced urinalysis as a screening test for urinary tract infection. Pediatrics 1993;91:1196-9.

3. Hoberman A, Wald ER, Reynolds EA, Penchansky L, Charron M. Pyuria and bacteriuria in catheterized urine specimens obtained from young children with fever. J PEDIATR 1994; 124:513-9.
4. Pylkkanen J, Vilska J, Koskimies O. Diagnostic value of symptoms and clean-voided urine specimen in childhood urinary tract infection. Acta Paediatr Scand 1979;68:341-4.
5. Kass EH. Asymptomatic infections of the urinary tract. Trans Assoc Am Physicians 1956;69:56-64.
6. Hoberman A, Wald ER, Reynolds EA, Charron M. Oral versus intravenous therapy for acute pyelonephritis in children 1-24 months [Abstract]. Pediatr Res 1994;35:143A.
7. Pylkkanen J, Vilska J, Koskimies O. The value of level diagnosis of childhood urinary tract infection in predicting renal injury. Acta Paediatr Scand 1981;70:879-83.

Local reactions to luteinizing hormone releasing hormone analog therapy

To the Editor:

Neely et al.[1] and Manasco et al.[2] observed repeated local reactions to depot leuprolide therapy, causing the failure of hormone suppression in one case.[1] We have treated 20 patients with precocious puberty, using two long-acting analogs of luteinizing hormone releasing hormone (LHRH), and observed local reactions in two of them.

A 9-year-old boy received triptorelin, a D-Trp-6-LHRH analog available in Europe, 3.75 mg (0.08 mg/kg body weight) every 4 weeks, and had local induration resembling a foreign body reaction (he could, however, continue the treatment effectively). A 10-year-old girl with nesidioblastosis and precocious puberty received leuprolide, 3.75 mg every 4 weeks (0.09 mg/kg body weight); in this patient we observed three local reactions. The first lesion (third injection) was local induration with a large area of erythema; the third and sixth administrations were followed by sterile abscesses in two different sites. The first abscess contained a dense serous liquid, similar to that injected. Although suppression had initially been complete, after the start of local reactions the pubertal development recommenced, thereby suggesting failure of the therapy. In the ninth month the patient, despite therapy, had pubertal progression from Tanner stage PH2 B2 to stage PH4 B4, significant sonographic increase in the ovarian volume, and vaginal blood spotting. The therapy was discontinued.

The prevalence of induration and abscess in our cases is, respectively, 10% and 5%, similar to the estimates of Manasco et al.[2] and Neely et al.,[1] who used leuprolide alone, in both long-acting and daily preparations. In our experience the reactions followed the administration of two different analogs, each in a long-acting preparation containing copolymer of lactic and glycolic acids. This observation supports the hypothesis that the vehicle, rather than the peptide, is responsible for local reactions, at least in some cases.

We consider our experience useful because it confirms that local reactions, like those reported by Neely and by Manasco, especially when recurring, can hinder the effect of the drug. If this is important in the treatment of precocious puberty, how much more so is it when the disease is a prostatic or a breast cancer?

Giorgio Tonini, MD
Stefano Marinoni, MD,
Vincenzo Forleo, MD,
Department of Paediatrics
Mariangela Rustico, MD
Department of Obstetrics and Gynecology
Childhood Institute "Burlo Garofolo"
Istituto di Ricovero e Cura a Carattere Scientifico
Trieste, Italy
9/35/60558

REFERENCES

1. Neely EK, Hintz RL, Parker B, et al. Two-year results of treatment with depot leuprolide acetate for central precocious puberty. J PEDIATR 1992;121:634-40.
2. Manasco PK, Pescovitz OH, Blizzard RM. Local reactions to depot leuprolide therapy for central precocious puberty [Letter]. J PEDIATR 1993;123:334-5.

Reply

To the Editor:

Our earlier publication[1] described a girl with central precocious puberty (CPP) in whom a sterile abscess developed at the site of depot gonadotropin releasing hormone (GnRH) analog injection, followed by obvious escape from the intended gonadotropin suppression. Many pediatric endocrinologists by now have encountered this complication of depot injection, and our earlier calculation of the incidence of local reactions (including erythema, induration, and sterile abscess) in 5% of patients still seems a reasonable estimate.[2] Reactions are seemingly idiosyncratic; they have occurred at any time during the first year of therapy, may be intermittent, or may never recur. Although it is crucial that the depot microcapsules be mixed with the appropriate diluent vehicle and be administered intramuscularly, there is usually no mechanical explanation for the local reaction. Fortunately, there have been no reports of systemic responses. Inexplicably, reactions appear to be more prevalent in children than in adults. It is not surprising that the depot formulation of triptorelin, available only in Europe (as Decapeptyl Depot) and also using a lactic/glycolic acid copolymer, results in similar local inflammatory responses when used for CPP. However, it is odd that other reports have not already reached the literature; it may be that the frequency of reactions to triptorelin is either lower or simply underreported.

As experience with depot leuprolide increases, injection reactions without obvious therapeutic failure have become more troublesome. These reactions can result in follow-up gonadotropin levels that are neither clearly suppressed nor elevated into the pubertal range. GnRH-stimulated luteinizing hormnore (LH) levels are usually suppressed during therapy to ≤ 1 IU/L (measured by the new double monoclonal assays). It is perplexing to interpret treatment LH levels in the range of 2 to 4 IU/L, which are normal prepubertal values and well below pretreatment levels. Is this degree of suppression sufficient? In these situations, investigators have increased the dosage in the hope that more drug will be absorbed, or have altered dose frequency to every 3 weeks, although there are no data to substantiate the efficacy of either strategy.

Despite the occasional injection reactions, the convenience and excellent clinical and biochemical suppression promptly attained in 95% of cases make this the drug of choice for CPP. Depot leuprolide, for whatever mix of medical and marketing reasons, has now captured virtually all of the U.S. market for treatment of CPP (a small market in comparison with that for prostate cancer). Leuprolide is the only GnRH analog in depot and daily forms in the United States, whereas other analogs are available only as daily injections (histrelin, deslorelin) or nasal spray (nafarelin). These are excellent alternatives when local reactions are persistent and efficacy is diminished.

The approach to managing CPP with depot leuprolide described by Tonini and colleagues, and seemingly prevalent in Europe, diverges in potentially problematic ways from that in the United States. Standard practice here is to use at least 7.5 mg at the start of therapy, but at least some European and Japanese practitioners are using the lower dose of 3.75 mg. Although there is evidence that doses less than 7.5 mg can be effective after therapy is initiated,[3] such a reduced dose certainly mandates scrupulous monitoring of hormone levels. Because depot GnRH analog therapy is not completely suppressive in 100% of cases, we hope that clinicians in both the United States and Europe will continue to survey gonadotropin levels during therapy, particularly in patients with a history of injection reactions.

E. Kirk Neely, MD
Darrell M. Wilson, MD
Department of Pediatrics
Stanford University
Stanford CA 94305
9/35/60557

REFERENCES

1. Neely EK, Hintz RL, Parker B, et al. Two-year results of treatment with depot leuprolide acetate for central precocious puberty. J PEDIATR 1992;121:634-40.
2. Neely EK, Wilson DM, Hintz RL. Local reactions to depot leuprolide acetate for central precocious puberty [Letter reply]. J PEDIATR 1993;123:335.
3. Parker KL, Baens-Bailon RG, Lee PA. Depot leuprolide acetate dosage for sexual precocity. J Clin Endocrinol Metab 1991;73:50-2.

Hypotension in preterm infants

To the Editor:

The article by Klarr et al.[1] on the use of dopamine versus dobutamine for treatment of hypotension in preterm infants with respiratory distress syndrome during the first 24 hours of life raised several questions. First, what was the incidence of the patent ductus arteriosus (PDA) in the two treatment groups? These data were not reported, but a PDA influences both the mean arterial blood pressure and the pulse pressure.[2] In addition, it may affect the responses to the two agents if there are relatively different effects on the systemic and pulmonary vascular resistances, as noted in the discussion. Second, was there prenatal and/or postnatal exposure to prostaglandin synthase inhibition? Finally, was there prenatal and/or postnatal exposure to corticosteroids, which are known to enhance vascular responses to noradrenaline?[3] This may be particularly important at higher doses of dopamine.

I have a pet peeve about solely reporting the blood pressure in terms of mean arterial blood pressure. Multiple different pulsatile pressure waveforms can yield the same mean arterial blood pressure. The analog signal of the blood pressure has tremendous information content. For example, the area under the systolic portion of the analog signal is proportional to the stroke volume.[4] In addition, the rate of diastolic pressure decay is a function of both vascular resistance and compliance, but for most vascular beds, resistance is the major determinant.[5] Such information may provide some insight regarding the derangements responsible for the hypotension, which, in turn, may be predictive of the responses to inotropic and vasoactive agents or to volume expansion. Therefore I encourage inspection of the analog signal as opposed to the mean arterial blood pressure alone, because of the information content.

Jay M. Milstein, MD
Division of Neonatology
Research Laboratory-TB 193
University of California
Davis, CA 95616-8646
9/35/60560

REFERENCES

1. Klarr JM, Faix RG, Pryce CJE, Bhatt-Mehta V. Randomized, blind trial of dopamine versus dobutamine for treatment of hypotension in preterm infants with respiratory distress syndrome. J PEDIATR 1994;125:117-22.
2. Milstein JM, Riemenschneider TA, Goetzman BW, George L, Wennberg RP. Assessment of patent ductus arteriosus shunting using diastolic pressure analysis. J PEDIATR 1979;94:122-6.
3. Walker BR, Connacher AA, Webb DJ, Edwards RW. Glucocorticoids and blood pressure: a role for the cortisol/cortisone shuttle in the control of vascular tone in man. Clin Sci 1992;83:171-8.
4. Bourgeois MF, Gilbert BK, Bernuth GV, Wood EH. Continuous determination of beat-to-beat stroke volume from aortic pressure pulses in the dog. Circulation Res 1976;39:15-24.
5. Milstein JM, Juris AL. Aortic diastolic pressure decay in congenital arteriovenous malformations. Pediatr Cardiol 1993; 14:204-7.

Reply

To the Editor:

No hemodynamically significant patent ductus arteriosus was detected by clinical examination (including pulse pressure determination), chest radiography, or echocardiography in either group during the relatively brief duration of the study protocol, although echocardiography was not performed in all patients. After completion of the study protocol, 6 of 31 dopamine and 10 of 32 dobutamine recipients ($p = 0.39$) eventually had a significant patent ductus arteriosus that required indomethacin therapy or surgical ligation before hospital discharge. This information was contained in the original manuscript but was deleted from the revision. No infant in either group was exposed to indomethacin tocolysis or received that drug postnatally before or during the study drug protocol. We have no information about maternal consumption of over-the-counter prostaglandin synthase inhibitors (e.g., aspirin, ibuprofen) before admission to the labor and delivery suite. Antenatal corticosteroid therapy was received by four dopamine and two dobutamine recipients ($p = 0.32$). As indicated in the Results section of the published article, no infant in either group received postnatal dexamethasone (or other glucocorticoid) before or during the study drug infusions.

We agree that mean arterial blood pressure is only one indicator of hemodynamic performance and that clinically important supplemental information can be derived from many other sources, including (but not limited to) arterial pressure waveform. Such additional information may be useful for therapeutic decisions. We selected mean arterial blood pressure as the primary end point for our trial because (1) it is an index that can be measured easily and reproducibly in most neonatal intensive care units, (2) it has been used in many other reports addressing the treatment of hypotension in preterm infants (references 1 and 2, for example), and (3) other authors have noted the significant association of low mean arterial blood pressure with adverse neurologic outcomes in preterm infants.[3]

Roger G. Faix, MD
Associate Professor of Pediatrics
Director of Newborn Services and
Neonatal-Perinatal Fellowship Program
Division of Neonatology
Mott Children's Hospital
Ann Arbor, MI 48109-0254
9/35/60559

REFERENCES

1. Roze JC, Tohier C, Maingueneau C, Lefevre M, Mouzard A. Response to dobutamine and dopamine in the hypotensive very preterm infant. Arch Dis Child 1993;69:59-63.
2. Miall-Allen VM, Whitelaw AG. Response to dopamine and dobutamine in the preterm infant of less than 30 weeks' gestation. Crit Care Med 1989;17:1166-9.
3. Miall-Allen VM, de Vries L, Whitelaw AG. Mean arterial pressure and neonatal cerebral lesions. Arch Dis Child 1987;62:1068-9.

Terbutaline powder for acute asthma

To the Editor:

We read with interest the article by Laberge et al.,[1] who pointed out the necessity of testing the efficacy of a dry powder inhaler in children with acute moderate asthma. We have compared the efficacy of 0.5 mg of terbutaline inhaled either with a Turbuhaler (Astro Draco AB, Sweden) or with a metered-dose inhaler attached to a spacer (Nebuhaler, Astra Draco AB) in 30 5- to 14-year old children with acute wheezing. These children with asthma were included in an open, randomized parallel group study (15 children in each group). Administration of the drug was similar to that in the study by Laberge et al. We measured the following parameters before and 15 and 30 minutes after inhalation: specific airway resistance (in centimeters of water displaced per liter per second; body plethysmograph mode I 2800, Physiosystem, Noisy Le Grand, France), forced expiratory volume in 1 second in milliliters; Pulmonet III, Gould Medical, Runois, France), and peak expiratory flow rate (in liters per minute; mini Wright).

Table. Bronchodilator response to terbutaline: Percentage of improvement from baseline (mean ± SD)

	Dry powder inhaler	Metered-dose inhaler with spacer
At 15 min		
Specific airway resistance (cm H_2O/L/sec)	−51.1 ± 12.9	−47.7 ± 10.9
Forced expiratory volume in 1 second (ml)	+16.4 ± 14.2	+23.2 ± 19.1
Peak expiratory flow rate (L/min)	+26.6 ± 20.7	+16.0 ± 10.8
At 30 min		
Specific airway resistance (cm H_2O/L/sec)	−52.9 ± 14.3	−54.2 ± 7.8
Forced expiratory volume in 1 second (ml)	+19.8 ± 13.6	+27.0 ± 13.4
Peak expiratory flow rate (L/min)	+30.4 ± 24.2	+26.7 ± 24.5

Basal obstruction was similar in both groups (dry powder inhaler, 14.2 ± 3.7 cm H_2O/L per second; metered-dose inhaler with a spacer, 14.0 ± 3.3 cm H_2O/L per second). The Table shows that both inhalational techniques improved lung functions compared with baseline ($p < 0.01$). There was no difference between treatments at any time (Mann-Whitney U test). Clinical efficacy and tolerance were excellent. These results[2] confirm our preliminary study[3] and demonstrate the efficacy of terbutaline powder in children older than 5 years of age who have acute moderate asthma.

P. Rufin, MD
M. R. Benoist, MD
J. de Blic, MD
P. Scheinmann, MD
Departments of Pneumonology and Pediatric Allergy
Hôpital des Enfants Malades
Paris, France
9/35/60736

REFERENCES

1. Laberge S, Spier S, Drblik SP, Turgeon JP. Comparison of inhaled terbutaline administered by either the Turbuhaler dry

powder inhaler or a metered-dose inhaler with spacer in preschool children with asthma. J PEDIATR 1994;124:815-7.
2. Rufin P, Benoist MR, Panqueva P, Brouard JJ, de Blic J, Scheinmann P. Efficacité d'un inhalateur de poudre (Turbuhaler) dans la crise d'asthme modérée de l'enfant. Rev Mal Respir 1993;10:545-50.
3. Rufin P, Benoist MR, de Blic J, Braunstein G, Scheinmann P. Terbutaline powder in asthma exacerbations [Letter]. Arch Dis Child 1991;66:1465-6.

Familial Guillain-Barré syndrome subsequent to *Campylobacter jejuni* enteritis

To the Editor:

Guillain-Barré (GB) syndrome is characterized by the acute onset of symmetric limb weakness and absence of tendon reflexes. There are few reports of familial GB syndrome. Saunders and Rake[1] reported a brother and sister in whom muscle weakness developed 4 years apart. MacGregor[2] reported a father with GB syndrome and a daughter with an acute febrile illness with painful sensory neuropathy. The brother reported by Saunders and Rake[1] and the daughter reported by MacGregor[2] would not have fulfilled the diagnostic criteria of the National Institute of Neurodegenerative Diseases and Stroke for GB syndrome. Ropper et al.[3] described two patients who had had first-order relatives (a father and a sister, respectively) with GB syndrome many years previously. Davidson et al.[4] described a father and son in whom GB syndrome developed 9 years apart. *Campylobacter jejuni*, a gram-negative bacterium that frequently causes acute enteritis, is one of the most common infections preceding GB syndrome. We recently described two children who had Fisher syndrome (a variant of GB syndrome) after *C. jejuni* infection.[5] We here describe two siblings who had GB syndrome after *C. jejuni* enteritis.

Patient 1. A 19-month-old girl had diarrhea that resolved during a period of 8 days. On the next day (day 1), she was unable to stand up or sit down by herself. On day 2, muscle weakness developed in the upper limbs and she was admitted to Ohtemae Hospital. Neurologic examination showed flaccid tetraplegia and areflexia with no sensory signs or symptoms. The cerebrospinal fluid protein concentration was 70 mg/dl on day 4, and 112 mg/dl on day 12, with normal cellularity on both days. Her stool cultures grew *C. jejuni* on days 2 and 3, but there was no growth on day 11. The bacterial serotype belonged to PEN 19: LIO 7. On day 5, esotropia and dysphagia developed and on day 6 dysarthria and nuchal weakness. On day 7, she could neither swallow nor move her neck. Both eyeballs became completely fixed. On day 8, she was not fully conscious and could not talk. Ocular and nuchal movements began to improve on days 13 and 17, respectively. On day 23, she was able to talk. On day 35, limb weakness gradually began to abate. On day 117, she could walk without support.

Patient 2. A $3\frac{10}{12}$-year old girl, the older sister of patient 1, had diarrhea 10 days after the onset in patient 1, and cough the next day. One week later (day 1), she could not stand up or walk. The next day she was admitted to the hospital because of dysarthria and flaccid tetraplegia associated with areflexia; sensory function was intact. The cerebrospinal fluid protein concentration was 106 mg/dl on day 8 with normal cellularity. *C. jejuni* grew from stool cultures taken on days 2 and 6. On day 3, cyanosis developed and the patient required a respirator. She became drowsy, and corneal reflexes were absent; on day 7 she was comatose. On day 16, voluntary respiration reappeared. On day 22, she regained consciousness. Marked blepharoptosis and external ophthalmoplegia were present. She could open her eyes on day 31, and her mouth on day 41. Limb weakness abated gradually from day 41. On day 46, endotracheal intubation was discontinued. On day 92, dysphagia disappeared. On day 166, she could walk without support.

Both patients met the clinical criteria for GB syndrome. We believe that this is the first report of the occurrence of GB syndrome in family members at the same time and after infection by *C. jejuni*.

Nobuhiro Yuki, MD, PhD
Department of Biochemistry
Faculty of Medicine
Tokyo Medical and Dental University
Bunkyo-ku, Tokyo, Japan

Yoshihiro Tsujino, MD
Department of Pediatrics
Ohtemae Hospital
Chuo-ku, Osaka, Japan
9/35/60556

We thank Drs. Kahiko Saito and Masaki Takahashi (Department of Microbiology, Tokyo Metropolitan Research Laboratory of Public Health) for the *C. jejuni* serotyping. This research was supported in part by grants-in-aid from the Uehara Memorial Foundation and the Ichiro Kanehara Foundation.

REFERENCES

1. Saunders M, Rake M. Familial Guillain-Barré syndrome. Lancet 1965;2:1106-7.
2. MacGregor GA. Familiar Guillain-Barré syndrome [Letter]. Lancet 1965;2:1296.
3. Ropper AH, Wijdicks EFM, Trumax BT. Guillain-Barré syndrome. Philadelphia: FA Davis, 1991:30.
4. Davidson DLW, O'Sullivan AF, Morley KD. HLA antigens in familial Guillain-Barré syndrome [Letter]. J Neurol Neurosurg Psychiatry 1992;55:508-9.
5. Yuki N, Ichikawa H, Doi A. Fisher syndrome after *Campylobacter jejuni* enteritis: human leukocyte antigen and the bacterial serotype. J PEDIATR (in press).

THE JOURNAL OF PEDIATRICS

FEBRUARY 1995 *Volume 126* *Number 2*

MEDICAL PROGRESS

Allergic colitis in infants

Robert D. Odze, MD, FRCP(C), Barry K. Wershil, MD, Alan M. Leichtner, MD, and Donald A. Antonioli, MD

From the Departments of Pathology, Brigham and Women's Hospital, Children's Hospital, and Beth Israel Hospital; the Department of Medicine, Children's Hospital; and Harvard Medical School, Boston, Massachusetts

BACKGROUND INFORMATION AND PREVALENCE

Allergic colitis is a condition characterized by inflammatory changes in the rectum and colon as a result of immune-mediated reactions to ingested foreign proteins.[1, 2] The condition predominantly affects infants in the first months of life, who have rectal bleeding (with or without diarrhea) and who generally recover promptly after elimination of the allergen from their diet.[3-5] The antigens are usually derived from proprietary formulas or may be found in human milk as a result of the maternal diet.[6]

Chong et al.[7] suggested that only a small percentage of children (20%) with colitis in this age group have AC; they emphasize that colitis in infants is a heterogeneous group of disorders, including infections, enterocolitis complicating Hirschsprung disease, inflammatory bowel disease, and Behçet syndrome.[7] Although cow milk–induced allergy is relatively common, with a prevalence estimated at between 2.0% and 7.5% in otherwise normal infants, the exact prevalence of AC is not known.[8-11] Jenkins et al.[12] suggested that AC accounts for most, if not all, cases of colitis in the first year of life.

Reprint requests: Robert Odze, MD, Department of Pathology, Division of Gastrointestinal Pathology, Brigham and Women's Hospital, 75 Francis St., Boston, MA 02115.

THE JOURNAL OF PEDIATRICS 1995;126:163-70

0022-3476/95/$3.00 + 0 **9/18/61123**

ETIOLOGY

Many foods have been associated with the development of AC, including wheat, eggs, corn, fish, seafood, and nuts.[13] However, by far the most common antigens implicated in AC are present in cow milk and soy formulas. Food antigens, regardless of their source, usually are small proteins with a molecular weight of 10,000 to 40,000 daltons, although antigens as large as 78,000 daltons have been reported.[14, 15] These antigens tend to be glycoproteins or acid proteins resistant to thermal and enzymatic denaturation,[16, 17] and their specific molecular architecture may also confer antigenic stability in vivo.

AC	Allergic colitis
GM-CSF	Granulocyte monocyte–colony-stimulating factor
IL	Interleukin
PAF	Platelet-activating factor

Cow milk contains more than 25 potentially immunogenic proteins, of which whey protein (β-lactoglobulin) is the most common offending antigen and has the greatest potential to induce immune reactions.[10] Soy formulas also possess strong antigenic properties both in vitro and in vivo[5, 9, 18-20]; some studies suggest that soy is even more allergenic than cow milk.[20-22] Furthermore, approximately 10% to 30% of infants with proven cow-milk sensitivity also have intolerance to soy proteins.[5, 20]

Breast-fed infants are also susceptible to the development of allergic gastrointestinal illnesses. In a prospective study of 20 infants with AC, 45% of cases occurred in exclusively breast-fed infants.[4] Potentially immunogenic proteins in the maternal diet, including cow milk–derived β-lactoglobulin, can be transferred into the milk[23] and may induce AC in nursing infants.[6, 21, 24-27]

CLINICAL FEATURES

Patient population. Most patients with AC have the onset of disease within the first few months of life.[3-5] The prevalence decreases with advancing age, so that by age 1 to 2 years most affected infants have become tolerant of the inciting milk-protein allergen.[9, 28] In a prospective study, we found that the mean age of symptom onset was 66 days, and none of the infants was more than 10 months of age at the time symptoms began.[4] Rarely, preterm babies, neonates less than 1 week of age, and even older children and adults may be affected. The onset of AC in infants less than 1 week of age may be the result of transplacental sensitization of the fetus by exposure to bovine milk antigens in utero.[29]

Symptoms and signs. Rectal bleeding is the most common sign of AC.[3, 4, 30] However, the gradual or sudden onset of loose mucus-containing stools, or even overt diarrhea, may dominate the clinical picture.[3, 30] Most patients do not have major constitutional or extraintestinal symptoms or signs, such as fever, weight loss, or anemia.

The onset of AC may be acute (<6 to 12 hours after the first feeding of the offending substance) but is more often insidious, showing a prolonged latent interval between the introduction of cow milk and the onset of symptoms.[3] In our prospective study, most mothers reported that the symptoms began soon after the introduction of milk or soy formula.[4] However, the mean duration from the development of symptoms to the time of diagnosis was approximately 25 days; in some infants, it was up to 6 months.

It has been suggested that the early exposure to cow milk proteins may cause a more acute or fulminant illness.[9] However, we found no relation between the intensity of symptoms or severity of tissue reaction and any of the clinical or demographic data. We did find that breast-fed infants tended to be older at diagnosis, have a longer time between symptom onset and clinical diagnosis, and have less severe histologic findings.[4] Cow milk protein in the mother's diet that is transferred into her milk may be altered both qualitatively and quantitatively; this may explain, at least in part, the milder symptoms in breast-fed infants.[6, 25, 26] However, other studies have not substantiated this finding.[12]

Diagnosis. The clinical diagnosis of AC can be difficult. Although a careful history detailing the relation of symptom onset to feeding (as well as a personal or family history of allergies) may be helpful, the presence or absence of these features has not been proved to have any predictive value in identifying infants with AC.[31] No single laboratory or biochemical test is either sensitive enough or specific enough to be diagnostic of AC.[1, 3, 32-34] However, the finding of either peripheral eosinophilia or eosinophils in stool samples stained with Wright stain is suggestive of AC.

Other diagnostic considerations include infections, enterocolitis complicating Hirschsprung disease, and inflammatory bowel disease. Both a stool culture and an examination of the stool for ova and parasites are essential because a variety of bacterial and parasitic infections can cause similar signs and symptoms. Enterocolitis complicating Hirschsprung disease or inflammatory bowel disease can be manifested as colitis in infants. However, the characteristic clinical, radiographic, endoscopic, and pathologic features of these conditions will usually differentiate them from AC.

Because the use of indirect tests for AC creates problems, the most definitive clinical approach to establish a diagnosis of food-induced hypersensitivity is the response to specific food elimination and rechallenge, as defined by Goldman et al.[35] This approach relies on the demonstration of a reproducible clinical response to oral challenges with milk allergens under controlled clinical conditions. However, the use of repeated oral challenges for diagnosis has not met with widespread clinical acceptance because the procedure is expensive and time-consuming and may elicit severe, life-threatening reactions in some infants.[5, 22, 25, 27]

Because of the difficulties associated with the Goldman diagnostic method, Powell[5] suggested confirming the clinical diagnosis of food allergy by a positive response to a trial of antigen withdrawal, followed by a single rechallenge under standardized conditions. However, the most practical approach is a positive response to an elimination diet alone. Sigmoidoscopy in conjunction with the evaluation of multiple mucosal biopsy specimens may be helpful in confirming the diagnosis, particularly in patients with a severe case and in patients whose condition does not improve after the start of an elimination diet.

PATHOLOGIC FEATURES

Knowledge of the pathologic features of AC is based primarily on information gained by endoscopy and the evaluation of mucosal biopsy specimens. Sigmoidoscopy, with a small-caliber, flexible endoscope, is the best method of assessing the extent and severity of AC, and is safe and well tolerated.[3, 4]

Lesions in AC may involve any segment of the colon.[3, 6, 9] However, the rectosigmoid segment is the most commonly involved area, and the changes are usually most severe in this region.[3, 4, 9] Endoscopic features most often identified

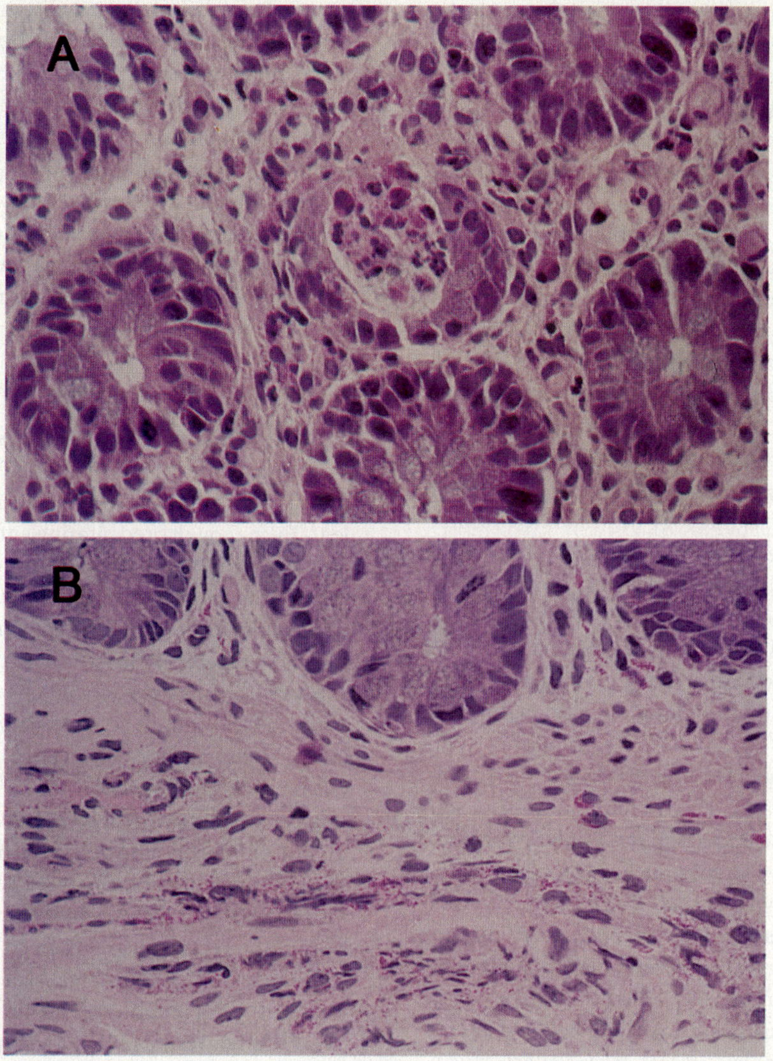

Fig. 1. Histologic features of AC. Eosinophils typically infiltrate the surface epithelium, mix with neutrophils to form crypt abscesses (**A**), aggregate at the periphery of mucosal lymphoid follicles, and infiltrate and degranulate within the muscularis mucosae (**B**). In the absence of other histologic abnormalities and in the appropriate clinical setting, this constellation of findings is essentially diagnostic of AC. (Hematoxylin-eosin stain; original magnification, ×400.)

are focal erythema, a friable-appearing mucosa, and an increased nodularity suggestive of lymphoid hyperplasia. Abnormal areas are typically separated by intervening zones of entirely normal-appearing mucosa. In addition, more severe cases may show decreased mucosal vascularity, multiple superficial erosions (aphthous type with erythematous margins), or, rarely, frank ulcerations with surface exudate mimicking the endoscopic features of infectious colitis.[12, 22, 24, 25] Neither the diffusely hemorrhagic, friable, and ulcerated mucosa seen in ulcerative colitis nor the cobblestone, linear, and serpiginous ulcerations characteristic of Crohn disease have ever been described in AC.[22] Enterocolitis complicating Hirschsprung disease may show mild, nonspecific or subtle endoscopic features similar to those of AC.[29] However, the absence of histologically identifiable ganglion cells in suction biopsy specimens is pathognomonic of this disorder.

Microscopically, the overall architecture of the mucosa in AC is well maintained,[3, 4, 30] without features of chronicity typical of inflammatory bowel disease, such as distorted, branched, or atrophic crypts, Paneth cell metaplasia, basally located lymphoid aggregates, or diffuse plasmacytosis.

The most striking and characteristic histologic feature is the presence of focal infiltrates of eosinophils in all mucosal compartments, but particularly in the lamina propria.[4] In our analysis of 60 biopsy specimens taken at 4, 8, and 12 cm from the anal verge, eosinophil accumulation varied not only among the three biopsy specimens but within individual biopsy samples. Only 60% of patients had abnormalities at all three biopsy sites; the others had one or two of the three specimens categorized as entirely normal.[4]

Although a prospective, controlled study comparing the histologic features of AC with other causes of colitis has not been performed, a retrospective study by Winter et al.[30] showed that AC can be distinguished from infectious colitis by histologic analysis. A particularly characteristic feature of AC is the presence of a large number of eosinophils in the lamina propria (≥60 eosinophils per 10 high-power fields), as well as numerous intact or degranulated eosinophils located at the base of the mucosa and interspersed among muscle fibers of the muscularis mucosae.[3, 4] This finding, which was not seen in the cases of infectious colitis reported by Winter et al.,[30] helps to distinguish AC from infectious colitis.[4, 36] Furthermore, crypt abscesses, when present in AC, are typically composed of both neutrophils and eosinophils[4, 30] (Fig. 1).

When all the histologic features described above are present, it is relatively easy to confirm the clinical suspicion of AC. On the basis of the findings in the Winter retrospective and in our prospective studies, we have proposed histologic criteria that strongly support the diagnosis of AC when the condition is encountered in the appropriate clinical setting.[4] These criteria are (1) an increase in the number of eosinophils in the lamina propria (≥60 per 10 high-power fields), often seen in close association with lymphoid aggregates; (2) epithelial (crypt or surface) or muscularis mucosae eosinophil infiltration (≥1 eosinophil per high-power field); (3) a mixture of eosinophils and neutrophils in crypt abscesses; and (4) the absence of other specific histologic features (parasites, ova, crypt architectural abnormalities) that suggest an alternative diagnosis. Because the histologic findings are focal, multiple mucosal biopsy specimens should be obtained and several levels of each specimen should be examined to obtain the maximal diagnostic yield. The use of these guidelines should offer a rapid confirmation of the clinical diagnosis of AC.

TREATMENT

The mainstay treatment of AC is elimination of the offending antigen from the diet. This approach usually requires changing the diet from milk or a proprietary formula to a more "hypoallergenic" formula. Current recommendations include hydrolyzed casein or whey formulas. In some infants, an elemental diet, consisting of free amino acids as the protein source, may be necessary.[25, 37] Soy formulas must be used with caution because up to 30% of infants who are sensitive to cow milk protein will also be sensitive to soy proteins.[5, 20] For infants who are breast-fed, maternal food elimination, starting with cow milk, is usually effective.[24] However, some studies have shown a highly variable response to maternal protein restriction.[6] The role of pharmacotherapy in the treatment of AC not responsive to changes in diet, with agents such as corticosteroids, has not been studied.

NATURAL HISTORY

Allergic colitis is a transient disorder; most affected infants can tolerate milk by 1½ to 2 years of age.[8, 25] In infants sensitive to cow milk protein, the prognosis is excellent. Even though precipitating antibodies to milk allergens may persist in more than 30% of patients, they do not correlate with ongoing gastrointestinal complaints.[38] Cautious reintroduction of milk in small amounts and at regular intervals is recommended at approximately 1 year of age.[7]

Several epidemiologic studies have suggested a relation between cow milk hypersensitivity at an early age and the later development of ulcerative colitis or proctitis.[39, 40] Glassman et al.[39] reported that a significantly higher percentage of adult patients with ulcerative colitis had a history of childhood cow milk sensitivity in comparison with those without inflammatory bowel disease. Patients with ulcerative proctitis have a higher fraction of IgE-containing cells in the rectal mucosa than do normal control subjects, and some of these patients benefit from topical or oral treatment with antiallergic medications, such as cromoglycate.[41, 42] However, Hill et al.[9] reported that of 13 infants with eosinophilic (presumably allergic) colitis, none acquired symptoms of inflammatory bowel disease in a 5- to 10-year follow-up. Therefore the knowledge concerning possible long-term clinical and pathologic consequences in infants with AC is limited and must await the results of further prospective studies.

NEW MECHANISMS OF PATHOGENESIS

The gastrointestinal tract is uniquely adapted to prevent luminal antigens from crossing the epithelium ("mucosal barrier" function) and to control the systemic immune response to foreign proteins (oral tolerance). The fact that food hypersensitivity reactions are more common in the pediatric population, and tend to decrease in incidence with increasing age, suggests that immaturity of the intestinal barrier function, immaturity of the mucosal immune system, or both are important in the pathogenesis of these con-

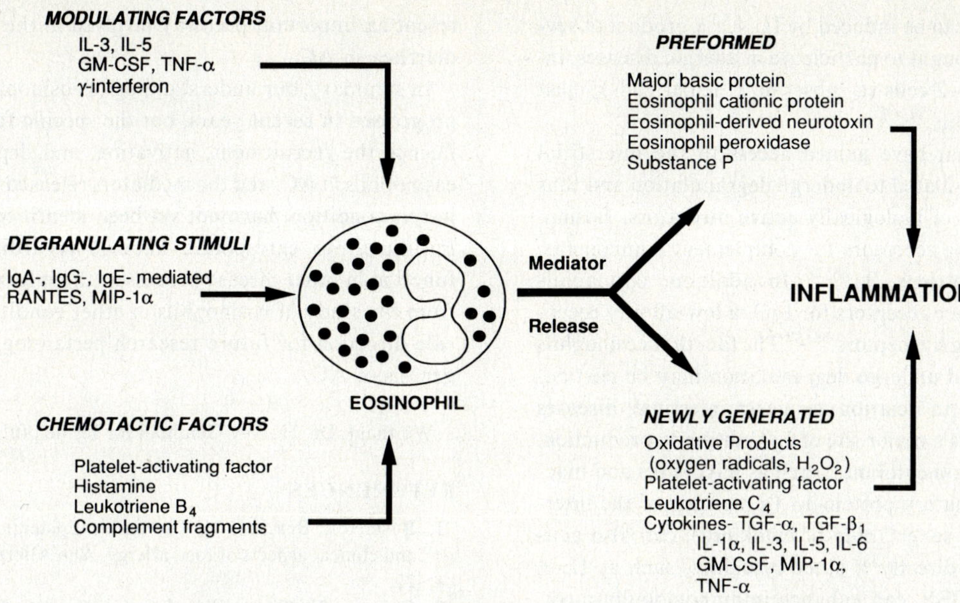

Fig. 2. Potential mechanisms involved in the pathogenesis of AC. Many factors have chemotactic properties for eosinophils and may be important for the recruitment of eosinophils into the colon during the development and evolution of AC. In addition, specific ingested antigens may elicit eosinophil degranulation and mediator release by specific immunoglobulin-mediated mechanisms, or by the generation of cytokines such as RANTES or macrophage inflammatory protein-1α *(MIP-1α)*, which can activate eosinophils. Preformed and newly synthesized mediators released by eosinophils may then promote the colonic inflammation typical of AC. *TNF-α*, Tumor necrosis factor-α; *TGF*, transforming growth factor (α and β_1).

ditions.[43, 44] However, the precise mechanisms that result in AC are not known.

The consequence of exposure to milk antigens in a sensitized infant is a complex reaction that may involve a combination of types I, III, and IV hypersensitivity responses.[44] However, it is difficult to determine to what degree each of these specific mechanisms may contribute to tissue injury, because very few studies have examined a carefully defined patient population. Nevertheless, the immune response leads to the infiltration of inflammatory cells, particularly eosinophils, and the destruction of epithelial cells, which may cause diarrhea and rectal bleeding. At the present time, it is believed that eosinophils, the histologic hallmark of AC, may be directly responsible for much of the tissue injury in this disease.[44] Thus a consideration of the rapidly expanding field of eosinophil biology may shed some light on the pathogenesis of AC.

Eosinophils develop and differentiate in the bone marrow under the influence of at least three cytokines: granulocyte-monocyte colony-stimulating factor, interleukin-3, and interleukin-5.[45, 46] Although GM-CSF and IL-3 can influence the development of multiple hematopoietic cell lineages, IL-5 appears to be more specific for eosinophils.[47] In addition to producing eosinophilia, GM-CSF, IL-3, and IL-5 act to change the morphologic, biochemical, and functional characteristics of eosinophils by inducing cellular activation.[45, 46] Other mediators, such as platelet-activating factor, can also "activate" eosinophils.[48, 49] "Activated" eosinophils typically have a lower density than "resting" eosinophils (so-called light-density, or hypodense, eosinophils) and are more metabolically active.[45, 46]

Eosinophils released from the bone marrow must then circulate and emigrate into relevant tissue sites. A fundamental process involved in the infiltration of eosinophils into tissues is their interaction with vascular endothelium. This interaction promotes the adhesion and subsequent migration of the eosinophil into the interstitial space. To accomplish this process, eosinophils express a variety of adhesion molecules on their cell surface that recognize counterligands expressed on the endothelial cell (reviewed in references 45 and 46). Cell surface molecules such as CD11/CD18 have been shown to participate in eosinophil adhesion, but this mechanism is not unique for eosinophils[50] and more recent evidence suggests that other adhesion molecules may also be involved. For example, eosinophils, but not neutrophils, express the β_1-integrin, termed very late antigen 4,[51] which recognizes vascular cell adhesion molecule-1 on the surface of endothelial cells.[52] The expression of this molecule can be induced by IL-4,[53] a product of several cell types thought to participate in allergic diseases, including T-helper–2 cells (a subset of T helper cells), mast cells, and basophils.[54, 55]

Eosinophils that have gained access to the interstitial space can be stimulated to undergo degranulation and thus release a variety of biologically active mediators. Eosinophils have surface receptors for complement components, PAF, and leukotriene B_4.[45, 46] In addition, eosinophils express cell surface receptors for IgG, a low-affinity receptor for IgE, and IgA receptors.[56, 57] The fact that eosinophils can bind IgA and undergo degranulation may be particularly important in relation to gastrointestinal diseases because the gut is a major site of IgA antibody production. In addition, certain cytokines, such as RANTES and macrophage inflammatory protein-1α (a member of the intercrine-chemokine superfamily of cytokines), can also activate eosinophils directly[58]; other cytokines, such as IL-3, IL-5, and GM-CSF, can enhance immunoglobulin-mediated degranulation.[59]

The degranulation of eosinophils results in the release of granule-associated mediators and the generation of newly synthesized mediators (Fig. 2). The major granule constituents of eosinophils are major basic protein, eosinophil-derived neurotoxin, eosinophilic cationic protein, and eosinophilic peroxidase.[45, 46] Although all the functions of these proteins are not known, the release of these granule-associated proteins is probably important in parasite killing and may be cytotoxic to a variety of normal mammalian cells, including the epithelium. In addition, eosinophils can also produce other mediators, such as PAF, leukotriene C_4, and the neuropeptide substance P (reviewed in references 45 and 46). The production of PAF by eosinophils may be particularly relevant to AC because PAF has been shown to induce bowel injury in experimental animals.[60]

In addition to the generation of lipid mediators, eosinophils produce a variety of multifunctional cytokines. Human eosinophils have been shown to produce messenger ribonucleic acid and/or protein for IL-1, IL-3, IL-5, IL-6, GM-CSF, tumor necrosis factor alpha, macrophage inflammatory protein-1α, transforming growth factor-α, and transforming growth factor-β_1 (reviewed in reference 61). Although little is known about the cytokines produced by eosinophils in AC, cytokines such as tumor necrosis factor-α have been associated with intestinal injury and increased intestinal permeability.[62, 63] At the present time, the role of eosinophil mediator–cytokine production is speculative, but a recent study showed that eosinophil-derived mediators can stimulate a secretory response from epithelial cells in vitro.[64] The precise mediator(s) responsible for this response has not been identified, but these findings may represent an important pathway involved in the production of diarrhea in AC.

In summary, our understanding of eosinophil biology has progressed in recent years, but the specific factors that influence the recruitment, activation, and degranulation of eosinophils in AC, and the mediators released by eosinophils in this condition, have not yet been identified. Although it is difficult to extrapolate findings regarding eosinophil function in other disease processes, the information gained from the study of eosinophils in other conditions may provide direction for future research pertaining to the pathogenesis of AC.

We thank Dr. Harvey Goldman for his helpful suggestions.

REFERENCES

1. Businco L, Benincor N, Cantani A. Epidemiology, incidence and clinical aspects of food allergy. Ann Allergy 1984;53:615-22.
2. Goldman H. Allergic disorders. In: Ming SC, Goldman H, eds. Pathology of the gastrointestinal tract. Philadelphia: WB Saunders 1992:182-4.
3. Goldman HG, Proujansky R. Allergic proctitis and gastroenteritis in children: clinical and mucosal biopsy features in 53 cases. Am J Surg Pathol 1986;10:75-86.
4. Odze RD, Bines J, Leichtner AM, Goldman H, Antonioli DA. Allergic proctocolitis in infants: a prospective clinical-pathologic biopsy study. Hum Pathol 1993;24:668-74.
5. Powell GK. Milk- and soy-induced enterocolitis of infancy: clinical features and standardization of challenge. J PEDIATR 1978;93:553-60.
6. Lake AM, Whitington PF, Hamilton SR. Dietary protein-induced colitis in breast-fed infants. J PEDIATR 1982;101:906-10.
7. Chong SKF, Blackshaw AJ, Morson BC, Williams CB, Walker-Smith JA. Prospective study of colitis in infancy and early childhood. J Pediatr Gastroenterol Nutr 1986;5:352-8.
8. Dannaeus A, Johansson SGO. A follow-up study of infants with adverse reactions to cow milk. Acta Paediatr Scand 1979;68:377-82.
9. Hill DJ, Ford RP, Shelton MJ, Hosking CS. A study of 100 infants and young children with cow milk allergy. Clin Rev Allergy 1984;2:125-42.
10. Sampson HA, Buckley RH, Metcalfe DD. Food allergy. JAMA 1987;258:2886-90.
11. Wilson NW, Hamburger RN. Allergy to cow milk in the first year of life and its prevention. Ann Allergy 1988;61:323-7.
12. Jenkins HR, Pincott JR, Soothill JF, Milla PJ, Harries JT. Food allergy: the major cause of infantile colitis. Arch Dis Child 1984;59:326-9.
13. Sampson HA. IgE-mediated food intolerance. J Allergy Clin Immunol 1988;81:495-504.
14. Kniker WT. Immunologically mediated reactions to food: state of the art. Ann Allergy 1987;59:60-70.
15. Langeland T, Harbitz O. A clinical and immunological study of allergy to hen's egg white. V. Purification and identification of a major allergen (antigen 22) in hen's egg white. Allergy 1983;38:131-9.
16. Aas K. Antigens in food. Nutr Rev 1984;42:85-91.

17. Metcalfe DD. Food allergens. Clin Rev Allergy 1985;3:331-49.
18. Iyngkaran N, Yadav M, Looi LM, et al. Effect of soy protein on the small bowel mucosa of young infants recovering from acute gastroenteritis. J Pediatr Gastroenterol Nutr 1988;7:68-75.
19. Eastham EJ, Lichauco T, Pang K, Walker WA. Antigenicity of infant formulas and the induction of systemic immunological tolerance by oral feeding: cow milk versus soy milk. J Pediatr Gastroenterol Nutr 1982;1:23-8.
20. Eastham EJ, Lichauco T, Grady MI, Walker WA. Antigenicity of infant formulas: role of immature intestine on protein permeability. J PEDIATR 1978;93:561-4.
21. Perisic VN, Filipovic D, Kokai G. Allergic colitis with rectal bleeding in an exclusively breast-fed neonate. Acta Paediatr Scand 1988;77:163-4.
22. Halpin TC, Byrne WJ, Ament ME. Colitis, persistent diarrhea, and soy protein intolerance. J PEDIATR 1977;91:404-7.
23. Kilshaw PJ, Cant AJ. The passage of maternal dietary proteins into human breast milk. Int Arch Allergy Appl Immunol 1984;75:8-15.
24. Pittschieler K. Cow milk protein–induced colitis in the breast-fed infant. J Pediatr Gastroenterol Nutr 1990;10:548-9.
25. Wilson NW, Self TW, Hamburger RN. Severe cow milk–induced colitis in an exclusively breast-fed neonate. Clin Pediatr 1990;29:77-80.
26. Lovegrove JA, Osman DL, Morgan JB, Hamptom SM. Transfer of cow milk β-lactoglobulin to human serum after a milk load: a pilot study. Gut 1993;34:203-7.
27. Lifschitz CH, Hawkins HK, Guerra C, Byrd N. Anaphylactic shock due to cow milk protein hypersensitivity in a breast-fed infant. J Pediatr Gastroenterol Nutr 1988;7:141-4.
28. Jakobsson I, Lindberg T. A prospective study of cow milk allergy in Swedish infants. Acta Paediatr Scand 1979;68:853-9.
29. Harrison CJ, Puntis JWL, Durbin GM, Gornall P, Booth IW. Case report: atypical allergic colitis in preterm infants. Acta Paediatr Scand 1991;80:1113-6.
30. Winter HS, Antonioli DA, Fukagawa N, Marcial M, Goldman H. Allergy-related proctocolitis in infants: diagnostic usefulness of rectal biopsy. Mod Pathol 1990;3:5-100.
31. Bock SA. Natural history of food sensitivity. J Allergy Clin Immunol 1982;69:173-7.
32. Peterson RDA, Good RA. Antibodies to cow milk: their presence and significance. Pediatrics 1963;31:209-21.
33. May CD, Remigio L, Bock SA. Usefulness of measurement of antibodies in serum in diagnosis of sensitivity to cow milk and soy proteins in early childhood. Allergy 1980;35:301-10.
34. Richards DG, Somers S, Issenman RM, Stevenson GW. Cow milk protein/soy protein allergy gastrointestinal imaging. Radiology 1988;167:721-3.
35. Goldman AS, Anderson DW Jr, Sellers WA. Saperstein S, Kniker WT, Halpern SR. Milk allergy. I. Oral challenge with milk and isolated milk proteins in allergic children. Pediatrics 1963;32:425-43.
36. Goldman H, Antonioli DA. Mucosal biopsy of the rectum, colon and distal ileum. Hum Pathol 1982;13:981-1012.
37. Finberg L, Bell EF, Hatch RE, et al. Hypoallergenic infant formulas. Pediatrics 1989;83:1068-9.
38. Verkasalo M, Kuitunen P, Savilahti E, Tiilikainen A. Changing pattern of cow milk intolerance: an analysis of the occurrence and clinical course in the 60s and mid-70s. Acta Paediatr Scand 1981;70:289-95.
39. Glassman MS, Newman LJ, Berezin S, Gryboski JD. Cow milk protein sensitivity during infancy in patients with inflammatory bowel disease. Am J Gastroenterol 1990;85:838-40.
40. Catlett JB. Ulcerative colitis in an allergic person: case report. Virginia Medical 1988;115:434-5.
41. Rosekrans PCM, Meijer CJLM, Van der Wal AM, Lindeman J. Allergic proctitis, a clinical and immunopathological entity. Gut 1980;21:1017-23.
42. Gould SR, Buckell NA, Day DW, Edwards AM, Lennard-Jones JE. Controlled trial of disodium cromoglycate in chronic persistent colitis. Gut 1978;19:1140-3.
43. Crowe SE, Perdue MH. Gastrointestinal food hypersensitivity: basic mechanisms of pathophysiology. Gastroenterology 1992;103:1075-95.
44. Wershil BK, Walker WA. The mucosal barrier, IgE-mediated gastrointestinal events, and eosinophilic gastroenteritis. Gastroenterol Clin North Am 1992;21:387-404.
45. Weller PF. The immunobiology of eosinophils. N Engl J Med 1991;324:1110-8.
46. Gleich GJ, Adolphson CR, Leiferman KM. The biology of the eosinophilic leukocyte. Annu Rev Med 1993;44:85-101.
47. Clutterbuck EJ, Hirst EM, Sanderson CJ. Human interleukin-5 (IL-5) regulates the production of eosinophils in human bone marrow cultures: comparison and interaction with IL-1, IL-3, IL-6, and GM-CSF. Blood 1989;73:1504-12.
48. Yukawa T, Kroegel C, Evans P, Fukuda T, Chung KF, Barnes PJ. Density heterogeneity of eosinophil leucocytes: induction of hypodense eosinophils by platelet-activating factor. Immunology 1989;68:140-3.
49. Rothenberg ME, Owen WF Jr, Silberstein DS, Soberman RJ, Austen KF, Stevens RL. Eosinophils cocultured with endothelial cells have increased survival and functional properties. Science 1988;237:645-7.
50. Springer TA. Adhesion receptors of the immune system. Nature 1990;346:425-7.
51. Bochner BS, Luscinskas FW, Gimbrone MA Jr, et al. Adhesion of human basophils, eosinophils and neutrophils to interleukin-1–activated human vascular endothelial cells: contribution of endothelial cell adhesion molecules. J Exp Med 1991;173:1553-62.
52. Elices MJ, Osborn L, Takada Y, et al. VCAM-1 on activated endothelium interacts with the leukocyte integrin VLA-4 at a site distinct from the VLA-4/fibronectin binding site. Cell 1990;60:577-83.
53. Moser R, Fehr J, Bruijnzeel PLB. IL-4 controls the selective endothelium-driven transmigration of eosinophils from allergic individuals. J Immunol 1992;149:1432-8.
54. Mosmann TR, Coffman RL. TH1 and TH2 cells: different patterns of lymphokine secretion lead to different functional properties. Annu Rev Immunol 1989;7:145-73.
55. Galli SG, Gordon JR, Wershil BK. Cytokine production by mast cells and basophils. Curr Opin Immunol 1991;3:865-73.
56. Abu-Ghazaleh RI, Fujusawa T, Mestecky J, Kyle RA, Gleich GJ. IgA-induced eosinophil degranulation. J Immunol 1989;142:2393-400.
57. Monteiro RC, Hostoffer RW, Cooper MD, et al. Definition of immunoglobulin A receptors on eosinophils and their enhanced expression in allergic individuals. J Clin Invest 1993;92:1681-5.
58. Rot A, Krieger M, Brunner T, Bischoff SC, Schall TJ, Dahinden CA. RANTES and macrophage inflammatory protein 1

induce the migration and activation of normal human eosinophil granulocytes. J Exp Med 1992;176:1489-95.
59. Fujisawa T, Abu-Ghazaleh R, Kita H, Sanderson CJ, Gleich GJ. Regulatory effect of cytokines on eosinophil degranulation. J Immunol 1990;144:642-6.
60. Sun XM, Hsueh W. Platelet-activating factor produces shock, in vivo complement activation, and tissue injury in mice. J Immunol 1991;147:509-14.
61. Galli SJ, Gordon JR, Wershil BK, et al. Mast cell and eosinophil cytokines in allergy and inflammation. In: Gleich GJ, Kay AB, eds. Eosinophils: immunological and clinical aspects. New York: Marcel Dekker, 1994:255-80.
62. Heyman M, Darmon N, Dupont C, et al. Mononuclear cells from infants allergic to cow milk secrete tumor necrosis factor α, altering intestinal function. Gastroenterology 1994;106:1514-23.
63. Torimoto K, Sato N, Okubo M, et al. Development of multiple necrotizing enteritis induced by a tumor necrosis factor–like cytokine from lipopolysaccharide-stimulated peritoneal macrophages in rats. Am J Pathol 1990;137:1103-11.
64. Resnick MB, Colgan SP, Patapoff TW, et al. Activated eosinophils evoke chloride secretion in model intestinal epithelia primarily via regulated release of 5′-AMP. J Immunol 1993;151:5716-23.

ORIGINAL ARTICLES

Enhanced adrenomedullary response and increased susceptibility to neuroglycopenia: Mechanisms underlying the adverse effects of sugar ingestion in healthy children

Timothy W. Jones, MD, Walter P. Borg, MD, Susan D. Boulware, MD, Gregory McCarthy, PhD, Robert S. Sherwin, MD, and William V. Tamborlane, MD

From the Departments of Pediatrics, Internal Medicine, and Neurosurgery and the General Clinical Research Centers, Yale University School of Medicine, New Haven, Connecticut

Objective: **Eating simple sugars has been suggested as having adverse behavioral and cognitive effects in children, but a physiologic mechanism has not been established. This study was performed to address this issue.**
Design: **Metabolic, hormonal, and symptomatic responses to a standard oral glucose load (1.75 gm/kg; maximum, 120 gm) were compared in 25 healthy children and 23 young adults, and the hypoglycemic clamp, together with measurements of P300 auditory evoked potentials, was used to assess whether children are more vulnerable than adults to neuroglycopenia.**
Setting: **Children's Clinical Research Center, Yale University School of Medicine.**
Results: **Baseline and oral glucose–stimulated plasma glucose and insulin levels were similar in both groups, including the nadir glucose level 3 to 5 hours after oral administration of glucose (3.4 ± 0.1 mmol/L (61 ± 1.8 mg/dl) in children and 3.5 ± 0.1 mmol/L (63 ± 1.8 mg/dl) in adults). The late glucose decrease stimulated a rise in plasma epinephrine levels that was twofold higher in children than in adults (2260 ± 289 vs 1031 ± 147 pmol/L (407 ± 52 vs 186 ± 26 pg/ml), $p<0.01$) and a significant increase in hypoglycemic symptom scores in children ($p<0.01$), but not in adults. During control experiments, in which six of the healthy children ingested a sugar-free drink, there were no significant changes in plasma glucose levels, hormone concentrations, or hypoglycemic symptom scores. During the hypoglycemic clamp, P300 potentials did not change in any of eight adult subjects until the plasma glucose concentration was lowered to 3.0 mmol/L (54 mg/dl), whereas similar changes in P300 potentials were observed in six of seven children at glucose levels 3.6 to 4.2 mmol/L (65 to 75 mg/dl).**
Conclusion: **Enhanced adrenomedullary responses to modest reductions in plasma glucose concentration and increased susceptibility to neuroglycopenia may be important contributing factors to adverse behavioral and cognitive effects after sugar ingestion in healthy children. (J PEDIATR 1995;126:171-7)**

Supported by grants RR06022, RR00125, DK20495, and HD30671 from the National Institutes of Health and by a grant from the Juvenile Diabetes Foundation International.

Submitted for publication Sept. 6, 1994; accepted Oct. 26, 1994.

Reprint requests: William V. Tamborlane, MD, Department of Pediatrics, Yale University School of Medicine, 333 Cedar St., New Haven, CT 06510-8064.

0022-3476/95/$3.00 + 0 **9/20/61576**

The question of whether refined sugar adversely affects the behavior or cognitive functions of healthy children is a continuing source of controversy. Whereas parents and clinicians have frequently reported that even healthy children are prone to the development of behavioral changes and cognitive defects after eating simple sugars, the outcomes of research studies have been complex and discrepant.[1-4] In addition, possible physiologic mechanisms for enhanced sensitivity to dietary sugar during childhood have not been clear. The presumed negative reactions to sugar have been attributed to an early rise or late fall in the plasma glucose concentration, and to an immunologic response to sucrose.[5] Unfortunately, given the lack of consistent objective data to substantiate these assumptions, all these hypotheses remain open to question.

The results of our previous studies of counterregulatory responses to hypoglycemia in children[6, 7] prompted us to propose a new hypothesis to explain the mechanisms underlying adverse effects of sugar ingestion in children. We hypothesized that, although the changes in plasma glucose levels after sucrose ingestion do not differ between adults and children, the children would show enhanced adrenomedullary and symptomatic responses to these changes in comparison with those of adults. Several lines of evidence support this hypothesis. Although sugar ingestion does not normally cause severe reductions in plasma glucose levels in the late postprandial period in children,[8, 9] our previous study showed that plasma epinephrine responses to identical, modest insulin-induced reductions in plasma glucose are twofold greater in healthy children than in healthy adults.[6] In addition, the plasma glucose level that triggers epinephrine release and symptoms is substantially higher in children than in adults,[7] reaching values (plasma glucose levels 4.4 to 3.4 mmol/L [80 to 61 mg/dl]) that are commonly observed 3 to 5 hours after oral glucose ingestion.

See related article, p. 178.

To test our hypothesis, we compared the metabolic, hormonal, and symptomatic responses of healthy children and healthy young adults with a standardized, large glucose load. In addition, the hypoglycemic clamp technique was combined with serial measurements of cortical auditory evoked potentials to assess whether young subjects are more susceptible to the adverse effects of reduced glucose availability on cognitive function.

METHODS

Subjects. Forty-eight nonobese subjects (25 children, 23 adults) were studied. To be eligible, the subjects had to be healthy, taking no medications, and have no history of diabetes or carbohydrate intolerance. The children included eight boys and 17 girls between 8 and 16 years of age; the adults included 9 men and 14 women between 20 and 30 years of age. Subjects with attentional, behavioral, or psychiatric problems or with a history of unusual sensitivity to sugar were excluded from the study. All subjects were consuming weight-maintaining diets containing at least 115 gm/m^2 body surface area of carbohydrates per day before the study. Of the 25 children, eight were prepubertal (Tanner stage I), and the other 17 had Tanner stage II to IV development. Body mass index (mean ± SD) averaged 18.2 ± 2.2 kg/m^2 in the children and 22.6 ± 2.8 in the adults. The study was approved by the Yale University School of Medicine Human Investigation Committee, and informed written consent was obtained from all subjects and their parents (for the children).

Procedures. All subjects were admitted to the Yale General Clinical Research Center, where a history was obtained and a physical examination performed. The studies were started between 8 and 8:30 AM, after the subjects had been fasting for 10 to 12 hours overnight. With all procedures, an intravenous catheter was inserted in a vein of a hand or distal portion of a forearm for blood sampling, and that hand was kept in a heated box (60° to 65° C) to "arterialize" the blood.

Oral glucose loading. All subjects took part in the oral glucose loading study. They were allowed to rest for at least 30 minutes after insertion of the blood sampling catheter before baseline measurements were obtained. Glucose was ingested in a dosage of 1.75 gm/kg body weight to a maximum of 120 gm (actual amount, 110 ± 5 gm in adults and 86 ± 6 gm in children [mean ± SD]) with a decaffeinated cola preparation (General Medical Corp., Richmond, Va.). Blood samples were obtained every 10 minutes from −30 to 300 minutes for measurement of the plasma glucose concentration, and every 30 minutes for measurement of plasma levels of insulin, catecholamines, and other counterregulatory hormones (growth hormone, cortisol, and glucagon).

Each of the subjects rated a list of symptoms before and every 60 minutes after glucose ingestion, as previously described. Symptoms (recorded on a lap-top computer) were rated on a scale of 1 (not at all) to 7 (extreme). The eight hypoglycemic symptoms included pounding heart, feeling shaky, feeling weak, having difficulty concentrating, headaches, feeling anxious, slowed thinking, and feeling sweaty. The sum of these symptoms at each observation point constituted the total hypoglycemic symptom score at that time. In addition, four filler items (earache, pain in joints, watery eyes, and ringing in ears) were included to account for nonspecific effects not referable to glucose and antiinsulin hormones.

Control experiments were also performed in three boys and three girls, aged 10 ± 3 years (mean ± SD), who had participated in the oral glucose loading studies. These control experiments were performed as described above; however, the oral glucose load was replaced by an equal volume of sugar-free decaffeinated cola drink (Coca-Cola Co., Atlanta, Ga.).

Hypoglycemic clamping. Eight of the children, aged 11 ± 2 years (mean ± SD), and eight of the adults, aged 24 ± 2 years, who had taken part in oral glucose loading experiments participated in the clamp protocol. However, the cortical evoked potentials of one of children could not be analyzed because of technical problems and was not included in the analysis of electrophysiologic data.

The methods used for the hypoglycemic clamp have been described in detail elsewhere.[10] For this procedure, a second catheter was inserted in an antecubital vein in the arm opposite to the blood-sampling hand for administration of exogenous glucose and insulin.

After a 30-minute rest period, three blood samples were obtained during a 40-minute interval for measurement of baseline glucose and hormone levels. A primed continuous infusion of rapid-acting human insulin (Novolin; Novo Nordisk, Princeton, N.J.) was then begun at a continuous rate of 480 pmol $\cdot$ m^{-2} $\cdot$ min^{-1}.

After the insulin infusion was begun, the desired plasma glucose level was achieved by varying the rate of 20% glucose infusion on the basis of measurements of plasma glucose obtained at 5-minute intervals. Blood samples for measurement of insulin and epinephrine were taken at 20-minute intervals throughout the study. In all subjects, plasma glucose was initially maintained at fasting euglycemic levels for 60 minutes and then reduced in hourly ~0.56 mmol/L (10 mg/dl) steps to a nadir of 3.0 mmol/L (54 mg/dl). The subjects were masked to plasma glucose levels during the study.

Electrophysiologic recordings were obtained during the last 10 to 15 minutes of each glycemic plateau. Scalp electrodes were placed at the C_z and P_z positions, with a reference electrode placed on one ear and the ground electrode placed on the opposite ear. A bipolar pair of electrodes was placed above and below the right eye to monitor for ocular artifacts. The P300 evoked potentials were obtained with an auditory categorization ("oddball") task in which subjects were required to count silently the number of soft clicks delivered in a train consisting of a random mix of frequent loud and infrequent soft clicks. The loud clicks were presented to the ear ipsilateral to the reference electrode, and the soft clicks were delivered to the ear contralateral to the reference electrode. The proportion of soft clicks varied between 10% and 20% of 200 clicks, and subjects reported their count of soft clicks at the end of each run. Two replications were obtained at each baseline (before insulin infusion) and at each plasma glucose plateau.

Determinations. Plasma glucose was measured in duplicate at the bedside with a glucose analyzer (Beckman Instruments Inc., Fullerton, Calif.). Epinephrine and norepinephrine were measured with a radioenzymatic assay (Amersham Corp., Arlington Heights, Ill.), glucagon (ICN Biomedicals, Inc., Costa Mesa, Calif.), cortisol (Diagnostic Products Corp., Los Angeles, Calif.), and growth hormone (Kallestad Diagnostic Inc., Chaska, Minn.) were determined by radioimmunoassay. The intraassay coefficients of variation for these assays were as follows: for epinephrine, 20.2% at 175 pmol/L (31.5 pg/ml) and 6.7% at 1168 pmol/L (210 pg/ml); for growth hormone, 6.2% at 3.5 μg/L (3.5 ng/ml); for glucagon, 9% at 122 ng/L (122 pg/ml); and for cortisol, <2%. Plasma insulin was measured by double-antibody radioimmunoassay (Binax Inc., South Portland, Maine).

Statistical methods and analyses. Glucose and hormone responses to orally administered glucose and during clamp studies were compared between groups by analysis of variance with repeated measures design. Other comparisons were made by analysis of variance, unpaired Student *t* test, and chi-square analysis where appropriate. The p values <0.05 are reported as significant.

Group differences in symptom scores after glucose ingestion were examined with time and at the plasma glucose nadir. For the latter comparison, the symptom assessment that occurred at or immediately after the nadir plasma glucose level in each subject was used. During the hypoglycemic clamp procedure, the plasma glucose threshold for epinephrine release in each individual subject was defined as the glucose level at which a sustained elevation of >410 pmol/L (74 pg/ml) above basal values was observed, as previously described.[7] The glycemic threshold for changes in P300 potentials in individual subjects during the clamp procedure was defined as the plateau plasma glucose level at which a 30% or greater reduction in P300 amplitude was observed. Demographic data are presented as mean ± SD, whereas other data are presented as mean ± SEM.

RESULTS

Glucose ingestion. Basal plasma glucose levels and plasma insulin levels (55 ± 5 pmol/L [8.8 ± 0.8 μU/ml] in children; 60 ± 5 pmol/L [9.6 ± 0.8 μU/ml] in adults) were similar in both groups, and the glucose and insulin profiles were similar in children and adults after glucose

Table I. Basal and nadir plasma glucose and basal and peak hormone concentrations (mean ± SEM) after glucose load

	Children	Adults
Plasma/glucose (mmol/L)		
Basal	4.6 ± 0.1	4.8 ± 0.1
Peak	7.5 ± 0.3	8.1 ± 0.4
Nadir	3.4 ± 0.1	3.5 ± 0.1
Plasma epinephrine (pmol/L)		
Basal	229 ± 27	191 ± 27
Peak	2260 ± 289*	1031 ± 147
Plasma growth hormone (μg/L)		
Basal	1.7 ± 0.3	1.1 ± 0.2
Peak	19.5 ± 2.5	18.3 ± 2.8
Plasma glucagon (ng/L)		
Basal	94 ± 12	120 ± 18
Peak	201 ± 31	180 ± 25

To convert to metric units: multiply glucose value by 18, epinephrine value by 0.18, growth hormone value by 1.0, and glucagon value by 1.0.
*p <0.01 versus adults.

ingestion (data not shown). Peak and nadir plasma glucose levels observed in the postprandial period in individual subjects determined by frequent sampling (every 10 minutes) were virtually identical in children and adults (Table I).

Baseline plasma epinephrine levels were similar, and mean epinephrine concentrations rose in both groups in response to the late postprandial fall in plasma glucose (Table I). However, the rise in the plasma concentration of epinephrine was significantly greater in the children, reaching peak values that were nearly twofold higher in the children than in the adults (p <0.01) (Table I). On the other hand, peak postprandial plasma growth hormone and glucagon levels did not differ between the groups. Basal plasma concentrations of cortisol and norepinephrine were similar in healthy children and adults, and levels of these hormones did not change significantly in either group after oral glucose (data not shown). Results of subgroup analyses failed to demonstrate a significant effect of gender or pubertal stage on the rise in epinephrine levels after glucose ingestion by the 25 healthy children.

Total hypoglycemic and filler (control) symptom scores were similar in both groups at baseline (Table II), and the symptom scores remained unchanged in the adults after glucose ingestion. In contrast, total hypoglycemic symptom scores rose sharply in the children in association with the late fall in plasma glucose concentration (p <0.01 vs baseline). As in the adults, filler (control) symptom scores did not change in the children throughout the study. The change in hypoglycemic symptom scores in the children was mainly due to significantly increased reporting of feeling shaky (from 1.7 ± 0.2 to 3.2 ± 0.6), sweaty (1.5 ± 0.2 to 2.8 ± 0.5), or weak (1.9 ± 0.3 to 3.8 ± 0.5), or having a pounding heart 1.7 ± 0.2 to 2.5 ± 0.5) (p <0.05 vs baseline).

Table II. Total hypoglycemic and filler (control) symptom scores at baseline and at the postprandial glucose nadir

	Children		Adults	
	Baseline	Glucose nadir	Baseline	Glucose nadir
Total hypoglycemic scores				
Mean	12.8	22.0*	10.0	13.0
SE	1.0	3.0	0.5	1.7
Filler (control) scores				
Mean	5.0	5.5	5.0	5.2
SE	0.5	0.6	0.4	0.5

*p <0.01 versus baseline.

In contrast to the response to glucose ingestion, no changes in plasma epinephrine levels were observed after the sugar-free cola drink. As a result, plasma epinephrine levels were significantly higher after glucose ingestion versus control values at 240 minutes and 270 minutes (p <0.05) in these subjects (Fig. 1). Total hypoglycemic symptom scores also did not change from baseline values (11 ± 2) during the control study, in contrast to the increase in hypoglycemic symptoms in these subjects (11 ± 2 to 25 ± 4) after glucose ingestion.

Hypoglycemic clamp studies. As shown in Fig. 2, the plasma glucose concentration was gradually reduced in nearly identical 0.56 mmol/L (10 mg/dl) steps from 4.8 to 3.0 mmol/L (86 mg/dl to 54 mg/dl) in both children and adults during the 240-minute hypoglycemic clamp procedure. As expected,[7] this controlled reduction in the plasma glucose concentration stimulated an exaggerated rise in the plasma epinephrine concentration in children, in comparison with that in adults (e.g., 4830 ± 334 vs 2365 ± 311 pmol/L [870 ± 60 vs 426 ± 56 pg/ml] at 240 minutes; p <0.01]. The plasma glucose level that stimulated a rise in epinephrine was also significantly higher in children than in adults (3.6 ± 0.1 vs 3.0 ± 0.1 mmol/L [65 ± 1.8 vs 54 ± 1.8 mg/dl]; p <0.01), even though steady-state plasma insulin levels achieved during the insulin infusion were similar in both groups (903 ± 48 pmol/L [144.5 ± 7.6 μU/ml] in children vs 857 + 42 pmol/L [137 ± 6.7 μU/ml] in adults).

At baseline (before the start of the insulin infusion) the P300 amplitude was not significantly greater in the children than in the adults (11.7 ± 1.5 vs 9.7 ± 1.4, respectively), and no change in either group was observed at the end of the initial euglycemic period (plasma glucose level, 4.8 mmol/L [86 mg/dl]) (Fig. 3). Most important, no change

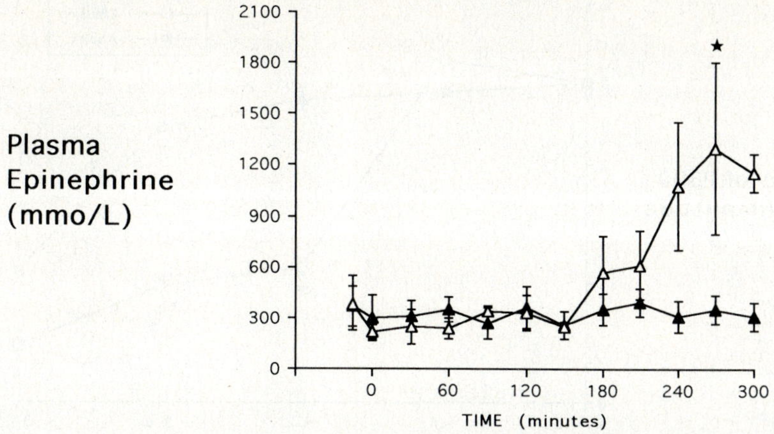

Fig. 1. Plasma epinephrine levels (mean ± SEM) in six of the healthy children before and after ingestion of oral glucose (△) and a sugar-free cola drink (▲). *Asterisk* indicates significant difference in values between oral glucose and control experiments (p <0.05). To convert to metric units, multiply epinephrine value by 0.18.

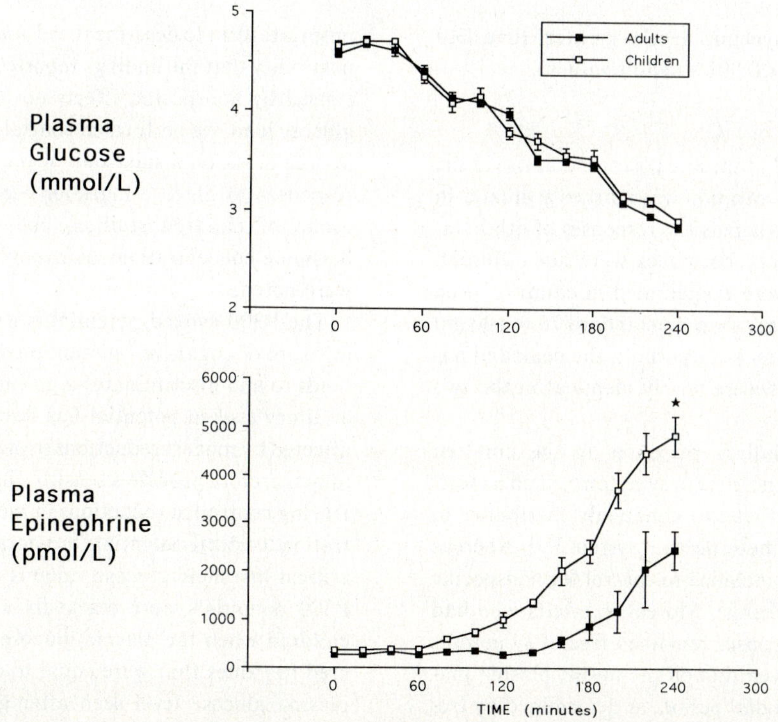

Fig. 2. Plasma glucose and epinephrine levels (mean ± SEM) during hypoglycemic clamp studies in children (□) and adults (■). *Asterisk* indicates significant difference (p <0.01) versus corresponding value in adults. To convert to metric units, multiply glucose value by 18, and epinephrine value by 0.18.

in P300 potentials was observed in any of the adults until the plasma glucose concentration was lowered to the last step (3.0 mmol/L [54 mg/dl]). In contrast, in the children the P300 amplitude was significantly reduced when the glucose concentration was lowered to 4.2 mmol/L (75 mg/dl) (p <0.05 vs baseline) and the P300 amplitude remained significantly reduced throughout the remainder of the study. All but one of the children had alterations in cortical

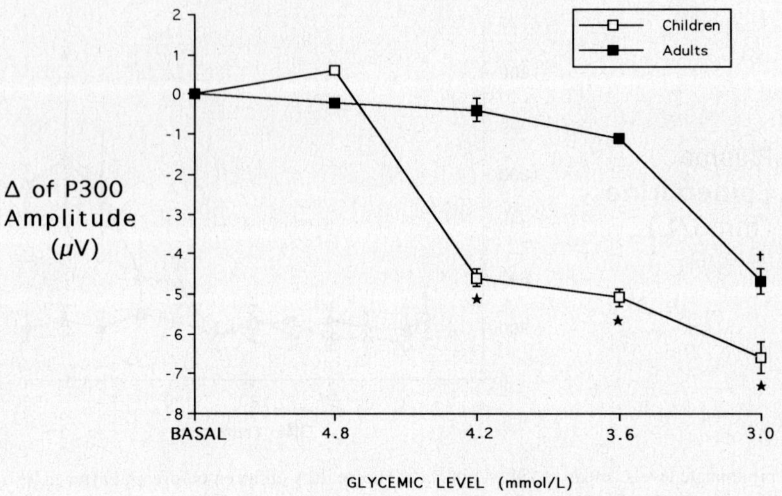

Fig. 3. Delta of P300 amplitude during each glycemic plateau in children (□) and adults (■). *Asterisks* indicate significant differences versus euglycemia in the children (*$p < 0.05$). *Dagger* (†) indicates significant difference versus euglycemia in adults ($p < 0.01$).

evoked potentials at glycemic levels greater than 3.0 mmol/L (54 mg/dl) ($p < 0.002$ vs adult values).

DISCUSSION

Our findings indicate that the late postprandial rise in the plasma epinephrine concentration was markedly greater in children than in adults, whereas the responses of other antiinsulin, counterregulatory hormones were not different. Epinephrine responses were exaggerated in children, even though a glucose load larger than the standard 75 to 100 gm was given to adults and, more important, the peak and nadir plasma glucose levels were nearly identical in the two groups.

Enhanced adrenomedullary responses in the children were associated with an increase in symptoms, such as feeling shaky and sweaty, that are commonly attributed to stimulation of the sympathetic nervous system,[11, 12] whereas the scores on filler items included to control for nonspecific fatigue effects did not change. Moreover, adults who had blunted epinephrine responses remained free of symptoms throughout the study, even though the lowest plasma glucose level in the postprandial period, as determined by frequent measurements, was nearly identical in the two groups. These data suggest that discrepancies in symptom awareness of the late fall in the plasma glucose concentration after an oral glucose load are more likely related to differences in epinephrine responses than to the absolute plasma glucose level achieved. The plasma glucose concentration fell to only 3.4 ± 0.1 mmol/L (61 ± 1.8 mg/dl) in the children, so "enhanced adrenomedullary responsiveness," rather than "reactive hypoglycemia," might be a more appropriate term to describe these phenomena. To exclude the possibility that the findings reported above might have been caused by nonspecific effects not connected with the oral glucose load, we performed control experiments with a sugar-free drink on a subgroup of the healthy children whose responses to glucose ingestion were typical of the entire group of children studied, and no changes in plasma hormone concentrations or hypoglycemic symptom scores were noted.

The P300 evoked potential is a neuroelectrophysiologic measure of cognitive function produced when a subject attends to and discriminates a given stimulus.[13] The cortical auditory evoked potential has been shown to be adversely affected by modest reductions in plasma glucose levels[14] and may therefore provide a sensitive index of neuroglycopenia. During controlled reductions in the plasma glucose concentration, cortical potentials are normally maintained until a critical threshold glucose value is reduced.[15] In this study, P300 potentials were markedly altered in almost all the children when the plasma glucose concentration was lowered to values that were equal to or higher than the nadir plasma glucose level seen after glucose ingestion in this group. On the other hand, in adults P300 potentials were preserved until the plasma glucose concentration was lowered to 3.0 mmol/L (54 mg/dl), values rarely observed in either group after glucose ingestion. These data suggest that healthy children are more vulnerable to the effects of hypoglycemia on cognitive function than are adults. Because release of epinephrine in response to a fall in the plasma glucose concentration appears to be mediated through the central nervous system,[16, 17] increased susceptibility to neuroglycopenia may, in turn, account for the higher plasma glucose level that triggered release of epinephrine in the children.

The putative adverse effects of dietary sugar on behavior and cognitive function in children have been the subject of marked controversy.[18-20] Previous studies in this area that have been focused on children with attention deficit disorder have tended to make exaggerated claims regarding the global effects of sugar and other food additives on their behavioral problems. Kinsbourne[21] noted that the problems caused by dietary sugar appear to be much less severe or prevalent than some studies suggest. On the other hand, we have shown in this study that consumption of glucose in an amount roughly equivalent in carbohydrate content to two 12-ounce cans of Coca-Cola is followed by a fall in the plasma glucose concentration sufficient to induce hormonal, symptomatic, and neurophysiologic changes in healthy children. However, the rise in the plasma epinephrine concentration and in associated adrenergic symptoms was acute and self-limited, and occurred only in the late postprandial period. These data do not indicate that dietary sugar is the cause of hyperactivity problems, but they emphasize that most children could benefit from eating mixed meals that include protein, fat, complex carbohydrate, and fiber to limit postprandial reductions in plasma glucose levels and increases in plasma epinephrine levels. In keeping with this conclusion, Wolraich et al.[1] were unable to demonstrate any effects on behavior and cognitive function in preschool and school-age children by adding or subtracting sucrose from a balanced diet.

REFERENCES

1. Wolraich ML, Lindgren SD, Stumbo PJ, Stegink LD, Appelbaum MI, Kiritsy MC. Effect of diets high in sucrose or aspartame on the behavior and cognitive performance of children. N Engl J Med 1994;330:301-7.
2. Milich R, Wolraich M, Lindgren SD. Sugar and hyperactivity: a critical review of empirical findings. Clinical Psychology Review 1986;6:493-513.
3. Crook WG. Food allergy: the great masquerader. Pediatr Clin North Am 1957;22:227-38.
4. Rapp DJ. Does diet affect hyperactivity? Journal of Learning Disabilities 1978;11:383-9.
5. Wender E. Review of research of the relationship of nutritive sweeteners and behavior. In: Diet and behavior. Washington, D.C.: National Center for Nutrition and Dietetics, 1991:65-80.
6. Amiel SA, Simonson DC, Sherwin RS, Lauritano AA, Tamborlane WV. Exaggerated epinephrine responses to hypoglycemia in normal and insulin dependent diabetic children. J Pediatr 1987;110:832-7.
7. Jones TW, Boulware SD, Kraemer DT, Caprio S, Sherwin RS, Tamborlane WV. Independent effects of youth and poor diabetes control on responses to hypoglycemia in children. Diabetes 1991;40:358-63.
8. Rosenbloom AL, Wheeler L, Bianchi R, Chin FT, Tiwary CM, Gorgic A. Age-adjusted analysis of insulin responses during normal and abnormal glucose tests in normal children and adolescents. Diabetes 1975;24:820-8.
9. Grant DB. Serum-insulin levels in children during glucose tolerance tests. Acta Paediatr Scand 1968;57:297-9.
10. Amiel SA, Simonson DC, Tamborlane WV, DeFronzo RA, Sherwin RS. Rate of glucose fall does not affect counterregulatory hormone responses to hypoglycemia in normal and diabetic humans. Diabetes 1987;36:518-22.
11. Cryer PE, Binder C, Bolli GB, et al. Hypoglycemia in IDDM. Diabetes 1989;38:1193-9.
12. Heller SR, Herbert M, MacDonald IA, Tattersall RB. Influence of sympathetic nervous system on hypoglycemic warning symptoms. Lancet 1987;2:359-63.
13. Sutton S, Tueting P, Zubin J, John ER. Information delivery and the sensing evoked potential. Science 1976;155: 1436-9.
14. DeFeo P, Gallai V, Mazzotta G, et al. Modest decrements in plasma glucose concentrations cause early impairment in cognitive function and later activation of glucose counterregulation in the absence of hypoglycemic symptoms in normal man. J Clin Invest 1988;82:436-44.
15. Jones TW, McCarthy G, Tamborlane WV, et al. Mild hypoglycemia and impairment of brain stem and cortical evoked potentials in healthy subjects. Diabetes 1990;39:1550-5.
16. Borg WP, During MJ, Sherwin RS, Borg MA, Brines ML, Shulman GI. Ventromedial hypothalamic lesions in rats suppress counterregulatory responses to hypoglycemia. J Clin Invest 1994;93:1677-82.
17. Biggers DW, Myers SR, Neal D, et al. Role of brain in counterregulation of insulin-induced hypoglycemia. Diabetes 1989;38:7-16.
18. Rosen LA, Booth SR, Bender ME, McGrath ML, Sorrel S, Drabman RS. Effects of sugar (sucrose) on children's behavior. J Consult Clin Psychol 1988;57:583-9.
19. Goldman JA, Lerman RH, Contois JM, Udall JN. Behavioral effects of sucrose on preschool children. J Abnorm Child Psychol 1986;14:565-77.
20. Wender EH, Solanto MV. Effects of sugar on aggressive and inattentive behavior in children with attention deficit disorder with hyperactivity and normal children. Pediatrics 1991; 88:960-6.
21. Kinsbourne M. Sugar and the hyperactive child. N Engl J Med 1994;330:355-6.

Effects of acute hyperglycemia on mental efficiency and counterregulatory hormones in adolescents with insulin-dependent diabetes mellitus

Sylvia Gschwend, MD, Christopher Ryan, PhD, Joy Atchison, MD, Silva Arslanian, MD, and Dorothy Becker, MBBCh
From the Departments of Pediatrics and Psychiatry, University of Pittsburgh School of Medicine, Pittsburgh, Pennsylvania

Objective: To determine whether acute hyperglycemia adversely affects mental efficiency to the same extent as acute mild hypoglycemia.
***Study design*: We administered a battery of cognitive tests to adolescents studied at hyperglycemic (20 mmol/L (360 mg/dl)), hypoglycemic (3.3 mmol/L (60 mg/dl)), or euglycemic (5.5 mmol/L (100 mg/dl)) targets, which were maintained by an insulin-glucose clamp. The study included 36 children, 9 to 19 years of age (mean = 14.7 years), with diabetes duration more than 2 years (mean = 6.9 years).**
***Results*: Cognitive test performance did not deteriorate during hyperglycemia. In contrast, there was a significant decline in performance on all cognitive tests during mild hypoglycemia. Autonomic symptoms did not change significantly during hyperglycemia or during the rapid return from hyperglycemia to euglycemia. Although significant increments in epinephrine and pancreatic polypeptide levels occurred during mild hypoglycemia, no changes in counterregulatory hormones occurred during hyperglycemia. An exploratory regression analysis demonstrated that changes in mental efficiency were best predicted by increases in pancreatic polypeptide, a marker of autonomic activation.**
***Conclusion*: These results confirm our previous finding that mild hypoglycemia causes transient decrements in cognitive function. In contrast, neither hyperglycemia, nor the rapid drop from acute hyperglycemia to euglycemia, affected symptoms, cognitive function, or counterregulatory hormone secretion. (J Pediatr 1995;126:178-84)**

Increasing evidence suggests that children with insulin-dependent diabetes mellitus may be more sensitive than adults to the effects of changes in plasma glucose levels. In a previous study, we examined the effects of experimentally induced mild hypoglycemia on cognitive functioning in adolescents with diabetes and found that large decrements in performance appeared on a variety of cognitive measures when serum glucose values were lowered to 3.3 to 3.6 mmol/L (60 to 65 mg/dl).[1] Adults, by contrast, rarely have

See related article, p. 171.

IDDM	Insulin-dependent diabetes mellitus
RT	Reaction time

Supported in part by National Institutes of Health grant 5 M01 RR00084, Diabetes Action Research and Education Foundation grant 001, and the Renziehausen Fund.
Submitted for publication July 29, 1994; accepted Oct. 6, 1994.
Reprint requests: Christopher M. Ryan, PhD, Department of Psychiatry, Western Psychiatric Institute and Clinic, University of Pittsburgh School of Medicine, 3811 O'Hara St., Pittsburgh, PA 15213.

0022-3476/95/$3.00 + 0 **9/20/61099**

such large, widespread performance decrements until serum glucose values fall into the moderate hypoglycemia range (2.5 to 2.8 mmol/L; [45 to 50 mg/dl]).[2, 3-8] Differences between adults and children are also apparent in the glycemic threshold for release of counterregulatory hormones and for the occurrence of symptoms of hypoglycemia.[9] Elevated circulating epinephrine levels (and concomitant reports of symptoms) occur at a serum glucose level that is significantly higher in adolescents with diabetes (4.9 mmol/L [88 mg/dl]) than in healthy adolescents (3.8 mmol/L [68 mg/dl]); both of those glycemic levels are higher than those found in healthy adults (3.1 mmol/L [56 mg/dl]),[9] or in adults with diabetes (3.3 mmol/L [59 mg/dl]).[10]

Many patients with IDDM have reported that they can tell when they are in a hyperglycemic state because they "feel different." Although one study of adults with diabetes produced mental slowing when blood glucose levels were increased to 16.7 mmol/L (300 mg/dl),[11] others failed to find a relation between hyperglycemia and mental slowing in adults.[2, 12] To test the hypothesis that acute hyperglycemia in children with diabetes produces a reduction in mental efficiency similar to that occurring during hypoglycemia, we experimentally induced hyperglycemia in a group of children with IDDM. Measures of cognitive test performance, autonomic symptoms, and counterregulatory hormones were obtained periodically and compared with values from groups of demographically similar children with IDDM whose serum glucose levels were clamped at either mild hypoglycemia or euglycemia for the same period. In addition, these responses were evaluated during a rapid return from hyperglycemic to euglycemic levels.

METHODS

Subjects. This study included 36 children with IDDM who were being followed at Children's Hospital of Pittsburgh (CHP) and were admitted for either research purposes, routine diabetes education, or assessment of subclinical complications and metabolic control. All subjects were between the ages of 9 and 19 years and had had diabetes for at least 2 years. Three clamp studies were conducted serially, for a 4-year period, with the hypoglycemia studies completed first and the hyperglycemia studies completed last. The three groups of subjects did not differ significantly in age, sex ratio, Full Scale IQ, duration of diabetes, or the mean glycosylated hemoglobin value in the year before this study (Table I). Cognitive test data from 9 of the 13 subjects participating in the hypoglycemic clamp study were reported previously.[1] Two subjects in the hypoglycemic group and one in the hyperglycemic group were taking L-thyroxine for Hashimoto thyroiditis and were euthyroid at the time of evaluation. This research protocol was

Table I. Demographic characteristics of subjects participating in the three clamp studies

	Hypoglycemia (n = 13)	Euglycemia (n = 10)	Hyperglycemia (n = 13)
Female (%)	54	70	54
Age (yr)	14.4 ± 2.6	15.1 ± 2.9	14.8 ± 2.5
Duration (yr)	6.7 ± 3.1	6.8 ± 4.2	7.2 ± 3.5
HbA_{1c} (%)	10.3 ± 1.4	10.8 ± 1.2	10.8 ± 1.5
Full Scale IQ	106.6 ± 12.8	99.9 ± 10.9	102.0 ± 8.1

Values (except gender) are expressed as mean ± SD.
HbA_{1c}, Glycosylated hemoglobin.

approved by the CHP Human Rights Committee. Informed consent and assent were obtained from the parents and subjects, respectively.

Procedures. Subjects were admitted to the CHP General Clinical Research Center at least 24 hours before the study. All intermediate-acting insulin was omitted the day before the clamp, and metabolic control was maintained with preprandial doses of regular insulin. In the evening before the study, two intravenous catheters, one for blood sampling (dorsal hand vein) and one for infusion of glucose and insulin (antecubital vein), were inserted in the nondominant arm. To achieve overnight euglycemia, we started a variable-rate intravenous infusion of regular pork insulin at 10 PM. The serum glucose concentrations, measured hourly from 2 to 8 AM, ranged from 4.7 to 7.4 mmol/L (mean ± SD, 5.5 ± 1.6 mmol/L) (85 to 133 mg/dl [99 ± 29 mg/dl]). All studies were performed after a 10-hour overnight fast. At 8 AM the intravenous insulin infusion was increased to 0.1 U/kg per hour for the entire duration of the clamp procedure. The serum glucose was maintained at the targeted level with an intravenous infusion of 10% dextrose in water (hypoglycemic or euglycemic clamp studies) or 12.5% dextrose in water (hyperglycemia study). Stable baseline euglycemia was maintained for 45 minutes, and the first cognitive function session was performed during the last 15 minutes (session 1), at least 60 minutes after the insulin infusion rate was increased.

For the hyperglycemia study, hyperglycemia was induced immediately after completion of session 1 by giving an intravenous dose of 25% dextrose in water and increasing the infusion rate of 12.5% dextrose in water. After 15 to 20 minutes, the serum glucose target of 19.4 mmol/L (350 mg/dl) was reached and a second battery of cognitive function tests was completed (session 2). Hyperglycemia was maintained for a total of 60 minutes, and a third session of cognitive tests was performed in the last 15 minutes (session 3). Afterward, the serum glucose concentration was decreased to euglycemia for a 45-minute period by decreasing the infusion rate of dextrose in water. The cognitive function tests were repeated when euglycemia was reached (session 4).

A similar procedure was used for subjects participating in the hypoglycemic clamp. After completion of the baseline (session 1) assessment, the serum glucose concentration was decreased to a target of 3.3 mmol/L (60 mg/dl) by decreasing the intravenous glucose infusion during a 20-minute period; this level was maintained for at least 15 minutes before the cognitive tests were repeated (session 2). For the first six subjects studied, the initial serum glucose target was 3.6 mmol/L (65 mg/dl); it was then lowered further to 3.1 mmol/L (55 mg/dl) for 15 minutes before session 3. Because the results from the two groups did not differ, their data were combined. All subjects were returned to euglycemia during a 15-minute period by increasing the glucose infusion rate. Cognitive tests were repeated (session 4) as soon as the plasma glucose concentration reached 5.0 to 5.5 mmol/L (90 to 100 mg/dl).

In subjects participating in the euglycemia clamp condition, a serum glucose concentration of 5.5 mmol/L (100 mg/dl) was maintained throughout the study, and the subjects were examined at the same time points as subjects in the other two experimental conditions.

For all subjects, blood was obtained from a heated nondominant hand vein at 5-minute intervals for determination of arterialized serum glucose concentrations. Every 15 minutes, blood was obtained for measurement of plasma free insulin, epinephrine, norepinephrine, and pancreatic polypeptide concentrations. Immediately before each test session, subjects were queried with a standard series of questions assessing autonomic and neuroglycopenic symptoms of hypoglycemia. All subjects were masked as to their actual serum glucose levels throughout the studies, and all but the first six subjects studied were unaware of whether they would be participating in a hypoglycemic, hyperglycemic, or euglycemic clamp study.

Assessment measures. Mental efficiency was assessed with three previously validated cognitive tasks: Simple Reaction Time, Choice Reaction Time, and Trail Making. Subjects were given practice with each measure before the baseline assessment in an effort to bring them to a "steady state" level of performance and thereby reduce the practice effects associated with repeated testing. To reduce practice effects further, we used four alternative versions of the Trail Making test; they were randomly distributed across test sessions.

Simple Reaction Time and Choice Reaction Time. Reaction time to visual stimuli was measured with a Lafayette Reaction Time Apparatus (Lafayette Instruments Co. Inc., Lafayette, Ind.). Each trial began with an auditory warning signal, followed by the onset of a colored light. The task was to press a key under the light as quickly as possible. Two blocks of trials (10 blue; 10 green) were presented, with the order of blocks randomized across trials. For the Simple RT task, subjects were informed in advance that the block of trials would be blue or green. This task provides a simple measure of vigilance. For the Choice RT test, subjects were not informed in advance of the color of the stimulus. Ten blue stimulus trials were randomly intermixed with 10 green stimulus trials. This task provides a measure of decision-making efficiency. The median RT in milliseconds was calculated from the 20 Simple RT trials and from the 20 Choice RT trials.[1]

Trail Making test. Mental flexibility and psychomotor efficiency were measured with Part B of this test.[13] The subject was shown 25 circled numbers and letters, randomly placed on a page, and told to draw a line, alternating sequentially between the numbers and letters (e.g., 1-A-2-B). Completion time (in seconds) is the primary outcome measure.

Symptoms. Symptoms of hyperglycemia and hypoglycemia were ascertained before each cognitive test. Subjects indicated the presence or absence of eight symptoms (shaky, sweaty, dizzy, sleepy, hungry, thirsty, heart racing, blurred vision), guessed whether their blood sugar was high, low, or normal, and estimated their blood sugar value.

Laboratory methods. Serum glucose was measured by the glucose oxidase method with a YSI glucose analyzer (Yellow Springs Instrument Co., Inc., Yellow Springs, Ohio). Free insulin levels were measured by treating plasma samples with polyethylene glycol within minutes of blood withdrawal to precipitate antibody-bound insulin.[14] Pancreatic polypeptide was measured with a charcoal radioimmunoassay modified from that of Chance et al.[15] Plasma levels of epinephrine and norepinephrine were determined by a high-pressure liquid chromatographic electrochemical method (LCEC capsule N-46; Bioanalytical Systems Inc., Lafayette, Ind.).[16] Stable glycosylated hemoglobin values were also measured by high-performance liquid chromatography (Diamat; Bio-Rad Laboratories, Chemical Division, Richmond, Calif.). The normal range for our method is 4.9% to 7.3%; the mean value for our IDDM population is 10.1%.

Statistical analyses. Changes in cognitive test scores and hormone levels were examined across the four assessment sessions for the three subject groups with a mixed-model, repeated-measures analysis of variance procedure. If statistically significant interactions were found, analyses of simple main effects were conducted. These were supplemented by single *df* (degrees of freedom) comparisons, when appropriate.[17] All statistical analyses were conducted with *z* scores, which were computed by using the baseline mean and standard deviation values for each of the three clamp groups. To examine the relation between changes in

Table II. Levels of plasma glucose, free insulin, pancreatic polypeptide, and counterregulatory hormones at each assessment session, for each of three clamp conditions

	Session 1	Session 2	Session 3	Session 4
Plasma glucose (mmol/L)*				
Hypoglycemia	5.1 ± 0.1	3.5 ± 0.1	3.3 ± 0.1	5.3 ± 0.1
Euglycemia	5.5 ± 0.2	5.4 ± 0.2	5.2 ± 0.1	5.2 ± 0.1
Hyperglycemia	5.8 ± 0.1	21.1 ± 0.8	20.7 ± 0.4	5.9 ± 0.2
Free insulin (pmol/L)†				
Hypoglycemia	491 ± 33	520 ± 39	499 ± 34	501 ± 31
Euglycemia	517 ± 47	517 ± 43	540 ± 46	532 ± 45
Hyperglycemia	575 ± 56	578 ± 39	569 ± 40	643 ± 55
Pancreatic polypeptide (pmol/L)‡				
Hypoglycemia	15.4 ± 2.9	41.9 ± 13.2	82.3 ± 25.5	34.7 ± 7.9
Euglycemia	15.5 ± 2.1	16.2 ± 1.8	17.5 ± 2.6	18.8 ± 2.5
Hyperglycemia	12.2 ± 2.6	10.4 ± 1.4	14.9 ± 2.2	18.3 ± 3.1
Epinephrine (pmol/L)§				
Hypoglycemia	1138 ± 184	1617 ± 336	2407 ± 424	1363 ± 204
Euglycemia	1293 ± 163	1394 ± 289	1165 ± 154	1526 ± 193
Hyperglycemia	1251 ± 119	1179 ± 98	1131 ± 58	1088 ± 50
Norepinephrine (nmol/L)‖				
Hypoglycemia	1.57 ± 0.21	1.55 ± 0.13	1.59 ± 0.16	1.63 ± 0.12
Euglycemia	2.03 ± 0.47	1.73 ± 0.38	2.17 ± 0.54	2.13 ± 0.58
Hyperglycemia	1.57 ± 0.80	1.44 ± 0.07	1.43 ± 0.05	1.21 ± 0.08

Values are expressed as mean ± SE.
*Conversion to milligrams per deciliter: 18.0.
†Conversion to microunits per milliliter: 0.167.
‡Conversion to picograms per milliliter: 4.18.
§Conversion to picograms per milliliter: 0.183.
‖Conversion to picograms per milliliter: 169.

hormone release and changes in mental efficiency, we conducted exploratory stepwise regression analyses. All data analyses were run on BMDP (PC-90[18]) statistical software. Unless otherwise noted, values are presented as mean ± SE.

RESULTS

Serum glucose levels. Glucose values for each of the three experimental clamp conditions, at each of the four assessment sessions, are summarized in Table II.

Plasma free insulin. Values for free insulin are also listed in Table II. There were no significant differences between groups or across sessions, nor was there a significant interaction between group and session (all p values >0.15).

Pancreatic polypeptide. Significant increases in pancreatic polypeptide (Table II) were restricted to subjects in the hypoglycemic clamp condition ($p < 0.0001$). Further analyses showed that those subjects had a significant increase in pancreatic polypeptide between sessions 1 and 2 ($p = 0.05$) and between sessions 2 and 3 ($p = 0.03$). Although there was a significant decrease between sessions 3 and 4 ($p = 0.02$), the value at session 4 was higher than the value of pancreatic polypeptide at baseline ($p = 0.009$).

Epinephrine. Only subjects in the hypoglycemia clamp condition had a significant increase in epinephrine release (Table II) ($p < 0.0001$). Specifically, epinephrine levels increased significantly between sessions 2 and 3 ($p = 0.0009$), and decreased significantly between sessions 3 and 4 ($p = 0.008$). By session 4, epinephrine values had returned to baseline levels.

Norepinephrine. Significant changes in norepinephrine release (Table II) were restricted to subjects in the hyperglycemic condition ($p < 0.0001$). Further analyses demonstrated that those changes occurred between sessions 3 and 4 ($p = 0.01$). By session 4, norepinephrine levels were significantly lower than baseline values ($p = 0.006$).

In summary, free insulin values remained stable across sessions for all groups of subjects. The pattern of release for both pancreatic polypeptide and epinephrine differed between hypoglycemic clamp conditions and either the euglycemic or hyperglycemic clamps. Hypoglycemia was associated with a sharp increase in pancreatic polypeptide and epinephrine, followed by a sharp decline when euglycemia was restored. In contrast, during the hyperglycemia clamp, there was no increase in release of either pancreatic polypeptide or epinephrine as glucose levels changed. There was, however, a significant decline in norepinephrine levels between the end of the hyperglycemic plateau and the restoration of euglycemia. During the euglycemic clamp, there were no changes in counterregulatory hormone release across time.

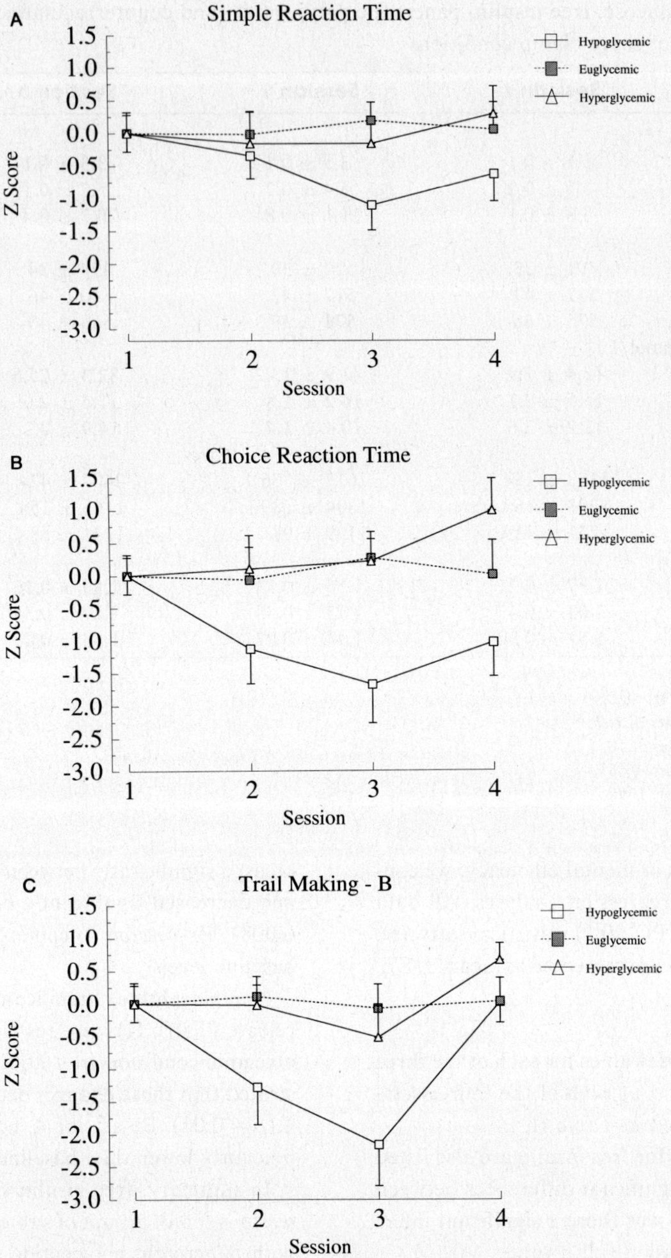

Fig. 1. Effects (mean ± SE) of three different clamps (hypoglycemic; euglycemic; hyperglycemic) on three cognitive tests (**A,** Simple RT; **B,** Choice RT; **C,** Trail Making, Part B) at four assessment periods. Raw scores have been converted into *z* scores, with mean and SD data from all subjects at session 1.

Simple reaction time (Fig. 1). A significant slowing in response time was limited to subjects in the hypoglycemic clamp condition ($p = 0.02$). Within that group, the only significant change in performance occurred between sessions 2 and 3 ($p = 0.0001$). That is, by the end of the hypoglycemic nadir, Simple RT scores were significantly slower than at baseline ($p = 0.0002$). At the return to euglycemia (session 4), performance continued to be slower than at baseline ($p = 0.05$). Hyperglycemia had no effect on performance.

Choice reaction time (Fig. 1). Changes in performance occurred in both the hypoglycemic clamp condition ($p = 0.001$) and the hyperglycemic clamp condition ($p = 0.05$). Contrasts within the hypoglycemic group indicated that performance became significantly slower between sessions 1 and 2 ($p = 0.007$). At session 4, subjects in the hypogly-

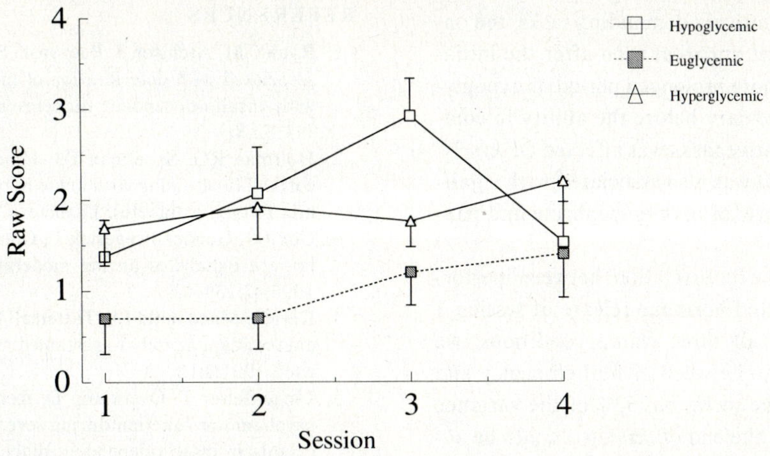

Fig. 2. Effects (mean ± SE) of three different clamps (hypoglycemic; euglycemic; hyperglycemic) on mean number of symptoms reported by subjects at each of four assessment periods.

cemic clamp condition continued to perform more slowly than they did at baseline ($p = 0.01$), even though glucose levels had been restored to the baseline euglycemia values. Contrasts within the hyperglycemic group indicated *improvement* in performance between sessions 3 and 4 ($p = 0.05$).

Trail Making, Part B (Fig. 1). Significant changes across sessions occurred in both the hypoglycemia study ($p < 0.00001$) and the hyperglycemia study ($p = 0.05$). Within-group contrasts indicated a significant decrement in performance for subjects in the hypoglycemic condition between sessions 1 and 2 ($p = 0.02$), and a significant improvement from session 3 to 4 ($p = 0.003$). By session 4, performance had recovered to baseline values ($p = 0.90$). Within the hyperglycemic group, a significant improvement in performance was noted between sessions 3 and 4 ($p = 0.008$). Nevertheless, performance during session 4 was not significantly faster than at baseline ($p = 0.10$).

Relation between cognitive test scores and metabolic measures. Two exploratory stepwise regression analyses were undertaken to determine whether changes in cognitive efficiency from baseline to session 3 (indexed by *z* scores at session 3) were associated with changes in free insulin, pancreatic polypeptide, or catecholamine levels. Change in Choice RT was found to be predicted best by change in pancreatic polypeptide level ($R^2 = 0.377$; $p < 0.0001$) and by change in epinephrine level ($R^2 = 0.07$; p 0.05). Together, those two predictor variables accounted for 44.7% of the variance in the Choice RT change at session 3. Change in Trail Making, Part B, performance could be best predicted by change in pancreatic polypeptide level ($R^2 = 0.42$; $p < 0.00001$) and by the child's age (R^2 change $= 0.18$; $p < 0.0001$). Those two variables explained 60.3% of the variance in the Part B change at session 3.

Symptoms. In general, the number of symptoms detected for any group was very small. Although there were significant changes in symptoms across sessions ($p = 0.02$), there were no significant differences between groups ($p = 0.08$), nor was there a significant group × session interaction ($p > 0.10$) (Fig. 2). All subjects were also asked whether they felt "different" (low; high). By session 3, 11 of 13 subjects in the hypoglycemic clamp study reported feeling "low"; in contrast, only one euglycemic clamp subject and only one hyperglycemic clamp subject reported feeling "different."

DISCUSSION

We found no compelling support for the hypothesis that acute hyperglycemia is associated with a transient decline in mental efficiency in children. Similarly, experimental hyperglycemia was not associated with an increase in the number of autonomic symptoms reported. However, restoration of euglycemia was associated with a significant *improvement* in mental efficiency; this finding is somewhat difficult to interpret because the initiation of hyperglycemia was not associated with a significant decline in performance. Given the absence of a significant change in performance across sessions within the euglycemic clamp condition, it is unlikely that this improvement within the hyperglycemic group is a consequence of practice effects. The only notable metabolic change was a significant decrease in norepinephrine levels, which occurred between the end of the hyperglycemic plateau and restoration of euglycemia. There was no evidence of counterregulatory hormone release nor symptoms suggestive of hypoglycemia. Moreover, there was no deterioration in cognitive function during the rapid drop from hyperglycemia to euglycemia.

On the other hand, as we reported previously,[1] mild hypoglycemia was associated with a significant reduction in mental efficiency. For cognitively demanding tasks, the onset of this change was most apparent soon after the initiation of hypoglycemia. A more prolonged period of hypoglycemia appeared to be necessary before the ability to complete less demanding cognitive tasks was affected adversely. The onset of hypoglycemia was also associated with significant increases in the release of both epinephrine and pancreatic polypeptide.

When we examined the interrelation between performance on cognitive tests and hormone release at session 3 for subjects drawn from all three clamp conditions, we found a robust relationship between mental efficiency and counterregulatory hormone secretion; 60% of the variance in Trail Making scores at the end of session 3 could be accounted for by the subject's age and the magnitude of increase in pancreatic polypeptide between the euglycemia baseline and the end of the hypoglycemia nadir. Younger subjects who had a relatively large increase in pancreatic polypeptide secretion were most likely to have the greatest deterioration on this cognitive test. Similarly, Choice RT was also influenced significantly by pancreatic polypeptide release. Although a significant relation was also found between epinephrine release and Choice RT scores, the magnitude of this effect was very small. Because of the exploratory nature of these regression analyses (i.e., conducted post hoc, with a relatively small sample and the use of a relatively large number of predictor variables), we are hesitant to overinterpret these findings. However, there does appear to be a relation between markers of autonomic nervous system activation and cognitive function. This requires further study and explanation.

In our previous study,[1] patients served as their own control subjects; performance during hypoglycemia was compared with the individual's performance during a euglycemic baseline. In this study, we compared performance during hypoglycemia with that of a demographically similar group of patients who were maintained at a euglycemic level for the same period. This paradigm, which controls for practice and fatigue effects, again demonstrates that even mild hypoglycemia can produce significant decrements in mental efficiency. In contrast, we found no effect of acute hyperglycemia or the rapid drop from acute hyperglycemia to euglycemia on symptoms, cognitive function, or counterregulatory hormone secretion. We therefore conclude that acute hyperglycemia (or the rapid excursion from hyperglycemia to euglycemia) causes no symptoms in this population.

We thank Theresa Williams, Pat Way, and Tomi Waters for technical assistance, and the nursing staff of the CHP General Clinical Research Center for excellent assistance during glucose clamps.

REFERENCES

1. Ryan CM, Atchison J, Puczynski S, et al. Mild hypoglycemia associated with deterioration of mental efficiency in children with insulin-dependent diabetes mellitus. J PEDIATR 1990; 117:32-8.
2. Hoffman RG, Speelman DJ, Hinnen DA, et al. Changes in cortical functioning with acute hypoglycemia and hyperglycemia in type I diabetes. Diabetes Care 1989;12:193-7.
3. Cox DJ, Gonder-Frederick L, Clarke W. Driving decrements in type I diabetes during moderate hypoglycemia. Diabetes 1993;42:239-43.
4. Kerr D, Macdonald IA, Tattersall RB. Patients with type I diabetes adapt acutely to sustained mild hypoglycaemia. Diabet Med 1991;8:123-8.
5. Lingenfelser T, Overkamp D, Renn W, et al. Cognitive and psychomotor function during severe insulin-induced hypoglycaemia in insulin-dependent diabetic patients. Neuropsychobiology 1992;25:161-5.
6. Widom B, Simonson DC. Glycemic control and neuropsychologic function during hypoglycemia in patients with insulin-dependent diabetes mellitus. Ann Intern Med 1990;112:904-12.
7. Wirsén A, Tallroth G, Lindgren M, Agardh C-D. Neuropsychological performance differs between type I diabetic and normal men during insulin-induced hypoglycaemia. Diabet Med 1992;9:156-65.
8. Mokan M, Mitrakou A, Veneman T, et al. Hypoglycemia unawareness in insulin-dependent diabetes mellitus. Diabetes Care 1994;17:1397-1403.
9. Jones TW, Boulware SD, Kraemer DT, et al. Independent effects of youth and poor diabetes control in responses to hypoglycemia in children. Diabetes 1991;40:358-63.
10. Boyle PJ, Schwartz NS, Shah SD, Clutter WE, Cryer PE. Plasma glucose concentrations at the onset of hypoglycemic symptoms in patients with poorly controlled diabetes and in nondiabetics. N Engl J Med 1988;318:1487-92.
11. Holmes CS, Hayford JT, Gonzalez JL, Weydert JA. A survey of cognitive functioning at different glucose levels in diabetic persons. Diabetes Care 1983;6:180-5.
12. Holmes CS, Koepke KM, Thompson RG. Simple versus complex performance impairments at three blood glucose levels. Psychoneuroendocrinology 1986;11:353-7.
13. Boll TJ, Barth JT. Halstead-Reitan neuropsychology battery. In: Filskov SB, Boll TJ, eds. Handbook of clinical neuropsychology. New York: John Wiley & Sons, 1981:577-607.
14. Nakagawa S, Nakayama H, Sasaki T, et al. A simple method for the determination of serum free insulin levels in insulin-treated patients. Diabetes 1973;22:590-600.
15. Chance RE, Moon NE, Johnson MG. Human pancreatic polypeptide (HPP) and bovine pancreatic polypeptide (BPP). In: Jaffe BM, Behrman HR, eds. Methods of hormone radioimmunoassay. New York: Academic Press, 1979:657-72.
16. Lin PYT, Bulawa MC, Wong P, et al. The determination of catecholamines, indoleamines, metabolites, and related enzymatic activities using three micron liquid chromatography columns. J Liquid Chromatogr 1984;7:509-38.
17. Keppel G. Design and analysis: a researcher's handbook. New Jersey: Prentice-Hall, 1973.
18. Dixon WJ, Brown MB, Engleman L, Jennrich RI. BMDP statistical software manual; vol 2. Berkeley: University of California Press, 1990.

Subsequent insect stings in children with hypersensitivity to Hymenoptera

Pia Hauk, MD, Katrin Friedl, Klaus Kaufmehl, MD, Radvan Urbanek, MD, and Johannes Forster, MD

From University Children's Hospitals, Freiburg, Germany, and Vienna, Austria

To investigate the risk of life-threatening reactions to future stings, we sequentially challenged 113 children (aged 2 to 17 years) allergic to insect stings with a sting by the relevant insect. The time interval between the challenges varied from 2 to 6 weeks. The history of the index stings was a large local reaction (LR) in 16% and a systemic reaction (SR) in 84% of the test subjects. On the first challenge, 76% had a normal LR, 11% a large LR, and 13% an SR. On the second challenge, 78% of the children had a normal LR, 5% a large LR, and 17% an SR. Thirty-nine of the untreated children were exposed to a field sting during the subsequent 3-year follow-up period. In comparison with other diagnostic evaluations such as skin-prick tests, determinations of specific IgE and IgG antibodies, and single-sting exposure, the dual sting challenge scheme appears to be the best predictor of reactions to subsequent stings. It also appears to be helpful in selecting patients with an uncertain sensitization status for venom immunotherapy. (J Pediatr 1995;126:185-90)

In childhood, allergy to Hymenoptera venom is mainly caused by stings of honeybees and wasps. In Europe, yellow jackets are known as "wasps," whereas in the United States, Polistes wasps are known as "wasps."[1] Between 0.4% and 4% of the population have systemic allergic reactions to insect stings.[2-4] The incidence of systemic reactions to subsequent stings is lower in children and adolescents than in adults.[5-8] Prospective observations of the natural course of insect allergy show that adults have a risk of 27% to 57%[3, 9-11] of having repeated systemic allergic reactions, in comparison with a risk of 10% to 20% in children.[4-6, 8] Therefore venom immunotherapy should be indicated less frequently in children.[8] In vitro assays and risk scores provide only limited help in identifying those patients at risk of having further life-threatening allergic reactions. Numerous studies[12-15] have been unsuccessful in showing a correlation between the standard diagnostic methods—mainly skin-prick tests and measurements of specific IgE and IgG antibodies—and the reactions to subsequent insect stings. Treatment recommendations based only on those criteria typically lead to an overestimation of the number of children who require venom immunotherapy.[6, 8, 16]

Although single diagnostic sting challenges give additional information, there is increasing concern about the possible booster effect. From the natural history of bee venom allergy, we know that one sting followed by another 2 to 4 weeks later will result in the highest incidence of systemic reactions. We tried to mimic this naturally occurring event by subjecting test subjects to sequential sting challenges to detect the group of patients at highest risk. Those who did not react and therefore were not assigned to receive venom immunotherapy were followed for up to 3 years for life-threatening events after natural stings.

See commentary, p. 257.

AU	Arbitrary unit(s)
LR	Local reaction
SR	Systemic reaction

Submitted for publication April 15, 1994; accepted Aug. 10, 1994.

Reprint requests: Johannes Forster, MD, University Children's Hospital, Mathildenstr. 1, D-79106 Freiburg, Germany.

0022-3476/95/$3.00 + 0 **9/20/59779**

Table I. Score estimating the risk of subsequent sting reactions used for recommendation of venom immunotherapy[17]

	Risk points	
	1	2
Reaction to index sting	Large LR, moderate SR	Severe SR
Skin-prick test (100 μg/ml venom)	Wheal diameter <3 mm	Wheal diameter ≥3 mm
Specific IgE (RAST)	Class 1	Classes 2-4

Recommendation for venom immunotherapy: ≥5 points.
RAST, Radioallergosorbent test.

Table II. Baseline characteristics of patients

Index sting reaction	n	Age (yr): median; range	Male/ female	Risk score ≥5 points
Large LR	18	9; 2-17	12/6	4
Moderate SR	57	8; 3-16	33/24	12
Severe SR	38	9; 3-15	26/12	21
TOTAL	113			37*

*Scored (37/91) as "at higher risk" of having a life-threatening reaction at first visit.

METHODS

From 1988 to 1991, a total of 71 boys and 42 girls aged 2 to 17 years (median, 9 years) with "insect allergy" were recruited from the outpatient clinic to undergo sequential sting challenges. Only children with large local reactions and systemic but not life-threatening reactions were included in this study. The initial evaluation consisted of a medical and allergic history with emphasis on prior insect sting reactions, a physical examination, venom skin testing, and venom-specific IgE and IgG antibody measurements. Furthermore, the patients were graded according to their risk score[17] (Table I), on which recommendations for venom immunotherapy are based in Germany.[18]

Venom skin testing. Skin-prick testing was performed with purified bee and wasp venom (ALK-prick SQ; ALK/Scherax, Hamburg, Germany) on the flexor surface of the forearm at concentrations of 0.1, 1, 10, and 100 μg/ml. Negative (diluent) and positive (histamine, 10 mg/ml) controls were also applied. The diameter of the wheal present 20 minutes after administration was measured. At a venom concentration of 100 μg/ml, a wheal diameter of <3 mm was considered a positive result and ≥3 mm a strongly positive result.

Antibody measurements. IgE antibodies to whole bee and wasp venom were measured by the radioallergosorbent test (Pharmacia AB, Uppsala, Sweden) and were expressed as classes 1 to 4. IgG antibodies were measured with enzyme-linked immunosorbent assay.[19] Results were expressed as low (bee venom <400 AU; wasp venom <25 AU) or high (bee venom ≥400 AU; wasp venom ≥25 AU). Blood samples for the determination of IgE and IgG antibodies were taken from each patient on the days on which the first and second challenge stings were performed.

Classification of hypersensitivity reaction. Depending on the clinical history, sensitized patients (positive skin-prick test result or specific IgE antibodies to bee or wasp venom) were placed into one of the following categories: large LR: an LR with redness and swelling >10 cm in diameter and lasting longer than 24 hours; moderate SRs: skin symptoms (general urticaria, redness, itching), angioedema, and gastrointestinal symptoms; and severe SRs: respiratory symptoms (wheezing, shortness of breath) and mainly cardiovascular symptoms (hypotension, collapse, cardiac arrhythmias).

Sequential sting challenges. The sting challenges were carried out by placing live insects on the flexor side of the forearm during intensive medical observation and with an intravenous line already in place. The second challenge was performed 2 to 6 weeks after the first challenge. A second challenge was omitted and venom immunotherapy was started if the patient had a severe SR on the first challenge and his or her parents agreed with the recommendation for treatment.

The procedure was approved by the medical ethics committee of the university, and informed consent was obtained from the parents, in particular with respect to the possible booster effect.

Follow-up. During the summer of 1992, all the patients and their parents underwent a structured telephone interview regarding reactions to subsequent field stings. Patients of both groups and their family doctors were instructed to send a serum sample for the determination of specific IgE and IgG antibodies 4 weeks after a subsequent insect sting. Only eight patients not undergoing immunotherapy sent serum samples irregularly, between 1 month and 3 years after the sequential challenge, when they were restung. All 11 patients undergoing venom immunotherapy treatment sent serum samples every 3 to 6 months.

Statistical analysis. We carried out statistical analysis with the SPSS-PC program (chi-square test of Pearson, Kruskal-Wallis test, one-way analysis of variance, logistic regression analysis) (SPSS Inc., Chicago, Ill.). The data obtained were compared to establish statistically significant differences ($p < 0.05$) between groups of patients showing different types of reactions.

Table III. Severity and number of clinical reactions to sting challenges in comparison with the index sting

Clinical reaction	Index sting reported	Bee and wasp sting challenges	
		First challenge	Second challenge
Normal LR	–	95	98
Severe LR	18	14	6
Moderate SR	57	14	10
Severe SR	38	2	11
Total	113	125	125

RESULTS

Baseline characteristics of patients are shown in Table II. Patients who had shown different types of index sting reactions had no significant differences in the results of skin-prick tests and measurements of specific IgE and IgG antibody levels (data not shown). Of 113 subjects, the tests of 91 could be scored according to the described risk score (Table I): 41% (37/91) were classified as at risk, with a score of ≥5 points. Thirty percent (34/113) had been sensitized to bee venom, 5% (6/113) to wasp venom, and 65% (73/113) to both. Sixteen percent of the children (18/113) had reported large LRs and 84% (95/113) SRs to the index sting.

Sting challenges. Monosensitized patients were sequentially challenged with the relevant insect only. In 61 of 73 doubly sensitized children, the sequential challenge was performed with the insect of clinical relevance on the basis of the history, the more prominent reaction to the skin-prick test, or a higher specific IgE concentration. Of the 73 patients, 12 were sequentially challenged by a bee and a wasp on 2 consecutive days.

First challenge. The time interval between the index sting and the first challenge varied from 2 weeks to 73½ months. This interval was not correlated with the reaction to the challenge.

One hundred thirteen patients were challenged with 125 stings (Table III). Of the bee venom–allergic patients, 69.2% (63/91) had a normal LR, 13.2% (12/91) a large LR, and 17.6% (16/91) an SR. The wasp challenges resulted in local reactions only. None of the children with large LRs or moderate SRs, or both, received venom immunotherapy after the first challenge, and therefore all of them were included in the second-challenge study group. In two children who had a severe SR, venom immunotherapy was advised but the recommendation was not accepted. At their parents' request, both were stung a second time.

Second challenge. The second challenge was performed 2 to 6 weeks after the first challenge. The time interval between the first and the second challenge did not influence the reaction to the second challenge.

Table IV. Severity and number of clinical reactions to subsequent field stings in children without immunotherapy 2 weeks to 35 months (median, 14½ months) after the sequential challenges in comparison with the index sting

Grade of clinical reaction	Index sting reported	Field sting reactions*
Normal LR	–	35
Severe LR	18	2
Moderate SR	57	1
Severe SR	38	1†
Total	113	39

*According to the standardized interview.
†Mild respiratory symptoms.

One hundred thirteen patients again were challenged with 125 stings (Table III). After the second challenge sting, 72.5% (66/91) of the bee venom–allergic patients had a normal LR and 6.6% (6/91) a large LR. In 20.9% (19/91) a systemic reaction occurred, which in 10 cases (11%) was severe. Only two SRs (6%) occurred among the wasp venom–allergic children, one of which was severe (3%). Those 11 children with a severe SR to the second challenge underwent subsequent venom immunotherapy. Of these 11 patients, 8 had a history of severe SRs and repeated severe SRs in the second challenge. Both children who had a severe SR to the first challenge had a local reaction to the second challenge. Once again, their parents refused venom immunotherapy.

Children not recommended for venom immunotherapy were carefully instructed in the use of emergency self-treatment kits containing clemastine tablets or syrup and an epinephrine inhaler.

We found no correlation between the grade of the reactions to sting challenges and the results of the initial skin-prick test, the initial IgE and IgG antibody concentrations, and the levels of specific antibodies during the challenges (data not shown).

Field stings. Between 2 weeks and 35 months after the challenge procedure, 45 (40%) of the 113 challenged children were stung in the field by the relevant insect. Of the patients who received venom immunotherapy, one had a moderate SR with only urticaria, which was treated with orally administered clemastine. The other five had LRs only. One of these used clemastine locally, and one orally for an extended swelling. Of the 39 patients not assigned to receive venom immunotherapy, only two had SRs (Table IV). One girl who had a history of severe SRs before the sequential challenge was restung on the foot 16 months after the second challenge. She was treated by a physician with

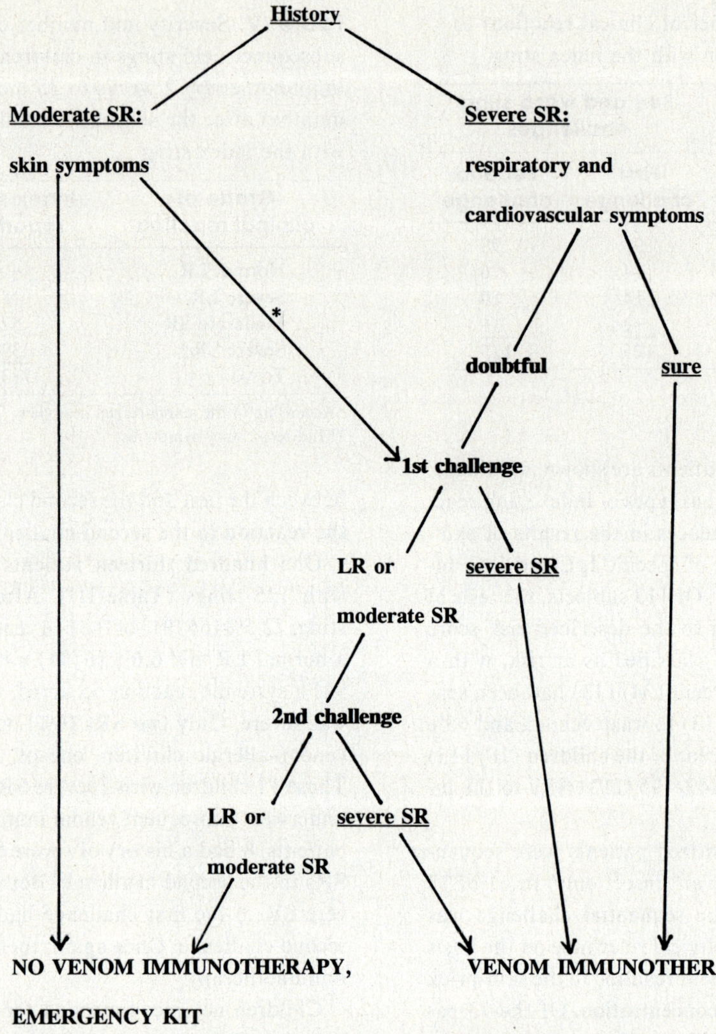

Figure. Diagnostic and therapeutic procedure in sensitized insect sting–allergic children and adolescents (positive skin-prick test result and/or specific IgE) with previous SRs. *Asterisk* indicates patient's request.

orally administered clemastine for urticaria 30 minutes after the sting. The other child had a history of moderate SRs and was restung on the forearm 14 months after the second provocation. This child was treated after 10 minutes with orally administered clemastine and subcutaneously administered terbutaline, because urticaria and mild respiratory symptoms developed. Venom immunotherapy was commenced subsequently.

The reaction to the first challenge was not predictive of the reaction either to the second challenge or to field stings. On the basis of the reaction to the second challenge, one of 39 patients had been misclassified as belonging to the group not recommended for venom immunotherapy. Thus the prediction that a severe systemic reaction would not occur was correct in 38 children (97.4% = negative predictive value; 95% confidence interval, 86.5 to 99.9).[20]

Doubly sensitized children were not more likely to have severe reactions to subsequent field stings. Whether those individuals were sensitized to multiple insects or had a cross-reactivity among venom proteins was not investigated.

Follow-up of sensitization markers. Patients receiving venom immunotherapy had a typical course of specific IgE and IgG antibodies[21] during the treatment. Patients who received no immunotherapy had changes in specific IgE and IgG antibodies dependent on subsequent stings that were not correlated with the sting reaction (data not shown).

DISCUSSION

In childhood, the benign natural history of allergy to Hymenoptera stings and the lack of correlation between the index sting and standard diagnostic methods leave the treating physician without precise criteria in determining whether an individual child should receive venom immunotherapy. We tried to separate the endangered insect venom–allergic children from those with a mild or transient hypersensitivity by subjecting them to sequential insect sting challenges within a period of 2 to 6 weeks. This particular period was chosen to include a possible booster effect of the first sting in the evaluation of individual reactivity. Mueller et al.[22] have shown that the highest grade of sensitization in terms of specific IgE levels is to be expected 2 to 4 weeks after a sting event. Therefore an additional sting at this time is the most dangerous situation that can arise for an insect venom–allergic person. Our patients faced such situations under ideal medical surveillance; consequently, none of them had any acute or permanent sequelae. Sequential challenge stings are generally not recommended in adults because they pose a higher risk of severe SRs in older patients.[10, 14]

In agreement with others who have investigated the natural course of insect allergy by prospective observations[5-8] or single-challenge tests,[11, 12] we demonstrated a lower frequency of subsequent SRs than expected on the basis of history or predicted by in vitro sensitization markers, or both. Valentine et al.[8] found that children whose allergic SRs had been only cutaneous have a risk of about 10% of having SRs to future stings, which was comparable to our data.

After the index sting, 16% of our bee and wasp venom–allergic children had a large LR and 84% an SR. In the sequential challenge, reversed percentages were obtained, and this result was confirmed with the second bee sting challenge. In the first challenge, all wasp sting–allergic children had LRs only; on the second provocation, SRs occurred in 6%. Thus wasp sting–allergic children were less likely to have repeated SRs. The latter finding might be at least partly explained by the different amount of venom applied by one wasp sting. This difference seems to be more pronounced in wasp stings than in bee stings,[23] because wasps are able to sting several times. Although there were more severe reactions in the group of children who required immunotherapy according to our assessment, no significant correlation could be detected between the reactions to the index sting and to the challenge stings, or between the reactions to the index sting and to the field sting.

We also confirmed the results of other studies,[12-15] which revealed the disappointing correlation between standard diagnostic methods—mainly skin-prick tests and measurement of specific IgE and IgG antibodies—and the reactions of an allergic individual to further insect stings. Because the level of specific IgE and IgG antibodies did not correlate with the concomitant sting reaction at any time during the study or the follow-up period, we have not shown these data in detail. Neither was it possible to use these tests to determine whether one or more subsequent stings could have induced immunity in the subjects. There is no in vitro test to examine the possibility of stimulating a protective state by administering sequential sting challenges; thus clinical immunity can be demonstrated only by the clinical reactions to subsequent field stings by patients not receiving venom immunotherapy.

Methods of treating insect-sting allergy recommended by the committee on insects of the European Academy of Allergy and Clinical Immunology[24] are based on standard diagnostic methods. Venom immunotherapy is recommended for those sensitized patients who have had a systemic allergic reaction more severe than skin symptoms only. This criterion corresponds to the result of the risk score mentioned above. Considering the previous reaction to the index sting and the results of skin-prick tests and venom-specific IgE measurements as criteria for the recommendation of venom immunotherapy, 41% of the scored bee venom– and wasp venom–allergic children would have been assigned to this treatment, but only 9% received venom immunotherapy as a result of the clinical reaction to the second challenge. Although this procedure may appear very invasive, children eventually benefit because the risk and inconvenience of 3 to 5 years of immunotherapy can be avoided in four of five current candidates for venom immunotherapy. The reliability of the sequential challenge procedure was evaluated by assessment of the reactions to subsequent stings in children who were not assigned to venom immunotherapy (large LR and moderate SR to second challenge). In our patients, this test had a negative predictive value of 97.4% (confidence interval, 86.5 to 99.9) for subsequent life-threatening reactions. Although this is not a 100% safety record, we believe that the sequential insect sting challenge performed in the hospital represents the safest and most informative method of eliminating unnecessary venom immunotherapy in children having mild to moderate SRs to an index sting. However, the procedure should be performed only by well-trained staff with intensive care facilities at hand.

On the basis of the data presented, we suggest the following diagnostic and therapeutic procedures for children up to 16 years of age: Sensitized patients, identified by a positive skin-prick test result or specific IgE finding, who had only a large LR to the index sting, need neither a challenge sting nor venom immunotherapy. However, if parents insist on treatment, the challenge can be used in an effort to convince them that venom immunotherapy is not necessary. In sensitized patients with a previous moderate SR with generalized skin symptoms, sting challenges and venom immunotherapy are not indicated, but these patients should carry an emergency kit.[6, 8] All sensitized patients who have life-threatening SRs should undergo venom immunotherapy without previous challenges. However, the challenge procedure can be offered to estimate the patient's individual risk to demonstrate the necessity of venom immunotherapy (Figure). Patients who are not sensitized to any insect venom according to standard tests but who have had a systemic allergic reaction to an insect sting should in any case be challenged to reveal their risk of having life-threatening reactions to the insect in question.

REFERENCES

1. Schmidt JO. Let's not forget crawling Hymenoptera. Clin Exp Allergy 1994;24:511-4.
2. Golden BK, Marsh DG, Kagey-Sobotka A, et al. Epidemiology of insect venom sensitivity. JAMA 1989;262:240-4.
3. Kampelmacher MJ, van der Zwan JC. Provocation test with a living insect as a diagnostic tool in systemic reactions to bee or wasp venom: a prospective study with emphasis on clinical aspects. Clin Allergy 1987;17:317-27.
4. Settipane GA, Chafee FH. Natural history of allergy to Hymenoptera. Clin Allergy 1979;9:385-90.
5. Graft DF, Schuberth KC, Kagey-Sobotka A, et al. A prospective study of the natural history of large local reactions after Hymenoptera stings in children. J PEDIATR 1984;104:664-8.
6. Schuberth KC, Lichtenstein LM, Kagey-Sobotka A, Szklo M, Kwiterovich KA, Valentine MD. Epidemiologic study of insect allergy in children. II. Effect of accidental stings in allergic children. J PEDIATR 1983;102:361-5.
7. Valentine MD, Golden DBK. Diagnosis of insect allergy. In: Levine MI, Lockey RF, eds. Monograph on insect allergy. Pittsburgh: Lambert Association, 1986;6:39-43.
8. Valentine MD, Schuberth KC, Kagey-Sobotka A, et al. The value of immunotherapy with venom in children with allergy to insect stings. N Engl J Med 1990;323:1601-3.
9. Hunt KJ, Valentine MD, Sobotka AK, Benton AW, Amodio FJ, Lichtenstein LM. A controlled trial of immunotherapy in insect hypersensitivity. N Engl J Med 1978;299:157-61.
10. Reisman RE, Dvorin DJ, Randolph CC, Georgitis JW. Stinging insect allergy: natural history and modification with venom immunotherapy. J Allergy Clin Immunol 1985;76:735-40.
11. Van der Linden PWG, Struyvenberg A, Kraaijenhagen RJ, Hack CE, Van der Zwan JK. Anaphylactic shock after insect-sting challenge in 138 persons with a previous insect-sting reaction. Ann Intern Med 1993;118:161-8.
12. Blaauw PJ, Smithuis LOMJ. The evaluation of the common diagnostic methods of hypersensitivity for bee and yellow jacket venom by means of an in-hospital insect sting. J Allergy Clin Immunol 1985;75:556-62.
13. Heinig JH, Engel T, Weeke ER. Allergy to venom from bee or wasp: the relation between clinical and immunological reactions to insect stings. Clin Allergy 1988;18:71-8.
14. Parker JL, Santrach PJ, Dahlberg MJE, Yuninger JW. Evaluation of Hymenoptera-sting sensitivity with deliberate sting challenges: inadequacy of present diagnostic methods. J Allergy Clin Immunol 1982;69:200-7.
15. Reisman RE, Lazell M, Arbesman CE. Insect venom allergy: a prospective case showing the lack of correlation between immunologic reactivity and clinical sensitivity. J Allergy Clin Immunol 1981;68:406-8.
16. Forster J, Eckes A, Hauk P, Urbanek R. Spezielle Probleme der Insektengift-Allergie im Kindesalter. Allerg Immunol 1991;37:59-62.
17. Urbanek R. Criteria for starting and stopping venom-immunotherapy. In: Bostroem H, Ljungstedt N, eds. Theoretical and clinical aspects of allergic diseases. Stockholm, Sweden: Almgvist & Wiksell, 1982:289-96.
18. Ring J, Forck G, Frosch P, et al. Richtlinien für die Diagnose und Behandlung von Überempfindlichkeitsreaktionen auf Bienen- und Wespenstiche. Allergologie 1989;1:43-5.
19. Forster J, Urbanek R. Enzyme-linked immunosorbent assay of allergen-specific IgG antibodies in bee sting allergic patients hyposensitized with pure bee venom. Klin Wochenschr 1979; 57:421-2.
20. Wissenschaftliche Tabellen Geigy. 8th ed. Basel: Ciba Geigy, 1980:91.
21. Thurnheer U, Mueller U, Stoller R, Lanner A, Hoigné R. Venom immunotherapy in Hymenoptera sting allergy. Allergy 1983;38:465-75.
22. Mueller U, Spiess J, Roth A. Serological investigations in Hymenoptera sting allergy: IgE and haemagglutinating antibodies against bee venom in patients with bee sting allergy, beekeepers and nonallergic blood donors. Clin Allergy 1977;7:57-64.
23. Schumacher MJ, Schmidt JO, Egen NB, Dhillon KA. Biochemical variability of venom from individual European and Africanized honeybees *(Apis mellifera)*. J Allergy Clin Immunol 1992;90:59-65.
24. Mueller U, Mosbech H, and other members of the Subcommittee on Insect Venom Allergy, European Academy of Allergy and Clinical Immunology. Immunotherapy with Hymenoptera venoms [Position paper]. Allergy 1993;48(suppl 14):37-46.

Relation between infant feeding and infections during the first six months of life

Micheline Beaudry, PDt, MNS, PhD, Renée Dufour, MSc, and Sylvie Marcoux, MD, PhD

From the Département de nutrition humaine et de consommation, Faculté des sciences de l'agriculture et de l'alimentation, and the Département de médecine sociale et préventive, Faculté de médecine, Université Laval, Sainte-Foy, Québec, Canada

We assessed the effect of the method of feeding on respiratory and gastrointestinal illnesses during the first 6 months of life among 776 infants born in New Brunswick, Canada. During a 1-year period, these infants were drawn from the offspring of a population of primiparous women in the province who, after at least 36 weeks of pregnancy, gave birth to one normal infant weighing 2500 gm or more. Data were collected by means of a self-administered standardized questionnaire mailed to every mother a week before her infant reached 6 months of age. The crude incidence density ratio (IDR) revealed a protective effect of breast-feeding on respiratory illnesses (IDR = 0.66; 95% confidence interval (CI), 0.52 to 0.83), on gastrointestinal illnesses (IDR = 0.53; 95% CI, 0.27 to 1.04) and on all illnesses (IDR = 0.67; 95% CI, 0.54 to 0.82). The protective effect of breast-feeding on respiratory illnesses persisted even after adjustment for age of the infant, socioeconomic class, maternal age, and cigarette consumption (adjusted IDR = 0.78; 95% CI, 0.61 to 1.00). Moreover, if we distinguished ear infection from other respiratory illnesses, we observed a separate protective effect for these two types of events. The results of this retrospective cohort study suggest a protective effect of breast-feeding in our population during the first 6 months of life. (J Pediatr 1995;126:191-7)

There is now general agreement that breast-feeding prevents infantile gastrointestinal infections in all settings.[1, 2] Although breast-feeding has been associated with significant reductions in nongastrointestinal infections, including pneumonia, otitis media, bacteremia, and meningitis, as well as in hospitalization,[2] an articulate minority doubts its importance in industrial nations.[3] This ambivalence may be due in part to the failure of both investigators and practitioners to consider several methodologic issues related to such studies.[3, 4] The problem of confounding factors related to both the choice of the method of feeding and the outcome measure, and the likelihood that the health benefits attributable specifically to breast-feeding may be modest in comparison with those in developing countries, could mean that studies to detect the effects of breast-feeding on the health of infants in the general population of developed countries would have to be large, with limited prospects for conclusive outcome. Kovar et al.[4] therefore suggested that such studies not receive high priority; rather, they suggested that when research on any aspect of infant health is undertaken for other reasons, and the study design is one that permits some judgment to be made about the effect of infant feed-

CI	Confidence interval
IDR	Incidence density ratio

Supported in part by grant No. 6604-1031-43 from the National Health and Research Development Program of Health and Welfare Canada.

Submitted for publication March 7, 1994; accepted Aug. 24, 1994.

Reprint requests: Micheline Beaudry, PhD, Nutrition Cluster, UNICEF, 3 UN Plaza, New York, NY 10017.

0022-3476/95/$3.00 + 0 **9/20/60181**

ing on infant health, consideration be given to including the collection of related information as part of that study.

It is in this context that the results discussed in this article were obtained, the data having been collected as part of a larger study of infant feeding in the province of New Brunswick, Canada[5-7]; the total study was designed by a team from the University of Moncton, with the provincial ministry of health, to provide information needed for the development of an infant nutrition and health program. Because of the large, population-based sample, we also sought to assess the effect of infant feeding on infectious illnesses during the first 6 months of life.

METHODS

Sampling and data collection. The population consisted of all infants born in New Brunswick in 1982 and 1983 to primiparous women who, after at least 36 weeks of pregnancy, gave birth to one normal infant who weighed 2500 gm or more and was still alive at the time of the study. Participating babies were selected by modified cluster sampling. Each cluster comprised all births in the province in a given month; four clusters were selected, the first one at random and the others every third month thereafter. All primiparous mothers who met our criteria in a given cluster were invited to participate when their baby was approximately 4 months of age by means of a bilingual letter from the provincial ministry of health. This invitation was sent only once. A week before the infant reached 6 months of age, mothers who had indicated their agreement received a questionnaire through the mail, in the language of their choice, to be completed and returned in a stamped, preaddressed envelope. Data were collected between December 1982 and September 1983.

Definition of variables

Feeding method. Breast-feeding was defined as the period of breast-feeding from birth until the infant was totally weaned, even if other foods were offered; the breast-feeding group therefore included both infants who were exclusively breast-fed (i.e., who received no complement of water, other milk, or other foods) and infants who received some breast-feeding complemented with either water, other milk, or other foods. Infants still breast-fed at the time of the study were considered to have been breast-fed for 26 weeks. The term *bottle feeding* referred to no breast-feeding but, rather, to the use of an infant formula or cow milk. Each infant was classified every week into either the breast-feeding or the bottle-feeding group.

Infectious illnesses. We studied gastrointestinal and respiratory illnesses because they had been previously associated with the method of infant feeding. All other illnesses, other than trauma, were included in a third category. The identification of events and their duration were based on answers provided by the mother to the following question: Has your baby been ill since birth? If yes, please indicate the name, the approximate duration (in days), and the age of the baby (in weeks) for each illness. The same question was then asked for hospitalizations, and appropriate spaces for answering were provided. Symptoms or illnesses reported by the mother were classified as follows, without knowledge of the mode of feeding: an event of gastrointestinal illness included episodes reported as diarrhea, colic, vomiting, gastroenteritis, or gastric influenza. An event of respiratory illness consisted of an episode of otitis, ear infection, cold, influenza, pneumonia, bronchopneumonia, chest cold, bronchitis, throat infection, pharyngitis, tonsillitis, whooping cough, croup, or any illness accompanied with wheezing. Episodes of respiratory illness accompanied with vomiting or diarrhea were considered as respiratory events; the rationale was that cough or fever associated with a respiratory illness could provoke vomiting, whereas the inverse is unlikely. Other illnesses mostly included episodes of other infectious illnesses, allergy, or anemia. We also studied the total number of events of illness for each infant and the number of hospital admissions. Episodes lasting less than 3 days were not considered as illnesses, as in the recent study by Howie et al.[8]

Potential confounding variables considered in the analysis referred either to the infant (age, birth weight, month of birth, and day care situation) or to the mother (age, cigarette consumption, and socioeconomic status). Socioeconomic status was assessed by the Hollingshead scale of social classes on the basis of the mother's education and occupation[9]; the five categories were regrouped into three for the analysis: upper, medium, and lower.

Statistical analysis. Every infant was classified each week as breast or bottle fed and thus contributed to a total of 26 infant-weeks of observation, some being "breast-feeding infant-weeks" and others being "bottle-feeding infant-weeks." An episode of illness was associated either with breast-feeding or bottle feeding according to the method of feeding used in the week during which the episode occurred (if an infant became ill during the week of weaning, the episode of illness was considered as a breast-feeding event).

The rate (or incidence density) of illness in breast-fed infants was computed as follows: The numerator of the rate of a specified type of illness corresponded to the total number of episodes of that illness reported while infants were breast-fed. More than one episode could be reported for each infant. The denominator was the number of "breast-feeding infant-weeks" contributed by all infants. The rate of illnesses in bottle-fed infants was obtained similarly.

To compare the rates of illnesses in breast-fed and bottle-fed infants, we computed incidence density ratios, which corresponded to the rate of a given illness among breast-fed

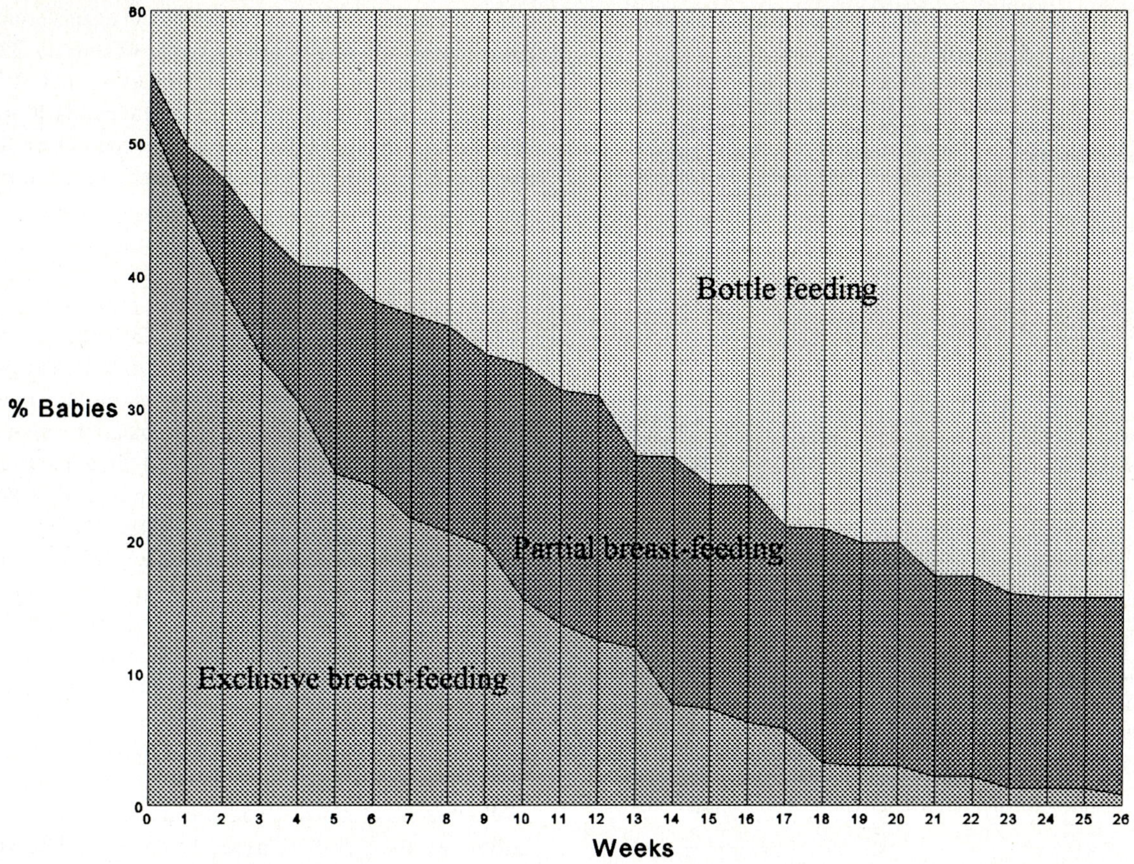

Figure. Distribution (%) of babies by method of feeding at each age in weeks.

infants divided by the rate of that type of illness among bottle-fed infants. Therefore, when equal to one, the IDR indicated no association between the method of feeding and the rate of illness. When less than one, the IDR indicated a protective effect of breast-feeding. The precision and the statistical significance of the IDR is given for the 95% confidence interval. The association is statistically significant at the 0.05 level if the interval does not overlap with the value of one.

To control for individual confounding variables, we carried out a stratified analysis and adjusted IDRs according to the Mantel-Haenszel procedure. Simultaneous adjustment of IDRs for several potential confounders was performed by means of the Poisson regression. The risk of hospitalization was adjusted by means of a logistic regression analysis. Analysis was done with the Statistical Analysis Systems (SAS Institute, Inc., Cary, N.C.) and a generalized linear interactive model (GLIM; NAG, Downers Grove, Ill.).

RESULTS

Among the 1387 eligible mothers, 864 (62%) agreed to participate and 780 (56% of those eligible, or 90% of those who had agreed to participate) returned a valid questionnaire. Three subjects were lost in a data transfer, and the age at the time of a disease (a cold) was unknown for one subject. The 776 remaining subjects were distributed evenly in the four clusters (Table I). Mothers who had agreed to participate but did not return the questionnaire were not different in socioeconomic status or cultural group (French, English, mixed, or other) from those who did.

The population and their feeding practices are described extensively elsewhere.[5,6] The majority of mothers and infants belong either to the English cultural group (55%) or to the French one (31%), the two major groups in the province and both predominantly white. Infants breast-fed at birth came from a higher socioeconomic status and had older mothers than those who were fed infant formula (Table I). Infants from the bottle-fed group had mothers who smoked more cigarettes. The two groups did not differ in birth weight or in the number of children sharing day care facilities with the index child. The mean age of infants at the time of study was 6.3 months (SD 0.76).

The Figure illustrates the distribution of infants by their method of feeding at each age in weeks. The prevalence of

Table I. Characteristics of study participants according to feeding method at birth

Characteristics	Breast-feeding group (n = 430)	Bottle-feeding group (n = 346)
Month of birth (%)		
December	24	24
March	25	26
June	25	22
September	27	28
Socioeconomic status (%)*		
High	22	5
Medium	39	25
Low	39	70
Mother's age (%)		
≤19 yr	7	24
20-24 yr	39	46
25-29 yr	46	23
≥30 yr	9	7
Mother's cigarette consumption (%)		
Nonsmokers	77	60
1-12 cigarettes/day	9	15
≥13 cigarettes/day	14	25
Birth weight (gm)		
Mean ± SD	3487 ± 460	3429 ± 473
Range†	2495-5330	2523-5245
Number of children sharing same day care facility (%)		
0	67	75
1-2	23	20
3-5	9	4
≥6	2	1

*Socioeconomic status was assessed with the Hollingsead scale of social classes.[9]

†Some hospitals report the weight in pounds and not in grams. The 5 lb 8 oz cutoff point for low birth weight was translated by the computer into 2495 gm.

exclusive breast-feeding was very low after the first few weeks, reaching 13% at 3 months and 1% at 6 months. Fifty-six percent of infants were breast-fed at birth; the percentage decreased to 31% at 3 months and 16% at 6 months. Babies classified as bottle fed were not receiving any amount of human milk. Forty-four percent of babies were never breast-fed. By 6 months of age, more than 80% of babies were completely bottle fed and all babies had received at least one complement of milk other than water. Half of the babies had received juice or solids before the age of 3 months (65% among those never breast-fed and 25% among those breast-fed for 14 weeks or more).[6]

A total of 530 episodes of illnesses were observed in the 776 infants, and 47% had at least one episode of illness. These infants had, on average, 1.45 (SD 0.75) episodes each. Respiratory illnesses accounted for 80% of the episodes; among respiratory illnesses, 13% were classified as ear infection.

The crude incidence density analysis revealed a significant protective effect of breast-feeding against total illnesses during the first 6 months of life (Table II). The incidence density for gastrointestinal illnesses was 47% lower in breast-fed infants than in bottle-fed infants (IDR = 0.53; 95% CI, 0.27 to 1.04). The IDRs, adjusted in turn for socioeconomic status, infant's age, mother's age, and maternal cigarette consumption, were virtually similar to the crude IDR, which indicates no confounding by the aforementioned factors (Table III).

The crude incidence density for respiratory illnesses was 34% lower in breast-fed infants than in bottle-fed infants (IDR = 0.66; 95% CI, 0.52 to 0.83) (Table II). The protective effect of breast-feeding on respiratory illnesses persisted after individual adjustment for the potential confounders shown in Table IV. When we adjusted simultaneously for the effect of the four variables by means of a Poisson regression, we obtained an adjusted IDR of 0.78 (CI, 0.61 to 1.00). In addition, if we distinguished ear infection from other respiratory illnesses, we observed a protective effect for ear infection as for other types of respiratory events. After adjustment for potential confounding variables individually, the Mantel-Haenszel adjusted IDRs (and 95% CIs) varied from 0.42 (0.20 to 0.87) to 0.57 (0.28 to 1.18) for ear infection and from 0.69 (0.54 to 0.88) to 0.76 (0.59 to 0.97) for other respiratory illnesses.

We then reexamined the data, considering only episodes lasting less than 21 days, as did Rubin et al.,[10] to exclude potentially insignificant illnesses such as loose stools resulting from dietary change or chronic cough resulting from allergic causes. With this definition, the crude IDR (with 95% CI) was 0.63 (0.31 to 1.32) for gastrointestinal illnesses, 0.71 (0.56 to 0.89) for all respiratory illnesses, 0.52 (0.26 to 1.06) for ear infection, 0.73 (0.57 to 0.94) for other respiratory illnesses, and 0.89 (0.47 to 1.68) for other illnesses.

We also reexamined the data, including data on episodes lasting less than 3 days, to make sure that we had not excluded episodes of otitis or pneumonia that had responded quickly to antibiotic therapy and that were thought to have lasted only 2 days. This added a total of five episodes of gastrointestinal illnesses and 23 episodes of respiratory illnesses. Crude IDRs (with 95% CIs) remained essentially unchanged: 0.53 (0.28 to 1.02) and 0.68 (0.55 to 0.85) for gastrointestinal illnesses and respiratory illnesses, respectively. Furthermore, if we again distinguished ear infection and other respiratory illnesses, the respective IDRs were 0.44 (0.22 to 0.87) and 0.72 (0.57 to 0.91).

Finally we considered the effect of the method of feeding on the severity of respiratory illnesses as judged by related hospital admissions. Only one hospital admission occurred for respiratory illnesses during breast-feeding weeks, in comparison with 51 hospital admissions during bottle-feed-

Table II. Crude incidence density ratios and 95% confidence intervals for specified illnesses

Illness	Breast-feeding group: No. of events	Breast-feeding group: Incidence density (×10⁻³)	Bottle-feeding group: No. of events	Bottle-feeding group: Incidence density (×10⁻³)	IDR (95% CI)
Gastrointestinal illness	10	1.6	44	3.1	0.53 (0.27,1.04)
Respiratory illness	93	15.3	329	23.3	0.66 (0.52,0.83)
Other illnesses	15	2.5	39	2.8	0.89 (0.49,1.62)
TOTAL	118	19.5	412	29.2	0.67 (0.54,0.82)

Table III. Specific and adjusted incidence density ratios and 95% confidence intervals for gastrointestinal illness* according to infant's age and socioeconomic status, and mother's age and cigarette consumption

Adjustment variable	Breast-feeding group: Infant-weeks	Breast-feeding group: Incidence density ($\times 10^{-3}$)	Bottle-feeding group: Infant-weeks	Bottle-feeding group: Incidence density ($\times 10^{-3}$)	IDR (95% CI)
Infant's age (wk)					
0-4	1519	4.6	1585	6.3	0.73 (0.28, 1.91)
5-9	1492	2.0	2388	5.0	0.40 (0.12, 1.36)
10-13	1005	1.0	2099	4.3	0.23 (0.03, 1.54)
14-17	783	2.5	2321	5.6	0.45 (0.11, 1.94)
18-21	633	3.2	2471	4.9	0.65 (0.15, 2.87)
22-26	636	3.1	3244	4.6	0.68 (0.16, 2.95)
Adjusted IDR†					*0.53 (0.30, 0.90)*
Socioeconomic status					
High	1634	1.2	1278	3.1	0.39 (0.08, 2.01)
Medium	2197	0.9	4459	4.3	0.21 (0.06, 0.80)
Low	2237	3.1	8371	3.0	1.05 (0.45, 2.42)
Adjusted IDR					*0.56 (0.30, 1.06)*
Mother's age (yr)					
≤19	364	2.7	2548	3.5	0.78 (0.10, 6.11)
20-24	2079	2.9	6397	3.3	0.89 (0.36, 2.18)
25-29	3023	3.3	4179	3.3	0.10 (0.02, 0.51)
≥30	602	5.0	984	4.1	1.23 (0.27, 5.46)
Adjusted IDR					*0.53 (0.26, 1.09)*
Mother's cigarette consumption‡					
Nonsmokers	5012	1.4	9002	3.0	0.47 (0.21, 1.05)
Smokers	1042	2.9	5068	3.3	0.86 (0.25, 2.93)
Adjusted IDR					*0.56 (0.28, 1.09)*

*Gastrointestinal illness consists of diarrhea, colic, vomiting, gastroenteritis or gastric influenza.
†Adjusted according to the Mantel-Haenszel procedure.
‡Data on two subjects were deleted because of missing information about their cigarette consumption.

ing weeks. The crude IDR for hospital admission for all respiratory illnesses was 0.05 (0.01 to 0.18). A logistic regression analysis comparing the probability of hospital admission during the first 6 months of life according to the mode of feeding at birth showed an adjusted odds ratio of 0.32 (95% CI, 0.14 to 0.72) (adjusted for mother's age, cigarette consumption, and socioeconomic status).

DISCUSSION

The results of this retrospective cohort study suggest a protective effect of breast-feeding against respiratory illnesses, as well as against gastrointestinal illnesses, during the first 6 months of life. We also observed a protective effect for ear infection, thus corroborating results from Duncan et al.[11] These results were obtained even though we grouped together infants who were exclusively breast-fed and those who received complements of water, other milk, or other foods if they still received some human milk. The fact that we did not specifically look at infants who were exclusively breast-fed could dilute all the observed effects.

Our study was planned before the recommendations of Kovar et al.[4] and Bauchner et al.[3] were published, but our design did try to improve on some of the methodologic issues that they raised. We were able to control for the im-

Table IV. Specific and adjusted incidence density ratios and 95% confidence intervals for respiratory illness* according to infant's age and socioeconomic status, and mother's age and cigarette consumption

	Breast-feeding group		Bottle-feeding group		
Adjustment variable	Infant-weeks	Incidence density ($\times 10^{-3}$)	Infant-weeks	Incidence density ($\times 10^{-3}$)	IDR (95% CI)
Infant's age (wk)					
0-4	1519	8.6	1585	13.2	0.65 (0.30, 1.35)
5-9	1492	12.7	2388	23.0	0.55 (0.31, 0.95)
10-13	1005	21.9	2099	21.4	1.02 (0.58, 1.74)
14-17	783	21.7	2321	22.8	0.95 (0.52, 1.67)
18-21	633	14.2	2471	25.9	0.55 (0.24, 1.11)
22-26	636	20.4	3244	28.1	0.73 (0.37, 1.31)
Adjusted IDR†					*0.73 (0.58, 0.92)*
Socioeconomic status					
High	1634	14.1	1278	24.3	0.58 (0.32, 1.03)
Medium	2197	15.9	4459	22.9	0.70 (0.46, 1.03)
Low	2237	15.6	8371	23.4	0.67 (0.45, 0.96)
Adjusted IDR					*0.66 (0.52, 0.84)*
Mother's age (years)					
≤19	364	27.5	2548	27.5	1.00 (0.46, 1.95)
20-24	2079	15.4	6397	20.5	0.75 (0.49, 1.11)
25-29	3023	14.9	4179	26.1	0.57 (0.39, 0.81)
≥30	602	10.0	984	19.3	0.52 (0.17, 1.34)
Adjusted IDR					*0.67 (0.53, 0.84)*
Mother's cigarette consumption‡					
Nonsmokers	5012	14.2	9002	20.9	0.68 (0.51, 0.90)
Smokers	1042	21.1	5068	27.8	0.76 (0.46, 1.19)
Adjusted IDR					*0.70 (0.55, 0.88)*

*Respiratory illness consisted of otitis, ear infection, cold, influenza, pneumonia, bronchopneumonia, chest cold, bronchitis, throat infection, pharyngitis, tonsillitis, whooping cough, croup, or any illness accompanied with wheezing.
†Adjusted according to the Mantel-Haenszel procedure.
‡Data on two subjects were deleted because of missing information about their cigarette consumption.

portant confounding variables either (1) by sampling only singleton first-born children weighing more than 2500 gm after 36 weeks of pregnancy, and thus controlling for infant birth weight, family size, and number of siblings, or (2) by controlling for infant's age, family's social class, mother's age, and maternal cigarette consumption. We also controlled for seasonal exposure to illness through selection of subjects all year round.

The statistical analysis based on person-time methods best handles the common problems that arise in such studies because it takes into account the facts that (1) the outcome may be recurrent in one individual, (2) the duration of breast-feeding is associated with the infant's age, and (3) the incidence of illnesses is also age related. Furthermore, we studied events per week instead of events per month, as Rubin et al.[10] had done, and thus obtained more accurate information about exposure.

The method that we used to collect data relied on the mother's report of the child's illnesses, and not on illnesses defined through medical reports. Thus, even if breast-feeding mothers were to seek medical care less often for their infant than bottle-feeding mothers, as some may suggest, such would not likely affect their own reporting of illness. If there were differential detection, we could argue that breast-feeding mothers might report illnesses more easily because of a closer link to their infant; they could also be more likely to report diarrhea in their infant because breast-fed infants tend to have more frequent and looser stools. This circumstance would therefore underestimate the protective effect of breast-feeding. The fact that only one hospitalization occurred for respiratory illness during breast-feeding weeks, in comparison with 51 in bottle-feeding weeks, suggests either less severity of illness, or less inclination of breast-feeding mothers to allow hospitalization to take place, or a combination of both. In any case, it points to a decreased risk of hospitalization for respiratory illnesses for the breast-fed infant. Leventhal et al.[12] also concluded that breast-feeding protects infants from hospitalization.

The definitions of illnesses reported by the mother were not checked with an algorithm on the basis of the presence of several symptoms. Mothers could have misdiagnosed problems. It is unlikely, however, that a gastrointestinal event would be misclassified into a respiratory event or vice versa. The misclassification by the mother more likely would relate to the specific problem within a global category and would therefore not likely affect our results.

The infants were 6 months of age when the mothers were asked to recall their infant's illnesses since birth and, for breast-fed infants, the age at total weaning. We did not use active surveillance to detect infectious illnesses nor age at weaning. Had data been reported prospectively, we might have had more complete and precise information; 6 months may be a long period on which to report. However, there is no reason to think that recall may be affected differently among breast feeders and bottle feeders. In addition, the first 6 months of a first baby's life are a very special and intense period of a mother's life, when she is very interested in her baby and in sharing every event. As evidence, the mothers in our study readily responded to a very lengthy questionnaire to which many added several comments, including letters and their baby's picture. Leventhal et al.[12] checked the accuracy of the mothers' recall against the records of a primary care center and in 111 cases found only one discrepancy in how the infants' feeding was classified. These interviews were conducted 8 to 15 months after birth.

We conclude that breast-feeding was protective against respiratory illnesses, including ear infection, and against gastrointestinal illnesses. Breast-feeding also protected against hospitalizations for respiratory illnesses. The internal consistency of the data, the strength of the association, and the stability of the IDRs across analyses support these conclusions. This study thus reinforces the benefits of breast-feeding for the health of infants in our society, and highlights the usefulness of taking advantage of research on other aspects of infant health to include the collection of related information as part of that study.

We thank Diane Potvin and Chantal Guimont for their valuable contribution to the statistical analysis.

REFERENCES

1. Report of the Task Force on the Assessment of the Scientific Evidence Relating to Infant-Feeding Practices and Infant Health. Pediatrics 1984;74(suppl):579-762.
2. Cunningham AS, Jelliffe DB, Jelliffe EFP. Breast-feeding and health in the 1980s: a global epidemiologic review. J PEDIATR 1991;118:659-66.
3. Bauchner H, Leventhal JM, Shapiro ED. Studies of breast-feeding and infections: how good is the evidence? JAMA 1986;256:887-92.
4. Kovar MG, Serdula MK, Marks JS, Fraser DW. Review of the epidemiological evidence for an association between infant feeding and infant health. Pediatrics 1984;74(suppl):615-38.
5. Beaudry M, Aucoin-Larade L. Who breastfeeds in New Brunswick: when and why? Can J Public Health 1989;80:166-72.
6. Beaudry M, Aucoin-Larade L. L'alimentation des nourrissons de 0 à 6 mois au Nouveau-Brunswick. J Can Diet Assoc 1991;52:24-9.
7. Beaudry M, Dufour R. Facteurs de réussite de l'allaitement maternel au Nouveau-Brunswick: information et conditions de travail compatibles. Can J Public Health 1991;82:325-30.
8. Howie PW, Forsyth JS, Ogston SA, Clark A, du V Florey C. Protective effect of breast-feeding against infection. BMJ 1990;300:11-6.
9. Hollingshead AB. Two factor index of social position (c1957). Privately printed, 1965, Yale Station, New Haven, Connecticut. Reprinted in: Miller DC. Handbook of research design and social measurement. 4th ed. New York: Longman, 1983.
10. Rubin DH, Leventhal JM, Krasilnikoff PA, et al. Relationship between infant feeding and infectious illness: a prospective study of infants during the first year of life. Pediatrics 1990;85:464-71.
11. Duncan B, Ey J, Holberg CJ, Wright AL, Martinez FD, Taussig LM. Exclusive breast-feeding for at least 4 months protects against otitis media. Pediatrics 1993;91:867-72.
12. Leventhal JM, Shapiro ED, Aten CB, Berg AT, Egerter SA. Does breast-feeding protect against infections in infants less than 3 months of age? Pediatrics 1986;78:896-903.

Effect of neonatal immunization with diphtheria and tetanus toxoids on antibody responses to *Haemophilus influenzae* type b conjugate vaccines

Jay M. Lieberman, MD, David P. Greenberg, MD, Victor K. Wong, MD, Susan Partridge, RN, Swei-Ju Chang, MS, Chung-Yin Chiu, MS, and Joel I. Ward, MD

From the Division of Pediatric Infectious Diseases, University of California, Los Angeles, Center for Vaccine Research, Harbor-UCLA Medical Center, Torrance, and the Kaiser Foundation Hospitals and Medical Clinics, Southern California

We randomly assigned 150 newborn infants to receive diphtheria and tetanus toxoids (DT) or Hib oligosaccharide conjugate (HbOC) at birth to determine whether exposure to the *Haemophilus influenzae* type b (Hib) conjugate vaccines' carrier proteins would enhance immune responses to subsequent administrations of HbOC or PRP-tetanus toxoid conjugate (PRP-T) at 2, 4, and 6 months of age. Their antibody responses were compared with those of 100 children immunized with HbOC or PRP-T beginning at 2 months of age. No serious adverse reactions were associated with neonatal vaccination. Administration of HbOC at birth did not lead to earlier or higher antibody levels. Newborn immunization with DT did not prime children for enhanced antibody responses. Moreover, Hib antibody levels were lower in DT-primed children than in children immunized beginning at 2 months of age. Diphtheria antibody levels, but not tetanus antibody levels, were also lower in children immunized with DT at birth. We conclude that neonatal immunization with Hib conjugate vaccines is not a means to provide earlier protection against invasive Hib disease. Newborn DT administration does not enhance subsequent antibody responses to Hib conjugate vaccines, and may lead to suppression of Hib and diphtheria antibody responses. (J Pediatr 1995;126:198-205)

The four licensed *Haemophilus influenzae* type b conjugate vaccines differ in composition, structure, and the immune responses they induce. PRP-D (ProHIBit; Connaught Laboratories, Swiftwater, Pa.) was the first Hib conjugate vaccine licensed for use in children, but it is the least immunogenic in infants and is approved for use only in children ≥12 months of age. The other three vaccines, PRP-OMP (PedvaxHIB; Merck & Co., West Point, Pa.), HbOC (HibTITER; Lederle–Praxis Biologics, Pearl River, N.Y.), and PRP-T (ActHIB; Pasteur Merieux, Lyon, France) are immunogenic in infants and are licensed in the United States for use beginning at 2 months of age.[1, 2] PRP-OMP stimulates a significant antibody response after the first dose administered at 2 months of age,[3] and clinical trials suggest that it provides protection with the initial dose.[4] In contrast, antibody responses in infants to the first dose of HbOC or PRP-T are negligible. Even after a second dose of these vaccines, not all infants attain antibody levels considered to

Supported by the National Institutes of Health (N01-AI-15124) and Connaught Laboratories.

Presented in part at the meeting of the Society for Pediatric Research, Washington, D.C., May 5, 1993.

Submitted for publication April 5, 1994; accepted Aug. 17, 1994.

Reprint requests: Jay M. Lieberman, MD, Harbor-UCLA Medical Center, 1124 West Carson St. E-6, Torrance, CA 90502.

0022-3476/95/$3.00 + 0 **9/20/59999**

See related article, p. 206.

CRM_{197}	Cross-reacting mutant of diphtheria toxin
DT	Diphtheria and tetanus toxoids
DTP	Diphtheria and tetanus toxoids and pertussis vaccine
ELISA	Enzyme-linked immunosorbent assay
HbOC	*Haemophilus influenzae* type b oligosaccharide conjugate vaccine
Hib	*Haemophilus influenzae* type b
PRP	Polyribosylribitol phosphate
PRP-D	PRP–diphtheria toxoid conjugate vaccine
PRP-OMP	PRP–outer-membrane protein conjugate vaccine
PRP-T	PRP–tetanus toxoid conjugate vaccine

be protective. After three doses, high levels of antibody are achieved[5, 6] and few vaccine failures have been reported.[7, 8]

A leading hypothesis as to why three doses of HbOC and PRP-T are required in infants to induce optimal immunity is that the infants' T cells must be adequately primed to the carrier protein. The protein carriers of HbOC (CRM_{197}—a nontoxic variant of diphtheria toxin) and PRP-T (tetanus toxoid) are also given as part of routine childhood immunizations. Priming is presumably accomplished by prior or simultaneous exposure to diphtheria and tetanus toxoids, or to the smaller amount of carrier protein contained in the Hib-conjugate vaccine itself. The importance of carrier priming has been suggested by observations of the adverse effect of withholding DT immunization on the antibody response to HbOC. Infant rhesus monkeys immunized with HbOC at birth and at 4 and 8 weeks of age did not respond to immunization unless diphtheria toxoid was administered concomitantly.[9] Similarly, data from human infants indicate that DT vaccination is required for optimal immune response to HbOC vaccine.[10]

Carrier priming has not been well studied in human subjects. We conducted this study to determine whether immunizing newborn infants with DT vaccine might enhance immune responses to subsequent immunizations with HbOC or PRP-T, compared with the responses of infants immunized with these vaccines beginning at 2 months of age. We also evaluated the immunogenicity of HbOC administered at birth. We did not evaluate giving PRP-T at birth because an earlier study did not demonstrate any benefit.[11] Our goals were to explore ways to provide earlier protective Hib immunity and to investigate the importance of carrier priming.

METHODS

Population and study design. There were five study groups (Table I): three groups recruited at birth and two groups recruited at 2 months of age. To be eligible for participation, infants had to be in good health and a parent had to sign informed consent. Infants were excluded if gestational age was less than 37 weeks, if they had received any blood product or immune globulin preparation, if there was a known or suspected impairment of neurologic function or a seizure disorder, if they had an acute febrile illness, if there was a severe congenital defect or major organ dysfunction, or if there was known maternal immunodeficiency or human immunodeficiency virus infection.

One hundred fifty newborn infants were recruited within the first 3 days of life from a Southern California Kaiser Permanente hospital and randomly assigned to one of three study groups. Two groups were immunized in the newborn nursery with DT vaccine and the third group with HbOC vaccine. They then received doses of either HbOC or PRP-T at 2, 4, and 6 months of age.

The control groups consisted of 100 children recruited at 2 months of age who were randomly assigned to receive a series of three doses of either HbOC or PRP-T as participants in a concurrently run trial.[12] These children were enrolled at two clinic sites, including the site where all newborn study participants received their follow-up care.

Nurses who administered the vaccines knew to which group the infants had been assigned, but parents and research personnel who collected the safety data and who assayed the serum specimens were masked. Cord blood was obtained from all newborn infants enrolled in the study, and serum (1 to 3 ml) was collected by venipuncture immediately before each vaccine dose at 2, 4, and 6 months of age, and again at 7 months of age.

Vaccines. A single lot of DT (Connaught Laboratories) and three lots of HbOC (M130HA, M140HF, M04JH) were obtained from commercial sources. Each 0.5 ml dose of HbOC consists of 10 μg of purified Hib capsular polysaccharide and 25 μg CRM_{197} protein. Two lots of PRP-T (S2372, S2760), consisting of 10 μg PRP and 20 μg tetanus toxoid per 0.5 ml dose, were obtained from Connaught Laboratories.

Each dose of HbOC, PRP-T, and DT vaccine was administered by intramuscular injection into the anterior portion of the thigh. Study vaccines were given at 2-month intervals in conjunction with regularly scheduled childhood immunizations (hepatitis B, DTP, and oral polio vaccines). Concurrent vaccines were administered by separate injection at a different site.

Safety evaluation. A brief medical history and physical examination were performed on enrollment into the study and at each vaccination visit. Each child was observed for 15 minutes after the immunization. Parents were given a thermometer with instructions for use, and a diary in which to record the child's temperature and information concern-

Table I. Tetanus antibody results

	Vaccine		Tetanus antibody levels (unit/ml)		
Group	Birth	2-4-6 mo*	Birth	2 mo	7 mo†
1	—	HbOC		0.34	2.97 (2.42, 3.64)
2	HbOC	HbOC	0.89	0.16	2.11 (1.69, 2.63)
3	DT	HbOC	0.97	0.27	2.50 (2.15, 2.91)
4	—	PRP-T		0.19	1.83 (1.36, 2.45)
5	DT	PRP-T		0.25	2.17 (1.77, 2.64)

*All participants received DTP at 2, 4, and 6 months of age.
†Numbers in parentheses represent 95% confidence intervals.

ing local and systemic reactions for the 72 hours after immunization. Parents were then called 3 to 7 days after each immunization to collect the data from the diary. At each visit, parents were interviewed to elicit information concerning interval adverse reactions. Information was also obtained through review of Kaiser medical records on all hospitalizations, outpatient visits, seizures, or invasive bacterial diseases of study participants.

Serologic studies. All serologic studies were performed in our laboratory. Total antibody to PRP was measured by a standardized radioimmunoassay using a modified Farr method.[13] The lower limit of detection of anticapsular antibody was 0.025 μg/ml. Tetanus and diphtheria antibodies were measured by methods described previously.[14] Briefly, tetanus antibodies were measured by enzyme-linked immunosorbent assay using tetanus immune globulin (Hyper-Tet [Cutter Biological], 400 IU/ml) as a standard and a best-fit curve to quantitate antibody levels. Diphtheria antibodies were similarly measured, with human serum immune globulin (Gamastan; Cutter Biological) used as a standard that was arbitrarily assigned a value of 1000 ELISA units/ml of anti-diphtheria antibody. The lower limit of detection of tetanus antibody was 0.02 IU/ml, and the lower limit of detection of diphtheria antibody was 1.57 ELISA units/ml.

Statistical methods. The primary analyses consisted of comparing the immune responses to PRP, tetanus toxoid, and diphtheria toxoid among groups by analysis of covariance. Specifically, the results in infants immunized at birth with DT or HbOC were compared with the results in infants given HbOC or PRP-T beginning at 2 months of age. For statistical analysis, PRP antibody levels less than 0.025 μg/ml were assigned a value of 0.012 μg/ml, tetanus antibody levels less than 0.02 unit/ml were assigned a value of 0.01 unit/ml, and diphtheria antibody levels below 1.57 units/ml were assigned a value of 0.78 unit/ml. The frequency of adverse reactions was compared among vaccine groups with the Cochran-Mantel-Haenszel test.

RESULTS

The ethnic backgrounds of the study participants reflect the diversity of Los Angeles County. Overall, 45% of the infants' mothers were Hispanic, 26% white, 19% black, 9% Asian, and 1% other. Fifty-one percent of the infants were female. There were no significant differences among the groups by gender or maternal race. There were very minor differences in some groups with regard to the ages at which vaccination was given; for example, group 1 received the third dose of HbOC at a mean age of 6.4 months, compared with 6.7 months for group 3 ($p < 0.04$).

Safety. Immunization with DT or HbOC in the newborn period was not associated with any immediate adverse effects. In the 72 hours after newborn immunization, one DT recipient had a temperature >38.5° C, and three other DT recipients and one HbOC recipient had temperatures ≥38.0° C. Four of these five neonates had also received hepatitis B vaccine. Local reactions after newborn vaccination were unusual, occurring in less than 4% of vaccinees, and there were no significant differences among the groups. Infants who were immunized as neonates were no more likely to have fever or local reactions after subsequent immunizations than were infants immunized beginning at 2 months of age (data not shown).

Of the 150 newborn infants, four were hospitalized in the first month of life. Only one of these hospitalizations was possibly related to immunization; an infant immunized with DT and hepatitis B vaccines at 1 day of age had fever the following day and was hospitalized for possible neonatal sepsis. Another infant had tachypnea 1 day after receiving HbOC and was briefly hospitalized for evaluation. The other two hospitalizations occurred 19 days (rule out sep-

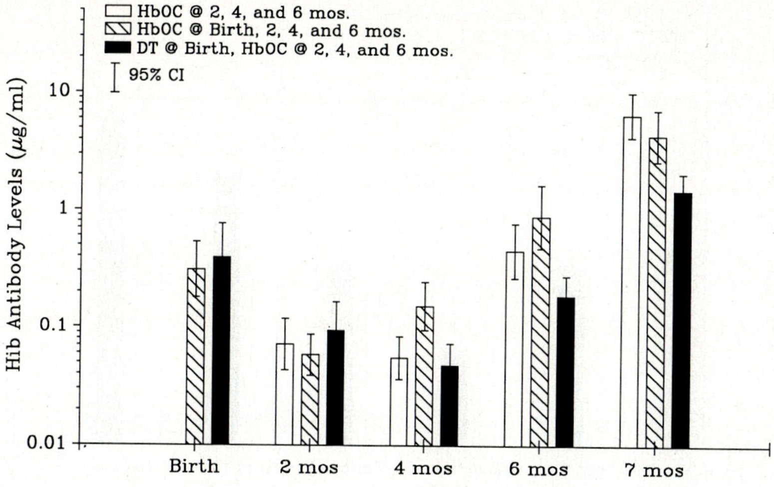

Fig. 1. Hib antibody results in children given HbOC vaccine. Children immunized with HbOC at birth had significantly higher antibody levels at 4 months of age than did children immunized with HbOC beginning at 2 months of age ($p = 0.002$). Children vaccinated with DT at birth had significantly lower antibody levels at 6 ($p = 0.01$) and 7 months of age ($p < 0.0001$) than did children immunized beginning at 2 months of age.

sis) and 25 days (aseptic meningitis) after HbOC and DT immunization, respectively. Results of bacterial cultures from all four patients were negative.

Hib antibodies

Neonatal HbOC immunization (Fig. 1). Newborn infants immunized with HbOC at birth had antibody levels at 2 months of age similar to those in infants not immunized at birth. In infants immunized with HbOC at birth and at 2 months, antibody levels were significantly higher at 4 months of age than in infants who received their first dose of HbOC at 2 months of age ($p = 0.002$). This advantage was not sustained, however, and antibody levels at 6 and 7 months of age in children given HbOC beginning at birth were similar to those in children immunized with HbOC beginning at 2 months of age, even though the former group had received an extra dose of Hib vaccine.

Neonatal DT immunization. Neonatal DT immunization did not result in higher Hib antibody levels in infants given HbOC as the primary Hib vaccine (Fig. 1). At 6 and 7 months of age, Hib antibody levels were significantly lower in infants given DT at birth than in infants not immunized at birth ($p = 0.01$ and $p < 0.0001$, respectively). This difference may be clinically significant because, at 7 months of age, 61% of DT-primed infants, compared with 90% of unprimed infants ($p = 0.004$), had antibody levels ≥ 1 μg/ml, a level thought to indicate long-term protection.

In infants immunized with DT at birth and subsequently immunized with PRP-T, Hib antibody levels were not significantly ($p = 0.08$) higher at 4 months of age than in those not given DT at birth (Fig. 2). There was no difference in antibody levels between the two groups after the second dose of PRP-T. After the third dose of PRP-T, antibody levels were significantly lower in the DT-primed children ($p = 0.014$), although this difference is probably not clinically important, because 92% of DT-primed children and 100% of unprimed children ($p = 0.24$) had antibody levels ≥ 1.0 μg/ml.

Evaluation of vaccine lots. Three lots of HbOC were used in the study, and we therefore evaluated immunogenicity by lot. In the control children, lot M130HA accounted for 73% of all doses administered and lot M140HF for the remainder. In the newborn group, the second lot, M140HF, accounted for 94% of all doses administered; a third lot (M04JH) was used for the remaining doses. Analysis of the two lots used in the control groups revealed that children who received three doses of M130HA (n = 32) had a geometric mean PRP antibody level of 7.72 μg/ml, compared with 3.50 μg/ml for children (n = 9) who received three doses of M140HF ($p = 0.13$). Two of the nine children who received lot M140HF failed to achieve an antibody level ≥ 1 μg/ml, compared with 2 of 32 who received lot M130HA ($p = 0.20$).

Two lots of PRP-T were used in the study. All control children received lot S2372, which also accounted for 94% of doses in the newborn immunization group. A second lot, S2760, was used as a third dose for 18 children. A comparison among children who received different lots as their third dose showed no significant difference in antibody levels.

Diphtheria and tetanus antibodies. Children immunized with tetanus toxoid at birth, even though they received an extra dose of vaccine, did not have higher tetanus antibody

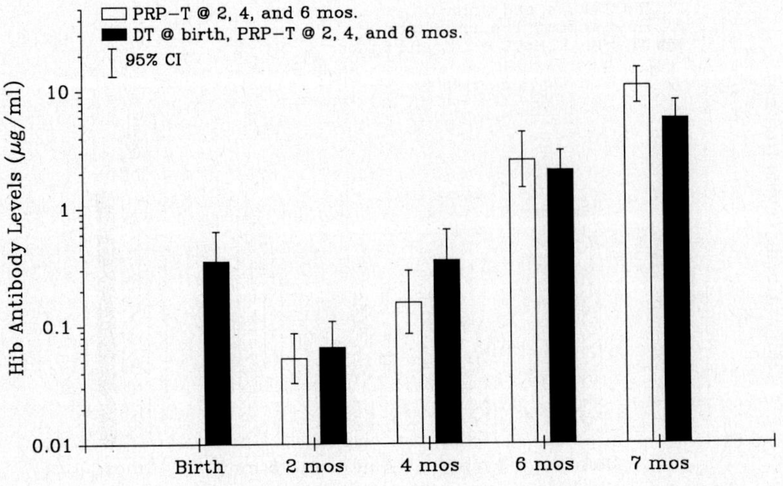

Fig. 2. Hib antibody results in children given PRP-T vaccine. Children given DT at birth had significantly lower antibody levels at 7 months of age ($p = 0.014$) than did children immunized beginning at 2 months of age.

levels at 7 months of age than children immunized beginning at 2 months of age (Table I). However, infants given diphtheria toxoid at birth had significantly lower diphtheria antibody levels at 7 months of age than those immunized beginning at 2 months of age (Table II), whether HbOC or PRP-T was administered subsequently.

DISCUSSION

The first vaccine licensed to prevent Hib disease, the purified polysaccharide (PRP) vaccine, was not immunogenic in infants, was not reliably immunogenic even in children >18 months of age, and provided variable protection for older children.[15] Polysaccharide antigens, such as PRP, function as thymus-independent (T-independent) antigens—they evoke weak primary antibody responses, particularly in infants and young children, and fail to elicit true booster responses with repeated administrations. For improvement of immunogenicity, the PRP polysaccharide antigen (hapten) was covalently linked (conjugated) to various protein carriers, to confer on the polysaccharide the T-dependent immunologic characteristics of the carrier protein. The immune response to polysaccharide-protein conjugate vaccines is characterized by (1) an enhanced response compared with that after plain polysaccharide vaccines, especially in infants and young children, (2) booster responses on readministration of the vaccine, (3) maturation of the response as indicated by a predominance of IgG antibody, and (4) carrier priming (i.e., the immune response is potentiated when there is prior or concurrent administration of the carrier protein).

We evaluated the possibility of taking advantage of this last feature of T-dependent antigens by immunizing newborn infants with DT in the hope that this might induce higher levels of antibody at an earlier age. In addition, we evaluated newborn immunization with one of the Hib conjugate vaccines (HbOC). We chose to evaluate newborn immunization because an effective newborn immunization strategy might improve compliance.

Newborn immunization with HbOC led to a slightly earlier antibody response but did not lead ultimately to higher antibody levels, even with the extra vaccine dose. A similar study of neonatal PRP-T immunization in Finland[11] also did not show evidence of earlier or enhanced protection. Newborn immunization with either HbOC or PRP-T did not, however, appear to have an adverse effect on later antibody responses to these vaccines. In contrast, Native Alaskan infants immunized with PRP-OMP at birth had significantly lower antibody levels after subsequent immunizations with PRP-OMP than did infants immunized beginning at 2 months of age, a finding that suggests immune tolerance.[16] Thus neonatal administration of Hib conjugate vaccines does not induce a substantial immune response, nor does it prime the infant for enhanced antibody responses to subsequent doses; in the case of PRP-OMP vaccine, it may be harmful. Neonatal immunization with Hib conjugate vaccines is not a means of providing earlier protection.

Neonatal immunization with the carrier proteins of the Hib conjugate vaccines also did not result in earlier or higher Hib antibody responses. Moreover, immunization with DT at birth may have suppressed the subsequent immune responses to HbOC and, to a lesser extent, to PRP-T. Carrier priming has been evaluated in a number of animal and human models with various conjugate vaccines. It is now apparent that the effect of carrier priming cannot be predicted a priori and that prior immunization with carrier protein can either enhance[17, 18] or suppress[17-20] the immune

Table II. Diphtheria antibody results

Group	Vaccine		Diphtheria antibody levels (units/ml)		
	Birth	2-4-6 mo*	Birth	2 mo	7 mo†
1	—	HbOC		8.1	347.2 (269.7, 447.0)
2	HbOC	HbOC	27.3	6.0	262.3 (201.7, 341.0)
3	DT	HbOC	18.6	9.4	191.1‡ (155.2, 235.4)
4	—	PRP-T		6.5	211.0 (159.7, 278.9)
5	DT	PRP-T		10.2	114.8§ (94.7, 139.2)

*All participants received DTP at 2, 4, and 6 months of age.
†Numbers in parentheses represent 95% confidence intervals.
‡$p = 0.0007$ (3 vs 1).
§$p = 0.0007$ (5 vs 4).

response to the hapten after subsequent immunization with conjugate vaccine. The outcome is dependent on multiple variables, including when priming occurs, the age at administration, the specific carrier protein, the priming dose of carrier protein,[18, 21] and the specific hapten.[17]

One type of suppression seen after carrier priming is called "carrier-specific epitopic suppression."[21] The suppression is carrier-specific (i.e., after being primed with carrier protein, the immune response is suppressed for a new antigenic epitope [hapten] presented on that carrier). When this occurs, the immune response to the hapten can remain suppressed even if the hapten is later administered separately from the carrier.[19] Carrier-specific epitopic suppression is not related to a suppressed immune response to the carrier protein; a normal secondary antibody response to the carrier is generally observed.[19, 21] In our study, however, the antibody response to the carrier was suppressed; antibody levels against diphtheria were lower in infants immunized at birth than in those immunized beginning at 2 months of age. In a previous study,[22] we did not observe tolerance to diphtheria toxoid in infants immunized with DTP at birth; perhaps the added pertussis component acted as an adjuvant to abrogate the tolerance. In a mouse model, coadministration of pertussis vaccine at the time of carrier priming abolished carrier-specific epitopic suppression.[23]

Because immune responses to both diphtheria and PRP were suppressed, we did not observe carrier-specific epitopic suppression. The induction of tolerance to diphtheria toxoid may have resulted in a reduced response to the Hib component of HbOC vaccine. Responses to PRP-T were also slightly diminished in infants primed with DT at birth, although we did not detect differences in the response to tetanus toxoid.

Two other studies have evaluated the possibility of priming infants to enhance the response to Hib conjugate vaccines. Granoff et al.[24] demonstrated that priming infants with DT at 1 month of age led to enhanced Hib antibody responses to both HbOC and PRP-T vaccines. Similarly, Barington et al.[25] reported that giving DTP 1 month before a first dose of PRP-T at 5 months of age resulted in higher Hib antibody levels than if DTP was administered simultaneously or subsequent to PRP-T. We do not believe that our study contradicts the findings of the other studies, which attempted priming at a later age. There is rapid development of the immune response in newborn and young infants, but the neonate's immune system is immature in a number of ways, and the lack of carrier priming may reflect the absence of memory T cells at this young age.[26] Although the mechanisms of neonatal immune tolerance are not fully understood, tolerance may result when certain antigens are presented to the maturing immune system before development of a competent T-cell repertoire.

In adults who were immunized with diphtheria or tetanus toxoid 4 weeks before immunization with PRP-D or PRP-T, respectively, antibody responses to both Hib and the carrier were depressed, although all subjects mounted an antibody response.[27] The mechanism of the suppressed antibody response is likely very different from that seen in our study, because the adults had high levels of antibody against the carrier, which presumably interfered with the subsequent immune response to the conjugate vaccine. This is further evidence of our need to understand better the role that preexisting immunity plays in modulating the response to conjugate vaccines.

Some aspects of the study design raise potential questions about our findings. The newborn infants enrolled in the study were not randomly selected to be immunized at birth or to begin immunization at 2 months of age; instead, control infants were recruited separately at 2 months of age. Conceivably, the groups might not be comparable, although analysis of maternal race and gender reveal no significant differences, nor are there differences in Hib antibody levels at 2 months of age. In addition, there were slight but significant differences between the groups with regard to the age at vaccine administration. However, when the results were age adjusted, all differences between antibody levels remained significant.

Of particular concern is that three lots of HbOC were used. Analysis of Hib antibody levels in control infants first immunized at 2 months of age did not show a significant difference in immunogenicity among lots, but suggested that the lot used as the primary vaccine in neonates might be less immunogenic than the lot primarily given to control infants. Therefore it is possible that the apparent Hib antibody suppression observed in DT-primed infants reflects receipt of a less immunogenic lot of HbOC. Infants immunized beginning at birth with the potentially less immunogenic lot had higher Hib antibody levels than did DT-primed infants, but the higher levels could represent the response to an extra dose of HbOC. Therefore we cannot say with absolute confidence that DT priming of newborn infants suppressed the subsequent immune response to HbOC, although the lower responses in DT-primed infants given PRP-T suggest that the suppression is real.

Our results, and the data on carrier priming from animal models, have implications for the future use of polysaccharide conjugate vaccines. They demonstrate that one cannot easily predict the effect that changes in the immunization schedule might bring. As new vaccines are developed, new combinations of vaccines are manufactured, and new schedules are introduced, there may be unforeseen adverse consequences for the recipient's immune response. Investigational conjugate vaccines against *Streptococcus pneumoniae* and *Neisseria meningitidis* are modeled after the Hib conjugate vaccines and employ the same carriers. We cannot be sure of the effect on the immune response of giving repeated doses of protein carrier, and the limited number of protein antigens being used as carriers may adversely affect the response to new synthetic vaccines. In addition, our understanding of the newborn infant's immune response is limited. If neonatal immunization is to be a cornerstone of future vaccine schedules, research must focus on learning more about the ontogeny of the neonate's immune response.

We gratefully acknowledge the dedication of the clinical research nurses who immunized and monitored the safety of the study participants: Gloria Leon, Victoria Nunez, and particularly Linda Gutierrez, who enrolled the newborn infants. We also thank Carolyn Garcia and Christina Laurel for data management, and Millie Badar, Misbah Siddiqui, and Patty Takahashi for performing the PRP, diphtheria, and tetanus antibody assays.

REFERENCES

1. Committee on Infectious Diseases. *Haemophilus influenzae* type b conjugate vaccines: recommendations for immunization with recently and previously licensed vaccines. Pediatrics 1993; 92:480-8.
2. Centers for Disease Control and Prevention. Recommendations for use of *Haemophilus* b conjugate vaccines and a combined diphtheria, tetanus, pertussis, and *Haemophilus* b vaccine. MMWR 1993;42(No. RR-13):1-15.
3. Santosham M, Hill J, Wolff M, et al. Safety and immunogenicity of a *Haemophilus influenzae* type b conjugate vaccine in high-risk American Indian population. Pediatr Infect Dis J 1991;10:113-7.
4. Santosham M, Wolff M, Reid R, et al. The efficacy in Navajo infants of a conjugate vaccine consisting of *Haemophilus influenzae* type b polysaccharide and *Neisseria meningitidis* outer-membrane protein complex. N Engl J Med 1991;324: 1767-72.
5. Madore DV, Johnson CL, Phipps DC, et al. Safety and immunologic response to *Haemophilus influenzae* type b oligosaccharide-CRM_{197} conjugate vaccine in 1- to 6-month-old infants. Pediatrics 1990;85:331-7.
6. Fritzell B, Plotkin S. Efficacy and safety of a *Haemophilus influenzae* type b capsular polysaccharide–tetanus protein conjugate vaccine. J PEDIATR 1992;121:355-62.
7. Vadheim CM, Greenberg DP, Eriksen E, et al. Eradication of *Haemophilus influenzae* type b disease in Southern California. Arch Pediatr Adolesc Med 1994;148:51-6.
8. Holmes SJ, Osterholm MT, Granoff DM, et al. *Haemophilus influenzae* type b (Hib) disease in infants vaccinated with Hib conjugate vaccine at <12 months [Abstract 976]. Program and Abstracts of the 32nd Interscience Conference on Antimicrobial Agents and Chemotherapy, Anaheim, California, 1992.
9. Vella PP, Ellis RW. Immunogenicity of *Haemophilus influenzae* type b conjugate vaccines in infant rhesus monkeys. Pediatr Res 1991;29:10-3.
10. Granoff DM, Rathore MH, Holmes SJ, Granoff PD, Lucas AH. Effect of immunity to the carrier protein on antibody responses to *Haemophilus influenzae* type b conjugate vaccines. Vaccine 1993;11:S46-51.
11. Kurikka S, Käyhty H, Peltola H, Saarinen L, Eskola J, Mäkelä PH. Neonatal immunization: response to *Haemophilus influenzae* type b–tetanus toxoid conjugate vaccine. Pediatrics (in press).
12. Greenberg DP, Lieberman JM, Marcy SM, et al. Enhanced antibody responses in infants given different sequences of heterogeneous *Haemophilus influenzae* type b conjugate vaccines. J PEDIATR 1995;126:206-11.
13. Greenberg DP, Ward JI, Burkart K, Christenson PD, Guravitz L, Marcy SM. Factors influencing immunogenicity and safety of two *Haemophilus influenzae* type b polysaccharide vaccines in children 18 and 24 months of age. Pediatr Infect Dis J 1987;6:660-5.
14. Greenberg DP, Vadheim CM, Partridge S, et al. Immunogenicity of *Haemophilus influenzae* type b tetanus toxoid conjugate vaccine (PRP-T) in young infants. J Infect Dis 1994; 170:76-81.
15. Ward JI, Lieberman JM, Cochi S. *Haemophilus influenzae*

vaccines. In: Plotkin S, Mortimer E, eds. Vaccines. 2nd ed. Philadelphia: WB Saunders, 1994:337-86.
16. Ward JI, Bulkow L, Wainwright R, Chang S. Immune tolerance and lack of booster responses to *Haemophilus influenzae* (Hib) conjugate vaccination in infants immunized beginning at birth [Abstract 987]. Programs and Abstracts of the 32nd Interscience Conference on Antimicrobial Agents and Chemotherapy, Anaheim, California, 1992.
17. Lise LD, Mazier D, Jolivet M, Chedid L, Schlesinger D. Enhanced epitopic response to a synthetic human malarial peptide by preimmunization with tetanus toxoid carrier. Infect Immun 1987;55:2658-61.
18. Peeters CCAM, Tenbergen-Meekes AM, Poolman JT, Beurret M, Zegers BJM, Rijkers GT. Effect of carrier priming on immunogenicity of saccharide-protein conjugate vaccines. Infect Immun 1991;59:3504-10.
19. Herzenberg LA, Tokuhisa T, Herzenberg LA. Carrier-priming leads to hapten-specific suppression. Nature 1980;285: 664-7.
20. DiJohn D, Torres JR, Murillo J, et al. Effect of priming with carrier on response to conjugate vaccine. Lancet 1989;2:1415-18.
21. Schutze MP, Leclerc C, Jolivet M, Audibert F, Chedid F. Carrier-induced epitopic suppression, a major issue for future synthetic vaccines. J Immunol 1985;135:2319-22.
22. Dengrove J, Lee EU, Heiner DC, et al. IgG and IgG subclass specific antibody responses to diphtheria and tetanus toxoids in newborns and infants given DTP immunization. Pediatr Res 1986;20:735-9.
23. Vogel FR, Leclerc C, Schutze MP, et al. Modulation of carrier-induced epitopic suppression by *Bordetella pertussis* components and muramyl peptide. Cell Immunol 1987;107:40-51.
24. Granoff DM, Holmes SJ, Belshe RB, Osterholm MT, McHugh JE, Anderson EL. Effect of carrier protein priming on antibody responses to *Haemophilus influenzae* type b conjugate vaccines in infants. JAMA 1994;272:1116-21.
25. Barington T, Gyhrs A, Kristensen K, Heilmann C. Opposite effects of actively and passively acquired immunity to the carrier on responses of human infants to a *Haemophilus influenzae* type b conjugate vaccine. Infect Immun 1994;62:9-14.
26. Wilson CB. The ontogeny of T-lymphocyte maturation and function. J Pediatr 1991;118:S4-9.
27. Barington T, Skettrup M, Juul L, Heilmann C. Non-epitope-specific suppression of the antibody response to *Haemophilus influenzae* type b conjugate vaccines by preimmunization with vaccine components. Infect Immun 1993;61: 432-8.

Enhanced antibody responses in infants given different sequences of heterogeneous *Haemophilus influenzae* type b conjugate vaccines

David P. Greenberg, MD, Jay M. Lieberman, MD, S. Michael Marcy, MD, Victor K. Wong, MD, Susan Partridge, RN, Swei-Ju Chang, MS, Chung-Yin Chiu, MS, and Joel I. Ward, MD

From the Division of Pediatric Infectious Diseases, Harbor-UCLA Medical Center, University of California at Los Angeles Center for Vaccine Research, Torrance, and the Kaiser Foundation Hospitals and Medical Clinics, Panorama City and Downey, California

To evaluate the safety and immunogenicity of differing sequences of heterogeneous *Haemophilus influenzae* type b (Hib) conjugate vaccines, we randomly assigned 300 infants to one of six vaccination schedules. At 2, 4, and 6 months of age, subjects were given single or heterogeneous vaccines: Hib polysaccharide (PRP) conjugated to mutant diphtheria toxin (HbOC), PRP conjugated to outer-membrane protein of *Neisseria meningitidis* (PRP-OMP), or PRP conjugated to tetanus toxoid (PRP-T). No serious reactions were attributable to immunization with heterogeneous vaccines, and there were few significant differences in the rates of minor adverse reactions among groups. PRP-OMP was the only vaccine that induced an antibody response after the first dose, but significant booster responses were not seen after the second and third doses. Subjects given PRP-T vaccine responded well after two doses, but three doses of HbOC vaccine were needed for an equivalent antibody response. All the Hib vaccine schedules evaluated were immunogenic, and schedules initiated by PRP-OMP vaccine at 2 months of age, followed by two doses of either HbOC or PRP-T vaccine at 4 and 6 months of age, induced the highest antibody levels after each dose. Such schedules may be the best for protecting infants and children who are at greatest risk of having invasive Hib disease, such as American Indian children. (J PEDIATR 1995;126:206-11)

The widespread use of *Haemophilus influenzae* type b polysaccharide (polyribosylribitol phosphate) conjugate vaccines has led to a significant (up to 95%) decrease in the incidence of invasive Hib infections in infants and children in the United States and elsewhere.[1-4] Despite the success of Hib conjugate vaccines, failures of immunization occur.[2, 3, 5-10] In two large population-based studies of Hib conjugate vaccine failures in the United States, approximately 88% of HbOC (HibTITER, Praxis Biologics, Rochester, N.Y.) vaccine failures occurred after the first or second dose,[3, 10] consistent with the lack of antibody responses after the first two doses of the vaccine.[10] The antibody response to a PRP–tetanus toxoid vaccine, PRP-T (ActHIB or OmniHIB; Pasteur Merieux, Lyon, France), in infants is similar to that to HbOC, with little antibody response until after the second or third dose.[11] In contrast, a PRP–outer-membrane protein vaccine, PRP-OMP (PedvaxHIB, Merck & Co., West Point, Pa.), typically induces a good antibody

Supported by the National Institutes of Health (RO1-AI-31580 and NO1-AI-15124) and Connaught Laboratories.

Submitted for publication April 5, 1994; accepted Aug. 17, 1994.

Reprint requests: David P. Greenberg, MD, Harbor-UCLA Medical Center, 1124 W. Carson St., Bldg. E-6, Torrance, CA 90502.

0022-3476/95/$3.00 + 0 **9/20/60007**

See related article, p. 198.

CRM	Cross-reacting mutant
HbOC	PRP oligosaccharide polymers coupled to a nontoxic variant of diphtheria toxin, CRM_{197}
Hib	*Haemophilus influenzae* type b
PRP	Polyribosylribitol phosphate
PRP-D	PRP polymers coupled to diphtheria toxoid
PRP-OMP	PRP polymers coupled to outer-membrane protein vesicles of *Neisseria meningitidis* group B
PRP-T	PRP polymers coupled to tetanus toxoid

response after the first dose at 2 months of age, although only modest increases in antibody levels are seen with subsequent doses at 4 and 6 months of age.[12]

The primary goal of this study was to evaluate antibody responses to several different sequences of heterogeneous Hib conjugate vaccines compared with responses induced by conventional schedules of single Hib vaccines. Because it would be difficult to evaluate all possible sequences of heterogeneous vaccines (n = 27), we restricted the study to three of the possible schedules. For two of the schedules, our hypothesis was that an initial dose of PRP-OMP vaccine, followed by two doses of HbOC or PRP-T vaccines, might induce higher antibody levels than any of the vaccines given alone. In addition, some infants inadvertently receive sequences of heterogeneous Hib conjugate vaccines from different health care providers, so we wanted to evaluate the potential interchangeability of Hib conjugate vaccines. The third schedule was chosen to evaluate the interchangeability of HbOC and PRP-T vaccines—specifically, administration of one dose of HbOC vaccine followed by two doses of PRP-T vaccine.

METHODS

Subjects and vaccine schedule. Three hundred healthy infants 6 to 12 weeks of age were recruited from two Kaiser Permanente pediatric clinics in Southern California. Infants were excluded if they had (1) a history of invasive Hib disease, (2) a major congenital birth defect affecting overall health, (3) a progressive neurologic disease or seizure disorder, (4) suspected immune dysfunction, or (5) received any immune globulin preparation or blood product. Immunizations were deferred for acute febrile illnesses (>38.3° C).

The study was approved by the Harbor-UCLA Research and Education Institute and Kaiser Permanente human subject committees, and informed consent was obtained from the parents of each infant before enrollment. During the first 6 months of the study, infants were randomly assigned in blocks of 30 to one of three vaccine schedule groups (HbOC–HbOC–HbOC group; PRP-OMP–PRP-OMP–PRP-OMP group; and PRP-OMP–HbOC–HbOC group). During the final 8 months of the study, after PRP-T vaccine was provided by Connaught Laboratories, three additional groups were added (PRP-T–PRP-T–PRP-T group; PRP-OMP–PRP-T–PRP-T group; and HbOC–PRP-T–PRP-T group), and infants were randomly assigned to one of six groups (a total of 50 infants per group). The sample size was chosen to achieve the maximal number of evaluable vaccine schedules while completing enrollment of all subjects within 1 year. Because each of the vaccines were distinguishable, the research nurses administering the vaccines were not masked to the infant's assignment. However, different research personnel ascertained safety and immunogenicity data, and they, along with the parents and Kaiser clinic personnel, were masked throughout the study as to the vaccine assignments. Concurrent vaccines were administered at separate sites and included diphtheria-tetanus-pertussis vaccine (2, 4, and 6 months of age), trivalent oral polio vaccine (2, 4, and an optional dose at 6 months of age), and occasionally hepatitis B vaccine (15 infants received one or more doses concurrently).

Overall, 46% of the 300 subjects were male, 25% white, 13% black, 49% Hispanic, and 12% other races. The mean age at the time of the first dose was 2.17 months; second dose, 4.41 months; and third dose, 6.50 months. There were few significant differences of gender, race, or age at vaccination between study groups, and when these demographic factors were used to adjust Hib antibody levels, there was no significant effect on the comparisons among groups.

Vaccines. Two lots of HbOC vaccine (lots M130HA and M140HF), containing 10 μg Hib oligosaccharide and 25 μg CRM_{197} protein per 0.5 ml dose, were obtained commercially. Two lots of PRP-OMP vaccine (lots 0498T and 1228T), supplied by Merck Research Laboratories, contained 15 μg capsular polysaccharide and 250 μg meningococcal outer-membrane protein complex per 0.5 ml dose. One lot of PRP-T vaccine (lot S2372), supplied by Connaught Laboratories, contained 10 μg capsular polysaccharide and 20 μg tetanus toxoid per 0.5 ml dose. All doses were administered intramuscularly in the anterior thigh.

Serum collection and antibody assays. Serum specimens were obtained from study subjects by venipuncture at 2, 4, 6, and 7 months of age. Total antibody to Hib capsular polysaccharide was measured by a standardized radioimmunoassay.[13] Tritiated PRP (Connaught Laboratories) and the U.S. Food and Drug Administration serum standard (Office of Biologics Research and Review, 70 μg/ml PRP antibody) were used. The lowest limit of detection for anticapsular antibody was 0.025 μg/ml.

Safety evaluation. Parents were instructed to complete an adverse reaction report card after each Hib vaccine dose. In

Table. Antibody responses to conventional and heterogeneous schedules of three Hib conjugate vaccines

Vaccine schedule	Subjects (No.)	Geometric mean PRP antibody level (μg/ml) Preimmunization (2 mo)	After 1 dose (4 mo)	After 2 doses (6 mo)	After 3 doses (7 mo)
H-H-H	43	0.07	0.06*	0.45†	6.49‡
O-O-O (PRP-OMP lot 0498T)§	24	0.10	0.40	0.38†	0.59‖
O-O-O (PRP-OMP lot 1228T)§	17	0.07	1.95¶	3.60	5.89**
T-T-T	36	0.05	0.16	2.55	10.88
O-H-H (PRP-OMP lot 0498T)	23	0.09	0.48	2.72	12.73
O-H-H (PRP-OMP lot 1228T)	16	0.08	2.37¶	3.98	11.75
O-T-T (PRP-OMP lot 1228T)	39	0.07	3.17¶	6.36††	14.84
H-T-T	39	0.11	0.10*	3.28	11.88

H, HbOC vaccine; *O*, PRP-OMP vaccine; *T*, PRP-T vaccine.
*The H-H-H and H-T-T groups were less immunogenic than all other groups (p <0.01), except that the responses to H-T-T were not significantly different from the responses to T-T-T.
†The H-H-H and O-O-O (lot 0498T) groups were less immunogenic than all other groups, p <0.0001.
‡The H-H-H group was less immunogenic than the O-H-H (PRP-OMP lots 0498T and 1228T, combined), O-T-T, and H-T-T groups, p <0.03.
§For the O-O-O schedule with lot 0498T, subjects received one, two, or three doses of a poorly immunogenic lot; for the O-O-O schedule with lot 1228T, subjects received all three doses of a lot, with expected immunogenicity.
‖The O-O-O (lot 0498T) group was less immunogenic than all other groups, p <0.0001.
¶The O-O-O (lot 1228T), O-H-H (PRP-OMP lot 1228T), and O-T-T groups were more immunogenic than all other groups, p <0.01.
**The O-O-O (lot 1228T) group was less immunogenic than the T-T-T, O-H-H (PRP-OMP lots 0498T and 1228T, combined), O-T-T, and H-T-T groups, p <0.05.
††The O-T-T group was more immunogenic than the T-T-T, O-H-H (PRP-OMP lot 0498T), and H-T-T groups, p <0.05.

addition to recording a rectal temperature (thermometer and instructions provided), parents answered questions about local and systemic reactions that occurred by 6, 24, 48, and 72 hours after vaccination. A research assistant telephoned the parents 3 to 4 days after each vaccination to obtain the responses to the report card questions. At each scheduled visit, the research nurse interviewed the parents and reviewed the child's medical record for information about interval illnesses, clinic visits, and hospitalizations.

Statistical analysis. Frequencies of adverse reactions were compared by means of the Cochran-Mantel-Haenszel test. The rates of some adverse reactions were more frequent in children followed at one Kaiser clinic than at the other, so there was an adjustment for the clinic in the analyses. The PRP antibody levels were log transformed before antibody responses were compared with analyses of variance. The antibody levels were also evaluated after stratification for gender, race, and Kaiser clinic, and after adjustment for the age at each dose. For statistical analyses, antibody levels less than 0.025 μg/ml were assigned a value of 0.012 μg/ml.

RESULTS

Of 300 infants enrolled in the study, 238 received all three doses of Hib conjugate vaccine and had blood specimens drawn. Reasons for discontinuations were parental request (31 infants), loss of Kaiser insurance or transferral of child's care to another clinic (26), and noncompliance with the protocol schedule (5). A greater number of infants left the group given three doses of PRP-T vaccine (n = 14) than the other groups (n = 7 to 11), but the number who left because of parental request did not differ in this group (n = 6) from the number in the other groups (n = 4 to 7). None of the discontinuations were for adverse reactions to vaccination.

The rates of minor local and systemic adverse reactions occurring within 3 days of vaccination were similar to rates we have observed in other studies of infants given concurrent Hib conjugate and diphtheria-tetanus-pertussis vaccines.[14] There were few significantly different rates of adverse reactions among the six vaccine groups. Fussiness occurred slightly more often in the group given three doses of PRP-OMP vaccine (68.2%) than in three of the other groups (range, 56.3% to 59.7%; $p \leq 0.05$). Pain at the injection site occurred more often in the group given PRP-OMP, PRP-T, and PRP-T (31.8%) than in the group given HbOC, PRP-T, and PRP-T (19.9%, p = 0.02). There were no serious adverse events thought to be related to vaccination.

Shown in the Table are antibody responses after each dose for the different vaccination groups. For statistical analysis, the original six study groups were further divided into eight groups because we learned that one of the PRP-OMP vaccine lots (lot 0498T) was significantly less immunogenic than the other (lot 1228T).[15] Infants given three doses of PRP-OMP vaccine were thus stratified into two groups: (1) those who received one or more doses of lot 0498T and (2) infants who received all three doses with the normally immunogenic lot (lot 1228T). Subjects given one dose of PRP-OMP vaccine, followed by two doses of HbOC vaccine, were also stratified into two groups depending on the PRP-OMP lot. All the infants given PRP-OMP vaccine, followed by two doses of PRP-T, received PRP-OMP lot 1228T.

After the first vaccine dose, only groups given PRP-OMP (lot 1228T) had mean antibody levels >1.0 μg/ml ($p < 0.01$ compared with all other groups). Two doses of PRP-T vaccine and three doses of HbOC vaccine were needed to achieve antibody levels comparable to that after one dose of PRP-OMP vaccine. After the second dose, all the groups had antibody rises except for the groups given two doses of HbOC or PRP-OMP lot 0498T ($p < 0.0001$). After three doses, the geometric mean antibody levels were >1.0 μg/ml in all groups except for the group given PRP-OMP lot 0498T (0.59 μg/ml; $p < 0.0001$). In addition, all infants had PRP antibody levels >1.0 μg/ml, except for some infants given three doses of HbOC or one or more doses of PRP-OMP lot 0498T (90% and 44% >1.0 μg/ml, respectively). After two doses of PRP-OMP vaccine (only two doses are recommended for primary immunization of infants), 94% of subjects given lot 1228T but only 35% of subjects given lot 0498T had antibody levels >1.0 μg/ml ($p = 0.0005$).

After each dose, subjects given the PRP-OMP–HbOC–HbOC sequence had significantly higher antibody levels than those given HbOC vaccine alone ($p < 0.03$). Similarly, after the first and second doses, infants given the PRP-OMP–PRP-T–PRP-T sequence had significantly higher antibody levels than those given PRP-T vaccine alone ($p < 0.01$). After the third dose, infants given these sequences of heterogeneous vaccines had significantly higher antibody levels than infants given three doses of PRP-OMP vaccine ($p < 0.03$). Subjects given the HbOC–PRP-T–PRP-T sequence had antibody levels comparable to those given PRP-T vaccine alone, and after the second and third doses, this group had higher antibody levels than the group given HbOC vaccine alone ($p < 0.03$). For each study group, PRP antibody levels were not appreciably different when the group members were stratified by gender, race, or Kaiser clinic, nor when the levels were adjusted for the age at each dose.

DISCUSSION

We evaluated two issues regarding the use of Hib conjugate vaccines in clinical practice. The first was whether the immunologic advantages of each vaccine might be used to design schedules to provide even better protection than is now observed, especially in children less than 6 months of age. We postulated that giving PRP-OMP vaccine at 2 months of age would induce an initial good antibody response and that subsequent doses of HbOC or PRP-T vaccine might induce even higher booster responses. The second important issue was the interchangeability of Hib vaccines during primary immunization of infants. The likelihood of inadvertently receiving a sequence of heterogeneous Hib conjugate vaccines has increased with the licensure of PRP-T and two different combination vaccines. To evaluate whether all possible schedules of heterogeneous Hib vaccines are as safe and immunogenic as conventional vaccine schedules, one would have to evaluate at least 27 different sequences. Although this was not possible, we wanted to evaluate the interchangeability of the most clinically useful schedules, some of which are distinct from those being addressed by other investigators.[16, 17]

We found few significant differences in the rates of local or systemic adverse reactions between groups given different schedules of Hib vaccines. The differences of adverse reactions were minor, and no serious adverse reactions were attributable to the different vaccine schedules. Although more infants would have to be studied for a definitive statistical comparison, it does not appear that schedules of heterogeneous Hib vaccines lead to increased rates of adverse reactions.

For the subjects given conventional schedules of the three Hib conjugate vaccines, our results confirmed previously published data.[12, 18-20] One lot of PRP-OMP was the only vaccine immunogenic after the first dose at 2 months of age, but only modest increases of antibody were seen after a second or third dose. In contrast, two doses of PRP-T vaccine and three doses of HbOC vaccine were required to induce similar high levels of antibody. After three doses, the geometric mean antibody titer of the group given PRP-T (but not HbOC) was greater than that of the group given PRP-OMP vaccine.

The group given PRP-T vaccine alone had significantly greater geometric mean antibody levels after the first and second doses (but not after the third dose) than the group given HbOC vaccine alone. The clinical significance of these differences is unknown. Invasive Hib disease has developed in infants after one or two doses of HbOC vaccine,[2, 3, 10] but there has not been sufficient experience with PRP-T to know whether similar cases will occur after this vaccine.

Of particular interest are the results of the following two schedules of heterogeneous Hib vaccines: the PRP-OMP–HbOC–HbOC schedule, and the PRP-OMP–PRP-T–PRP-T schedule. Infants given these schedules had higher geometric mean antibody levels than infants given any of the three Hib conjugate vaccines alone. After the first dose, 82% of the infants given one lot of PRP-OMP vaccine had antibody levels >1.0 μg/ml (generally considered protective), compared with only 2% and 17% of the infants given HbOC and PRP-T vaccines, respectively. Moreover, after three doses, these two heterogeneous vaccine schedules induced significantly higher antibody levels than PRP-OMP vaccine alone; PRP-OMP primed vaccinees for subsequent booster responses with the other Hib conjugate vaccines. Heterogeneous schedules may provide protection early in infancy and contribute to sustained high antibody levels and protection. Such schedules may be especially useful in populations with a high risk of Hib disease (e.g., Alaskan Eskimos and American Indians) and in populations with high rates of incomplete immunizations (e.g., inner-city populations).

As a test of interchangeability, we evaluated the heterogeneous HbOC–PRP-T–PRP-T vaccine schedule. The antibody levels induced with this schedule were comparable to those induced with three doses of PRP-T, and were significantly higher than the antibody levels induced by three doses of HbOC vaccine. This schedule was therefore comparable to, or better than, either of the vaccines given in conventional schedules.

One of the PRP-OMP vaccine lots used in this study was later identified as one of several that had impaired potency.[21] In the Table, which shows geometric mean antibody levels, the results for infants given one, two, or three doses of lot 0498T were combined. However, when further analyzed, the antibody responses correlated inversely with the number of doses of the poorly immunogenic lot. At 7 months of age, the geometric mean antibody levels were 1.45 μg/ml, 0.57 μg/ml, and 0.15 μg/ml for infants given one, two, and three doses of lot 0498T, respectively.

Unexpectedly, we found that infants given the poorly immunogenic PRP-OMP vaccine lot, followed by two doses of HbOC, achieved antibody responses comparable to those in infants given the same heterogeneous vaccine schedule but initially given the normally immunogenic PRP-OMP lot. Therefore, although the weakly immunogenic PRP-OMP lot did not induce high antibody levels, it appears to have primed infants for booster responses to HbOC; in fact, there was better priming than with the homologous vaccine, HbOC.

We know of two other studies evaluating the interchangeability of Hib conjugate vaccines for primary immunization.[16, 17] As in our study, even with a poorly immunogenic lot of PRP-OMP vaccine, infants given vaccine on the PRP-OMP–HbOC–HbOC schedule had significantly higher antibody responses than infants given PRP-OMP or HbOC vaccines alone.[16] In the second study, infants given a poorly immunogenic lot of PRP-OMP vaccine, followed by two doses of PRP-T, achieved antibody levels after the third dose that were comparable to those in infants given three doses of PRP-T vaccine alone.[17] In addition, infants given a poorly immunogenic lot of PRP-OMP vaccine, followed by two doses of PRP-D vaccine (Connaught Laboratories, Swiftwater, Pa.), had higher antibody responses than would be expected for infants given PRP-D alone[17] (PRP-D is not licensed for use in infants in the United States). These data confirm that even poorly immunogenic lots of PRP-OMP vaccine prime infants to respond to booster doses of other Hib conjugate vaccines.

We conclude that heterogeneous schedules of PRP-OMP, HbOC, and PRP-T vaccines given in infancy were as safe and immunogenic as schedules of single Hib conjugate vaccines. Immunization schedules consisting of a first dose of PRP-OMP vaccine, followed by two doses of HbOC or PRP-T vaccines, induced higher antibody levels than other schedules tested.

We acknowledge and express our profound thanks to the Southern California Kaiser Permanente pediatricians, family practitioners, nurse practitioners, nurses, and other clinic personnel at the Panorama City and Imperial (Downey) Medical Offices who contributed to this project, without whose help this study would not have been possible. We also thank the clinical research nurses who enrolled, immunized, and monitored the safety of the study subjects (Deanna Bundy, Linda Gutierrez, Pamela Johnson, and Gloria Leon); Millie Badar for assaying the serum specimens for PRP antibody; and Christina Laurel and Caroline Garcia for data entry and verification.

REFERENCES

1. Murphy TV, White KE, Pastor P, et al. Declining incidence of *Haemophilus influenzae* type b disease since introduction of vaccination. JAMA 1993;269:246-8.
2. Black SB, Shinefield HR. Immunization with oligosaccharide conjugate *Haemophilus influenzae* type b (HbOC) vaccine on a large health maintenance organization population: extended follow-up and impact on *Haemophilus influenzae* disease epidemiology. Pediatr Infect Dis J 1992;11:610-3.
3. Vadheim CM, Greenberg DP, Eriksen E, et al. Eradication of *Haemophilus influenzae* type b disease in Southern California. Arch Pediatr Adolesc Med 1994;148:51-6.
4. Peltola H, Kilpi T, Anttila M. Rapid disappearance of *Haemophilus influenzae* type b meningitis after routine childhood immunisation with conjugate vaccines. Lancet 1992;340:592-4.
5. Santosham M, Rivin B, Wolff M, et al. Prevention of *Haemophilus influenzae* type b infections in Apache and Navajo children. J Infect Dis 1992;165(suppl 1):S144-51.
6. Black SB, Shinefield HR, Fireman B, Hiatt R. Safety, immunogenicity, and efficacy in infancy of oligosaccharide conjugate *Haemophilus influenzae* type b vaccine in a United States population: possible implications for optimal use. J Infect Dis 1992;165(suppl 1):S139-43.
7. Eskola J, Peltola H, Kayhty H, Takala AK, Makela PH. Finnish efficacy trials with *Haemophilus influenzae* type b vaccines. J Infect Dis 1992;165(suppl 1):S137-8.
8. Frasch CE, Hiner EE, Gross TP. *Haemophilus* b disease after vaccination with *Haemophilus* b polysaccharide or conjugate vaccine. Am J Dis Child 1991;145:1379-82.
9. Holmes SJ, Lucas AH, Osterholm MT, Froeschle JE, Granoff DM. Immunoglobulin deficiency and idiotype expression in children developing *Haemophilus influenzae* type b disease

after vaccination with conjugate vaccine. JAMA 1991;266:1960-5.

10. Holmes SJ, Osterholm MT, Granoff DM, Vaccine Failure Group. *Haemophilus influenzae* type b (Hib) disease in infants vaccinated with Hib conjugate vaccine at <12 months [Abstract 976]. Thirty-second Interscience Conference of Antimicrobial Agents and Chemotherapy, Anaheim, California October 11, 1992.
11. Fritzell B, Plotkin S. Efficacy and safety of a *Haemophilus influenzae* type b capsular polysaccharide–tetanus protein conjugate vaccine. J PEDIATR 1992;121:355-62.
12. Granoff DM, Anderson EL, Osterholm MT, et al. Differences in the immunogenicity of three *Haemophilus influenzae* type b conjugate vaccines in infants. J PEDIATR 1992;121:187-94.
13. Greenberg DP, Ward JI, Burkart K, Christenson PD, Guravitz L, Marcy SM. Factors influencing immunogenicity and safety of two *Haemophilus influenzae* type b polysaccharide vaccines in children 18 and 24 months of age. Pediatr Infect Dis J 1987;6:660-5.
14. Vadheim CM, Greenberg DP, Partridge S, Jing J, Ward JI. Effectiveness and safety of an *Haemophilus influenzae* type b conjugate vaccine (PRP-T) in young infants. Pediatrics 1993;92:272-9.
15. Immunization Practices Advisory Committee (ACIP). Update: report of PedvaxHIB lots with questionable immunogenicity. MMWR Morb Mortal Wkly Rep 1992;41:878-9.
16. Anderson EL, Decker MD, Edwards KM, Englund JA, Belshe RB. Interchangeability of conjugated *Haemophilus influenzae* type b (Hib) vaccines in infants [Abstract 493]. Pediatr Res 1993;33:85A.
17. Daum RS, Milewski WM, Ballanco GA. Interchangeability of *H. influenzae* type b vaccines for the primary series (mix and match): a preliminary analysis [Abstract 976]. Pediatr Res 1993;33:166A.
18. Kayhty H, Eskola J, Peltola H, et al. Antibody responses to four *Haemophilus influenzae* type b conjugate vaccines. Am J Dis Child 1991;145:223-7.
19. Decker MD, Edwards KM, Bradley R, Palmer P. Comparative trial in infants of four conjugate *Haemophilus influenzae* type b vaccines. J PEDIATR 1992;120:184-9.
20. Bulkow LR, Wainwright RB, Letson GW, Chang SJ, Ward JI. Comparative immunogenicity of four *Haemophilus influenzae* type b conjugate vaccines in Alaska Native infants. Pediatr Infect Dis J 1993;12:484-92.
21. Greenberg DP, Vadheim CM, Partridge S, et al. Post-licensure evaluation of PRP-OMP vaccine lots with less than expected immunogenicity [Abstract 996]. Pediatr Res 1993;33:169A.

Pediatric Investigators Collaborative Network on Infections in Canada (PICNIC) prospective study of risk factors and outcomes in patients hospitalized with respiratory syncytial viral lower respiratory tract infection

Elaine E. L. Wang, MDCM, Barbara J. Law, MD, Derek Stephens, MS, and other members of PICNIC[a]

From the Clinical Epidemiology Unit, Hospital for Sick Children, Toronto, Ontario, Canada

Objective: **To provide information on disease attributable to respiratory syncytial viral lower respiratory tract infection (RSV LRI) and to quantify the morbidity associated with various risk factors.**

Design: **Prospective cohort study.**

Subjects: **Patients hospitalized with RSV LRIs at seven centers were eligible for study if they were younger than 2 years of age, or hospitalized patients of any age if they had underlying cardiac or pulmonary disease or immunosuppression.**

Measurements and results: **Enrolled (n = 689) and eligible but not enrolled (n = 191) patients were similar in age, duration of illness and proportion with underlying illness, use of intensive care, and ventilation. Of the enrolled patients, 156 had underlying illness. The isolates from 353 patients were typeable: 102 isolates were subgroup A, 250 were subgroup B, and one isolated grouped with both antisera. The mean hospital stay attributable to respiratory syncytial virus (RSV) was 7 days; 110 patients were admitted to intensive care units, 63 were supported by mechanical ventilation, and 6 patients died. Regression models were developed for the prediction of three outcomes: RSV-associated hospital duration, intensive care unit admission, and ventilation treatment. In addition to previously described risk factors for an increased morbidity, such as underlying illness, hypoxia, prematurity and young age, three other factors were found to be significantly associated with complicated hospitalization: aboriginal race (defined by maternal race), a history of apnea or respiratory arrest during the acute illness before hospitalization, and pulmonary consolidation as shown on the chest radiograph obtained at admission. The RSV subgroup, family income, and day care attendance were not significantly associated with these outcomes.**

Supported by a grant from Lederle, Canada Inc.

Presented in part at the Society for Pediatric Research Meeting, Seattle, Washington, May 2, 1994.

Submitted for publication May 23, 1994; accepted Aug. 10, 1994.

Reprint requests: Elaine E. L. Wang, MCDM, Clinical Epidemiology Unit, Hospital for Sick Children, 555 University Ave., Toronto, Ontario, M5G 1X8, Canada.

[a]The list of participating members and institutions is provided at the end of the text.

0022-3476/95/$3.00 + 0 **9/20/59781**

Conclusions: **Hypoxia on admission, a history of apnea or respiratory arrest, and pulmonary consolidation should be considered in the management of children with RSV LRIs. Vaccine trials should target patients with underlying heart or lung disease or of aboriginal race. (J PEDIATR 1995;126:212-9)**

A recent 3-year retrospective study demonstrated an improved outcome of respiratory syncytial virus infection in high-risk groups.[1] The mortality rate attributed to RSV in subjects with underlying heart or lung disease was only 3%, a tenfold reduction compared with previously described rates.[2-4] Because data were obtained by chart review,[1] it was not possible to separate the morbidity that could be attributed to RSV infection from that caused by the underlying disease.

This study was conducted to obtain comparative data on morbidity and death in children hospitalized with RSV in high-risk groups and in children without known risk factors. Data were collected prospectively to describe morbidity directly attributable to RSV infection. In addition, if a group at high risk of complicated hospitalization could be identified on admission, they might be considered for treatment with ribavirin[5] and other interventions such as high titers of RSV immune globulin.[6] Thus we wished to determine whether prognostic indicators could be defined at the time of admission.

See related article, p. 220.

LRI	Lower respiratory tract infection
RSV	Respiratory syncytial virus

METHODS

Patients. The study population consisted of children admitted between Jan. 1 and April 30, 1993, to one of the following seven pediatric tertiary care hospitals in Canada: Izaak Walton Killam Hospital, Halifax; Le Centre Hospitalier de l'Université Laval, Québec City; Montreal Children's Hospital, Montreal; Children's Hospital of Eastern Ontario, Ottawa; Hospital for Sick Children, Toronto; Winnipeg Children's Hospital, Winnipeg; and British Columbia's Children's Hospital, Vancouver. Because of the delayed season in Winnipeg, where the peak infection rate occurred after April, patient enrollment there continued until June 30, 1993. All patients younger than 2 years of age, and those older than 2 years of age with underlying heart or lung disease or with immunosuppression, who were hospitalized with RSV lower respiratory tract infection were eligible. Patients older than 2 years of age who had only asthma were excluded, as were patients who had only RSV upper respiratory tract infections.

At all centers, a nasopharyngeal specimen was obtained from patients with symptoms suggestive of LRI, including cough, wheezing, dyspnea, tachypnea, or apnea. In addition, admission lists were monitored by study nurses to ensure that a nasopharyngeal specimen was submitted from any patient meeting enrollment criteria with the above symptoms or who had wheezing, bronchiolitis, pneumonia, pneumonitis, or a respiratory problem. Specimens were also usually obtained from patients in whom such symptoms or diagnoses developed after hospitalization during respiratory viral season (at the request of infection control personnel).

Once an eligible patient was identified by RSV antigen detection in the nasopharyngeal specimen, consent for enrollment was sought from parents by study personnel. After enrollment, data on patient demographic characteristics, clinical assessment, oximetry, and the results of a chest radiograph were entered on standard data collection forms. Chest radiographs were obtained by attending physicians as indicated by clinical symptoms, and the results from the radiograph obtained within 24 hours of admission were entered into prognostic models. Patients were assessed daily and their management was noted in the data collection form. At these assessments, the reason for continuation of hospitalization was indicated in a hierarchic classification as follows: patient receiving drug treatment for RSV LRI; patient receiving oxygen supplementation or parenteral fluids because of RSV LRI; patient hospitalized because of underlying illness only; patient hospitalized because of an uncertain home environment or awaiting transportation home. Thus the first reason on the list that applied to the patient was recorded. The underlying cardiac or pulmonary conditions could lead to supportive or drug treatment of RSV LRI because they may contribute to the underlying physiologic derangement. The hospital stay that was attributed to RSV disease consisted of the number of days for which either of the first two reasons was recorded. Similarly, for the outcomes of receipt of intensive care and mechanical ventilation, only those that were associated with RSV infection were included in the analysis. In patients with underlying conditions, the duration of the hospital stay attributed to RSV disease was counted from the day when there was an increase in the supportive therapy from the baseline requirement until the day of return to baseline requirement. The study was approved by the institutional review board at each participating hospital.

Patients were grouped according to the presence or absence of each of the following: congenital heart disease,

Table I. Laboratory methods by study center

Center No.	Patients (No.)	Type of NP specimen	Type of rapid diagnosis	Patients with positive culture results No. (%)	A/B/nontypeable infection (No.)	A subtype (%)
1	85	Wash	EIA,DFA	68 (80)	51/17/0	75
2	90	Aspirate	EIA	67 (74)	28/39/0	42
3	146	Swab	DFA,EIA	16 (11)	1/4/11	6
4	152	Aspirate	DFA	116 (76)	13/103/0	11
5	82	Aspirate	DFA	63 (77)	3/54/6	5
6	85	Aspirate	EIA	29 (34)	1/28/0	3
7	49	Aspirate	EIA	14 (29)	5/5/4	35

DFA, Direct immunofluorescence; *EIA*, enzyme immunoassay; *NP*, nasopharyngeal.

chronic lung disease (includes bronchopulmonary dysplasia, cystic fibrosis, congenital pulmonary anomaly), immunocompromise (includes immunodeficiency, immunosuppressant therapy, and use of corticosteroids), other multisystemic disease, gestation less than 37 weeks, or postnatal age younger than 6 weeks. Patients could have more than one underlying problem. Thus a patient who was both premature and had chronic lung disease of prematurity would have been included in both of those groups.

Oximetry. Oxygen saturation was determined daily in room air whenever possible with a portable Nellcor oximeter (model N10A; Nellcor Inc., Hayward, Calif.). Patients were examined when they were awake and quiet. A probe was placed on either a finger or toe, and oxygen saturation and pulse rate were recorded for at least 5 minutes. The study nurse then estimated the saturation on the basis of this recording as described below. All study nurses had received training with the respiratory therapy team in their hospitals before the study and moderate interobserver reliability for this measure had been demonstrated (kappa, 0.61). In patients who were receiving oxygen supplementation of less than 35% oxygen, the amount of supplementation was reduced by decrements of 10% by the study nurse. If the oxygen saturation fell below 90% during this time, the oxygen supplementation was returned to the original level and the oxygen saturation was considered to be less than 90% in room air. If patients were supported by mechanical ventilation or if the amount of supplementation was >35%, no attempt was made to alter the amount of oxygen supplementation and the saturation was considered to be less than 90% in room air. Oxygen saturation was categorized as <90%, ≥90% to 95%, and >95%. Because the outcomes of patients in the intermediate group were the same as those with oxygen saturation >95%, these two groups were combined, those with oxygen saturation <90% were considered to be hypoxic. Measurements taken in the emergency department or on admission to the ward were used in the prognostic model.

Virologic studies. Nasopharyngeal specimens were obtained according to the usual protocols at each hospital (Table I). Viral antigen detection was performed by direct immunofluorescence microscopy using RSV monoclonal antibodies (from Ortho Diagnostic Systems, Raritan, N.J. [centers 1 and 4], Frappier Diagnostic SNC, Ville De Laval, Quebec, Canada [center 3], or Chemicon International, Temecula, Calif. [center 5]). In addition, the enzyme immunoassay, Test Pack (Abbott Laboratories, Abbott Park, Ill.) was performed (centers 1, 2, 3, 6 and 7). At two centers, inoculation of cell cultures for viral isolation was performed only when antigen had been detected. At other centers, all specimens were cultured. At all centers, at least two cell lines were used. Cells from cultures in which RSV was isolated were fixed on glass slides and sent to the Cadham Provincial Laboratory, Winnipeg, Manitoba, for virus subgrouping by fluorescent microscopy with monoclonal antibodies A9-21 and 102-10B provided by Dr. L. Anderson.[7]

Statistical analysis. Patients were grouped according to the presence of risk factors as follows: (1) those with underlying illness, (2) those who were born prematurely or those younger than 6 weeks of age on admission, and (3) those without known risk factors. In this way, patients were counted only once in the analysis. Thus a patient who was both premature and had chronic lung disease would be considered only in the group with underlying illness. Because the duration of hospital stay attributable to RSV had a skewed distribution, Kruskal-Wallis analysis was used to compare across the above subgroups. Proportions of patients within each group who were supported by mechanical ventilation or who received intensive care were compared. The proportion of patients receiving different treatments was recorded for each center.

Demographic variables including age, maternal race, family income, smoking in the home, day care, breast-feeding, a history of underlying illness, and hospital data were recorded for all enrolled patients. The association between each independent variable was determined for the main outcomes of interest: hospital duration attributable to RSV, admission to intensive care, and mechanical ventilation. These independent variables included demographic variables, a history of apnea or respiratory arrest, oxygen saturation on admission, chest radiograph on admission, nosocomial infection versus community-acquired infection, and virus subgroup. An infection was considered nosocomial if symptoms appeared more than 48 hours after hospitalization. Candidate predictors statistically associated with the outcome at a value of $p \leq 0.25$ were included in the multiple regression models. A multiple regression model was developed to predict for the natural logarithm of the duration hospital stay attributable to RSV. Logistic regression models were developed for admission to intensive care and mechanical ventilation.

RESULTS

A total of 698 children were enrolled from Jan. 1 to April 30, 1993, at all centers except Winnipeg Children's Hospital, where enrollment continued until June 30, 1993. Nine patients were excluded because they did not have lower respiratory tract illness associated with the RSV infection. Thus 689 patients were included in the analysis.

There was variation in the type of nasopharyngeal specimen submitted for diagnosis. In addition, there was variation in the ability to isolate and subgroup viruses. Overall, subgroupable viruses were isolated from 353 (51%) of the total samples. Viruses were isolated from only 11% of patients enrolled at study center 3, the only center that used the specimen obtained by nasopharyngeal swab as the preferred specimen. Of the subgroupable isolates, 102 were subgroup A, 250 were subgroup B, and one isolated grouped with both antisera. There was a predominance of subgroup B infections at all except two centers.

During the same period 191 eligible children were not enrolled (21.7%) of all eligible subjects); of these, 37 were admitted during the study period when the specific hospital was not yet enrolling patients for the study; 64 were discharged before study personnel were aware of the diagnosis; consent could not be obtained for 77 patients because parents refused or were unavailable, or there was a language barrier; and 13 had other reasons. Those who were enrolled were similar to nonenrolled patients (Table II). However, three patients who died had not been enrolled. Two of these patients had congenital heart disease; one also had chronic lung disease. The third patient was prematurely born and younger than 6 weeks of age at the time of admission.

For the enrolled patients, the age range was 6 days to 18.4 years (mean and median age, 9.1 months and 4.9 months, respectively); 156 patients had underlying illness. Forty-three (6%) of the infections were nosocomially acquired. Patient characteristics are summarized by center in Table III.

Table II. Comparison of enrolled and nonenrolled patients

Feature	Study population	Non-enrolled
Patients (No.)	689	191
Proportion with underlying illness (%)	22.6	28.1
Age (mean, mo)	9.08	8.42
Duration hospital stay (mean, days)	6.98	6.59
Proportion admitted to ICU (%)	16.0	9.4
Proportion receiving mechanical ventilation (%)	9.1	5.2
Deaths: No. (%)	6 (0.9)	3 (1.6)

ICU, Intensive care unit.

The mean duration of hospital stay attributable to RSV was 7 days (range, 1 to 47 days); 110 (16%) patients received intensive care, 63 (9.1%) were supported by mechanical ventilation, and 6 (0.9%) patients died. The morbidity associated with groups of patients with different risk factors is shown in Table IV. To prevent double counting of patient data, patients were divided into three subgroups: those with underlying illness, those who were premature or younger than 6 weeks of age on admission, and those without known risk factors. There was a significant prolongation of hospital stay attributable to RSV in patients with underlying illness (median, 9.5 days; range, 2 to 47 days) compared with those who were premature or younger than 6 weeks of age on admission (median, 6.0 days; range, 2 to 22 days; Kruskal-Wallis, $p < 0.0001$), which was longer than in those without known risk factors (median, 5 days; range, 1 to 35 days; $p < 0.001$). Although there was no difference in the proportion receiving intensive care or ventilatory support in the groups with risk factors, these proportions were significantly higher than in those without known risk factors (chi-square analysis, $p < 0.0001$). Four of the patients who died had underlying illness, two had either been premature or were younger than 6 weeks of age, and none had no risk factors. The mortality rates also varied significantly across all groups (Fisher Exact Test, $p < 0.005$).

The administration of different drugs varied among centers. Bronchodilators were used in 77.6% to 95.3% of patients at each center. The use of corticosteroids ranged from 8.2% to 37.7%, ribavirin from 2.4% to 17.1%, and antibiotics from 57% to 81%.

Table III. Proportions of patients with risk factors across centers

	Center No.							
	1 (N = 85)	2 (N = 90)	3 (N = 146)	4 (N = 152)	5 (N = 82)	6 (N = 85)	7 (N = 49)	All centers (N = 689)
Cardiac disease	7	14	10	5	5	12	4	8
Chronic lung disease	19	7	11	11	16	8	8	11
Immunocompromise	1	1	5	5	0	1	8	3
Other disease	9	11	8	5	7	5	10	8
Gestation <37 wk	22	23	16	19	30	19	31	21
Age <6 wk	24	13	16	15	12	9	12	15
None of above risk factors	42	49	53	59	55	65	51	54
Hospital days (mean)	7.7	7.5	7.2	5.7	7.1	7.8	6.5	7.0

N, Total number of patients.

Table IV. Measures of morbidity in different subgroups

	Cardiac disease	Chronic lung disease	Immuno-compromised	Other disease	Gestation <37 wk	Age <6 wk	No known risk factors
Patients (No.)	57	79	21	52	148	101	372
Hospital stay (median, days)	11	10	10	10	7	6	5
Patients in ICU (%)	31.6	36.7	19.1	34.6	25.0	28.7	7.3
Days in ICU (median)*	6.5	7	4	8	6	4	3
Patients receiving mechanical ventilation (%)	19.3	25.3	14.3	21.2	18.2	16.8	3.2
Days of ventilation (median)*	5	8	5	8	5	4	5.5
Days of oxygen supplementation (median)*	7	6	3	6.5	4	3	2
Death (No.)	3	4	1	3	5	1	0

ICU, Intensive care unit.
*For patients with ≥1 day of this treatment.

The multiple regression models are summarized in Table V. A history of apnea, hypoxia on admission, and pulmonary consolidation contributed to models for all three outcomes: duration of hospital stay, admission to intensive care, and mechanical ventilation. In addition, aboriginal race, age <6 weeks, and underlying pulmonary disease were significant risk factors for the first two outcomes. Prematurity, congenital heart disease, and immunosuppression were also significantly associated with duration of hospitalization. Additionally, the specific hospital was associated with each of the outcomes independently of the variables listed in the table. Income, day care attendance, maternal smoking, and breast-feeding did not contribute further to the predictive capability of the models.

DISCUSSION

In our previous retrospective study, it was not possible to separate morbidity attributable to RSV infection from that caused by underlying disease.[1] Thus this prospective study was performed to determine morbidity attributable to RSV. In addition, we wished to compare prospectively the morbidity in those with underlying illness with that in patients without underlying disease.

The reduced morbidity in a population with underlying heart and lung disease noted in our previous retrospective study,[1] compared with that described in older reports,[2-4] was confirmed in this study. The disease duration attributable to RSV was shorter than total hospitalization for such patients because it excluded hospitalization for the underlying illness. Nevertheless, this duration was still significantly longer than that in patients without underlying illness. Other measures of morbidity, such as admission to intensive care and mechanical ventilation, may be less biased than hospital stay. However, the higher rate of admission to intensive care and use of mechanical ventilation than in those without risk factors confirmed the validity of separating high-risk groups. There was a gradation in risk in that patients with underlying heart and lung disease had

Table V. Results of regression analysis

Independent variable	Dependent variables: Prolonged hospitalization (days)	Admission to ICU (OR)	Ventilation (OR)
Aboriginal race (native Indian or Inuit)	1.2* (1.1-1.4)	3.1 (1.0-9.2)	NS (0.3-2.3)
History of apnea/respiratory arrest	1.3 (1.1-1.4)	6.5 (3.0-14.1)	8.8 (3.2-24.0)
Age <6 wk	1.2 (1.1-1.3)	3.8 (1.8-8.0)	NS (0.9-7.4)
Prematurity	1.1 (1.0-1.3)	NS (0.6-2.2)	NS (0.7-3.6)
Congenital heart disease	1.4 (1.2-1.6)	NS (0.8-4.0)	NS (0.7-5.2)
Underlying lung disease	1.2 (1.1-1.4)	2.7 (1.2-6.0)	NS (0.9-7.0)
Immunosuppression	1.7 (1.4-2.2)	NS (0.5-10.2)	NS (0.6-25.5)
Hypoxia on admission	1.3 (1.2-1.5)	2.9 (1.1-5.9)	9.6 (4.1-22.6)
Pulmonary consolidation on radiograph	1.2 (1.1-1.3)	3.7 (1.9-6.9)	3.9 (1.6-9.5)

ICU, Intensive care unit; *OR*, odds ratio; *NS*, not significant.
*Estimate and (95% confidence intervals).

a longer hospital stay and a higher incidence of receiving intensive care and mechanical ventilation, compared with those who were premature or younger than 6 weeks of age; the latter group, in turn, had greater morbidity than those who had no such risk factors. The immunocompromised patients had a long hospital stay associated with RSV, but this was not accompanied by receipt of intensive care; this finding was previously observed in the retrospective study.[1] The overall mortality rate of <1% also was similar to that observed in previous reports. The mortality rates in each of the subgroups with underlying disease were similar to those in the retrospective study, and all subjects who died had known risk factors.

Most previous studies have described risk factors in a univariate analysis.[8-11] Without a multiple regression analysis, it is not possible to separate the independent effect of different risk factors. Two studies that used regression models have either excluded subjects with underlying disease[12] or used an empiric severity index.[13] Some prognostic factors included in this study, such as underlying condition, young age, prematurity and hypoxia, have previously been reported to affect outcome.[8-13] The use of a multiple regression model allows estimations of the independent effects of these factors. In addition to the factors that have been reported previously, a worse prognosis was observed in aboriginal patients and in patients with a history of apnea or respiratory arrest, or with pulmonary consolidation on chest radiograph.

The observation of more severe disease in aboriginal patients may reflect referral bias. Such patients were often transferred to tertiary care centers from remote communities because of their severe condition and therefore may not be representative of RSV LRIs seen in those communities; 61% were from communities other than that of the tertiary care center. Further study is needed to determine whether native Indians and Inuits with RSV LRIs are at increased risk of adverse outcomes.

The patient's hospital was significantly associated with all three outcomes in the multiple regression models. This may reflect both variation in severity of illness in the patients and the use of different interventions. Threefold to tenfold variation in rates of hospitalization for LRI has been observed previously.[14] The difference in use of medications across centers described here confirms a previous observation by this multicenter group.[15] Conclusions from multicenter studies should therefore be more generalizable because they incorporate variation in admission and management practices. Although all centers are tertiary care centers, they are also the main pediatric facility in their community. Thus it is likely that morbidity observed in children without known risk factors can be generalized to risks in children hospitalized in community hospitals.

There was variation across centers in the ability to isolate virus. Of particular concern is that virus was isolated from only 11% of specimens that contained antigen in center 3. This likely reflects the suboptimal choice of specimen at that site.[16] At center 6, where the isolation rate was 34%, the virology laboratory was located in a different hospital, and there was delay in inoculation of the specimen onto cell culture. At center 7, a second specimen was obtained for culture after the first culture specimen yielded a positive result by enzyme immunoassay. Because enrollment into the study depended on antigen detection and not viral isolation, the lack of ability to isolate the virus should not bias the study unless antigen detection capabilities were also altered. Furthermore, if data from the three centers with the lowest viral isolation rate are excluded, there was no change in the absolute odds ratios for prolonged hospital stay.

The isolates detected in the study were predominantly subgroup B. Some researchers have observed that RSV subgroup A is associated with increased disease severity,[13, 17, 18] whereas others have not.[19-21] However, most studies have observed years in which subgroup A was predominant.[17, 19-25] Thus the subgroup B predominance observed during this respiratory viral season may reduce the study's generalizability. Continuation of this study through a second RSV season with viral subgrouping may help to validate the regression models that have been developed.

A bias of the study is caregiver awareness of the previously described risk factors. The presence of risk factors may have affected the decision to admit the patient or may have altered the management of certain patients. However, there is no evidence that the usual supportive therapy of RSV LRI, such as bronchodilators, use of corticosteroids, and oxygen supplementation, alters the outcomes examined in this study. Ribavirin was used in only 12% of patients and is therefore unlikely to have substantially affected the outcomes. Nevertheless, concern that a patient's condition may worsen may alter the duration of hospital stay and a decision to transfer a patient to an intensive care unit. This expectation bias would be less likely to affect the initiation of mechanical ventilation, for which there are more standardized criteria. For mechanical ventilation, the only significant risk factors were a history of apnea or respiratory arrest, the presence of hypoxia, and the presence of pulmonary consolidation on the chest radiograph. These items could easily be incorporated into any decision rules about management and be included in stratification in future treatment trials.

The fact that this study included only hospitalized patients, an extreme end of the spectrum of RSV LRI, limits the generalizability of conclusions to this population. Although maternal smoking, income, breast-feeding and use of day care were not found to be significantly associated with morbidity in this patient population, they may affect the need for hospitalization versus management in an ambulatory setting.[26, 27] The mothers of 34.4% of patients smoked, for example, whereas the proportion of current smokers in Canadian women in 1990 is 28%.[28]

We conclude that patients with underlying diseases and, possibly, those of aboriginal race should be targeted for RSV vaccine trials. A history of apnea or respiratory arrest, or other findings at the time of admission such as hypoxia or pulmonary consolidation on chest radiograph, should be included when considering patients for novel therapies. Additionally, these factors may better delineate the group of patients for whom ribavirin therapy should be considered. Given the good outcomes in the study patients despite the relatively limited usage of ribavirin, however, further randomized trials of this intervention are needed before making stronger recommendations for its use in RSV LRIs.

We thank the dedicated research nurses who enrolled and followed all study patients.

The Pediatric Investigators Collaborative Network on Infections in Canada (PICNIC) for this study consists of the following members: Francois Boucher, MD, and Michel Couillard, PhD, Centre Hospitalier de l'Université Laval, Québec City, Québec; Simon Dobson, MBBS, and Eva Thomas, MD, PhD, British Columbia's Children's Hospital, Vancouver, British Columbia; Joanne Langley, MD, and Spencer Lee, PhD, Izaak Walton Killam Hospital, Halifax, Nova Scotia; Jane McDonald, MD, and Patrick Quennec, RT, Montreal Children's Hospital, Montreal, Québec; Noni MacDonald, MD, Francisco Diaz Mitoma, MD, PhD, and Helen Miller, MSc, Children's Hospital of Eastern Ontario, Ottawa; Elaine E. L. Wang, MDCM, Derek Stephens, MSc, and Martin Petric, PhD, Hospital for Sick Children, Toronto, Ontario; Barbara J. Law, MD, and Volia de Carvalho, MD, Winnipeg Children's Hospital, Winnipeg, Manitoba; Gregory Hammond, MD, Cadham Provincial Laboratory, Winnipeg, Manitoba.

REFERENCES

1. Navas L, Wang E, de Carvalho V, Robinson J, PICNIC. Improved outcome of respiratory syncytial virus infections in a high-risk hospitalized population of Canadian children. J PEDIATR 1992;121:348-54.
2. MacDonald NE, Hall CB, Suffin SC, Alexson C, Harris PJ, Manning JA. Respiratory syncytial virus infection in infants with congenital heart disease. N Engl J Med 1982;307:397-400.
3. Groothuis JR, Gutierrez KM, Lauer BA. Respiratory syncytial virus infection in children with bronchopulmonary dysplasia. Pediatrics 1988;82:199-203.
4. Groothuis JR, Salbenblatt CK, Lauer BA. Severe respiratory syncytial virus infection in older children. Am J Dis Child 1990;144:346-8.
5. Ribavirin therapy of respiratory syncytial virus. In: Peter G, ed. Red book: Report of the Committee on Infectious Diseases, 22nd ed. Elk Grove Village, Illinois: American Academy of Pediatrics, 1991:581-7.
6. Groothuis JR, Simoes EAF, Levin MJ, et al. Prophylactic administration of respiratory syncytial virus immune globulin to high-risk infants and young children. N Engl J Med 1993; 329:1524-30.
7. Anderson LJ, Hierholzer JC, Tsou C, et al. Antigenic characterization of respiratory syncytial virus strains with monoclonal antibodies. J Infect Dis 1985;151:626-33.
8. McMillan JA, Tristram DA, Weiner LB, Higgins AP, Sandstrom C, Brandon R. Prediction of the duration of hospitalization in patients with respiratory syncytial virus infection: use of clinical parameters. Pediatrics 1988;81:22-6.

9. Meert K, Heidemann S, Lieh-Lai M, Sarnaik AP. Clinical characteristics of respiratory syncytial virus infections in healthy versus previously compromised host. Pediatr Pulmonol 1989;7:167-70.
10. Stretton M, Ajizian SJ, Mitchell I, Newth CJL. Intensive care course and outcome of patients infected with respiratory syncytial virus. Pediatr Pulmonol 1992;12:143-50.
11. Tissing WJE, van Steensel-Moll HA, Offringa M. Risk factors for mechanical ventilation in respiratory syncytial virus infection. Eur J Pediatr 1993;152:125-7.
12. Green M, Brayer AF, Schenkman KA, Wald ER. Duration of hospitalization in previously well infant with respiratory syncytial virus infection. Pediatr Infect Dis J 1989;8:601-5.
13. McConnochie KM, Hall CB, Walsh EE, Roghmann KJ. Variation in severity of respiratory syncytial virus infections with subtype. J Pediatr 1990;117:52-62.
14. Perrin JM, Homer CJ, Berwick DM, Woolf AD, Freeman JL, Wennberg JE. Variations in rates of hospitalization of children in three communities. N Engl J Med 1989;320:1183-7.
15. Law BJ, Carvalho V, PICNIC. Respiratory syncytial virus infections in hospitalized Canadian children: regional differences in patient populations and management practices. Pediatr Infect Dis J 1993;12:659-63.
16. Ahluwalia G, Embree J, McNicol P, Law B, Hammond GW. Comparison of nasopharyngeal aspirate and nasopharyngeal swab specimens for respiratory syncytial virus diagnosis by cell culture, indirect immunofluorescence assay, and enzyme-linked immunosorbent assay. J Clin Microbiol 1987;25:763-7.
17. Hall CB, Walsh EE, Schnabel KC, et al. Occurrence of groups A and B of respiratory syncytial virus over 15 years: associated epidemiologic and clinical characteristics in hospitalized and ambulatory children. J Infect Dis 1990;162:1283-90.
18. Taylor CE, Morrow S, Scott M, Young B, Toms GL. Comparative virulence of respiratory syncytial virus subgroups A and B. Lancet 1989;1:777-8.
19. Hendry RM, Pierik LT, McIntosh K. Prevalence of respiratory syncytial virus subgroups over six consecutive outbreaks: 1981–1987. J Infect Dis 1989;160:185-90.
20. Stark JM, Fatemi SH, Amini SB, Huang YT. Occurrence of respiratory syncytial virus subtypes in hospitalized children in Cleveland, Ohio from 1985 to 1988. Pediatr Pulmonol 1991;11:98-102.
21. Monto AS, Ohmit S. Respiratory syncytial virus in a community population: circulation of subgroups A and B since 1965. J Infect Dis 1990;161:781-3.
22. Anderson LJ, Hendry RM, Pierik LT, Tsou C, McIntosh K. Multicenter study of strains of respiratory syncytial virus. J Infect Dis 1991;163:687-92.
23. Thomas E, Margach MJ, Orvell C, Morrison B, Wilson E. Respiratory syncytial virus subgroup B dominance during one winter season between 1987 and 1992 in Vancouver, Canada. J Clin Microbiol 1994;32:238-42.
24. Tsutsumi H, Onuma M, Suga K, et al. Occurrence of respiratory syncytial virus subgroup A and B strains in Japan, 1980 to 1987. J Clin Microbiol 1988;26:1171-4.
25. Mufson MA, Orvell C, Rafnar B, Norrby E. Two distinct subtypes of human respiratory syncytial virus. J Gen Virol 1985;66:2111-24.
26. Pullan CR, Toms GL, Martin AJ, Gardner PS, Webb JKG, Appleton DR. Breast-feeding and respiratory syncytial virus infection. Br Med J 1980;281:1034-6.
27. McConnochie KM, Roghmann KJ. Parental smoking, presence of older siblings and family history of asthma increase risk of bronchiolitis. Am J Dis Child 1986;140:806-12.
28. Pederson LL. Smoking. In: Stephens T, Fowler Graham D, eds. Canada's health promotion survey 1990 technical report. Ottawa: Health and Welfare Canada, 1993.

Hospitalization for lower respiratory tract illness in infants: Variation in rates among counties in New York State and areas within Monroe County

Kenneth M. McConnochie, MD, MPH, Klaus J. Roghmann, PhD, and Gregory S. Liptak, MD, MPH

From the Department of Pediatrics, University of Rochester School of Medicine, Rochester, New York

Objective: **Lower respiratory tract illness (LRI) is the most common serious illness in childhood and the most common reason for hospitalization of infants beyond the neonatal period. This study assessed the potential for cost savings from reduction in hospitalization for LRI.**
Setting and sample: **LRI hospitalization rates for children in the first 2 years of life (infants) were studied for the 62 counties of New York State and six socioeconomic areas within Monroe County (Rochester) for the years 1985 through 1991.**
Design: **Analysis of small area variations.**
Results: **LRI accounted for 51.2% of infant hospitalizations in New York State. The overall LRI hospitalization rate for New York's 62 counties was 27.0 per 1000 child-years and ranged, among the 18 most populous counties, from 10.7 for Monroe County to 39.3 for the Bronx. Unemployment rate was the strongest predictor of LRI hospitalization rates for counties, explaining 29% of the variance in multiple regression analysis. Within Monroe County, LRI hospitalization rates followed a geographic gradient from the inner city (22.5) to the rest of the city (12.2), and to the suburbs (7.3). Deaths from LRI were uncommon (0.36% of state LRI hospitalizations) and varied little between inner city (0.42%) and suburbs (0.51%). If LRI hospitalization rates for Monroe County suburban children prevailed for the entire state, 10,439 hospitalizations and $32,916,000 would be saved annually.**
Conclusions: **A large portion of the increased cost of health care for children living in poverty is attributable to hospitalization for LRI in infants. Physician discretion in decision making and factors associated with socioeconomic status are probably major determinants of variation. Well-coordinated follow-up of acute illness visits, home monitoring by visiting nurses, and empirically based clinical guidelines for management of LRI might yield both substantial cost savings and better service to families. (J Pediatr 1995;126:220-9)**

Supported in part by grant No. 2802-4 from the Thrasher Research Fund.
Submitted for publication May 24, 1994; accepted Sept. 15, 1994.
Reprint requests: Kenneth M. McConnochie, MD, MPH, Box 777, Department of Pediatrics, University of Rochester Medical Center, 601 Elmwood Ave., Rochester, NY 14642.

0022-3476/95/$3.00 + 0 **9/20/60614**

Lower respiratory tract infection is the most common serious illness in childhood and the most common reason for hospitalization of infants beyond the neonatal period. Approximately 30% of children have at least one LRI in the first year of life,[1-5] and yet management varies widely. Studies of geographic variation in hospitalization for LRI in children have found sixfold differences in hospitalization

See related article, p. 212.

DRG	Diagnosis-related groups
ICD	International Classification of Diseases (9th revision)
LRI	Lower respiratory tract illness

for bronchiolitis (a diagnosis of infants almost exclusively) among communities in Vermont[6] and 15-fold differences for LRI in children of all ages covered by Medicaid.[7] Hospitalization rates for infants of 13.5 per 1000 child-years have been reported in England[8] and 20.0 per 1000 child years in Seattle, Wash.[9] These rates are twofold to threefold greater than the rate of 6.3 per 1000 child years observed among infants in suburban Monroe County (Rochester), New York in the early 1970s.[5]

Hospitalization accounts for a large proportion of costs attributable to this common illness. In a suburban Rochester pediatric practice serving primarily middle-class families, hospitalization accounted for 56% of total direct costs attributable to LRI, although hospitalization occurred in only 1.7% of LRI episodes for these infants, who had ready access to primary care.[5] Hospitalization probably accounts for substantially more than 56% of the direct cost of LRI in many communities. The national hospitalization rate for all conditions in childhood was 2.4-fold greater than the rate for all conditions in Rochester,[10,11] and hospitalization rates for asthma in Boston and New Haven were 3.8- and 2.3-fold greater, respectively, than in Rochester.[11]

Our analysis was conducted to investigate geographic variation in rates of hospitalization for LRI among children in the first 2 years of life (infants); to assess the potential for cost savings from avoidance of hospitalization; and to assess risk of LRI based on the diagnosis of respiratory failure and on deaths among children admitted with LRI. In addition, relationships among sociodemographic variables, health system characteristics, and hospitalization rates were examined.

METHODS

Samples. Hospital discharge data for New York State counties and for areas within Monroe County (Rochester) for the years 1985 through 1991 were obtained. Data for New York State came from the Statewide Planning and Research Cooperative System data set. For Monroe County, data came from the Rochester Hospitals Data Base, a data set developed and maintained cooperatively by all Rochester area hospitals. Key data common to both data sets included International Classification of Diseases and diagnosis-related group codes, insurance type, mortality, and place of residence. Residence for New York State data was identified by county. For Monroe County, it was identified by zip code. Data available for New York State were already aggregated by county and diagnostic group. Specific ICD and DRG codes were available only for Monroe County. Denominators for estimating hospitalization rates were based on birth records. Expressed as child-years at risk, denominators were estimated for each year and for each geographic area as the sum of births for the preceding 2 years.

For Monroe County, zip codes and birth certificate data were used to divide the county into inner city, rest of city, and suburban areas. *Inner city* was defined as zip codes for which the largest proportion of births was covered by Medicaid. *Rest of city* was defined by zip codes not in the inner city but with the majority of births to city dwellers. The *suburbs* included remaining areas in the county. Each area was then divided further into an eastern and western section by the Genesee River, which runs from the southern border of Monroe County, through the center of Rochester, and into Lake Ontario, which borders the county on the north. Eastern and western divisions for each area were analyzed separately because there are geographic, demographic, and health care system differences between them.

For Monroe County, small differences between population estimates and LRI frequencies based on New York State and Monroe County data sources were noted. Based on state data, total child-years at risk for Monroe County were 154,138 and total LRIs were 1656, whereas on the basis of county data, these values were 154,100 and 1664, respectively. The impact of these minor differences on results was trivial.

Definitions. *LRI* was defined by ICD codes indicating bronchitis, bronchiolitis, pneumonia, asthma, and respiratory failure. Table I displays specific ICD codes defining LRI and indicates their frequency among the first five diagnoses listed for each of the hospital discharge records for Monroe County. Pertussis (033.) and pneumonia caused by *Haemophilus influenzae* (482.2) were excluded from the LRI classification because they were included in a classification of vaccine-preventable disease. This had little impact on the total number of LRI hospitalizations, as indicated by observations for Monroe County. The codes 482.2 and 033. appeared only 8 and 54 times, respectively, among the 2055 LRI diagnoses applied to the 1826 Monroe County LRI hospitalizations.

Hospitalization for LRI was defined as a hospitalization for which an LRI appeared as any of the first five discharge diagnoses listed in the hospital discharge record. This definition allowed determination of rates that were not influenced by variation in assignment of diagnoses to position (first through fifth) in discharge records. Further, it pro-

Table I. ICD codes and diagnosis included in the classification of LRI and their distribution among 1824 Monroe County LRI hospitalizations

ICD code	Diagnosis	Frequency among first 5 diagnoses: No.	Dx 1-5* (%)	LRI† (%)
Bronchiolitis and bronchitis				
466.	Acute bronchitis/bronchiolitis	2	0.10	0.11
466.0	Acute bronchitis	61	2.97	3.34
466.1	Acute bronchiolitis	601	29.25	32.91
490.	Bronchitis, NOS	14	0.68	0.77
	TOTAL	678	32.99	37.13
Viral pneumonia				
480.	Viral	1	0.05	0.05
480.1	Respiratory syncytial viral	98	4.77	5.37
480.2	Parainfluenza viral	1	0.05	0.05
480.8	Viral NEC	15	0.73	0.82
480.9	Viral NOS	166	8.08	9.09
487.0	Influenza with pneumonia	4	0.19	0.22
	TOTAL	285	13.87	15.61
Bacterial pneumonia				
481.	Pneumococcal	21	1.02	1.15
482.0	*Klebsiella pneumoniae*	1	0.05	0.05
482.3	Streptococcal	10	0.49	0.55
482.4	Staphylococcal	6	0.29	0.33
482.8	Bacterial NEC	3	0.15	0.16
482.9	Bacterial NOS	15	0.73	0.82
483.	Bacterial organism NEC	2	0.10	0.11
484.3	Pneumonia in whooping cough	1	0.05	0.05
	TOTAL	59	2.87	3.23
Pneumonia, organism unclassified				
485.	Bronchopneumonia organism NOS	6	0.29	0.33
486.	Pneumonia, organism NOS	231	11.24	12.65
484.8	Pneumonia in infectious disease NEC	1	0.05	0.05
	TOTAL	238	11.58	13.03
Asthma				
493.	Asthma	4	0.19	0.22
493.0	Extrinsic asthma	8	0.39	0.44
493.0	Extrinsic asthma, status	10	0.49	0.55
493.1	Intrinsic asthma	1	0.05	0.05
493.9	Asthma	438	21.31	23.99
493.9	Asthma, status	295	14.36	16.16
	TOTAL	756	36.79	41.40
Respiratory failure				
518.8	Respiratory failure	39	1.90	2.14
TOTAL		**2055**	**100.00**	**112.54**

NOS, Not otherwise specified; *NEC*, not elsewhere classified.
*Proportion accounted for by this diagnosis among the 2055 LRI diagnoses appearing as the first through fifth diagnoses among the 1826 hospital discharges for LRI.
†Proportion for which the diagnosis was noted as one or more of the first five discharge diagnoses among the 1826 LRI hospital discharges. Total is greater than 100% because multiple LRI diagnoses appeared for some LRI discharges.

vided maximal estimates in attribution of death to LRI. An alternative approach of attributing hospitalization to LRI only if an LRI appeared as the first diagnosis would have produced results very similar to those presented. The total number of LRI hospitalizations for New York State, based on the first diagnosis only, was 91,776 (24.59/1000 children at risk), whereas the total number of hospitalizations based on diagnoses 1 through 5 was 100,699 (26.98/1000 children at risk).

Mortality rate. Any death for which an LRI diagnosis was included as one of the first five diagnoses was counted as a death caused by LRI. This ensures a complete count of deaths attributable to LRI, but may overestimate the LRI mortality rate because underlying problems (e.g., congen-

Table II. Risk of LRI hospitalization in New York State counties

County	Child-years at risk	LRI as Dx1 to Dx5: Admittances	Rate per 1000	Standard error*	Relative risk of LRI admittance
Monroe (Rochester)	154,138	1,656	10.74	0.26	1.00
Nassau	223,776	2,742	12.25	0.23	1.14
Erie (Buffalo)	188,317	2,665	14.15	0.27	1.32
Albany	51,746	767	14.82	0.54	1.38
Onondaga (Syracuse)	100,373	1,595	15.89	0.40	1.48
Suffolk	258,937	4,295	16.59	0.25	1.54
Rockland	53,350	896	16.79	0.56	1.56
Westchester	159,254	2,762	17.34	0.33	1.61
Dutchess	48,242	888	18.41	0.62	1.71
Broome (Binghamton)	41,051	786	19.15	0.68	1.78
Oneida	50,558	1,007	19.92	0.63	1.85
Richmond (Staten Island)	76,860	1,783	23.20	0.55	2.16
Queens	390,729	9,496	24.30	0.25	2.26
New York (Manhattan)	282,045	8,595	30.47	0.33	2.84
Kings (Brooklyn)	594,315	21,420	36.04	0.25	3.35
Orange	65,757	2,532	38.51	0.77	3.58
Bronx	327,775	12,886	39.31	0.35	3.66
Niagara	43,193	1,862	43.11	1.00	4.01
TOTAL: counties above	3,110,418	78,633	25.28	0.09	2.35
TOTAL: all other counties	622,373	22,066	35.45	0.24	3.30
STATE TOTAL	3,732,790	100,699	26.98	0.09	2.51

The 18 most populous counties (>40,000 child-years at risk, 1985 through 1991) are listed in order of increasing risk.
*Standard error for rate, based on Poisson distribution.

ital heart disease, neuromuscular disorder) may be a more fundamental reason for some of these deaths. Any bias introduced by this approach would be conservative.

Comparison diagnoses. For purposes of comparison, variations in rates of hospitalization for surgical procedures and acute, undifferentiated febrile illness (febrile illness) were also studied for Monroe County. Surgical procedures were identified by DRG classifications. Febrile illness was defined by ICD codes for bacteremia, septicemia, unexplained fever, and unspecified viral illness.

Characteristics of geographic areas. For New York State's 62 counties, the 1990 United States Census was the basis for information on population density, racial and ethnic distribution, unemployment rates, and per capita income.[12] Data from the New York State Department of Social Services on the number of children in each county eligible for Aid to Dependent Children[12] provided the numerator for an index of poverty in each county. The total number of children less than age 19 years served as the denominator for this index, which was termed the *Aid to Dependent Children rate.* The proportion of the population covered by Medicaid was termed the *Medicaid rate* and served as another measure of poverty. Indexes for access to health care services and supply of hospital beds included *physician density* (per 1000 persons in the population) and *hospital bed density* (acute care beds per 1000 persons in the population). Numerators for these indexes were based on the number of nonfederal, office-based physicians in 1985[13] and the number of acute-care hospital beds in each county in 1992.[14]

For the six areas within Monroe County, sociodemographic information available from the 1990 United States Census by zip codes[15] was supplemented by data based on county birth certificate records for 1988 through 1990.

Cost estimates. To provide an estimate for cost of LRI hospitalization that is generalizable to current health care financing throughout the United States, reimbursement rates based on the 1992 federal prospective payment program were used. Diagnosis-related groups were assigned to all hospitalizations in the Monroe County database with the eleventh version of the federal classification system. To estimate the cost of each hospitalization, weight factors for specific DRGs were multiplied by $3568, the national standard reimbursement rate for large urban hospitals.[16] Standard reimbursement rates for other urban hospitals and rural hospitals, the other two standard categories, were $3511 and $3341, respectively.

Analysis. Analysis was primarily descriptive. Secondary analysis explored relationships among sociodemographic variables, health system characteristics, and hospitalization

Table III. Monroe County hospital admissions: 1985 through 1991

		All admissions				LRI: Dx1 to Dx5				
Area	Child-years at risk	Admitted (No.)	Rate per 1000 No.	Deaths Admitted	Deaths No.	Admitted (No.)	Rate per 1000	Standard error*	Deaths No.	Deaths % LRI
Inner city	31,663	2636	83.3	17	0.64	714	22.5	0.84	3	0.42
Rest of city	43,182	2228	51.6	29	1.30	525	12.2	0.53	3	0.57
Suburbs	79,631	3068	38.5	35	1.14	583	7.3	0.30	3	0.51
Missing Zips	2,111	37	17.5	0	0.00	9	4.3	1.42	0	0.00
TOTAL	156,587	7969	50.9	81	1.02	1831	11.7	0.27	9	0.49

*Standard error for the rate, based on Poisson distribution.

rates with the use of simple linear regression. Rates are presented as events per 1000 child-years ± 1 standard error. The formula used for calculation of standard errors is based on the Poisson distribution, as appropriate for rare events.

RESULTS

As indicated in Table II, the New York State hospitalization rate for LRI among infants was 27.0 (±0.09) per 1000 child-years. This indicates that 2.7% of children were hospitalized for LRI in the first 2 years of life. LRI hospitalizations accounted for 51.2% of all hospitalizations for children in this age group. Based on the New York State data set, the Monroe County LRI hospitalization rate was 10.7 per thousand, and LRI hospitalizations accounted for 40.8% of infant hospitalizations in the county.

Etiology. Bacterial lower respiratory tract infection was uncommon, and was identified by any of the first five diagnoses for only 3.2% of the 1826 Monroe County LRI hospitalizations. As expected, the distribution for specific LRI diagnoses (Table I) suggested that the vast majority of LRI hospitalizations were precipitated by self-limited respiratory virus infections. Bronchiolitis or bronchitis, almost exclusively viral infection in infants, was the first diagnosis for 32.6% of the 1826 LRI admissions, viral pneumonia was the first diagnosis on an additional 12.9%, and asthma, usually precipitated by respiratory virus infection in the age group studied, accounted for 33.2%. Assuming that three fourths of the unclassified-organism pneumonia was viral in origin, one may conservatively estimate that about 85% of LRI admissions were attributable to respiratory viruses.

Outcomes. Observations from both New York State and Monroe County indicated that severe LRI was a rare event. For New York, among the 100,699 admissions with LRI among the five diagnoses, death occurred in 363 (0.36%). As suggested by observations in the Monroe County data set, many of these deaths attributed to LRI were attributable to other causes as well. Among the 1826 LRI hospitalizations in the Monroe County data set, death occurred in 9 (0.49%). Underlying conditions in the 9 infants who died included congenital heart disease (3 infants), chronic liver disease (1), urinary tract infection (2), and chronic renal disease (2). Respiratory failure was also rare, recorded for 39 (2.3%) of the LRI hospitalizations in Monroe County.

The mortality rate associated with LRI hospitalization ranged from 0 to 2.78 per 100 LRI admissions for all counties, and from 0.05 to 1.07 for the 18 most populous counties, defined as those with more than 40,000 child-years at risk (Table II). Correlations between LRI hospitalization rates and LRI mortality rates, whether defined as deaths per admission or deaths per child in the population, were not statistically significant.

Variation in LRI hospitalization rate within New York State. The Figure maps all of New York's counties and indicates the quintile ranking of their LRI hospitalization rates. As a simplification of the graphic presentation, the two quintiles representing the highest hospitalization rates have been collapsed into one level (range, 33.9 to 142.8). Rates of hospitalization for LRI, death from LRI, and hospitalization for all reasons are available from the authors for all 62 counties in the state. Analysis of risk of hospitalization focused on the 18 counties with more than 40,000 child-years at risk (Table II). These counties accounted for 83.3% of the total 3,732,790 child-years at risk, and 78.1% of the 100,699 LRI admissions. Among the 18 counties, Monroe and Nassau counties had the lowest LRI hospitalization rates, 10.7 and 12.3, respectively, whereas Bronx and Niagara counties had the highest at 39.3 and 43.1. If the lowest rate, that for Monroe County, is defined as baseline, risks of hospitalization (relative risks) with LRI varied among counties more than 3.5-fold.

Hospitalization rates for less populous counties were generally greater (35.5) than those for the 18 larger counties (25.3). The highest rate observed was 142.7 (Montgomery County), 43-fold greater than that for Schoharie County (3.3), the lowest in the state.

Variation in LRI hospitalization rate within Monroe County. Because there was little difference in hospitaliza-

LRI: Dx1 only		Febrile illness: DX1 to Dx5				Surgical procedures	
				Deaths			
Admitted (No.)	Rate per 1000	Admitted (No.)	Rate per 1000	No.	%	Admitted (No.)	Rate per 1000
651	20.6	494	15.6	3	0.61	277	8.7
475	11.0	390	9.0	3	0.77	380	8.8
535	6.7	408	5.1	1	0.25	734	9.2
7	3.3	4	1.9	0	0.00	10	4.7
1668	10.7	1296	8.3	7	0.54	1401	8.9

tion rates between eastern and western sections of Monroe County areas, sections were combined in final analysis. A stepwise increase in LRI hospitalization rates was observed (Table III) from suburbs (7.3 ± 0.30) to rest-of-city areas (12.2 ± 0.53) to the inner city (22.5 ± 0.84). The rate for the eastern section of the inner city (23.7) was highest among Monroe County areas but was comparable to rates falling in the second lowest quintile for New York State counties. Defining the suburban rate of 7.3 as baseline, risks of hospitalization with LRI increased 1.66-fold from suburbs to rest-of-city areas and 3.08-fold from suburbs to inner city areas.

On the basis of the DRGs assigned to each hospitalization, costs for all hospitalizations and for LRI hospitalizations were estimated. Mean cost per LRI hospitalization was $3061 and, as expected with prospective payment reimbursement, varied little among geographic areas. Mean costs per LRI admission were $2977, $3137, and $3117 for the inner city, rest-of-city areas, and the suburbs, respectively. In contrast, costs per child-year attributable to LRI hospitalization varied substantially. Mean costs per child-year for the inner city, rest-of-city areas, and the suburbs were $67, $38, and $23, respectively, and the LRI hospitalization rate accounted for 27.8%, 23.6%, and 17.4% of overall hospitalization costs.

Hospitalization for comparison conditions within Monroe County. Table III also indicates that rates for the next most common reasons for hospitalization in Monroe County, surgical procedures (8.9) and febrile illness (8.3), were substantially lower than for LRI. There was virtually no variation in rates of surgical procedures among areas, whereas variation in admission rates for febrile illness was similar to that for LRI. The overall mortality rate for febrile illness hospitalizations in the county as a whole (0.54%) was virtually identical to that for LRI (0.49%).

Predicting LRI hospitalization rates in New York's counties. In bivariate analysis for the 62 counties, variables with a statistically significant ($p < 0.05$) Pearson correlation with LRI hospitalization rate included unemployment rates (0.54), per capita income (−0.33), physician density (−0.30), and Medicaid rate (0.26). Correlations for the proportion of children eligible for Aid to Dependent Children (0.03), hospital bed density (0.01), proportion of population that was black (0.18), proportion of population that was Hispanic (0.05), and population density (−0.04) were not significant.

Relationships for variables that were significant in bivariate analysis were assessed further in multiple regression analysis. In stepwise analysis, only two variables entered the regression model—unemployment rate, a highly significant predictor ($p < 0.0001$), and Medicaid-covered population proportion, a marginally significant predictor ($p = 0.09$). Unemployment rate, alone, explained 29% of the variance in LRI hospitalization rate. Overall, this model explained 33% of the variance in LRI hospitalization rate.

Predicting LRI hospitalization rates in Monroe County areas. Striking differences were noted in many sociodemographic attributes between the inner city and the suburbs. In addition, there was a distinct, stepwise gradient in moving from the inner city, to rest-of-city areas, and to the suburbs, but relatively little difference between western and eastern sections of each of these areas. The most notable difference between eastern and western sections of any area was that 22.8% of births from the eastern section of the inner city were Hispanic, compared with only 6.0% in the western section. Between areas, a gradient in poverty was reflected in the fact that 65% of inner-city births were covered by Medicaid, whereas Medicaid, whereas Medicaid covered 27% and 6% of rest-of-city and suburban births. The proportion of births without insurance coverage was very small in all areas, ranging from 1.0 (suburbs) to 1.7% (inner city). The proportion of black infants varied from 63% among inner-city births, and 21% among rest-of-city births, to 3% among suburban births. The proportion of mothers with less than a high school education at the time they gave birth was 43%, 20%, and 5%; and the proportion of mothers reporting smoking during pregnancy was 29%, 24%, and 14% for the inner city, rest-of-city areas, and the suburbs, respectively. Finally, for households in Monroe County areas, lack of a telephone was reported for 13%, 4%, and 1%, and lack of an automobile was reported for 42%, 19%, and 5%. In bivariate analysis, each of these attributes was highly correlated (0.85 or higher) with LRI hospitalization rates for the six Monroe County areas. Maternal education had the highest correlation (0.99). Because of the small number of areas in this data set, multiple regression was not meaningful.

DISCUSSION

Impact of LRI in infants. The overall hospitalization rate for LRI for the state was 27.0 per 1000 child-years. On the basis of the New York State hospitalization rate, and the national population estimate,* infant LRI admissions were estimated at 224,600 annually. This estimate represents 31.8% of LRI admissions for children less than 15 years of age and 9.2% of admissions for all reasons for children less than 15 years of age.[17] On the basis of the 224,600 LRI admissions and a cost of $3137 per admission (the mean DRG-based cost estimate for admissions in Monroe County), the total national annual direct cost of LRI hospitalizations in the first 2 years of life may be estimated at $705 million.

Analysis of specific diagnoses for Monroe County indicated that the hospitalization rate for LRI was substantially greater than that for the next most common medical reason for hospitalization, febrile illness. Development of clinical guidelines for management of febrile illness has received much attention, and recently developed guidelines have been disseminated widely.[18-23] Similar attention directed at management of LRI for infants may substantially benefit children, families, and the economy.

Variation in rates. On the basis of an extended study period and large sample sizes, rates derived from this analysis are reliable and precise. Their wide variation and magnitude are important. Although the large suburban population in Monroe County contributed substantially to the low rate for this county, many of the 18 most populous counties had rates greater than that for Monroe County's inner city. The proportion of infants living in poverty in the Monroe County inner city was similar to that for counties with some of the highest LRI hospitalization rates in the state. Medicaid coverage for LRI hospitalizations from inner-city Monroe County was 71.2%. Similar proportions were observed for Bronx (74.6%), Kings (67.9%), and New York (71.2%) counties.

Uncertainty and physician discretion. Variation in rates may be due to physician discretion, health system differences, or biologic or environmental factors that produce differences in incidence or severity. The prevailing view in the health services literature explains small area variations on the basis of differences in physician response to uncertainty surrounding the effectiveness of medical care. Uncertainty gives rise to divergent practice styles,[25, 26] which, in turn, produce high and low rates.[27-29] A wide variation in rates is generally believed to identify resource utilization decisions involving high levels of physician discretion, and high rates are believed to reflect overuse of resources.[30-32]

Although explaining variation was not the primary focus of this analysis, several observations suggest a significant role for physician discretion. Adverse outcomes of LRI in infants have a low probability but are valued very negatively, attributes that may engender uncertainty. Although most LRIs are mild and managed without hospitalization, severe illness may occur. Risks of greatest concern to physicians caring for infants with LRI include respiratory failure and apnea.[33, 34] The impression that disastrous events, particularly apnea, may occur suddenly and unexpectedly may weigh heavily in the decision to hospitalize a baby. Variation in hospitalization rates may be influenced by variation in physician estimates of the risk of not hospitalizing a child and by variation in the tolerance for risk. In the absence of reliable information about the risk of nonhospitalization, physician discretion may play an important role in the decision to hospitalize.

No variation in rates of surgical admissions occurred within Monroe County. This suggests that access to scheduled surgical procedures and incidence rates of surgical conditions did not vary within the county. In contrast, admission for febrile illness varied in a pattern similar to that for LRI. We speculate that hospitalization decision making for febrile illness in infants—another acute illness for which adverse outcome has a low probability but a high negative value—is similar to that for LRI.

Health system differences. Although physician discretion may play an important role in variation in LRI hospitalization rates, we expect that health system attributes and family characteristics also influence physician decision making and hospitalization rates substantially. Access to care, physician-family relationships, characteristics of telephone and after-hours coverage systems, and transportation systems may influence physician decision making and patterns of utilization for acute illness.

The health services system may function differently for affluent and for impoverished families. Sociodemographic differences between inner-city and suburban areas of Mon-

*In deriving a denominator for estimating national impact of LRI, we used 4.2 million births, the total for 1990,[24] and an infant mortality rate of 9.0 per 1000 live births. To estimate the total number of children less than 24 months of age, we doubled the number of births and made adjustment for the infant mortality rate, which yielded an estimate of 8,324,000.

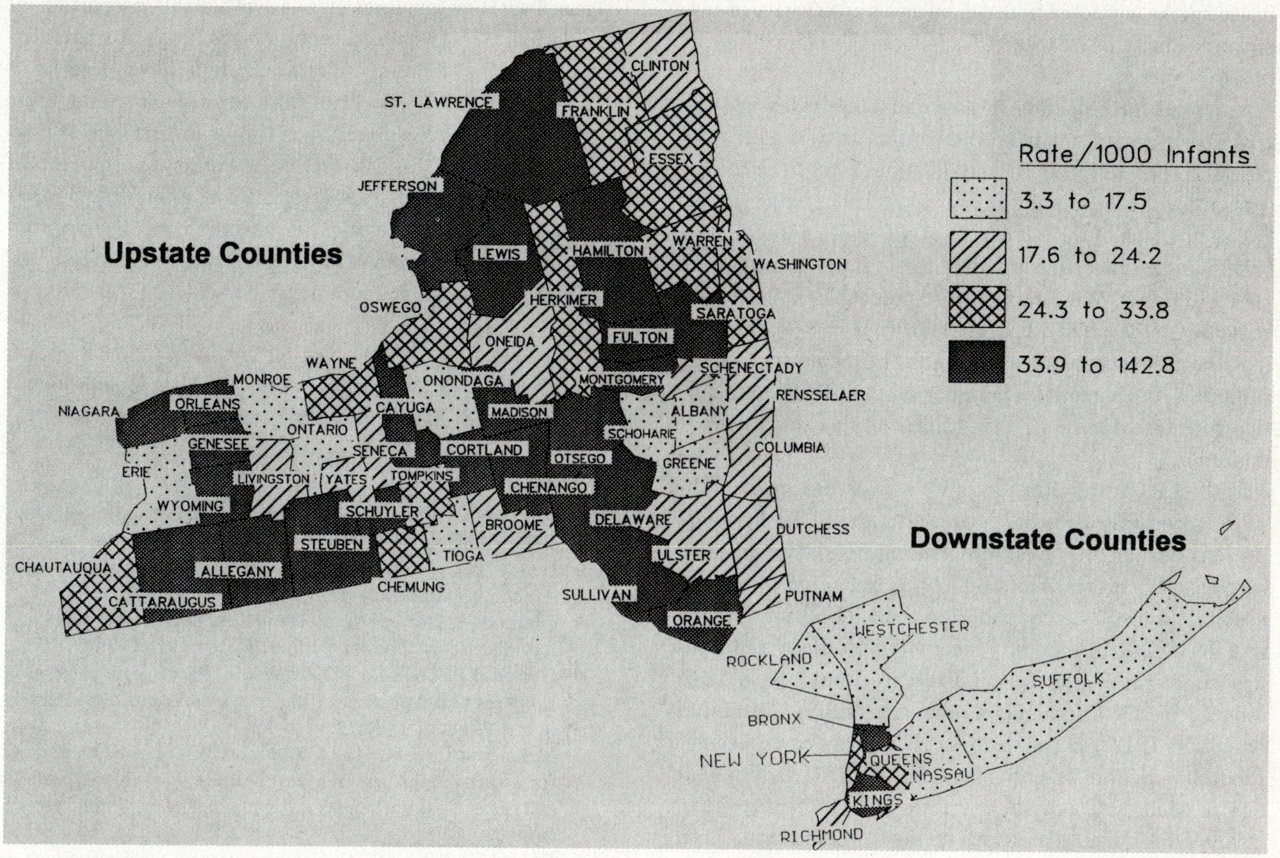

Figure. LRI hospitalization rates in New York State.

roe County are striking. Sociodemographic differences paralleled gradients in LRI hospitalization rates and were highly correlated with them. Maternal education less than high school was the strongest predictor of LRI hospitalization. These observations are consistent with explanations for the gradient in hospitalization rates within Monroe County that lie in the domains of health system functioning, family–health system interactions, or both.

The health services system may also function differently in rural and urban areas. Physician density (physicians per 1000 persons), highly correlated with population density (0.50), was a moderately strong predictor (0.30) of LRI hospitalization in New York counties. One plausible explanation for high rates in rural areas is an inability to evaluate illness in an infant during an extended treatment and observation period before deciding on hospitalization. Although this is common practice in many urban settings, lack of pediatric training for personnel in rural emergency departments may preclude this approach.

The strongest predictor of county hospitalization rates in multivariate analysis was unemployment rate, followed by proportion of the population covered by Medicaid. Physician density did not achieve statistical significance in a stepwise multiple regression model in which these variables had been included. These observations are consistent with the hypothesis that social and economic factors are the most important determinants of variation among counties. There was no correlation between county LRI hospitalization rate and hospital bed density.

Although the issue was not addressed in analysis, the Figure demonstrates that upstate counties with academic medical centers had substantially lower rates than surrounding counties. These counties included Erie (Buffalo), Monroe (Rochester), Onondaga (Syracuse), and Albany. This observation, similar to findings of Goodman et al.[35] warrants further investigation.

Biologic, genetic, and environmental differences. The possibility that biologic, genetic, or environmental factors might play a major role in the wide variation in LRI hospitalization rates is less likely, although the possibility that modifiable environmental conditions play some role should not be ignored. For example, widespread use of woodstoves in rural areas might contribute to the higher LRI hospitalization rate for rural areas,[36] or industrial air pollution might contribute to elevated rates in some urban counties. The sensitivity of infants to the effects of environmental tobacco smoke, reflected in the incidence and severity of respiratory illness in infants,[37-39] supports the plausibility of this hypothesis.

Potential for reduction in hospitalization rates and for cost savings. Variation in hospitalization rates suggests the possibility of reducing hospitalization rates if effective measures exist for bringing the rates toward baseline values. A large portion of the increased cost of health care for children living in poverty is attributable to hospitalization for LRI in infants. We estimated the potential for statewide reduction in hospitalization rates for LRI in two ways, using the LRI hospitalization rate for Monroe County suburbs as the potential minimum and the LRI hospitalization rate for Monroe County's inner city as the potential minimum.

If the LRI hospitalization rate for Monroe County suburbs had prevailed for the entire state, total LRI hospitalizations during the 7-year observation period would have been 27,249, rather than 100,699, a reduction of 10,493 hospital admissions per year. Had the LRI hospitalization rate for the Monroe County inner city prevailed for the entire state, total LRI hospitalizations would have been reduced by 2387 admissions each year, still a substantial reduction. If LRI hospitalization rates for Monroe County suburban children and the mean cost per LRI hospitalization in Monroe County had prevailed for the entire state, estimated annual statewide savings would have been $32,916,000. True potential savings may have been even greater. Leape et al.[40] noted that rates of inappropriate care tend to be high even in areas of low utilization.

Implications. According to the prevailing interpretation of small area variation, the forces producing variation will diminish when uncertainty is reduced. Information provided by this study—(1) risk of respiratory failure and death from LRI is low, (2) mortality rates are unrelated to hospitalization rates, and (3) a small proportion (3.2%) of LRI hospitalizations involve bacterial infection—reduces and quantifies uncertainty. Empirically based guidelines, identifying LRI episodes safely managed at home because they are unlikely to become severe, will further reduce uncertainty. Uncertainty in the home management of LRI in infants might be reduced still further through health service improvements and innovations. Readily accessible telephone coverage that is well integrated with primary care for illness might yield substantial reduction in hospitalization rates. Nurse home-visitors, reassuring anxious physicians with oximetry and respiratory rate measurements, might also yield substantial cost savings as a relatively inexpensive alternative to hospitalization for management of selected episodes of LRI.

Prevailing explanations of small area variations have been challenged recently by findings suggesting that physician discretion explains a relatively small proportion of variation.[40-43] Although several observations of small area variations in childhood hospitalization have been published,[7, 11, 35] relatively little work toward explaining these variations has been done. The relative importance of physician uncertainty and discretion and other determinants of variation in hospitalization for LRI is unknown. Further work in explaining reasons for variation in LRI hospitalization, including individual level analysis, may be essential before substantial reduction can be achieved.

We thank Jeffry Mailloux and Jill Szyolowski, of the Rochester Healthcare Information Group Inc., for providing Monroe County and New York State hospital discharge data in timely fashion.

REFERENCES

1. Denny FW. Acute respiratory infections in children: etiology and epidemiology. Pediatrics in Review 1987;9:135-46.
2. Denny W, Clyde WA. Acute lower respiratory tract infections in nonhospitalized children. J Pediatr 1986;105:635-46.
3. Glezen WP, Denny FW. Epidemiology of acute lower respiratory disease in children. N Engl J Med 1973;288:498-505.
4. Glezen WP, Loda FA, Clyde WA. Epidemiologic patterns of acute respiratory disease of children in a pediatric group practice. J Pediatr 1971;78:397-406.
5. McConnochie KM, Hall CB, Barker WH. Lower respiratory tract illness in the first two years of life: epidemiologic patterns and costs in a suburban pediatric practice. Am J Public Health 1988;78:34-9.
6. Wennberg J, Kim SYS. Common uses of hospitals: a look at Vermont. In: Developing a better health system for children; vol 2. Cambridge, Mass: Ballinger, 1977:353-82. (Harvard Child Health Project.)
7. Connell FA, Day RW, LoGerfo JP. Hospitalization of Medicaid children: analysis of small area variations in admission rates. Am J Public Health 1981;71:606-13.
8. Martin AJ, Gardner PS, McQuillen J. Epidemiology of respiratory viral infection among pediatric inpatients over a six-year period in northeast England. Lancet 1978;2:1035-8.
9. Foy HM, Cooney MK, Maletsky AJ, et al. Incidence and etiology of pneumonia, croup, and bronchiolitis in preschool children belonging to a prepaid medical care group. Am J Epidemiol 1973;97:80-92.
10. Kozak LJ, Norton C, McManus, McCarthy E. Hospital use patterns for children in the United States, 1983 and 1984. Pediatrics 1987;80:481-90.
11. Perrin JM, Homer CJ, Berwick DM, et al. Variations in rates of hospitalization of children in three urban communities. N Engl J Med 1989;320:1183-7.
12. U.S. Department of Commerce, Bureau of the Census. County and City Data Book, 1988. Washington, D.C.: U.S. Government Printing Office.
13. U.S. Department of Commerce, Bureau of the Census. USA Counties [Compact disc]. Washington, D.C.: The Department, June 1993.
14. American Hospitals Association. AHA Guide to the Health Care Field. Chicago: The Association, 1994.
15. U.S. Department of Commerce, Bureau of the Census. 1990 Census of Population and Housing [Summary tape file 3B;

compact disc: CD90-3B-01]. Washington, D.C.: The Department, July 1993.
16. Calculation of prospective payment rates for FY 1992. Federal Register 1991;56:43248-73.
17. Graves EJ. Detailed diagnoses and procedures, National Hospital Discharge Survey, 1990. National Center for Health Statistics. Vital Health Stat 13(113), 1992.
18. McCarthy PL, Fink HD, Baron MA, et al. Observation, history and physical exam in identifying serious illnesses in febrile children less than 24 months. J PEDIATR 1987;110:26-30.
19. McCarthy PL, Sharpe MR, Spiesel SZ, et al. Observation scales to identify serious illness in febrile children. Pediatrics 1982;70:802-9.
20. Klein J, Schlesinger P, Karasic R. Management of the febrile infant three months of age or younger. Pediatr Infect Dis 1984;3:75-9.
21. Dagan R, Sofer S, Phillip M, Shachak E. Ambulatory care of febrile infants younger than 2 months of age classified as being at low risk for having serious bacterial infections. J PEDIATR 1988;112:355-60.
22. American College of Emergency Physicians. Clinical policy for the initial approach to children under the age of 2 years presenting with fever. Ann Emerg Med 1993;22:628-37.
23. Baraff LJ, Bass JW, Fleisher GR, et al. Practice guidelines for the management of infants and children 0 to 36 months of age with fever without source. Pediatrics 1993;92:1-12.
24. U.S. Department of Commerce, Bureau of the Census. Statistical Abstract of the United States, 1992. 112th ed. Washington, D.C.: The Department, 1993.
25. Wennberg JE, Barnes BA, Zubkoff M. Professional uncertainty and the problem of supplier-induced demand. Soc Sci Med 1982;15:811-24.
26. Eddy DM. Variations in physician practice: the role of uncertainty. Health Affairs 1984;3:74-89.
27. Wennberg JE. Factors governing utilization of hospital services. Hosp Pract 1979;14:115-7.
28. Wolfe BL, Detmer DE. The economics of surgical signatures. Hospital Medical Staff 1984;13:2-9.
29. Roos LL. Supply, workload and utilization: a population-based analysis of surgery. Am J Public Health 1983;73:414-21.
30. Roos NP, Wennberg JE, McPherson K. Using diagnosis-related groups for studying variations in hospital admissions. Health Care Financing Review 1988;9:53-62.
31. Paul-Shaheen P, Clark JD, Williams D. Small area analysis: a review and analysis of the North American literature. J Health Polit Policy Law 1987;12:741-809.
32. Wennberg JE, Freeman RM, Shelton RM, Bubholz TA. Hospital use and mortality among Medicare beneficiaries in Boston and New Haven. N Engl J Med 1989;321:1168-73.
33. Anas N, Boettrich C, Hall CB, Brooks JG. The association of apnea and respiratory syncytial virus infection in infants. J PEDIATR 1982;101:65-8.
34. Church NR, Anas NG, Hall CB, Brooks JG. Respiratory syncytial virus–related apnea in infants: demographics and outcome. Am J Dis Child 1984;138:247-50.
35. Goodman DC, Fisher ES, Gittelsohn A, Chang CH, Fleming C. Why are children hospitalized? The role of nonclinical factors in pediatric hospitalizations. Pediatrics 1994;93:896-902.
36. Honicky RE, Osborne JS, Akpom CA. Symptoms of respiratory illness in young children and the use of wood-burning stoves for indoor heating. Pediatrics 1984;75:587-93.
37. Colley JRT, Holland WW, Corkhill RT. Influence of passive smoking and parental phlegm on pneumonia and bronchitis in early childhood. Lancet 1974;2:1031-4.
38. McConnochie KM, Roghmann KJ. Parental smoking, presence of older siblings, and family history of asthma increase risk of bronchiolitis. Am J Dis Child 1986;140:806-12.
39. Young S, LeSouef PN, Geelhoed GC, Stick SM, Landau LI. The influence of a family history of asthma and parental smoking on the level of airway responsiveness in infants soon after birth. N Engl J Med 1991;324:1168-73.
40. Leape LL, Park RE, Solomon DH, Chassin MR, Kosecoff J, Brook RH. In reply. JAMA 1990;263:3150.
41. Roos NP. Hospitalization style of physicians in Manitoba: the disturbing lack of logic in medical practice. Health Serv Res 1992;27:361-84.
42. Lomas J. Holding back the tide of caesareans: publishing recommendations is not enough to stop the rise. BMJ 1988;297:569-70.
43. Leape LL, Park RE, Solomon DH, Chassin MR, Kosecoff J, Brook RH. Does inappropriate use explain small-area variations in the use of health care services. JAMA 1990;263:669-72.

Binding of *Pseudomonas aeruginosa* to respiratory epithelial cells from patients with various mutations in the cystic fibrosis transmembrane regulator

Heather Zar, MBBCh, Lisa Saiman, MD, Lynne Quittell, MD, and Alice Prince, MD

From the Department of Pediatrics, College of Physicians and Surgeons, Columbia University, New York, New York

***Objective*: To determine whether there is an association between mutations of the cystic fibrosis transmembrane regulator (CFTR) and the predilection of patients with cystic fibrosis (CF) for *Pseudomonas aeruginosa* infection.**
***Method:* We quantified the adherence of *P. aeruginosa* PA01, labeled with sulfur 35–methionine, to epithelial monolayers derived from nasal scrapings of patients with specific CFTR mutations, and of carriers and normal subjects.**
***Results:* Adherence of *P. aeruginosa* to epithelial cells from patients with CF was significantly greater than to cells from either carriers ($t = 2.94$; $p = 0.009$) or normal subjects ($t = 3.32$; $p = 0.004$). Adherence to epithelial cells from patients with CF who were homozygous for the ΔF508 mutation ranged from 12% to 35% (mean, 23.7%) of the added inoculum, which was significantly greater than the binding to cells from patients with other mutations, which ranged from 3% to 18% (mean, 9.4%; $t = 3.71$; $p = 0.002$), from heterozygote carriers (3% to 11%; mean, 7.9%; $t = 4.87$; $p = 0.002$), or from normal subjects (2% to 10%: mean, 7.0%; $t = 5.21$; $p = 0.002$).**
***Conclusion:* Adherence to *P. aeruginosa* can be correlated with homozygosity for the Δ508 mutation; CFTR dysfunction may be one of the factors involved in the pathogenesis of pulmonary infection in CF. (J PEDIATR 1995;126:230-3)**

Approximately 90% of patients with cystic fibrosis become infected with *Pseudomonas aeruginosa*, but the age at colonization and the subsequent course of the pulmonary disease are highly variable.[1,2] Unlike the relation between pancreatic sufficiency and CF genotype,[3] no clear correlation between the clinical manifestations of pulmonary disease and CF genotype has been established.[4,5] An association between cystic fibrosis transmembrane regulator dysfunction and *P. aeruginosa* infection has been suggested by in vitro studies showing that CF epithelial cells in primary culture bound approximately twice as many *P. aeruginosa* organisms as did comparable cells from normal subjects.[6] Furthermore, CF respiratory cells expressed significantly more of the GalNAc$_{\beta1\text{-}4}$Gal receptor, which binds *P. aeruginosa* pilin, than did epithelial cells from control subjects.[7] The GalNAc$_{\beta1\text{-}4}$Gal receptor is a component of asialylated glycolipids; thus CFTR dysfunction, by diminishing sialyltransferase activity,[8] may result in an increased

CF	Cystic fibrosis
CFTR	Cystic fibrosis transmembrane regulator
GalNAc$_{\beta1\text{-}4}$Gal	*N*-Acetylgalactosamine–galactose

Supported by U.S. Public Health Service grant DK36963 (Dr. Prince) and by the Cystic Fibrosis Foundation Research Development Program at Columbia University.

Submitted for publication June 20, 1994; accepted Aug. 17, 1994.

Reprint requests: Alice Prince, MD, Pediatric Infectious Diseases, Columbia University, 650 W. 168th St., New York, NY 10032.

0022-3476/95/$3.00 + 0 **9/20/60006**

proportion of glycoconjugates that are not fully sialylated and could potentially serve as receptors for *P. aeruginosa* pili.[7] Thus epithelial cells from patients with CF whose mutations are relatively severe would have fewer sialylated glycolipids and consequently would have increased numbers of receptors available for *P. aeruginosa* binding.

To test this hypothesis, we compared the adherence of *P. aeruginosa* PAO1 to respiratory epithelial cells in primary culture from patients with diverse mutations in CFTR, from their heterozygote parents, and from normal subjects.

METHODS

Subjects. Nasal epithelial cells were obtained from 15 patients with CF, 15 normal subjects, and 10 parents of patients with CF (obligate heterozygotes). All patients with CF were colonized with *P. aeruginosa* as defined by positive results of sputum cultures for this organism for at least 6 months. The extent of pulmonary disease was evaluated with the Shwachman-Kulczycki scoring system.[9] All but one patient had evidence of pancreatic insufficiency and received replacement enzyme therapy. Normal subjects were medical students and laboratory workers who did not have chronic lung disease; none had had an upper respiratory tract infection within the preceding 6 weeks. The patients with CF had not had a pulmonary exacerbation for at least 1 month before the study. Informed consent was obtained in all cases.

Cystic fibrosis genotyping of the patients was performed in the laboratory of Dr. W. E. Highsmith, University of North Carolina, Chapel Hill, with the polymerase chain reaction to screen for the five commonest North American CF genotypes. If necessary, further testing for the presence of an additional 13 rare mutations was performed.[10]

Epithelial cell culture. Respiratory epithelial cells were obtained by gentle scraping of the inferior nasal turbinates, by the methods developed by Knowles et al.,[11] to obtain approximately 5.0×10^5 epithelial cells. The cells were placed in a 0.1% protease solution of Dulbecco modified Eagle medium/F12 at 37° C for 1 hour, resuspended in M3 medium containing 10% fetal calf serum, and plated at a concentration of 1×10^6 cells/ml in 96-well flat-bottomed microtiter plates coated with human type IV collagen. Cells were fed twice a week and confluent monolayers were obtained within 2 weeks.

Bacterial adherence assay. The number of *P. aeruginosa* organisms binding to the monolayers was quantified, as previously reported, with the use of PAO1 labeled with sulfur 35–methionine.[6] This is a piliated nonmucoid laboratory strain, representative of initial clinical *P. aeruginosa* isolates. For comparative purposes, the number of adherent bacteria was expressed as a percentage of the initial inoculum added to the monolayers, standardized to 5×10^8 colony-forming units per milliliter per well. All experiments were done in triplicate.

Statistical analysis. One-way analysis of variance was used to compare adherence to epithelial cells from normal subjects, carriers, patients with CF who were homozygous for ΔF508, and patients with other CF mutations. Post hoc *t* tests were conservatively two tailed. All statistics were calculated with the Statistical Package for the Social Sciences (SPSS Inc., Chicago, Ill.).

RESULTS

Patient population. The study patients with CF represented a diverse group in terms of both their genotypes and the extent of pulmonary disease (Table I). Within the group of seven patients homozygous for ΔF508 were four patients with mild disease (Shwachman-Kulczycki score >80) and three patients with moderate disease (Shwachman-Kulczycki score 50 to 80). The eight patients with "other" mutations included a 43-year-old, fully functional professional woman with moderate pulmonary disease and a 60-year-old man who had had pancreatic sufficiency, infertility, and mild pulmonary symptoms throughout his life but was given a diagnosis of CF only when he reached 60 years of age. More than half of the patients in this group had mild pulmonary disease.

Adherence of *P. aeruginosa*. Adherent *P. aeruginosa*, expressed as the mean percentage of a standard inoculum, varied from 3% to 35% for CF monolayers; for carriers and normal subjects this range was 3% to 11% and 2% to 10%, respectively. The mean binding of PAO1 to CF, carrier, and normal epithelial cells was 16.1%, 7.9%, and 7.0%, respectively, and was significantly greater to CF epithelial cells than to epithelial cells of carriers ($p = 0.009$) and normal subjects ($p = 0.004$). There was no significant difference in adherence to carrier and to normal epithelia.

Adherence of *P. aeruginosa* to ΔF508 homozygous cells was 12% to 35%, with a mean adherence of 23.7%. This was significantly greater than the binding to monolayers from patients with other mutations, which ranged from 3% to 18%, with a mean adherence of 9.4% ($p = 0.002$), as well as significantly greater than the binding to cells from heterozygotes ($p = 0.002$) or normal subjects ($p = 0.002$). The *P. aeruginosa* adherence to the epithelial cells from each of the patients homozygous for ΔF508 mutation was greater than the adherence to cells from any of the normal subjects or carriers. Binding of PAO1 to monolayers from patients with mutations other than those homozygous for ΔF508 did not differ significantly from the binding to monolayers from carriers and normal subjects. Although several of the patients with non-ΔF508 CFTR mutations had both mild pulmonary disease and a low percentage of *P. aeruginosa*

Table. Correlation of cystic fibrosis genotype, pulmonary disease, and *P. aeruginosa* (PA01) adherence to CF epithelial cells

Patient No.	Age (yr)	Sex	Genotype	Mutation defect	Pulmonary disease*	Shwachman-Kulczycki score	Adherence (%)
1	13	F	ΔF508/ΔF508	Processing	Mild	80	35
2	21	F	ΔF508/ΔF508	Processing	Mild	83	33
3	13	M	ΔF508/ΔF508	Processing	Mild	87	26
4	15	M	ΔF508/ΔF508	Processing	Mild	87	22
5	15	F	ΔF508/ΔF508	Processing	Moderate	60	21
6	28	M	ΔF508/ΔF508	Processing	Moderate	50	17
7	15	F	ΔF508/ΔF508	Processing	Moderate	60	12
8	29	M	ΔF508/3849 + 10	Processing/protein synthesis	Moderate	55	7
9	43	F	W1282X/W1282X	Protein synthesis	Moderate	60	3
10	13	F	ΔF508/W1282X	Processing/protein synthesis	Mild	88	13
11	16	M	Unknown	Unknown	Mild	82	6
12	22	F	ΔF508/G551D	Processing/regulation	Mild	80	4
13	19	M	ΔF508/G551D	Processing/regulation	Mild	80	18
14	12	M	G542X/3849 + 10	Protein synthesis	Mild	87	18
15	60	M	W1282X/unknown	Protein synthesis	Moderate	75	5

*Severity of pulmonary disease was measured with the Shwachman-Kulczycki scoring system.

binding, there was no significant correlation between pulmonary status and the quantity of adherent bacteria.

DISCUSSION

This study attempted to establish a relationship between CF genotype and *P. aeruginosa* infection by focusing on a single measurement relevant to the pathogenesis of infection, namely, the avidity of epithelial cells for *P. aeruginosa* binding. Our results indicate that *P. aeruginosa* PAO1 binds significantly more to the epithelial cells of patients homozygous for the ΔF508 mutation than to those of patients with other CF mutations, heterozygote carriers, or normal subjects. However, no correlation between the quantity of *P. aeruginosa* binding to these cells and the clinical status of the patients was found.

Increased *P. aeruginosa* adherence to epithelial cells homozygous for ΔF508 may be a reflection of larger numbers of asialylated glycolipids, which serve as receptors for *Pseudomonas* pilin on the surface of these cells.[7] The CFTR dysfunction, by limiting Cl^- and H^+ transport into the *trans*-Golgi complex, may result in decreased sialyltransferase activity and production of a greater proportion of asialyated surface glycolipids.[8] Receptor density or duration of contact with receptors may be important as this ubiquitous organism is transiently inhaled but promptly cleared from normal airways. However, it is difficult to attribute the initial acquisition of this organism solely to the properties of bacterial receptors because normal epithelial cells express sites for *P. aeruginosa* binding, and not all CF mutations could be correlated with increased *P. aeruginosa* attachment. Furthermore, other bacteria not associated with infection in CF also recognize the GalNAc$_{\beta 1\text{-}4}$Gal receptor,[12] which indicates that additional characteristics of *P. aeruginosa* may be important in the pathogenesis of this infection.

A possible limitation of this study is that all our patients were colonized with *P. aeruginosa*. It would be of interest to study adherence to ΔF508 homozygotes not infected with *P. aeruginosa*, but we have been unable to recruit such patients, because most have *P. aeruginosa* by the time they are old enough to allow nasal scrapings to be performed. To our knowledge, the respiratory epithelium of noncolonized patients has not been shown to have different characteristics from that of colonized patients.

A clear correlation between CF genotype and the extent of pulmonary involvement has not been established. Genotypes that result in defective CFTR synthesis or aberrant processing may be responsible for phenotypes that are more severe than mutations that produce abnormal regulation of a potentially functional chloride channel.[13, 14] Pancreatic insufficiency has been associated with earlier acquisition of *P. aeruginosa*[13] and rapid deterioration in clinical status.[1] Other studies suggest, however, that the pulmonary function of *P. aeruginosa*–colonized patients with CF gradually declines.[2] The majority of patients who have mutations associated with a failure of CFTR function and pancreatic insufficiency have highly variable pulmonary disease.[4, 5] Difficulties in correlating CFTR mutations with the severity of pulmonary disease have led some investigators to suggest that other genetic loci may be involved in modulating the phenotypes currently attributed to abnormalities in CFTR alone.[15] Furthermore, multiple other factors, such as environmental variables, the host's immune response, and infections with other organisms, may affect the clinical expression of lung disease.

We thank Jack Gorvoy, MD, Director, Long Island Jewish Medical Center Cystic Fibrosis Center, New Hyde Park, N.Y., Celia Ores, MD, Babies Hospital, New York, N.Y., and Jack Jacoby, MD, St. Vincent's Hospital Medical Center, New York, N.Y., for allowing us to study their patients, and Qais Al-Awqati, MD, for many helpful discussions.

REFERENCES

1. Hudson VL, Wielinski CL, Regelmann WE. Prognostic implications of initial oropharyngeal bacterial flora in patients with cystic fibrosis diagnosed before the age of two years. J PEDIATR 1993;122:854-60.
2. Kerem E, Corey M, Gold R, Levison H. Pulmonary function and clinical course in patients with cystic fibrosis after pulmonary colonization with *Pseudomonas aeruginosa.* J PEDIATR 1990;116:714-9.
3. Kristidis P, Bozon D, Corey M, et al. Genetic determinants of exocrine pancreatic function in cystic fibrosis. Am J Hum Genet 1992;50:1178-84.
4. Kerem E, Corey M, Kerem B, et al. The relationship between genotype and phenotype in cystic fibrosis: analysis of the most common mutation (ΔF508). N Engl J Med 1990;323:1517-22.
5. Johansen HK, Nir M, Hoiby N, Koch C, Schwartz M. Severity of cystic fibrosis in patients homozygous and heterozygous for ΔF508 mutation. Lancet 1991;337:631-4.
6. Saiman L, Cacalano G, Gruenert D, Prince A. Comparison of adherence of *P. aeruginosa* to respiratory epithelial cells from cystic fibrosis patients and healthy subjects. Infect Immun 1992;60:2808-14.
7. Saiman L, Prince A. *Pseudomonas aeruginosa* pili bind to asialoGM1, which is increased on the surface of cystic fibrosis epithelial cells. J Clin Invest 1993;92:1875-80.
8. Barasch J, Kiss B, Prince A, Saiman L, Gruenert D, Al-Awqati Q. Acidification of intracellular organelles is defective in cystic fibrosis. Nature 1991;352:70-3.
9. Shwachman H, Kulczycki LL. Long-term study of 105 patients with cystic fibrosis. Am J Dis Child 1958;96:6-15.
10. Friedman KJ, Highsmith WE, Silverman LM. Detecting multiple cystic fibrosis mutations by polymerase chain reaction–mediated site-directed mutagenesis. Clin Chem 1991; 37:753-5.
11. Knowles MR, Carson JL, Collier AM, Gatzy JT, Boucher RC. Measurements of transepithelial electric potential differences in normal subjects in vivo. Am Rev Respir Dis 1981;124:484-90.
12. Krivan HC, Roberts DD, Ginsburg V. Many pulmonary pathogenic bacteria bind specifically to the carbohydrate sequence GalNAc beta 1-4Gal found in some glycolipids. Proc Natl Acad Sci USA 1988;85:6157-61.
13. Kubesch P, Dork T, Wulbrand U, et al. Genetic determinants of airways' colonization with *Pseudomonas aeruginosa* in cystic fibrosis. Lancet 1993;341:189-93.
14. Welsh MJ, Smith AE. Molecular mechanisms of CFTR chloride channel dysfunction in cystic fibrosis. Cell 1993;73:1251-4.
15. Santis G, Osborne L, Knight RA, Hodson M. Independent genetic determinants of pancreatic and pulmonary status in cystic fibrosis. Lancet 1990;336:1081-4.

FELLOWSHIPS

Fellowships available in pediatric subspecialties and those for general academic pediatric training are listed once a year, in **January,** in THE JOURNAL OF PEDIATRICS. Each **June,** forms for listing fellowships available for the academic year beginning 18 months after publication are sent to the Chairman of the Department of Pediatrics at major hospitals in the United States and Canada. In addition, **a copy of the application form appears in the July, August, and September issues** of THE JOURNAL (please use the current form). Should you desire to list fellowships, a separate application must be made *each* year for *each* position. All applications must be returned to Mosby–Year Book, Inc., by **October 15** preceding the listing year to ensure publication. Additional forms will be supplied on request from the Journal Editing Department, Mosby–Year Book, Inc., 11830 Westline Industrial Drive, St. Louis, MO 63146-3318/800-325-4177, ext. 4317, or 314-453-4317.

Expanded spectrum of herpes simplex encephalitis in childhood

Yechiel Schlesinger, MD, Richard S. Buller, PhD, Janice E. Brunstrom, MD, Christopher J. Moran, MD, and Gregory A. Storch, MD

From the Departments of Pediatrics, Neurology, Radiology, Medicine, and Molecular Microbiology, Washington University School of Medicine, St. Louis, Missouri

We designed a polymerase chain reaction method to detect herpes simplex virus (HSV) DNA in spinal fluid from patients with encephalitis. The polymerase chain reaction amplified a 211 base-pair segment of the HSV DNA polymerase gene. Applying this method, we diagnosed HSV type 1 infection in three young children, aged 7 to 13 months, who had atypical forms of the illness. On the basis of magnetic resonance imaging, their disease was diffuse or multifocal in two cases and, in all three, lacked the temporal lobe involvement considered characteristic of HSV encephalitis beyond the neonatal period. Most of the diffuse or multifocal abnormalities detected by magnetic resonance imaging were not apparent by computed tomography. Restriction enzyme analysis of the polymerase chain reaction products from all three patients indicated that their disease was caused by HSV type 1. We conclude that in preschool-age children beyond the neonatal period, the spectrum of HSV encephalitis includes multifocal or diffuse involvement of the brain, which may be detected most efficiently by magnetic resonance imaging. The polymerase chain reaction method has the potential for providing an early diagnosis, but further studies are required to define the sensitivity and specificity of the polymerase chain reaction before it can be used for routine clinical decision making. (J Pediatr 1995;126:234-41)

Herpes simplex virus is the most common cause of sporadic encephalitis in the United States.[1] The clinical spectrum of HSV encephalitis includes two distinct entities. In adults and children beyond the neonatal period, temporal and, less often, frontal lobe localization is characteristic, and the cause is HSV type 1. In neonates, widespread involvement of the brain is present and the cause is usually HSV type 2.[2, 3] Although the diagnosis of the neonatal form can sometimes be made by isolating HSV from the cerebrospinal fluid,[4] viral cultures of the CSF are typically negative in older children and adults.[5] In these patients, brain biopsy has been the only way to obtain early laboratory confirmation of the diagnosis,[5-7] but the need for brain biopsy has been questioned because of potential morbidity and the widespread practice of providing empiric acyclovir therapy.[8] In many cases in which empiric therapy is used, a certain diagnosis is never established.

CSF	Cerebrospinal fluid
CT	Computed tomography
EBV	Epstein-Barr virus
HSV	Herpes simplex virus
MRI	Magnetic resonance imaging
PCR	Polymerase chain reaction

Two recent technologic developments may alter the approach to diagnosis and treatment of the patient with suspected HSV encephalitis. On the basis of reports of small numbers of cases, magnetic resonance imaging may be more sensitive than other imaging techniques for detecting abnormalities in the brain early in the course of HSV encephalitis.[9-11] Other reports suggest that the diagnosis can be confirmed early in the course by using the polymerase chain

Supported in part (Dr. Schlesinger) by the American Physician Fellowship, Inc., for Medicine in Israel.

Submitted for publication Dec. 3, 1992; accepted Feb. 5, 1993.

Reprint requests: Gregory A. Storch, MD, Department of Pediatrics, Washington University School of Medicine at Children's Hospital, One Children's Place, St. Louis, MO 63110.

0022-3476/95/$3.00 + 0 **9/20/46186**

reaction to detect HSV DNA in CSF.[12-15] We recently applied these techniques to the diagnosis of three children, 7 to 13 months of age, who had atypical forms of encephalitis.

METHODS

Polymerase chain reaction (DNA polymerase gene). The PCR was performed on 10 μl untreated CSF. Two 18-base oligonucleotides were selected from regions of homology in the published sequences of the DNA polymerase genes of HSV types 1 and 2.[16-18] The primer sequences were 5′GACTACCTGGAGATCGAG′3 and 5′TGAACCCG-TACACCGAGT′3. These primers amplify a 211 base-pair segment corresponding to bases 56,057 through 56,250 (genomic number) in HSV-1 strain 17.[17] Within this segment there is greater than 90% homology between HSV-1 and HSV-2 but no homology with Epstein-Barr virus, cytomegalovirus, or varicella zoster virus. The PCR was carried out in a reaction volume of 100 μl containing 50 mmol/L KCl, 10 mmol/L Tris-HCl (pH 8.35), 1.5 mmol/L MgCl, 0.01% gelatin, 15% glycerol, 200 μmol (each) deoxynucleoside triphosphate, 50 pmol of each oligonucleotide primer, and 5.0 units of *Taq* polymerase (Perkin-Elmer Corp., Norwalk, Conn.). The reaction was performed in Perkin-Elmer DNA Thermal Cycler 480. After 5 minutes at 95° C, 40 cycles, consisting of 1 minute of denaturation at 94° C, 1 minute of annealing at 51° C, and 1 minute of elongation at 72° C, were performed. The final cycle was followed by 7 minutes at 72° C. The assay was able to detect 10^1 to 10^2 copies of the plasmid pMC122,[19] which contains the HSV DNA polymerase gene of HSV-1, strain KOS (gift of Paul Olivo, MD, PhD, Washington University School of Medicine, St. Louis, Mo.), with either ethidium bromide or Southern blot detection. A negative control tube, in which water was substituted for CSF, was also included in each PCR run. Specimens from patients with disease processes other than HSV encephalitis were tested simultaneously as negative control specimens. Recommended precautions for avoiding PCR contamination were followed,[20] including the use of positive-displacement pipettes for samples containing nucleic acids and analysis of PCR products in a room separate from that in which specimens were processed and reactions were set up. All reaction tubes and components (except for the specimens, primers, and *Taq* polymerase) were ultraviolet irradiated at 300 mjoules with an ultraviolet Stratalinker 1800 oven (Strategene, La Jolla, Calif.).

Polymerase chain reaction (glycoprotein D gene). Specimens also were tested according to the PCR method of Aurelius et al.[12] In this method, two sets of "nested primers" are used to amplify a 137 base-pair segment of the glycoprotein D gene of HSV-1. This segment shares partial homology with HSV-2 and has no homology with the DNA of EBV, cytomegalovirus, or varicella zoster virus. This PCR was also performed on 10 μl untreated CSF.

Analysis of PCR products. The PCR reaction products were analyzed by electrophoresis through a 3% agarose gel (3:1 NuSieve:agarose; FMC BioProducts, Rockland, Me.) and detected by staining with ethidium bromide (0.5 μg/ml). After electrophoresis, the gel was washed for 30 minutes in water and photographed. The identity of the amplified reaction product was confirmed by Southern blotting[21] with a blotting unit (Bios Corp., New Haven, Conn.) and Biosbrane membrane BMB-2020 (Bios Corp.). Oligonucleotide probe 5′GCCATGCGAAAGCAGATC-CGCTCGCGGAT3′, labeled with phosphorus 32 and located within the amplified segment of the DNA polymerase gene (bases 56,152 to 56,180),[17] was used. This segment is 100% homologous to the published sequences of HSV-1 and HSV-2[16-18] but has no homology with other herpes viruses. The identity of the product of the glycoprotein-D PCR reaction was also confirmed by Southern blotting with the probe described by Aurelius et al.[12]

Differentiation between HSV types 1 and 2. For differentiation between HSV-1 and HSV-2, the DNA polymerase PCR product was digested with the restriction enzymes *Hinf*I and *Bam*HI. The amplified segment of HSV-1 but not HSV-2 contains a *Hinf*I site that yields products of 122 and 89 base pairs. The amplified segment of HSV-2 but not HSV-1 contains a *Bam*HI site that yields products of 121 and 90 base pairs. A 35 μl aliquot of the PCR reaction mixture was digested under the conditions recommended by the manufacturer (Promega Inc., Madison, Wis.). The digested products were analyzed by electrophoresis through a 3% 3:1 NuSieve:agarose gel and stained with ethidium bromide.

This method was validated by restriction enzyme digestion of PCR products of lysates of cell cultures infected by known isolates of HSV-1 and HSV-2. Six primary rabbit kidney–cell cultures infected with HSV-1 and six infected with HSV-2 were tested. The isolates were provided by the diagnostic virology laboratory of Washington University Department of Pediatrics. The isolates were typed by fluorescent antibody staining with monoclonal antibodies specific for HSV-1 and HSV-2 (Syva Corp., San Jose, Calif.).

Antibody studies in CSF and serum. The HSV antibody levels in CSF and serum were determined by enzyme-linked immunosorbent assay (Herpes Stat; Whittaker Bioproducts, Inc., Walkersville, Md.). Serial dilutions were tested and the results were graphed as plots of absorbance versus log dilution. The linear portion of each curve was used to estimate the dilution of CSF and serum giving the same absorbance at an outside diameter of 405 nm. These dilutions were used to calculate the CSF/serum ratios of HSV antibodies. This ratio was compared with the "albumin index,"

Table I. Summary of patient data

Patient No.	Age (mo)	Major symptoms and signs	Day*	CSF Erythrocytes (mm³)	CSF Leukocytes (mm³)	CSF % Neutrophils	CSF Protein (mg/dl)	CSF Glucose (mg/dl)	PCR†
1	13	Fever, generalized seizure activity continued neurologic deterioration	2	4	5	75	21	65	ND‡
			10	11	47	1	104	66	+
			38	6250	10	11	62	46	−
2	11	Fever, left focal seizures, continued neurologic deterioration, movement disorder	1	0	0	—	<10	50	ND‡
			5	1684	56	4	46	50	+§
			8	460	110	0	65	56	+
			13	2720	20	7	94	63	−
			14	556	34	1	64	55	−
			32	10	7	0	18	57	−
3	7	Generalized tonic-clonic seizure without fever, left hemiplegia, complete resolution	1	0	0	0	<13	67	ND‡
			4	220	16	61	<13	61	+

ND, Not done.
*Day of illness.
†Specimens were tested with PCR protocols for the DNA polymerase and glycoprotein D genes, except where indicated.
‡Specimens were not available for PCR.
§Glycoprotein D gene only.

Table II. Summary of HSV antibody results

Patient No.	Day*	Serum anti-HSV IgG†	Serum anti-HSV IgM‡	CSF anti-HSV IgG†	CSF antibody index§
1	11	1.19	ND	ND	NA
	29	5.57	ND	1.36	1.45
2	9	2.67	2.5	ND	NA
	36	4.16	ND	0.48	5.7

ND, Not done; *NA*, not available.
*Day of illness.
†Values given as a ratio of optical density at 405 nmol/L between tested specimen and a known low positive control. Values greater than 1.0 are considered positive. A ratio of values greater than 1.47 is considered equivalent to a fourfold or greater change.
‡Values given as enzyme immunoassay (EIA) units. Values greater than 1.10 are considered positive.
§The CSF antibody index is defined as the ratio of CSF to serum HSV antibody divided by the ratio of CSF to serum albumin.

the CSF/serum albumin ratio, which serves as a measure of blood-brain barrier integrity.[22] Serum and CSF albumin concentrations were measured by rocket electroimmunodiffusion, and the CSF/serum ratio was calculated. The "CSF antibody index" was calculated by dividing the CSF/serum HSV antibody ratio by the CSF/serum albumin ratio. Values greater than 1.91 are considered unequivocal evidence of intrathecal synthesis of HSV antibodies.[22]

RESULTS

Selected clinical and laboratory data from the three patients are summarized in Table I. Serologic data from patients 1 and 2 are summarized in Table II.

Case reports

Patient 1. Patient 1 was a 13-month-old, previously healthy black female infant who had fever and generalized seizures. The CSF on the second day of illness had 4 · 10⁶ erythrocytes/L (4 erythrocytes/mm^3) and 5 · 10^6 leukocytes/L (5 leukocytes/mm^3) with 75% neutrophils, protein 0.21 gm/L (21 mg/dl), and glucose 3.6 mmol/L (65 mg/dl) (Table I). Bacterial and viral cultures were negative. The seizure activity persisted, and the infant was admitted to an outside hospital; anticonvulsant therapy was started. Despite antibiotic therapy, her level of consciousness declined. Acyclovir therapy was instituted on the third day of illness. A lumbar puncture performed on the same day revealed no significant changes. An electroencephalogram showed generalized slowing with bilateral periodic lateralizing epileptiform discharges. A computed tomographic scan of the head without and with contrast material was normal. An MRI scan of the head 3 days later demonstrated several swollen gyri in both frontal and parietal lobes in the paracentral region, as well as in the occipital lobes, with adjacent edema. The inferior frontal and temporal lobes were spared (Fig. 1). The infant was transferred to St. Louis Children's Hospital on the fifth day of illness when she required tracheal intubation for deteriorating neurologic status.

On admission the infant was febrile to 39.5° C and comatose with a stiff neck and intermittent generalized seizures. Her hemoglobin level was 94 gm/L (9.4 gm/dl), leukocyte count 7.1 · 10^9/L (7100/mm^3) with a normal differential cell count and a platelet count of 683 · 10^9/L (683,000/mm^3). Paired serum specimens had no detectable antibodies to arboviruses, *Mycoplasma pneumoniae*, and *Toxoplasma gondii*. Serologic tests showed no evidence of infection with measles virus, hepatitis A, B, and C viruses, or human immunodeficiency virus and no evidence of antinuclear antibodies or rheumatoid factor. The titer of IgG antibodies to the EBV capsid antigen was 1:1280. Antibodies to the EBV early antigen were present at a titer of 1:40. Results of tests for antibodies to the EBV nuclear antigen and IgM antibodies to the viral capsid antigen were negative. The serum HSV IgG antibody titer showed an increase equivalent to a four-fold or greater rise in specimens obtained on days 11 and 29 of illness (Table II). Despite continued treatment with intravenously administered acyclovir (16 days at 30 to 50 mg/kg per day), her course was marked by recurrent fever and seizures and progressive functional and structural neurologic damage.

Patient 2. Patient 2 was an 11-month-old black female infant with no underlying disease who had fever to 38.6° C and lethargy. A lumbar puncture on the first day of illness revealed normal CSF (Table I). Her fever continued and she had left focal seizures. On admission to the hospital, her neurologic examination was notable for generalized seizures beginning on the left side, irritability, and preferential use of the right arm. Her leukocyte count was 12.1 · 10^9/L (12,100 leukocytes/mm^3). Serum electrolytes, blood urea nitrogen, creatinine, calcium, and magnesium values were within normal limits. Therapy with acyclovir, 30 mg/kg per day, was started within 8 hours of admission to the hospital. An electroencephalogram was normal. Computed tomography of the head demonstrated a wedge-shaped low-density region involving the cortex in both paracentral regions, which was not enhanced by contrast administration. Three days later, MRI of the head showed more extensive involvement. The paracentral gyri were swollen and the involved cortical surfaces intensely enhanced after administration of intravenous contrast material (gadopentetate dimeglumine). Increased signal was also present in both thalami. The inferior frontal and temporal lobes were normal. A second MRI scan after 8 days showed progression of the lesions. Additional lumbar punctures showed persistent pleocytosis that gradually improved (Table I). All bacterial, fungal, and viral cultures of the CSF were negative for pathogens. Acute and convalescent antibody titers revealed no evidence of infection by arboviruses or *M. pneumoniae.* Results of a rapid plasma reagin test and tests for antinuclear antibodies and rheumatoid factor were negative. The titers of IgG antibodies to the EBV capsid antigen were less than 1:10 on day 9 and 1:80 on days 20, 37, and 40 of illness. Results of tests for IgM antibodies to the EBV capsid antigen and antibodies to the early antigen and nuclear antigen were negative. The patient was treated with acyclovir for 10 days with gradual clinical improvement, including resolution of fever and control of seizures. Shortly after the acyclovir therapy was stopped, seizures recurred and were controlled with the addition of phenytoin. Sixteen days after completing her first course of acyclovir, she was readmitted with increased seizure activity and decreased level of activity. A lumbar puncture on the day of readmission revealed 26 · 10^6 leukocytes/L (26 leukocytes/mm^3), all mononuclear, and normal protein and glucose concentrations. Despite an additional 15-day course of acyclovir, 30 mg/kg per day, that was begun on the ninth hospital day, the patient had progressive neurologic deterioration with increased seizure activity, persistent choreoathetoid movements, and a decline in the level of consciousness to the extent that, although conscious, she had no response to visual or auditory stimuli.

Levels of HSV antibodies were measured by enzyme-linked immunosorbent assay in serum specimens from days 9 and 36 of illness. The increase in the enzyme-linked immunosorbent assay value was equivalent to a more than fourfold increase in titer. The HSV-specific IgM antibodies were demonstrated in serum specimens from days 9 and 15 of illness (Table II).

Patient 3. Patient 3 was a 7-month-old previously healthy black female infant with generalized tonic-clonic seizures without fever. Examination findings after the seizures were entirely normal except for a left Babinski sign and macrocephaly. A lumbar puncture yielded no cells, a protein value less than 0.13 gm/L (13 mg/dl), and a glucose value of 3.7 mmol/L (67 mg/dl). Phenobarbital therapy was initiated. On the following day the patient had a prolonged (>15 minutes) episode of left facial twitching with brief, intermittent generalized convulsive activity of all extremities. The seizures resolved after intravenous administration of phenytoin, after which she had a residual left hemiplegia, a left Babinski sign, and an apparent left visual field defect manifested by inattentiveness to the left visual field. An electroencephalogram was normal. An MRI scan of the head demonstrated swollen gyri in the right paracentral region that caused a slight mass effect. Administration of contrast material (gadopentetate dimeglumine) slightly enhanced the involved area. The inferior frontal and temporal lobes were normal. On the following day a CT scan of the head demonstrated extensive low density in the right parietal area that was larger than the MRI abnormality. A second lumbar puncture on day 4 of illness revealed 220 · 10^6 erythrocytes/L (220 erythrocytes/mm^3), 16 · 10^6 leukocytes/L (16 leukocytes/mm^3) with

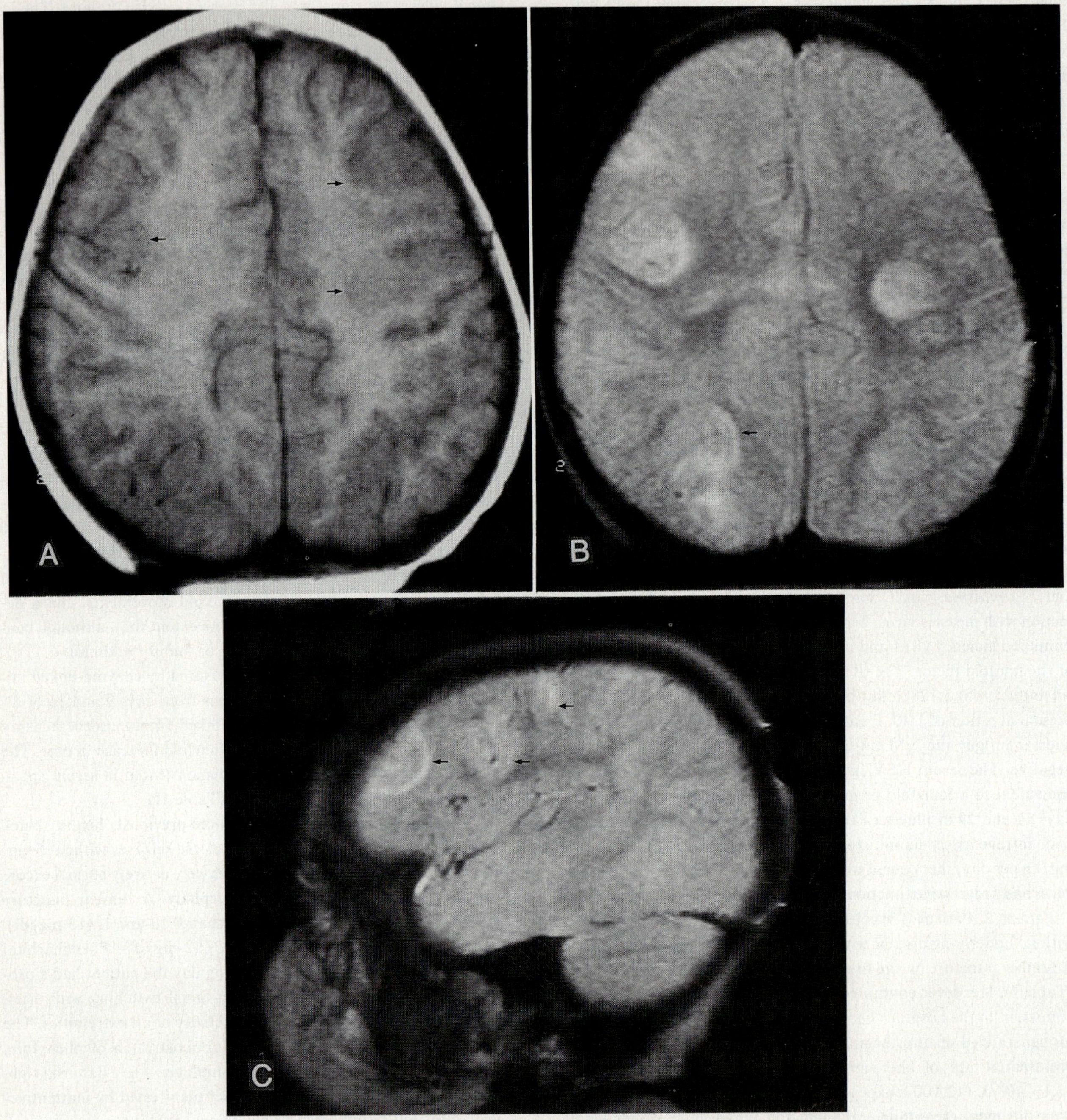

Fig. 1. Patient 1: MRI of head performed 6 days after onset of illness. **A,** Axial T1-weighted image shows several swollen frontal and parietal gyri *(arrows)*. **B,** T2-weighted image shows swollen frontal and parietal gyri with high signal intensity. Another area of involvement is present in right parieto-occipital region *(arrow)*. **C,** Sagittal T2-weighted image demonstrates involvement of right frontal convexity *(arrows)* with sparing of inferior right frontal lobe and right temporal lobe.

61% neutrophils and 39% lymphocytes, protein concentration less than 0.13 gm/L (13 mg/dl), and glucose concentration 3.4 mmol/L (61 mg/dl). The CSF bacterial and viral cultures remained negative for pathogens. Treatment with acyclovir, 30 mg/kg per day, was started on day 5 and continued for 10 days. The patient's seizures were controlled with anticonvulsants. An additional MRI scan 10 days later showed progression of the original lesion. Because the scans were interpreted as compatible with infarction, as well as encephalitis, an extensive evaluation for causes of stroke was performed; no abnormalities were found. After 2 weeks of therapy, the patient's general clinical condition improved and she was discharged, seizure free, with a residual left hemipare-

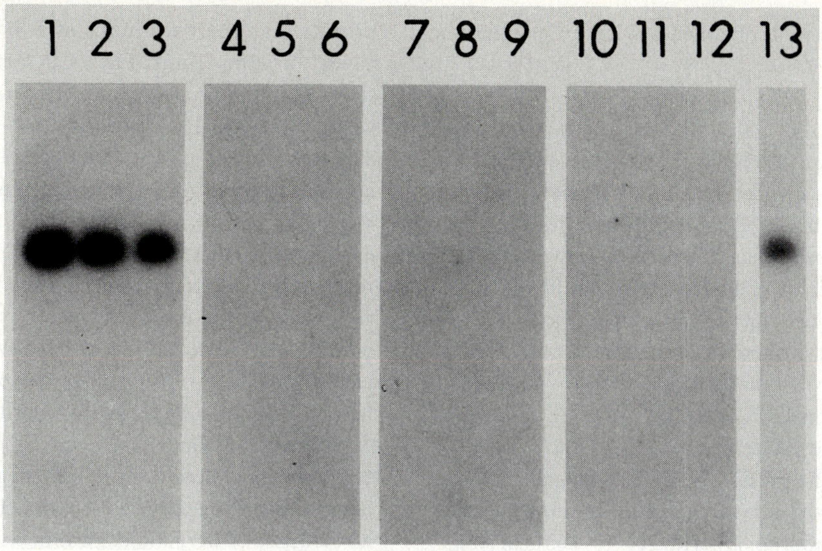

Fig. 2. Southern blot of PCR products from spinal fluid specimens of selected patients with primers specific for HSV-1 and HSV-2 DNA polymerase gene. PCR procedure and Southern blotting were performed as described in text. *Lanes 1* through *3*, patients 1 through 3; *lanes 4* through *6*, patients with enteroviral meningitis; *lanes 7* through *9*, patients with human immunodeficiency virus infection and cytomegalovirus central nervous system disease; *lanes 10* through *12*, patients with herpes febrilis and no evidence of HSV central nervous system disease; *lane 13*, 10^2 copies of plasmid pMC122 containing HSV DNA polymerase gene.

sis involving predominantly the upper extremity and persistent inattentiveness to the left side.

Cerebrospinal fluid PCR (DNA polymerase gene). Each of the three patients was subsequently found to have HSV DNA in CSF as detected by PCR for the DNA polymerase gene. A CSF specimen from patient 1, obtained on day 10 of her illness was positive for HSV (Fig. 2). A subsequent CSF specimen obtained 1 month later was negative for the organism. A CSF specimen from patient 2, obtained on day 8 of illness, was positive (Fig. 2); specimens from the thirteenth, fourteenth, and thirty-second days were negative (Table I). A CSF specimen from patient 3 on the fourth day of illness was positive (Fig. 2). Each of the positive reactions was detected by both ethidium bromide staining and Southern blot.

All nine CSF specimens from patients with disease processes other than HSV encephalitis had no detectable HSV DNA (Fig. 2). These patients included three with confirmed enteroviral meningitis, three with human immunodeficiency virus infection and cytomegalovirus disease of the central nervous system, and three with peripheral HSV lesions and no clinical evidence of HSV neurologic disease.

Cerebrospinal fluid PCR (glycoprotein D gene). Each of the specimens with HSV detectable by the DNA polymerase amplification protocol also had HSV DNA detectable by PCR for amplification of the HSV glycoprotein D gene (Table I). In addition, a specimen from patient 2, obtained on day 5 of illness and not available for testing with the DNA polymerase PCR assay, was also positive for HSV. The PCR products from patients 1 and 2 were detected by both ethidium bromide staining and Southern blot. The reaction product from patient 3 was not visible by ethidium bromide staining but Southern blot results were positive. In the same run, 12 CSF specimens from patients with disease processes other than HSV encephalitis had no detectable HSV. These cases included five of culture-proved enteroviral meningitis and one case each of group B streptococcal meningitis, organic solvent intoxication, febrile seizures, convulsive disorder, brain infarct, human immunodeficiency virus–associated lymphoma, and human immunodeficiency virus–associated progressive multifocal leukoencephalopathy.

Viral typing. Restriction enzyme analysis of the DNA polymerase gene PCR products from the three patients with HSV encephalitis was consistent with HSV-1 in all three cases (data not shown). Results for the 12 lysates of cell cultures infected with HSV-1 and HSV-2 were in agreement with typing by the fluorescent antibody staining method.

Cerebrospinal fluid HSV antibodies. Appropriate convalescent CSF and serum specimens were available for retrospective serologic testing in two of the three patients. Patient 1 had antibodies to HSV in a CSF specimen obtained on day 29 of illness; patient 2 had HSV IgG antibodies in a CSF specimen obtained on day 36 of illness (Table II).

DISCUSSION

These patients illustrate the importance of two techniques, MRI and PCR, which together provide new insight into the clinical spectrum of HSV encephalitis in this age group. The MRI revealed diffuse or multifocal involvement of the brain in two patients and a frontoparietal lobe lesion in the third. These patients lacked the temporal lobe localization thought to be characteristic of the nonneonatal form of HSV encephalitis. Nevertheless, PCR revealed the presence of HSV DNA in the CSF of each of the three patients.

Recent reports suggest excellent sensitivity and specificity of PCR for the diagnosis of HSV encephalitis.[12-15] However, because of the unusual clinical findings in our patients, we sought additional evidence to confirm the diagnosis. We used two independent PCR methods that detect two unrelated genes to ensure that the PCR findings were not spurious. In addition, we attempted to demonstrate intrathecal synthesis of HSV antibodies, a technique that has been widely used to make a diagnosis of HSV encephalitis.[5, 22, 23] The clinical value of this approach is limited because the results are usually not diagnostic until relatively late in the illness, but the technique can be useful for retrospective confirmation of the diagnosis. Appropriate convalescent CSF and serum specimens from two of the three patients were available for retrospective testing. In one of our patients, evidence of intrathecal synthesis of HSV antibodies was strong; in the other it was suggestive rather than diagnostic.

Our three cases illustrate the possible association of HSV encephalitis in young children beyond the neonatal period with widespread involvement of the brain; the clinical picture may resemble the neonatal rather than the adult form of the disease. The finding that the PCR product was HSV-1 in all three cases indicates that they represent the lower end of the age distribution of the "adult" form of the disease, rather than the upper end of the neonatal form, which is usually associated with HSV-2. Multifocal or diffuse involvement in children beyond the neonatal age has also been noted in reports of CT findings in children with HSV encephalitis[24-27]; all but one of the children with multifocal or diffuse involvement were 5 years of age or less. The concept that HSV encephalitis in young children may not be localized to the temporal lobe is especially pertinent because of the increasing use of MRI, which may have greater sensitivity than CT for revealing the widespread involvement of the brain. Further studies comparing MRI and CT findings early in the course of HSV encephalitis in very young children are required to clarify this issue.

Although we believe that PCR will prove to be useful in providing an early diagnosis of HSV encephalitis, several caveats are important. The PCR method is still not a routine laboratory procedure, and its sensitivity and specificity when applied in the clinical setting remain to be defined. The risk of false-positive PCR results is well known, and elaborate precautions are required to avoid this danger.[20] Although positive results have been reported as early as 2 days after the first symptoms,[12-12b, 12d, 13-15] false-negative results also have been reported when testing was performed very early in the disease course.[12, 12c, 12d, 13, 14] Treatment with acyclovir also may cause negative results.[12-12c, 13, 14] A particular concern is whether the presence of peripheral herpetic lesions such as herpes febrilis could be associated with detectable HSV DNA in CSF in the absence of central nervous system disease. The negative results reported here from three patients with peripheral herpetic lesions and no evidence of herpetic central nervous system disease are reassuring, but additional patients should be tested before this concern can be laid aside. If carefully used, with scrupulous attention to details of performance and appropriate positive and negative controls, PCR has the potential to improve the clinical recognition of HSV infection of the central nervous system.

We are indebted to Dr. Paul Olivo for providing us with plasmid pMC122, as well as numerous useful suggestions, Dr. John Trotter for his help with the CSF serology, and Dr. John Sninsky, Roche Molecular Systems, for technical suggestions regarding the PCR assay. Monique Gaudreault-Keener provided expert technical assistance, Colleen Haug provided the typed HSV isolates, and Antoinette Campbell performed the CSF serologic testing. Drs. Phillip R. Dodge and Dan M. Granoff provided helpful comments on the manuscript.

REFERENCES

1. Center for Disease Control. Encephalitis surveillance: annual summary 1978. Washington, DC: US Department of Health and Human Services, 1981:24-5.
2. Nahmias AJ, Whitley RJ. Herpes simplex virus encephalitis in pediatrics. Pediatr Rev 1981;2:259-66.
3. Whitley RJ, Soong SJ, Linneman C Jr, Liu C, Pazin G, Alford CA, NIAID Collaborative Antiviral Study Group. Herpes simplex encephalitis: clinical assessment. JAMA 1982;247: 317-20.
4. Frank AL, Tucker G. Isolation of herpes simplex type 1 from ventricular fluid of an infant with encephalitis. J Pediatr 1978;92:601-2.
5. Nahmias AJ, Whitley RJ, Visintine AN, Takei Y, Alford CA Jr, Collaborative Antiviral Study Group. Herpes simplex virus encephalitis: laboratory evaluations and their diagnostic significance. J Infect Dis 1982;145:829-36.
6. Whitley RJ, Cobbs CG, Alford CA, et al. Diseases that mimic herpes simplex encephalitis: diagnosis, presentation and outcome. JAMA 1989;262:234-9.
7. Kohl S, James AR. Herpes simplex virus encephalitis during

childhood: importance of brain biopsy diagnosis. J PEDIATR 1985;107:212-5.

8. Whitley RJ, Gnann JW Jr. Drug therapy: acyclovir: a decade later. N Engl J Med 1992;327:782-9.
9. Zimmerman RD, Haimes AB. The role of MR imaging in the diagnosis of infections of the central nervous system. Curr Clin Top Infect Dis 1989;10:82-108.
10. Albertyn LE. Magnetic resonance imaging in herpes simplex encephalitis. Australas Radiol 1990;34:117-21.
11. Gasecki AP, Steg RE. Correlation of early MRI with CT scan, EEG, and CSF: analysis in a case of biopsy-proven herpes simplex encephalitis. Eur Neurol 1991;31:372-5.
12. Aurelius E, Johansson B, Skoldenberg B, Staland A, Forsgern M. Rapid diagnosis of herpes simplex encephalitis by nested polymerase chain reaction assay of cerebrospinal fluid. Lancet 1991;337:189-92.

12a. Kimura H, Aso K, Kuzushima K, Hanada N, Shibata M, Morishima T. Relapse of herpes simplex encephalitis in children. Pediatrics 1992;89:891-4.

12b. Ando Y, Kimura H, Miwata H, Kudo T, Shibata M, Morishima T. Quantitative analysis of herpes simplex virus DNA in cerebrospinal fluid of children with herpes simplex encephalitis. J Med Virol 1993;41:170-3.

12c. Troendle-Atkins J, Demmler GJ, Buffone GJ. Rapid diagnosis of herpes simplex virus encephalitis by using the polymerase chain reaction. J PEDIATR 1993;123:376-80.

12d. Uren EC, Johnson PDR, Montanaro J, Gilbert B, Gilbert GL. Herpes simplex virus encephalitis in pediatrics: diagnosis by detection of antibodies and DNA in cerebrospinal fluid. Pediatr Infect Dis J 1993;12:1001-6.

12e. DeVincenzo JP, Thorne G. Mild herpes simplex encephalitis diagnosed by polymerase chain reaction: a case report and review. Pediatr Infect Dis J 1994;13:662-4.

13. Rozenberg F, Lebon P. Amplification and characterization of herpesvirus DNA in cerebrospinal fluid from patients with acute encephalitis. J Clin Microbiol 1991;29:2412-7.
14. Klapper PE, Cleator MG, Dennet C, Lewis AG. Diagnosis of herpes encephalitis via southern blotting of cerebrospinal fluid DNA amplified by polymerase chain reaction. J Med Virol 1990;32:261-4.
15. Kimura H, Futamura M, Kito H, et al. Detection of viral DNA in neonatal herpes simplex virus infections: frequent and prolonged presence in serum and cerebrospinal fluid. J Infect Dis 1991;164:289-93.
16. Gibbs JS, Chiou HC, Hall JD, et al. Sequence and mapping analysis of herpes simplex virus DNA polymerase gene predict a C-terminal substrate binding domain. Proc Natl Acad Sci USA 1985;82:7969-73.
17. McGeoch DJ, Dalrymple MA, Davison AJ, et al. The complete DNA sequence of the long unique region in the genome of herpes simplex virus type 1. J Gen Virol 1988;69:1531-74.
18. Tsurumi T, Maeno K, Nishiyima Y. Nucleotide sequence of the DNA polymerase gene of herpes simplex type 2 and comparison with the type 1 counterpart. Gene 1987;52:129-37.
19. Challberg MD. A method for identifying the viral genes required for herpesvirus DNA replication. Proc Natl Acad Sci USA 1986;83:9094-8.
20. Kwok S, Higuchi R. Avoiding false positives with PCR. Nature 1989;339:237-8.
21. Southern EM. Detection of specific sequences among DNA fragments separated by gel electrophoresis. J Mol Biol 1975; 98:503-17.
22. Klapper PE, Laing I, Longson M. Rapid non-invasive diagnosis of herpes encephalitis. Lancet 1981;2:607-9.
23. Koskiniemi M, Vahery A, Taskinen E. Cerebrospinal fluid alterations in herpes simplex virus encephalitis. Rev Infect Dis 1984;6:608-18.
24. Schauseil-Zipf U, Harden A, Hoare RD, et al. Early diagnosis of herpes simplex encephalitis in childhood: clinical, neurophysiological and neuroradiological studies. Eur J Pediatr 1982;138:154-61.
25. Sugimoto T, Woo M, Okazaki H, et al. Computed tomography in young children with herpes simplex virus encephalitis. Pediatr Radiol 1985;15:372-6.
26. McCrossin DB, Gwendolyn LG. Herpes simplex virus encephalitis in children. Med J Aust 1986;144:711-3.
27. Taccone A, Gambaro G, Ghizori M, et al. Computed tomography (CT) in children with herpes simplex encephalitis. Pediatr Radiol 1988;19:9-12.

Lipid abnormalities in Turner syndrome

Judith L. Ross, MD, Penelope Feuillan, MD, Lauren M. Long, RN,
Karen Kowal, PA, Harvey Kushner, PhD, and Gordon B. Cutler, Jr., MD

From the Department of Pediatrics, Thomas Jefferson University, Philadelphia, Pennsylvania, the Developmental Endocrinology Branch, National Institute of Child Health and Human Development, National Institutes of Health, Bethesda, Maryland, and the Department of Statistics, Hahnemann University, Philadelphia, Pennsylvania

Turner syndrome is associated with insulin resistance, increased incidence of type II diabetes, and hypertension, all of which are cardiovascular risk factors. The purpose of this study was to evaluate the lipid profile of girls with untreated Turner syndrome, (aged 5 to 14 years; 68% 45,XO) and age-matched, normal girls. A total of 137 girls with Turner syndrome and 70 normal girls had lipid profile measurements, including cholesterol, high-density lipoprotein cholesterol, and triglycerides. Older girls with Turner syndrome (>11.0 years) had increased cholesterol levels (*p* <0.01), compared with control values (190 ± 38 vs 165 ± 26 mg/dl). Cholesterol levels were elevated in older subjects with Turner syndrome versus normal subjects, after adjustment for age, karyotype, and body mass index *z* score effects (*p* = 0.01). In the subjects with Turner syndrome but not the normal subjects, serum cholesterol values correlated with age, weight, and body mass index *z* score (*p* <0.02). We conclude that adolescent girls with untreated Turner syndrome have significantly increased cholesterol levels, independent of age, body mass index *z* score, or karyotype, and that these precede any treatment with exogenous estrogen or growth hormone. (J Pediatr 1995;126:242-5)

Turner syndrome is associated with insulin resistance, increased incidence of type II diabetes, and hypertension,[1-3] all of which are cardiovascular risk factors. Previous studies have demonstrated insulin resistance in young girls with Turner syndrome (10.8 ± 0.8 years), independent of estrogen replacement or body mass index.[4] Girls with TS have an increased risk of obesity, impaired glucose tolerance, and type II diabetes mellitus. Hyperinsulinemia has been independently associated with hypercholesterolemia,[5] another cardiovascular risk factor. The purpose of this study was to examine the hypothesis that girls with TS (aged 5 to 14 years) have elevated lipid levels before any estrogen replacement therapy or growth hormone treatment.

Supported in part by Eli Lilly and Company.

Submitted for publication May 27, 1994; accepted Aug. 25, 1994.

Reprint requests: Judith L. Ross, MD, Department of Pediatrics, Thomas Jefferson University, 1025 Walnut St., Philadelphia, PA 19107.

9/20/60184

METHODS

The study was approved by the human studies committees at the National Institute of Child Health and Human Development, National Institutes of Health (NIH), and at Thomas Jefferson University. All subjects and their parents gave informed assent and consent. No child with documented hyperlipidemia in one or both parents was included.

BMI	Body mass index
HDL	High-density lipoprotein
LDL	Low-density lipoprotein
TS	Turner syndrome

Subjects

Normal control subjects. The 70 normal female control subjects were recruited through the normal volunteer office at the National Institutes of Health, and through the Philadelphia school system. All the girls had heights and weights between the 5th and 95th percentiles. Each girl had pubertal Tanner staging according to the method of Mar-

Table I. Comparison of anthropometric and lipid measurements

	Turner syndrome		Normal subjects		
	Age 5-10.9 yr (n = 99)	Age 11.0-14.9 yr (n = 38)	Age 5-10.9 yr (n = 27)	Age 11.0-14.9 yr (n = 43)	p (TS vs normal subjects)
Age (yr)	7.4 ± 2.0	12.0 ± 0.6	8.7 ± 1.2	12.3 ± 1.0	0.0001
Height z score	−2.5 ± 0.8	−3.1 ± 1.0	−0.3 ± 1.0	0.0 ± 1.1	0.0001
BMI	17.3 ± 3.5	21.0 ± 3.9	16.9 ± 2.3	19.0 ± 2.7	0.80
BMI z score	0.3 ± 1.2	0.5 ± 1.2	0.0 ± 1.0	−0.2 ± 0.8	0.005
Cholesterol (mg/dl)	166 ± 29	190 ± 38*	167 ± 31	165 ± 26	0.01
HDL cholesterol (mg/dl)	50 ± 11	55 ± 14	47 ± 9	45 ± 12	0.007
LDL cholesterol (mg/dl)	101 ± 28	116 ± 34*	115 ± 23	101 ± 24	0.83
Triglycerides (mg/dl)	78 ± 56	94 ± 53	91 ± 42	102 ± 69	0.08

*$p \leq 0.01$, two-way analysis of variance, older TS age group versus control subjects.

Table IIA. Correlation between lipid levels and anthropometric measures in Turner syndrome

	Cholesterol	HDL cholesterol	LDL cholesterol	Triglycerides
Age	0.33†	0.12	0.31†	0.14
Height z score	0.13	0.03	0.13	0.03
Weight	0.40‡	0.12	0.36‡	0.27*
BMI z score	0.28†	0.17	0.21†	0.25*
Cholesterol	1.00	0.20	0.91‡	0.39‡
LDL	0.91‡	0.06	1.00	0.16
Triglycerides	0.39‡	0.29†	0.16	1.00

*$p < 0.02$.
†$p < 0.002$.
‡$p < 0.0001$.

Table IIB. Correlation between lipid levels and anthropometric measures in control girls

	Cholesterol	HDL cholesterol	LDL cholesterol	Triglycerides
Age	0.02	0.10	0.29	0.03
Height z score	0.26	0.16	0.22	0.09
Weight z score	0.05	0.08	0.09	0.07
BMI z score	0.15	0.03	0.22	0.16
Cholesterol	1.00	0.40*	0.71‡	0.33*
LDL	0.71‡	0.05	1.00	0.46†
Triglycerides	0.33*	0.11	0.46†	1.00

*$p < 0.02$.
†$p < 0.002$.
‡$p < 0.0001$.

shall and Tanner.[6] The racial composition of the control group was white 86%, black 9%, Hispanic 4%, and other 1%. The pubertal stages for breast development were Tanner I 47%, Tanner II 13%, Tanner III 10%, Tanner IV 17%, and Tanner V 13%. The girls were grouped according to chronologic age of 5 to 10.9 years or 11.0 to 14.9 years.

Subjects with Turner syndrome. Study subjects included 137 girls with TS between the ages of 5 and 14 years. Their karyotypes were as follows: 68% 45,XO, 26% mosaic, and 6% monosomic partial deletion of the second X chromosome. Ninety-three percent of the subjects with TS had Tanner stage I breast development and 7% had Tanner II breast development. Hypothyroidism had been diagnosed in 25 children, all of whom were taking thyroid replacement at the time of this evaluation, and were euthyroid. All the study subjects were euthyroid, according to thyroid studies done within the preceding 6 months. Nine patients had received prior treatment with growth hormone or estrogen for less than 12 months but had stopped these treatments for a minimum of 6 months before being studied. All subjects with TS had normal fasting glucose and glycosylated hemoglobin levels. The racial composition of the Turner syndrome group was white 85%, black 6%, Hispanic 6%, and other 3%, which was not statistically different from the racial composition of the control subjects.

Two thirds of the subjects with TS and all the control subjects had lipids measured at the NIH, and one third of the subjects with TS had lipids measured at another reference laboratory (Scicor, Indianapolis, Ind.). Cholesterol was measured with identical photometric methods on Hitachi analyzers (NSA Hitachi, Mountain View, Calif.) at both sites. An analysis of 19 samples measured in both laboratories (Scicor and NIH) showed a highly significant correlation ($r = 0.99$; $p < 0.001$) and no statistically significant difference in the paired means ($t = 1.29$; $p > 0.20$). The mean lipid and anthropometric measurements for the

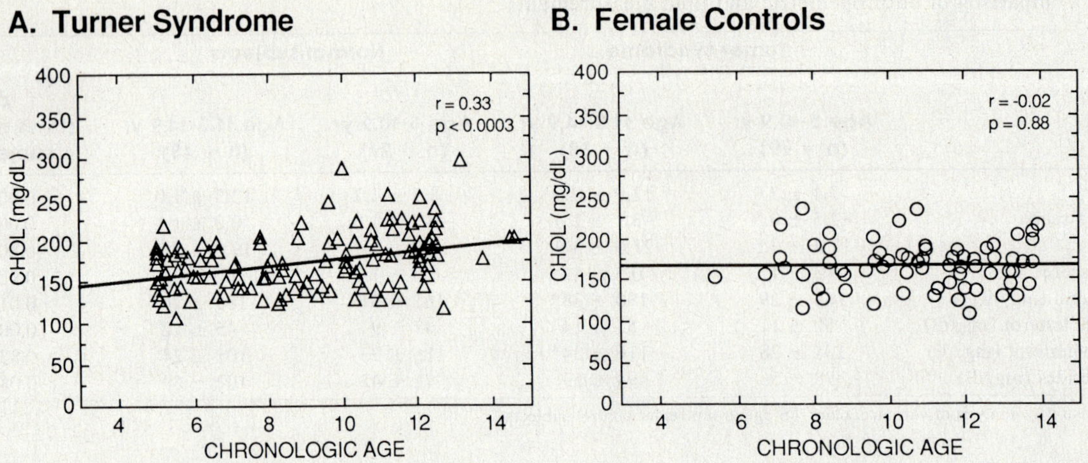

Figure. **A,** Total cholesterol levels in girls with TS, according to chronologic age. **B,** Total cholesterol levels in healthy girls, according to chronologic age.

two groups with TS were similar, and consequently the data were merged for the analyses discussed in this article.

Clinical protocol. All subjects underwent fasting for 6 to 12 hours after midnight or an early meal (before 7 AM). Samples from the TS and control populations were collected concurrently. All subjects had measurement of serum cholesterol, high-density lipoprotein cholesterol, and triglycerides. Low-density lipoprotein cholesterol was calculated according to the method of Friedewald et al.[7] (= total cholesterol − HDL cholesterol − triglycerides/5).

Body mass index was used as a measure of obesity and was calculated by dividing the weight (in kilograms) by the height (in meters) squared. Body mass index z scores were calculated from published norms.[8] Height z scores were calculated from National Center for Health Statistics.

Statistics. Analytic methods used included two-way analysis of variance, analysis of covariance, and simple Pearson correlations. Multiple regression analysis was also performed when indicated. Results were considered statistically significant for $p < 0.05$. All means are presented as mean ± SD.

RESULTS

The population with TS was somewhat younger than the control subjects. The girls with TS were significantly shorter, and the older girls, in particular, had increased BMI z scores ($p < 0.005$). Lipid levels were compared in the two populations after analysis of covariance was performed with BMI z score and age as covariates; thus adjustment was made for the analysis for differences in BMI z score or chronologic age. In addition, two-way analysis of variance was performed to examine the interaction of age and the diagnosis of TS versus control subjects. The older girls with TS (≥11.0 years of age) had significantly increased total, HDL, and LDL cholesterol levels, compared with age-matched, normal female subjects (Table I; analysis of covariance). Levels of triglycerides were similar in the two groups. Mean lipid values for girls with 45,XO versus mosaic karyotypes did not differ (data not shown).

Total cholesterol and LDL cholesterol levels tended to rise as chronologic age increased in subjects with TS (Figure; Table IIA; $p < 0.0003$). HDL and triglyceride levels were not related to age in the subjects with TS ($p = 0.12$, 0.14). In contrast, cholesterol in the normal control subjects did not show the same age-related changes ($r = -0.02$; $p = 0.87$; Figure). Multiple regression analysis was performed with age and diagnosis (TS vs normal) as the independent variables and cholesterol level as the dependent variable. The relation between cholesterol and age in the TS versus the control subjects was significantly different (regression coefficient [slope] ± SE [slope]: 3.2 ± 0.8 for age and 13.4 ± 4.8 for diagnosis; $p < 0.0002$ and $p < 0.006$, respectively).

We examined Pearson correlations among all anthropometric and lipid measurements for subjects with TS and control subjects separately. The subjects with TS had the following statistically significant ($p < 0.05$) correlations (Table IIA): Cholesterol levels were correlated with age, weight, BMI z score, LDL cholesterol, and triglyceride levels. HDL cholesterol levels were correlated with total cholesterol ($p < 0.04$) and triglyceride levels. Triglyceride levels correlated with weight, glucose level, insulin level, BMI z score, and total cholesterol. The LDL cholesterol level correlated with age, weight, BMI z score, and total cholesterol levels.

In contrast, control subjects had no significant correlations between serum lipids and age, height z score, weight, or BMI z score (Table IIB).

DISCUSSION

Adolescent girls with TS have significantly elevated cholesterol levels compared with normal values. This elevation may be explained, in part, by their increased HDL cholesterol levels. The elevation in total cholesterol persisted, even after adjustment for age. Girls with TS have increased obesity (as measured by BMI *z* score) compared with normal control subjects, but plasma lipids in the older girls with TS were elevated compared with normal subjects even when the groups were matched for BMI. Obesity in normal girls is associated with a decrease in HDL cholesterol.[9] Wilson et al.[10] reported normal lipid levels in TS without any significant correlation with age or body mass; additional measurement variation may have been present in these observations because the measurements were performed at 11 different centers.

There are several potential causes of these lipid abnormalities. Girls with TS have ovarian failure and therefore do not have significant ovarian estrogen production. Estrogen, in general, lowers lipid levels in girls and women. Normal girls have a drop in total and LDL cholesterol levels during adolescence[10]; HDL levels do not change to any significant extent.[11] Amenorrheic adolescent athletes have increased cholesterol, LDL cholesterol, and HDL cholesterol levels, compared with eumenorrheic athletes.[12] These increased levels are presumed to be secondary to the estrogen-deficient state. The LDL cholesterol levels are higher in the lower-estrogen, follicular phase of the menstrual cycle than in the luteal phase, and higher after menopause than before menopause.[13, 14]

Another major contributing factor to these lipid abnormalities in girls with TS may be their insulin resistance.[4] Hypercholesterolemia and relative hyperinsulinism have been found in adult subjects with type IIa hypercholesterolemia, even after control for age, gender, body mass, and glucose tolerance.[5]

Adolescent girls with TS appear to express two metabolic alterations at an early age: relatively increased lipid levels and insulin resistance. This association in girls lacking an X chromosome raises a question about genetic linkage of hypercholesterolemia and hyperinsulinemia. It is not clear whether insulin resistance influences the lipid profile, whether hyperlipidemia increases the insulin resistance, or whether another factor influences both derangements. Insulin stimulates cholesterol synthesis in vitro, and hyperinsulinism stimulates lipid synthesis in arterial walls of animal models.[15, 16] The contribution of these metabolic alterations to the incidence of cardiovascular disease in TS is not known. Future studies will examine the natural history of hyperlipidemia in TS, as well as the effects of estrogen replacement and growth hormone treatment.

REFERENCES

1. Forbes AP, Engel E. The high incidence of diabetes mellitus in 41 patients with gonadal dysgenesis and their close relatives. Metabolism 1963;12:420-36.
2. Nielsen J, Johansen K, Yale H. The frequency of diabetes mellitus in patients with Turner's syndrome and pure gonadal dysgenesis. Acta Endocrinol (Copenh) 1969;62:251-8.
3. Lippe BM. Primary ovarian failure. In: Kaplan SA, ed. Clinical pediatric endocrinology. Philadelphia: WB Saunders, 1990.
4. Caprio S, Boulware S, Diamond M, et al. Insulin resistance: an early metabolic defect of Turner's syndrome. J Clin Endocrinol Metab 1991;72:832-6.
5. Paolisso G, Ferrannini E, Sgambato S, Varricchio M, D'Onofrio F. Hyperinsulinemia in patients with hypercholesterolemia. J Clin Endocrinol Metab 1992;75:1409-12.
6. Marshall WA, Tanner JM. Variations in patterns of pubertal changes in girls. Arch Dis Child 1969;44:291-303.
7. Friedewald WT, Levy RI, Fredrickson DS. Estimation of the concentration of LDL cholesterol in plasma. Clin Chem 1972; 18:499-502.
8. Hammer LD, Kraemer HC, Wilson DM, Ritter PL, Dornbusch SM. Standardized percentile curves for body-mass index for children and adolescents, AJDC 1991;145:259-63.
9. Freedman DS, Srinivasan SR, Harsha DW, et al. Relation of body fat patterning to lipid and lipoprotein concentration in children and adolescents: the Bogalusa Heart Study. Am J Clin Nutr 1989;50:930-9.
10. Wilson DM, Frane JW, Sherman B, Johanson AJ, Hintz RL, Rosenfeld RG. Carbohydrate and lipid metabolism in Turner syndrome: effect of therapy with growth hormone, oxandrolone, and a combination of both. J PEDIATR 1988;112:210-7.
11. Kwiterovich PO Jr. Plasma lipid and lipoprotein levels in childhood. Annals of the NY Academy of Sciences 1991;623: 90-119.
12. Friday KE, Drinkwater BL, Bruemmer B, Chesnut C, Chait A. Elevated plasma low-density lipoprotein and high-density lipoprotein cholesterol level in amenorrheic athletes: effects of endogenous hormone status and nutrient intake. J Clin Endocrinol Metab 1993;77:1605-9.
13. Kim HJ, Kalkhoff RK. Changes in lipoprotein composition during the menstrual cycle. Metabolism 1979;28:663-8.
14. Walsh BW, Schiff I, Rosner B, Greenberg L, Ravnikar V, Sacks FM. Effects of postmenopausal estrogen replacement on the concentrations and metabolism of plasma lipoproteins. N Engl J Med 1991;325:1196-204.
15. Chait A, Bierman EL, Albers JJ. Low-density lipoprotein receptor activity in cultured human skin fibroblasts: mechanisms of insulin-induced stimulation. J Clin Invest 1979;64:1309-19.
16. Stout RW. The effect of insulin and glucose on sterol synthesis in cultured rat arterial smooth muscle cells. Atherosclerosis 1977;27:271-8.

Lysinuric protein intolerance characterized by bone marrow abnormalities and severe clinical course

Giancarlo Parenti, MD, Gianfranco Sebastio, MD, Pietro Strisciuglio, MD, Barbara Incerti, MD, Carmine Pecoraro, MD, Luigi Terracciano, MD, and Generoso Andria, MD

From the Departments of Pediatrics and Pathology, Federico II University, Naples, and the Department of Pediatrics, University of Reggio Calabria, Catanzaro, Italy

***Study objective*: To evaluate phenotypic variability of lysinuric protein intolerance in a cohort of nine Italian patients.**
***Design*: Retrospective analysis of patient records.**
***Subjects*: Nine Italian patients (seven independent families), all originating from southern Italy, observed during the last 14 years.**
***Results*: Some of the patients had unique clinical features, including bone marrow abnormalities featuring erythroblastophagocytosis (five patients) and acute pancreatitis (two patients). Severe complications, known to affect the clinical course and the outcome of the disease, have also been observed: respiratory involvement was present in five cases, with a lethal picture of "alveolar proteinosis" in one. Severe kidney involvement, with both glomerular and tubular damage and rapidly progressing to chronic renal failure, has been observed in one case.**
***Conclusion*: Lysinuric protein intolerance may cause severe multisystem involvement, which requires early and careful monitoring. Some peculiar clinical findings observed in Italian patients point to a genetic heterogeneity of lysinuric protein intolerance. (J Pediatr 1995;126:246-51)**

Lysinuric protein intolerance is an inborn error of metabolism because of a defective transport of cationic amino acids at the basolateral membrane of enterocytes, renal tubular cells, hepatocytes, and fibroblasts.[1, 2] The most likely basic defect involves the carrier system called "y^+," a system that is Na^+ independent, trans-stimulated, saturable, and stereospecific.[3] The reduced intestinal absorption and the increased renal clearance of cationic amino acids lead to a depletion of their pools and, as a consequence, to impaired functioning of the urea cycle with hyperammonemic crises. Most of the symptoms of LPI appear related to the metabolic derangement and include aversion to protein-rich foods, gastrointestinal symptoms, osteoporosis, failure to thrive, and episodes of stupor and coma. The disease has been considered relatively benign when appropriately treated with citrulline supplementation and a low-protein diet. During the past few years, however, other manifestations have been reported, and they have suggested multisystem involvement and raised some concern about the final outcome of the disease in these patients.[4-7]

LPI	Lysinuric protein intolerance

Here we describe the clinical findings observed in nine patients, referred to us during the past 14 years, and focus on their unusual manifestations, some of which have been observed only in Italian patients.

Supported in part by Ministero della Sanità, "Progetto Gaslini Nord e Sud—Malattie genetiche—1991," Rome, Italy, and in part by Telethon Italy (grant No. E.09).

Submitted for publication May 18, 1994; accepted Aug. 26, 1994.

Reprint requests: Generoso Andria, MD, Department of Pediatrics, Federico II University, Via S. Pansini 5, 80131 Naples, Italy.

0022-3476/95/$3.00 + 0 **9/20/60161**

Table. Clinical data on the Italian patients affected by LPI

	Patient No.									
	1	2	3	4	5	6	7	8	9	Total
Sex	M	M	M	M	F	M	F	M	M	7M/2F
Region of origin	Campania	Campania	Campania	Campania	Campania	Campania	Campania	Calabria	Calabria	
Parental consanguinity	+	+	–	–	–	–	+	–	+	
Age at onset	2 yr	6 mo	6 mo	*	9 mo	4 mo	10 mo	3 mo	Neonatal	
Age at diagnosis	6½ yr	†	4 yr	1 mo	14 yr	9 mo	15 mo	9 yr	9 mo	
Outcome	Alive	Dead	Dead	Alive	Alive	Alive	Alive	Dead	Alive	
Age at last observation or age of death	24 yr	6½ yr	10½ yr	7 yr 8 mo	25 yr	11 yr 9 mo	8 yr 10 mo	11 yr	6 yr 10 mo	
Presentation										
Visceromegaly	+	+	+	+	+	+	+	+	+	9/9
Vomiting and GI symptoms	+	+	+	–	+	+	+	–	–	6/9
Failure to thrive	+	+	+	–	+	–	+	+	–	6/9
Protein aversion	+	+	+	–	+	+	+	+	–	7/9
Lethargy and coma	+	+	+	–	–	–	–	+	–	4/9
Osteoporosis	+	–	–	–	+	–	–	–	–	2/9
Joint laxity	+	+	–	–	–	–	–	–	–	2/9
Hyperammonemia	+	np	+	–	–	–	–	+	–	3/8
Bone marrow abnormalities	+	+	–	np	+	+	+	np	np	5/6
Pancreatitis/recurrent abdominal pain	+	–	–	–	+	–	+	–	–	3/9
Lung involvement										
Abnormal standard x-ray film	+	np	np	+	+	+	+	+	–	6/7
Abnormal CT scan	+	np	np	np	+	–	–	+	–	3/6
Abnormal histologic findings	np	np	np	np	np	np	np	+	np	1/1
Kidney involvement										
Proteinuria	–	np	–	+	+	+	+	–	–	4/8
Tubular dysfunction	–	np	–	–	+	–	–	–	–	1/8
Glomerular dysfunction	–	np	–	–	+	–	–	–	–	1/8
Abnormal histologic findings	np	np	np	np	+	np	np	np	np	1/1
Psychomotor delay	–	–	–	–	–	–	–	+ (IQ 61)	–	1/9
Seizures	–	–	–	–	–	–	–	+	–	1/9

GI, Gastrointestinal; *np*, not performed; *CT*, computed tomography.
*Younger brother of patient 3. Diagnosis established in the first month of life, before the onset of symptoms.
†Elder brother of patient 1; presumptive diagnosis made posthumously on the basis of his clinical and family history.

CASE REPORTS

All nine patients (Table), from seven families, were born in two regions of southern Italy, Campania (seven) or Calabria (two). In all families the patients' parents originated from the same geographic area; consanguinity was confirmed in three families. In two families remote consanguinity can be supposed because of the presence of common last names in the maternal and paternal ancestries. The diagnosis of LPI relied on both clinical and biochemical criteria. In all patients, biochemical confirmation of the diagnosis was based on the presence of at least three of the following findings: low plasma levels of cationic amino acids; increased urinary clearance of cationic amino acids; increased oroticaciduria; hyperammonemia and oroticaciduria after protein loading tests (1 gm/kg), prevented by oral administration of citrulline; and reduced intestinal absorption of cationic amino acids after an oral loading test.[8] Results of routine biochemical tests were in all cases consistent with those observed in patients with LPI, including elevated plasma levels of lactate dehydrogenase, thyroxine, and ferritin.

Clinical onset of the disease occurred at ages ranging from 3 months to 2 years; the age at diagnosis ranged from 1 month to 14 years. All patients, except patient 2, have been treated with a low-protein diet and oral citrulline supplementation. Patients 1, 3, 5, and 6 were initially treated with arginine, which was later replaced by citrulline. Six patients are presently alive (age range, 7½ to 25 years); three died at the ages of 6½, 10, and 11 years.

The main features observed in our patients are summarized in the Table. Two patients (Nos. 5 and 8) showing some peculiarities are described in detail.

Patient 5. The patient[9] was breast-fed until 12 months of age, when failure to thrive and aversion to protein-rich foods became

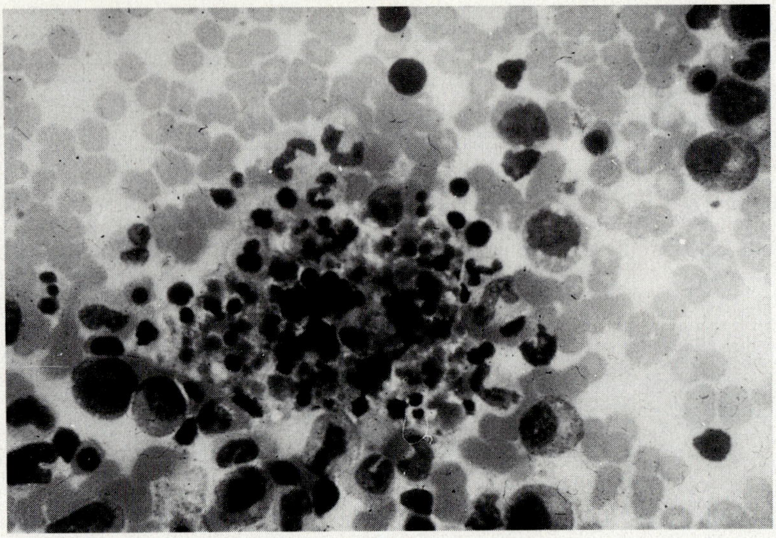

Fig. 1. May-Grünwald-Giemsa staining of bone marrow smear from patient 5, showing erythroblastophagocytosis.

evident. She was referred to our hospital at the age of 7 years because of visceromegaly, short stature, and malar flush. Other remarkable findings included reticulonodular infiltration on chest roentgenograms, and kidney dysfunction with proximal tubular disease and reduced glomerular filtration rate. A bone marrow smear showed cells resembling "sea-blue histiocytes." A diagnosis of Niemann-Pick disease type B was initially proposed; however, several lysosomal hydrolase activities (including sphingomyelinase), assayed in her leukocytes and fibroblasts, were in the normal range. LPI was considered because of the reported aversion to protein-rich food, her origin from the same geographic area as patients 1 to 4, and poor correlation between a high plasma creatinine concentration and a relatively low blood urea nitrogen level. The diagnosis, hampered by the presence of generalized aminoaciduria, was definitely confirmed by abnormal results on arginine and lysine oral loading tests, whereas intestinal absorption of citrulline was normal. Therapy was started at that time. A reevaluation of the bone marrow smear revealed erythroblastophagocytosis (Fig. 1), as in patients 1 and 2.

The patient's follow-up was marked by clinical and biochemical signs of progressive nephropathy, leading to both glomerular and proximal tubular damage. Her glomerular filtration rate decreased to 6.5 ml/min per 1.73 m^2 body surface area, with a parallel increase of creatininemia to 710 μmol/L (8 mg/dl); the blood urea nitrogen level was 35.5 mmol/L (100 mg/dl). Findings consistent with a complex proximal tubular disease (Fanconi syndrome) were also present, with glycosuria, generalized hyperaminoaciduria, reduced tubular reabsorption of phosphate (as corrected for glomerular filtration rate), biochemical signs of rickets, and progressive bone deformities at the lower limbs. Renal histologic examination showed both normal and sclerosed glomeruli; hypertrophy and lipid inclusions were observed in the endothelial cells on electron microscopy (Fig. 2). The patient's subsequent clinical history was characterized by frequent episodes of abdominal pain. At the age of 15 years, she had intestinal obstruction. Laparatomy showed diffuse infiltration of the intestinal wall and omentum by an undefined storage material; liponecrosis was observed; the pancreas and kidneys were firm and reduced in size. When the patient was 25 years of age, a high-resolution computed tomography scan of the lung showed interstitial involvement. She is presently a short woman with bone deformities of the lower limbs and chronic renal failure.

Patient 8. The patient was seen during the first few months of life with failure to thrive, anorexia, vomiting, mild visceromegaly, and hypotonia. Later he had recurrent generalized seizures, mostly occurring after meals, and an episode of coma. Several admissions to various hospitals did not lead to a definitive diagnosis. At 4 years of age, a myopathy was suspected because of mild psychomotor retardation and increased levels of lactate dehydrogenase (2800 U/L) and creatine kinase (280 U/L); however, electrophysiologic studies were inconclusive. In two instances, urinary organic acids showed increased excretion of α-ketoglutarate by gas chromatography–mass spectrometry.

The patient was first admitted to our hospital at the age of 6 years 10 months because of short stature and aversion to protein-rich foods. At that time, mental retardation, impairment of learning abilities, and dyspraxia were observed. The diagnosis of LPI was made and therapy was started.

At the age of 10 years the patient had partial seizures that were treated with carbamazepine and clobazam. Electroencephalography did not show evidence of focal activity. Magnetic resonance imaging of the brain suggested possible anoxic damage. At that time a chest x-ray study showed moderate reticulonodular opacities.

At the age of 11 years, during an intercurrent respiratory illness with mild fever and cough, the patient had progressive dyspnea and arterial oxygen desaturation. Massive perihilar densities, detected by standard chest roentgenograms and computed tomography scan, were evident within the diffuse reticulonodular pattern. Despite corticosteroid, antibiotic, and oxygen therapy, his condition pro-

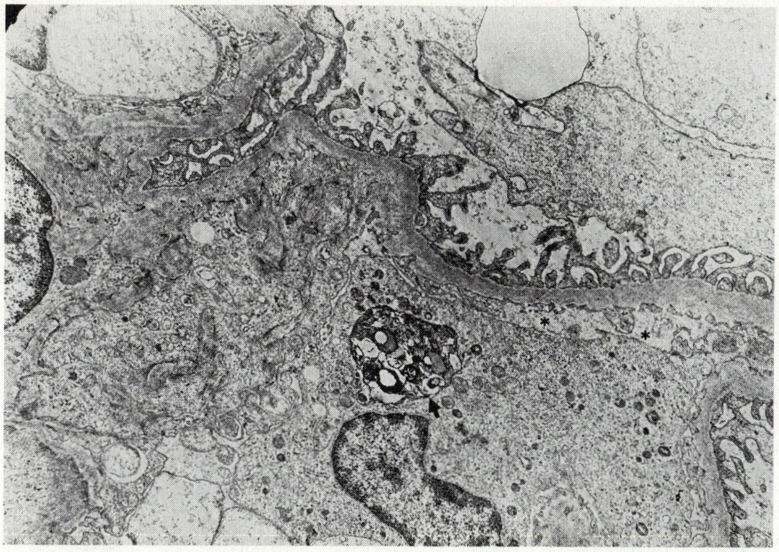

Fig. 2. Electron microscopy of a renal biopsy specimen from patient 5, showing hypertrophy of endothelial cells, with a cytoplasmic lipid inclusion *(arrow)*, and thickening of the basal membrane with subendothelial deposition of electron-lucent material *(asterisks)*. (Courtesy Dr. L. Torri Tonelli, Institute of Anatomy, University of Milan, Italy.)

gressively worsened and he died 2 months later. Light microscopic examination of a lung biopsy specimen showed findings consistent with "alveolar proteinosis," with total alveolar infiltration of amorphous material showing positive results on periodic acid–Schiff staining, cholesterol crystals, macrophages, and lymphocytes (Fig. 3, *A*). Electron microscopic examination of the lung specimen revealed the presence of amorphous material and multilamellar bodies within the alveolar space (Fig. 3, *B*).

DISCUSSION

Approximately half of the patients with LPI have been described in Finland, where the disease has a prevalence of about 1:60,000. LPI appears to be much more rare in other populations, where only sporadic cases have been found.[10] In Italy, however, a multicenter study has recently collected 17 cases, including those described here.[5] Three additional cases have recently been referred to our attention (Magazzù G, Dionisi Vici C, Rizzoni G: personal communication, 1994). All subjects came from southern Italy; a cluster of patients with LPI have been found in a small area around Naples, where we have diagnosed seven cases. Italian patients have some unique features, namely bone marrow abnormalities and pancreatic involvement, which suggests the existence of genetic heterogeneity of LPI in different ethnic groups.

Bone marrow abnormalities are one of the peculiar findings in the Italian patients. In an earlier report[11] we described the occurrence of bone marrow abnormalities in two siblings affected by LPI. This finding was later confirmed among our patients (five of six examined). The most frequent feature is erythroblastophagocytosis; in one patient, findings resembling "sea-blue histiocytosis" were present. Similar findings have been documented in three other Italian patients[5] and in a Turkish patient,[12] but not in the few Finnish patients whose bone marrow has been examined.[10]

Bone marrow abnormalities have been responsible for initial misdiagnoses, as outlined in the Italian multicenter study.[5] In most instances the initial diagnosis, a lysosomal storage disease, was based on the association of the bone marrow findings with hepatosplenomegaly and interstitial pneumopathy.

The reason for the occurrence of symptoms reminiscent of a lysosomal storage disease is not clear. The observation of intracellular lipid droplets or granulations and, occasionally, fatty degeneration in liver biopsy specimens has been reported, and nonspecific lysosomal damage caused by the possible expression of the basic defect of LPI at the lysosomal membrane has been proposed.[10] However, the genetic control of the known carriers for cationic amino acids at the lysosomal membrane differs from that of the y^+ system, which is likely involved in LPI.[13]

Two of our patients were seen during the second decade of life with clinical signs of pancreatitis and increased amylase levels. In one patient, surgical treatment was required; in this patient both pancreatic fibrosis, suggesting chronic involvement, and liponecrosis, pointing to acute damage, were detected at laparoscopy. Pancreatitis has been re-

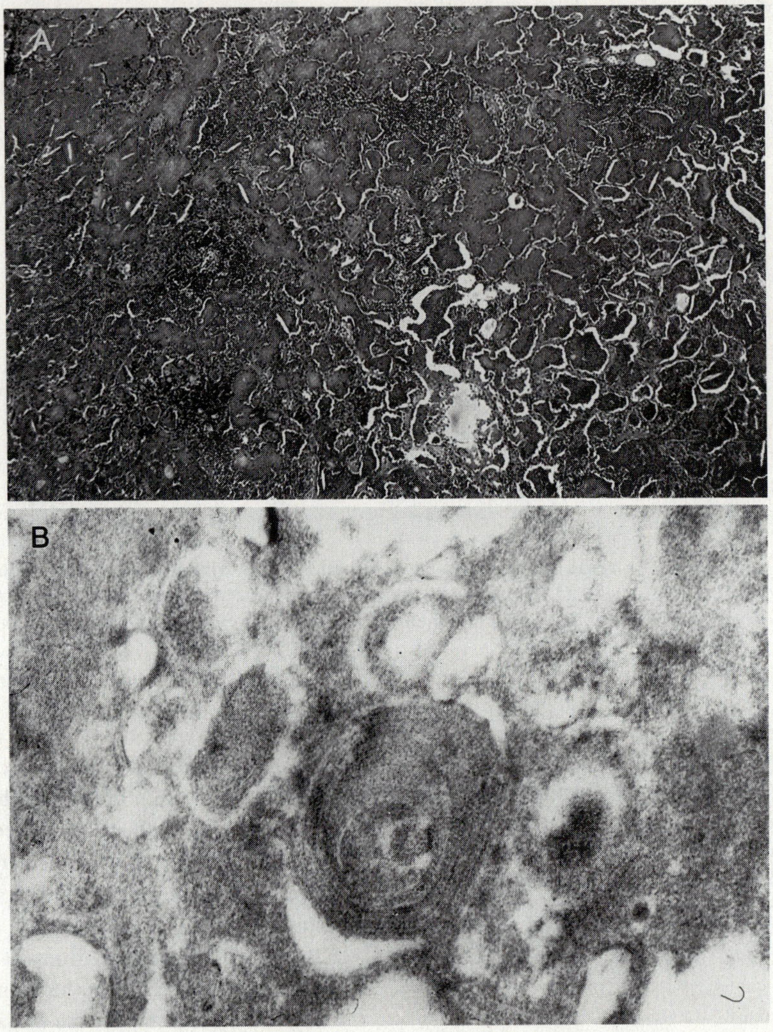

Fig. 3. Light microscopy (A) of a lung biopsy specimen from patient 8, showing interstitial infiltration and alveolar spaces completely filled with amorphous material. This material showed positive staining (not shown) by periodic acid–Schiff reagent. Electron microscopy (**B**) showing multilamellar bodies within the alveolar space.

ported in association with other metabolic disorders and may represent a nonspecific finding in LPI. To our knowledge, there is only a single autopsy report of pancreatic involvement in LPI, characterized by duct obstruction by material showing positive staining by periodic acid–Schiff reagent.[7] It should be clarified whether episodes of abdominal pain, as observed in our patient 7, are due to chronic pancreatitis or result from intestinal cationic amino acid malabsorption.

Respiratory involvement is the most threatening complication of LPI. Severe lung disease has been described in six Finnish patients[14] (four children with a lethal course and two affected by "adult respiratory distress syndrome"), in three Italian patients,[4] and in single Saudi Arabian,[6] Japanese, Moroccan, and North American patients.[10] In our cohort the clinical expression of this complication ranged from clinically silent roentgenographic abnormalities to alveolar proteinosis that progressed rapidly to death. Alveolar proteinosis, a heterogeneous entity associated with different disorders, should be considered a typical end stage of lung disease in LPI.

Little is known about the events promoting lung disease in LPI. Hallman et al.[15] demonstrated a higher concentration of cationic amino acids in bronchoalveolar lavage fluid from two patients, suggesting that the basic defect of LPI is expressed in the lung and may play a role in initiating lung damage. However, the Hallman data have not been confirmed in subsequent studies.[4] The onset and clinical course of the respiratory complication seem to be poorly influenced by therapy with citrulline. Age appears critical; patients at the end of their first decade have the worst prognosis.[14]

Chronic renal failure is another potentially life-threatening complication of LPI.[4, 7] The basic defect affects the basolateral membrane of different cells, including renal tubular cells. The clinical findings in our patient 5, however, are not explained by the biochemical defect of the disease. She had signs of both glomerular and tubular involvement, an association recorded only in another Italian patient.[4] Mild proteinuria, observed in four of our nine patients, may represent an initial sign of renal disease and should be carefully monitored. Tubular dysfunction with generalized aminoaciduria, masking the presence of cationic aminoaciduria, can be particularly misleading during the initial diagnostic evaluation.

We conclude that LPI is an intriguing disease with multisystem involvement. Further investigations are needed to understand the mechanisms involved in the damage to lung, kidney, bone marrow, and possibly pancreas. The identification of the molecular defect of LPI will help to clarify the genetic basis for the clinical variability.

We thank Dr. R. Sartorio, Dr. M. Ghezzi and Dr. D. Sperli, who have been involved in the follow-up of patients and Prof. C. Borrone for referring to us patient 9; Dr. F. Santamaria, Prof. M. Sofia, and Dr. P. Carratù for their help in the respiratory assessment of patient 8.

REFERENCES

1. Rajantie J, Simell O, Perheentupa J. Basolateral membrane transport defect for lysine in lysinuric protein intolerance. Lancet 1980;1:1219-21.
2. Smith DW, Scriver CR, Tenenhouse HS, Simell O. Lysinuric protein intolerance mutation is expressed in the plasma membrane of cultured skin fibroblasts. Proc Natl Acad Sci USA 1987;84:7711-5.
3. White MF, Christensen HN. The two-way flux of cationic amino acids across the plasma membrane of mammalian cells is largely explainable by a single transport system. J Biol Chem 1982;257:10069-80.
4. Di Rocco M, Garibotto G, Rossi GA, et al. Role of haematological, pulmonary and renal complications in the long-term prognosis of patients with lysinuric protein intolerance. Eur J Pediatr 1993;152:437-40.
5. Incerti B, Andria G, Parenti G, et al. Lysinuric protein intolerance: studies on 17 Italian patients. Am J Hum Genet 1993; 53(suppl):908A.
6. Kerem E, Elpeg ON, Shalev RS, Rosenman E, Bar Ziv Y, Branski D. Lysinuric protein intolerance with chronic interstitial lung disease and pulmonary cholesterol granulomas at onset. J PEDIATR 1993;123:275-8.
7. Parto K, Kallajoki M, Aho H, Simell O. Pulmonary alveolar proteinosis and glomerulonephritis in lysinuric protein intolerance: case reports and autopsy finding of four pediatric patients. Hum Pathol 1994;25:400-7.
8. Andria G, Sebastio G, Sartorio R, Sannolo N. Arginine supplementation in lysinuric protein intolerance. J Inher Metab Dis 1982;5(suppl 1):61-2.
9. Andria G, Sebastio G, Parenti G, et al. Un caso di intolleranza alle proteine con lisinuria con presentazione ed anomalie ematologiche insolite. Ital J Pediatr 1982;8:634A.
10. Simell O. Lysinuric protein intolerance and other cationic aminoacidurias. In: Scriver CR, Beaudet AL, Sly WS, Valle D, eds. The metabolic basis of inherited disease. New York: McGraw-Hill, 1989:2497-513.
11. Andria G, Sebastio G, Strisciuglio P, Del Giudice E. Lysinuric protein intolerance: possible genetic heterogeneity? J Inher Metab Dis 1981;4:151-2.
12. Behbehani AW, Gahr M, Schroter W. Lysinuric protein intolerance. Monatsschr Kinderheilkd 1983;131:784-7.
13. Pisoni RL, Thoene JG, Lemons M, Christensen HN. Important differences in cationic amino acid transport by lysosomal system c and system y+ of the human fibroblast. J Biol Chem 1987;262:15011-8.
14. Parto K, Svedstrom E, Majurin ML, Harkonen R, Simell O. Pulmonary manifestations in lysinuric protein intolerance. Chest 1993;104:1176-82.
15. Hallman M, Maasilta P, Sipila I, Tahvanainen J. Composition and function of pulmonary surfactant in adult respiratory distress syndrome. Eur Respir J 1989;2(suppl 3):104-8.

Long-term reduction in bone mass after severe burn injury in children

Gordon L. Klein, MD, David N. Herndon, MD, Craig B. Langman, MD, Thomas C. Rutan, MSN, William E. Young, MS, Gregory Pembleton, CNMT, Martin Nusynowitz, MD, Joseph L. Barnett, BSN, Lyle D. Broemeling, PhD, Dawn E. Sailer, MS, and Robert L. McCauley, MD

From the Departments of Pediatrics, Surgery, and Nuclear Medicine, University of Texas Medical Branch and Shriners Burns Institute, Galveston, and the Division of Nephrology Mineral Metabolism Laboratory, Children's Memorial Hospital and Northwestern University Medical School, Chicago, Illinois

Objective: **Because burn victims are at risk of having bone loss, a cross-sectional study was undertaken to determine whether severe burn injury had acute and long-term effects on bone mass or on the incidence of fractures in children.**
Methods: **Dual-energy x-ray absorptiometry of the lumbar portion of the spine was performed on 68 children: 16 moderately burned (15% to 36% of total body surface area) and 52 age-matched severely burned (≥40% of total body surface area). Twenty-two severely burned children were hospitalized and studied within 8 weeks of their burn, and 30 others were studied approximately 5 years after discharge. In the severely burned group, both hospitalized and discharged, serum and urine were analyzed for calcium, phosphorus, intact parathyroid hormone, osteocalcin, and type I collagen telopeptide.**
Results: **Sixty percent of severely burned patients had age-related *z* scores for bone density less than −1, and 27% of severely burned patients had age-related *z* scores for bone density less than −2 (p <0.005, for each). In the moderately burned group, 31% of patients had *z* scores less than −1 (p <0.005 vs normal distribution), but only 6% had *z* scores less than −2 (p value not significant). There was evidence of increased incidence of fractures after discharge in the severely burned patients. Biochemical studies were compatible with a reduction in bone formation and an increase in resorption initially, and with a long-term persistence of low formation.**
Conclusion: **We conclude that acute burn injury leads to profound and long-term bone loss, which may adversely affect peak bone mass accumulation. (J PEDIATR 1995;126:252-6)**

Supported in part by a grant from the Shriners Hospitals for Crippled Children (SHCC 15877) (Dr. Klein) and an unrestricted grant from the Otto Sprague Memorial Fund, and in part by the General Clinical Research Center (grant RR00048), National Institutes of Health (Dr. Langman).

Presented in part at the Third Sino-American Conference on Burns and Trauma, Canton, China, Aug. 16 to 19, 1993, and at the Fifteenth Annual Meeting of the American Society for Bone and Mineral Research, Tampa, Fla., Sept. 18 to 22, 1993.

Submitted for publication April 8, 1994; accepted Aug. 18,1994.

Reprint requests: Gordon L. Klein, MD, Pediatric Gastroenterology Division, Children's Hospital, Rm C353, University of Texas Medical Branch, Galveston, TX 77555-0352.

0022-3476/95/$3.00 + 0 **9/20/62556**

The long-term effects of major thermal injuries on growth and development of children are now receiving significant attention. Rutan and Herndon[1] reported significant growth delays in children for up to 3 years after survival from thermal injury, and permanent stunting of linear growth. However, little attention has been directed to the effects of such injury on bone metabolism.

Recently we identified the acute onset of alterations in bone turnover associated with burn injury in young adults. As demonstrated by bone biopsy, this abnormality consisted of a marked reduction in bone formation combined with a decreased area of unmineralized osteoid; changes in bone resorption were inconsistent.[2] The disproportionate reduction in bone formation suggests that burned patients are at risk of having bone mineral loss within the first 2 months after burn injury. The pathogenesis of the lesion may include such factors as immobilization,[2] increased endogenous production of corticosteroids,[2] aluminum loading,[2] and the production of bone resorptive cytokines such as interleukin-1[3] and interleukin-6.[4,5]

TBSA	Total body surface area

Despite the early presence of this burn-associated bone abnormality, neither its duration nor its clinical significance is known. Therefore our present study was designed to determine whether a deficit in bone mass persisted after recuperation from burn injury, and whether the reduction in bone mass was associated with an increase in fractures in this population.

METHODS

Patients. We studied 68 children and adolescents recruited from the inpatient acute care unit or the reconstructive surgery clinic at the Shriners Burns Institute, Galveston, Tex., from November 1992 through April 1994. The patients were divided initially into two groups on the basis of the severity of thermal injury.[6,7] Burns in patients with less than 40% of their total body surface area burned were classified as moderate (range, 15% to 36%; n = 16), and burns in those with burns >40% of TBSA were classified as severe (range, 40% to 100%; n = 52). Clinical features of all patients are shown in Table I.

The Shriners Burns Institute, Galveston Unit, is a referral hospital whose patients come from the southwestern United States. The ethnic backgrounds of the study patients were 60% white, 30% Hispanic, and 10% black.

Severely burned patients were subdivided by inpatient or outpatient status. The inpatients (n = 22) were studied during their hospitalization, which usually was during the first 8 weeks after the burn; the outpatients (n = 30) were studied after discharge when they returned to the reconstructive surgery clinic (Table I). We matched sequentially, during a 17-month period, the ages and percentage TBSA burn of the discharged patients to those of the hospitalized patients (12.4 ± 4.2 years vs 11.1 ± 3.5 years [mean ± SD], respectively).

Nutritional support of hospitalized patients consisted of a daily nasogastric infusion of milk, usually beginning in the first 24 hours, to achieve between 1500 and 1800 kcal/m^2 body surface area plus an additional 1500 to 2000 kcal/m^2 surface area burned.[6] The milk provided 1.8 mg of elemental calcium per kilocalorie delivered; thus hospitalized patients received a calculated minimum of 2.7 gm of elemental calcium per square meter daily during the acute burn period. All discharged patients were eating regular diets and pursued unrestricted activities; many participated electively in competitive sports.

Procedures. Patients in each group underwent measurements of bone mass of the lumbar vertebrae (L1 to L4) by dual-energy x-ray absorptiometry with the QDR 1000W absorptiometer (Hologic Inc., Waltham, Mass.). During the period of the study, the coefficient of variation of the spine phantom in repeated measurements was 0.31%. The bone mass measurements were transformed into *z* scores, with the use of data on 219 children and adolescents studied by Southard et al.[8]

Heights and weights were determined in all discharged patients at the time of their bone mass measurements. Heights in the hospitalized patients were obtained at admission, and weights were obtained at the time of bone mass measurement.

From the 22 hospitalized patients, we obtained 24-hour urine collections for the determination of calcium and phosphate concentrations (n = 12), and blood for determination of serum levels of total calcium, phosphorus, intact parathyroid hormone (n = 22), and serum osteocalcin and type I collagen telopeptide (n = 21). From 12 of the 30 discharged severely burned patients, we obtained blood for serum levels of intact parathyroid hormone, osteocalcin, and type I collagen telopeptide. Calcium and phosphorus were analyzed colorimetrically on an Ektachrome 700 analyzer (Eastman Kodak Co., Rochester, N.Y.). Serum intact parathyroid hormone,[9] osteocalcin,[10] and type I collagen telopeptide[11] were measured as previously described.

Additionally, the moderately burned and severely burned patients discharged from the hospital, and their parents, were asked whether the patients had had fractures after release from the initial hospitalization for burn, the location of such fractures, and the circumstances under which the fractures occurred.

This study was approved by the institutional review board of the University of Texas Medical Branch, and the form for informed consent was reviewed and approved by the Shriners Hospitals for Crippled Children, Tampa, Fla.

RESULTS

In our study, the age at which the discharged patients acquired their burn did not differ in the moderately and the severely burned groups (Table I). However, the hospitalized severely burned patients were significantly older at injury ($p < 0.002$). All patients were of comparable age when studied (Table I). Moderately burned patients underwent bone mass determination a mean (±SD) of 5.8 ± 4.4 years (range, 0.3 to 16.2 years) after the injury; discharged, severely burned patients underwent bone mass determination 5.5 ± 3.7 years (range, 0.4 to 13 years) after the injury. Hospitalized severely burned patients underwent bone mass determination 37 ± 14 days (range, 18 to 59 days) after the burn. The heights and weights of the three groups were not significantly different.

The percentage of patients with moderate burns (31%; 5/16) and the percentage of those with severe burns (60%; 31/52) who had a *z* score for bone mass ≤ -1 were increased ($p < 0.005$) (Figure). In the severely burned group, 27% (14/52) of the patients had a bone mass *z* score ≤ -2, which differed significantly from the normal distribution ($p < 0.005$).

Table I. Patient characteristics

	Patients (No.)		Age at burn (yr)		Age at study (yr)		Weight* (% ile for age)		Height† (% ile for age)	
	M	F	M	F	M	F	M	F	M	F
Moderate burn (<40%)										
Discharged	9	7	5.4 (±4.0)	4.8 (±3.7)	11.1 (±4.2)	10.5 (±4.4)	60 (±31)	66 (±20)	46 (±34)	53 (±31)
Severe burn (>40%)										
Hospitalized	14	8	11.4‡ (±3.4)	10.8‡ (±4.1)	11.4 (±3.4)	10.8 (±4.1)	64 (±29)	76 (±29)	52 (±35)	62 (±34)
Discharged	15	15	6.9 (±5.4)	7.1 (±4.7)	12.9 (±4.8)	12.0 (±4.4)	39 (±30)	47 (±33)	32 (±22)	39 (±29)

All values except number of patients are given as mean (±SD).
*Obtained at the time of bone mass determination.
†Obtained at the time of bone mass determination in discharged patients and at the time of admission in hospitalized patients.
‡p <0.02 versus moderately burned and discharged severely burned groups.

Table II. Serum levels of osteocalcin and type I collagen telopeptide in severely burned hospitalized and discharged patients

	Hospitalized (n = 21)	Discharged (n = 12)
Osteocalcin (μg/L)		
Mean	3.1 ± 2.2*	6.3 ± 2.9
Range	0.5-7.6	0.8-12.3
Normal (for age)		
<12 yr	10-25	
>12 yr	2-8	
Type I collagen telopeptide (μg/L)		
Mean	82.2 ± 43.1	18.4 ± 9.0†
Range	23.9-186.5	9.7-44.1
Normal (all ages)	<30	

*Mean ± SD.
†$p < 0.05$ compared with hospitalized patients.

We performed linear regression analysis on the bone mass z score as a function of the percentage of TBSA burned and determined that when the moderate and severe groups were combined, there was a weak but significant correlation ($r = -0.3$; $p = 0.001$). We did not find a relation between the time after burn injury and the bone mass z score.

There had been no fractures in the moderate burn group. Ten patients (3 girls, 7 boys) in the discharged severe burn group had had fractures; 8 fractures were appendicular (of a limb or digit) and 2 were axial (1 of the hip, 1 of the ribs). All but one of the fractures were from trauma incurred as a result of age-appropriate physical activity; one ankle fracture was pathologic. The extrapolated fracture incidence in the discharged severely burned group was 76.3/1000 boys per year and 40.8/1000 girls per year. Incidence of fracture for age-matched healthy children are 41 to 43/1000 boys per year and 27 to 30/1000 girls per year,[12, 13] which suggests that the incidence of fractures in this severely burned group may be higher than normal, although the number of patients was too small to perform statistical analysis in comparison with the large population studies on which the normative data are based.

Hospitalized severely burned patients (n = 12) had daily urinary calcium excretion of 50.4 ± 30.4 mmol (202 ± 122 mg) (range, 11.4 to 118.3 mmol [46 to 474 mg]) or, expressed on a body mass basis, 1.22 ± 0.81 mmol/kg (4.89 ± 3.24 mg/kg) (range, 0.19 to 2.77 mmol/kg [0.77 to 11.10 mg/kg]).[14] However, the extent of the hypercalciuria correlated neither with bone mass z scores ($r = -0.2$) nor with the percentage of TBSA burned ($r = 0.42$). Daily urinary phosphate excretion ranged from 3.2 to 77.5 mmol (0.1 to 2.4 gm).

Serum total calcium concentrations in the hospitalized, severely burned group were low on admission (range, 1.8 to 2.1 mmol [7.2 to 8.6 mg/dl]), and rose to the normal range (2.1 to 2.4 mmol [8.5 to 9.6 mg/dl]), by 1 week later. Serum phosphorus and intact parathyroid hormone concentrations remained normal throughout the burn period. Serum osteocalcin concentrations were low for age in 86% (18/21) of the patients, and type I collagen telopeptide concentrations were elevated in 90% (19/21) of the patients (Table II).

In the discharged severely burned group, serum osteocalcin levels were reduced for age in 50% (6/12) and normal in the others. Serum type I collagen telopeptide concentrations were normal in 92% (11/12) of the patients. Serum intact parathyroid hormone concentrations were normal in all 12 patients.

DISCUSSION

Our study demonstrates that in children who sustain a severe thermal burn injury, acute loss of bone mass occurs and is maintained. The pathogenesis remains incompletely understood, but our study has added the information that bone formation, as assessed indirectly by serum osteocalcin levels, may be reduced from normal, and bone resorption as assessed indirectly by serum type I collagen telopeptide and urinary calcium excretion may be increased. This disorder of bone homeostasis may increase the susceptibility of burned children to appendicular or axial fractures long after the acute thermal injury. Our

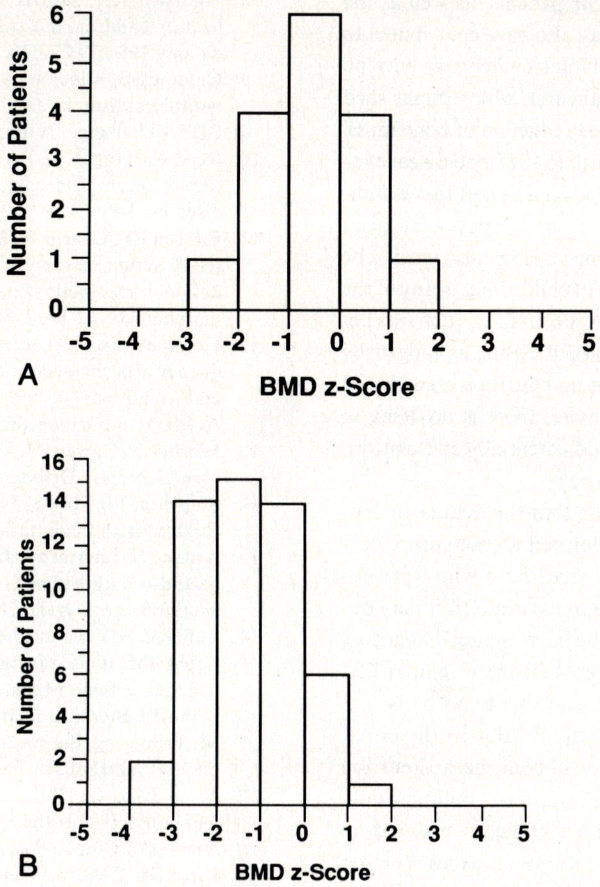

Figure. A, Distribution of bone mineral density *(BMD) z* scores in relation to number of patients in the moderately burned group. **B,** Distribution of bone mass *(BMD) z* scores in relation to number of patients in the severely burned group.

data on bone turnover are consistent with previously published findings in adults with comparable thermal injury.[2]

A variety of factors may contribute to the acute bone loss detected in our patients, although roles played by these factors have not been investigated in depth. Immobilization after burn injury may contribute to an acute reduction in bone formation and a reduction in bone mass. Thus Arnaud et al.[15] found a reduction in bone formation in normal young adults at bed rest for only a week, and LeBlanc et al.[16] reported that young adults at bed rest for 17 weeks lost up to 10% of their bone mass. Because of the necessity of confining a patient to bed after severe burn injury, it is not possible to determine whether reduced bone formation can occur in patients in the absence of immobilization.

Increased production of endogenous corticosteroids may contribute to reduced bone formation,[17] although the rapidity and the extent to which they may do so are currently unknown. Corticosteroids may also contribute to increased bone resorption by decreasing intestinal calcium absorption and thus producing secondary hyperparathyroidism,[17] a finding that we did not observe in our patients. Moreover, corticosteroids may increase bone resorption by stimulating production of bone-resorbing cytokines, such as interleukin-6.[18]

Aluminum loading is another well-described cause of reduced bone formation[19] and has been reported to occur in thermal injury.[2] However, we found no evidence in our previous work[20] that aluminum-induced bone disease persists after withdrawal of aluminum-contaminated parenteral solutions, such as albumin or calcium gluconate.[21] Furthermore, neither the rapidity with which aluminum can reduce bone formation nor the quantity of aluminum needed to produce those changes is clear. Thus the reduction in bone formation in adults treated with total parenteral nutrition delivering an aluminum load of 60 μg/kg per day[22] occurred by approximately 8 weeks after initiation of total parenteral nutrition.[23] This quantity was about tenfold greater than that calculated to be received by adult burn patients.[2]

The origin of hypercalciuria in the acute postburn period in our patients is not clear. Hypercalciuria may simply be a manifestation of increased bone resorption as reflected in the elevated serum telopeptide levels. However, the large amounts of dietary protein[24-26] received by our patients, as well as the high intake of dietary calcium,[19] may also have contributed to the pathogenesis of hypercalciuria. Unfortunately, we have no data on the duration of the hypercalciuria, which might shed more light on its role in the sustained reduction of bone mass.

Other factors that may contribute to the bone disease include altered body biomechanics produced by soft tissue damage caused by the burn injury. The role of specific surgical techniques in contributing to the bone loss may also need to be investigated. There was no evidence of child abuse in any of the patients participating in the study. Acute malnutrition was not present in any of the severely burned patients, as judged by weight for age, so it is unlikely that malnutrition contributed significantly to bone loss. Furthermore, there is no delay in puberty in burned children that could potentially cause misinterpretation of the bone mass *z* score.[27]

Our cross-sectional data showing that the acute osteopenia is maintained indicates that children do not completely recover from the acute insult and that those who were entering the period of peak bone mass accumulation may develop lifelong osteoporosis. Thus the burn-induced bone loss may be a forerunner of early-onset osteoporosis in later life. A longitudinal study is needed to test this hypothesis.

Cross-sectional studies are of limited value in the provision of data on the rate and direction of bone mass alteration during acute thermal injury and long-term recuperation. However, we have demonstrated a significant problem in such patients with significant clinical consequences. Further studies will address intervention to prevent the acute bone loss, and longitudinal study of other patients with burn-associated osteoporosis will provide insights into the pathophysiologic mechanism.

REFERENCES

1. Rutan RL, Herndon DN. Growth delay in postburn pediatric patients. Arch Surg 1990;125:392-5.
2. Klein GL, Herndon DN, Rutan TC, et al. Bone disease in burn patients. J Bone Miner Res 1993;8:337-45.
3. Kupper FJ, Deitch EA, Biker CC, Wong W. The human burn wound as primary source of interleukin-1 activity. Surgery 1986;100:409-15.
4. Guo Y, Dickerson C, Chrest FJ, et al. Increased levels of circulating interleukin-6 in burn patients. Clin Immunol Immunopathol 1990;54:361-71.
5. Ishimi Y, Miyaurh C, Jin CH, et al. IL-6 is produced by osteoblasts and induces bone resorption. J Immunol 1990; 145:3297-303.
6. Herndon DN, Rutan RL, Alison WE Jr, Cox CC Jr. Management of burn injuries. In: Eichelberger MR, ed. Pediatric trauma prevention acute care, rehabilitation. St Louis: Mosby–Year Book, 1993:568-90.
7. Rutan TC, Herndon DN, Van Osten T, Abston S. Metabolic rate alterations in early excision and grafting versus conservative treatment. J Trauma 1986;26:140-2.
8. Southard RN, Morris JD, Mahan JD, et al. Bone mass in healthy children: measurements with quantitative DXA. Radiology 1991;179:735-8.
9. Gidding SS, Minciotti A, Langman CB. Unmasking of hyperparathyroidism in familial partial DiGeorge syndrome by EDTA challenge. N Engl J Med 1988;319:1589-91.
10. Reed A, Haugen M, Pachman LM, Langman CB. Abnormalities of serum osteocalcin in children with chronic rheumatic diseases. J Pediatr 1990;116:574-80.
11. Eriksen EF, Charles P, Melsen F, Mosekide L, Risteli L, Risteli J. Serum markers of type I collagen formation and degradation in metabolic bone disease: correlation with bone histomorphometry. J Bone Miner Res 1993;8:127-32.
12. Holbrook TL, Grazier K, Kelly JL, Stauffer RN. The frequency of occurrence, impact and cost of selected musculoskeletal conditions in the United States. Chicago: American Academy of Orthopedic Surgeons, 1984:73-135.
13. Worlick P, Stower M. Fracture patterns in Nottingham children. J Pediatr Orthop 1986;6:656-60.
14. Stapleton FB, Roy S, Noe HN, Jerkins G. Hypercalciuria in children with hematuria. N Engl J Med 1984;310:1345-8.
15. Arnaud S, Sherrard DJ, Maloney N, et al. Effects of 1-week head-down tilt bed rest on bone formation and the calcium endocrine system. Aviat Space Environ Med 1992;63:14-20.
16. LeBlanc AD, Schneider VS, Evans HJ, Engelbretson DA, Krebs JM. Bone mineral loss and recovery after 17 weeks of bed rest. J Bone Miner Res 1990;5:843-50.
17. Hahn TJ. Steroid and drug-induced osteopenia. In: Favus MJ, ed. Primer on the metabolic bone diseases and disorders of mineral metabolism. New York: Raven Press, 1993:250-5.
18. Mastorakos G, Chrousos GP, Weber JS. Recominant interleukin-6 activates the hypothalamic-pituitary-adrenal axis in humans. J Clin Endocrinol Metab 1993;77:1690-4.
19. Klein GL, Coburn JW. Parenteral nutrition: effect on bone and mineral homeostasis. Annu Rev Nutr 1991;11:93-119.
20. Vargas JH, Klein GL, Ament ME, et al. Metabolic bone disease of total parenteral nutrition, course after changing from casein to amino acids in parenteral solutions with reduced aluminum content. Am J Clin Nutr 1988;48:1070-8.
21. Sedman AB, Klein GL, Merritt RJ, et al. Evidence of aluminum loading in infants receiving intravenous therapy. N Engl J Med 1985;312:1337-43.
22. Klein GL, Alfrey AC, Shike M, Sherrard DJ. Parenteral drug products containing aluminum as an ingredient or a contaminant: response to FDA notice of intent. Am J Clin Nutr 1991; 53:399-402.
23. Klein GL, Targoff CM, Ament ME, et al. Bone disease in parenteral nutrition. Lancet 1980;2:1041-4.
24. Margen S, Chu JY, Kaufmann NA, Calloway DH. Studies in calcium metabolism 1: the calciuretic effect of dietary protein. Am J Clin Nutr 1974;27:584-9.
25. American Academy of Pediatrics Committee on Nutrition. Pediatric nutrition handbook. Elk Grove Village, Illinois: American Academy of Pediatrics, 1985:354.
26. Neer RM. Calcium and inorganic phosphate homeostasis. In: De Groot L, ed. Endocrinology. Philadelphia: Saunders, 1989:927-53.
27. Rutan RL, Moore M, Alvarado MI, Blakeney PE, Herndon DN. Growth and development following thermal injury [Abstract]. Proceedings of the 3rd Sino-American Conference on Burns and Trauma, Canton, China, 1993, p. 171.

EDITOR'S COLUMN

Venom immunotherapy: Who should receive it?

In this issue of THE JOURNAL, Dr. Pia Hauk and colleagues recount their experience with 113 children, aged 2 to 17 years, who had large local or non-life-threatening systemic reactions to Hymenoptera stings.[1] This is the second article to be published in the United States in the past year concerning deliberate Hymenoptera stings in patients allergic to them, and the first dealing with direct Hymenoptera stings in children. After the investigators established the identity of the offending insect with radioallergosorbent tests or skin tests or both, the children were admitted to the University Children's Hospital Clinical Research Center and, with an intravenous line in place, were restung by the insect identified as the one that had induced the reaction (with appropriate emergency equipment on hand). Thirteen percent of the children had a systemic reaction. Two to six weeks later, a second challenge was carried out to be certain that the children were not further sensitized to the first sting. Seventeen percent had a systemic allergic reaction to the second sting (4% had only had a large local reaction to the first sting), which indicated that a few children did become further sensitized. In the subsequent 3 years, 39 children who had not been not treated with venom immunotherapy had a wild sting. Only two reacted, one with hives and one with hives and mild respiratory symptoms. The authors recommended immunotherapy for only 13 of 113 children. They further noted that the skin test, per se, or the values obtained by radioallergosorbent tests, did not identify those to whom immunotherapy should be administered.

This article complements one by van der Linden et al.[2]; 324 adult patients with a history of yellow jacket or honeybee sting anaphylaxis were admitted to the intensive care unit, had appropriate monitoring with a continuous intravenous infusion, and were restung by the appropriate *Vespula* species or *Apis mellifera*. The majority of the patients who were restung either had less severe reactions than originally or had normal reactions. In 27% of the patients sensitive to honeybees and 11% of those sensitive to yellow jackets, the reaction after challenge was similar to that after the previous field sting. Most patients with normal reactions, or with only moderate local reactions, were not given venom immunotherapy. Thus only 17% of those who would have been candidates for immunotherapy by standard criteria were obliged to have it. Again, the authors noted that neither the absolute grades of skin tests nor plasma levels of specific IgE or IgG4 predicted the clinical response to a sting challenge in individual patients. They also found that more of the patients sensitive to honeybees than to yellow jackets reacted, possibly because the honeybee injected more venom (similar to the findings in the Hauk study.) Van der Linden et al. thought that only those with pulmonary or cardiovascular symptoms needed to be given venom immunotherapy. In an accompanying editorial from the Johns Hopkins Asthma and Allergy Center, Dr. Lawrence Lichtenstein[3] noted that this study suggests that we must reconsider the approach to deciding who should receive immunotherapy.

See related article, p. 185.

It would be valuable to do a similar study with American children, but it would be impossible to get this pediatric protocol through a U.S. institutional review board and receive parental permission for children to receive direct in-hospital stings, unless a study of U.S. adults showed a compelling reason for doing so.[4] However, there is evidence from American studies of direct sting procedures that only a minimal number of children react to a second sting. For instance, Harry Mueller,[5] after treating his patients with whole body extract (which was subsequently found not to be effective),[6] encouraged the children to have a sting or multiple stings by wild insects. Very few of his patients reacted, which he took as evidence that immunotherapy with whole body extracts was effective (Mueller HL: personal communication, 1974). Now, from the German-Austrian article, we know that it was the natural course of Hymenoptera stings which induced the attenuated reaction.[1]

THE JOURNAL OF PEDIATRICS 1995;126:257-8

0022-3476/95/$3.00 + 0 **9/21/61756**

This finding is in keeping with a study by the Johns Hopkins group,[7] which showed that of children who were not treated, only 9.2% had a systemic reaction to a wild sting, most having a reaction less severe than to the first sting; two reactions were of similar severity and none was more severe. The investigators concluded that immunotherapy is unnecessary for most children who react allergically to Hymenoptera stings.

Thus we have a paradoxical situation. Although initial reports suggested that all children who had systemic or large local reactions after a Hymenoptera sting should be immunized with venom from the offending insect,[8] many children received venom immunization who did not need it. These include children with large local reactions, which do not progress to systemic reactions; treatment with corticosteroids and antihistamines should control these local reactions. Those with cutaneous systemic reactions (such as erythema or hives) after a sting probably do not require immunotherapy[9]; they should, though, have an anaphylaxis emergency treatment kit with epinephrine and also an antihistamine on hand for such stings. However, if parents insist on immunotherapy, their child should receive it. Those who have pulmonary or cardiovascular reactions to the sting (the group not tested by Hauk et al.) should receive venom immunotherapy. Only 30% to 40% of venom-sensitive children would require immunotherapy if these criteria were applied. The result would be a tremendous saving in time, pain, and expense for the children who previously had been candidates for several years of immunotherapy. Emergency equipment (injectable epinephrine and antihistamine) should still be on hand. However, those who have had a systemic reaction with airway or cardiovascular involvement should additionally receive venom immunotherapy.

C. Warren Bierman, MD
Division of Allergy, Department of Pediatrics
University of Washington School of Medicine
Seattle, WA 98195

REFERENCES

1. Hauk P, Friedl K, Kaufmehl K, Urbanek R, Forster J. Subsequent insect stings in children with hypersensitivity to Hymenoptera. J PEDIATR 1995;126:185-90.
2. van der Linden PW, Hack CE, Stuyvenberg A, van der Zwan JK. Insect sting challenges in 324 subjects with a previous anaphylactic reaction: current criteria for insect-venom hypersensitivity do not predict the occurrence and the severity of anaphylaxis. J Allergy Clin Immunol 1994;94:151-9.
3. Lichtenstein LM. A reappraisal of sting challenges: to whom should we offer venom immunotherapy? J Allergy Clin Immunol 1994;94:137-8.
4. Reisman RE. Intentional diagnostic sting challenges: a medical and ethical issue [Letter]. J Allergy Clin Immunol 1993; 91:1100.
5. Mueller HL. Further experiences with severe allergic reactions to insect stings. N Engl J Med 1959;261:374-7.
6. Schwartz HL. Skin sensitivity in insect allergy. JAMA 1965;194:703-5.
7. Valentine MD, Schuberth KC, Kagey-Sobotka A, et al. The value of immunotherapy with venom in children with allergy to insect stings. N Engl J Med 1990;323:1601-3.
8. Schuberth KC, Lichtenstein LM, Kagey-Sobotka A, et al. Epidemiologic study of insect allergy in children. J PEDIATR 1983;102:361-5.
9. Graft DF, Schuberth KC, Kagey-Sobotka A, et al. Assessment of prolonged venom immunotherapy in children. J Allergy Clin Immunol 1987;80:162-9.

Critical illness neuromuscular disease in children manifested as ventilatory dependence

Raj D. Sheth, MD, William E. M. Pryse-Phillips, MD, Jack E. Riggs, MD, and John B. Bodensteiner, MD

From the Departments of Neurology and Pediatrics, West Virginia University Health Sciences Center, Morgantown, and the Department of Medicine (Neurology), Memorial University of Newfoundland, St. John's, Canada

Four children with prolonged dependency on a ventilator were found to have reversible quadriparesis, muscle wasting, and hyporeflexia after 8 to 20 days of assisted ventilation for life-threatening sepsis or respiratory failure. Critical illness neuromuscular disease, which was recently recognized as a distinct clinical syndrome in adults, may also be manifested in children by prolonged ventilatory dependency. (J Pediatr 1995;126:259-61)

Prolonged dependence on a ventilator occurs in 30% of adults recovering from sepsis and multiple organ failure[1] and was initially attributed to nutritional or steroid myopathy, toxic effects of gentamicin or pancuronium bromide, acute inflammatory demyelinating polyneuropathy, or pancreatic dysfunction.[2] Subsequently a distinctive syndrome involving an underlying polyneuropathy or myopathy was identified,[3] which is herein referred to as critical illness neuromuscular disease. Similar problems have not been well characterized in children.

METHODS

The medical records of all patients who underwent electrophysiologic studies for failure to be weaned from ventilatory support in a tertiary care pediatric intensive care unit during a 6-year period were reviewed. Many patients had difficulty being weaned from ventilatory support during this period, but only four patients had electrophysiologic studies.

CASE REPORTS

Patient 1. A 15-year-old girl had septic shock as a result of group C *Neisseria meningitidis*, and she had associated bilateral adrenal hemorrhages. Two days later acute kidney failure necessitated peritoneal dialysis for 72 hours. Medications administered included midazolam, cefotaxime, dopamine, and methylprednisolone. Intermittent doses of vecuronium, 0.03 mg/kg, provided neuromuscular blockade for 48 hours. Although the patient's mental status returned to normal, she could not undergo extubation until 6 days after vecuronium was discontinued because she had profound hyporeflexic muscle weakness. Serum creatine kinase activity (116 mmol/L) and results of cerebrospinal fluid analysis (protein, 0.39 gm/L; no cells) were normal. Electrophysiologic studies on day 8 demonstrated small compound muscle action potentials over the abductor pollicis brevis muscle. Median and peroneal motor nerve conduction velocities were normal. Electromyography of the deltoid muscle demonstrated a poor recruitment pattern. Additional electromyography on day 16 demonstrated prominent fibrillations in the first dorsal interosseous muscle with a slight excess of polyphasic units of increased duration. The patient's strength returned to normal 6 weeks after the onset of illness.

Patient 2. A 15-year-old boy with septic shock as a result of group B *N. meningitidis* required vigorous fluid resuscitation and ventilatory support. He received ampicillin, chloramphenicol, midazolam, dopamine, and methylprednisolone. Intermittent doses of vecuronium, 0.04 mg/kg, provided neuromuscular blockade for 5 days. The patient's mental status was normal when vecuronium was discontinued. An extubation attempt on day 8 was unsuccessful because of severe quadriparesis. Diffuse muscle atrophy was present, and muscle stretch reflexes were absent. Serum creatine kinase activity (116 mmol/L) and results of cerebrospinal fluid analysis (protein, 0.29 gm/L; no cells) were normal. Cranial computed tomography and abdominal ultrasonography findings were normal. Three days later a second attempt at extubation was successful. A gradual return to normal muscle strength occurred during the next 3 months, although hyporeflexia remained. Seventeen months later, the patient's reflexes were normal. At that time, motor nerve conduction velocities were normal in the median and common peroneal nerves, although compound muscle action potentials were dispersed. Electromyography demonstrated motor unit potential amplitudes to 11 mV in the tibialis anterior, vastus lateralis, and extensor digitorum communis muscles, suggesting

Submitted for publication July 20, 1994; accepted Sept. 6, 1994.
Reprint requests: Raj D. Sheth, MD, West Virginia University Health Science Center, Box 9180, Morgantown, WV 26506-9180.

0022-3476/95/$3.00 + 0 **9/22/60449**

Table. Differentiating features of the critical illness neuromuscular disease in children

Features	Critical illness polyneuropathy	Acute myopathic syndrome	Hopkins syndrome
Age group	Elderly (reports in children)	Adolescents	Young child
Antecedent	Multiorgan failure/sepsis	Acute steroid use	Status asthmaticus
Timing	>2 wk	Variable	<2 wk
Limbs affected	Quadriparesis	Quadriparesis	Monoparesis
Pain	Unusual	Muscular tenderness	Severe
Reflexes	Absent or ↓	↓	Normal in unaffected limbs
Creatinine kinase	Less than twice upper normal value	↑↑↑	Normal
Electromyography	Neuropathic	Myopathic	Localized neuropathic
Spinal fluid	Normal	Not reported	Pleocytosis
Muscle biopsy	Grouped atrophy	Type II atrophy	Not reported
Recovery	Good	Good	Poor

denervation with reinnervation. Results of repetitive nerve stimulation studies were normal.

Patient 3. A 17-year-old girl with a 9-year history of asthma was admitted to the hospital with fever, status asthmaticus, and pneumonia. She required assisted ventilation and was treated with ampicillin, cefotaxime, cimetidine, hydrocortisone, salbutamol, and aminophylline. Bilateral pneumothoraces developed, and required the placement of chest tubes. Intermittent doses of vecuronium, 0.02 mg/kg, were administered for 8 days. Although the bronchospasm and pneumonia resolved, the patient remained dependent on a ventilator. She was alert but quadriplegic, and communicated by using eye and minimal head movements. Sensation and sphincter functions were normal. She had marked muscle wasting distally in the arms and legs. Muscle stretch reflexes were absent. Multiple bacterial cultures of blood, urine, and cerebrospinal fluid, obtained after antibiotic therapy had been initiated, showed negative results. Mycoplasma antibody, antinuclear antibody, erythrocyte sedimentation rate, serum creatine kinase activity (98 mmol/L), and results of cerebrospinal fluid analysis (protein, 0.25 gm/L; no cells) were absent or normal. On the tenth hospital day, median and ulnar nerve conduction velocities and distal latencies were normal, but the amplitudes of the compound muscle action potentials were reduced; F waves were unobtainable. On electromyography, fibrillations were found in the biceps and tibialis anterior muscles. No voluntary units were recruited. Sensory conduction velocities were normal. The patient continued to receive assisted ventilation via tracheostomy for an additional 6 weeks and slowly regained normal strength during the next 4 months.

Patient 4. A 6-year-old girl with alveolar proteinosis (confirmed by lung biopsy) had pneumonia and ventilatory failure. She was treated with ceftriaxone and six doses of vecuronium, 0.02 mg/kg for a 48-hour period; corticosteroids were not used. Her respiratory status improved, but she had quadriparesis and could not be weaned from ventilatory support. Twenty-one days after admission to the hospital she was hyporeflexic, markedly weak, and able to move only her fingers and toes. Serum creatine kinase activity (88 mmol/L) was normal. Electromyography showed fibrillations in the deltoid, quadriceps, and tibialis anterior muscles, and an excess of polyphasic units. Nerve conduction studies showed mild slowing of motor velocity in the common peroneal nerve. Six months later, the patient continued to require nocturnal ventilatory support.

DISCUSSION

Witt et al.[1] prospectively studied critically ill adults and found evidence of polyneuropathy in 70% of the subjects, 30% of whom had difficulty in being weaned from assisted ventilation. A spectrum of neuromuscular disease with reversible flaccid weakness in critically ill adults is now recognized.[4] Critical illness polyneuropathy, motor neuropathy, disuse (cachectic) myopathy, necrotic myopathy, pyomyositis, and acute myopathy are delineated entities included in the syndrome of critical illness neuromuscular disease.[3] Electrophysiologic studies have been helpful in differentiating these entities.[5] Serum creatine kinase activity is elevated in necrotic myopathy,[6] pyomyositis,[7] and acute myopathy.[8, 9]

Hopkins syndrome occurs in children recovering from asthma.[10] However, unlike Hopkins syndrome, in which weakness is permanent and restricted to one or two limbs,[11] patients in this case series had severe diffuse weakness that was reversible. A neuromuscular transmission defect induced by vecuronium, particularly in the presence of kidney failure, may result in diffuse weakness.[12] Diffuse weakness may also be seen in children with acute myopathy[13] or "disuse atrophy."[14-16] The clinical course, electrophysiologic studies, and normal serum creatine kinase levels in our patients do not support either a neuromuscular transmission defect or a myopathy (Table). Rather, the findings suggest the diagnosis of critical illness polyneuropathy,[3] a condition not previously reported in children.

Failure to be weaned from assisted ventilation despite cardiopulmonary recovery in children is a perplexing, challenging, and not infrequent clinical problem. In this patient series, electrophysiologic studies had been performed in four patients who could not be weaned and in each case provided valuable diagnostic information. Increased awareness and recognition of critical illness neuromuscular disease in children will, as in adults, facilitate advances in understanding the frequency, natural history, and pathogenesis of this syndrome.

REFERENCES

1. Witt NJ, Zochodne DW, Bolton CF, et al. Peripheral nerve function in sepsis and multiple organ failure. Chest 1991; 99:176-84.
2. Goldstein RL, Hyde RW, Lapham LW, Gazioglu K, dePapp ZG. Peripheral neuropathy presenting with respiratory insufficiency as the primary complaint: problem of recognizing alveolar hypoventilation due to neuromuscular disorders. Am J Med 1974;56:443-9.
3. Bolton CF, Young GB, Zochodne DW. Neurological changes during severe sepsis. In: Dobbs GJ, ed. Current topics in intensive care number 1. Philadelphia: W B Saunders, 1994:180-217.
4. Chad DA, Lacomis D. Critically ill patients with newly acquired weakness: the clinicopathological spectrum. Ann Neurol 1994;35:257-9.
5. Bolton CF. Electrophysiologic studies of critically ill patients. Muscle Nerve 1987;10:129-35.
6. Zochodne DW, Ramsay DA, Saly V, Shelley S, Moffatt S. Acute necrotizing myopathy of intensive care: electrophysiological studies. Muscle Nerve 1994;17:285-92.
7. Adamski GB, Garin EH, Ballinger WE, et al. Generalized non-supparitive myositis with staphylococcal septicemia. J Pediatr 1980;96:694-7.
8. Lacomis D, Smith TW, Chad DA. Acute myopathy and neuropathy in status asthmaticus: case report and literature review. Muscle Nerve 1993;16:84-90.
9. Hirano M, Ott BR, Raps EC, et al. Acute quadriplegic myopathy: a complication of treatment with steroids, nondepolarizing blocking agents, or both. Neurology 1992;42:2082-7.
10. Shapiro GG, Chapman JT, Pierson WE, Bierman CW. Poliomyelitis-like illness after acute asthma. J Pediatr 1979; 94:767-8.
11. Shahar EM, Hwang PA, Niesen CE, Murphy EG. Poliomyelitis-like paralysis during recovery from acute bronchial asthma: possible etiology and risk factors. Pediatrics 1991; 88:276-9.
12. Segredo V, Caldwell JE, Matthay MA, et al. Persistent paralysis in critically ill patients after long-term administration of vecuronium. N Engl J Med 1992;327:524-8.
13. Kaplan PW, Rocha W, Sanders DB, D'Souza B, Spock A. Acute steroid-induced tetraplegia following status asthmaticus. Pediatrics 1986;78:121-3.
14. Torres CF, Maniscalco MA, Agostinelli T. Muscle weakness and atrophy following prolonged paralysis with pancuronium bromide in neonates [Abstract]. Ann Neurol 1985;18:403.
15. Pascucci RC. Prolonged weakness after extended mechanical ventilation in a child. Crit Care Med 1990;18:1181-2.
16. Rutledge ML, Hawkins EP, Langston C. Skeletal muscle growth failure induced in premature newborn infants by prolonged pancuronium treatment. J Pediatr 1986;109:883-6.

Transient elevation of sweat chloride concentration in a malnourished girl with the Mauriac syndrome

Fernando P. Polack, MD, David J. Transue, MD, William M. Belknap, MD, Bishara J. Freij, MD, and David J. Aughton, MD

From the Department of Pediatrics, William Beaumont Hospital, Royal Oak, Michigan

Elevated sweat chloride concentration in a patient with Mauriac syndrome has been reported only once. The authors of that report regarded their patient's underlying malnutrition, and not Mauriac syndrome per se, as the cause of the elevated sweat chloride concentration. We describe a second example of transient elevation of sweat chloride concentration, which confirms that the malnutrition intrinsic to Mauriac syndrome, rather than the syndrome itself, was the probable cause of elevated sweat chloride values. (J Pediatr 1995;126:261-3)

Submitted July 5, 1994; accepted Sept. 9, 1994.

Reprint requests: David J. Aughton, MD, Division of Genetics, Department of Pediatrics, William Beaumont Hospital, 3601 W. Thirteen Mile Rd., Royal Oak, MI 48073.

0022-3476/95/$3.00 + 0 **9/22/60450**

In 1979, Rosenfeld et al.[1] reported transiently elevated sweat chloride concentration in a 6-year-old girl with Mauriac syndrome (hepatomegaly, glycogen infiltration of the liver, and short stature in children with diabetes mellitus treated with insufficient amounts of insulin and an inappropriate diet). They attributed the elevated sweat chloride concentration to "the state of malnutrition and not the underlying disease," and there have been no subsequent reports of the concurrence of Mauriac syndrome and elevated sweat chloride values. Nevertheless, many standard reference books list Mauriac syndrome (in addition to malnutrition) among the conditions other than cystic fibrosis in which elevations of sweat chloride may be encountered.[2-6] Only one of these references notes that the concurrence has been reported but once[5]; the reader of the other references would reasonably infer that this "association" is well established through multiple observations.

We report the second case of a child with Mauriac syndrome who had a transiently elevated sweat chloride concentration.

CASE REPORT

An 8-year-old white girl with a 2-year history of type I diabetes mellitus was seen for evaluation of growth failure and hepatomegaly associated with poor control of diabetes. A diagnosis of Mauriac syndrome was made, and the patient was admitted to the hospital for improved management of diabetes. Examination revealed that she was malnourished and without edema. She weighed 22 kg (5th percentile; unchanged from 10 months earlier) and was 125 cm tall (10th percentile; an increase of 0.7 cm in 10 months). The patient had two alopecic patches of the scalp, white plaques consistent with moniliasis on the oropharyngeal and vaginal mucosas, a liver edge 6 cm below the right costal margin, a scabious eruption on the trunk and extremities, and reduced muscle mass. Laboratory results included hemoglobin A_{1c}, 0.218 (21.8%) (normal, 0.04 to 0.08 [4 to 8]); hemoglobin, 98 gm/L; total protein, 66 gm/L; albumin, 44 gm/L; and globulins, 22 gm/L. Blood glucose values fluctuated between 8.3 mmol/L (150 mg/dl) and 19.4 mmol/L (350 mg/dl), without evidence of ketosis. A sweat chloride level (determined with the Gibson-Cooke method) on day 2 of hospitalization was 55 mmol/L (normal, 5 to 40 mmol/L).

The patient was provided with a 2000 kcal American Diabetes Association diet, and a twice-daily insulin regimen was begun. The diet was eventually increased to 2500 kcal. The patient's body weight increased by 4 kg during her 17-day hospitalization, and the hepatomegaly resolved. The scabies infestation responded to permethrin, and the moniliasis quickly resolved without specific antifungal treatment. New hair growth was observed by the end of the patient's hospital stay. The sweat chloride concentration on day 8 was 68 mmol/L, and on day 16 was normal (40 mmol/L).

Results of a celiac antibody panel, levels of triiodothyronine, thyroxine, and thyroid-stimulating hormone, 24-hour measurement of fecal fat, three stools for ova and parasites, and determinations of antithyroid, antiadrenal, antiparietal cell, antinuclear, and antismooth muscle antibodies were normal. The patient had normal serum IgM and IgA concentrations, but her IgG levels were low (3.68 gm/L [normal, 6.88 to 15.33 gm/L]). IgG subclass measurements showed IgG1 deficiency (2.52 gm/L [normal, 3.50 to 9.00 gm/L]), with normal levels of IgG2, IgG3, and IgG4.

Within 1 month of her release from the hospital, the patient's hemoglobin A_{1c} was 0.117 (11.7%). Total protein, albumin, and globulin levels were not significantly changed. Levels of IgG2, IgG3, and IgG4 remained normal, and the IgG1 level was 4.13 gm/L; however, total IgG levels remained low (4.97 gm/L). Results of DNA amplification and direct mutation analysis for cystic fibrosis–associated mutations (Henry Ford Hospital, Detroit, Mich.) were negative. Mutations that were tested included ΔF508, ΔI507, G542X, G551D, R553X, N1303K, R560T, 621+1, 1717-1, R117H, and W1282X.

DISCUSSION

Several conditions considered to be associated with an elevated sweat chloride concentration were found concurrently in our patient, including Mauriac syndrome, malnutrition,[7, 8] and low IgG1 levels.[9] Her history was also suggestive of other conditions associated with an elevated sweat chloride concentration, including psychosocial neglect and depression,[10, 11] although these conditions were not demonstrated to be present. Despite her low IgG1 level,[12] our patient had no history of lung disease and no clinical evidence of gastrointestinal dysfunction. With restitution of a proper insulin regimen and diet, her sweat chloride concentration fell to the upper range of normal during her hospital stay. In this respect, our patient's course was very similar to that of the previously reported patient with Mauriac syndrome and a transiently elevated sweat chloride concentration.[1]

Malnutrition has also been described in association with hypogammaglobulinemia-associated elevated sweat chloride concentration.[13] The association of elevated sweat chloride concentration with hypogammaglobulinemia was described in patients who had low IgG and IgM serum concentrations and serum IgA that was consistently absent.[9, 13] It is likely that the sweat chloride concentration elevation noted in patients with hypogammaglobulinemia is also related more to the malnutrition found in association with the chronic illness of these patients than to the hypogammaglobulinemia itself.

There is no basis for the common belief that Mauriac syndrome is an independent cause of elevated sweat chloride concentrations. Our patient's case provides further evidence that malnutrition is the proximate cause of the elevation of the sweat chloride concentration that is sometimes observed in these patients.

REFERENCES

1. Rosenfeld R, Spigelblatt L, Chicoine R. False positive sweat test, malnutrition, and the Mauriac syndrome. J PEDIATR 1979;94:240-2.
2. Boat TF, Welsh MJ, Beaudet AL. Cystic fibrosis. In: Scriver CR, Beaudet AL, Sly WS, Valle D, eds. The metabolic basis of inherited disease. 6th ed. New York: McGraw-Hill, 1989: chap 108.

3. Rajkumar S, Toback C. Principles and practice of ambulatory pediatrics. New York: Plenum Publishing, 1988:672.
4. Kessler CJ, Lebenthal E. The exocrine pancreas. In: Silverberg M, Daum F, eds. Textbook of pediatric gastroenterology. 2nd ed. Chicago: Year-Book Medical Publishers, 1988: chap 16.
5. Lloyd-Still JD. Cystic fibrosis. In: Lebenthal E, ed. Textbook of gastroenterology and nutrition in infancy. New York: Raven Press, 1989: chap 62.
6. Rosenstein BJ. Cystic fibrosis. In: Oski FA, ed. Principles and practice of pediatrics. Philadelphia: J B Lippincott, 1990: chap 72.
7. Mace JW, Schanberger JE. Elevated sweat chlorides in a child with malnutrition. Clin Pediatr 1971;10:285-6.
8. Beck R, Durie PR, Hill JG, Levison H. Malnutrition: a cause of elevated sweat chloride concentration. Acta Paediatr Scand 1986;75:639-44.
9. Corkey CWB, Gelfand EW. Hypogammaglobulinemia and antibody deficiency in patients with elevated sweat chloride concentrations. J PEDIATR 1982;100:420-2.
10. Christoffel KS, Lloyd-Still JD, Brown G, Shwachman H. Environmental deprivation and transient elevation of sweat electrolytes. J PEDIATR 1985;107:231-4.
11. Pelteret RM. Depressive illness and abnormal sweat electrolytes. S Afr Med J 1990;77:107-8.
12. Papadea C, Check IJ. Human immunoglobulin G and immunoglobulin G subclasses: biochemical, genetic, and clinical aspects. Crit Rev Clin Lab Sci 1989;27:27-58.
13. Rosario NA, Neto RS, Nitta A, Marinoni LP. Hypogammaglobulinemia and elevated sweat chloride values. J PEDIATR 1983;102:163.

Transformation of congenital neutropenia into monosomy 7 and acute nonlymphoblastic leukemia in a child treated with granulocyte colony-stimulating factor

Mark E. Weinblatt, MD, Philip Scimeca, MD, Anne James-Herry, MD, Indira Sahdev, MD, and Joseph Kochen, MD, PhD

From the Department of Pediatrics, Division of Pediatric Hematology/Oncology, North Shore University Hospital–Cornell University Medical College, Manhasset, New York

A cytogenetically normal infant with Kostmann syndrome (severe congenital granulocytopenia) was treated with granulocyte colony-stimulating factor, which resulted in a rapid improvement in his neutrophil count and a resolution of recurrent infections. After 11 months of therapy, splenomegaly developed, with thrombocytopenia, anemia, circulating nucleated erythrocytes, and acquired monosomy 7, which evolved during a period of 7 months into acute nonlymphoblastic leukemia. The use of granulocyte colony-stimulating factor in patients with congenital marrow failure disorders may induce or hasten the onset of a malignant transformation. (J PEDIATR 1995;126:263-5)

Kostmann syndrome, also known as severe neutropenia of infancy, is a rare, inherited disorder with onset very early in life. It is characterized by recurrent umbilical granulomas, pyogenic skin infections (usually caused by *Staphylococcus aureus*), otitis media, and pneumonia. Septicemia, peritonitis, and abscesses ultimately develop in most affected children. Circulating granulocytes are either rare or entirely absent, even in the presence of serious infections. The bone marrow usually shows early maturation arrest, and untreated patients usually succumb to infection within the first year of life. Until recently, the only successful treatment has been transplantation of healthy bone marrow from a donor with compatible HLA.

G-CSF	Granulocyte colony-stimulating factor
HLA	Human leukocyte antigen

Submitted for publication July 8, 1994; accepted Sept. 9, 1994.
Reprint requests: Mark Weinblatt, MD, Department of Pediatrics, Division of Pediatric Hematology/Oncology, North Shore University Hospital, 300 Community Dr., Manhasset, NY 11030.

0022-3476/95/$3.00 + 0 **9/22/60451**

During the past few years, children with chronic neutropenia have been treated successfully with granulocyte colony-stimulating factor[2-4]; daily injections have raised the granulocyte count in most patients, and as a result infections have been prevented and growth and development have improved. Except for mild splenomegaly, no significant adverse effects have been noted. We now describe a child with Kostmann syndrome in whom monosomy 7 and nonlymphoblastic leukemia developed during long-term treatment with G-CSF.

CASE REPORT

Shortly after birth, respiratory distress developed in a neonate born at term, and he was found to have severe neutropenia and monocytosis. His hemoglobin concentration was 163 gm/L, his platelet count was 398×10^9/L (398,000/mm^3), and his leukocyte count was 8.1×10^9/L (8100/mm^3) with no granulocytes, 69% lymphocytes, and 25% monocytes. Despite resolution of the respiratory problems with antibiotic therapy, his neutrophil count did not improve. He subsequently had recurrent umbilical granulomas, staphylococcal skin infections, and otitis media, and his neutrophil count did not improve. Bone marrow examination revealed an absence of granulocyte precursors, with normal megakaryocyte and erythroid activity. Kostmann syndrome was diagnosed, and the patient was treated with G-CSF at a dosage of 10 to 15 μg/kg per day, which raised his granulocyte count into the normal range within 3 weeks and resulted in a resolution of the infections. His absolute granulocyte count remained greater than 1×10^9/L (1000/mm^3) despite a lower dose of G-CSF, and this count did not change as he continued to grow and do well without infection. His spleen was not palpable, and a routine sonogram at age 13 months revealed a normal-sized spleen. Both language development and gross motor development were several months behind those appropriate for his chronologic age.

When the patient reached 15 months of age, marked tonsillar hypertrophy, moderate splenomegaly, leukocytosis, and thrombocytopenia were found. His spleen continued to enlarge, which caused discomfort and clinical signs of hypersplenism. Despite cessation of G-CSF therapy, his clinical findings did not change; the absolute neutrophil count remained greater than 3×10^9/L (3000/mm^3), and a progressive decrease in platelets and erythrocytes necessitated transfusion therapy. A complete blood cell count at this time included a hematocrit of 0.22 with 2% reticulocytes and a platelet count of 40×10^9/L (40,000/mm^3), and his leukocyte count was 45.7×10^9/L (45,700/mm^3), with 26% monoblast cells and 10% blast cells. Fetal hemoglobin value was 4.6%. Leukocyte alkaline phosphatase was 200 U/L (normal, 25 to 100 U/L). Serum lactic dehydrogenase was 693 U/L (normal, 60 to 200 U/L). The bone marrow was markedly hypercellular, with ample granulocyte precursors and normal maturation in all cell lines; cytogenetic analysis of blood and bone marrow confirmed the presence of monosomy 7. No increase in chromosome fragility could be elicited by diepoxybutane challenge. Polymerase chain reaction testing of the DNA from blood smears obtained during the first few months of life found both No. 7 chromosomes present.

At age 18 months the patient underwent a splenectomy without complications, which resulted in a rise in his platelet count into the normal range and no further requirement for either erythrocyte or platelet transfusions. Enlarged tonsils and adenoids caused problems with eating and breathing; they were removed, and tympanostomy tubes were placed to treat recurrent otitis media. The patient was hospitalized on several occasions for treatment of pneumonia or multifocal staphylococcal cellulitis of the extremities and pneumonia, despite an absolute granulocyte count of greater than 2×10^9/L (2000/mm^3). Increasing leukocytosis with peripheral blast cells was noted, and pronounced hepatomegaly developed. A compatible bone marrow donor could not be located within the immediate and extended family or through a computer search of marrow registries. Aside from a brief trial of hydroxyurea, the family elected to use no further treatment options, including that of a partially mismatched bone marrow transplantation. A second cytogenetic evaluation revealed new chromosome abnormalities, with two clones having new monosomy and marker chromosomes: 46,XY,−7,+frag, and 46,XY,−7,−18,+frag. The patient's peripheral leukocyte count rose as high as 300×10^9/L (300,000/mm^3), with numerous blast cells, nucleated erythrocytes, and atypical monocytes on peripheral smear. No medications other than antibiotics are being administered, according to the family's wishes.

DISCUSSION

Severe congenital granulocytopenia of infancy is one of several early childhood disorders caused by defective marrow cell lines, which results in decreased numbers of circulating blood cells. Patients with Kostmann syndrome have severe deficiencies of granulocytes, Blackfan-Diamond syndrome is characterized by severe anemia, and patients with thrombocytopenia–absent radius syndrome have severe thrombocytopenia. In all three of these disorders, patients have normal chromosome patterns at the time of diagnosis, whereas Fanconi anemia is characterized by aplastic anemia, increased chromosome breaks, and poor DNA repair.

Because of success attained in the treatment of patients with chemotherapy-induced neutropenia, clinical trials of G-CSF have been broadened to include patients with bone marrow failure who have neutropenia and infections, with good results. Patients receiving long-term injections of G-CSF have generally tolerated the treatments well. Splenomegaly, probably resulting from splenic extramedullary hematopoiesis, has been noted, and one death was reported after splenic rupture.[5] Sweet syndrome has been seen,[6] with resolution after cessation of drug therapy. Therapy has also been associated with one case of interstitial pneumonitis[7] and sporadic cases of leukocytoclastic vasculitis.[8]

A serious concern in patients with congenital marrow disorders has been a propensity toward malignant disease, particularly acute leukemia. The risk of malignancy in patients with Kostmann syndrome has been difficult to evaluate because most patients formerly succumbed to serious infections and few have lived long enough to be observed for increased risk of malignancy. However, acute nonlymphoblastic leukemia developed in a few patients who survived into their teenage years,[9] which suggests that patients with this disorder might also be predisposed to malignancy.

A theoretical concern regarding the use of G-CSF in patients with acute nonlymphoblastic leukemia has been the possibility of stimulation of the malignant clone; many leukemic cells express receptors for cytokines, and cytokines can support in vitro survival and proliferation of these cells.[4] Myelodysplasia and leukemia have occurred in patients treated for aplastic anemia with G-CSF,[10] and in one child with nonconstitutional aplastic anemia treated with G-CSF, monosomy 7 and, ultimately, acute myeloid leukemia developed.[11] There have been recent sporadic reports of myelodysplastic syndrome and monosomy 7, some evolving into leukemia, in patients with congenital neutropenia treated with G-CSF.[5, 12] Kostmann syndrome might predispose patients like ours to leukemic transformation; the acquired monosomy 7 might have been induced by cytokine stimulation of a defective myeloid precursor cell.

Although the exact relation between myelodysplastic disorders and congenital neutropenia remains unclear, caution should be exercised in the treatment and follow-up of patients with marrow failure syndromes. Careful surveillance of cytogenetics and changes in the hematologic profile (thrombocytopenia and circulating nucleated erythrocytes) should be maintained. It is unknown whether a myeloproliferative transformation, if induced by G-CSF, is reversible on cessation of therapy. Families of affected children should be made aware of this association and its implications, and the possibility of bone marrow transplantation should be entertained before G-CSF is administered, particularly if an HLA-matched sibling is available. Prudence might warrant initiation of treatment only for patients who already have severe neutropenia and recurrent infections until there is further elucidation of the interaction of G-CSF and marrow failure syndromes, as well as clarification of the mechanism of evolution into malignant disease.

We thank Dr. Kevin Shannon for his assistance in DNA analysis of the patient's blood and marrow specimens and his invaluable advice regarding our patient's cytogenetic abnormalities. We also thank Dr. P. R. K. Koduru and those at his laboratory for the cytogenetic analysis of our patient's blood and marrow.

REFERENCES

1. Rappeport JM, Parkman R, Newburger P, et al. Correction of infantile agranulocytosis (Kostmann's syndrome) by allogeneic bone marrow transplantation. Am J Med 1980;68:605-9.
2. Bonilla MA, Gillio AP, Ruggeiro M, et al. Effects of recombinant human granulocyte colony-stimulating factor on neutropenia in patients with congenital agranulocytosis. N Engl J Med 1989;320:1574-80.
3. Dale DC, Bonilla MA, Davis MW, et al. A randomized controlled Phase III trial of recombinant human granulocyte colony-stimulating factor (Filgastrin) for treatment of severe chronic neutropenia. Blood 1993;81:2496-502.
4. Gillio AP, Gabrilove JL. Cytokine treatment of inherited bone marrow failure syndromes. Blood 1993;81:1669-74.
5. Zimmer BM, Berdel WE, Ludwig WD, et al. Fatal splenic rupture during induction chemotherapy with rh GM-CSF priming for acute monocytic leukemia. Leuk Res 1993;17:277-83.
6. Park JW, Mehotra B, Barnett BO, et al. The Sweet syndrome during therapy with granulocyte colony stimulating factor. Ann Intern Med 1992;116:996-8.
7. Katoh M, Shikoshi K, Takadam M, et al. Development of interstitial pneumonitis during treatment with granulocyte colony stimulating factor. Ann Hematol 1993;67:201-2.
8. Yang YM, Mankad UN, Manci E. Granulocyte colony stimulating factor associated leukocytoclastic vasculitis mimicking Henoch-Schonlein Purpura. Pediatr Hematol Oncol 1993;10:193-5.
9. Wong W, Williams D, Slovak ML, et al. Terminal acute myelogenous leukemia in a patient with congenital agranulocytosis. Am J Hematol 1993;43:133-8.
10. Kojima S, Tsuchida M, Matsuyama T. Myelodysplasia and leukemia after treatment of aplastic anemia with G-CSF. N Engl J Med 1992;326:1294-5.
11. Kojima S, Matsuyama T. Stimulation of granulopoiesis by high-dose recombinant human granulocyte colony-stimulating factor in children with aplastic anemia and very severe neutropenia. Blood 1994;83:1474-8.
12. Zeidler C, Reiter A, Yakisan E, et al. Long-term treatment with recombinant human granulocyte colony stimulating factor in patients with severe congenital neutropenia. Klin Padiatr 1993;205:264-71.

Painful keratoderma and photophobia: Hallmarks of tyrosinemia type II

Linda G. Rabinowitz, MD, Lynn R. Williams, MD, MPH, Carol E. Anderson, MD, Alice Mazur, RN, MS, and Paige Kaplan, MB,BCh

From the Departments of Pediatrics and Dermatology, Medical College of Wisconsin, Milwaukee, the Department of Dermatology, Case Western Reserve University, Cleveland, Ohio, the Department of Medical Genetics, Jefferson Medical College, Philadelphia, Pennsylvania, and the Department of Pediatrics, Division of Biochemical Development and Molecular Diseases, University of Pennsylvania, Philadelphia

Tyrosinemia type II (Richner-Hanhart syndrome), which is caused by a deficiency of hepatic tyrosine aminotransferase, results in elevated plasma and urinary tyrosine concentrations. We describe a young boy who was seen at 6 months of age with red eyes, photophobia, and eye pain that were not suspected to be caused by tyrosinemia II until painful plantar keratoderma developed at 2½ years of age. Treatment with a diet low in tyrosine and phenylalanine reversed the manifestations of the disease. (J Pediatr 1995;126:266-9)

Tyrosinemia type II is a rare autosomal recessive disorder of tyrosine metabolism that is clinically distinct from the more severe hepatorenal form of tyrosinemia, type I, and the benign transient form seen in newborn infants.[1] The tyrosinemias are characterized by elevated plasma tyrosine levels; however, the clinical spectrum is broad. Tyrosinemia type II is the only form manifested by characteristic cutaneous lesions. In addition, this form is associated with various ocular abnormalities that include photophobia and corneal ulcerations.

CASE REPORT

A 2½-year-old boy was seen in the pediatric dermatology clinic for evaluation of painful warty plantar lesions that had developed acutely 3 weeks earlier and prevented him from walking. Previous treatment with antifungal and corticosteroid creams was unsuccessful. The patient had a history of intermittent "red eyes" and tearing since 6 months of age. By age 16 months his eye problems were persistent, and it was determined that he had photophobia accompanied by screaming episodes. Ophthalmologic examinations, including use of a slit lamp, revealed no abnormalities. Results of computed tomography of the brain were normal. Congenital esotropia was surgically corrected at 1 year of age. The patient was not taking any medications and had no allergies. He had been delivered by cesarean section at 35 weeks of gestation because of placenta previa.

The patient's developmental history included floppiness during early infancy that resolved by 4 months of age, and mild gross motor delay (he walked at age 14 months). His parents described him as "slightly hyperactive." In addition, he refused to eat meat, chicken, and fish, and maintained a vegetarian diet that included dairy products. His physicians and parents thought that the problem was psychologic.

The family history was unremarkable except for various mild atopic conditions. A healthy 4-year-old brother had no skin or eye problems. There was no history of consanguinity. The parents were of Irish, Italian, and Dutch descent. There was no family history of tyrosinemia, mental retardation, or metabolic, eye, or skin disease.

Physical examination revealed an alert, friendly, cooperative boy. His weight was 14.4 kg (50th percentile), his height was 92.6 cm (50th to 75th percentile), and his head circumference was 52 cm (95th percentile). Sharply demarcated yellowish white hyperkeratotic papules and plaques surrounded by erythema were located on the plantar surfaces of both feet (Fig. 1); the right foot was more involved than the left foot. The lesions were localized to pressure points but were asymmetrical (Fig. 2). There appeared to be subtle vesiculation within the keratotic papules. His palms were unaffected. Results of ophthalmologic and neurologic examinations were grossly normal.

The patient's plasma tyrosine concentration was 2300 nmol/ml (normal, <100 nmol/ml), his urinary tyrosine concentration was 5860 nmol/ml (normal, <600 nmol/ml), and his urinary metabolites, *p*-hydroxyphenyl acetate and *p*-hydroxyphenyl lactate, were 688 and 6283 mg per gram of creatinine (normal, <20 mg per gram of creatinine), respectively. Results of a complete blood cell count with differential cell count, urinalysis, blood chemistry panel, and liver function tests were within normal limits.

Submitted for publication July 19, 1994; accepted Aug. 25, 1994.
Reprint requests: Linda G. Rabinowitz, MD, MACC Fund Research Center, 8701 Watertown Plank Rd., Milwaukee, WI 53226.

0022-3476/95/$3.00 + 0 **9/22/60183**

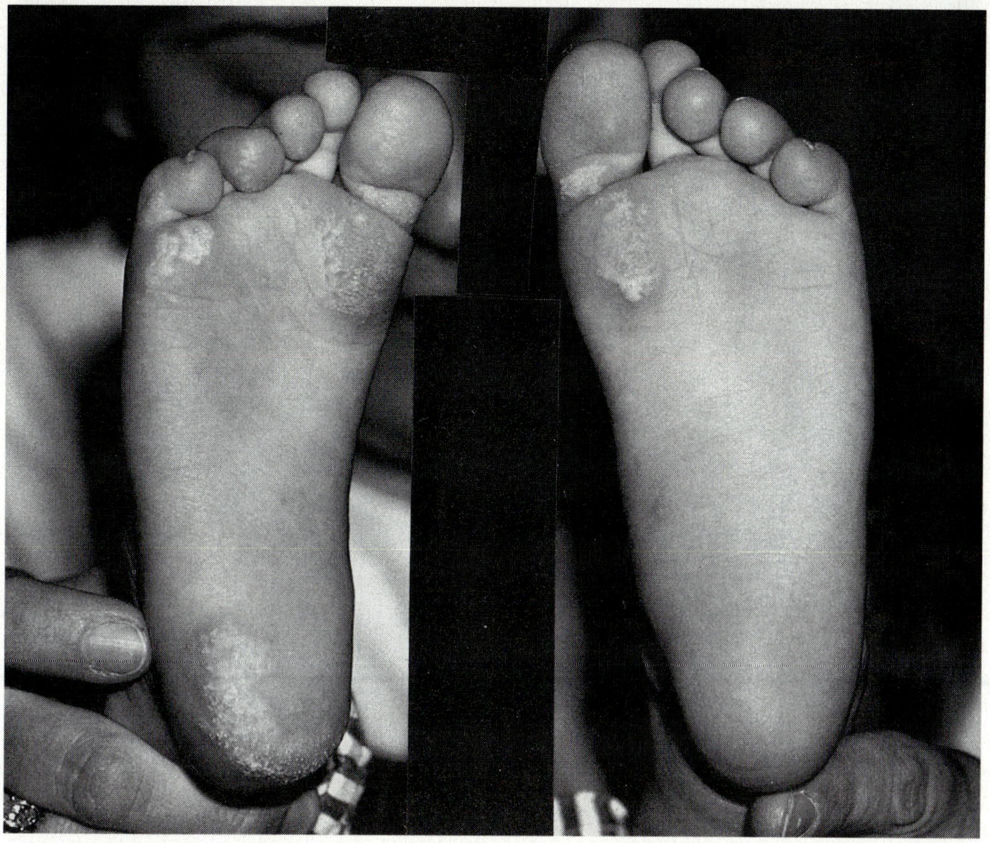

Fig. 1. Thick, yellowish white hyperkeratotic plaques surrounded by erythema on both plantar surfaces.

Our patient was started on a diet low in protein and dairy products immediately after initial blood and urine specimens were obtained. Within 3 days the photophobia and eye pain disappeared. His plantar keratoderma cleared completely within 10 to 14 days. In addition, his parents reported that his speech was clearer and that he was using longer sentences. On the Bayley Scales of Infant Scales Development, performed 2 weeks after the low protein diet was initiated, his motor score was one standard deviation below normal and showed that he had difficulty in balancing and changing direction.

After referral to the division of metabolism, Children's Hospital of Philadelphia, the patient was started on a strict diet low in tyrosine and phenylalanine. Tyrosine intake was limited to 45 mg/kg per day. Maxamaid, an orange-flavored dietary supplement, was administered as a source of tyrosine-free protein and extra calories. Tyrosine levels were monitored closely. Two weeks after the boy's initial visit to the dermatology clinic, his plasma tyrosine concentration had decreased to 450 nmol/ml. Despite stringent dietary control, his plasma tyrosine levels continue to range from 600 to 650 nmol/ml.

Currently, at 6 years of age, this boy remains somewhat hyperactive. Formal evaluations show normal speech and a mild language disorder; the total language score was 79, the expressive score was 85, and the receptive score was 75 (normal = 100 ± 15). His skin lesions and eye symptoms have never recurred. Tyrosinemia type II was diagnosed in a sister born in February 1994. Although her cord blood tyrosine level was normal, at 1½ days it was 1300 nmol/ml. After she received a low tyrosine diet for 1 to 2 days, her tyrosine level was 108 nmol/ml. With strict dietary control, subsequent levels have ranged from 100 to 294 nmol/ml.

DISCUSSION

Tyrosinemia type II (also known as oculocutaneous tyrosinemia and Richner-Hanhart syndrome) is a distinct clinical syndrome characterized by skin and eye lesions and, occasionally, mental retardation.[2] Plasma tyrosine levels are elevated because of a deficiency of hepatic tyrosine aminotransferase. The typical dermatologic findings include well-demarcated hyperkeratotic papules and plaques of the palms and soles. These lesions, which may begin as bullae and erosions that progress to crusted, hyperkeratotic plaques, are painful and often associated with hyperhidrosis.[3] The pain associated with the plantar lesions can be severe enough to cause refusal to walk. Few dermatologic

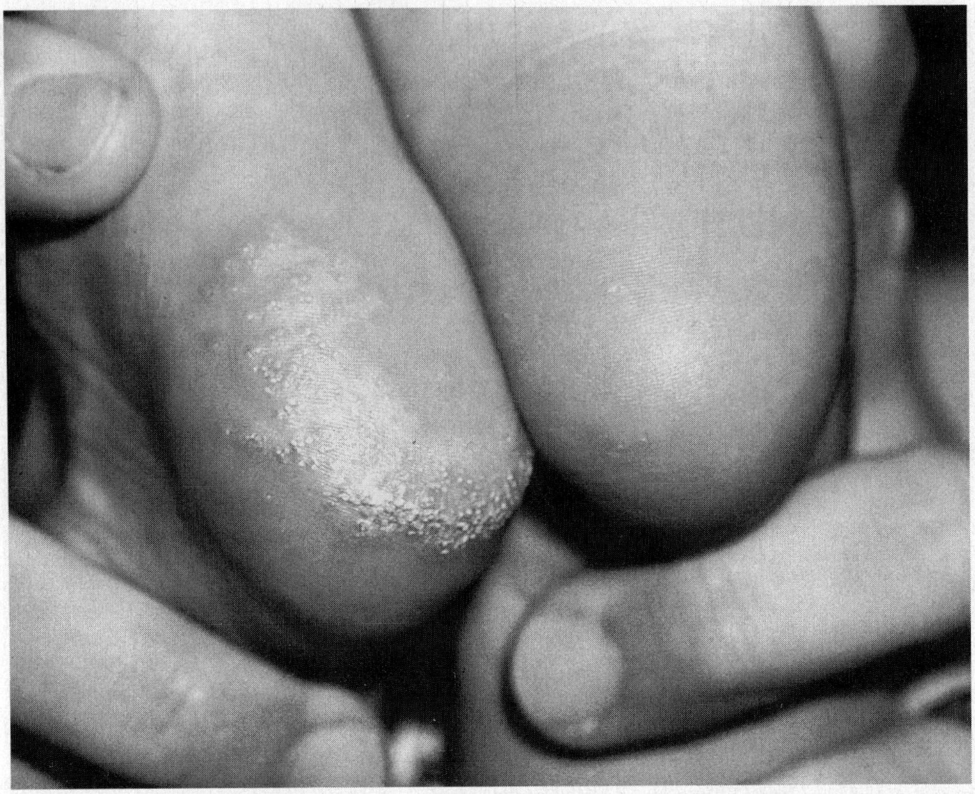

Fig. 2. Close-up view of hyperkeratotic plaque on right heel.

disorders occurring at these sites are accompanied by such intense pain. The hyperkeratosis is usually limited to pressure points on the soles, fingertips, and thenar and hypothenar eminences. A diagnosis of tyrosinemia type II can be made without palmar involvement, as in our patient. The pathogenesis of these skin lesions and the reason they occur in this particular distribution are unclear. Age at onset of skin lesions can range from the first few weeks of life to the second decade.[4]

Ophthalmologic features of tyrosinemia type II typically occur before skin lesions develop; the early signs consist of excessive tearing, redness, pain, and photophobia. Skin and ocular lesions may occur simultaneously or independently.[5] Eye symptoms can develop as early as 2 weeks of age. Late signs include corneal clouding with central or paracentral opacities, neovascularization, dendritic ulcers, and scarring. Deposition of tyrosine crystals in the cornea is responsible for the ocular changes and has been reported to occur in other forms of tyrosinemia as well.[6,7] In our patient, excessive tearing, redness, pain, and photophobia developed at 6 months of age. However, no abnormalities were detected on repeated ophthalmologic examinations despite the long duration of his symptoms.

Mental retardation and neurologic abnormalities are highly variable features of tyrosinemia type II.[1,4] Our patient had mild gross motor delays, hyperactivity, and a mild language disorder. The relationship between his behavioral problem and tyrosinemia II is unclear.

Dietary restriction of phenylalanine and tyrosine is the key to managing tyrosinemia type II.[8] Our patient was unusual because of his self-selected vegetarian-type diet; protein aversion has been reported in other inborn errors of metabolism. Although he has been adhering to a diet low in phenylalanine and tyrosine for 3 years, he has never been able to achieve normal plasma tyrosine levels. Because he has remained without symptoms, his current levels of 600 to 650 nmol/ml have been deemed to be acceptable. Ocular and skin lesions may become evident only when a certain threshold is exceeded. Because the special diet is difficult to follow, patients in whom there are no ocular or central nervous system abnormalities may be treated with etretinate, an aromatic retinoid that has been reported to control the hyperkeratotic skin lesions; however, long-term outcome has not been studied.[3]

Tyrosinemia type II is an autosomal recessive disorder. The tyrosine aminotransferase gene has been localized on human chromosome 16.[9] Perhaps in the future, with DNA analysis, heterozygotes (carriers) could be detected and prenatal diagnosis would be possible if requested.

Tyrosinemia type II, an easily treatable condition, should be considered in the differential diagnosis of eye pain and photophobia, especially if accompanied by painful palmoplantar keratoderma. When these features are present, a search for other hallmarks of the disease, such as corneal ulcerations and neurologic involvement, should be initiated. Early institution of a diet low in phenylalanine and tyrosine will promptly reverse ocular and cutaneous abnormalities. The effect of early dietary intervention on prevention of neurologic manifestations is unknown.

REFERENCES

1. Goulden KJ, Moss MA, Cole DE, et al. Pitfalls in the initial diagnosis of tyrosinemia: three case reports and a review of the literature. Clin Biochem 1987;20:207-12.
2. Goldsmith LA, Kang E, Bienfang DC, et al. Tyrosinemia with plantar and palmar keratosis and keratitis. J PEDIATR 1973; 83:798-805.
3. Fraser NG, MacDonald J, Griffiths WA, et al. Tyrosinemia type II (Richner-Hanhart syndrome): report of two cases treated with etretinate. Clin Exp Dermatol 1987;12:440-3.
4. Colditz PB, Yu JS, Billson FA, et al. Tyrosinaemia II. Med J Aust 1984;141:244-5.
5. Heidemann DG, Dunn SP, Bawle EV, et al. Early diagnosis of tyrosinemia type II. Am J Ophthalmol 1989;107:559-60.
6. Goldsmith LA. Tyrosinemia II: lessons in molecular pathophysiology. Pediatr Dermatol 1983;1:25-34.
7. Driscoll DJ, Jabs EW, Alcorn D, et al. Corneal tyrosine crystals in transient neonatal tyrosinemia. J PEDIATR 1988;113: 91-3.
8. Machino H, Miki Y, Kawatsu T, et al. Successful dietary control of tyrosinemia II. J Am Acad Dermatol 1983;9:533-9.
9. Natt E, Kao FT, Rettenmeier R, et al. Assignment of the human tyrosine aminotransferase gene to chromosome 16. Hum Genet 1986;72:225-8.

Loss of detectable antibody to hepatitis B surface antigen in immunized patients with hemophilia but without human immunodeficiency virus infection

John M. Maris, MD, Regina B. Butler, RN, and Alan R. Cohen, MD

From the Division of Hematology, Children's Hospital of Philadelphia, and the Department of Pediatrics, University of Pennsylvania School of Medicine, Philadelphia

We investigated the loss of detectable antibody directed against the hepatitis B surface antigen after immunization with hepatitis B vaccine in 55 patients who were seronegative for the human immunodeficiency virus and had hemophilia. Twenty percent of patients lost detectable antibody at a mean of 4.6 years after completion of immunization. Monitoring of hepatitis B serostatus or routine revaccination may be necessary. (J PEDIATR 1995;126:269-71)

Immunization against hepatitis B has become standard care for children with hemophilia.[1] Several studies have reported excellent seroconversion rates with either the plasma-derived or the recombinant vaccines in children and adults with factor VIII or IX deficiency who were seronegative for the human immunodeficiency virus.[2-5] Anti-hepatitis B surface antigen levels are achieved at high titer with intramuscular,[2] intradermal[6] or subcutaneous injection.[2, 7] Patients with hemophilia who have HIV infection are much less likely to mount an initial immune response,[3, 5, 8] and if one is achieved, it is commonly short lived.[8, 9]

HepB	Hepatitis B
HepBsAg	Hepatitis B surface antigen
HIV	Human immunodeficiency virus
EIA	Enzyme-linked immunoassay

Little information exists on the duration of the immune

Submitted for publication July 26, 1994; accepted Sept. 15, 1994.

Reprint requests: John M. Maris, MD, Division of Hematology, Children's Hospital of Philadelphia, 34th St. and Civic Center Blvd., Philadelphia, PA 19104.

0022-3476/95/$3.00 + 0 **9/22/60613**

Table. Patient characteristics

	No loss of antibody	Loss of antibody
No. of patients	44	11
Factor deficiency		
Severe VIII	33	6
Severe IX	4	1
Moderate VIII	4	3
Moderate IX	3	0
Mild VIII	0	1
Age at completion of immunization (yr)	1.68 ± 0.88	1.67 ± 1.03
Duration of follow-up (yr)	6.15 ± 2.98	5.99 ± 2.57
Number of anti-HepBsAg assays	6.00 ± 2.31	6.27 ± 1.79
Plasma-derived vaccine	31	6
Recombinant vaccine	13	5

response to HepB vaccination in children who have hemophilia but not HIV infection. We therefore conducted a retrospective study to determine the frequency and timing of the loss of detectable humoral immunity to HepB after children with hemophilia were administered primary immunization with the HepB vaccine.

METHODS

A chart review was conducted on all patients with factor VIII or IX deficiency who were receiving regular care in the Children's Hospital of Philadelphia Hemophilia Comprehensive Care Program between Jan. 1, 1980, and Dec. 31, 1990. All 55 patients had no detectable HepBsAg and repeatedly had no antibody against HIV on annual screenings. Each child had received a complete primary immunization series against HepB before the age of 4 years according to the recommendations of the manufacturers and the Centers for Disease Control and Prevention.[1] A plasma-derived vaccine (Heptavax; Merck Sharpe & Dohme, West Point, Pa.) was used at a dose of 10 μg until 1989. Thereafter a recombinant preparation (Recombivax; Merck Sharpe & Dohme) was used at a dose of 5 μg. All children received three doses. Patients received the initial does as soon as possible after the coagulation disorder was diagnosed and received subsequent doses 1 and 6 months later. The vaccines were administered subcutaneously into the anterior thigh with a 26-gauge needle.

Antibody directed toward HepBsAg was qualitatively assayed every 6 to 12 months by the enzyme-linked immunoassay technique[10] with the AUSAB kit (Abbott Laboratories, Abbott Park, Ill.). This EIA is sensitive to an anti-HepBsAg titer of 2 to 3 mIU/ml,[11] which indicates that a loss of detectable antibody by EIA correlates with an anti-HepBsAg titer less than the assumed minimal protective level of 10 mIU/ml.

Numeric values are presented as means ± SD. Statistical analysis was performed with either the Fisher Exact Test or the Student two-tailed *t* test.

RESULTS

Patient characteristics are presented in the Table. Of the 55 patients, 11 (20%) lost detectable antibody directed toward HepBsAg after having had an adequate primary immune response. Seroconversion was documented by positive results on at least two EIAs after the primary series was completed. The time to detection of the loss of antibody, as characterized by a negative EIA result and confirmed in six patients by a second negative EIA result, was 4.6 ± 2.2 years (median, 3.7 years; range, 1.8 to 7.9 years). The duration of follow-up for those patients who have not lost detectable antibody is 6.1 ± 3.0 years (median, 6.1 years; range, 1.0 to 11.2 years).

Patients who lost antibody and those who continued to have detectable antibody did not differ significantly in age at completion of immunization, serologic response (100% in both groups), duration of follow-up, or number of assays ($p \geq 0.95$ by Student *t* test). Moreover, no difference was found between the two groups when the age at completion of immunization was analyzed according to both yearly intervals ($p = 0.70$ by Fisher Exact Test) and immunization before and after 15 months of age ($p \geq 0.95$ by Fisher Exact Test). Loss of antibody was not related to the type of vaccine administered ($p = 0.45$ by Fisher Exact Test). No patient has had clinical or serologic evidence of HepB infection.

Of 11 patients who lost detectable antibody, 10 were reimmunized with one dose of vaccine and one patient had a series of three vaccinations. Each patient who was revaccinated had a serologic response that was demonstrated by a positive result on an anti-HepBsAg EIA and that has persisted during a mean follow-up period of 1.9 years (range, 0.5 to 2.7 years).

DISCUSSION

Although levels of antibody directed against HepBsAg wane with time after immunization with either plasma-derived or recombinant vaccine, the exact duration of seropositivity induced by the HepB vaccines remains uncertain.[12] Mannucci et al.[8] reported that 100% of 65 patients with hemophilia but without HIV infection, after four doses of plasma-derived vaccine, had detectable antibody at 4 years but progressively declining titers. Drake et al.,[9] investigating the alterations that HIV imposes on HepB immunity, reported a loss of detectable antibody in 7% of their patients who did not have HIV; however, neither the duration of immunity nor that of follow-up was specified. Our finding that one fifth of all children with hemophilia lost detectable anti-HepBsAg within a relatively short time after vaccination suggests that either heightened surveillance of anti-HepBsAg serostatus or periodic booster immunization should be part of routine clinical care in this high-risk group.

The amount of anti-HepBsAg wanes with time, but on rechallenge with vaccine a marked anamnestic response is seen.[13] It is possible that loss of detectable antibody by EIA has little bearing on the host's resistance to HepB infection because of prolonged immunologic memory.[14] However, no data are available to support the hypothesis that patients with loss of detectable antibody continue to be protected against HepB infection.

Many reasons exist for the decreasing incidence of HepB infection in persons with hemophilia, other than vaccination. These reasons include improved donor screening, viral inactivation of plasma-derived factor concentrates, and the introduction of recombinant factor VIII products. However, patients with hemophilia remain at increased risk of acquiring HepB, which indicates a need for diligent protection against this preventable disease. Until the duration of humoral immunity and the role of immunologic memory are better defined, children with hemophilia who have been immunized against HepB may benefit from periodic screening for anti-HepBsAg or from routine booster administration.

REFERENCES

1. Hepatitis B virus: a comprehensive strategy for eliminating transmission in the United States through universal childhood vaccination. Recommendations of the Immunization Practices Advisory Committee (ACIP). MMWR CDC Surveill Summ 1991;40:1-25.
2. Buchanan GR, Richards N, Sexauer CL, Stevens B. Serologic response to hepatitis B vaccine in children receiving multiple blood transfusions. Pediatr Infect Dis J 1986;5:68-70.
3. Zanetti AR, Mannucci PM, Tanzi E, et al. Hepatitis B vaccination of 113 hemophiliacs: lower antibody response in anti-LAV/HTLV-III–positive patients. Am J Hematol 1986;23: 339-45.
4. Mannucci PM, Gringeri A, Morfini M, et al. Immunogenicity of a recombinant hepatitis B vaccine in hemophiliacs. Am J Hematol 1988;29:211-4.
5. Chan W, Petric M, Wang E, Koren G, Read S, Blanchette V. Response to hepatitis B immunization in children with hemophilia: relationship to infection with human immunodeficiency virus type 1. J Pediatr 1990;117:427-30.
6. Parish DC, Muecke HW, Joiner TA, Pope WT, Hadler SC. Immunogenicity of low-dose intradermal recombinant DNA hepatitis B vaccine. South Med J 1991;84:426-30.
7. Janco RL. Immunogenicity of subcutaneous hepatitis B vaccine in hemophiliacs [Letter]. J Pediatr 1985;107:316.
8. Mannucci PM, Zanetti AR, Gringeri A, et al. Long-term immunogenicity of a plasma-derived hepatitis B vaccine in HIV seropositive and HIV seronegative hemophiliacs. Arch Intern Med 1989;149:1333-7.
9. Drake JH, Parmley RT, Britton HA. Loss of hepatitis B antibody in human immunodeficiency virus–positive hemophilia patients. Pediatr Infect Dis J 1987;6:1051-4.
10. Hildebrand RL. Elisa (Enzyme-Linked Immunosorbent Assay). In: Rytel MN, ed. Rapid diagnosis in infectious disease. New York: CRC Press, 1979.
11. Wolters G, Nelissen P, Kuijpers L. Improved ELISA for the detection of HBsAg. J Virol Methods 1985;10:299-305.
12. Greenberg DP. Pediatric experience with recombinant hepatitis B vaccines and relevant safety and immunogenicity studies. Pediatr Infect Dis J 1993;12:438-45.
13. Milne A, Krugman S, Waldon JA, et al. Hepatitis B vaccination in children: five year booster study. N Z Med J 1992; 105:336-8.
14. Resti M, Di Francesco G, Azzari C, Rossi ME, Vierucci A. Anti-HBs and immunological memory to HBV vaccine: implication for booster timing [Letter]. Vaccine 1993;11:1079.

Effect of maternal glucocorticoid exposure on risk of severe intraventricular hemorrhage in surfactant-treated preterm infants

Jeffery S. Garland, MD, SM,[a] Rosanne Buck, MSN, CNNP, and Alan Leviton, MD, SM

From the Joint Program in Neonatology and the Department of Neurology, Harvard Medical School, and Children's Hospital, Boston, Massachusetts

Objective: **To determine whether the reduced risk of severe intraventricular hemorrhage (SIVH) that follows antenatal maternal glucocorticoid (AMG) receipt is mediated by an AMG effect on blood pressure or improved respiratory function in infants who receive artificial surfactant as rescue therapy.**
Design: **Retrospective cohort study.**
Setting: **Two level III neonatal intensive care units, Boston, Mass.**
Participants: **Two hundred twenty-five infants ≤32 weeks of gestational age and ≤1.7 kg birth weight, treated with surfactant.**
Main findings: **SIVH occurred in 10% (10/102) of infants who were exposed to AMG, compared with 23% (25/111) of infants not exposed (odds ratio, 0.4; 95% confidence interval, 0.2 to 0.8). Hypotension and need for colloid or dopamine were associated with both SIVH and the absence of AMG exposure ($p \leq 0.03$). Logistic regression models of SIVH risk and AMG exposure, with adjustment for antenatal potential confounders, were altered by the addition of measures of hypotension. Most clinical measures of pulmonary function, both before and after surfactant receipt, were not associated with reduced risk of SIVH and did not appear to account for the increased risk of SIVH in babies not exposed to AMG.**
Conclusion: **The reduced risk of SIVH in preterm newborn infants whose mothers received AMG was associated with normal blood pressures. The association between AMG and SIVH was not consistently enhanced by respiratory function improvement after surfactant therapy. (J PEDIATR 1995;126:272-9)**

Antenatal maternal glucocorticosteroid treatment before the delivery of high-risk preterm infants decreases the incidence and severity of respiratory distress syndrome and also appears to reduce the incidence of periventricular-intraventricular hemorrhage.[1-9] Some authors have postulated that the risk of PIVH can be reduced by reducing the risk of RDS.[10]

In this observational study, we wanted to identify how AMG reduced the risk of severe intraventricular hemorrhage, defined as intraventricular hemorrhage filling much of the lateral ventricle or intraventricular hemorrhage, with acute dilation. We considered two possible mechanisms. One was through improvement in lung function and lowered likelihood of increased intrathoracic pressure (i.e., less grunting or "bucking the respirator") and, consequently, a

Supported in part by a grant from the Medical Foundation, Boston, Massachusetts.

Submitted for publication Dec. 20, 1993; accepted Aug. 12, 1994.

Reprint requests: Jeffery S. Garland, MD, SM, 5000 West Chambers St., Milwaukee, WI 53210.

[a]Now at St. Joseph's Hospital, Milwaukee, Wis.

0022-3476/95/$3.00 + 0 **9/23/59940**

See related article, p. 317.

a/A	Arterial/alveolar [ratio]
AMG	Antenatal maternal glucocorticoidsteroid
OI	Oxygenation index
PIVH	Periventricular-intraventricular hemorrhage
RDS	Respiratory distress syndrome
SIVH	Severe intraventricular hemorrhage
VEI	Ventilatory efficiency index

lowered probability of increased cerebral venous pressure. Another was by reducing the risk of hypotension and the need for volume expanders, both of which have been associated with PIVH. A third mechanism, which could not be evaluated in this sample, was that AMG enhanced the maturation of intracranial vessels traversing areas of the germinal matrix.

METHODS

Subjects. The population for this retrospective cohort study included all infants who were ≤32 weeks of gestational age (≤1700 gm), had received rescue artificial surfactant (Exosurf [Burroughs Wellcome]) therapy for RDS within the first 24 hours of life, had no major congenital anomalies, and had been cared for at one of two special care nurseries between November 1989 and April 1992. The study population was further limited to infants who had at least one cranial ultrasound study during the first 14 days of life. Care at both nurseries was provided by the same group of neonatology fellows and attending physicians.

Between November 1989 and August 1990, rescue surfactant therapy was administered in two doses, 12 hours apart, to infants who had radiographs compatible with respiratory distress syndrome, required mechanical ventilation, and had arterial/alveolar ratios of ≤0.22 before the first dose of artificial surfactant. After U.S. Food and Drug Administration approval of Exosurf in August 1990, criteria for surfactant therapy were liberalized and infants with RDS were eligible for Exosurf if they required a mean airway pressure of ≥7 cm H_2O and a fractional inspiratory oxygen concentration of at least 0.40 to maintain acceptable arterial blood gas values.

Exposures. Data were collected from infant and maternal records by two of us (R.B. and J.S.G.). The gestational age of 63% of babies was determined by a first-trimester sonogram. Maternal dates (13%) or Ballard evaluation[11] (23%) was used to determine gestational age when early sonograms were not available. Glucocorticoids were given to women in preterm labor at the discretion of attending obstetricians; AMG treatment consisted of either two doses of betamethasone separated by 24 hours or four doses of dexamethasone 12 hours apart. A course was considered complete if there was at least a 24-hour, but not more than a 7-day, delay between the last dose and delivery. A second complete course was defined in a similar fashion. A partial course of AMGs was defined by at least one dose of glucocorticoids before delivery but less than a complete course.

Data collected from each record included demographics and information pertaining to the pregnancy, delivery room events, and the clinical course before artificial surfactant treatment and for the subsequent 24 hours. Data on ventilator settings, clinical measures of pulmonary function, and changes with time in these measures were also collected from each record. These clinical measures of severity of pulmonary disease included oxygenation index[12, 13] (mean airway pressure × fraction of inspired oxygen/arterial oxygen tension), a/A oxygen tension ratio,[12-16] and ventilatory efficiency index[17] [3800/(positive inspiratory pressure − positive expiratory pressure) × respiratory rate × arterial carbon dioxide tension]. Because most PIVHs occur during the first 48 hours of life,[18-21] we limited our study to the interval between birth and 24 hours after the first dose of artificial surfactant, which was invariably given between 1 and 24 hours of life.

Whenever possible, exposures were dichotomized into clinically relevant strata that have been used in past studies.[3, 13] For clinical measures of pulmonary function improvement, we compared infants in the upper quartile of improvement with those in the lower three quartiles.

Outcomes. Cranial sonograms were obtained at the discretion of the clinicians; in 60% of infants (134/225) the first scan was obtained within the first 24 hours of life. Subsequent scans were obtained most often on postnatal days 3, 7, 14, and 28. Cranial sonograms were obtained with a DS-30 Diasonics real-time unit (Diasonics Inc., Milpitas, Calif.) with either a 5, 6, or 7.5 MHz transducer (Children's Hospital) or a Mark-100 unit (Advanced Technology Laboratories, Inc., Bothell, Wash.) with a 5 or 7.5 MHz transducer (Brigham and Women's Hospital). These scans were evaluated by ultrasonographers at each institution who had no knowledge of each child's AMG exposure. Severe intraventricular hemorrhage was defined as an intraventricular hemorrhage filling much of a lateral ventricle, or intraventricular hemorrhage with acute ventricular dilation. Parenchymal hemorrhages unaccompanied by SIVH were excluded from the analysis.

Data analysis. Three hypotheses were evaluated:

1. Among babies who require rescue surfactant, those exposed to AMG are at lower risk of having SIVH than those not so exposed.
2. The reduced risk of SIVH associated with AMG in babies who require rescue surfactant is accompanied by reduced risk of hypotension and reduced need of

Table I. Percentage of infants with (n = 35) and those without (n = 178) SIVH who had each maternal or neonatal characteristic

	SIVH		
	(+)	(−)	*p*
Maternal factors			
Outborn	20	10	0.08
Pregnancy-induced hypertension	6	25	**0.01**
Rupture of membranes ≥24 hr	9	19	0.1
Chorioamnionitis	3	8	0.5
Cesarean section	54	72	**0.04**
Cesarean section for fetal distress	37	46	0.5
Any maternal glucocorticoids	29	52	**0.01**
Infant characteristics			
Male	66	56	0.3
Birth weight ≤1.0 kg	49	47	0.8
Gestational age ≤28 wk	71	57	0.1
Apgar score (at 5 min) <5	20	8	0.06
Nursery course/treatment *before* surfactant			
Sodium bicarbonate for acidosis	14	4	**0.03**
Mean arterial blood pressure <30 mm Hg	74	54	**0.03**
Dopamine for hypotension	31	18	0.08
Albumin ≥10 ml/kg for hypotension	46	25	**0.02**
Mean airway pressure at ≥10 cm H_2O	50	36	0.1
a/A ratio ≤0.15	66	52	0.07
VEI ≤0.15	59	31	**0.002**
OI ≥0.25	13	7	**0.03**
Positive inspiratory pressure ≥25 cm H_2O	40	27	0.1
Nursery course/treatment *after* surfactant receipt			
Average mean blood pressure <30 mm Hg			
At 0-12 hr	38	40	0.9
At 12-24 hr	29	25	0.6
Albumin requirements for hypotension ≥10 ml/kg	46	39	0.4
Dopamine for hypotension	26	24	0.8
Mean airway pressure ≥10 cm H_2O*	47	23	**0.02**
Positive inspiratory pressure ≥25 cm H_2O*	57	58	**0.04**
Pulmonary function improvements from baseline*			
VEI: ≤77%	77	71	0.2
a/A ratio: ≤150%	66	76	0.2
OI: ≤65%	93	88	0.7
PIP: no improvement	88	78	0.2

PIP, Positive inspiratory pressure.
*Assessed 24 hours after surfactant.

colloid or dopamine infusion before rescue receipt of surfactant.

3. The reduced risk of SIVH associated with AMG is not appreciably influenced by the magnitude of pulmonary function improvement after surfactant therapy.

After correlates of SIVH were identified (Table I), correlates of AMG were considered (Table II). Rate ratios were then evaluated among infants exposed and those not exposed to AMG, stratified by the presence or absence of measures of physiologic characteristics associated with both SIVH and AMG (Table III). These stratified analyses were examined to determine to what extent the AMG effect on SIVH risk might have been influenced by covariates. Only covariates associated with both SIVH and AMG at a *p* level of ≤0.25 were evaluated.

In another attempt to identify variables that might explain how AMG reduces SIVH risk, we first modeled SIVH risk with logistic regression analysis, adjusting for five maternal or infant variables unalterable by subsequent nursery therapies (i.e., pregnancy-induced hypertension, cesarean delivery, rupture of membranes ≥24 hours before delivery, delivery in a hospital without a level III nursery, and gestational age ≤28 weeks). We then compared the AMG regression coefficient (an index of AMG effect on SIVH risk) in this model with the coefficient in models that also included selected, individual postnatal measures of

Table II. Percentage of infants exposed (n = 102) and those not exposed (n = 111) to AMG who had each maternal and neonatal characteristic to surfactant

	AMG*		
	(+)	(−)	p
Maternal factors			
Outborn	1	22	**0.001**
Rupture of membranes ≥24 hr	30	6	**0.001**
Chorioamnionitis	9	6	0.5
Cesarean section	65	73	0.2
Cesarean section for fetal distress	37	46	0.4
Pregnancy-induced hypertension	25	19	0.3
Infant characteristics			
Male	60	56	0.6
Birth weight ≤1.0 kg	49	45	0.6
Gestational age ≤28 wk	63	57	0.4
Apgar score at 5 min: <5	7	14	0.1
Nursery course/treatment *before* surfactant			
Dopamine for hypotension	9	32	**0.001**
Mean arterial blood pressure <30 mm Hg	46	68	**0.001**
Albumin for hypotension ≥10 cc/kg	15	41	**0.001**
Sodium bicarbonate for metabolic acidosis	4	7	0.3
Mean airway pressure ≥10 cm	27	48	**0.003**
a/A ratio ≤0.15	44	64	**0.004**
VEI ≤0.15	30	41	0.1
Positive inspiratory pressure ≥25 cm H_2O	25	33	0.2
OI ≥0.25	5	11	0.2
Nursery course/treatment *after* surfactant receipt			
Average mean blood pressure <30 mm Hg			
At 0-12 hr	35	44	0.2
At 12-24 hr	25	27	0.6
Albumin requirement for hypotension: ≥10 ml/kg	27	51	**0.001**
Dopamine for hypotension	20	29	0.1
Mean airway pressure ≥10 cm H_2O	20	39	**0.004**
Positive inspiratory pressure ≥25 cm H_2O	30	51	**0.002**
Pulmonary function improvements from baseline*			
VEI: ≤75%	71	72	0.9
a/A: ≤150%	82	66	**0.009**
OI: ≤65%	85	92	0.1
PIP: no improvement	83	76	0.2

PIP, Positive inspiratory pressure.
*Assessed 24 hours after surfactant therapy.

respiratory function and blood pressure. We separately evaluated eight characteristics identified before surfactant receipt and nine characteristics after receipt of surfactant. Finally we added groups of those postnatal variables that individually most changed the AMG coefficient.

RESULTS

Of 280 infants who received artificial surfactant from November 1989 to April 1992, a total of 241 received rescue artificial surfactant during the first 24 hours of life; 225 of these infants had at least one cranial sonogram during the first 14 days of life. We excluded 12 infants who had a parenchymal hemorrhage but did not satisfy the study criteria for SIVH, leaving 213 infants for the final analysis.

Timing of the first cranial sonogram in relation to the first dose of artificial surfactant or birth time was not associated with AMG exposure, birth weight, or final SIVH status. Infants ≤28 weeks of gestational age were more likely than older infants to have ultrasonographic examination of the head during the first 24 postnatal hours ($p = 0.01$). No measure of pulmonary function before or improvement after surfactant therapy was associated with the timing of the first cranial sonogram.

Seventeen percent (36/213) of infants died, 12 during the first week of life. We obtained at least two cranial sonograms of 8 of these infants before their death. Of the 12 infants who died during the first week of life, 6 had been exposed to AMG.

Table III. Percentage of infants who had SIVH (n = 35), presented separately for strata of sample classified by both AMG exposure and selected characteristics

Potential effect modifier	AMG (+)	AMG (−)	Odds ratio (95% CI)
Gestational age			
Age ≤28 wk	13	27	**0.4 (0.2-0.98)**
Age >28 wk	5	17	0.3 (0.06-1.4)
Apgar score (at 5 min)			
<5	29	33	0.8 (0.1-5.7)
≥5	8	21	**0.4 (0.1-0.8)**
Dopamine before surfactant	22	26	0.8 (0.1-4.8)
No dopamine before surfactant	9	21	**0.4 (0.1-0.9)**
VEI at time of surfactant*			
≤0.15	17	34	0.4 (0.1-1.3)
>0.15	7	14	0.5 (0.2-1.5)
a/A ratio at time of surfactant			
≤0.15	14	26	0.5 (0.2-1.3)
>0.15	7	18	0.4 (0.1-1.3)
a/A ratio improvement			
≤150% improvement	13	19	0.6 (0.3-1.6)
>150% improvement	0	36	**0.0†**
Positive inspiratory pressure improvement			
No improvement	10	26	**0.3 (0.1-0.8)**
Any improvement	6	12	0.5 (0.05-5.2)
Positive inspiratory pressure at 24 hr			
≥25 cm H_2O	13	29	0.4 (0.1-1.3)
<25 cm H_2O	9	17	0.5 (0.2-1.4)

Percentages are specific for each row and column.
CI, Confidence interval.
*Newborn infants with missing value not included.
†Confidence interval cannot be calculated.

Severe intraventricular hemorrhage developed in 16% (35/213) of the infants. Because SIVH risk was similar for infants who exposted to a complete or partial course of glucocorticoids (10% [6/59] vs 9% [4/43]), the groups were combined. Ten percent (10/102) of infants who were exposed to any AMG had SIVH, compared with 23% (25/111) of infants who were not (odds ratio, 0.4; 95% confidence interval, 0.2 to 0.8).

Physiologic characteristics and their correlates before artificial surfactant that were associated with increased SIVH risk included sodium bicarbonate infusion (p = 0.03), hypotension (defined as a mean arterial blood pressure <30 mm Hg) (p = 0.03), hypotension treated with more than 10 ml/kg of colloid (p = 0.02), VEI ≤0.15 (p = 0.002), and OI ≥0.25 (p = 0.03) (Table I). Of nine potential risk factors for SIVH during the 24 hours after surfactant therapy, only a high mean airway pressure (≥10 cm H_2O) and a high positive inspiratory pressure (defined as ≥25 cm H_2O) were associated with an increased risk of SIVH (p ≤0.04).

Pulmonary function improvement (i.e., percentage change in OI, VEI, or a/A ratio) was not associated with SIVH (Table I). When the a/A ratio improvement was stratified by the level of a/A ratio before surfactant, infants with low a/A ratios (≤0.15) had similar (20% vs 23%; p = 0.7) rates of SIVH whether or not their a/A ratio improved after surfactant. Infants with a/A ratios >0.15 before surfactant whose a/A ratios improved ≥150% after surfactant were more likely to have SIVH than were infants showing less improvement (38% [3/8] vs 9% [8/85]; p = 0.05).

Before surfactant therapy, infants exposed to any AMG were less likely than infants not so exposed to become hypotensive (p = 0.001) or to receive dopamine (p = 0.001) or colloid infusions (p = 0.001) for blood pressure support (Table II). Infants exposed to any AMG were also less likely to require a high mean airway pressure (p = 0.003) and have a low a/A ratio (p = 0.004). After artificial surfactant therapy, infants exposed to any AMG required less colloid support (p ≤0.04) and were less likely to require a high positive inspiratory pressure (≥25 cm H_2O; p = 0.002) or mean airway pressure (≥10 cm H_2O; p = 0.004). Infants exposed to AMG were also less likely to show a great improvement (i.e., ≥150% improvement from baseline) in their a/A ratios after artificial surfactant therapy (p ≤0.009).

The reduced risk of SIVH in infants exposed to AMG was most prominent among babies with 5-minute Apgar scores ≥5 and for babies who did not receive dopamine before surfactant therapy (Table III). Hypotensive episodes and colloid infusion appeared to influenced the AMG/SIVH relation in a fashion similar to dopamine infusion (data not shown). SIVH risk differences between neonates exposed to AMG and those not exposed were not consistently influenced by pulmonary function improvement after surfactant therapy. Reduction in SIVH associated with AMG was greatest among infants showing the greatest improvement (>150%) in a/A ratio after surfactant therapy. On the other hand, SIVH risk reduction associated with AMG was more apparent in infants showing no improvement with respect to positive inspiratory pressure after surfactant therapy than in infants who showed any improvement in positive inspiratory pressures (Table III). Measures of pulmonary function improvement after surfactant that were determined primarily by the level of ventilatory support, such as percentage of change in OI or VEI, were not analyzed because they were not associated with either AMG (change in VEI) or SIVH (change in OI). Analyses limited to infants ≤28 weeks of gestational age (data not shown) demonstrated similar findings.

In logistic regression models that adjusted for five maternal or infant characteristics evident by the time of birth (gestational age, pregnancy-induced hypertension, birth in hospital without level III nursery, cesarean birth, rupture of membranes >24 hours), the use of AMG was associated with a reduced risk of SIVH (odds ratio, 0.5; 95% confidence interval, 0.2 to 1.1). The regression coefficient for AMG was altered most by the addition of individual or groups of postnatal correlates of low blood pressure and less by individual or groups of clinical measures of respiratory illness before surfactant therapy (Table IV). Adding correlates for hypotension occurring after surfactant therapy to the regression model did not reduce the association between AMG and SIVH (data not shown). Adding individual or groups of measures of pulmonary function that exhibited little change after surfactant therapy accentuated the apparent protective effect of AMG on SIVH risk (regression coefficient for AMG increased by up to 28%; data not shown).

Table IV. Risk of SIVH among newborn infants exposed to AMG as a function of the risk among newborn infants not so exposed

Postnatal variable before surfactant therapy	Odds ratio* (95% CI)	Percentage change in AMG
Apgar score at 5 min: <5	0.5 (0.2, 1.3)	−18
Sodium bicarbonate for acidosis	0.5 (0.2, 1.3)	−12
Dopamine infusion	0.5 (0.2, 1.2)	−3
Mean arterial blood pressure <30 mm Hg	0.5 (0.2, 1.2)	−11
Albumin ≥10 ml/kg	0.5 (0.2, 1.3)	−11
a/A ratio ≤0.15	0.5 (0.2, 1.2)	−8
VEI ≤0.15	0.5 (0.2, 1.2)	−6
Positive inspiratory pressure ≥25 cm H_2O	0.5 (0.2, 1.2)	−6
Sets of variables		
Correlates of hypotension: Albumin ≥10 ml/kg, Sodium bicarbonate for acidosis	0.5 (0.2, 1.3)	−17
Measures of respiratory illness severity: a/A ratio ≤0.15, VEI ≤0.15	0.5 (0.2, 1.3)	−9
Both sets of variables	0.5 (0.2, 1.4)	−15

All values are adjusted for five antenatal variables (pregnancy-induced hypertension, abdominal delivery, rupture of membranes ≥24 hours, gestational age, birth in hospital without level III nursery). Additional adjustment was made for the postnatal variable listed on the left. The percentage change in the AMG coefficient compares logistic regression models with and without the variable on the left.
*Point estimate (95% confidence interval).

DISCUSSION

This study had four main findings. First, in agreement with prior studies, AMG receipt is associated with a reduced risk of SIVH. Second, a partial course of AMG administration appears to be as effective as a full course. Third, the SIVH protective effects of AMG appear to be explained by or correlated with avoidance of hypotension. Fourth, marked improvement in clinical measures of pulmonary function after surfactant therapy did not appear to enhance the beneficial effects of AMG on SIVH risk.

If AMG produced much of its SIVH reduction via improved pulmonary function during the first hours of life, thereby reducing the need for surfactant, the babies who most prominently responded to AMG would be excluded from this sample. Thus our finding of an AMG effect on SIVH risk even in babies with significant respiratory distress treated with surfactant therapy adds to the evidence that much of the SIVH risk reduction caused by AMG is not a consequence of improved pulmonary function.

Some have found, as did we, that hypotension is associated with increased risk of intracranial hemorrhage,[22-25] whereas others have not.[26, 27] Receipt of volume expanders also appears to be associated with increased risk of intracranial hemorrhage.[28, 29] In the beagle puppy, both hypotension and subsequent volume expansion appear to be required to induce intraventricular hemorrhage.[30]

As we did, Moise et al.[21] found that "antenatal steroids reduce the need for blood pressure support in extremely premature infants." In addition, mean blood pressure in preterm sheep appears to be stabilized by exposure to AMG.[31] In our data set, some of the SIVH risk information conveyed by hypotension and volume expansion is appropriated by the AMG variable. This suggests that some of the SIVH reduction by AMG might be achieved through reduced risk of hypotension and the need for volume expansion.

In stratified analyses, the SIVH reduction capability of AMG was more obvious in babies who had good Apgar scores and in those who did not receive dopamine or albumin before surfactant therapy. Thus, although AMG was associated with less dopamine or albumin use for hypotension and may thereby contribute to reducing the risk of SIVH, the SIVH risk reduction in those who did not receive dopamine suggests that another mechanism might be involved. For example, it is possible that AMG enhances maturation of blood vessels within the ganglionic eminence,[32] thereby improving their capacity to withstand transmural pressures and other influences thought to contribute to PIVH.[33] We were unable to evaluate this hypothesis.

This study has several limitations. First is the method of ascertaining gestational age. Although 63% of babies had gestational age determined by a first-trimester sonogram, Ballard evaluations served as the measure of gestational age in approximately 23% of infants. Second, as in other studies,[5] we do not know when many of the hemorrhages occurred. Thus we cannot establish an exact temporal relation between SIVH and receipt of surfactant.

Others have reported that low birth weight infants who

receive AMG are at reduced risk of having intracranial hemorrhage,[2, 3, 5-8, 34, 35] even after partial courses.[1, 4, 5] This, however, has not always been the case.[34] The apparent effectiveness of partial courses has been evident only since the availability of surfactants. Many other changes in the care of women at risk of undergoing preterm delivery have also been made since then. Although others have suggested that surfactant may potentiate some of the intracranial beneficial effects of AMG,[5] we were unable to demonstrate that a marked improvement in pulmonary function after surfactant therapy enhanced the association between AMG and SIVH. Our findings may differ from those recently reported because of differences in study design, study populations, definition of outcomes, or surfactant preparations.

The evidence that AMG reduces the risk of PIVH satisfies all the epidemiologic criteria of causation.[36] The strength criterion is met by the finding that in most studies the odds ratio is close to 0.5. Because AMG receipt antedates the vast majority of PIVH, the temporal order criterion is also satisfied. An expanding literature about the effects of corticosteroids on fetal lung, heart, and cerebral blood vessels provides support for the biologic plausibility criterion.[31, 37, 38] Most impressive, however, is support for the experiment criterion. Five of six randomized clinical trials demonstrated that preterm newborn infants whose mothers received AMG had a prominently reduced risk of PIVH.[39] Our data support the hypothesis that some of the SIVH protection provided by AMG is mediated by the reduced occurrence of hypotension, reduced need for blood pressure support (including volume expansion), or closely related phenomena.

We conclude that AMG exposure reduces SIVH risk in newborn infants who require artificial surfactant therapy. This appears to be true for both gestationally younger and gestationally older infants. Although AMG was associated with the reduced occurrence of hypotension, the beneficial effects of AMG on SIVH were evident even among preterm infants with acceptable blood pressure levels. Measures of pulmonary function improvement after surfactant therapy, especially those related to ventilatory requirements, did not appear to enhance the protective effect that AMG had on SIVH risk.

REFERENCES

1. Jobe AH, Mitchell BR, Gunkel JH. Beneficial effects of the combined use of prenatal corticosteroids and postnatal surfactant on preterm infants. Am J Obstet Gynecol 1993;168:508-13.
2. Garite TJ, Rumney P, Briggs GG, et al. A randomized, placebo-controlled trial of betamethasone for prevention of respiratory distress syndrome at 24 to 48 weeks' gestation. Am J Obstet Gynecol 1993;166:646-51.
3. Leviton A, Kuban KC, Pagano M, et al. Antenatal corticosteroids appear to reduce the risk of postnatal germinal matrix hemorrhage in intubated low birth weight babies. Pediatrics 1993;91:1083-8.
4. Andrews EB, White AD, Weinberg JM, et al. Antenatal steroids and neonatal outcomes in infants receiving surfactants in Exosurf treatment IND [Abstract]. Pediatr Res 1992;31:241A.
5. Kari M, Hallman M, Eronen M, et al. Prenatal dexamethasone treatment in conjunction with rescue therapy of human surfactant: a randomized, placebo-controlled, multicenter study. Pediatrics 1994;93:730-6.
6. Doran TA, Sawyer P, MacMurray B, et al. Results of a double-blind controlled study on the use of betamethasone in prevention of respiratory distress syndrome. Am J Obstet Gynecol 1980;136:313-20.
7. Morales WJ, Diebel D, Lazar A, Zadrozny D. The effect of antenatal dexamethasone administration the prevention of respiratory distress syndrome in preterm gestations with premature rupture of membranes. Am J Obstet Gynecol 1986; 154:591-5.
8. Gamsu HR, Mullinger BM, Donnai P, Dash CH. Antenatal administration of betamethasone to prevent respiratory distress syndrome in preterm infants: report of a UK multicenter trial. Br J Obstet Gynaecol 1989;96:401-10.
9. O'Shea M, Savitz DA, Hage ML, Feinstein KA. Prenatal events and the risk of subependymal/intraventricular hemorrhage in very low birth weight neonates. Paediatr Perinat Epidemiol 1992;6:352-62.
10. Volpe JJ. Intraventricular hemorrhage in the premature infant: current concepts. Part I. Ann Neurol 1989;25:3-11.
11. Ballard JL, Novack KK, Driver A. A simplified score assessment of fetal maturation of newly born infants. J PEDIATR 1979;95:769-84.
12. Fujiwara T, Kouishi M, Chida S, et al. Surfactant replacement therapy with a single postventilatory dose of a reconstituted bovine surfactant in preterm neonate with respiratory distress syndrome: final analysis of a multicenter, double-blind, randomized trial and comparison with similar trials. Pediatrics 1990;86:753-64.
13. Hallman M, Merritt TA, Jarvenpaa AL, et al. Exogenous human surfactant for treatment of severe respiratory distress syndrome: a randomized prospective clinical trial. J PEDIATR 1985;106:963-9.
14. Hallman M, Merritt TA, Kristina B, Berry C. Association between neonatal care practices and efficacy of exogenous human surfactant: results of a bicenter randomized trial. Pediatrics 1993;91:552-60.
15. Horbar JD, Soll RF, Schachinger H, et al. A European multicenter randomized controlled trial of single-dose surfactant therapy for idiopathic respiratory distress syndrome. Eur J Pediatr 1990;149:416-23.
16. Horbar JD, Soll RF, Sutherland JM, et al. A multicenter randomized placebo-controlled trial of surfactant therapy for respiratory distress syndrome. N Engl J Med 1989;320:959-65.
17. Kwong MS, Egan EA, Notter RH, Shapiro DL. Double-blind clinical trial of calf lung surfactant extract for the prevention of hyaline membrane disease in extremely premature infants. Pediatrics 1985;76:585-91.
18. Paneth N, Pinto-Martin J, Gardiner J, et al. Incidence and timing of germinal matrix/intraventricular hemorrhage in low birth weight infants. Am J Epidemiol 1993;137:1167-76.
19. Ment LR, Duncan CC, Ehrenbranz RA, et al. Intraventricu-

lar hemorrhage in the preterm neonate: timing and cerebral blood flow changes. J PEDIATR 1984;104:419-25.
20. Perlman JM, Volpe JJ. Intraventricular hemorrhage in extremely small premature infants. Am J Dis Child 1986; 140:1122-4.
21. Moise AA, Wearden ME, Kozinetz CA, et al. Antenatal steroids reduce the need for blood pressure support in extremely premature infants [Abstract]. Am J Perinatol 1994;11:171.
22. McDonald MM, Koops BL, Guggenheim MA, et al. Timing and etiology of neonatal intracranial hemorrhage. Pediatrics 1984;74:32-6.
23. Miall-Allen VM, de Vries LS, Dubowitz LMS, Whitelaw AGL. Blood pressure fluctuation and intraventricular hemorrhage in the preterm infants of less than 31 weeks gestation. Pediatrics 1989;83:657-61.
24. Watkins AMC, West CR, Cooke RWI. Blood pressure and cerebral haemorrhage and ischaemia in very low birth weight infants. Early Hum Dev 1989;19:103-10.
25. Bada HS, Korones SB, Perry EH, et al. Mean arterial blood pressure changes in premature infants and those at risk for intraventricular hemorrhage. J PEDIATR 1990;117:607-14.
26. Pryds O, Greisen G, Lou H, Friis-Hansen B. Heterogeneity of cerebral vasoreactivity in preterm infants supported by mechanical ventilation. J PEDIATR 1989;115:638-45.
27. Perry EH, Bada HS, Ray JD, et al. Blood pressure increases birth weight dependent stability boundary and intraventricular hemorrhage. Pediatrics 1990;85:727-32.
28. Goldberg RN, Chung D, Goldman SL, Bancalari E. The association of rapid volume expansion and intraventricular hemorrhage in the preterm infant. J PEDIATR 1980;96:1060-3.
29. Murton LJ, Butt WW, Mackay JR, et al. Perinatal factors periventricular haemorrhage and mortality in very low birth weight infants. Austr Pediatr J 1985;21:39-43.
30. Goddard-Finegold J, Armstrong DL, Zeller RS. Intraventricular hemorrhage following volume expansion after hypovolemic hypotension in the newborn beagle. J PEDIATR 1982; 100:796-9.
31. Stein HM, Oyama K, Martinez A, et al. Effects of corticosteroids in preterm sheep on adaption and sympathoadrenal mechanisms at birth. Am J Physiol 1993;264 (Endocrinol Metab) 27:E763-9.
32. Kitchens CS, Pendergast JF. Human thrombocytopenia is associated with structural abnormalities of the endothelium that are ameliorated by glucocorticoid administration. Blood 1986; 67:203-6.
33. Sotrel A, Lorenzo AV. Ultrastructure of blood vessels in the ganglionic eminence of premature rabbits with spontaneous germinal matrix hemorrhages. J Neuropathol Exp Neurol 1989; 48:462-82.
34. Ment LR, Oh W, Philip AGS, et al. Risk factors for early intraventricular hemorrhage in low birth weight infants. J PEDIATR 1992;121:776-83.
35. Eronen M, Kari A, Pesonen E, Hallman M. The effect of antenatal dexamethasone administration on the fetal and neonatal ductus arteriosus: a randomized double-blind study. Am J Dis Child 1993;147:187-92.
36. Susser M. What is a cause and how do we know one? a grammar for pragmatic epidemiology. Am J Epidemiol 1991;133: 635-48.
37. Meyer JS. Biochemical effects of corticosteroids on neural tissues. Physiol Rev 1985;65:946-1020.
38. Ikegami M, Berry D, Elkady T, et al. Corticosteroids and surfactant change lung function and protein leaks in the lungs of ventilated premature rabbits. J Clin Invest 1987;79:1371-8.
39. Crowley P. Update of the antenatal steroid meta-analysis: current knowledge and the future research needs [Appendix to report of the Panel for Consensus Development Conference on Effect of Corticosteroids for Fetal Maturation on Perinatal Outcomes]. Bethesda, Maryland: Office of Medical Applications of Research, National Institute of Health, 1994.

Reducing blood donor exposures in low birth weight infants by the use of older, unwashed packed red blood cells

David A. Lee, MD, Terri A. Slagle, MD, Thomas M. Jackson, MD, and Cherie S. Evans, MD

From the Departments of Neonatology and Pathology, California Pacific Medical Center, San Francisco, and the Blood Bank of the Alameda–Contra Costa Medical Association, Oakland, California

We performed a prospective, randomized masked trial to determine whether the use of dedicated units of packed red blood cells equipped with seven satellite bags would reduce donor exposures in infants with birth weights <1500 gm. We also examined the use of unwashed and older red blood cells. Red blood cells given to the study group were used without washing and until their expiration date (35 to 42 days). Changes in blood pH, potassium, ionized calcium, and hemoglobin were determined with each transfusion and compared with data collected from a control group that received washed, younger red blood cells. There was a 64% reduction in donor exposures in the study group. Changes in infants' blood pH and calcium levels with transfusion were the same in the two groups. There was a clinically unimportant difference in potassium levels. A greater rise in hemoglobin values occurred when washed cells were used. There was no correlation between changes in the blood levels measured and the age of unwashed cells infused. We conclude that the use of red blood cells from satellite bag–equipped dedicated units decreases donor exposures, and that the practices of using only younger red blood cells and of saline washing of red blood cells before infusion, are unwarranted. (J Pediatr 1995;126:280-6)

Although expanded blood bank screening programs have increased the safety of blood transfusions, there is still a risk of infection that is proportional to the number of donor units to which an infant is exposed. Because the volume of each transfusion is small, many neonatal intensive care nurseries provide blood from shared units that are changed daily. As a result, infants often receive an additional donor exposure with each transfusion. Attempts to limit donor exposures in infants have included the use of walking donor programs[1] and dedicated units (units set aside for the use of an individual patient).[2] Some of the problems encountered by these programs were high cost, difficulty in recruiting donors, the low number of transfusions yielded per donation, the infrequency with which donors were allowed to donate, and compliance with testing regulations.[1, 2]

This prospective, randomized, blind trial examined a method to decrease donor exposures that overcame many of these obstacles. We hypothesized that donor exposures would be reduced in premature infants without affecting their blood pH or their ionized calcium or potassium concentration by using unwashed red blood cells from dedicated units equipped with satellite bags until their expiration date.

NICU	Neonatal intensive care unit
VLBW	Very low birth weight

Presented in part at the Western Society for Pediatric Research meetings, February 1993, Carmel, California and the 46th Annual Meeting of the American Association of Blood Banks, October 1993, Miami, Florida.

Submitted for publication May 28, 1993; accepted Aug. 16, 1994.

Reprint requests: David A. Lee, MD, Neonatology, California Pacific Medical Center, 3850 California St., San Francisco, CA 94118.

0022-3476/95/$3.00 + 0 **9/23/59944**

METHODS

The California Pacific Medical Center Neonatal Intensive Care Unit is a level III referral center with both inborn and transport admissions. There are approximately 450 admissions per year; 25% of these infants have birth weights <1500 gm. All infants admitted to our NICU who met the following criteria were eligible to be entered into the study: (1) birth weight <1500 gm, (2) no previous red blood cell transfusions, and (3) initial red blood cell transfusion ordered during the first week of life.

At the time of the first transfusion, study infants were randomly assigned by hospital blood bank personnel into one of two groups. Patients in the eight-pack group received type-specific packed red blood cells from dedicated units equipped with seven satellite bags. The satellite bags (14-9732-150/14-9732R; Miles Inc., Cutter Biological, Elkhart, Ind.) were attached at the central blood bank (Irwin Memorial Blood Centers, San Francisco, Calif.) with a sterile docking device (Terumo SCD 312; Haemonetics Corp., Braintree, Mass.). Patients in the control group received packed red blood cells from units divided into three split packs shared with other infants who also needed transfusions. Units from volunteer community donors were collected in citrate-phosphate-dextrose-adenine anticoagulant preservative and had a shelf life of 35 days. Infants in both groups could receive red blood cells from individuals recruited by their families who donated blood specifically for their infant ("directed" donation).[3] These directed donations were processed into eight-packs or split packs on the basis of study group assignment. Directed-donor red blood cells were collected in citrate-phosphate-dextrose anticoagulant preservative and stored in adenine in saline anticoagulant preservative, and had a shelf life of 42 days. All red blood cells used in our NICU were drawn from donors with no cytomegalovirus antibodies and were irradiated before shipment from Irwin Memorial Blood Centers to the hospital blood bank.

Transfusions were ordered by primary caretakers who were masked to study group assignments. Red blood cells were processed by hospital blood bank personnel and sent to the NICU in syringes unmarked as to study group assignment. When transfusions were ordered for an infant in the eight-pack group, the amount of red blood cells needed for that transfusion was drained by gravity from the main unit into a satellite bag. The satellite bag was then sealed off and detached. Red blood cells for infusion were removed from the satellite bag to a syringe via a filter to remove microaggregates (SQ40SN; Pall Corp., Biomedical Products Division, East Hills, N.Y.). Once all seven satellite bags were used, the final transfusion aliquot or aliquots were removed directly from the main unit via a filter. Any blood remaining in an individual bag >24 hours after the bag was entered was discarded. Red blood cells from the eight-packs were not washed before administration and had hematocrits of 68% to 75%. Packed red blood cells given to the control group were washed (IBM-COBE Blood Processor 2991; COBE Laboratories, Inc., Lakewood, Colo.), resuspended in saline solution to a hematocrit of 80% to 85% and then filtered to remove microaggregates. Unused red blood cells were discarded 24 hours after being processed. Red blood cell infusions were given for a period of 2 to 4 hours with a syringe pump (model 2001; Medfusion Systems, Inc., Duluth, Ga.).

The infants' whole blood pH, potassium, ionized calcium, and hemoglobin values were measured just before and 1 hour after each transfusion. Blood for analysis was obtained by percutaneous arterial or venous sampling or from indwelling catheters. All blood samples were analyzed immediately after collection with a CIBA-Corning 288 blood gas analyzer (Ciba-Corning Diagnostics Corp., Medfield, Mass.).

The infants' temperature, heart rate, respiratory rate, and blood pressure at the beginning of, 15 minutes into, at the end of, and 1 hour after each transfusion were recorded to monitor for transfusion reactions.

The study period ended when the infant either was discharged home, was transferred to another facility, or died. The following data were collected for each infant: birth weight, gestational age, sex, length of hospital stay, days of mechanical ventilation, days of supplemental oxygen use, whether the infant required surgery, age and weight at each transfusion, the reason for the transfusion, the volume of red blood cells infused with each transfusion, the time span between transfusion episodes, and the number of transfusions received. Blood bank records were reviewed to ascertain the age of the red blood cells used for each transfusion, the number of donor exposures each infant received, and the number of transfusions yielded by each unit.

The Mann-Whitney U test for nonparametric data and the chi-square test were used to analyze patient and transfusion data. Comparison of changes in laboratory data between groups was analyzed with the unpaired t test. Comparison of pretransfusion and posttransfusion laboratory data within groups was done with the paired t test. Changes in blood laboratory values and time between transfusion episodes, as related to the age of the red blood cells infused, were analyzed by linear regression. Statistical significance was set at $p < 0.05$. Values are presented as mean ± SD (range) or as indicated.

On average, infants with birth weights <1500 gm who receive transfusions of red blood cells in our NICU have five donor exposures.[4] A power analysis using a projected reduction in exposures from five to two estimated that a total of 34 infants would need to be entered for a two-tailed

Table I. Patient information

	8-Pack group	Control group*
Number	13	8
Birth weight (gm)†	905 ± 238 (430-1230)	787 ± 271 (460-1170)
Gestational age (wk)†	26.6 ± 2.0 (24-31)	26.3 ± 2.4 (24-31)
Male/female (No.)	9/4	3/5
Deaths (No.)	2	2
Surgery (No.)	4	3
Duration of hospital stay (days)†	63 ± 31 (10-107)	88 ± 62 (11-190)
Days of mechanical ventilation†	12.2 ± 8.5 (0-24)	21.8 ± 15.2 (4-45)
Days of supplemental oxygen†	39.2 ± 28.8 (7-87)	53.0 ± 47.0 (10-111)

*All comparisons statistically nonsignificant: $p > 0.05$.
†Values are expressed as mean ± SD (range).

Table II. Changes in pretransfusion and posttransfusion blood chemistry values

	8-Pack group	Control group
ΔpH*	−0.01 ± 0.06 (−0.30-0.11)	−0.01 ± 0.07 (−0.17-0.27)
ΔIonized calcium (mmol/L)*	−0.01 ± 0.89 (−2.5-3.1)	0.07 ± 0.72 (−2.1-2.3)
ΔPotassium (mmol/L)*	0.14 ± 0.53 (−0.97-1.40)	−0.15 ± 0.46 (−1.12-1.08)†

Values are expressed as mean ± SD (range).
*Calculated as posttransfusion minus pretransfusion values.
†$p = 0.002$; all others not significant.

alpha of 0.05 and a power of 0.80. A quality control and safety check was prospectively scheduled for the time when half of the required infants had completed their hospital course. The study was closed at that time because a statistically significant reduction in donor exposures had been reached. Infants who had not completed the study at the time of closure were allowed to finish the study before final analysis.

This study was approved by the California Pacific Medical Center Research Committee, and informed parental consent was obtained for all participating infants.

RESULTS

During the entry period, 66 infants with a birth weight <1500 gm were admitted to the NICU. Forty-nine infants (74%) received at least one transfusion and 32 of these infants met entry criteria. The parents of six of the eligible infants refused to allow them to participate. Two other eligible infants had antibodies in their serum that necessitated the use of washed group O blood, and were ruled ineligible for random assignment to treatment. One eligible infant had a transfusion before consent could be obtained. Twenty-three infants were entered into our study. Of these, two (a set of twins) were withdrawn from the study by parental request because only one directed donor could be found and the infants could not share this unit and remain in the study. A total of 21 infants completed the study: 13 were randomly assigned to the eight-pack group, and 8 to the control group.

The two groups were similar with respect to birth weight, gestational age, sex distribution, rate of survival, duration of hospital stay, days of mechanical ventilation, need for supplemental oxygen, and the number of infants who required surgery (Table I). One infant in each group died of necrotizing enterocolitis and related complications, one infant in the eight-pack group died of sepsis, and one in the control group died of pulmonary insufficiency as a result of immaturity.

Fifty percent of all red blood cell transfusions in each group were given during the first 2 weeks of life. The majority of these were given to replace blood withdrawn from the infants for laboratory testing and/or to maintain a hematocrit >0.40 while the infant was being supported with mechanical ventilation. A few transfusions were given to treat shock. Indications for red blood cell transfusions administered after the first 2 weeks of life included replacement of blood removed for laboratory testing and treatment of infants with clinical signs of anemia (lethargy, poor weight gain, apnea) with a hematocrit <0.30. No infant received an exchange transfusion.

Eighty-six transfusions were received by infants in each of the two study groups (6.0 vs 7.5 per infant [median, eight-pack vs control]; $p = 0.25$). Infants in the eight-pack group had less than half the number of donor exposures (2.0 vs 5.5 per infant [median, eight-pack vs control]; $p = 0.0002$). The mean age of red blood cells given to the eight-pack group was greater (Fig. 1). There were no differences between groups in the age of the infants when transfusions were given, in the volume of blood infused with

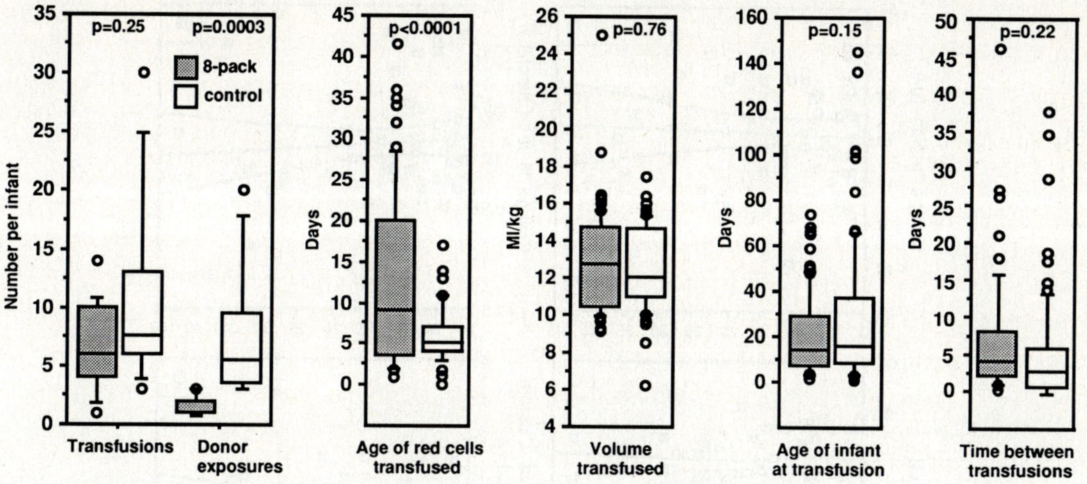

Fig. 1. Comparison of transfusion-related data. The *shaded boxes* denote data from the eight-pack group, the *open boxes* the control group. The *outline* of the boxes denotes the 75th and 25th percentiles, the *middle crossbar* the median, the *outer crossbars* the 90th and 10th percentiles, and the *circles* the values that fall at <10th or >90th percentiles.

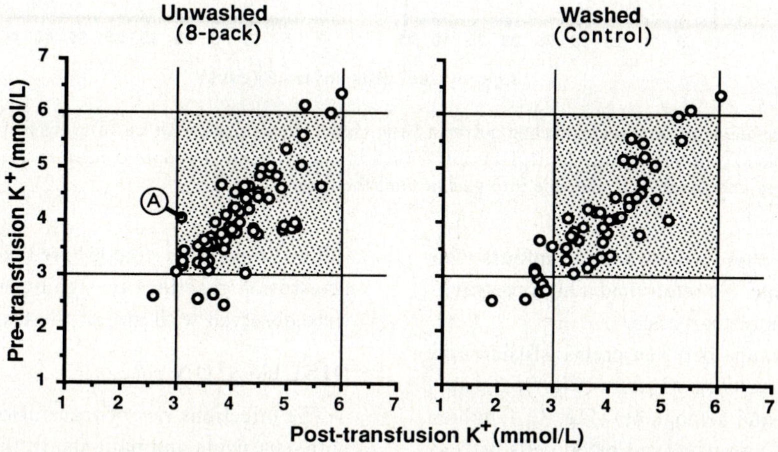

Fig. 2. Pretransfusion and posttransfusion potassium values for each transfusion. Pretransfusion values are plotted along the *y*-axis, posttransfusion values along the *x*-axis (example: *point A* denotes a transfusion episode in which the infant had a pretransfusion potassium level of 4.2 mmol/L and a posttransfusion level of 3.1 mmol/L). *Shaded areas* denote pretransfusion and posttransfusion potassium values of 3.0 to 6.0 mmol/L.

each transfusion, or in the number of days between transfusions (Fig. 1). The number of transfusions that each unit of blood yielded was similar in the eight-pack group (4.0 ± 2.6 [1 to 10]) and the control group (3.6 ± 1.5 [1 to 7]; $p = 0.60$). (Red blood cells received by the control group were from units shared with other infants; the number of transfusions per unit includes transfusions given to nonstudy patients.)

Paired data on pretransfusion and posttransfusion pH, ionized calcium, potassium, and hemoglobin were obtainable for 125, 118, 121, and 106 of all transfusions, respectively. Data were not available for the other transfusions, either because blood samples were not obtained for analysis or were drawn incorrectly (i.e., at the wrong time or by heel stick), or because there was a processing problem in the clinical laboratory.

There was a mean increase in the serum potassium concentration of 0.14 mmol/L (0.14 mEq/L) with unwashed blood compared with a net drop in the potassium concentration of 0.15 mmol/L with washed red blood cells; pretransfusion and posttransfusion values for pH and ionized calcium were similar in the two groups (Table II). A similar number of infants in each group had markedly elevated potassium levels (>5.5 mmol/L) before transfusion

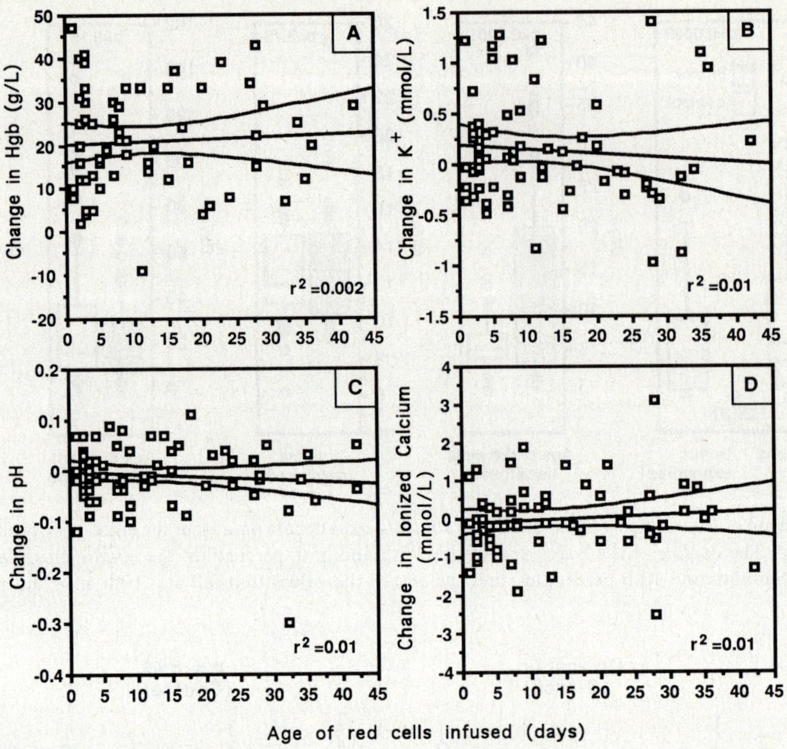

Fig. 3. Differences between pretransfusion and posttransfusion laboratory values, with transfusions plotted versus the age of unwashed red blood cells infused. **A,** Hemoglobin. **B,** Potassium. **C,** pH value. **D,** Ionized calcium. *Regression lines* are shown for the mean and the 95% confidence intervals around the mean.

(Fig. 2); the majority of these values were in infants who were less than 7 days of age. No infant had a high pretransfusion potassium level more than once.

Figure 3 shows the change between pretransfusion and posttransfusion pH (Fig. 3, *C*), potassium (Fig. 3, *B*), ionized calcium (Fig. 3, *D*), and hemoglobin (Fig. 3, *A*) values with each transfusion of unwashed red blood cells plotted versus the age of the red blood cells given. There was no correlation between the age of the infused unwashed red blood cells and any of the changes in the infants' blood values or the time between transfusion episodes (regression analysis, $r^2 = 0.07$). There were no differences in the changes in blood pH, ionized calcium, potassium, or hemoglobin values between infants who received red blood cells that were <7 days of age versus those who received red blood cells ≥7 days of age, nor were there any differences in these measurements in the infants who received red blood cells <14 days of age versus those who received red blood cells ≥14 days of age. There were also no differences in those infants who received red blood cells that were <7 days of age versus those who received red blood cells >28 days of age.

Significant increases in hemoglobin levels were seen with both unwashed (21 ± 12 gm/L; $p < 0.0001$) and washed (30 ± 14 gm/L; $p < 0.0001$) red blood cell transfusions. No transfusion reactions or significant changes in vital signs were observed with any of the transfusions.

DISCUSSION

The infectious risk of transfusions is a major concern of both caregivers and patients. In theory, this risk is directly related to the number of different donors to whom an infant is exposed. Infants with birth weights <1500 gm commonly receive multiple red blood cell transfusions, with at least 5 to 10 donor exposures, during their course in the NICU.[5-7] The small volumes used in transfusions given to VLBW infants and the advent of sterile connecting device techniques allow the provision of multiple transfusions from a single donation and support strategies to reduce donor exposures. By using units dedicated to individual infants, with multiple satellite bags attached, we were able to reduce donor exposures by 64%; 38% of the infants in the eight-pack group received only a single donor exposure, despite having received an average of five transfusions. To achieve this reduction in donor exposures, we made two significant changes in our neonatal transfusion policies: (1) the use of unwashed rather than washed red blood cells, and (2) the use of red blood cells until their expiration date, rather than only red blood cells less than 14 days of age. Although these policies are common,[8] they are based only on concern for theoretical risks.

Proponents of blood washing are concerned about the infusion of potassium that has leaked from the red blood cells into the plasma-preservative solution[9, 10] and about the possible effects of the anticoagulant preservative solution on an infant's pH and calcium levels.[11] Saline washing before infusion removes essentially all of the plasma-preservative solution and any leaked potassium from red blood cell preparations. Opposition to the use of blood washing was summarized by Strauss.[12, 13] He and others[11, 14] argue that the small-volume transfusions that newborn infants receive contain such small amounts of plasma-preservative solution that the amount of potassium and anticoagulant preservative infused is clinically insignificant.[11-13] In addition, washing of red blood cells requires increased handling and processing time, and some red blood cells are lost during the procedure. This not only increases cost but may also result in blood wastage and a longer delay from the time when the decision to give a transfusion is made to the time when the red blood cells are ready for infusion.

There have been several reports that the use of unwashed red blood cells for small-volume transfusion in neonates did not result in significant changes in serum potassium levels,[15-19] pH, or calcium levels.[19] These studies, however, were either retrospective,[17, 18] utilized younger red blood cells (less than 4 to 10 days of age),[16, 19] or did not have well-controlled infant blood sampling.[16-18] Our data support the premise that washing red cells before infusion into VLBW infants is unwarranted. There were no changes in the infants' pretransfusion and posttransfusion whole blood pH or ionized calcium levels regardless of whether washed or unwashed red blood cells were used. There was a clinically unimportant increase in potassium levels after the infusion of unwashed red blood cells and a small decrease when washed cells were given.

All the red blood cells used in this study were irradiated at the blood collection site before shipment to the hospital. Irradiation-induced membrane injury results in progressive leakage of potassium with increasing storage time.[10, 20, 21] Infants who received unwashed red blood cells that were near or at the maximum time of storage did not have a significant rise in blood potassium levels with transfusion. There was also no difference in the change in blood potassium levels in the infants who received younger versus older unwashed red blood cells.

The infants who received washed cells had a greater rise in hemoglobin increment than those who received unwashed cells. This did not correlate with a difference in the transfusion volume nor with the age of the blood infused, and was probably due to a difference in the hematocrit of the red blood cells infused. During the process of washing, red blood cells are concentrated to a hematocrit of 0.85, which is substantially higher than the usual 0.68 to 0.75 hematocrit found in unwashed packed red blood cell preparations. It is not clear whether the greater rise in hemoglobin after the transfusion of washed cells is important. Infants who received unwashed red blood cells did not require more transfusions than the infants who received washed cells, nor was there a difference in the time between transfusions. This difference in hemoglobin rise, however, may indicate that units with higher hematocrits should be used or that a larger volume per kilogram should be transfused when unwashed red blood cells are used.

Many neonatologists advocate the use of red blood cells less than 7 to 14 days of age for VLBW infants.[8] Three theoretical reasons are given for this practice: (1) posttransfusion recovery and subsequent survival of red blood cells may be reduced by prolonged storage; (2) older red blood cell preparations may have an adverse effect on infant pH and potassium levels because of increased levels of potassium[10, 20, 21] and a lower pH in the storage solution[20-22]; and (3) the level of 2,3-diphosphoglycerate in stored red blood cells decreases significantly after 7 days and is totally depleted by 21 days.[20, 22-24] The method used in the eight-pack group is not in conflict with the concern that critically ill infants may need to receive fresh blood. The majority of transfusions in this study occurred during the first 2 weeks of life. Freshly collected units were assigned at the time of the first transfusion; transfusions given to infants in the eight-pack group during the first 2 weeks of their lives had a maximum storage time of 2 weeks. These early transfusions, given during the time when the infants were more likely to be severely ill, employed red blood cells at their best in terms of function, posttransfusion survival, and 2,3-diphosphoglycerate content.

Although there were no statistically significant differences between the two groups, the somewhat longer hospital stay and the higher number of days of ventilatory and oxygen support might indicate that the control group contained sicker patients and therefore may have needed more transfusions, resulting in a greater number of donor exposures. Analysis of data showed that the differences in the outcome variables between the two groups were largely due to a single patient in the control group who received 30 transfusions with 20 donor exposures. Reanalysis of the data without this patient eliminated the small differences between the two groups.

Because of concerns over irradiation-induced membrane injury resulting in progressive leakage of potassium during storage and decreased posttransfusion survival, the U.S. Food and Drug Administration has recently changed its maximum storage recommendations for irradiated red blood cells from 42 days to 28 days.[25] With this change, an alternative strategy will be needed to make use of the full shelf life of red blood cell units. One method would be to irradiate only a portion of the unit, use that portion until it is exhausted or the 28-day expiration date has been reached, and then irradiate the remaining portion for subsequent transfusions. Another method would be to irradiate each aliquot immediately before infusion. These approaches would be cumbersome unless irradiation facilities were available at the hospital. However, reanalysis of our data with a 28-day expiration date for the eight-pack units shows a nearly identical number of donor exposures compared with the actual number (2.0 vs 1.8, respectively; $p = 0.2$). Thus the same reduction in donor exposures using eight-pack units would have been realized even if a 28-day maximum storage time had been used rather than the 42-day expiration date.

We conclude that the use of dedicated eight-packs of red blood cells reduced donor exposures in infants with birth weights <1500 gm, and yet was technically simple. Adoption of this strategy required only a sterile connecting device and revision of our policies on neonatal transfusion. Demands on our blood supply were not increased by this technique. Our data show no evidence that the practices of washing red blood cells and of using only younger red blood cells for neonatal transfusions are warranted.

We thank the personnel in the blood bank who entered infants into our study and gave them random treatment assignments, the laboratory technicians who performed blood level determinations, and the NICU nurses who collected the blood samples needed to accomplish this study. We also thank Irwin Memorial Blood Centers, San Francisco, Calif., and its staff for providing the blood used in this study and for technical and financial support.

REFERENCES

1. Blankenship WJ, Goetzman BW, Gross S, Hattersley PG. A walking donor program for the intensive care nursery. J PEDIATR 1975;86:583-5.
2. Minifee PK, Daescher CW III, Griffen MP, Allison PL, Zwischenberger JB. Decreasing blood donor exposure in neonates on extracorporeal membrane oxygenation. J Pediatr Surg 1990;25:38-42.
3. Paul Gann Blood Safety Act, California Health and Safety Code, Section 1645, 1989 (revised 1991).
4. Lee DA, Evans CS, Slagle TA. The use of designated donor blood does not decrease donor exposures in the intensive care nursery [Abstract]. Clin Res 1992;40:86A.
5. Strauss RG. Transfusion therapy in neonates. Am J Dis Child 1991;145:904-11.
6. Sacher RA, Luban NLC, Strauss RG. Current practice and guidelines for the transfusion of cellular blood components in the newborn. Trans Med Rev 1989;3:39-54.
7. Donowitz LG, Turner RB, Searcy MAM, et al. The high rate of blood donor exposure for critically ill neonates. Infect Control Hosp Epidemiol 1989;10:509-10.
8. Levy GJ, Strauss RG, Hume H, et al. National Survey of Neonatal Transfusion Practices. I. Red blood cell therapy. Pediatrics 1993;91:523-9.
9. Ramirez AM, Woodfield DG, Scott R, et al. High potassium levels in stored irradiated blood [Letter]. Transfusion 1987; 27:444-5.
10. Rivet C, Baxter A, Rock G. Potassium levels in irradiated blood [Letter]. Transfusion 1989;29:185.
11. Luban NLC, Strauss RG, Hume HA. Commentary on the safety of red cells preserved in extended-storage media for neonatal transfusions. Transfusion 1991;31:229-35.
12. Strauss RG. Routinely washing irradiated red cells before transfusion seems unwarranted. Transfusion 1990;30:675-7.
13. Strauss RG. Neonatal anemia: pathophysiology and treatment. In: Wilson SM, Levitt JS, Strauss RG, eds. Improving practice for pediatric patients. Arlington, Virginia: American Association of Blood Banks, 1991:1-17.
14. Strauss RG, Sacher RA, Blazina JF, et al. Commentary on small-volume red cell transfusions for neonatal patients. Transfusion 1990;30:565-70.
15. Friedman KD, Backstrom C, Armon M. Newborn tolerance of the potassium load from simple transfusion of stored irradiated red blood cells [Abstract]. Transfusion 1992;32(suppl):10S.
16. Stroupe TK, Hanrahan JB, Lantzy A, et al. The effects of high plasma potassium in neonatal transfusions [Abstract]. Transfusion 1983;23:430.
17. Fong K, Malott R. "Older" directed donor blood in neonates [Abstract]. Transfusion 1988;28:7S.
18. Patten E, Robbins M, Vincent J, et al. Use of red blood cells older than five days for neonatal transfusion. J Perinatol 1991;11:37-40.
19. Tan KL, Wong LY. Effect of blood transfusion on acid-base, glucose and electrolyte status in very low birth weight infants. Biol Neonate 1991;59:373-80.
20. Moroff G, Dende D. Characterization of biochemical changes occurring during storage of red cells: comparative studies with CPD and CPDA-1 anticoagulant–preservative solutions. Transfusion 1983;23:484-9.
21. Heaton A, Miripol J, Aster R, et al. Use of Adsol preservation solution for prolonged safety of low-viscosity AS-1 red blood cells. Br J Haematol 1984;57:467-78.
22. Moore GL, Ledford ME. Effects of 4,000 rad irradiation on the in vitro storage properties of packed cells. Transfusion 1985; 25:583-5.
23. Heaton A, Keegan T, Holme S. In vivo regeneration of red cell 2,3-diphosphoglycerate following transfusion of DPG-depleted AS-1, AS-3, and CPDA-1 red cells. Br J Haematol 1989;71: 131-6.
24. Valeri CR, Valeri DA, Gray A, et al. Viability and function of red blood cell concentrates stored at 4° C for 35 days in CPDA-1, CPDA-2 or CPDA-3. Transfusion 1982;22:210-6.
25. Quinnan GV Jr. Recommendations regarding license amendments and procedures for gamma irradiation of blood products. Washington, D.C.: U.S. Department of Health and Human Services, Center or Biologics Evaluation and Research, Food and Drug Administration, July 22, 1993.

Effects of parenteral L-carnitine supplementation on fat metabolism and nutrition in premature neonates

Cynthia M. Bonner, MD, Karan L. DeBrie, RD, George Hug, MD, Evelyn Landrigan, BS, and Bonnie J. Taylor, MD

From the Department of Pediatrics, University of Arkansas for Medical Sciences, and Arkansas Children's Hospital, Little Rock, and the Department of Pediatrics, University of Cincinnati, and Division of Enzymology, Children's Hospital Medical Center, Cincinnati, Ohio

The effects of parenteral L-carnitine supplementation on fat metabolism, nutrient intake, and plasma and erythrocyte carnitine concentrations were studied in 43 very low birth weight infants. Infants were randomly assigned to control or carnitine-supplemented (50 μmol/kg per day) groups within two weight categories: group 1, 750 to 1000 gm, and group 2, 1001 to 1500 gm. Plasma total, free, and acyl carnitine levels, erythrocyte carnitine levels, serum β-hydroxybutyrate and triglyceride levels, and total fat intake were monitored weekly until 50% of total caloric intake was met enterally. Neonates receiving carnitine had higher plasma carnitine levels than control groups (total carnitine: group 1, 75.2 ± 22.9 vs 9.6 ± 2.7 mmol/ml; group 2, 61.6 ± 31.2 vs 13.0 ± 9.2 nmol/ml). Levels of β-OH-butyrate decreased from baseline in control neonates (group 1, 0.12 ± 0.06 to 0.03 ± 0.02 mmol/L; group 2, 0.11 ± 0.03 to 0.05 ± 0.02 mmol/L); they remained unchanged in supplemented groups. Thus ketogenesis appeared less impaired in infants receiving supplements. Supplemented group 2 tolerated more fat than control group 2; triglyceride levels remained acceptable in all groups. Carnitine group 2 had greater weight gain than control group 2 during the first 2 weeks of life. We conclude that very low birth weight infants requiring prolonged parenteral nutrition have carnitine deficiency with impaired ketogenesis. Parenteral administration of carnitine appears to alleviate this metabolic disturbance. (J Pediatr 1995;126:287-92)

Premature infants have limited fat stores and often require parenteral nutrition for extended periods. Parenteral nutrition includes emulsified lipids to supply calories for growth and essential fatty acids. Carnitine, β-hydroxy-γ-trimethylaminobutyric acid, facilitates transport of fatty acids across the inner mitochondrial membranes through an acyltransferase enzyme system[1, 2] and is required in fatty acid metabolism. Neonates have limited free fatty acid oxidative capacity, which may relate to their low acylcarnitine and free carnitine levels.[3-6] Carnitine is synthesized in human liver and kidney[7] from the essential amino acids lysine and methionine.[8] Previous studies have shown that neonates receiving parenteral nutrition devoid of carnitine are unable to synthesize sufficient carnitine to maintain plasma concentrations equivalent to values found in healthy newborn infants, older children, or adults,[3, 4, 6, 9-11] despite the presence of these amino acids in parenteral nutrition fluids. Therefore infants must rely on dietary intake of carnitine to maintain adequate carnitine stores.

Depletion of tissue carnitine stores has been reported in neonates who received parenteral nutrition devoid of carnitine for at least 15 days.[12] Studies evaluating carnitine supplementation have yielded varying results regarding fat

Submitted for publication April 5, 1994; accepted Aug. 17, 1994.

Reprint requests: Cindy Bonner, MD, Department of Pediatrics, Arkansas Children's Hospital, 800 Marshall St., Little Rock, AR 72202.

0022-3476/95/$3.00 + 0 **9/23/60000**

metabolism. Some have reported enhanced ketogenesis,[9, 13] whereas others have demonstrated no effect.[14, 15] There have been no reported studies of carnitine supplementation and its effect on fat metabolism during the slower, more prolonged fat infusion that is normally used in intensive care nurseries, as opposed to evaluation during a fat tolerance test. We prospectively investigated the changes in carnitine status and fat metabolism of very low birth weight infants receiving intravenous infusions of L-carnitine.

METHODS

Patients. Forty-three premature neonates admitted to the Arkansas Children's Hospital Neonatal Intensive Care Unit at less than 48 hours of age were studied. The study was approved by the University of Arkansas for Medical Sciences Institutional Review Board. The statistical basis for determining the specific numbers of patients to be enrolled was a power analysis with a detectable difference of 40% to 50% and an anticipated standard deviation of 25% to 30% in the measurements.[16] Given those requirements, each group would have had to contain from 4 to 16 patients. Ten patients were then chosen as the sample size for each group on the basis of an anticipated enrollment during 1 year. Informed consent was obtained from a parent or guardian before enrollment into the study. The infants were classified into weight groups according to their birth weight (group 1, 751 to 1000 gm; group 2, 1001 to 1500 gm) and then were randomly assigned to receive either intravenous infusions of L-carnitine (50 μmol/kg per day) or no supplementation within their respective weight category. Eligible infants who were not enrolled included five infants whose disease was so severe that they were not expected to survive >48 hours, four infants who had received erythrocyte transfusions before initial laboratory studies were obtained, and two infants who were not expected to receive parenteral nutrition for more than 1 week. The study was not masked so that safety of the parenteral form of carnitine, which was not licensed by the U.S. Food and Drug Administration at the time of this study, could be followed more closely. Patient characteristics were recorded, including birth weight, sex, estimated gestational age by Dubowitz[17] examination, weight gain during study, the duration of enrollment in the study until 50% caloric intake (60 kcal/kg per day) was met enterally with human milk or a carnitine-containing formula, and duration of hospitalization. A clinical severity score,[18] which summarizes the severity of a patient's clinical illness, also was used to ensure group equality. Daily intake and output records were maintained.

Nutritional regimens. Patients received parenteral nutrition beginning on postnatal day 2 or 3; on the next day, intravenous infusion of lipid emulsion (Intralipid; Kabi Pharmacia, Clayton, N.C.), given continuously for 20 to 24 hours, was begun. Lipid intake was started at 0.5 to 1.0 gm/kg per day and advanced by 0.25 to 0.5 gm/kg per day. Lipid intake was not advanced if the serum triglyceride concentrations were ≥1.7 mmol/L (150 mg/dl), but was not decreased if the serum triglyceride level was <2.25 mmol/L (200 mg/dl). Serum triglyceride values were monitored daily while intravenous infusion of lipids was advanced to a maximum of 3.0 gm/kg per day and then monitored weekly. The patients who had been randomly assigned to the carnitine groups received L-carnitine, 50 μmol/kg per day, as a continuous infusion beginning at the institution of parenteral nutrition. At the neonatologist's discretion, enteral feedings were begun when the clinical condition was deemed stable, and were advanced in volume and concentration as tolerated.

Laboratory studies. On admission to the hospital, and then weekly as long as the patient remained enrolled in the study, blood was obtained for carnitine levels (plasma total, free, and acyl carnitine, and erythrocyte carnitine), serum ketone (β-OH butyrate) levels, and serum triglyceride concentrations. Blood was collected in heparinized tubes and immediately placed on ice, and then the plasma was separated by centrifugation. Aliquots of plasma were immediately frozen (plasma carnitine and β-OH-butyrate). Carnitine levels were assayed according to the Cederblad-Lindstedt method.[19] Triglycerides were measured by an enzymatic assay with correction for free glycerol.[20] Ketone bodies were determined by spectrophotometric enzymatic assays.[21] All reported laboratory measurements were performed in the same laboratory (carnitine in the Cincinnati Children's Hospital Medical Center Division of Enzymology; lipid indexes at Arkansas Children's Hospital). Routine biochemical and hematologic tests were done as a part of our usual clinical monitoring. Two-week values are reported here because previous work has shown tissue carnitine levels to be decreased after at least 2 weeks of parenteral nutrition devoid of carnitine.[12]

Statistical analysis. Mann-Whitney U tests[22] were performed to determine whether differences existed in means between and within groups for patient characteristics, nutrient intake, lipid indexes (β-OH-butyrate and triglyceride), and carnitine levels. Statistical significance was established at $p < 0.05$.

RESULTS

There was no significant difference for any demographic variable between carnitine and control groups within each weight category. Diagnoses and clinical severity scores were similar within and between groups. There were no documented cases of sepsis or other infections. Nutrient intake of each group was similar (Table I), with the exception of fat intake in group 2. There was no difference in the

Table I. Average daily nutrient intake of very low birth weight infants during first 2 weeks of life

	Group 1 (751-1000 gm)		Group 2 (1001-1500 gm)	
	Control	Carnitine	Control	Carnitine
Calories (kcal/kg/day)	74 ± 14	71 ± 10	67 ± 9	72 ± 8
Protein (gm/kg/day)	2.1 ± 0.3	1.8 ± 0.6	1.7 ± 0.4	1.9 ± 0.2
Fat (gm/kg/day)	2.3 ± 0.5	2.1 ± 0.4	2.0 ± 0.6	2.5 ± 0.4*

Values are expressed as mean ± SD. Nutrient intake represents combined parenteral and enteral intake.
*p <0.05, compared with control values.

Table II. Fractionated carnitine levels of very low birth weight infants on parenteral nutrition regimen with or without intravenous carnitine supplementation

Duration of regimen, by group	Free (nmol/ml)	SC (nmol/ml)	RBC total (nmol/mgh)
Child normal values*	(43.5 ± 13.3)	(15.4 ± 9.1)	(NA)
Group 1, control (n = 11)			
Initial	20.0 ± 12.5	7.9 ± 2.7	0.17 ± 0.06
After 2 wk	5.8 ± 2.0[b]	3.7 ± 1.5[b]	0.05 ± 0.02[b]
Group 1, carnitine (n = 11)			
Initial	17.3 ± 8.8	5.3 ± 2.4	0.18 ± 0.06
After 2 wk	56.8 ± 19.5[b, d]	18.4 ± 6.5[b, d]	0.07 ± 0.05[b]
Group 2, control (n = 10)			
Initial	18.0 ± 8.7	5.6 ± 3.3	0.13 ± 0.06
After 2 wk	8.7 ± 6.4[b]	4.1 ± 3.0	0.04 ± 0.02[b]
Group 2, carnitine (n = 11)			
Initial	17.0 ± 8.7	4.9 ± 2.7	0.14 ± 0.07
After 2 wk	50.1 ± 23.9[a, d]	14.1 ± 4.9[a, d]	0.10 ± 0.06[c]

Values are expressed as mean ± SD.
SC, Short chain; *RBC*, red blood cells; *mgh*, milligrams of hemoglobin; *NA*, not available.
*Normal values were established in the reference laboratory where assays were performed.
[a]p <0.05 from baseline.
[b]p <0.01 from baseline.
[c]p <0.01 from control.
[d]p <0.001 from control.

percentage of nutrient intake provided enterally when carnitine-supplemented infants were compared with control infants within each weight category.

On entering the study, all infants had carnitine levels that were 50% below the published normal values for children and adults, but were similar to values reported previously for premature infants.[23] Plasma total carnitine levels decreased from their low baseline to 20% to 25% of normal in both control groups (p <0.01), and rose to within the normal range in both carnitine groups (p <0.05; Fig. 1). Plasma carnitine levels were significantly higher in the infants given carnitine than in the control infants of the same weight classification after 2 weeks of parenteral nutrition (p <0.001). Erythrocyte carnitine levels decreased in both control groups and in the smaller infants given carnitine (group 1). However, the larger infants receiving carnitine (group 2) had a significantly higher erythrocyte carnitine level than control group 2 after at least 2 weeks on a parenteral nutrition regimen (p <0.01; Table II). The plasma carnitine levels in the control infants in each weight classification rose significantly once enteral feedings were established (Table III). Levels of β-OH-butyrate decreased significantly from baseline in both control groups (p <0.05),

Table III. Total carnitine values of control very low birth weight infants on parenteral nutrition regimen before and after institution of enteral feeding

Group	Duration of enteral nutrition	Total carnitine (nmol/ml)	Enteral intake (%)
Group 1 (n = 11)	Initial	7.3 ± 4.5	
	1 Wk	12.2 ± 5.9*	38 ± 12
	2 Wk	37.2 ± 39.6*	78 ± 26
Group 2 (n = 10)	Initial	10.8 ± 7.2	
	1 Wk	14.9 ± 9.3*	43 ± 16
	2 Wk	25.7 ± 13.3*	82 ± 22

Values are expressed as mean ± SD.
*p <0.05 from baseline.

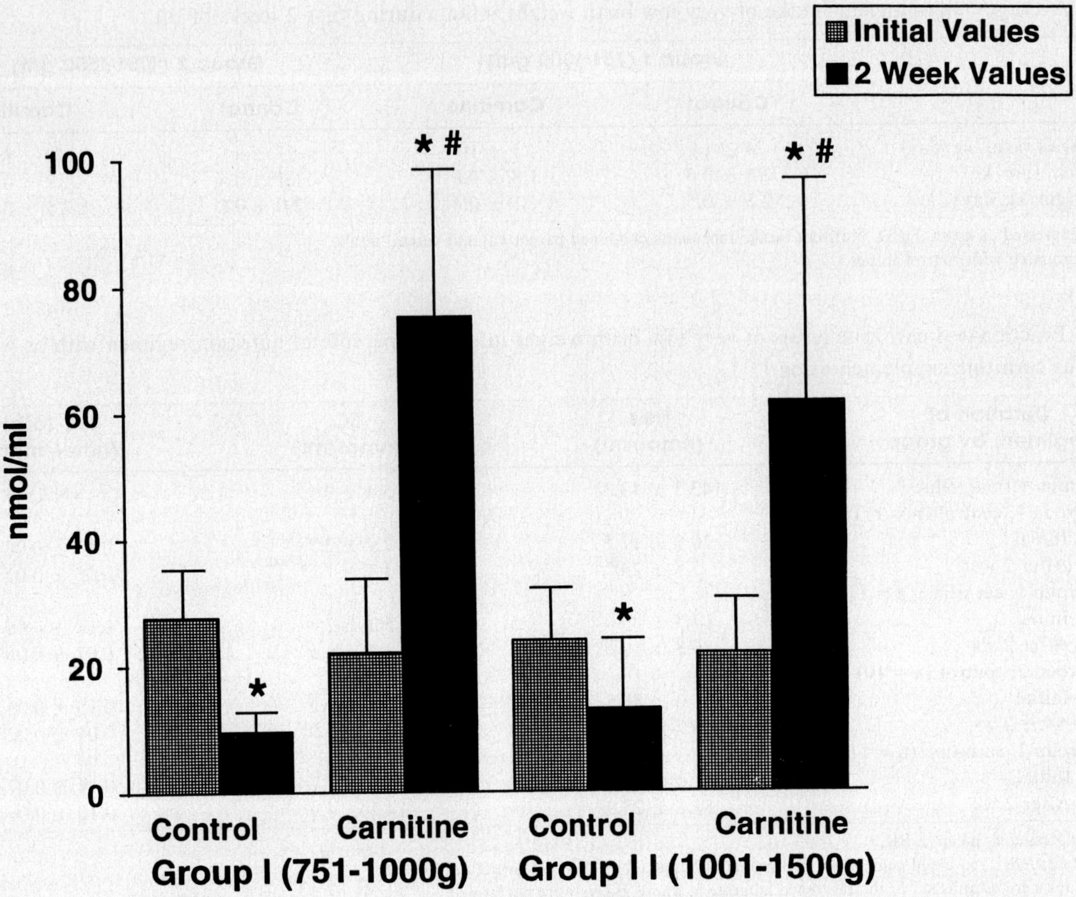

Fig. 1. Total carnitine levels (in nanomoles per milliliter; mean ± SD) of very low birth weight infants receiving parenteral nutrition with or without intravenous carnitine supplementation. In group 1: control n = 11, carnitine n = 11; in group 2, control n = 10, carnitine n = 11. Values at entry to the study (initial) are shown as *shaded bars*. Values after 2 weeks of parenterally administered nutrition with or without carnitine supplementation (2 weeks) are shown as *dark solid bars*. *p <0.05 from baseline; #p <0.001 from control.

and remained unchanged in both carnitine groups (Fig. 2). Carnitine group 2 tolerated significantly more lipid than control group 2 during the study period (p <0.05; Table I). The serum triglyceride level remained acceptable regardless of group or supplementation status. Carnitine group 2 had a significantly greater weight gain per day (6.9 ± 5.9 vs 1.3 ± 7.1 gm/day) than control infants in this weight category during the first 2 weeks of life (p <0.05).

DISCUSSION

We have demonstrated, as have others,[3-6, 9-11, 13] that maintenance of plasma carnitine levels is dependent on an exogenous supply of carnitine in the premature neonate. Although neonates requiring prolonged parenteral nutrition receive the essential precursors lysine and methionine[8] for synthesis, plasma carnitine levels fall to levels consistent with systemic carnitine deficiency within 2 weeks and continue to decrease or remain low until carnitine is supplied exogenously. Reduced capacity for biosynthesis of carnitine appears to be secondary to low activities of several enzymes.[24] Plasma carnitine levels increased when feedings with carnitine-containing human milk or premature formula were begun. Neonates who received parenterally administered carnitine had normal plasma carnitine levels within 2 weeks. This dose of carnitine was chosen to correlate with the minimal amount normally found in human milk, and to be comparable to the amount used in previous studies. We evaluated the different fractions of plasma carnitine and found that all fractions were decreased in nonsupplemented infants and rose to within the normal range in supplemented infants.

The erythrocyte carnitine levels at the beginning of our study were slightly lower than previously reported values[25, 26] for preterm neonates, but decreased as previously described[25] with increasing postnatal age. However, carnitine group 2 had no significant decrease in their erythro-

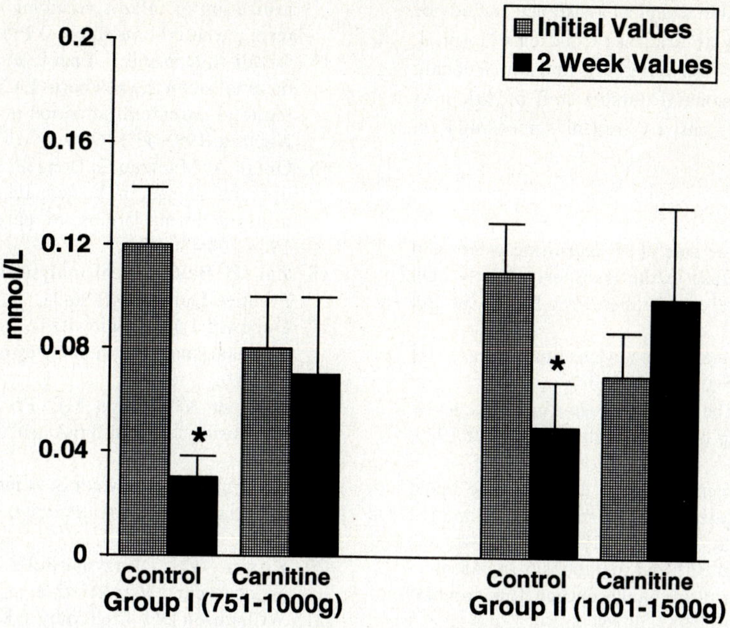

Fig. 2. Levels of β-OH-butyrate (in millimoles per liter; mean ± SEM) of very low birth weight infants receiving parenteral nutrition with or without intravenous carnitine supplementation. In group 1: control n = 11, and carnitine n = 11. In group 2: control n = 10, and carnitine n = 11. Values at entry to the study *(Initial)* are shown as *shaded bars*. Values after 2 weeks of parenterally administered nutrition with or without carnitine supplementation (2 weeks) are shown as *dark solid bars*. **p* <0.05 from baseline.

cyte carnitine content during a 2-week period. Erythrocytes may serve a transport function for carnitine.[27] If such a transport system exists, erythrocyte carnitine may be an important indicator of tissue availability of carnitine. If so, these results suggest insufficient tissue stores in our smallest weight group despite supplementation.

We demonstrated that premature neonates receiving parenterally administered nutrition devoid of carnitine had significantly decreased β-OH-butyrate levels, and that parenteral carnitine supplementation resulted in increased levels. Most previous studies investigating fatty acid metabolism with carnitine supplementation used fat tolerance tests[9, 10] to demonstrate effects of carnitine on fat metabolism. We infused the lipid for 20 to 24 hours, the routine schedule for fat administration in our nursery. Perhaps because the lipid was not infused rapidly, β-OH-butyrate levels were twofold to fivefold lower than those reported in other studies.

Carnitine group 2 tolerated significantly more fat than the control subjects in this weight group. There was no difference in the amount of heparin used between the groups in each weight classification. Therefore heparin-induced lipoprotein lipase activity[28] should not have affected the results of triglyceride clearance. Although increased weight gain occurred in the supplemented infants in the larger birth weight group, this finding may not be clinically significant because weight gain during the initial 2 weeks of life was minimal in all groups. The only other study evaluating changes in growth rate in very low birth weight infants revealed an increase in growth only after increasing the dose of parenterally administered L-carnitine to 100 μmol/kg per day.[10] No adverse side effects of carnitine supplementation, such as diarrhea or foul odor, which have been reported with oral supplementation,[29] were noted.

In summary, intravenous carnitine supplementation resulted in increased plasma carnitine levels and enhanced ketogenesis in premature infants maintained on a regimen of prolonged parenteral nutrition devoid of carnitine (at least 2 weeks). Our results suggest that preterm neonates have limited carnitine reserves and that parenteral carnitine supplementation may increase these stores. Erythrocyte carnitine, amount of lipid tolerated, and weight gain were improved with parenteral carnitine supplementation at the current dose (50 μmol/kg per day) in the larger premature neonates (>1000 gm). These findings suggest that intravenous carnitine supplementation along with parenterally administered nutrition may allow for more rapid growth and better fat utilization in the larger group of very low birth weight infants. Additional studies are needed in smaller neonates to see whether more pronounced benefits are achieved with larger doses of intravenously administered L-carnitine.

We acknowledge the invaluable technical assistance and advice from the metabolics laboratory at Arkansas Children's Hospital, including Dr. Marge Brewster, Fran Soderberg, and Jan Woodall, and the assistance from the neonatal nursing staff at Arkansas Children's Hospital Neonatal Intensive Care Unit, especially Pam McMillan, RN.

REFERENCES

1. Fritz IB, Marquis NR. The role of acylcarnitine esters and carnitine palmitoyltransferase in the transport of fatty acyl groups across mitochondrial membranes. Proc Natl Acad Sci USA 1965;54:1226-33.
2. Pande S. A mitochondrial carnitine acylcarnitine translocase system. Natl Acad Sci USA 1975;72:883-7.
3. Schiff D, Chan G, Seccombe D, et al. Plasma carnitine levels during intravenous feeding of the neonate. J PEDIATR 1979; 95:1043-6.
4. Schmidt-Sommerfeld E, Penn D, Wolf H. Carnitine blood concentrations and fat utilization in parenterally alimented premature newborn infants. J PEDIATR 1982;100:260-4.
5. Takahanshi M, Sawaguchi S. Lipid metabolism in parenterally alimented neonates: carnitine blood concentrations and fat utilization. Indian J Pediatr 1983;50:161-8.
6. Yeh Y, Cooke RJ, Zee P. Impairment of lipid emulsion metabolism associated with carnitine insufficiency in premature infants. J Pediatr Gastroenterol Nutr 1985;4:795-8.
7. Rebouche CJ, Engel AG. Tissue distribution of carnitine biosynthetic enzymes in man. Biochim Biophys Acta 1980;630: 22-9.
8. Tanphaichitr V, Broquist HP. Role of lysine and *N*-trimethyllysine in carnitine biosynthesis. II. Studies in the rat. J Biol Chem 1973;248:2176-81.
9. Schmidt-Sommerfeld E, Penn D, Wolf H. Carnitine deficiency in premature infants receiving parenteral nutrition: effect of L-carnitine supplementation. J PEDIATR 1983;102: 931-4.
10. Helms RA, Mauer EC, Hay WW, Christensen ML, Storm MC. Effect of intravenous L-carnitine on growth parameters and fat metabolism during parenteral nutrition in neonates. JPEN J Parenter Enteral Nutr 1990;14:448-53.
11. Smith RB, Sachan DS, Plattsmier J, Feld N, Lorch V. Plasma carnitine alterations in premature infants receiving various nutritional regimes. JPEN J Parenter Enteral Nutr 1988;12:37-42.
12. Penn D, Schmidt-Sommerfeld E, Pascu F. Decreased tissue carnitine concentrations in newborn infants receiving total parenteral nutrition. J PEDIATR 1981;98:976-8.
13. Helms RA, Whitington PF, Mauer EC, et al. Enhanced lipid utilization in infants receiving oral L-carnitine during long-term parenteral nutrition. J PEDIATR 1986;109:984-8.
14. Orzali A, Donzelli F, Enzi E, et al. Effect of carnitine on lipid metabolism in the newborn. I. Carnitine supplementation during total parenteral nutrition in the first 48 hours of life. Biol Neonate 1983;43:186-90.
15. Orzali A, Maetzke G, Donzelli F, et al. Effect of carnitine on lipid metabolism in the neonate. II. Carnitine addition to lipid infusion during prolonged parenteral nutrition. J PEDIATR 1984;104:436-40.
16. Zar JH. Biostatistical analysis. Englewood Cliffs, New Jersey: Prentice-Hall, 1984:126-31.
17. Dubowitz LMS, Dubowitz D, Goldberg C. Clinical assessment of gestational age in the newborn infant. J PEDIATR 1970; 77:1-10.
18. Scheiner AP, Sexton ME. Prediction of developmental outcome using a perinatal risk inventory. Pediatrics 1991;88:1135-43.
19. Cederblad G, Lindstedt S. A method for the determination of carnitine in the picomole range. Clin Chim Acta 1972;37:235-43.
20. Kreutz FH. Enzymatische Glyzerinbestimmung. Klin Wochenschr 1962;40:362-3.
21. Williamson DH, Mellamby J, Krebs HA. Enzymatic determination of D-β-hydroxybutyric acid and acetoacetic acid in blood. Biochem J 1962;82:90-6.
22. Hollander M, Wolfe DA. Nonparametric statistical methods. New York: John Wiley & Sons, 1973:71-3.
23. Sheard N. Carnitine deficiency. In: Blackburn GL, Bell SJ, Mullen JL, eds. Nutritional medicine: a case management approach. Philadelphia: WB Saunders, 1989:92-5.
24. Rebouche CJ. Recent advances in carnitine biosynthesis and transport. In: Borum PR, ed. Clinical aspects of human carnitine deficiency. New York: Pergamon Press, 1986:1-15.
25. Mares-Perlman JA, Farrell PM, Gutcher GR. Changes in erythrocyte and plasma carnitine concentrations in preterm neonates. Am J Clin Nutr 1986;43:77-84.
26. Shenai JP, Borum PR, Mohan P, Donlevy SC. Carnitine status at birth of newborn infants of varying gestation. Pediatr Res 1983;17:579-82.
27. Borum PR, York CM. Red cell carnitine binding protein [Abstract 1559]. Fed Proc 1982;41:537.
28. Hamosh M, Hamosh P. Lipoprotein lipase, hepatic lipase and their role in lipid clearing during total parenteral nutrition. In: Lebenthal E, ed. Total parenteral nutrition. New York: Raven Press, 1986:29-58.
29. Fernandez C, La Menza B, Pola P. Trials clinici difase IV e di farmacobigilanza-nuobe ipotesi matodologiche-il terzo trial Ance. JAMA [Italian edition] 1985;9.

Clinical and laboratory observations

Congenital cytomegalovirus infection as a result of nonprimary cytomegalovirus disease in a mother with acquired immunodeficiency syndrome

Kay Schwebke, MD, Keith Henry, MD, Henry H. Balfour, Jr., MD, Douglas Olson, MD, R. Thomas Crane, MS, and M. Colin Jordan, MD

From the Departments of Medicine and Pathology, St. Paul-Ramsey Medical Center, St. Paul, Minnesota, and the Departments of Medicine, Laboratory Medicine and Pathology, and Pediatrics, University of Minnesota Medical School, Minneapolis

A pregnant woman with acquired immunodeficiency syndrome had nonprimary cytomegalovirus (CMV) viremia and died of complications from *Pneumocystis carinii* pneumonia and CMV sinusitis and pneumonitis. A boy was delivered by cesarean section at 34 weeks of gestation as the mother's health deteriorated and fetal distress developed. The infant died soon after delivery of interstitial pneumonitis and hyaline membrane disease with invasive CMV disease that affected the kidneys, adrenal glands, and placenta; the CMV strains from the mother and neonate were identical. (J Pediatr 1995;126:293-5)

Although in utero infection with cytomegalovirus is common, the occurrence of severe, invasive CMV disease is rare.[1] It occurs most often when the mother has primary CMV infection during gestation. We report a case of nonprimary CMV infection in a pregnant woman with acquired immunodeficiency syndrome in which in utero transmission of CMV resulted in disseminated disease in her premature neonate.

CASE REPORT

A 21-year-old pregnant (32 weeks) white woman was admitted to the hospital and a diagnosis of *Pneumocystis carinii* pneumonitis was made by histologic examination of broncheoalveolar lavage washings; additional samples of the bronchoalveolar lavage fluid were sent for further studies, and CMV was detected by the rapid "shell vial" assay. During treatment for the PCP, the mother's clinical condition deteriorated, necessitating tracheal intubation on hospital day 7. On day 11 a cesarean section was performed because of further compromise in the mother's health and concern about fetal distress. The baby boy died of interstitial pneumonitis and hyaline membrane disease soon after delivery. Autopsy studies revealed evidence of invasive CMV disease that affected the kidney tubules, adrenal glands, and placenta with no other findings suggestive of cytomegalic inclusion disease.

Intravenous ganciclovir therapy was added to the mother's medical regimen soon after delivery. A maternal blood culture sent the day of delivery grew CMV on hospital day 19. Despite all efforts, the mother died on hospital day 23 as a result of multiple complications. Autopsy findings confirmed PCP, splenic candidiasis, CMV sinusitis and pneumonitis, and hemorrhagic pancreatitis.

Virologic and serologic data. Virologic results are summarized in the Table. The samples obtained from the mother 2 weeks before hospitalization and on hospital day 13 both contained CMV IgG antibody at a titer of 1:8. Testing of a stored plasma sample from 1990 revealed positive CMV IgM and IgG antibody indexes. The CMV strains isolated from blood samples from the mother, infant, and laboratory strain AD169 were analyzed at four amplified gene

CMV	Cytomegalovirus
HIV	Human immunodeficiency virus
PCP	*Pneumocystis carinii* pneumonia

Supported by grants AI27761 and AI30456 from the National Institutes of Health.

Submitted for publication May 24, 1994; accepted Aug. 8, 1994.

Reprint requests: Keith Henry, MD, St. Paul-Ramsey Medical Center, HIV Programs Office, 640 Jackson St., Suite 125, St. Paul, MN 55101.

0022-3476/95/$3.00 + 0 **9/24/59699**

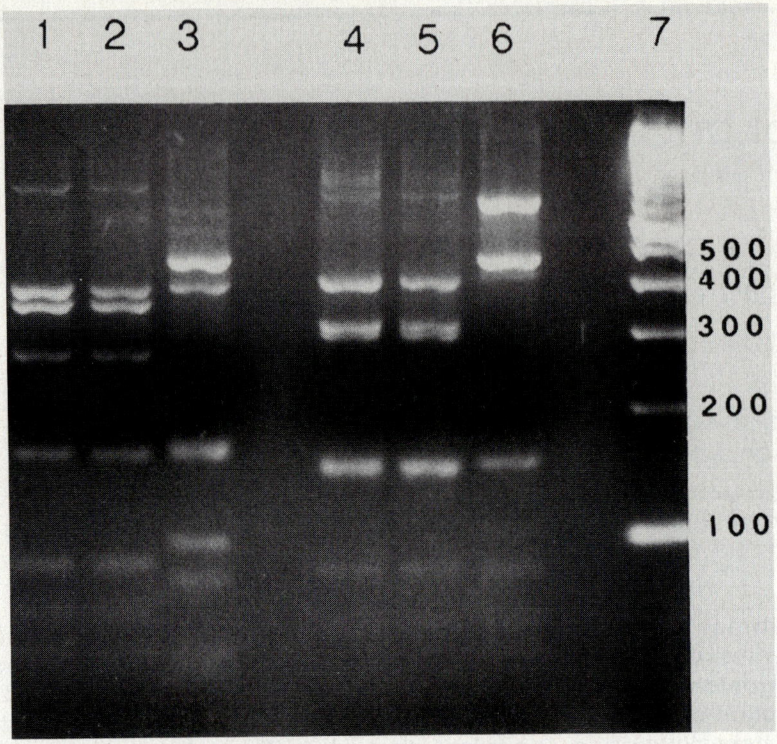

Figure. Polymerase chain reaction–amplified products of the gH region digested with restriction enzymes for mother and infant CMV isolates. *Lanes 1 to 3* show digestion of viral DNA with *Hae* II for the mother, infant, and AD169 strains, respectively. *Lanes 4 to 6* show digestion with *Hha* I for the mother, infant, and AD169 strain, respectively. *Lane 7* is the molecular weight ladder. All patterns were identical for CMV strains recovered from the mother and infant for all enzyme and primer combinations.

Table. Summary of virologic results from mother and neonate.

	Date of sampling				
	1990	7/6/92	8/3/92	8/5/92	8/15/92
Mother					
CMV IgM	1.126*	<1:10†		<1:10†	
CMV IgG	105.6*	1.8‡		1.8‡	
CMV blood culture			+		
CMV inclusions					+ Lung, sinus
HIV antibody	+				
Neonate					
CMV blood culture			+		
CMV inclusions			+ Adrenal, kidney, placenta		

Positive signs denote positive test results.
*Antibodies to CMV were tested by microparticle enzyme immunoassay (Abbott Laboratories). A CMV IgM antibody index ≥0.600 U/ml and a CMV IgG index >15.0 antibody units/ml is considered a positive result.
†Antibodies to CMV were tested by indirect fluorescent antibody method (Biowhittaker, Inc., Walkersville, Md.).
‡Antibodies to CMV were tested by complement fixation (Zeus Scientific, Branchburg, N.J.).

regions (viral polymerase, major immediate-early, and glycoproteins B and H) by restriction endonuclease digestion according to the method of Chou.[2,3] The CMV strains from the mother and infant were identical at all four gene regions, in contrast to the differences seen with the laboratory control strain AD169 (Figure). Antibodies to human immunodeficiency, virus were not detected in cord blood from the neonate (by enzyme immunoassay and Western blot), and test results for HIV (by HIV blood culture) and for

HIV DNA (by HIV polymerase chain reaction) were also negative.

DISCUSSION

Nonprimary CMV infection during gestation rarely causes serious congenital CMV infection.[4] Several cases of symptomatic congenital CMV infection after recurrent maternal infection have been reported,[5] but this is the first instance, to our knowledge, of such transmission from a mother with acquired immunodeficiency syndrome. Maternal CMV viremia apparently resulted in intrauterine transmission to the fetus. The mother had CMV antibodies 2 years before her pregnancy and at the time also had a positive CMV IgM titer, suggesting that she might have had her primary CMV infection in 1990. Evidently maternal immunity sufficient to modify congenital CMV infection when the mother and baby are immunologically intact was not adequate in this instance to protect the mother and infant from overwhelming viral disease.

The infant had invasive CMV infection of the kidneys and adrenal glands that may have contributed to his death. He had no evidence of HIV infection but this cannot be excluded.[6] The mother's PCP did not respond to standard therapy despite the absence of poor prognostic factors at the onset of illness, leading us to speculate that management of her pulmonary disease was complicated by CMV infection in the lungs. The use of corticosteroids for the treatment of the mother's PCP may have contributed to the activation of CMV disease.[7]

Although much attention has been focused on the risk of HIV infection among children born to HIV-infected women, there has been relatively little discussion about the risk of mother-to-child transmission of HIV-related opportunistic pathogens.[8, 9] Recent observations suggest that congenital CMV infection among children born to HIV-infected women may emerge as a serious problem.[10] In addition to CMV, other common HIV-related pathogens that may pose a particular threat to the fetus or neonate include toxoplasmosis and herpes simplex, so that fetal/neonatal prophylaxis may evolve as an important issue. The pharmacokinetics of maternal-fetal distribution of drugs used for treatment and prophylaxis of HIV-related infections has also received little study. For example, we observed placental transfer of pentamidine when plasma samples were analyzed for pentamidine concentration from this pregnant mother and the cord blood from her neonate.[11]

Concern also exists that CMV infection might promote vertical transmission of HIV,[12, 13] accelerate the course of pediatric HIV disease, or both. More information is needed to determine the level of risk in this setting and appropriate measures for counseling, monitoring, prophylaxis, and treatment for CMV infection in pregnant women with HIV infection.

REFERENCES

1. Pass RF, Stagno S, Myers GJ, Alford CA. Outcome of symptomatic congenital cytomegalovirus infection: results of long-term longitudinal follow-up. Pediatrics 1980;66:758-62.
2. Chou S. Differentiation of cytomegalovirus strains by restriction analysis of DNA sequences amplified from clinical specimens. J Infect Dis 1990;162:738-42.
3. Saltzman RI, Quirk MR, Jordan MC. Disseminated cytomegalovirus infection: molecular analysis of virus and leukocyte interactions in viremia. J Clin Invest 1988;81:75-81.
4. Fowler KB, Stagno S, Pass RF, Britt WJ, Boll TJ, Alford CA. The outcome of congenital cytomegalovirus infection in relation to maternal antibody status. N Engl J Med 1992;326:663-7.
5. Morris DJ, Sims D, Chiswick M, Das VK, Newton V. Symptomatic congenital cytomegalovirus infection after maternal recurrent infection. Pediatr Infect Dis J 1994;13:61-4.
6. El-Sadr W, Oleske JM, Agins BD, et al. Diagnosis of HIV infection in infants and children: evaluation and management of early HIV infection. Clinical practice guideline no. 7:82-5. Washington, D.C.: U.S. Department of Health and Human Services, January 1994.
7. Nelson MR, Erskine D, Hawkins DA, Gazzard BG. Treatment with corticosteroids—a risk factor for the development of clinical cytomegalovirus disease in AIDS. AIDS 1993;7:375-8.
8. Boyer P, Dillon M, Navaie M, et al. Factors predictive of maternal-fetal transmission of HIV-1. JAMA 1994;271:1925-30.
9. Thomas P, Weedon J, Krasinski K, et al. Maternal predictors of perinatal human immunodeficiency virus transmission. Pediatr Infect Dis J 1994;13:489-95.
10. Saenz M, Leist T, Fallo A, Hutto C. Congenital CMV infection in infants born to HIV infected mothers [Abstract 1201]. In: Program and abstracts of the 33rd Interscience Conference on Antimicrobial Agents and Chemotherapy, American Society of Microbiology, New Orleans, Louisiana, October 17-20, 1993.
11. Schwebke K, Fletcher C, Acosta E, Henry K. Pentamidine pharmacokinetics in a neonate and his mother with AIDS: case report. Clin Infect Dis (in press).
12. Cooper ER, Schwartz T, Brena A, Regan AM, Pelton SI. Cytomegalovirus as a cofactor in transmission and progression of perinatal HIV infection. Pediatr AIDS HIV Infect 1992;3:302-7.
13. Tovo P, Riva C, Palomba E, et al. Herpesvirus infections do not influence the course of perinatal HIV-1 infection. Pediatric AIDS HIV Infect 1994;3:180-3.

THE BOOK SHELF **André D. Lascari,** *Editor*

Book reviews

Guidebook for pediatric hypertension

Hohn AR, Mount Kisco, New York: Futura, 1994. 278 pages. $55.

This book presents a panoramic and in-depth view of arterial hypertension in childhood. Such a multifaceted and fascinating subject may sometimes lack specific causes; conversely, clearcut etiologies emerge in other instances. Thus differentiation between primary and secondary blood pressure disorders can become a highly complex problem that may tax the mind and stretch considerably the capabilities and the imagination of pediatricians and internists. Moreover, arterial hypertension remains unprecisely defined in children. At this age, appropriate determination of blood pressure levels, implementation of diagnostic techniques, use of antihypertensive medications and/or corrective surgery are necessary goals to effect adequate control or complete cure.

In recent years, understanding of arterial hypertension's regulatory mechanisms in general, and in pediatrics in particular, has experienced a "quantum leap." The momentum created by this knowledge has enhanced awareness about an ailment that was not in the vanguard of pediatric interests. By stimulating pediatricians to look for earlier developmental stages of the disorder, a more aggressive therapeutic and preventive posture to control a "silent killer" has evolved. All this and much more is clearly, thoroughly, and elegantly discussed, and "distilled" by Dr. Hohn in his eminently clinical book. Its 10 chapters cover topics ranging from blood pressure regulation to measurement techniques and normal values, to the epidemiology of the disorder in young people and their risk factors for development of hypertension. Cardiac, renal, and endocrine-related hypertension problems are extensively discussed. The subject of neonatal hypertension and its intricacies is expertly handled. Finally, clinical evaluation and therapeutic principles for hypertension in the young conclude the main body of the book. A small appendix listing "other causes of hypertension, and texts" on the subject bring this work to a conclusion.

In this comprehensive, scholarly—yet highly practical—book, Dr. Hohn has successfully assembled a large body of updated literature. More importantly, however, he has imparted his personal, "cardiologic," and highly experienced approach to the study and management of pediatric hypertension. The text's terse style is fully reinforced with useful tables, illustrations, and references. We highly recommend this fine-quality teaching book to individuals at all levels of training in general pediatrics and the subspecialties.

Rod E. Urizar, MD
Professor of Pediatrics
Associate Professor of Medicine
Director, Pediatric Dialysis Service
Department of Medicine, Division of Nephrology
Albany Medical College
Albany, NY 12208

Practitioner's guide to developmental and psychological testing

Aylward GP. New York: Plenum, 1994. 258 pages. $37.50.

The author, a psychologist, has written this guide for physicians and other health care professionals to improve their ability to deal with developmental evaluations, learning disabilities, and other clinical problems often requiring application of developmental assessment instruments. Interpretation of psychologic test results requires that the nonpsychologist have some knowledge of the strengths and weaknesses of each test, the range of normal, and the range of variation among children with delays or disabilities.

The initial chapter deals with terminology and standard statistical concepts. The second chapter covers developmental screening and briefly describes commonly used instruments, some familiar (Denver Developmental Screening Test[s], Bayley Scales of Infant Development) and others less so. Subsequent chapters discuss evaluation of language and of behavioral/adaptive function, cognitive/intellectual (IQ) testing, and assessment of academic achievement. An entire chapter is devoted to attention/concentration, but rating scales that measure attention-deficit problems are included in the chapter on behavioral assessment. The discussion of school performance problems provides guidance regarding the overall assessment of the many factors that can contribute to learning difficulties, including limited intellect, attention deficits, and behavior problems. The final chapter contains practical advice regarding many clinical issues, such as counseling parents and explaining the need for medications to children.

This book is generally free of psychologic jargon and written in a way that makes it easy for a physician to read. The descriptions of the various assessment instruments are probably more detailed than many physicians will want, but are valuable for those interested in child development. Figures illustrate the approach to some of the commonly encountered initial complaints. I believe that this book would be a good addition to pediatric departmental libraries and to the personal collections of health care workers dealing with problems of delayed development, poor school achievement, or behavior.

Joseph M. Garfunkel, MD
Editor

Growth and the growth hormone axis in prepubertal children with asthma

Suzanne Crowley, MRCP, Peter C. Hindmarsh, MD, David R. Matthews, MD, and Charles G. D. Brook, MD

From the Endocrine Unit, Middlesex Hospital, Mortimer Street, London, and the Diabetes Research Laboratories, Radcliffe Infirmary, Woodstock Road, Oxford, United Kingdom

To determine the influence of asthma and its treatment with inhaled corticosteroids on growth, linear growth velocity, and the growth hormone axis in prepubertal children, we performed a longitudinal study for 12 months in 56 children with asthma, aged between 4.4 and 11.7 years. Height, weight, skin-fold thickness, and lung function were measured every 3 months and bone age at entry to and exit from the study. A 24-hour serum growth hormone concentration profile and fasting insulin-like growth factor I levels were measured halfway through the year. Seventy-four percent of boys and 62% of girls had heights below the 50th percentile. Growth velocity in the nonsteroid-treated control group (n = 13) was normal; 10 of 20 children taking beclomethasone grew slowly (14/20 used a dry powder device), and 4 of 19 children taking budesonide grew slowly (15/19 used a spacer). Three of four children using inhaled steroids and prednisolone grew slowly. In none of the treatment groups were measures of growth hormone secretion or levels of radioimmunoassayable serum insulin-like growth factor I affected. We conclude that slow growth in steroid-treated children with asthma does not appear to be associated with major perturbations in the growth hormone axis. (J Pediatr 1995;126:297-303)

Delay in growth and puberty is a feature of asthma,[1, 2] eczema,[3, 4] and rhinitis,[5] suggesting an association between atopy and growth delay. Growth retardation may occur independently of asthma severity[5] but is exaggerated in those with severe disease and chronic hypoxemia,[6] by oral treatment with corticosteroids in a dose- and duration-dependent manner,[7] and by the emergence of symptoms before the age of 3 years.[6]

Inhaled glucocorticoids are commonly used for the treatment of moderate and severe asthma[8]; the two most commonly used in this country are beclomethasone dipropionate and budesonide. Several long-term studies[9-11] have concluded that treatment with up to 600 μg BDP daily does not suppress growth velocity in mid-childhood, although late prepubertal growth may be adversely affected.[11] It has been suggested that treatment with up to 1600 μg BDP or budesonide daily will permit normal growth velocity, provided that symptoms are well controlled.[12] By contrast, significant retardation of linear growth has been demonstrated in prepubertal children receiving 200 to 800 μg BDP in dry powder form,[13] and assessment of tibial growth by knemometry for short periods (up to 56 days) has demonstrated significant inhibition of linear growth velocity with a daily dose of 800 μg budesonide delivered through a large-volume

BA	Bone age
BDP	Beclomethasone dipropionate
FEV_1	Forced expiratory volume in 1 second
GH	Growth hormone
IGF-I	Insulin-like growth factor I
OC_{95}	Observed threshold concentration at or below which hormone concentrations are measured 95% of the time
SDS	Standard deviation score

Supported in part by Children Nationwide and by Novo Nordisk, Gentofte, Denmark (Dr. Crowley), and Kabi Pharmacia, Stockholm (Dr. Hindmarsh).

Submitted for publication May 17, 1994; accepted Aug. 16, 1994.

Reprint requests: Charles Brook, MD, Endocrine Unit, Middlesex Hospital, Mortimer St., London W1N 8AA, United Kingdom.

0022-3476/95/$3.00 + 0 **9/25/59945**

spacer.[14] Thus the potential of inhaled steroids to retard growth exists, but the dose at which this is likely to occur may depend on the type of delivery device used,[15] the age of the child,[11] and individual susceptibility to steroid-induced side effects. The endocrine events accompanying growth delay and steroid-mediated growth suppression have not been elucidated in children with asthma. The few reports of growth hormone secretion in children treated for asthma, with or without steroids, suggest that stimulated GH secretion is not less than in normal subjects.[16-19] Serum levels of insulin-like growth factor I are normal in steroid-treated adults with asthma.[20] To clarify the relationship between asthma and its treatment with growth and the GH axis, we studied 56 prepubertal children with asthma.

METHODS

Patients. Children were selected on the basis of age (range, 4.4 to 11.7 years) from the asthma clinics of three London teaching hospitals (Hammersmith Hospital, Royal Brompton National Heart and Lung Hospital, and King's College Hospital) and from a district general hospital (Kingston-upon-Thames, Surrey). Patients were excluded if there were signs of puberty, coexisting rhinitis, and/or eczema requiring treatment with topical application of steroids, low birth weight, parental heights <3rd percentile, or a history of psychologic difficulties requiring treatment. A total of 141 patients were invited to participate; 58 declined and 83 (59%) were recruited to the study. Those who did not enroll were measured. The study protocol was approved by the ethics committee of each participating hospital. Informed parental consent and patient assent were obtained in each case.

A detailed history of asthma symptoms and drug use, physical examination, and measurement of height (Harpenden stadiometer), weight, subscapular and triceps skin-fold thickness (Holtain calipers), and pubertal stage were recorded at each 3-monthly visit throughout the observation period of 12 months. Measurement of height was made without knowledge of the previous measurement. Lung function was assessed with a portable Vitalograph analyzer (Vitalograph Medical Instruments Ltd., Buckingham, United Kingdom) measuring forced expiratory volume in 1 second and forced vital capacity. Inhaler technique was checked by one of us (S.C.) or by a trained clinic nurse. Bone age was estimated by the method of Tanner and Whitehouse at the beginning and end of the study. Patients taking inhaled steroids must have been stable on their treatment for at least 1 month before recruitment, but dosage was increased to cover any exacerbation of symptoms during the observation year. Any increase was included in the calculations of mean annual dose. Assessment of treatment compliance was based on patient and parental information.

Fifty-two children were admitted to the hospital for a 24-hour GH profile approximately halfway through their observation year. Sampling for GH commenced after an overnight period of acclimatization, and blood was withdrawn at 20-minute intervals through an indwelling heparinized intravenous cannula, commencing at 7 AM. At 6 AM on the following morning, blood was withdrawn for estimation of fasting IGF-I concentration. Normal daily activity was encouraged during the sampling period, and the usual asthma treatment was taken. A 5-day dietary diary (Salford University "Microdiet" System, Salford University, Manchester, United Kingdom) was completed as soon as possible after admission to the hospital.

Hormone assays. The samples from each patient were spun, separated, and stored at −20° C before assay. Serum GH concentration was measured with the Tandem-R immunoradiometric kit (Hybritech, Liege, Belgium). The interassay coefficients of variation were 10.5%, 7.2%, and 5.4% at serum GH concentrations of 6.0, 13.2, and 33.3 mU/L, respectively, and the intraassay coefficients of variation were 10.6%, 4.9%, and 5.2% at serum GH concentrations of 1.4, 3.4, and 26.4 mU/L, respectively. The sensitivity of the assay was 0.5 mU/L. Serum IGF-I concentration was measured with a polyclonal radioimmunoassay.[21] The sensitivity of the assay was 0.07 U/ml. The interassay coefficients of variation were 10.5% and 5.1% at concentrations of 0.38 and 3.73 U/ml, respectively, and the intraassay coefficients of variation were 11.3% and 4.7% at concentrations of 0.32 and 3.77 U/ml, respectively.

Analysis of growth. All anthropometric data are presented as standard deviation scores.[22] Linear growth velocity was determined by linear regression of height measurements against age for each child. This method minimizes inaccuracies in measurement by including all intervening observations, rather than just the initial and final ones.

Analysis of growth hormone secretion. Two methods of analysis were applied to each 24-hour GH profile. First, the profiles were analyzed by Fourier transformation to determine the dominant oscillatory frequency (relative spectral power).[23] Second, the method of observed concentration was used to determine alterations in "peak" and "trough" concentrations.[24] The 72-serum GH concentration values from each profile were arranged in ascending order and allocated to log-distributed GH intervals (bins) as a cumulative percentage value of the profile. These percentage values were then assigned values as linear probits and plotted against the log-transformed bin values, to yield a straight line. From the resulting equation, an estimate of the "peak" value (OC_{95}—the observed concentration for 95%), which is defined as the threshold concentration at or below which the hormone concentrations are measured 95% of the time, was derived. Conversely, the OC_5 yields an estimate of trough values, and OC_{50} an estimate of mean values.

Assessment of lung function. Lung function was assessed at each clinic visit with the portable Vitalograph to measure FEV_1 and forced vital capacity. The best values from three attempts were taken. There was less than 15% variability in the results.

Analysis of dietary data. Five-day nutrient intakes were compared with 1991 dietary reference values for boys and girls aged 7 to 10 years. These are presented as percentage values of the recommended daily intake for energy, protein, carbohydrate, and fat.

Statistical analysis. The children were grouped according to treatment as follows: group 1, non-steroid-dependent (n = 13); group 2, budesonide (n = 19); group 3, beclomethasone (n = 20); and group 4, inhaled steroid and prednisolone (n = 4). For 95% power at a 5% level of significance, at least 12 patients were required in each of groups 1, 2, and 3 to detect a difference in linear growth velocity of 0.8 SDS (approximately 0.75 cm/yr).[25] Group comparisons of GH, IGF-I, and auxologic and dietary data were made with one-way analysis of variance, with the Newman-Keuls aftertest applied to assess significance between the groups. Multiple analysis of variance was used to examine influences on height achieved. The Student t test was used to examine differences between steroid-treated and non-steroid-treated patients, and nonparametric statistics were used when data were not normally distributed. Data are presented as mean (SD), and 95% confidence limits are used when normal population data are not available.

RESULTS

Patients and treatment. Thirty-five boys and 21 girls completed the study; four children refused blood sampling. The overall mean (range) age was 8.3 (4.4 to 11.7) years; group means did not differ significantly. The most common reason given for refusal to participate in the study was the dislike of hospital admission and blood sampling (18/58); three gave "normal growth" as a reason. Of the 83 patients recruited, 17 (20%) dropped out during the observation year and 10 were excluded on the grounds of poor treatment compliance or the onset of pubertal development. The children who were treated with steroids had asthma symptoms at age 1.9 versus 3.3 years for the control group ($p = 0.19$). The mean doses of inhaled steroid in groups 2 and 3 was similar (762 [525] and 560 [281] $\mu g/m^2$ per day for budesonide and BDP, respectively; $p = 0.15$). Fifteen of nineteen children and 4 of 20 children in the budesonide and BDP groups, respectively, used a large-volume spacer device, reflecting general prescribing habits. All patients receiving inhalation steroids used a twice-daily treatment regimen, with the exception of one patient who used BDP four times daily. One patient in group 2 used nebulized budesonide, 2.43 mg/m^2 per day; two patients in group 4 were taking nebulized budesonide in doses of 2.5 and 2.4 mg/m^2 per day, respectively, in addition to prednisolone by mouth in doses ranging from 4.5 to 20 mg/m^2 on alternate days. A third child taking budesonide, 1070 $\mu g/m^2$ per day, delivered as a dry powder through a dry-powder inhalation device (Turbohaler; Lund, Sweden), received four short courses (3 days) of prednisolone (30 mg/m^2 per day) for infective exacerbations during winter months. Her endocrine profile was assessed before any prednisolone was taken. The remaining child took BDP, up to 1470 $\mu g/m^2$ per day, via a large-volume spacer and a mean dose of prednisolone of 20 mg/m^2 per day.

Anthropometry. The height SDS for study patients was −0.37 compared with −0.03 for the 58 nonparticipants ($p = 0.09$). When the height SDS of nonparticipants and study patients was compared according to treatment, no significant difference emerged: height SDS for BDP patients was −0.17 versus −0.66 ($p = 0.10$) and for budesonide patients −0.04 versus −0.36 ($p = 0.5$), respectively. When all groups were considered, including those nonparticipants for whom no treatment information was available (n = 14), no height SDS difference emerged ($p = 0.6$). Of those completing the study, 7 (20%) of 35 boys, and 3 (15%) of 21 girls had heights at or below the 3rd percentile, whereas 26 (74%) of 35 boys and 13 (62%) of 21 girls had heights below the 50th percentile. Boys had a height SDS of −0.61 compared with −0.08 for girls ($p = 0.1$). This trend was not due to boys' being clustered around the peripubertal period, when growth velocity may be slow in the presence of growth delay; 11 of 35 boys were aged 10 years or older, and their height SDS was −0.60 (1.01) compared with −0.61 (1.21) for those aged less than 10 years.

Mean linear growth velocity SDS was significantly lower in the beclomethasone- and prednisolone-treated groups (−1.04 [0.99] and −1.58 [1.01], respectively) in comparison with the non-steroid-treated group (0.03 [0.90]) and the budesonide-treated group (−0.20 [0.99], $p < 0.001$) (Figure). Of 39 children receiving inhaled steroids, 14 (36%) grew slowly (GV SDS < -0.8); 4 (29%) of 14 children were taking budesonide and 10 (71%) of 14 were taking BDP (7 dry powder). Among the 10 BDP-treated patients growing slowly, the largest homogeneous group comprised seven using dry powder, at a mean dose of 655 (200) $\mu g/m^2$ per day. Of the remaining three children, two were using a metered-dose inhaler (310 and 355 $\mu g/m^2$ per day) and one was using a large-volume spacer (1000 $\mu g/m^2$ per day). Of the four budesonide-treated patients growing slowly, two were using a large-volume spacer (985 and 1555 $\mu g/m^2$ per day)

Table. Measures of 24-hour growth hormone secretion in children with asthma, expressed as "peak" (OC_{95}), average (OC_{50}), and "trough" (OC_5) values, and serum insulin-like growth factor I concentrations according to treatment and growth rate

Group	GH OC_{95} (mU/L)	GH OC_{50} (mU/L)	GH OC_5 (mU/L)	IGF-I (U/ml)
1 (nonsteroid)	27.2 (14.5)	1.38 (0.81)	0.12 (0.14)	0.58 (0.27)
2 (budesonide)	16.3 (11.9)	1.27 (0.82)	0.17 (0.28)	0.53 (0.30)
3 (BDP)	21.5 (10.9)	1.11 (0.76)	0.87 (0.09)	0.57 (0.29)
4 (prednisolone)	18.4 (12.4)	1.52 (2.18)	0.27 (0.41)	0.90 (0.02)
	(p = 0.12)	(p = 0.82)	(p = 0.26)	(p = 0.25)
GV SDS <−0.8	17.9 (12.2)	1.05 (0.78)	0.10 (0.14)	0.70 (0.31)
GV SDS >−0.8	22.6 (13.0)	1.37 (0.99)	0.16 (0.24)	0.53 (0.26)
	(p = 0.20)	(p = 0.21)	(p = 0.26)	(p = 0.06)

Data are presented as mean (SD).
GV, Growth velocity (linear).

and two a dry-powder device (Turbohaler) (630 and 565 $\mu g/m^2$ per day).

The weight SDS and the triceps and subscapular skin-fold thickness SDS were similar to standard values.

Bone age. Mean (SD) bone age was not significantly delayed by steroid use (mean BA delay −0.52 [1.19] and −1.05 [1.56] in non-steroid-treated and steroid-treated children, respectively (p = 0.20). When height was expressed according to BA (height SDS for BA), the children's heights matched those of the general population and were not diminished by steroid use: height SDS BA = 0.75 (1.24) and 0.68 (1.23), respectively; p = 0.86.

Lung function and growth. Mean (±SD) FEV_1 (percentage of the predicted value) did not differ among the groups (group 1, 88% ± 12%; group 2, 89% ± 13%; group 3, 92% ± 11%; group 4, 88% ± 12%; p = 0.8) and showed no correlation with linear growth velocity (r = −0.11; p = 0.44).

GH secretion and IGF-I. The modal GH pulse frequency assessed by Fourier transformation was 200 minutes in the non-steroid-treated group. Pulse frequency was significantly faster in the beclomethasone group (140 minutes) ($p < 0.025$) but not in the budesonide (160 minutes) or in the prednisolone (180 minutes) group.

There were no significant group differences in quantitative measures of GH secretion (Table). There was no difference in $OC_{95, 50, 5}$ values in those growing slowly compared with normal growers (Table).

There were no significant group differences in IGF-I values (Table). In non-steroid-treated children, IGF-I was significantly correlated with chronologic and bone age (r = 0.66, p = 0.02 and r = 0.67, p = 0.01, respectively), but this relationship was lost with steroid treatment: r = 0.18, p = 0.27 and r = 0.21, p = 0.20, respectively.

Dietary analysis. Thirty-eight of the returned diaries were suitable for analysis. There were no group differences in daily energy intake or proportion of energy derived from protein, fat, and carbohydrate (data not shown).

DISCUSSION

This study demonstrates that inhaled steroids influence the growth rates of children with asthma but that this effect is not reflected in major quantitative changes in GH secretion or the generation of immunoreactive IGF-I. Each patient had one 24-hour GH profile during the study year, and although individual values may vary from day to day, group data are known to be reproducible.[26] The study took into account nutrition and lung function, both of which may influence growth rate. Our dietary assessments and the weight and skin-fold thickness measures did not indicate that inadequate nutrition was responsible for the slow growth; in such a situation, we would expect IGF-I levels to be low and the GH pulsatility to be abnormal.[27] Increased GH pulse frequency, as demonstrated in group 3, is a recognized glucocorticoid effect.[28] The possible tendency for IGF-I levels to be higher in slowly growing children suggests a degree of resistance to its action. The lack of group differences in mean FEV_1 values and the absence of correlation with growth rates indicate that poor lung function was not responsible for the observed differences in linear growth velocity.

The remaining major variables are disease severity and treatment.[7] The effects of these variables are difficult to separate because patients with more severe disease will require more intensive treatment. Categorization of asthma is based on frequency, chronicity, and severity of symptoms; when possible, lung function measurements provide a more objective assessment.[8] The promotion of catch-up growth when patients with asthma are converted from a daily to an alternate-day steroid regimen[29] suggests that when symptoms are controlled, prednisolone rather than disease severity is more likely to be responsible for slow growth. Growth

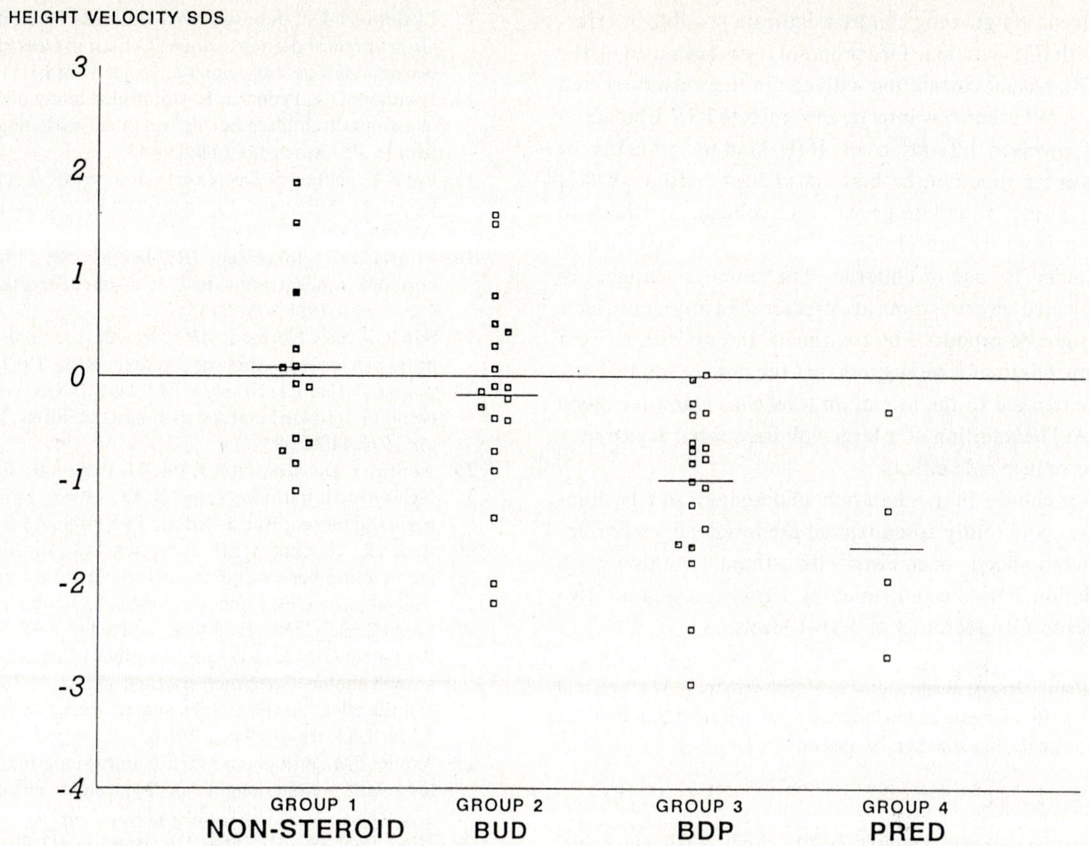

Figure. Linear growth velocity expressed as an SDS for each treatment group. *Bar* represents mean values. *BUD*, Budesonide treatment; *BDP*, beclomethasone therapy; *PRED*, treatment with prednisolone.

delay was present in the non-steroid-treated children but was more marked in the steroid-treated children, suggesting a cumulative effect of both treatment and disease.

Within the steroid-treated groups, differences in growth rate were observed. In groups 2 and 3, this may have been due to the use of large-volume spacer devices in group 2, which reduced the incidence and severity of systemic side effects,[30] although pharmacologic differences between the two drugs may be more important.[31] Approximately 60% to 70% of swallowed BDP in powdered form is absorbed from the gut,[32] and its 17-α-monopropionate metabolite is largely responsible for systemic side effects. The use of a volumatic spacer-device in adult volunteers reduces oropharyngeal deposition of salbutamol labeled with technetium 99m[33]; the same device reduces the incidence of adrenal suppression.[15, 30] Ideally, all patients in the study would have been using the same drug delivery device, but at the time of its inception the importance of the device in relation to side effects was only beginning to be recognized.

The mechanism of glucocorticoid-induced growth suppression is not clear. Glucocorticoids exert a dual influence on GH, enhancing the pituitary content[34] while inhibiting its release.[35] The latter is thought to be mediated by an increase in somatostatin tone,[35] and glucocorticoid-treated rats grow better when passively immunized with somatostatin antibodies.[36] Patients with Cushing syndrome have a blunted GH response to insulin-induced hypoglycemia,[37] but the GH response to hypoglycemia is normal in steroid-treated children with asthma,[16-19] which suggests a dose-dependent inhibition of GH release. Steroids may exert their effects more locally on bone and cartilage, because glucocorticoid receptors have been found on osteoblasts and osteoclasts.[38] The lack of significant quantitative changes in GH secretion in the children using inhaled steroids or prednisolone or both indicates that the latter mechanism may be more important.

Glucocorticoid effects on bone are numerous, but their mechanism of action on skeletal growth is not understood. IGF-I mediates the promotion of skeletal growth by GH, and immunoreactive levels of IGF-I in steroid-treated adult patients with asthma do not differ from those of non-steroid-treated subjects with asthma.[20] The lack of group difference in IGF-I levels in our study patients despite significant differences in growth rates, and the tendency toward higher levels in slowly growing children, indicate possible interference with IGF-I action. This proposal is strengthened by the loss of the usual correlation with age in the steroid-treated patients. Whether this interference affects IGF-I bioactivity or involves alteration of IGF binding proteins or postreceptor function, or both, is unclear. Although GH treatment can stimulate growth and collagen synthesis in glucocorticoid-treated children,[39] there is no evidence to recommend its use in children. The potential dangers of uncontrolled severe asthma are greater than any side effects that might be produced by treatment. In line with current recommendations,[8] we suggest that the dose of inhaled steroid be titrated to the minimum level that maintains good control. The addition of a large-volume spacer device may help to reduce side effects.

We conclude that inhalation budesonide and beclomethasone, and orally administered prednisolone, retard linear growth velocity in children with asthma, but this growth retardation is not accompanied by significant quantitative changes in GH secretion or IGF-I levels.

We thank Drs. A. Bush, J. Price, M. Silverman, J. Warner, and R. Wilson for allowing us to study their patients, and Sandra Gardiner for analyzing the dietary diaries.

REFERENCES

1. Spock A. Growth patterns in 200 children with bronchial asthma. Ann Allergy 1965;23:608-15.
2. Hauspie R, Susanne C, Alexander F. Maturational delay and temporal growth retardation in asthmatic boys. J Allergy Clin Immunol 1967;59:200-6.
3. Kristmundsdottir F, David TJ. Growth impairment in children with atopic eczema. J R Soc Med 1987;80:9-12.
4. Pike MG, Chang CL, Atherton DJ, Carpenter RG, Preece MA. Growth in atopic eczema: a controlled study by questionnaire. Arch Dis Child 1989;64:1566-9.
5. Ferguson AC, Murray AB, Tze WJ. Short stature and delayed skeletal maturation in children with allergic disease. J Allergy Clin Immunol 1982;69:461-6.
6. Murray AB, Fraser BM, Hardwick DF, Pirie GE. Chronic asthma and growth failure in children. Lancet 1976;2:197-8.
7. Chang KC, Miklich DR, Barwise G, Chai H, Miles-Lawrence R. Linear growth of chronic asthmatic children: the effects of disease and various forms of steroid therapy. Clin Allergy 1982;12:369-78.
8. Asthma: a follow-up statement from an international paediatric asthma consensus group. Arch Dis Child 1992;67:240-8.
9. Kerrebijn KF. Beclomethasone dipropionate in long-term treatment of asthma in children. J Pediatr 1976;89:821-6.
10. Godfrey S, Balfour-Lynn L, Tooley M. A three- to five-year follow-up of the use of the aerosol steroid, beclomethasone dipropionate, in childhood asthma. J Allergy Clin Immunol 1978;62:335-9.
11. Balfour-Lynn L. Growth and childhood asthma. Arch Dis Child 1986;61:1049-55.
12. Ninan T, Russell G. Asthma, inhaled corticosteroid treatment, and growth. Arch Dis Child 1992;67:703-5.
13. Littlewood JM, Johnson AW, Edwards PA, Littlewood AE. Growth retardation in asthmatic children treated with inhaled beclomethasone dipropionate. Lancet 1988;1:115-6.
14. Wolthers OD, Pedersen S. Controlled study of linear growth in asthmatic children during treatment with inhaled glucocorticoids. Pediatrics 1992;89:839-42.
15. Prahl P, Jensen T. Decreased adrenocortical suppression utilizing the Nebuhaler for inhalation of steroid aerosols. Clin Allergy 1987;17:393-8.
16. Morris HG, Jorgensen JR, Jenkins SA. Plasma growth hormone concentration in corticosteroid-treated children. J Clin Invest 1968;47:427-35.
17. Sanders SS, Norman AP. Growth hormone secretion in growth-retarded asthmatic children. BMJ 1969;3:25-6.
18. Nigam P, Laungia S, Goyal BM, Dutt B. Growth hormone secretion in growth retarded asthmatic children. Indian J Pediatr 1977;44:315-9.
19. Amirav I, Dowdeswell RJ, Plit M, Panz VR, Joffe BI, Seftel HC. Growth hormone response to exercise in asthmatic and normal children. Eur J Pediatr 1990;149:443-6.
20. Reid IR, Gluckman PD, Ibbertson HK. Insulin-like growth factor 1 and bone turnover in glucocorticoid-treated and control subjects. Clin Endocrinol 1989;30:347-53.
21. Morrell DJ, Dadi H, More J, Taylor AM, Dabestani A, Buchanan CR. A monoclonal antibody to human insulin-like growth factor 1: characterisation, use in radioimmunoassay and the effect on the biological activities of the growth factor. J Mol Endocrinol 1989;2:201-6.
22. Tanner JM, Whitehouse RH. Clinical longitudinal standards for height, weight, height velocity, weight velocity, and stages of puberty. Arch Dis Child 1976;51:170-9.
23. Hindmarsh PC, Matthews DR, Brook CGD. Growth hormone secretion in children determined by time series analysis. Clin Endocrinol 1988;29:35-4.
24. Matthews DR, Hindmarsh PC, Pringle PJ, Brook CGD. A distribution method for analysing the baseline of pulsatile endocrine signals as exemplified by 24-hour growth hormone profiles. Clin Endocrinol 1991;35:245-52.
25. Day SJ, Graham DF. Sample size and power for comparing two or more treatment groups in clinical trials. BMJ 1989;299:663-5.
26. Saini S, Hindmarsh PC, Matthews DR, et al. Reproducibility of 24-hour serum growth hormone profiles in man. Clin Endocrinol 1991;34:455-62.
27. Ho KY, Veldhuis JD, Johnson ML, et al. Fasting enhances growth hormone secretion and amplifies the complex rhythms of growth hormone secretion in man. J Clin Invest 1988;81:968-75.
28. Pralong FP, Miell JP, Corder R, Gaillard RC. Dexamethasone treatment in man induces changes in 24-hour growth hormone (GH) secretion profile without altering total GH released. J Clin Endocrinol Metab 1991;73:1191-5.
29. Byron MA, Jackson J, Ansell BM. Effect of different corticosteroid regimens on hypothalamic-pituitary-adrenal axis and growth in juvenile chronic arthritis. J R Soc Med 1983;76:452-7.
30. Brown PH, Blundell G, Greening AP, Crompton GK. Do large volume spacer devices reduce the systemic effects of high-dose inhaled corticosteroids? Thorax 1990;45:736-9.
31. Harris DM. Some properties of beclomethasone dipropionate and related steroids in man. Postgrad Med J 1975;51(suppl 4):20-5.

32. Martin LE, Tanner RJN, Clark TJH, Cochrane GM. Absorption and metabolism of orally administered beclomethasone dipropionate. Clin Pharmacol Ther 1973;15:267-75.
33. Matthys H, Eltschka R, App EM. Deposition of a radioactively labelled beta$_2$-sympathomimetic aerosol. Atemw.-Lungenkrkh 1988;14:485-8.
34. Wehrenberg WB, Baird A, Ling N. Potent interaction between glucocorticoids and growth hormone-releasing hormone in vivo. Science 1983;221:556-7.
35. Wehrenberg WB, Janowski BA, Piering AW, Culler F, Jones KL. Glucocorticoids: potent inhibitors and stimulators of growth hormone secretion. Endocrinology 1990;126:3200-3.
36. Wehrenberg WB, Bergman PJ, Stagg L, Ndon J, Giustina A. Glucocorticoid inhibition of growth in rats: partial reversal with somatostatin antibodies. Endocrinology 1990;127:2705-8.
37. Krieger DT, Glick SM. Growth hormone and cortisol responsiveness in Cushing's syndrome. Am J Med 1972;52:25-40.
38. Chen TL, Feldman D. Glucocorticoid receptors and actions in subpopulations of cultured rat bone cells: mechanism of dexamethasone potentiation of parathyroid hormone–stimulated cyclic AMP production. J Clin Invest 1979;63:650-8.
39. Allen DB, Goldberg BD. Stimulation of collagen synthesis and linear growth by growth hormone in glucocorticoid-treated children. Pediatrics 1992;89:416-21.

Corticosteroid therapy for ventricular tachycardia in children with silent lymphocytic myocarditis

Toshihiro Ino, MD, Mataichi Okubo, MD, Katsumi Akimoto, MD, Kei Nishimoto, MD, Keijiro Yabuta, MD, Sachio Kawai, MD, and Ryozo Okada, MD

From the Department of Pediatrics and Cardiovascular Pathology Laboratory, Juntendo University School of Medicine, Tokyo, Japan

Objective: **The objective of our study was to describe the efficacy of corticosteroids for ventricular tachycardia in four children with structurally normal hearts in whom endomyocardial biopsy revealed histologic changes of lymphocytic myocarditis.**

Patients: **The four patients had unexplained ventricular tachycardia. Three dysrhythmias were sustained, and one was inducible by exercise. Patient ages ranged from 4 months to 12 years. Three of the four patients had no symptoms. In two of them, ventricular tachycardia was identified by mass screening for heart disease. Two patients received oral steroids and two received pulse steroid therapy.**

Results: **In all four patients, significant underlying diseases were not found by noninvasive evaluation. Right ventricular endomyocardial biopsy revealed abnormal histologic findings of chronic lymphocytic myocarditis in all patients. Steroid therapy was effective in all four patients, two of whom received methylprednisolone pulse therapy.**

Conclusions: **We conclude that unexplained ventricular tachycardia may be the only manifestation of clinically silent myocarditis. Steroid therapy should therefore be considered if conventional antiarrhythmic medication is not effective and histologic findings confirm the presence of lymphocytic myocarditis. (J Pediatr 1995;126:304-8)**

Ventricular tachycardia is a relatively uncommon arrhythmia in children with structurally normal hearts. Mass screening for heart disease is available for Japanese children, and arrhythmias are sometimes detected unexpectedly.[1] In these children the characteristics of ventricular tachycardia are usually considered to be benign because of slow ventricular rate, nonsustained duration, and the absence of obvious associated heart disease.[2] However, these conditions are potentially life-threatening and may be related to sudden death during exercise. According to previous reports, more than half of patients with unexplained ventricular tachycardia have histologic myocardial abnormalities such as myocarditis or dilated cardiomyopathy.[3-5]

During an 8-year period, we encountered 10 patients with unexplained ventricular tachycardia. In 4 of these 10 cases, lymphocytic myocarditis was confirmed by endomyocardial biopsy and treatment with prednisolone was effective. We report the clinical and laboratory characteristics of these 4 patients.

Submitted for publication Jan. 27, 1994; accepted Aug. 26, 1994.

Reprint requests: Toshihiro Ino, MD, Department of Pediatrics, Juntendo University School of Medicine, 2-1-1 Hongo, Bunkyo-ku, Tokyo 113 Japan.

0022-3476/95/$3.00 + 0 **9/25/60159**

METHODS

During the period from January 1985 to December 1993, we identified 10 consecutive patients with unexplained ventricular tachycardia. The age of these patients ranged from

Table. Clinical and laboratory details of four patients with unexplained ventricular tachycardia

	Patient 1	Patient 2	Patient 3	Patient 4
Age at presentation	4 mo	10 mo	6 yr	12 yr
Sex	Male	Male	Male	Male
Tachycardia				
Type	S, LBBB	S, RBBB	LBBB	S, LBBB
Rate (/min)	150-170	250-300	120-140	120-140
EPS performed	(−)	(−)	(+)	(−)
24 hr ECG	(+)	(+)	(+)	(+)
Symptoms	(−)	Poor sucking	(−)	Palpitations
Cardiothoracic ratio (%) on chest x-ray film	45%	65%	54%	55%
Echocardiography				
Fractional shortening (%)	35%	21%	32%	36%
Ventricular dilation	(−)	Slight	(−)	(−)
Creatine kinase (U/L)	48	38	52	51
Abnormal viral titer	(−)	Coxsackievirus A3, B7	(−)	(−)
Catheter data				
LV contractility	Normal	Slightly reduced	Normal	Normal
LV end-diastolic pressure (mm Hg)	5	10	5	3
Coronary artery	Normal	Normal	Normal	Normal
Histologic findings	Chronic myocarditis	Chronic myocarditis	Chronic myocarditis	Chronic myocarditis
Treatment before steroid therapy	Propranolol Verapamil	Pilsicainide hydrochloride Dysopyramide Verapamil Mexiletine	None	Mexiletine
Follow-up period (yr)	3.4	5.0	3.2	1.9

S, Sustained; *LBBB*, left bundle-branch block; *RBBB*, right bundle-branch block; *EPS*, electrophysiologic study; *ECG*, electrocardiogram; *LV*, left ventricular.

4 months to 17.9 years (median, 9.6 years), and the male/female ratio was 8/2. Two of the patients were less than 1 year of age. In five of them, ventricular tachycardia was identified by mass screening for heart disease available in Tokyo, which consisted of simplified electrocardiography (leads I, aVF, V_1, and V_6) and phonocardiography (at second and fourth intercostal spaces of left sternal border). The results of clinical and noninvasive examinations (chest x-ray study, resting and exercise electrocardiography, 24-hour ambulatory electrocardiography, and two-dimensional echocardiography) were reviewed, and the cause of the ventricular tachycardia could not be definitely established. According to our policy, cardiac catheterization, angiography, and endomyocardial biopsy were performed for any of the following reasons: (1) asymptomatic ventricular tachycardia inducible by exercise stress electrocardiography, (2) sustained tachycardia, (3) right bundle-branch block pattern, or (4) two-dimensional echocardiogram showing abnormal left ventricular wall motion. Ventricular tachycardia was defined as sustained in patients with spontaneous ventricular arrhythmia of uniform QRS configuration lasting >30 seconds or requiring termination because of hemodynamic compromise; it was defined as nonsustained in patients with uniform broad QRS complexes lasting for >3 beats for <30 seconds and terminating spontaneously without hemodynamic compromise.

Myocardial biopsy. Myocardial tissue was obtained by percutaneous transvenous techniques; two or three specimens were obtained from different sites within the right ventricle in each patient. The specimens were immediately fixed in 2.5% phosphate-buffered formalin in the catheterization room, and were preserved in paraffin blocks for light microscopic examination with hematoxylin-eosin, azan, and elastic–van Gieson stains. Two cardiac pathologists independently examined each specimen by light microscopy. Myocarditis was diagnosed on the basis of the histologic criteria (so-called Dallas criteria) proposed by Aretz et al.[6]

Corticosteroid therapy. Corticosteroid therapy was initiated when lymphocytic myocarditis was suspected on the basis of histologic examinations. Initially, prednisolone at a dose of 1 to 2 mg/kg per day was administered orally after the withdrawal of conventional antiarrhythmic medication. After 1 week, the dose of prednisolone was slowly decreased for a period of 4 to 6 weeks until a maintenance dose of 0.1 to 0.3 mg/kg per day was attained. Maintenance therapy was then continued for at least 3 months. When oral prednisolone therapy proved ineffective, pulse therapy with 30 mg methylprednisolone per kilogram body weight was

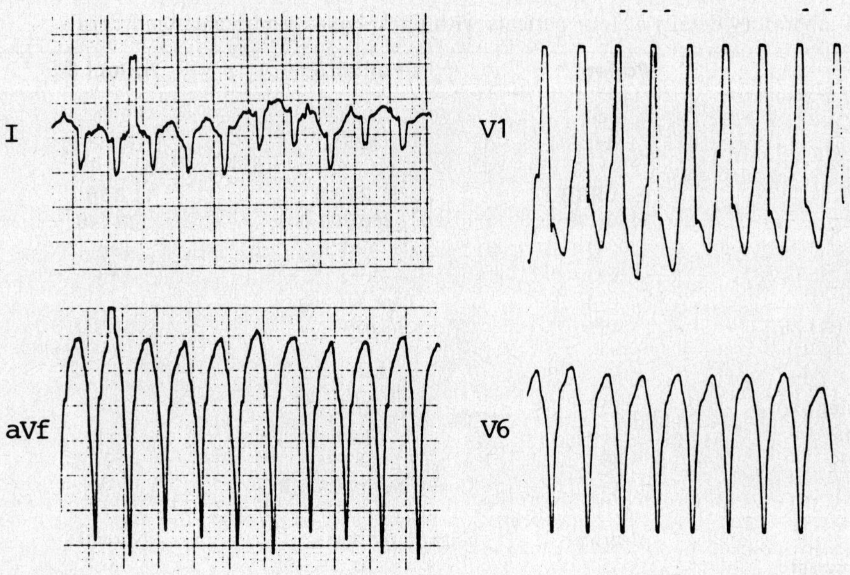

Fig. 1. Sustained ventricular tachycardia of right bundle-branch block type on standard electrocardiogram obtained on admission. Heart rate exceeded 300 beats/min.

instituted and continued for 3 days. The effect of corticosteroid therapy on ventricular tachycardia was assessed by standard and 24-hour ambulatory electrocardiograms. Effective treatment was defined as complete or >90% suppression of sustained tachycardia. Partially effective treatment was defined as a 60% to 90% reduction of sustained tachycardia or as a decrease in heart rate during persistent tachycardia to normal rates for age.

RESULTS

On the basis of histologic examination results, corticosteroid therapy was eventually instituted in four patients with lymphocytic myocarditis (Table).

Clinical and laboratory data. Two of the four patients had no symptoms. One patient had poor sucking because of ventricular tachycardia, and another had palpitations. None of the patients had abnormal erythrocyte sedimentation rate or C-reactive protein values, or significant elevations of myocardial enzymes (including creatine kinase). The ventricular tachycardia was of the left bundle-branch block type in three patients and the right bundle-branch block type in one, and was sustained in three of the four patients. The ventricular rate exceeded 300 beats/min in one patient (Fig. 1). Two-dimensional echocardiography revealed no structural abnormalities in all patients but disclosed a slightly dilated left ventricle in patient 2; the left ventricular dilation in this patient might be attributable to abnormal ventricular filling arising from ventricular tachycardia per se. Only patient 2 had slightly elevated antibody titers to coxsackieviruses A and B and to echovirus during the convalescent stage. All the patients underwent cardiac catheterization with left ventriculography and coronary angiography. Three patients had normal ejection fractions; the other had slightly reduced left ventricular contractility. Coronary arterial anatomy was normal in all patients. There was no significant elevation of left ventricular end-diastolic pressure in any patient.

Results of myocardial biopsy. Chronic lymphocytic myocarditis (Fig. 2) was histologically confirmed in all four patients. Histologic examination in these patients revealed slight mononuclear cell infiltration with moderate perivascular and interstitial fibrosis. The number of mononuclear cells was five or more times normal per high-power field in each specimen of all four patients. There was also evidence of mild but significant myocellular hypertrophy with unformed nuclei.

Results of corticosteroid therapy. Three of the four patients received prednisolone after ineffective antiarrhythmic treatment; the remaining patient received prednisolone as an initial treatment because at that time we had already confirmed the effectiveness of corticosteroids in previous patients. Ineffective drug treatment before prednisolone therapy consisted of propranolol, mexiletine, verapamil, and pilsicainide hydrochloride (Ic group antiarrhythmic drug). Oral administration of prednisolone was effective in two of the four patients, and pulse corticosteroid therapy was effective in two patients, one of whom had been ineffectively treated by oral corticosteroid therapy before pulse therapy. Follow-up 24-hour ambulatory electrocardiography revealed complete disappearance of ventricular

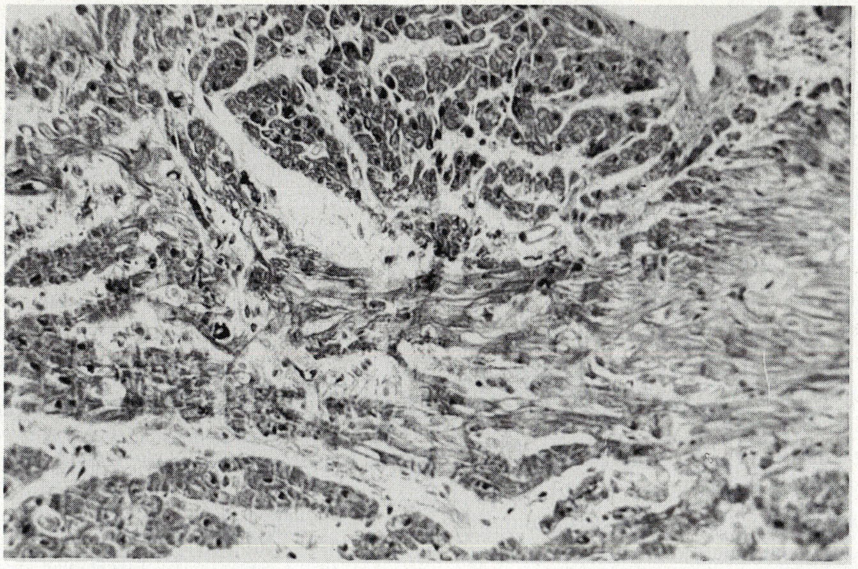

Fig. 2. Azan-stained right ventricular endomyocardial biopsy specimen from the same patient as in Fig. 1. Mild lymphocytic infiltration with interstitial fibrosis was noted. Some myocytes were slightly hypertrophic with uniform nuclei.

tachycardia in three patients and only sporadic ventricular premature beats in one patient. No significant complications related to corticosteroid therapy were observed.

DISCUSSION

The most common diseases underlying ventricular tachycardia in children are congenital heart disease, hypertrophic and dilated cardiomyopathy, myocardial tumor, arrhythmogenic right ventricular dysplasia, mitral valve prolapse, and postsurgical complications.[7-13] However, nonsustained and asymptomatic ventricular tachycardia with a structurally normal heart is sometimes encountered during electrocardiographic screening of schoolchildren.[1] The underlying disease often cannot be ascertained by noninvasive examinations alone, and therefore endomyocardial biopsy may be required for precise diagnosis. Vignola et al.[14] and Sugrue et al.[15] demonstrated by endomyocardial biopsy that 50% to 90% of unexplained ventricular tachycardia in adults is associated with histologic abnormalities of clinically silent myocarditis or cardiomyopathy. Wiles et al.[16] found similar results in 33 children with unexplained ventricular ectopic rhythm, approximately 50% of whom had abnormal histologic findings. Our studies also revealed histologic findings similar to those of subclinical lymphocytic myocarditis, and support previous reports to the effect that ventricular tachycardia may be the sole clinical manifestation in children with clinically silent myocarditis.

Long-term follow-up studies have revealed that sudden, unexpected death occurs exclusively among children with symptoms of ventricular tachycardia and underlying cardiac disease.[17, 18] Symptom-free children with nonsustained ventricular tachycardia may have a good long-term prognosis if underlying heart disease is absent.[19, 20] Nevertheless, one cannot guarantee that sudden death will not occur in some patients with benign ventricular tachycardia. In our study, no patients had apparent cardiac disease on noninvasive examinations, but abnormal histologic findings of subclinical lymphocytic myocarditis were detected in all. Furthermore, ventricular tachycardia was inducible by exercise electrocardiography in the two older children. Antiarrhythmic treatment and limitation of strenuous exercise might therefore be indicated for such patients to prevent sudden death.[1]

Little information exists regarding immunosuppressive treatment for unexplained ventricular tachycardia. Vignola et al.[14] and Wiles et al.[16] reported that corticosteroid therapy for nonsustained ventricular tachycardia was effective in a few patients in whom chronic myocarditis was confirmed by right ventricular endomyocardial biopsy. However, the efficacy of corticosteroid pulse therapy has not been reported. Previous experimental studies have suggested that neoantigens produced by viruses from myocardial protein may be a cause of chronic myocarditis[21, 22]; an immunologic process mediated by cytotoxic T cells directed against these neoantigens may be related to the pathogenic mechanism.[23, 24] Immunosuppressive therapy may therefore constitute a reasonable strategy because of its antiinflammatory effect. In our study, corticosteroid therapy was effective in the treatment of ventricular tachycardia per se in all patients, although the population studied was small.

In two patients treated by pulse therapy, ventricular tachycardia completely resolved without any complications during the month after initiation of corticosteroid administration. In contrast to the histologic results, the favorable response to corticosteroid treatment suggests that unexplained ventricular tachycardia detected by electrocardiographic screening may be related to some immunologic inflammatory process. However, the long-term prognosis of steroid-treated patients remains unknown. During the mean 3.4-year follow-up period in our study, no patient had a recurrence of ventricular tachycardia, had dilated cardiomyopathy, or died suddenly. Further long-term follow-up is required to elucidate the natural history of steroid-treated patients.

We conclude that unexplained ventricular tachycardia may be the only clinical feature of chronic silent lymphocytic myocarditis related to some immunologic inflammatory process. We recommend that endomyocardial biopsy be performed when the type of ventricular tachycardia is exercise induced, sustained, or has a right bundle-branch block pattern, and/or when a two-dimensional echocardiogram shows abnormal left ventricular wall motion. Corticosteroid therapy should be considered in the treatment of ventricular tachycardia when conventional antiarrhythmic drugs are ineffective and histologic examination by endomyocardial biopsy reveals subacute or chronic myocarditis.

REFERENCES

1. Ino T, Yabuta K, Yamauchi T. Japanese mass screening for heart disease [Letter]. BMJ 1993;306:1128.
2. Fulton DR, Chung KJ, Tabakin BS, Keane JF. Ventricular tachycardia in children without heart disease. Am J Cardiol 1985;55:1328-31.
3. Deal BJ, Miller SM, Scagliotti D, Prechel D, Gallastegui JL, Hariman RJ. Ventricular tachycardia in a young population without overt heart disease. Circulation 1986;73:1111-8.
4. Garson A, Gillette PC, Porter CJ, McNamara DG. Ventricular tachycardia in children with a normal heart [Abstract]. Circulation 1982;66:II-170.
5. Strain JE, Grose RM, Factor SM, Fisher JD. Results of endomyocardial biopsy in patients with spontaneous ventricular tachycardia but without apparent structural heart disease. Circulation 1983;68:1171-81.
6. Aretz TH, Billingham ME, Edwards WD, et al. Myocarditis: a histopathologic definition and classification. Am J Cariovasc Pathol 1986;1:3-14.
7. Paul T, Marchal C, Garson A Jr. Ventricular couplets in the young: prognosis related to underlying substrate. Am Heart J 1990;119:577-82.
8. Bricker JT, Traweek MS, Smith RT, Moak JP, Vargo TA, Garson A Jr. Exercise-related ventricular tachycardia in children. Am Heart J 1986;112:186-8.
9. Rocchini AP, Chun PO, Dick M. Ventricular tachycardia in children. Am J Cardiol 1981;47:1091-7.
10. Bisset GS III, Schwartz DC, Meyer RA, James FW, Kaplan S. Clinical spectrum and long-term follow-up of isolated mitral valve prolapse in 119 children. Circulation 1980;62:423-9.
11. Garson A Jr, Smith RT, Moak JP, et al. Incessant ventricular tachycardia in infants: myocardial hamartomas and surgical cure. J Am Coll Cardiol 1987;10:619-26.
12. Dunnigan A, Pierpont E, Smith SA, Breningstall G, Benditt DG, Benson DW. Cardiac and skeletal myopathy associated with cardiac dysrhythmias. Am J Cardiol 1984;53:731-7.
13. Pederson DH, Zipes DP, Foster PR, Troup PJ. Ventricular tachycardia and ventricular fibrillation in a young population. Circulation 1979;60:985-97.
14. Vignola PA, Aonuma K, Swaye PS, et al. Lymphocytic myocarditis presenting as unexplained ventricular arrhythmias. J Am Coll Cardiol 1984;4:812-9.
15. Sugrue DD, Holmes DR, Gersh BJ, et al. Cardiac histologic findings in patients with life-threatening ventricular arrhythmias of unknown origin. J Am Coll Cardiol 1984;4:952-7.
16. Wiles HB, Gillette PC, Harley RA, Upshur JK. Cardiomyopathy and myocarditis in children with ventricular ectopic rhythm. J Am Coll Cardiol 1992;20:359-62.
17. Bergdahl DM, Stevenson JG, Kawabori I, Guntheroth WG. Prognosis of primary ventricular tachycardia in the pediatric patient. Circulation 1980;62:897-901.
18. Garson A Jr, Smith RT, Moak JP, Ross BA, McNamara DG. Ventricular arrhythmias and sudden death in children. J Am Coll Cardiol 1985;5:130B-3B.
19. Garson A Jr, McNamara OG. Sudden death in a pediatric cardiology population, 1958 to 1983: relation to prior arrhythmias. J Am Coll Cardiol 1985;5:134B-7B.
20. Yabek SM. Ventricular arrhythmias in children with an apparently normal heart. J Pediatr 1991;119:1-11.
21. Cambridge G. Antibodies to Coxsackie B viruses in congestive cardiomyopathy. Br Heart J 1979;41:692-6.
22. Laufer A. Human and experimental myocarditis: the possible role of immune processes in pathogenesis. Isr J Med Sci 1975; 11:37-66.
23. Jacobs B, Matsuda Y, Deoddhar S, Shirey E. Cell-mediated cytotoxicity to cardiac cells of lymphocytes from patients with primary myocardial disease. Am J Clin Pathol 1979;72:1-4.
24. Eckstein R, Mempel W, Bolt HD. Reduced suppressor cell activity in congestive cardiomyopathy and in myocarditis. Circulation 1982;65:1224-9.

A randomized comparison of intravenously administered granisetron versus chlorpromazine plus dexamethasone in the prevention of ifosfamide-induced emesis in children

Karel Hählen, MD, PhD, Erica Quintana, MD, C. Ross Pinkerton, MD, DCH, FRCPI, and Eve Cedar, MSc

From the Department of Pediatrics, Division of Hematology/Oncology, Sophia Children's Hospital, Rotterdam, the Netherlands; the Pediatric Department, Institute Curie, Paris, France; the Department of Pediatric Oncology, Royal Marsden Hospital, Sutton, United Kingdom; and SmithKline Beecham, Harlow, United Kingdom

***Purpose*: To compare the efficacy and safety of intravenously administered granisetron with those of chlorpromazine plus dexamethasone in the prevention of ifosmamide-induced emesis in children with malignant disease.**
***Patients and methods*: Eighty-eight children, aged 2 to 17 years, were scheduled for ifosfamide therapy ($\geq$3 gm/m^2) for 2 or 3 consecutive days. On each day, children received granisetron, 20 μg/kg intravenously, before ifosfamide therapy, plus up to two more doses within 24 hours if required, or chlorpromazine, 0.3 to 0.5 mg/kg intravenously, every 4 to 6 hours, plus dexamethasone, 2 mg/m^2 intravenously every 8 hours.**
***Results*: During the initial 24 hours, significantly fewer episodes of vomiting were recorded after granisetron administration (median number, 1.5 vs 7.0; p = 0.001), and the percentages of children having no more than one vomiting episode (51% granisetron vs 21% chlorpromazine-dexamethasone) and no worse than mild nausea (67% granisetron vs 38% chlorpromazine-dexamethasone) were lower after granisetron therapy (p <0.01). Fewer children had sedation with granisetron (2 vs 19; p <0.001); there were no extrapyramidal reactions during granisetron therapy compared with two during control therapy.**
***Conclusion*: Granisetron was superior to chlorpromazine-dexamethasone antiemetic therapy for children receiving ifosfamide therapy and deserves further study during other chemotherapy regimens. (J Pediatr 1995;126:309-13)**

Control of chemotherapy-induced emesis in children poses particular problems because antiemetic agents are often poorly effective and may be associated with dose-limiting side effects. Although high-dose metoclopramide therapy is of benefit for adults, its neurologic toxicity tends to limit its use in children. The phenothiazines, given alone or in combination, have been widely prescribed as antiemetics for children. Chlorpromazine has been more effective than conventional low doses of metoclopramide and of similar efficacy to methylprednisolone in randomized studies in children,[1, 2] but is commonly associated with sedation, which limits patient acceptance.

Several open studies indicate that selective 5-hydroxytryptamine (serotonin$_3$) receptor antagonists offer particular promise for use in children, showing a high level of ef-

Submitted for publication April 27, 1994; accepted Aug. 24, 1994.
Reprint requests: Eve Cedar, MSc, SmithKline Beecham, New Frontiers Science Park, Third Avenue, Harlow, Essex CM19 5AW, United Kingdom.

0022-3476/95/$3.00 + 0 **9/25/60182**

ficacy without extrapyramidal side effects or sedation.[3-8] Although these agents are now the antiemetics of choice for adults receiving chemotherapy, comparative clinical studies in children are lacking. We report the results of a prospective, randomized study comparing a selective serotonin$_3$ receptor antagonist, granisetron, against a commonly used conventional combination regimen, chlorpromazine plus dexamethasone, in children undergoing high-dose ifosfamide chemotherapy.

METHODS

This study was conducted in accordance with Good Clinical Practice guidelines, and informed consent was obtained from parents or legal guardians (and children when possible) after the nature and purpose of the study had been explained. The study was approved by local ethics committees at participating centers.

Patients. Eighty-eight children (aged 2 to 17 years) were recruited by 19 pediatric oncology centers within France, The Netherlands, and the United Kingdom. All children were scheduled to receive ifosfamide ($\geq$3 gm/m^2 per day) for 2 or 3 consecutive days for treatment of malignant disease. Other cytostatic agents were permitted to be given concurrently during or after completion of ifosfamide administration. Patients were eligible if they were naive or nonnaive to chemotherapy but were excluded if they had any nausea or vomiting at any time in the previous week. Patients were also excluded if they had marked hepatic or renal dysfunction, congestive heart failure, a primary or secondary brain tumor, or a history of seizures in the previous year. Patients were not permitted to take antiemetics other than study medication or to receive concomitant corticosteroids (except as part of the chemotherapy regimen or study medication) or radiotherapy during the chemotherapy period.

The study was planned to recruit 100 patients (50 per group), sufficient to detect a 26% difference between groups in complete response rates (no vomiting and no worse than mild nausea) with 90% power at 5% level of significance. The study was terminated after recruitment of 88 patients because of the emerging evidence of the superior effectiveness and tolerability of granisetron over the control therapy.

Antiemetic therapy. Children were assigned on a single-blind basis, according to a computer-generated randomization code, to receive one of two antiemetic treatments for the duration of the ifosfamide treatment period (2 or 3 days). The randomization was stratified to ensure that 2- and 3-day ifosfamide treatments were evenly represented in the two study treatment groups: group 1 and group 2.

Group 1. On each treatment day, granisetron, 20 μg/kg in 20 ml saline solution, was infused intravenously for 5 minutes; after the completion of 5 minutes, the ifosfamide infusion was begun. Two further intravenous doses of granisetron, 20 μg/kg per dose, were permitted within each 24-hour period for any patient having moderate or severe nausea or any vomiting. No more than 60 μg of granisetron per kilogram of body weight was allowed in 24 hours.

Group 2. Dexamethasone, 2 mg/m^2, was infused intravenously 30 minutes before the start of ifosfamide therapy each day, followed by further dexamethasone doses (2 mg/m^2) 8 and 16 hours later. Chlorpromazine was initially given as an intravenous dose of 0.5 mg/kg at 4 to 6 hourly intervals throughout ifosfamide therapy, the infusion starting 25 minutes before commencement of the ifosfamide infusion. However, the dosage was subsequently reduced to a loading dose of 0.3 mg/kg, followed by doses of 0.3 to 0.5 mg/kg at 4 to 6 hourly intervals, after reports of unacceptable levels of sedation in some children receiving the higher dose.

At the end of ifosfamide treatment, patients in both treatment groups were discharged with standard antiemetic treatment of the clinician's choice. Granisetron was not administered to patients after discharge from the hospital.

Assessment of antiemetic efficacy and safety. Nausea and vomiting assessments were completed by hospital staff every 6 hours on each day of ifosfamide treatment. At each assessment, the severity of nausea in the preceding 6-hour period was recorded as none, mild, moderate, or severe. The number of episodes of vomiting or retching during the same period was also noted. Patients whose symptoms were not adequately controlled by study treatment were withdrawn from the study and offered alternative antiemetics. At the end of the treatment period, the clinician made a subjective global assessment of overall clinical response to antiemetic therapy on a 5-point scale (very good; good; average; poor; very poor).

Blood pressure and pulse rate were recorded every 6 hours throughout the study. Blood samples were taken for routine hematology and clinical chemistry studies before the initial infusion of study medication and on completion of the ifosfamide treatment. Adverse experiences were recorded at the end of each 24-hour period and at a follow-up visit between 7 and 28 days after the last dose of antiemetic treatment.

Statistical analysis. All primary analyses of interest were performed during the first 24 hours. These were (1) the percentage of patients obtaining complete response defined as no worse than mild nausea, no vomiting, no rescue antiemetics required (including additional doses of granisetron), and not withdrawn from the study, (2) the total number of vomiting episodes, (3) the percentage of patients having no nausea or only mild nausea, and (4) the percentage of patients having at most one vomiting episode. In addition, distribution of times to first occurrence of vomiting and moderate to severe nausea during a 72-hour period were examined by means of survival analyses. Patients with-

Table I. Overall results of antiemetic therapy

	Granisetron (n = 46)	Chlorpromazine/ dexamethasone (n = 42)	*p*
Efficacy for 24 hours			
Complete response	21.7%	9.5%	0.118
None or one vomiting episode	50.0%	21.4%	0.005
None or mild nausea	67.4%	38.1%	0.006
Median number of vomiting episodes	1.5	7.0	0.001
Median time to first vomit (hr)	11.5	4.5	NS
Median time to first moderate to severe nausea (hr)	49.7	24.0	NS
Clinicians' rating "good" or "very good"	63.0%	31.0%	0.019

NS, Not significant.

drawn but having no symptoms were censored at the time of withdrawal.

All statistical tests (two-tailed) were performed at a significance level of 5%. The chi-square test was used for differences in percentages between treatment groups; if patient numbers were small, the Fisher Exact Test was used. Differences between treatment groups in the total number of vomiting episodes were compared with the Mann-Whitney U test. The Cox Log Rank test was employed for differences between treatment groups in survival distributions for 72 hours. Patients scheduled to receive only 2 days of ifosfamide treatment were censored at 48 hours for 72-hour survival analyses unless the critical event had already occurred.

RESULTS

A total of 88 children participated in this study. The groups were matched for gender, age, weight, primary disease site, and prior chemotherapy exposure. Approximately half the children in both groups were female. The mean age was approximately 9.5 years, and there was a similar age distribution in the two treatment groups (data not shown). The majority of children had soft tissue sarcomas. In most cases, ifosfamide was given for 3 consecutive days, usually in combination with other agents (e.g., dactinomycin, doxorubicin, and vincristine). Ifosfamide was administered at a mean dose of 3 gm/m^2 on each treatment day in both groups; three children (granisetron, 1; chlorpromazine-dexamethasone, 2) were treated with ifosfamide at doses

Table II. Most commonly reported adverse events

	Granisetron (n = 46)	Chlorpromazine/ dexamethasone (n = 42)
Any event	28 (60.9%)	33 (78.5%)
Somnolence	2	19*
Fever	8	8
Headache	8	5
Abdominal pain	8	5
Leukopenia	7	5

*$p < 0.001$.

less than 3 gm/m^2 in violation of the protocol. Approximately two thirds of children in both groups had received prior chemotherapy. All children were included in efficacy and safety evaluations presented below.

Assessment of antiemetic response (Table I). Granisetron was superior to the comparator in terms of the percentage of children having one vomiting episode or fewer in 24 hours ($p = 0.005$) and no worse than mild nausea in 24 hours ($p = 0.006$). Children in the granisetron group also had significantly fewer vomiting episodes ($p = 0.001$). During the first 24 hours, 34.8% of children in the granisetron group received only one dose of granisetron, 50.0% received two doses, and 15.2% received three doses. Symptoms were reported as "resolved" or "improved" in 93.3% of children receiving the second dose and 100% of children after the third dose. Alternative antiemetic agents were required during hospitalization by 28.3% of patients in the granisetron group and 52.4% receiving chlorpromazine-dexamethasone ($p = 0.02$). At the end of the ifosfamide treatment period, overall response to antiemetic treatment was rated by clinicians as "good" or "very good" in a higher percentage of children given granisetron ($p = 0.019$).

Subgroup analyses were performed to examine the influence of gender, age, and prior chemotherapy exposure on antiemetic response during the first 24 hours. For granisetron, 24-hour complete response rates were similar in male (20.8%) and female (22.7%) subjects, whereas a numerically higher complete response rate was noted in male (13.0%) than female (5.3%) subjects receiving chlorpromazine-dexamethasone. In the granisetron group, younger children (aged 2 to 6 years) had a complete response rate of 30.8% compared with 15.0% in adolescents (aged >12 years). No trend was detected to suggest that previous chemotherapy exposure influenced complete response rates in either treatment group.

Assessment of safety (Table II). The overall percentage of children having any events was similar in both groups. Granisetron was well tolerated, and there were no serious or unexpected adverse experiences suspected to be related to granisetron; the most commonly reported events after treatment with granisetron were headache, fever, and abdominal pain. Headaches were of mild to moderate severity and of short duration. No cases of fever or abdominal pain were considered to be related to granisetron. Somnolence was reported with a significantly higher frequency after chlorpromazine-dexamethasone and was described as severe in seven cases. There were no reports of extrapyramidal reactions in the granisetron group, compared with two cases after chlorpromazine-dexamethasone therapy (severe ocular-buccal dyskinesia; moderate choreoathetosis).

No children were withdrawn from granisetron therapy because of adverse experiences. Chlorpromazine-dexamethasone therapy was discontinued in five children because of chlorpromazine intolerance.

DISCUSSION

Conventional antiemetic therapies are far from ideal for children undergoing intensive chemotherapy regimens because of inconsistent efficacy and troublesome, dose-limiting side effects. The new selective serotonin$_3$ receptor antagonists are of particular interest for children because they do not cause extrapyramidal side effects or sedation, two of the major drawbacks to traditional antiemetic therapy. Granisetron has been an effective and well-tolerated antiemetic for adults[9, 10] but experience in children is limited.[3, 11, 12]

Antiemetic studies are difficult to perform in children with cancer because of the small number of available subjects, complex and often lengthy cytostatic regimens, and the wide variety of disease diagnoses. To overcome some of these difficulties, we conducted our study as a collaborative effort in several pediatric oncology centers. Entry to the study was restricted to children scheduled for high-dose ifosfamide regimens, one of the most emetogenic agents in common use in pediatric oncology practice. To aid recruitment, we studied both chemotherapy-naive and nonnaive patients provided that no anticipatory emesis had occurred in the preceding week. Thus the study compared the two antiemetic regimens in a reasonably homogeneous group of children under extreme conditions.

The results demonstrate that granisetron was superior to a combination of chlorpromazine plus dexamethasone in terms of efficacy, tolerability, and convenience of administration. The difference between treatment groups in the median number of vomiting episodes within 24 hours further confirmed the superiority of granisetron in this population. Granisetron was well tolerated; mild to moderate headache was the only adverse event probably attributable to the compound. No patient was withdrawn from the granisetron group because of poor tolerability.

It could be argued that an inappropriately high dose of chlorpromazine was given to the control group, thus accounting for the poor tolerability observed. The chlorpromazine dose initially chosen (0.5 mg/kg) has been widely used by pediatric oncologists[5] and previously was shown to be significantly more effective than the same dose of metoclopramide, without inducing an unacceptable degree of sedation.[5] In our study, however, severe sedation occurred among the first few patients given 0.5 mg/kg, and it proved necessary to reduce the initial dose to 0.3 mg/kg for subsequent patients. Chlorpromazine-induced sedation remained a common problem even after the dose reduction.

Despite the superior response to granisetron, the percentage of children attaining complete response was lower than predicted from similar studies in adult patients. It is difficult to extrapolate from children to adults because chemotherapy regimens utilized in the childhood population are often more intensive than those used to treat adult cancers. However, the possibility exists that children may have a greater susceptibility to chemotherapy-induced emesis than adults. Future studies should investigate whether efficacy can be further enhanced by administration of higher granisetron doses or combination with a corticosteroid.

Control of emesis was more difficult to achieve in adolescents than in young children treated with granisetron. An age-related difference is consistent with earlier surveys in which adolescents reported more severe nausea than children.[13, 14] This finding may simply reflect the difficulties in assessing subjective symptoms, such as nausea, in young children but may also indicate that chemotherapy-induced nausea and vomiting are a "learned response" that develops with age.[13] Although it has been reported that female subjects in adult and pediatric populations have poorer responses to antiemetics than male subjects,[14] there was no clear gender-related difference in this study. Additionally, there was no evidence to indicate that antiemetic outcome was influenced by previous chemotherapy exposure.

We conclude that intravenously administered granisetron represents an improvement over chlorpromazine plus dexamethasone for control of ifosfamide-induced emesis in children. Further studies of differing doses and regimens seem justified in children enrolled in other intensive chemotherapy protocols.

We are grateful to the following investigators who also participated in this study: Dr. A. Babin-Boilletot, Strasbourg, France; Dr. B. Bui, Bordeaux, France; Dr. M. Brunat-Mentigny, Lyon, France; Dr. M. Demaille, Lille, France; Dr. E. Le Gall, Rennes, France; Prof. J. Lemerle, Paris, France; Dr. I. Lewis, Leeds, U.K.; Dr. G. Marguerite, Montpellier, France; Dr. F. Mechinaud-Lacroix, Nantes, France; Dr. E. Plouvier, Besançon, France; Prof. C. Raybaud, Marseilles, France; Prof. A. Robert, Toulouse, France; Prof. D. Sommelet, Nancy, France; Dr. M. Stevens, Birmingham, U.K.; Prof. A. Thyss, Nice, France; and Dr. E. Van Leeuwen, Amsterdam, The Netherlands.

REFERENCES

1. Graham-Pole J, Weare J, Engel S, Gardner R, Mehta P, Goss S. Anti-emetics in children receiving cancer chemotherapy: a double-blind prospective randomised study comparing metoclopramide with chlorpromazine. J Clin Oncol 1986;4: 1110-3.
2. Mehta P, Gross S, Graham-Pole J, Gardner R. Methylprednisolone for chemotherapy-induced emesis: a double-blind randomised trial in children. J PEDIATR 1986;108:774-6.
3. Lemerle J, Amaral D, Southall DP, et al. Efficacy and safety of granisetron in the prevention of chemotherapy-induced emesis in paediatric patients. Eur J Cancer 1991;27:1081-3.
4. Hachimi-Idrissi S, De Schepper J, Maurus R, Otten J. Prevention of emesis by ICS 205-930 in children receiving cytotoxic chemotherapy. Eur J Cancer 1993;29A:854-6.
5. Sullivan MJ, Abbott GD, Robinson BA. Ondansetron antiemetic therapy for chemotherapy- and radiotherapy-induced vomiting in children. N Z Med J 1992;105:369-70.
6. Pinkerton CR, Williams D, Wootton C, Meller ST, McElwain TJ. 5-HT_3 antagonist ondansetron: an effective outpatient antiemetic in cancer treatment. Arch Dis Childh 1990;65: 822-5.
7. Jurgens H, McQuade B. Ondansetron as prophylaxis for chemotherapy and radiotherapy-induced emesis in children. Oncology 1992;49:279-85.
8. Hewitt M, McQuade B, Stevens R. The efficacy and safety of ondansetron in prophylaxis of cancer chemotherapy–induced nausea and vomiting in children. Clin Oncol 1993;5:11-4.
9. Chevallier B. The control of acute cisplatin-induced emesis A comparative study of granisetron and a combination regimen of high-dose metoclopramide and dexamethasone. Br J Cancer 1993;68:176-80.
10. Soukop M. A dose-finding study of granisetron, a novel antiemetic in patients receiving high-dose cisplatin. Supportive Care in Cancer 1994;2:177-83.
11. Jacobson SL, Shore RW, Nishimura L, Mee D, Chan H, Spielberg SP. The efficacy and safety of granisetron in pediatric cancer patients who failed standard antiemetic therapy during anticancer chemotherapy. Am J Pediatr Hematol Oncol 1994;16/3:231-5.
12. Pinkerton CR, Jacobson SJ, Leclerc JM, Cohn R, Cedar E. IV granisetron in children receiving highly emetogenic chemotherapy: A double-blind dose-ranging study. Eur J Cancer 1993;29A(suppl 6):S200 (abstract 1118).
13. Frick SB, GuzziDelpo EG, Keith JA, Davis MS. Chemotherapy-associated nausea and vomiting in pediatric oncology patients. Cancer Nurs 1988;11:118-24.
14. LeBaron S, Zeltzer LK, LeBaron C, et al. Chemotherapy side effects in pediatric oncology patients: drugs, age and sex as risk factors. Med Pediatr Oncol 1988;16:263-8.

Clinical and laboratory observations

Short-term use of amoxicillin-clavulanate during upper respiratory tract infection for prevention of acute otitis media

Terho Heikkinen, MD, Olli Ruuskanen, MD, Thedi Ziegler, PhD,[a] Matti Waris, PhD,[a] and Heikki Puhakka, MD

From the Departments of Pediatrics, Virology, and Otolaryngology, University of Turku, and the Department of Otolaryngology, University of Tampere, Finland

We performed a randomized, double-blind, placebo-controlled study to determine whether acute otitis media could be prevented by antibiotic therapy initiated promptly after the appearance of symptoms of upper respiratory tract infection. One hundred four children aged 1 to 4 years received a 7-day course of either amoxicillin-clavulanate or placebo. Acute otitis media developed in 9 (18%) of the 50 children receiving amoxicillin clavulanate and in 12 (22%) of the 54 children receiving placebo ($p = 0.59$). (J PEDIATR 1995;126:313-6)

Supported by grants from the Pediatric Research Foundation and the Medical Council of the Academy of Finland.

Submitted for publication May 17, 1994; accepted Aug. 26, 1994.

Reprint requests: Terho Heikkinen, MD, Department of Pediatrics, Turku University Hospital, FIN-20520 Turku, Finland.

[a]Now at the Influenza Branch (Dr. Ziegler) and the Respiratory and Enteric Viruses Branch (Dr. Waris), Division of Viral and Rickettsial Diseases, National Center for Infectious Diseases, Centers for Disease Control and Prevention, Atlanta, GA 30333.

0022-3476/95/$3.00 + 0 **9/26/60160**

Several placebo-controlled clinical trials have demonstrated the efficacy of long-term antimicrobial prophylaxis for recurrent acute otitis media in children.[1] Because a reduction by ~60% of attacks of AOM has been achieved by the daily use of sulfonamides or amoxicillin, antimicrobial prophylaxis has been recommended as the initial intervention for children with recurrent AOM.[2] However, long-term antimicrobial prophylaxis is associated with potential problems such as adverse drug reactions, emergence of resistant strains of bacteria, suppression of symptoms of infection without affecting the disease process itself, and poor compliance.[2] Most of these problems could possibly be avoided by limiting medication to periods of upper respiratory tract infection. To date, no study has reliably evaluated the efficacy of intermittent antimicrobial prophylaxis versus placebo to prevent AOM. We conducted a randomized, double-blind, placebo-controlled study to determine whether development of AOM could be prevented by short-term amoxicillin-clavulanate treatment of children with URI.

METHODS

Patients. This study was carried out at a private otologic center in Turku, Finland. On the basis of repeated surveys among day-care center children younger than 4 years of age, all children with a history of ≥3 attacks of AOM, of which ≥1 had occurred during the preceding 6 months, or ≥2 during the preceding 6 months, were invited to participate in the study; children with previous adenoidectomy or placement of tympanostomy tubes, or allergy to penicillin or amoxicillin, were excluded. Informed consent was obtained from the parents of 215 children. The study protocol was approved by the ethics committee of Turku University Hospital.

AMCL	Amoxicillin-clavulanate
AOM	Acute otitis media
MEF	Middle-ear fluid
URI	Upper respiratory tract infection

Study design. The parents were asked to bring their children to the study office free of charge whenever fever or signs of URI appeared. The clinical examinations were performed by otologists all of whom are validated otoscopists experienced in the use of tympanocentesis. In addition to a standard otoscopic examination, a tympanogram was obtained to rule out otitis media. At the first visit the time of the onset of respiratory symptoms was recorded and a nasopharyngeal aspirate specimen was obtained for detection of viruses. In the presence of URI, medication with AMCL or placebo was started if the children met the following criteria: normal middle-ear status; no other need for antimicrobial therapy; and no antimicrobial therapy during the preceding 4 weeks. The dose of AMCL was 40 mg/kg per day, divided in two daily doses; the volume of the placebo syrup was similar. Administration of the study medication was continued for 7 days, after which the children were reexamined; an earlier reexamination was performed whenever the parents suspected the development of AOM. Compliance was determined by measuring the amount of drug remaining in the bottles, and was judged acceptable if more than 80% of the expected amount of the drug was used.

When AOM was diagnosed, the use of the study medication was discontinued and appropriate antimicrobial therapy was started. With the consent of the parent, tympanocentesis was performed and the middle-ear fluid was cultured for pathogenic bacteria and viruses. If during the study another infection developed and required antimicrobial therapy, use of the study medication was terminated and appropriate therapy was started. Such an episode was excluded from the analysis.

Sample size and randomization. Acute otitis media was estimated to develop in 30% of children receiving placebo. Full-dose, twice-daily medication with good compliance was anticipated to provide an efficacy exceeding that of long-term prophylaxis (~60%), so a 75% reduction in the frequency of AOM among children receiving AMCL was judged to be clinically significant. At the significance level of 95% and with a power of 80% to detect the desired efficacy, the minimum number of children required in each group was calculated to be 46. Thus the enrollment of new patients was to be stopped after 100 children had completed the study.

Equal amounts of bottles containing AMCL and placebo were randomly put in order in blocks of four according to a computer-based randomization scheme. In consecutive order of study entry, the participants were given the next available bottle of medication.

Definitions. The diagnosis of URI was made if the child had acute rhinitis either alone or together with cough and/or fever, or if the child had cough with fever and no signs of a lower respiratory tract infection. The duration of symptoms of URI was recorded as whole days; a part of a 24-hour period was defined as 1 day. The diagnosis of AOM was based on signs and symptoms of acute infection, together with bulging or opacity of the tympanic membrane, the mobility of which to pneumatic otoscopy was either absent or markedly decreased.

Virologic studies. Detection of viruses in the nasopharyngeal aspirates and MEFs was performed by virus culture, and by direct detection of viral antigens by time-resolved fluoroimmunoassay as described earlier.[3]

Statistical analysis. Significance testing was performed by means of the standard chi-square test, the Mann-Whitney U test, and the two-sample t test.

Table I. Characteristics of the study children

Variable	AMCL (n = 50)	Placebo (n = 54)
Age (yr)*	2.6 ± 0.9	2.6 ± 0.8
Male, No. (%)	23 (46)	23 (43)
Total No. of previous AOM attacks†	3 (2-15)	4 (2-12)
No. of AOM attacks during preceding 6 mo†	2 (1-4)	2 (1-6)
Duration of respiratory symptoms before study medication, (days)†	2 (1-5)	2 (1-3)

*Values are expressed as mean ± SD.
†Values are expressed as median (range).

Table II. Duration of symptoms of URI before commencement of use of medication and corresponding occurrence of AOM in study groups

	AMCL		Placebo	
Duration of URI (days)	Children (No.)	AOM No. (%)	Children (No.)	AOM No. (%)
1	24	4 (17)	24	5 (21)
2	18	4 (22)	22	5 (23)
3	5	1 (20)	8	2 (25)
4	2	0 (0)	0	0
5	1	0 (0)	0	0
TOTAL	50	9 (18)	54	12 (22)

RESULTS

A total of 115 children received the study medication. Of those, 11 failed to complete the study and were excluded from the analysis (7 AMCL, 4 placebo). Of the 104 children who acceptably completed the study, 50 received AMCL and 54 placebo. The characteristics of the children in the groups were comparable (Table I).

In the group receiving AMCL, AOM developed in nine (18%) of the 50 children, compared with 12 (22%) of the 54 children in the placebo group (relative risk, 0.81; 95% confidence interval, 0.37 to 1.76; $p = 0.59$). The duration of symptoms of URI before commencement of the use of medication showed no significant influence on the occurrence of AOM in the groups (Table II).

The viral cause of the URIs could be determined in 31 (30%) of the 104 children; respiratory syncytial virus, influenza virus type A, and rhinovirus were the most common viruses detected. No significant differences were observed in the occurrences of AOM related to different viruses in the groups.

Tympanocentesis was performed in four children receiving AMCL. None of these MEF specimens yielded bacterial growth; influenza B virus was detected in one. In the placebo group, MEF was obtained from nine children. *Haemophilus influenzae* was cultured from one and *Moraxella catarrhalis* from two specimens; in one specimen without bacterial growth, respiratory syncytial virus was detected.

DISCUSSION

The results of this study suggest that antibiotic treatment of URI does not prevent the development of AOM, although such practice might appear logical in light of the efficacy of long-term antimicrobial prophylaxis. The rate of occurrence of AOM in the group who received AMCL did not significantly differ from the rate in the placebo group, even though AMCL has good activity against all the common bacteria that cause AOM,[4] the dose was that used in the treatment of AOM, and medication was started at an early stage of the URI, when the middle ear status was normal.

The discrepancy between the efficacy of long-term antimicrobial prophylaxis and the results of this study raises many questions. According to our present understanding of the pathogenesis of AOM, viral infection of the respiratory tract causes eustachian tube dysfunction and negative middle ear pressure, which lead to accumulation of middle ear secretions and proliferation of microbial pathogens in the secretions.[5] Our findings suggest that the ultimate pathogenesis of AOM may be more complicated. Some studies have suggested that virus-induced polymorphonuclear leukocyte dysfunction may contribute to the pathogenesis of AOM.[6] Further, viral infection of the respiratory tract induces a local release of inflammatory mediators, the role of which (and of the entire immune system in otitis media) remains unclear.[7]

The fact that antimicrobial therapy initiated soon after the appearance of symptoms of URI could not prevent the development of AOM also calls into question the overall value of antibiotic therapy for AOM. The high rate of spontaneous recovery from AOM without antimicrobial treatment has been well established.[8, 9] It is possible that in our study antibiotic treatment prevented bacterial growth in the MEF, but from a clinical point of view this was unimportant because the antibiotic failed to prevent the development of AOM (i.e., accumulation of fluid in the middle ear cavity, together with symptoms of acute infection). The results of this study are in accordance with the conclusions from the clinical trials investigating the efficacy of antibiotic treatment of URI in the prevention of pneumonia.[10]

The occurrence of AOM (22%) among the children in our study who received placebo was lower than expected, but the study had a power of 70% to detect the desired 75% prophylactic efficacy. Exclusion of a lower efficacy of antimicrobial prophylaxis would require a much larger sample size.

We conclude that the natural history of viral URIs—at least the progression to acute otitis media—cannot be modified by short-term use of antimicrobial agents. That long-term antimicrobial prophylaxis has been shown to be beneficial in preventing AOM indicates that other mechanisms of disease may exist. Information derived from recent studies on the pathogenesis and resolution of AOM suggest, however, an important role for respiratory viruses and inflammatory mediators.[7, 11, 12]

We are grateful to our colleagues and all the staff members at Korvacenter and at the Department of Virology for their good collaboration.

REFERENCES

1. Williams RL, Chalmers TC, Stange KC, Chalmers FT, Bowlin SJ. Use of antibiotics in preventing recurrent acute otitis media and in treating otitis media with effusion: a meta-analytic attempt to resolve the brouhaha. JAMA 1993;270:1344-51.
2. Paradise JL. Antimicrobial prophylaxis for recurrent acute otitis media. Ann Otol Rhinol Laryngol 1992;101(suppl 155):33-6.
3. Arola M, Ruuskanen O, Ziegler T, et al. Clinical role of respiratory virus infection in acute otitis media. Pediatrics 1990;86:848-55.
4. Marchant CD, Shurin PA, Johnson CE, et al. A randomized controlled trial of amoxicillin plus clavulanate compared with cefaclor for treatment of acute otitis media. J PEDIATR 1986;109:891-6.
5. Bluestone CD, Klein JO. Otitis media in infants and children. Philadelphia: WB Saunders, 1988:15-29.
6. Abramson JS, Giebink GS, Quie PG. Influenza A virus–induced polymorphonuclear leukocyte dysfunction in the pathogenesis of experimental pneumococcal otitis media. Infect Immun 1982;36:289-96.
7. Ruuskanen O, Ogra PL. Respiratory syncytial virus. Curr Probl Pediatr 1993;23:50-79.
8. Marchant CD, Carlin SA, Johnson CE, Shurin PA. Measuring the comparative efficacy of antibacterial agents for acute otitis media: the "Pollyanna phenomenon." J PEDIATR 1992;120:72-7.
9. Rosenfeld RM, Vertrees JE, Carr J, et al. Clinical efficacy of antimicrobial drugs for acute otitis media: metaanalysis of 5400 children from thirty-three randomized trials. J PEDIATR 1994;124:355-67.
10. Gadomski AM. Potential interventions for preventing pneumonia among young children: lack of effect of antibiotic treatment for upper respiratory infections. Pediatr Infect Dis J 1993;12:115-20.
11. Ruuskanen O, Arola M, Heikkinen T, Ziegler T. Viruses in acute otitis media: increasing evidence for clinical significance. Pediatr Infect Dis J 1991;10:425-7.
12. Chonmaitree T, Owen MJ, Patel JA, Hedgpeth D, Horlick D, Howie VM. Effect of viral respiratory tract infection on outcome of acute otitis media. J PEDIATR 1992;120:856-62.

Antenatal corticosteroid therapy to prevent respiratory distress syndrome

Ten years ago, Mary Ellen Avery[1] argued that failure to accept antenatal corticosteroids as an essential intervention to prevent neonatal respiratory distress syndrome, on the basis of the accumulated evidence at that time, constituted poor medical practice. In 1990, Crowley et al.[2] carried out an overview of all published reports of controlled trials of antenatal corticosteroid use and analyzed data from 12 controlled trials involving more than 3000 women who fulfilled all of their inclusion criteria. Their metaanalysis demonstrated that antenatal corticosteroid administration was associated with a 50% reduction of neonatal respiratory distress (typical odds ratio, 0.49; 95% confidence interval, 0.41 to 0.60), and that this effect was more marked when delivery occurred after 24 hours and within 7 days of drug administration. They noted that babies born outside this interval also benefited (OR, 0.69; 95% CI, 0.50 to 0.94), and that corticosteroid administration after premature rupture of the membranes was also associated with a reduction in respiratory morbidity of a similar magnitude. Their review also determined that antenatal steroid therapy reduced the odds of both periventricular hemorrhage and necrotizing enterocolitis by between 10% and 80%, and that data from the two appropriate follow-up studies indicated that neurologic abnormalities might be less frequent among babies whose mothers received steroids (OR, 0.61; 95% CI, 0.34 to 1.08). They did not find any evidence of increased risk of fetal death, maternal infection, or fetal or neonatal infection.

More recently, Maher et al.[3] reviewed outcome in infants of 32,658 women participating in the March of Dimes Multicenter Prematurity Prevention Program, of whom 432 were delivered at 26 to 31 weeks. Infants of women given betamethasone before delivery had a lower incidence of RDS in the 26- to 28-week and the 29- to 31-week gestational groups ($p = 0.008$; $p = 0.003$), and a rate of intraventricular hemorrhage that was possibly lower in the 26- to 28-week gestational group (15.4% vs 32.3%; $p = 0.17$) and significantly lower for the 29- to 31-week group (3.1% vs 16.5%; $p = 0.029$). Antenatal betamethasone treatment was associated with a lowered OR for respiratory distress of 0.20 (CI, 0.10 to 0.42), for intraventricular hemorrhage 0.26 (CI, 0.08 to 0.90), and for neonatal death 0.14 (CI, 0.02 to 1.09). Thus this study confirmed the review by Crowley et al.[2]

Despite these observations, the majority of which were published before 1990, use of ANS treatment was infrequent in recently published studies evaluating distended pressure for extubation (11.3%),[4] multiple doses of surfactant (6.5%),[5] and the incidence of bronchopulmonary dysplasia after antenatal indomethacin therapy (10.3%).[6] The use of ANS was equally infrequent (mean, 12%; range, 0.3% to 80%) in 13 international trials of neonatal surfactant published during the past 5 years that included ANS in their analyses (Table).[7-19] In the study of Phibbs et al.,[13] 80% of women received ANS; this may represent the achievable standard because it is not always possible to achieve 100% compliance with a minimum of 24 hours' exposure to ANS as a result of coexisting fetomaternal conditions. In these same studies, the use of tocolysis was greater than the use of ANS in all cases for which information was available. Even in the Canadian randomized trial of tocolysis in preterm labor,[20] fewer than half of the women received ANS (Moutquin J, Canadian Preterm Investigators Group: personal communication May 1994). In view of the known inefficacy of tocolysis to inhibit labor beyond 48 hours,[21] we agree with Liggins,[22] who stated that "reluctance to use corticosteroids based on reservations about the safety of tocolytics can be respected, but not the practice of some centers in which tocolytics are used and corticosteroids withheld."

ANS	Antenatal steroids
CI	Confidence interval
OR	Odds ratio
RDS	Respiratory distress syndrome

Kari et al.[23] recently conducted a placebo-controlled, randomized, double-blind trial to determine whether prenatal dexamethasone treatment improved outcome in preterm infants during the surfactant era. They demonstrated that neonates born within 1 to 14 days after dexamethasone therapy had a lower incidence of RDS and a lower requirement for surfactant, with shorter duration of ventilatory support and oxygen therapy, and a higher rate of neonatal

THE JOURNAL OF PEDIATRICS 1995;126:317-9

0022-3476/95/$3.00 + 0 **9/34/61101**

Table. Antenatal use of antenatal corticosteroids in surfactant studies (1989–1994)

Author	Year	Location	Birth weight or gestation	Control group receiving ANS		Surfactant group receiving ANS	
				No.	(%)	No.	(%)
Horbar et al.[7]	1989	United States	750-1750 gm	19/81	(23)	13/78	(17)
Bose et al.[8]	1990	United States	700-1350 gm	63/193	(32)	66/192	(34)
Dunn et al.[9]	1990	Canada	30-36 wk	10/24	(22)	13/51	(26)
Dunn et al.[10]	1991	Canada	24-30 wk	26/60	(43)	59/122	(48)
Segerer et al.[11]	1991	Sweden	700-1499 gm	No control		21/35	(60)
Kendig et al.[12]	1991	United States	<30 wk	66/235	(34)	84/244	(28)
Phibbs et al.[13]	1991	United States	700-1350 gm	27/38	(71)	29/36	(80)
Long et al.[14]	1991	United States	700-1350 gm	14/213	(7)	15/206	(7)
Long et al.[15]	1991	United States/Canada	>1250 gm	57/622	(9)	50/615	(8)
Corbet et al.[16]	1991	United States	700-1100 gm	46/222	(21)	44/224	(20)
Stevenson et al.[17]	1992	United States	500-699 gm	11/109	(10)	18/106	(17)
OSIRIS Group[18]	1992	Worldwide	Preterm	No control		1615/9447	(17)
Konishi et al.[19]	1992	Japan	500-1500 gm	No control		1/32	(0.3)

survival. Steroid-treated infants also had higher mean blood pressures during the first 3 days of life, and infants treated with dexamethasone had a lower incidence of intraventricular hemorrhage and periventricular leukomalacia, a reduction that was even more impressive in infants treated with exogenous human surfactant. They concluded that prenatal steroid therapy combined with exogenous human surfactant therapy markedly reduces morbidity and cerebral complications. This study provides the additional information that ANS, in combination with postnatal surfactant, provides optimal management with improved outcomes for premature neonates.

SUMMARY

The recent National Institutes of Health Consensus Development Conference[24] on ANS was strongly supportive of the use of ANS, even for 24 hours but, if possible, for 48 hours, in all fetuses between 24 and 34 weeks of gestation and at risk of preterm delivery regardless of race, gender, or the availability of surfactant replacement. For preterm rupture of membranes at less than 30 to 32 weeks, the use of ANS was also recommended in the absence of amnionitis, and patients eligible for tocolytic therapy were also deemed eligible for ANS. Thus the currently available literature indicates that pediatricians should encourage obstetricians to provide ANS in high-risk pregnancies, as outlined in the proposed National Institutes of Health guidelines. Even if a full 48-hour course of ANS cannot be achieved, ANS given less than 24 hours before delivery is associated with a decreased incidence of intraventricular hemorrhage and periventricular leukomalacia. In addition, we propose that investigators, reviewers, and editors ensure uniformly high maternal ANS exposure, consistent with the realities of clinical practice, when designing, evaluating, and publishing clinical trials with outcomes (e.g., RDS, intraventricular hemorrhage, periventricular leukomalacia, bronchopulmonary dysplasia, and death) that can be significantly affected by ANS. Otherwise, studies will continue to be performed on infants who, as fetuses, were deprived of treatment that may have prevented or ameliorated the disorder being assessed. Studies with an infrequent use of ANS may not be applicable or generalizable to an era when the use of ANS is an essential part of perinatal practice. Future trials should document both ANS use and the reasons for failure to achieve an acceptable level of such treatment.

C. Anthony Ryan, MB, FRCPC
Department of Pediatrics
University College Cork
Cork Regional Hospital
Cork, Ireland

Neil N. Finer, MD, FRCPC
Department of Newborn Medicine
Royal Alexandra Hospital
10240 Kingsway
Edmonton, Alberta T5H 3V9, Canada

REFERENCES

1. Avery ME. The argument for prenatal administration of dexamethasone to prevent respiratory distress [Editorial]. J PEDIATR 1984;104:240.
2. Crowley P, Chalmers I, Keirse MJNC. The effects of corticosteroid administration before preterm delivery: an overview of the evidence from controlled trials. Br J Obstet Gynecol 1990;97:11-25.
3. Maher JE, Cliver SP, Goldenberg RL, et al. The effect of corticosteroid therapy in the very premature infant. Am J Obstet Gynecol 1994;170:869-73.
4. Annibale DJ, Hulsey TC, Engstrom PC, Wallin LA, Ohning

BL. Randomized, controlled trial of nasopharyngeal continuous positive airway pressure in the extubation of very low birth weight infants. J PEDIATR 1994;124:455-60.
5. Berry DD, Pramanik AK, Phillips JB, et al. Comparison of the effect of three doses of a synthetic surfactant on the alveolar-arterial oxygen gradient in infants weighing <1250 gm with respiratory distress syndrome. J PEDIATR 1994;124:294-301.
6. Eronen M, Pesonen E, Kurki T, Teramo K, Ylikorkala O, Hallman M. Increased incidence of bronchopulmonary dysplasia after antenatal administration of indomethacin to prevent preterm labor. J PEDIATR 1994;124:782-8.
7. Horbar JD, Soll RF, Sutherland JM, et al. A multicenter randomized, placebo-controlled trial of surfactant therapy for respiratory distress syndrome. N Engl J Med 1989;320:959-65.
8. Bose C, Corbet A, Bose G, et al. Improved outcome at 28 days of age for very low birth weight infants treated with a single dose of a synthetic surfactant. J PEDIATR 1990;117:947-53.
9. Dunn MS, Shennan AT, Possmayer F. Single- versus multiple-dose surfactant replacement therapy in neonates of 30 to 36 weeks' gestation with respiratory distress syndrome. Pediatrics 1990;86:564-71.
10. Dunn MS, Shennan AT, Xayack D, Possmayer F. Bovine surfactant replacement in neonates of less than 30 weeks' gestation: a randomized controlled trial of prophylaxis versus treatment. Pediatrics 1991;87:377-86.
11. Segerer H, Stevens P, Schadow B, et al. Surfactant substitution in ventilated very low birth weight infants: factors related to response types. Pediatr Res 1991;30:591-6.
12. Kendig JW, Notter RH, Cox C, et al. A comparison of surfactant as immediate prophylaxis and as rescue therapy in newborns of less than 30 weeks' gestation. N Engl J Med 1991; 324:865-71.
13. Phibbs RH, Ballard RA, Clements JA, et al. Initial clinical trial of Exosurf, a protein-free synthetic surfactant, for the prophylaxis and early treatment of hyaline membrane disease. Pediatrics 1991;88:1-9.
14. Long W, Thompson T, Sundell H, et al. Effects of two rescue doses of a synthetic surfactant on mortality rate and survival without bronchopulmonary dysplasia in 700- to 1350-gram infants with respiratory distress syndrome. J PEDIATR 1991; 118:595-605.
15. Long W, Corbet A, Cotton R, et al. A controlled trial of synthetic surfactant in infants weighing 1250 g or more with respiratory distress syndrome. N Engl J Med 1991;325:1696-703.
16. Corbet A, Bucciarelli R, Goldman S, et al. Decreased mortality rate among small premature infants treated at birth with a single dose of synthetic surfactant: a multicenter controlled trial. J PEDIATR 1991;118:277-84.
17. Stevenson D, Walther F, Long W, et al. Controlled trial of a single dose of synthetic surfactant at birth in premature infants weighing 500 to 600 grams. J PEDIATR 1992;120:S1-S12.
18. The OSIRIS Collaborative Group [Open Study of Infants at High Risk of or With Respiratory Insufficiency—the Role of Surfactant]. Early versus delayed neonatal administration of a synthetic surfactant—the judgement of OSIRIS. Lancet 1992;340:1363-87.
19. Konishi M, Fujiwara T, Chida S, et al. A prospective, randomized trial of early versus late administration of a single dose of surfactant-TA. Early Hum Dev 1992;29:275-82.
20. Canadian Preterm Investigators Group. Treatment of preterm labor with the beta-adrenergic agonist ritodrine. N Engl J Med 1992;327:308-12.
21. Higby K, Wenakis EMJ, Pauerstein CJ, Harbert GM, et al. Do tocolytic agents stop preterm labor? A critical and comprehensive review of efficacy and safety. Am J Obstet Gynaecol 1993;168:1247-59.
22. Liggins GC. Obstetric and paediatric collaboration to reduce morbidity after preterm birth. Br J Obstet Gynaecol 1990; 97:1-3.
23. Kari MA, Hallman M, Eronen M, et al. Prenatal dexamethasone treatment in conjunction with rescue therapy of human surfactant: a randomized, placebo-controlled multicenter study. Pediatrics 1994;93:730-6.
24. National Institutes of Health Consensus Development Conference. Statement on the effect of corticosteroids for fetal maturation on perinatal outcomes. February 28 to March 2, 1994, National Institutes of Health, Bethesda, Maryland.

THE BOOK SHELF **André D. Lascari,** *Editor*

Book reviews

Water and electrolytes in pediatrics: Physiology, pathophysiology and treatment

Finberg L, Kravath RE, Hellerstein S. Philadelphia: WB Saunders, 1993. 270 pages. $49.

This book discusses and critically reviews pediatric water and electrolyte abnormalities and their therapy. This revised version has maintained the original four sections. As in the 1982 edition, it encompasses concepts on the physiology of body fluids, the pathophysiology and clinical manifestations of the disease processes, and their diagnostic evaluation. Last, but not least, a detailed account of the management of water and mineral metabolism disorders follows. The 35 chapters, including an introduction, comprise this rich, terse, and concise text. The authors dissect the body's fluid composition, the fluid abnormalities, and the mechanism of distribution within compartments of individual ions and organic molecules. Furthermore, they present experienced views on how to analyze and interpret clinical and laboratory data and how to treat specific problems, namely, dehydration, diarrhea, and their effects on the central nervous system. Excellent chapters thoroughly address the physiologic, pathophysiologic, and therapeutic issues related to kidney, adrenal gland, heart, and liver disease, diabetes mellitus, cystic fibrosis, and asthma, to mention a few. Two useful and interesting appendixes conclude this work.

This remarkably well-organized and scholarly book is a useful and comprehensive compendium of complicated biochemistry, acid-base balance, and water and electrolyte diseases in children. It provides clear and commonsense yet highly sophisticated knowledge of encyclopedic proportions, despite its small size. The authors present logical and sequential approaches to study situations that dovetail perfectly with problem-solving examples. The net result is an outstanding "teaching . . . and reference" instrument of the finest quality. Those of us who believe that teaching and management of water and electrolyte disorders in pediatrics is truly in the realm of the general pediatrician and not only of the subspecialist highly recommend this most complete and practical text on the subject. Individuals involved in the care of children, particularly nurses, house officers, pediatricians, and subspecialists, should read this book. It will enrich their knowledge about frequent and potentially serious pediatric disorders and will provide a solid foundation to understand their therapeutic principles.

Rod E. Urizar, MD
Professor of Pediatrics
Associate Professor of Medicine
Medical Director, Pediatric Dialysis Service
Department of Medicine, Division of Nephrology
Albany Medical College
Albany, NY 12208

The epidemiology of childhood disorders

Pless IB, ed. New York: Oxford University Press, 1994. 531 pages. $75.

More than a basic epidemiology text in which principles and methods are described, this informative reference book provides a stimulating and thorough epidemiologic discussion of many pediatric disorders. This should come as no surprise because of the editor's collaboration with an impressive array of internationally recognized contributors, who together present a comprehensive review of pediatric epidemiology.

Two introductory chapters cover fundamental epidemiologic concepts, terms, and methods, and the role of longitudinal studies. Part 1 then reviews perinatal disorders such as prematurity, birth defects, and genetic disorders. Infectious disorders discussed in Part 2 include congenital and respiratory infections, gastroenteritis, and communicable diseases. Chapters on mental and behavioral disorders in Part 3 examine mental retardation, emotional and behavioral problems, and suicide. Part 4 concentrates on violence and injuries, both intentional and unintentional. The last part focuses on chronic disorders—asthma, malignancies, cerebral palsy, and the prediction of adult disease, particularly heart disease and respiratory illness. Most chapters include historical epidemiologic data and a discussion of study limitations in establishing causes of disease. As with many epidemiology texts, this one is full of tables and graphs, most of which are well labeled and easy to understand. At the end of each chapter, the author(s) provide(s) an extensive list of references.

Both the generalist and the subspecialty pediatrician will find this text interesting and informative, as will medical students, residents, and other health care professionals. Readers may initially want to use the text as a quick reference but will soon find themselves immersed in extra reading and reviewing cited references.

The choice of topics presented is timely. However, a noted and disappointing absence from the communicable disease section is a much-needed discussion of the epidemiology of human immunodeficiency virus infection in children.

Elaine E. Schulte, MD, MPH
Assistant Professor of Pediatrics
Albany Medical College
Albany, NY 12208

Usefulness of cerebrospinal fluid bacterial antigen tests

To the Editor:

We found the recent article[1] attempting to quantify the clinical utility of the cerebrospinal fluid (CSF) Directigen test (Becton Dickinson Microbiology Systems, Cockeysville, Md.) very interesting. This study addresses issues of cost containment that are vital to providing quality care in a managed care environment. If a diagnostic study or therapeutic intervention is without utility, it should be abandoned. We applaud the authors for having the intellectual courage to examine the usefulness of CSF bacterial studies in that light.

Of the 901 reviewed circumstances in which a CSF Directigen test was obtained, 29 antigen test results were positive and 872 results were negative. The authors describe in detail the negligible impact that the positive test result had on the management of the 29 patients with positive results, but are curiously silent about the 872 patients with negative results, except to say that results for 6 patients were deemed falsely negative. Is it possible that the real benefit of the Directigen test is in the true-negative results? How many of these patients would have been hospitalized and given intravenously administered antibiotics (with all of the costs involved) had it not been for the negative Directigen test result? Preventing only a few needless admissions each year could more than offset the cost savings of not performing the test.

Given that the purpose of the study was to try to find ways to cut costs without decreasing the quality of care rendered, have the authors considered eliminating the routine ordering of determinations of CSF protein and glucose levels? On the basis of our understanding of their protocol, the results of these determinations apparently never affected the clinical decisions made for patients in whom a diagnosis of meningitis was suspected. At a cost of $54 per test, not obtaining these studies in the 901 subjects would have saved nearly $49,000 during the study period. Perhaps the utility of those tests should be the focus of a future clinical review.

In this era of changes in health care delivery, all health care professionals are obligated to seek opportunities to cut costs. Provided our efforts serve to eliminate the "dead wood" and preserve the "good wood," we can be assured that we are making progress; however, it is incumbent on us to consider the value of a negative test result when we make those determinations. This article serves an admirable purpose in focusing our attention toward the goal of practicing quality, cost-conscious medicine, but until all of the potential cost benefits of a negative test result are included in the equation, the author's conclusion that the Directigen test not be used is premature.

C. R. Warren, DO
W. R. Kiser, MD, MA
Department of Family Practice
Naval Hospital
2080 Child St.
Jacksonville, FL 32214-5227
9/35/61127

REFERENCE

1. Maxson S, Lewno MJ, Schultze GE. Clinical usefulness of cerebrospinal fluid bacterial antigen studies. J PEDIATR 1994; 125:235-8.

Reply

To the Editor:

In our institution, a decision to admit a patient from the clinic or emergency department has never been based on the results of a cerebrospinal fluid bacterial antigen test. Therefore we cannot comment on its role in keeping patients out of the hospital. As for determinations of cerebrospinal fluid protein and glucose levels, we believe that their role is very useful. The first part of our suggested protocol states that ". . . two groups of patients with bacterial meningitis could benefit from having CSF antigens tested." Patients with bacterial meningitis are implied to have abnormal protein and glucose values. We understand that bacterial antigen testing has a different role at different institutions. We believe, however, that the *routine* use of these tests for every patient who has a lumbar puncture is not cost effective.

M. Suzanne Maxson, MD
Fellow, Pediatric Infectious Diseases
Mary Jo Lewno, BS
Chief Technical Director
Microbiology Laboratory
Gordon E. Schutze, MD
Assistant Professor of Pediatrics and Pathology
Pediatric Infectious Diseases/Immunology
Arkansas Children's Hospital
800 Marshall St.
Little Rock, AR 72202-3591
9/35/61126

Infectious hazards of immune globulin

To the Editor:

I read with interest the article by Karna et al., "Passive Transfer of Hepatitis Antibodies During Intravenous Administration of Immune Globulin."[1] The authors found no clinical or laboratory evidence of transmission of hepatitis B or C, despite passive transfer of hepatitis B and C antibodies in the majority of the 10 premature neonates studied. However, the small number of infants studied does not preclude a type II error. Lest complacency develop regarding the safety of U.S. preparations of intravenously administered immune globulin, a recent outbreak of acute hepatitis C infections in 112 recipients of licensed intravenous immune globulin preparations serves as a reminder of the infectious hazards of all biologic preparations.[2]

Leslie L. Barton, MD
Department of Pediatrics
Section of Infectious Diseases
University of Arizona Health Sciences Center
Steele Memorial Children's Research Center
Tucson, AZ 85724
9/35/61305

REFERENCES

1. Karna P, Murray DL, Valduss D, Mattarella N, Dyke JW, Maier GA. Passive transfer of hepatitis antibodies during intravenous administration of immune globulin. J PEDIATR 1994; 125:463-5.
2. CDC. Outbreak of hepatitis C associated with intravenous immunoglobulin administration—United States, October 1993-June 1994. MMWR Morb Mortal Wkly Rep 1994;43: 505-9.

Reply

Intravenous immune globulin preparations have enjoyed a very successful track record in this country for safety from infectious diseases. As mentioned in our article, initial preparations of intravenously administered immune globulin in Europe were associated with non-A, non-B hepatitis.[1] Testing for hepatitis C (non-A, non-B hepatitis) is not 100% sensitive at this time. We agree with Dr. Barton that the recent problem with intravenously administered immune globulin is disturbing and should cause physicians to use such preparations cautiously.

Padmani Karna, MD
Dennis L. Murray, MD
John W. Dyke, PhD
Michigan State University and Sparrow Hospital
Lansing, MI 48909-7980
9/35/61304

REFERENCES

1. Ochs MD, Fischer SH, Virant FS, et al. Non-A, non-B hepatitis after intravenous immunoglobulin. Lancet 1986;1:322-3.

Differences in clinical significance of maternal-infant blood group incompatibility in mothers with blood type O, A, or B

To the Editor:

I read with interest the article by Ozolek et al.,[1] which is an elegant study of a very large population base. I was disappointed, however, to find that there was no mention of the physiologic basis of their findings. I was also surprised to find that a standard pediatric hematology textbook also does not mention the physiologic basis for their results.

On the other hand, a standard adult hematology textbook states "Antibodies of the ABO system are 'naturally occurring,' suggesting immunization against cross-reactive antigens that are widespread on cell types of other organisms such as bacteria. Anti-A and anti-B are predominantly IgM in group B or A individuals, whereas the serum of group O subjects contains significant amounts of anti-A and anti-B that is also of the IgG class. This difference in immune response remains unexplained." [2] Although the cause for these differences remains unexplained, the fact that they do occur provides a simple and logical explanation for the findings of Ozolek et al. Mothers with blood type A or B whose anti-B or anti-A antibodies are predominantly of the IgM class, which do not cross the placenta, would be far less likely to encounter complications of incompatibility than mothers with blood type O, in whom a significant amount of anti-A and anti-B antibody is of the IgG class, which readily crosses the placenta. This is consistent with the findings of Ozolek et al. that "type A or B mothers were 5.5 times less likely to have a positive Coombs test result than type O mothers."

Although individuals with blood type O have a significant amount of IgG isoantibodies, the exact amount or percentage probably varies in each person with blood type O. This is probably a major reason for the observed clinical variability, even in O-A and O-B incompatibilities. One might hope that this knowledge of the antibodies of the ABO system will become as common in the pediatric literature as it is in the adult literature.

Harold Perl, MD
Division of Neonatology
Hackensack Medical Center
Hackensack, NJ 07601
9/35/61299

REFERENCES

1. Ozolek JA, Watchko JF, Mimouni F. Prevalence and lack of clinical significance of blood group incompatibility in mothers with blood type A or B. J PEDIATR 1994;125:87-91.
2. Silberstein LE, Spitalnick SL. Human blood group antigens and antibodies. In: Hoffman R, Benz EJ Jr, Shattel SJ, Furie B, Cohen HJ, eds. Hematology: basic principles and practice. New York: Churchill Livingstone, 1991:1548-56.

Reply

To the Editor:

Contrary to Dr. Perl's impression, the pediatric hematology literature does address the pathophysiology of ABO incompatibility in the newborn infant and specifically the role of different antibody classes in this phenomenon. In *Hematologic Problems in the Newborn*, by Oski and Naiman,[1] the explanation cited for cases of hemolytic disease of the newborn as a result of ABO incompatibility is that natural anti-A and anti-B of mothers with blood group O are of the IgG class and can cross the placenta, whereas those of mothers with blood type A or B are predominantly IgM and cannot cross the placenta. The original work describing the predominance of 19S (IgM) globulin in B anti-A and A anti-B donors was reported by Abelson and Rawson in 1961.[2] We did not discuss the possible pathophysiology of our findings because that was beyond the scope of our study. To our knowledge, however, several interesting questions remain regarding the immunology of ABO incompatibility. We know that the normal immunologic response to antigens is the appearance of IgM, followed by IgG, which provides lifelong protection. Why does B anti-A and A anti-B antibody remain as IgM? Why does IgM not disappear and IgG appear? The A and B substance is very prevalent in foods and bacteria; why do all infants with blood type A or B born to mothers with blood type O not have evidence of antibody as detected by a direct or indirect Coombs test? As we have shown, not all infants with blood type A or B born to mothers with blood type O have a positive Coombs test (direct or indirect) result, and of those infants with a positive direct Coombs test result, only approximately 20% have clinically significant jaundice. Dr. Perl is correct in stating that the amount of IgG isoantibody varies in each person with blood type O. This is one part of the explanation for the clinical variability among O-A and O-B incompatibilities.[3] This may also be related in part to strength, number, and type of the A antigen on neonatal erythrocytes, and even the subclass of IgG produced against the A or B antigens.

John A. Ozolek, MD
Department of Pediatrics
Jon F. Watchko, MD
Associate Professor of Pediatrics,
Obstetrics, Gynecology and
Reproductive Sciences
Department of Pediatrics
Magee-Womens Hospital
Pittsburgh, PA 15213

Francis B. Mimouni, MD
Professor of Pediatrics
Director, Division of Neonatology
Department of Pediatrics
Maimonides Medical Center
Brooklyn, NY 11219
9/35/61300

REFERENCES

1. Oski FA, Naiman JL. Erythroblastosis fetalis. Hematologic problems in the newborn, 3rd ed. Philadelphia: WB Saunders, 1982:283-346.
2. Abelson NM, Rawson AJ. Studies of blood group antibodies. V. Fractionation of examples of anti-B, anti-A,B, anti-M, anti-P, anti-Jk^a, anti-Le^a, anti-D, anti-CD, anti-K, anti-Fy^a, anti-s and anti-Good. Transfusion 1961;Mar-Apr:116-23.
3. Grundbacher FJ. The etiology of ABO hemolytic disease of the newborn. Transfusion 1980;20:563-8.

Screening neonates for intrauterine cocaine exposure

To the Editor:

Ryan et al.[1] provide data on the association between intrauterine cocaine exposure and other variables in their population. However, they overstep their data when they make clinical recommendations on screening for cocaine exposure. They are ambiguous about screening criteria, although poor prenatal care, low socioeconomic status, decreased gestational age, and sexually transmitted diseases are noted as "most meaningful" factors. They also ignore basic principles for designing a screening program.

The investigators argue that adherence to specific guidelines can avoid bias in ordering toxicology tests, yet such guidelines may also be used to formalize systematic bias. All four "meaningful" factors are strongly biased by social class and access to medical care. The common practice of overscreening newborn infants of poor women of color is justified by their guidelines. In an effort to lessen such social bias in referring drug-exposed infants for child neglect, in 1991 the New York State Department of Social Services eliminated lack of prenatal care and extrahospital births as sufficient criteria for toxicology testing.[2]

The investigators advocate screening without considering recommended criteria for such a program.[3] They do not define the problem to be detected; is it simply cocaine exposure or specific conditions related to such exposure? Current research has shown that most cocaine-exposed newborn infants have normal behavior and development.[4] Is there effective treatment or amelioration available, including drug treatment and support programs for parents? Is asymptomatic treatment more effective? Is there a procedure to communicate results to the family and to minimize negative labeling? Are the risks and costs of screening, diagnosis, and treatment justifiable? Are there procedures to protect confidentiality?

In addition to these questions, parental consent must be considered. Maternal drug use alone is not sufficient grounds for neglect and must be accompanied by other evidence of neglectful parenthood to determine child maltreatment in New York state.[2] Without independent evidence for neglect or abuse, parental consent for newborn toxicology testing should be strongly considered. More careful attention to screening criteria is needed to avoid further social and racial stigmatization related to perinatal substance exposure.

Daniel R. Neuspiel, MD, MPH
Associate Professor of Pediatrics and
of Epidemiology and Social Medicine
Albert Einstein College of Medicine and
Montefiore Medical Center
Bronx, NY 10467
9/35/61585

REFERENCES

1. Ryan RM, Wagner CL, Schultz JM, et al. Meconium analysis for improved identification of infants exposed to cocaine in utero. J PEDIATR 1994;125:435-40.
2. Neuspiel DR, Zingman TM, Templeton VH, DiStabile P, Drucker E. Custody of cocaine-exposed newborns: determinants of discharge decisions. Am J Public Health 1993; 83:1726-9.
3. Hoekelman RA, Friedman SB, Nelson NM, Seidel HM, eds. Primary pediatric care. 2nd ed. St. Louis: Mosby–Year Book, 1992.
4. Neuspiel DR. Behavior in cocaine-exposed infants and children: association versus causality. Drug Alcohol Depend 1994; 36:101-7.

Reply

To the Editor:

We agree that there is little "hard" evidence to support the postnatal identification of an infant who underwent intrauterine cocaine exposure. Our study was not designed to address this issue. When scientific evidence is lacking, each physician must use his or her own clinical judgment. We report that if one wishes to screen for intrauterine cocaine exposure, (1) meconium testing is superior to urine sampling, and (2) screening criteria culled from the literature and based largely on experience in large urban populations performed well in our population.

We also agree that there are sensitive issues involved. Our original screening criteria (see Methods[1]) do not specify race or socioeconomic status. The factors obtained by regression analysis (which included socioeconomic status but not race) did not provide better screening guidelines; we elected to keep our original criteria. We believe it is unreasonable to eliminate poor prenatal care as a screening criterion; almost one third of mothers with poor prenatal care had cocaine-exposed infants. If identification of cocaine-exposed infants is desired, and the increased expense of universal screening is to be avoided, it is necessary to include some factors that are associated with illegal drug use.

We agree with Dr. Neuspiel that there are many unanswered questions regarding identification of drug-exposed newborn infants. At our institution, we have a protocol (available on request) that includes the procedure to be followed in these situations regarding communication to the family and other physicians; our approach is to keep the infant with his or her mother and to provide support for the mother as much as possible.

Rita M. Ryan, MD
Assistant Professor of Pediatrics
Dale L. Phelps, MD
Professor of Pediatrics
Division Chief of Neonatology
Department of Pediatrics
University of Rochester Medical Center
601 Elmwood Ave., Box 651
Rochester, NY 14642
9/35/61584

REFERENCE

1. Ryan RM, Wagner CL, Schultz JM, et al. Meconium analysis improves identification of intrauterine cocaine exposed infants. J PEDIATR 1994;125:435-40.

Accuracy of aural infrared temperature device

To the Editor:

Your July 1994 issue contained findings of a study[1] using the Sherwood IMS FirstTemp Genius (model 3000A) aural thermometer (Intelligent Medical Systems, Carlsbad, Calif.). We have examined the data for causes of the unexpected results.

In addition to the reported >0.3° C discrepancy between rectal and aural readings, the following statements describe the data:

1. Thirty readings differed by 1° to 2.44° C.
2. Same-ear measurements differed by an average of 0.14° C (±0.50°) and by up to 2.45° C, suggesting inconsistent technique.
3. Repeatability differed by study sites, perhaps because one site declined our in-service training.
4. No outliers were discarded. Even when two same-ear readings differed by >1° C, or the rectal temperature was recorded as 35.8° C and both aural readings were 38° C, the data were not questioned.

We reanalyzed the data, using the *highest* of the two *aural* readings to reduce operator error effect. Data sets with a difference >±1.12° C between *aural* and rectal temperature were not included (n = 19). In the remaining data (n = 215), the mean difference between *aural* and rectal temperature recording was only 0.12° C (±0.45° C).

These additional points about the article are noteworthy:

1. Simple linear regression presupposes linearity of site-to-site temperature differences, which vary widely among human beings. The appropriate statistical analysis for this study is described by Bland and Altman.[2]

2. The authors concluded that "no prediction of the actual rectal temperature could be made." Prediction of temperature at one site made on the basis of a reading taken at another is not possible. Our use of the term *equivalence* may contribute to this misunderstanding. Nevertheless, our product literature states that prediction is not our purpose. *Equivalences* serve to provide users with familiar scales for interpreting aural temperature readings.

3. Interoperator reliability was not addressed; thus inconsistent technique may have caused discrepancies.

The FirstTemp Genius device is recommended for use in all ages. However, training and consistent operation are essential.

Naja E. McKenzie, RN, MN
Senior Clinical Specialist
Sherwood IMS
Carlsbad, CA 92009
9/35/61583

REFERENCES

1. Petersen-Smith A, Barber N, Coody DK, West MS, Yetman RJ. Comparison of aural infrared with traditional rectal temperatures in children from birth to age three years. J PEDIATR 1994;125:83-5.
2. Bland JM, Altman DG. Statistical methods for assessing agreement between two methods of clinical measurement. Lancet 1986;1:307-10.

Reply

To the Editor:

Ms. McKenzie raises some interesting points regarding our recent article in the JOURNAL. The technique used to collect the data was sound. Investigators at one site received in-service training by

Sherwood personnel before beginning the study; investigators at the other site declined such training because they had multiple years of experience with the device. Therefore "inconsistent technique" is probably not the answer to the differences noted between the glass-mercury and the aural thermometers.

Reevaluation of the data by Sherwood IMS to exclude outliers and reanalysis of the data with the highest of the two aural readings taken resulted in a lower group mean difference between the aural and the rectal temperature of ±0.12° C. These group means are not helpful with the individual patient, in whom the standard deviation by their own calculations was ±0.45° C. This degree of variability may be small for an older child but may prove to be significant for younger children. Regardless of the statistical technique used (that of Bland and Alman vs simple linear regression), a large number of subjects remain with unacceptably large divergence in temperatures by the two modalities.

We agree with Ms. McKenzie's statement that use of the term *equivalence* by Sherwood IMS may be misleading. The aural thermometer provides very quick, painless measurements of temperature that are likely *different* from oral or rectal sites. For instance, rectal lag (the tendency of the rectum to resist temperature changes readily measurable at other sites) is only one such factor that renders the sites different.

Until the "aural" temperature is established as a *different* site and clinicians develop experience with temperatures taken with an aural device in its "core" mode (without adjustments to make measurements "equivalent" to either oral or rectal temperatures), generalizability of this potentially helpful technique to all age groups will continue to be questioned.

Robert Yetman, MD
Associate Professor of Pediatrics
Department of Pediatrics
University of Texas-Houston Medical School
Houston, TX 77030-1503
9/35/61582

New books received

Pediatric disease (fourth series) test and syllabus
Siegel BA, Proto AV, eds. Reston, Virginia: American College of Radiology, 1993. 836 pages. No price listed.

A guide to the practice of paediatric endocrinology
Brook CGD. New York: Cambridge University Press, 1993. 181 pages. $49.95.

Perspectives in pediatric cardiology; vol. 4.
Ferenz C, Rubin JD, Loffredo CA, Magee CA. Mount Kisco, New York: Futura Publishing Company, 1993. 353 pages. $75.

Review of mainstream CFIDS research in the USA
Dayger K. Rochester, New York: CFIDS Rochester Research Project, 1993. 271 pages. $18.50.

Depression in children and adolescents
Koplewicz HS, Klass E. Langhorne, Pennsylvania: Harwood Academic Publishers, 1993. 254 pages. $28.

Handbook of pediatric neurology and neurosurgery
Gaskill SJ, Marlin AE. Boston: Little, Brown, 1993. 242 pages. $32.95.

Molecular genetics of sex determination
Watchel SS. New York: Academic Press, Inc., 1994. 518 pages. No price listed.

Early supplementary feeding and cognition
Pollitt E, Gorman KS, Engle PL, Martorell R, Rivera J. Chicago: University of Chicago Press, 1993. 122 pages. $14.

Bedside cardiology. 4th ed.
Constant J. Boston: Little, Brown, & Co., 1993. 360 pages. $51.95.

The psychoanalytic study of the child; vol. 48.
Solnit AJ, Neubauer PB, Abrams S, Dowling S. New Haven, Connecticut: Yale University Press, 1994. 408 pages. $55.

Medical genetics: A self-instruction guide and workbook
McKusick VA. Baltimore, Maryland: Johns Hopkins University Press, 1993. 125 pages. $30.

Child abuse: Medical diagnosis and management
Reece RM. Malvern, Pennsylvania: Lea & Febiger, 1994. 466 pages. $69.50.

Life span motor development
Haywood KM. Champaign, Illinois: Human Kinetics Publishers, 1993. 416 pages. $48.50.

Laboratory activities for life span motor development
Haywood KM. Champaign, Illinois: Human Kinetics Publishers, 1993. 168 pages. $22.

Perez on medicine
Perez J, Spence WR. Waco, Texas: WRS Group, Inc., 1993. 64 pages. $29.95.

Toddlers and their mothers
Furman E. Madison, Connecticut: International Universities Press, Inc., 1993. 243 pages. $24.95.

Issues and reviews in teratology
Kalter H, ed. New York: Plenum Publishing, 1993.234 pages. $75.

The many meanings of play
Solnit AJ, Cohen DJ, Neubauer PB, eds. New Haven, Connecticut: Yale University Press, 1993. 322 pages. $35.

Précis de médecine foetale et néonatale
Schlaeder G, Messer J, Haddad J, Langer B. Paris: Springer-Verlag France, 1993. 400 pages. No price listed.

Textbook of prematurity: antecedents, treatment, and outcome
Witter FR. Boston: Little, Brown, 1993. 406 pages. $85.

Molecular genetics for the clinician
Brock DJH. New York: Cambridge University Press, 1993. 289 pages. $64.95 (paper $24.95).

Iodine deficiency in Europe: A continuing concern
Delange F, Dunn JT, Glinoer D, eds. New York: Plenum Publishing Corporation, 1993. 492 pages. $125.

Essential paediatrics
Hull D, Johnston DJ. New York: Churchill Livingston, Inc., 1993. 365 pages. $35.

Dino Mites declare war
New York: Family Vision Press, 1993. 80 pages. $8.95.

REVIEWERS

Acknowledgment of reviewers

Once again it is my happy responsibility to express our gratitude to the hundreds of individuals who helped with the review of manuscripts during 1994. This is my thirtieth year of association with THE JOURNAL, and I never cease to be amazed at the willingness of the scientific community to spend so much time and effort in the evaluation of the work of others, without recompense and with no recognition except for inclusion in a list such as the one appended. The peer review system is not perfect (nor is any human endeavor), but we believe that its strengths far outweigh its weaknesses.

In our continuing effort to ensure fairness of the peer review process, we plan to participate in a multijournal study designed to determine whether masking the reviewers to the origins of papers will improve the quality of the reviews by eliminating one possible source of bias. During the next few months, some reviewers will be asked to evaluate manuscripts from which obvious identification has been removed; the review process will not otherwise be affected in any way. Our hope is that definitive conclusions will be possible because of the number of journals and the large number of manuscripts that will be involved in the study. We respectfully urge our reviewers to cooperate if they are asked to participate.

Because of my retirement, this will be my last acknowledgment of the contribution made by reviewers to the work of the editorial staff. As this note is being written, a search for a new editor is under way; perhaps by the time this is published, the identity of the new editor will be known. It has been a great privilege to have served as editor of THE JOURNAL, and my debt to literally thousands of reviewers is enormous. Thank you.

Joseph M. Garfunkel, MD
Editor

A

Carolyn L. Abitbol, MD
Steven H. Abman, MD
Jon S. Abramson, MD
Pasquale Accardo, MD
Frank J. Accurso, MD
Robert Adams, MD
Robert Adler, MD
Stuart P. Adler, MD
Javeed Akhter, MD
Steven R. Alexander, MD
Walter C. Allan, MD
David B. Allen, MD
Marilee C. Allen, MD
Uri S. Alon, MD
Estella M. Alonso, MD
Brad E. Alpert, MD
Bruce S. Alpert, MD
Blanche P. Alter, MD
Dale C. Alverson, MD
Charles M. Anderson, MD, PhD
Donald C. Anderson, MD
Warren A. Andiman, MD
Sharon P. Andreoli, MD
Maureen Andrew, MD
Gerald S. Arbus, MD
Robert Arceci, MD, PhD
Ronald L. Ariagno, MD
Silva Arslanian, MD
Ann M. Arvin, MD
Stephen Ashwal, MD
Balu H. Athreya, MD
Stephanie A. Atkinson, PhD
Theodore W. AvRuskin, MD
Felicia B. Axelrod, MD
Glen P. Aylward, PhD
Elia M. Ayoub, MD
Richard Azizkhan, MD

B

Henrietta Bada, MD
Philip Bagnell, MD
Sami L. Bahna, MD, PhD
Carol J. Baker, MD
Donald Baker, PharmD
Robert Baldassano, MD
Jill E. Baley, MD
J. Williamson Balfe, MD
Henry H. Balfour, MD
Jeanne L. Ballard, MD
Mark Ballow, MD
Eduardo H. Bancalari, MD
Linda G. Bandini, RD, PhD
Emmalee S. Bandstra, MD
Elaine S. Barefield, MD
Pierre Barker, MD
Ann B. Barnet, MD
John A. Barranger, MD
Keith J. Barrington, MB,ChB
Karyl S. Barron, MD
Leslie L. Barton, MD
James W. Bass, MD
Mark L. Batshaw, MD
Daniel G. Batton, MD
Charles R. Bauer, MD
Stephen Baumgart, MD
Richard N. Baumgartner, MD
Bonnie Bean, MD
David V. Beard, MD
Arthur L. Beaudet, MD
Dorothy Becker, MB,BCh
Jonathan Becker, MD
John W. Belmont, MD
George Benzing, MD
Barry B. Bercu, MD
Robert A. Berg, MD
Melvin Berger, MD, PhD
Abraham Bergman, MD
Ira Bergman, MD
Jerry M. Bergstein, MD
Jay E. Berkelhamer, MD
Bram H. Bernstein, MD

THE JOURNAL OF PEDIATRICS 1995;126:327-32
9/37/62093

Jay Bernstein, MD
David D. Berry, MD
Gerard T. Berry, MD
Carol Lynn Berseth, MD
Jatinder J.S. Bhatia, MBBS
Vinod Kuman Bhutani, MD
Diana W. Bianchi, MD
C. Warren Bierman, MD
W. Douglas Biggar, MD
Jeffrey A. Biller, MD
Dennis D. Black, MD
Ingeborg Blancquaert, MD
Julie Blatt, MD
Thomas A. Blondis, MD
Charles D. Bluestone, MD
Jeffrey L. Blumer, MD, PhD
S. Allan Bock, MD
Desmond J. Bohn, MB
William A. Bonadio, MD
Charlotte Boney, MD
W. Clay Bordley, MD
William Borkowsky, MD
Michael Borzy, MD
Carl L. Bose, MD
Laurence A. Boxer, MD
Robert J. Boyle, MD
Jane E. Brazy, MD
Charles Brill, MD
Pim Brouwers, PhD
Mark S. Brown, MD
D. Spencer Brudno, MD
Saul W. Brusilow, MD
A. Charles Bryan, MD
George R. Buchanan, MD
E. Stephen Buescher, MD
Neil R. Buist, MD
A. Wesley Burks, MD
Jane C. Burns, MD
Barbara K. Burton, MD
James B. Bussel, MD
Nancy Butte, MD
J. Decker Butzner, MD
Peter H. Byers, MD
William J. Byrne, MD
Craig J. Byrum, MD

C

Mitchell S. Cairo, MD
Peter R. Camfield, MD
Charles E. Canter, MD
Michael S. Caplan, MD
Waldemar A. Carlo, MD
Susan E. Carlson, PhD
Thomas O. Carpenter, MD
Patrick H. Casey, MD
William J. Cashore, MD
James T. Cassidy, MD
Maureen Cassidy Riski, MD
Salvador Castells, MD
Valerie Castle, MD
Anita Cavallo, MD
Stephen Cederbaum, MD
Stuart Chalew, MD
Gary M. Chan, MD
H. Peter Chase, MD
Ira J. Chasnoff, MD
Subhash Chaudhary, MD
Allen R. Chauvenet, PhD, MD
Steven Chernausek, MD
Victor Chernick, MD
Bart Chernow, MD
James D. Cherry, MD
Nancy Chescheir, MD
P. Joan Chesney, MD
Russell W. Chesney, MD
Pamela Ching, RD, ScD
J. Julian Chisolm, MD
Sechin Cho, MD
Robert D. Christensen, MD
Cameron Chumlea, MD
Joseph A. Church, MD
D. Wade Clapp, MD
Reese H. Clark, MD
Sterling K. Clarren, MD
Thomas G. Cleary, MD
William J. Cochran, MD
Alan R. Cohen, MD
Albert M. Collier, MD
James W. Collins, MD, MPH
Susan B. Conley, MD
Dennis A. Conrad, MD
Felix A. Conte, MD
James Conway, MD
Michael Cooperstock, MD
Donna R. Copeland, PhD
Mary Corey, PhD
Jean A. Cortner, MD
Andrew T. Costarino, MD
Gertrude Costin, MD
Robert F. Covert, MD
Morton Cowan, MD
Richard M. Cowett, MD
J. Carl Craft, MD
W. Hugh Craft, MD
Robert E. Cross, MD
Dennis T. Crouse, MD
Allan S. Cunningham, MD
Richard G. Curless, MD
Leona Cuttler, MD
Steven J. Czinn, MD

D

O'Neill D'Cruz, MD
Denis Daneman, MD
Stephen Daniels, MD, PhD
Richard J. David, MD
Pedro De Alarcon, MD
Richard J. Deckelbaum, MD
Ralph B. Dell, MD
Scott C. Denne, MD
Penelope H. Dennehy, MD
Barbara A. Dennison, MD
Floyd Denny, MD
Ruthmary K. Deuel, MD
Salvatore DiMauro, MD
Macdonald Dick, MD
William H. Dietz, MD, PhD
John Diliberti, MD
David L. Donaldson, MD
Terry Doran, MD
Deborah J. Dotters, MD
Stephen M. Downs, MD, MS
Amelia F. Drake, MD
Willa H. Drummond, MD
Stephen C. Duck, MD
John W. Duckett, MD
Peter Durie, MD
Jean H. Dussault, MD

E

Kathryn M. Edwards, MD
Morven S. Edwards, MD
Robert M. Ehrlich, MD
Louis J. Elsas, MD
S. Jean Emans, MD
Barbara Engelhardt, MD
William A. Engle, MD
B. Keith English, MD
Janet A. Englund, MD
Ruth Etzel, MD, PhD
William E. Evans, PharmD

F

James B. Fahner, MD
Frank Falkner, MD
Henry C. Farrar, MD
Laura Fehrs, MD
Stephen A. Feig, MD
Sandor Feldman, MD
Marianne E. Felice, MD
Gerald W. Fernald, MD
Paul M. Fernhoff, MD
John M. Fiascone, MD
Michael Fiedler, MD
David Finegold, MD
Neal N. Finer, MD
Jordon Finkelstein, MD
Debra H. Fiser, MD
David E. Fisher, MD
Marvin A. Fishman, MD
David E. Fixler, MD
Alan R. Fleischman, MD
David R. Fleisher, MD
Gary R. Fleisher, MD
Thomas P. Foley, MD
J. Dennis Fortenberry, MD
Mary Glenn Fowler, MD
Julie Francis, MD
Uta Francke, MD
Lee Frank, MD, PhD
Robert C. Franks, MD

Ivan D. Frantz, MD
S. Douglas Frasier, MD
Doren D. Fredrickson, MD
Gary Freed, MD
Sharon P. Freedman, MD
John Freeman, MD
Deborah K. Freese, MD
Eugene B. Freid, MD
Frank S. French, MD
Timothy C. Frewen, MD
Ilona J. Frieden, MD
Henry S. Friedman, MD
Virginia Frisk, MD
Donald P. Frush, MD
Bradley P. Fuhrman, MD

G

Peter Gal, PharmD
Richard E. Garcia, MD
Cynthia Garcia-Coll, PhD
Arthur Garson, MD, MPH
Mitchell E. Geffner, MD
Robert Geggel, MD
Harry K. Genant, MD
Myron Genel, MD
Michael K. Georgieff, MD
Michael A. Gerber, MD
Jeffrey S. Gerdes, MD
Tilo O. Gerhardt, MD
John Germak, MD
Anne A. Gershon, MD
Welton M. Gersony, MD
Joseph M. Gertner, MD
Fayez K. Ghishan, MD
James B. Gibson, MD
Samuel S. Gidding, MD
G. Scott Giebink, MD
Joan Gill, MD
Paul C. Gillette, MD
Peter H. Gilligan, PhD
Matthew W. Gillman, MD
Janet R. Gilsdorf, MD
Jeannine L. Gingras, MD
Laurence B. Givner, MD
Bertil E. Glader, MD, PhD
Joy H. Glaser, MD
W. Paul Glezen, MD
Philip L. Glick, MD
Mary P. Glode, MD
Allen I. Goldberg, MD
Ronald N. Goldberg, MD
Neville H. Golden, MD
Sidney Goldfischer, MD
Armond S. Goldman, MD
Steven L. Goldman, MD
Edward D. Gomperts, MD
Stephen I. Goodman, MD
Paul Goodyer, MD
Allen M. Goorin, MD
Gerald V. Goresky, MD
Jeffrey B. Gould, MD, MPH
Clarence W. Gowen, MD
Gregory A. Grabowski, MD
John M. Graham, MD, ScD
Michael L. Graham, MD
Barry M. Gray, MD
Leonard J. Graziani, MD
Carol L. Greene, MD
Walter Greene, MD
Robert S. Greenwood, MD
Frank R. Greer, MD
Patricia M. Griffin, MD
Anne Marie Griffiths, MD, FRCP
Steven J. Gross, MD
William C. Gruber, MD
Joyce D. Gryboski, MD
Lawrence J. Grylack, MD
Christian Guilleminault, MD
Eva C. Guinan, MD
Shumei Guo, MD
Robert D. Guthrie, MD

H

Maureen Hack, MD
Joseph R. Hageman, MD
Daniel E. Hale, MD
Colin D. Hall, MD
Robert T. Hall, MD
Neal A. Halsey, MD
K. Michael Hambidge, MD
Stanley R. Hamilton, MD
Margit Hamosh, PhD
James W. Hansen, MD
Nancy Hansen, MD
Kenneth Harkavy, MD
Andrew P. Harris, MD
Glenn D. Harris, MD
Mary C. Harris, MD
Gail G. Harrison, PhD
Robert H.A. Haslam, MD
Terry F. Hatch, MD
Gregory F. Hayden, MD
Anthony R. Hayward, MD, PhD
Thomas A. Hazinski, MD
Diane Hebert, MD, FRCP
Thomas Hegyi, MD
Douglas C. Heiner, MD, PhD
William C. Heird, MD
Stanley Hellerstein, MD
Leslie Hendeles, PharmD
Frederick W. Henderson, MD
Richard C. Henderson, MD, PhD
Robin Henderson, PhD
J. Owen Hendley, MD
Jay Herman, MD
Henry G. Herrod, MD
Seth V. Hetherington, MD
James E. Heubi, MD
Michael A. Heymann, MD
Harry R. Hill, MD
Malcolm Hill, PharmD
Craig A. Hillemeier, MD
Karen J. Hofman, MB,BCh
Lindsay Hofman, PhD
Lewis B. Holmes, MD
Philip G. Holtzapple, MD
Ronald B. Holtzman, MD
Richard Hong, MD
Paul J. Honig, MD
Stephen R. Hooper, PhD
Michael J. Horgan, MD
William A. Horton, MD
Margaret K. Hostetter, MD
Valera Hudson, MD
George Hug, MD
Walter T. Hughes, MD
Carl E. Hunt, MD
Carol A. Huseman, MD
Jeffrey S. Hyams, MD

I

Susan T. Iannaccone, MD
Norman T. Ilowite, MD
David Ingram, MD
J. Nevin Isenberg, MD, PhD

J

Jerry C. Jacobs, MD
Marc S. Jacobson, MD
Robert M. Jacobson, MD
Paula K. Jaudes, MD
Jerri Ann Jenista, MD
John C. Jennette, MD
Hal B. Jenson, MD
John P. Johnson, MD
Helen S. Johnstone, MD
Deborah P. Jones, MD
Gary R. Jones, MD

K

Marilyn Kacica, MD
Stephen G. Kahler, MD
David Kalwinsky, MD
Stephen R. Kandall, MD
William P. Kanto, MD
Lilly Ching-Chung Kao, MD
Bernard S. Kaplan, MB,BCh
Edward L. Kaplan, MD
M. Karmali, MD
W. Karp, PhD, DMD
Sudesh Kataria, MD
John Kattwinkel, MD
Ben Z. Katz, MD
Anne E. Kazak, PhD
Gregory L. Kearns, PharmD
Thomas G. Keens, MD
Richard I. Kelley, MD, PhD
Dorothy Kelly, MD
Kevin J. Kelly, MD
Thomas L. Kennedy, MD
Douglas Kerr, MD

L. Lyndon Key, MD
Sigmund J. Kharasch, MD
Vikram Khoshoo, MD, PhD
Thomas R. Kimball, MD
Gail King, MD
Lowell R. King, MD
Nancy M. King, JD
John P. Kinsella, MD
C. Thomas Kisker, MD
Niranjan Kissoon, MD
Gordon L. Klein, MD, MPH
Jonathan Klein, MD, MPH
Leonard I. Kleinman, MD
Ronald E. Kleinman, MD
William J. Klish, MD
Matthew E. Knight, MD
Richard Koch, MD
William Koch, MD
Joseph A. Kochen, MD, PhD
Peter Kollros, MD
Diane M. Komp, MD
Arthur E. Kopelman, MD
Gideon Koren, MD
David N. Korones, MD
Robert V. Kotas, MD
Jonathan B. Kotch, MD
Stella Kourembanas, MD
Boris G. Kousseff, MD
A. Avinoam Kowarski, MD
Richard E. Kravath, MD
Ernest N. Kraybill, MD
Deborah W. Kredich, MD
Richard E. Kreipe, MD
Jonathan B. Kronick, MD, PhD
Mark A. Kummer, MD
Stuart Kupfer, MD
Joanne Kurtzberg, MD
Jan A. Kylstra, MD

L

Craig F. LaForce, MD
Stephen LaFranchi, MD
Richard J. Labotka, MD
Stuart R. Lacey, MD
Stephan Ladisch, MD
Parviz Lalezari, MD
Edward J. Lammer, MD
Peter A. Lane, MD
Beverly Lange, MD
Leonard O. Langer, MD
Diane L. Langkamp, MD
Craig B. Langman, MD
Carole Lannon, MD
Andre D. Lascari, MD
Stephen T. Lawless, MD
Ronald Laxer, MD
Michael H. LeBlanc, MD
Charles T. Leach, MD
Fred D. Ledley, MD
Haesoon Lee, MD
Peter A. Lee, MD, PhD
Vicky A. Legrys, DA
Thomas J.A. Lehman, MD
Harold P. Lehmann, MD, PhD
Margaret Leigh, MD
Stanley Lemon, MD
Martha Lepow, MD
Barry M. Lester, MD
Daniel L. Levin, MD
Henry Levison, MD
Lynne L. Levitsky, MD
Harvey L. Levy, MD
David B. Lewis, MD
Steven Lichtman, MD
Jay M. Lieberman, MD
Edward A. Liechty, MD
Helen G. Liley, MD
Wilma A. Lim, MD
Tsu-Hui Lin, MD
Calvin Linnemann, MD
Michael A. Linshaw, MD
Barbara Lippe, MD
Steven Lipshultz, MD
Mark Lipson, MD
John J. Lipuma, MD
Robert H. Listernick, MD
John D. Lloyd-Still, MD
Vera A. Loening-Baucke, MD
Jennifer Loggie, MD
Jacob A. Lohr, MD
Kenneth A. Lombard, MD
Sarah S. Long, MD
John M. Lorenz, MD
Andrea Lotze, MD
Betsy Lozoff, MD
Naomi L.C. Luban, MD
Frederick L. Lueder, MD

M

C. Charlton Mabry, MD
William MacLean, PhD
William C. MacLean, MD
Michael L. Macknin, MD
Larry Mahoney, MD
Lynn Mahony, MD
J. Jeffrey Malatack, MD
John I. Malone, MD
Penelope Manasco, MD
Thomas J. Mancuso, MD
Scott Mandel, MD
M. Joan Mansfield, MD
Colin D. Marchant, MD
Margaret Marcon, MD, FRCP
Carole L. Marcus, MB,BCh
Peter A. Margolis, MD, PhD
Milton Markowitz, MD
Morri E. Markowitz, MD
Keith H. Marks, MD, PhD
Richard A. Marlar, MD
Gerard R. Martin, MD
Richard J. Martin, MD
Thomas R. Martin, MD
Lois Martyn, MD
Reuben Matalon, MD
David O. Matson, MD, PhD
Alvin M. Mauer, MD
S. Michael Mauer, MD
John Mazur, MD
Edward R.B. McCabe, MD, PhD
Paul L. McCarthy, MD
Richard E. McClead, MD
Kenneth M. McConnochie, MD
Kristine McCulloch, MD
Anthony F. McDonagh, PhD
Paul T. McEnery, MD
Charles P. McKay, MD
Ross E. McKinney, MD
Anna T. Meadows, MD
Herman C. Meissner, MD
Jon N. Meliones, MD
Eli O. Meltzer, MD
Stanley A. Mendoza, MD
James A. Menke, MD
Laura Ment, MD
William C. Mentzer, MD
T. Allen Merritt, MD
David F. Merten, MD
Hrair-George Mesrobian, MD
Richard A. Meyer, MD
Michael V. Miles, PharmD
Denis R. Miller, MD
Martha J. Miller, MD
Francis Mimouni, MD
Frank W. Moler, MD
Wayne V. Moore, MD
Bruce Z. Morgenstern, MD
Akira Morishima, MD
C. Richard Morris, MD
Mary Ellen Mortensen, MD, MS
Hugo W. Moser, MD
Thomas Moshang, MD
John C. Moskop, PhD
Sue Moyer, MD
Virginia A. Moyer, MD, MPH
Joseph Muenzer, MD, PhD
Jody Reed Murph, MD
Anne M. Murphy, MD

N

J. Lawrence Naiman, MD
Don K. Nakayama, MD
Michael N. Needle, MD
Allen H. Neims, MD, PhD
Eliot W. Nelson, MD
Karin B. Nelson, MD
Mark E. Nesbit, MD
Elizabeth F. Neufeld, MD
Richard W. Newcomb, MD
David G. Nichols, MD
John F. Nicholson, MD
Michael E. Norman, MD
Daniel A. Notterman, MD

Eliezer Nussbaum, MD
Robert L. Nussbaum, MD

O

John S. O'Brien, MD
Margaret E.D. O'Flynn, MD
P. Pearl O'Rourke, MD
T. Michael O'Shea, MD
Sharon E. Oberfield, MD
Judith Ochs, MD
Karen Olness, MD
Enrique M. Ostrea, MD
Harry Ostrer, MD
Nancy K. Ostrom, MD
Gary D. Overturf, MD

P

Lauren M. Pachman, MD
Seymour Packman, MD
Roberta A. Pagon, MD
Michael J. Painter, MD
Judith S. Palfrey, MD
Amy S. Paller, MD
Howard Panitch, MD
Richard Parad, MD
Jack L. Paradise, MD
Jan E. Paradise, MD
Yong D. Park, MD
Samuel K. Parrish, MD
John B. Paton, MD
Edward N. Pattishall, MD
Arnall Patz, MD
Andrew T. Pavia, MD
David B. Peden, MD
Paul B. Pencharz, MB,ChB
Gilberto R. Pereira, MD
Carlos R. Perez, MD
Max Perlman, MD
Jay A. Perman, MD
Georges Peter, MD
Charles Peters, MD
Raymond D.A. Peterson, MD
Stephannie Phelps, PharmD
Alistair G.S. Philip, MD, FRCP
Larry K. Pickering, MD
Arthur S. Pickoff, MD
William W. Pinsky, MD
Sergio Piomelli, MD
Ivan B. Pless, MD
Martin Polinsky, MD
Constantin Polychronakos, MD
Darlene F. Powars, MD
Dwight A. Powell, MD
Geraldine K. Powell, MD
Keith R. Powell, MD
Greg E. Prazar, MD
Wayne Price, MD
Neil S. Prose, MD
Roy Proujansky, MD

Q

Qutub H. Qazi, MD, PhD
Paul G. Quie, MD
Charmian A. Quigley, MD
John J. Quinn, MD

R

Tonse N. K. Raju, MD
Rajam S. Ramamurthy, MD
Madu Rao, MD
Madjid Rasoulpour, MD
Alok Rastogi, MD, MRCP
Charles J. Rebouche, PhD
Ann M. Reed, MD
Michael D. Reed, PharmD
Warren E. Regelmann, MD
J. Rautt Reigart, MD
Edward O. Reiter, MD
Mark D. Reller, MD
Mary V. Relling, PharmD
Steven Resnick, MD
George Z. Retsch-Bogart, MD
Philip J. Rettig, MD
Peter D. Reuman, MD
John W. Reynolds, MD
William J. Rhead, MD, PhD
Karen Rheuban, MD
Marc Rhoads, MD
Douglas Richardson, MD
Robert A. Richman, MD
Donald A. Riopel, MD
Stephen D. Rioux, MD
William Rizzo, MD
Michael W. Roberts, DDS
Alexander F. Robertson, MD
Albert P. Rocchini, MD
Lance E. Rodewald, MD
John H. Rodman, PharmD
William J. Rodriguez, MD, PhD
Charles R. Roe, MD
Walter J. Rogan, MD
Chaim M. Roifman, MD
Nancy Roizen, MD
Carolyn A. Romshe, MD
Allen W. Root, MD
John F. Rosen, MD
Ron G. Rosenfeld, MD
Harley A. Rotbart, MD
Joanne P. Rovet, PhD
Jonelle C. Rowe, MD
Thomas W. Rowland, MD
Anne H. Rowley, MD
Shane Roy, MD
Arye Rubinstein, MD
Barry H. Rumack, MD
Carol W. Runyan, PhD
Desmond Runyan, MD, DrPH

S

Paul H. Saenger, MD
David J. Sahn, MD
Saroj Saigal, MD
Alan Salamy, PhD
Stephen E. Sallan, MD
Isidro B. Salusky, MD
Hugh A. Sampson, MD
Marilyn R. Sanders, MD
Adrian Sandler, MD
Harvey B. Sarnat, MD
Frank T. Saulsbury, MD
John W. Scanlon, MD
Richard J. Schanler, MD
Daniel V. Schidlow, MD
Richard M. Schieken, MD
David Schiff, MD, PhD
Richard I. Schiff, MD, PhD
Alicia Schiffrin, MD
Eberhard Schmidt-Sommerfeld, MD
Rachel Schneerson, MD
John Schreiber, MD
Michael D. Schreiber, MD
Seth L. Schulman, MD
Richard Schwartz, MD
Kathleen B. Schwarz, MD
Sarah J. Schwarzenberg, MD
W. Frederick Schwenk, MD
John P. Scott, MD
Charles R. Scriver, MD
Ruth A. Seeler, MD
Mouin G. Seikaly, MD
Gerald A. Serwer, MD
Carolyn Seymore Ashworth, MD
Penelope G. Shackelford, MD
Mary-Ann B. Shafer, MD
Stanley G. Shaffer, MD
Thomas H. Shaffer, PhD
Kevin Shannon, MD
Eugene D. Shapiro, MD
Harvey L. Sharp, MD
Salley E. Shaywitz, MD
Danny Shen, PhD
Jayant P. Shenai, MD
Jerry L. Shenep, MD
I. Ronald Shenker, MD
Joseph R. Sherbotie, MD
James M. Sherman, MD
Philip M. Sherman, MD
Ann O. Shigeoka, MD
Vivian E-an Shih, MD
Benjamin Shneider, MD
John M. Shoffner, MD
Dorothy Shulman, MD
Robert J. Shulman, MD
Stanford T. Shulman, MD
David B. Shurtleff, MD
Richard L. Siegler, MD
Janet H. Silverstein, MD
Jean M. Silvestri, MD
Lynn Singer, PhD

Bernhard H. Singsen, MD, MPH
Charles Sklar, MD
John Sleasman, MD
Alfred E. Slonim, MD
Barry T. Smith, MD
Bryan W. Smith, MD
Charles V. Smith, PhD
David S. Smith, MD
Jean C. Smith, MD
A. Rebecca Snider, MD
Selma Snyderman, MD
Scott J. Soifer, MD
Ronald J. Sokol, MD
Judith M. Sondheimer, MD
Robert M. Spear, MD
Bonnie L. Specker, PhD
Barbara B. Specter, MD
David P. Speert, MD
Alan R. Spitzer, MD
Brian Stabler, PhD
Virginia A. Stallings, MD
Charles A. Stanley, MD
F. Bruder Stapleton, MD
Ann R. Stark, MD
Jeffrey R. Starke, MD
Barbara A. Stechenberg, MD
B. T. Steele, MD
Russell W. Steele, MD
John L. Stefano, MD
Leonard Stein, MD
Mark A. Stein, PhD
Ruth E.K. Stein, MD
Lynne S. Steinbach, MD
Curt Steinhart, MD
Mark C. Steinhoff, MD
Robert C. Stern, MD
David K. Stevenson, MD
Clinton F. Stewart, PharmD
Jane Stewart, MD
James A. Stockman, MD
Barbara S. Stonestreet, MD
Sylvan E. Stool, MD
Rainer Storb, MD
Victor C. Strasburger, MD
Jose Strauss, MD
Cyril F. Strife, MD
Gerald L. Strope, MD
Robert C. Strunk, MD
Terrence L. Stull, MD
Raymond A. Sturner, MD
Harris R. Stutman, MD
Frederick J. Suchy, MD
John L. Sullivan, MD
Dennis M. Super, MD, PhD
James L. Sutphen, MD
Lawrence Sweetman, PhD
Virginia P. Sybert, MD
Stanley J. Szefler, MD

T

Glenn S. Takata, MD, MS
David T. Tanaka, MD
Manuel E. Tancer, MD
Kenneth J. Tarnowski, PhD
Lesli A. Taylor, MD
David W. Teele, MD
Michael B. Tennison, MD
Stuart W. Teplin, MD
Robert Tepper, MD
Andrew Tershakovec, MD
Donald W. Thibeault, MD
Jess G. Thoene, MD
Jerry Thompson, PhD
Paul S. Thornton, MD
John M. Thorp, MD
James D. Thullen, MD
Jeffrey A. Towbin, MD
Doris A. Trauner, MD
Joel Tsevat, MD, MPH
William R. Turk, MD
Ronald B. Turner, MD
Eileen Tyrala, MD
Jon E. Tyson, MD

U

Ricardo Uauy, MD, PhD

V

Mary Ann Vaccarello-Cruz, MD
Jimmie L. Valentine, PhD
Robert Valley, MD
Russell Van Dyke, MD
Johan Van Hove, MD
Linda J. Van Marter, MD
Rao Varada, MD
Jorge H. Vargas, MD
Surendra Varma, MD
Kathryn N. Vedder, MD, MPH
V. Matti Vehaskari, MD
Pankaje S. Venkataraman, MBBS
Frank S. Virant, MD
Betty R. Vohr, MD

W

Ellen R. Wald, MD
F. Bryson Waldo, MD
Paul G. Walfish, CM, MD
Michael A. Wall, MD
Philip A. Walravens, MD
James K. Walsh, PhD
Michele C. Walsh-Sukys, MD
Philip D. Walson, MD
Bradley Warady, MD
Joel I. Ward, MD
Kent E. Ward, MD
Russell E. Ware, MD, PhD
Reginald L. Washington, MD
Jon F. Watchko, MD
John B. Watkins, MD
Kristi L. Watterberg, MD
David J. Weber, MD
Debra E. Weese-Mayer, MD
Kristen A. Weigle, MD
William B. Weil, MD
Miles M. Weinberger, MD
Peggy S. Weintrub, MD
Thomas R. Welch, MD
Rita Wellens, PhD
Robert C. Welliver, MD
Thomas G. Wells, MD
Richard P. Wennberg, MD
Steven L. Werlin, MD
David L. Wessel, MD
Carl W. White, MD
Neil H. White, MD
William Whitehead, PhD
Peter F. Whitington, MD
Richard J. Whitley, MD
J. Kenneth Whitt, PhD
Michael P. Whyte, MD
Joseph M. Wiley, MD
Catherine Wilfert, MD
Christine L. Williams, MD
Thomas Williams, MD
David Willis, MD
Robert W. Wilmott, MD
Christopher B. Wilson, MD
Darrell M. Wilson, MD
Don A. Wilson, MD
John T. Wilson, MD
Thomas A. Wilson, MD
Jerry A. Winkelstein, MD
Harland S. Winter, MD
Jeremy S.D. Winter, MD
William E. Winter, MD
Thomas E. Wiswell, MD
Barry Wolf, MD, PhD
Grace Wolff, MD
Mark L. Wolraich, MD
Richard Womer, MD
William W. Wong, PhD
Gordon Worley, MD
Anne Wright, PhD
Robert J. Wyatt, MD
Robert Wyllie, MD

Y

Steven M. Yabek, MD
Robert J. Yetman, MD
Mervyn C. Yoder, MD
Robert H. Yolken, MD
Thomas Young, MD
Marc Yudkoff, MD

Z

Elaine H. Zackai, MD
Arno Zaritsky, MD
Ekhard E. Ziegler, MD
Jerry J. Zimmerman, MD
William H. Zinkham, MD
Basil J. Zitelli, MD
Barry S. Zuckerman, MD
Robert J. Zwiener, MD

THE JOURNAL OF
PEDIATRICS

MARCH 1995 Volume 126 Number 3

MEDICAL PROGRESS

Cardiovascular, renal, and endocrine actions of dopamine in neonates and children

Istvan Seri, MD, PhD

From the Division of Neonatology, Department of Medicine, Children's Hospital of Philadelphia, Philadelphia, Pennsylvania

Dopamine has been widely used in pediatric and neonatal intensive care for the treatment of hypotension or oliguria in sick preterm[1-6] and term neonates[2, 7] and in children.[8] Through stimulation of the adrenergic and dopaminergic receptors, dopamine exerts dose-dependent cardiovascular, renal, and endocrine effects that combat the clinical manifestations of shock. Despite the extensive use of the drug in pediatric and neonatal clinical practice, only recently have advances in the fields of molecular biology and cellular physiology resulted in a better understanding of the mechanisms of these cardiovascular, renal, and hormonal actions of dopamine. The present review summarizes the impact of this recently accumulated knowledge on the clinical management of the sick neonate and child requiring pressor support.

The following discussion first briefly describes the physiology of the dopaminergic system in the central nervous system and on the periphery, and reviews the structure, distribution, postreceptor mechanisms, and function of the peripheral dopamine receptors. The relevant cardiovascular, renal, and endocrine effects of dopamine and their clinical implications in the neonatal and pediatric patient population are then discussed in detail.

Reprint requests: Istvan Seri, MD, PhD, Division of Neonatology, Department of Medicine, Children's Hospital of Philadelphia, 34th St. and Civic Center Blvd., Philadelphia, PA 19104.

THE JOURNAL OF PEDIATRICS 1995;126:333-44

0022-3476/95/$3.00 + 0 **9/18/61903**

PHYSIOLOGY OF THE CNS AND PERIPHERAL DOPAMINERGIC SYSTEM

Dopamine, in addition to being a precursor of norepinephrine and epinephrine, is a naturally occurring endogenous catecholamine. In the CNS, dopaminergic modulation of ion fluxes regulate emotion, activity, behavior, and nerve conduction. In the CNS and peripheral adrenergic system,

ADH	Antidiuretic hormone
ATPase	Adenosinetriphosphatase
GFR	Glomerular filtration rate
P_i	Inorganic phosphate

and in certain endocrine organs, dopamine also regulates the release of other hormones, including prolactin,[9, 10] thyrotropin,[9, 10] growth hormone,[11] gonadotropins,[9] antidiuretic hormone,[12] renin,[13, 14] and aldosterone.[15] In the kidney, endogenous dopamine plays an important role in the physiologic regulation of ion transport along the nephron.[3, 16, 17] Nonneuronal dopamine, produced in the proximal tubule cells by the uptake and decarboxylation of filtered L-dopa,[18] regulates renal sodium[3, 16, 17] and phosphorus[19] excretion. Thus, when used as a therapeutic agent to improve deranged cardiovascular activity and renal hemodynamics, dopamine also exerts significant effects on renal tubular[3, 16, 17] and endocrine functions.[9-15] These actions in turn may then modulate the desired hemodynamic effects of dopamine contingent on the underlying disease process, fluid-electrolyte balance, and age of the patient.

STRUCTURE, DISTRIBUTION, POSTRECEPTOR MECHANISMS, AND FUNCTION OF THE PERIPHERAL DOPAMINE RECEPTORS

Dopamine receptors belong to a large family of seven transmembrane domain-containing G-protein–coupled cell surface hormone receptors.[20] On the basis of pharmacologic criteria, two subtypes of both the CNS and peripheral dopamine receptors have been identified and are designated as D_1 and D_2, and as DA_1 and DA_2, respectively.[16, 17, 20, 21]Peripheral dopamine receptors are dopamine receptors present outside the CNS in the cardiovascular system,[17] adrenergic nerve endings,[22] renal tubules,[21] and certain endocrine organs.[12, 14, 16]

In the CNS, the molecular structures of two D_1-type and four D_2-type dopamine receptors have been characterized.[21] Some of the peripheral dopamine receptors are central dopamine receptors expressed on the periphery[21]; other peripheral dopamine receptors are thought to have similar but not identical molecular structures as their CNS counterparts.[21, 23] However, this remains to be proved because complete molecular characterization of the peripheral dopamine receptors has been unsuccessful.[21, 24]

Developmental studies in animals have found maturation-dependent increases in the expression and integrity of the cardiovascular and renal tubular dopamine receptors and postreceptor events.[25-28] Recent observations in the human preterm neonate suggest a more advanced functional maturity of these receptors than expected on the basis of the findings in most of the animal studies.[1, 2, 4-6]

DA_1-type peripheral dopamine receptors. The DA_1 receptors are almost exclusively postsynaptic in location and are positively coupled to adenylate cyclase or phospholipase C.[16, 21] In the cardiovascular system, these receptors are most abundant in the renal vasculature, and in the mesenteric and coronary arteries[16, 17]; the extracerebral vessels[29] and the pulmonary circulation[30] express DA_1 receptors at lower densities. Stimulation of the vascular DA_1 receptors causes vasorelaxation via a cyclic adenosine monophosphate–dependent and protein kinase A–mediated decrease in the sensitivity of vascular smooth muscle to intracellular calcium.[31]

In the kidney, nonvascular DA_1 receptors are present in the brush-border and basolateral membranes of the proximal tubule, and in the juxtaglomerular cells, the thick ascending limb, and the distal tubule and cortical collecting duct.[16, 21] As described in the section on the renal effects of dopamine, stimulation of these receptors induces changes in tubular ion fluxes and increases renin release.[3, 16, 17, 21]

DA_2-type peripheral dopamine receptors. Peripheral DA_2 receptors are presynaptic[16] or postsynaptic[17, 22, 32] in location; stimulation of these receptors inhibits adenylate cyclase activity[16, 17, 21, 22] or polyphosphoinositide turnover.[21] The coupling mechanisms of some of the cloned CNS D_2 receptors seem to depend not only on their molecular structure but also on the cellular environment.[33]

Adrenergic nerve varicosities and terminals surrounding the renal and mesenteric vascular beds[16, 17, 22] are especially abundant in presynaptic DA_2 receptors. Through inhibition of adenylate cyclase activity,[17, 21] activation of these receptors inhibits norepinephrine release, resulting in a decrease in sympathetic discharge and thus vasodilation of these vessels.[17] Vascular postsynaptic DA_2 receptors are found mostly in the intimal layer of the renal, mesenteric, and cerebral vasculature,[34] and their stimulation may cause vasodilation by influencing the release of endothelial vasoactive factors.

In the kidney, poorly characterized nonvascular postsynaptic DA_2 receptors are present along the nephron and in the juxtaglomerular apparatus.[16, 21] In the inner medulla, a unique postsynaptic DA_2 receptor, termed $DA_{2k'}$, has recently been characterized and shown to be coupled to prostaglandin E_2 production through stimulation of phospholipase A.[35] Activation of this receptor attenuates the effect of ADH and inhibits Na^+,K^+-ATPase activity in the distal part of the nephron.[21, 36]

Among the endocrine organs, postsynaptic DA_2 receptors are found in the adrenal cortex[16] and pituitary gland,[12] where they inhibit the release of aldosterone[15] and certain pituitary hormones,[9-12] respectively. Postsynaptic DA_2 receptors are also expressed in the carotid bodies; these receptors play an important role in the peripheral regulation of breathing.[37]

CARDIOVASCULAR, RENAL, AND ENDOCRINE ACTIONS OF DOPAMINE

Irrespective of the cause of the cardiovascular collapse, dopamine has been widely used in the treatment of shock in children[8] and in term[2, 7] and preterm neonates.[1-6] Exogenous dopamine exerts its complex effects almost exclusively by the dose-dependent stimulation of the dopaminergic, the α- and β-adrenergic and the serotonin receptors.[3, 16, 17, 38, 39] The ability of dopamine also to stimulate other aminergic receptors appears to be related to the flexibility of the side chain and to the freedom of rotation of the benzene ring, which allows conformational changes that fit many different receptors.[38, 39] In adults and children, at low doses (0.5 to 2 μg/kg per minute), the effects of stimulation of peripheral dopamine receptors in the cardiovascular system, kidneys, adrenergic nerve endings, and certain endocrine organs dominate the clinical response. At medium doses (2 to 6 μg/kg per minute), the effects of cardiac β_1- and β_2-adrenergic receptor stimulation also become apparent. Finally, at doses beyond 6 to 10 μg/kg per minute, the dopamine-induced activation of the cardiovascular α_1- and α_2-adrenergic receptors and serotonin receptors begins to influence the clinical response. However, in preterm neonates, because of developmental differences in the maturation of the adrenergic receptor system and in metabolic clearance rates,[6] signs of activation of cardiovascular α receptors occur at lower doses, preceding some of the clinical signs of β-receptor stimulation.[1-6]

Dopamine undergoes complex metabolic and elimination processes.[40, 41] In the plasma, a portion of the drug is protein bound; the free form is taken up and distributed by the peripheral tissues to its sites of action. Dopamine is then either metabolized by catechol *O*-methyltransferase, taken up by the peripheral sympathetic neurons, or diffused back into the plasma.[40, 41] In the sympathetic nerve endings, dopamine is either converted to norepinephrine, stored in vesicles, or degraded by monoamine oxidase. Approximately 25% of the infused dopamine is converted to norepinephrine.[42] The released norepinephrine, especially at high dopamine doses, significantly contributes to the cardiovascular actions of the drug.[8, 25, 38] Irreversible metabolism of dopamine takes place mostly in the liver, kidney, and pulmonary endothelium by catechol *O*-methyltransferase.[40, 41] Reversible sulfoconjugation in the plasma also occurs, and may contribute to norepinephrine production from dopamine-3-0-sulfate and to the prolonged half-life of the drug observed in some cases.[40] Some unmetabolized dopamine is also excreted by the kidneys.[39, 41] Not surprisingly, dopamine clearance rates are decreased in the presence of liver or kidney failure.[41]

Recent findings also indicate that sick preterm neonates have decreased plasma dopamine clearance rates during the first days of life[6, 43]; the effectiveness of lower doses of dopamine to combat hypotension and oliguria in these patients[1, 2, 4-6] may, at least in part, be a consequence of the decreased drug metabolism and elimination.[6]

Cardiovascular effects of dopamine. At low doses (0.5 to 2 μg/kg per minute), the dopamine-induced stimulation of the peripheral DA_1 and DA_2 receptors results in significant augmentation of renal,[3, 16, 17, 38, 44] mesenteric,[22, 38, 44] and coronary[38] blood flow with less pronounced cerebral[6, 17, 29, 45] and pulmonary[30] vasodilation. These effects are largely independent of changes in cardiac output.

At medium doses (2 to 6 μg/kg per minute), activation of the cardiac adrenergic receptors leads to increases in myocardial contractility through a β_1- and α-receptor–mediated direct effect,[8, 25, 38, 46] and through an indirect action via a mostly β_2-receptor–induced release of stored norepinephrine from cardiac adrenergic nerve endings.[8, 25, 38] Approximately 50% of dopamine's effect on myocardial contractility is due to its indirect, norepinephrine-releasing action.[47] Depletion of intracardiac norepinephrine stores is influenced by the underlying myocardial abnormality, age, and maturation[25, 38, 39]; differences in the dopamine-induced increases in myocardial contractility may occur accordingly. At medium and high doses, the drug also induces dose-dependent increases in heart rate through the activation of β_1 and β_2 receptors, which influence sinus node activity, and through a β_1-receptor–mediated enhancement of conduction velocity.[8, 39]

At doses beyond 6 to 10 μg/kg per minute,[8, 38, 39] activation of vascular α_1 and α_2 receptors results in vasoconstriction and thus in dose-dependent increases in total peripheral vascular resistance and afterload. However, stimulation of serotonin and α-adrenoreceptors also causes venoconstriction and thus a decrease in venous capacitance, so high doses of dopamine also enhance venous return to the heart.[8, 38, 39] The decrease in venous capacitance may be beneficial in infants and children with hypovolemic or septic shock. However, attention should be paid to this effect of high-dose dopamine treatment in cardiogenic shock, because the resultant increases in ventricular filling pressure may adversely affect the impaired myocardial function of these patients. Table I summarizes the cardiovascular effects of dopamine therapy.

In contrast to dopamine, dobutamine's effect on myocardial contractility does not depend on the release of stored norepinephrine.[48] Dobutamine also exerts a less limiting effect on the enhancement of coronary blood flow associated with increased myocardial oxygen demand. Therefore dobutamine is the drug of choice in patients with primary myocardial dysfunction, especially when myocardial norepinephrine stores are likely to be depleted.[39] However, when an increase in renal and mesenteric blood flow or total peripheral vascular resistance, or both, is also necessary to achieve hemodynamic stability, the addition of dopamine to dobutamine is recommended.

Epinephrine and norepinephrine, like dobutamine, exert a mostly direct inotropic effect by the stimulation of cardiac β and α receptors linked to increases in intracellular generation of cyclic adenosine monophosphate and calcium availability, respectively.[31] However, the overwhelming stimulatory effect of epinephrine and norepinephrine on the vascular α receptors limits their clinical use to conditions not responding to therapy with dopamine or dobutamine or both, and to those in which peripheral vasodilation is a major component of the pathophysiologic mechanism of the circulatory collapse, as in septic shock.[39, 49]

Table I. Cardiovascular effects of dopamine*

Dose (μg/kg/min)	Receptors	Vascular effects	Cardiac effects
Low dose (0.5-2)	Dopamine	↑↑↑ Coronary blood flow ↑↑↑ Renal cortical/medullary blood flow ↑↑↑ Mesenteric blood flow ↑ Cerebral and pulmonary blood flow	↑ Myocardial workload capacity
		↓ Or no change in TPVR →	↑ Or no change in cardiac output no change in blood pressure
Medium dose (2-6)	Dopamine	↑↑↑ Coronary, renal, mesenteric blood flow	
	β	↑ Or no peripheral vasodilation	↑↑ Myocardial contractility ↑ HR, ↑ conduction velocity ↑ Venous return, ↑ myocardial contractility
	α (serotonin)	↑ Peripheral vasoconstriction and venoconstriction	
		↑ Or no change in TPVR →	↑↑/↑↑↑ Cardiac output ↑/↑↑ Blood pressure
High dose (>6-10)	Dopamine	↑↑/↑↑↑ Coronary, renal, mesenteric blood flow	
	β	↑ Or no peripheral vasodilation	↑↑ Myocardial contractility ↑ HR, ↑ conduction velocity ↑ Venous return, ↑ myocardial contractility
	α (serotonin)	↑↑ / ↑↑↑ Peripheral vasoconstriction and venoconstriction	
		↑↑ / ↑↑↑ TPVR →	↑ / ↑↑ / ↑↑↑ Cardiac output* ↑↑ / ↑↑↑ Blood pressure

See text for details.
TPVR, Total peripheral vascular resistance; *HR*, heart rate; ↑, increase; ↓, decrease.
*The magnitude of ↑ in cardiac output may be influenced by the significant rise in afterload (TPVR).

Animal studies on the cardiovascular effects of dopamine during development have shown that its positive inotropic effect and selective vasodilatory actions in the different regional circulations are maturation dependent.[25-27, 30] However, in the human preterm neonate, clinical studies have demonstrated greater increases in stroke volume[2] and glomerular filtration rate[6, 50] in response to dopamine administration than expected from the findings of the developmental animal studies. Thus functional cardiovascular β-adrenergic and dopaminergic receptors exist, at least beyond 24 weeks of gestation, in the heart and the renal circulation of the human neonate.[2, 5, 6, 50] Moreover, in hypotensive preterm infants during the first few days of life, medium-dose dopamine therapy may be more effective in combating hypotension than volume expansion[51] or dobutamine treatment.[52, 53] These findings indicate that in this patient population, in contrast to older age groups, hypotension is more frequently due to poor peripheral vasoregulation than to primary volume depletion or myocardial dysfunction.[1, 51, 54]

Preterm neonates are also prone to the development of intraventricular hemorrhage or periventricular leukomalacia or both in association with sustained systemic hypotension and with sudden changes in blood pressure.[55] Even small changes in systemic blood pressure may temporarily and adversely influence cerebral perfusion in preterm infants during the first few days of life.[6] Thus, to avoid the persistence of hypotension and to minimize sudden changes in systemic hemodynamics, one should give dopamine early and at low doses to the immature, hypotensive preterm neonate, and the dose should be very carefully tailored to the cardiovascular and renal response of the patient.[6] Older patients with structural maturity and presumably intact autoregulation of cerebral blood flow are unlikely to have such complications, even with very high doses of the drug.[8, 39]

The most frequent adverse effect of dopamine treatment is localized severe vasoconstriction after extravasation of the infusion.[8, 39] If noted early in its course, this side effect is usually successfully treated with infiltration of the affected area with an α receptor antagonist, phentolamine. Cardiac arrhythmia[8, 39] and gangrene[39] are uncommon complications of dopamine therapy and generally occur in patients with diseased myocardium and sepsis, respectively.

The effect of dopamine on pulmonary vascular resistance depends on the balance between the vasodilatory actions of the pulmonary DA_1 receptors and the vasoconstrictive effects of the pulmonary α-adrenergic receptors, and on the presence or absence of preexisting pulmonary hypertension. Studies in infants and adults with preexisting pulmonary hypertension[8, 56] have demonstrated that higher doses of dopamine may increase pulmonary artery pressure; in adults with respiratory distress syndrome, dopamine decreases rather than increases pulmonary vascular resistance.[57] The pulmonary vascular response to dopamine is of particular interest to neonatologists, who almost uniformly use the drug in the treatment of neonates with persistent pulmonary hypertension. Although it is assumed that, especially with higher dopamine doses, pulmonary vasoconstriction could occur in this patient population, no such adverse effect has been documented.[58]

In term neonates and in infants and children, but not in preterm neonates,[1, 51, 54] cardiovascular shock is most frequently due to decreased preload caused by intravascular volume depletion. Therefore, for restoration of ventricular filling pressure and for optimal catecholamine action on myocardial contractility, appropriate volume support should in most instances precede pressor therapy.[39, 59] However, fluid loss is frequently accompanied by vasoregulatory distrubance[1, 51, 54] or myocardial dysfunction or both[39]; the addition of dopamine in these cases will further improve myocardial performance, systemic blood pressure, and tissue perfusion. Dopamine therapy should be started soon after volume loading and, in pediatric patients with renal and hepatic dysfunction and in preterm neonates during the first days of life, at lower starting doses. The dose of the drug should then be titrated to the desired hemodynamic and renal response rather than attempting to predict an effect based on textbook dosage recommendations. If necessary, pressor support and fluid replacement should be increased in series and in a stepwise manner until hemodynamic stability is achieved. At this point, improved coronary blood flow and tissue perfusion may result in spontaneous improvement in myocardial contractility, and the dose of the drug may be carefully decreased. However, especially after long-term dopamine administration, down-regulation and desensitization of cardiac adrenergic receptors may slow the pace of weaning.[60] In summary, thorough monitoring of the patient's renal and cardiovascular status, including right and, in some cases, left atrial pressure measurements, together with appropriate frequent adjustments in volume administration and dopamine dosage, is the cornerstone of optimal support with the drug.

Renal actions of dopamine. As long as renal perfusion pressure is within the autoregulatory range, the direct tubular rather than the renal hemodynamic actions of dopamine are mostly responsible for the diuretic and saluretic effects of the drug[3, 6, 16] (Fig. 1). These effects are brought about by activation of the renal tubular dopamine receptors along the nephron.[16, 21] Available data indicate the presence and functional integrity of these receptors and postreceptor mechanisms in the human kidney from as early as week 24 of gestation.[4-6, 50, 61] Stimulation of the tubular α receptors by norepinephrine or by very high doses of dopamine may exert an opposing effect on sodium and water handling, resulting in increases in sodium and water reabsorption, mostly in the proximal tubule.[62, 63]

Through selective activation of the renal vascular DA_1 and DA_2 receptors, low doses of dopamine induce an approximately 20% to 40% increase in renal blood flow[16, 17, 26, 38, 64] without significantly influencing systemic blood pressure.[16, 17, 38] Whole-kidney GFR shows a variable, approximately 5% to 20% rise.[16, 50, 64] Findings of micropuncture studies indicate that the mechanism of the drug-induced increase in the GFR is the enhancement of glomerular ultrafiltration pressure caused by a more pronounced vasodilation of the afferent than the efferent arteriole.[32] However, in isolated glomeruli, dopamine induces an afferent and efferent vasodilation of similar magnitude.[65] The most likely explanation for this apparent contradiction is found in the renal hemodynamic effects of the dopamine-stimulated[13, 14] renin-angiotensin system in the intact animal.[66] The dopamine-induced increase in local angiotensin production results in preferential efferent vasoconstriction,[66] which in turn attenuates the efferent but not the afferent dopaminergic vasodilation and leads to increases in glomerular ultrafiltration pressure. Enhancement of medullary blood flow by dopamine results in the "urea washout" phenomenon,[50] a vascular effect that decreases urea recycling and hyperosmolality of the renal medulla. This vascular effect contributes to the diminished urine-concentrating capacity of the dopamine-treated patient.[6, 16, 50]

At the brush-border membrane of the proximal tubule, stimulation of tubular DA_1 receptors inhibits the activity of the Na^+/H^+ antiporter,[67] resulting in decreased sodium entry from the lumen into the proximal tubule cell. The extrusion of H^+ by this transporter is one of the key steps in the process of proximal tubular HCO_3^- reabsorption, and patients treated with dopamine may show signs of proximal tubular acidosis. This dopaminergic effect may be more pronounced in extremely low birth weight preterm neonates, who are born with an underlying but transient proximal tubular acidosis.[68] Furthermore, dopamine, like parathyroid hormone, inhibits the P_i/Na^+ cotransporter at the brush-border membrane of the proximal tubule,[69] which results in significant increases in urinary excretion of phosphorus.[3, 6, 16, 19, 69]

At the basolateral membrane of the proximal tubule,[70-73]

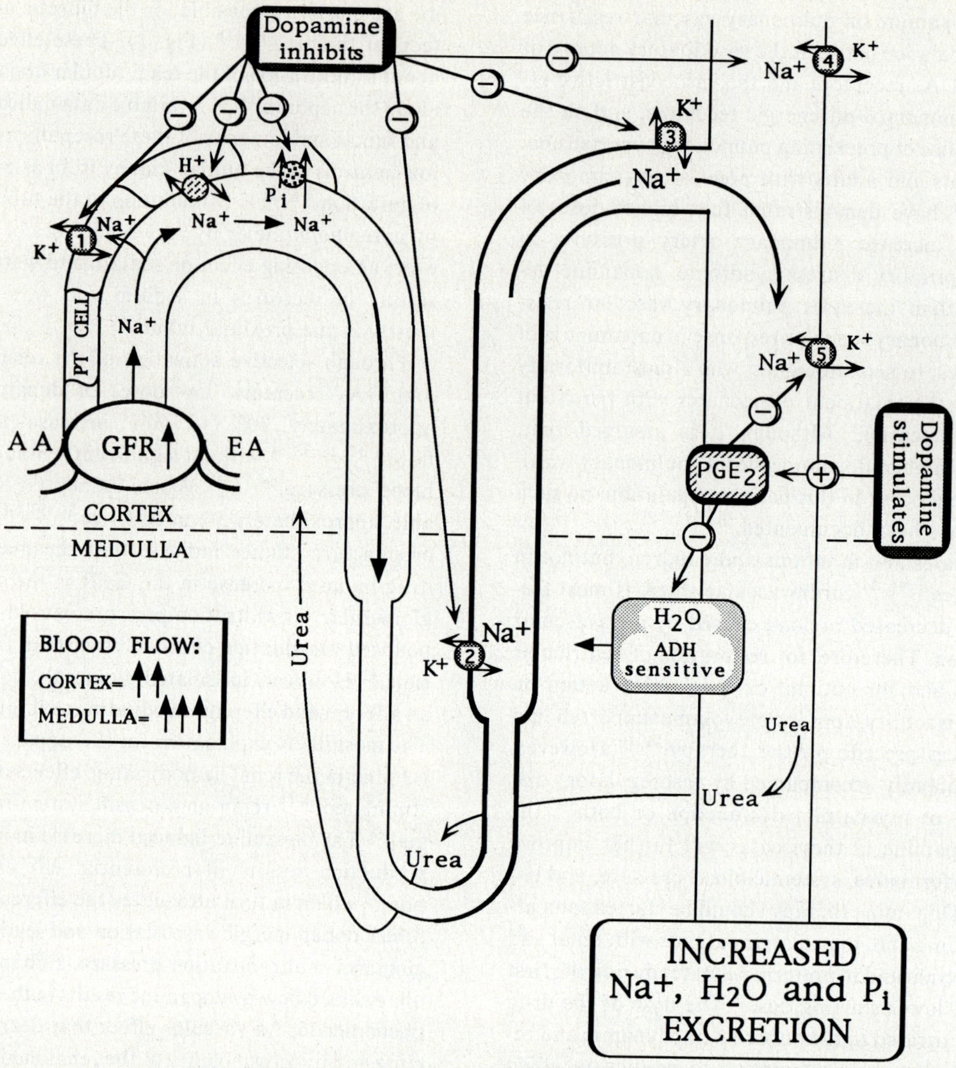

Fig. 1. Hemodynamic and direct tubular effects of dopamine in the kidney. Dopamine increases renal cortical and medullary blood flow as well as GFR. An important consequence of the increased medullary blood flow is the resulting enhanced transport of urea out of the inner medulla, which results in decreases in medullary hyperosmolality and thus in concentrating capacity ("urea washout"). Dopamine directly inhibits Na^+,K^+-ATPase activity at the basolateral membrane in the proximal tubule *(PT) (1)*, the ascending loop of Henle *(2)*, the distal tubule *(3)*, and the cortical collecting duct *(4)*. At the brush-border membrane in the proximal tubule, the Na^+/H^+ exchanger and Na^+/P_i cotransporter are also directly inhibited by dopamine. Through increases in local prostaglandin E_2 *(PGE_2)* generation, dopamine attenuates the effect of ADH and inhibits Na^+,K^+-ATPase activity in the inner medullary collecting duct *(5)*. These actions of dopamine result in enhanced excretion of Na^+, water, and P_i and decreased concentrating capacity. (See text for details.) *AA*, Afferent arteriole; *EA*, efferent arteriole.

thick ascending limb,[74] distal tubule, and cortical collecting duct,[75] dopamine also inhibits Na^+,K^+-ATPase activity. Figure 2 summarizes the proposed intracellular mechanisms of the inhibitory effect of dopamine on the enzyme along the nephron. In the proximal tubule, the majority of sodium absorption is driven by the activity of Na^+,K^+-ATPase[76]; thus a 10% to 30% inhibition of enzyme activity[71, 72] results in a significant enhancement of sodium delivery to the distal parts of the nephron. Moreover, the activity of the facilitated transporters is also governed by the tubular Na^+,K^+-ATPase,[76] so the magnitude of the direct dopaminergic inhibition of the Na^+/H^+ antiporter and the P_i/Na^+ cotransporter at the brush-border membrane is indirectly enhanced by the simultaneous inhibition of Na^+,K^+-ATPase activity at the basolateral membrane. The major result of these effects of dopamine is a significant increase in re-

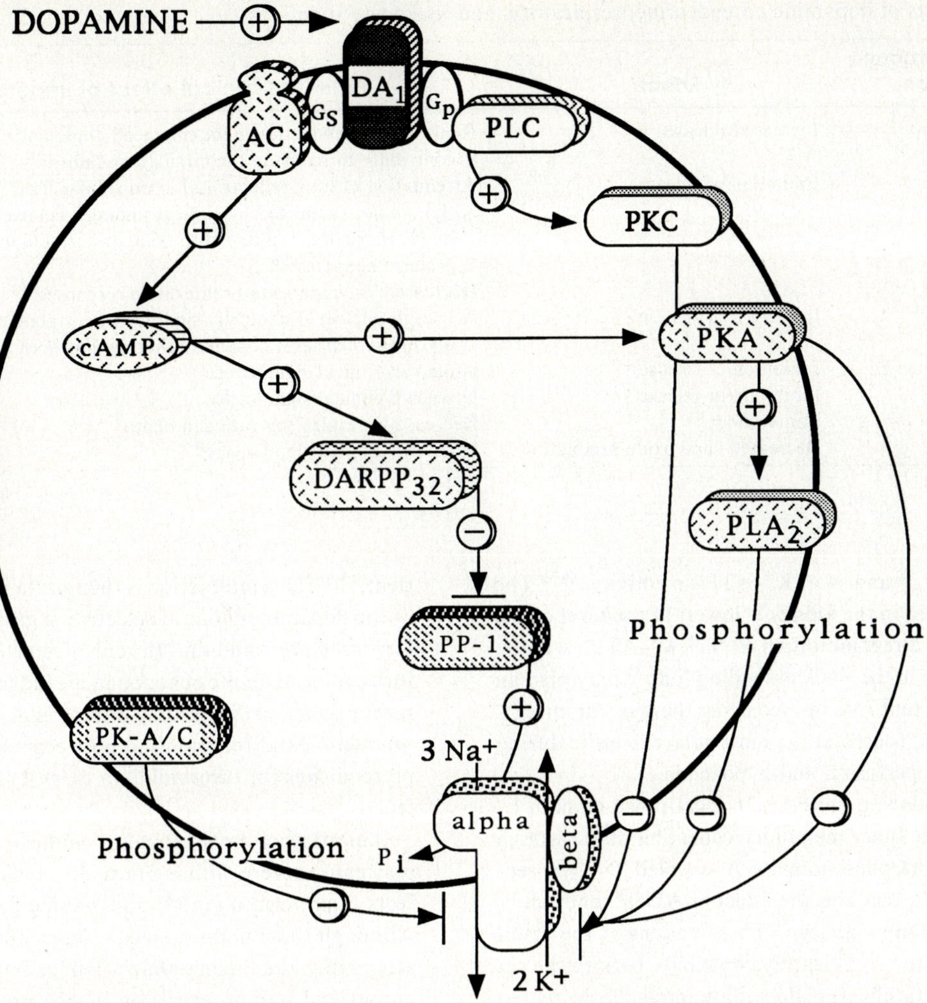

Fig. 2. Suggested intracellular mechanisms of short-term regulation of Na^+,K^+-ATPase activity by dopamine in the kidney. Phosphorylation of the alpha subunit of Na^+,K^+-ATPase by protein kinase A or C or both decreases enzyme activity,[21, 63] whereas dephosphorylation by protein phosphatase-1 activates the enzyme.[63] In a given cell, a balance exists between the two processes and baseline Na^+,K^+-ATPase activity is maintained accordingly. In the thick ascending limb, stimulation of adenylate cyclase–coupled DA_1 receptors increases intracellular cyclic adenosine monophosphate *(cAMP)* concentration.[74] This in turn activates $DARPP_{32}$', a protein phosphatase-1 inhibitor,[63] resulting in a decrease in the rate of dephosphorylation and thus in Na^+,K^+-ATPase activity.[63, 74] Proximal tubule, distal tubule, and cortical collecting duct cells do not express $DARPP_{32}$.[74] At these sites, stimulation of phospholipase C– and adenylate cyclase–coupled DA_1 receptors activates protein kinase C and protein kinase A enzymes (with or without subsequent phospholipase A_2 stimulation). Activation of these protein kinases then increases the rate of alpha subunit phosphorylation and thus inhibits Na^+,K^+-ATPase activity.[21, 63] Findings of developmental studies suggest that the inhibitory effect of dopamine on renal Na^+,K^+-ATPase is fully developed even in the immature animal.[28] Similar intracellular mechanisms have been proposed for the inhibition of Na^+,K^+-ATPase activity by dopamine in the central nervous system.[63] (See text for details.) *AC*, Adenylate cyclase; G_p, PLC stimulatory G protein; G_s, AC stimulatory G protein; *PKA*, protein kinase A; *PKC*, protein kinase C; *PLA_2*, phospholipase A_2; *PLC*, phospholipase C; *PP-1*, protein phosphatase-1.

nal sodium and phosphorus excretion. Another very important clinical consequence of the dopamine-induced renal tubular Na^+,K^+-ATPase inhibition is the resulting significant decrease in cellular oxygen consumption.[71, 72] A decrease in cellular energy demand increases the resistance of the cells to hypoxemia.[77] Therefore the benefit of early treatment of impending shock by dopamine may lie not only in the stabilization of blood pressure and enhancement of renal blood flow and thus oxygen supply[16, 17, 38, 64] but also in the reduction of oxygen demand by the inhibition of Na^+

Table II. Effects of dopamine on endocrine, respiratory, and leukocyte functions

Affected hormone or function	Effect	Potential clinical effect or importance
Renin[13, 14]	Increased release	Renin release and subsequent enhanced angiotensin production may contribute to relieving the circulatory failure[13]
Prolactin[9, 10]	Inhibition of release	Attenuation of intracellular and extracellular fluid retention*
		Although not supported by clinical findings, decreased prolactin levels, in theory, could lead to delayed surfactant maturation in preterm neonates[96]*
		Decreased T-lymphocyte proliferative responses[98]
Thyrotropin[9, 10]	Inhibition of release	Although unclear if clinically significant, postpone neonatal thyroid-screen until dopamine therapy has been discontinued*
Growth hormone[11]	Inhibition of release	Unknown clinical significance
Gonadotropins[9]	Inhibition of release	Unknown clinical significance
Carotid bodies	Stimulation	Decrease in respiratory rate and depth[37]*
Leukocyte[91]	Decreased superoxide production	Unknown clinical significance*

*See text for details.

absorption[3, 6, 16, 38] and Na^+,K^+-ATPase activity.[70-75] The hypoxic threshold in the kidney is lowest at the level of the loop of Henle[78]; direct inhibition of Na^+,K^+-ATPase activity by dopamine in the thick ascending limb[74] may play an especially important role in increasing the hypoxic threshold of renal tubular cells at the most vulnerable site during episodes of hypoperfusion and hypoxemia.

Finally, by inducing increases in local prostaglandin E_2 production in the inner medullary collecting duct through stimulation of the phospholipase-A–coupled DA_{2k} receptor,[35] dopamine attenuates the effect of ADH[36] and inhibits Na^+,K^+-ATPase activity.[21] These actions at the distal part of the nephron significantly contribute both to the saluretic and diuretic effects of dopamine and to the decreased concentrating capacity of the kidney of the dopamine-treated patient.

Hyponatremia is the most frequent renal adverse effect of dopamine administration.[1] Although hypophosphatemia and proximal tubular acidosis have not been reported in the pediatric population, theoretically they may also occur, especially after long-term dopamine treatment. Although these side effects are transient, they are clinically important and should be prevented with appropriate supplementation therapy.

In cases of aminoglycoside toxicity, dopamine, by increasing renal blood flow and GFR, may be useful in facilitating renal excretion of these antibiotics. Dopamine also modifies the renal effects of furosemide[79, 80] and indomethacin.[81, 82] The recently discovered mechanisms of the renal actions of dopamine[3, 6, 16, 21] enable us to better understand the cellular basis and nature of these interactions.

Independent of age and maturation, dopamine enhances the diuretic effect of furosemide in the anuric-oliguric patient.[79, 80] This interaction is thought to be the consequence of the dopamine-induced selective augmentation of medullary circulation and thus the enhancement of the delivery of furosemide to its site of action in the kidney.[80] Furthermore, recent data[83] indicate that intact renal tubular dopamine production and receptor and postreceptor function may be prerequisites for furosemide to exert its full natriuretic effect.

Inhibition of prostaglandin synthesis by indomethacin may cause severe, although usually transient, renal side effects in preterm infants[84] and volume-depleted children.[85] Although these findings need to be confirmed,[86] dopamine attenuates the indomethacin-induced decrease in urine output and sodium excretion in sick preterm infants with patent ductus arteriosus.[81, 82] However, the renal vasoconstrictive actions of indomethacin have not been reported to be influenced by dopamine.[81, 82] Dopamine interacts with the renal prostaglandin system mainly at the tubular level,[36, 87] and it is not surprising that the renal tubular but not the vascular actions of indomethacin are attenuated by the drug. In contrast, furosemide, by stimulating prostaglandin synthesis at both vascular and tubular sites in the kidney,[88] prevents the occurrence of both the renal hemodynamic and the tubular side effects of indomethacin.[89] However, long-term furosemide administration also increases the occurrence of patent ductus arteriosus in preterm infants,[90] so extensive use of this drug may not be prudent in preterm neonates treated with indomethacin to close their duct.[81, 90]

Effects of dopamine on endocrine, respiratory, and leukocyte functions. As discussed earlier, dopamine regulates the release of certain hormones in the pituitary[9-12] and adrenal[15] glands and in the kidney.[13, 14] Furthermore, dopamine plays a role in the peripheral regulation of breathing[37] and also influences some aspects of leukocyte function.[91] The nature and clinical importance of these effects are summarized in Table II.

Renin-angiotensin-aldosterone system. The enhancement of renin release by dopamine[13, 14] may play an important role in the mechanism of the drug-induced increase in GFR.[32] However, despite activation of the renin-angiotensin system, aldosterone secretion does not significantly change during dopamine administration[13, 15] because aldosterone release is under the tonic inhibitory control of locally generated dopamine in the zona glomerulosa of the adrenal gland.[15, 92] Even with low-dose dopamine infusion, plasma dopamine concentrations are at least 500-fold higher than the pretreatment values[6, 41, 43]; thus the tonic inhibitory effect of dopamine on aldosterone secretion is maintained during drug administration despite the simultaneous dopamine-induced activation of the renin-angiotensin system.

Prolactin. Another clinically important endocrine effect of dopamine administration is the drug-induced inhibition of prolactin release.[9-11] Prolactin is a modulator of the actions of aldosterone and ADH, hormones involved in the physiologic regulation of sodium and water homeostasis, respectively.[93] It has also been suggested that prolactin directly regulates tissue water homeostasis during intrauterine and early extrauterine development.[94] All these actions of prolactin result in increased intracellular and extracellular water and sodium stores.[93, 94] Thus, by decreasing prolactin release, dopamine attenuates intracellular and extracellular fluid retention in patients with hyperprolactinemia. Although hyperprolactinemia rarely occurs in children, preterm infants uniformly have developmentally regulated increases in prolactin production during the first weeks of life.[95] Therefore, in the preterm neonate, the dopamine-induced inhibition of prolactin release indirectly contributes to the diuretic effect of the drug.[10] Furthermore, although the point is debated, fetal prolactin may play a permissive role in the maturation of surfactant synthesis.[96] Thus, by inhibiting prolactin secretion in the sick preterm infant with hyaline membrane disease, dopamine treatment may further delay maturation of surfactant production. However, no data are available to suggest any effect of dopamine administration on the rate of recovery of preterm infants with hyaline membrane disease. Moreover, medium to high doses of dopamine also activate the β-adrenergic receptors, so dopamine is likely to directly stimulate pulmonary surfactant production and release.[97] Finally, dopamine or the drug-induced inhibition of prolactin release[98] may lead to decreased T-lymphocyte proliferative responses. The cellular mechanisms and the clinical importance of this observation need to be clarified.

Thyrotropin, growth hormone, and gonadotropins. Dopamine also inhibits the secretion of other pituitary hormones, including thyrotropin,[10] growth hormone,[11] and the gonadotropins.[9] Critically ill patients usually have depressed thyroid hormone levels, and inhibition of thyrotropin release by dopamine further interferes with the physiologic regulation of thyroid function in these patients. Although it is unclear whether long-term dopamine therapy results in a hypothyroid state in neonates and children, postponing the neonatal thyroid screening test until dopamine therapy has been discontinued is strongly recommended. It is also not known whether the dopamine-induced inhibition of the other pituitary hormones bears any clinical significance.

Carotid bodies. Stimulation of the DA_2 receptors in the carotid bodies decreases respiratory rate and depth.[37] This effect of dopamine is clinically most important for the neonatologist who treats spontaneously breathing preterm babies who are prone to the development of apnea and bradycardia. Theoretically, in these patients, administration of dopamine could increase the number and severity of spells. However, dopamine-treated premature babies not given ventilatory support have not been reported to have worsening of apnea and bradycardia. The most likely explanations for this observation are that in preterm infants, unlike in older age groups, dopamine crosses the blood-brain barrier and alters the monoamine metabolism of the brain,[99] and that the carotid bodies of preterm neonates play a less important role in the physiologic regulation of breathing during the first few weeks of life.[100]

Leukocytes. Finally, dopamine, without altering leukocyte mobility or bactericidal ability, also decreases superoxide anion production in these cells.[91] Whether this action of dopamine might have a clinical impact by reducing oxygen-induced tissue damage in critically ill patients, especially in preterm neonates, remains an intriguing question.

CONCLUSIONS

This review has summarized the recent discoveries of the cellular and molecular mechanisms of the dopaminergic effects in the developing and mature cardiovascular system, kidney, and certain endocrine organs. These insights have direct clinical applications; the thoughtful clinician will apply this knowledge accordingly and consider the many potential effects of dopamine when using the drug and evaluating the efficacy of therapy.

I thank Drs. Roberta R. Ballard and Judy C. Bernbaum for their critical review of the manuscript.

REFERENCES

1. Seri I, Tulassay T, Kiszel J, Machay T, Csömör S. Cardiovascular response to dopamine in hypotensive preterm infants

with severe hyaline membrane disease. Eur J Pediatr 1984; 142:3-9.

2. Padbury JF, Agata Y, Baylen BG, et al. Dopamine pharmacokinetics in critically ill newborn infants. J Pediatr 1986; 110:293-8.
3. Seri I. Dopamine and natriuresis: mechanism of action and developmental aspects. Am J Hypertens 1990;3:82S-6S.
4. Cuevas L, Yeh TF, John EG, Cuevas D, Plides RS. The effect of low-dose dopamine infusion on cardiopulmonary and renal status in premature newborns with respiratory distress syndrome. Am J Dis Child 1991;145:799-803.
5. Emery EF, Greenough A. Efficacy of low-dose dopamine infusion. Acta Paediatr 1993;82:430-2.
6. Seri I, Rudas G, Bors ZS, Kanyicska B, Tulassay T. Effects of low-dose dopamine on cardiovascular and renal functions, cerebral blood flow, and plasma catecholamine levels in sick preterm neonates. Pediatr Res 1993;34:742-9.
7. DiSessa TG, Leitner M, Ti CC, Gluck L, Coen R, Friedman WF. The cardiovascular effects of dopamine in the severely asphyxiated neonate. J Pediatr 1981;99:772-6.
8. Zaritsky A, Chernow B. The use of catecholamines in pediatrics. J Pediatr 1984;105:341-50.
9. Leblanc H, Lachelin GCL, Abu-Fadil S, Yen SSC. Effects of dopamine infusion on pituitary hormone secretion in humans. J Clin Endocrinol Metab 1976;43:668-74.
10. Seri I, Tulassay T, Kiszel J, et al. Effect of low-dose dopamine infusion on prolactin and thyrotropin secretion in preterm infants with hyaline membrane disease. Biol Neonate 1985; 47:317-22.
11. de Zegher F, Van den Berghe G, Devlieger H, Eggermont E, Veldhuis JD. Dopamine inhibits growth hormone and prolactin secretion in the human newborn. Pediatr Res 1993; 34:642-5.
12. Pittman QJ, Lawrence D, Lederis K. Presynaptic interactions in the neurohypophysis: endogenous modulators of release. In: Cross BA, Leng G, eds. The neurohypophysis: structure, function and control. Amsterdam: Elsevier, 1983:319-32.
13. Sulyok E, Seri I, Tulassay T, Kiszel J, Ertl T. The effect of dopamine administration on the activity of the renin-angiotensin-aldosterone system in sick preterm infants. Eur J Pediatr 1985;43:191-3.
14. Kurtz AR, Bruna D, Pratz J, Cavero I. Rat juxtaglomerular cells are endowed with DA-1 dopamine receptors mediating renin release. J Cardiovasc Pharmacol 1988;12:658-63.
15. Carey RM, Thorner MD, Ortt BM. Effects of metoclopramide and bromocriptine on the renin-angiotensin-aldosterone system in man: dopaminergic control of aldosterone. J Clin Invest 1979;63:727-35.
16. Felder RA, Felder CC, Eisner GM, Jose PA. The dopamine receptor in adult and maturing kidney. Am J Physiol 1989; 257:F315-27.
17. Lokhandwala MF, Hedge SS. Cardiovascular dopamine receptors: role of renal dopamine and dopamine receptors in sodium excretion. Pharmacol Toxicol 1990;66:237-43.
18. Chan YL. Cellular mechanisms of the renal tubular transport of L-dopa and its derivatives in the rat: microperfusion studies. J Pharmacol Exp Ther 1976;199:17-24.
19. Cuche JL, Marchand DR, Greger RF, Lang FC, Knox FG. Phosphaturic effect of dopamine in dogs: possible role of intrarenally produced dopamine on phosphate regulation. J Clin Invest 1976;58:71-6.
20. Kebabian JW, Calne DB. Multiple receptors for dopamine. Nature 1979;277:93-6.
21. Jose PA, Raymond JR, Bates MD, Aperia A, Felder RA, Carey, RM. The renal dopamine receptors. J Am Soc Nephrol 1992;2:1265-78.
22. Willems JL, Buylaert WA, Lefebvre RA, Bogaert MG. Neuronal dopamine receptors on autonomic ganglia and sympathetic nerves and dopamine receptors in the gastrointestinal system. Pharmacol Rev 1985;37:165-216.
23. Sidhu A, Felder RA, Jose PA, Fishman PH. Comparison of the central and renal $dopamine_1$ receptor. Am J Hypertens 1990;3:37S-9S.
24. Seri I, Simmons CF, Gullans SR. Partial molecular characterization of a peripheral D_1-type dopamine receptor in the rat kidney [Abstract]. J Am Soc Nephrol 1993;4:500.
25. Driscoll DJ, Gillette PC, Ezrailson EG, Schwartz A. Inotropic response of the neonatal canine myocardium to dopamine. Pediatr Res 1978;12:42-5.
26. Pelayo JC, Fildes RD, Jose PA. Age-dependent renal effects of intrarenal dopamine infusion. Am J Physiol 1984; 247:R212-6.
27. O'Laughlin MP, Fisher DJ, Dreyer WJ, Smith EO. Augmentation of cardiac output with intravenous catecholamines in unanesthetized hypoxemic newborn lambs. Pediatr Res 1987;22:667-74.
28. Fryckstedt J, Svensson LB, Linden M, Aperia A. The effect of dopamine on adenylate cyclase and Na^+,K^+-ATPase activity in the developing rat renal cortical and medullary tubule. Pediatr Res 1993;34:308-11.
29. Amenta F, Cavalloti C, DeRossi M, Mione MF. Dopamine-sensitive cAMP generating system in rat extracerebral arteries. Eur J Pharmacol 1984;97:105-9.
30. Polak MJ, Drummond WH. Systemic and pulmonary vascular effects of selective dopamine (DA_1) receptor blockade in lambs. Pediatr Res 1993;33:181-4.
31. Morgan JP, Perreault CL, Morgan KG. The cellular basis of contraction and relaxation in cardiac and vascular smooth muscle. Am Heart J 1991;121:961-8.
32. Seri I, Aperia A. Contribution of $dopamine_2$ receptors to the dopamine-induced increase in glomerular filtration rate. Am J Physiol 1988;254:F196-201.
33. Vallar L, Muca C, Magni M, Albert P, Bunzow J, Meldolesi J, Civelli O. Differential coupling of dopaminergic D_2 receptors expressed in different cell types. J Biol Chem 1990; 265:10320-6.
34. Amenta F, Collier WL, Ricci A. Autoradiographic localization of vascular dopamine receptors. Am J Hypertens 1990;3:34S-6S.
35. Huo T, Ye MQ, Healy DP. Characterization of a dopamine receptor (DA_{2K}) in the kidney inner medulla. Proc Natl Acad Sci USA 1991;88:3170-4.
36. Huo TL, Grenader A, Blandina P, Healy DP. Prostaglandin E_2 production in rat IMCD cells. II. Possible role for locally formed dopamine. Am J Physiol 1991;261:F655-62.
37. Welsh MJ, Heistad DD, Abboud FM. Depression of ventilation by dopamine in man: evidence for an effect on the chemoreceptor reflex. J Clin Invest 1978;61:708-13.
38. Goldberg LI. Cardiovascular and renal actions of dopamine: potential clinical applications. Pharmacol Rev 1972;24:1-29.
39. Bhatt-Mehta V, Nahat MC. Dopamine and dobutamine in pediatric therapy. Pharmacotherapy 1989;9:303-14.

40. Zaritsky A, Miles M. Too much pharmacokinetics? Crit Care Med 1993;21:1620-2.
41. Zaritsky A, Lotze A, Stull R, Goldstein DS. Steady-state dopamine clearance in critically ill infants and children. Crit Care Med 1988;16:217-20.
42. Goodall MC, Alton H. Metabolism of 3-hydroxy-tyramine (dopamine) in human subjects. Biochem Pharmacol 1968; 17:905-10.
43. Bhatt-Mehta V, Nahata MC, McClead RE, Menke JA. Dopamine pharmacokinetics in critically ill newborn infants. Eur J Clin Pharmacol 1991;40:593-7.
44. Seri I, Eklöf AC, Aperia A. Role of dopamine$_2$-receptors in mediating renal vascular response to low dose dopamine infusion in the rat. Acta Physiol Scand 1987;130:563-9.
45. Rennie JM. Cerebral blood flow velocity variability after cardiovascular support in premature babies. Arch Dis Child 1989;64:897-901.
46. Schümann HJ, Wagner J, Knorr A, Reidemeister C, Sadony V, Schramm G. Demonstration in human atrial preparations of α-adrenoreceptors mediating positive inotropic effects. Naunyn Schmiedebergs Arch Pharmacol 1978;302:333-6.
47. Lass NA, Glock D, Goldberg LI. Cardiovascular and renal hemodynamic effects of intravenous infusions of the selective DA_1 agonist, fenoldopam, used alone or in combination with dopamine and dobutamine. Circulation 1988;78:1310-5.
48. Tuttle RR, Mills J. Dobutamine: development of a new catecholamine to selectively increase cardiac contractility. Circ Res 1975;36:185-96.
49. Meadows D, Edwards JD, Wilkins RG, Nightingale P. Reversal of intractable septic shock with norepinephrine therapy. Crit Care Med 1988;16:663-6.
50. Tulassay T, Seri I, Machay T, Kiszel J, Varga J, Csömör S. Effects of dopamine on renal functions in premature infants with respiratory distress syndrome. International Journal of Pediatric Nephrology 1983;4:19-23.
51. Gill AB, Weindling AM. Randomized controlled trial of plasma protein fraction versus dopamine in hypotensive very low birthweight infants. Arch Dis Child 1993;69:284-7.
52. Greenough A, Emery AF. Randomized trial comparing dopamine and dobutamine in preterm infants. Eur J Pediatr 1993;152:925-7.
53. Klarr JM, Faix RG, Pryce CJE, Bhatt-Mehta V. Randomized, blind trial of dopamine versus dobutamine for treatment of hypotension in preterm infants with respiratory distress syndrome. J PEDIATR 1994;125:117-22.
54. Barr PA, Bailey PE, Sumners J, Cassady G. Relation between arterial blood pressure and blood volume and effect of infused albumin in sick preterm infants. Pediatrics 1977;60:282-9.
55. Van Bel F, Van de Bor M, Stijnen T. Aetiological role of cerebral blood flow alterations in development and extension of peri-intraventricular haemorrhage. Dev Med Child Neurol 1987;29:601-14.
56. Lang P, Williams RG, Norwood WI, Castaneda AR. The hemodynamic effects of dopamine in infants after corrective cardiac surgery. J PEDIATR 1980;96:630-4.
57. Malloy WD, Dobson K, Girling L, Greenberg ID, Prewitt RM. Effects of dopamine on cardiopulmonary function and left ventricular volume in patients with acute respiratory failure. Ann Rev Respir Dis 1984;130:396-9.
58. Keeley SR, Bohn DJ. The use of inotropic and afterload-reducing agents in neonates. Clin Perinatol 1988;15:467-89.
59. Driscoll DJ. Use of inotropic and chronotropic agents in neonates. Clin Perinatol 1987;14:931-49.
60. Bristow MR, Hershberger RE, Port JD, et al. Beta-adrenergic pathways in nonfailing and failing human ventricular myocardium. Circulation 1990;82:I12-25.
61. Perez CA, Reimer JM, Schreiber MD, Warburton D, Gregory GA. Effect of high-dose dopamine on urine output in newborn infants. Crit Care Med 1986;14:1045-9.
62. Beach RE, Schwab SJ, Brazy PC, Dennis VW. Norepinephrine increases Na^+,K^+-ATPase activity and solute transport in rabbit proximal tubules. Am J Physiol 1987;252:F215-20.
63. Ibarra F, Aperia A, Svensson LB, Eklöf AC, Greengard P. Bidirectional regulation of Na^+,K^+-ATPase activity by dopamine and an alpha-adrenergic agonist. Proc Natl Acad Sci USA 1993;90:21-4.
64. McDonald RH, Goldberg LI, McNay JL, Tuttle E. Effect of dopamine in man: augmentation of sodium excretion, glomerular filtration rate, and renal plasma flow. J Clin Invest 1964;43:1116-24.
65. Steinhausen M, Weis S, Fleming J, Dussel R, Parekh N. Responses of in vivo renal microvessels to dopamine. Kidney Int 1986;30:361-70.
66. Hall JE. Regulation of glomerular filtration rate and sodium excretion by angiotensin II. Fed Proc 1986;45:1431-7.
67. Felder CC, Campbell T, Albrecht F, Jose PA. Dopamine inhibits Na^+-H^+ exchanger activity in renal BBMV by stimulation of adenylate cyclase. Am J Physiol 1990;259:F297-303.
68. Jones DP, Chesney RW. Development of tubular function. In: Bailie MD, ed. Clinics in perinatology. 1992;19:33-58.
69. Perrichot R, Garcia-Ocana A, Couette S, Comoy E, Vrtovsnik F, Friedlander G. Endogenous dopamine (DA) modulates $Na-P_i$ cotransport in proximal tubule cells (PTC) [Abstract]. J Am Soc Nephrol 1993;4:713.
70. Aperia A, Bertorello A, Seri I. Dopamine causes inhibition of Na^+,K^+-ATPase activity in proximal convoluted tubule segments. Am J Physiol 1987;252:F39-45.
71. Seri I, Kone BC, Gullans SR, Aperia A, Brenner BM, Ballermann BJ. Locally formed dopamine inhibits Na^+,K^+-ATPase activity in rat renal cortical tubule cells. Am J Physiol 1988;255:F666-73.
72. Seri I, Kone BC, Gullans SR, Aperia A, Brenner BM, Ballermann BJ. Influence of Na^+ intake on the dopamine-induced inhibition of renal cortical Na^+,K^+-ATPase. Am J Physiol 1990;258:F52-60.
73. Bertorello A, Aperia A. Inhibition of proximal tubule Na^+,K^+-ATPase activity requires simultaneous activation of DA_1 and DA_2 receptors. Am J Physiol 1990;F924-8.
74. Meister B, Fryckstedt J, Schalling M, et al. Dopamine- and cAMP-regulated phosphoprotein (DARRP-32) and dopamine DA_1 agonist-sensitive Na^+,K^+-ATPase in renal tubule cells. Proc Natl Acad Sci USA 1989;86:8068-72.
75. Takemoto F, Cohen HT, Staoh T, Katz AI. Dopamine inhibits Na^+,K^+-ATPase in single tubules and cultures cells from distal nephron. Pflugers Arch 1992;421:302-6.
76. Weinstein AM. Sodium and chloride transport: proximal nephron. In: Seldin DW, Giebisch G, eds. The kidney: physiology and pathophysiology. New York: Raven Press, 1992: 1925-73.
77. Duke GJ, Bernsten AD. Dopamine and renal salvage in the critically ill patient. Anaesth Intensive Care 1992;20:277-302.

78. Epstein FH. Hypoxia of the renal medulla. Q J Med 1985; 224:807-10.
79. Lindner A. Synergism of dopamine plus furosemide in diuretic-resistant, oliguric renal failure. Nephron 1983; 33:121-6.
80. Tulassay T, Seri I. Interaction of dopamine and furosemide in acute oliguria of preterm infants with hyaline membrane disease. Acta Paediatr Scand 1986;75:420-4.
81. Seri I, Tulassay T, Kiszel J, Csömör S. The use of dopamine for the prevention of the renal side effects of indomethacin in premature infants with patent ductus arteriosus. Intern J Pediatr Nephrol 1984;5:209-14.
82. Cochran J, Reddy R, Devaskar U. Effect of indomethacin vs indomethacin + dopamine on serum BUN and creatinine, urinary output and the closure of patent ductus arteriosus in preterm neonates with hyaline membrane disease [Abstract]. Pediatr Res 1989;25:211A.
83. Nowicki S, Enero MA. Role of $dopamine_1$-receptors in mediating renal responses to furosemide in the rat. Gen Pharmacol 1991;22:459-563.
84. Cifuentes RF, Olley PM, Balfe JW, Radde IC, Soldin SJ. Indomethacin and renal function in premature infants with persistent patent ductus arteriosus. J PEDIATR 1979;95:583-7.
85. Dunn MJ, Zambraski EJ. Renal effects of drugs that inhibit prostaglandin synthesis. Kidney Int 1980;18:609-22.
86. Fajardo Ca, Whyte RK, Steele BT. Effect of dopamine on failure of indomethacin to close the patent ductus arteriosus. J PEDIATR 1992;121:771-5.
87. Seri I, Hajdu J, Tulassay T, Kiszel J, Aperia A. The effect of low-dose dopamine infusion on urinary PGE_2 excretion in sick preterm infants. Eur J Pediatr 1988;147:616-20.
88. Gerber JG. Role of prostaglandins in the hemodynamic and tubular effects of furosemide. Fed Proc 1983;42:1707-10.
89. Yeh TF, Wilks A, Singh J, Betrekur MV, Lilien L, Pildes RS. Furosemide prevents the renal side effects of indomethacin therapy in premature infants with patent ductus arteriosus. J PEDIATR 1982;101:433-7.
90. Green TP, Thompson TR, Johnson D, Lock JE. Furosemide promotes patent ductus arteriosus in premature infants with the respiratory distress syndrome. N Engl J Med 1983; 308:743-8.
91. Matsuoka T. A sedative effect of dopamine on the respiratory burst in neonatal polymorphonuclear leukocytes. Pediatr Res 1990;28:24-7.
92. Buu NT, Lussier C. Origin of dopamine in the rat adrenal cortex. Am J Physiol 1990;258:F287-91.
93. Horrobin DF. Prolactin as a regulator of fluid and electrolyte metabolism. Fed Proc 1980;39:2567-70.
94. Coulter DM. Prolactin: a hormonal regulator of the neonatal tissue water reservoir. Pediatr Res 1983;17:665-8.
95. Perlman M, Schenker J, Glassman M, Ben-David M. Prolonged hyperprolactinemia in preterm infants. J Clin Endocrinol Metab 1978;47:894-7.
96. Lucas A, Baker BA, Cole TJ. Plasma prolactin and clinical outcome in preterm infants. Arch Dis Child 1990;65:977-83.
97. McDonald JV Jr, Gonzales LW, Ballard PL, Pitha J, Roberts JM. Lung β-adrenoreceptor blockade affects perinatal surfactant release but not lung water. J Appl Physiol 1986; 60:1727-33.
98. Devins SS, Miller A, Herndon BL, O'Toole L, Reisz G. Effects of dopamine on T-lymphocyte proliferative responses and serum prolactin concentrations in critically ill patients. Crit Care Med 1992;20:1644-9.
99. Seri I, Tulassay T, Kiszel J, et al. Effect of low-dose dopamine therapy on catecholamine values in cerebrospinal fluid in preterm neonates. J PEDIATR 1984;105:489-91.
100. Spitzer AR, Shaffer TH, Fox WW. Assisted ventilation: physiologic implications and complications. In: Polin RA, Fox WW, eds. Fetal and neonatal physiology. WB Saunders, 1992:894-913.

ORIGINAL ARTICLES

Definition and application of the discretionary screening indicators according to the National Cholesterol Education Program for Children and Adolescents

Philip M. Diller, MD, PhD, Gertrude A. Huster, MHS, Alan D. Leach, MS, Peter M. Laskarzewski, PhD, and Dennis L. Sprecher, MD

From the Department of Family Medicine, the Lipid Research Program, Department of Internal Medicine, and the Department of Pediatrics, Children's Hospital Medical Center, University of Cincinnati, Cincinnati, Ohio

Objectives: **(1) To propose definitions for the discretionary screening indicators described by the National Cholesterol Education Program for Children and Adolescents (NCEP-Peds); (2) to examine the relative prevalence of major screening indicators (family history of premature heart disease and parental plasma cholesterol concentration ≥6.21 mmol/L (240 mg/dl)) and discretionary screening indicators (excessive consumption of fat or cholesterol or both, smoking, diabetes, hypertension, and steroid use) in a family population; and (3) to evaluate the relative value of the major and the discretionary indicators in detecting high serum levels of low-density lipoprotein–cholesterol (LDL-C) (≥3.36 mmol/L (≥130 mg/dl)).**

Design: **Control cohort from a case-control study.**

Setting: **Lipid research clinic.**

Participants: **White children and adolescents <20 years of age from 232 nuclear families who participated in the Cincinnati Myocardial Infarction Hormone Study.**

Main outcome measures: **(1) Number of children who have major and discretionary screening indicators; (2) sensitivity and specificity of the major and the discretionary screening indicators in identifying children with LDL-C concentrations >3.36 mmol/L (130 mg/dl) (high LDL-C).**

Results: **With cutoff points of the 90th percentile for blood pressure, the 85th percentile for obesity, and the 80th percentile for dietary fat and cholesterol, and self-report for diabetes, smoking, and corticosteroid use, 54% of the 232 children in the cohort had one or more discretionary indicators. Additionally, applying the major screening indicators raised the percentage of children identified to 74%. Twenty-eight percent had both major and discretionary indicators. Having a discretionary screening indicator did not increase the probability of having a major indicator. Applying both discretionary and major screening indicators**

Supported by the Cincinnati Lipid Clinic Research Fund, grant NIH HD-18281-08, "Genetic Epidemiology of Sex Hormones and Lipoproteins."

Submitted for publication July 7, 1994; accepted Sept. 20, 1994.

Reprint requests: Philip M. Diller, MD, PhD, Lipid Research Program, Department of Internal Medicine, University of Cincinnati, 231 Bethesda Ave., ML 540, Cincinnati, OH 45267-0540.

0022-3476/95/$3.00 + 0 **9/20/60735**

to the cohort identified 96% of the children who had a high concentration of LDL-C; 30% of the children with high LDL-C levels were discovered solely by the discretionary indicators. Similar sensitivity and specificity were noted between the major and the discretionary indicators. Children with high LDL-C concentrations were more likely to have multiple screening indicators.
***Conclusion*: Discretionary and major screening indicators suggested by the National Cholesterol Education Program for Children and Adolescents identify different subsets of children at risk of having premature cardiovascular disease. Both major and discretionary indicators contribute to the identification of children with high LDL-C concentrations. (J Pediatr 1995;126:345-52)**

Factors contributing to the development of atherosclerosis in children include elevated plasma lipid concentrations,[1, 2] smoking,[1] and hypertension.[2, 3] Children with these risk factors and/or obesity,[4, 5] diabetes,[6, 7] or a family history of heart disease[8-10] are believed to be at higher risk of having cardiovascular disease in the future. During the last decade, expert panels and committees from the American Heart Association, the National Institutes of Health, and the American Academy of Pediatrics have advocated the use of family history to identify and treat individuals at risk of having premature CVD.[11, 12] Investigators have subsequently shown that family history is not a sufficiently sensitive screening tool because it misses a large number of children with elevated serum cholesterol values.[7, 13-17]

In response to this newer information, the Expert Panel for the National Cholesterol Education Program for Children and Adolescents published revised recommendations for identifying children at high risk of having CVD.[18] According to the NCEP-Peds, children should be screened for elevated plasma cholesterol concentrations if they have a family history of premature CVD (age ≤55 years), and also if the parental serum cholesterol levels are ≥6.21 mmol/L (240 mg/dl). In addition to these major screening criteria, a child may be screened for an elevated plasma cholesterol concentration at the physician's discretion if the family history is unknown or if the child has other risk factors for CVD, including obesity; cigarette use; consumption of a high-fat, high-cholesterol diet; diabetes; hypertension; or current use of lipid-raising medication such as corticosteroids. This screening strategy is based on the theory that a child's propensity to develop clinically significant CVD as an adult is the result of genetic factors, nutritional practices, and lifestyle characteristics that are established in the context of the family and that persist into adulthood.[19] However, these discretionary indicators are not clearly defined in the guidelines, and little information is available to understand their contribution relative to the major screening indicators for identifying "at risk" subjects according to the new guidelines.

CVD	Cardiovascular disease
LDL-C	Low-density lipoprotein–cholesterol
NCEP-Peds	National Cholesterol Education Program for Children and Adolescents

The primary objective of this study was to define each discretionary screening indicator and apply these definitions to a cohort of well-characterized nuclear families to estimate the number of children who are screened by means of the NCEP-Peds major and discretionary screening indicators. A second objective was to test whether the presence of the major screening indicators are independent of the discretionary screening indicators. A final objective was to determine whether the number of major as well as the number of discretionary screening indicators increased the probability of detecting a high concentration of low-density lipoprotein–cholesterol in screened children.

METHODS

Subjects. The Cincinnati Myocardial Infarction and Hormone (CIMIH) Family Study was an epidemiologic study funded by the National Institutes of Health and done by trained staff members who were instructed in uniformity and consistency of data collection. A description of the recruitment of subjects for the CIMIH Family Study and their clinical characteristics was reported separately.[20] In brief, white male subjects (probands) selected to represent the population at large ("control cohort") were recruited from the Cincinnati metropolitan area in 1988 and 1989. Patients were recruited through media advertising, the database of a previously completed boy's maturation study, a local blood donation center, and area food stores. The availability of a proband, a spouse, and one natural child living in the household was required for inclusion in the original study. For this report, only the "control cohort" families that had children <20 years of age were analyzed. Thus we studied 241 families, and 501 children between the ages of 2 and 19 years. To eliminate the effect of familial clustering of risk factors, we randomly selected for study only one child from each family. Nine children had missing lipid values and were not included in the analysis, which yielded a final population of 232. The mean age (±SD) of the children was 13.2 (±4.0) years, and the age range was 5 to 19 years. Fifty-seven percent were male. The mean age of the fathers and mothers was 43.8 years and 41.9 years, respectively.

Lipid determination and NCEP-Peds LDL-C definitions. Total serum cholesterol and LDL-C in the children were determined in a Centers for Disease Control and Prevention–National Heart, Lung, and Blood Institute standardized laboratory.[21] A single lipid profile was obtained for each child and parent. Total cholesterol values were missing in 3.9% of the fathers and 0.9% of the mothers.

The NCEP-Peds defines an LDL-C value <2.84 mmol/L (<110 mg/dl) as *acceptable*, an LDL-C value ≥2.84 and <3.36 mmol/L (110 to 130 mg/dl) as *borderline*, and an LDL-C value ≥3.36 mmol/L (≥30 mg/dl) as *high*. Children with both borderline and high LDL-C concentrations are described herein as having an *elevated* LDL-C value.

Screening indicator and risk factor definitions

Major screening indicators. The NCEP-Peds Expert Panel defines *family history of premature heart disease* as a history in parents or grandparents of documented myocardial infarction, angina pectoris, peripheral vascular disease, sudden death, angiographically demonstrated coronary artery disease, balloon angioplasty, or coronary artery bypass grafting before the age of 56 years. This information was obtained from parents by a questionnaire administered by a staff interviewer. No attempt was made to validate this information by examining participants' medical records. A genetic basis for hyperlipidemia was considered when the parental cholesterol concentration was ≥6.21 mmol/L (240 mg/dl).

Discretionary screening indicators. The NCEP-Peds Expert Panel did not explicitly define the levels at which a screening for cholesterol would be initiated with the presence of additional risk factors. For this analysis, the discretionary screening indicators have been defined as follows:

hypertension systolic or diastolic blood pressure at ≥90th percentile for age and sex, by National Task Force on Pediatric Hypertension standards—Korotkoff sound, type 4, for children ≤12 years of age and Korotkoff sound, type 5, for children >12 years were used.[22]

obesity overweight[23] as indicated by Quetelet index (weight/height^2 × 1000) ≥85th percentile (Second National Health and Nutrition Examination Survey [NHANES II]) for age and gender, as used by Frisancho[24] and Kuczmarski.[25]

diabetes use of insulin or identified by self-report.

smoking ≥10 cigarettes per day, according to self-report.

lipid-raising medications all oral corticosteroids and isotretinoin identified through self-report from children and parents.

high-fat, high-cholesterol diet ≥400 mg cholesterol per day or ≥40% calories as fat or both. Forty percent of calories as fat or ≥400 mg cholesterol consumed per day represents the amount of fat, as calories and cholesterol, consumed by the 80th and 84th percentiles, respectively, of the CIMIH pediatric population. Estimations of dietary fat and cholesterol intake were made on the basis of information obtained through the food frequency questionnaire developed by Block et al.[26] All parents' and children's responses to the self-administered questionnaire were verified by a University of Cincinnati Lipid Research Clinic registered dietitian, who reviewed the self-recorded dietary information with the participants. Although the Block questionnaire has not been validated for use in children, the levels of 40% of calories as fat or ≥400 mg cholesterol consumed per day are in agreement with the 80th percentile for intake of total fat and cholesterol obtained in NHANES II.[27]

Statistical methods. *Sensitivity* was calculated as the percentage of children with high LDL-C values who had the screening indicator (true positive rate). *Specificity* was calculated as the percentage of children with acceptable LDL-C values who did not have a screening indicator (true negative rate). *Positive predictive value* was the probability of having a high LDL-C concentration when a child had a screening indicator; the *negative predictive value* was the probability of not having a high LDL-C concentration when a child did not have a screening indicator.

The chi-square statistic was used to test for independence of the major and discretionary screening indicators.

A logistic regression model, $E(y) = 1/[1 + e^{-(B_0+B_1x_1)}]$, was also constructed; it modeled the risk of having a high LDL-C or an elevated LDL-C concentration as a function of the number of screening indicators present (0, 1, 2, or ≥3). This analysis determined whether there was an increased risk of having a high or an elevated LDL-C concentration when the number of screening indicators increased. A quantitative estimate of the increase in the risk of having high or elevated LDL-C values per increase in the number of screening indicators was derived from the indicator estimate of the logistic regression (β). The risk of having high or elevated LDL-C values, for individuals with no screening indicators, was multiplied by a factor of e^β with each added screening indicator.[28]

RESULTS

Number of children screened by definitions of screening indicators. Based on the definitions of the major and the discretionary screening indicators provided in the guidelines and herein, the prevalence of the major NCEP-Peds screening indicators was 47.8% and of the discretionary indicators 54.7% (Table I). After sequential application of the major and the discretionary indicators to the CIMIH pediatric population, a total of 74.5% of the sample had at least one indicator, either major or discretionary; 19.8% had only major indicators, 26.7% had only discretionary indicators, and 28.0% had both. Fifty-nine children had no screening indicators; 86, 56, 27, 3, and 1 had a combination of 1, 2, 3, 4, and 5 screening indicators, respectively.

Table I. Prevalence of screening indicators in the CIMIH pediatric population and percentage of children screened

Screening indicator*	Prevalence (n = 232) No.	Prevalence (n = 232) %	% Screened sequentially (%)
Major indicator			
Family history of premature CVD	57	24.6	24.6
Parental cholesterol ≥240 mg/dl	68	29.3	47.8
TOTAL	111	47.8	47.8
Discretionary indicator			
High-fat, high-cholesterol diet	76	32.8	32.8
Hypertension (SBP or DBP ≥90%)	44	19.0	44.4
Obesity (Quetelet index ≥85%)	34	14.7	51.3
Smoker (≥10 cigarettes/day)	12	5.2	53.0
Steroid/medication	5	2.2	54.7
Diabetes	0	0.0	54.7
TOTAL	127	54.7	54.7

SBP, Systolic blood pressure; *DBP*, diastolic blood pressure.
*Major and discretionary indicators = 74.5%.

Table II. Number of screening indicators present in subjects with elevated LDL-C concentrations*

	Total No. of indicators present			
	0	1	2	≥3
Subjects with ≥1 major indicator	0	13	8	14
(Parent cholesterol, ≥240 mg/dl)	(0)	(9)	(8)	(13)
Subjects with ≥1 discretionary indicator	0	10	12	16
(Diet present)	(0)	(7)	(10)	(12)

*Elevated LDL-C concentrations: ≥110 mg/dl.

Of 232 children studied, we observed 111 (47.8%) with a major screening indicator; 65 (58.6%) of the 111 had at least one discretionary screening indicator present. Similarly, 127 children (54.7%) had at least one discretionary screening indicator present, and 65 (51.2%) of the 127 also had at least one major indicator. The presence of a major or a discretionary indicator was independent of the other; no one indicator was associated with any other (chi-square value = 1.25; $p = 0.26$).

Lipid measurements according to NCEP-Peds and clustering of screening indicators in children with elevated LDL-C concentrations. In this cohort, 9.9% had high LDL-C and 15.1% had borderline LDL-C levels. Therefore 25% of the 232 children had elevated LDL-C levels. More children with acceptable LDL-C levels had no or one screening indicator (n = 115) than children with two or more screening indicators (n = 59) (Figure). For those children with elevated LDL-C levels, 30 had no or one screening indicator, in comparison with 28 children who had two or more screening indicators. In addition, only 12% of the children with elevated LDL-C levels had no screening indicators, in comparison with 30% of the children with acceptable LDL-C levels. This clustering of individuals with multiple screening indicators and elevated LDL-C levels was significant when analyzed by logistic regression analysis (elevated LDL-C levels, $p = 0.0006$; high LDL-C levels, $p = 0.03$). Each screening indicator increased the risk of having an elevated LDL-C concentration by 1.70 (β parameter = 0.533) and the risk of having a high LDL-C concentration by 1.64 (β parameter = 0.497).

Parental cholesterol concentration and a high-fat, high-cholesterol diet were the primary factors associated with elevated LDL-C values (Table II). Of the 58 children with elevated LDL-C values, 7 had no identifiable screening indicators, 38 had at least one of the discretionary indicators, and 37 had at least one of the major indicators. Diet alone would have identified 29 children with elevated LDL-C values; parental cholesterol concentrations ≥6.21 mmol/L (240 mg/dl) alone would have identified 31 children with elevated LDL-C values (Table II).

Ability of specific screening indicators to identify children with high LDL-C concentrations (Table III). Individually, each screening indicator was more specific than sensitive (i.e., the absence of an individual screening indicator was associated with an acceptable LDL-C value between 74% to 98% of the time). However, very few children with high LDL-C values were detected by a single screening indicator; thus the sensitivity was low—none more than 60.9%.

The major indicators were modestly more sensitive and more specific than the discretionary indicators. In total, the major and the discretionary indicators were more sensitive than specific (i.e., applied as a group they detected children with high LDL-C values 95.7% [elevated LDL-C values 88%, data not shown] of the time, but they also identified 71% of the children with acceptable LDL-C values). In addition, as a group they had a high negative predictive value (i.e., the absence of the screening indicators indicated a 98.3% probability of not having a high LDL-C concentration).

DISCUSSION

The NCEP-Peds Expert Panel chose to recommend selective screening, instead of universal screening, primarily

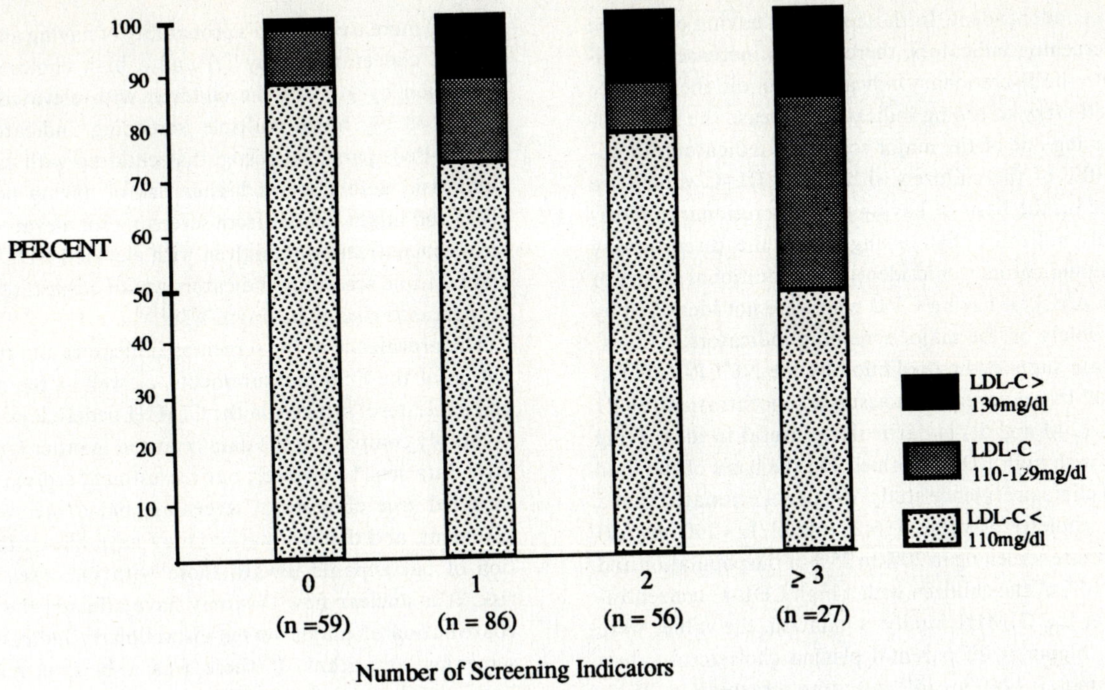

Figure. Percentage of children with 0, 1, 2, and ≥3 screening indicators and their LDL-C levels. Children with elevated LDL-C levels had significantly more screening indicators than children with acceptable LDL-C levels (logistic regression: $p < 0.001$; for high LDL-C levels; $p < 0.03$).

Table III. Sensitivity and specificity of individual screening indicators in identifying children with high LCL-C concentrations

Screening indicator	SENS	SPEC	PPV	NPV
Major indicator				
Family history of premature CVD	17.4	74.6	7.0	89.1
Parent cholesterol ≥240 mg/dl	60.9	74.2	20.6	94.5
BOTH MAJOR INDICATORS	73.9	55.0	15.3	95.0
Discretionary indicator				
High-fat, high-cholesterol diet	47.8	68.9	14.5	92.3
Hypertension	13.0	80.4	6.8	89.4
Obesity	17.4	85.7	11.8	90.4
Smoker	8.7	95.2	16.7	90.5
Steroid/medication	4.4	98.1	20.0	90.3
ALL DISCRETIONARY INDICATORS	65.2	46.4	11.8	92.4
ALL INDICATORS (MAJOR AND DISCRETIONARY)	95.7	27.8	12.7	98.3

SENS, Sensitivity (%); *SPEC*, specificity (%); *PPV*, positive predictive value (probability); *NPV*, negative predictive value (probability) as defined in the Statistical Methods section.

focusing on serum cholesterol elevation occurring in the family, and secondarily on individuals with additional screening indicators. These latter indicators can be used at the discretion of the physician to screen children for elevated serum cholesterol. We determined that the discretionary indicators as defined herein, when applied to our nuclear family data set, capture a slightly greater percentage of children (27%) than the major familial factors (19.8%), with an estimated overlap of 28%. The use of both major and discretionary indicators in the CIMIH cohort results in identification of 75% of children screened, a percentage that is probably inflated by the availability of complete nuclear families and possible recruitment bias. We doubt that the full application of the NCEP-Peds screening guidelines to a clinical practice would ever exceed this estimated level, because few physicians have all the screening indicator data, as we do for this cohort.

The major and the discretionary screening indicators appear to be independent. In those subjects having one of the major screening indicators, there was no increased association with the discretionary indicators. Nor did the presence of discretionary screening indicators increase the probability of having one of the major screening indicators. In addition, 30% of the children with high LDL-C values are identified on the basis of having only discretionary indicators. This indicates that asking about the discretionary screening indicators would identify an additional subset of children at risk of having CVD who were not identified by reliance solely on the major screening indicators.

The data support the prediction by the NCEP-Peds Expert Panel that a parental cholesterol concentration ≥6.21 mmol/L (240 mg/dl) is particularly useful in identifying children with high LDL-C values. On the basis of the lipid research clinic prevalence study, the panel estimated that a parental cholesterol value ≥6.21 mmol/L (240 mg/dl) would initiate screening in 20% to 25% of the population and identify 40% of the children with a high LDL-C concentration.[18] For the CIMIH family population, the values were modestly higher, with parental plasma cholesterol values ≥6.21 mmol/L (240 mg/dl) initiating screening in 29.3% and identifying 61% of the children with a high LDL-C concentration. This result would have been predicted on the basis of the availability of nuclear families in the CIMIH population, not necessarily the case in the data set of the lipid research clinic. These values are consistent with those of Benuck et al.,[29] who recently reported that parental plasma cholesterol values ≥6.21 mmol/L (240 mg/dl) identified 50% of the children from 160 white families with high LDL-C values.

Among the discretionary screening indicators, the consumption of a high-fat, high-cholesterol diet resulted in the screening of 33% of the cohort, and significantly enhanced the number of children with elevated LDL-C concentrations who were identified. Multiple epidemiologic studies have demonstrated the influence of dietary fat and cholesterol on mean serum cholesterol values,[30, 31] and dietary changes are the cornerstone of intervention for the NCEP-Adult and NCEP-Peds recommendations.[18, 32] Children identified as having elevated LDL-C concentrations as a result of consuming a high-fat, high-cholesterol diet may be particularly susceptible to dietary intervention. However, dietary evaluation of children is currently time-consuming and impractical in a busy primary care office; the simpler dietary instruments being developed for children may ultimately be helpful.[33-35]

Our data also show that a clustering of screening indicators is observed more frequently in children with elevated LDL-C values. Clustering of risk factors and elevated cholesterol in adults have been reported previously.[36-40] In our cohort, having a screening indicator (major, discretionary, or both) increased a child's probability of having an elevated LDL-C concentration by 1.7 and a high cholesterol concentration by 1.6. Of the children with elevated LDL-C levels, 48.3% have multiple screening indicators. The NCEP-Peds panel suggested that children with cardiovascular risk factors are at higher risk of having premature CVD and might benefit from screening for elevated cholesterol concentrations. Children with elevated LDL-C levels and multiple screening indicators would constitute a subset at increased risk of having CVD.[1-10]

The prevalence of the screening indicators and the distribution of the lipid measurements, as well as the mean fat and cholesterol intakes, in the CIMIH pediatric population favorably compare to the data reported in other large pediatric data sets.* However, our recruitment strategy, which included free cholesterol screening, blood pressure measurement, and diet evaluation, may have biased the selection of participants toward those with increased cardiac risk. It is unclear how this may have affected the relative contribution of major versus discretionary indicators to a screening algorithm. If there was a bias, it may have increased the contribution of family history. However, the prevalence of a family history of CVD in the CIMIH population is within the range reported by other investigators.[42-46]

The NCEP-Peds guidelines provide definitions for the major indicators. The relative contributions of the discretionary indicators are clearly dependent on the definition of each factor. The definition utilized herein for hypertension is fairly well accepted,[22] but a universal definition for childhood obesity is lacking. The Quetelet index has been the most commonly used index of obesity during the last decade[47] and is closely related to body fatness in white persons.[48] The age- and gender-specific 85th percentile captures both moderately and severely obese children and has been used previously.[24, 25] The definition for smoking (≥10 cigarettes per day) could be considered too restrictive in children. Redefining smoking as any cigarette use during the previous year would raise the prevalence from 5.2% to 11.6% of the cohort, but none of these additional children had an elevated LDL-C concentration. Finally, our definition of a high-fat, high-cholesterol diet (i.e., consumption of ≥400 mg cholesterol per day or ≥40% calories as fat or both) is only at the 80th percentile in normative distributions[27] but is considered high within the NCEP framework, which recommends a prudent diet for the American population with <30% calories as fat and <300 mg cholesterol consumed per day.[18, 31] Nonetheless, higher dietary percentage cutoff points would have reduced the overall screening contribution of the discretionary indicators.

*References 18, 24, 27, 29, 31, 41, and 42.

We conclude that despite the overlap in identified populations, each group of screening indicators targeted a subset of subjects whom the other did not; major and discretionary indicators were independent. A physician cannot choose to use only the major indicators and assume that the majority of those with other screening indicators will be found; one in three children with high LDL-C concentrations will go undiscovered. However, absence of the data for the major familial screening indicators still allows for some reasonable screening by full use of the discretionary indicators. Knowing a parent's cholesterol level appears to be particularly useful in identifying children with a high LDL-C level, and this information should be sought in clinical practice. Finally, the high negative predictive value observed in this cohort suggests that children without any screening indicators are at very low risk of having a high LDL-C concentration (<2%).

We greatly appreciate the assistance of Loretta A. Simbartl for statistical support.

REFERENCES

1. PDAY Research Group. Relationship of atherosclerosis in young men to serum lipoprotein cholesterol concentrations and smoking: a preliminary report from the Pathobiological Determinants of Atherosclerosis Group. JAMA 1990;265:3018-24.
2. Newman WP III, Wagigney W, Berenson GS. Autopsy studies in U.S. children and adolescents: relationship of risk factors to atherosclerotic lesions. Ann NY Acad Sci 1991;623:16-25.
3. Newman WP III, Freedman DS, Voors AW, et al. Relation of serum lipoproteins and systolic blood pressure to early atherosclerosis: the Bogalusa Heart Study. N Engl J Med 1986; 314:138-44.
4. Freedman DS, Burke GL, Harsha DW, et al. Relationship of changes in obesity to serum lipid and lipoprotein changes in childhood and adolescence. JAMA 1985;254:515-20.
5. Burns TL, Moll PP, Lauer RM. Increased familial cardiovascular mortality in obese schoolchildren: the Muscatine Ponderosity Family Study. Pediatrics 1992;89:262-8.
6. Sarlund H, Laakso M, Voutilainen E, Penttila I, Pyorala K. Familial aggregations of non-insulin-dependent, diabetes and coronary heart disease are accompanied by different effects on serum lipids, lipoproteins and apolipoproteins. Atherosclerosis 1991;31:17-29.
7. Dennison BA, Kikuchi DA, Srinivasan SR, Webber LS, Berenson GS. Parental history of cardiovascular disease as an indication for screening for lipoprotein abnormalities in children. J Pediatr 1989;115:186-94.
8. Schrott HG, Clarke WR, Wiebe DA, et al. Increased coronary mortality in relatives of hypercholesterolemic schoolchildren: the Muscatine study. Circulation 1979;59:320-6.
9. Moll PP, Sing CF, Weidman WH, et al. Total cholesterol and lipoproteins in schoolchildren: prediction of coronary heart disease in adult relatives. Circulation 1983;67:127-34.
10. Glueck CJ, Fallat RW, Tsang R, Buncher CR. Hyperlipidemia in progeny of parents with myocardial infarction before age 50. Am J Dis Child 1974;127:70-5.
11. Committee on Atherosclerosis and Hypertension of the Council on Cardiovascular Disease in the Young and the Nutrition Committee, American Heart Association. A joint position statement for physicians: diagnosis and treatment of primary hyperlipidemia in childhood. Circulation 1986;74:1181A-8A.
12. American Academy of Pediatrics Committee on Nutrition. Indications for cholesterol testing in children. Pediatrics 1989; 83:141-2.
13. Meyerson DA, Santanello NC. Pediatric lipid screening based upon criteria of high-risk family history fails to identify two-thirds of higher-risk children. Circulation 1988;78(suppl II):II-383.
14. Dennison BA, Kikuchi DA, Srinivasan SR, Webber LS, Berenson GS. Serum total cholesterol screening for the detection of elevated low-density lipoprotein in children and adolescents: the Bogalusa Heart Study. Pediatrics 1990;85:472-9.
15. Garcia RE, Moodie DS. Routine cholesterol surveillance in childhood. Pediatrics 1989;84:751-5.
16. Griffin TC, Christoffel KK, Binns HJ, McGuire PA (Pediatric Practice Research Group). Family history evaluation as a predictive screen for childhood hypercholesterolemia. Pediatrics 1989;84:365-73.
17. Davison DM, Van Camp J, Iftner CA, Landry SM, Bradley BJ, Wong ND. Family history fails to detect the majority of children with high capillary blood total cholesterol. J Sch Health 1991;61(2):75-80.
18. National Cholesterol Education Program. Report of the Expert Panel on Blood Cholesterol Levels in Children and Adolescents. (National Institutes of Health publication No. 91-2732.) Bethesda, Maryland: National Heart, Lung, and Blood Institute, September 1991:1-119.
19. Lauer RM. A family history of risk factors and cardiovascular diseases [Editorial]. Circulation 1991;84:1445-6.
20. Rice TR, Sprecher DL, Borecki IB, Mitchell LE, Laskarzewski PM, Rao DC. The Cincinnati Myocardial Infarction and Hormone (CIMIH) Family Study: family resemblance for dehydroepiandrosterone sulfate (DHEAS) in control and MI families. Metabolism 1993;42:1284-90.
21. Lipid Research Clinics Program. Manual of laboratory operations, lipid and lipoprotein analysis. In: Hainline A, Karon J, Lippel K, eds. (U.S. Department of Health, publication No. [NIH] 75-628 [revised]; (U.S. Government Printing Office No. 1982-361-132:678.) Bethesda, Maryland: National Heart, Lung, and Blood Institute, 1982.
22. Task Force on Blood Pressure Control in Children. Report of the Second Task Force on Blood Pressure Control in Children—1987. Pediatrics 1987;79:1-25.
23. Najjar MF, Rowland M. Anthropometric reference data and prevalence of overweight: United States, 1976-80. (Vital and Health Statistics, Series 11, No. 238.) Washington, D.C.: U.S. Department of Health and Human Services, 1987.
24. Frisancho AR. Anthropometric standards for the assessment of growth and nutritional status. Ann Arbor: University of Michigan Press, 1990:168.
25. Kuczmarski R. Prevalence of overweight and weight gain in the United States. Am J Clin Nutr 1992;55:495s-502s.
26. Block G, Hartman AM, Dresser CM, Carroll MD, Gannon J, Gardner L. A data-based approach to diet questionnaire design and testing. Am J Epidemiol 1986;124:453-69.
27. Human Nutrition Information Service. Nationwide food consumption survey: continuing survey of food intakes by individuals, women 19-50 years and their children 1-5 years, 4 days,

1986. (CSFII report No. 1988;86-3.) Hyattsville, Maryland: U.S. Department of Agriculture, 1988.
28. Kleinbaum DG, Kupper LL, Morgenstern H. Epidemiologic research: principles and quantitative methods. Belmont, California: Lifetime Learning Publications (Wadsworth), 1982: 299.
29. Benuck I, Gidding SS, Donovan M, Traisman ES, Traisman HS. Usefulness of parental serum total cholesterol levels in identifying children with hypercholesterolemia. Am J Cardiol 1992;69:713-7.
30. Keys A. Coronary heart disease in seven countries. Circulation 1970;40(suppl 1):1-199.
31. Simon LA. Interrelations of lipids and lipoproteins with coronary artery disease mortality in 19 countries. Am J Cardiol 1986;57(suppl G):5-10.
32. Expert Panel on Detection, Evaluation, and Treatment of High Blood Cholesterol in Adults. Summary of the Second Report of the National Cholesterol Education Program (NCEP) Expert Panel on Detection, Evaluation, and Treatment of High Blood Cholesterol in Adults (Adult Treatment Panel II). JAMA 1993;269:3015-36.
33. Hunninghake DB, Quiter ES, Brekke DE, Harper DE, Mullis RM. Reliability testing of a self-administered eating pattern assessment tool: presented at the First National Cholesterol Conference, November 9-11, 1988, Arlington, Virginia.
34. Dennison BA, Jenkins PL, Chan J, Pearson TA. Food habits questionnaire to assess dietary cholesterol and saturated fatty acid (SFA) intakes in 2-year-old children. Circulation 1992;86:I-311a.
35. Gans KM, Sundaram SG, McPhillips JB, et al. Rate your plate: an eating pattern assessment and educational tool used at cholesterol screening and education programs. J Nutr Educ 1993;25(1):29-36.
36. Kannel WB, Neaton JD, Wentworth D, et al. Overall and coronary heart disease mortality rates in relation to major risk factors in 325,348 men screened for MRFIT. Am Heart J 1986;112:825-36.
37. Criqui MH, Cowan LD, Heiss G, et al. Frequency and clustering of nonlipid coronary risk factors in dyslipoproteinemia: the Lipid Research Clinics Prevalence Study. Circulation 1986;73(suppl I):I-40–50.
38. Gordon T, Kannel WB. Multiple risk functions for predicting coronary heart disease: the concept, accuracy, and application. Am Heart J 1982;103:1031-9.
39. William RR, Hunt SC, Hopkins PN, et al. Familial dyslipidemic hypertension: evidence from 58 Utah families for a syndrome present in approximately 15% of patients with essential hypertension. JAMA 1988;259:3579-86.
40. Berenson GS, Srinivasan SR, Hunter SM, et al. Risk factors in early life as predictors of adult heart disease: the Bogalusa Heart Study. Am J Med Sci 1989;298(3):141-151.
41. National Heart, Lung, and Blood Institute. The Lipid Research Clinics Population Studies Data Book; volume I: The prevalence study. (National Institutes of Health publication No. 80-1527.) Bethesda, Maryland: The Institute, July 1980.
42. Barrett-Connor E, Khaw K. Family history of heart attack as an independent predictor of death due to cardiovascular disease. Circulation 1984;69:1065-9.
43. Dennison BA, Jenkins PL, Pearson TA. The NCEP pediatric guidelines: how many children require cholesterol screening [Abstract]? Circulation 1991;84(suppl):131a.
44. Deutscher S, Epsterin FH, Keller JB. Relationships between familial aggregation of coronary heart disease and risk factors in the general population. Am J Epidemiol 1969;89:510-20.
45. Kannel WB, Feinleib M, McNamara PM, Garrison RJ, Castelli WP. An investigation of coronary heart disease in families. Am J Epidemiol 1979;110:281-90.
46. Morrison JA, Horvitz R, Khoury P, et al. Parental history of coronary heart disease, hypertension, diabetes, and stroke: relationship to coronary heart disease risk factor variables in their adult children. Prev Med 1980;9:773-86.
47. Guo S, Salisbury S, Roche AF, Chumlea WC, Siervogel RM. Cardiovascular disease risk factors and body composition: a review. Nutrition Research 1994;14:1719-76.
48. Roche AF, Siervogel RM, Chumlea WC, Webb P. Grading body fatness from limited anthropometric data. Am J Clin Nutr 1981;34:2831-8.

Relation of activity levels to body fat in infants 6 to 12 months of age

Ruowei Li, MD, PhD, Lisa O'Connor, MEd, Donna Buckley, BA, and Bonny Specker, PhD
From the Department of Pediatrics, University of Cincinnati Medical Center, Cincinnati, Ohio

We examined longitudinally the relation between body fatness and physical activity, adjusting for energy intake, in 31 healthy white infants. Measures of physical activity, dietary intake, and body composition were obtained at 6, 9, and 12 months of age. The percentage of body fat was inversely related to activity level, an association that became stronger with increasing age and remained significant after adjustment for dietary energy intake. The percentage of body fat was not related to energy consumed per lean body mass regardless of high or low activity level, nor was energy consumed related to physical activity. We conclude that the percentage of body fat in infants may be related more to their activity levels than to their energy intake. (J PEDIATR 1995;126:353-7)

Initially it was thought that excessive energy intake was the primary cause of obesity and that heavy people merely overindulge in food consumption. However, it has been reported that obesity can develop because of a reduction in total energy expenditure below normal values rather than an excessive energy intake.[1-3] Zurlo et al.[4] showed that a lower physical activity in adults might be responsible for the reduced total energy expenditure in the development of obesity. In addition, because increased physical activity allows a higher energy consumption without risk of weight gain,[5] the association between percentage body fat and energy intake also may be influenced by the activity levels of the infant.

Because of the possibility that body composition during infancy may have implications with respect to obesity during childhood and adult life, it is important to identify factors that influence body composition during infancy and to evaluate the cause-and-effect relationship. We therefore investigated whether the level of body fatness was related to physical activity in a cohort of infants enrolled in a longitudinal study.

Supported by National Institutes of Health grant ROI-AR40169.
Submitted for publication April 4, 1994; accepted Sept. 15, 1994.
Reprint requests: Bonny Specker, PhD, University of Cincinnati Medical Center, Department of Pediatrics, 231 Bethesda Ave. (ML 0541), Cincinnati, OH 45267-0541.

0022-3476/95/$3.00 + 0 **9/20/60610**

METHODS

Subjects. All 31 healthy white infants (16 female) participating in a longitudinal study of activity and bone mineral content were included in this study. They were recruited from 12 child care centers before 6 months of age and satisfied the following criteria: (1) born at term, (2) not small for gestational age,[6] (3) free of cardiac, respiratory, hematologic, hepatic, gastrointestinal, or bone disease, and (4) consent obtained for participation in longitudinal study of activity and bone mineralization. All infants were supplied with the same formula from at least 6 to 12 months of age. In addition, the infants were permitted to receive either commercially prepared or homemade supplemental foods. Physical activity, dietary intake, and body composition were measured at 6, 9, and 12 months of age by a 6-hour direct observation, three 24-hour diet diaries, and dual-energy x-ray absorptiometry. The protocol was approved by Cincinnati Children's Hospital Medical Center Institutional Review Board, and informed consent was obtained.

CARS	Children's Activity Rating Scale

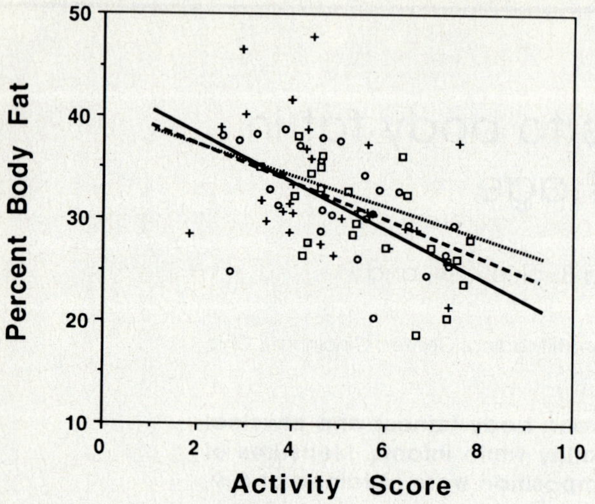

Figure. Relation between percentage of body fat and activity scores (*dotted line and plus signs*, 6 months: $r = -0.36$; $p = 0.049$; $y = 40.32 - 1.54x$; *dashed line and clear circles*, 9 months: $r = -0.47$, $p = 0.010$, $y = 40.16 - 1.83x$; *solid line and clear squares*, 12 months: $r = -0.61$; $p = 0.001$, $y = 40.90 - 2.09x$).

Table I. Body composition, energy consumption, and activity levels at 6, 9, and 12 months of age

	Age (mo)		
	6	9	12
Weight (kg)	8.2 ± 0.9	9.3 ± 0.9	10.5 ± 1.2
Percentage of body fat (%)	33 ± 6	31 ± 6	29 ± 5
Total energy consumed (kJ/day)	2803 ± 483	3334 ± 608	4022 ± 859
Energy consumed per LBM (kJ/kg/day)	534 ± 83	535 ± 84	575 ± 149
Activity score	4.4 ± 1.4	5.1 ± 1.4	5.6 ± 1.3

Values are expressed as mean ± SD.
LBM, Lean body mass.

Physical activity. Direct observation of spontaneous activity was conducted at the day care centers by the study coordinators, who were masked to the percentage of body fat of the infants. Habitual activity of the infants was observed for the first minute of every 15 minutes for a total of 6 hours, usually from 8 AM until 2 PM. When infants slept during this period, the activity was scored as zero and the sleeping time was noted. A modified Children's Activity Rating Scale was used to record activity. The CARS has been validated in several studies of preschool children[7, 8] and encompasses a wide range of energy expenditure; the percentage of agreement between observers for paired observations with the CARS in children is 84%. Activities are scored with a scale ranging from 1 to 5 and based on the amount of body movement (1 = no movement; 2 = stationary, with movement; 3 = translocation, slow and easy; 4 = translocation, medium or moderate; and 5 = translocation, fast or very fast, and strenuous). Because the CARS was established for young children and activity levels of infants are lower than those of young children, we modified the CARS slightly to have a broader range for infants in the low activity levels. We utilized a scale ranging from 0 to 5 (none, minimal, light, moderate, vigorous, maximal activity levels). In addition, we determined the activity levels for each region of the body; the movements of the arms, legs, head, and trunk were each assigned a score. The scores for the four body parts during the observation time were summed, and the average score was calculated as the sum of the scores divided by the number of entries observed. Each 6-hour observation period was scored by one person. Two observers were trained with the modified CARS by the same person using videotapes of infants performing various levels of activity. They scored activity independently and a Pearson correlation coefficient of 0.83 ($p < 0.001$) was observed.

Dietary intake. Three 24-hour diet diaries were completed at 6, 9, and 12 months of age; two of them were done on consecutive weekdays and one on the following weekend. The quantities of all the foods eaten by the infants were recorded in household measures, and the brand or recipe of each food was also noted. On weekdays, diet information was collected from child care centers by care providers and reviewed by a registered dietitian. Standard forms were used to record intake. A separate form was supplied to parents for recording foods consumed at home in the evenings. On one weekend day, a 24-hour diary was completed by the parents and the forms were returned to the dietitian for review; if there were questions, the parents were contacted by phone. Dietary intakes of energy and other nutrients were determined with the nutrient database from the University of Minnesota Nutrition Coding Center (version 2.3).

Body composition. Body composition was measured by a total body scan with dual-energy x-ray absorptiometry (Hologic QDR 1000W, Pediatric Software V5.56, Waltham, Mass.). A form pillow with Velcro straps was used to restrain the infants. The percentage of body fat was calculated as whole body fat mass divided by total body mass. The accuracy of DXA has been evaluated in infants.[9, 10] Our coefficients of variation, determined from duplicate scans in 17 infants 3 to 17 months of age, is 7.0% for total body fat and 6.2% for percentage of body fat; we

Table II. Multiple regression parameter estimates, standard errors, and *p* values for the model assessing the relation between percentage of body fat and activity levels at 6, 9, and 12 months of age

	Parameter estimate			SEE			*p*		
	6	9	12	6	9	12	6	9	12
Intercept	41.95	35.64	41.24	7.47	6.21	5.09			
Activity score	−1.52	−2.12	−2.11	0.76	0.69	0.59	0.056	0.005	0.002
Energy consumed per LBM (kJ/kg/day)	−0.003	0.011	−0.000	0.013	0.114	0.005	0.805	0.332	0.944

LBM, Lean body mass.

previously found that triceps skin-fold thickness correlated with percentage of body fat measured by DXA at 6 ($r = 0.78$), 9 ($r = 0.72$), and 12 ($r = 0.68$) months of age.[11]

Statistical analysis. All statistical analyses were done with the Statistical Analysis Systems SAS/PC program.[12] The relation between percentage of body fat and physical activity, between percentage of body fat and daily energy intake, and between dietary energy intake and physical activity levels were assessed by calculating a Pearson correlation coefficient. To evaluate the effects that potential confounders might have on the apparent relation between percentage of body fat and physical activity levels, we considered multiple regression models. To determine whether the relation between percentage of body fat and energy intake was influenced by activity levels, we included the interaction term of energy intake and activity level in the general linear model.

RESULTS

Mean body weight, percentage of body fat, total energy consumed, energy consumed per lean body mass, and activity scores for each age are provided in Table I. There were no gender differences in percentage of body fat or activity level at 6, 9, or 12 months of age; therefore male and female infants were grouped together. Percentage of body fat was correlated with body weight at 6 months ($r = 0.372$; $p = 0.04$) and 9 months of age ($r = 0.461$; $p = 0.01$), but not at 12 months ($r = 0.170$; $p = 0.4$). Percentage of body fat was inversely related to activity level, and the magnitude of the effect and its significance became stronger with increasing age (Figure). When both activity and energy consumed were included in a multiple regression model, activity remained inversely related to percentage of body fat (Table II).

Further analyses showed that activity levels at 12 months of age were associated with both body fat mass and percentage of body fat at 6 months of age ($r = -0.45$ and $p = 0.013$; $r = -0.49$ and $p = 0.006$, respectively). Similar associations were found between the activity levels at 12 months of age and both fat mass and percentage of fat at 9 months of age. No significant relationships were observed between fat mass at 12 months of age or continuing changes in body fat and activity levels at 6 months of age. We expressed changes in body fat with time as an absolute rate (fat mass at 12 months − fat mass at 6 months or percentage of body fat at 12 months − percentage of body fat at 6 months) and as percentage of initial fat mass [(fat mass at 12 months − fat mass at 6 months)/fat mass at 6 months]. These results indicate that fatter babies are less active later in infancy, but low activity levels in early infancy (at least at 6 months of age) are not good predictors of higher body fatness in later infancy.

The interaction terms of activity and energy consumption, based on both variables as continuous values, were not significant at any age. Thus the relation between percentage of body fat and energy consumption per lean body mass was similar at different activity levels. Dietary energy consumed per lean body mass was not related to the activity levels at any age, nor was percentage of body fat related to energy consumed per lean body mass.

DISCUSSION

Regardless of the causes of obesity, it must be a result of an increased energy supply relative to requirements. Theoretically, physical activity has an impact on body composition by modulating energy expenditure or energy intake or both. Results of a study by Rose and Mayer[5] indicated that high physical activity levels in 4- to 6-month-old infants may allow a higher energy consumption without increased body fat, as measured by skin-fold thicknesses. Because no studies have assessed physical activity in relation to body fatness among infants older than 6 months of age, our results can be compared only with those for total daily energy expenditure of infants. Two prospective studies on the contribution of low total energy expenditure to excessive weight gain in infants have been reported,[1, 13] and the results conflict. Roberts et al.[1] selected two cohorts of newborn infants whose mothers were either obese or nonobese, and showed that total daily energy expenditure among infants who become overweight by 1 year of age was significantly lower than that of infants who remained lean. However, Davies et al.,[13] in a cohort study of 33 healthy term infants, did not support the hypothesis that a reduced total daily energy expenditure is related to the development of infant obesity.

Our results confirm the speculation of Roberts et al.[1] that obesity, or level of fatness, is associated with decreased physical activity in infants. Our data also are consistent with reports from other age groups indicating that physical activity is reduced in persons who are already overweight;[14-17]; we found that activity levels at 12 months of age were significantly related to both fat mass and percentage of body fat at 6 or 9 months of age. Although babies who were less active at 12 months of age had a higher percentage of body fat at 6 and 9 months of age, differences in earlier physical activity in relation to later body fatness and its changes could not be detected. Therefore it appears that increased body fatness came first, with inactivity as the consequence.

Low activity levels at 6 months of age did not lead to higher body fatness at 12 months of age. One explanation is that activity at 6 months is a poor indicator of the activity between 6 and 12 months of age. Six-month-old infants are just becoming more active and may not yet have established an activity pattern. Another explanation is that higher body fatness is caused not only by lower physical activity but also by other factors. In future studies, infants with reduced physical activity should be followed to evaluate the future occurrence of increased body fatness.

Our finding of no association between percentage of body fat and level of energy intake is in agreement with results of previous studies.[14, 15, 18-21] Perhaps it is not the total energy content of the diet that is contributing to body fatness but, rather, the diet composition.[20-22] Because dietary fat is stored in the body more efficiently than is carbohydrate and protein, and because the human body has a much greater capacity for fat storage, excessive consumption of dietary fat may be a more important determinant of obesity than excessive consumption of either carbohydrate or protein.[23, 24] Because increased physical activity allows higher energy consumption without risk of weight gain,[5] the association between percentage of body fat and energy intake may also be influenced by the activity levels of the infant. In other words, a more significant positive relationship may exist between percentage of body fat and energy intake among children with low activity levels, whereas there may be no relation among children with high activity levels. We found that percentage of body fat was not related to energy intake regardless of the activity levels.

We conclude that in a normal infant, body fatness is related more to activity levels than to energy intake. Although we cannot infer from this study that the decreased physical activity is the cause of increased body fatness in infants, our findings do indicate that the babies with higher body fatness early tend to become less active later. More attention should therefore be paid to babies with high body fat, and physical activity may need to be encouraged early in life.

We thank Gemma Uetrecht for dual-energy x-ray scans, Susan Krug-Wispe for assisting in diet diaries, Mono Ho for assisting in data analysis, and the parents for participating in the study.

REFERENCES

1. Roberts SB, Savage J, Coward WA, Chew B, Lucas A. Energy expenditure and intake in infants born to lean and overweight mothers. N Engl J Med 1988;318:461-6.
2. Ravussin E, Lilliga S, Knowler WC, et al. Reduced rate of energy expenditure as a risk factor for body weight gain. N Engl J Med 1988;318:467-72.
3. Bandini LG, Schoeller DA, Dietz WH. Energy expenditure in obese and nonobese adolescents. Pediatr Res 1990;27:198-203.
4. Zurlo F, Ferraro RT, Fontvieilie AM, Rising R, Bogardus C, Ravussin E. Spontaneous physical activity and obesity: cross-sectional and longitudinal studies in Pima Indians. Am J Physiol 1992;263:E296-300.
5. Rose HE, Mayer JM. Activity, calorie intake, fat storage, and the energy balance of infants. Pediatrics 1968;41:18-29.
6. Usher R, Mclean F. Intrauterine growth of live-born Caucasian infants at sea-level: standards obtained from measurements in 7 dimensions of infant born between 25 and 44 weeks of gestation. J PEDIATR 1969;74:901-10.
7. Puhl J, Greaves K, Hoyt M, Baranowski T. Children's Activity Rating Scale (CARS): description and calibration. Res Q Exerc Sport 1990;61(1):26-36.
8. Baranowski T, Thompson WO, DuRant RH, Baranowski J, Puhl J. Observations on physical activity in physical locations: age, gender, ethnicity, and month effects. Res Q Exerc Sport 1993;64:127-33.
9. Chan G. Performance of dual-energy x-ray absorptiometry in evaluating bone, lean body mass and fat in pediatric subjects. J Bone Miner Res 1992;7:369-74.
10. Brunton JA, Bayley HS, Atkinson SA. Validation and application of dual-energy x-ray absorptiometry to measure bone mass and body composition in small infants. Am J Clin Nutr 1993;58:839-45.
11. Buckley D, O'Connor L, Ho M, Kalkwarf H, Specker B. How do anthropometric measurements of body composition compare with DEXA in infancy [Abstract]? J Am Coll Nutr 1993;12:606.
12. SAS institute. SAS/STAT user's guide; vol 2. Version 6, 4th ed. Cary, North Carolina: The Institute, 1989.
13. Davies PSW, Day JME, Lucas A. Energy expenditure in early infancy and later body fatness. Int J Obesity 1991;15:727-31.
14. Johnson ML, Burke BS, Mayer J. Relative importance of inactivity and overeating in the energy balance of obese high school girls. Am J Clin Nutr 1956;4:37-44.
15. Stefanik PA, Heald FP, Mayer J. Caloric intake in relation to energy output of obese and nonobese adolescent boys. Am J Clin Nutr 1959;7:55-62.
16. Brownell KD, Stunkard AJ. Physical activity in the develop-

ment and control of obesity. In: Stunkard AJ, ed. Obesity. Philadelphia: WB Saunders, 1980:300-24.
17. Gardner AW, Poehlman ET. Physical activity is a significant predictor of body density in women. Am J Clin Nutr 1993;57:8-14.
18. Goth E. Etiological factors in obesity. Proc Nutr Soc 1973; 32:175-9.
19. Kromhout D. Energy and macronurient intake in lean and obese middle-aged men (the Zutphen Study). Am J Clin Nutr 1983;37:295-9.
20. Romieu I, Willett WC, Stampfer MJ, et al. Energy intake and other determinants of relative weight. Am J Clin Nutr 1988;47:406-12.
21. Dreon DM, Frey-Hewitt B, Ellsworth N, Williams PT, Terry RB, Wood PD. Dietary fat: carbohydrate ratio and obesity in middle-aged men. Am J Clin Nutr 1988;47:995-1000.
22. Gazzaniga JM, Burns TL. Relationship between diet composition and body fatness, with adjustment for resting energy expenditure and physical activity, in preadolescent children. Am J Clin Nutr 1993;58:21-8.
23. Flatt JP. Energetics of intermediary metabolism. In: Garrow JS, Halliday D, eds. Substrate and energy metabolism in man. London: John Liberty, 1985:58-69.
24. Bray GA. Appetite control in adults. In: Fernstorm JD, Miller GD, eds. Appetite and body weight regulation: sugar, fat, and macronutrient substitutes. Boca Raton, Florida: CRC Press, 1994:17-34.

A cross-sectional study of catheter-related thrombosis in children receiving total parenteral nutrition at home

Maureen Andrew, MD, Velma Marzinotto, RN, Paul Pencharz, MD, Stanley Zlotkin, MD, PhD, Patricia Burrows, MD, Joanne Ingram, RN, Margaret Adams, and Robert Filler, MD

From the Divisions of Hematology, Clinical Nutrition, and Surgery, Hospital for Sick Children, Toronto, Ontario, Canada

We performed a cross-sectional evaluation of deep vein thrombosis (DVT) related to the use of central venous lines (CVLs) in all pediatric patients receiving home total parenteral nutrition at our institution (N = 12). All children (5 months to 17 years of age) were examined with bilateral upper limb venography. All CVLs were flushed daily with heparin (200 units). At the time of evaluation, 49 CVLs had been placed in the 12 children. Of the 39 CVLs removed, 27 (66%) were blocked; venograms had not been previously obtained except of one child. Eight children had clinical evidence of superficial collateral circulation in the upper portion of the chest and the upper extremities; five had intermittent symptoms of superior vena cava obstruction. On venography, 8 of the 12 children had extensive evidence of DVT; two were unilateral and six bilateral. Five children were treated with warfarin (0.12 to 0.28 mg/kg per day) to achieve an international normalized ratio of 1.4 to 1.8. Neither bleeding nor further CVL-related DVT has occurred. We conclude that the risk of CVL-related DVT in children requiring home total parenteral nutrition is high, and that venography should be performed early in the event of CVL blockage. A multicenter, controlled trial assessing optimal warfarin therapy in this patient population is indicated. (J Pediatr 1995;126:358-63)

Cuffed, tunneled silicone rubber central venous lines, as pioneered by Broviac et al.[1] and adapted by Hickman et al.,[2] have revolutionized the management of patients requiring prolonged venous access, particularly for chemotherapy or total parenteral nutrition. Unfortunately, these intravascular devices are not without risks, of which sepsis and thrombotic occlusion are the most frequent and clinically significant.

A coordinated children's thrombophilia program was established at the Hospital for Sick Children, Toronto, Canada, in 1991 for the investigation and management of children with thrombotic complications. One child receiving long-term home TPN was referred for evaluation because of significant CVL blockage; a venogram showed complete obstruction of the venous system in the upper part of the body. This experience prompted a review of the other 11

CVL	Central venous line
DVT	Deep vein thrombosis
INR	International normalized ratio
TPN	Total parenteral nutrition

Supported by a grant-in-aid from the Medical Research Council of Canada. Dr. Andrew holds a Career Investigator Award from the Heart and Stroke Foundation of Canada.

Submitted for publication Jan. 5, 1994; accepted Sept. 21, 1994.

Reprint requests: Maureen Andrew, MD, Hamilton Civic Hospitals Research Centre, Henderson General Division, 711 Concession St., Hamilton, Ontario L8V 1C3, Canada.

0022-3476/95/$3.00 + 0 **9/20/60784**

Table I. Clinical information at time of evaluation

Patient No.	Age	Duration	Clinical findings	Total CVL No.	Use of local UK	CVL removed Blocked/Other	Venogram Right/Left
1	14 yr	65	SVC, C	4	10	3/0	+/+
2	17 yr	136	C	5	6	4/0	+/+
3	6 yr	89	C	8	15	5/2	+/+
4	1 yr	32	SVC, C	3	9	1/1	−/+
5	5 mo	25	SVC, C	2	4	1/0	+/+
6	1 yr	14	SVC, C	3	2	2/0	+/+
7	15 mo	31	SVC, C	3	3	1/1	−/+
8	4 yr	66	Normal	3	14	1/1	−/−
9	9 yr	118	C	7	4	4/2	+/+
10	6 yr	56	Normal	4	17	2/1	−/−
11	6 yr	97	Normal	5	3	1/3	−/−
12	6 mo	11	Normal	2	0	0/1	−/−
TOTAL				49	87	25/12	6 Bilateral DVT 2 Unilateral DVT

UK, Urokinase; *SVC*, symptoms of superior vena cava syndrome; *C*, collateral circulation in the skin.

children receiving home TPN through a CVL. The histories of having numerous CVLs, requirements for urokinase to remove CVL blockages, and clinical findings of superficial collateral circulation resulted in the decision to examine all 12 children in the home TPN program with venography to determine the frequency of CVL-related deep venous thrombosis. The results of this cross-sectional evaluation are presented in this report.

METHODS

Patient population. All children followed by the clinical nutrition program at the Hospital for Sick Children, Toronto, Canada, and receiving home TPN through a CVL were assessed clinically and by venography. Comprehensive demographic information was obtained for each patient.

Central venous line information. All CVLs were inserted in the operating room with the patient under general anaesthesia, by surgeons following well-established techniques. The CVL tip was positioned at the superior vena caval–right atrial junction during electrocardiographic monitoring. All CVLs were single-lumen, thick-walled silicone rubber tubing of varying lengths and diameters (ROKA catheters; Dr. Andre Bahoric, Hospital for Sick Children, Toronto).[3, 4]

All CVLs were flushed with saline solution at the initiation of the daily administration of TPN, and by saline solution, followed by heparin (200 units), at the completion of the daily administration of TPN. When a blockage occurred in a CVL, a standard protocol was followed. If a saline flush failed to restore patency, 2 ml of urokinase (5000 units/ml) was instilled into the CVL and left in place for 2 to 4 hours. If urokinase therapy failed to restore normal flow, either the CVL was removed or urokinase was infused locally (150 units/kg per hour for 24 hours).

Radiographic evaluation. All prior radiographic evaluations of the current and previous CVLs were reviewed. Patency of the upper venous system was evaluated in each child by means of bilateral venography. In patients subsequently treated with warfarin therapy, additional venograms were obtained if the CVL required treatment with urokinase for blockage or was removed because of sepsis.

Laboratory evaluation. When therapy with warfarin was instituted, prothrombin times were measured and expressed as an international normalized ratio. The prothrombin times were measured in community and hospital laboratories where the children lived. However, the doses of warfarin administered were monitored centrally by members of the children's thrombophilia program. Target INR values were 2.0 to 3.0 for full-dose therapy and 1.3 to 1.8 for low-dose therapy.

RESULTS

Patient population. At the time of evaluation, six girls and six boys were receiving home TPN (Table I). The age range was 5 months to 17 years, with a median age of 5 years. The primary diagnoses included severe combined immunodeficiency syndrome (1 patient), hollow viscous myopathy (1), gastroschisis (2), aganglionosis (1), short gut (3), villous atrophy (2), intestinal pseudo-obstruction (1), and duodenal atresia (1). The direct consequences of CVL-related DVT in our patients included 55 general-anesthesia procedures to place new CVLs, complete loss of venous access in the upper system (n = 6), intermittent superior vena cava syndrome (n = 5), chylothorax (n = 1), early signs of postphlebitic syndrome (n = 8), and probable pulmonary embolism (n = 2). Eight children had superficial venous collateral circulation in the upper portion of the chest and in the neck, face, and shoulder, and the upper arm.

Status before evaluation. A total of 49 CVLs had been

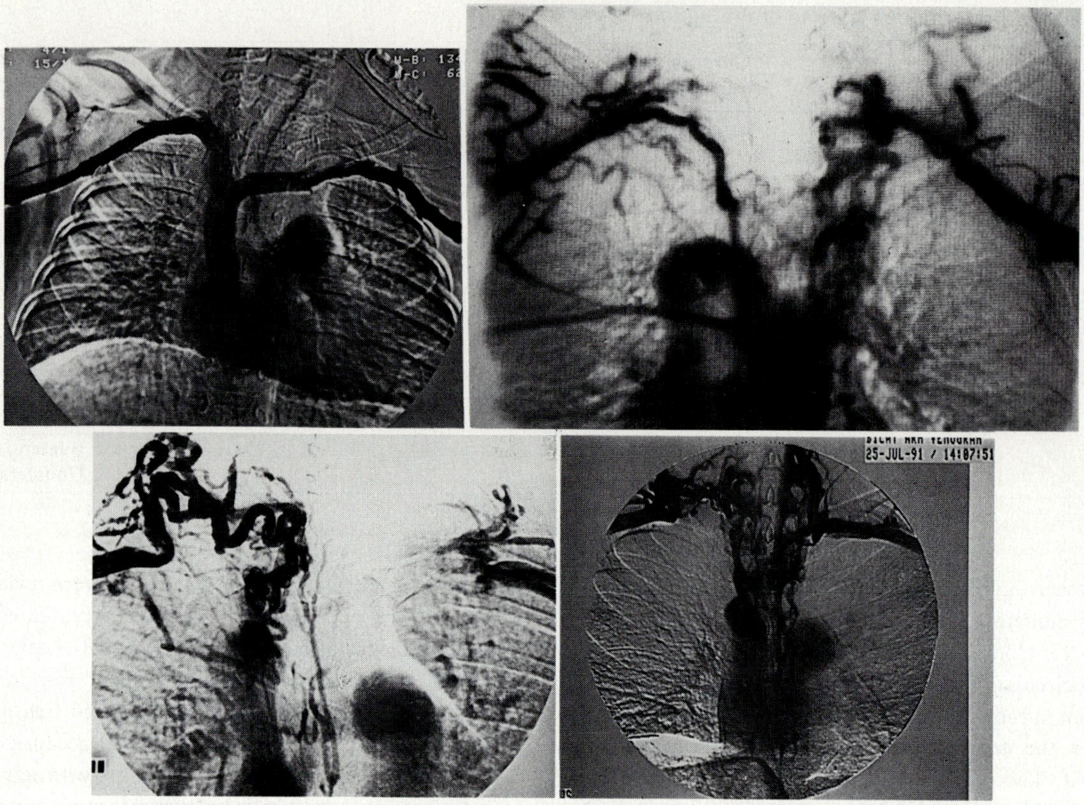

Figure. Four bilateral venograms of patients receiving home TPN. The *upper left* venogram is normal, whereas the other three show varying degrees of venous occlusion with collateral circulation.

placed in the 12 children before the time of evaluation. The number of CVLs placed per child ranged from 2 to 8 with a median of 3.5. Local instillation of urokinase was used repeatedly in all but one child. Twenty-five of the CVLs (68%) were removed because of blockage that had not resolved with urokinase instillation. The remaining CVLs were removed because of sepsis (n = 9), leaks (n = 1), or dislodgment (n = 2).

Before the cross-sectional study, radiographic evaluation had consisted of the use of a "lineogram" (obtained by instilling nonionic contrast medium [Omnipaque] into the CVL under continuous fluoroscopy to determine the potency end position of the CVL; the term is unique to the Hospital for Sick Children, in Toronto, Canada) (n = 46), duplex ultrasonography (n = 16), venography (n = 1), and ventilation/perfusion scintigraphy (n = 2). The venogram in patient 1 demonstrated extensive CVL-related DVT, which resulted in referral to our service.

Radiographic results of the cross-sectional study. Bilateral venography was performed in all 12 children (Table I). Six children had bilateral large-vessel thrombosis in the upper system (Figure), two children had unilateral disease, and four children had normal venograms. Children with bilateral disease had complete replacement of large vessels in the upper system, with small collateral vessels draining through the paravertebral vessels into the azygous system.

Anticoagulation therapy. Five children with extensive CVL-related DVT were treated with warfarin. Full-dose warfarin therapy (INR 2 to 3) was given to 2 of 5 children who had no further accessible vessels for CVL. Of the 3 remaining children, 2 were treated with full doses of warfarin for 6 months, followed by low doses of warfarin to achieve an INR of 1.3 to 1.8, and 1 patient received low-dose warfarin therapy only. There were no bleeding complications or CVL-related DVT during warfarin administration. Three CVLs were replaced in these 5 children, 1 for sepsis, 1 for a leak, and 1 for blockage. There was no evidence of a DVT on a second venogram in the child with the blocked CVL. After the use of urokinase, a second venogram of 3 of the 4 remaining children receiving warfarin was obtained; there was no evidence of new CVL-related DVT. The total duration of CVL life spans per child without new CVL-related DVT ranged from 19 to 27 months (Table II).

DISCUSSION

The clinical histories of our patients were remarkably similar. First, the CVLs did not give blood return, and pressures

Table II. Current clinical status

Patient No.	Warfarin	Status	CVL placements since evaluation	Local UK	Reason for CVL removal	Catheter life span: Total before warfarin* (mo)	CVL before warfarin†	CVL after warfarin (mo)
1	Yes	Deceased	1	0	Block‡	38	7 days	27
2	Yes§	Alive/TPN	0	0	—	113	19 mo	23
3	Yes	Alive/TPN	0	0	—	25	3 mo	64
4	Yes	Alive/TPN	1	0	Leak	11	11 days	21
5	Yes	Alive/TPN	1	2	Sepsis	6	6 mo	19

UK, Urokinase.
*"Total life span" refers to all previous CVL placements.
†"Catheter life span before warfarin" refers to the last CVL placement.
‡There was no evidence of further large vessel thrombi on venography at the time that the CVLs became blocked.
§Intravenous infusion of warfarin.

increased during infusion. Second, the CVLs required repeated urokinase instillation to remove a blockage, and some required a short infusion of a thrombolytic agent. Third, lineograms were obtained to assess the position of the CVLs and to determine whether thrombi were present. Fourth, when the CVLs remained blocked, they were replaced without visualization of the deep venous system. Fifth, the life span of subsequent CVLs decreased; some functioned for only a few days or weeks. Finally, a venogram was obtained and extensive DVT was documented. The reasons for delays in diagnosing the extent of the thrombotic disease in these children were not entirely clear but reflected, in part, the misconception that CVLs are blocked only at the tip. A recent registry has established that CVL-related thrombotic complications are the most frequent cause of DVT in pediatric patients.[5] It is important to identify patients at high risk of having thrombotic occlusion of a CVL, because potentially effective prophylactic anticoagulant therapy is available and may prevent both short-term and long-term problems.[6] This study has shown that children receiving home TPN are at particularly high risk of having clinically important CVL-related DVT.

Early studies showed that cuffed, tunneled silicone rubber catheters provided venous access for nearly twice as long as other catheters for patients receiving home TPN.[1, 2] More recently, totally implantable devices have achieved popularity because of a decreased risk of infection and the greater acceptability of the devices to patients.[7] At the Hospital for Sick Children, Toronto, the ROKA CVL has for many years been used exclusively for children requiring home TPN. The use of only one type of CVL removes an important variable in comparisons of the life spans of CVLs in a small group of children, both before and after warfarin therapy.

A MEDLINE search of the English-language literature from 1976 to 1993 identified 25 publications describing CVL-related thrombotic complications in children older than 1 month of age who were receiving TPN. Of these 25 publications, 14 were case reports involving 15 children (references available on request), 2 were prospective case series,[8, 9] 3 retrospective case series,[10-12] and 6 probable retrospective case series.[13-18] Of the 11 case series, the percentage of children with documented CVL-related DVT ranged from 1% to 35%: 8 studies reported an incidence of 7% or less. The differences between the 11 case series and our study probably reflect the frequency of radiographic testing, the choice of radiographic test, and the diverse patient populations. Radiographic testing in the 11 case series was triggered by clinical symptoms that varied in severity, thereby affecting the detection rate of CVL-related DVT. In one study the inability to draw blood samples from CVLs prompted the use of radiographic evaluation; the DVT detection rate was 35%.[17] In other studies, symptoms of obstruction of the superior vena cava were required, and the result was a detection rate of less than 5%. In contrast, we systematically examined every patient receiving home TPN with venography.

The choice of radiographic test also influenced the observed frequency of CVL-related DVT. In none of the 11 studies was venography uniformly used, even though it is the reference test for adults. Lineograms were commonly used. In our 12 patients, 46 lineograms had been obtained without detection of the extensive obstruction present in the deep venous system. Although lineograms are useful for determining the location of the catheter tip, their low sensitivity in our patients precludes our recommending lineograms for the detection of CVL-related DVT.

A second radiographic test commonly used was ultrasonography, presumably because of its high sensitivity and specificity in the diagnosis of proximal DVT in adult patients.[19, 20] However, compressibility of the vein or lack thereof confers a high positive predictive value in proximal

DVT in adults, and compressibility is not possible for the proximal portion of the upper venous system, which was the location of all thrombi in our patients. Recently, magnetic resonance imaging has been used to diagnose DVT. However, there are no comparison studies of MRI and venography in children with DVT. On the basis of the literature and our study, venography (not lineography) should be considered the reference test for the diagnosis of CVL-related DVT in the upper system until future studies demonstrate a high predictive value for other imaging procedures.

Our results in pediatric patients are similar to the experience with adult patients. Four large series of CVL-related cases of DVT in adults receiving TPN reported incidences of 9%, 20%, 30%, and 76%.[21-24] The available evidence suggests that the risk of CVL-related DVT is higher when TPN fluids are infused. The TPN solutions, particularly the amino acid and hypertonic dextrose components, induce endothelial cell procoagulant activity in vitro.[25, 26]

Although the risk of symptomatic and asymptomatic CVL-related DVT is not known, one cannot assume that either is benign. Besides loss of venous access, complications include pulmonary embolism,[15, 27] chylothorax,[28] superior vena cava syndrome,[29-31] postphlebitic syndrome,[32, 33] and death. The frequency, seriousness, and predictability of CVL-related DVT in children receiving TPN at home justify programs directed at prevention and early detection, with institution of effective treatment when present. Our results support the early examination of patients with CVL blockage.

Flushing catheters with heparin, the most common form of prophylaxis, was insufficient in our patients. We identified only one published randomized, controlled trial of anticoagulant prophylaxis for CVL.[6] Prophylactic fixed-dose warfarin therapy in adults reduced CVL-related DVT diagnosed by venography from 37.5% to 9.5%[6]; the treated group received only 1 mg of warfarin, which did not prolong the INR. Low-dose warfarin therapy has also been demonstrated to provide good prophylaxis for other high-risk disorders in adult patients.[34] Together, these trials provided the basis for choosing low-dose warfarin prophylaxis for our patients. The relatively small number of patients and the very high incidence of thrombosis precluded a randomized trial. The results of low-dose warfarin therapy in our patients are promising but must be considered as preliminary.

We conclude that children requiring long-term home TPN are at very high risk of having CVL-related DVTs that are serious and frequent enough to compromise venous access. A multicenter randomized, controlled trial in new patients requiring home TPN is feasible and is justified to determine the role of low-dose warfarin prophylaxis.

REFERENCES

1. Broviac JW, Cole JJ, Scribner BH. A silicone rubber atrial catheter for prolonged parenteral alimentation. Surg Gynecol Obstet 1973;136:602-6.
2. Hickman RO, Buckner CD, Clift RA, Sanders JE, Stewart P, Thomas E. A modified right atrial catheter for access to the venous system in marrow transplant recipients. Surg Gynecol Obstet 1979;148:871-5.
3. Hoffman MA, Langer JC, Pearl RH, et al. Central venous catheter—no x-rays needed: a prospective study in 50 consecutive infants and children. J Pediatr Surg 1988;23:1201-3.
4. Bahoric A, Filler RM, Perlman K, Jackman WS, Albisser AM. New devices and methods for long-term vascular access for blood sampling and insulin infusion. Diabetes Care 1980;3:338-44.
5. David M, Andrew M. Venous thromboembolism complications in children: a critical review of the literature. J Pediatr 1993;123:337-46.
6. Bern MM, Lokich JJ, Wallach SR, et al. Very low doses of warfarin can prevent thrombosis in central venous catheters: a randomized prospective trial. Ann Intern Med 1990;112:423-8.
7. Strum S, McDermed J, Korn A, Joseph C. Improved methods for venous access: the Port-a-Cath, a totally implanted catheter system. J Clin Oncol 1986;4:596-603.
8. Stenzel JP, Green TP, Fuhrman BP, Carlson PE, Marchessault RP. Percutaneous central venous catheterization in a pediatric intensive care unit: a survival analysis of complications. Crit Care Med 1989;17:984-8.
9. Stenzel JP, Green TP, Fuhrman BP, Carlson PE, Marchessault RP. Percutaneous femoral venous catheterizations: a prospective study of complications. J Pediatr 1989;114:411-5.
10. Maksimak M, Ament ME, Fonkalsrud EW. Comparison of the pediatric Broviac Silastic catheter with a standard No. 3 French Silastic catheter for central venous alimentation. J Pediatr Gastroenterol Nutr 1982;1:227-31.
11. Effmann EL, Ablow RC, Touloukian RJ, Seashore JH. Radiographic aspects of total parenteral nutrition during infancy. Radiology 1978;127:195-201.
12. Moukarzel A, Azancot-Benisty A, Brun P, Vitoux C, Cezard JP, Navarro J. M-mode and two-dimensional echocardiography in the routine follow-up of central venous catheters in children receiving total parenteral nutrition. JPEN J Parenter Enteral Nutr 1991;15:551-5.
13. Fonkalsrud EW, Ament ME, Berquist WE, Burke M. Occlusion of the vena cava in infants receiving central venous hyperalimentation. Surg Gynecol Obstet 1982;154:189-92.
14. Strobel CT, Byrne WJ, Fonkalsrud EW, Ament ME. Home parenteral nutrition: results in 34 pediatric patients. Ann Surg 1978;188:394-403.
15. Mulvihill SJ, Fonkalsrud EW. Complications of superior versus inferior vena cava occlusion in infants receiving central total parenteral nutrition. J Pediatr Surg 1984;19:752-7.
16. Curnow A, Idowu J, Behrens E, Toomey F, Georgeson K. Urokinase therapy for Silastic catheter–induced intravascular thrombi in infants and children. Arch Surg 1985;120:1237-40.
17. Bagnall HA, Gomperts E, Atkinson JB. Continuous infusion of low-dose urokinase in the treatment of central venous catheter thrombosis in infants and children. Pediatrics 1989;83:963-6.
18. Fonkalsrud EW, Berquist W, Burke M, Ament ME. Long-

term hyperalimentation in children through saphenous central venous catheterization. Am J Surg 1982;143:209-11.
19. Heijboer H, Buller HR, Lensing AWA, Turpie AGG, Colly LP, ten Cate JW. A comparison of real-time compression ultrasonography with impedance plethysmography for the diagnosis of deep-vein thrombosis in symptomatic outpatients. N Engl J Med 1993;329:1365-9.
20. Verstraete M. The diagnosis and treatment of deep-vein thrombosis. N Engl J Med 1993;329:1418-20.
21. Padberg FT, Ruggiero J, Blackburn GL, Bistrian BR. Central venous catheterization for parenteral nutrition. Ann Surg 1981;193:264-70.
22. Valerio D, Hussey JK, Smith FW. Central vein thrombosis associated with intravenous feeding: a prospective study. JPEN J Parenter Enteral Nutr 1981;5:240-2.
23. Wolfe BM, Ryder MA, Nishikawa RA, Halsted CH, Schmidt BF. Complications of parenteral nutrition. Am J Surg 1986;152:93-9.
24. Brismar B, Hardstedt C, Malmborg AS. Bacteriology and phlebography in catheterization for parenteral nutrition. Acta Chir Scand 1980;146:115-9.
25. Wakefield A, Cohen Z, Craig M, et al. Thrombogenicity of total parenteral nutrition solutions. I. Effect on induction of monocyte/macrophage procoagulant activity. Gastroenterology 1989;97:1210-9.
26. Wakefield A, Cohen Z, Rosenthal A, et al. Thrombogenicity of total parenteral nutrition solutions. II. Effect on induction of endothelial cell procoagulant activity. Gastroenterology 1989;97:1220-8.
27. Rockoff MA, Gang DL, Vacanti JP. Fatal pulmonary embolism following removal of a central venous catheter. J Pediatr Surg 1984;19:307-9.
28. Kramer SS, Taylor GA, Garfinkel DJ, Simmons MA. Lethal chylothoraces due to superior vena caval thrombosis in infants. Am J Radiol 1981;137:559-63.
29. Dhande V, Kattwinkel J, Alford B. Recurrent bilateral pleural effusions secondary to superior vena cava obstruction as a complication of central venous catheterization. Pediatrics 1983;72:109-13.
30. Graham L Jr, Gumbiner CH. Right atrial thrombus and superior vena cava syndrome in a child. Pediatrics 1984;73:225-8.
31. Bertrand M, Presant CA, Klein L, Scott E. Iatrogenic superior vena cava syndrome: a new entity. Cancer 1984;54:376-8.
32. Tilney NI, Griffiths HJG, Edwards EA. Natural history of major venous thrombosis of the upper extremity. Arch Surg 1970;101:792-6.
33. Painter TD, Karpf M. Deep venous thrombosis of the upper extremity, five years' experience at a university hospital. Angiology 1984;35:743-9.
34. Poller L, McKernan A, Thomson JM, Elstein M, Hirsch PJ, Jones JB. Fixed minidose warfarin: a new approach to prophylaxis against venous thrombosis after major surgery. BMJ 1987;295:1309-12.

Precocious puberty in children with neurofibromatosis type 1

Reema Habiby, MD, Bernard Silverman, MD, Robert Listernick, MD, and Joel Charrow, MD

From the Department of Pediatrics, Northwestern University Medical School, and the Divisions of Endocrinology, General Academic and Emergency Pediatrics, and Genetics, Children's Memorial Hospital, Chicago, Illinois

We undertook a comprehensive study of children with neurofibromatosis type 1 (NF-1) cared for in a large multidisciplinary clinic to determine the prevalence of precocious puberty and its relationship to optic pathway tumors (OPTs). Precocious puberty was diagnosed in 7 of 219 children with NF-1 (5 boys and 2 girls) examined between Jan. 1, 1985, and April 20, 1993. All seven children had OPTs involving the optic chiasm; they represented 39% of children with NF-1 and chiasmal tumors (95% confidence interval, 17% to 64%). Eleven prepubertal children (aged 2 to 10 years) with NF-1 and OPTs, and age- and sex-matched NF-1 control subjects without OPTs, underwent luteinizing hormone–releasing hormone (LH-RH) stimulation tests. Two boys with OPTs had pubertal luteinizing hormone (LH) responses, and testosterone levels >10 ng/dl. Basal LH levels were also elevated in these two boys when tested with a very sensitive immunochemiluminometric assay. None of the children without an OPT had either a pubertal response to LH-RH or an elevated basal LH level. We conclude that precocious puberty in children with NF-1 is found exclusively in those who have OPTs involving the optic chiasm; it is a common complication in those children. With the use of a highly sensitive LH assay, biochemical evidence of hypothalamic-pituitary-gonadal axis activation may be demonstrated, even without provocative testing. (J Pediatr 1995;126:364-7)

Early maturation of the hypothalamic-pituitary-gonadal axis, leading to precocious puberty, is a recognized complication of neurofibromatosis type 1 in childhood.[1-5] Precocious puberty has been reported primarily in those children with NF-1 who have optic pathway tumors.[5-8] Although there are several reports of precocious puberty in children with NF-1 in the absence of such tumors, they are flawed by imprecise definitions of NF-1 and the absence of sensitive neuroimaging techniques.[3, 4]

Supported in part by the National Center of Research Resources and General Clinical Research Centers Program, RR00078, and a grant from the Children's Memorial Institute for Education and Research.

Presented in part at the Midwest Society for Pediatric Research, Nov. 4, 1992, Chicago, Ill., and the Fourth Joint Meeting of the Lawson Wilkins Pediatric Endocrine Society and the European Society for Pediatric Endocrinology, June 1993, San Francisco, Calif.

Submitted for publication June 10, 1994; accepted Sept. 30, 1994.

Reprint requests: Joel Charrow, MD, Division of Genetics—59, Children's Memorial Hospital, 2300 Children's Plaza, Chicago, IL 60614.

0022-3476/95/$3.00 + 0 **9/20/60907**

FSH	Follicle-stimulating hormone
LH	Luteinizing hormone
LH-ICMA	Luteinizing hormone immunochemiluminometric assay
LH-RH	Luteinizing hormone–releasing hormone
NF-1	Neurofibromatosis type 1
OPT	Optic pathway tumor

We undertook a comprehensive study of children with NF-1 being cared for in a large multidisciplinary clinic to determine the prevalence of precocious puberty and its relationship to OPTs. This report consists of both a retrospective review of all cases of precocious puberty seen in our

Table I. Prevalence of precocious puberty in children with NF-1 who underwent neuroimaging

	No tumor	Nonchiasmatic OPT	Chiasmatic OPT	Total
Girls	0/63	0/12	2/10	2/85
Boys	0/75	0/3	5/8	5/86
TOTAL	0/138	0/15	7/18	7/171

Cases of precocious puberty/number of children with neuroimaging in each category.

program and a controlled, prospective study of the function of the hypothalamic-pituitary-gonadal axis in prepubertal children with NF-1 and OPTs.

METHODS

The Children's Memorial Hospital Neurofibromatosis Clinic is a multidisciplinary clinic that provides consultation services to assist in the diagnosis and management of neurofibromatosis in children. All children are seen at least annually and are examined by a general academic pediatrician, a geneticist, and a pediatric ophthalmologist at each visit. Patients seen in this clinic between Jan. 1, 1985, and April 20, 1993, were the subjects of this study. NF-1 was diagnosed in each subject on the basis of the criteria established by the National Institutes of Health Consensus Development Conference.[9] During the period of study we routinely recommended neuroimaging, using a special imaging protocol for the diagnosis of OPTs, once the diagnosis of NF-1 was confirmed. Before 1988, computed tomography was performed; magnetic resonance imaging has been used exclusively thereafter. Optic pathway tumors were diagnosed on the basis of accepted criteria.[10] Neuroimaging was not repeated in children without OPTs or other tumors unless neurologic, ophthalmologic, or neuroendocrine symptoms appeared.

We reviewed the neurofibromatosis clinic records of all children seen during the study period to identify children with precocious puberty. The diagnosis of precocious puberty was based on the appearance of breast development before age 8 years in girls or on testicular enlargement before age 9 years in boys, and a pubertal luteinizing hormone response after intravenous injection of LH–releasing hormone (see below).

We prospectively examined all prepubertal children (Tanner stage I[11]) between the ages of 2 and 10 years who had an OPT. Children were excluded if they had received radiation or chemotherapy (one child). Age- and sex-matched control subjects were recruited for each child with an OPT who was enrolled in the study. All control subjects had NF-1, normal neuroimaging, and a complete ophthalmologic evaluation no more than 2 years before entry, and were matched for age (±6 months) and gender.

Table II. Growth and maturation in children with optic pathway tumors and paired control subjects

	OPT	No OPT
Height (cm)	118.0 (93.4-135.3)	106.0 (93.2-124.5)
Height standard score	−0.69 (−1.5-2.12)	−1.13 (−2.71-0.46)
Bone age–height age (yr)	−0.055 (−2.06-3.03)	−0.88 (−2.17-0.50)
Mid-parental height (cm)	163.7 (152.0-173.5)	165.0 (157.3-172.6)

Values are expressed as median (range); the two pairs of subjects in which one member of the pair had a pubertal LH-RH response are excluded.

The study protocol was approved by the institutional review board of the Children's Memorial Institute for Education and Research and was conducted at the Northwestern University Medical School Clinical Research Center. Signed, informed consent was obtained from one or both parents of each subject. The following data were obtained from each subject: stadiometer height, weight, Tanner stage, parental heights, radiograph of the left hand and wrist for bone age, and gonadotropin levels. Height standard scores were calculated by the anthropometric program of the Centers for Disease Control and Prevention.[12] Bone ages were derived with the method of Tanner et al.[13] by an investigator who was unaware of the clinical history.

Pituitary gonadotropin response to LH-RH was determined after intravenous injection of 100 μg LH-RH (gonadorelin hydrochloride [Factrel]). Serum samples for determination of LH and follicle-stimulating hormone were obtained before injection of LH-RH and 15, 30, 45, and 60 minutes after injection. Testosterone was measured in boys and estradiol in girls before LH-RH injection and 60 minutes after injection. We measured LH by a standard double-antibody radioimmunoassay to the LH β-subunit (Amerlex LH RIA Kit, Amersham Corp., Arlington Heights, Ill.). The lower limit of sensitivity of this assay is 2.5 mIU/ml. Using this assay, our laboratory has established that a peak LH level >20 mIU/ml is a pubertal response to LH-RH. The LH was also measured with a new, very sensitive LH immunochemiluminometric assay (normal range, 0.02 to 0.3 mIU/ml),[14] which allows improved discrimination between unstimulated prepubertal and pubertal LH levels. The FSH, testosterone, and estradiol levels were measured by radioimmunoassay with established methods.

RESULTS

Two hundred nineteen children with NF-1 were examined during the period of study, and precocious puberty was

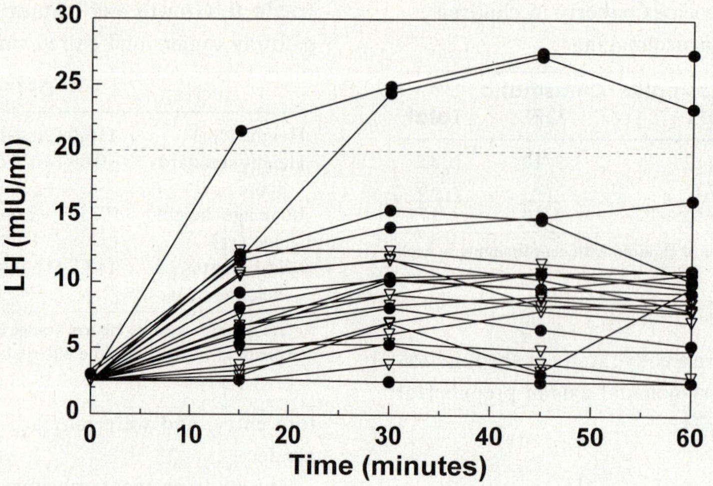

Figure. Serum LH levels (measured by radioimmunoassay) after intravenous injection of 100 μg LH-RH in 11 children with OPTs *(dark circles)* and their age- and sex-matched control subjects *(clear triangles)*.

diagnosed in seven of them (3%). All seven children who had precocious puberty had abnormal LH-RH test results. Of the 219 children, 171 underwent neuroimaging. All the children with precocious puberty had tumors involving the optic chiasm (Table I); they represented 39% of children with chiasmal tumors (95% confidence interval, 17% to 64%). Fifty-seven percent of the children without OPTs and 64% of the children with OPTs were younger than the cutoff age for precocious puberty (8 years for girls, 9 years for boys) when last seen in the clinic, and precocious puberty could conceivably still develop. The male/female ratio was 5:2 among children with precocious puberty, and 11:22 among children with OPTs (Fisher Exact Test; $p = 0.145$).

Eleven prepubertal children with OPTs who were between the ages of 2 and 10 years (9 girls and 2 boys), and their age- and sex-matched control subjects were examined prospectively. None of the children without an OPT had a pubertal LH response to LH-RH. Two boys with OPTs had pubertal LH responses (Figure). In one, the tumor was confined to the optic chiasm, and an accelerated growth rate was noted at the time of evaluation; no other clinical signs of puberty were apparent. The other boy, who was 9.9 years of age at the time of testing, had a tumor confined to the intraorbital portion of the optic nerve. During the next 6 months he underwent normal pubertal maturation.

Basal serum LH concentrations in the two boys with pubertal LH responses to LH-RH were ≤2.5 mIU/ml, the lower limit of assay sensitivity by radioimmunoassay, similar to those in the prepubertal subjects. When the same specimens were analyzed by the LH-ICMA method, basal LH concentrations were elevated only in these same two boys (0.76 and 0.88 mIU/ml, respectively). Peak LH-ICMA concentrations in response to LH-RH in these two subjects were 12.0 and 13.0 mIU/ml, compared with 1.9 ± 0.8 mIU/ml (mean ± SD; range, 0.6 to 4.0 mIU/ml) in the prepubertal children.

Testosterone concentration was >10 ng/dl only in the two boys with pubertal LHRH responses. Estradiol levels were <0.5 ng/dl in all girls. The FSH levels did not differ in children with OPTs, in comparison with those in their matched control subjects (analysis of variance, $p > 0.05$).

The mid-parental height for children with OPTs did not differ from that for control subjects (paired *t* test, $p = 0.87$). The median height of children with OPTs (excluding the two pubertal children) was 118 cm, and the median height of the control subjects was 106 cm (paired *t* test comparing height standard scores, $p = 0.09$; Table II). There was no significant difference in the discrepancy between bone age and height age.

DISCUSSION

The main finding of this study is that precocious puberty was found exclusively in those children with NF-1 who had OPTs involving the optic chiasm. Previous reports of this association in the absence of OPTs may have erroneously included children with McCune-Albright syndrome, in whom café au lait spots and precocious puberty may also occur. Saxena[3] reported two examples of precocious puberty occurring in NF-1 without tumors of the optic chiasm, but neither computed tomography nor magnetic resonance imaging was available at that time, which leaves open the possibility of undetected tumors. Laue et al.[4] described four children with NF-1 and precocious puberty, three of whom had optic gliomas. No information is given as to how the absence of a tumor was conclusively proved in the fourth child.

Precocious puberty occurred in 3% of our entire population of children with NF-1, markedly greater than its incidence in the general population of about 0.06%.[15,16] Precocious puberty developed in 39% of the children with NF-1 who had tumors of the optic chiasm; this may underrepresent the true incidence, because many of the children in whom precocious puberty may develop are still very young. We believe that these figures are generalizable and that our children with NF-1 are representative of the NF-1 population at large, because most were referred because of the presence of multiple café au lait spots rather than for the more serious complications. In addition, 76% of the OPTs were discovered by screening neuroimaging rather than by the presence of symptoms.[8, 10] These data indicate that such children should be followed very closely for the early signs of puberty, such as linear growth acceleration. We were able to identify one subject with precocious puberty before the development of obvious clinical signs. Conversely, we previously described two children with NF-1 in whom such signs led to the discovery of tumors of the optic chiasm.[17]

The relationship of precocious puberty to the exact location of the tumor is unknown and has not been commented on in previous studies. All the children with clinical precocious puberty in our study had tumors involving the optic chiasm. Although almost half of our patients with optic pathway gliomas had tumors confined to the optic nerves, precocious puberty developed in none of them. This observation is consistent with the currently accepted theory that lesions located near the hypothalamus interfere with tonic central nervous system inhibition of the hypothalamic-pituitary-gonadal axis, resulting in the premature onset of puberty.[18, 19] However, one of the two patients with a pubertal LH-RH test was a 9-year-old boy with a glioma confined to the intraorbital optic nerve; puberty developed shortly after study completion. Although his age- and sex-matched control subject did not have a pubertal response to LH-RH, this boy's relatively early entrance into puberty may have been physiologic rather than the result of the tumor.

Previous studies of precocious puberty have involved children who already had clinical manifestations of puberty. The earliest hormonal manifestations of precocious puberty have never been studied. We identified two children in whom the development of precocious puberty was a risk because of the presence of OPTs; before obvious pubertal signs developed, these children had pubertal LH responses to LH-RH, elevated basal LH-ICMA concentrations, and elevated levels of testosterone. In contrast, none of the control children had abnormal LH-RH tests. Thus the preponderance of evidence is that the precocious onset of puberty is due to the presence of OPTs rather than to NF-1 itself.

We conclude that precocious puberty is found exclusively in children with NF-1 who have OPTs involving the optic chiasm. Precocious puberty will develop in at least 39% of such children. With the use of a highly sensitive LH assay, biochemical evidence of premature activation of the hypothalamic-pituitary-gonadal axis may be found before overt signs of puberty, without the need for provocative testing with LH-RH. Children with NF-1 who have OPTs should be followed closely for signs of premature sexual development.

We thank Mark Stene, PhD, of Endocrine Sciences, for the LH-ICMA measurements.

REFERENCES

1. Listernick R, Charrow J. Neurofibromatosis type 1 in childhood. J PEDIATR 1990;116:845-53.
2. Riccardi VM. Type 1 neurofibromatosis and the pediatric patient. Curr Probl Pediatr 1992;22:66-106.
3. Saxena KM. Endocrine manifestations of neurofibromatosis in children. Am J Dis Child 1970;120:265-71.
4. Laue L, Comite F, Hench K, Loriaux L, Cutler GB, Pescovitz OH. Precocious puberty associated with neurofibromatosis and optic gliomas. Am J Dis Child 1985;139:1097-100.
5. Tertsch D, Schoen R, Ulrich FE, et al. Pubertas praecox in neurofibromatosis of the optic chiasm. Acta Neurochir Suppl (Wien) 1979;28(suppl):413-5.
6. Brauner R, Malandry F, Rappaport R, et al. Growth and endocrine disorders in optic glioma. Eur J Pediatr 1990;149:825-8.
7. Iraci G, Gerosa M, Scanarini M, et al. Anterior optic gliomas with precocious or pseudoprecocious puberty. Childs Brain 1980;7:314-24.
8. Listernick R, Charrow J, Greenwald M, Mets M. The national history of optic pathway tumors in children with neurofibromatosis type 1: a longitudinal study. J PEDIATR 1994;125: 63-6.
9. National Institutes of Health Consensus Development Conference Statement: Neurofibromatosis. Bethesda, Maryland: The Institute, 1987:6.
10. Listernick R, Charrow J, Greenwald MJ, Esterly NA. Optic gliomas in children with neurofibromatosis type 1. J PEDIATR 1989;114:788-92.
11. Tanner JM. Growth at adolescence. Oxford: Blackwell, 1962.
12. CDC anthropometric software package, edition 3.0. Atlanta, Georgia: Centers for Disease Control, 1987.
13. Tanner JM, Whitehouse RH, Cameron N, Marshall WA, Healy MJR, Goldstein H. Assessment of skeletal maturity and prediction of adult height (TW2 method). 2nd ed. London: Academic Press, 1983.
14. Stene MA, Mayes D, Neely EK, Wilson DM. Usefulness of highly sensitive chemiluminescent gonadotropin assays in the diagnosis and treatment of central precocious puberty [Abstract]. Endocrinology 1993;132(suppl):92A.
15. Marshall WA, Tanner JM. Variations in pattern of pubertal changes in girls. Arch Dis Child 1969;44:291-303.
16. Marshall WA, Tanner JM. Variation in the pattern of pubertal changes in boys. Arch Dis Child 1970;45:13-23.
17. Listernick R, Charrow J, Greenwald M. Emergence of optic pathway gliomas in children with neurofibromatosis type 1 after normal neuroimaging results. J PEDIATR 1992;121: 584-7.
18. Grumbach MM, Kaplan SL. The neuroendocrinology of human puberty: an ontogenetic perspective. In: Grumbach MM, Sizonenko PC, Aubert ML, eds. Control of the onset of puberty. Baltimore: Williams & Wilkins, 1990:1-68.
19. Stein DT. Southwestern Internal Medicine Conference. New developments in the diagnosis and treatment of sexual precocity. Am J Med Sci 1992;303:53-71.

Immunologic characterization of children vertically infected with human immunodeficiency virus, with slow or rapid disease progression

Alessandra Viganó, MD, Nicola Principi, MD, Maria Luisa Villa, MD, Chiara Riva, PharmD, Lina Crupi, MD, Daria Trabattoni, BS, Gene M. Shearer, PhD, and Mario Clerici, MD

From the Cattedra di Pediatria IV, H. L. Sacco, Milan, Italy, the Cattedra di Immunologia, and the Clinica delle Malattie Infettive, Universitá degli Studi di Milan, Milan, Italy, and the Experimental Immunology Branch, National Cancer Institute, National Institutes of Health, Bethesda, Maryland

Cytokine production of unstimulated and mitogen-stimulated peripheral blood mononuclear cells of 31 children vertically infected with human immunodeficiency virus type 1 (HIV) and with different patterns of disease progression was evaluated to establish possible correlations between the immunologic and the clinical findings. Production of interferon gamma and interleukin-2 (type 1 cytokines), and of interleukin-4 and interleukin-10 (type 2 cytokines), was analyzed in seven symptom-free patients (Centers for Disease Control and Prevention class P-1B), 10 patients with mild symptoms (class P-2A), and 14 patients with severe symptoms (class P-2B-F). Cytokine production was compared with that of 10 age- and sex-matched control subjects who were seronegative for HIV. The HIV-infected patients produced significantly fewer type 1 cytokines and significantly more type 2 cytokines than the uninfected control subjects. No differences in the production of interferon gamma and interleukin-2 were detected among the different clinical categories of HIV-infected patients. In contrast, interleukin-4 production was augmented in the patients with class P-2A (*p* <0.05) and class P-2B-F HIV infection (*p* <0.03), in comparison with the children with class P-1B infection. The increase in interleukin-4 production was paralleled by an increase in the number of children with hyperimmunoglobulinemia E in each of the clinical groups (0% in class P-1B; 40% in class P-2A; and 71% in class P-2 B-F infection). Similarly, interleukin-10 production was increased both in patients with class P-2A and in those with class P-2B-F infection, in comparison with the children with class P-1B disease (*p* <0.006 and <0.04, respectively). These data indicate (1) that vertically acquired HIV infection results in decreased production of type 1 cytokines and in increased production of type 2 cytokines, and (2) that an increased production of type 2 cytokines correlates with hyperimmunoglobulinemia E and is present in, and may be characteristic of, the symptomatic phases of childhood HIV infection. (J PEDIATR 1995;126:368-74)

Supported by grants from Istituto Superiore di Sanitá "VI Progetto AIDS 1993 and VII Progetto AIDS 1994," Nos. 9202-11, 9204-31, and 9206-09.

Submitted for publication July 11, 1994; accepted Sept. 26, 1994.

Reprint requests: Mario Clerici, MD, Cattedra di Immunologia, Universitá degli Studi di Milano, Via Venezian, 1, 20133 Milan, Italy.

9/20/60908

Infection with the human immunodeficiency virus type 1 in adults can result in different clinical outcomes.[1] The majority of adult patients with HIV seropositivity progress toward the acquired immunodeficiency syndrome, but a minority do not have signs of disease and maintain stable CD4+ lymphocyte counts.[1] Vertically (i.e., perinatally) acquired HIV infection can cause either extremely rapid symptomatic disease, with death in early childhood,[2, 3] or a chronic condition with varying patterns of disease.[4-9] The factors that influence the evolution of HIV infection, and therefore determine the natural history of the disease in each patient, are currently unknown but are likely to include both viral factors and host factors.

Two of us (M.C. and G.M.S.) recently proposed the hypothesis that cell-mediated immunity could be more protective than humoral immunity in the progression of HIV infection.[10, 11] CMI is stimulated mainly through the production of the type 1 cytokines interferon gamma, interleukin-2, and IL-12, whereas humoral immunity is enhanced mainly through the production of IL-4, IL-5, IL-6, and IL-10.[12-14] Because of the cross-regulatory properties of some of these cytokines, the production of type 1 and type 2 cytokines can be mutually exclusive.[15, 16] On the basis of a series of observations,[17-27] we proposed that a strong type-1–weak type-2 cytokine production pattern would be associated with a slower progression of HIV infection.[10, 11] Thus we decided to measure mitogen-stimulated production of type 1 and type 2 cytokines in a cohort of vertically infected children surviving after early childhood with slow or rapid progression of HIV disease.

See related article, p. 375.

AIDS	Acquired immunodeficiency syndrome
CMI	Cell-mediated immunity
ELISA	Enzyme-linked immunosorbent assay
HIV	Human immunodeficiency virus (type 1)
IFN-γ	Interferon gamma
IL	Interleukin
NS	Not significant
PBMC	Peripheral blood mononuclear cells
PCD	Programmed cell death
PHA	Phytohemagglutinin

METHODS

Selection of patients. Thirty-one children infected vertically with HIV, aged 44 months to 12 years, were studied. The diagnosis of HIV infection was based on the detection of serum HIV-specific IgG antibodies by ELISAs and a positive Western blot test result. The clinical status of the 31 children was defined according to the Centers for Disease Control and Prevention (CDC) classification for children on the basis of all symptoms evident at the time of the study.[28] All the children in the class P-2 categories (subclasses A to F) were receiving antiretroviral therapy at the time of the study, as follows: children with class P-2A infection received zidovudine, 600 mg/m^2 per day, and children with class P-2B-F infection received zidovudine, 600 mg/m^2 per day, or didanosine, 270 mg/m^2 per day. These same children were also treated with immune globulins (Immuno Sandoz, 400 mg/kg per month). During the 4 weeks before evaluation, none of the children had any evidence of opportunistic and bacterial infections.

Ten children without HIV infection (aged 8.2 ± 1.3 years), matched by sex to those in the experimental group and admitted to pediatric department IV, University of Milan, for minor surgical procedures, were used as healthy control subjects. Informed consent was obtained by the parents or legal guardians of the patients and of the healthy children.

Processing of blood. Whole blood from HIV-infected individuals and uninfected control subjects was drawn by venipuncture in Vacutainer tubes containing heparin (Becton Dickinson and Co., Rutherford, N.J.). Peripheral blood mononuclear cells were separated by flotation on lymphocyte separation medium (LSM; Organon Teknika Corp., Durham, N.C.), washed twice in phosphate-buffered saline solution, and resuspended at 3×10^6/ml in RPMI 1640 culture medium (Gibco Laboratories, Grand Island, N.Y.) containing 0.5% penicillin, 0.5% streptomycin, 1% glutamine and HEPES biologic buffer (*N*-hydroxyethylpiperazine–*N*′-ethanesulfonic acid), 10 mmol/L. Viable cell counts were determined by trypan blue exclusion.

Lymphocyte subsets and immunoglobulin concentrations. The determination of lymphocyte subsets was based on results of immunofluorescence assays. The levels of serum IgG, IgA, and IgM were determined by immunoturbidimetry (Specific Instruments, Kone, Helsinki, Finland) after antigen-antibody complex formation (Orion Antibodies antisera, Helsinki, Finland). The serum concentrations of IgE were determined by immunocapture (CAP System IgE radioimmunoassay; Pharmacia, Uppsala, Sweden). The reference values for normal immunoglobulin concentrations during childhood were based on previously published data.[29, 30]

Production of IFN-γ, IL-2, IL-4, and IL-10. The ability of PBMC to produce mitogen-stimulated IL-2, IL-4, IL-10, and IFN-γ was determined by culturing PBMC, 3×10^6/well, in 24-well LINBRO plates (Flow Laboratories, Inc., McLean, Va.) at 37° C in a moist, 7% carbon dioxide atmosphere. PBMC either were unstimulated or were stimulated with phytohemagglutinin diluted 1:100 (Gibco). The cultures were also supplemented with 5% pooled AB+ hu-

Table I. Demographic and laboratory characteristics of 31 HIV-infected children

	Clinical status according to CDC classification		
Characteristics	**Class P-1B**	**Class P-2A**	**Class P-2B-F**
Gender ratio (M/F)	2/5	3/7	8/6
Age (yr)			
Mean (SD)	8.7 (2.9)	5.6 (1.3)	7.4 (1.7)
Range	3.6-11	4.0-6.8	4.6-11.0
$CD4^+$ cell count (cells/mm³)			
Mean (SD)	629 (138)	724 (297)	295 (267)
Range	428-824	394-1278	22-879
$CD8^+$ cell count (cells/mm³)			
Mean (SD)	916 (358)	1271 (546)	1295 (1170)
Range	591-1654	452-1933	40-1951
$CD4^+/CD8^+$ ratio			
Mean (SD)	0.70 (0.31)	0.70 (0.53)	0.31 (0.30)
Range	0.40-1.20	0.20-1.2	0.006-0.80

man serum or plasma (Sigma Diagnostics, St. Louis, Mo.). Supernatants were harvested after 48 hours of culture, because kinetic studies indicated that 48 hours was the optimal time for assessing lymphokine production. Supernatants were frozen and stored at −20° C until assayed for cytokine production. The production of PHA-stimulated cytokine was evaluated with commercially available ELISA assays as follows: for IFN-γ, human IFN-γ (Intertest γ; Genzyme, Cambridge, Mass.); for IL-2, human IL-2 (Quantikine; R&D Systems, Inc., Minneapolis, Minn.); for IL-4, human IL-4 (Intertest-4; Genzyme); and for IL-10, human IL-10 ELISA (Bender MedSystems, Vienna, Austria). The procedures suggested by the manufacturers were followed. Values for all the cytokines were calculated from a standard curve of the corresponding recombinant human cytokine according to the instructions of the manufacturers.

Statistical analysis. Statistical analyses were performed with a Macintosh computer (Macintosh, Cupertino, Calif.) and with the Microsoft Excel version 4.0 analysis program (Microsoft Co., Redmond, Wash.). The analytic procedures followed were based on a t test for two samples, with equal variances assumed. All the values shown are derived from the results of a two-tailed statistical analysis.

RESULTS

Demographic and clinical laboratory characterization of children with HIV infection. Of the 31-HIV-infected children, 7 were considered to have CDC class P-1B infection (asymptomatic infection and abnormal immune function); 10 were considered to have CDC class P-2A infection (presence of moderate, nonspecific general symptoms); and 14 were considered to have CDC class P-2B-F infection (severe manifestations). There were no significant differences with regard to age between children in CDC class P-1B and those in class P-2B-F. In contrast, patients in CDC class P-2A were younger than those in the two previous groups (P-2A vs P-1B: $p < 0.01$ by two-tailed Student t test; P-2A vs P-2B-F: $p < 0.01$) (Table I).

Whereas no differences were detected in $CD8^+$ lymphocyte counts among the three CDC classes of HIV-infected children, the $CD4^+$ lymphocytes counts were significantly reduced in the patients in CDC class P-2B-F compared with both patients in CDC class P-1B and those in class P-2A (P-2B-F vs P-1B: $p < 0.005$; P-2B-F vs P-2A: $p < 0.001$). Finally, the $CD4^+/CD8^+$ ratios were significantly reduced in the class P-2B-F group compared with both the class P-1B and the class P-2A groups (P-2B-F vs P-1B: $p < 0.01$; P-2B-F vs P-2A: $p < 0.003$) (Table I).

Analysis of type 1 cytokine production by PBMC from HIV-infected individuals and from uninfected control subjects. The mean amount of IFN-γ produced by each of the groups was as follows: uninfected control group, 71 pg/ml; P-1B group, 54.2 pg/ml (control vs P-1B group: $p < 0.05$ by two-tailed Student t test); P-2A group, 17.9 pg/ml (control vs P-2A group: $p < 0.001$; P-1B vs P-2A group: not significant); and P-2B-F group, 27.8 pg/ml (control vs P-2B-F group: $p < 0.02$; P-1B vs P-2B-F group: NS; P-2A vs P-2B-F group: NS). The mean amount of IL-2 produced by each of the groups was as follows: control group, 72 pg/ml; P-1B group, 18 pg/ml (control vs P-1B group: $p < 0.02$); P-2A group, 25.1 pg/ml (control group vs P-2A group: $p < 0.03$; P-1B vs P-2A group: NS); and P-2B-F, 33.4 pg/ml (control vs P-2B-F group: $p < 0.04$; P-1B vs P-2B-F group: NS; P-2A vs P-2B-F group: NS) (Figure). All the HIV-infected clinical groups produced a decreased amount of both IFN-γ and IL-2, in comparison with values for the control group. No differences were evident when the mean production of IFN-γ and IL-2 by symptom-free children with seropositivity for HIV was compared with that by the infected patients with symptoms.

Analysis of type 2 cytokine production by PBMC from HIV-infected individuals and uninfected control subjects. The mean amount of IL-4 produced by each of the groups was as follows: control group, 53.5 pg/ml; P-1B group, 143.1 pg/ml (control vs P-1B group: $p < 0.001$); P-2A group, 254.4 pg/ml (control vs P-2A group: $p < 0.0004$; P-1B vs P-2A group: $p < 0.05$); and P-2B-F group, 298.4 pg/ml (control vs P-2B-F group: $p < 0.0001$; P-1B vs P-2B-F group: $p < 0.03$; P-2A vs P-2B-F group: NS). The mean amount of IL-10 produced by each of the groups was as follows: control group, 51.1 pg/ml; P-1B group, 30.1 pg/ml (control vs P-1B group: NS); P-2A group, 114.7 pg/ml (control vs P-2A group: NS; P-1B vs P-2A group: $p < 0.04$);

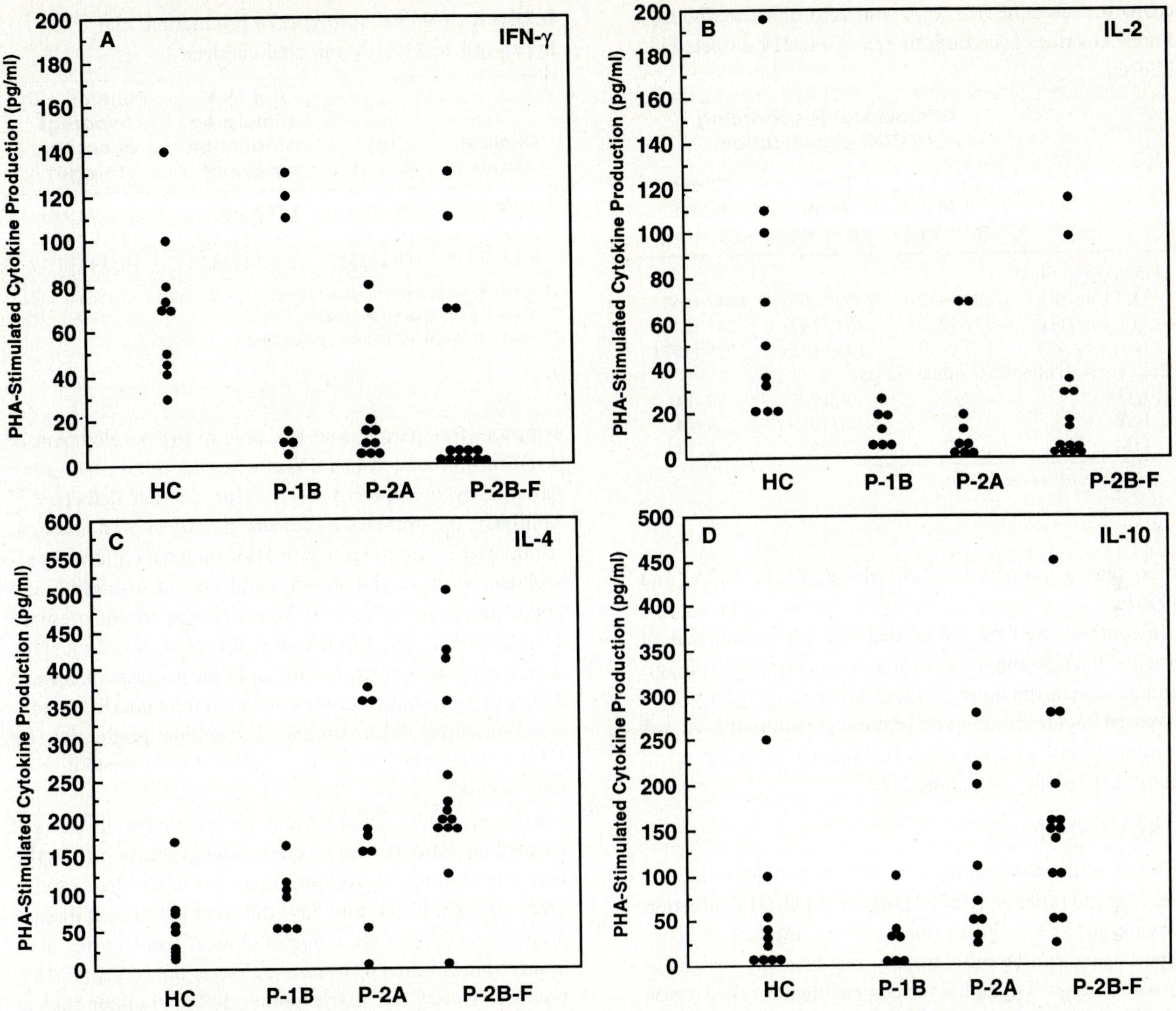

Figure. PHA-stimulated cytokine production by PBMC from 10 uninfected control subjects *(HC)*, or from 31 HIV-infected individuals with CDC classification as follows: P-1B (n = 7); P-2A (n = 10); or P-2B-F (n = 14). Each *dark circle* represents the results obtained from one individual. Values for IFN-γ **(panel A)**, IL-2 **(panel B)**, IL-4 **(panel C)**, and IL-10 **(panel D)** are shown.

and P-2B-F group, 163.3 pg/ml (control vs P-2B-F group: $p < 0.01$; P-1B vs P-2B-F group: $p < 0.006$; P-2A vs P-2B-F group: NS) (Figure). All the HIV-infected clinical groups produced significantly increased amounts of IL-4 in comparison with the healthy control group; the production of IL-10 by the P-2B-F group, but not that by the P-2A or the P-1B group, was significantly increased in comparison with that of the healthy control group. There was a gradual augmentation in both IL-4 and IL-10 production that paralleled the worsening of clinical conditions; the most severely diseased patients had a slightly greater than twofold increase in IL-4 production, and a slightly greater than fivefold increase in IL-10 production, above that of the symptom-free patients with seropositivity for HIV.

Analysis of changes in the serum levels of immunoglobulins in HIV-infected pediatric patients. As shown in Table II, no significant differences were detected between HIV-infected children in the three CDC classes with respect to serum levels of IgG, IgM, and IgA. Whereas most children had increased concentrations of serum IgG in comparison with the normal values for each given age group, fewer had increases in the serum concentrations of IgM and IgA. Nevertheless, the proportion of children with abnormally elevated serum concentrations of IgG, IgM, and IgA did not

Table II. Levels of IgG, IgA, and IgM and fraction of abnormal values according to age in 31 HIV-infected children

	Clinical status according to CDC classification		
	Class P-1B (n = 7)	Class P-2A (n = 10)	Class P-2B-F (n = 14)
Immunoglobulins*			
IgG (mg/dl)	2291 (422)	2309 (600)	1842 (661)
IgA (mg/dl)	231 (220)	264 (147)	247 (215)
IgM (mg/dl)	189 (150)	195 (182)	165 (177)
Patients with abnormal values for age			
IgG	7/7	9/10	10/14
IgA	2/7	6/10	8/14
IgM	2/7	3/10	5/14

*Values expressed as mean (SD).

differ among patients in CDC classes P-1B, P-2A, and P-2B-F.

In contrast, we detected an increase in the incidence of patients having abnormally high concentrations of IgE compared with the normal values for that age group. The increased incidence of hyperimmunoglobulinemia E was correlated both with the clinical stage and with the mean concentration of IL-4 (Table III).

DISCUSSION

Better understanding of viral and immunologic factors that relate to rapid or delayed progression of HIV infection has emerged as an urgent priority.[1-9] The immune response to pathogens can be differentially regulated by two functionally distinct T-lymphocyte compartments called "type 1," which mainly induce CMI through the production of IFN-γ, IL-2, and IL-12, and "type 2," which primarily activate B lymphocytes and the generation of antibodies through the production of IL-4, IL-5, IL-6, and IL-10.[12-16] Additionally, because some of these cytokines have cross-regulatory properties, the production of type 1 and type 2 cytokines, and hence CMI and humoral immunity, can be preferentially stimulated.[15, 16] We therefore evaluated the relative efficacy of CMI and humoral responses by measuring the production of IFN-γ and IL-2, and of IL-4 and IL-10, respectively. Thus we observed that HIV infection in adults is characterized by decreased production of IL-2[17] accompanied by increased production of both IL-4[19] and IL-10[21]; others have shown that IL-12[18] is diminished and IL-6[31] is augmented. Although detected by in vitro assays, these findings have important clinical implications. The decline in CD4$^+$ lymphocyte counts, the duration of the symptom-free period, and the time to the development of AIDS are predicted in HIV-infected, symptom-free adult patients by the severity of IL-2 production defects.[23, 24] Similarly, the presence of defects in antigen- and mitogen-stimulated IL-2 production in HIV-infected children is associated with an increased incidence of bacterial and opportunistic infection.[25, 26] To verify whether the presence of a dominant type 1 cytokine profile over type 2 cytokine profile could be a protective factor in the progression toward AIDS in symptom-free, HIV-infected individuals, we analyzed in vitro PHA-stimulated cytokine production by HIV-infected pediatric patients with slow or rapid disease progression.

Table III. Clinical status, IL-4 production, and hyper-IgE in 31 HIV-infected children

Clinical status	IgE (KIU/L)*	IL-4 PHA-stimulated production (pg/ml)*	Patients with hyper-IgE according to age†
P-1B	43 (16)	143.1 (38)	0/7 (0%)
P-2A	102 (52)	254.4 (125.8)	4/10 (40%)
P-2B-F	369 (153)	298.4 (128.7)	10/14 (71%)

Hyper-IgE, Hyperimmunoglobulinemia E; *KIU*, kilo international units.
*Values expressed as mean (SD).
†Values expressed as fraction (percentage).

Previous studies[2, 3] of perinatally infected children have focused on patients with a severe clinical course during the first years of life. A substantial number of children survive after early childhood and have different patterns of disease progression.[7, 8] A wide range of clinical features has been observed in children who survived longer than 5 years[9]: 15% were completely free of symptoms, 30% had minor clinical manifestations, and 55% had severe disease, with 30% of them meeting the definition for AIDS. The definition of rapid or slow disease progression in HIV-infected adults is based on the slope of decline in CD4$^+$ lymphocyte counts and on the presence of AIDS-defining conditions. A similar definition of childhood AIDS is not yet well delineated, because standards for T-lymphocyte subsets based on percentiles are available only for the first 4 years of life.[32] Because all the children in this study were older than 4 years of age, their classification as rapid or slow progressors was based on clinical manifestations. Nevertheless, the mean age was comparable in the symptom-free P-1A group and in the P-2B-F group, whose symptoms were severe, and the CD4$^+$ lymphocyte counts were significantly lower in the group with symptomatic infection.

We report here that (1) production of IL-2, but not of IFN-γ, is reduced in HIV-infected patients compared with that in uninfected control subjects, but is not significantly different among HIV-infected patients with and without symptoms; (2) IL-4 production by all groups of HIV-infected children is increased compared with that by control subjects; (3) IL-10 production by children with class P-2B-F infection is increased compared with that by control subjects; and (4) children with symptomatic P-2A and P-2B-F infection produce augmented quantities of PHA-stimulated IL-4 and IL-10 compared with symptom-free P-1B patients. Thus the healthy control subjects differ from HIV-infected children because the control individuals produce higher levels of type 1 cytokines and lower amounts of type 2 cytokines, whereas vertically infected patients with symptomatic disease differ from symptom-free patients in that the patients with symptoms have augmented production of the type 2 cytokines, IL-4 and IL-10. The defective production of type 1 cytokines in children with P-1B asymptomatic infection is in agreement with previous data[25] and could be a characteristic feature of vertically acquired HIV infection. The observed differences in cytokine production are not dependent on age differences—the ages of the healthy control subjects and of the patients with P-1B and the P-2B-F infection were comparable. Furthermore, these differences are not due to the immaturity of the immune response; T lymphocytes and antigen-presenting cells are fully functional by 24 months after birth, and none of our patients was younger than 2 years of age.[33]

Increased levels of IgE have been recognized as an unfavorable prognostic factor in both adult[34, 35] and childhood[36] HIV infection. IL-4 is the main cytokine favoring the isotopic switch from IgG to IgE,[37] and, as expected, we observed that the increase in PHA-stimulated IL-4 production, which parallels the worsening of clinical classification, was reflected by an increase of hyperimmunoglobulinemia E. Therefore the characterization of vertically infected patients with symptoms appears to include both the augmented production of IL-4 and IL-10, and the presence of hyperimmunoglobulinemia E.

The dominant production of type 2 cytokines in children with symptomatic infection could theoretically account for a more rapid progression to AIDS in at least two ways. The PBMC of HIV-infected patients are particularly susceptible to programmed cell death after antigen recognition through their T cell receptor.[38, 39] We recently observed that the in vitro addition of exogenous type 1 cytokines—IFN-γ, IL-2, and IL-12—blocks T-lymphocyte PCD; in contrast, two type 2 lymphokines, IL-4 and IL-10, enhance in vitro T cell PCD.[40] Therefore an increase in the concentration of type 2 cytokines could induce increased PCD, resulting in a more rapid reduction in $CD4^+$ cells in children with symptomatic HIV infection. Furthermore, augmented secretion of type 2 cytokines could have a stimulating effect on HIV replication because the combination of IL-4 and IL-10 enhances in vitro HIV replication in a monocytic cell line.[41]

We conclude that there is an imbalance in type 1 and type 2 cytokine production in HIV-infected children. We also identified a correlation between faster disease progression and both augmented IL-4 and IL-10 production and the presence of hyperimmunoglobulinemia E. On the basis of these results, we suggest that in both childhood and adult HIV infection, therapy for the purpose of counteracting the effects of type 2 cytokines might enhance T-cell immunity,[42] resulting in clinical immunologic benefit for the patients.

We are grateful to Prof. Massimo Galli, Dr. Claudia Balotta, and the staff of the Laboratorio della Clinica delle Malattie Infettive, Universitá degli Studi di Milano, Milan, Italy, for helpful discussions and continuous support.

REFERENCES

1. Levy JA. HIV pathogenesis and long-term survival. AIDS 1993;7:1401-10.
2. Blanche S, Rouzioux C, Guihard Moscato ML, et al. A prospective study of infants born to women seropositive for human immunodeficiency virus type 1. N Engl J Med 1989;320:1643-8.
3. Scott GB, Hutto C, Mackuch RW, et al. Survival in children with perinatally acquired human immunodeficiency virus type 1 infection. N Engl J Med 1989;321:1791-6.
4. Blanche S, Tardieu M, Duliega AM, et al. Longitudinal study of 94 HIV symptomatic infants with materno-foetal HIV infection: evidence for a bimodal expression of clinical and biological symptoms. Am J Dis Child 1990;144:1210-5.
5. Auger I, Thomas P, De Gruttola V, et al. Incubation period for pediatric AIDS patients. Nature 1988;336:575-7.
6. Johnson JP, Nair P, Hines SE, et al. Natural history and serologic diagnosis of infants born to human immunodeficiency virus–infected women. Am J Dis Child 1989;143:1147-53.
7. Thomas P, Singh T, Williams R, Blum S. Trends in survival for children with maternally transmitted acquired immunodeficiency syndrome in New York City, 1982–1989. Pediatr Infect Dis J 1992;11:34-9.
8. Tovo PA, de Martino M, Gabiano C, et al. Prognostic factors and survival in children with perinatal HIV-1 infection. Lancet 1992;339:1249-53.
9. Italian Register for HIV Infection in Children. Features of children perinatally infected with HIV-1 surviving longer than 5 years. Lancet 1994;343:191-5.
10. Clerici M, Shearer GM. Is HIV associated with a TH1→TH2 switch? Immunol Today 1993;14:107-11.
11. Clerici M. Immune responses to HIV. AIDS 1993;7:S135-41.
12. Mossmann TR, Coffman RI. Two types of mouse T helper cell clone: implications for immune regulation. Immunol Today 1987;8:223-6.
13. Mossmann TR, Coffman RI. TH1 and TH2 cells: different pattern of lymphokine secretion lead to different functional properties. Annu Rev Immunol 1989;7:145-68.

14. Romagnani S. Human TH1 and TH2 subsets: doubt no more. Immunol Today 1991;12:256-7.
15. Fiorentino DF, Bond MW, Mosmann TR. Two types of mouse T helper cell. IV. Th2 clones secrete a factor that inhibits cytokine production by Th1 clones. J Exp Med 1989;170:2081-98.
16. Scott P, Kaufmann SHE. The role of T-cell subsets and cytokines in the regulation of infection. Immunol Today 1991;12: 346-8.
17. Clerici M, Stocks NI, Zajac RA, et al. Detection of three distinct patterns of T helper cell dysfunction in asymptomatic, human immunodeficiency virus–seropositive patients: independence of $CD4^+$ cell numbers and clinical staging. J Clin Invest 1989;84:1892-9.
18. Chehimi J, Trinchieri G, Frank I. IL-12 deficiency in HIV-infected patients. J Exp Med 1994;179:1361-6.
19. Clerici M, Hakim FT, Venzon DJ, et al. Changes in interleukin-2 and interleukin-4 production in asymptomatic, HIV-seropositive individuals. J Clin Invest 1993;91:759-65.
20. Benjamin D, Knobloch TJ, Dayton MA. Human B-cell interleukin-10: B-cell lines derived from patients with AIDS and Burkitt lymphoma constitutively secrete large quantities of interleukin-10. Blood 1992;80:1289-99.
21. Clerici M, Wynn TA, Berzofsky JA, et al. Role of interleukin-10 (IL-10) in T helper cell dysfunction in asymptomatic individuals infected with the human immunodeficiency virus (HIV-1). J Clin Invest 1994;93:768-775.
22. Barcellini W, Rizzardi GP, Borghi MO, et al. TH1 and TH2 cytokine production by peripheral blood mononuclear cells from HIV-infected patients. AIDS 1994;8:757-62.
23. Lucey DR, Melcher GP, Hendrix CW, USAF HIV Study Group. The U.S. Air Force HIV study 1985–1990: immunological analyses, seroconversion and the potential utility of a T-helper functional assay to predict change in $CD4^+$ T-cell counts during early stage HIV infection. J Infect Dis 1991; 164:631-7.
24. Dolan MJ, Melcher GP, Clerici M, Shearer GM. A T cell functional assay combined with measurement of $CD4^+$/$CD29^{bright}$ cells is predictive of death in HIV infection [Abstract WS A 13-4]. XI International Conference on AIDS, Berlin, Germany, June 6-11, 1993.
25. Roilides E, Clerici M, DePalma L, Rubin M, Pizzo PA, Shearer GM. T helper cell responses in children infected with human immunodeficiency virus type 1. J PEDIATR 1991;118: 724-30.
26. Shearer GM, Clerici M. Abnormalities of immune regulation in human immunodeficiency virus infection. Pediat Res 1993;33(suppl):S71-5.
27. Clerici M, Roilides E, Butler KM, et al. Changes in T helper cell function in human immunodeficiency virus infected children during dideoxyinosine therapy as a measure of antiretroviral activity. Blood 1992;80:2196-202.
28. Revision of the CDC surveillance case definition for acquired immunodeficiency syndrome. MMWR 1987;36:1S-15S.
29. Nelson WE. Textbook of pediatrics. Philadelphia: WB Saunders, 1992:1813-4.
30. Bjorksten B, Weeke B. New developments in serum IgE measurement. Allergy 1985;40(suppl IV):117-23.
31. Boue FC, Goujard C, et al. HIV induces IL-6 production by human B lymphocytes: role of IL-4. J Immunol 1992;148: 3661-7.
32. European Collaborative Study. Age-related standards for T lymphocyte subsets based on uninfected children born to HIV-1 infected women. Pediatr Infect Dis J 1992;11: 1018-26.
33. Clerici M, DePalma L, Roilides E, Baker R, Shearer GM. Analysis of T helper and antigen presenting cell functions in cord blood and peripheral blood leukocytes from healthy children of different ages. J Clin Invest 1993;91:2829-36.
34. Wright DN, Nelson RP, Ledford DK, et al. Serum IgE and human immunodeficiency virus (HIV) infection. J Allergy Clin Immunol 1990;85:445-52.
35. Israel-Biet D, Labrousse F, Tourani JM, et al. Elevation of IgE in HIV-infected subjects: a marker of poor prognosis. J Allergy Clin Immunol 1992;89:68-75.
36. Viganó A, Principi N, Crupi L, et al. Elevation of IgE in HIV-infected children and its correlation with the progression of the disease. J Allergy Clin Immunol (in press).
37. Paul WE, Ohara J. B-cell stimulatory factor-1/interleukin 4. Annu Rev Immunol 1987;5:429-60.
38. Ameisen JC, Capron A. Cell dysfunction and depletion in AIDS: the programmed cell death hypothesis. Immunol Today 1991;12:102-6.
39. Kabelitz D, Pohl T, Pechhold T. Activation-induced cell death (apoptosis) of mature peripheral T lymphocytes. Immunol Today 1993;14:338-42.
40. Clerici M, Sarin A, Coffman RL, et al. Type 1/type 2 cytokine modulation of T cell programmed cell death as a model for HIV pathogenesis. Proc Natl Acad Sci (USA) 1994; 91:11811-5.
41. Poli G, Kinter AL, Weismann D, Fauci AS. TH2-specific cytokines IL-4 and IL-10 regulate HIV expression in monocytic cells [Abstract WS A 08-2]. XI International Conference on AIDS. Berlin, Germany, June 6-11, 1993.
42. Cohen J. T cell shift: key to AIDS therapy? Science 1993; 1262:175-6.

Cognitive assessment of school-age children infected with maternally transmitted human immunodeficiency virus type 1

Marc Tardieu, MD, Marie-Jeanne Mayaux, BA, Nathalie Seibel, PsyD, Isabelle Funck-Brentano, PsyD, Elisabeth Straub, PsyD, Jean-Paul Teglas, PhD, and Stéphane Blanche, MD

From the Service de Neurologie, Département de Pédiatrie, the Unité INSERM U292, Hôpital de Bicêtre, and the Unité d'Immuno-Hématologie, Hôpital des Enfants-Malades, Paris, France

Thirty-three children vertically infected with human immunodeficiency virus type 1 (HIV-1), who were born before 1985, were followed in a single center, and had reached the age of 6 years, were studied and tested for school achievement. Of these 33 children, 24 were also tested for cognitive abilities, fine motor and language skills, and emotional adaptation. Of the 33 patients, 22 (67%) had normal school achievement at a mean age of 9.5 ± 1.6 years. The mean IQ was 95 ± 11, but 54% of the patients (13/24) had abnormal results on visual-spatial and time orientation tests, 44% had speech and/or language delay or articulation disorders, and 29% of the children and 42% of the parents had psychoaffective disturbances of intermediate or high severity. Normal school performance was positively correlated with results of the different cognitive tests and to a lesser extent with the absence of psychoaffective symptoms, but was independent of the mode of maternal infection or the parents' educational level. Children with normal school achievement had a higher percentage of circulating $CD4^+$ lymphocytes during the course of infection. We conclude that children whose HIV-1 infection is maternally acquired have better cognitive abilities and school achievement than was initially thought, and that the percentage of circulating $CD4^+$ lymphocytes during the first years of life appears to be predictive of future school adaptation or cognitive abilities. (J Pediatr 1995;126:375-9)

Two thirds of the children infected with human immunodeficiency virus type 1 by mothers with HIV-1 seropositivity are alive and apparently well at the age of 6 years.[1-4] Early reports suggested that they frequently had cognitive impairment and reduced performance at school.[5-12] Our initial experience was not similar: progressive encephalopathy (corresponding to the U.S. Centers for Disease Control and Prevention (CDC) class P-2, subclass B) was usually observed before the age of 3 years, and most patients died before the age of 6 years, whereas patients alive at 6 years

See related article, p. 368.

GAF	Global Assessment of Functioning [Scale]
HIV-1	Human immunodeficiency virus type 1
NEMI	Nouvelle Echelle Métrique de l'Intelligence
WISC-R	Wechsler Intelligence Scale for Children—Revised

Supported by the Agence Nationale de Recherche sur le SIDA (ANRS), and by a grant from the Banque Nationale de Paris.

Submitted for publication April 29, 1994; accepted Sept. 26, 1994.

Reprint requests: Marc Tardieu, MD, Service de Neurologie, Département de Pédiatrie, Hôpital de Bicêtre, 94275 Le Kremlin-Bicêtre Cedex, France.

0022-3476/95/$3.00 + 0 **9/20/60906**

Table I. Clinical and biologic characteristics of the 33 patients

	At first referral	At time of neuropsychologic tests (proposed)	At cutoff date*
Age (mo)	50 ± 25	82 ± 12	114 ± 19
CDC class P-1/P-2, subclass A (%)†	82	58	58
$CD4^+$ lymphocytes (%)	22 ± 16	14 ± 12‡	13 ± 10

Age and percentage of $CD4^+$ lymphocytes expressed as mean ± SD.
*Two children died during the course of the study.
†Percentage of patients in CDC class P-1 or class P-2, subclass A.
‡Of the 33 patients, 9 had less than 5% circulating $CD4^+$ lymphocytes. The p24 titers were highly variable (42% positive; among them the p24 titer was 363 ± 591 pg/ml).

were usually neurologically normal and able to attend elementary school.[1] We consequently decided to evaluate the cognitive abilities, fine motor and language skills, emotional adaptation, and school achievements of all HIV-1–infected children followed in our center who had reached 6 years of age.

METHODS

Study design. All children infected by maternal-fetal transmission of the virus, followed at our center and born before Aug. 31, 1985, were included in the study (n = 57). The children were routinely followed by both an immunologist and a neurologist throughout the study. The usual clinical and biologic evaluations were obtained serially.[1] The time of the first evaluation was recorded, as was the start of antiviral treatment or the time of death.

Among the 57 HIV-1–infected children, 33 were examined. Of the others, 15 died before 6 years of age, 5 either died after 6 years but before the start of the study or were in very poor condition at that time, and 4 were lost to follow-up. Of the 33 patients, 2 died during the course of the study. Evaluations were performed at the end of the 1992–1993 academic year, when the patients were at a mean age of 9.5 ± 1.6 years.

Of the 33 patients, 24 had neurologic, neuropsychologic, language, and psychoaffective evaluations at a mean age of 6.8 ± 1.0 years; the parents of the other 9 refused the formal tests but accepted the clinical and academic evaluation.

Academic achievement. School achievement was evaluated by using regular school reports, examining schoolwork (most of the teachers did not know of the infection), and administering tests to evaluate learning (Borel Maisonny test for reading and spelling[13]; Nouvelle Batterie de Mathématiques for mathematics[14]). Achievement was rated as normal (grade usual for age and performance in the normal range), borderline (poor performance either in normal grade for age or held back 1 year), school failure (held back 2 years or repeated 1 year with very poor achievement, or special education).

Neuropsychologic and language assessments. Three rationales guided the choice of tests and subtests to be given: (1) to use classic tests routinely administered with established standardization for age, (2) to put emphasis on the adaptation and success of children at school, a point of social importance, and (3) to administer all the tests within two 2-hour sessions (one for neuropsychologic evaluation and the other for language evaluation). For these reasons, we chose the Nouvelle Echelle Métrique de l'Intelligence (Stanford-Binet test, third revision)[15-17] to assess the global intellectual level. From the Wechsler Intelligence Scale for Children—Revised (French version) the Similarities and Block Design subtests were administered.[18] The Block Design subtest of the WISC-R, the Bender Visual-Motor Gestalt test,[19] the Rey-Osterrieth Complex Figure test (at and after the age of 8 years), and a general evaluation of the child's strategies during the tests, were used to appraise visual-spatial organization. Temporal orientation was studied with items about concepts of time, some of which are included in the NEMI. Fine motor abilities were studied by the Stamback test[20] and facial motoricity by the Kwint test.[20] Phonologic maturation, expressive and receptive language, and verbal memory were evaluated through the Examen pour l'Evaluation du Langage (with 10 standardized items).[21] Tests were administered by a trained psychologist and a speech therapist. Most of the children took all the tests; in a few cases, one of the subtests was not administered because of fatigue or because the child refused to take it.

Social and psychoaffective evaluation. Psychoaffective evaluation of the children used a semistructured interview with the child and three drawings (a free drawing, a self body image, and a family drawing). The Child Behavior Checklist[22] was used to provide a standardized description, as reported by the parents, of the children's behavioral problems during the previous 6 months. A psychologic evaluation of the parents was also obtained during an interview with them (or with foster parents if the child had been staying at their home for more than 3 years). Any persistent disorder was rated from 90 to 1 according to the Global Assessment of Functioning Scale.[23] The cultural-educational level was determined by the highest academic degree obtained by one of the two parents.

Statistical analysis. Proportions were compared by chi-square analysis or the Fisher Exact Test for cell counts less than 5. The 95% confidence limits for relative risks were es-

Table II. Results of psychometric tests in HIV-1–infected children

Test result	NEMI (n = 24)	WISC-R* Similarities (n = 22)	WISC-R* Block Design (n = 22)	Bender (n = 24)
Mean ± SD	95 ± 11	11 ± 3	9 ± 4	—
No. of children in range†				
Superior range	2	9	8	2
Median range	17	8	2	11
Lower range	4	4	8	11
Pathologic range	1	1	4	

*Maximum score on either WISC-R test = 19.

†Superior range: 25% of the population, score >+0.66 SD; median range: 50% of the population, score between −0.66 and +0.66 SD; lower range: 20% of the population, score between −0.66 and −1.66 SD; pathologic range: 5% of the population score <−1.66 SD (i.e., for the NEMI IQ at, respectively, ≥110, 109 to 91, 90 to 76, and ≤75). For the Bender test: superior, 25% of the population; median, 50%; and inferior, 25%.

timated according to the Mantel-Haenszel method for prospective studies. Quantitative variables are expressed as means ± SD. Nonparametric tests were used to compare means (Wilcoxon test) and to compute the coefficients of correlation (Kendall rank correlation coefficients). All p values were two tailed, and the threshold of significance was set at 0.05. Analysis was performed with software from BMDP Statistical Software, Inc., Los Angeles, Calif.

RESULTS

Medical evaluation. By August 1993, the cutoff date, 58% of the patients were in CDC class P-1/P-2, subclass A and all patients were ambulatory (Table I). Neurologic findings, including head circumference, were normal in 30 patients. One child had, from the age of 5 years, a pseudobulbar syndrome with buccolingual dyspraxia and unexpressive facies. Another had multiple brain metastases of a leimyosarcoma, and one patient had a generalized cytomegalovirus infection. The last two patients died during the course of the study at 9 and 7 years of age, respectively. All but four patients had been receiving zidovudine for a mean of 4.4 ± 1.6 years. Absence of treatment was justified by a good clinical and biologic condition in one and by rejection of zidovudine treatment by three families.

Social and cultural description of the families. The educational level was elementary school for 12 of the parents and end of high school and university level for the other 16 (no family belonged to the intermediate category). One child had been in a foster care center for more than 3 years, and the educational level of four parents was unknown. Fifteen children were living with both parents at home, 9 with only 1 of the 2 parents (usually the mother), and 4 with grandparents; 5 were in foster care (3 in foster families and 2 in institutions).

The mode of infection of mothers was heterosexual contact in 17 (11 mothers from central Africa or Haiti and 6 from France), intravenous use of street drugs in 10 (but none of the children was living with a mother still using street drugs), and contaminated blood transfusion before pregnancy in 6.

Academic achievement. At a mean age of 9.5 ± 1.6 years, 21 children were performing normally at school and 1 had good school performance until her death at 7 years of age; 5 children performed in the borderline range, and 6 were considered to have failed (including a patient who died at 9 years of age but had failed since 6 years).

Neuropsychologic, language, and psychoaffective evaluations. Of the 33 patients, 24 were tested at a mean age of 6.8 ± 1.0 years. They did not differ from the 9 other patients in any variable available in this analysis.

The mean results on the NEMI and the Similarities subtest of the WISC-R were normal, and the distribution of individual results showed only one child with abnormal results on the NEMI and another one for the Similarities subtest (Table II). The number of children obtaining abnormal results on either the Block Design subtest or the Bender test or on both was higher than expected from the standardization of the test (Table II). Evaluation of visual-spatial and temporal orientations was normal in only 11 patients (46%). Ten patients had impairment of visual-spatial organization, 10 were disoriented with respect to concepts of time, and 7 (29%) had both visual-spatial and time orientation deficits. Results of the other tests (especially fine motor abilities) were normal.

The results of 3 of the 10 tests for language assessments showed a distribution of performances that differed from the expected (Table III). No patient had severe abnormalities of oral language such as dysphasia, but 2 had isolated articulation disorders, associated with speech and/or language delay in 4, sequelae of speech delay in 3, and stutter-

Table III. Results of language assessment in HIV-1–infected children

	Test		
	Facial motoricity (n = 23)	Phonemics (n = 23)	Vocabulary (n = 23)
Test result (range*)			
Superior range	19	6	4
Median range	3	6	6
Lower range	0	5	7
Pathologic range	1	6	6

*Superior range: score >+0.66 SD; median range: score between −0.66 and +0.66 SD; lower range: score between −0.66 and −1.66 SD; pathologic range: score <−1.66 SD.

ing in 1. Abnormal results for vocabulary and delay in speech and langage were more frequent in the 7 patients living in a bilingual home environment.

None of the 24 children and only one of the parents in the study had severe psychoaffective symptoms (30 or less on the GAF Scale). Seven children and 9 parents (in 4 cases, parents and child within the same family) had symptoms of intermediate severity (between 50 and 31 on the GAF Scale), and 17 children and 14 parents had no or mild symptoms (more than 51 on the GAF Scale). Symptoms were related to anxiety, depression, behavioral problems, or pervasive developmental disorders in the children. Depression, neurosis, or antisocial personalities were found in the parents.

Correlations between school performance and neuropsychologic evaluation, and clinical or biologic factors. School performance was positively correlated, in the 24 children who received the formal tests, with NEMI scores (normal school results vs others: 100 ± 7 vs 87 ± 12; $p < 0.02$), the Similarities subtest (12 ± 3 vs 8 ± 3; $p < 0.03$), the Block Design subtest (10 ± 3 vs 7 ± 4; $p < 0.03$), and tests for visual-spatial and/or temporal orientation (69% of normal values in children with normal school performance vs 0% in others; $p < 0.002$). School performance was not significantly linked to the psychoaffective findings (57% of school difficulties in children with scores between 50 and 31 on the GAF Scale vs 24% in others; $p = 0.17$); no correlation was observed between the psychoaffective findings in the children and the NEMI score, the Block Design subtest score, and the Similarities subtest score.

The risk of school failure was not significantly related to the following maternal characteristics: geographic origin (school failure: 24% in European vs 45% in African or Haitian [relative risk, 1.9; 95% confidence interval, 0.7 to 5.2]), mode of infection (20% for intravenous drug abuse vs 36% for others [relative risk, 0.6; 95% confidence interval, 0.1 to 2.1]), educational level, or psychologic status (data not shown). The same was true for the risk of abnormal results on tests of visual-spatial and temporal orientation (data not shown).

Children with subsequently normal school achievement were compared with others three times during the course of the disease: (1) when the earliest $CD4^+$ lymphocyte count was obtained for the greatest number of children (at 4.3 ± 0.25 years (n = 22)), (2) when treatment was started (at 5.0 ± 2.0 years), and (3) when neuropsychologic and language tests were proposed (at 6.8 ± 1.0 years). The mean age of the two groups of children did not differ at the three chosen times. At each time, the percentage of $CD4^+$ lymphocytes was significantly higher in children with subsequently normal school achievement than in the others (for example 24 ± 11 vs 15 ± 16 [$p = 0.05$] for the earliest). The same was true when percentages of $CD4^+$ lymphocytes were compared with results of visual-spatial and temporal orientation tests (data not shown).

Children with normal academic achievement had been treated with zidovudine for a longer period (with an earlier age at onset) than those with abnormal results ($p = 0.05$). However, interpretation was difficult because of the preexisting early difference in the percentage of circulating $CD4^+$ lymphocytes between the two groups of children.

DISCUSSION

The survival rate at 6 years of age of the patients whom we studied was similar to that of the patients from the French Prospective Study,[24] which supports the conclusion that the population of children studied was representative of perinatally HIV-1–infected children at school age. Two thirds of the children followed had normal performance in elementary school, and most had normal results on tests evaluating general abilities, language, and motor functions; these results are in opposition to initial findings suggesting a high rate of mental retardation in HIV-1–infected children.[5-12] Our patients, however, more frequently had difficulties or failed at school than the general population (10% to 15% is the usual rate) and more frequently had visual-spatial impairment and time-orientation deficits than the population used for standardization of tests. In the standard population, the percentage of children of African or Haitian origin was probably lower than that of the children whom we studied, but the risk of school failure and of abnormal results for visual-spatial and time-orientation tests was not significantly related in this study to the geographic origin of the mothers.

The educational level of the families that we studied was somewhat higher than that of the families described earlier. Another major difference is that we decided to test children after 6 years of age to ensure a more homogeneous group; this eliminated patients with early and severe disease who had progressive encephalopathy and mental retardation (CDC class P-2, subclass B) and died early. Levenson et al.[25] found that 44% of HIV-1–infected children (age 5 ± 1.7 years) scored in the mental retardation range, and that neurologically normal HIV-1–infected children had results similar to those of children with seroreversion,[25] an observation similar to our findings.

The influence of the stage of disease on cognitive abilities and school achievement is difficult to analyze in a relatively small population, but there was a trend toward poorer academic achievement or poorer results on visual-spatial or temporal orientation tests because the children had lower percentages of circulating $CD4^+$ lymphocytes. Moreover, the percentage of circulating $CD4^+$ lymphocytes obtained at the age of 4 years was already higher in patients who subsequently had normal school achievement several years later. Poorer academic achievement and low results on cognitive tests were not merely the reflection of a poorer general condition of the patients, because no decrease in fine motor abilities or motor speed was observed. A predictive effect of the percentage of $CD4^+$ lymphocytes (obtained several years before) on future school adaptation or cognitive abilities is suggested by our results. A progressive decrease of cognitive abilities may be associated with the decrease of $CD4^+$ lymphocytes, and could depend on an increasing viral load within the brain and an increasing level of activation of brain macrophages, inducing neurotoxic effects.[26]

REFERENCES

1. Blanche S, Tardieu M, Duliège AM, et al. Longitudinal study of 94 symptomatic infants with materno-foetal HIV infection: evidence for a bimodal expression of clinical and biological symptoms. Am J Dis Child 1990;144:1210-5.
2. Tovo P, De Martino M, Gabiano C, et al. Prognostic factors and survival in children with perinatal HIV-1 infection. Lancet 1992;339:1249-53.
3. Turner BJ, Denison M, Eppes SC, et al. Survival experience of 789 children with the acquired immunodeficiency syndrome. Pediatr Infect Dis J 1993;12:310-20.
4. Belman AL. AIDS and the child's central nervous system. Pediatr Clin [Pediatric Neurology] 1992;39:691-714.
5. Belman AL, Ultmann MH, Horouplan D, et al. Neurologic complications in infants and children with acquired immune deficiency syndrome. Ann Neurol 1985;18:560-6.
6. Epstein LG, Sharer LR, Joshi VV, et al. Progressive encephalopathy in children with acquired immune deficiency syndrome. Ann Neurol 1985;17:488-96.
7. Ultmann MH, Belman AL, Ruff HA, Novick BE, et al. Developmental abnormalities in infants and children with acquired immune deficiency syndrome (AIDS) and AIDS-related complex. Dev Med Child Neurol 1985;27:563-71.
8. Ultmann MH, Diamond GW, Ruff HA, et al. Developmental abnormalities in children with acquired immunodeficiency syndrome (AIDS): a follow-up study. Int J Neurosci 1987; 32:661-7.
9. Epstein LG, Sharer LR, Oleske JM, et al. Neurologic manifestations of human immunodeficiency virus infection in children. Pediatrics 1986;78:678-87.
10. Belman AL, Diamond G, Dickson D, et al. Pediatric AIDS: neurologic syndromes. Am J Dis Child 1988;142:29-35.
11. Diamond GW, Gurdin P, Wiznia AA, et al. Effects of congenital HIV infection on neurodevelopmental status of babies in foster care. Dev Med Child Neurol 1990;32:999-1005.
12. Diamond GW. Developmental problems in children with HIV infection. Ment Retard 1989;4:213-7.
13. Girolami-Boulinier A. Les niveaux actuels dans la pratique du langage oral et écrit. Paris: Masson, 1984.
14. Rabreau J. Echelle d'évaluation mathématique. Paris: Establissement d'application psychotechnique, 1989.
15. Zazzo R, Gilly M, Verba-Rad M. Nouvelle Echelle Métrique de 'Intelligence. Paris: Colin-Bourrelier, 1966.
16. Zazzo R, Dague P, Schmelk MA, Rossi P. WISC et NEMI: premiers résultats d'une étude comparative. Enfance 1975;2: 253-71.
17. Terman LM, Merrill MA. Standford-Binet intelligence scale. 3rd rev. Boston: Houghton-Mifflin, 1973.
18. Wechsler D. Manual for the Wechsler Intelligence Scale for Children—Revised. New York: Psychological Corp., 1974.
19. Koppitz EM. The Bender Gestalt Test for Young Children; vol 2. New York: Grune & Stratton, 1975.
20. Zazzo R. Manuel pour l'examen psychologique de l'enfant. Paris: Delachaux et Niestlé, 1979.
21. Chevrie Muller C. Epreuves pour l'examen du langage. Paris: Edition Centre de Psychologie Appliquée, 1981.
22. Achenbach TM. Child Behavior Checklist 1983. French adaptation by Fombonne E. Paris: Département de recherche centre Alfred Binet, 1986.
23. Diagnostic and statistical manual of mental disorders. 3rd ed, revised [DSMIII-R]. Washington, D.C.: American Psychiatric Association, 1987.
24. Blanche S, Mayaux M-J, Rouzioux C, et al. Relation of the course of HIV infection in children to the severity of the disease in their mothers at delivery. N Engl J Med 1994;330:308-12.
25. Levenson RL Jr, Mellins CA, Zawadzki R, Kairam R, Stein Z. Cognitive assessment of human immunodeficiency virus–exposed children. Am J Dis Child 1992;146:1479-83.
26. Gendelman HE, Lipton SE, Tardieu M, et al. The neuropathogenesis of HIV-1 infection. J Leukoc Biol 1994;56:589-98.

Long-term effects of L-thyroxine therapy for congenital hypothyroidism

Joanne F. Rovet, PhD, and Robert M. Ehrlich, MD, FRCP(C)

From the Department of Pediatrics (Endocrinology Division) and the Department of Psychology, University of Toronto and Hospital for Sick Children, Toronto, Canada

Objective: To study the effects of initial and concurrent dose levels of L-thyroxine on ability and behavior in children with congenital hypothyroidism.
Methods: An existing database, involving a large cohort of children with congenital hypothyroidism detected by neonatal screening, was analyzed retrospectively. There were 94 children: 89 were assessed at age 7 years for intelligence and selective cognitive abilities, and 87 at age 8 years for behavior, achievement, and selective abilities.
Results: Subjects were stratified by median split into low and high starting dose groups. The high-dose group performed better on indexes of intelligence, verbal ability, and memory but had more behavior problems reflecting increased anxiety, social withdrawal, and poorer concentration. The dose of L-thyroxine at age 8 years was negatively correlated with memory task performance.
Conclusion: A higher starting dose of L-thyroxine is beneficial for subsequent intellectual outcome in children with congenital hypothyroidism but may be associated with internalizing behavior problems. (J PEDIATR 1995;126:380-6)

Recently there has been considerable interest in determining the ideal starting dose of L-thyroxine for later physical[1, 2] and intellectual[3-5] development of children with congenital hypothyroidism. Present guidelines recommend a relatively high starting dose level (10 to 15 μg/kg) to achieve rapid normalization and minimize the period during which the brain is lacking thyroid hormone.[6-8] Follow-up studies, based mainly on global intelligence indexes, indicate that although lower dose levels (7 to 10 μg/kg) are sufficient to ensure normal intelligence,[4] higher doses may be necessary for more severe hypothyroidism.[5] Although a set dose is no longer recommended for later replacement,[9, 10] current guidelines suggest levels of L-thyroxine that maintain T_4 in the upper normal range but ensure normal levels of thyrotropin.[7] Adequate long-term therapy sustains normal intelligence and school achievement[11]; however, behavioral difficulties,[12] as well attention and arithmetic problems,[13] may occur when circulating T_4 is elevated.

See related article on p. 389.

CBCL	Child Behavior Checklist
CH	Congenital hypothyroidism
FSIQ	Full Scale Intelligence Quotient
HDG	High-dose group
LDG	Low-dose group
T_4	Thyroxine
VMI	Visuomotor Integration
WISC-R	Wechsler Intelligence Scale for Children—Revised

We explored the effects of initial and subsequent L-thyroxine dose levels on a variety of cognitive abilities and on behavior in children with CH. During the period of recruitment, two modifications were made to the initial treatment protocol: (1) from a dose of 2.5 to 5 μg/kg per day to a dose of 5 to 7 μg/kg per day and (2) from a dose of 5 to 7 μg/kg

Supported in part by research grants to Drs. Rovet and Ehrlich from the Ontario Mental Health Foundation and the Ontario Ministry of Health.

Submitted for publication July 29, 1994; accepted Oct. 31, 1994.

Reprint requests: Joanne F. Rovet, PhD, Department of Psychology, Hospital for Sick Children, 555 University Ave., Toronto, Ontario M5G 1X8, Canada.

0022-3476/95/$3.00 + 0 **9/20/61659**

per day to a dose of 7 to 10 μg/kg per day. These modifications therefore provided a "natural experiment" to study initial dose effects, which could not readily have been achieved ethically.

METHODS

Sample. Subjects were 65 female and 29 male children born between 1976 and 1985 with CH detected by one of two screening programs.[14, 15] These children represented more than 90% of a larger cohort that was participating in a long-term prospective study to evaluate outcome after screening, most since the age of 1 year.[16] Nonparticipants included 5 children who moved, 2 with transient hypothyroidism, and 4 dropouts; one child with an IQ less than 60, unrelated to his thyroid hormone deficiency, was eliminated from this study. For the remaining 94 children, technetium scans or ultrasonography at the time of diagnosis revealed that there were 26 with athyrosis, 24 with dyshormonogenesis, usually with goiter, and 44 with an ectopic gland in a lingual or sublingual position. The mean age at the start of treatment was 15.8 ± 15.4 days (range, 3 to 145 days). A total of 91 children were examined at age 7 years and 88 at age 8 years.

The initial dose given to the first five patients, who were screened between 1976 and 1978, when there were few established guidelines, was 2.5 to 5 μg/kg per day. In 1978, this was increased to 5 to 7.0 μg/kg per day[17] and after 1983, to 7 to 10 μg/kg per day.[5] Doses were rounded to the nearest 25, 37.5, or 50 μg tablet. For children born before 1978, the mean starting dose of L-thyroxine was 5.1 ± 1.3 μg/kg; between 1978 and 1983, 7.9 ± 1.1 μg/kg; and after 1983, 9.1 ± 1.4 μg/kg. Ten children born after 1983 received starting doses of 10 μg/kg or higher. The mean age for the start of L-thyroxine therapy for children born before 1983 was older than that for later-born children (18.3 ± 18.9 vs 12.0 ± 3.5 days; $p < .01$). No other disease or treatment factors differentiated the two cohorts.

Tests and measures. In the long-term prospective study, children were assessed annually, usually near the time of their birthday and coincident with their annual endocrine clinic appointment. They received a battery of age-appropriate psychologic tests, which varied by age according to a protocol established when the project began. The rationale for using different tests was to ensure that the findings would not be affected by repetition and practice effects, and to study systematically a comprehensive range of cognitive and behavioral functions. At age 7 years, the assessment evaluated intelligence, selective cognitive abilities, and achievement, and at age 8 years behavior, selective cognitive abilities, and achievement. The cognitive abilities included language, auditory discrimination, visuomotor integration, and memory. Informed consent was obtained from parents at the child's first evaluation, usually 12 months of age. Verbal assent was provided by the child at 7 and 8 years of age.

At age 7 years, children were assessed with the Wechsler Intelligence Scale for Children—Revised,[18] the Carrow Language Scales,[19] the Wepman Test of Auditory Discrimination,[20] the Beery Developmental Test of Visual Motor Integration,[21] McCarthy Scales of Children's Abilities (Memory subscale),[22] and the Wide Range Achievement Test—Revised.[23] When the children were 8 years of age, parents completed the Child Behavior Checklist,[24] and the Conners Parent Hyperactivity Scale[25]; the Wepman, VMI, McCarthy Memory, Wide Range Achievement Test—Revised, and Woodcock Reading Mastery—Revised Passage Comprehension subtest[26] were given to the children. Socioeconomic status was measured with the Hollingshead scale.[27]

The medical variables evaluated cause, confirmatory T_4 level, bone age at time of diagnosis, age at start of treatment, and age at normalization of T_4 values; 7- and 8-year T_4, thyrotropin, and dose levels were also available. Normalization age was computed by interpolation from the linear relationships between the age and T_4 level at diagnosis and the age at the visit when T_4 level was reported to be greater than 128 nmol/L (10.9 μg/dl), the exact day when the T_4 level would have reached 128 nmol/L.[28] All assays were performed in the Hospital for Sick Children Department of Clinical Chemistry.

Data analysis and statistics. Children were stratified into two groups with a median split procedure based on starting dose levels of L-thyroxine. Those children who initially received 7.7 μg/kg or less were assigned to the low-dose group; those with starting doses of 7.8 μg/kg or more were assigned to the high-dose group. Eighty percent of children in the LDG were born before 1983; 92% in the HDG were born after 1983. We used *t* tests and analyses of variance and covariance to compare the groups, with the Bonferroni *p* correction applied to all multiple indexes at the same level of a test (e.g., all verbal subtests of the WISC-R, all narrow-band internalizing scales of the CBCL). Pearson product-moment correlations facilitated determination of the relationships between starting and later doses of L-thyroxine and test performance. Because of the large number of correlations, the *p* value was set at 0.01.

RESULTS

The results were initially analyzed to compare the effects of low and very low starting doses of L-thyroxine given to the first patients in the study. A comparison of children started with an L-thyroxine dose of 5.0 μg/kg or less and with 5.1 to 7.7 μg/kg indicated no differences. Similarly, comparisons between the HDG and all children

Table I. Medical demographic information of low (<7.8 μg/kg) and high (≥7.8 μg/kg) starting dose groups

	LDG		HDG			
	Mean	**SD**	**Mean**	**SD**	***t***	***p***
Birth						
Bone age (wk)	37.4	1.8	36.4	2.6	1.87	
Confirmation T_4 (nmol/L)	54.0	42.4	68.2	52.8	−1.40	
Treatment age (days)	20.2	20.8	11.6	4.0	2.80	0.01
Starting dose (μg/kg)	6.4	1.1	9.0	1.1	−11.58	0.0001
Normalization age (days)	82.7	78.8	35.2	23.2	4.00	0.0001
Age 3 mo						
T_4 at 3 mo (nmol/L)	149.8	55.8	168.3	42.4	1.79	
Age 7 yr						
T_4 (nmol/L)	163.3	27.0	143.0	25.5	3.63	0.001
TSH (mU/L)	3.5	3.3	6.8	9.4	−2.14	0.05
Dose (μg/kg)	3.6	0.9	3.3	0.8	1.95	0.05
Age 8 yr						
T_4 (nmol/L)	159.4	30.1	137.9	21.9	3.62	0.001
Thyrotropin (mU/L)	3.8	3.7	5.8	6.9	−1.63	
Dose (μg/kg)	3.4	1.0	2.9	0.8	2.68	0.01

receiving the lower dose versus only those receiving a moderate dose (i.e., "knocking out" the lowest doses) also indicated no differential effects. Therefore all children started on a dose less than 7.8 μg/kg were compared with those started at a dose of 7.8 μg/kg or more.

The LDG and HDG differed in age at the start of therapy and when normalization was achieved (Table I); the LDG presumably started therapy later because screening and recall procedures were not as efficient in the earlier years and children born after 1983 were discharged earlier. They did not differ in onset or severity of hypothyroidism. At age 7 years the LDG had higher circulating T_4 and lower thyrotropin concentrations; at age 8 years the LDG had higher levels of circulating T_4. At both ages, the LDG was receiving a higher dose of L-thyroxine. The groups did not differ in sex distribution (percentage female: LDG = 65.2; HDG = 72.9), etiologic composition (percentage with athyrosis: LDG = 28.3; HDG = 27.1), or socioeconomic status (LDG = 37.88; HDG = 41.4).

Shown in Table II are the *t* test results of the LDG and the HDG at age 7 years; analyses of covariance, with treatment age as a covariate, yielded essentially identical findings. The HDG had higher Full Scale IQ and Verbal IQ scores. With the Bonferroni correction applied, the HDG also scored significantly higher on the WISC-R verbal comprehension factor and on the Similarities and Arithmetic subtests. No differences were observed on indexes of speech, auditory discrimination, visuomotor coordination, memory, or school achievement. There were no significant correlations between performance on these measures and starting dose level, which for tests involving significant group differences suggests that the relationship is not linear.

A comparison of children whose doses were at or greater than 10.0 μg/kg with those whose doses were between 7.8 and 10.0 μg/kg indicated no difference in FSIQ: all four children with FSIQ scores greater than 125 had starting doses between 5.0 and 9.5 μg/kg.

At age 8 years the HDG scored higher on the McCarthy Memory subtest and the Passage Comprehension subtest of the Woodcock Reading Mastery—Revised test (Table III). Examination of the individual McCarthy Memory Scale subtests revealed that the largest difference occurred on Verbal Memory II (LDG = 6.44; HDG = 7.23; $p = 0.057$), which requires retelling a story. On behavioral indexes, parents rated the HDG higher on the Internalizing Problems subtest. With the Bonferroni correction applied, the HDG received higher scores on the Social Withdrawal, Anxious/Depressed, Social Problems, Delinquency, and Aggression subscales. On the Conners Scale, the HDG received higher ratings on the Conduct Problems subscale and had a higher Hyperactivity Index. Among the HDG, the only score that was clinically significant was on the Impulsivity/Hyperactivity subscale of the Conners Scale. Of the 15 children (17%) whose individual CBCL Internalizing behavior problems scores were in the clinical range for the test ($t \geq 63$),[24] 14 were from the HDG. For all three children (3.4%) with CBCL scores in the "psychopathologic range" (>2 SD or $t \geq 70$),[24] starting doses were more than 10.0 μg/kg.

To address the issue of whether a higher starting dose had a greater benefit on cognitive skills of children more severely hypothyroid at birth, we computed two-factor analyses of variance on data from 7 years, with bone age at diagnosis (>36 or <36 weeks)[27] and starting dose as independent

Table II. Seven-year test results in LDG (n = 45) and HDG (n = 46)

	LDG		HDG			
	Mean	SD	Mean	SD	t	p
WISC-R						
Full Scale IQ	100.0	12.7	107.6	12.2	−2.53	0.01
Verbal IQ	98.6	13.6	106.3	13.2	−2.73	0.01
Performance IQ	103.8	12.7	108.2	12.4	−1.68	NS
Verbal Comprehension*	10.0	2.4	11.1	2.3	−2.19	0.03
Perceptual Organization*	10.9	1.9	11.6	1.9	−1.63	NS
Freedom Distractibility*	9.6	2.1	10.3	1.9	−1.77	NS
Information*	9.7	3.0	11.0	2.7	−2.07	0.04
Similarities*	10.3	3.0	12.2	2.9	−3.13	0.002
Arithmetic*	9.5	2.4	11.2	2.5	−3.08	0.01
Vocabulary*	9.6	2.4	10.1	2.6	−1.01	NS
Comprehension*	9.7	2.9	10.5	2.7	−1.12	NS
Digit Span*	10.2	2.8	11.1	2.3	−1.69	NS
Picture Completion*	10.4	2.4	11.5	2.4	−2.09	0.04
Picture Arrangement*	10.9	2.8	11.7	3.4	−0.97	NS
Block Design*	11.3	3.1	11.8	2.8	−0.80	NS
Object Assembly*	11.2	2.1	11.3	2.8	0.31	NS
Coding*	9.4	3.0	9.6	2.7	0.26	NS
Carrow Language Inventory†,[19]	65.3	32.6	75.0	26.6	−1.41	NS
Wepman Auditory Discrimination Test†,[20]	60.8	31.0	65.5	25.6	−0.77	NS
VMI†	52.2	27.8	53.0	23.6	−0.16	NS
McCarthy Memory‡,[22]	49.4	8.0	51.7	7.6	−1.28	NS
WRAT-R†						
Reading	40.5	28.1	44.2	33.1	−0.56	NS
Spelling	39.1	28.0	40.5	32.1	−0.22	NS
Arithmetic	42.4	25.9	42.4	26.0	−0.16	NS
WRM-R Passage Comprehension†	58.4	23.9	59.1	25.6	−0.13	NS

NS, Not significant; *WRAT-R*, Wide Range Achievement Test—Revised; *WRM-R*, Woodcock Reading Mastery—Revised.
*Scale score (mean = 10; SD = 3).
†Percentile score.
‡*T* score (mean = 50; SD = 10).

variables. For bone age, significant main effects were observed for FSIQ ($p <0.01$), Verbal IQ ($p <0.05$), performance IQ ($p <0.01$), Freedom from Distractibility ($p <0.01$), McCarthy Memory ($p <0.05$), and VMI ($p <0.01$) tests: children with bone ages greater than 36 weeks at diagnosis obtained higher scores. For the starting dose, significant effects were observed for FSIQ ($p <0.001$), verbal IQ ($p <0.01$), Verbal Comprehension ($p <0.01$), Freedom from Distractibility ($p <0.01$), McCarthy Memory ($p <0.01$), and Carrow Language ($p <0.05$) tests. The VMI test was the only task providing a significant ($p <0.01$) interaction, in which children in the HDG with delayed bone ages scored equivalent to children without delayed bone ages, whereas children in the LDG with delayed bone ages scored significantly below those without delayed bone ages. By contrast, the differences in FSIQ between delayed and nondelayed groups on FSIQ were constant regardless of which starting dose was given.

There were no significant correlations between dose at age 7 years and concurrently assessed intelligence or achievement. At age 8 years, concurrent dose correlated negatively with McCarthy Memory task performance ($r[85] = -0.31$; $p <0.01$); this correlation was significantly different ($p <0.001$), and in the opposite direction, from that between starting dose and performance on this task ($r[85] = 0.19$; $p <0.10$).

DISCUSSION

These findings indicate that, in the treatment of CH, better intellectual outcome is associated with a higher starting dose of L-thyroxine. Particularly affected are verbal and memory competencies, as well as reading comprehension; perceptual skills are generally less affected. The relationships are not linear, but a threshold effect is indicated: children at the lowest dose levels (<5.0 μg/kg) did not differ from those with moderately low levels, whereas those at the highest dose levels (>10.0 μg/kg) did not differ from those with moderately high levels. Except for

Table III. Eight-year test results in LDG (n = 44) and HDG (n = 44)

	LDG		HDG			
	Mean	SD	Mean	SD	t	p
Wepman Auditory Discrimination Test*,[20]	68.8	29.6	72.4	28.6	−0.56	NS
Beery VMI*,[21]	46.4	21.6	47.4	26.0	−0.20	NS
McCarthy Memory†,[22]	46.6	8.4	53.8	14.2	−2.84	0.01
WRAT-R*						
Reading	38.0	25.8	47.6	31.8	−1.55	NS
Spelling	39.3	29.1	42.7	32.3	−0.52	NS
Arithmetic	33.5	25.8	22.8	27.6	−0.04	NS
Woodcock Passage Comprehension*,[26]	50.1	20.9	59.3	20.4	−2.04	0.05
CBCL*						
Social Competence	47.9	10.5	49.8	10.2	−0.84	NS
Behavior Problems	51.3	8.3	54.7	12.3	−1.48	NS
Internalizing Problems	50.2	7.8	53.4	12.0	−2.33	0.02
Externalizing Problems	51.7	9.1	54.5	11.1	−1.27	NS
Social Withdrawn	53.4	6.9	59.1	7.8	−3.57	0.001
Somatic Complaints	54.8	6.8	60.4	9.1	−3.19	0.002
Anxious/Depressed	54.8	6.9	57.9	7.1	−2.01	0.05
Social Problems	55.2	5.7	60.8	7.3	−3.89	0.0001
Thought Problems	54.4	7.3	59.8	8.2	−3.19	0.002
Attention Problems	55.9	7.8	59.5	7.8	−2.17	0.03
Delinquency	57.8	5.3	61.1	6.2	−2.62	0.01
Aggression	51.6	9.6	58.4	6.4	−3.84	0.0002
Sex Problems	57.5	4.6	59.1	5.1	−1.52	NS
Conners Rating Scales‡,[25]						
Conduct Problems	0.29	0.30	0.46	0.33	−2.46	0.01
Learning Problems	0.39	0.35	0.66	.58	−2.22	0.03
Psychosomatic Problems	0.13	0.26	0.17	0.27	−0.72	NS
Impulsive/Hyperactive	0.78	0.67	1.05	0.67	−1.66	NS
Anxiety	0.48	0.28	0.69	0.51	−2.10	0.04
Hyperactivity Index	0.46	0.28	0.69	0.51	−2.01	0.04

NS, Not significant; *WRAT-R*, Wide Range Achievement Test—Revised.
*Percentile score.
†*T* score (mean = 50; SD = 10).
‡*z* score (mean = 0; SD = 1).

the VMI task, a differential benefit of starting dose level for children with more severe and long-standing hypothyroidism at birth was not observed, in contrast to the findings of Dubuis et al.,[5] who studied much younger children. Regarding dose at time of testing, the only effect was a negative association with Memory task performance.

Despite improved cognitive skills when a higher starting dose was given, there were more behavior problems in later childhood. These included increased social withdrawal, anxiety, social problems, conduct problems, and hyperactivity, consistent with our earlier observation of greater temperamental difficulty in infants with higher circulating T_4 levels in the preceding months.[12] Although only a few children obtained scores that were clinically significant, those who did almost invariably came from the HDG; all the children with Internalizing Problems scores warranting immediate professional attention had starting doses greater than 10.0 μg/kg.

An unexpected finding was that children who initially received lower doses of L-thyroxine had higher T_4 levels at 7 and 8 years of age. This outcome appears to be dose related, but there is no obvious explanation for the higher doses subsequently given to these children. Because dose at time of testing was not correlated with any behavioral indexes, it is unlikely that our results reflect a side effect of L-thyroxine. Attention problems, found to be correlated with circulating T_4 at the time of testing (Rovet JF and Alvarez M: unpublished observations), were similarly not associated with dose.

The finding that euthyroidism was achieved earlier when starting doses were higher, and that a higher dose was associated with improved verbal and memory abilities, may indicate that periods of sensitivity to thyroid hormone for verbal skills differ from those for nonverbal skills. The critical period of thyroid hormone effects for verbal and memory skills appears to be the first 2 months or so of life. In contrast, the critical period for visuospatial or visuomotor skills seems to be prenatal; hence these skills, which differ significantly from those of control subjects[29] are less affected by starting dose.

The observation that performance on the McCarthy Memory scale correlated positively with starting dose and negatively with current dose may signify different activities of thyroid hormone at different stages of development. Regarding starting dose, the association may reflect an organizational effect of thyroid hormone during a period when the brain's "hardware" is being formed: pharmacologic, albeit therapeutic, manipulations of thyroid hormone may modulate structural changes in brain development during critical periods of thyroid hormone receptivity.[30, 31] By contrast, the inverse correlation between current dose and memory may signify an activational effect of thyroid hormone on neurotransmitter functions, which affect memory and attentional processing.[32, 33] Our observation that the memory task requiring children to retell a story was the most sensitive to early and subsequent dose effects may have clinical relevance in that performance on this task correlates with academic progress: children who do more poorly on it also tend to have greater difficulty at school in following oral directions and remembering homework assignments.

The limitations of this study include (1) its retrospective design, (2) small sample sizes in the extreme high and low dose ranges, (3) use of different tests at different ages, (4) most tests performed only once, and (5) reliance on behavioral questionnaire data without a parent interview or teacher rating. Because recruitment for this study took place during an extended 8-year period and lower starting doses were given mainly before 1983, it is conceivable that the lower scores by the LDG may signify either normally occurring improvements in intelligence that occur with time[34, 35] or a cohort effect. However, there are no specific events or other factors that explain why children born before 1983 have lower intelligence than children born after. Regarding single testing, the behavioral findings observed in children with CH at age 8 years were in fact replicated at age 7 years in a subgroup of children whose parents additionally completed the CBCL and Conners scales. The behavioral tests used in this study are among those most commonly used in pediatric psychology research with other chronic illnesses,[36] but they may not take into account the altered perceptions of parents after an early screening diagnosis[37]; thus the negative associations between behavior and starting dose should be interpreted cautiously. Although direct interviews were not obtained with parents, teachers' ratings on those children in our study who have now reached the sixth grade at school indicate that children with lower starting doses were perceived by their teachers as having fewer behavior problems.

We conclude that a higher starting dose of L-thyroxine is associated with better cognitive outcome, particularly in the areas of verbal ability and verbal memory. However, a higher starting dose of L-thyroxine may also be associated with more behavior problems, particularly if starting dose levels are >10.0 μg/kg. These findings therefore indicate that a dose between 7.5 and 10.0 μg/kg may be sufficient to improve outcome and prevent later behavior problems associated with increased anxiety, social withdrawal, and poor concentration. The finding of a negative association between current dose and memory suggests the need to consider behavior, as well as levels of thyroid hormone, in adjusting dose levels. A prospective study of the effects of different starting dose levels on outcome is warranted.

Special thanks to Miguel Alvarez, who provided the impetus for this article and set the groundwork during his stay as a RESTRACOM Visiting Scientist funded by the Hospital for Sick Children Foundation. We also acknowledge Deborah Altmann and Donna Sorbara for their many contributions to the project.

REFERENCES

1. Germak J, Foley TP. Longitudinal assessment of L-thyroxine therapy for congenital hypothyroidism. J PEDIATR 1990;117:211-9.
2. Kooh S, Brnjac L, Ehrlich R, Krishnan S. Bone mass in children with congenital hypothyroidism (CHT) [Abstract]. Pediatr Res 1994;35:102A.
3. Toublanc JE, Job JC, Chaussain JL, Canlorbe P. Traitement des hypothyroidies congenitales par la L-thyroxine en solution. Arch Fr Pediatr 1983;40:379-83.
4. Campos S, Sandberg D, Barrick C, Voorhess M, MacGillivray M. Outcome following lower L-thyroxine dose for treatment of congenital hypothyroidism [Abstract]. Pediatr Res 1994;35:95A.
5. Dubuis JM, Richer F, Glorieux J, Deal C, Dussault J, Van Vliet G. Should all patients with congenital hypothyroidism (CH) be treated with 10-15 μg/kg · day of levothyroxine(T_4) [Abstract]? Pediatr Res 1994;35:98A.
6. American Academy of Pediatrics Committee on Genetics. Newborn screening for congenital hypothyroidism: recommended guidelines. Pediatrics 1987;80:745-9.
7. American Academy of Pediatrics. Newborn screening for congenital hypothyroidism: recommended guidelines. Pediatrics 1993;91:1203-9.
8. Grüters A, Delange F, Giovannelli G, et al. Guidelines for neonatal screening programmes for congenital hypothyroidism. Eur J Pediatr 1993;152:974-5.
9. Rezvani I, Di George AM. Reassessment of the daily dose of oral thyroxine for replacement therapy in hypothyroid children. J PEDIATR 1977;90:291-7.
10. Abassi V, Aldridge C. Evaluation of sodium L-thyroxine (T_4) requirements in replacement therapy of hypothyroidism. J PEDIATR 1990;117:211-9.
11. New England Congenital Hypothyroidism Collaborative. Correlation of cognitive test scores and adequacy of treatment in adolescents with congenital hypothyroidism. J PEDIATR 1994;124:383-7.

12. Rovet JF, Ehrlich R, Sorbara D. The effect of thyroid hormone on temperament in infants with congenital hypothyroidism detected by newborn screening. J PEDIATR 1989;114:63-9.
13. Rovet JF, Ehrlich RM, Donner E. Long-term neurodevelopmental correlates of treatment adequacy in screened hypothyroid children. Pediatr Res 1993;33(5, suppl):S91.
14. Walfish PG. The best way to screen for neonatal hypothyroidism. Diagn Med 1989;321:13-6.
15. Peter F. Screening for congenital hypothyroidism with the TSH test. Proceedings of the Fourth National Newborn Screening Symposium. Columbus, Ohio: 1988:147-56.
16. Rovet JF. A prospective investigation of children with congenital hypothyroidism identified by neonatal thyroid screening in Ontario. Can J Public Health 1986;77:164-73.
17. Guyda HJ. Therapy of congenital hypothyroidism: evoluation of biochemical parameters. In: Burrow GN, Dussault JH, eds. Neonatal thyroid screening. New York: Raven Press, 1980.
18. Wechsler D. The Wechsler Intelligence Scale for Children—Revised. New York: The Psychological Corporation, 1974.
19. Carrow E. Carrow Elicited Language and Inventory—Manual. Austin, Texas: Learning Concepts, 1974.
20. Wepman JM. Auditory Discrimination Test. Los Angeles, California: Western Psychological Services, 1973.
21. Beery KE, Buktenica NA. The VMI Develomental Test of Visual Motor Integration. Cleveland: Modern Curriculum Press, 1989.
22. McCarthy D. McCarthy Scales of Children's Abilities. New York: The Psychological Corporation, 1970.
23. Jastak S, Wilkinson GS. Wide Range Achievement Test—Revised. Wilmington: Jastak Associates, 1984.
24. Achenbach TM. The Child Behavior Checklist. Burlington: University of Vermont, 1991.
25. Conners KC. Conners' Rating Scales Manual. Toronto: Multi-Health Systems, 1990.
26. Woodcock RN. Woodcock Reading Mastery Tests—Revised. Circle Pines, Minnesota: American Guidance Service, 1987.
27. Hollingshead AB. Four-factor index of social status. Department of Sociology, Yale University, New Haven, Connecticut, 1975.
28. Rovet JF, Ehrlich R, Sorbara D. Intellectual outcome in children with fetal hypothyroidism. J PEDIATR 1987;110:700-4.
29. Rovet JF. Neurodevelopmental outcome in infants and preschool children following newborn screening for congenital hypothyroidism. J Pediatr Psychol 1992;17:187-213.
30. Strait KA, Schwartz HL, Perez-Castillo A, Oppenheimer JH. Relationship of c-erbA mRNA content to tissue triiodothyronine nuclear binding capacity and function in developing and adult rats. J Biol Chem 1990;265:10514-21.
31. Munoz A, Rodriguez-Pena A, Perez-Castillo A, Ferreiro B, Sutcliffe JG, Bernal J. Effects of neonatal hypothyroidism on rat brain gene expression. Mol Endocrinol 1991;5:273-80.
32. Savard P, Merand Y, DiPaolo T, Dupont A. Effects of thyroid state on serotonin, 5-hyroxyindolacetic acid and substance P contents in discrete brain nuclei of adult rats. Neuroscience 1983;10:1399-404.
33. Puymirat J. Effects of dysthyroidism on central catecholaminergic neurons. Neurochem Int 1985;17:969-77.
34. Brand C. Keeping up with the times. Nature 1987;328:761.
35. Lynn R, Sampson SL, Mullineux JC. A long-term increase in the fluid intelligence of English children. Nature 1987;328:797.
36. Lavigne JV, Faier-Routman J. Psychological adjustment to pediatric physical disorders: a meta-analytic review. J Pediatr Psychol 1992;17:133-58.
37. Rovet JF. Does newborn screening increase the risk of the vulnerable child syndrome? Proceedings of the 8th National Neonatal Screening Symposium and XXI Birth Defects Symposium, Washington, D.C.: Association of State and Territorial Public Health Directors, 1992:211-8.

EDITOR'S COLUMN

Adolescent medicine 1995

As I departed from the Editorial Board in May 1994 after 7 years of service, I asked Dr. Garfunkel if I could follow the lead taken by my predecessor, George Comerci (December 1986), and comment on progress in the field of adolescent medicine. During my tenure, much has changed in adolescent medicine and medicine in general. Major crises confront the status of youth in contemporary American society, including high levels of intentional and nonintentional injury, depression, substance abuse, sexually transmitted diseases including human immunodeficiency virus infection, and teen pregnancy, among others. Many of these problems occur in all adolescent populations, but they are most prevalent within economically and socially disadvantaged groups, including poor, minority, and inner-city teens. Addressing many of the new morbidities presents a major challenge to pediatricians. Programs designed to address these risks have often received categorical funding, such as family planning, sexually transmitted diseases, or substance abuse; the need to provide or fund comprehensive services has often not been recognized. Research has frequently focused on surveys and assessments rather than on rigorous evaluations of the programs undertaken and interventions initiated.

Several key factors have come together to provide more advocacy to address adolescent health care needs. In 1992 the American Medical Association promulgated the new Guidelines for Adolescent Preventive Services (GAPS), a framework for preventive services for adolescents that included a comprehensive annual visit for health guidance and screening. The delineation of services made it clear that health delivery for teens requires more than a 10 to 15-minute visit and that episodic care for acute illnesses is not sufficient. At the same time, the establishment of adolescent medicine as a subspecialty under the American boards of internal medicine and of pediatrics (with the first examination given in November 1994) began the process of recognition of the distinctive training, body of knowledge, and research opportunities in this field. Specialists in adolescent medicine now occupy the unique roles of providing primary care for adolescents and serving as consultants to pediatricians, internists, and others. The training of adolescent medicine specialists bodes well for augmenting the training of all primary care physicians in pediatrics, internal medicine, obstetrics and gynecology, and family practice. From THE JOURNAL's perspective, the research requirement for specialty certification under the American Board of Pediatrics should bring forth important new research efforts by faculty and fellows in these programs. It is unfortunate that funding remains a major barrier to significant improvement in the quality and amount of research in the field. Currently the Maternal and Child Health Bureau (U.S. Department of Health and Human Services) funds seven interdisciplinary adolescent health programs in the United States, two more than in the previous decade. Additional adolescent medicine programs are desperately in need of federal and foundation support to augment training opportunities, research, and continuing education at medical centers with pediatric and internal medicine residency training.

Specialists in adolescent medicine can look proudly to the selection of two well-known adolescent medicine specialists by the American Academy of Pediatrics: Joe Sanders as executive director and George Comerci as president. In 1994 a new institute for health policy, the National Adolescent Health Information Center, located in San Francisco, was funded by the Maternal and Child Health Bureau. The Society for Adolescent Medicine is a vibrant, expanding organization. Advocacy groups and foundations have helped fill many of the gaps in health services for teens.

So where are the problems in 1995? From a clinical point of view, adolescents are frequently lost in the health care reform debate. Issues of confidentiality and access for poor teens, the need for annual comprehensive preventive services, and adequate reimbursement for time (not procedures) are rarely heard in the halls of Congress. Adolescent medicine has no technical procedures to charge to insurers, and the extra time needed to provide health guidance and counseling about sexually transmitted diseases, family planning, nutrition, and violence prevention, as well as to provide gynecologic services to young women, is poorly compensated. The switch to capitated care in many areas of the country assumes that adolescents will not use health care services; the low reimbursement discourages preventive care and benefits physicians in the short run for not asking questions about eating disorders, substance abuse, risk of infection with the human immunodeficiency virus,

THE JOURNAL OF PEDIATRICS 1995;126:387-8

0022-3476/95/$3.00 + 0 **9/21/62436**

and sexuality; positive answers have the potential to lead to referral for mental health, nutrition, gynecologic, and other services. Laboratory tests for Papanicolau smears and screening for sexually transmitted diseases are not inexpensive, and the "don't ask, don't need to do" strategy may appear attractive at a time when asking questions and providing confidential services have financial consequences. The change to lessened reimbursement occurs at a time when many pediatric and internal medicine programs are earnestly working with adolescent medicine specialists to improve primary care training and to help residents feel more comfortable with adolescent health care issues. Even today, some pediatricians believe that once an adolescent has become sexually active, he or she must be an adult. The internist is often not prepared to deal with the issues of growth and development, and the style of adolescents may not fit the model of health care delivery expected in adult institutions. Adolescents may continue to "fall through the cracks."

What else is problematic in 1995? From my perspective as a reviewer, there are insufficient numbers of adolescent health research papers submitted to THE JOURNAL that clearly delineate hypothesis, research design, and conclusions. Admittedly, it is always a difficult task to assess the quality of some of the research presented. Budgets for projects are often far less than what is needed to answer the more global questions posed. More funding is needed so that less energy is devoted to small surveys and more energy to large surveys, especially to the creation and evaluation of individual and public health interventions based on theoretical models. Health services research is needed to assess new models of care, particularly for special-needs and high-risk youth. Research is also needed to examine the utilization and impact of a myriad of new curricula in adolescent health care designed to augment the training of medical students and residents in primary care.

My hope for the next 5 years is that the new adolescent medicine fellowship opportunities will be funded and will attract some of the brightest minds in medicine. This would open the possibility that more high-quality research will be funded by large and small foundations, and by state and federal government agencies. It would be heartening to see investigators think of THE JOURNAL OF PEDIATRICS as the premier place to send their research and to find several articles in the Adolescent Medicine section in every issue of THE JOURNAL. I also hope that, in the next few years, THE JOURNAL and other pediatric journals will ensure that whenever a disease or drug is reviewed, the author is expected to take note of the implications in adolescents who may have an unplanned pregnancy, have effects on reproductive function, or suffer the consequences of interactions with medications such as oral contraceptives and antidepressants.

Perhaps I am a dreamer, but so much has occurred in my 7-year tenure on the Editorial Board at THE JOURNAL that I continue to believe that the future is bright. I will miss Joe Garfunkel and all that he has done for THE JOURNAL.

S. Jean Emans, MD
Co-Chief, Division of Adolescent Medicine
Children's Hospital, Boston
Associate Professor of Pediatrics
Harvard Medical School
Boston, MA 02115

Brain metabolite changes on in vivo proton magnetic resonance spectroscopy in children with congenital hypothyroidism

Rakesh K. Gupta, MD, Vijayalakshmi Bhatia, MD, Harish Poptani, MSc, and Ratni B. Gujral, MD

From the Magnetic Resonance Section, Departments of Radiology and Endocrinology, Sanjay Gandhi Postgraduate Institute of Medical Sciences, Lucknow, India

Localized in vivo proton magnetic resonance spectroscopy and imaging were performed in five children with untreated congenital hypothyroidism to look for biochemical markers of abnormal myelin and neuronal development. The patients had high levels of choline-containing compounds, which returned to normal with euthyroidism. These metabolic alterations may reflect blocks in myelin maturation that are reversible by thyroid hormone replacement throughout childhood. (J PEDIATR 1995;126:389-92)

Lack of thyroxine during the "critical period" of central nervous system responsiveness to this hormone results in delay of myelination, dendritic arborization, synapse formation, and neuronal migration. Thyroid hormone regulates protein synthesis in the brain, which affects the maturation of enzymes necessary for the aforementioned processes.[1] Magnetic resonance spectroscopy is an excellent noninvasive tool for studying metabolic changes in vivo. Phosphorus 31 spectroscopy has been successfully used to study energy metabolism in muscle and brain in patients with hypothyroidism[2,3]; proton magnetic resonance spectroscopy, which identifies peaks of the myelin precursor choline-containing compounds and *N*-acetyl aspartate, a neuronal marker, has been useful in studying various demyelinating and degenerative brain disorders.[4] We therefore used PMRS to study metabolic abnormalities in five children with congenital hypothyroidism before and after thyroxine replacement.

METHODS

Patients. Our study included five consecutively seen children, 6 to 15 years of age, with untreated congenital hypothyroidism. All of the children had a history of delayed development, constipation, and growth retardation. Physical examination revealed short stature, a large tongue, dry skin, and a low IQ. One patient with dyshormonogenesis had a soft goiter; the remainder had impalpable thyroid glands. All the patients had hormonal biochemistry findings that were diagnostic of primary hypothyroidism. Four patients had sporadic hypothyroidism. One patient was born and lived during early childhood in an endemically iodine-deficient region; at the time of the study, his iodine intake was normal. Thyroxine was undetectable in four patients and measured 40.5 nmol/L in one patient (normal, 70 to 170 nmol/L). Thyroid-stimulating hormone measured more than 50 mIU/L in all patients (normal, 0.2 to 5 mIU/L). Undernutrition was excluded in all the patients by detailed physical examination and standard anthropometric criteria.

All the patients underwent a baseline MR imaging and spectroscopic study within 2 days of confirmation of the di-

See related article, p. 380.

Cho	Choline-containing compounds
Cr	Total creatine
mI	*myo*-Inositol
MR	Magnetic resonance
NAA	*N*-Acetyl aspartate
PMRS	Proton magnetic resonance spectroscopy
TE	Echo time
TI	Inversion time
TM	Mixing time
TR	Repetition time

Supported by an intramural grant from the Sanjay Gandhi Postgraduate Institute of Medical Sciences.

Submitted for publication May 23, 1994; accepted Sept. 2, 1994.

Reprint requests: Rakesh K. Gupta, MD, Magnetic Resonance Section, Department of Radiology, Sanjay Gandhi Postgraduate Institute of Medical Sciences, Lucknow, 226014, India.

0022-3476/95/$3.00 + 0 **9/22/60327**

Table. Ratios of Cho, mI, and NAA to Cr in patients (before and after treatment) and in age-matched control subjects

	Patients		
Ratio	Before treatment	After treatment	Control subjects
Cho/Cr	0.93 ± 0.09*†	0.69 ± 0.14‡	0.72 ± 0.05
NAA/Cr	1.51 ± 0.29	1.31 ± 0.14	1.54 ± 0.23
mI/Cr	0.71 ± 0.18	0.62 ± 0.15	0.66 ± 0.13

*Mean ± SD.
†p <0.001 versus control.
‡p <0.008 versus pretreatment.

agnosis. Spectroscopy was repeated after 6 weeks and again after 3 months of thyroxine replacement, at which time all the patients were euthyroid. Oral sedation was given in appropriate doses before the examination when necessary.

Five age-matched healthy control subjects (volunteers or children whose short stature was evaluated but found to be normal) underwent imaging and spectroscopy for comparison. Informed consent was given for all the MR studies.

Magnetic resonance imaging. Magnetic resonance imaging and spectroscopy were performed with a 2-tesla superconducting system (Magnetom; Siemens, Erlangen, Germany) operating at 1.5 T with use of a circularly polarized head coil. T1- and T2-weighted imaging was performed with an inversion recovery sequence (TR/TI/TE = 3000/25/30) in the axial plane with a 7 mm slice thickness, a 0.7 mm interslice gap, and a 256 × 256 matrix.

Magnetic resonance spectroscopy. Localized, in vivo PMRS was performed with the stimulated echo acquisition mode (STEAM) sequence,[5, 6] with three water suppression chemical shift selective pulses (band width, 60 Hz). A volume of 2.4 cm^3 was selected from the left parietal region, which included gray matter, white matter, and the junctional zone. Selection of the volume was based on the maximal biochemical and structural changes documented in the cerebral cortex in experimental animals.[7] The dominant hemisphere was chosen arbitrarily. The spectroscopic measurements included the following: TR/TE/TM/number of acquisition = 5000/20/29.5/128. Voxel shimming yielded a line width (full width, half maximum) of 2 to 4 Hz. Postprocessing of the free induction decay was performed with use of zero filling (4k data points) and gaussian multiplication for resolution enhancement. The time domain spectrum was Fourier transformed and phase corrected. The real part of the spectrum was extracted, and no baseline correction was performed.

The coordinates of the volume selected were rechecked at the end of the measurement by performing imaging in three orthogonal planes to ensure that the data were obtained from the same preselected volume. Every effort was made to obtain additional spectra from the same volume with use of known anatomic landmarks on the image.

The peaks for NAA, *myo*-inositol, Cho, and total creatine, with chemical shifts of 2.02, 3.56, 3.22, and 3.02 ppm,[5] were quantified by peak integration. The ratios of NAA to Cr, mI to Cr, and Cho to Cr were calculated. The Cr value was chosen as the reference value because the total amount of Cr in brain tissue appears to be constant under different metabolic conditions.[8] Reproducibility of spectral patterns under baseline conditions was tested by performing measurements on the same volume on three different occasions in five adult volunteers.

Statistical analysis. Results were expressed as mean ± SD. One-way analysis of variance was used for comparison between groups.

RESULTS

Magnetic resonance imaging revealed that signal intensities from various white matter areas were comparable in untreated patients and control subjects. There was also no change in signal intensities after thyroxine replacement. All patients had mild cerebral cortical atrophy in the frontal and parietal lobes.

Proton MR spectroscopy revealed a high pretreatment Cho peak in patients, with a decline to normal values as euthyroidism was achieved (Figure). The Table shows the ratios of Cho, NAA, and mI to Cr in patients and control subjects. Patients had a significantly high mean pretreatment Cho/Cr ratio compared with control subjects (p <0.001). The mean Cho/Cr ratio also declined to a significantly lower mean level after thyroxine replacement in the patient group (p <0.008 vs pretreatment ratio). The level after treatment was comparable with the values obtained in the control group. Before and after treatment ratios of mI to Cr and NAA to Cr in the patient group were comparable with control values.

DISCUSSION

A prominent Cho resonance on PMRS, accounted for by choline, phosphocholine, and glycerophosphocholine,[4, 9-10] characterizes the neonatal brain. The gradual decline in this peak with increasing age has been attributed to the myelin maturation process[10, 11]; mature myelin is largely composed of galactolipids and sphingomyelin, which do not contribute to the Cho signal on PMRS.[4, 9-11] Thyroid hormone is essential for normal myelinogenesis. Studies in neonatally hypothyroid rats have shown suppressed formation of sphingomyelin and galactolipids, cerebroside, and sulfatide.[1] The high Cho levels in our patients could therefore be a reflection of delayed myelin maturation in the absence of thyroid hormone. Tzika et al.,[2] who used phosphorus 31 spectroscopy in neonatally hypothyroid rats, also showed a delay in the progressive rise of

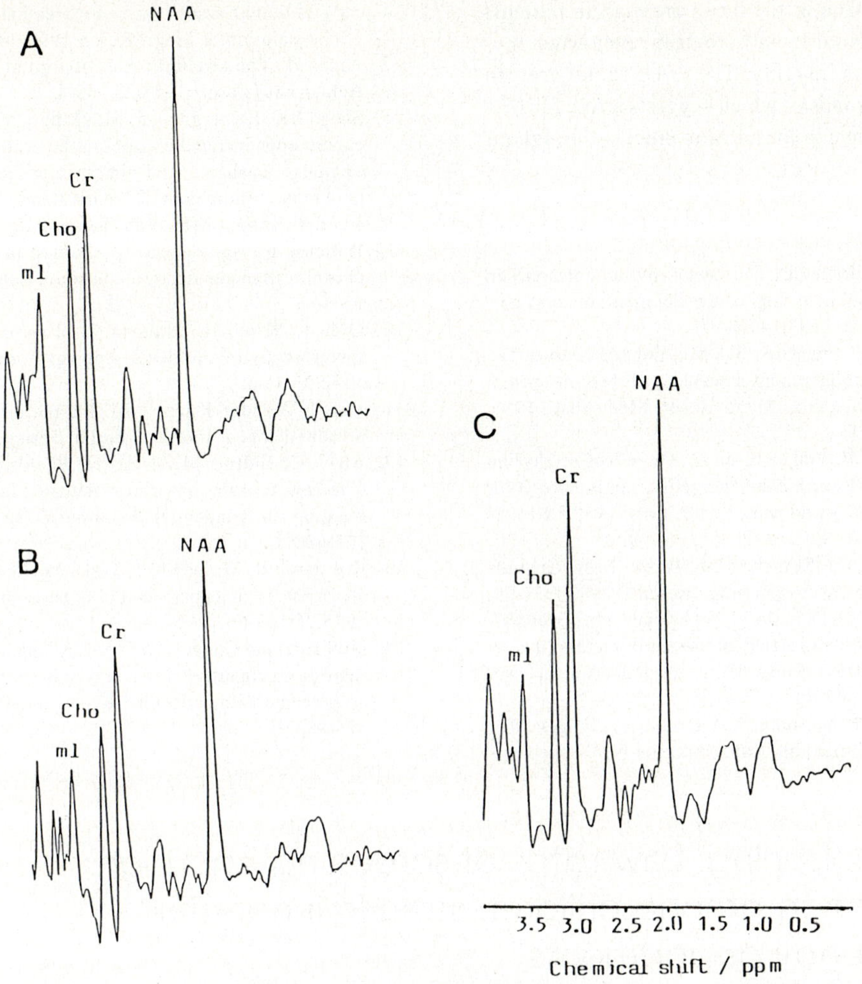

Figure. In vivo proton spectra at stimulated echo acquisition mode, 20 msec. **(A)**, Before treatment; **(B)**, 6 weeks after thyroxine replacement; **(C)**, 3 months after treatment (note gradual decrease in Cho resonance compared with Cr).

phosphodiester seen in the hypothyroid state, possibly reflecting delay in myelin maturation.

The prompt normalization of Cho levels with thyroxine replacement suggests that myelin maturation processes may be responsive to thyroid hormone throughout childhood. Magnetic resonance imaging was reported to have identified a delay in myelination in a 14-month-old girl with untreated congenital sporadic hypothyroidism; improvement was documented after thyroxine replacement.[12] In contrast, the myelin pattern of our untreated patients, who were older, was comparable with that of age-matched control subjects on MR imaging. This finding may be explained by the fact that myelin begins to be laid down at a later stage, even in the face of continuing thyroid hormone deficiency.[13] It appears that beyond the "critical period" of myelin formation, thyroid hormone is not essential for the process of myelination to begin.[1] However, our spectroscopic studies suggest that thyroid hormone may be essential throughout childhood for the completion of myelin maturation; MR imaging is probably not sensitive enough to study these processes. Although further studies in children and adults with hypothyroidism are necessary, our findings assume greater significance in the light of recent suggestions that thyroid hormone levels are directly proportionate to psychometric testing scores in poorly compliant adolescents with sporadic hypothyroidism who were treated optimally in early childhood.[14]

Our patients had NAA/Cr ratios comparable with those of the control subjects. NAA is a marker of neuronal maturation; its concentration reflects the number of axons, dendrites, and synaptic connections. Although congenitally hypothyroid rats have delayed dendritic arborization and synapse formation, they also have increased neuronal density in the cerebral cortex,[1] which could result in a normal NAA signal from the volume evaluated and mask the effect of decreased neuronal number and maturation.

We conclude that Cho in the brain are high in patients with untreated congenital hypothyroidism, even when myelin appears normal on imaging. The levels rapidly return to normal with euthyroidism, which suggests a role for thyroid hormone in the myelin maturation process throughout childhood.

REFERENCES

1. Porterfield SP, Hendrich CE. The role of thyroid hormones in parental and neonatal neurological development: current perspectives. Endocr Rev 1993;14:94-106.
2. Tzika A, Chew WM, Engelsted BL, Moseley ME, James TL, Timiras PS. Brain development assessed by NMR in normal and hypothyroid state. Soc Magn Reson Med Abstr 1985: 114-5.
3. Argov Z, Renshaw P, Boden B, et al. The effect of thyroid hormone on skeletal muscle bioenergetics: an in vivo 31-P NMR study of humans and rats. J Clin Invest 1988;81:1695-701.
4. Howe FA, Maxwell RJ, Saunders DE, Brown MM, Griffiths JR. Proton spectroscopy in vivo. Magn Reson Q 1993;9:31-59.
5. Michalis T, Merboldt KD, Hanicke W, Gyngell ML, Bruhn H, Frahm J. On the identification of cerebral metabolites in localized proton NMR spectra of the normal brain in vivo. NMR Biomed 1991;4:90-8.
6. Frahm J, Michalis T, Merboldt KD, Bruhn H, Gyngell ML, Hanicke W. Improvement in localized proton NMR spectroscopy of human brain, water suppression, short echo time and 1 ml resolution. J Magn Reson 1990;90:465-73.
7. Eagrs JT. The cerebral cortex of normal and hypothyroid rats. Acta Anat (Basel) 1955;25:160-4.
8. Siesjo BK, Folbergrova J, MacMillan V. The effect of hypercapnia upon intracellular pH in the brain, evaluated by the bicarbonate-carbonic acid method and from the creatine phosphokinase equilibrium. J Neurochem 1971;119:2483-95.
9. Vander Knaap MS, Van Rijan PC, Faber JAJ, Valk J, Willeuse K. Age dependent changes in localized proton and phosphorus spectroscopy of the brain. Radiology 1990;176:509-15.
10. Hida K, Kwell IL, Nakoda T. In vivo 1-H and 31-P NMR spectroscopy of the developing rat brain. Magn Reson Med 1992;23:31-6.
11. Valk J, Vander Knapp MS. Magnetic resonance of myelin, myelination and disorders. Berlin: Springer-Verlag, 1989:9-21.
12. Alves C, Eidson M, Engle H, Sheldon J, Cleveland WW. Changes in brain maturation detected by magnetic resonance imaging in congenital hypothyroidism. J PEDIATR 1989; 115:600-3.
13. Rosman NP, Malone MJ, Szoke M. Reversal of delayed myelinogenesis in experimental hypothyroidism. J Neurol Sci 1975;26:159-66.
14. New England Congenital Hypothyroidism Collaborative. Correlation of cognitive test scores and adequacy of treatment in adolescents with congenital hypothyroidism. J PEDIATR 1994; 124:383-7.

Lead poisoning: Low rates of screening and high prevalence among children seen in inner-city emergency departments

James F. Wiley II, MD, Louis M. Bell, MD, Lisa S. Rosenblum, MD, MPH, Jayne Nussbaum, MPA, Richard Tobin, MS, and Fred M. Henretig, MD

From the Section of Emergency Medicine, St. Christopher's Hospital for Children, Department of Pediatrics, Temple University School of Medicine, Philadelphia, Pennsylvania; the Section of Emergency Medicine and Division of General Pediatrics, Children's Hospital of Philadelphia, Department of Pediatrics, University of Pennsylvania School of Medicine; the Centers for Disease Control and Prevention, U.S. Department of Health and Human Services, Atlanta, Georgia; and the Philadelphia Childhood Lead Poisoning Prevention Program, Department of Public Health, Philadelphia, Pennsylvania

Of 254 children who were 1 to 6 years of age and were tested at two major inner-city emergency departments, 65% had no record of previous lead screening in the previous 30 months, and 71% (97/137) and 50% (58/117), respectively, had blood lead levels ≥0.48 μmol/L (10 μg/dl). The emergency department may be an appropriate resource for lead screening of selected inner-city children. (J PEDIATR 1995;126:392-5)

Supported in part by the Centers for Disease Control and Prevention, U.S. Department of Health and Human Services (OMB No. 0990-0115).

Presented in part at the American Academy of Pediatrics, Emergency Medicine Section Meeting, San Francisco, California, October 9, 1992.

Submitted for publication May 2, 1994; accepted Oct. 14, 1994.

Reprint requests: James F. Wiley II, MD, Section of Pediatric Emergency Medicine, St. Christopher's Hospital for Children, Front St. at Erie Ave., Philadelphia, PA 19134.

9/22/61271

The Centers for Disease Control and Prevention recommends blood lead screening of all children between the ages of 6 months and 6 years except in communities where large numbers of children have been screened and found not to have lead poisoning.[1] Although much recent literature has focused on defining what constitutes a low-prevalence community and on developing questionnaires to identify high-risk children for targeting lead screening in low-prevalence areas,[2,3] high prevalences of childhood lead poisoning persist in many communities (primarily inner cities).[4,5] Two recent reports from major cities suggest that many inner-city children may not have been screened for lead poisoning.[6,7] The main objective of this study was to determine the prevalences of having been screened for lead and having an elevated blood lead level in an inner-city pediatric emergency department population.

METHODS

From Oct. 21, 1991, to Nov. 3, 1991, venous blood lead screening was offered between 12 noon and 10 PM to children 1 to 6 years of age who were residents of Philadelphia and who were patients or children accompanying these patients in the EDs of St. Christopher's Hospital for Children and Children's Hospital of Philadelphia. These hospitals have 110,000 annual ED visits. Of 600 patients 1 to 6 years of age seen in the EDs during the study period, 240 were enrolled in our study. Exclusions occurred primarily as a result of limited staff to facilitate enrollment; some parents declined to participate because they believed that their children had undergone previous lead screening or because they preferred to have their children screened by their primary health care provider. In addition 50 children who accompanied the 240 patients were enrolled.

ED	Emergency department
EPSDT	Early Periodic Screening, Diagnosis, and Treatment
PCLPPP	Philadelphia Childhood Lead Poisoning Prevention Program

After informed consent was obtained from a parent or guardian, a phlebotomist performed venipuncture and used precautions to avoid specimen contamination. The Philadelphia Department of Public Health Lead Laboratory, the central laboratory for the city, analyzed the blood samples by atomic absorption spectrophotometry by the graphite furnace technique. Each specimen was run in duplicate, and the average of the two results was recorded. The standard deviation was ± 0.0483 μmol/L (1 μg/dl) for each test, with a minimal detectable value of 0.0966 μmol/L (2 μg/dl). Quality control measurements with standard samples were run on a regular basis (Dr. R. Chiuri, Director, Philadelphia Department of Public Health Lead Laboratory: personal communication, September 1991).

Referrals were made for medical management, and necessary follow-up and environmental investigations were administered through the Philadelphia Childhood Lead Poisoning Prevention Program in accordance with published guidelines.[1] Computerized records of the ED study population and of the PCLPPP (January 1989 to October 1991) were linked to determine whether the children in the ED had been previously screened for lead. The outcome of the computerized match was validated. Finger-stick tests for erythrocyte protoporphyrin or blood lead levels were considered as previous screening. During the study period the Philadelphia lead laboratory provided blood lead analysis at no charge for Philadelphia residents and therefore performed almost all blood lead screening for the area.

A questionnaire was administered to a parent or guardian by a trained epidemiologist to obtain information on the patient's age, race or ethnicity, sex, history of screening, contact with programs that offer lead screening (such as Early Periodic Screening, Diagnosis, and Treatment; Supplemental Food Program for Women, Infants, and Children; and Headstart), the principal site of primary health care, and the expected principal source of payment for the patient's current health care visit. Information on source of payment was not obtained for children accompanying these patients. Demographic information was validated with ED records and PCLPPP computer records.

The Pearson chi-square method was used to analyze categoric variables ($p < 0.05$). For odds ratios, the 95% confidence intervals were calculated with an exact method.[8] This protocol was reviewed and accepted by the institutional review boards of the participating institutions.

RESULTS

Of the 240 enrolled pediatric patients and the 50 children who accompanied them, 206 and 48, respectively, completed questionnaires and provided blood specimens. Thus the study population consisted of 254 children.

Of the participants, 50% were 1 to 2 years of age (mean, 3 years). Most were male (56%), had Medicaid as their expected principal source of payment for health care (72%), and received primary health care at a hospital clinic (52%). Fifty-four percent of participants were enrolled at site 1 (137/254). Participants at the two sites did not differ by age, gender, principal source of health care, number with Medicaid as primary source of payment, number with previous lead screening, number in Headstart, or number in the EPSDT program. Site 1 had more black participants (88% vs 46%; $p < 0.001$), and site 2 had more Latino participants (46% vs 4%; $p < 0.01$). Seventy-one percent of children at site 1 and 50% of children at site 2 had blood lead levels ≥ 0.48 μmol/L (10 μg/dl), and 7% at each site had blood lead levels ≥ 1.20 μmol/L (25 μg/dl).

Screening status. Of the 254 children, 164 (65%) had no record of previous lead screening. Factors significantly associated with having a record of lead screening were having as the principal source of primary health care a hospital medical clinic (57/133 screened vs 7/53 whose principal source was a pediatrician or family doctor; odds ratio 4.9, confidence interval 2.0 to 13.8), contact with EPSDT (75/177 screened vs 15/73; odds ratio 2.8, confidence interval 1.5 to 5.8), and contact with the Headstart program (28/54 screened vs 59/195; odds ratio 2.5, confidence interval 1.3 to 4.8). Factors not associated with having a previous record of screening were age, sex, race, and a blood lead level ≥0.48 μmol/L (10 μg/dl).

Of 360 children who received health care in the ED during the study period but who were not enrolled in the study, 238 (66%) had no record of lead screening. No significant difference was seen in the prevalence of past lead screening between those enrolled in the study and those not; this finding held true for all age groups.

Because health department records used to ascertain the status of previous lead screening were available for only 34 months, we tested whether older children might be less likely to have received screening after computerization of records by comparing screening rates among children younger than 34 months with rates among those older than 34 months. However, the proportion of children with no record of screening among those 12 to 34 months of age (85/131;65%) was similar to that among children 35 to 72 months of age (79/123; 64%).

DISCUSSION

In these two large, pediatric, inner-city EDs, most of the children who were 1 to 6 years of age had blood lead levels ≥0.48 μmol/L (10 μg/dl, 71% at site 1 and 50% at site 2) compared with an estimated 8.9% among children in the general U.S. population in 1991.[9] Sixty-one percent of the children seen in the EDs had not been screened previously for lead poisoning. Children who received services from EPSDT or Headstart or who received health care at a hospital were more likely to have been screened for lead burden than were other children. Some differences existed between the study sites, which reflected a difference in ethnic composition and suggested a higher prevalence of children with blood lead levels between 0.48 and 0.72 μmol/L at site 1. However, no difference in screening rates was seen between the two sites.

Limitations of our study include the availability of only 34 months of health department records to ascertain whether a child had had previous lead screening. However, when analyses were restricted to children less than 35 months of age, the study findings held true. Another limitation was that the enrollment included only 40% of children 1 to 6 years of age seen in the ED; however, no evidence showed that selection bias accounted for these findings. No difference was seen in the proportion of children in the ED who had been screened previously between those enrolled in the study and those not enrolled.

Our data indicate that lead screening in inner-city EDs identifies many children at high risk of having lead poisoning who had not been screened previously. Although most children seen in the ED had contact with primary care providers and other potential lead screening venues, such as EPSDT and the Supplemental Food Program for Women, Infants, and Children, most had not been screened for lead. Many U.S. children without health insurance may receive their only medical care in EDs. If a health care system that ensures access to care and universal coverage were instituted, EDs would probably not continue to serve as a source of primary health care for children. Until that time, screening children in EDs may be a useful adjunct to routine health care channels used to identify children with lead poisoning.

Some have expressed concern about the provision of primary health care activities in EDs because of expense, inefficiency, and negative impact on seeking subsequent primary care.[10] Proponents of limited primary care activities in the ED argue that real barriers to primary care still exist for poor urban children; they suggest a partnership between primary care and emergency care providers that would allow use of the ED as an adjunct source of primary care for underprivileged children, particularly in urban areas.[11] The ED may serve as a source of lead screening for selected inner-city children as long as central tracking of screening results, linkage to primary care service, and medical management of lead poisoning occur.

REFERENCES

1. Centers for Disease Control. Preventing lead poisoning in young children: A statement by the Centers for Disease Control, 1991. Atlanta: Centers for Disease Control, 1991.
2. Geller GA, Wagner GA, Maxwell RM, et al. Lead poisoning among low income children in Orange County, California: a need for regionally differentiated policy. JAMA 1993;270:69-71.
3. Binns HJ, Lebailly SA, Poncher J, et al. Is there lead in the suburbs? risk assessment in Chicago suburban pediatric practices. Pediatrics 1994;93:164-71.
4. Rifai N, Cohen G, Wolf M, et al. Incidence of lead poisoning in young children from inner-city, suburban, and rural communities. Ther Drug Monit 1993;15:71-4.
5. Centers for Disease Control and Prevention. Blood lead levels among children in high-risk areas—California, 1987-1990. MMWR Morb Mortal Wkly Rep 1992;41:291-4.
6. Campbell JR, Weitzman M, McConnochie K. Lead screening opportunities missed among urban children [Abstract]. Am J Dis Child 1992;146:477.
7. Wiley JF, Henretig FM, Selbst SM. Blood lead levels in children with foreign bodies. Pediatrics 1992;89:593-6.
8. Mehta CR, Patel, Gray R. Computing an exact confidence in-

terval for the common odds ratio in several 2 × 2 contingency tables. Journal of the American Statistical Association 1985; 80:969-73.
9. Brody DJ, Pirkle JL, Kramer RA, Flegal KM, et al. Blood lead levels in the US Population: phase 1 of the third National Health and Nutrition Examination Survey (NHANES III, 1988-1991). JAMA 1994;272:277-83.
10. Barton LL, Binkiewicz A, Ey J, Eicher M. Primary care in the emergency department [Letter]. Pediatrics 1994;94:406-7.
11. Bell LM. Providing primary care to children in the emergency department: a problem or a missed opportunity? [Editorial]. Pediatr Emerg Care 1991;7:124.

Resolution of breath-holding spells with treatment of concomitant anemia

Kenneth F. Colina, MD, and Herbert T. Abelson, MD
From the Department of Pediatrics, University of Washington School of Medicine and the Children's Hospital and Medical Center, Seattle

We describe two children who had breath-holding spells that were accelerating in frequency and severity and in one case had recrudesced. Both patients had signs, symptoms, and laboratory findings of severe anemia. With correction of anemia the breath-holding spells promptly and completely resolved in each case. We conclude that in some patients anemia may be a factor contributing to breath-holding spells and that correction of concomitant anemia may produce amelioration or remission of the spells. (J PEDIATR 1995;126:395-7)

Breath-holding spells occur to some degree in up to 27% of typical children. DiMario[1] noted that the term is a misnomer that implies a voluntary action resulting in a prolonged inspiration, whereas in actuality the spells are involuntary, reflexive, and occur during expiration. Although BHS are generally benign in nature and prognosis, some children sustain physical trauma during these events, and the spells cause both parental alarm and use of medical services. Both the pathophysiology and the treatment of BHS remain controversial. An association between anemia and BHS has previously been recognized, but published reports are few and are not general pediatric knowledge. We report two children with typical BHS who were found to be profoundly anemic and whose BHS resolved after treatment of their anemia.

CASE REPORTS

Patient 1. A 32-month-old white girl was seen for evaluation of "passing out when she cries." She had a 1-month history of episodes occurring two or three times a day in which she would vigorously cry without inhaling, pass out, and fall to the floor for 1 to 2 minutes, often with cyanosis. She would then arouse, be groggy for about 30 seconds, and then resume playing normally. She would occasionally stiffen while on the floor, but she usually was limp; no history of tonic-clonic activity was reported. The parents noted that these episodes had been increasing in frequency during the preceding weeks and that the patient had increasing fatigue and decreasing activity, and had been more pale than usual during the preceding month. They had begun giving her iron pills 3 days before the visit to treat the pallor. No recent illnesses were reported.

Between the ages of 12 and 18 months the patient had episodes of breath holding and passing out. At that time she was treated for "anemia" with orally administered iron by her physician; both the breath-holding episodes and the anemia resolved by 18 months. The medical history was otherwise noncontributory. Her diet was appropriate for her age.

BHS	Breath-holding spells
TIBC	Total iron-binding capacity

Physical examination revealed a very pale, well-nourished, playful girl with a hyperdynamic precordium and a grade 3/6 systolic ejection murmur at the base. The liver edge was 1.5 cm below the right costal margin, and the spleen tip was just palpable in the left upper abdominal quadrant. Examination findings were otherwise unremarkable.

The complete blood cell count showed hemoglobin 48 gm/L, hematocrit 0.15, mean cell volume 62 fl, mean cell hemoglobin 20 pg, mean cell hemoglobin concentration 320 gm/L, red cell distribution width 16.2%, erythrocytes, $2.4 \times 10^{12}/L$, platelets $507 \times 10^9/L$, and leukocytes $5.7 \times 10^9/L$ with neutrophils 42%, bands 1%, lymphocytes 46%, monocytes 6%, eosinophils 4%, and myelocytes 1%. The raw reticulocyte count was 4.9%; the doubly corrected re-

Submitted for publication July 5, 1994; accepted Sept. 13, 1994.
Reprint requests: Kenneth F. Colina, MD, Scott and White Clinic, 7700 Fish Pond Rd., Waco, TX, 76710.

0022-3476/95/$3.00 + 0 **9/22/60609**

ticulocyte count was 0.7%. The smear showed many hypochromic cells, few microcytes, few teardrops, few erythrocyte fragments, moderate elliptocytes, and moderate polychromatophilic erythrocytes. Iron study findings were all within the normal range: serum iron 17 μmol/L (97 μg/dl), total iron-binding capacity 53 μmol/L (297 μg/dl), and ferritin 42 ng/ml. Hemoglobin electrophoresis revealed hemaglobin A, increased hemoglobin F, and increased hemoglobin A_2 at 4.7%, compatible with β-thalassemia trait. The zinc protoporphyrin level was normal: 93 μmol/mol heme. On the basis of these results, the β-thalassemia trait and either intercurrent transient erythroblastopenia of childhood or viral suppression were diagnosed.

The patient received an erythrocyte transfusion of 10 ml/kg which raised the hematocrit to 0.25. The BHS resolved completely after the transfusion. One week later her hematocrit was 0.28 (doubly corrected reticulocyte count 2.4%), and 2 weeks later it was 0.32 (doubly corrected reticulocyte count 1.2%) without further treatment. Nine months later she continued to have no BHS.

Patient 2. A 19-month-old Southeast Asian girl was referred by her family physician for evaluation of a 4-month history of BHS that had been increasing markedly in frequency and severity for the previous 2 months. At the time of evaluation, episodes were occurring up to 10 times/day whenever the patient cried vigorously. The patient would cry, then stop breathing, have either perioral cyanosis or pallor, and then fall to the ground and frequently have tonic-clonic movements of the upper and lower extremities. She would typically remain unresponsive for 1 to 5 minutes and would then resume activity. Pallor and fatigue had been noted by the parents, and they had started therapy with orally administered iron 1 week previously.

The patient's diet consisted of 1200 to 2400 ml whole cow milk/day and some cereal but rarely any other foods. The medical history was unremarkable.

Physical examination revealed an extremely pale well-nourished girl who was very irritable. A grade 2/6 systolic ejection murmur was heard along the upper left sternal border. The examination was otherwise unremarkable. An episode of breath holding and unresponsiveness occurred during the examination and was consistent with severe BHS.

The complete blood cell count showed hemoglobin 51 gm/L, hematocrit 0.18, mean cell volume 51 fl, mean cell hemoglobin 15 pg, mean cell hemoglobin concentration 280 gm/L, red cell distribution width 32.8%, erythrocytes 3.5×10^{12}/L, platelets 467×10^9/L, leukocytes 15.2×10^9/L with neutrophils 26%, lymphocytes 69%, eosinophils 4%, and basophils 1%. The raw reticulocyte count was 7.5%; the doubly corrected reticulocyte count was 1.9%. The smear showed moderate hypochromic cells, many microcytes, few teardrops, few erythrocyte fragments, moderate elliptocytes, and moderate polychromatophilic erythrocytes. Iron studies showed serum iron concentration 4 μmol/L (21 μg/dl) (normal, 4 to 22 μmol/L), TIBC 65 μmol/L (364 μg/dl) (normal, 45 to 72 μmol/L), and ferritin 3 ng/ml (normal, 15 to 160 ng/ml). Hemoglobin electrophoresis revealed hemoglobin A and A_2, with 1.8% A_2. Brilliant cresyl blue preparation was negative for α-thalassemia. Zinc protoporphyrin was >200 μmol/mol heme. Stool had occult blood on two separate specimens. Iron deficiency anemia (partially treated) caused by excessive cow milk intake, with occult blood loss in the stool and probable insufficient dietary iron intake, was diagnosed.

Chest x-ray findings were normal. An echocardiogram revealed a left atrial membrane (cor triatriatum) without evidence of pulmonary venous obstruction (flow velocity through the mitral valve ring, 1.7 m/sec), mild concentric left ventricular hypertrophy, and a small pericardial effusion. A 24-hour Holter monitor study revealed bradycardia associated with BHS but no other arrhythmia.

The patient was treated with orally administered iron and responded with a rise in hematocrit to 0.23 within 8 days. The parents succeeded in decreasing the milk intake and broadening the child's diet. Within 2 months her hematocrit had risen to 0.34, her BHS had completely resolved, and her activity level had increased to normal. Results of tests for stool occult blood became negative. Follow-up echocardiogram showed lower-flow velocity (1.2 m/sec) across the left atrial membrane, normal cardiac dimensions and function, and resolution of the pericardial effusion.

DISCUSSION

The final event leading to loss of consciousness in BHS is cerebral anoxia.[1, 2] In a retrospective case-control study, Holowach et al.[3] demonstrated that children with severe BHS had significantly lower hemoglobin values than did children in a control group. They speculated that children with anemia have decreased cerebral oxygen tension at baseline and that these children were thus more susceptible to the chain of events leading to loss of consciousness during BHS. Other controlled studies during the 1960s did not find significant differences in hemoglobin concentrations between children with and those without BHS.[4, 5]

A recent prospective study in India[6] found that children with BHS seen in an outpatient immunization clinic had significantly lower hemoglobin and serum iron values, a lower percentage of saturation of transferrin, and higher TIBC than did a control group (although the mean serum iron and TIBC values were in the normal range for both groups). These investigators demonstrated that all anemic children with BHS had a decrease in severity and frequency of BHS with oral iron therapy, paralleling a rise in hemoglobin levels to $\geq$ 110 gm/L in 82% of cases. (However, they did not treat nonanemic children with BHS with iron.) In a recent review DiMario[1] speculated that "anemia cannot contribute significantly to the cause of BHS, but may be an additional influence in individual children," and mentioned anecdotal experience of improvement of BHS with resolution of anemia in one child. Others have included similar cases in their reports.[2, 3]

The irritability of children with iron deficiency is well known, and this factor alone may contribute to the frequency of BHS, causing more instances of emotional upset and crying, which serve as initiating events for BHS. Resolution of the irritability of iron deficiency thus may account for some decrease in BHS but not their complete cessation: all children cry and are emotionally upset at times, and one would not expect the initiating events of BHS to resolve completely. Indeed, BHS occur commonly in children without iron deficiency. Anemia from causes other than iron deficiency appears to exert an effect on BHS, as demonstrated by our first patient, who was severely anemic but iron replete.

Our second patient had cor triatriatum and a small pericardial effusion but no evidence of pulmonary venous congestion. With resolution of the anemia the flow velocity across the left atrial membrane diminished, consistent with resolution of the high output state of anemia. The patient's spells ceased with resolution of the anemia, but the cardiac findings changed only minimally (and these changes were consistent with resolution of the anemic state), indicating that the anemia rather than the cardiac disease was the factor contributing to BHS. Whether the combination of anemia and congenital heart disease further predisposed this patient to severe BHS is not known.

On the basis of our findings and those reported in the literature, it is prudent to consider the diagnosis of anemia in children with BHS. Because BHS generally occur at an age when both iron deficiency anemia and elevated lead levels are common, it may be reasonable to screen all children with BHS for anemia. Certain children with BHS warrant special consideration for evaluation: those with a suggestive history or physical findings such as fatigue, irritability, or pallor; those with severe or accelerating events; those with recrudescent BHS; and those at risk of having anemia because of genetic, dietary, or other factors.

The precise relation between anemia and BHS awaits further large prospective investigations. Our experience adds to the anecdotal evidence that children with BHS benefit from treatment of concomitant anemia.

REFERENCES

1. DiMario FJ. Breath-holding spells in childhood. Am J Dis Child 1992;146:125-31.
2. Lombroso CT, Lerman P. Breathholding spells (cyanotic and pallid infantile syncope). Pediatrics 1967;39:563-81.
3. Holowach J, Thurston DL. Breath-holding spells and anemia. N Engl J Med 1963;268:21-3.
4. Laxdal T, Gomez MR, Reiher J. Cyanotic and pallid syncopal attacks in children (breath-holding spells). Dev Med Child Neurol 1969;11:755-76.
5. Maulsby R, Kellaway P. Transient hypoxic crisis in children. In: Kellaway P, ed. Neurological and electroencephalographic correlative studies in infancy. New York: Grune & Stratton, 1964:349-60.
6. Bhatia MS, Singhal PK, Dhar NK, Nigam VR, Malik SC, Mullick DN. Breath holding spells: an analysis of 50 cases. Indian Pediatr 1990;27:1073-9.

Overinterpretation of gastroduodenal motility studies: Two cases involving Munchausen syndrome by proxy

Howard I. Baron, MD, David C. Beck, MD, Jorge H. Vargas, MD, and Marvin E. Ament, MD

From the Departments of Pediatrics and Psychiatry, University of California at Los Angeles Center for the Health Sciences

Two children were thought to have an atypical gastroduodenal motility disorder because of the history and clinical course; both had received parenteral alimentation because of claims of inability to tolerate enteral feedings, and both continued to have unusual medical problems during parenteral alimentation. Both children had motility studies that were interpreted by a pediatric gastroenterologist to be "abnormal" and "diagnostic" of a motility disorder, but each was eventually shown to have a behavioral abnormality related to Munchausen syndrome by proxy. (J Pediatr 1995;126:397-400)

Submitted for publication June 27, 1994; accepted Oct. 11, 1994.

Reprint requests: Howard I. Baron, MD, 3196 Maryland Parkway, Suite 309, Las Vegas, NV 89109.

0022-3476/95/$3.00 + 0 9/22/61301

Clinical gastroenterologists use water-perfused and solid-state catheters to evaluate possible gastrointestinal motility disorders in patients with a large spectrum of complaints referable to the gastrointestinal tract. However, much remains to be learned about what makes up a "normal" gastrointestinal motility pattern and what clinical conditions can be conclusively said to have "abnormal" patterns. If a parent exaggerates, distorts, or fabricates a child's symptoms, a gastroenterologist may unwittingly overinterpret the results of motility studies by correlating false history with nonspecific findings. As illustrated in the following case reports, assigning patients a diagnosis of a motility disorder solely on the basis of pattern recognition or abstract measures such as a motility index can be a great disservice to the patient and may perpetuate a form of child abuse.

CASE REPORTS

Patient 1. A 2½-year-old boy was referred to the University of California at Los Angeles Center for the Health Sciences for elective evaluation and treatment of "visceral hyperalgesia" and an "enteric neuromuscular disorder." He was born at 37 weeks of gestational age by cesarean section for placenta accretia. His birth weight was 3.1 kgs. He had multiple episodes of pneumonia beginning early in infancy and vomiting that was initially managed with metoclopramide and a variety of aerosol medications after an upper gastrointestinal tract x-ray series revealed gastroesophageal reflux. The child had been examined by a pulmonologist, a gastroenterologist, an immunologist, a pediatrician, and finally a surgeon, who performed a Nissen fundoplication and gastrostomy at 9 months of age. Subsequently the patient was described as being in "constant pain" when fed through his gastrostomy tube, even when formula was given as a continuous drip. By his mother's report he had sweating, gagging, choking, cramping, screaming, thrashing, and retching. A central venous catheter was placed at 16 months of age for parenteral nutritional support. Attempts at enteral feeding via the gastrostomy or even a gastrojejunal tube resulted in behaviors interpreted as severe pain. Cisapride was given without significant change in clinical symptoms. Eventually even manipulation of the gastrostomy resulted in episodes of screaming and crying.

MSP	Munchausen syndrome by proxy
TPN	Total parenteral nutrition

The patient underwent gastroduodenal motility evaluation with the mother present and had complaints of pain during duodenal phase III episodes. He also had postprandial duodenal hypomotility, which was indicated by lack of the usual disorganized postprandial activity in the duodenum. He had symptoms during the postprandial period that included pain, retching behavior, diaphoresis, and lethargy. Colonic manometry was also performed, and results were interpreted as normal.

The family history as reported by the mother included hypoglycemia in the patient's father and diabetes mellitus on his side of the family. The maternal grandmother reportedly had porphyria, and a maternal aunt had a bipolar disorder. The patient's mother described immunologic problems in herself and in her teenage son from a previous marriage, and she reported that he had had an extensive medical evaluation for severe allergies and intestinal problems including testing for Hirschprung disease. The mother reported that she slept with the patient in the living room rather than with her husband because of concern about the patient's medical problems.

Because of the manometric findings the patient was admitted to the hospital for pain management. This treatment included epidural catheter placement and an attempt at ablation of visceral sensory afferent pathways, which might then allow enteral feedings. However, observations of the maternal-child interaction by nursing staff, residents, and faculty members during the first 24 to 48 hours of hospitalization suggested a strong behavioral component to his symptoms and overintrusive maternal behavior in response to these symptoms. The epidural catheter was removed (only one dose of medication had been given), and the mother was encouraged to leave the hospital to see whether the child's behavior would change while the father provided parental support. The patient then had a substantial decrease in the frequency of pain. The father, who had previously not been involved with the patient's medical care, quickly adapted to the caregiver role and with coaching was able to distract the patient from the pain, which was extinguished within 1 week. During that time the parenteral nutrition was tapered off and enteral feedings were begun (first by gastrostomy, then by mouth). By the twenty-third day of hospitalization the patient was receiving oral feeding only and the central venous catheter and gastrostomy were removed. His parents were coached to redirect his (and their) attention away from his body.

Toward the end of the hospitalization the mother was reintroduced to the caregiver role and again reported severe pain and diaphoresis episodes in the patient while he was being observed by other members of the health care team. They did not agree with her assessment, and the mother was repeatedly asked to alter her intrusive approach to her son's symptoms. All caregivers agreed that the mother fit the typical maternal profile for Munchausen syndrome by proxy. Although no evidence of purposeful covert induction of medical illness was obtained during the hospitalization, the mother's history of illness fabrication in herself (her reports of immunologic problems had no basis when reviewed with her doctors) and her witnessed overreporting of symptoms in her son, in combination with his recovery during her absence, indicated a need for close supervision and psychotherapy for this family, and this intervention had been arranged at the time of hospital discharge.

Patient 2. An 18-month-old boy was referred to the University of California at Los Angeles Center for the Health Sciences with the clinical diagnosis of chronic intestinal pseudoobstruction syndrome dependent on parenteral nutrition. He had had an unusual history of recurrent episodes of gram-negative and gram-positive sepsis in the 5 months before his admission, which had kept him hospitalized for most of that time. The patient had been born at 32 weeks of gestational age and weighed 2012 gm at birth. He was born with respiratory distress that required 1 week of mechanical ventilation, but he had no evidence of chronic lung disease. He had poor weight gain and was spitting up, and an x-ray study of the upper gastrointestinal tract revealed an episode of gastroesophageal reflux that was initially managed with positioning and later metoclopramide, bethanecol, and cimetidine. Recurrent admissions for respiratory illnesses, vomiting, and failure to thrive led to endoscopy and biopsy of the upper gastrointestinal tract. On two occasions these tests revealed mild esophageal inflammation. The patient's mother continued to report vomiting, and the patient stopped gaining weight, which prompted a Nissen fundoplication and gastrostomy. After this procedure was done, the patient had "severe gagging" whenever he was fed, even by continuous drip. The patient was readmitted at 14 months of age, and a third upper endoscopy was performed; biopsy specimens were "improved but showing some features of mild reflux esophagitis." Finally, after continuous-drip elemental formula failed because of retching, a central venous catheter was placed for nighttime parenteral nutrition.

After the central venous catheter was placed, the patient had sepsis on multiple occasions; blood cultures revealed multiple gram-positive and gram-negative organisms. Each episode of sepsis was treated with appropriate antibiotics for 2 to 4 weeks, and yet each time antibiotic therapy was stopped, sepsis recurred within hours or days, even when the patient was hospitalized. The central venous catheter was replaced on two occasions, but infections quickly recurred. Results of an evaluation of the patient's immune system were normal, and an attempt at treatment of presumed intestinal bacterial overgrowth failed to decrease the infection rate. The mother always insisted on providing all central line care herself, even when the patient was hospitalized. Because of the great difficulty in providing TPN, an attempt at promoting gut motility was made with cisapride for a total of 6 weeks, but no improvement occurred in the patient's ability to tolerate enteral feedings. Other studies performed included renal ultrasonography, suction rectal biopsies, x-ray studies (with barium) of the upper gastrointestinal tract, and a gastric emptying study, all of which showed normal findings.

At this point the patient was referred to our health care center to obtain another opinion. Because of the pattern of illness and the history, the diagnosis of MSP was suspected, and transfer of this patient to the pediatric intensive care unit was arranged, with one-to-one nursing and close monitoring of any contact between mother and patient. The patient spent 18 days in the intensive care unit. The hospitalization was structured to demonstrate that the patient could be successfully fed by mouth; he had no need for TPN or gastrostomy tube feedings. On the patient's admission, blood cultures were obtained and all antibiotics were stopped. The patient (who had never remained afebrile for more than 1 week in the 5 months before admission) remained afebrile with no signs of sepsis during his hospitalization. The nursing staff never allowed the mother to be alone with the child and did not allow her to administer care or food to the child. The patient's TPN regimen was initially continued and the patient was offered oral elemental formula as desired. A gastric emptying study performed with a liquid meal revealed that only 38% of the radiolabeled meal remained in the stomach after 90 minutes. Results of an esophageal motility study were normal, and a 24-hour intraesophageal pH study revealed no episodes of reflux longer than 2 minutes and no retching episodes. Intraesophageal pH was less than 4 for only 3% of the entire study. Feedings were then begun as a continuous drip by gastrostomy and were rapidly advanced, which allowed complete discontinuation of TPN within 48 hours. A gastroduodenal motility study revealed normal fasting motility patterns in phases I, II, and III, and a meal was followed by conversion to the usual disorganized "fed" pattern in the antrum and duodenum.

The patient was given intermittent feedings via the gastrostomy and was then given oral feedings. After a normal lactose breath hydrogen test result, milk products were introduced. The gastrostomy and the central venous catheter were removed, and the patient began a "diet for age" before hospital discharge. The nursing staff noted that in the mother's absence the patient would happily play with food and put it into his mouth, but in her presence he would spit it out and hold his abdomen, shouting "owee, owee." The social history strongly supported the diagnosis of MSP. When confronted with the steady improvement in her child during his hospital stay, the mother expressed no relief or satisfaction. The mother was suspected to have purposely contaminated the blood via the central venous catheter, causing the recurrent sepsis. The child was discharged to foster care, where he continued to thrive, with none of the symptoms or difficulties previously noted.

A legal battle ensued regarding foster placement of this patient, and argument by experts in the field of pediatric gastrointestinal motility disorders centered around whether the gastroduodenal manometry findings were normal, because the "motility index" was seemingly lower than "normal" in the postprandial phase of the study. The motility index (MI) is an arithmetic expression of the postprandial phasic pressure response of a portion of the gastrointestinal tract and is obtained by the following formula[1]: $MI = \log_e$ (Sum of amplitudes × Number of waves + 1).

DISCUSSION

These two cases illustrate how overinterpretation of intraluminal gastrointestinal motility studies can cause clinicians to ignore more salient features of a set of symptoms. In both examples the patients had a multitude of symptoms that seemed improbable or bizarre. Both patients had mothers who fit the classically described profile of a parent with MSP. Both patients recovered promptly when isolated from maternal interventions, completely losing symptoms that had been thought to originate in the gastrointestinal tract. In both cases, gastrointestinal motility patterns were judged to be abnormal, and a cause-effect relationship was inferred by experts in the field. Although intraluminal gastroduodenal motility testing has become the vogue among academic centers across the United States, much remains to be learned regarding what constitutes a "normal" versus an "abnormal" result. Distinctive patterns have been delineated in both the fasting and fed states,[2, 3] but normative data have not been published for children because of an inability to obtain sanction by hospital ethics committees to perform invasive manometric testing on healthy children. This lack of information leaves the clinician who performs gastroduodenal motility studies devoid of any reference ranges for frequency of migrating motor complexes, duration of its constituent phases, rate of propagation of the migrating motor complex, and even more abstract arithmetic measurements such as motility index. The interpatient and intrapatient variability in these studies, which has been described for healthy adults,[4, 5] likely applies to children also.[6]

In our first patient a motility study was interpreted to show postprandial duodenal hypomotility. This entity has been described in a child with cystic fibrosis[7] whose postprandial motility pattern became quiescent for 1 hour after ingestion of a meal and whose symptoms responded to the prokinetic agent cisapride. Our patient did not realize any benefit from cisapride and did not have his motility study performed in the absence of his mother. Stress has been implicated as a major factor contributing to the results of motility tests,[8-10] and it is impossible to determine what effect stress may have had on the outcome of this child's study. Nonetheless the interpretation of the motility study prompted unnecessary and invasive medical evaluation and transiently diverted the focus of the evaluation away from the psychosocial aspects of the case.

In patient 2 a strong suspicion of MSP prompted a thorough, controlled evaluation, which included a gastroduodenal motility study as part of a global attempt to document "normalcy" in the absence of the mother. Although initial interpretation of this study was that findings were normal, considerable time and attention was focused on the study results during the custody hearing by expert witnesses who claimed that the motility index was abnormally low. Motility index ranges have been established in healthy adult control groups,[1] but no studies of typical children have been published. Because of interequipment variability, normal ranges need to be established for each motility laboratory; our laboratory has no normative data for pediatric patients. The court eventually concluded that the motility index was an uninterpretable and insignificant factor. The manometry study may have hindered the eventual resolution of this case more than it helped, and given the clinical course of the patient, the motility study should have been deferred, especially in the presence of normal gastric emptying.

It is natural for physicians to desire objective data to prove or disprove physical illness, but a test such as gastroduodenal manometry probably cannot differentiate between organic disease and MSP. Nonetheless, centers with the most experience in pediatric motility disorders frequently receive referrals of patients with gastrointestinal symptoms to rule out MSP with manometry.[6] Our two cases demonstrate the pitfalls in believing that gastroduodenal motility testing can differentiate MSP from organic causes, and we recommend a moratorium on manometric testing for this purpose. We also suggest caution in interpretation of pediatric motility patterns as abnormal, until normal data are available.

REFERENCES

1. Malagelada J, Camilleri M, Stanghellini V. Manometric diagnosis of gastrointestinal motility disorders. New York: Thieme, Inc, 1986:57.
2. Wingate DL. Backward and forwards with the migrating complex. Dig Dis Sci 1981;26:641-64.
3. Sarna SK. Cyclic motor activity: migrating motor complex: 1985. Gastroenterology 1985;189:894-913.
4. Dooley CP, diLorenzo C, Valenzuela JF. Variability of the migrating motor complex in the human. Dig Dis Sci 1992; 37:723-8.
5. Quigley EMM, Donovan JP, Lane MJ, Gallagher TF. Antroduodenal manometry: usefulness and limitations as an outpatient study. Dig Dis Sci 1992;37:10-3.
6. Hyman PE, Napolitano JA, Diego A, et al. Antroduodenal manometry in the evaluation of chronic functional gastrointestinal symptoms. Pediatrics 1990;86:39-44.
7. Hyman PE. Absent postprandial duodenal motility in a child with cystic fibrosis; correction of the symptoms and manometric abnormality with cisapride. Gastroenterology 1986;90: 1274-9.
8. Camilleri M, Neri M. Motility disorders and stress. Dig Dis Sci 1989;34:1777-86.
9. Wingate DL. The brain-gut link. Viewpoints Dig Dis 1985; 17:17-20.
10. Welgan P, Meshkinpour H, Beeler M. Effect of anger on colon motor and myoelectric activity in irritable bowel syndrome. Gastroenterology 1990;94:1150-6.

A missense mutation in a patient with guanosine triphosphate cyclohydrolase I deficiency missed in the newborn screening program

N. Blau, PhD, H. Ichinose, PhD, T. Nagatsu, PhD, MD, C. W. Heizmann, PhD, F. Zacchello, MD, and A. B. Burlina, MD

From the Division of Clinical Chemistry, Department of Pediatrics, University of Zurich, Zurich, Switzerland; the Division of Molecular Genetics (II) Neurochemistry, Institute for Comprehensive Medical Science, Fujita Health University, Toyoake, Japan; and the Department of Pediatrics, University of Padua, Padua, Italy

A patient with guanosine triphosphate cyclohydrolase I deficiency passed the newborn phenylketonuria screening program. The characteristic clinical phenotype developed in a 5-month-old patient; elevated plasma phenylalanine, undetectable urinary pterins, and absence of the enzyme activity in a liver biopsy were present. A point mutation that results in an amino acid substitution from methionine to isoleucine at position 211 was proposed to be the cause for this new phenotypic expression of guanosine triphosphate cyclohydrolase I deficiency. (J Pediatr 1995;126:401-5)

Deficiency of guanosine triphosphate cyclohydrolase I (McKusick 233910) is an autosomal recessive disorder caused by a defect in the biosynthesis of tetrahydrobiopterin.[1] The variable but common symptoms are mental retardation, convulsions, disturbance of tone and posture, abnormal movements, hypersalivation, and swallowing difficulties. Most of the patients were screened for hyperphenylalaninemia between 4 and 11 days of age and had plasma phenylalanine levels between 300 and 800 μmol/L.[1-4] BH_4 is the natural cofactor of the aromatic amino acid monooxygenases[5] and nitric oxide synthase.[6] GTPCH catalyzes the first reaction in BH_4 biosynthesis and is regulated by feedback inhibition of BH_4.[7] GTPCH deficiency is less common compared with other forms of BH_4 deficiencies; only eight patients have been described.[8] We describe a mutation analysis of a patient with GTPCH deficiency.

Supported by the Swiss National Science Foundation (grant 31-33897.92) and the Helmut Horten Research Foundation (both to Dr. Blau), and by the Sandoz Foundation (Dr. Heizmann).

Submitted for publication July 25, 1994; accepted Sept. 16, 1994.

Reprint requests: N. Blau, PhD, Division of Clinical Chemistry, Department of Pediatrics, University of Zurich, Steinwiesstrasse 75, 8032 Zurich, Switzerland.

0022-3476/95/$3.00 + 9/22/60733

CASE REPORT

An infant boy, the second child of healthy nonconsanguineous parents, was born at term after a normal pregnancy. His birth weight was 3700 gm, and Apgar scores were 10 at 1 and 5 minutes. At birth, slight hypotonia of the neck and limbs was observed. The phenylketonuria screening Guthrie test showed normal values (<120 μmol/L).

The patient was breast-fed, and his weight gain was normal during the first few months of life. He had no feeding problems. When he was 4 months of age, developmental delay was noted; the objective neurologic findings were generalized hypotonia, clonic movements, and tendon reflexes in the upper limbs. The patient was admitted to another hospital where routine biochemical investigations (including plasma ammonia and lactate) and instrumental investigations (electroencephalography and cerebral magnet resonance imaging) were done; all findings were negative.

BH_4	Tetrahydrobiopterin
CSF	Cerebrospinal fluid
5-HIAA	5-Hydroxyindoleacetic acid
GTPCH	GTP cyclohydrolase I
HVA	Homovanillic acid

At the age of 4½ months the patient was referred to us. A physical examination confirmed the neurologic delay in development with generalized hypotonia and dystonic Parkinson-like movements with wide-ranging tremors, especially of the upper limbs and the head. Electroencephalography showed slight asymmetry in the right hemisphere; brain-stem auditory-evoked potential studies pointed to an alteration in the central components. Plasma amino

Table. Biochemical data and therapy protocols in our patient with a GTPCH deficiency

	CSF						
Age (mo)	**Neopterin (nmol/L)**	**Biopterin (nmol/L)**	**Phenylalanine (μmol/L)**	**Tyrosine (μmol/L)**	**5-HIAA (nmol/L)**	**HVA (nmol/L)**	**5-MTHF nmol/L**
5	0	7.5	94	14	92	50	ND
6	ND	ND	ND	ND	ND	ND	ND
7	ND	ND	ND	ND	ND	ND	ND
9	ND	ND	ND	ND	ND	ND	ND
10	0	5.8	14	16	262	192	ND
12½	0	0	24	12	154	163	45
16	0	4.5	10	14	191	306	86
18	0	6.8	126	19	93	43	74
25	0.5	4.0	12	16	203	423	93
33	0.8	9.3	21	10	188	310	92
Control subjects							
0-1 yr	9-20	10-34	<20	<25	114-336	295-932	64-182
2-4 yr					105-299	211-871	62-111

ND, Not determined; *5-MTHF*, 5-methyltetrahydrofolic acid; *5-HTRP*, 5-hydroxytryptophan.

acid analysis, performed during the period of exclusive breast-feeding, revealed an increase of phenylalanine concentrations up to 418 μmol/L. Analysis of the organic urinary acids showed no abnormal metabolites. To rule out any deficit in the BH_4 cofactor, we performed a dihydropteridine reductase assay (normal results), BH_4 loading test (positive results), and urinary pterin analysis (characteristic pattern for GTPCH deficiency). Moreover dopamine and serotonin metabolites (5-hydroxyindoleacetic acid and homovanillic acid) in the cerebrospinal fluid were lower than the lower limit of the normal range. The initial CSF phenylalanine level was 94 μmol/L (normal, <20 μmol/L). The assay for enzyme activity confirmed the diagnosis of GTPCH deficiency.

When the patient was 9 months of age, BH_4 and neurotransmitter replacement therapy was started (Table), and the low-phenylalanine diet was stopped. One month later a reduction in the intention tremors and dystonic movements was observed, but axial hypotonia persisted. The neurophysiologic examination (visual-evoked and brain-stem auditory-evoked potentials) revealed an improvement in stimulus conduction. When the patient was 15 months of age, after he had undergone therapy for 6 months, slight axial hypotonia persisted, but the intention tremors and the dystonic movements had completely disappeared.

When the patient was 33 months of age, largely autonomous walking had been achieved with a slight ataxic gait; intention tremors and dystonia were no longer observed, but slight mental retardation remained.

METHODS

(*6R,S*)-Tetrahydrobiopterin dichloride tablets were purchased from Milupa AG (Friedrichsdorf, Germany). Measurement of pterins in urine and CSF was performed after oxidation was done with manganese dioxide; high-performance liquid chromatography was done with fluorescence detection.[9] We measured 5-HIAA and HVA by ion-pair high-performance liquid chromatography with electrochemical detection as described previously.[10] Fresh random urine samples were collected on filter paper,[11] and CSF was collected in ethylenediamine tetraacetic acid tubes and frozen immediately at −20° C. The activity of GTPCH in liver biopsy tissue was measured as described elsewhere,[12] except that chromatography of the neopterin triphosphate formed was done on a 4.6 × 12 cm column of 3 μm ODS-Hypersil (Shandon Ltd., Cheshire, U.K.). Amino acid analysis was performed by ion-exchange chromatography.

Polymerase chain reaction and direct nucleotide sequencing. Amplification of genomic DNA was performed in a reaction mixture of 25 μl containing 100 ng genomic DNA, 10 pmol of each primer, 10 mmol/L Tris-HCl (pH 8.3), 50 mmol/L KCl, 1.5 mmol/L $MgCl_2$, 5% dimethylsulfoxide, 0.2 U Perfectmach (Stratagene, La Jolla, Calif.), and 1.25 U Taq polymerase (Perkin-Elmer, Norwalk, Conn.). After the reaction mixture was heated at 94° C for 3 minutes, it was cycled according to the following program: 30 cycles of 30 seconds at 94° C, and 1 minute at 60° C, and a final extension at 60° C for 6 minutes. The primer sequence used for detection of a mutation in the patient was a sense primer, 5′-ACCAAACCAGCAGCTGTCTACTTT-3′ and an antisense primer, 5′-AATGCTACTGGCAGTACGATCGG-3′. The polymerase chain reaction products were sequenced directly with the same primers as for amplification by use of an automatic DNA sequencer (model 373A; Perkin-Elmer) and a Taq Dye Deoxy terminator Cycle sequencing kit (Applied Biosystems, Division of Perkin-Elmer, Rotkrenz, Switzerland). Mutated sequences were confirmed on both identical and complementary strands.

Plasma		Therapy			
Phenylalanine (μmol/L)	Tyrosine (μmol/L)	BH_4 (mg/kg/day)	L-Dopa (mg/kg/day)	5-HTRP (mg/kg/day)	Diet (mg/kg/day)
1488	71	0	0	0	—
85	40	0	0	0	Phenylalonine ↓
251	55	0	0	0	Phenylalonine ↓
140	90	0	0	0	Phenylalonine ↓
49	43	3.5	5.8	3.0	—
39	43	3.0	5.3	2.6	—
44	58	3.0	5.0	2.5	—
72	110	3.8	5.7	2.3	—
40	71	3.3	15.0	3.0	—
50	44	3.0	13.4	2.8	—
<120	<70				

RESULTS

Analysis of pterins. Urinary total neopterin and total biopterin were barely detectable in urine spots on filter paper when the patient was 6 months of age. The pterin pattern was similar to that found previously in patients with GTPCH deficiency; the excretion increased slightly 1 month later to neopterin, 0.06 mmol/mol creatinine (controls, 0.40 to 1.71), biopterin, 0.14 mmol/mol creatinine (controls, 0.78 to 1.67). Repeated measurements showed values 10 times less than control values. The percentage of neopterin to biopterin (69%) was in the normal range (49% to 74%). The CSF neopterin was not detectable, and biopterin levels were less than the lower normal range (Table). Substitution with BH_4 (10 mg/kg per day) did not restore the CSF biopterin levels to normal.

Analysis of neurotransmitter metabolites. Levels of 5-HIAA and HVA in the CSF were low at the time of diagnosis and increased after the substitution with neurotransmitter precursors L-dopa and 5-hydroxytryptophan (Table). 5-Methyltetrahydrofolic acid was always in the normal range.

Analysis of amino acids. When the patient was 4 days of age a routine Guthrie test was performed; the results were normal and were later confirmed. When the patient was 5 months of age, plasma amino acids were normal except for high concentrations of phenylalanine in plasma and CSF, 418 μmol/L and 101 μmol/L, respectively (Table). Another examination done 1 month later, when the patient was fed cow milk, showed a plasma phenylalanine concentration of 1488 μmol/L, which increased to 1506 μmol/L after feeding. After a challenge with phenylalanine (180 mg/kg body weight) the level rose to 1746 μmol/L. Introduction of a low-phenylalanine diet (35 mg/kg per day) resulted in normalization of the plasma phenylalanine levels within a few days. Introduction of the diet resulted in a decrease of the plasma phenylalanine concentration to less than 80 μmol/L.

Challenge with BH_4. The effect of BH_4 administration (7.5 mg/kg body weight) was significant. The elevated phenylalanine level in plasma fell from 250 to 157, 89, 61, and 39 μmol/L after 1, 2, 4, and 6 hours, respectively, whereas plasma tyrosine concentrations remained nearly constant: from 49 to 62, 44, 51, and 57 μmol/L. The excretion of total neopterin remained unchanged, whereas the excretion of total biopterin increased sharply. The highest values were at 6 hours after loading (data not shown). A combination phenylalanine (100 mg/kg) and BH_4 (20 mg/kg) loading test was also positive.[13]

Enzymatic analysis. The activity of dihydropteridine reductase in erythrocytes from a Guthrie card was 2.8 mU/mg hemoglobin (controls, 2 to 5 mU/mg hemoglobin). Activity of GTPCH was not detectable in a liver biopsy specimen (7 mg) from the patient (less than 3% of the mean control value).

Mutation analysis. We discovered a single-base change that suggests nonconservative amino acid substitution. A transition from G to A in the patient substituted the isoleucine residue for methionine residue at position 211 (Met 211 Ile). This patient was homozygous in terms of this mutation, and no other mutations were found in the coding region of the GTPCH gene. No mutation was found on 30 other chromosomes from unrelated typical individuals.

DISCUSSION

A diagnosis of hyperphenylalaninemia is usually based on the plasma phenylalanine levels obtained with a normal diet after a positive Guthrie test result. Breast or formula feeding for as little as 24 hours is sufficient to raise the baby's blood phenylalanine concentration sufficiently to trigger a positive test result (>240 μmol/L). Consequently screening for BH_4 deficiency should be done in all newborn infants with plasma phenylalanine values exceeding this cutoff point. Deficiency of BH_4 can easily be detected by the analysis of pterins in urine and by measurement of dihydropteridine activity in blood from Guthrie cards. This patient with BH_4 deficiency was not identified by the newborn screening program. Repetitive measurements of initial blood samples confirmed the normal phenylalanine levels when the patient was 6 days of age.

The goals of treatment of GTPCH deficiency are to control the hyperphenylalaninemia and to correct the neurotransmitter deficiencies.[14] Administration of BH_4 appears to be the most efficient therapy for controlling increased blood phenylalanine levels. Relatively low doses of BH_4 normalized the blood phenylalanine levels in our patient and offered a practical alternative to a phenylalanine-restricted diet. Simultaneously L-dopa and 5-hydroxytryptophan administration in combination represents a common therapeutic approach for controlling the CSF neurotransmitter levels in all BH_4 deficiency variants. Monitoring of the treatment in a patient with GTPCH deficiency by analysis of 5-HIAA and HVA documented the efficacy of such therapy. Interruption of the treatment resulted in a prompt decrease of the CSF metabolites.

The urinary excretion of neopterin and biopterin and of isoxanthopterin and pterin (data not shown) was very low, although the relative proportion of pterins was normal. In CSF of patients with GTPCH deficiency, neopterin and biopterin, as well as the neurotransmitter metabolites 5-HIAA and HVA, are usually very low.[14] In our patient, levels of biopterin in the CSF were in the subnormal range. Obviously some residual GTPCH activity was sufficient for the synthesis of the small amounts of dihydroneopterin triphosphate, a substrate for the enzyme 6-pyruvoyl-tetrahydropterin synthase. The relatively heat-stable and magnesium-dependent GTPCH is the rate-limiting enzyme in BH_4 biosynthesis in mammals[15, 16] but probably not in human beings. The human enzyme has been cloned, and the DNA sequence has been reported.[17] Three species of messenger ribonucleic acid corresponding to the three complementary DNAs were detected in human liver by analysis of reverse transcription polymerase chain reaction.[17] In GTPCH deficiency the rate-limiting step would be the conversion of GTP to dihydroneopterin triphosphate, which is then converted completely to BH_4 by 6-pyruvoyl-tetrahydropterin synthase and sepiapterin reductase.

The GTPCH gene is composed of six exons (Ichinose H, et al.: unpublished observations). Because we already knew the sequences around the exons except for the boundary between exon 3 and exon 4, we were able to amplify exons, including splicing junctions from genomic DNAs by polymerase chain reaction. The antisense primer for the amplification of exon 3 was set in the coding region (19 nucleotides). Amplified DNA fragments were directly sequenced with an automated DNA sequencer. With our primer set we determined 97.5% (731/750) of the nucleotides in the coding sequence. The amino acid substitution in our patient (Met 211 Ile) affects a highly conserved amino acid residue of GTPCH. Gene expression studies, gene transfection studies, and kinetic experiments with the mutant enzyme will give more information about catalytic and conformational consequences of this missense mutation. This report documents the potential risk of missing some patients with BH_4 deficiency by the routine Guthrie test for newborn infants. The late onset of neurologic signs may be an important indication of the presence of hyperphenylalaninemia caused by GTPCH deficiency. We suggest reevaluation for BH_4 disorders of any neonate or infant with neurologic problems of unknown origin.

We thank Lucja Kierat, Udo Redweik, Sönke Holm, and Sabrina Piovan for skillful technical assistance, Tamae Ohye for the DNA analysis, and Margrith Killen for editorial help.

REFERENCES

1. Niederwieser A, Blau N, Wang M, Joller P, Atares M, Cardesa Garcia J. GTP cyclohydrolase I deficiency, a new enzyme defect causing hyperphenylalaninemia with neopterin, biopterin, dopamine, and serotonin deficiencies and muscular hypotonia. Eur J Pediatr 1984;141:208-14.
2. Matalon R. Neopterin deficiency: a cause for hyperphenylalaninemia. Pediatr Res 1984;18:223A.
3. Dhondt JL, Farriaux JP, Boudha A, Largilliere C, Ringel J, Roger MM, Leeming RJ. Neonatal hyperphenylalaninemia presumably caused by guanosine triphosphate-cyclohydrolase deficiency. J PEDIATR 1985;106:954-6.
4. Naylor EW, Ennis D, Davidson AG, Wong LT, Applegarth DA, Niederwieser A. Guanosine triphosphate cyclohydrolase I deficiency: early diagnosis by routine urine pteridine screening. Pediatrics 1987;79:374-8.
5. Kaufman S. New tetrahydrobiopterin-dependent systems. Annu Rev Nutr 1993;13:261-86.
6. Marletta MA. Nitric oxide synthase structure and mechanism. J Biol Chem 1993;268:12231-4.
7. Harada T, Kagamiyama H, Hatakeyama K. Feedback regulation mechanisms for the control of GTP cyclohydrolase I activity. Science 1993;260:1507-10.
8. Blau N, Thöny B, Heizmann CW, Dhondt JL. Tetrahydro-

biopterin deficiency: from phenotype to genotype. Pteridines 1993;4:1-10.
9. Niederwieser A, Staudenmann W, Wetzel E. High-performance liquid chromatography with column switching for the analysis of biogenic amine metabolites and pterins. J Chromatogr 1984;290:237-46.
10. Blau N, Kierat L, Matasovic A, Leimbacher W, Heizmann CW, Guardamagna O, Ponzone A. Antenatal diagnosis of tetrahydrobiopterin deficiency by quantification of pterins in amniotic fluid and enzyme activity in fetal and extrafetal tissue. Clin Chim Acta 1994;226:159-69.
11. Blau N, Kierat L, Heizmann CW, Endres W, Giudici T, Wang M. Screening for tetrahydrobiopterin deficiency in newborns using dried urine on filter paper. J Inherit Metab Dis 1992; 15:402-4.
12. Blau N, Niederwieser A. Guanosine triphosphate cyclohydrolase I assay in human and rat liver using high-performance liquid chromatography of neopterin phosphates and guanine nucleotides. Anal Biochem 1983;128:446-52.
13. Ponzone A, Ferraris S, Spada M, Blau N, Piovan S, Burlina AB. Combined phenylalanine-tetrahydrobiopterin loading test in GTP cyclohydrolase I deficiency [Letter]. Eur J Pediatr 1994;153:616.
14. Blau N. Inborn errors of pterin metabolism. Annu Rev Nutr 1988;9:185-209.
15. Cha KW, Jacobson KB, Yim JJ. Isolation and characterization of GTP cyclohydrolase I from mouse liver: comparison of normal and the hph-1 mutant. J Biol Chem 1991;266:12294-300.
16. Nomura T, Ichinose H, Sumi-Ichinose C, Nomura H, Hagino Y, Fujita K, Nagatsu T. Cloning and sequencing of cDNA encoding mouse GTP cyclohydrolase I. Biochem Biophys Res Commun 1993;191:523-7.
17. Togari A, Ichinose H, Matsumoto S, Fujita K, Nagatsu T. Multiple mRNA forms of human GTP cyclohydrolase I. Biochem Biophys Res Commun 1992;187:359-65.

New books received

Hypnosis in the relief of pain
Hilgard ER, Hilgard JR. New York: Brunner/Mazel Publishers, 1994. 312 pages. $28.95.

Handbook for adolescent inpatient psychiatric treatment
Ghuman HS, Sarles RM. New York: Brunner/Mazel Publishers, 1994. 336 pages. $40.95.

Annual progress in child psychiatry and child development, 1993 (vol. 26)
Hertzig ME, Farber EA. New York: Brunner/Mazel Publishers, 1994. 590 pages. $62.95.

Toward active living
Quinney HA, Gauvin L, Wall AET, eds. Champaign, Illinois: Human Kinetics Publishers, 1994. 287 pages. No price listed.

Atypical cognitive deficits in developmental disorders
Broman SH, Grafman J. Hillsdale, New Jersey: Lawrence Erlbaum Associates, 1993. 336 pages. $65.

A doctor's guide to chronic fatigue syndrome
Bell DS. Reading, Massachusetts: Addison-Wesley, 1994. 275 pages. $21.

Bronchial asthma: Principles of diagnosis and treatment. 3rd ed.
Gershwin ME, Halpern GM. Totowa, New Jersey: Humana Press, 1994. 767 pages. $125.

Bridging early services for children with special needs and their families
Rosenkoetter SE, Hains AH, Fowler SA. Baltimore, Maryland: Brookes Publishing, 1993. 208 pages. $22.

Child and adolescent mental health consultation in hospitals, schools, and courts
Fritz GK, Mattison RE, Nurcombe B, Spirito A. Washington, D.C.: American Psychiatric Press, 1993. 316 pages. $35.

Interviewing the sexually abused child
Jones DPH. Washington, D.C.: American Psychiatric Press, 1992. 67 pages. $15.

Psychiatric hospitalization of school-age children
Dalton R, Forman MA. Washington, D.C.: American Psychiatric Press, 1992. 203 pages. $23.50.

Handbook of mucosal immunology
Ogra PL, et al, eds. New York: Academic Press, 1994. 766 pages. Price not listed.

Pediatric Aids. 2nd ed.
Pizzo PA, Wilfert CM, eds. Baltimore: Williams & Wilkins, 1994. 1040 pages. Price not listed.

You don't have to suffer
Lang SS, Patt SB. New York: Oxford University Press, 1994. 366 pages. $25.

Common problems in pediatric pathology
Joshi VV. New York: Igaku-Shoin Medical Publishers, 1994. 524 pages. $125.

Pediatric and adolescent gynecology
Sanfilippo JS, Muram D, Lee PA, Dewhurst J. Philadelphia: WB Saunders, 1994. 744 pages. $95.

Prevention and early intervention: Individual differences as risk factors for the mental health of children
Carey WB, McDevitt SC. New York: Brunner/Mazel Publishers, 1994. 328 pages. $38.95.

Death to dust: What happens to dead bodies?
Iserson KV. Tucson, Arizona: Galen Press, 1994. 709 pages. $38.95.

The pharmacologic approach to the critically ill patient. 3rd ed.
Chernow B. Baltimore: Williams & Wilkins, 1994. 1220 pages. Price not listed.

Improved oxygenation during synchronized intermittent mandatory ventilation in neonates with respiratory distress syndrome: A randomized, crossover study

John P. Cleary, MD, Graham Bernstein, MD, Frank L. Mannino, MD, and Gregory P. Heldt, MD

From the Division of Neonatology, Department of Pediatrics, University of California, San Diego, School of Medicine

In a randomized, crossover study, we compared arterial partial pressure of oxygen and of carbon dioxide between consecutive periods of conventional and synchronized intermittent mandatory ventilation (SIMV). We studied spontaneously breathing infants with an endotracheal tube in place. The infants were <12 hours of age, had a diagnosis of respiratory distress syndrome, and had an arterial/alveolar oxygen ratio of <0.25. The infants had a mean birth weight of 1077 gm and gestational age of 28 weeks. The mean rate of asynchrony on intermittent mandatory ventilation (IMV) was 52% (range, 36% to 76%), and on SIMV was <1%. Infants were randomly assigned to IMV or SIMV as their initial ventilator mode and underwent ventilation for four 15-minute periods, and crossed over to the alternate mode after each period. Ventilator settings and the fraction of inspired oxygen were not changed between modes. At the end of each period, arterial blood gas measurements were obtained; 26 paired comparisons were made between modes. The mean arterial partial pressure of oxygen was significantly higher during SIMV than during IMV (mean, 61.5 vs 53.3 mm Hg; *p* <0.01). The mean arterial partial pressure of carbon dioxide was slightly lower during SIMV than during IMV (mean, 42.7 vs 41.3 mm Hg; *p* <0.05). The improvement in oxygenation demonstrated with SIMV may allow a reduction in ventilator pressure or oxygen exposure in this group of infants, who are at risk of having complications of ventilation. (J PEDIATR 1995;126:407-11)

The interaction of spontaneous breathing with mechanical ventilation in neonates has been the subject of ongoing study.[1] During conventional intermittent mandatory ventilation, ventilator breaths that occur late in spontaneous inspiration or early in expiration are likely to cause active expiratory effort against the ventilator breath.[2, 3] This asynchrony of spontaneous and ventilator breaths has been associated with decreased oxygenation,[4, 5] increased barotrauma,[6, 7] and increased use of sedation or paralysis.[4, 5, 7] In addition, asynchrony has been associated with increased cerebral blood flow variability, which may be associated with intraventricular hemorrhage.[8-10] These prob-

IMV	Intermittent mandatory ventilation
$Paco_2$	Arterial partial pressure of carbon dioxide
Pao_2	Arterial partial pressure of oxygen
SIMV	Synchronized intermittent mandatory ventilation

Presented in part at the annual meeting of the Society for Pediatric Research, Washington, D.C., May 1993.

Submitted for publication June 6, 1994; accepted Sept. 26, 1994.

Reprint requests: John P. Cleary, MD, The Med Center—Memorial, 119 Belmont St., Worcester, MA 01605.

0022-3476/95/$3.00 + 0 **9/23/60904**

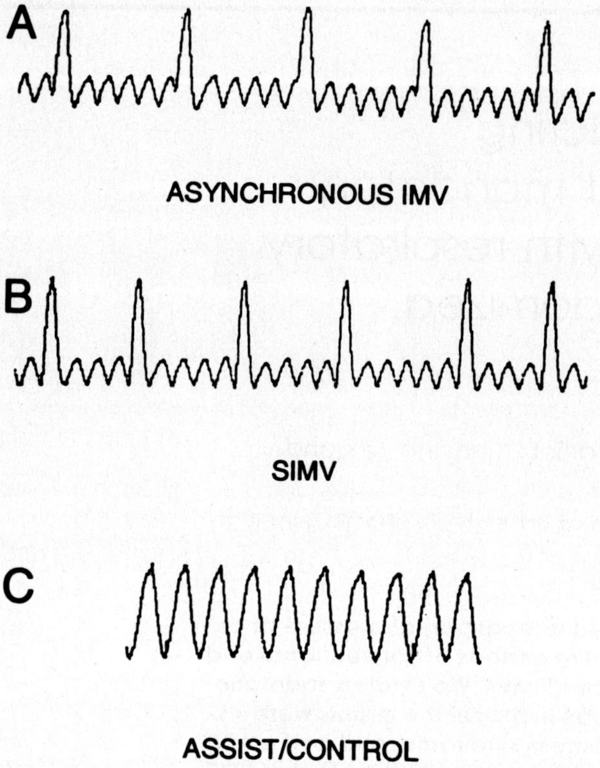

Fig. 1. Tidal volume tracings (inspiration = upward) demonstrating three patterns of ventilator interaction with spontaneous breathing. In illustration, tidal volume of spontaneous breaths is less than that of ventilator breaths. **A,** Asynchronous IMV with ventilator breaths delivered during spontaneous expiration. During IMV, ventilator breaths occur at a constant rate with random timing with respect to spontaneous breaths. **B,** SIMV with ventilator breaths delivered early in selected spontaneous inspirations. During SIMV, ventilator breaths occur more irregularly, but the ventilator delivers the set rate synchronously with spontaneous breaths. **C,** Assist/control mode, with ventilator breaths delivered early in all spontaneous inspirations. The assist/control mode delivers ventilator breaths synchronously with all spontaneous breaths and may lead to increased ventilation.

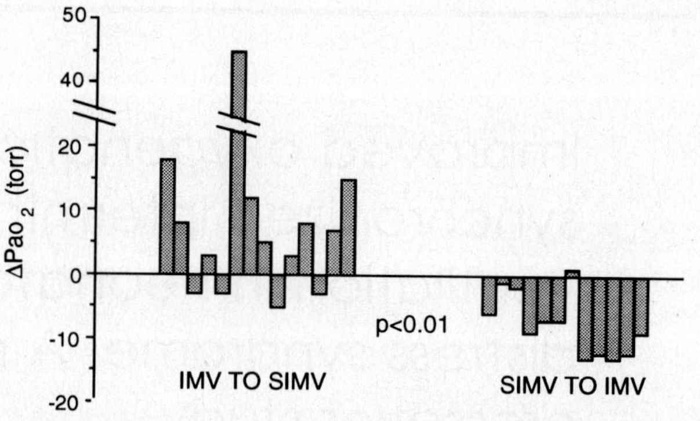

Fig. 2. Change in PaO_2 at each crossover. The value improved by 7.9 ± 3.4 mm Hg when crossover was from IMV to SIMV, and decreased by 6.4 ± 1.4 when crossover was from SIMV to IMV.

lems have led to efforts to synchronize ventilator breaths with spontaneous breathing by matching the rate and inspiratory time of the conventional ventilator with the patient's spontaneous breathing (synchronous ventilation)[11-13] or by using patient-triggered ventilation.[14-20]

Patient-triggered ventilators are designed to deliver a mechanical breath each time a spontaneous breath occurs in the assist/control mode, or to deliver a mechanical breath on selected spontaneous breaths at a rate set in the synchronized intermittent mandatory ventilation mode. Tidal volume recordings during these modes and during asynchronous IMV are shown in Fig. 1. Previous studies of the effect of synchrony on gas exchange have used the assist/control mode[14-20] or synchronous ventilation.[12] Both of these modes use higher ventilator rates, minute ventilation, and mean airway pressure than would be used during asynchronous IMV.

The objective of this study was to evaluate the short-term effects on oxygenation and ventilation of SIMV compared with asynchronous IMV. We chose to compare SIMV with asynchronous IMV at identical ventilator rates and pressures to evaluate the effects of synchrony per se on gas exchange.

METHODS

Patient population. Infants were eligible for study if their birth weight was less than 1750 gm, gestational age was <32 weeks, and chronologic age was <12 hours. All had radiographic evidence of respiratory distress syndrome, had an arterial line inserted for routine monitoring, were breathing spontaneously on a ventilator, and had an arterial/alveolar oxygen ratio <0.25. The ratio of arterial to alveolar partial pressure of oxygen was calculated with the fraction of inspired oxygen and the arterial oxygen and carbon dioxide tensions measured within 30 minutes of entry.[21] The PaO_2 and $PaCO_2$ values were determined with a model 288 blood gas system (Ciba Corning Diagnostics Corp., Medfield, Mass.) The study protocol was approved by the University of California, San Diego, Committee on Human Subjects, and informed written consent was obtained from the parents of each subject.

Infants were studied between 3 and 6 hours after administration of artificial surfactant (Exosurf Neonatal, Burroughs Wellcome Co., Research Triangle Park, N.C.). Ventilator settings and fraction of inspired oxygen were those thought to produce optimal gas exchange by the attending neonatologist, and were not changed during the study unless the PaO_2 was <35 or >100 mm Hg.

Infants were given ventilatory support with an Infant Star ventilator with the Star Sync module (Infrasonics Inc.,

San Diego, Calif.) to deliver both IMV and SIMV. The ventilator uses an abdominal pressure capsule (Graseby Dynamics Ltd., Herts, United Kingdom) to detect the outward movement of the abdomen at the start of spontaneous inspiratory effort. We previously reported a response time of 53 ± 13 msec and reliability of 98.8% ± 0.4% during SIMV with this system.[22] All ventilator settings were the same during IMV and during SIMV; transitions between IMV and SIMV were made by changing the mode setting on the Star Sync module and did not require disconnecting the ventilator or handling the infant.

Determination of asynchrony. Before the crossover study of gas exchange, we performed 1-minute airway flow recordings to determine the rate of asynchrony on IMV and SIMV. Airway flow and pressure were recorded with a Fleisch size 00 pneumotachometer (OEM Medical, Richmond, Va.) placed between the endotracheal tube and ventilator, and the Star Calc pulmonary function testing system (Infrasonics). Our objective was to compare asynchronous IMV to SIMV, so only those infants with more than 30% asynchrony during IMV were included in the study (one infant was excluded).

Crossover design. Infants were randomly assigned to IMV or SIMV as the initial ventilator mode. They underwent ventilation for four 15-minute periods, crossing over to the alternate mode after each period. At the end of each period of ventilation, blood gas tensions were determined.

Data analysis. To establish the percentage of asynchrony during IMV and SIMV, airway flow recordings of all ventilator breaths were reviewed. The inspiratory time of the spontaneous breath preceding a ventilator breath was used to determine the timing of each ventilator breath. Asynchronous ventilator breaths were defined as beginning during the second half of spontaneous inspiration or during expiration. The differences in Pa_{O_2} and Pa_{CO_2} associated with each crossover were compared by paired two-tailed *t* tests, and comparisons grouped by the direction of crossover used unpaired *t* tests (Statview SE+, Abacus Concepts Inc., Berkeley, Calif.). Statistical significance was considered at $p < 0.05$. Differences in Pa_{O_2} and Pa_{CO_2} are expressed as mean ± SEM.

RESULTS

Ten infants meeting initial entry criteria were enrolled in the study. The airway flow recording showed one infant to have a rate of asynchrony <10% during IMV, and he was therefore excluded from further study. The rate of synchrony achieved during SIMV was >98%.

Three paired comparisons of Pa_{O_2} and Pa_{CO_2} between IMV and SIMV were possible for each patient. Twenty-six comparisons were made in the nine infants who completed the study; one comparison was excluded because the ventilator settings were decreased between blood gas measurements when the Pa_{O_2} increased to 126 mm Hg with the first transition from IMV to SIMV.

Table. Infant characteristics and ventilator settings at entry

	Mean	Range
Birth weight (gm)	1077	430-1550
Gestational age (wk)	28	25-30
Chronologic age (hr)	6	4-10
Asynchrony during IMV (%)	53	36-76
Asynchrony during SIMV (%)	<1	0-2
MAP (cm H_2O)	10	7-16
Inspiratory time (sec)	0.39	0.30-0.50
Ventilator rate	43	29-66
F_{IO_2}	0.65	0.45-1.0
a/A P_{O_2}	0.13	0.07-0.22

MAP, Mean airway pressure; *F_{IO_2}*, fraction of inspired oxygen; *a/A*, arterial/alveolar ratio.

The characteristics of the infants and ventilator settings are shown in the Table. The mean Pa_{O_2} was significantly higher during SIMV than during IMV (61.5 ± 3.7 vs 53.3 ± 2.4 mm Hg; $p < 0.01$). There were 14 comparisons changing modes from IMV to SIMV, and 12 comparisons changing from SIMV to IMV. The change in Pa_{O_2} was significant whether crossover was from IMV to SIMV or from SIMV to IMV (7.9 ± 3.4 vs −6.4 ± 1.4 mm Hg; $p < 0.01$). The paired changes in Pa_{O_2} for all 26 crossover comparisons are shown in Fig. 2. A small decrease in Pa_{CO_2} was seen between IMV and SIMV (42.7 ± 1.0 vs 41.3 ± 0.9 mm Hg; $p < 0.05$).

DISCUSSION

We demonstrated an improvement in Pa_{O_2} and a small increase in ventilation between IMV and SIMV in low birth weight infants with moderate to severe respiratory distress syndrome. A mean rate of asynchrony of 53% was seen during IMV despite what was thought to be optimal ventilator support based on gas exchange and no visible evidence that the infant was "fighting the ventilator." Asynchrony was essentially eliminated during SIMV.

Asynchrony has been associated with active expiration,[2, 3] reduced ventilator tidal volume,[23, 24] decreased oxygenation,[4, 5] pneumothoraces,[6, 7] and intraventricular hemorrhages.[8-10] SIMV has been shown to limit active expiration,[24] improve ventilator tidal volume,[23, 24] and reduce cerebral blood flow velocity variability,[25] which has been associated with intraventricular hemorrhage.[9] We believe that comparing IMV and SIMV at identical ventilator settings is the most valid way to evaluate the effects of synchrony.

Asynchrony can be eliminated by interventions other

than SIMV. These measures include matching the rate of IMV with the spontaneous respiratory rate, using a patient-triggered ventilator to augment each spontaneous breath in the assist/control mode, and eliminating spontaneous breathing through paralysis. Achieving synchrony with rate matching or with the assist/control mode leads, in our experience, to a higher mean airway pressure and minute ventilation than those obtained during SIMV. Strategies for weaning a patient from ventilation are limited because the ventilator rate is determined by the spontaneous respiratory rate. Rate matching also requires frequent adjustment of the ventilator rate to maintain synchrony as the spontaneous rate changes.[12] In contrast, SIMV ensures synchrony across a wide range of ventilator settings, which is especially important during weaning.

Eliminating asynchrony through paralysis with pancuronium reduces the incidence of pneumothoraces,[7] improves oxygenation and mortality rates,[4] and reduces cerebral blood flow variability and intraventricular hemorrhage.[9] Eliminating asynchrony by means of SIMV may be preferable to paralysis, because the contribution to ventilation of spontaneous breathing effort is maintained and potential complications of paralysis, such as fluid retention and growth failure, are avoided.[26] Moreover, paralysis may result in an increase in oxygen requirement in small infants.[27]

Several previous studies have compared gas exchange during IMV with that during patient-triggered ventilation with the assist/control mode.[14-20] Because the ventilator settings were not identical between patient study groups, the cause of differences in gas exchange were not due simply to synchrony. In most of these studies the assist/control period followed the period of IMV to which it was compared[15-17, 20]; thus an improvement in underlying lung disease could have been responsible for the change in gas exchange attributed to synchrony. Moreover, the results of these studies have been variable. Greenough and Pool[15] showed improved oxygenation between conventional IMV and flow-triggered assist/control ventilation. Infants with the greatest increase in ventilator rate between modes had the most significant improvement in oxygenation, which suggests that changes may have been due to the difference in ventilator rate rather than to synchrony. Servant et al.[14] also showed improved oxygenation during assist/control periods; however, minute ventilation and mean airway pressure were increased in the assist/control group. Hird and Greenough[20] were unable to demonstrate improved oxygenation in infants born at less than 29 weeks of gestation; the ventilator used in this study (Draeger Babylog 8000, with its original software; North American Drager, Telford, Pa.) has since been shown to have had a high rate of failure in the assist/control mode, and asynchrony may not have been apparent visually.[22] Another study by Hird and Greenough[16] showed assist/control ventilation to be associated with deterioration in blood gas values. However, a ventilator with an unacceptably high rate of failure (only 4 of 13 patients in the assist/control group had synchronized ventilation) was compared with IMV at rates between 61 and 120 breaths/min—a range likely to lead to synchronous ventilation.[11]

We studied low birth weight infants because they are at high risk of having complcations of ventilation, and successful patient-triggered ventilation in infants of low birth weight and early gestation has been questioned.[28, 29] Asynchrony during IMV and successful delivery of SIMV were documented before the study. Infants were studied in the first 12 hours of life, a time when compilications of asynchronous ventilation, such as air leak and intraventricular hemorrhage, are common. The multiple crossover design and the randomization of initial assignment limited the potential confounding variables. SIMV and IMV were compared at identical ventilator settings; synchrony was the only variable studied. In addition, arterial blood gas studies were done, rather than less exact measures such as transcutaneous oxygen monitoring or oxygen saturation.

Our demonstration that SIMV improves oxygenation could be explained physiologically by a number of mechanisms. Increased tidal volume and more consistent flow-volume relationships have been shown with SIMV.[23, 24] This finding is compatible with improved distribution of ventilation, which could improve ventilation/perfusion matching. A reduction in oxygen consumption as a result of decreased work of breathing could also lead to an increase in Pa_{O_2}. We previously showed that SIMV reduces inspiratory diaphragmatic electromyographic amplitude and duration.[24] It also reduces active expiration, which should decrease oxygen consumption.

Few investigators using patient-triggered ventilators have addressed long-term outcome variables. Two studies in which the assist/control mode was used resulted in a shorter duration of mechanical ventilation.[18, 19] One nonrandomized study showed a decreased incidence of grade 3 or 4 intraventricular hemorrhage.[18] The results of a randomized multicenter trial comparing SIMV with IMV are being analyzed.[30] Findings to date include a decreased duration of ventilation as well as a decreased percentage of low birth weight infants requiring oxygen at 35 weeks of postconceptional age.

We conclude that significant improvement in gas exchange was achieved during SIMV versus IMV in low birth weight infants with respiratory distress syndrome. We speculate that increased synchrony and reduced oxygen or ventilator pressure exposure could reduce the incidence of complications of ventilation. Further randomized trials will be required to determine the benefits and optimal clinical uses of patient-triggered ventilators.

We thank the staff of the University of California, San Diego, Infant Special Care Unit. Doug G. Elmore, CRTT, and James K. Goody, RRT, CPFT, provided valuable technical assistance.

REFERENCES

1. Heldt GP, Bernstein G. Patient initiated mechanical ventilation. In: Boynton BR, Carlo WA, Jobe AH, eds. New therapies for neonatal respiratory failure: a physiologic approach. New York: Cambridge University Press, 1994:152-70.
2. Greenough A, Morley CJ, Johnson P. An active expiratory reflex in preterm ventilated infants. In: Jones CT, Nathanielsz PW, eds. The physiological development of the fetus and newborn. New York: Academic Press, 1985:259-62.
3. Field D, Milner AD, Hopkin IE. Manipulation of ventilator settings to prevent active expiration against positive pressure inflation. Arch Dis Child 1985;60:1036-40.
4. Henry GW, Stevens CS, Schreiner RL, Grosfeld JL, Ballantine TVN. Respiratory paralysis to improve oxygenation and mortality in large newborn infants with respiratory distress. J Pediatr Surg 1979;14:761-6.
5. Stark AR, Bascom R, Frantz ID. Muscle relaxation in mechanically ventilated infants. J PEDIATR 1978;94:439-43.
6. Greenough A, Morley CJ, Davis JA. Interaction of spontaneous respiration with artificial ventilation in preterm babies. J PEDIATR 1983;103:769-73.
7. Greenough A, Wood S, Morley CJ, Davis JA. Pancuronium prevents pneumothoraces in ventilated premature babies who actively expire against positive pressure ventilation. Lancet 1984;1:1-3.
8. Rennie JM, South M, Morley CJ. Cerebral blood flow velocity variability in infants receiving assisted ventilation. Arch Dis Child 1987;62:1247-51.
9. Perlman JM, Goodman S, Kreusser KL, Volpe JJ. Reduction in intraventricular hemorrhage by elimination of fluctuating cerebral blood-flow velocity in preterm infants with respiratory distress syndrome. N Engl J Med 1985;312:1353-7.
10. Perlman JM, McMenamin JB, Volpe JJ. Fluctuating cerebral blood-flow velocity in respiratory distress syndrome. N Engl J Med 1983;309:204-9.
11. South M, Morley CJ. Synchronous mechanical ventilation of the neonate. Arch Dis Child 1986;61:1190-5.
12. Amitay M, Etches PC, Finer NN, Maidens JM. Synchronous mechanical ventilation of the infant with respiratory disease. Crit Care Med 1993;21:118-24.
13. Greenough A. The premature infant's respiratory response to mechanical ventilation. Early Hum Dev 1988;17:1-5.
14. Servant GM, Nicks JJ, Donn SM, Bandy KP, Lathrop C, Dechert RE. Feasibility of applying flow-synchronized ventilation to very low birthweight infants. Respir Care 1992;37:249-53.
15. Greenough A, Pool J. Neonatal patient triggered ventilation. Arch Dis Child 1988;63:77-8.
16. Hird MF, Greenough A, Chan V. Randomized trial of patient-triggered ventilation versus high-frequency positive-pressure ventilation in acute respiratory distress. J Perinat Med 1991;19:471-6.
17. Greenough A, Hird MF, Chan V. Airway pressure triggered ventilation for preterm neonates. J Perinat Med 1991;19:471-6.
18. Vishveshwara N, Freeman B, Peck M, Caliwig W, Shook S, Rajani K. Patient-triggered synchronized assisted ventilation of newborns. J Perinatol 1991;11:347-54.
19. Donn SM, Nicks JJ, Becker MA. Flow-synchronized ventilation of preterm infants with respiratory distress syndrome. J Perinatol 1994;14:90-4.
20. Hird MF, Greenough A. Patient-triggered ventilation using a flow-triggered system. Arch Dis Child 1991;66:1140-2.
21. West JB. Pulmonary pathophysiology: the essentials. 4th ed. Baltimore: Williams & Wilkins, 1992;28.
22. Bernstein G, Cleary JP, Heldt GP, Rosas JF, Schellenberg LD, Mannino FL. The response time and reliability of three neonatal patient triggered ventilators. Am Rev Respir Dis 1993;148:358-64.
23. Bernstein G, Heldt GP, Mannino FM. Increased and more consistent tidal volumes during synchronized intermittent mandatory ventilation in newborn infants. American Journal of Respiratory and Critical Care Medicine 1994;150:1444-8.
24. Rosas JF, Cleary JP, Mannino FL, Bernstein G, Heldt GP. Diaphragmatic effort and lung mechanics on conventional and synchronized intermittent mandatory ventilation (IMV/SIMV) [Abstract]. Pediatr Res 1992;32:148-0.
25. Govindaswami B, Bejar R, Bernstein G, Heldt GP. Reduction in cerebral blood flow velocity (CBFV) variability in infants <1500 gm during synchronized intermittent mandatory ventilation [Abstract]. Pediatr Res 1993;33:1258-50.
26. Shaw NJ, Cooke RWI, Gill AB, Saeed M. Randomized trial of routine versus selective paralysis during ventilation for neonatal respiratory distress syndrome. Arch Dis Child 1993;69:479-82.
27. Runkle B, Bancalari E. Acute cardiopulmonary effects of pancuronium bromide in mechanically ventilated newborn infants. J PEDIATR 1984;104:614-7.
28. Mitchell A, Greenough A, Hird MF. Limitations of patient triggered ventilation in neonates. Arch Dis Child 1989;64:924-7.
29. Hird MF, Greenough A. Causes of failure of neonatal patient-triggered ventilation. Early Hum Dev 1990;23:101-8.
30. Bernstein G, Mannino FL, Heldt GP, et al. Prospective randomized multicenter trial comparing synchronized and conventional ventilation (SIMV and IMV) in neonates [Abstract]. Pediatr Res 1994;35:216A.

Partial liquid ventilation in premature lambs with respiratory distress syndrome: Efficacy and compatibility with exogenous surfactant

Corinne Lowe Leach, MD, PhD, Bruce Holm, PhD, Frederick C. Morin III, MD, Bradley P. Fuhrman, MD, Michele C. Papo, MD, David Steinhorn, MD, and Lynn J. Hernan, MD

From the Divisions of Neonatology and Critical Care, Department of Pediatrics, and the Department of Obstetrics and Gynecology, Children's Hospital of Buffalo, State University of New York at Buffalo

Objective: **To determine the efficacy of partial liquid ventilation (PLV) by means of a medical-grade perfluorochemical liquid, perflubron (LiquiVent), in premature lambs with respiratory distress syndrome (RDS). Further, to determine the compatibility of perflubron with exogenous surfactant both in vitro and in vivo during PLV.**
Design: **Prospective, randomized, controlled study, with in vitro open comparison.**
Subjects: **Twenty-two premature lambs with RDS.**
Interventions: **In vitro assays were conducted on three exogenous surfactants before and after combination with perflubron. We studied four groups of lambs, which received one of the following treatment strategies: conventional mechanical ventilation (CMV); surfactant (Exosurf) plus CMV; PLV; or surfactant plus PLV.**
Measurements and main results: **In vitro surface tension, measured for three exogenous surfactants, was unchanged in each animal after exposure to perflubron. Lung mechanics and arterial blood gases were serially measured. All animals treated with PLV survived the 5 hours of experiment without complication; several animals treated with CMV died. During CMV, all animals had marked hypoxemia and hypercapnia. During PLV, arterial oxygen tension increased sixfold to sevenfold within minutes of initiation, and this increase was sustained; arterial carbon dioxide tension decreased to within the normal range. Compliance increased fourfold to fivefold during PLV compared with CMV. Tidal volumes were increased during PLV, with lower mean airway pressure. Resistance was similar for both CMV and PLV; there was no difference with surfactant treatment.**
Conclusions: **We conclude that PLV with perflubron improves lung mechanics**

Supported by Alliance Pharmaceutical Corp, American Lung Association, Women and Children's Research Foundation, and HL RO1 41387. Drs. Leach and Fuhrman are paid consultants to Alliance Pharmaceutical Corp.

Submitted for publication Aug. 15, 1994; accepted Dec. 2, 1994.

Reprint requests: Corinne L. Leach, MD, PhD, Division of Neonatology, Children's Hospital of Buffalo, 219 Bryant St., Buffalo, NY 14222.

0022-3476/95/$3.00 + 0 **9/23/62527**

and gas exchange in premature lambs with RDS, that PLV is compatible with exogenous surfactant therapy, and that, as a treatment for RDS in this model, PLV is superior to the surfactant studied. (J PEDIATR 1995;126:412-20)

Ventilation with perfluorochemical liquids has been shown to improve gas exchange and lung mechanics in models of surfactant deficiency and surfactant dysfunction.[1-10] One technique, partial liquid ventilation (perfluorocarbon-associated gas exchange [PAGE]) employs a conventional ventilator to deliver gas tidal volumes into a lung with liquid functional residual capacity.[11] More recently, a medical-grade perfluorochemical liquid, perflubron (LiquiVent; Alliance Pharmaceutical Corp., San Diego, Calif.) has become available; it is distinguished from other perfluorochemicals by high wetting or spreading properties and by low vapor pressure. We thus undertook to determine whether PLV with perflubron could improve lung mechanics and gas exchange in premature lambs with respiratory distress syndrome in which conventional ventilation has failed.

In addition, although exogenous surfactant replacement reduces mortality rates in infants with RDS,[12] it is not uniformly effective.[13-16] We questioned whether PLV may represent a treatment for patients with RDS who have also received exogenous surfactant replacement, and examined the compatibility of PLV with exogenous surfactant before treatment in this same model.

ANOVA	Analysis of variance
CMV	Conventional mechanical ventilation
FRC	Functional residual capacity
Pa_{CO_2}	Arterial carbon dioxide tension
Pa_{O_2}	Arterial oxygen tension
PEEP	Positive end-expiratory pressure
PIP	Peak inspiratory pressure
PLV	Partial liquid ventilation
RDS	Respiratory distress syndrome

METHODS

In vitro assays. To assess biochemical compatibility of exogenous surfactant and perflubron, we studied the surface-tension–lowering ability of three exogenous surfactant preparations after combination with perflubron in vitro, using the precision bubble apparatus.[17] Dynamic surface pressure of concentrations (5 mg/ml) of Exosurf (Burroughs Wellcome, Research Triangle Park, N.C.), Infasurf (ONY Inc., Amherst, N.Y.), and Survanta (Ross Laboratories, Columbus, Ohio) was measured by the pulsating-bubble technique. Each surfactant was then mixed for 30 minutes with equal parts by volume of perflubron, and allowed to stand for 1 hour. The surfactant was decanted and then studied again. The test was performed in triplicate in separate samples and mean values were calculated.

Animal preparation. Twenty-two premature lambs with a gestational age of 125 to 127 days (term, 145 days) were delivered by cesarean section. A 4.0 OD endotracheal tube and carotid and jugular catheters were placed as described previously.[4]

At delivery, each animal was connected to a Siemens Servo 500 ventilator (Siemens-Elema Ventilator Systems, Shaumburg, Ill.), the cord was clamped and cut, and the animal was placed in the supine position and dried. Ventilator settings included pressure-controlled ventilation with a fraction of inspired oxygen of 1.0, peak inspiratory pressure of 30 to 38 cm H_2O, positive end-expiratory pressure of 4 cm H_2O, inspiratory time of 0.33 to 0.5 second, and respiratory rate of 50 to 60 breaths/min. Anesthesia was maintained with ketamine, 5 mg/kg, supplemented as needed. Temperature and hemodynamic stability, and fluid and electrolyte homeostasis, were maintained as described previously.[4] This study was approved by the State University of New York at Buffalo Laboratory Animal Care Committee, and the care and handling of the animals were in accord with National Institutes of Health guidelines.

Experimental design. All animals initially underwent ventilation by conventional mechanical ventilation, and were prospectively randomly assigned to one of four groups. Group 1 (CMV; n = 5) continued with CMV for the experimental period. Group 2 (surfactant plus CMV; n = 5) received Exosurf, 5 mg/kg administered according to package insert directions at 30 minutes of life, and continued with CMV. Group 3 (PLV; n = 7) was switched to PLV at 30 minutes. Group 4 (surfactant plus PLV; n = 5) received Exosurf at 30 minutes, as did group 2, and was switched to PLV at 45 minutes. This study was concluded 5 hours after birth. Lambs were killed with a ketamine overdose and a potassium chloride injection. The lungs were removed and examined grossly for evidence of barotrauma.

PLV technique. PLV was initiated with a combination rapid infusion–slow infusion technique to establish the perflubron liquid FRC. Perflubron was preoxygenated with 100% O_2 and warmed to 39° C. The lamb's endotracheal tube was disconnected from the ventilator, and perflubron, 5 to 7 ml/kg, was instilled with a syringe into the trachea for 30 to 60 seconds. During this period of apnea, the ventilator settings were adjusted to a rate of 20 to 25 breaths/

Table. Surface tension (mean ± SEM) of three exogenous surfactant preparations (5 mg/ml) in pure form and after exposure to perflubron

	Surface tension (dynes/cm^2)	
Surfactant (trade name)	**Pure form**	**Perflubron exposed**
Exosurf	27.3 ± 1.3	24.5 ± 5.3
Infasurf	0.1 ± 0.1	0.4 ± 0.3
Survanta	0.9 ± 0.4	2.3 ± 1.5

min, with an inspiratory time of 0.75 second, and PIP of 30 cm H_2O. At the completion of the liquid infusion, the endotracheal tube was reconnected to the ventilator and the remaining volume of perflubron was slowly infused via a side port adapter at the proximal endotracheal tube during ventilation. Filling was performed at a rate slow enough to allow uptake by the lung, thus avoiding premature complete filling of the endotracheal tube with liquid. This ensured that tidal volume delivered by pressure-limited support was not significantly decreased by high airway resistance during instillation. PIP often had to be decreased during this period of filling to maintain tidal volume at less than or equal to 12 ml/kg. Instillation was considered complete when a meniscus of fluid was consistently visible in the endotracheal tube at end-expiration without PEEP. The filling process took 5 to 15 minutes. After filling was completed to physiologic FRC, PLV was performed with PIP adjusted to achieve arterial carbon dioxide tension in the range of 40 to 55 mm Hg (5 to 7 kPa). During PLV, animals were maintained in the supine position. Every 30 minutes, each animal was rotated to both the right and left lateral decubitus positions for 30 to 60 seconds. To compensate for evaporative loss of perflubron and maintain constant FRC, we replaced perflubron at a rate of 2.5 ml/kg per hour every 30 minutes by means of instillation into the endotracheal tube.

Measurements. Serial measurements of lung mechanics, hemodynamics, and arterial blood gases were performed. Arterial blood pressure, transthoracic pressure, inspiratory and expiratory gas flow, and tidal volume were simultaneously monitored as previously described,[4] and compliance, resistance, and time constants were calculated. Arterial pH, carbon dioxide and oxygen tensions, percentage of hemoglobin saturation, and hemoglobin concentration were measured by an automated blood gas analyzer (ABL 2; Radiometer America, Westlake, Ohio).

Data analysis. Within-group differences were analyzed by ANOVA with repeated measures, with comparisons between points by a paired two-tailed *t* test with a Bonferroni correction. The ANOVA was performed for all points until the first death in the group. For comparison between groups, significant differences were tested by ANOVA at each time point, followed by an unpaired two-tailed *t* test with a Bonferroni correction for comparison between individual groups. Significance was accepted at the 95% confidence interval.

RESULTS

In vitro surface tension–reducing activity of three surfactants, before and after exposure to perflubron, is shown in the Table. At a concentration of 5 mg/ml, Exosurf had limited in vitro activity, which was unchanged after exposure to perflubron. Survanta and Infasurf lowered surface tension at this concentration, and this surface tension–lowering capability was unaltered after exposure to perflubron.

Mean gestational age for all animals was 126.3 ± 0.2 days, with no difference between groups. All animals in the PLV and surfactant-plus-PLV groups survived the 5 hours of the experiment. In the groups receiving CMV, there was one death by 2 hours (CMV group), and two deaths by 3 and 4 hours (surfactant-plus-CMV group), respectively.

Figure 1 depicts representative tracings of airway pressure during CMV and PLV in one animal. In contrast to the monophasic curve seen during CMV, the airway pressure curve was often biphasic during PLV. The first phase was spiked, followed by a lower, plateau phase. The presence and magnitude of the spike varied inversely with the level of PEEP and directly with filling volumes.

Partial liquid ventilation was initiated and conducted without complication for all animals. There was no cyanosis, bradycardia, hypotension, or acidosis associated with the initiation or conduct of PLV. The use of PLV improved gas exchange and mechanics in both groups receiving it (Figs. 2 to 6). The PLV and surfactant-plus-PLV groups showed similar responses (i.e., prior treatment with Exosurf did not change the effect of PLV on gas exchange and mechanics).

Mean arterial oxygen tension at 30 minutes of life during CMV was less than 60 mm Hg (8 kPa) for all groups (Fig. 2). Pa_{O_2} increased sixfold to sevenfold within minutes of the initiation of PLV in the PLV group, and this increase was maintained. Pa_{O_2} increased similarly during PLV in the surfactant-plus-PLV group of animals; this response, however, was delayed. In the CMV groups, Pa_{O_2} remained low, and was unchanged by Exosurf.

Mean Pa_{CO_2} ranged from 79 to 101 mm Hg (10.5 to 13.4 kPa) at 30 minutes of life during CMV for all groups (Fig. 3) and continued to increase for both groups receiving CMV. Pa_{CO_2} decreased to within the normal range within minutes of the initiation of PLV; pH changes paralled Pa_{CO_2} changes. There was mild ongoing metabolic acidosis, which was corrected with sodium bicarbonate in all animals; there was no difference in the base deficit among groups.

Dynamic compliance was markedly low in all animals in

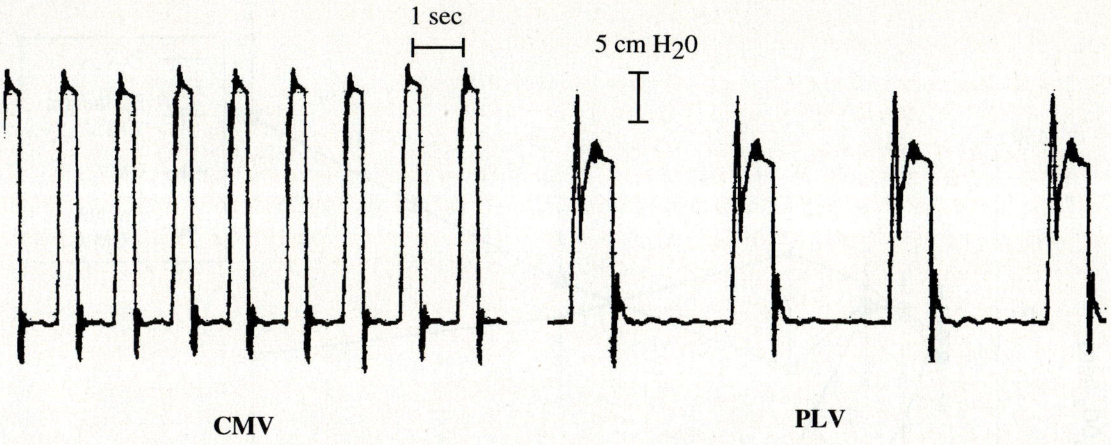

Fig. 1. Airway pressure tracing during CMV and PLV in one animal from the PLV group. Note the pressure spike early in inspiration during PLV, which is suggestive of liquid refluxing into large airways during expiration. PEEP was titrated to minimize this spike.

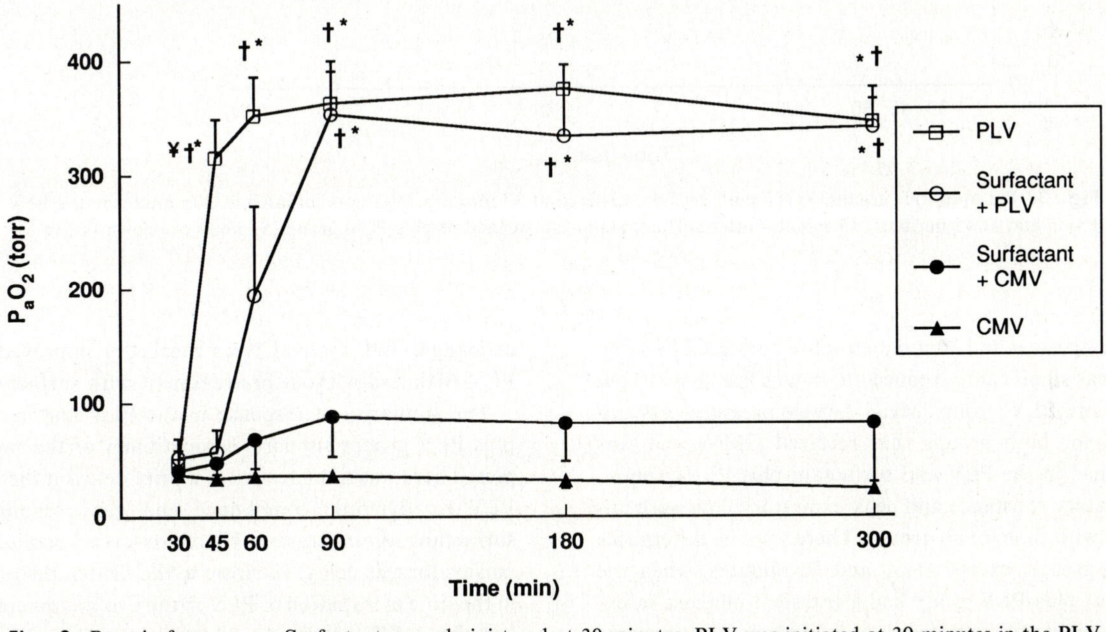

Fig. 2. PaO_2 in four groups. Surfactant was administered at 30 minutes. PLV was initiated at 30 minutes in the PLV group and at 45 minutes (15 minutes after surfactant) in the surfactant-plus-PLV group. *$p < 0.05$ compared with baseline value within group; †$p < 0.008$ compared with the CMV group at the same time point; ¥$p < 0.008$ compared with the surfactant-plus-CMV group at the same time point.

the first 30 minutes of life during CMV (Fig. 4). Within minutes of initiation, compliance increased fourfold in the PLV group. Compliance was increased as well in the surfactant-plus-PLV group, although the response to PLV appeared delayed; there was no significant increase until 90 minutes had elapsed. There was no difference overall between the PLV and surfactant-plus-PLV groups. Compliance remained low in the CMV groups, and was not affected by surfactant.

During the initial CMV period for all animals, mean tidal volume ranged from 3.6 to 4.9 ml/kg at maximal pressure support (Fig. 5). Tidal volume increased during PLV up to means of 11.8 ml/kg for both the PLV and surfactant-plus-PLV groups. Again, the improvement in tidal volume appeared delayed for the surfactant-plus-PLV group. Tidal volume did not improve in either group receiving CMV. Minute ventilation was similar for all groups.

Mean airway pressure ranged from means of 13 to 17 cm

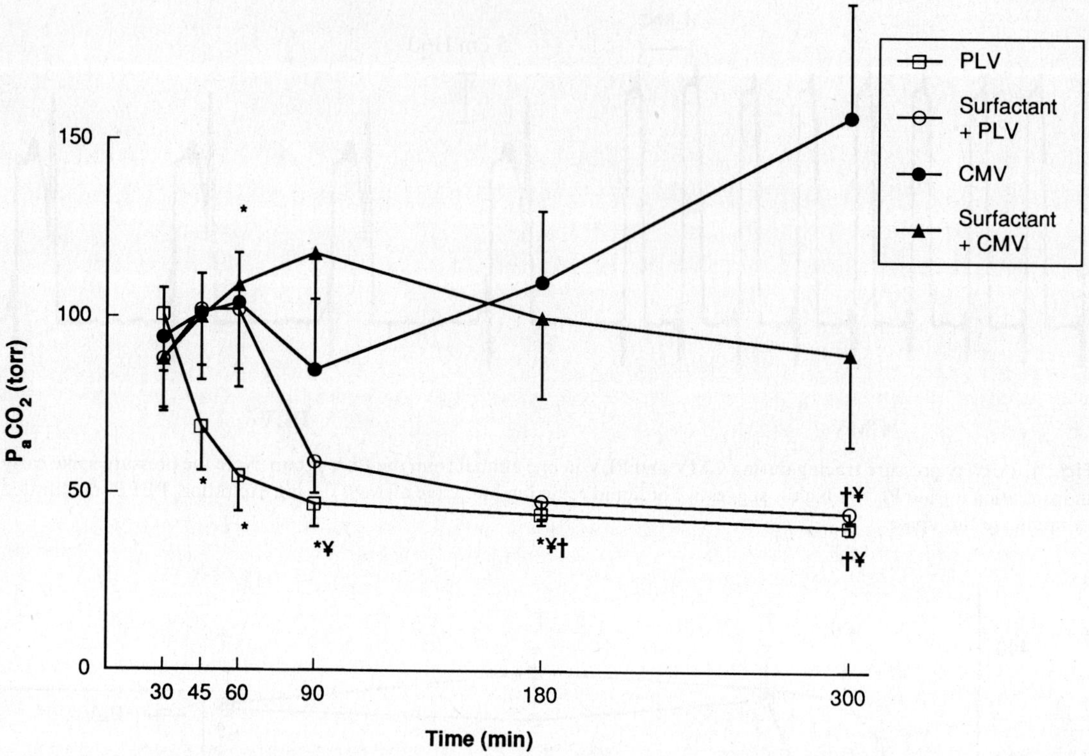

Fig. 3. Pa_{CO_2} in four groups. Surfactant was administered at 30 minutes. PLV was initiated at 30 minutes in the PLV group and at 45 minutes (15 minutes after surfactant) in the surfactant-plus-PLV group. Symbols as shown in Fig. 2.

H_2O during the initial 30 minutes of life during CMV (Fig. 6) and was significantly reduced to means less than 10 cm H_2O in the PLV group. Mean airway pressure was unchanged for both groups that received CMV, and was higher than in the PLV and surfactant-plus-PLV groups.

Expiratory resistance and peak expiratory flow were unchanged with time for all groups. There were no differences between groups, except at 60 and 90 minutes, when the surfactant-plus-PLV group had a transient increase in expiratory resistance and decrease in peak expiratory flow, compared with others. As predicted from the increased compliance with PLV, expiratory time constants increased threefold to fourfold in both the PLV and surfactant-plus-PLV groups, whereas the CMV and surfactant-plus-CMV groups showed no change with time.

There was no evidence of barotrauma associated with PLV (i.e., no parenchymal cysts or hemorrhages were seen on gross examination of the lungs post mortem).

DISCUSSION

This study demonstrated the efficacy of PLV with perflubron, both alone and in conjunction with Exosurf, in the premature lamb with RDS. Lung mechanics, gas exchange, and survival were markedly improved during PLV with and without pretreatment with surfactant.

The similarity of response in the PLV and surfactant-plus-PLV groups supports compatibility of the two therapies. There was a tendency for a brief delay in the effect of PLV on dynamic compliance and gas exchange after surfactant administration. There are several possible mechanisms for this delay. Intrinsic to the model, the difference in the time of initiation of PLV in the two groups could have permitted different levels of lung injury. Disproportionate volumes of surfactant regionally[18-20] may have caused deflection of perflubron, temporarily limiting its range of reduced surface tension and alveolar recruitment. The transient increase in expiratory resistance in the surfactant-plus-PLV group supports delayed distal migration of perflubron because surfactant remained in the small airways and alveolar ducts. Dynamic compliance is frequency dependent, and the increased resistance may have produced an artifactual decrease in compliance in the surfactant-plus-PLV group. It appears that for both gas exchange and mechanics, within an additional 15 minutes, the PLV effect in the surfactant-plus-PLV group was virtually indistinguishable from that in the PLV group. This finding lends

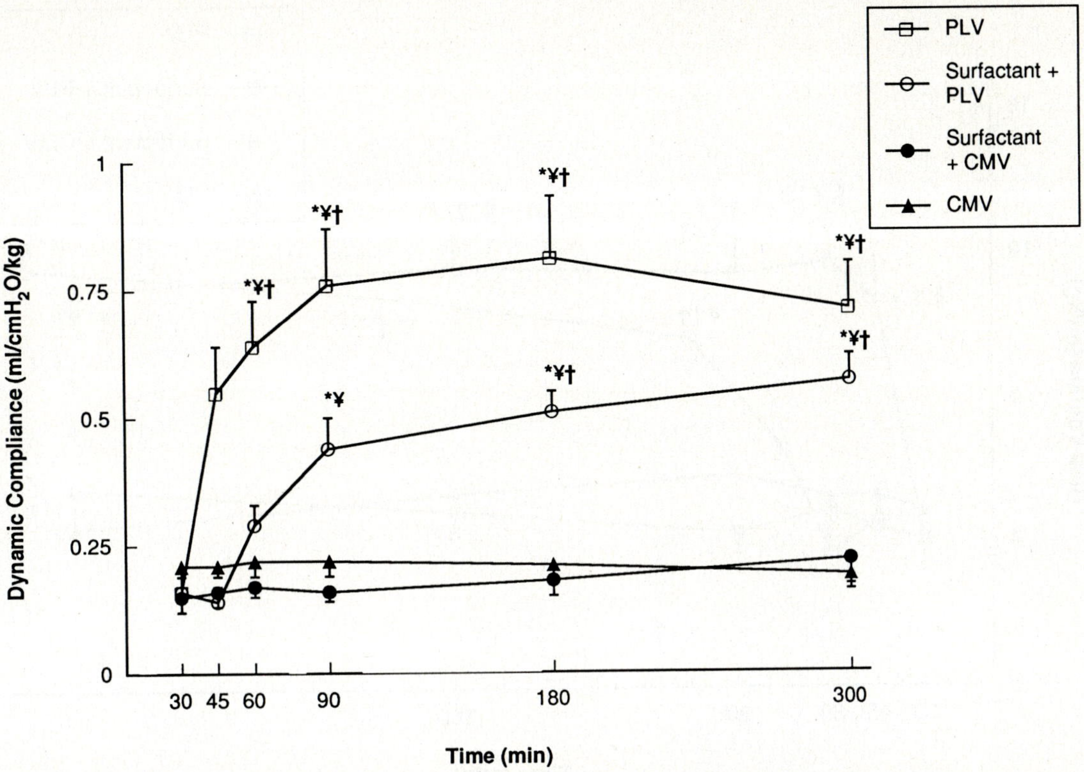

Fig. 4. Dynamic compliance in four groups. Surfactant was administered at 30 minutes. PLV was initiated at 30 minutes in the PLV group and at 45 minutes (15 minutes after surfactant) in the surfactant-plus-PLV group. Symbols as shown in Fig. 2.

further support to mechanical interference as the cause of a delayed response in the surfactant-plus-PLV group. Biochemical interaction between perflubron and Exosurf as a contribution to the delayed effect in the surfactant-plus-PLV group is less likely in light of both the transient nature of the effect and the in vitro compatibility of surfactants with perflubron. This is consistent with a previous study which showed that ventilation with a perfluorochemical liquid neither washed out nor altered the surface tension properties of endogenous surfactant.[21]

The lack of efficacy of Exosurf, chosen for its status as the only open-label surfactant at the time of initiation of this study, is consistent with previous reports in animals.[22] Its modest physiologic activity in this study, however, restricts complete extrapolation of these results to the effects of combination treatment of PLV with a more surface-active surfactant preparation. Although the in vitro results support the lack of interaction between three surfactants and perflubron, further studies would be required to determine whether other, less specific pulmonary effects might occur with the combination of two surface-active drugs in the lung.

As a modification of total liquid ventilation, PLV is distinguished from total liquid ventilation by several factors. PLV involves the primary establishment of liquid FRC with continuing gas ventilation, and does not require the delivery of liquid tidal volumes at any point. In PLV, the liquid FRC is maintained by supplementation with liquid for the duration of the procedure. The liquid is continually oxygenated and ventilated within the lung of the patient by gas tidal volumes, in contrast to the extracorporeal oxygenation of liquid by a separate membrane during total liquid ventilation. The in vivo oxygenation that occurs through an FRC of liquid in PLV, in comparison with the larger end-inspiratory volume of liquid in total liquid ventilation, may permit a shorter diffusion distance of gas from the airway to the alveolar-capillary interface, where gas exchange occurs. This may contribute to the greater oxygenation achieved with PLV in this model than that found in previous studies employing total liquid ventilation.[3, 23]

There are several approaches to the initiation of PLV. In this study, liquid FRC was established by a combination rapid-infusion, slow-infusion technique. The small initial dose rapidly cleared the large airways and established the improved mechanics, enabling us to make early ventilatory adjustments. Full liquid FRC was completed during venti-

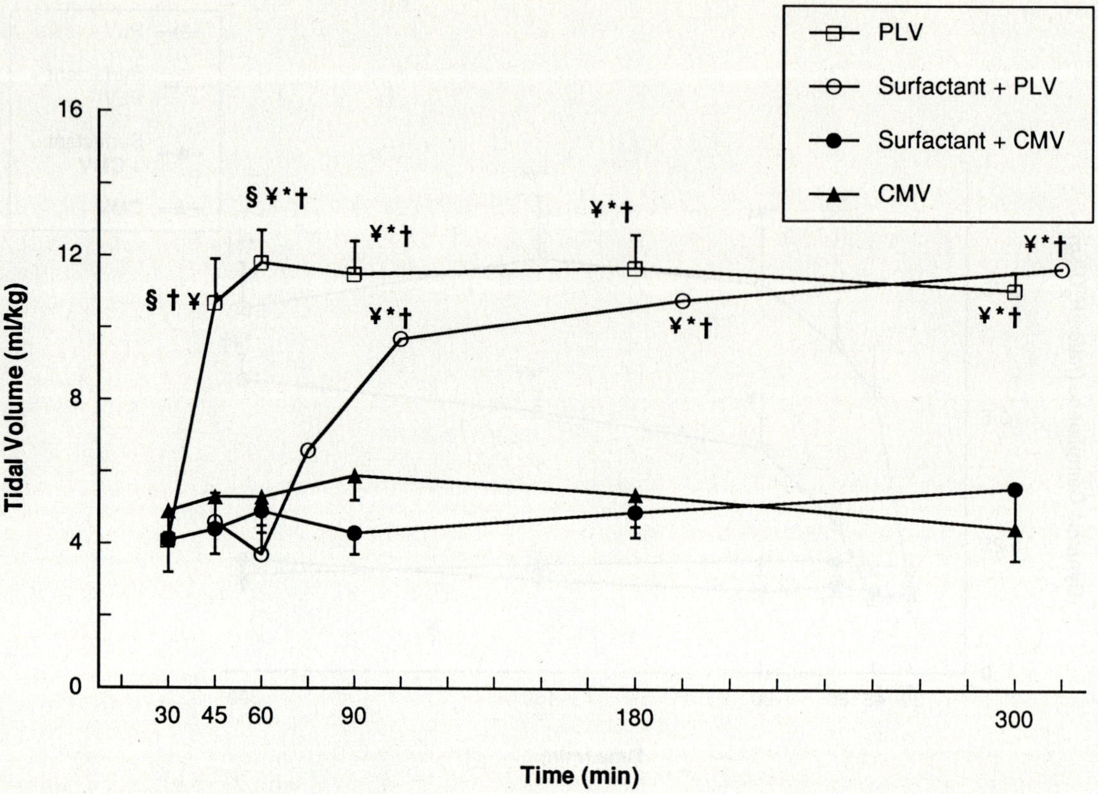

Fig. 5. Tidal volume in four groups. Surfactant was administered at 30 minutes. PLV was initiated at 30 minutes in the PLV group and at 45 minutes (15 minutes after surfactant) in the surfactant-plus-PLV group. Symbols (except section [§] symbol) as shown in Fig. 2. §Compared with the surfactant-plus-PLV group at the same time point.

lation, while tidal volume was carefully maintained during pressure support. Three other techniques to initiate PLV have been described: single liquid infusion during apnea followed by gas tidal volumes,[11] single liquid infusion during apnea with a brief period of total liquid ventilation followed by gas tidal volumes,[4] and multiple small doses during intermittent apnea and gas tidal volumes.[6] Although successful in adult animal models, a single large infusion of liquid immediately followed by conventional gas tidal volumes in premature lambs with aerated lungs frequently resulted in pneumothorax in pilot studies in our laboratory.

The ventilatory scheme for PLV reflected the improved lung mechanics and the increased diffusion time of gases in liquid[24] by employing reduced respiratory rates and long inspiratory time. The use of PEEP in PLV differs from its use in CMV in that it functions not to establish FRC (this is accomplished by the liquid) but to maintain the upper airways clear of liquid, so as to reduce airway resistance and dynamic ventilatory pressures. The biphasic airway pressure curve during PLV likely represents an acute pressure pulse caused by perfluorochemical liquid refluxing into the large airways during expiration. The pressure pulse resets to a lower plateau as the fluid moves to smaller airways with a greater cross-sectional area and therefore lower resistance. The valley between the two peaks probably reflects the time response of the Servo 500 ventilator to compensate or regulate pressure with rapidly changing airway mechanics. The presence and height of the spike varied inversely with the level of PEEP, which was generally titrated to achieve a near monophasic curve.

An important mechanism of action of PLV in surfactant-deficient states is the reduction of surface tension through replacement of the alveolar membrane gas-liquid interface with a liquid-liquid interface.[25] This "surfactant-like activity" of perfluorochemical liquids is exhibited when they are administered in small doses,[6, 26, 27] as well as in larger volumes approximating FRC.[4, 28] However, PLV differs from surfactant replacement in several ways. Surfactants exert their effect in part by changing the aqueous phase of the alveolar membrane and thus reducing the high surface tension of membrane water. During PLV, perfluorochemicals, which have low surface tension, interface with the membrane water unchanged but have, instead, created a new, or second, gas-liquid interface of lower surface tension.

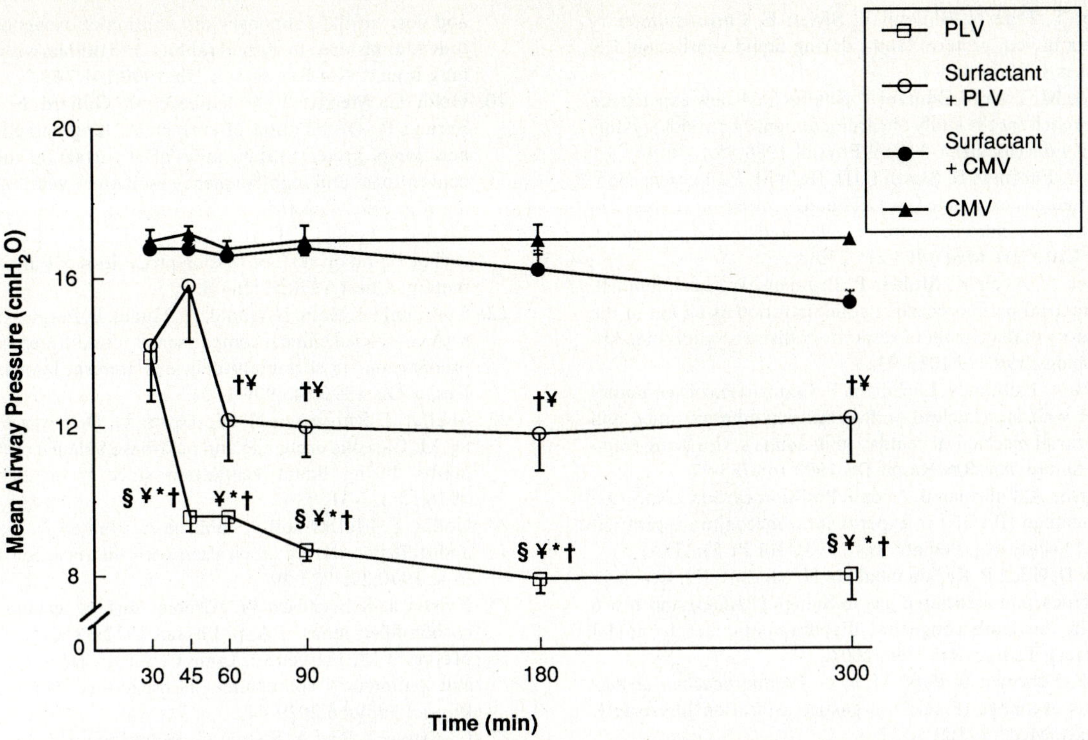

Fig. 6. Mean airway pressure in four groups. Surfactant was administered at 30 minutes. PLV was initiated at 30 minutes in the PLV group and at 45 minutes (15 minutes after surfactant) in the surfactant-plus-PLV group. Symbols (except section [§] symbol) as shown in Fig. 2. §Compared with the surfactant-plus-PLV group at the same time point.

The exact nature and interplay of these various surface tension interfaces are not well understood. A second mechanism of action of PLV, distinct from that of surfactant, is its stabilization of alveoli by bulk distention with a noncompressible liquid.[29]

In this model of surfactant deficiency, PLV quickly and markedly improved compliance. In contrast, exogenous surfactants generated modest, gradual improvement in compliance in both animal and human trials.[15, 30-33] The increased FRC coupled with improved compliance suggests that extensive alveolar recruitment occurs during PLV, whereas regional overdistention may account for the increase in FRC and gas exchange during surfactant replacement therapy.[34] In addition, one of the more striking pnenomena associated with PLV is its virtual uniformity of response in this model of RDS (i.e., there were no individual animals who had clinical deterioration or responded marginally to the technique). This is in contrast to surfactant therapy, in which there is often significant variability of response.[13-15] As an inert fluid, perflubron is not subject to inactivation by protein, as occurs with surfactant in both advanced RDS and adult RDS.[35, 36] Likewise, the maldistribution that occurs with surfactant[18, 20] is less of an issue with PLV because large volumes are insufflated relative to the dose of exogenous surfactant tolerable.[19] Even small amounts of perflubron may confer the advantage of improved distribution because of its unique wettability.[6] Perflubron has a very high spreading coefficient, a number related to interfacial tension between two liquids, and is able to spread over the respiratory membrane. This is in contrast to the poor spreading capability of phospholipids in exogenous surfactant, which may contribute to its maldistribution. PLV therefore might be particularly advantageous in the treatment of established RDS and adult RDS, when exogenous surfactant has failed or has been of limited efficacy.

We conclude that PLV with perflubron improves lung mechanics and gas exchange in premature lambs with RDS, that PLV is compatible with exogenous surfactant, and that, as a treatment for RDS in this model, PLV is superior to the surfactant studied.

We thank Mark Rath, Daniel Swartz, Cynthia Maloney and June Sokolowski for their expert technical assistance.

REFERENCES

1. Shaffer T, Douglas P, Lowe C, Bhutani V. Liquid ventilation: improved gas exchange and lung compliance in preterm lambs. Pediatr Res 1983;17:303-6.

2. Shaffer T, Tran N, Bhutani V, Sivieri E. Cardiopulmonary function in very preterm lambs during liquid ventilation. Pediatr Res 1983;17:680-4.
3. Wolfson M, Tran N, Bhutani V, Shaffer T. A new experimental approach for the study of cardiopulmonary physiology during early development. J Appl Physiol 1988;65:1436-43.
4. Leach C, Fuhrman B, Morin F III, Rath M. Perfluorocarbon-associated gas exchange (partial liquid ventilation) in respiratory distress syndrome: a prospective, randomized, controlled study. Crit Care Med 1993;21:1270-8.
5. Tutuncu A, Akpir K, Mulder P, Erdmann W, Lachmann B. Intratracheal perfluorocarbon administration as an aid in the ventilatory management of respiratory distress syndrome. Anesthesiology 1993;79:1083-93.
6. Tutuncu A, Faithful N, Lachmann B. Comparison of ventilatory support with intratracheal perfluorocarbon administration and conventional mechanical ventilation in animals with acute respiratory failure. Am Rev Respir Dis 1993;148:785-92.
7. Thompson A, Fuhrman B, Allen J. Perfluorocarbon-associated gas exchange (PAGE) in experimental meconium aspiration (MAS) [Abstract]. Pediatr Res 1993;33(4 Pt 2):239A.
8. Wilcox D, Glick P, Karamanoukian H, Morin F III, Leach C. Perfluorocarbon associated gas exchange (PAGE) and nitric oxide in the lamb congenital diaphragmatic hernia model [Abstract]. Pediatr Res 1994;260A.
9. Nesti F, Fuhrman B, Papo M, et al. Perfluorocarbon-associated gas exchange (PAGE) in gastric aspiration [Abstract]. Crit Care Med 1993;21:S157.
10. Papo M, Paczan P, Burak B, et al. A medical grade perfluorocarbon used during PAGE improves oxygenation and ventilation in a model of ARDS [Abstract]. Crit Care Med 1993;21(4 suppl):S288.
11. Fuhrman B, Paczan P, DeFranc M. Perfluorocarbon-associated gas exchange. Crit Care Med 1991;19:712-22.
12. Halliday H. Clinical experience with exogenous natural surfactant. Dev Pharmacol Ther 1989;13:173-81.
13. Fujiwara T, Konishi M, Chida S. Surfactant replacement therapy with a single postventilatory dose of a reconstituted bovine surfactant in preterm neonates with respiratory distress syndrome: final analysis of a multicenter, double-blind, randomized trial and comparison with similar trials. Pediatrics 1990;86:753-64.
14. Charon A, Taeusch H, Fitzgibbon C, Smith G, Treves S, Phelps D. Factors associated with surfactant treatment response in infants with severe respiratory distress syndrome. Pediatrics 1989;83:348-54.
15. Hallman M, Pohjavuori M, Bry K, Merritt T. Human surfactant from amniotic fluid in the treatment of respiratory distress syndrome. In: Lachmann B, ed. Surfactant replacement therapy in neonatal and adult respiratory distress syndrome. Berlin: Springer-Verlag, 1988:136-42.
16. Segerer H, Stevens P, Schadow B, et al. Surfactant substitution in ventilated very low birth weight infants: factors related to response types. Pediatr Res 1991;30:591-6.
17. Notter R. Biophysical behavior of lung surfactant: implications for respiratory physiology and pathophysiology. Semin Pernatol 1988;12:180-212.
18. Jobe A, Ikegami M, Jacobs H, Jones S. Surfactant and pulmonary blood flow distributions following treatment of premature lambs with natural surfactant. J Clin Invest 1984;73:848-56.
19. Gilliard N, Richman P, Merritt T, Spragg R. Effect of volume and dose on the pulmonary distribution of exogenous surfactant administered to normal rabbits or to rabbits with oleic acid lung injury. Am Rev Respir Dis 1990;141:743-7.
20. Heldt G, Merritt T, Golembeski D, Gilliard N, Bloor C, Spragg R. Distribution of surfactant, lung compliance, and aeration of preterm rabbit lungs after surfactant therapy and conventional and high-frequency oscillatory ventilation. Pediatr Res 1992;31:270-5.
21. Modell J, Gollan F, Giammona S, Parker D. Effect of fluorocarbon liquid on surface tension properities of pulmonary surfactant. Chest 1970;57:263-5.
22. Cummings J, Holm B, Hudak M, Hudak B, Ferguson W, Egan E. A controlled clinical comparison of four different surfactant preparations in surfactant-deficient preterm lambs. Am Rev Respir Dis 1992;145:999-1004.
23. Shaffer T, Rubenstein S, Moskowitz G, Delivoria-Papdopoulos M. Gaseous exchange and acid-base balance in premature lambs during liquid ventilation since birth. Pediatr Res 1976;10:227-31.
24. Gollan F, McDermott J, Johnson A, Namon R. Compliance and diffusion during respiration with fluorocarbon fluid. Fed Proc 1970;29:1725-30.
25. Kylstra J, Schoenfisch W. Alveolar surface tension in fluorocarbon-filled lungs. J Appl Physiol 1972;33:32-5.
26. Mercurio M, Fiascone J, Lima C, Jacobs H. Surface tension and pulmonary compliance in premature rabbits. J Appl Physiol 1989;66:2039-44.
27. Gladstone I, Ray A, Salafia C, Perez-Fontan J, Mercurio M, Jacobs H. Effect of artificial surfactant on pulmonary function in preterm and full-term lambs. J Appl Physiol 1990;69:465-72.
28. Shaffer T, Douglas P, Lowe C, Bhutani V. The effects of liquid ventilation on cardiopulmonary function in preterm lambs. Pediatr Res 1983;17:303-6.
29. Leach C, Fuhrman B, Morin F III, Rath M. Perfluorocarbon-associated gas exchange (partial liquid ventilation) in respiratory distress syndrome: a prospective, randomized, controlled study. Crit Care Med 1993;21:1270-8.
30. Armsby D, Bellon G, Carlisle K, et al. Delayed compliance increase in infants with respiratory distress syndrome following synthetic surfactant. Pediatr Pulmonol 1992;14:206-13.
31. Davis J, Veness-Meehan K, Notter R, Bhutani V, Kendig J, Shapiro D. Changes in pulmonary mechanics after the administration of surfactant to infants with respiratory distress syndrome. N Engl J Med 1988;319:476-9.
32. Pfenninger J, Aebi C, Bachmann D, Wagner B. Lung mechanics and gas exchange in ventilated preterm infants during treatment of hyaline membrane disease with multiple doses of artificial surfactant (Exosurf). Pediatr Pulmonol 1992;14:10-5.
33. Couser R, Ferrara T, Ebert J, Hoekstra R, Fangman J. Effects of exogenous surfactant therapy on dynamic compliance during mechanical breathing in preterm infants with hyaline membrane disease. J PEDIATR 1990;116:119-24.
34. Goldsmith L, Greenspan J, Rubenstein S, Wolfson M, Shaffer T. Immediate improvement in lung volume after exogenous surfactant: alveolar recruitment versus increased distention. J PEDIATR 1991;119:424-8.
35. Kobayashi T, Nitta K, Ganzuka M, Inui S, Grossman G, Robertson B. Inactivation of exogenous surfactant by pulmonary edema fluid. Pediatr Res 1991;29:353-6.
36. Ikegami M, Jobe A, Jacobs H, Lam R. A protein from airways of premature lambs that inhibits surfactant function. J Appl Physiol 1984;57:1134-42.

Efficacy and cost analysis of treating very low birth weight infants with erythropoietin during their first two weeks of life: A randomized, placebo-controlled trial

Robin K. Ohls, MD, Karen A. Osborne, RN, and Robert D. Christensen, MD
From the Division of Neonatology, University of Florida, Gainesville, and the Division of Human Development and Aging, University of Utah School of Medicine, Salt Lake City

***Objective:* We hypothesized that using a higher dose of erythropoietin (Epo) and starting treatment on the first day of life would reduce the transfusion requirements of ventilator-dependent and non-ventilator-dependent very low birth weight (VLBW) infants. Moreover, we hypothesized that this treatment would be cost-effective.**
***Methods:* We randomly assigned 20 ill newborn VLBW infants to receive either Epo (200 units/kg per day) or placebo during their first 2 weeks of life. The caregivers were unaware of the treatment assignments, and erythrocyte transfusions were administered according to hematocrit and signs of anemia.**
***Results:* On day 1, reticulocyte counts and hematocrits were similar in the two groups. During the subsequent 2 weeks, reticulocyte counts of the placebo recipients fell significantly below those of the Epo recipients, but hematocrits in the two groups did not differ. More transfusions were received by the placebo recipients (mean = 1.4 per patient) than by the Epo recipients (mean = 0.2 per patient; *p* <0.01). No adverse effects of Epo were noted, and the costs in the placebo group exceeded those in the Epo group.**
***Conclusions:* We conclude that administration of Epo to VLBW infants during the first 2 weeks of life results in fewer transfusions and is cost-effective. (J PEDIATR 1995;126:421-6)**

Diminishing the number of transfusions administered to preterm neonates is widely maintained to be a desirable goal.[1, 2] Large trials on three continents have shown that treatment with erythropoietin can reduce such transfusions.[3-5] By beginning the administration of Epo on the third or fourth day of life, Maier et al.[3] sought to reduce transfusions that result predominantly from phlebotomy losses. By waiting until approximately 2 to 4 weeks of age to begin treatment, Phibbs and Keith[5] and Meyer et al.[4] sought to reduce transfusions that result predominantly from the "anemia of prematurity." The results of these trials are encouraging, but many questions remain regarding the use of Epo in preterm very low birth weight infants. One question relates to the potential effectiveness of Epo in ventilator-

Epo	Recombinant erythropoietin
PDA	Patent ductus arteriosus
VLBW	Very low birth weight

Supported by grants HD-00988 and HL-44951 from the National Institutes of Health, grant RR-00064 from the National Center for Research Resources, and an award from the Children's Miracle Network Telethon.

Submitted for publication June 23, 1994; accepted Sept. 15, 1994.

Reprint requests: Robin K. Ohls, MD, Division of Neonatology, University of Florida College of Medicine, P.O. Box 100296, JHMHC, Gainesville, FL 32610-0296.

0022-3476/95/$3.00 + 0 **9/20/60611**

supported, ill preterm VLBW infants during their first days and weeks of life, who generally require repeated laboratory tests for management.[6] A second question relates to the cost of Epo treatment.[7]

With these issues in mind, we conducted a single-center, placebo-controlled, randomized trial to determine whether administering Epo to ill VLBW infants, beginning on the first or second day of life, would reduce blood transfusions and be cost-effective.

METHODS

Infants were eligible for study if they required intensive care, were less than 48 hours of age, weighed between 750 and 1500 gm at birth, were born at ≥27 weeks of gestation, and had hematocrits between 0.40 and 0.60. Infants were ineligible for study if hemolytic or hemorrhagic disease was documented, or if, during mechanical ventilation, more than 80% oxygen was required for the preceding 4 hours. Infants were also ineligible if congenital heart disease or disease requiring immediate surgical intervention was present.

Infants were randomly selected in a double-blind fashion to receive either Epo, 200 units/kg per day,[8] or placebo (an equivalent volume of the diluent, 0.9% saline solution) intravenously for a 4-hour period, for 14 consecutive days. We chose to give Epo as a 4-hour infusion to more closely mimic the pharmacokinetics of subcutaneous dosing, which has been effective in preterm infants[3-5] but requires injections. The Epo or placebo was diluted in 2 ml of protein-containing parenteral alimentation fluid or 2 ml of 5% albumin, if parenteral alimentation had not been started. The Epo was suspended in protein-containing solution to meet or surpass the protein concentration of the original solution (Epo is formulated in solution containing 0.25% human albumin). Infants in both groups received iron, 2 mg/kg per day orally, when they were taking 70 ml/kg per day enterally. Oral iron supplementation was increased to 6 mg/kg per day when the infants were receiving enteral feedings of more than 100 ml/kg per day.

Heart rate, respiratory rate, and blood pressure were monitored, and infants were observed for adverse events by a study nurse during the infusion. Hematocrit, platelet count, leukocyte count with differential counts, absolute reticulocyte count, and blood lactate concentration were measured on days 1, 3, 6, 10, 14, and 20. Lactate values were measured as previously described.[9] The number and volume of transfusions were recorded, as was the volume of blood withdrawn.

All caregivers and investigators were masked to the treatment groups, and transfusions were administered only according to protocol. Specifically, transfusions were given during the first 3 weeks of life if the hematocrit was <0.33, and if the infant had one or more symptoms thought to be due strictly to anemia. Symptoms were defined as tachycardia (heart rate >160 beats/min, calculated as the average of all heart rates recorded by the bedside nurse during the preceding 24-hour period), an increasing oxygen requirement (an increase in fraction of inspired oxygen of >0.20 during a 24-hour period), "lethargy" as assessed by the primary caregiver, or an increase in the number of episodes of bradycardia requiring stimulation to increase the heart rate from less than 60 beats/min (an increase of such episodes by 3 or more per day). The assessments described above were performed according to each infant's schedule; no attempt was made to make all observations uniform with regard to feeding or sleep-wake states. Infants in both groups whose hematocrits were >0.33 and yet whose phlebotomy losses exceeded 10 ml/kg body weight received an infusion of 5% albumin, administered in aliquots of not less than 10 ml/kg. The intent of this treatment was to aid in the prevention of hypovolemia[10] when the phlebotomy losses were considerable, and yet the hematocrit was above the criteria for transfusion. Infants were not given transfusions if they were free of symptoms, even if the hematocrit fell to less than 0.33.

In addition, we compared the number of transfusions given to study patients with those given to other infants concomitantly in the intensive care unit who met all of the study eligibility criteria but were not entered into this protocol because of parental refusal or their participation in a different study. Informed consent was obtained from parents of the study infants, and the study was approved by the institutional review boards of the University of Utah Hospital and the Primary Children's Medical Center.

A power analysis (using a two-sided significance level of 0.05 and a power of 80%) determined that a sample size of approximately 32 infants was needed to show a difference of 2 ± 2 transfusions. A single interim analysis was planned after entry of 16 patients. Demographic data were compared with an unpaired t test. Laboratory data were compared with two-tailed, paired, or unpaired t tests. When data were not parametrically distributed, the Wilcoxon signed rank test was performed. The Fisher Exact Test was used to assess differences in the number of transfusions between groups, and to assess differences in intercurrent events between groups.

RESULTS

After the interim analysis, the study was discontinued because of significant differences between groups in number of transfusions. Twenty patients were enrolled. There were no differences between groups in birth weight, gestational age, or age at the time of study entry (Table I). There were also no differences between groups in hematocrit, absolute reticulocyte count, or blood lactate concentration.

Changes in absolute reticulocyte count are shown in the

Table I. Characteristics of the study infants

	Epo	Placebo
Birth weight (gm)	1229 ± 51	1241 ± 76
Gestation (wk)	30.0 ± 0.4	29.3 ± 0.3
Age (hr)	27 ± 4	27 ± 5
Hematocrit (L/L)	0.49 ± 0.02	0.46 ± 0.01
Lactate (μmol/gm)	1.3 ± 0.4	1.2 ± 0.1
Absolute reticulocyte count (×10⁹/L)	357 ± 38	410 ± 28

Values represent mean ± SEM.

upper panel of the Figure. Reticulocyte counts in the Epo recipients declined on days 3 and 6 but increased to the range observed at birth by days 10 and 14 (Figure). Reticulocyte counts in the placebo recipients decreased significantly from day 3 to day 20. Reticulocyte counts were greater in the Epo recipients than in the placebo recipients on days 6, 10, 14, and 20.

Hematocrits declined in both groups (Figure). Hematocrits in the Epo recipients were greater than hematocrits in the placebo recipients on days 3, 6, and 10. There were no differences in hematocrits between the groups on days 1, 14, and 20.

There were no significant changes in platelet count or absolute neutrophil count between groups during the study (data not shown). No infant acquired neutropenia (absolute neutrophil count, $\leq 1.0 \times 10^9/L$) in either group. Two infants in the placebo group had neutrophilia on day 20 (absolute neutrophil counts, 37.4×10^9 and $18.9 \times 10^9/L$). One infant in the placebo group had thrombocytopenia (platelet count, $66 \times 10^9/L$) on day 20.

Lactate values gradually decreased in both groups during the 14 day treatment period, but increased to 1.1 ± 0.9 in the placebo recipients by day 20 (vs 0.7 ± 0.2 in the Epo recipients; $p < 0.05$). There were no significant changes overall in heart rate, respiratory rate, or blood pressure in either group during the study.

Phlebotomy losses were similar in the two groups (Table II). During the 20-day study period, 2 of 10 Epo recipients and 7 of 10 placebo recipients received transfusions ($p < 0.01$). Epo recipients received fewer transfusions per patient ($p < 0.01$) and also received less blood per kilogram of body weight ($p < 0.05$) than placebo recipients. During the study period a matched population of preterm infants not enrolled in the study (birth weight 1127 ± 52 gm, gestational age 28.7 ± 0.4 weeks) received 2.8 ± 0.5 transfusions and 42.1 ± 5.5 ml packed erythrocytes per kilogram of body weight. A higher percentage of Epo recipients (40%) than placebo recipients (20%, $p < 0.05$) received no transfusions during their hospitalization, and Epo recipients received fewer transfusions per patient during their hospitalization than did placebo recipients (1.9 ± 0.9 vs

Table II. Phlebotomy losses and transfusions given during the study

	Epo recipients (n = 10)	Placebo recipients (n = 10)
Phlebotomy losses during first 20 days (ml/kg)	23 ± 4	29 ± 4
Patients who received transfusions during first 20 days	20%*	70%
Transfusions per patient	0.2 ± 0.1*	1.4 ± 0.4
Transfusions per transfused patient	1 ± 0*	2.0 ± 0.4
(Range)	(1)	(1-3)
Blood transfused per patient (ml/kg)	13.4 ± 0.9*	28.7 ± 4.7

Values (except percentage of patients who received transfusions during first 20 days) represent mean ± SEM.
*$p < 0.05$ versus placebo.

Table III. Charge comparison

Therapy and unit charge		No.	Total	Charge per patient
Epo recipients				
Epo*	$100.00	10	1000.00	
Transfusion†	$145.00	2	290.00	
TOTAL			$1290.00	$129.00
Placebo recipients				
Transfusion	$145.00	14	$2030.00	$255.55

*Based on pharmacy-derived multiuse vials.
†Based on charge of blood products, type and screen, intravenous setup, and nursing charge.

2.7 ± 1.1; $p < 0.05$), whereas 94% of matched preterm infants not enrolled in the study were given a transfusion one or more times, for an average of 5.6 ± 2.1 transfusions during their hospital stay.

There were no differences between the Epo and the placebo recipients in the number of infants with respiratory distress syndrome, bronchopulmonary dysplasia, intraventricular hemorrhage, or necrotizing enterocolitis (data not shown). Five of the placebo recipients had a patent ductus arteriosus treated with indomethacin (three patients) or surgery (two). None of the Epo recipients received therapy for a PDA ($p < 0.005$). Of 16 infants in the nonstudied group, 10 required therapy for a PDA (four indomethacin, six surgery). There were no differences in duration of hospital stay or of mechanical ventilation.

The charges associated with administration of an erythrocyte transfusion included type and crossmatch, the charges for blood products, setup charges, and nursing charges. The cost analysis did not include the charge for irradiating blood, screening for cytomegalovirus, or treating transfu-

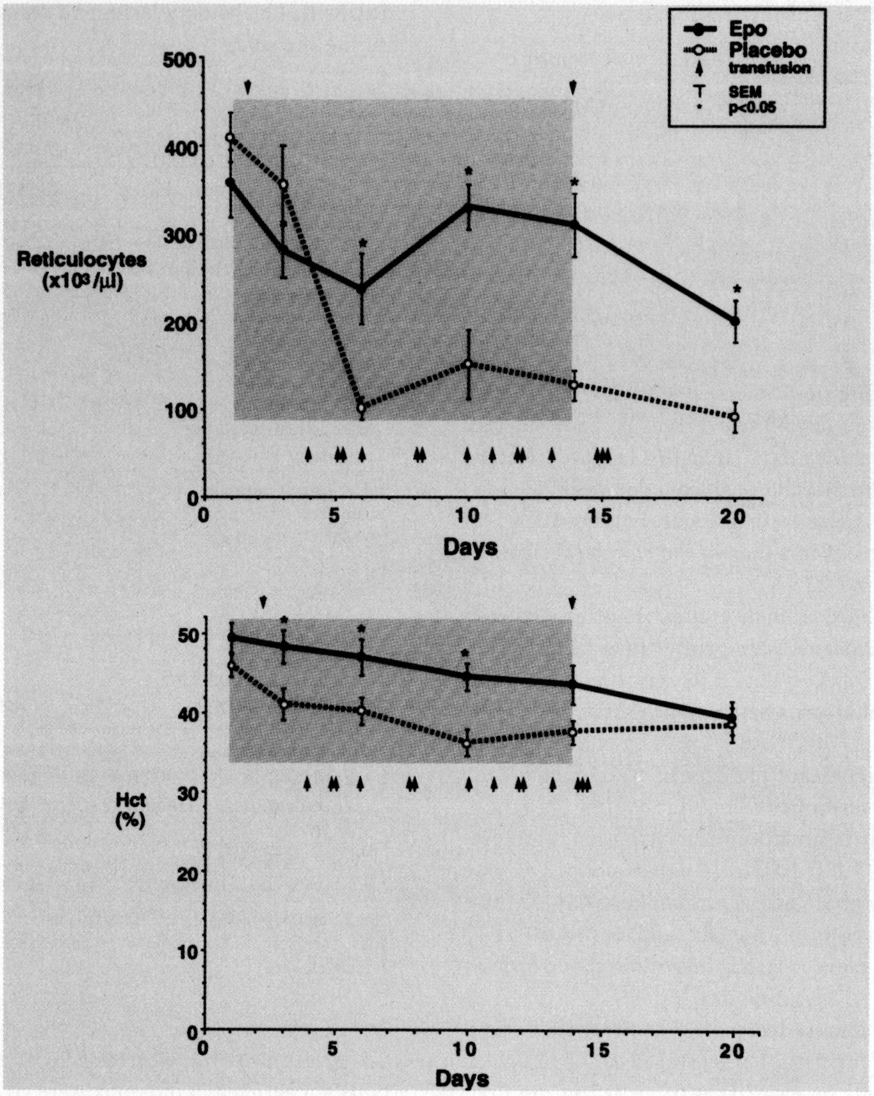

Figure. Changes in reticulocyte count *(upper panel)* and hematocrit *(lower panel)* for Epo recipients *(solid line)* and placebo recipients *(dashed line)*. *Shaded area* represents 14-day treatment period. The *two arrows* above the graph represent transfusions given to Epo recipients, and the *multiple arrows* below the graph represent transfusions given to placebo recipients. *p <0.05 versus placebo.

sion-acquired infection with cytomegalovirus, hepatitis C, or human immunodeficiency virus. The charges for 14 days of Epo therapy, including the pharmacy setup (with vials divided into sterile, multidose units) and the charge for two 1 ml vials of Epo, were approximately $100. During the study, the charge per patient for transfusions and Epo was $129 for the Epo recipients and $256 for the placebo recipients. The charge for transfusions in the nonstudied group for the same period was $399 per patient.

DISCUSSION

After blood loss, adult subjects promptly increase production of endogenous erythropoietin, and the subsequent acceleration in erythropoiesis restores the erythroid mass.[11] A limited capacity to increase serum concentrations of erythropoietin during anemia appears to render VLBW infants less capable of compensating for blood loss.[12, 13] The number of transfusions given to VLBW infants in the first few weeks of life remains a significant problem.[1] One recently studied alternative to transfusions is the use of human recombinant erythropoietin. In previous studies we have shown Epo to be safe, efficacious, and cost-effective for use in older preterm infants with symptomatic anemia.[8, 14] In the present study the administration of Epo to VLBW infants, beginning in the first 2 days of life, was associated with a maintenance of reticulocyte counts greater than those in the placebo group, and with fewer transfusions.

Carnielli et al.[15] evaluated the use of Epo in preterm infants, starting in the first 2 days of life. They randomly selected infants to receive either 400 units of Epo per kilogram three times a week, or no treatment. In addition, the infants receiving Epo received iron, 20 mg/kg intravenously once a week. The Epo recipients had a significant increase in reticulocytes and required fewer transfusions. However, the lack of a placebo group may have influenced transfusion decisions. In addition, the intravenous iron replacement dose of 20 mg/kg is generally not the standard dose or typical route of administration in this country.

Previous studies evaluated iron stores in Epo recipients,[3, 4] and both groups noted increased iron requirements in infants receiving Epo, as evidenced by diminished ferritin concentrations and elevated numbers of hypochromic red cells, despite iron doses of 6 mg/kg per day. More evaluation is required to determine the optimal dose and route of administration of iron in preterm infants receiving Epo.[16]

Maier et al.[3] completed a randomized, multicentered trial involving 241 infants, in which the use of Epo was compared with no treatment in diminishing the number of transfusions given to VLBW infants. They found a significant decrease in the number of transfusions given to Epo recipients, but the lack of a placebo group may have affected the transfusion practices of the caregivers. Because transfusion practices vary so widely from one institution to another (and from one caregiver to another), we incorporated a standardized transfusion protocol into our study. Even our placebo recipients were given fewer transfusions than were comparable infants in our neonatal intensive care unit who were not enrolled in this study.

The transfusion-associated charges per patient were significantly lower for the Epo recipients than for the placebo recipients. Given the risks of transfusions, such as transmission of hepatitis, cytomegalovirus, and human immunodeficiency virus, and the possible development of graft-versus-host disease,[17-19] treatment of these patients with Epo appears to be safer and more cost-effective. A recent study evaluating the cost-effectiveness of Epo versus transfusions to treat the anemia of prematurity[7] showed a cost benefit of Epo if two or more doses were obtained from each vial, as was done in our study. This can also be accomplished by using a single vial each day for all infants receiving Epo.

We observed no adverse effects of Epo administration; hypertension, rashes, or infusion reactions to the Epo were not seen. The Epo recipients had no increase in morbidity or adverse outcome measures in comparison with the placebo recipients or with infants outside the study. The fewer infants requiring therapy for a PDA requires further study before any hypotheses can be tested. Katoh et al.[20] reported increased endothelin-1 production when cells were stimulated with Epo in vitro. Because endothelin has vasoconstrictive effects in fetal animals,[21] this might explain the fewer PDAs requiring intervention in the Epo-treated group. In the Meyer study,[4] a PDA developed in 2 of 40 infants in the Epo group and 7 of 40 in the placebo group.

We previously reported the development of neutropenia in a group of preterm neonates who were treated with Epo for the anemia of prematurity.[14] The kinetic mechanism appeared to involve reduced production of neutrophils from granulocytic progenitors.[22, 23] The reason that neutropenia did not develop in these small preterm infants in the first weeks of life is unknown. The cause may involve total numbers of progenitors and a depletion of those progenitors in slightly older preterm infants.

Multicentered trials are required to evaluate the possible association of Epo administration with PDA closure, and to evaluate the long-term effects of Epo. In addition, the effectiveness of Epo on the transfusion requirements of extremely low birth weight infants (<750 gm) remains to be determined. Moreover, the evolution of clinical practice in the care of VLBW infants continues to affect the number of transfusions given to these infants. For example, decreasing the volume of blood lost through phlebotomy[24] and instituting standardized transfusion guidelines[25] results in a decrease in the transfusion requirements of VLBW infants.

We conclude that the VLBW infants treated with Epo in the first 2 weeks of life require fewer transfusions. Further, for this study population, the charges associated with Epo therapy were less than the charges associated with transfusions. We speculate that Epo administration, in combination with instituting more rigorous and standardized transfusion criteria and diminishing the volume of blood lost through phlebotomy, will have the greatest impact in decreasing transfusion requirements in VLBW infants.

REFERENCES

1. Strauss RG. Erythropoietin and neonatal anemia. N Engl J Med 1994;330:1227-8.
2. Christensen RD. Recombinant erythropoietic growth factors as an alternative to erythrocyte transfusion for patients with "anemia of prematurity." Pediatrics 1989;83:793-6.
3. Maier RF, Obladen M, Scigalla P, et al. The effect of epoetin beta (recombinant human erythropoietin) on the need for transfusion in very low birth weight infants. N Engl J Med 1994;330:1173-8.
4. Meyer MP, Meyer JH, Commerford A, et al. Recombinant human erythropoietin in the treatment of the anemia of prematurity: results of a double-blind, placebo-controlled study. Pediatrics 1994;93:918-23.
5. Phibbs RH, Kieth JF. Recombinant human erythropoietin (r-HuEPO) stimulates erythropoiesis and reduces transfusions in preterm infants [Abstract]. Pediatr Res 1994;35:248A.
6. Blanchette VS, Zipursky A. Assessment of anemia in newborn infants. Clin Perinatol 1984;11:489-510.
7. Shireman TI, Hilsenrath PE, Strauss RG, Widness JA, Mutnick AH. Recombinant human erythropoietin vs transfusions

in the treatment of the anemia of prematurity: a cost-benefit analysis. Arch Pediatr Adolesc Med 1994;148:582-8.
8. Ohls RK, Hunter DD, Christensen RD. A randomized, placebo-controlled trial of recombinant erythropoietin as treatment for the anemia of bronchopulmonary dysplasia. J PEDIATR 1993;123:996-1000.
9. Kimura RE, LaPine TR, Gooch WM III. Portal venous aortic glucose and lactate changes in a chronically catheterized rat. Pediatr Res 1988;23:325-40.
10. Bifano EM, Smith F, Borer J. Relationship between determinants of oxygen delivery and respiratory abnormalities in preterm infants with anemia. J PEDIATR 1992;120:292-6.
11. Erslev AJ, Wilson J, Caro J. Erythropoietin titers in anemic, nonuremic patients. J Lab Clin Med 1987;109:429-33.
12. Stockman JA III, Graeber JE, Clark DA, McClellan K, Garcia JF, Kavey REW. Anemia of prematurity: determinants of the erythropoietin response. J PEDIATR 1984;105:786-92.
13. Brown MS, Garcia JF, Phibbs RH, Dallman PR. Decreased response of plasma immunoreactive erythropoietin to "available oxygen" in anemia of prematurity. J PEDIATR 1984; 105:793-8.
14. Ohls RK, Christensen RD. Recombinant erythropoietin compared with erythrocyte transfusion in the treatment of anemia of prematurity. J PEDIATR 1991;119:781-8.
15. Carnielli V, Montini G, Da Riol R, Dall'Amico R, Cantarutti F. Effect of high doses of human recombinant erythropoietin on the need for blood transfusions in preterm infants. J PEDIATR 1992;121:98-102.
16. Ehrenkrantz RA, Sherwonit EA, Nelli CM, Janghorbani M. Recombinant human erythropoietin (r-HuEPO) stimulates incorporation of absorbed iron (Fe) into RBC's in VLBW infants [Abstract]. Pediatr Res 1994;35:311A.
17. Tipple M, Bland LA, Murphy JJ, et al. Sepsis associated with transfusion of red cells contaminated with *Yersinia enterocolitica*. Transfusion 1990;30:207-13.
18. DePalma L, Luban NLC. Blood component therapy in the perinatal period: guidelines and recommendations. Semin Perinatol 1990;14:403-15.
19. Holland PV. Prevention of transfusion-associated graft-versus-host disease. Arch Pathol Lab Med 1989;113:285-91.
20. Katoh K, Mizuno K, Hashimoto S, et al. Direct evidence for erythropoietin-induced release of endothelin from peripheral vascular tissue. Life Sci 1994;54:253-9.
21. Bonvallet ST, Oka M, Yano M, McMurtry IF, Stelzne TJ. An endothelin receptor antagonist attenuates endothelin-1 (ET-1) induced vasoconstriction in the rat pulmonary circulation. J Cardiovasc Pharmacol 1993;22:39-43.
22. Christensen RD, Liechty KW, Koenig JM, Schibler KR, Ohls RK. Administration of erythropoietin to newborn rats results in diminished neutrophil production. Blood 1991;78: 1241-5.
23. Christensen RD, Rothstein G. Erythropoietin affects the maturation pattern of fetal G-CSF–responsive progenitors. Am J Hematol 1992;39:108-12.
24. Keith JF, Phibbs RH. Effects of phlebotomy losses on transfusions in preterm infants treated with recombinant human erythropoietin [Abstract]. Pediatr Res 1994;35:233A.
25. Bifano EM, Miggiani WP, Parker PR. Impact of transfusion guidelines on transfusion practices in premature infants [Abstract]. Pediatr Res 1994;35:216A.

Neonatal mortality rate: Is further improvement possible?

Alistair G. S. Philip, MD, FRCPE

From the Division of Neonatology, Maine Medical Center, Portland, Maine

Objective: **To determine whether improvement in neonatal and infant mortality rates is possible or likely.**
Setting: **Regional neonatal intensive care unit.**
Methods: **Experience during a decade (1982–1991) was evaluated. We determined postnatal age at death and birth weight–specific and gestational age–specific mortality rates. Neonatal deaths (deaths before discharge) were categorized as "possibly preventable" or "probably unpreventable."**
Results: **Deaths occurring after 28 days ("postponed" deaths) contributed 9% of the total for the decade, and 5% for those with extremely low birth weight (ELBW; <1000 gm) during the last 6 years; 47% of all deaths and 65% of deaths of ELBW infants occurred within 24 hours of birth. Congenital malformations accounted for 7%, 54%, and 66% of deaths when birth weight was 500 to 1499 gm, 1500 to 2499 gm, and ≥2500 gm, respectively. In infants with birth weight ≥1000 gm, probably unpreventable deaths (predominantly from congenital malformations, but also including hydrops and inborn errors of metabolism) accounted for 61% of deaths. Of deaths of ELBW infants, extreme prematurity (500 to 750 gm) accounted for 58%; major malformations and pulmonary hypoplasia contributed an additional 9%.**
Conclusion: **During the decade, the gestational age at which there was a 50% survival rate fell from 26 weeks to 24 weeks and a marked increase in the survival rate occurred at birth weights <1500 gm (VLBW) after the introduction of exogenous surfactant therapy. The number of possibly preventable deaths is now very small. For any substantial impact on mortality rates, it will be necessary to lower VLBW and ELBW rates. (J Pediatr 1995;126:427-33)**

There has been a steady but slow decline in infant mortality rates in the United States in the past decade.[1,2] However, in comparison with other industrialized nations, the United States has not gained ground and may even have lost a little.[1,2] Low rates in Scandinavia and Japan may be attributed to low rates of low birth weight and particularly very low birth weight.[1-3] Preliminary evidence from 1990 suggests that mortality rates for neonates with a birth weight of 601 to 1300 gm abruptly decreased after the availability of exogenous surfactants increased,[4] but similar improvement would be expected in the other developed nations. It is doubtful that the United States can improve its position in the "international rankings" without major societal changes. Nevertheless, there may be ways of lowering infant mortality rates further.

ELBW	Extremely low birth weight (<1000 gm)
LBW	Low birth weight (500 to 2499 gm)
NICU	Neonatal intensive care unit
RDS	Respiratory distress syndrome
VLBW	Very low birth weight (<1500 gm)

Attempts to use death certificates to identify the cause of death do not necessarily reveal the initiating cause,[5] especially among VLBW infants. To identify strategies to decrease neonatal mortality rates, there is a need to look

Submitted for publication June 1, 1994; accepted Sept. 1, 1994

Reprint requests: Alistair G. S. Philip, MD, Division of Neonatal and Developmental Medicine, Department of Pediatrics, Stanford University School of Medicine, 750 Welch Rd., Suite 315, Palo Alto, CA 94304.

0022-3476/95/$3.00 + 0 **9/23/60326**

Table I. Birth weight–specific neonatal mortality rates (deaths before discharge) for infants admitted to the Maine Medical Center NICU during the years 1982 to 1991

Birth weight (gm)	Inborn (planned)		Inborn (MFT)		Outborn		Total NMR		Deaths from congenital anomaly	Corrected NMR
	No.	%	No.	%	No.	%	No.	%		
500-749	38/54*	70	51/95	54	17/27	63	106/176	60	3	60
750-999	16/58	28	40/133	30	14/43	33	70/234	30	6	28
1000-1249	8/71	11	18/154	12	5/58	9	31/283	11	4	10
1250-1499	3/78	4	9/148	6	4/47	9	16/273	6	3	5
Total	65/261	(25)	118/530	(22)	40/175	(23)	223/966	(23)	16	(22)
1500-1999	14/233	6	7/328	2	9/113	8	30/674	4	14	2
2000-2499	10/222	5	10/218	5	13/187	7	33/627	5	20	2
Total	24/455	(5)	17/546	(3)	22/300	(7)	63/1301	(5)	34	(2)
2500-3499	15/381	4	14/152	9	62/538	12	91/1071	8	63	3
3500-4499	7/216	3	4/44	9	26/289	9	37/549	7	22	3
>4500	2/16	13	0/5	0	3/26	12	5/47	11	3	5
Total	24/613	(4)	18/201	(9)	91/853	(11)	133/1667	(8)	88	(3)

MFT, Maternal-fetal transfer; *NMR*, neonatal mortality rate.
*Deaths/total admitted.

more carefully at whether neonatal deaths are potentially preventable or apparently unpreventable. This report deals with a review of admissions to and deaths in a regional neonatal intensive care unit during a decade (1982–1991). In keeping with other reports, "neonatal deaths" are defined as deaths before discharge,[6-8] the inverse of which is survival to discharge.[9]

METHODS

Data on all infants admitted to the NICU of the Maine Medical Center in the years 1982 through 1991 were evaluated. The hospital is the only tertiary-level facility in the state of Maine, and throughout the period, 60% to 70% of all VLBW (<1500 gm) infants born in the state were delivered at the Maine Medical Center. Another 10% or so of the state's VLBW infants were transferred to the NICU after birth. All neonatal surgical problems and almost all serious cardiac problems from the state were transferred to the NICU.

Neonatal deaths were defined as any death of a live-born infant, either in the delivery room (if birth weight was ≥500 gm) or before discharge from the hospital, after admission to the NICU during the first 28 days after birth. Late admissions usually involved congenital abnormalities. Almost all live-born infants with birth weights between 400 and 500 gm were admitted to the NICU for care, although a few died in the delivery room. There were no deaths outside either the delivery room or the NICU.

Gestational age assessment was performed, with the use of the Ballard modification of the Dubowitz score, on every baby admitted to the NICU.[10] When the estimate based on the mother's last menstrual period was confirmed postnatally, that gestational age was used. If there was clear disagreement between the stated gestational age based on the last menstrual period and the postnatal evaluation of gestational age, the latter estimate was used. The discrepancy was usually 4 weeks. If any bias exists in these data, it is in the direction of overestimating gestational age.

Monthly conferences were held throughout the period for the purpose of evaluating the cause of death of each baby who died, and incorporating the findings of a pediatric pathologist. The time of death was also recorded and annual reports were prepared.

RESULTS

Birth weight–specific mortality rates and congenital malformations. Birth weight–specific mortality rates were prepared according to whether the mother planned to deliver at Maine Medical Center (inborn, planned), was transferred for delivery (inborn, maternal-fetal transfer), or delivered elsewhere with the baby transferred after birth (outborn). These data are displayed in Table I for birth weights of 500 gm or more. There were no substantial differences among the three categories (inborn, planned; inborn maternal-fetal transfer; and outborn) that cannot be explained by congenital malformations. The denominators were reliable for inborn infants who weighed <1500 gm at birth, but for overall mortality rates for infants who weighed >1500 gm, the denominators would be much larger and the mortality rates much lower than indicated. For instance, all 791 inborn VLBW infants were admitted to the NICU, but only 1001 of 1880 infants with birth weights of 1500 to 2499

Table II. Comparison of birth weight–specific and gestational age–specific mortality rates for low birth weight infants by time interval at Maine Medical Center NICU

	1982–1985		1986–1989		1990–1991	
	No.	% (corrected)	No.	% (corrected)	No.	% (corrected)
Birth weight (gm)						
500-749	45/70	64 (64)*	47/71	66 (66)	14/35	40 (38)
750-999	37/97	38 (37)	27/80	34 (31)	6/57	11 (9)
1000-1249	12/99	12 (11)	15/121	12 (12)	4/62	6 (3)
1250-1499	8/106	8 (7)	7/113	6 (5)	1/54	2 (2)
1500-1749†	8/121	7 (4)	6/144	4 (2)	3/67	4 (2)
1750-1999†	6/107	6 (4)	4/140	3 (1)	3/97	3 (2)
2000-2249†	5/91	5 (2)	6/163	4 (1)	2/62	3 (2)
2250-2499†	8/106	8 (4)	8/148	5 (1)	4/59	8 (4)
GA (wk)						
≤25	51/66	77	53/82	65	17/56	30
26-27	32/87	37	26/93	28	2/44	5
28-29	12/112	11	13/122	11	2/60	3
30-31	9/128	7	7/143	5	6/75	8
32-33	15/193	8	6/255	2	4/140	3
34-35	4/139	3	6/178	3	3/84	4

GA, Gestational age.
*Figures in parentheses indicate corrected mortality rates after exclusion of deaths from congenital anomaly.
†Denominators for these categories are much larger than stated, since many (or most) do not go to NICU.

gm, and only 814 of 25,280 infants with birth weights ≥2500 gm, required admission to the NICU. In addition, of a total of 26 infants with birth weights <500 gm who were admitted to the NICU, only two survived (mortality rate, 92%), at 24 and 28 weeks of gestation. A large proportion of babies with birth weights >2500 gm died as a result of congenital malformations (88/133, 66%). For infants who weighed >1500 gm and <4500 gm at birth, were admitted to the NICU, and did not have congenital malformations, the neonatal mortality rate was 2% to 3%.

Low birth weight infants. Birth weight–specific and gestational age–specific mortality rates for different time intervals for low birth weight infants are displayed in Table II. There was very little improvement between the first (1982–1985) and second (1986–1989) periods, but substantial improvement in the 1990–1991 interval for all groups weighing <1500 gm at birth or <30 weeks of gestational age. Before 1984, there were no survivors born at or before 24 weeks of gestation, so the designation ≤25 weeks was initiated. In 1990 and 1991, survival of infants born at gestational ages >25 weeks appeared to be 95%. Therefore a more detailed analysis of extremely low birth weight infants was performed.

Extremely low birth weight infants. A detailed breakdown by birth weight and gestational age categories for infants with birth weights <1000 gm is provided in the Figure, where an additional year's experience has been added to provide more equal numbers for comparison across time intervals.* The survival rate was 90% at 26 weeks of gestation in 1990 to 1992. No infant born at less than 23 weeks of gestational age survived, and very few between 23 and 24 weeks of gestational age (one each in 1984, 1985, 1990, and 1991, of 41 infants with birth weights >500 gm). However, the gestational age with a 50% survival rate dropped from 26 weeks in the 1982–1985 interval to 25 weeks in the 1986–1989 interval, and to 24 weeks in the 1990–1992 interval.

Causes of death. Table III describes the major causes of death in infants with birth weights ≥1000 gm, divided into possibly preventable and probably unpreventable causes. The former accounted for 39% of deaths. The leading cause of these deaths was the respiratory distress syndrome and its complications. However, in the 1990–1991 interval, there was only one death in this category: that of a 1500 gm baby who had severe pulmonary interstitial emphysema and could not be given adequate ventilatory support. For inborn infants with birth weights ≥1000 gm, there were 121 deaths among 27,611 births (4.38/1000); 39% of the deaths were considered possibly preventable, and the probably unpreventable group represented 2.67 per 1000 live births.

In Table IV are listed the conditions associated with death in infants with birth weights between 500 and 999 gm. A division was made into "probably unpreventable" and

*Details on specific birth-weight and gestational-age cells are available from the author.

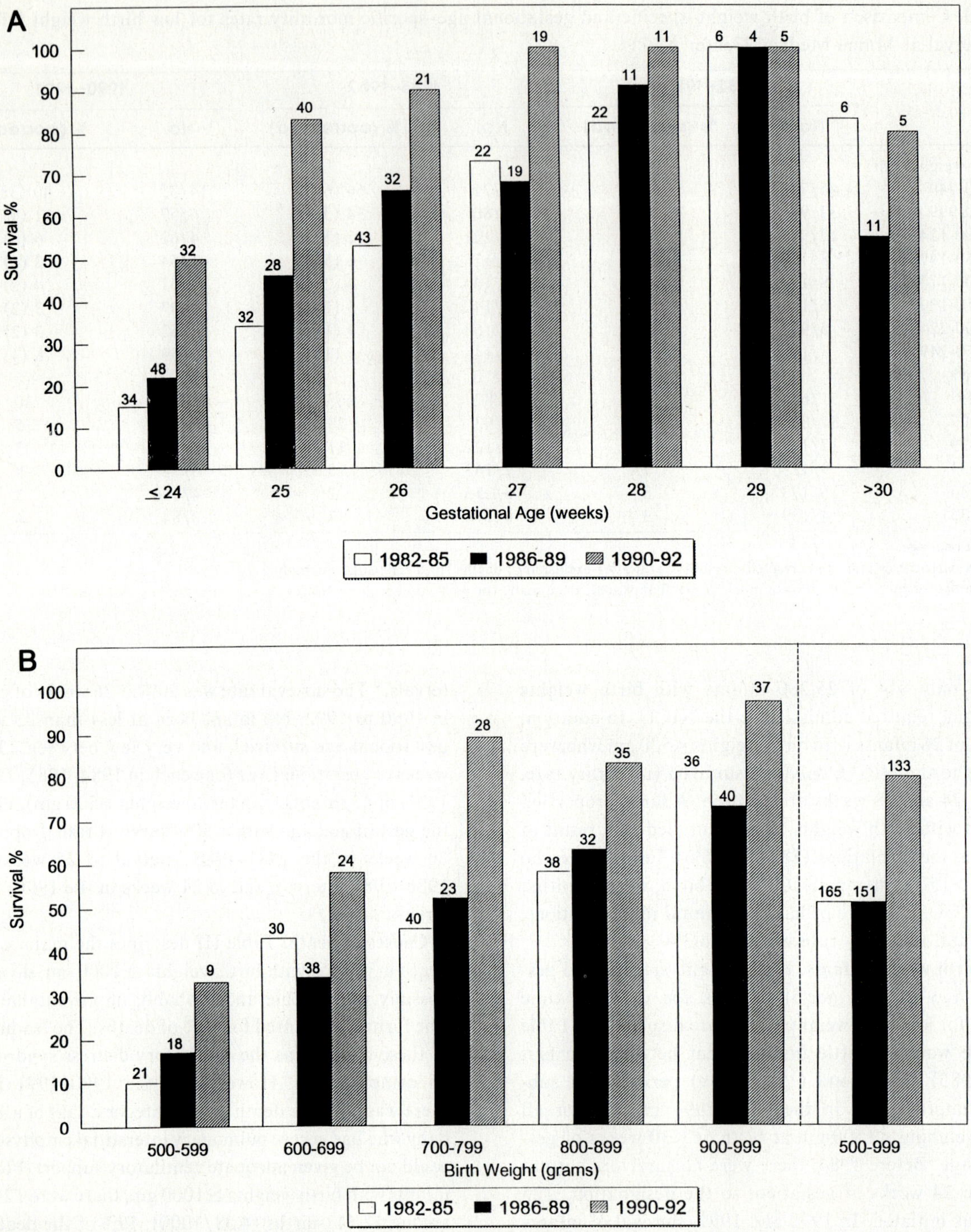

Figure. Survival rates (%) of ELBW infants in the Maine Medical Center NICU, compared, with time (1982 through 1992), by gestational age (**A**) and by birth weight (**B**), showing a marked improvement from 1990 through 1992. The *numbers above each column* indicate the denominator from which the percentages were derived in each category.

"possibly preventable" deaths, but it is difficult to be certain what proportion should have been characterized as probably unpreventable. The majority of those who died within 24 hours (114/176; 65%) probably should fall into that category. The six cases of pulmonary hypoplasia were in infants with birth weights 750 to 999 gm whose mothers had had rupture of the membranes before 22 weeks of gestation but were able to sustain the pregnancy for a few more weeks.

Table III. Maine Medical Center NICU, 1982–1991: Deaths with birth weight ≥1000 gm

Diagnosis	Deaths (No.)	Age at death: <24 hr No. (%)	1-7 days No. (%)	7-28 days No. (%)	>28 days No. (%)
Possibly preventable					
RDS, complications	22	6	9	7	—
Hypoxic-ischemic encephalopathy	17	3	11	3	—
Bacterial infection (sepsis)	15	7	5	3	—
Persistent pulmonary hypertension	13	3	9	—	1
Meconium aspiration syndrome	9	4	5	—	—
Bronchopulmonary dysplasia	9	—	—	—	9
Intracranial hemorrhage	3	—	1	2	—
Herpes simplex infection	2	—	1	1	—
Hemolytic disease of the newborn	1	—	1	—	—
Late PIE	1	—	—	—	1
TOTAL	92	23 (25%)	42 (46%)	16 (17%)	11 (12%)
Probably unpreventable					
Complex congenital heart disease	40	5	16	14	5
Congenital diaphragmatic hernia	14	8	4	2	—
Trisomies	14	5	3	5	1
Pulmonary hypoplasia	13	9	4	—	—
Multiple anomalies (without CHD)	12	3	3	3	3
Major renal anomalies	12	12	—	—	—
Hydrops fetalis	12	11	—	1	—
CNS malformations	11	5	3	2	1
Ventral wall defects	3	—	—	3	—
Inborn errors of metabolism	3	—	2	—	1
Miscellaneous	11	2	5	3	1
TOTAL	145	60 (41%)	40 (28%)	33 (23%)	12 (8%)

PIE, Pulmonary interstitial emphysema; *CHD*, congenital heart disease.

Table IV. Maine Medical Center NICU, 1982–1991: Deaths with birth weight 500 to 999 gm

Diagnosis	Deaths (No.)	Age at death: <24 hr No. (%)	1-7 days No. (%)	7-28 days No. (%)	>28 days No. (%)
Possibly preventable					
Complications of RDS etc. (PIE, severe PV-IVH)	43	23	14	6	0
Bronchopulmonary dysplasia	9	—	—	—	9
Bacterial infection	7	4	0	3	—
Probably unpreventable					
Extreme prematurity (<600 gm)	44	32	7	0	5
Extreme prematurity (601-750 gm)	58	43	10	4	1
Major malformations	9	7	1	1	—
Pulmonary hypoplasia	6	5	1	—	—
TOTAL	176	114 (65%)	33 (19%)	14 (8%)	15 (9%)

PIE, Pulmonary interstitial emphysema; *PV-IVH*, periventricular-intraventricular hemorrhage.

Age at death. Tables III and IV also show the age at death of those with birth weights ≥1000 gm and of ELBW infants, respectively. In both categories, late deaths (occurring after 28 days) accounted for 9% of the deaths; particularly in the ELBW group, late deaths accounted for a smaller percentage of the total in recent years (5% to 6% for the 1986–1991 interval).

Stillbirths. In addition to the 121 deaths of inborn, liveborn infants who weighed ≥1000 gm, there were 114 stillbirths of infants who weighed ≥1000 gm. An additional 42

stillborn infants (7 of whom had major malformations) weighed 500 to 999 gm, compared with 141 neonatal deaths of inborn infants in this birth weight category.*

DISCUSSION

The state of Maine has a very homogeneous population and a low LBW rate compared with the national figure, although it does reflect the rate for white infants in the United States.[1,2] Although there are many areas of poverty in Maine, the distribution of obstetric care is good, and a high percentage of mothers receive appropriate prenatal care. Data from the Maine Medical Center are representative of the state because of the high proportion of LBW infants born there. They are also probably representative of other NICUs in rural states and may be broadly representative, because survival figures for the early years (1982–1985) are similar to data from Australia in extremely premature infants at about the same time[11] and somewhat better than national data from the Netherlands in 1983.[12] The data for the 1982–1985 interval are also similar to combined data from several university centers in the United States from 1982 through 1986.[13]

Evaluation of when and why infants die should allow an appraisal of what strategies might be used to lower infant mortality rates further. The ability to determine the underlying cause of death from death certificates is unsatisfactory and frequently minimizes the impact of short gestation.[5] Because death certificates are "frequently incomplete and imprecise," it has been suggested that "health professionals should rely more on local review of causes of infant mortality."[5] This report was the result of that approach. The term "probably unpreventable" was preferred to "nonpreventable,"[14,15] because the birth weight and the gestational age at which 50% of infants survive have declined markedly in the past decade, and many deaths of extremely premature or tiny babies were considered "nonpreventable" in the past.

Concern has been expressed that a more aggressive approach to VLBW infants and particularly ELBW infants has resulted in infants' having their lives prolonged, only to succumb later, but at enormous expense.[16,17] Our data do not support that contention. In the ELBW category, 65% of deaths occurred within 24 hours of delivery and fewer than 10% after 28 days. Fewer than one fourth of all deaths occurred after 7 days.

The proportion of deaths attributable to congenital anomalies in the United States during this decade was 21% to 23% (see Wegman reports[2]). In Maine, congenital anomalies contributed an even larger proportion, accounting for 33% of all deaths. However, because of the high incidence of referrals to the tertiary care center, this percentage is probably consistent with the national figures. On the other hand, in a regional study from Finland, from 1968 through 1982, the proportion of neonates who died from lethal malformations was 27% for the whole period, but 37% from 1978 through 1982.[18] A study from the Netherlands[12] revealed that congenital malformations accounted for only 9% of deaths in VLBW infants. Data from more than 20 years ago[19] indicate that among infants with birth weights >2500 gm the proportion of deaths caused by congenital anomalies was 36%, compared with 66% in the present series. Congenital heart disease was and is the commonest category of lethal anomaly. More recently, in a regional study from Iowa,[15] the proportion of all deaths attributable to malformations increased from 21% in 1978 and 1979 to 31% in 1982 and 1983.

In Iowa, five disorders accounted for more than 90% of neonatal deaths.[15] In addition to lethal malformations, these disorders were ELBW (<750 gm), RDS, asphyxia, and bacterial sepsis. Comparable figures may be derived from the Maine experience.

Evidence provided in this report indicates a sharp fall in mortality rates after the introduction of exogenous surfactants for the treatment of RDS, in keeping with other recent reports.[4,20] There was only one death related to RDS among infants with birth weights ≥1000 gm who were born in 1990 or 1991. The birth weight–specific mortality rates declined significantly for each birth weight category <1500 gm in the 1990–1991 interval, and the survival rates improved for each week less than 29 weeks of gestation in ELBW infants born in 1990 and 1992. Thus there is evidence that in the next decade the leading cause of "possibly preventable" death in infants >1000 gm may be eliminated, and complications of RDS reduced in those <1000 gm. Nevertheless, with current technology, the limit of viability seems to be at 23 to 24 weeks of gestation.[21] Although exogenous surfactants do not significantly decrease the incidence of bronchopulmonary dysplasia, they may lessen its severity.[22] There were no deaths from this disorder in 1990 to 1991 in infants with birth weights >1000 gm *or* in infants with birth weights of 500 to 999 gm, in contrast to nine deaths in each group in the earlier years.

The remaining "possibly preventable" categories deal with hypoxic-ischemic injury and infection. Recent experience suggests that deaths from bacterial infection may also be decreasing,[23] possibly because of increased antenatal administration of antibiotics to mothers with preterm labor or premature rupture of membranes. This leaves hypoxic-ischemic encephalopathy, persistent pulmonary hypertension, and meconium aspiration syndrome, the last two being difficult to separate. However, with the use of extracor-

*Details of stillbirth rates and perinatal mortality rates are available from the author.

poreal membrane oxygenation and the promise of other strategies such as nitric oxide therapy,[24] these, too, may decline markedly in the next few years.

These data from a recent decade indicate that in infants with birth weights ≥1000 gm, we may be approaching an "irreducible minimum," a concept put forth by Usher[25] more than two decades ago; he calculated the irreducible minimum for the neonatal mortality rate to be 2.6 per 1000 live births for infants with birth weights >1000 gm. In this study an almost identical figure of 2.7 per 1000 for "probably unpreventable" deaths was found for infants ≥1000 gm. A reduction in the minimum could perhaps result from continuing research in human genetics, which might eliminate some of the congenital malformations.

The major unsolved problem in the context of neonatal and infant death is how to prevent prematurity,[26-28] particularly extreme prematurity. The VLBW rate strongly predicts the neonatal mortality rate in industrialized nations,[29] but LBW, VLBW, and ELBW rates have not changed substantially in Maine (and in the United States) during the past two decades. Achievement of further substantial decreases in infant mortality rates will require that all these rates be lower, but how this goal can be accomplished remains elusive.

I thank Douglas A. Dransfield for preparing information for the monthly conferences throughout this period.

REFERENCES

1. Wegman ME. Annual summary of vital statistics—1991. Pediatrics 1992;90:835-45.
2. Wegman ME. Annual summary of vital statistics—1992. Pediatrics 1993;92:743-54. [See also similar summaries published annually.]
3. Heinonen K, Hakulinen A, Jokela V. Survival of the smallest: time trends and determinants of mortality in a very preterm population during the 1980s. Lancet 1988;2:204-7.
4. Horbar JD, Wright EC, Onstad L, et al. Decreasing mortality associated with the introduction of surfactant therapy: an observational study of neonates weighing 601 to 1300 grams at birth. Pediatrics 1993;92:191-6.
5. Carver JD, McDermott RJ, Jacobson HN, et al. Infant mortality statistics do not adequately reflect the impact of short gestation. Pediatrics 1993;92:229-32.
6. Harper R, Rosenstein R, Sia C, et al. Should we continue to define neonatal mortality as death within the first 28 days of life [Abstract]? Pediatr Res 1979;13:390.
7. Philip AGS, Little GA, Polivy DR, Lucey JF. Neonatal mortality risk for the eighties: the importance of birth weight/gestational age groups. Pediatrics 1982;68:122-30.
8. Kitchen WH, Lissenden JV, Yu VYH, Bajuk B. Collaborative study of VLBW infants: techniques of perinatal care and mortality. Lancet 1982;1:1454-7.
9. Grögaard JB, Lindstrom DP, Parker RA, Culley B, Stahlman MT: Increased survival rate in very low birth weight infants (1500 grams or less): no association with increased incidence of handicaps. J PEDIATR 1990;117:139-46.
10. Ballard JL, Novak KK, Driver M. A simplified score for assessment of fetal maturation of newly born infants. J PEDIATR 1979;95:769-74.
11. Yu VYH, Orgill AA, Bajuk B, Astbury J. Survival and 2-year outcome of extremely preterm infants. Br J Obstet Gynaecol 1984;91:640-6.
12. Verloove-Vanhorick SP, Verwey RA. Project on preterm and small for gestational age infants in the Netherlands 1983. 's-Gravenhage, the Netherlands: J. H. Pasmans B.V., 1987.
13. Copper RL, Goldenberg RL, Creasy RK, et al. A multicenter study of preterm birth weight– and gestational age–specific neonatal mortality. Am J Obstet Gynecol 1993;168:78-84.
14. Usher R. Changing mortality rates with perinatal intensive care and regionalization. Semin Perinatol 1977;1:309-19.
15. Hein HA, Lathrop SS. The changing pattern of neonatal mortality in a regionalized system of perinatal care. Am J Dis Child 1986;140:989-93.
16. Buehler JW, Hogue CJR, Zaro SM. Postponing or preventing deaths? trends in infant survival, Georgia, 1974 through 1981. JAMA 1985;253:3564-7.
17. Turkel SB, Sims ME, Guttenberg ME. Postponed neonatal death in the premature infant. Am J Dis Child 1986;140:576-9.
18. Tenovuo A, Kero P, Piekkala P, Sillanpää M, Erkkola R. Advances in perinatal care and declining regional neonatal mortality in Finland, 1968–82. Acta Paediatr Scand 1986;75:362-9.
19. Valdes-Dapena MA, Arey JB. The causes of neonatal mortality: an analysis of 501 autopsies on newborn infants. J PEDIATR 1970;77:366-75.
20. Wegman ME. Annual summary of vital statistics—1990. Pediatrics 1991;88:1081-92.
21. Hack M, Fanaroff A. Outcomes of extremely immature infants: a perinatal dilemma. N Engl J Med 1993;329:1649-50.
22. Mercier CE, Soll RF. Clinical trials of natural surfactant extract in respiratory distress syndrome. Clin Perinatol 1993; 20:711-35.
23. Philip AGS. The changing face of neonatal infection experience at a regional medical center. Pediatr Infect Dis J 1994; 13:1098-102.
24. Walsh-Sukys M, Stork EK, Martin RJ. Neonatal ECMO: iron lung of the 1990s? J PEDIATR 1994;124:427-30.
25. Usher R. Clinical implications of perinatal mortality statistics. Clin Obstet Gynecol 1971;14:885-925.
26. Cole CH. Prevention of prematurity: can we do it in America? Pediatrics 1985;76:310-2.
27. Creasy RK. Preventing preterm birth. N Engl J Med 1991; 325:727-9.
28. Garbaciak JA Jr. Prematurity prevention: who is at risk? Clin Perinatol 1992;19:275-89.
29. Lee K, Paneth N, Gartner LM, Pearlman M. The very low birth weight rate: principal predictor of neonatal mortality in industrialized populations. J PEDIATR 1980;97:759-64.

Twenty-month outcome in ventilator-dependent, very low birth weight infants born during the early years of dexamethasone therapy

L. Furman, MD, M. Hack, MB,ChB, C. Watts, MD, E. Borawski-Clark, PhD, J. Baley, MD, S. Amini, PhD, and B. Hook, MD

From the Departments of Pediatrics and Epidemiology, Case Western Reserve University, Cleveland, Ohio

We sought to examine the effect of the introduction of dexamethasone therapy on health, growth, and neurodevelopmental outcome in very low birth weight (VLBW) infants at 20 months of age. We compared outcomes in all 86 VLBW infants (mean birth weight 871 gm, mean gestational age 26.4 weeks) who were ventilator dependent on day 21 of life during the 2 years preceding October 1988 (period 1), when dexamethasone therapy became accepted clinical practice in our unit, with outcomes in all 124 infants (mean birth weight 891 gm, mean gestational age 26.9 weeks) with similar ventilator status during the subsequent 2 years (period 2). In addition, we compared outcomes in infants who received dexamethasone during period 2 with those in a concurrent cohort of less ill infants who were not given dexamethasone. There were no significant differences between periods 1 and 2 in mortality rates after 21 days (17% vs 21%), need for home oxygen (23% vs 25%), oxygen dependence at 20 months of corrected age (11% vs 10%), rate of neurosensory impairment (24% vs 25%), and mean Bayley Mental scores (81.5 vs 77.2) or Psychomotor Development Index (81.6 vs 71.1). Infants who received dexamethasone during period 2 had significantly more severe lung disease and poorer respiratory, growth, and developmental outcomes. We conclude that VLBW infants with ventilator-dependent chronic lung disease have very poor outcomes, even when treated with dexamethasone. More information is needed from prospective, randomized trials before dexamethasone can be accepted as routine therapy for chronic lung disease. (J PEDIATR 1995;126:434-40)

The improved survival rates of very low birth weight infants in the late 1970s were accompanied by an increase in chronic lung disease.[1] Despite various ventilator modalities to prevent lung injury,[2] and the introduction of surfactant to prevent or treat respiratory distress syndrome,[3] there has been little change in the rate of chronic lung disease. Several pharmacologic strategies aimed at ameliorating chronic lung disease have been unsuccessful,[4-7] but dexamethasone therapy has improved short-term pulmonary mechanics and accelerated weaning from the ventilator.[8-12] Reports on outcomes in dexamethasone-treated infants have, with one exception,[8] not shown a significant decrease in duration of oxygen dependence, hospital stay, or later improvements in growth or development.[13-17]

VLBW	Very low birth weight, <1500 gm

Submitted for publication July 19, 1994; accepted Sept. 8, 1994.

Reprint requests: Maureen Hack, MD, Division of Neonatology, Rainbow Babies and Childrens Hospital, University Hospitals of Cleveland, 11100 Euclid Ave., Cleveland, OH 44106.

0022-3476/95/$3.00 + 0 **9/23/60453**

We sought to examine the impact of dexamethasone therapy on mortality and morbidity rates, growth, and developmental outcome in VLBW infants who were ventilator dependent at 21 days of life by comparing outcomes during the 2 years before and after the introduction of dexamethasone therapy in our unit.

METHODS

Population. Dexamethasone became accepted clinical therapy in our unit in October 1988. Four hundred five VLBW infants were admitted to the neonatal intensive care unit at Rainbow Babies and Childrens Hospital during the 2-year period preceding this time (period 1, October 1986 to September 1988), and 426 infants were admitted during the subsequent 2-year period (period 2, October 1988 to September 1990). Of the infants from each period, 330 (81%) and 353 (83%), respectively, survived to 21 days of age. The study population comprised 86 (26%) and 124 (35%) infants, respectively, who were receiving assisted ventilation on day 21 of life. During period 1, nine infants (10%) received compassionate rescue dexamethasone therapy for very severe chronic lung disease, whereas during period 2, 55 (44%) infants received dexamethasone as accepted clinical care, generally according to the Avery protocol.[11] Two additional infants who received dexamethasone were excluded from the study: one died before day 21 and the other had been weaned from the ventilator by day 21.

Procedures. We undertook a study of the impact of dexamethasone therapy, in which outcomes in VLBW infants who were ventilator dependent on day 21 of life during period 1 were compared with outcomes in infants with similar ventilator status during period 2. Period 2 was further examined to give a concurrent comparison of outcomes in infants who received dexamethasone with outcomes in those who had less severe lung disease and thus did not receive steroid therapy. Outcomes examined included death after 21 days of life, morbidity before and after discharge, and growth and neurodevelopmental outcome at 20 months of age.

The rationale for studying infants with oxygen and ventilator dependence at 21 days was twofold. First, preliminary data had revealed that 86% of VLBW infants with a Respiratory Index score (mean airway pressure × fraction of inspired oxygen) of 2.4 or more at 3 weeks of age required oxygen at 28 days of life (National Institute of Child Health and Human Development Neonatal Network: unpublished data). Second, during the years from 1988 to 1990, dexamethasone therapy was rarely given before day 21 of life.

Data collection. Data were obtained from our comprehensive neonatal database. Demographic data included maternal age, race, marital status, level of education, and a derived composite Social Risk score (marital status [married = 0; single = 1], race [white = 0; black = 1], and education [high school = 0; less than high school = 1]).[18] Neonatal data examined included duration of oxygen and ventilator dependence, episodes of sepsis (defined as a positive blood culture result with clinical symptoms of sepsis), meningitis, necrotizing enterocolitis, and rates of severe cranial ultrasonographic abnormality (defined as grade 3 or 4 hemorrhage,[19] periventricular leukomalacia, or ventricular dilation).

For examination of the use of dexamethasone therapy, additional information was obtained by hospital chart review. Measures of respiratory morbidity included duration of oxygen and ventilator dependence and the Respiratory Index score, recorded both on day 21 of life and before the administration of dexamethasone when applicable. Duration of oxygen dependence and duration of hospital stay were calculated to 20 months of corrected age for all infants, although some infants received oxygen beyond this time, and two infants remained hospitalized.

Postdischarge Follow-up. All infants were enrolled in the high-risk infant follow-up program and followed to 20 months of corrected age. A physical examination and neurologic assessment[20] were performed serially during the first year and at 20 months of corrected age. Neurosensory status at 20 months was defined as normal or abnormal (including hypotonia, spastic diplegia, hemiplegia, quadriplegia, unilateral or bilateral blindness, or deafness requiring a hearing aid). At 20 months, the Bayley Scales of Infant Development were also administered.[21] Information regarding rehospitalizations and postdischarge therapy was ascertained. Death was recorded up to 20 months of corrected age. The primary cause of death was classified as either respiratory failure caused by chronic lung disease, septicemia (complicating chronic lung disease), respiratory syncytial virus pneumonia, necrotizing enterocolitis, or other (including major congenital malformations and sudden unexplained death at home).

Informed consent was obtained from the parents of the study children.

Analysis of data. The *t* test was used for continuous measures and the chi-square test was used for categorical data to compare period 1 with period 2, and to compare infants who received dexamethasone with those who did not during period 2. The Wilcoxon Rank Sum Test was used to compare oxygen and ventilator dependence, duration of hospital stay, and duration of survival before death.

RESULTS

Demographic and birth data (Table I). A comparison of the demographic and birth data on infants who were ventilator dependent at 21 days of life during periods 1 and 2,

Table I. Infants ventilator dependent at 21 days: Maternal demographic and birth data

	Period 1* (n = 86)	Period 2† (n = 124)	*p*	Period 2: dexamethasone — Yes (n = 55)	Period 2: dexamethasone — No (n = 69)	*p*
Maternal demographic and perinatal data						
Maternal age (yr) (mean ± SD)	24.5 ± 6	25.9 ± 6	0.51	26 ± 6.6	25.9 ± 5.4	0.90
Maternal race, black: No. (%)	54 (63%)	75 (61%)	0.68	32 (58%)	43 (62%)	0.50
Outborn: No. (%)	29 (34%)	30 (24%)	0.13	17 (31%)	13 (19%)	0.12
Antenatal steroids: No. (%)	7 (18%)	23 (19%)	0.90	6 (11%)	17 (25%)	0.05
Birth data						
Birth weight (gm) (mean ± SD)	871 ± 195	891 ± 222	0.49	911 ± 225	876 ± 219	0.39
Gestational age (wk) (mean ± SD)	26.4 ± 1.8	26.9 ± 2.0	0.07	27.1 ± 2.2	26.7 ± 1.9	0.35
Sex, male: No. (%)	45 (52%)	70 (56%)	0.55	34 (62%)	36 (52%)	0.28
Multiple birth: No. (%)	13 (15%)	28 (23%)	0.18	8 (14%)	20 (29%)	0.06
Small for gestational age: No. (%)	14 (16%)	32 (26%)	0.10	15 (27%)	17 (25%)	0.74
Surfactant therapy: No. (%)	0 (0%)	33 (27%)	<0.001	15 (27%)	18 (26%)	0.88

*Period 1: October 1986 to September 1988.
†Period 2: October 1988 to September 1990.

Table II. Infants ventilator dependent at 21 days: Morbidity before discharge

	Period 1* (n = 86)	Period 2† (n = 124)	*p*	Period 2: dexamethasone — Yes (n = 55)	Period 2: dexamethasone — No (n = 69)	*p*
Respiratory data						
Respiratory Index Score at 21 days (mean ± SD)	3.9 ± 3	3.6 ± 3	0.38	4.9 ± 3	2.4 ± 1	<0.001
Oxygen use (days): median (range)	96 (25-1018)	80 (21-832)	0.07‡	119 (23-832)	53 (21-184)	<0.001‡
Ventilator use (days): median (range)	45 (22-455)	40 (19-463)	0.23‡	54 (19-463)	36 (21-116)	<0.001‡
Other data						
Patent ductus arteriosus: No. (%)	56 (65%)	77 (62%)	0.66	30 (54%)	47 (68%)	0.12
Necrotizing enterocolitis: No. (%)	5 (6%)	17 (14%)	0.07	4 (7%)	13 (19%)	0.06
Episodes of sepsis: No. (%)	31 (36%)	88 (71%)	<0.001	35 (64%)	53 (77%)	0.12
Meningitis: No. (%)	5 (6%)	7 (6%)	0.96	2 (4%)	5 (7%)	0.39
Severe abnormality on cranial ultrasound study: No. (%)	22 (26%)	43 (35%)	0.16	18 (33%)	25 (36%)	0.68
Duration of stay (days): median (range)	121.5 (24-990)§	110.5 (23-800)§	0.11‡	126 (23-800)§	101 (23-197)	<0.002‡

*Period 1: October 1986 to September 1988.
†Period 2: October 1988 to September 1990.
‡Mann-Whitney U test.
§One infant in both periods 1 and 2 remained in the hospital beyond 20 months of corrected age.

and of those within period 2 who did or did not receive dexamethasone, showed that maternal and birth data were similar. Within period 2, antenatal steroid therapy was given to 11% of the mothers of dexamethasone-treated infants, in comparison with 25% of mothers of untreated infants (p 0.05). Surfactant became available in our unit in December 1989, in the second half of period 2.

Neonatal complications of infants ventilator dependent at 21 days of life (Table II). There were no significant differences between periods 1 and 2 in the severity of lung disease as measured by the Respiratory Index score at 21 days of life, or by the median duration of ventilator or oxygen dependence before the initial hospital discharge. Additionally, there were no significant differences between periods 1 and

Table III. Infants ventilator dependent at 21 days: Postdischarge morbidity among survivors

	Period 1* (n = 70)	Period 2† (n = 98)	*p*	Period 2: dexamethasone Yes (n = 40)	Period 2: dexamethasone No (n = 58)	*p*
Measures of oxygen dependence						
Discharge on oxygen: No. (%)‡	17 (23%)	25 (25%)	0.86	22 (52%)	3 (5%)	<0.001
On oxygen at 20 mo corrected age: No. (%)	8 (11%)	10 (10%)	0.80	9 (22%)	1 (2%)	<0.001
Total oxygen dependence (days): median (range)§	97 (26-1018)	93 (22-1544)	0.49‖	231 (28-1544)	66 (22-865)	<0.001‖
Discharge						
Medication for chronic lung disease: No. (%)¶	27 (39%)	26 (27%)	0.12	23 (53%)	30 (24%)	<0.001
To chronic care facility: No. (%)	13 (18%)	12 (12%)	0.26	11 (26%)	1 (2%)	<0.001
Rehospitalizations						
One or more: No. (%)	46 (66%)	61 (62%)	0.64	29 (72%)	32 (55%)	0.08

*Period 1: October 1986 to September 1988.
†Period 2: October 1988 to September 1990.
‡Infants discharged alive, including those who died later.
§Includes oxygen dependence during hospital stay and after discharge.
‖Mann-Whitney U test.
¶Diuretics, steroids, and/or bronchodilators.

2 in the rates of severe cranial ultrasonographic abnormality or median duration of hospital stay. However, the rate of septicemia doubled from 36% during period 1 to 71% during period 2 (p <0.001).

Within period 2, dexamethasone-treated infants, in comparison with those not treated, had significantly more severe lung disease as evidenced by the Respiratory Index score at 21 days of life and by the median duration of both ventilator and in-hospital oxygen dependence. Their median duration of hospital stay was also significantly longer. There were no significant differences in their rates of either severe cranial ultrasound abnormality or septicemia. Forty-four percent (16/36) of septic episodes among dexamethasone-treated infants occurred before age 21 days, in comparison with 63% (34/54) of episodes among those not treated (p 0.08).

Details of dexamethasone therapy. The mean Respiratory Index score before dexamethasone therapy in the nine infants treated during period 1 was 6.5 ± 4; four infants died later. Because of the small population and high death rate, and because dexamethasone was considered last-resort rescue therapy during period 1, no further analyses of dexamethasone therapy during period 1 were undertaken. Mean age of initiation of therapy during period 2 was 34.8 ± 15 days, and the mean duration of the initial course was 43 ± 18 days. Of the 55 infants, 30 (54%) responded to dexamethasone, defined as having successful extubation within 8 days of the initiation of therapy. However, many of these infants subsequently required reintubation, and there was no difference between "responders" and "nonresponders" in their overall median duration of ventilator and oxygen dependence, duration of hospital stay, or overall mortality rate. Sixteen of the infants (29%) received a second course of steroids.

Mortality rates and causes of death. The post-21-day mortality rates were similar during periods 1 and 2 (19% and 21%, respectively). The median ages at death were 112 and 85 days in periods 1 and 2, respectively (p 0.10). The majority of deaths occurred before the initial hospital discharge. The most frequent cause of death was respiratory failure, followed by infection. Infection with respiratory syncytial virus accounted for the deaths of two infants in period 2 (one of whom had received dexamethasone) and three infants in period 2 (all of whom had received dexamethasone). Six infants, all during period 2, succumbed to necrotizing enterocolitis and its complications; five of these infants had not received dexamethasone. When only infants who died of respiratory failure or related infections were considered, the median ages at death were 123 and 119 days for periods 1 and 2, respectively (p 0.69).

Within period 2, 27% of dexamethasone-treated infants died, in comparison with 16% of untreated infants (p 0.12). The median age at death of the treated infants was significantly greater (124 vs 35 days; p <0.01); however, when only infants with death directly attributed to respiratory or infectious causes, or both, were considered, the ages at death were 124 days and 47 days, respectively (p 0.14).

Postdischarge morbidity (Table III). There were no significant differences between periods 1 and 2 in the various measures of postdischarge oxygen dependence. The num-

Table IV. Infants ventilator dependent at 21 days: Follow-up to 20 months of corrected age

	Period 1* (n = 62)	Period 2† (n = 83)	p	Period 2: dexamethasone Yes (n = 37)	Period 2: dexamethasone No (n = 46)	p
Bayley MDI (mean ± SD)	81.5 ± 21	77.2 ± 19	0.20	72.7 ± 20	80.1 ± 18	0.052
Bayley PDI (mean ± SD)	81.6 ± 18	77.1 ± 17	0.13	71.0 ± 18‡	82.4 ± 14§	0.003
MDI <70: No. (%)	20 (32%)	29 (35%)	0.63	17 (46%)	12 (26%)	0.03
Neurosensory abnormality: No. (%)‖	15 (24%)	21 (25%)	0.73	12 (32%)	9 (20%)	0.18
Cerebral palsy¶	4 (6%)	10 (12%)	0.26	5 (14%)	5 (11%)	0.71
Hypotonia	7 (11%)	8 (10%)	0.75	6 (16%)	2 (4%)	0.07
Shunted hydrocephalus	1 (1%)	1 (1%)	0.83	—	1 (2%)	0.37
Blindness**	1 (1%)	3 (4%)	0.47	2 (5%)	1 (2%)	0.43
Deafness**	1 (1%)	3 (4%)	0.47	1 (3%)	2 (4%)	0.69
Hypertonia	1 (1%)	2 (2%)	0.74	1 (1%)	1 (1%)	0.88
Impairment: No. (%)††	23 (37%)	35 (42%)	0.54	19 (51%)	16 (35%)	0.13

MDI, Mental Development Index; *PDI*, Psychomotor Development Index.
*Period 1: October 1986 to September 1988.
†Period 2: October 1988 to September 1990.
‡n = 35.
§n = 41.
‖Some children had more than one abnormality.
¶Spastic quadriplegia, diplegia, hemiplegia.
**Unilateral or bilateral.
††Bayley MDI <70 and/or neurosensory abnormality.

bers of infants receiving medication for chronic lung disease or discharged to a chronic care facility were similar. The rates of all the measures of postdischarge morbidity within period 2 were significantly greater among the dexamethasone-treated infants, most of whom had very severe chronic lung disease: 52% were discharged on a regimen of oxygen therapy, and 22% were still receiving oxygen at 20 months of corrected age.

There were no significant differences in the rates and causes of rehospitalizations between periods 1 and 2, or within period 2. At least 60% of infants required one rehospitalization. The primary cause of rehospitalization in the majority of cases was considered to be respiratory.

Neurodevelopmental outcome at 20 months of corrected age (Table IV). Eighty-six percent of surviving infants were followed to 20 months of corrected age. There were no significant differences between infants followed and those lost to follow-up in birth weight, gestational age, rates of severe cranial ultrasonographic abnormality, median days of ventilator dependence, or social risk scores. There were no significant differences in the rates of severe cranial ultrasonographic abnormality among survivors during periods 1 and 2 (27% vs 32%, respectively), or within period 2 (28% of dexamethasone-treated vs 35% of untreated infants). The level of social risk was similar during the two periods and within period 2.

Neurodevelopmental outcome as measured by the mean scores on the Bayley Scales of Infant Development, rates of neurosensory abnormality, and overall impairment (Bayley Mental Development Index <70 or neurosensory impairment or both) were similar during periods 1 and 2 (Table IV). Within period 2, infants given dexamethasone had significantly lower Bayley psychomotor scores and higher rates of subnormal (<70) Bayley Mental Development Index scores.

Growth. There were no significant differences between periods 1 and 2 in the rates of subnormal (<3%) weight, length, and head circumference.[22] Seventeen percent in each group had subnormal weight, 14% and 20% had subnormal length (p 0.31), and 23% and 13% had subnormal head circumference (p 0.1), respectively. Within period 2, the rate of subnormal weight was higher among dexamethasone-treated than untreated infants (30% vs 9%; $p < 0.01$); rates of subnormal length and head circumference were similar.

DISCUSSION

Dexamethasone therapy for ventilator-dependent chronic lung disease was rapidly introduced into clinical practice after its success in several small randomized trials, without full knowledge of its long-term efficacy. Although double-blinded, placebo-controlled, randomized trials are the gold standard by which new therapies are judged, the lack of information available on the long-term outcomes in children treated with steroids for chronic lung disease led us to examine our clinical experience. In the absence of a randomized, controlled trial, longitudinal observational studies such as this one can provide information on the clinical impact of a new therapy as it is integrated into clinical care.

During the 2 years before and after the introduction of dexamethasone therapy in our unit, we found no differences in the sequelae of chronic lung disease after 21 days of life, including duration of ventilator and oxygen dependence, and numbers of infants continuing to receive supplemental oxygen at 20 months of corrected age. Similarly, no differences were found in the rates of death after 21 days, causes of rehospitalization, or neurodevelopmental outcomes at 20 months of corrected age. Not surprisingly, those infants selected to receive dexamethasone had significantly more severe lung disease, and poorer respiratory, growth, and developmental outcomes.

In our population, 20% of all infants born between 1986 and 1990 who were ventilator dependent at 21 days, and 27% of infants receiving dexamethasone during period 2, subsequently died, the majority of respiratory failure. Of infants ventilator dependent at entry to the multicenter collaborative trial, at age 29 or 30 days, 25% of dexamethasone and 24% of placebo recipients died before hospital discharge.[12] A similar mortality rate among dexamethasone-treated infants has been reported by others, with a predominance of deaths caused by respiratory failure.[13, 14] In the multicenter collaborative trial, 18% of dexamethasone-treated infants and 22% of placebo recipients were sent home on a regimen of supplemental oxygen, similar to our overall rates. Their reported readmission rates by age 3 years were comparable to ours.[17]

Early childhood neurodevelopment and the growth of infants with chronic lung disease are seriously compromised by multiple factors, including the high rate of periventricular lesions in these immature infants, and the hypoxia and poor growth associated with chronic lung disease.[23-25] Information on outcomes in infants treated with dexamethasone is limited to the results of six studies, three reported as abstracts.[8, 13-17] Comparisons among studies are complicated by the small sample size in some studies, differing ages at follow-up, differing methods of assessment, and varying details published. With the exception of the small Cummings[8] study, neurodevelopmental outcomes in infants receiving dexamethasone have not improved. The rates of subnormal weight in dexamethasone-treated infants have ranged from 30% to 67%. Even in the randomized trials, untreated comparison infants have had lower rates of subnormal weight, which suggests a deleterious effect of dexamethasone on long-term weight gain.[8, 17] Length and head circumference do not appear to be consistently affected by dexamethasone therapy. (A detailed table comparing results of these studies is available from the authors on request.)

Our report has several weaknesses. The rate of sepsis increased from period 1 to period 2, which is a complicating factor that can interact with chronic lung disease and outcome, and thus complicate analysis of measures of morbidity, including weaning from the ventilator.[26] The increased rate of infection may have contributed to the significantly higher rate of 21-day ventilator dependence during period 2. However, our rates of chronic lung disease, severe ultrasound abnormality, and infection, even at their peak, are well within the reported ranges.[27-29] In the absence of a randomized clinical trial, treated and untreated infants necessarily differed, making any specific assessment of the efficacy of dexamethasone difficult. There is no evidence that dexamethasone therapy influenced the rate of septicemia or that infants receiving dexamethasone were disproportionately affected. Initial studies reported an increase in infectious complications during dexamethasone therapy,[11, 15] but later work has not confirmed this association.[8, 14, 30, 31]

Despite successful use in early trials, dexamethasone, as used in 1988 to 1990 in our nursery and others, has had little impact on long-term pulmonary or developmental outcome in infants with chronic lung disease. We and other investigators urge caution in its use.[13, 32, 33] Before dexamethasone can be accepted as routine therapy for chronic lung disease, more information is needed from prospective, randomized trials on optimal patient selection, timing, dosing, duration of therapy, and effects on postdischarge outcome.

Special thanks to Harriet Friedman, MA, Eloise Scott, Bonnie Siner, Kathleen Sweeney, Nancy Newman, and Janet Sterl for research assistance.

REFERENCES

1. Parker RA, Lindstrom DP, Cotton RB. Improved survival accounts for most, but not all, of the increase in bronchopulmonary dysplasia. Pediatrics 1992;90:663-8.
2. HiFi Study Group. High-frequency oscillatory ventilation compared with conventional mechanical ventilation in the treatment of respiratory failure in preterm infants. N Engl J Med 1989;320:88-93.
3. Jobe AH. Pulmonary surfactant therapy. N Engl J Med 1993; 328:861-8.
4. Hallman M, Bry K, Hoppu K, Lappi M, Pohjavuori M. Inositol supplementation in premature infants with respiratory distress syndrome. N Engl J Med 1992;326:1233-9.
5. Ehrenkranz RA, Bonta BW, Ablow RC, Warshaw JB. Amelioration of bronchopulmonary dysplasia after vitamin E administration. N Engl J Med 1978;299:564-9.
6. Shenai JP, Kennedy KA, Chytil F, Stahlman MT. Clinical trial of vitamin A supplementation in infants susceptible to bronchopulmonary dysplasia. J PEDIATR 1987;111:269-77.
7. Watterberg K, Murphy S, Neonatal Cromolyn Study Group. Failure of cromolyn sodium to reduce the incidence of bronchopulmonary dysplasia: a pilot study. Pediatrics 1993;91: 803-6.

8. Cummings JJ, D'Eugenio DB, Gross SJ. A controlled trial of dexamethasone in preterm infants at high risk for bronchopulmonary dysplasia. N Engl J Med 1989;320:1505-10.
9. Ohlsson A, Calvert SA, Hosking M, Shennan AT. Randomized controlled trial of dexamethasone treatment in very-low-birth-weight infants with ventilator-dependent chronic lung disease. Acta Paediatr 1992;81:751-6.
10. Ehrenkranz RA, Mercurio MR. Bronchopulmonary dysplasia. In: Sinclair JC, Bracken MB, eds. Effective care of the newborn infant. Oxford: Oxford University Press, 1992:399-424.
11. Avery GB, Fletcher AB, Kaplan M, Brudno DS. Controlled trial of dexamethasone in respirator-dependent infants with bronchopulmonary dysplasia. Pediatrics 1985;76:106-11.
12. Collaborative Dexamethasone Trial Group. Dexamethasone therapy in neonatal chronic lung disease: an international placebo-controlled trial. Pediatrics 1991;88:421-7.
13. O'Shea TM, Kothadia JM, Klinepeter KL, Goldstein DJ, Jackson B, Dillard RG. Follow-up of preterm infants treated with dexamethasone for chronic lung disease. Am J Dis Child 1993;147:658-61.
14. Ferrara TB, Couse RJ, Hoekstra RE. Side effects and long-term follow-up of corticosteroid therapy in very low birthweight infants with bronchopulmonary dysplasia. J Perinatol 1990;10:137-42.
15. Mammel MC, Fiterman C, Coleman M, Boros SJ. Short-term dexamethasone therapy for bronchopulmonary dysplasia: acute effects and 1-year follow-up. Dev Pharmacol Ther 1987;10:1-11.
16. Satish M, Schwartz P, Urrutia J, et al. Developmental outcome of dexamethasone treated infants [Abstract]. Pediatr Res 1991;29:1564A.
17. Jones RA, Wincott E, Elbourne D, Grant A. Collaborative placebo-controlled trial of dexamethasone for neonatal chronic lung disease: a 3-year follow up [Abstract]. Pediatr Res 1993;33:274A.
18. Hack M, Breslau N, Weissman B, Aram D, Klein N, Borawski E. Effects of very low birth weight and subnormal head size on cognitive abilities at school age. N Engl J Med 1991;325:231-7.
19. Papille LA, Burstein R, Koffler H. Incidence and evaluation of subependymal intraventricular hemorrhage: a study of infants with birth weights less than 1500 grams. J PEDIATR 1978;92:529-34.
20. Amiel-Tison C. A method for neurologic evaluation within the first year of life. In: Gluck L, ed. Current problems in pediatrics; vol 7. Chicago: Year Book Medical Publishers, 1976.
21. Bayley N. Bayley Scales of Infant Development. New York: Psychological Corp., 1969.
22. Wingerd J, Schoen EJ, Solomon IL. Growth standards in the first two years of life based on measurements of white and black children in a prepaid health care program. Pediatrics 1971;47:808-25.
23. Bregman J, Farrell E. Neurodevelopmental outcome in infants with bronchopulmonary dysplasia. Clin Perinatol 1992;19:673-94.
24. Skidmore MD, Rivers A, Hack M. Increased risk of cerebral palsy among very low-birthweight infants with chronic lung disease. Dev Med Child Neurol 1990;32:325-32.
25. Vohr B, Bell EF, Oh W. Infants with bronchopulmonary dysplasia: growth pattern and neurologic and developmental outcome. Am J Dis Child 1982;136:443-7.
26. Overstreet DW, Jackson JC, van Belle G, Truog W. Estimation of mortality risk in chronically ventilated infants with bronchopulmonary dysplasia. Pediatrics 1991;88:1153-60.
27. Hack M, Horbar JD, Malloy MH, Tyson JE, Wright L, Wright E. Very low birth weight outcomes of the National Institute of Child Health and Human Development neonatal network. Pediatrics 1991;87:587-97.
28. Avery ME, Tooley WH, Keller JB, et al. Is chronic lung disease in low birth weight infants preventable? a survey of eight centers. Pediatrics 1987;79:26-30.
29. Cooke RWI. Factors associated with chronic lung disease in preterm infants. Arch Dis Child 1991;66:776-9.
30. Ng PC, Thomson MA, Dear PRF. Dexamethasone and infection in premature babies: a controlled study. Arch Dis Child 1990;65:54-6.
31. Cordero L, Davis K, Morehead S, Ayers L. Factors affecting microbial colonization of the trachea and septicemia in mechanically ventilated neonates. Respir Care 1993;38:1355-63.
32. Ng PC. The effectiveness and side effects of dexamethasone in preterm infants with bronchopulmonary dysplasia. Arch Dis Child 1993;68:330-6.
33. Frank L. The use of dexamethasone in premature infants at risk for bronchopulmonary dysplasia or who have already developed chronic lung disease: a cautionary note [Letter]. Pediatrics 1992;87:413-4.

Postnatal attainment of intrauterine macromineral accretion rates in low birth weight infants fed fortified human milk

Richard J. Schanler, MD, and Steven A. Abrams, MD

From the U.S. Department of Agriculture/Agricultural Research Service Children's Nutrition Research Center, and the Section of Neonatology, Department of Pediatrics, Baylor College of Medicine, Houston, Texas

Hypothesis: **Provision of more bioavailable mineral sources as human milk supplements enables very low birth weight (VLBW) infants to meet the intrauterine accretion rate for calcium and phosphorus.**
Design: **Comparison of currently formulated human milk fortifier with previous formulation.**
Setting: **Neonatal level II and III nurseries**
Patients: **Twenty-six healthy, VLBW infants, whose mothers chose to breast-feed.**
Interventions: **We tested the effects of two formulations designed for VLBW infants as human milk supplements and differing primarily in their quantity and source of Ca, P, and magnesium. The study interval began with a milk intake of 100 ml · kg^{-1} · day^{-1} and ended when a body weight reached 2.0 kg.**
Main outcome measures: **Net absorption and retention of Ca, P, and Mg during a nutritional balance study conducted once during the study interval, growth during the entire study interval, and bone mineral content of the radius were measured at the beginning and end of the study interval.**
Results: **The newer Ca gluconate-glycerophosphate preparation (given to group CaGP) resulted in greater net absorption and retention of Ca and P (*p* <0.01) than in infants given Ca phosphate (group CaTB). Mg retention was greater than (in group CaGP) or equivalent to (in group CaTB) the intrauterine accretion rate. Radius bone mineral content was significantly greater in group CaGP than in group CaTB (*p* <0.001). Volumes of the fortified human milk preparation needed to meet the needs for gain in body weight were higher in group CaGP than in group CaTB (*p* <0.001).**
Conclusions: **Intrauterine accretion rates for Ca and P can be achieved when VLBW infants are fed human milk supplemented with Ca gluconate-glycerophosphate. Supplementation of human milk with Mg may not be indicated. In this study, greater intakes of Ca and P, and not improvements in bioavailability, result in improved net retention and bone mineral content of VLBW infants. (J PEDIATR 1995;126:441-7)**

Supported in part by the General Clinical Research Center, Baylor College of Medicine/Texas Children's Hospital Clinical Research Center, by grant No. MO1-RR-00188, National Institutes of Health, and Mead Johnson Nutritional Division, Evansville, Ind. Partial funding also has been provided from the U.S. Department of Agriculture/Agricultural Research Service under Cooperative Agreement No. 58-6250-1-003.

The contents of this publication do not necessarily reflect the views or policies of the U.S. Department of Agriculture, nor does mention of trade names, commercial products, or organizations imply endorsement by the U.S. Government.

Submitted for publication April 12, 1994; accepted Sept. 8, 1994.

Reprint requests: Richard J. Schanler, MD, Children's Nutrition Research Center, Baylor College of Medicine, 1100 Bates St., Houston, TX 77030.

0022-3476/95/$3.00 + 0 **9/23/60452**

The need for mineral and, perhaps, protein supplementation of human milk in the nutritional support of the very low birth weight infant is recognized.[1-5] The data indicate that without mineral supplementation during hospitalization, bone mineralization and long-term outcomes such as growth, particularly in length, are adversely affected.[6-8] We observed a "catch-up" period of bone mineral content of the distal radius by 2 years of corrected age in healthy, former VLBW infants who received *fortified* human milk during their hospitalization.[9] The methods used at that time to fortify human milk did not provide optimal retention of calcium and phosphorus.[10] We inferred from those data that had we improved the retention of Ca and P during the period of most rapid bone mineral accretion, catch-up mineralization would have been achieved earlier.[9, 11] Recently, investigators have suggested that supplemental Ca and P be continued beyond hospitalization for VLBW infants.[12-14] It is unclear whether continued supplementation is necessary if in-hospital efforts at providing appropriate net retention of Ca and P are optimal. Our previous studies, however, indicated lower bioavailability of calcium phosphate, compared with other sources, for use as a human milk fortifier.[10]

The objective of this investigation was to compare, under similar conditions, the net Ca and P retention in VLBW infants who received a newly formulated human milk fortifier containing calcium gluconate and glycerophosphate, with Ca and P retention when a previous formulation containing calcium phosphate was used as the principal mineral source. We hypothesized that more bioavailable mineral salts in the new preparation would improve absorption and promote Ca and P retention to meet intrauterine estimates.[15]

BMC	Bone mineral content
VLBW	Very low birth weight

METHODS

Subjects. Healthy VLBW infants admitted to the neonatal nurseries of Texas Children's Hospital were enrolled in the first week after birth if they were of appropriate size for gestational age, their mothers intended to breast-feed, and they were free from major cardiopulmonary and gastrointestinal disorders. Two separate cohorts were studied under similar conditions: 15 infants, who received the newer Ca gluconate-glycerophosphate preparation (group CaGP), were studied from 1991 to 1992, and 11 infants, who received Ca phosphate (group CaTB), were studied in 1988 and 1989. Informed written consent was obtained from parents and the protocol was approved by the review boards for human research at our institutions.

Study design. Growth, nutritional balance, serum indexes of mineral and protein status, and bone mineralization were compared in the two groups. The two studies represented the evaluations of current (group CaGP) and previous (group CaTB) formulations (Table I) of Enfamil Human Milk Fortifier (Mead Johnson Nutritional Group, Evansville, Ind.). The initiation of enteral nutrition was at the discretion of the attending neonatologist. The protocol for orogastric feeding began with unfortified human milk, 20 to 25 ml · kg^{-1} · day^{-1}, and advanced daily by that volume, as tolerated, on the basis of clinical examination results and gastric residual volume. When the intake reached 100 ml · kg^{-1} · day^{-1}, the volume was maintained for 2 days while the concentration was increased by the addition of two packets, and then four packets, of fortifier per 100 ml. Subsequently, the intake of fortified human milk was advanced daily to maintain adequate body weight gain. Infants received only their own mothers' milk, and not donor milk, throughout the study. Vitamin D, 400 IU/day, was given to infants after complete enteral nutrition was achieved in group CaTB. Vitamin D was not given to infants in group CaGP. All infants received elemental iron, 2 mg · kg^{-1} · d^{-1}, 2 weeks after complete enteral nutrition was achieved. The protocol for the lactation management of the mothers and the preparation of milk for feeding has been published previously.[16] The most recent milk available, either fresh or frozen, was used for fortification.

Anthropometric measurements were determined as the slope of serial determinations obtained during the interval beginning with a milk intake of 100 ml · kg^{-1} · day^{-1} and ending with a body weight of 2.0 kg. A 3- to 4-day nutritional balance study was initiated 2 to 3 weeks after complete enteral nutrition was achieved. One blood sample for the determination of Ca and P concentrations, alkaline phosphatase activity, blood urea nitrogen concentration, and albumin concentration was obtained during the week of the balance study. Bone mineral content of the distal one third of the left radius was measured at the start and the end of the study interval.

Analytic methods. Measurements of body weight were made with electronic scales, length with a rigid board providing immobile head support and adjustable foot support, head circumference with a flexible stainless steel measure, and skin-fold thickness with Lange calipers. The methods for the balance studies have been described.[1, 16] Carmine red (100 mg/kg) was given through an orogastric tube at the beginning and the end of the balance period to mark the fecal collection interval. Milk and feces were analyzed for energy by bomb calorimetry (Parr Instrument Co., Moline, Ill.) and for fat by gravimetric methods.[16] Nitrogen in milk, urine, and feces was analyzed by semiautomated Kjeldahl methods (Kjeltec; Tecator Inc., Herndon, Va.). Milk and feces were ashed in a muffle furnace at 440° C for 14 hours.

Table I. Nutrient composition of study human milk fortifiers (per 4 gm powder)*

	CaGP	CaTB
Protein (gm)	0.7	0.7
Carbohydrate (gm)	2.7	2.7
Sodium (mg)	7	7
Potassium (mg)	15.6	15.6
Chloride (mg)	17.7	17.7
Calcium (mg)	90	60
Phosphorus (mg)	45	33
Magnesium (mg)	1.0	0
Zinc (μg)	710	310
Copper (μg)	62	80
Manganese (μg)	4.7	9.0
Vitamin A (IU)	950	780
Vitamin D (IU)	210	260
Vitamin K (μg)	4.4	9.1
Biotin (μg)	2.7	0.8
Vitamin C (mg)	12	24

*From manufacturer's product manual.

Urine and ashed milk and fecal samples were analyzed for Ca and magnesium by atomic absorption spectrophotometry, and P colorimetrically.[1] Serum was analyzed for Ca, P, alkaline phosphatase activity, albumin, and blood urea nitrogen values by automatic analyzer (COBAS FARA II; Roche Diagnostic Systems, Inc., Montclair, N.J.). Bone mineral content of the distal one third of the left radius was determined by single-photon absorptiometry (SP-2 scanner; Lunar Radiation Corp., Madison, Wis.).

Data analyses. Group comparisons were made by one-way analysis of variance. Relationships between variables were tested by linear regression analysis. Confounding variables such as postnatal age, birth weight, gestation, vitamin intake, and time of initiation of enteral feedings were tested as potential covariates in the analyses. The level of statistical significance was set at $p < 0.01$. Data are expressed as mean ± SD.

RESULTS

Infants in the two studies were of similar birth weight and gestational age (Table II). There was no difference between groups in the age at which enteral feedings were initiated or when complete enteral feedings were achieved. The study interval duration (39 ± 15 vs 46 ± 9 days), rate of weight gain (20 ± 4 vs 19 ± 3 g $\cdot$ kg^{-1} $\cdot$ day^{-1}), and increments in length and head circumference were similar in the two groups. Differences between group CaGP and group CaTB were observed for the average of triceps, biceps, subscapular, and thigh skin-fold thicknesses: 0.15 ± 0.09 versus 0.36 ± 0.06 mm/wk ($p < 0.001$), respectively. Infants in group CaGP required greater fluid intake to achieve targeted growth rates (10 to 15 gm $\cdot$ kg^{-1} $\cdot$ day^{-1}) than did those in group CaTB ($p < 0.001$). The intake of parenteral nutrition and supplemental iron was similar in the two groups. Vitamin D intake differed between groups CaGP and CaTB: 550 versus 1000 IU/day, respectively. When tested as covariates, differences between groups in postnatal age, birth weight, gestation, vitamin intake, and time of initiation of enteral feedings did not affect subsequent analyses.

Table II. Infant characteristics

	Group CaGP (n = 15)	Group CaTB (n = 11)
Birth weight (gm)	1148 ± 263	1041 ± 117
Gestational age (wk)	28 ± 2	28 ± 1
Enteral feeding initiated (day)	10 ± 5	14 ± 7
Complete enteral feeding (day)	19 ± 6	22 ± 9
Balance study		
Postmenstrual age (days)	33 ± 2	34 ± 1
Body weight (gm)	1498 ± 250	1507 ± 166
Milk intake (gm $\cdot$ kg^{-1} $\cdot$ day^{-1})	172 ± 10*	159 ± 5

Values are expressed as mean ± SD
*$p < 0.001$.

At the time of the balance study, the two groups of infants were similar with respect to body weight and postmenstrual age (Table II). The groups had similar average heart and respiratory rates and carmine red fecal transit times during the balance study. Differences in the N, Ca, P, and Mg concentrations in the fortified human milk were reflected in differences in the net intake of these nutrients (Table III). Metabolizable energy intake (gross energy intake − fecal and urinary energy losses) was similar in the two groups. Differences between groups for fat absorption and the net retention of N, Ca, P, and Mg were significant (Table IV). The net N and Mg retention in group CaGP surpassed, and in group CaTB was equivalent to, the intrauterine accretion rate (N, 23 mmol, or 325 mg $\cdot$ kg^{-1} $\cdot$ day^{-1}; Mg, 0.11 mmol, or 2.7 mg $\cdot$ kg^{-1} $\cdot$ day^{-1}). The intrauterine accretion rate for Ca (2.5 to 3.0 mmol, or 100 to 120 mg $\cdot$ kg^{-1} $\cdot$ day^{-1}) was approximated and for P (2.3 mmol, or 70 mg $\cdot$ kg^{-1} $\cdot$ day^{-1}) was surpassed by infants in group CaGP, but in group CaTB both Ca and P retention were far below the intrauterine accretion rate.[15] No differences in Ca bioavailability were observed. The percentage of Ca absorption was similar in groups CaGP and CaTB: 60% ± 13% versus 59% ± 19%, respectively. The percentage of P absorption differed between groups CaGP and CaTB: 94% ± 6% versus 74% ± 12%, respectively; $p < 0.001$.

The percentage absorption of Ca was significantly correlated with the percentage absorption of Mg ($r = 0.71$; p

Table III. Intakes of energy and selected nutrients

	Group CaGP (n = 15)	Group CaTB (n = 11)	*p*	95% CI
Gross energy (kJ)	567 ± 95	515 ± 32	0.095	−3, 107
Nitrogen (mmol)	41 ± 6	33 ± 3	<0.001	5, 12
Fat (gm)	6.0 ± 1.3	5.0 ± 0.8	0.049	0.1, 2
Calcium (mmol)	4.6 ± 0.41	3.0 ± 0.3	<0.001	1.3, 1.8
Phosphorus (mmol)	4.1 ± 0.35	2.1 ± 0.27	<0.001	1.7, 2.2
Magnesium (mmol)	0.31 ± 0.03	0.25 ± 0.03	0.001	0.03, 0.08

Conversion factors: 1 kJ = 0.239 kcal; 1 mmol N = 14 mg N; 1 mmol Ca = 40 mg Ca; 1 mmol P = 31 mg P; 1 mmol Mg = 24 mg Mg.
Values (except *p* values and CIs) are expressed as mean ± SD and are in units per kilogram of body weight per day.
CI, Confidence interval of differences.

Table IV. Metabolizable energy, fat absorption, and retention of N, Ca, P, Mg

	Group CaGP (n = 15)	Group CaTB (n = 11)	*p*	95% CI
Metabolizable energy ($kJ \cdot kg^{-1} \cdot day^{-1}$)	449 ± 112	459 ± 38	0.800	−77, 58
Fat absorption (%)	64 ± 21	84 ± 12	0.007	6, 34
Net retention ($mmol \cdot kg^{-1} \cdot day^{-1}$)				
Nitrogen	28 ± 5	23 ± 3	0.016	1, 8
Calcium	2.6 ± 0.9	1.6 ± 0.4	0.003	0.4, 1.6
Phosphorus	3.2 ± 0.6	1.5 ± 0.3	<0.001	1.4, 2.1
Magnesium	0.1 ± 0.06	0.1 ± 0.04	0.068	−0.001, 0.1

Conversion factors: 1 kJ = 0.239 kcal; 1 mmol N = 14 mg N; 1 mmol Ca = 40 mg Ca; 1 mmol P = 31 mg P; 1 mmol Mg = 24 mg Mg.
Values (except *p* values and CIs) are expressed an mean ± SD.
CI, Confidence interval of differences.

<0.001) and fat ($r = 0.56$; $p = 0.003$) but not with age or the intake of Ca, P, Mg, fat, or vitamin D. The following factors significantly ($p < 0.01$) affected net Ca retention: Ca intake ($r = 0.62$), P retention ($r = 0.63$), Mg retention ($r = 0.80$), and fat absorption ($r = 0.48$). Fecal excretion of fat correlated significantly with fecal excretion of Ca ($r = 0.68$; $p < 0.001$) and Mg ($r = 0.62$; $p = 0.001$). As a proportion of intake, the urinary concentration of Ca was lower in group CaGP than in group CaTB: 3% ± 2% versus 7% ± 6%, respectively ($p = 0.02$); the urinary concentration of P was significantly greater in group CaGP than in group CaTB: 16% ± 9% versus 5% ± 6%, respectively ($p = 0.003$). Serum P and albumin concentrations differed between groups at the time of the balance study (Table V). Significant relationships were observed between net P retention and the serum P concentration ($r = 0.55$); $p < 0.004$). The range in serum Ca concentrations was 2.3 to 2.7 mmol/L (9.1 to 10.9 mg/dl). A serum Ca concentration >2.6 mmol/L (10.5 mg/dl) was observed in one infant in group CaGP and in three infants in group CaTB.

There was no difference between groups in bone mineral content at the start of the study interval. However, bone mineral content at hospital discharge differed between group CaGP and group CaTB: 42 ± 4 versus 31 ± 5 mg/cm (95% confidence interval of differences = 5 to 16 mg/cm), respectively ($p < 0.001$). The age at the time of the BMC differed (9 ± 3 vs 6 ± 1 wk in groups CaGP and CaTB, respectively; $p = 0.01$). When BMC was adjusted for age, the difference between groups remained significant ($p = 0.002$). The BMC obtained near hospital discharge correlated positively with net retention of Ca ($r = 0.58$; $p = 0.003$), P ($r = 0.78$; $p < 0.001$), and Mg ($r = 0.54$; $p = 0.006$).

DISCUSSION

These data suggest that newer formulations available for the fortification of human milk provide greater concentrations of Ca and P, and with greater intakes the intrauterine accretion rates now are approached more closely and even surpassed. The increased retention of Ca and P also was manifested by greater BMC of the radius in group CaGP than in group CaTB. Furthermore, the addition of Mg to human milk resulted in net retention of Mg significantly above intrauterine accretion rates.

Of concern to us was that despite greater fat intakes the efficiency of fat absorption in infants fed the newer formulation (group CaGP) was significantly lower than in group CaTB infants, and the larger fecal fat losses adversely affected mineral retention. We also observed that to achieve targeted growth rates, infants in group CaGP received sig-

Table V. Serum biochemical indexes

	Group CaGP (n = 15)	Group CaTB (n = 11)	*p*	95% CI
Sodium (mmol/L)	135 ± 2	135 ± 1	0.91	−2, 2
Total CO_2 (mmol/L)	20 ± 3	21 ± 2	0.48	−3, 2
Ca (mmol/L)	2.5 ± 0.1	2.6 ± 0.1	0.36	−0.1, 0.04
P (mmol/L)	2.3 ± 0.2	1.8 ± 0.2	<0.001	0.3, 0.7
APA				
(μkat/L)	6.6 ± 2.4	5.9 ± 0.9	0.32	0.8, 2.2
(IU/L)	396 ± 142	353 ± 53	0.32	−47, 134
Albumin (gm/L)	35 ± 4	28 ± 3	<0.001	3, 10
Hematocrit	0.28 ± 0.06	0.30 ± 0.05	0.57	−0.07, 0.04

Conversion factors: 1 mmol Ca = 40 mg Ca; 1 mmol P = 31 mg P.
Values (except *p* values and CIs) are expressed as mean ± SD.
CI, Confidence interval of differences; *APA*, alkaline phosphatase activity.

nificantly greater fluid intakes than those in group CaTB. Although similarities in weight, length, and head circumference measurements were observed, the greater fluid intakes prescribed to meet these growth rates may be a concern for the more compromised VLBW infant. It concerns us that volumes of milk in excess of 170 ml · kg^{-1} · day^{-1} were offered in an attempt to meet intrauterine needs for weight gain and for Ca and P. Although safe for healthy VLBW infants, nutritional recommendations must consider those infants whose fluid intakes are restricted and who are unable to tolerate the high volumes of milk used in this study.[17]

Although the groups in our study were not evaluated concurrently, the data on group CaTB serve as a framework to evaluate the newer formulation, CaGP. The comparisons are valid because similar environmental conditions, study population characteristics, and feeding patterns were practiced in the neonatal units between 1988 and 1992. The reported differences between groups in this study would not be affected by differences in times at which the study was conducted.

The net retention data on VLBW infants fed the earlier formulation (group CaTB) are similar to those published by Ehrenkranz et al.[18] That study demonstrated similarities in nutrient utilization between infants fed preterm formula and those fed fortified human milk; neither Ca nor P retention in infants fed fortified human milk approximated intrauterine accretion. The data, however, demonstrated greater Ca retention in the preterm formula-fed infants. The newer formulation of fortified human milk evaluated in our study provides a greater content of Ca and P, which results in a greater net mineral retention and BMC.

By improving bone mineralization, we expect to avoid the potential for fractures in VLBW infants.[19] The positive relation between radius BMC at hospital discharge and net mineral retention suggests that mineral supplementation is essential to the bone development of VLBW infants. Our findings confirm the data of Horsman et al.,[4] who reported increments in BMC with Ca and P supplementation of formula for hospitalized VLBW infants. We speculate that the differences in BMC are a result of the differences in Ca and P intakes between groups. It is unknown whether other differences, such as the Mg content of the two fortifiers, could account for these differences. Whether these differences will remain with long-term evaluation is unknown.

We observed that the high net retention of P in group CaGP surpassed the intrauterine accretion rate.[15] The urinary losses of P also were large but not out of line with those of other milk-fed VLBW infants.[1, 10] Contrary to the data on Ca, it appears that P bioavailability from the glycerophosphate salt is relatively high. Thus, in further modifications of the commercial fortifier, the Ca glycerophosphate portion may need to be reduced in conjunction with a proportional increment in the Ca gluconate component. The use of the glycerophosphate salt also should be considered in other hypophosphatemic states.

The interaction among Ca, Mg, and fat is of interest. Fat intakes were slightly greater in group CaGP because of greater volumes of milk consumed. The higher fat intake was associated with a lower percentage of fat absorption. In addition, the malabsorbed fat was associated with fecal losses of Ca and Mg. We speculate that the high concentration of minerals in the milk formulation bound with fatty acids and promoted fecal soap formation. Interactions between Ca and fatty acids have been reported during Ca supplementation of human milk for VLBW infants.[20] However, our data indicate differential effects of specific calcium salts on fat absorption. Whether this is an osmolar characteristic or a characteristic peculiar to Ca glycerophosphate awaits laboratory study.

The vitamin D intake also differed between study groups. It is unlikely that the greater vitamin D intake affected Ca absorption; both groups absorbed approximately 60% of the Ca intake. Bronner et al.[21] indicated that preterm infants absorb Ca through a vitamin D–independent mechanism; despite widely differing intakes of vitamin D, similarities in Ca absorption were observed. The data on the coefficient of Ca absorption in our study were similar to data summarized by Bronner et al. and also to data reported by Hillman et al.[22] Thus, for VLBW infants, further dosage increments beyond a usual vitamin D intake probably do not improve Ca absorption.

Our data indicate that given a bioavailable source of Ca, the VLBW infant apparently absorbs a maximum of 60% of Ca intake. Simply increasing intake will thus improve net Ca absorption and retention significantly. Alternatively, Ca absorption may be increased if fat absorption can be improved in VLBW infants. We did not observe a difference in the bioavailability of Ca from glycerophosphate compared with the tribasic phosphate salt. This was unexpected because initial observations in animals suggest that the organic salts, such as glycerophosphate, are highly soluble and bioavailable.[23] Studies of parenteral nutrition indicate that more Ca and P can be solubilized with the organic, glycerophosphate salt.[24]

Our data also readdress the optimal intake of Mg.[2] Group CaGP had greater Mg intake (because Mg was added to the newer formulation) and greater net Mg retention (significantly more than the intrauterine accretion rate), whereas net Mg retention in group CaTB was not significantly different from the intrauterine accretion rate. Although we have compared our data with estimates for intrauterine accretion, which, at least for Mg, have not been verified, we conclude that Mg supplementation of human milk for VLBW infants may not be necessary.

The average skin-fold thickness in group CaGP was significantly less than, and that of group CaTB was significantly greater than, published values for triceps skin-fold thickness measurements.[25] Body weight gain was similar in the two groups, and we speculate, therefore, that lean body mass was greater in group CaGP. The greater net N retention and serum albumin concentration in group CaGP support that speculation. These data further suggest that higher N intakes may be appropriate for growing VLBW infants.

We conclude that intrauterine accretion rates for Ca and P can be achieved while feeding VLBW infants fortified human milk. Newer formulations should be targeted to reduce the potential for fat malabsorption and promote better mineral utilization so that fluid intake can be minimized.

We thank Pamela Burns, RN, the neonatal nursery staff of the Neonatal Clinical Research Center and Texas Children's Hospital for their expertise, Charles Imo for laboratory assistance, and J. Kennard Fraley for database management.

REFERENCES

1. Schanler RJ, Garza C, Smith EO. Fortified mothers' milk for very low birth weight infants: results of macromineral balance studies. J PEDIATR 1985;107:767-74.
2. Atkinson SA, Radde IC, Anderson GH. Macromineral balances in premature infants fed their own mothers' milk or formula. J PEDIATR 1983;102:99-106.
3. Greer FR, McCormick A. Improved bone mineralization and growth in premature infants fed fortified own mother's milk. J PEDIATR 1988;112:961-9.
4. Horsman A, Ryan SW, Congdon PJ, Truscott JG, Simpson M. Bone mineral accretion rate and calcium intake in preterm infants. Arch Dis Child 1989;64:910-8.
5. Polberger SKT, Axelsson IA, Räihä NCR. Growth of very low birth weight infants on varying amounts of human milk protein. Pediatr Res 1989;25:414-9.
6. Abrams SA, Schanler RJ, Garza C. Bone mineralization in former very low birth weight infants fed either human milk or commercial formula. J PEDIATR 1988;112:956-60.
7. Lucas A, Brooke OG, Baker BA, Bishop N, Morley R. High alkaline phosphatase activity and growth in preterm neonates. Arch Dis Child 1989;64:902-9.
8. Abrams SA, Schanler RJ, Tsang RC, Garza C. Bone mineralization in former very low birth weight infants fed either human milk or commercial formula: one-year follow-up observation. J PEDIATR 1989;114:1041-4.
9. Schanler RJ, Burns PA, Abrams SA, Garza C. Bone mineralization outcomes in human milk-fed preterm infants. Pediatr Res 1992;31:583-6.
10. Schanler RJ, Abrams SA, Garza C. Bioavailability of calcium and phosphorus in human milk fortifiers and formula for very low birth weight infants. J PEDIATR 1988;113:95-100.
11. Congdon PJ, Horsman A, Ryan SW, Truscott JG, Durward H. Spontaneous resolution of bone mineral depletion in preterm infants. Arch Dis Child 1990;65:1038-42.
12. Friel JK, Andrews WL, Matthew JD, McKim E, French S, Long DR. Improved growth of very low birthweight infants. Nutr Res 1993;13:611-20.
13. Lucas A, Bishop NJ, King FJ, Cole TJ. Randomised trial of nutrition for preterm infants after discharge. Arch Dis Child 1992;67:324-7.
14. Chan GM. Growth and bone mineral status of discharged very low birth weight infants fed different formulas or human milk. J PEDIATR 1993;123:439-43.
15. Ziegler EE, O'Donnell AM, Nelson SE, Fomon SJ. Body composition of the reference fetus. Growth 1976;40:329-41.
16. Schanler RJ, Garza C, Nichols BL. Fortified mothers' milk for very low birth weight infants: results of growth and nutrient balance studies. J PEDIATR 1985;107:437-45.
17. American Academy of Pediatrics Committee on Nutrition: Nutritional needs of low-birth-weight infants. Pediatrics 1985;75:976-86.
18. Ehrenkranz RA, Gettner PA, Nelli CM. Nutrient balance studies in premature infants fed premature formula or fortified preterm human milk. J Pediatr Gastroenterol Nutr 1989;8:58-67.
19. Koo WWK, Sherman R, Succop P, et al. Sequential bone mineral content in small preterm infants with and without fractures and rickets. J Bone Miner Res 1988;3:193-7.
20. Chappell JE, Clandinin MT, Kearney-Volpe C, Reichman B, Swyer PW. Fatty acid balance studies in premature infants fed

human milk or formula: effect of calcium supplementation. J PEDIATR 1986;108:439-47.
21. Bronner F, Salle BL, Putet G, Rigo J, Senterre J. Net calcium absorption in premature infants: results of 103 metabolic balance studies. Am J Clin Nutr 1992;56:1037-44.
22. Hillman LS, Johnson LS, Lee DZ, Vieira NE, Yergey AL. Measurement of true absorption, endogenous fecal excretion, urinary excretion, and retention of calcium in preterm infants by using a dual-tracer, stable isotope method. J PEDIATR 1993;123:444-56.
23. Atkinson SA, Shah JK, Webber CE, Gibson IL, Gibson RS. A multi-element isotopic tracer assessment of true fractional absorption of minerals from formula with additives of calcium, phosphorus, zinc, copper, and iron in young piglets. J Nutr 1993;123:1586-93.
24. Hanning RM, Mitchell MK, Atkinson SA. In vitro solubility of calcium glycerophosphate versus conventional mineral salts in pediatric parenteral nutrition solutions. J Pediatr Gastroenterol Nutr 1989;9:67-72.
25. Georgieff MK, Amarnath UM, Mills MM. Determinants of arm muscle and fat accretion during the first postnatal month in preterm newborn infants. J Pediatr Gastroenterol Nutr 1989;9:219-24.

Clinical and laboratory observations

Diagnosis of neonatal enterovirus infection by polymerase chain reaction

Mark J. Abzug, MD, Michael Loeffelholz, PhD, and Harley A. Rotbart, MD
From the Departments of Pediatrics (Infectious Diseases) and Microbiology, University of Colorado School of Medicine and Children's Hospital, Denver; and Roche Molecular Systems, Branchburg, New Jersey

A 5-hour colorimetric polymerase chain reaction (PCR) assay was more sensitive than viral culture in identifying viral infection in initial serum (13/16 vs 5/16; $p = 0.008$) and urine (10/16 vs 5/16; $p = 0.2$) specimens from 16 enterovirus-infected newborn infants, and remained more sensitive throughout their illnesses. Combined sensitivity of serum and urine PCR was 14 of 16 (88%). Results of all acute-phase PCR assays of serum and urine from four neonates with cultures negative for enterovirus were also negative. PCR assay of serum and urine facilitates rapid, accurate diagnosis of neonatal enterovirus infections. (J PEDIATR 1995;126:447-50)

Neonatal enterovirus infections are a common cause of illness and hospitalization[1] with significant morbidity and mortality rates.[2] Distinguishing EV infection in a sick newborn infant from other infectious and noninfectious diseases that may have similar manifestations is challenging.[2] Currently, laboratory diagnosis depends on tissue culture isola-

Supported by grant RR-69 from the General Clinical Research Centers Program of the Division of Research Resources, National Institutes of health; the Kempe Research Center, Children's Hospital, Denver, Colo.,; and Roche Molecular Systems. Dr. Loeffelholz is a full-time employee of, and Dr. Rotbart a paid consultant for, Roche Molecular Systems, whose products were used for the work discussed in the article.
Presented in part at the 10th Annual Clinical Virology Symposium and Annual Meeting of the Pan American Group for Rapid Viral Diagnosis, Clearwater, FL, April 1994 and the 34th Interscience Conference on Antimicrobial Agents and Chemotherapy, Orlando, FL, Oct. 1994.
Submitted for publication July 22, 1994; accepted Sept. 15, 1994.
Reprint requests: Mark J. Abzug, MD, Infectious Diseases, Box B055, Children's Hospital, 1056 E. 19th Ave., Denver, CO 80218.

0022-3476/95/$3.00 + 0 **9/24/60612**

EV	enterovirus
CSF	cerebrospinal fluid
PCR	Polymerase chain reaction
RNA	Ribonucleic acid

tion of the virus, most commonly from mucosal sites or cerebrospinal fluid. This can be laborious and requires several days to ≥1 week,[3, 4] and mucosal cultures may not [2]distinguish infection from colonization.[1] Furthermore, certain EV serotypes will not grow in standard tissue culture. We investigated the potential utility of polymerase chain reaction assay of serum and urine specimens for rapid diagnosis of neonatal EV infections.

METHODS

Patients and specimen collection. Newborn infants ≤14 days of age seen between June and October with meningitis (CSF leukocyte count, >50 cells/mm^3), hepatitis (alanine aminotransferase value >100 IU/L), myocarditis (abnormal echocardiogram or electrocardiogram), or clinical sepsis without evident bacterial focus, and with a history and physical examination suggestive of EV infection (e.g., fever, family history consistent with EV infection, viral exanthem) were studied after informed consent was obtained from parents.

Throat specimens, rectum-and-stool specimens, CSF, serum, and urine (catheter or bag specimen) for viral culture, and serum and urine for EV PCR assay (frozen at −70° C), were collected at study entry. Bacterial cultures of blood, CSF, and urine were grown by standard methods.

Half of patients received one 750 mg/kg dose of intravenously administered immune globulin in a prospective, randomized treatment trial. Serial samples of serum and urine (generally bag specimens) for viral culture and PCR assay were subsequently obtained (and stored at −70° C) daily during the first 5 hospital days, at a follow-up visit within 4 days of discharge for patients hospitalized <5 days, on the last day of hospitalization for those with hospital stays >5 days, and approximately 1 and 4 months after onset (serum only).

Viral cultures. Initial CSF, serum, urine, throat, and rectal specimens were inoculated onto monkey kidney, HEp-2, Vero, and human lung fibroblast cells. Serial neonatal serum and urine specimens were inoculated onto Vero cells or human lung fibroblasts, depending on which yielded the patient's original isolate. Both lines were used if initial culture results were negative. A culture positive for a nonpoliovirus EV from any site at any time was accepted as evidence of EV infection. Serum obtained at 1 and 4 months was cultured on monkey kidney, HEp-2, and human lung fibroblast cell lines.

PCR assay. Antisense primer EV1b and sense primer EV2b, derived from MD90 and MD91 sequences,[5, 6] were biotin labeled, and antisense probe EV3, derived from the MD92 sequence.[5, 6] was bound, unlabeled, to the bottom of microwells by bovine serum albumin conjugated to the 5′ end.[7]

The ribonucleic acid was extracted from 100 μl of sample (serum or urine) with guanidine thiocyanate, glycogen, and dithiothreitol in Tris buffer; precipitated in isopropanol and 70% ethanol; and resuspended in 200 μl of diluent solution.[6] Resuspended specimen, 50 μl, was added to 50 μl of master mix containing uracil *N*-glycosylase (AmpErase; Roche Molecular Systems, Branchburg, N.J.), primers, deoxynucleotide triphosphates (deoxyuridine triphosphate in place of deoxythymidine triphosphate), and rTth enzyme (Roche Molecular Systems) in bicine buffer.[8] Samples were amplified in a thermal cycler, with a 50° C incubation for 2 minutes to activate uracil *N*-glycoslyase (which degrades amplified product inadvertently carried over from past PCR assays), followed by a 60° C 30-minute reverse transcription incubation and 35 amplification cycles.[6] A positive control tube (EV-derived RNA and nonspecific carrier RNA) and a negative control tube (buffer and nonspecific carrier RNA) were processed identically with tubes containing samples and amplified singly and in triplicate, respectively, with each run of 35 samples. After amplification, 100 μl of sodium hydroxide denaturing solution (Amplicor; Roche Molecular Systems) was added to each tube.

Twenty-five microliters of each denatured solution of amplified material was combined with 100 μl of hybridization buffer (Amplicor) in a well of a 96-microwell plate that contained prebound EV3 probe. After 1 hour at 37° C, wells were washed, 100 μl of avidin–horseradish peroxidase conjugate was added, wells were washed again, and 100 μl of substrate (hydrogen peroxide and tetramethylbenzidine) was added.[6] Optical density ≥0.35 determined on a plate reader at 450 mm was interpreted as positive for EV RNA. The entire PCR assay required 5 hours for completion.

Statistical analysis Comparisons were performed with the Fisher Exact Test and the McNemar Test.

RESULTS

Sixteen of the twenty neonates studied were shown by viral culture to be infected with EV; the remaining four had cultures negative for EV, with specimens obtained from all body sites at all times. The yield of viral cultures at study entry among EV-infected neonates and the mean time to positivity were as follows: serum, 5 of 16 neonates, 5.0 days; urine, 5 of 16 neonates, 6.0 days; throat, 10 of 16 neonates, 5.4 days; CSF, 12 of 14 neonates, 4.9

Table I. Results of polymerase chain reaction assay and viral culture of serum and urine during the acute illnesses of 20 neonates examined for possible enterovirus infection

Study group	Study day	Serum culture (+/No. tested)	Serum PCR assay (+/No. tested)	Urine culture (+/No. tested)	Urine PCR assay (+/No. tested)
EV infected	1	5/16	13/16	5/16	10/16
	2	3/16	9/16	2/16	5/16
	3	1/16	7/16	1/14	5/14
	4	1/11	9/11	0/9	2/9
	5	0/6	5/6	0/6	2/6
	6-8	0/9	7/9	1/8	2/8
Not infected	1	0/4	0/4	0/4	0/4
	2	0/4	0/4	0/4	0/4
	3	0/4	0/3	0/4	0/4
	4	0/4	0/4	0/4	0/4
	5	0/3	0/3	0/2	0/2
	6-8	0/3	0/3	0/2	0/2

+, Positive results.

Table II. Concordance of results of polymerase chain reaction assay and viral culture of serum and urine during the acute illnesses of 16 enterovirus-infected neonates

Specimen (n)	PCR+/culture+ (%)	PCR+/culture− (%)	PCR−/culture+ (%)	PCR−/culture− (%)
Serum (74)	8 (11)	42 (57)	2 (3)	22 (30)
Urine (69)	6 (9)	20 (29)	3 (4)	40 (58)

+, Positive results; −, negative results.

days; and rectum, 14 of 16 neonates, 5.2 days. The mean time to first positive culture of a specimen from any site for EV-infected neonates was 4.2 days (SD = 1.9 days). Viral isolates included echoviruses 6 (2), 9 (2), and 11 (3); coxsackie-viruses B2 (2) and B4 (5); and 2 nontypeable isolates. Results of bacterial cultures were negative for all infants, except for two contaminated urine specimens.

Serum and urine PCR assays were more sensitive than viral culture among EV-infected neonates at entry (13/16 vs 5/16 [$p = 0.008$] and 10/16 vs 5/16 [$p = 0.2$], respectively) and throughout the neonatal illness (Table I). Combined sensitivity of serum and urine PCR assay versus serum and urine viral culture at entry was 14 of 16 (88%) versus 9 of 16 (56%), ($p = 0.2$). Yield of the PCR assay was unaffected by intravenous administration of immune globulin (not shown). A relatively large number of serum and urine specimens obtained from EV-infected neonates during their acute illnesses had discordantly positive PCR results and negative culture results; very few specimens had positive culture results and negative PCR results (Table II). Results of all PCR assays of sera and urine obtained during the acute illnesses of the four EV-uninfected babies were negative (Table I). Positive and negative control tubes gave appropriate results in each PCR run.

No long-term follow-up sera had positive viral culture results. However, among originally EV-infected infant results were PCR positive in 2 of 13 sera obtained approximately 1 month after the onset of neonatal illness (range, 1 to 1¾ months) and in 3 of 11 sera at approximately 4 months (range, 3 to 5 months). One of four originally EV-uninfected infants had positive results on PCR assay of serum at the 1-month visit.

DISCUSSION

There are several advantages of PCR for diagnosis of neonatal EV infection over traditional tissue culture isolation of virus from rectum, CSF, and/or throat.[2, 9] The PCR assay described is more rapid (5 hours) than tissue culture—which took a mean of 4.2 days to reveal the earliest positive result for each patient—and is easy to perform, with an objective colorimetric end point. Rapid diagnosis of neonatal EV infections by PCR would be expected to reduce unnecessary treatment and hospitalization, a consequence similar to the impact of tissue culture and PCR diagnosis of EV meningitis on patient management.[4, 10] Recovery of an EV from a mucosal surface may represent asymptomatic shedding[1] or prolonged shedding after symptomatic infection.[11] In contrast, isolation of EVs from nonpermissive sites such as serum, aseptically collected urine, and CSF is unlikely to represent asymptomatic shedding. Studies in infants with symptomatic infection have demonstrated that rates of tissue culture positivity are lower for serum and urine (24% to 47%) than for mucosal sites.[2, 9, 11] In the current study, in which we applied EV PCR to serum and urine specimens, the sensitivity of serum and urine PCR exceeded that of tissue culture (of serum and urine) throughout the acute illness, with very high specificity.

Several patient's sera were positive for EV by PCR at 1- and 4-month visits, most likely representing new EV infections after the neonatal illnesses or vaccine-strain viremia after immunization with live poliovirus vaccine. The PCR assay used will amplify and detect vaccine-strain (and wild-type) polioviruses, a potentially confounding factor in infants of vaccination age, but generally not in neonates.

The application of the PCR assay to serum and urine provides rapid, easy, and accurate diagnosis of neonatal EV infection. Utilization of this test will facilitate management of sick newborn infants during the summer and fall months.

We thank Neva Murphy for her technical assistance; Dennis Luckey, PhD, for help with the statistical analyses; Dr. Mark Pallansch, Centers for Disease Control and Prevention, Atlanta, Ga., for serotyping the viral isolates; and the referring physicians, parents, and children who participated in this study.

REFERENCES

1. Jenista JA, Powell KR, Menegus MA. Epidemiology of neonatal enterovirus infection. J Pediatr 1984;104:685-90.
2. Abzug MJ, Levin MJ, Rotbart HA. Profile of enterovirus disease in the first two weeks of life. Pediatr Infect Dis J 1993;12:820-4.
3. Chonmaitree T, Ford C, Sanders C, Lucia HL. Comparison of cell cultures for rapid isolation of enteroviruses. J Clin Microbiol 1988;26:2576-80.
4. Chonmaitree T, Menegus MA, Powell KR. The clinical relevance of "CSF viral culture": a two-year experience with aseptic meningitis in Rochester, NY. JAMA 1982;247:1843-7.
5. Rotbart HA. Enzymatic RNA amplification of the enteroviruses. J Clin Microbiol 1990;28:438-42.
6. Rotbart HA, Sawyer MH, FAST S, et al. Diagnosis of enteroviral meningitis by using PCR with a colorimetric microwell detection assay. J Clin Microbiol 1994;32:2590-2.
7. Tung CH, Randolph MJ, Stein S. Preparation of oligonucleotide-peptide conjugates. Bioconjug Chem 1991;2:464-5.
8. Myers TW, Gelfand DH. Reverse transcription and DNA amplification by a *Thermus thermophilus* DNA polymerase. Biochemistry 1991;30:7661-6.
9. Lake AM, Lauer BA, Clark JC, Wesenberg RL, McIntosh K. Enterovirus infections in neonates. J Pediatr 1976;89:787-91.
10. Schlesinger Y, Sawyer MH, Storch GA. Enteroviral meningitis in infancy: potential role for polymerase chain reaction in patient management. Pediatrics 1994;94:157-62.
11. Dagan R, Jenista JA, Prather SL, Powell KR, Menegus MA. Viremia in hospitalized children with enterovirus infections. J Pediatr 1985;106:397-401.

Inhaled nitric oxide for premature infants after prolonged rupture of the membranes

Abraham Peliowski, MD, Neil N. Finer, MD, Philip C. Etches, MB, Anne J. Tierney, MB, and C. Anthony Ryan, MB

From the Departments of Newborn Medicine and Pediatrics, Royal Alexandra Hospital, University of Alberta, Edmonton, Alberta, Canada

We evaluated the use of inhaled nitric oxide in eight premature infants (520 to 1440 gm, 24 to 31 weeks of gestation) who failed to respond to conventional management and who had prolonged rupture of the membranes and oligohydramnios. All infants had a significant improvement in oxygenation and a fall in mean airway pressure with inhaled nitric oxide. Further studies are required to determine the safety and efficacy of this form of therapy. (J Pediatr 1995;126:450-3)

Submitted for publication April 18, 1994; accepted Sept. 9, 1994.

Reprint requests: Neil Finer, MD, Royal Alexandra Hospital, 10240 Kingsway, Edmonton, Alberta T5H 3V9, Canada.

0022-3476/95/$3.00 + 0 **9/24/60454**

Inhaled nitric oxide has been shown to improve oxygenation in term neonates with intractable hypoxemia and right-to-left shunting.[1-3] Premature infants with severe hyaline membrane disease have elevated pulmonary vascular resistance with low aortopulmonary pressure difference,[4] and

FIO_2	Fraction of inspired oxygen
HFO	High-frequency oscillation
INO	Inhaled nitric oxide
MAP	Mean airway pressure
NO	Nitric oxide
NO_2	Nitrogen dioxide
OI	Oxygenation index
PaO_2	Arterial oxygen tension
PROM	Prolonged rupture of the membranes

frequently a bidirectional ductal flow.[5] Recently, Abman et al.[6] administered INO to a premature infant with group B β-hemolytic streptococcal sepsis and demonstrated reversal of right-to-left ductal shunting after the use of INO. In view of these observations, we have used INO in premature infants who do not respond to maximal conventional therapy. We report our experience in treating eight such infants, all of whom had similar clinical findings with prolonged rupture of the membranes, oligohydramnios, and suspected hypoplastic lungs.

METHODS

Premature infants eligible to receive INO were infants whose condition was deteriorating and who were unresponsive to what was considered maximal therapy. All infants were receiving a fraction of inspired oxygen of 1.0, all were supported by conventional ventilation and/or high-frequency oscillation (Infant Star; Infrasonics Inc., San Diego, Calif.), and all were treated with either a bovine surfactant (bLES; bLES Biochemicals Inc., London, Ontario, Canada) or Exosurf (Burroughs Wellcome Co., Research Triangle Park, N.C.). All received ventilation with a mean airway pressure of $\geq$14 cm H_2O and had an oxygenation index [$OI = (MAP)(FIO_2)(100) \div PaO_2$] of 19 or more before treatment with INO. Whenever possible, echocardiography and cranial ultrasonography were performed before administration of INO.

Our method of INO administration has been reported.[3] In brief, NO was obtained as a gas in balance nitrogen in a certified concentration of 800 ppm ± 1% (Canadian Liquid Air, Montreal, Quebec, Canada) with <5 ppm nitrogen dioxide. Single-stage stainless-steel diffusion-free regulators were utilized. The NO mixture was connected at a pressure of 50 psi to a Matheson No. 603 flowmeter (Matheson Canada Inc., Edmonton, Alberta), and injected into the inspiratory line of a time-cycled, pressure-limited neonatal ventilator (Infant Star). The gas mixture was analyzed for NO, NO_2, and total oxides of nitrogen with a chemiluminescence analyzer (model 42H; Thermo Environmental Instruments, Franklin, Mass.) and an electrochemical sensor (Pulmonox, Tofield, Alberta). Exhaled gas was scavenged. The FIO_2 was measured with an on-line oxygen sensor (Ohmeda No. 5120; BOC Health Care, Madison, Wis.).

All infants were treated with an initial INO dose of 20 ppm; attempts were made to lower the dose within 2 hours of administration by reducing the concentration by 5 ppm to determine whether the infant tolerated such a reduction. The INO was continued until the infant's OIs were <10.

Infants who responded (increase in PaO_2 of $\geq$10 mm Hg) continued to receive the lowest dose of INO associated with improvement. Twenty-four hours later, and then every 24 hours, an attempt was made to wean the infant from INO. Every 15 minute the concentration of INO was decreased by 5 ppm and subsequently discontinued. If the PaO_2 fell by $\geq$10 mm Hg, the higher dose was reinstated. If the infant had an OI of <10 while not inhaling NO, the INO therapy was discontinued.

Methemoglobin concentration was measured every 8 hours (IL-282; Instrumentation Laboratory, Lexington, Mass.). If this concentration reached 5% on two measurements 30 minutes apart, the use of INO was discontinued.

This clinical trial was approved by the Royal Alexandra Hospital Investigational Review Committee and by the Canadian Health Protection Branch. Infants were treated with INO only after informed parental consent was given.

RESULTS

Eight premature infants were treated with INO after what was considered to be failure of conventional management. All infants were inborn; birth weights ranged from 520 to 1440 gm and gestations between 24 to 31 weeks (Table). All infants had an antepartum history of oligohydramnios and PROM for more than 3 days. The mothers of all infants had received dexamethasone and antibiotics antenatally. Four of the eight infants had a cranial ultrasound study before INO therapy, and all had findings reported as normal. All infants had severe oligohydramnios at delivery, with very low lung volumes on the initial chest x-ray studies. The pre-INO MAP was 16 ± 3.2 cm H_2O (range, 12 to 22 cm H_2O). In seven of the eight infants, HFO was initiated between 1 and 10 hours of age, and all infants first received INO between 2 and 11 hours of age. Five of the eight infants received INO during HFO. Pre-INO echocardiograms were obtained in five of the eight infants and showed evidence of pulmonary hypertension with right-to-left shunting at the ductal and, in some, at the foramen level, consistent with previous observations of infants who responded to INO.[1-3] The remaining three infants underwent their initial echocardiographic study while receiving INO, and for all three the ductal flow was left to right and the transcutaneous PaO_2 gradients were 20 mm Hg or greater between preductally and postductally placed probes at the time of the administration of INO. All infants responded to

Table. Clinical characteristics of studied infants

Patient No.	Weight (gm)/ GA (wk)	Amniotic fluid	MAP (cm H_2O) pre-NO	OI pre-NO	OI post-NO	Duration of NO (hr)	Outcome
1	770/25	PROM × 8 days; oligohydramnios	15	48	22	60	Died at 5 days; grade 1 IVH; *Candida* sepsis
2	1020/28	PROM × 21 days; oligohydramnios	19	19	12	64	Survived; no IVH
3	750/24	PROM × 42 days; oligohydramnios; amnionitis	22	73	33	24	Died at 5 days; Trx D/C; grade 4 IVH
4	1120/27	PROM × 12 days; oligohydramnios	14	47	28	137	Survived; grade 3 IVH
5	1435/31	PROM × 12 days; oligohydramnios; amnionitis	20	76	7	10	Survived; no IVH
6	520/24	PROM × 7 days; oligohydramnios	14	25	14	14	Died at 3 days; Trx D/C; grade 4 IVH
7	1440/30	PROM × 77 days; oligohydramnios	15	28	14	59	Survived; no IVH
8	860/25	PROM × 3 days; oligohydramnios	12	31	11	6	Survived; no IVH

GA, Gestational age; *IVH*, intraventricular hemorrhage; *Trx D/C*, treatment discontinued.

INO with an increase in postductal PaO_2 of 73 ± 94 mm Hg (range, 19 to 284 mm Hg).

All infants responded to INO, leading to a decrease in MAP and an improvement in oxygenation as demonstrated by a fall in the OIs (pre-INO OI 45.1 ± 22.8 vs post-INO OI 18.5 ± 4.3; $p = 0.015$). Five of these eight infants survived. Infant 1 died at 5 days of age with *Candida* sepsis and intraventricular hemorrhage. Therapy was discontinued for infants 3 and 6 because of massive intraventricular hemorrhage with severe parenchymal involvement.

Nitric oxide therapy was continued for an average of 47 hours with a range of 6 to 137 hours. No infant's methemoglobin level was more than 3%, and no infant's exposure to an NO_2 concentration was more than 2 ppm when NO_2 concentration was measured downstream of the injection site by the chemiluminescence or electrochemical analyzers.

DISCUSSION

Our observations add to the report by Abman et al.[6] that premature infants with severe respiratory disease, hypoxemia, and right-to-left shunting at the ductal and/or foramen level may have significant improvement in oxygenation after treatment with INO, a result that allows a reduction in MAP. All infants had received what we consider to be maximal ventilatory and other supportive therapy. The eight infants were thought to be at very high risk of having hypoplastic lungs because of the PROM for more than 1 week in seven of the eight infants.

The deaths of two infants were caused by significant intraventricular hemorrhage. These infants had had normal results on cranial ultrasonography 24 hours after the start of INO therapy, and the bleeding occurred after NO therapy was discontinued. Increases in bleeding time have been noted in normal adult subjects who have received INO.[7] More recently, increased bleeding time has also been reported in rabbits receiving as little as 3 ppm of INO.[8] It is thought that INO will come into contact with platelets in the pulmonary circulation and may decrease platelet adhesiveness and aggregation, and could contribute to bleeding disorders in such infants.

In addition, there is recent evidence that peroxynitrites, which form when NO combines with superoxide, can inhibit surfactant function.[9] There is no current information regarding the formation of peroxynitrites in human beings receiving INO or regarding potential toxic effects of this reaction.

Although methemoglobin is produced through the interaction of NO and hemoglobin, the levels in our babies remained well below 5%. With ≤20 ppm of INO, production of methemoglobin should not be a problem, even in premature infants who have low levels of methemoglobin reductase. Similarly, although NO_2 is thought to be a toxic byproduct of INO, the concentrations in our study were well below the currently accepted toxic limits (5 ppm per weighted 8-hour average).[10] To monitor the levels of NO and NO_2, we utilized both a chemiluminescence and an electrochemical analyzer. We tested both analyzers simultaneously and found an excellent correlation.

We believe that it was ethical to attempt to treat these infants with INO because all conventional management, including conventional mechanical ventilation, HFO, and surfactant therapy, had failed. In addition, OIs >15 in premature infants are associated with a high mortality rate, especially among infants who receive surfactant.[11]

The response to INO by our infants is consistent with the pathophysiology of severe respiratory distress with evidence of pulmonary hypertension and right-to-left shunting as initially described by Chu et al.[12] and Stahlman et al.[13] and recently confirmed by Walther et al.[4] The PROM that occurred in each of these pregnancies may have been an additional contributing factor; Bhutani et al.[14] reported right-to-left shunts in 8 of 15 premature infants with prolonged amniotic fluid leaks. Our observations suggest that INO therapy can result in improvements in oxygenation, with the ability to reduce the MAP and thus decrease barotrauma.

However, before the use of INO becomes an accepted form of therapy in premature infants, further studies are required to determine whether such therapy does alter coagulation, whether it is associated with the initiation or extension of intracranial or other hemorrhages, and whether such therapy has the potential to reduce exogenous or endogenous surfactant effectiveness. Because of the timing and acute nature of their deterioration, not all of our infants had cranial ultrasound evaluations before INO therapy, and we believe that any future study should include such an evaluation. Further studies are also necessary to evaluate the potential toxicity of INO and the role of INO therapy in premature infants with intractable respiratory failure and hypoxemia.

REFERENCES

1. Roberts JD, Polaner DM, Lang P, Zapol WM. Inhaled nitric oxide in persistent pulmonary hypertension of the newborn. Lancet 1992;340:818-9.
2. Kinsella JP, Neish SR, Dunbar I, Shaffer E, Abman SH. Clinical responses to prolonged treatment of persistent pulmonary hypertension of the newborn with low doses of inhaled nitric oxide. J PEDIATR 1993;123:103-8.
3. Finer NN, Etches PC, Kamstra B, Tierney AJ, Peliowski A, Ryan CA. Inhaled nitric oxide in infants referred for extracorporeal membrane oxygenation: dose response. J PEDIATR 1994; 124:302-8.
4. Walther FJ, Benders MJ, Leighton JO. Persistent pulmonary hypertension in premature neonates with severe respiratory distress syndrome. Pediatrics 1992;90:899-904.
5. Skinner JR, Boys RJ, Hunter S, Hey EN. Pulmonary and systemic arterial pressure in hyaline membrane disease. Arch Dis Child 1992;67:366-73.
6. Abman S, Kinsella JP, Schaffer MS, Wilkening RB. Inhaled nitric oxide in the management of a premature newborn with severe respiratory distress and pulmonary hypertension. Pediatrics 1993;92:606-9.
7. Hogman M, Frostell C, Arnberg H, Hedenstierna G. Bleeding time prolongation and NO inhalation. Lancet 1993;341: 1664-5.
8. Hogman M, Frostell C, Arnberg H, Sandhagen B, Hedenstierna G. Prolonged bleeding time during nitric oxide inhalation in the rabbit. Acta Physiol Scand 1994;151:125-9.
9. Haddad IY, Ischiropoulos H, Holm BA, Beckman JS, Baker JR, Matalon S. Mechanisms of peroxynitrite-induced injury to pulmonary surfactants. Am J Physiol 1993;265:L555-64.
10. National Institute for Occupational Safety and Health. NIOSH recommendations for occupational safety and health standards. MMWR 1988;37:21.
11. Hamvas A, Devine T, Cole FS. Surfactant therapy failure identifies infants at risk for pulmonary mortality. Am J Dis Child 1993;147:665-8.
12. Chu J, Clements JA, Cotton E, et al. The pulmonary hypoperfusion syndrome. Pediatrics 1965;35:733-42.
13. Stahlman M, Blankenship WJ, Shepard FM, et al. Circulatory studies in clinical hyaline membrane disease. Biol Neonate 1972;20:300-20.
14. Bhutani VK, Abbasi S, Weiner S. Neonatal pulmonary manifestations due to prolonged amniotic leak. Am J Perinatol 1986;3:225-30.

Administration of granulocyte colony-stimulating factor to neutropenic low birth weight infants of mothers with preeclampsia

Rita A. Makhlouf, MD, Mia W. Doron, MD, Carl L. Bose, MD, Wayne A. Price, MD, and Alan D. Stiles, MD

From the Division of Neonatal/Perinatal Medicine, Department of Pediatrics, University of North Carolina at Chapel Hill

Nine low birth weight infants with neutropenia born to mothers with preeclampsia were treated with granulocyte-colony stimulating factor, 10 μg/kg intravenously, within 24 hours of birth and at 24-hour intervals for a maximum of three doses if neutropenia persisted. The absolute neutrophil count increased significantly in eight of the nine infants within 6 hours, and neutrophilia was sustained for at least 72 hours after administration of a single dose of granulocyte-colony stimulating factor. (J Pediatr 1995;126:454-6)

Almost 50% of infants born to mothers with preeclampsia have neutropenia according to the Manroe reference values for normal neonatal neutrophil counts[1-4] and are at increased risk of having early-onset sepsis[5] and nosocomial infections.[1, 6] The low absolute neutrophil counts in these infants are partly the result of inhibited activity of granulocyte colony-stimulating factor, a hematopoietic growth factor that stimulates neutrophil production.[7] In neutropenic adults and children, recombinant human G-CSF increases circulating neutrophils and bone marrow neutrophil storage pools, improves neutrophil function, and results in fewer bacterial infections.[8, 9] We examined circulating neutrophil values after administration of G-CSF to neutropenic neonates of mothers with preeclampsia.

METHODS

Subjects were selected from low birth weight infants (<2500 gm) born to mothers with preeclampsia at the University of North Carolina Hospitals between Nov. 1, 1993, and May 31, 1994. Preeclampsia was defined as hypertension (diastolic blood pressure >90 mm Hg, or systolic blood pressure >140 mm Hg, or an increase from baseline blood pressure of ≥30 mm Hg systolic or ≥15 mm Hg diastolic) plus proteinuria, edema, elevated liver enzyme concentrations, or central nervous system signs and symptoms (headache, blurry vision, or seizures) in a pregnant woman with no other cause for the symptoms. Infants were included in the study if they had an ANC before 24 hours of age below the lower limit of the Manroe reference range.[2] Infants were excluded if they had multiple congenital anomalies or congenital infection or if their mothers had received medications that could cause neonatal neutropenia. The study protocol was approved by the institutional review board of the University of North Carolina at Chapel Hill.

See related article p. 457.

ANC	Absolute neutrophil count
G-CSF	Granulocyte colony-stimulating factor

The G-CSF was administered as an intravenous infusion, 10 μg/kg per dose,[10] for a 15-minute period. The first dose was given before 24 hours of age, and the medication was given at 24-hour intervals for a maximum of three doses if neutropenia persisted.

Complete blood cell counts were obtained before study entry (baseline) and at 6, 24, 48, 72, and 120 hours after G-CSF administration. Absolute neutrophil counts were performed with a Technicon H2 counter (Miles, Inc., Tarrytown, N.Y.) and were then corrected for the number of nucleated erythrocytes. Blood samples were taken from cap-

Supported by the University of North Carolina Neonatal/Perinatal Fellow Research Fund.

Submitted for publication July 25, 1994; accepted Oct. 13, 1994.

Reprint requests: Carl L. Bose, MD, Division of Neonatal/Perinatal Medicine, CB No. 7596, Fourth Floor, University of North Carolina Hospitals, University of North Carolina at Chapel Hill, Chapel Hill, NC 27599-7596.

0022-3476/95/$3.00 + 0 **9/24/61268**

Table. Change in ANC after G-CSF treatment

Time after G-CSF (hr)	ANC ($\times 10^9$/L)
0	1.81 ± 0.77
6	6.47 ± 2.70*
24	7.77 ± 3.35*
48	5.85 ± 1.61*
72	4.10 ± 1.60*
120	4.19 ± 2.53

Data presented as mean ± SD.
*p <0.001 compared with baseline ANC.

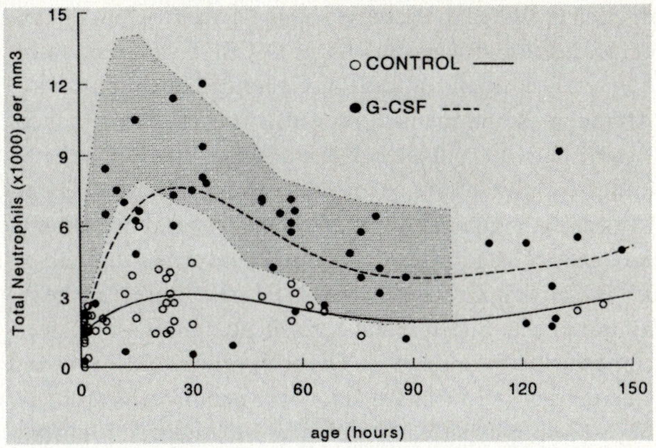

Figure. Absolute neutrophil count as a function of age in infants treated with G-CSF *(dark circles)* and control infants *(clear circles)*. A best-fit polynomial curve is shown for control infants *(solid line)* and for infants treated with G-CSF *(broken line)*. The Manroe criteria for neonatal neutrophil counts *(shaded area)* are adapted from Figure 1, Manroe BL, Weinberg AG, Rosenfeld CR, Browne R (J PEDIATR 1979;95:89-98).

illaries, arteries, or veins, and ANCs were adjusted for the source of blood sampled (for arterial samples, ANC was divided by 0.77; for venous samples, ANC was divided by 0.82).[11]

A cohort of infants born at the University of North Carolina Hospitals between July 1, 1987, and Dec. 31, 1992, who would have met eligibility criteria for the study was identified from hospital records. We selected one or two control infants from this cohort to match each study subject for gestational age, ANC in the first 12 hours of life ($\pm 0.5 \times 10^9$/L of the study infant's value), and birth weight.

Statistical analyses were performed with the chi-square test for categoric variables and the Student *t* test for continuous variables. Mean ANCs were initially compared by analysis of variance. Comparisons of baseline ANCs with subsequent neutrophil counts were then evaluated with paired *t* tests with a Bonferroni adjustment in significance for multiple comparisons.

RESULTS

Study infants (n = 9) were delivered at 26 to 33 weeks of gestation (mean, 31 ± 2 weeks); birth weights ranged from 800 to 1835 gm (mean, 1248 ± 306 gm). Control infants (n = 16) did not differ from study subjects with regard to gestational age, birth weight, size for gestational age, 5-minute Apgar score, race, gender, or delivery method. No infant had early-onset sepsis proved by positive blood culture results, but early-onset sepsis was presumed because of clinical signs of sepsis in one infant who received G-CSF and in two control infants. Severity of maternal preeclampsia, incidence of chorioamnionitis, maternal infection within 2 weeks before delivery, or antenatal treatment with corticosteroids or antibiotics did not differ between groups.

Initial ANCs of the study infants, obtained between 1 and 4 hours of age (mean, 2 hours), ranged from 0.25 to 2.70×10^9/L (mean, $1.81 \pm 0.77 \times 10^9$/L). Initial ANCs of the control infants, obtained between 1 and 7 hours of age (mean, 2 hours), ranged from 0 to 2.59×10^9/L (mean, $1.63 \pm 0.69 \times 10^9$/L) and were not significantly different from the ANCs of the study infants (p = 0.55).

The first G-CSF dose, given between 1 and 10 hours of age (mean, 6 hours), was followed by a significant increase in ANC by 6 hours after administration, which was sustained for at least 72 hours (p <0.001 by analysis of variance; individual comparisons shown in the Table). Absolute neutrophil counts by age in study and control infants are shown in the Figure. Absolute neutrophil counts were significantly higher in treated infants at 6 to 16 hours (p <0.05), 20 to 34 hours (p <0.001), and 48 to 90 hours (p <0.05) of age. Eight of nine infants had resolution of neutropenia within 24 hours of G-CSF administration, and ANCs remained within the Manroe normal range for the duration of the study. In contrast, ANCs of control infants did not reach normal levels until after 60 hours of age. Only one study infant had persistent neutropenia 24 hours after the first G-CSF dose; therefore the infant received two subsequent doses. This infant's ANC exceeded the lower limit of the Manroe range by 111 hours of age.

Mean blood concentrations of lymphocytes, eosinophils, monocytes, and platelets 72 to 120 hours after one dose of G-CSF remained within the normal reference range.[12] Only the infant who received three doses of G-CSF had a posttreatment monocyte count (4.5×10^9/L) higher than normal.

DISCUSSION

Low birth weight neutropenic infants born to mothers with preeclampsia have decreased bone marrow neutrophil storage pools, without evidence of increased neutrophil destruction or margination.[1] This disorder of neutrophil production is related to decreased biologic activity, but not decreased serum concentrations, of G-CSF because of an inhibitor of neutrophil production elaborated by the placenta.[7] Although the mechanism by which this inhibitor reduces G-CSF activity, and the half-life of the inhibitor in affected infants, are unknown, our results demonstrate that the effects of the inhibitor can be overcome by administration of exogenous G-CSF. Our findings indicate either that the biologic activity of exogenous G-CSF is not altered by the inhibitor or that higher blood concentrations of G-CSF overcome the inhibitor's action. The observations of Koenig and Christensen[7] that bone marrow progenitor cells from infants born to hypertensive mothers have normal proliferative responses to exogenous G-CSF in an in vitro, inhibitor-free culture medium support these conclusions.

The response to administration of G-CSF was rapid, with a significant increase in circulating neutrophils by 6 hours after G-CSF administration. After normal levels of neutrophils had been achieved, ANCs remained within the Manroe range for the duration of the study period, which indicates a sustained neutrophilic response. These results are consistent with the described early and late effects of G-CSF: induction of initial neutrophil release from the bone marrow storage pool, followed by an increase in neutrophil production that is sustained for approximately 4 to 7 days.[8-10]

No infant had clinical signs of acute toxic effects of G-CSF. Blood concentrations of eosinophils and lymphocytes remained stable, in contrast to the increase seen after administration of granulocyte-macrophage colony-stimulating factor.[8, 9] It is unclear whether the abnormally high monocyte count in the infant who received three doses of G-CSF constitutes an adverse effect.

Mouzinho et al.[13] published a revised reference range for neutrophil counts in healthy, very low birth weight ($\leq$1500 gm) neonates, which widened the Manroe range and decreased its lower boundary. We used the Manroe criteria to define neutropenia in this study because prior studies have established that low birth weight infants of preeclamptic mothers who have ANCs less than the Manroe lower limit are at increased risk of having both early-onset sepsis and nosocomial infections.[1, 5, 6]

We speculate that the early increase in circulating neutrophils, and possibly improved neutrophil function, after administration of G-CSF may lower the risk of infection in neutropenic infants of mothers with preeclampsia. Before G-CSF administration in this population becomes routine, however, a randomized, controlled study showing clinical efficacy, and further evaluating the potential toxic effects, should be performed.

We thank Pamela D. Reiter, PharmD, for her help in procuring and administering granulocyte colony-stimulating factor.

REFERENCES

1. Koenig J, Christensen R. Incidence, neutrophil kinetics, and natural history of neonatal neutropenia associated with maternal hypertension. N Engl J Med 1989;321:557-62.
2. Manroe BL, Weinberg AG, Rosenfeld CR, Browne R. The neonatal blood count in health and disease. I. Reference values for neutrophilic cells. J Pediatr 1979;95:89-98.
3. Brazy JE, Grimm JK, Little VA. Neonatal manifestations of severe maternal hypertension occurring before the thirty-sixth week of pregnancy. J Pediatr 1982;100:265-71.
4. Engle WD, Rosenfeld CR. Neutropenia in high-risk neonates. J Pediatr 1984;105:982-6.
5. Doron M, Makhlouf R, Katz V, Lawson E, Stiles A. Increased incidence of sepsis at birth in neutropenic infants of mothers with preeclampsia. J Pediatr 1994;125:452-8.
6. Cadnapaphorchai M, Faix R. Increased nosocomial infection in neutropenic low birth weight (2000 grams or less) infants of hypertensive mothers. J Pediatr 1992;121:956-61.
7. Koenig J, Christensen R. The mechanism responsible for diminished neutrophil production in neonates delivered of women with pregnancy-induced hypertension. Am J Obstet Gynecol 1991;165:467-73.
8. Lieschke G, Burgess A. Granulocyte colony-stimulating factor and granulocyte-macrophage colony-stimulating factor [first of two parts]. N Engl J Med 1992;327:28-35.
9. Lieschke G, Burgess A. Granulocyte colony-stimulating factor and granulocyte-macrophage colony-stimulating factor [second of two parts] N Engl J Med 1992;327:99-106.
10. Gillan E, Suen Y, Stringham D, et al. A randomized placebo controlled phase I/II trial of rhG-CSF in newborns with presumed sepsis: absence of toxicity and induction of significant neutrophilia and bone marrow storage and progenitor pools [Abstract]. Pediatr Res 1993;33:1724.
11. Christensen R, Rothstein G. Pitfalls in the interpretation of leukocyte counts of newborn infants. Am J Clin Pathol 1979;72:608-11.
12. Avery GB. Neonatology: pathophysiology and management of the newborn. Philadelphia: Lippincott, 1987;1359-60.
13. Mouzinho A, Rosenfeld C, Sanchez P, Risser R. Revised reference ranges for circulating neutrophils in very-low-birth-weight neonates. Pediatrics 1994;94:76-82.

Effect of granulocyte colony-stimulating factor on preeclampsia-associated neonatal neutropenia

Edmund F. La Gamma, MD, Oral Alpan, MD, and
Prabhakar Kocherlakota, MD

From the Department of Pediatrics and Neurobiology, State University of New York at Stony Brook

Absolute neutropenia lasting longer than 72 hours after birth occurred in four very low birth weight neonates with a maternal history of severe pregnancy-induced hypertension, and was treated with recombinant granulocyte colony-stimulating factor for 3 days. Absolute neutrophil counts increased nearly fourfold within 48 hours; maximal values were recorded on the ninth day after the infusion was started. Total leukocyte counts subsequently decreased but remained in the normal range. It appears that recombinant human granulocyte colony-stimulating factor promotes a rapid increase in circulating neutrophils in these patients despite the possible presence of a circulating preeclampsia-associated inhibitor of neutrophil production. (J PEDIATR 1995;126:457-9)

Neutropenia (absolute neutrophil count <1500/mm^3) is frequently observed in the newborn infant with birth asphyxia, extreme prematurity, or intrauterine growth retardation, or after a pregnancy complicated by preeclampsia.[1-7] Although 80% of preeclampsia-associated neutropenia resolves by 60 hours of postnatal age, neutropenia may persist for as long as 30 days.[1, 7] We identified four premature infants with intrauterine growth retardation and very low birth weight who were the products of pregnancies complicated by severe preeclampsia. Each neonate had persistent neutropenia for more than 72 hours after birth. We treated these infants with recombinant human granulocyte colony-stimulating factor to raise their neutrophil count.

CASE REPORTS

Three boys (536 gm, 593 gm, 905 gm) and one girl (637 gm) with gestational ages between 25 and 30 weeks were each delivered by cesarean section to women with severe preeclampsia (systolic blood pressures, 230 to 250 mm Hg; diastolic, 100 to 130 mm Hg). The hypertension was controlled with magnesium sulfate, hydralazine, and methyldopa. Neonatal management included mechanical ventilation, placement of vascular catheters, and empiric antibiotic therapy with ampicillin and gentamicin after culture of body fluids. All cultures subsequently showed no growth, and administration of antibiotics was discontinued on day 3. The initial ANC count in each patient was <1500 cells/mm^3 (Table). Two patients (boys) were given immune globulin (0.5 gm/kg intravenously; Sandoz) on an empiric basis for immunoprophylaxis. After a discussion with the parents regarding the risks of infection caused by the persistent neutropenia, a clinical trial of rhG-CSF (Amgen, Thousand Oaks, Calif.) was started on day 3 or 4 of life to increase the leukocyte count. One infant had *Staphylococcus epidermidis* sepsis at 3 weeks of age and later died during the sixth week of hospitalization of a cardiorespiratory arrest after an episode of aspiration pneumonia. A second infant had *Klebsiella pneumoniae* septicemia at 5 weeks of postnatal age after completing 2 courses of dexamethasone but was successfully treated with antibiotics. The girl's mother also received cyclosporine and azathioprine for systemic lupus erythematosus; this neonate was never infected and continues to do well. The fourth patient was weaned from positive airway pressure to room air by 9 days of age and was never infected.

See related article, p. 454.

ANC	Absolute neutrophil count
rhG-CSF	Recombinant human granulocyte colony-stimulating factor
VLBW	Very low birth weight

RESULTS

Granulocyte colony-stimulating factor was administered in three daily doses of 10 μg/kg per day[8-10] as a 2- or 4-hour

Submitted for publication Aug. 8, 1994; accepted Oct. 18, 1994.
Reprint requests: Edmund F. La Gamma, MD, Pediatrics/Neurobiology, State University of New York HSC 11-060, Stony Brook NY 11794-8111.

0022-3476/95/$3.00 + 0 **9/24/61401**

Table. Peripheral leukocyte response to rhG-CSF in four VLBW neonates with intrauterine growth retardation

Type of leukocyte	Absolute cell count before and at 3 time points after rhG-CSF infusion: At time zero	At 48 hr	At 72 hr	At 7-10 days	Peak value	Peak day*
PMN	582 ± 110	1709 ± 603	3366 ± 1428	5119 ± 1317	8074 ± 1488†	Day 9
Band cells	148 ± 49	1585 ± 597	2337 ± 963	2369 ± 747	2606 ± 735‡	Day 8
ANC total	747 ± 109	3320 ± 1202	5703 ± 2374	7494 ± 1559	11281 ± 1989‡	Day 9
Lymphocytes	2422 ± 438	3332 ± 708	2731 ± 889	4639 ± 1267	5761 ± 1688	Day 9
Monocytes	729 ± 263	1757 ± 696	2771 ± 1020	3531 ± 1271	3799 ± 894§	Day 8

Values represent mean ± SEM per cubic millimeter.
PMN, Polymorphonuclear leukocytes.
**Peak day* refers to the number of days after the first dose of rhG-CSF.
†$p < 0.01$ versus time zero by paired t test.
‡$p < 0.02$ versus time zero by paired t test.
§$p < 0.04$ versus time zero by paired t test.

intravenous infusion in 2 or 4 ml of 0.2% albumin and 5% glucose water (final concentration, 5 μg/ml). The response to rhG-CSF was nearly identical in each case. The total neutrophil count increased nearly fourfold within 48 hours of the start of the administration of rhG-CSF, and peaked at a value nearly 15-fold higher ($p < 0.02$) than at the initiation of therapy less than 1 week after it was discontinued (Table). The ratio of band cells to polymorphonuclear cells (i.e., the immature/total cell ratio) ranged from 1.0 to 5.0 (data not shown). As reported for adults,[11, 12] a transient increase in the absolute monocyte count ($p < 0.04$) but no change in the absolute lymphocyte count was observed (Table). In each case there was no evidence of worsening of respiratory function, skin reaction, irritability, electrolyte disturbance, or change in cardiovascular performance that could be attributed to the infusion of rhG-CSF. All cultures of body fluid obtained during the three daily infusions remained sterile.

DISCUSSION

Preeclampsia is the most commonly recognized condition associated with neonatal neutropenia; 6% of all pregnancies are complicated by pregnancy-induced hypertension, and nearly 50% of the infants delivered have an ANC below the lower limit of normal for postnatal age.[1-7] The significant hematopoietic response that we observed in our patients indicates that VLBW neonates who are at increased risk of having an infection because of their persistent neutropenia may benefit from rhG-CSF treatment. Of particular interest is recent evidence indicating that a circulating factor may suppress neonatal neutrophil proliferative and storage pools.[1, 7] Our findings suggest the possibility that the effects of this bone marrow inhibitor could be overcome by this cytokine.

The rhG-CSF treatment resulted in a rapid initial increase in the ANC by 48 hours after drug administration; this likely represents a sudden egress of neutrophils into the circulation from the bone marrow, rather than cell division. A larger late response occurred >7 days after completion of the infusion and is more likely a result of an increase in the progenitor cell pool, facilitated mitosis of neutrophil lineage, or both of these mechanisms. The coincident abrupt increase in the absolute band cell count, the marked change in the percentage of band cells to nearly 30% of all circulating leukocytes, and the fact that the immature/total neutrophil cell ratio increased promptly after drug treatment are each *atypical* for the recovering bone marrow in neonates with persistent preeclampsia-induced neutropenia.[1-6] Moreover, these apparent rhG-CSF effects exceeded the typical neonatal leukocyte responses to bacteremia.[6] Consequently, because our patients were not infected at the time of rhG-CSF treatment, we feel confident in attributing the changes in their neutrophil counts to the effects of the rhG-CSF administered.

Additional support for the specificity of the rhG-CSF effects comes from comparison with three other reports.[8-10] In the first, a VLBW patient received rhG-CSF at 3 months of postnatal age (because of recurrent *Staphylococcus aureus*, *S. epidermidis*, and group B streptococcus infections); yet the timing of his leukocyte cell responses paralleled those of our four patients.[8] In the second case, rhG-CSF was thought to contribute to the ultimate survival of a 1500 gm 1-day-old neonate with *Escherichia coli* sepsis and neutropenia.[9] Although the neutrophil count also appeared to increase in response to the rhG-CSF, he also received a granulocyte transfusion and intravenously administered immune globulin and antibiotics, which complicates interpretation of the rhG-CSF effects.[9] In the third case, Cairo et al.[13] showed similar increases in circulating neutrophils, as well as in the bone marrow neutrophil storage pool, in granulocyte-macrophage colony-forming units, and in granulocyte-erythrocyte-macrophage-megakaryocyte colony-forming units, but no changes in the neutrophil progenitor pool.

Our success in rapidly elevating the neutrophil cell count with rhG-CSF to a range presumed to be normal is significant, particularly for phagocytic cells with a half-life of just 7 hours.[12] Moreover, functional defects in neonatal neutrophil chemotaxis, killing capacity, and bone marrow egress in the presence of a reduced progenitor pool size[1, 13] all support use of rhG-CSF in these VLBW patients. Although neutrophil counts less than $1.0 \times 10^9/L$ ($1000/mm^3$) are associated with increased risk of bacterial sepsis, even in well infants,[3-6] it is not well established whether increased cell counts alone will reduce the incidence of infection in affected neutropenic neonates.[1-4] Until randomized trials are performed, the use of rhG-CSF in the neonatal intensive care unit should be considered experimental therapy.

We thank Drs. J. DeCristofaro, H. Fleit, R. Parker, and L. I. Kleinman for their helpful suggestions and comments in the preparation of this article.

REFERENCES

1. Koenig JM, Christensen RD. Incidence, neutrophil kinetics, and natural history of neonatal neutropenia associated with maternal hypertension. N Engl J Med 1989;321:557-62.
2. Mouzinho A, Rosenfeld CR, Sanchez PJ, Risser R. Effect of maternal hypertension on neonatal neutropenia and risk of nosocomial infection. Pediatrics 1992;90:430-5.
3. Cadnapaphornchai M, Faix RG. Increased nosocomial infections in neutropenic low birth weight (2000 gm or less) infants of hypertensive mothers. J Pediatr 1992;121:956-61.
4. Doran MW, Makhlouf RA, Katz VL, Lawson EE, Stiles AD. Increased incidence of sepsis at birth in neuropenic infants of mothers with preeclampsia. J Pediatr 1994;125:452-8.
5. Baley JE, Stork EK, Warkentin PI, Shurin SB. Neonatal neutropenia clinical manifestations, cause, and outcome. Am J Dis Child 1988;142:1161-6.
6. Rodwell RL, Taylor K, Tudehope DI, Gray PH. Hematologic scoring system in early diagnosis of sepsis in neutropenic newborns. Pediatr Infect Dis J 1993;12:372-6.
7. Koenig JM, Christensen RD. The mechanism responsible for diminished neutrophil production in neonates delivered of women with pregnancy-induced hypertension. Am J Obstet Gynecol 1991;165:467-73.
8. Roberts RL, Szelc CM, Scates SM, et al. Neutropenia in an extremely premature infant treated with recombinant human granulocyte colony-stimulating factor. Am J Dis Child 1991; 145:808-12.
9. Murray JC, McClain KL, Wearden ME. Using granulocyte colony-stimulating factor for neutropenia during neonatal sepsis. Arch Pediatr Adolesc Med 1994;148:764-6.
10. Gillan E, Christensen RS, Kuenn K, et al. A randomized placebo controlled trial of RhG-CSF in newborns with presumed sepsis: significant induction of peripheral and bone marrow neutrophilia. Blood 1994;84:1427-33.
11. Daifuku R, Andresen J, Morstyn G. Recombinant methionyl human granulocyte colony-stimulating factor for the prevention and treatment of non-neutropenic infectious diseases. J Antimicrob Chemother 1993;32(suppl A):91-7.
12. Nelson S. Role of granulocyte colony-stimulating factor in the immune response to acute bacterial infection in the nonneutropenic host: an overview. Clin Infect Dis 1994;18(suppl 2):S197-204.
13. Cairo MS, VandeVen C, Toy C, et al. Lymphokines: enhancement by granulocyte-macrophage and granulocyte colony-stimulating factors of neonatal myeloid kinetics and functional activation of polymorphonuclear leukocytes. Rev Infect Dis 1990;12(suppl 4):S492-7.

THE BOOK SHELF **André D. Lascari,** *Editor*

Book reviews

Respiratory illness in children

Phelan PD, Olinsky A, Robertson CF. London: Blackwell Scientific Publications, 1994. 414 pages. $125.

This text of pediatric pulmonary disorders covers the subject matter with two different approaches. Several of the chapters are organized according to symptoms and signs of disease, such as cough, respiratory noises, and clinical patterns of acute respiratory infections. Other chapters are disease oriented, such as those on asthma, cystic fibrosis, tuberculosis, and congenital malformations. There are epidemiologic data on almost every topic, much of which are from Britain or Australia. Some of the medications described (e.g., budesonide for asthma) are not approved for use in the United States.

The writing is very clear and easy to read, and the topics covered as thematic chapters are up-to-date and complete. However, the book fails as a reference tool for the clinician or student. For example, researching a topic such as "RSV bronchiolitis" would require reading from two or three separate chapters to cover the topic completely. Although there is little repetition among these sections, it is distracting to have to search through different sections on the same topic.

To the credit of the publishers, this text has the best-reproduced radiographs of many similar works. The topic of infection in the immunocompromised host, including lung disease caused by the human immunodeficiency virus, is well covered. The chapter on sleep-related disorders briefly touches the major aspects without much detail, whereas the chapter on congenital malformations is very detailed. This is an example of the imbalance of coverage of topics.

The place of this text in the field of pediatric pulmonary medicine is unclear. Readers wishing a more extensive treatment of many topics will have to look elsewhere; those reading in this field for the first time may become frustrated by the fragmentation of topics. For a slightly higher price, the market offers better texts covering pediatric pulmonology.

Robert A. Kaslovsky, MD
Associate Professor of Pediatrics
Assistant Director, Pediatric Pulmonary and Cystic Fibrosis Center
Albany Medical College
Albany, NY 12208

The clinical recognition of congenital heart disease. 4th ed.

Perloff JK. Philadelphia: WB Saunders, 1994. 797 pages. $110.

This textbook is devoted solely to congenital heart disease. Its coverage of the diagnostic aspects of the malformations exceeds in detail that of general textbooks of pediatrics and medicine. Often it gives even more information than a textbook of pediatric or adult cardiology. It is especially strong on the historical development of today's knowledge. Many early literature references that have disappeared from more conventional texts of pediatric cardiology are included. The book avoids the whole area of treatment and emphasizes the natural history of the untreated child and adult, valuable information for someone planning to practice in a developing country. Another great strength is the rational explanation of physical findings. It correlates the clinical with the laboratory findings very well.

The author makes a sincere effort to teach, and does so in a patient, somewhat ponderous style. After a relatively easy but fascinating chapter on normal and innocent murmurs, he shifts gears to a chapter on malpositions of the heart, one of the most confusing areas of congenital heart disease. This topic is handled more than adequately, with unflagging attention to the definition of terms and descriptions of clinical situations. This chapter sets the tone for a book that should appeal to scholarly individuals who have plenty of time for reading. Terse it is not. There are 32 chapters, and virtually every known lesion is given very thorough coverage. My only strong objection is that a chapter is devoted to "primary endocardial fibroelastosis" as though it were a disease entity, when it is known to be a pathologic reaction to myocardial malfunction of diverse origins. I hope the author will call it "fetal cardiomyopathy" in the next edition.

This is the fourth edition of a work first published in 1970, and being of single authorship, it has not changed its approach. Since the third edition, published in 1987, the echocardiographic sections relating to each lesion have been updated and many new references have been added. I believe that medical libraries should have this book, which provides much detail that is difficult to find. It is a useful reference for specialists, not a tool for a generalist needing to get the gist of a problem in a hurry.

Paul R. Lurie, MD
Professor of Pediatrics
Albany Medical College
Albany, NY 12208

Intravenous morphine pharmacokinetics in pediatric patients with sickle cell disease

Carlton D. Dampier, MD, B. N. Y. Setty, PhD, Joann Logan, BA, Jacqueline G. Ioli, MS, and Roger Dean, PharmD

From the Marian Anderson Sickle Cell Anemia Care and Research Center at St. Christopher's Hospital for Children and the Department of Pediatrics, Temple University School of Medicine, Philadelphia, Pennsylvania, and the Department of Pharmacy, University of Chicago Medical Center, Chicago, Illinois

To examine the pharmacokinetics of parenteral opioids, such as morphine, in patients with sickle cell disease, we determined the plasma morphine clearances in 18 patients (aged 6 to 19 years) who were receiving continuous intravenous infusions, and the pharmacokinetics of morphine in an additional six patients after single intravenous doses. Plasma morphine clearances ranged from 6.2 to 59.1 ml min^{-1} kg^{-1} (35.5 ± 12.4, mean ± SD) during steady-state infusions. There was a negative correlation between clearance values and age over the age range studied ($p = 0.013$). A significant difference ($p = 0.042$) was also observed in clearance values between patients who had serious adverse symptoms (23.4 ± 10.7 ml min^{-1} kg^{-1}) and those who had less serious symptoms (36.3 ± 6.4 ml min^{-1} kg^{-1}) when morphine was given at high dosage rates (≥0.15 mg kg^{-1} hr^{-1}). Pharmacokinetic modeling of plasma morphine concentrations adequately fit a two-compartment model with a short initial distribution phase (mean half-life = 4.5 minutes) and a rapid terminal elimination half-life (77.6 ± 19.2 minutes). These findings suggest that considerable individualization of morphine dosing may be necessary to achieve optimal analgesia and minimal adverse effects in these patients. (J Pediatr 1995;126:461-7)

The most common and debilitating complication of sickle cell disease is recurrent vaso-occlusive pain.[1] The typical frequency of hospital-treated pain in individuals with SCD is between 0.5 and 1.0 episodes per patient-year.[2] However, 5% of patients with sickle cell anemia have between 3 and 10 hospital visits for pain treatment each year. Treatment of such severe painful episodes has been largely empiric, and most studies have focused on pain treatment in the emergency department setting.[3-5] Those aimed at treatment of hospitalized patients have described the use of parenteral narcotics delivered by continuous infusion[6, 7] or by patient-controlled analgesia.[8-11] Some patients had treatment failures, or required much larger doses of narcotics than others to achieve adequate pain relief.

We sought to determine the pharmacokinetics of intravenously administered morphine in our pediatric patients with SCD within the context of their clinical care for painful episodes. We also wished to examine the relation between morphine infusion dosage rates (and plasma morphine concentration) and the subsequent incidence of drug-related side effects such as nausea, excessive sedation, uri-

AIC	Akaike information criterion
SCD	Sickle cell disease

Supported in part by a grant from the Gustavus and Louise Pfeiffer Research Foundation.

Submitted for publication April 5, 1994; accepted Oct. 3, 1994.

Reprint requests: Carlton Dampier, MD, Marian Anderson Sickle Cell Center, St. Christopher's Hospital for Children, Erie Avenue at Front Street, Philadelphia, PA 19134-1095.

0022-3476/95/$3.00 + 0 **9/25/61033**

Table. Patient characteristics

	Continuous infusion	Single dose
Age (yr)	14.7 ± 4.3	16.0 ± 4.9
Gender		
Male: No. (%)	10 (55.5)	1 (17)
Female	8 (45.5)	5 (83)
Hemoglobin level (gm dl^{-1})	85.1 ± 15.5	80.3 ± 11.2
Dose rate (mg kg^{-1} hr^{-1})	0.123 ± 0.042	NA
Plasma clearance (ml min^{-1} kg^{-1})	35.5 ± 12.4	34.4 ± 14.3
Terminal elimination half-life (min)	78.7 ± 21.5	77.6 ± 19.2

Values (except gender) expressed as mean ± SD.
NA, Not applicable.

nary retention, and clinically significant respiratory depression. A more thorough understanding of the dose-response relationship of these side effects would improve the safety of narcotic analgesic therapy in these patients.

METHODS

Patients who were hospitalized for vaso-occlusive pain and had normal renal and hepatic function were eligible for these studies. All patients studied were not tolerant to morphine or other narcotics, as judged from their history of prior narcotic usage, and were not currently receiving medications known to cross-react with our morphine assay (codeine, hydromorphone). Concurrent medications in most patients included acetaminophen, ibuprofen, and cefuroxime. Both studies had the approval of our local institutional review board, and informed consent was obtained from either the patient or the patient's parent or guardian.

We initially studied children and adolescents with SCD who were hospitalized for severe painful episodes and were given continuous infusions of morphine because of pain that was refractory to dosing every 2 hours. Most patients were studied within 24 to 48 hours of infusion initiation. However, some studies were done later to allow blood sampling at lower morphine dosage rates. Blood samples were obtained after the patient had been receiving a stable morphine dose for at least 24 hours, because little prior information was available that described morphine half-lives in this patient population. A routine hemoglobin determination was also done on one of these blood samples. Steady-state morphine concentrations were calculated as the average value for 2 to 4 separate samples taken 1 to 4 hours apart. Six patients were studied on successive days at different dose rates or during subsequent hospitalizations at the same or different dose rates. Four patients had hourly blood samples obtained after their morphine infusions were discontinued to determine the half-life of morphine under steady-state conditions. The presence or absence of adverse side effects was determined by patient self-report.

Six consecutive patients were given single intravenous morphine doses to characterize the pharmacokinetics of morphine given by intermittent dosing. Five patients were studied during a hospitalization for treatment of a painful episode, three of these during their first 2 hospital days and two on their last hospital day. Because of difficulty with intravenous access, one patient was studied as an outpatient 1 to 2 weeks after hospitalization. Patients having pain during these study periods were treated with either parenterally or orally administered meperidine depending on their pain intensity. Morphine sulfate at a dose of 0.15 to 0.20 mg kg^{-1} was given into a free-flowing intravenous line for 30 seconds, between 9 and 10 AM in the morning, after an overnight fast. Morphine doses were given no sooner than 2 hours after a previous meperidine dose. Patients remained recumbent in bed for the first 2 hours of the study, and a light lunch was allowed between 1 and 2 hours later. Blood samples were obtained from an indwelling catheter at 5, 10, 15, 20, 30, 45, 60, 90, 120, 180, 240, 300, and 360 minutes after injection of morphine. Pain intensity was assessed at these times by patient self-report with either a verbal 0 to 10 categorical scale or a written questionnaire consisting of visual analog and categorical scales[12, 13] until the patients requested remedication with additional narcotic analgesics.

Blood samples were placed in heparinized glass tubes, and plasma was obtained by centrifugation and stored at −70° C until analysis. Morphine plasma levels were measured with a highly specific radioimmunoassay (Coat-a-Count; Diagnostic Products Corp., Los Angeles, Calif.). Plasma samples of 25 μl were assayed in triplicate. Results were compared with logit plots of morphine standards by means of software provided with the Wallac Twin-Gamma gamma counter. The within and between assay coefficients of variance were 7% and 10%, respectively, at 140 to 175 nm L^{-1} (40 to 50 ng ml^{-1}). Data provided by the manufacturer indicated a cross-reactivity of 0.3% with morphine-3-glucuronide and of 0.15% with morphine-6-glucuronide, the two major morphine metabolites.

Morphine plasma clearance was calculated from the morphine dose rate and the steady-state morphine plasma concentration obtained from the continuous infusion studies. Pharmacokinetic parameters for single-dose studies were calculated with PCNONLIN version 4.2 software (SCI Software; ClinTrials, Inc., Lexington, Ky.). Appropriateness of the fit to the models was judged on the basis of calculated output parameters, including estimated standard errors of parameters, and on the basis of a calculated Akaike information criterion.[14] The results reported had AIC values in the range of 40 to 60 for a two-compartment

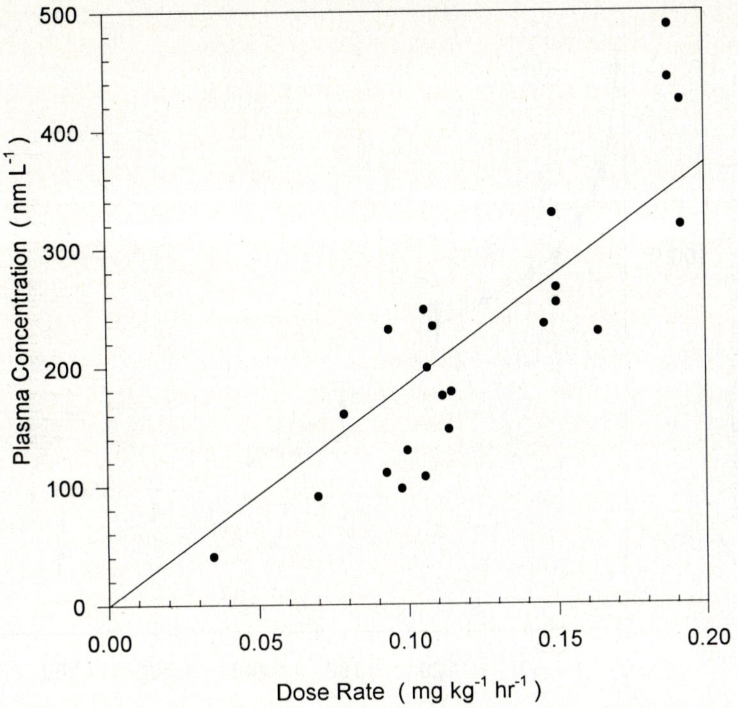

Fig. 1. Effect of dose rate on plasma concentration. Plasma morphine concentration as a function of continuous infusion dose rate over the range of dose rates studied (0.035 to 0.195 mg $kg^{-1}hr^{-1}$).

model. The relation between continuous variables such as morphine clearance and age or hemoglobin concentration, and between morphine plasma concentration and dose rate, were analyzed by regression analysis using a general linear model. Because the distribution of clearance values did not follow a normal distribution, comparison of mean clearance values in different groups was analyzed with the Mann-Whitney U test statistic from the Kruskal-Wallis procedure.

RESULTS

We studied 18 patients who received continuous infusions of morphine (Table). Although this group of patients represented a convenience sample, it included the majority of patients receiving this therapy in the 1990–1992 period at our institution. The morphine dose rates of 0.035 to 0.206 mg kg^{-1} hr^{-1} were similar or somewhat higher than those reported in other studies.[6]

Adverse symptoms sufficiently severe to require reduction of infusion dose rates occurred during five of six infusions with morphine levels >315 nm L^{-1} (90 ng ml^{-1}) and included excessive sedation, frequent emesis, or urinary retention. These occurred at dose rates of 0.15 mg kg^{-1} hr^{-1} or more, although some patients with rapid morphine clearances tolerated this dose rate without serious side effects. No clinically serious respiratory depression was noted (i.e., no hypopnea or bradycardia), but all patients at dose rates >0.15 mg kg^{-1} hr^{-1} required supplemental oxygen to maintain an oxygen saturation greater than 94%. End-tidal or arterial carbon dioxide tension were not measured. Some patients continued to report severe pain despite these adverse effects from high morphine levels.

As shown in Fig. 1, there was a linear relationship between the morphine dose rate and the plasma morphine concentration ($r = 0.45$; $p = 0.028$). This suggests that there were no dose-dependent changes in morphine pharmacokinetic parameters in the dosage range studied. The mean coefficient of variance for serial steady-state samples was 10%. Plasma clearance of morphine ranged from 6.2 to 59.1 ml min^{-1} kg^{-1} (35.5 ± 12.4, mean ± SD) in the 18 patients (Table). Six patients had morphine clearance remeasured; four studies were obtained during their next admission and two studies during subsequent admissions. The mean coefficient of variance of these additional clearance values was 12.1%.

There was no difference between mean clearance values for male patients (33.2 ± 13.0 ml min^{-1} kg^{-1}, mean ± SD) and those for female patients (42.2 ± 14.2 ml min^{-1} kg^{-1}, mean ± SD; $p = 0.182$). However, there was a significant negative correlation between morphine clearance values

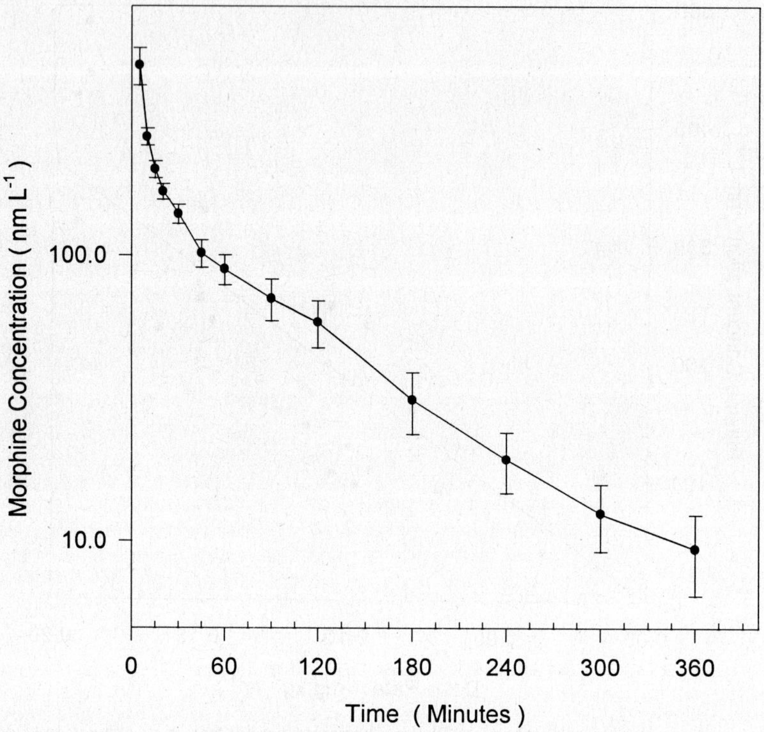

Fig. 2. Plasma concentrations from single-dose studies. Mean plasma morphine concentration from six patients, obtained after a single intravenous dose of morphine (data normalized to a dose of 0.2 mg kg^{-1}) as a function of time in minutes after dose was administered. The *error bars* represent the standard error of the mean for each time point.

and age within the age range of the patients studied ($r = -0.573$; $p = 0.013$). A similar relation was noted between morphine clearance and the hemoglobin concentration at the time of the clearance determination ($r = -0.513$; $p = 0.035$). When both hemoglobin concentration and age were incorporated into a multiple linear regression model, age appeared to be the dominant factor ($p = 0.033$ vs $p = 0.296$). Because all but two patients were homozygous for sickle hemoglobin, it was not possible to examine the relation between morphine clearance and type of hemoglobinopathy. Although there was considerable overlap in clearance values, a significant difference ($p = 0.042$) was observed between clearance levels in patients who had severe symptoms (23.4 ± 10.7 ml min^{-1} kg^{-1}, mean ± SD) and those in patients who had less severe symptoms (36.3 ± 6.4 ml min^{-1} kg^{-1}, mean ± SD) when given high morphine dose rates (≥0.15 mg kg^{-1} hr^{-1}) for very severe pain. There was no difference in age or hemoglobin concentration between the two groups that could predict the differences in clearance values. The elimination half-life of morphine under steady-state conditions was determined in four patients by obtaining serial blood samples after their constant infusions were discontinued. The mean elimination half-life was 78.7 ± 21.5 minutes (Table).

Single-dose morphine pharmacokinetics were studied in six patients at intravenous bolus doses of 0.15 to 0.21 mg kg^{-1} (Table). A two-compartment open model adequately fit the experimental data, according to the AIC for model assessment. Figure 2 displays the time course of mean plasma morphine levels obtained in this study and the line calculated from these data with a two-compartment open model. The initial distribution phase was short (mean half-life, 4.5 minutes). The mean terminal elimination half-life was 77.6 ± 19.2 minutes (mean ± SD). This value is similar to that obtained under steady-state conditions (Table), and is somewhat shorter than the ~120 minutes typically reported for normal individuals.[15, 16] Calculated mean clearance value was 34.4 ± 14.3 ml min^{-1} kg^{-1} (mean ± SD), which was similar to that obtained from the constant infusion data. The mean steady-state volume of distribution was 2.88 ± 0.76 L kg^{-1} (mean ± SD), a value consistent with morphine's known extensive tissue distribution.[15, 16] No adverse effects were reported during these single-dose studies. For the three patients in severe pain at the beginning of the study, the decrease in pain intensity peaked at 20 to 30 minutes. However, this represented only a 10% to 20% reduction from the initial pain intensity value. Pharmacodynamic modeling was not attempted on this small data set.

Figure 3 shows a computer simulation using a two-com-

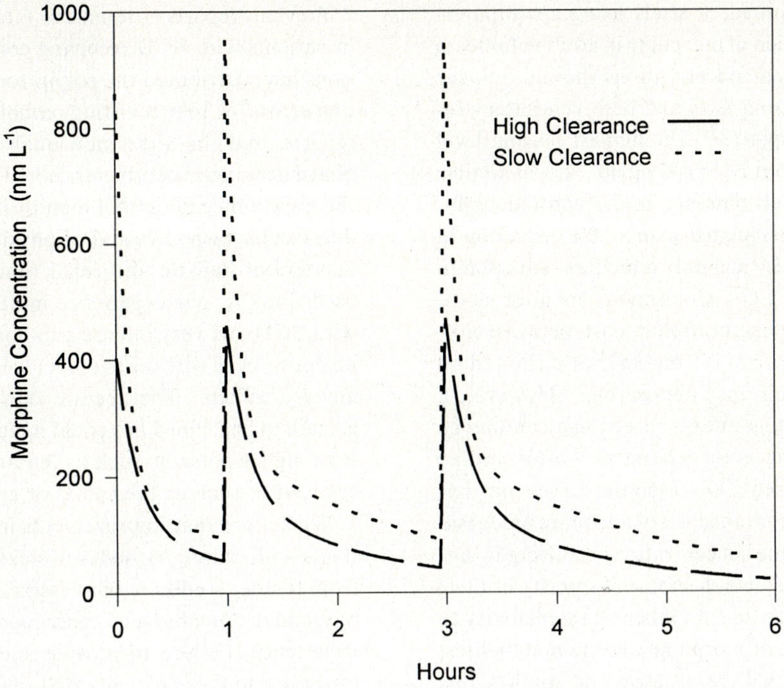

Fig. 3. Morphine concentrations in patients with slow versus high rates of clearance. Morphine plasma concentration versus time for an intravenous morphine dose, 0.15 mg kg^{-1}, at baseline and at 1 and 3 hours, obtained by computer simulation using PCNONLIN for a patient with a morphine clearance value of 27.5 ml min^{-1} kg^{-1} (slow clearance: *dotted line*) or a patient with a morphine clearance value of 56.7 ml min^{-1} kg^{-1} (high clearance: *dashed line*).

partment model of the plasma morphine concentrations that would be attained from a 0.15 mg kg^{-1} dose given intravenously at baseline and at 1 and 3 hours; the single-dose pharmacokinetic parameters for a patient with a slower, nearly normal clearance (27.5 ml min^{-1} kg^{-1}) were contrasted with those for a patient with a high plasma morphine clearance (56.7 ml min^{-1} kg^{-1}). The initial peak morphine plasma concentration is much lower and falls to lower values more quickly in the patient with the more rapid clearance.

DISCUSSION

Our data demonstrate a greater than eightfold range of morphine clearance values, which is consistent with the interpatient variability noted in other patient groups.[15, 16] Previous studies of children in the postoperative period[17] and of pediatric patients with cancer[18] who were receiving parenteral morphine therapy reported morphine plasma clearances of 22 to 25 ml min^{-1} kg^{-1}. In comparison, the plasma clearance of morphine in our patients with sickle cell anemia was substantially higher, whether measured during single-dose or steady-state conditions. This finding is similar to that of previous reported data on continuous infusions.[19] We observed differences in morphine clearances that were correlated with patient age and hemoglobin level, with patient age being the dominant factor. Our finding of increased morphine clearance in younger children is similar to a previously reported study of children with SCD.[19] Differences in the steady-state morphine levels associated with "toxicity," 315 nm L^{-1} (90 ng ml^{-1}) versus 105 nm L^{-1} (30 ng ml^{-1}), between our study and this previous study reflect differences in the severity of adverse symptoms required for this classification, rather than any apparent differences in drug effects. The high intensity of pain in many of our patients may also have antagonized some of the respiratory depression that might otherwise have been associated with these high morphine dose rates.

We believe that the increased morphine clearance is caused by disease- or anemia-related changes in physiologic variables, such as renal or hepatic blood flow, that could lead to accelerated renal excretion or metabolic (liver or kidney) clearance of morphine.[20, 21] It is also possible that these physiologic variables are further altered during painful episodes because of fever, worsening anemia, or concurrent medications. These same physiologic variables may also influence the pharmacokinetics of the principal morphine metabolites, morphine-3-glucuronide and morphine-6-glucuronide; the latter likely has analgesic activity.[22, 23] These disease-related changes may be superimposed on differences in morphine clearance related to ethnicity, as recently reported for individuals of Asian origin.[24]

Information about the dose-response relation for adverse

effects of morphine is limited. A study using a computer-controlled constant infusion of morphine in adult volunteers at several different plasma concentrations showed a linear relationship between plasma level and both ventilatory response and analgesic response.[25] The highest plasma level of morphine tested, 350 nm L^{-1} (100 ng ml^{-1}), was similar to the higher plasma levels obtained in our continuous-infusion studies, and was associated with a 50% reduction in experimental pain intensity and only a modest reduction in ventilatory response to CO_2. Continuous monitoring of end-tidal CO_2 and oxygen saturation in postoperative children receiving a single dose of 0.1 mg kg^{-1} also showed no clinically significant respiratory depression.[26] However, a study of newborn and young infants receiving a continuous morphine infusion yielding levels $\geq$20 ng ml^{-1} after cardiac surgery observed depressed CO_2-response curves and hypercapnia.[27] We believe that the lack of adequate analgesia in our patients at morphine concentrations resulting in significant adverse effects reflects the unusual severity of their vaso-occlusive pain, rather than an inherent insensitivity to the pharmacologic effect of morphine and its metabolites; however, further studies will be necessary to confirm this point.

There are several implications of the increased clearance in our patients with SCD. The slope of the dose-plasma morphine concentration curve for continuous infusions is likely to be less steep for patients with higher clearance values. Thus the steady-state plasma morphine concentration will be lower for a given morphine dosage, and increased dose rates will yield lower incremental increases in morphine concentration. This effect may cause a weaker analgesic response at a given dose or a poorer response to increasing dosages, potentially leading to a false clinical conclusion that the pain experienced by these patients is "not physiologic," or that the patient has a "tolerance" to the pharmacologic effect of morphine because of prior narcotic exposure. Rather, these patients require a larger dose to attain a similar morphine plasma concentration and hence a similar degree of analgesia.

Similar clearance effects are seen with intermittent dosing. Morphine administration on a more frequent dosing schedule in patients with a high clearance rate has little effect on the initial peak concentrations. The somewhat higher concentrations remaining after 1- or 2-hour intervals result in a higher plasma morphine concentration profile that is likely to provide somewhat more effective and consistent analgesia. Because the large tissue distribution and short elimination half-life in these patients cause a rapid fall in plasma morphine concentrations, patients with severe pain who require relatively high plasma concentrations of morphine for effective analgesia would receive more benefit from continuous infusions.

Previous reports of serious or fatal respiratory depression in patients with SCD receiving continuous morphine infusions have attributed the respiratory depression to medication errors[6] or to preexisting pathologic conditions.[28] These reports, and the wide individual variability in morphine pharmacokinetic parameters noted in our study, underscore the importance of careful monitoring of analgesic and cardiovascular responses and of physiologically important indicators of hepatic and renal function when this drug is used. Finally, our experience indicates that some patients with SCD and very intense pain may not achieve adequate analgesia even with doses of morphine that cause significant adverse effects. Therapeutic options for these patients remain to be defined but could include alternative narcotics with higher potency, such as fentanyl, or alternative delivery routes, such as the spinal or epidural route.[29]

We believe that improvements in the clinical care of patients with painful episodes in sickle cell disease can result from further studies of pain assessment, opioid pharmacology, and the psychosocial consequences of this complex pain experience. Failure to provide adequate analgesia does a disservice to these patients that may lead to significant adverse medical and psychologic sequelae.

REFERENCES

1. Shapiro BS. The management of pain in sickle cell disease. Pediatr Clin North Am 1989;36:1029-45.
2. Platt OS, Thorington BD, Brambilla DJ, et al. Pain in sickle cell disease: rates and risk factors. N Engl J Med 1991;325:11-6.
3. Wright SW, Norris RL, Mitchell TR. Ketorolac for sickle cell vaso-occlusive crisis pain in the emergency department: lack of a narcotic-sparing effect. Ann Emerg Med 1992;21:925-8.
4. Gonzalez ER, Bahal N, Hansen LA, et al. Intermittent injection vs patient-controlled analgesia for sickle cell crisis pain: comparison in patients in the emergency department. Arch Intern Med 1991;151:1373-8.
5. Friedman EW, Webber AB, Osborn HH, Schwartz S. Oral analgesia for treatment of painful crisis in sickle cell anemia. Ann Emerg Med 1986;15:787-91.
6. Cole TB, Sprinkle RH, Smith SJ, Buchanan GR. Intravenous narcotic therapy for children with severe sickle cell pain crisis. Am J Dis Child 1986;140:1255-9.
7. Sartori PCE, Gordon GJ, Darbyshire PJ. Continuous papaveretum infusion for the control of pain in painful sickling crisis. Arch Dis Child 1990;65:1151-3.
8. McPherson E, Perlin E, Finke H, Castro O, Pittman J. Patient-controlled analgesia in patients with sickle cell vaso-occlusive crisis. Am J Med Sci 1990;299:10-2.
9. Shapiro BS, Cohen DE, Howe CJ. Patient-controlled analgesia for sickle-cell–related pain. J Pain Symptom Manage 1993;8:22-8.
10. Schechter NL, Berrien FB, Katz SM. The use of patient-controlled analgesia in adolescents with sickle cell pain crisis: a preliminary report. J Pain Symptom Manage 1988;3:109-13.
11. Holbrook CT. Patient-controlled analgesia: pain management

for children with sickle cell disease. J Assoc Acad Minor Phys 1990:1:93-6.

12. Walco GA, Dampier CD. Pain in children and adolescents with sickle cell disease: a descriptive study. Pediatr Psychol 1990;15: 643-58.
13. Ballas SK, Delengowski A. Pain measurement in hospitalized adults with sickle cell painful episodes. Ann Clin Lab Sci 1993;23:358-61.
14. Akaike S, Yamoka K, Nakagawa T, Uno T. Application of the Akaike information criterion in evaluation of linear pharmacokinetic equations. J Pharmacokinet Biopharm 1978;6:165-70.
15. Glare PA, Walsh TD. Clinical pharmacokinetics of morphine. Ther Drug Monit 1991;13:1-23.
16. Brunk SF, Delle M. Morphine metabolism in man. Clin Pharmacol Ther 1974;16:51-7.
17. McRorie TI, Lynn AM, Nespeca MK, Opheim KE, Slattery JT. The maturation of morphine clearance and metabolism. Am J Dis Child 1992;146:972-6.
18. Greene RF, Miser AW, Lester CM, Balis FM, Poplack DG. Cerebrospinal fluid and plasma pharmacokinetics of morphine infusions in pediatric cancer patients and rhesus monkeys. Pain 1987;30:339-48.
19. Robieux IC, Kellner JD, Coppes MJ, et al. Analgesia in children with sickle cell crises: comparison of intermittent opioids vs. continuous intravenous infusion of morphine and placebo-controlled study of oxygen inhalation. Pediatr Hematol Oncol 1992;9:317-26.
20. Milne RW, Nation RL, Somogyi AA, Bochner F, Griggs WM. The influence of renal function on the clearance of morphine and its glucuronide metabolities in intensive-care patients. Br J Clin Pharmacol 1992;34:53-9.
21. Crotty B, Watson KJR, Desmond PV, et al. Hepatic extraction of morphine is impaired in cirrhosis. Eur J Clin Pharmacol 1989;36:501-6.
22. Portenoy RK, Thaler HT, Inturrisi CE, Friedlander-Klar H, Foley KM. The metabolite morphine-6-glucuronide contributes to the analgesia produced by morphine infusion in patients with pain and normal renal function. Clin Pharmacol Ther 1992;51:422-31.
23. Osborne R, Thompson P, Joel S, Trew D, Patel N, Slevin M. The analgesic activity of morphine-6-glucuronide. Br J Clin Pharmacol 1992;34:130-8.
24. Zhou HH, Sheller JR, Nu H, Wood M, Wood AJ. Ethnic differences in response to morphine. Clin Pharmacol Ther 1994;54:507-13.
25. Hill HF, Chapman CR, Saeger LS, et al. Steady-state infusions of opioids in human. II. Concentration-effect relationships and therapeutic margins. Pain 1990;43:69-79.
26. Hamunen K. Ventilatory effects of morphine, pethidine and methadone in children. Br J Anaesth 1993;70:414-8.
27. Lynn AM, Nespeca MK, Opheim KE, Slattery JT. Respiratory effects of intravenous morphine infusions in neonates, infants, and children after cardiac surgery. Anesth Analg 1993; 77:695-701.
28. Gerber N, Apseloff G. Death from a morphine infusion during a sickle cell crisis. J PEDIATR 1993;123:322-5.
29. Yaster M, Tobin JR, Billett C, Casella JF, Dover G. Epidural analgesia in the management of severe vaso-occlusive sickle cell crisis. Pediatrics 1994;93:310-5.

Combination treatment with growth hormone and gonadotropin-releasing hormone analogs in short normal girls

Giuseppe Saggese, MD, Graziano Cesaretti, MD, Stefania Barsanti, MD, and Anna Rossi, MD.

From the Chair of Preventive Pediatrics, Department of Pediatrics, University of Pisa, Pisa, Italy

To improve final adult height, we treated with growth hormone (0.65 ± 0.07 (mean ± SD) IU · kg^{-1} · wk^{-1}) and gonadotropin-releasing hormone analogs (66 ± 9 μg · kg^{-1} every 28 days) a group of seven short normal girls in early puberty with a chronologic age (CA) of 11.50 ± 0.95 years, predicted adult height (PAH) lower ($0.003 < p < 0.001$) than mean target height, and without any endocrine abnormalities. The results were compared with those obtained in a similar group of seven untreated girls considered as control subjects. The mean period of combined therapy was 2.01 ± 0.52 years; in two subjects treatment is still in progress. The value of height standard deviation score for bone age (BA) improved from −1.69 ± 0.47 to −1.04 ± 0.56 ($p = 0.001$); height age (HA)/BA ratio also increased from 0.83 ± 0.05 to 0.90 ± 0.04 ($p < 0.01$), as did PAH (from 146.8 ± 4.4 to 152.9 ± 3.6 cm; $p < 0.002$). The ratio of gain in HA to gain in BA was 2.08 ± 0.78. Pubertal stages showed an arrest in five cases and a regression in the other two girls. After administration of gonadotropin-releasing hormone analogs was interrupted, in four of five girls growth hormone was administered alone for a further period of 6 to 18 months to improve their physiologic growth spurt. The present height in five girls is higher than PAH before therapy. In the treated girls the height values for BA, for BA/CA and HA/BA ratios, and for PAH were higher ($0.002 < p < 0.04$) than those in control subjects. This preliminary study demonstrates that combination therapy with growth hormone and gonadotropin-releasing hormone analogs in short, endocrinologically normal girls may be useful in improving both height prognosis and predicted adult height. Further studies are necessary to reach definitive conclusions regarding the efficacy of this kind of therapy. (J Pediatr 1995;126:468-73)

One of the most common forms of growth delay is short normal stature, which includes those short children who, in the absence of growth hormone deficiency and other organic or nonorganic diseases, have both normal timing of pubertal development and a restricted predicted adult height. The results obtained with growth-promoting treatments in this kind of short stature have been disappointing. Recent preliminary data demonstrated that long-term GH therapy, administered for 7 years, gave unsatisfactory results,[1] probably because of an inappropriate progression in bone maturation; these subjects have grown faster but have reached a final stature no taller than that predicted before

BA	Bone age
CA	Chronologic age
GH	Growth hormone
GnRHa	Gonadotropin-releasing hormone analogs
HA	Height age
PAH	Predicted adult height

Submitted for publication June 1, 1994; accepted Oct. 6, 1994.

Reprint requests: Giuseppe Saggese, MD, Chair of Preventive Pediatrics, Department of Pediatrics, University of Pisa, Via Roma, 35, 56125 Pisa, Italy.

0022-3476/95/$3.00 + 0 **9/25/61100**

Table. Auxologic findings in examined subjects

	Treated subjects			Control subjects	
	Before therapy	After combination therapy	Actual	At start of study	Actual
CA	11.50 ± 0.95	13.42 ± 0.79	14.35 ± 1.16	11.26 ± 0.57	14.64 ± 1.45
BA	11.45 ± 0.84	12.46 ± 0.44	13.47 ± 0.64	10.97 ± 0.80	14.78 ± 1.41
Height SDS-CA	−1.76 ± 0.59	−1.86 ± 0.70	−1.27 ± 0.47	−1.47 ± 0.71	−1.68 ± 0.60
Height SDS-BA	−1.69 ± 0.47	−1.04 ± 0.56	−0.88 ± 0.31	−1.23 ± 0.54	−1.70 ± 0.54
Weight Δ%	+17.0 ± 16.5	+19.7 ± 15.7	+19.7 ± 8.0	+7.3 ± 10.9	+6.1 ± 6.5
HA/CA ratio	0.83 ± 0.06	0.84 ± 0.05	0.87 ± 0.05	0.85 ± 0.08	0.83 ± 0.07
BA/CA ratio	1.00 ± 0.05	0.93 ± 0.04	0.94 ± 0.04	0.97 ± 0.04	1.01 ± 0.02
HA/BA ratio	0.83 ± 0.05	0.90 ± 0.04	0.92 ± 0.03	0.87 ± 0.06	0.82 ± 0.06
PHA	146.8 ± 4.4	152.9 ± 3.6	156.1 ± 2.1	149.0 ± 4.5	152.0 ± 3.4
ΔHA/ΔBA		2.08 ± 0.78	0.87 ± 0.29		0.71 ± 0.27

SDS, Standard deviation score; Δ%, variation in percentage; *ΔHA/ΔBA*, change in HA/change in BA ratio.
Statistical analysis was as follows: For treated subjects (1) after combination therapy versus pretreatment values, (a) height SDS-CA, weight Δ%, and HA/CA ratio, p = not significant; (b) height SDS-BA, $p = 0.001$; (c) BA/CA ratio, $p < 0.001$; (d) HA/BA ratio, $p < 0.01$; and (e) PHA, $p < 0.002$; and (2) actual values versus the moment of interruption of GnRHa, (a) ΔHA/ΔBA, $p < 0.04$; and (b) all other values, p = not significant. For examined subjects versus control subjects (1) before therapy, all values, p = not significant; and (2) after combination therapy, (a) height SDS-CA, weight Δ%, and HA/CA ratio, p = not significant; (b) height SDS-BA, $p < 0.02$; (c) BA/CA ratio and ΔHA/ΔBA, $p < 0.002$; (d) HA/BA ratio, $p < 0.01$; and (e) PHA, $p < 0.04$.

the commencement of GH treatment. On the other hand, the administration of gonadotropin-releasing hormone analogs to slow bone maturation and delay puberty, so as to prolong prepubertal growth and thereby improve adult height, also produced disappointing results[2, 3] because of a concomitant decrease in growth velocity.

These data provide support for combining GH and GnRHa in the treatment of short children who have entered puberty at the usual age without GH deficiency and with a poor height prognosis; the impairment in GnRHa-induced growth velocity could be counterbalanced by the growth-promoting effect of GH administration.[2, 4] Few preliminary data on combination treatment with GH and GnRHa in short, endocrinologically normal children are available, and they have given contrasting results. Some authors showed an improvement in height prognosis after 12 to 18 months[5-7]; others did not show any beneficial effect on predicted growth compared with that with GH treatment alone.[8]

We evaluated the effect of combination therapy with GH and GnRHa in a group of short girls with onset of puberty at the usual age, with low PAH, and without GH deficiency, who were treated for almost 2 years and were subsequently followed. We compared results with those in a similar group of untreated girls who were considered as control subjects.

METHODS

We examined seven short girls with CA ranging from 10.19 to 13.04 years at the beginning of the combination therapy with GH and GnRHa (auxologic features are reported in the Table). The girls had had normal birth weight and length. GH deficiency was excluded on the basis of sufficient responses (peak higher than 10 μg/L) to two stimuli (L-dopa and insulin-induced hypoglycemia) and was confirmed by normal spontaneous secretion (24-hour mean GH concentration >3 μg/L). Psychosocial deprivation syndrome, celiac disease, and other endocrine or nonendocrine systemic diseases were ruled out; the karyotype examination was normal. No hypothalamic-pituitary structural abnormalities were detected by magnetic resonance imaging.

Height, expressed as a standard deviation score for chronologic age, was evaluated according to the method of Tanner et al.[9] Mean target height was calculated according to Tanner.[10] Bone age was determined according to the Greulich-Pyle method[11] by two assessors (G.C. and S.B.) without knowledge of the identity of the subjects; in the few cases in which a discrepancy occurred, the radiograph was evaluated by the other two authors as well. PAH was calculated by the Bayley-Pinneau method.[12] Height was expressed also as a standard deviation score for BA.

Height age was calculated on the basis of the Tanner method[10] and pubertal stage according to this method. Weight was expressed also as a variation percentage from ideal value for HA on the basis of data of Tanner et al.[9]

One subject had at least one parent with height at the 3rd percentile; another four girls had at least one parent with stature under the 25th percentile, and the other two girls had no identifiable causes of short stature. Pubertal stage was Ph_1B_2, Ph_2B_2, Ph_2B_3, Ph_3B_3, and Ph_4B_3 in 2, 2, 1, 1, and 1 patients, respectively. They had plasma estradiol values of 17.4 ± 6.2 pg/ml (mean ± SD), plasma luteinizing hormone values after gonadotropin-releasing hormone administration of 7.4 ± 1.9 mU/ml, ultrasonic ovarian volume of 1.74 ± 0.43 ml, and uterine length of 45.8 ± 5.2 mm.

The study was approved by the ethics committee of the

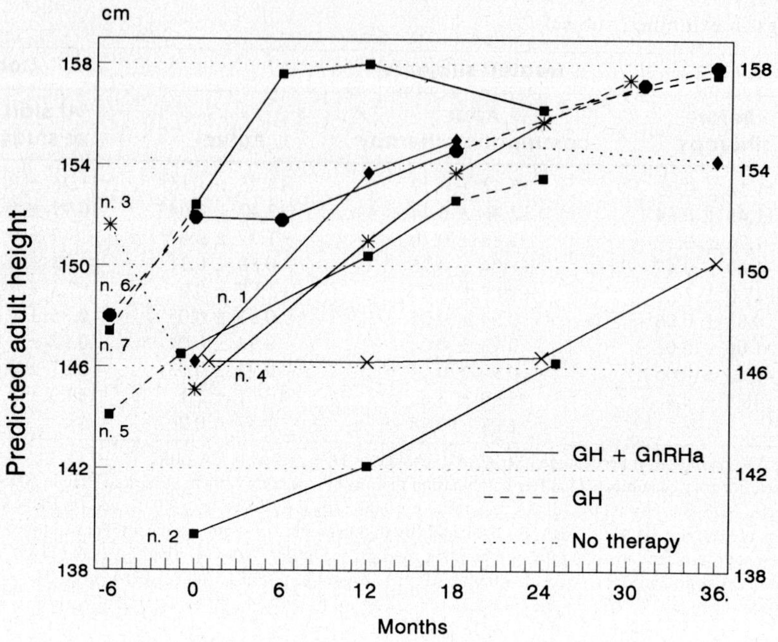

Fig. 1. Values of PAH in each patient during entire period of study.

University of Pisa Faculty of Medicine. Informed consent for the study was obtained from the children's parents. Treatment with GH and GnRHa was begun also on the basis of persistence of a discrepancy between PAH and mean target height (146.8 ± 4.4 vs 157.9 ± 3.3 cm; $p < 0.003$). The possible effects of the treatment, including the arrest or regression of pubertal development and the costs of the therapy, were discussed with patients and their parents after an accurate explanation of the girls' auxologic and endocrinologic patterns. The decision was then made jointly by patients and parents.

Growth hormone was given at the usual dose of 0.6 $IU \cdot kg^{-1} \cdot wk^{-1}$ divided into seven subcutaneous doses, and GnRHa (long-acting D-Trp-6-GnRH) was given at dose of 60 μg/kg intramuscularly every 28 days. Subjects 5, 6, and 7 had been treated with GH for a period of 6 months immediately before the beginning of GnRHa administration. As control subjects, we examined for a period of 3.09 ± 1.35 years a group of seven short girls with a PAH lower than mean target height (149.0 ± 4.5 vs 158.1 ± 4.6 cm; $p < 0.003$) and with no organic causes of short stature. During therapy, height, weight, and BA were evaluated every 6 months, as well as the following plasma values: estradiol, glucose, aminotransferases, cholesterol, triglycerides, leukocyte counts, thyroxin, and thyrotropin. In addition, ultrasonic examination of the ovaries and uterus was performed every 6 months.

Statistical methods employed to analyze the results were the paired and unpaired *t* tests.

RESULTS

The mean dose of GH was 0.65 ± 0.07 $IU \cdot kg^{-1} \cdot wk^{-1}$, and that of GnRHa was 66 ± 9 μg/kg every 28 days. The mean period of combined therapy was 2.01 ± 0.52 years: in subjects 2 and 4, treatment is still in progress. Auxologic features at the end of combination therapy (subjects 1, 3, 5 to 7) or at the time of the last examination (subjects 2 and 4) are reported in the Table.

The PAH values and the HA/BA ratio for each subject are reported in Figs. 1 and 2, respectively. During combination therapy, growth velocity was appropriate for CA, with an increase in HA of 1.80 ± 0.58 years. There was a slowing in bone maturation, so progression in BA was 1.01 ± 0.64 years. Increase in PAH was 3.95 ± 1.51 cm/yr of combination treatment. Pubertal stage showed an arrest in 5 girls and a regression in the other two. Ultrasonic measurements of the uterus and ovaries decreased significantly; plasma estradiol values fell to less than 10 pg/ml.

Subjects 3, 5, 6, and 7 underwent a further period of GH therapy of 6, 6, 18, and 12 months, respectively, after GnRHa administration; GH treatment is still in progress in patients 5, 6, and 7. Patient 1 did not accept GH administration: therefore, after interruption of the combination treatment, no further therapy was given. A progression in pubertal stage was noted in all girls; menarche appeared in subjects 5 and 6. Ultrasonic measurements of the uterus and ovaries increased, and plasma estradiol concentrations rose to 22.2 ± 6.2 pg/ml. BA maturation (increase of 1.03 ±

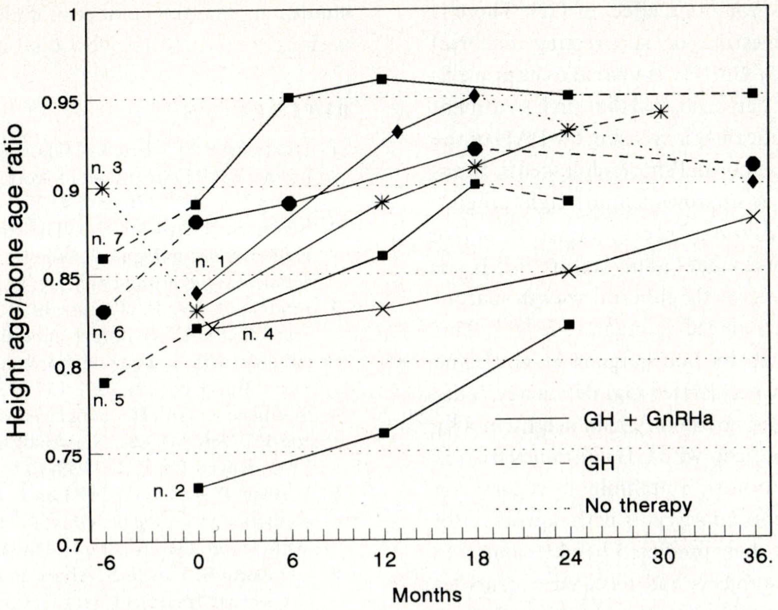

Fig. 2. Ratio of HA to BA in each patient during entire period of study.

0.47 years) was commensurate with progression in CA (0.98 ± 0.43 years) and with growth rate (increase in HA: 0.82 ± 0.24 years).

In five girls (Nos. 1, 3, 5-7) the height attained is already higher than PAH before therapy, and in subject 2 it is almost the same (−0.1 cm); subject 4 has a height of 141.5 cm, with a PAH before therapy of 146.2 cm, but her BA is only 12.25 years.

Treatment was well tolerated and no side effects were observed.

DISCUSSION

The pathophysiologic bases for combination treatment with GH and GnRHa come from the experiences acquired during treatment of isolated GH deficiency and precocious puberty. In patients with isolated GH deficiency, to improve the disappointing final results, we added GnRHa administration to GH therapy to delay the onset of puberty or to prolong the period of sexual development, or both.[13-16] The rationale for the addition of GnRHa to GH in these patients derived from findings showing a correlation between final height and the height attained at the onset of puberty; if pubertal development begins when stature is still insufficient, as often occurs in GH-deficient patients receiving GH therapy, final height will be short.[14, 17, 18] Furthermore, GH administration, especially when started late, may accelerate bone maturation, shortening the duration of pubertal development and, ultimately, the pubertal growth spurt.[4, 14, 19-21] On the other hand, in some girls with precocious puberty, GH treatment was proposed to balance the decreased growth rate caused by GnRHa administration, which is probably secondary to a rapid increase in BA. The final result may be a stature shorter than that predicted before treatment with GnRHa.[22-24]

Our preliminary data regarding combination treatment with GH and GnRHa in short normal subjects are encouraging. During the combination treatment, the PAH (evaluated by the Bailey-Pinneau method, which is probably the most reliable in such patients[3, 25] increased significantly, and the other prognostic measurements also improved (increase in HA/BA ratio, and the ratio of gain in HA to gain in BA higher than 1). Although the method of prediction of adult height is appropriate only for normal subjects, as in those we studied, final height will be the only reliable measure to evaluate the effectiveness of combination therapy. In this regard, after interruption of combination therapy, PAH increased further in the four girls in whom GH administration was continued, or remained higher than that predicted before combination therapy in the girl without GH therapy. In five of seven girls the height attained is already greater than the PAH before therapy, and in one case almost the same; the last girl has a BA of only 12.25 years. Furthermore, the comparison between treated girls and control subjects confirmed the favorable effect of therapy, but a randomized, controlled study will be necessary to confirm these preliminary findings.

The good results that we obtained may be attributed to the effects of the concomitant administration of GH and GnRHa: a GnRHa-induced block of pubertal development occurs with a slowing down of bone maturation, simultaneously with the growth-promoting effect of GH. There is evidence that either arresting or suppressing pubertal development by using only GnRHa is unable to improve final height; Lindner et al.[3] demonstrated that such treatment was not successful in significantly increasing the PAH or the HA/BA ratio in otherwise normal short adolescents. Stanhope and Brook[2] showed no improvement in height prognosis in children with constitutional short stature. Thus late puberty does not result in a higher adult stature if it is not accompanied by adequate growth; pubertal growth spurt of late onset is shorter and reduced in magnitude.[10, 26] This finding has been confirmed by Bourguignon et al.,[17] who showed that, in subjects with isolated GH deficiency, a delay in puberty induction did not modify final height, and by Stanhope and Brook[2] in subjects with GH deficiency treated with GnRHa alone. In contrast, a preliminary report[27] on a trial with GnRHa in short adolescents with normal onset of puberty indicates that their predicted height seemed to increase; however, some subjects had received concurrent GH therapy. Furthermore, GH treatment alone may shorten the duration of pubertal development in subjects with isolated GH deficiency[21] or with multiple pituitary deficiencies,[20] and in short normal subjects GH administration may induce the onset of puberty and therefore worsen the height prognosis.[4]

With regard to combination therapy with GH and GnRHa in short children with normal endocrine function, the available data are conflicting. Mathew et al.[5] reported an improvement in PAH in short children without GH deficiency. Gambotto et al.[6] described an increase in height prognosis in three subjects with advanced BA and low PAH treated with GnRHa and GH for 12 months, and then with GH alone for 6 months. On the other hand, Job and Landier[8] did not show any advantage of combination therapy for 2 years in a group of short adolescents treated subsequently with GH alone for another year, in comparison with GH treatment alone. However, patients must be followed to their final height before one can draw final conclusions.

Finally, the economic aspects of this kind of treatment should be considered, because the two drugs are very expensive. Therefore growth-promoting treatment in short children with normal endocrine function should be considered only after meticulous evaluation of the individual situation and accurate explanation of the possible effects of hormone therapy and its costs.

This pilot study has demonstrated that in a group of seven short normal girls who entered puberty at normal age with insufficient height and a poor PAH, a period of almost 2 years of treatment with GH combined with GnRHa was successful in improving height prognosis. This nonconventional treatment should be considered only when the requirement for improved stature is very pressing. Other studies, in a larger number of children treated for a longer period, are needed to allow final conclusions.

REFERENCES

1. Hindmarsh PC, Brook CGD. Long-term effects of growth hormone (GH) treatment in short normal children [Abstract]. Horm Res 1992;37(suppl 4):2.
2. Stanhope R, Brook CGD. The effect of gonadotropin releasing hormone analogue on height prognosis in growth hormone deficiency and normal puberty. Eur J Pediatr 1988;148:200-2.
3. Lindner D, Job JC, Chaussain JL. Failure to improve height prediction in short-stature pubertal adolescents by inhibiting puberty with luteinizing hormone–releasing hormone analogue. Eur J Pediatr 1993;152:393-6.
4. Stanhope R. GnRH analogues in short stature. In: Cavallo L, Job JC, New MI, eds. Growth disorders: state of the art. New York: Raven Press, 1991:99-103.
5. Mathew P, Redmond GP, Lee Y-J, Kelly P. Improved height prediction in very short children treated with the GnRH analogue leuprolide [Abstract]. Pediatr Res 1990;27:81A.
6. Gambotto S, Vanelli S, Altare F, Benso L. Effects on growth of one year treatment with GH combined with LHRHa. In: Cavallo L, Job JC, New M, eds. Growth disorders: state of the art. New York: Raven Press, 1991:293-9.
7. Veimo D. Combination therapy with gonadotrophin-releasing-analogue and growth hormone: a way of treating children in early puberty with low predicted final height [Abstract]. Acta Paediatr Scand 1993;suppl 388:132.
8. Job JC, Landier F. Growth of pubertal short normal children treated 3 years with growth hormone alone or associated with LHRH agonist [Abstract]. Pediatr Res 1993;33(suppl):S36.
9. Tanner JM, Whitehouse RH, Takaishi M. Standards from birth to maturity for height, weight, height velocity and weight velocity: British children 1965. Arch Dis Child 1966;41:454-71, 613-35.
10. Tanner JM. Foetus into man. Cambridge, Massachusetts University Press, 1978.
11. Greulich WW, Pyle SI. Radiograph atlas of skeletal development of the hand and wrist. 2nd ed. Stanford, California: Stanford University Press, 1959.
12. Bayley N, Pinneau SR. Tables for predicting adult height for skeletal age: evidence for use with the Greulich-Pyle hand standards. J PEDIATR 1952;40:423-41.
13. Toublanc JE, Couprie C, Garnier P, Job JC. The effects of treatment combining an agonist of gonadotropin-releasing hormone with growth hormone in pubertal patients with isolated growth hormone deficiency. Acta Endocrinol (Copenh) 1989;120:795-9.
14. Tanaka T, Yoshizawa A, Tanae A, Hibi I, Shizume K. Relationship between puberty and growth at adolescence in growth-hormone-deficient males: effect of growth hormone and of associated gonadal suppression therapy. Horm Res 1990;33(suppl 4):102-5.
15. Leheup B, Schaeffer L, Jeandel C, Pierson M. Agoniste de la LH-RH chez les sujets traités par hormone de croissance pour insuffisance somatotrope. Èvolution de la vélocité de croissance et des prédictions de taille. Pediatrie 1992;47:291-5.
16. Saggese G, Cesaretti G, Andreani G, Carlotti C. Combined treatment with growth hormone and gonadotropin-releasing hormone analogues in children with isolated growth hormone deficiency. Acta Endocrinol (Copenh) 1993;128:307-12.

17. Bourguignon JP, Vandeweghe M, Vanderschueren-Lodeweyckx M, et al. Pubertal growth and final height in hypopituitary boys: a minor role of bone age at onset of puberty. J Clin Endocrinol Metab 1986;63:376-82.
18. Frisch H, Schober E, Waldhauser F, Hausler G. Puberty in isolated growth hormone deficiency. In: Frisch H, Laron Z, eds. Induction of puberty in hypopituitarism. Serono Symposia Review 1988;16:49-65.
19. Job JC, Chaussain JL, Garnier P, Rolland A, Joab N. Dose response relationship in the treatment of hypopituitary children with human growth hormone: a retrospective study. Acta Paediatr Scand 1987;337(suppl):93-105.
20. Van der Werff ten Bosch JJ, Bot A. Does hGH treatment promote adult height of hypopituitary children? Neth J Med 1988;32:217-25.
21. Darendeliler F, Hindmarsh PC, Preece MA, Cox L, Brook CGD. Growth hormone increases rate of pubertal maturation. Acta Endocrinol (Copenh) 1990;122:414-6.
22. Brain CE, Stanhope R, Brook CGD. The effect of GH on the growth of girls with central precocious puberty treated with (D-Ser 6) GnRH analogue [Abstract]. Horm Res 1989;31(suppl 1):43.
23. Oostdijk W, Drop SLS, Odink RJH, Hummelink R, Partsch CJ, Sippel WG. Long-term results with a slow-release gonadotropin-releasing hormone agonist in central precocious puberty. Acta Pediatr Scand 1991;372(suppl):39-46.
24. Saggese G, Pasquino A, Battini R, Franchi G, Pucarelli C. GH administration improves growth in long-term LH-RH analog-treated children [Abstract]. Horm Res 1991;35(suppl 2):40.
25. Zachmann M, Sobradillo B, Frank M. Height predictions in normal children and in patients with various pathological conditions. J PEDIATR 1969;93:749-56.
26. Brook CGD. Growth assessment in childhood and adolescence. Oxford: Blackwell, 1982.
27. Municchi G, Rose RG, Barnes KM, Cassorla F, Cutler GB Jr. A double-blind, placebo-controlled trial of LHRH agonist treatment in patients with short stature and normal onset of puberty: preliminary results [Abstract]. Pediatr Res 1991; 29:82A.

Response to growth hormone therapy in patients with growth hormone deficiency who at birth were small or appropriate in size for gestational age

Antonio Balsamo, MD, Paola Tassoni, MD, Alessandra Cassio, MD, Cristina Colli, MD, Davide Tassinari, MD, Alessandro Cicognani, MD, and Emanuele Cacciari, MD
From the First Pediatric Clinic, University of Bologna and S. Orsola Hospital, Bologna, Italy

Objective: To determine long-term growth response to growth hormone (GH) therapy in patients with isolated GH deficiency who had been small for gestational age and in those who had been appropriate in size for gesttaional age.
Design: Longitudinal, case-control study.
Setting: Pediatric clinic, endocrinology center, University of Bologna, Italy.
Patients: Sixteen GH-deficient children, small for gestational age with unknown cause, and 16 GH-deficient children, appropriate in size for gestational age, who were matched for chronologic age, bone age, pubertal stage, and target height at the beginning of treatment and were treated for 36 months.
Intervention: Recombinant human GH given subcutaneously at a dose of 20 IU/m^2 per week in six doses per week for 36 months.
Measurements: Growth hormone levels (fluoroimmunoenzymatic method), levels of insulin-like growth factor I (radioimmunoassay), and complete 36-months auxologic follow-up.
Results: Patients who were small for gestational age had a modest improvement in height for chronologic age but no increase in predicted final height. Patients who were appropriate in size for gestational age had significantly better improvement in both measurements (multivariate analysis of variance: $F = 6.3$ ($p < 0.001$) and $F = 3.8$ ($p < 0.05$), respectively). Catch-up growth was similar during the first year of therapy for the two groups, after which the linear growth velocity decreased more rapidly in the small-for-gestational-age patients (multivariate analysis of variance: $F = 4.9$ ($p < 0.05$)).
Conclusions: The constitutional component of the statural deficiency of small-for-gestational-age children seemed to prevail over hormonal deficiency during treatment with GH. Further follow-up to final height is necessary to evaluate these different responses. (J PEDIATR 1995;126:474-7)

Small-for-gestational-age patients are generally characterized by a deficient subsequent growth pattern.[1,2] To improve these results, physicians have attempted treatment with growth hormone in these patients, regardless of whether there was a deficiency of GH.[3-5] However, long-term results have differed greatly, and generally there has been little improvement in the prognosis for height.[5]

Our study was intended to assess the long-term (36 months) response to replacement therapy with synthetic GH in patients who had been SGA and also had isolated GH

Submitted for publication March 3, 1994; accepted Oct. 16, 1994.
Reprint requests: Emanuele Cacciari, MD, Clinica Pediatrica I, Policlnico S. Orsola, via Massarenti 11, 40138 Bologna, Italy.

0022-3476/95/$3.00 + 0 **9/25/61097**

AGA	Appropriate in size for gestational age
GH	Growth hormone
IGF-I	Insulin-like growth factor I
IUGR	Intrauterine growth retardation
SGA	Small for gestational age

deficiency. Comparisons were made with a control group consisting of patients who had been appropriate in size for gestational age and had similar GH deficiency.

METHODS

This study involved 16 SGA children born at term (14 boys, 2 girls; mean [±SD] neonatal weight, 2226 ± 295 gm; mean [±SD] neonatal length, 43.6 ± 1.6 cm) and 16 AGA children born at term (14 boys, 2 girls; mean [±SD] neonatal weight, 3342 ± 507 gm; mean [±SD] neonatal length, 49.3 ± 1.1 cm).

The SGA patients were enrolled in the study at random and were considered SGA in accordance with the criteria of Battaglia and Lubchenko[6]; height at birth was lower than the 10th percentile for gestational age.[7] We prefer the term *SGA* rather than *intrauterine growth retardation* because, according to some authors,[8] the latter definition implies a documented variation in fetal growth rate, which was the case in only some of our patients. We chose idiopathic SGA children and excluded those with Silver-Russell syndrome and those with a history of neonatal asphyxia, intrauterine sepsis, dysmorphic features, or congenital and chromosomal abnormalities.

The patients in the AGA group had chronologic ages (SGA group, 10.1 ± 3.5 years; AGA group, 9.9 ± 4.2 years), bone ages (SGA group, 7.9 ± 3.8 years; AGA group, 7.5 ± 4.4 years), target heights (SGA group, 166.3 ± 4.6 cm [SD score, −1.03 ± 0.49]; AGA group, 167.0 ± 5.9 cm [SD score, −0.8 ± 0.58]), and pubertal stages similar to those in the SGA group.

All the patients were studied in our clinic for short stature (height ≤3rd percentile according to the Tanner standards) and had isolated GH deficiency. Two stimulation tests (arginine and L-dopa) produced abnormal results (GH peak, <8 ng/ml); seven patients in each group had severe GH deficiency (peak, <4 ng/ml), and nine had milder GH deficiency (peak, <8 ng/ml). The mean of the GH peaks (maximal peak of the two tests) was 4.3 ± 2.2 ng/ml for the SGA group and 4.6 ± 2.0 ng/ml for the AGA group. We reassessed the GH secretory status of nine SGA and eight AGA patients after completion of or during GH therapy (after 1-month suspension), repeating the arginine and L-dopa tests; all the subjects had deficient GH secretion (maximal peak of the two tests, 4.5 ± 2.8 ng/ml for SGA and 4.2 ± 2.1 ng/ml for AGA subjects). No patient had other endocrinopathies or chronic diseases. The patients were treated with biosynthetic GH subcutaneously at a dose of 20 IU/m^2 per week in six doses per week.

Growth was assessed during the year before treatment (12 months for 5 subjects, 6 months for 24 subjects, and 3 months for 3 subjects) and then every 6 months for both groups. We took into account only yearly periods of growth, for a total follow-up period of 36 months. Height was measured in the morning with a Harpenden stadiometer (mean of three measurements). Bone age was assessed by the same observer, who followed the Greulich and Pyle method.[9] The standards of Tanner et al.[10] were used to evaluate height, which was expressed in standard deviation scores for both chronologic and bone ages; height for age and linear growth velocity were expressed both as centimeters per year and as SD scores for bone age. Previous data were used to calculate the height age increment/bone age increment ratio. Target height was calculated on the basis of parental height, after Tanner[11]; predicted height was assessed with the Bayley-Pinneau method.[12] The latter value was statistically analyzed only for male patients because of the insufficient number of female subjects.

The rate of pubertal maturation, evaluated according to Marshall and Tanner,[13, 14] remained prepubertal during the entire study for six boys and for the two girls in both groups, progressed from Tanner stage G1 to G3 for two SGA and three AGA patients, and from Tanner stage G2 to G4 for six SGA and five AGA patients.

The GH levels were measured with a fluoroimmunoenzymatic method (Cybefluor Inc., Toronto, Canada). The intraassay and interassay coefficients of variation were 7.8% and 10.7%, respectively. Levels of insulin-like factor I were evaluated at yearly intervals by a radioimmunoassay method (RIA Kit, Nichols Institute Products, San Juan Capistrano, Calif.).[15] Results of magnetic resonance imaging of the sellar area, performed in four SGA and seven AGA patients, were normal.

Statistical analysis was performed with an IBM XT computer and an SPSS program (SPSS Inc., Chicago, Ill.). Variance analysis (multivariance analysis of variance) for repeated measures was used to compare the two groups with time, and the r correlation coefficient was used to relate the auxologic features to other measurements. The results are expressed as mean ± SD.

RESULTS

The height-for-chronologic-age SD score was similar in the two groups before therapy and increased significantly with time in both groups ($F = 46.6$; $p < 0.0001$), with a significantly greater increment in the AGA group ($F = 7.9$; $p < 0.0001$) (Figure). However, the height-for-bone-age SD score showed a difference between the two groups with time ($F = 3.9$; $p < 0.025$), with a significantly greater decrease in the SGA than in the AGA group ($F = 2.9$;

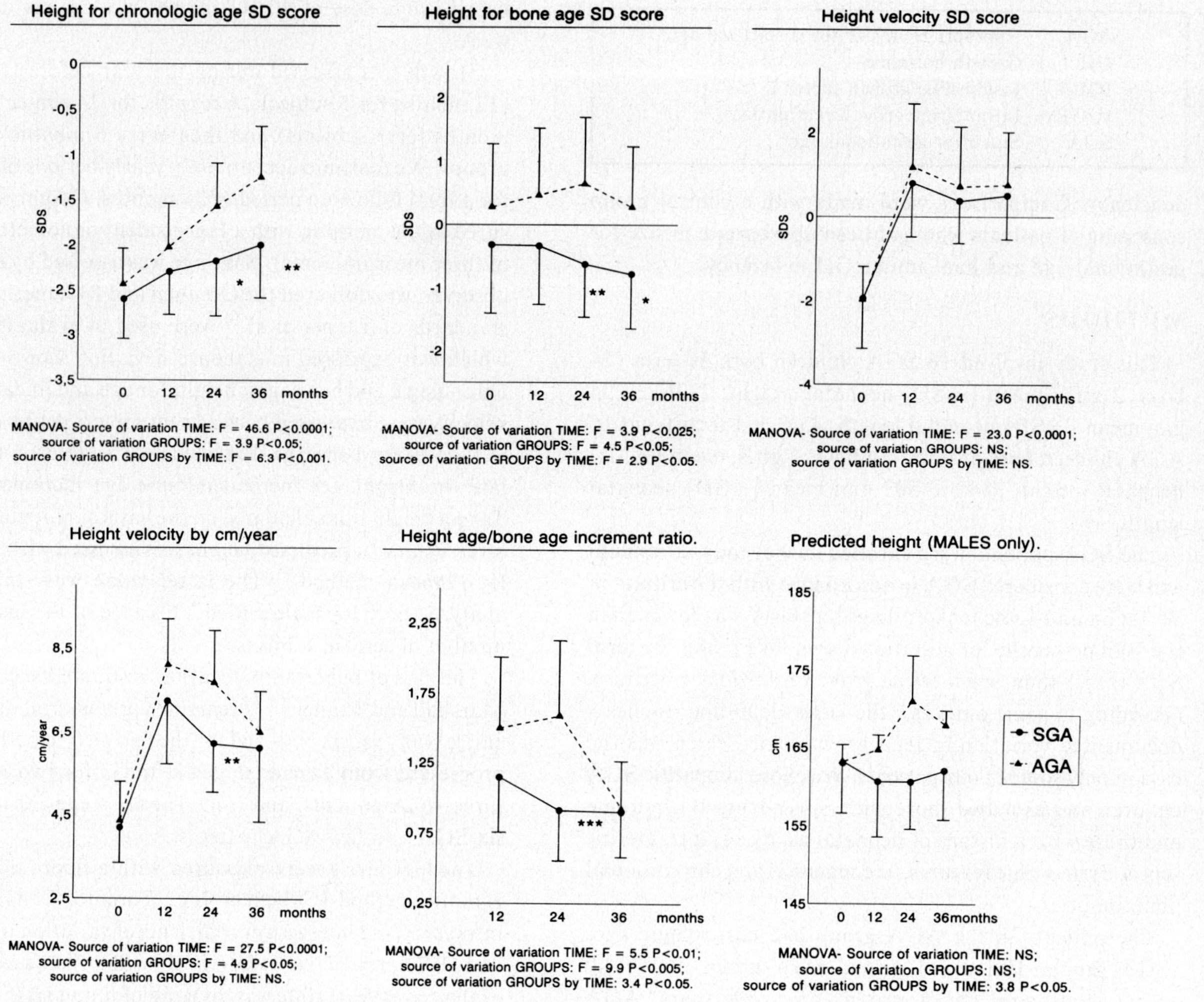

Figure. Auxologic features as function of time in the two groups. F is the value of the multivariate analysis of variance *(MANOVA)* for repeated measurements. The *asterisks* indicate points at which SGA and AGA groups were significantly different: $*p < 0.05$; $**p < 0.01$; $***p < 0.005$. *NS*, Not significant.

$p < 0.05$). On average, this measurement was negative for the SGA group and positive for the AGA group at the start of therapy, although there was no significant difference between the two groups (Figure).

Both the linear growth velocity SD score and the linear growth velocity, in centimeters per year increased significantly in the two groups during the therapy (F = 23.0 [$p < 0.0001$] and F = 27.5 [$p < 0.0001$], respectively), with a significant difference for linear growth velocity, in centimeters per year, between the two groups at month 24 in favor of the AGA group (F = 4.9; $p < 0.05$) (Figure).

The height age/bone age increment ratio increased for the AGA group and decreased for the SGA group with time (F = 5.5; $p < 0.01$) with a significant difference at month 24 between the two groups (F = 3.4; $p < 0.05$) (Figure). Predicted height (assessed only in boys) differed significantly in the two groups and increased significantly only in the AGA group (F = 3.76; $p < 0.05$).

The IGF-I levels were similar in the two groups before therapy (SGA 1.0 ± 0.5, AGA 1.1 ± 0.3 U/ml) and increased significantly (F = 11.8, $p < 0.0001$) after therapy with no differences between groups (SGA 2.3 ± 1.5, AGA 2.3 ± 1.2 U/ml at 36 months' therapy). There were no significant correlations between the linear growth response to GH therapy and GH maximum peak, IGF-I levels and birth length in either the SGA or AGA group.

DISCUSSION

These data show that GH therapy improves linear growth velocity in both SGA and AGA children with GH deficiency. Both groups also had a corresponding gain in height for chronologic age SD score. The mean standard gain of our SGA group was similar to that described by Albertsson-Wikland[3] (+0.68 SD) after 24 months of therapy in a group of patients with IUGR and highly variable GH secretion, which also included patients with Silver-Russell syndrome, and to those of Lanes et al.[4] (+0.60 SD), who gave GH to 19 non-GH-deficient prepubertal subjects with IUGR for two periods of 12 months. However, the overall gain after 36 months of therapy in our SGA group was less than in the AGA group. The latter reached an increment in their height score of +1.20 SD at month 36 of therapy, and their linear growth velocity as of month 12 decreased more slowly than in the SGA group.

When statural gain for bone age was assessed, the prognosis for final height in the SGA group was unfavorable, whereas the AGA group had an improved height-for-bone-age SD score until at least month 24 of therapy.

Both the height age/bone age increment ratio and the trend of predicted height in our SGA group are in concordance with previous observations of Stanhope et al.,[5] who found that these patients benefit little from GH therapy. Unlike our own study, these authors included patients with Silver-Russell syndrome, and only 25.8% of their patients had GH deficiency.

We conclude that even when the cause of IUGR is idiopathic and when there is isolated GH deficiency, SGA patients have modest improvement in height for chronologic age but no increase in predicted final height after 36 months of therapy with synthetic GH. Patients with similar hormonal deficiency but who were AGA have significantly better improvement in both measurements. Catch-up growth in SGA patients is similar to that in the AGA patients during the first year of therapy, after which their linear growth velocity decreases more rapidly than that of the AGA subjects, presumably because of the constitutional component in their statural deficiency.[1] Nevertheless, it will be necessary to assess the final height of patients in the two groups to determine whether GH therapy can have a positive influence on at least some SGA patients with GH deficiency.

REFERENCES

1. Westwood M, Kramer MS, Munz D, Lovett JM, Watters GV. Growth and development of full-term nonasphyxiated small-for-gestational-age newborns: follow-up through adolescence. Pediatrics 1983;71:376-82.
2. Davies PSW, Valley R, Preece MA. Adolescent growth and pubertal progression in the Silver-Russell syndrome. Arch Dis Child 1988;63:130-5.
3. Albertsson-Wikland K. Growth hormone secretion and growth hormone treatment in children with intrauterine growth retardation. Acta Paediatr Scand[Suppl]349:35-41.
4. Lanes R, Plotnick LP, Lee PA. Sustained effect of human growth hormone therapy on children with intrauterine growth retardation. Pediatrics 1979;63:731-5.
5. Stanhope R, Preece MA, Hamill G. Does growth hormone treatment improve final height attainment of children with intrauterine growth retardation? Arch Dis Child 1991;66:1180-3.
6. Battaglia FC, Lubchenko LO. A practical classification of newborn infants by weight and gestational age. J PEDIATR 1967;71:159-63.
7. Lubchenko LO, Honsman C, Boyd E. Intrauterine growth in length and head circumference as estimates from live birth and gestational age from 26 to 42 weeks. Pediatrics 1966;37:403-8.
8. Pollack RN, Divon MY. Intrauterine growth retardation: definition, classification, and etiology. Clin Obstet Gynecol 1992;35:99-107.
9. Greulich W, Pyle SI. Radiographic atlas of skeletal development of the hand and wrist. 2nd ed. Palo Alto, California: Stanford University Press, 1959.
10. Tanner JM, Whitehouse RH, Takaishi M. Standards from birth to maturity for height, weight, height velocity, and weight velocity: British children. Parts I and II. Arch Dis Child 1966;41:454-71.
11. Tanner JM. Growth at adolescence. 2nd ed. Oxford: Blackwell Scientific Publications, 1962.
12. Bayley N, Pinneau S. Tables for predicting adult height from skeletal age. J PEDIATR 1952;40:423-41.
13. Marshall WA, Tanner JM. Variations in the pattern of pubertal changes in girls. Arch Dis Child 1969;44:291-303.
14. Marshall WA, Tanner JM. Variations in the pattern of pubertal changes in boys. Arch Dis Child 1970;45:13-23.
15. Furlanetto RW, Underwood LE, Van Wyk JJ, D'Ercole AJ. Estimation of somatomedin-C in normals and patients with pituitary disease by radioimmunoassay. J Clin Invest 1977;60:648-57.

Clinical and laboratory observations

Effect of growth hormone therapy on final versus predicted height in short twelve- to sixteen-year-old boys without growth hormone deficiency

Paul B. Kaplowitz, MD

From the Department of Pediatrics, Medical College of Virginia, Virginia Commonwealth University, Richmond

The effect of growth hormone therapy on final height in 28 short boys without growth hormone deficiency was evaluated retrospectively. The boys had received growth hormone for at least 2 years and were close to final height when therapy was stopped. The mean estimated final height was very close to that predicted from the pretherapy bone age. The fact that bone age advanced a mean of 4.9 years during a mean of 3.5 years of therapy may account for the lack of effect on final height. (J Pediatr 1995;126:478-80)

Since biosynthetic growth hormone was introduced in 1985, enthusiasm has grown for the use of GH in short children with no defined cause of shortness (e.g., constitutional growth delay and "idiopathic" short stature) and with multiple nonhormonal causes. During the first year of therapy in short children without GH deficiency, linear growth velocity increases without an increased rate of skeletal maturation, which results in an improved height prediction[1]; this improvement is sustained for at least the first 3 years of therapy.[2] It has therefore been widely assumed that adult height will eventually be greater in such patients than if they had not received GH. At present, however, the only group of short children without GHD for whom improved final height has been documented is girls with Turner syndrome.[3]

Bierich et al.[4] described 13 boys and 2 girls (mean age, 12 years) with constitutional growth delay who were given GH for an average of 3 years. Mean final height was 170 cm, which was identical to that predicted by the Bayley-Pinneau method but was still 5 cm below target height based on parental height.[4] More recently Loche et al.[5] found that 4 to 10 years of GH therapy in a group of 10 boys and 5 girls without GHD (mean age, 10.5 years) resulted in a mean final height not significantly different from both the predicted height and the target height. A masked, placebo-controlled study of the effect of GH therapy on final height in healthy, short, 9 to 14-year-old children without GHD is under way at the National Institutes of Health, but final results will not be available for many years. To obtain information on this problem to help guide physicians in the interim, we looked retrospectively at the outcome of therapy in a group of short boys without GHD who have been treated with GH to near final height at various institutions in the United States and Canada, and whose growth data have been entered into a computerized database. The goal of the study was to see whether adult height in these children exceeded that which was predicted from bone age at the start of therapy.

GH	Growth hormone
GHD	GH deficiency
PAH	Predicted adult height

METHODS

The National Cooperative Growth Study is a database maintained by Genentech, Inc. (South San Francisco, Calif.), containing demographics and growth information before and during GH therapy on more than 16,000 patients

Submitted for publication May 2, 1994; accepted Sept. 14, 1994.

Reprint requests: Paul Kaplowitz, MD, Medical College of Virginia, PO Box 980140, Richmond, VA 23298-0140.

0022-3476/95/$3.00 + 0 **9/22/60608**

from the United States and Canada. Children who have normal GH testing results and no other obvious cause of growth retardation are coded as having "idiopathic short stature," a category that includes patients with constitutional growth delay and genetic short stature. The 28 boys in this study met the following criteria: (1) diagnosis of idiopathic short stature, (2) a documented peak GH concentration of >10 ng/ml, (3) an enrollment height of ≤−2 SD, (3) initial bone age of ≤13 years, (4) duration of GH therapy ≥2 years, and (5) at the last recorded visit, linear growth velocity ≤3 cm/yr (to ensure that patients were very close to their adult height). Patients were treated with different doses and schedules of GH according to the practice of each individual endocrinologist, but most were receiving a weekly dose of ≈0.3 mg/kg per week, divided into six or seven doses. Predicted adult height was estimated on the basis of bone age close to the time of initiation of GH therapy by the method of Bayley and Pinneau. Tanner target height was based on the heights of the parents and was available for 27 of 28 patients.

RESULTS

As shown in the Table, at the time of initiation of GH therapy the patients had a mean age of 14.1 years (range, 12.1 to 17.9 years—but only one boy was older than 16 years) and a mean bone age delay of 3 years. The stage of puberty was assessed by testicular volume; for 7 patients this volume was ≤3 ml, for 12 it was >3 to 6 ml, for 7 it was >6 to 10 ml, for 1 it was >10 ml, and for 1 the data were missing. This finding indicates that most patients were either prepubertal or in early puberty. Height averaged 2.9 SD below the mean, and both the Tanner target height and the PAH were significantly below the mean male adult height of 177 cm, indicating that genetic factors may have contributed to the short stature of these patients.

At the time GH therapy was discontinued, the mean patient age was 17.8 years and the mean duration of GH therapy was 3.7 years. Mean last linear growth velocity was 1.9 ± 0.8 cm/yr. The mean height at the last visit when GH therapy was stopped was 164.4 cm (4.2 cm less than the mean PAH), and the mean height SD had improved to −1.8. True final height is difficult to obtain outside a research protocol because patients are generally no longer seen after GH therapy is discontinued. To estimate final height, we took advantage of the fact that for 25 of 28 patients, a bone age was obtained at or very close to the time of the last visit. The mean bone age was 16 years, which according to the Bayley-Pinneau tables corresponds to 98.2% of completed height. Thus the estimated mean final height was 164.4/0.982 = 167.4 cm, still 1.2 cm less than the mean PAH. For the 25 patients with both pretherapy and end-of-therapy bone ages, the mean advance in bone maturation was 4.9 years during a mean of 3.5 years of GH treatment.

Table. Characteristics of patients at start and end of GH therapy

	At enrollment	At last visit
Age (yr)	14.1 ± 1.4	17.8 ± 1.2
Height (cm)	139.8 ± 6.9	164.4 ± 4.0
Height SD	−2.92 ± 0.72	−1.81 ± 0.62
Bone age (yr)	11.1 ± 1.4	16.0 ± 0.9* (n = 25)
Growth rate (cm/yr)	4.8 ± 1.9	1.9 ± 0.8
Predicted adult height (cm)	168.6 ± 5.2	167.4 ± 4.9
Tanner target height (cm)	171.1 ± 3.9	—

All values are expressed as mean ± SD.
*Mean age at which the last bone age was done was 17.6 years.

For the 25 boys who had bone ages obtained either at the end or 3 to 12 months before the end of therapy, final heights were estimated and compared with the enrollment PAH. For only one patient did estimated final height substantially surpass the PAH. This boy had an enrollment age of 13 years with a bone age of 11.5 years and a PAH of only 154.7 cm, well below his target height of 167.9 cm. His estimated final height was 167.8 cm, 13.1 cm above the PAH. (Bone age reading was not standardized; it is possible that an error in estimating the bone age could have caused an underestimation of his PAH.) For 3 boys the estimated final height was between 2 and 4 cm above PAH, for 6 it was within 2 cm of PAH, for 9 it was between 2.1 and 6 cm less than PAH, and for 4 it was more than 6 cm less than PAH. The boy who greatly exceeded his PAH was the only one in this study whose PAH was <160 cm.

DISCUSSION

This retrospective study has several limitations. One limitation was the lack of an untreated control group. Therefore the conclusion as to whether treated patients achieved final heights better than they would have without treatment rests entirely on the validity of the Bayley-Pinneau method of height prediction. Many studies have shown that in untreated boys with constitutional growth delay, final height is frequently less than the predicted height based on bone age alone. However, when the results of four different studies of boys with constitutional growth delay were pooled, the Bayley-Pinneau method overestimated final height by a mean of only 1.7 cm.[4] Therefore the error involved in predicting *mean* final height by this method in a group of 28 boys should not be large. A related problem is the inherent inaccuracy of individual bone age readings, which for patients enrolled in the National Cooperative Growth Study are done by a wide variety of individuals at different institutions. However, bone ages can be misread in either direction, and one would anticipate that these small errors in PAH would cancel out.

Another major limitation of this study is that these patients were older than many patients without GHD who are now receiving GH. The use of GH for idiopathic short stature increased rapidly after 1987, and at present only the oldest patients have completed their growth and have discontinued therapy. It is possible that better outcomes will be seen when children without GHD who began GH therapy between 8 and 12 years of age reach their final height, although even a recent study in which the mean pretreatment age was 10.5 years found no effect of GH on final versus predicted height.[5]

The apparent paradox of having increased growth during the initial years of GH therapy but no improvement in final height is best explained by the increased rate of bone maturation during GH therapy. The mechanism by which GH increases the rate of bone maturation is unknown, but other studies suggest that GH increases the rate of pubertal progression. In a retrospective study of children with isolated GHD who progressed through puberty spontaneously during GH therapy, the duration of puberty was shortened compared with the Tanner data in typical children.[6] This finding was confirmed in a subsequent prospective study in which both children with GHD and short children without GHD showed an increased rate of pubertal progression during GH therapy[7]; doubling the dose of GH at the onset of the pubertal growth spurt caused no improvement in growth rate, indicating that GH dose is probably not a limiting factor in pubertal growth. The fact that GH does increase final height in girls with Turner syndrome may be due to the absence of spontaneous puberty in most affected girls.

Although this study has failed to show an effect of GH on final height in a group of older boys who have completed their growth, several questions remain to be answered. It is possible that starting treatment at earlier ages and having a longer duration of therapy before the onset of puberty will result in a better outcome. Withdrawing therapy at the onset of the pubertal growth spurt may prevent the apparent rapid advancement of bone maturation during puberty and may also reduce the overall cost of GH therapy in children without GHD. A recent report suggests that delaying puberty during GH therapy with synthetic analogs of gonadotropin-releasing hormone in short pubertal children without GHD may improve final height.[8] Finally, GH therapy might be most beneficial in selected short children without GHD who have particularly poor predicted heights. The one child with a sustantially improved outcome in this study had a PAH of only 154.7 cm. Furthermore in nine girls with extremely poor PAH (mean, 140.9 cm) and bone age <13 years, GH therapy for an average of 2 years resulted in heights 7 cm above the PAH, whereas a group of eight similar but untreated girls showed no change in actual versus predicted height.[9]

It may be argued that even if GH therapy in older short boys without GHD does not improve final height, it is justified because of the positive psychologic effects of a short-term increase in growth rate. If short-term growth stimulation is desired, the use of a brief course of androgen therapy in older boys with delayed puberty is still a safe and inexpensive alternative to GH, and it has no adverse effect on adult height.[10] Until more data are available that document which subgroups of short patients without GHD are likely to derive long-term benefit from GH therapy, we should be very cautious about recommending treatment for this group of patients.

I thank Peter Compton, of Genentech, Inc., for assisting with the procurement and analysis of the data.

REFERENCES

1. Genentech Collaborative Study Group. Idiopathic short stature: results of a one-year controlled study of human growth hormone treatment. J PEDIATR 1989;115:713-9.
2. Hopwood NJ, Hintz RL, Gertner JM, et al. Growth response of children with non-growth-hormone deficiency and marked short stature during three years of growth hormone therapy. J PEDIATR 1993;123:215-22.
3. Rosenfeld RG, Frane J, Attie KM, et al. Six-year results of a randomized prospective trial of human growth hormone and oxandrolone in Turner syndrome. J PEDIATR 1992;121:49-55.
4. Bierich JR, Nolte K, Drews K, Brugmann G. Constitutional delay of growth and adolescence: results of short-term and long-term treatment with GH. Acta Endocrinol 1992;127:392-6.
5. Loche S, Cambiaso P, Carta D, Marini R, Borrelli P, Cappa M. Final height after growth hormone therapy in non-growth-hormone-deficient children with short stature. J PEDIATR 1994;125:196-200.
6. Darendeliler F, Hindmarsh PC, Preece MA, Cox L, Brook CGD. Growth hormone increases the rate of pubertal maturation. Acta Endocrinol 1990;122:414-6.
7. Stanhope R, Albanese A, Hindmarsh P, Brook CGD. The effects of growth hormone therapy on spontaneous sexual development. Horm Res 1992;38(suppl):9-13.
8. Municchi G, Rose SR, Pescovitz OH, Barnes KM, Cassorla FG, Cutler GB. Effect of deslorelin-induced pubertal delay on the growth of adolescents with short stature and normally timed puberty: preliminary results. J Clin Endocrinol Metab 1993;77:1334-9.
9. Leboeuf G. Biosynthetic hGH can improve significantly final heights of some short children without classical GH deficiency. Presented to the Seventh Annual National Cooperative Growth Study investigators meeting, Scottsdale, Arizona, October 28-31, 1993.
10. Richman RA, Kirsch LR. Testosterone treatment in adolescent boys with constitutional delay in growth and development. N Engl J Med 1988;319:1563-7.

Otitis media, hearing sensitivity, and maternal responsiveness in relation to language during infancy

Joanne Erwick Roberts, PhD, Margaret R. Burchinal, PhD, Lynn P. Medley, MS, Susan A. Zeisel, EdD, Martha Mundy, MS, Jackson Roush, PhD, Stephen Hooper, PhD, Donna Bryant, PhD, and Frederick W. Henderson, MD

From the Frank Porter Graham Child Development Center, the Division of Speech and Hearing Sciences, Department of Medical Allied Health, the Departments of Psychology, Psychiatry, and Pediatrics, and the Clinical Center for Study of Development and Learning, University of North Carolina at Chapel Hill

The relation of otitis media with effusion (OME) and associated hearing loss to language and cognitive skills at 1 year of age was studied to determine whether OME-related hearing loss had a direct association with language and cognitive outcomes at 1 year of age or an indirect association with these outcomes, as mediated by the child-rearing environment. Subjects were 61 black infants attending community-based child care programs. The presence of OME was assessed biweekly from 6 to 12 months of age by otoscopy and tympanometry. Hearing was assessed with visual reinforcement audiometry when children were well and when ill with OME. Language and cognitive skills and the child-rearing environment at home and in child care were examined. The results indicated a modest correlation between hearing loss associated with OME and receptive language. However, the direct association between OME-related hearing loss and all the language and cognitive measures was negligible. Hearing loss had an indirect association with receptive and expressive language, cognitive development, and overall communication as mediated by child-rearing factors. That is, children with more frequent hearing loss tended to have less responsive mothers and home environments, and this association was linked to lower performance on the infant assessments. (J Pediatr 1995;126:481-9)

During the past decade an increasing number of studies have reported that children with frequent or persistent otitis media with effusion during early childhood perform more poorly on measures of language than their peers without a significant history of OME.[1, 2] One explanation is that the mild to moderate fluctuating hearing loss associated with OME negatively affects language development during the formative years of language learning. The child whose hearing sensitivity changes may receive a partial or inconsistent auditory signal, thereby missing or confusing important auditory information. Persistent or frequent disruptions in auditory input, in turn, may impair the development of language skills.

Although the relation between early OME and later language and cognitive development is conceptually compelling, the results of studies examining language sequelae of OME have been inconsistent. Many studies have reported

Supported by Maternal and Child Health Program (MCJ-370599 and MCJ-370649, Title V, Social Security Act), Health Resources and Services Administration, U.S. Department of Health and Human Services.

Submitted for publication July 6, 1994; accepted Oct. 4, 1994.

Reprint requests: Joanne E. Roberts, PhD, Frank Porter Graham Child Development Center, University of North Carolina at Chapel Hill, CB 8180, 105 Smith Level Rd., Chapel Hill, NC 27599-8180.

0022-3476/95/$3.00 + 0 **9/73/61029**

CSBS	Communication and Symbolic Behavior Scales
dB HL	Decibels, hearing level
ECA	Expressive communication age
GFI	Goodness-of-fit index
HOME	Home Observation for Measurement of the Environment—Inventory for Infants
ITERS	Infant/Toddler Environment Rating Scale
MDI	Mental Development Index
NCATS	Nursing Child Assessment Teaching Scales
OME	Otitis media with effusion
PNP	Pediatric nurse practitioner
RCA	Receptive communication age
SICD-R	Sequenced Inventory of Communication Development—Revised

that children with frequent OME during the first few years of life score lower on language measures during infancy,[3] the preschool years,[1, 2] and into the school-age years.[4, 5] Other investigators have not demonstrated an association between OME and language during these same periods.[6-8] Methodologic problems may explain the discrepant findings in these studies; these include collection of OME data retrospectively, cross-sectional study designs, inadequate OME documentation both in subjects and controls, and failure to document hearing sensitivity.[6, 9, 10] Moreover, almost all previous studies examining the developmental sequelae of OME lacked consideration of the multiple factors influencing child development and considered only the consequences of OME or, in some studies, of hearing loss on children's language and learning. Recent models of child development, however, emphasize the dynamic, multifactorial nature of development within the child's environment.[11, 12]

From a transactional perspective,[12] children with frequent hearing loss associated with OME may miss or only partially hear communication around them and thus may be less responsive to caregivers. Caregivers, in turn, may modify their interaction styles, causing them to be less responsive and less likely to initiate interactions with the child. Less-than-optimal language development could result if caregiver-child interactions continue to be less frequent or less responsive after the child's OME has resolved. Further, even after OME episodes resolve, the caregiver may view the child as less linguistically skilled, and these beliefs may continue to influence patterns of interaction.[13, 14]

The purpose of this study was to use a prospective design to determine whether OME-related hearing loss showed direct or indirect associations with child outcomes at 1 year of age. We postulated that the mild to moderate fluctuating hearing loss associated with persistent OME during the formative years of language learning may be either directly associated with children's cognitive and language development, or indirectly associated with children's cognitive and language development, as mediated by changes in the caregiver-child interaction style.

METHODS

Study populations. Participants in this study were 61 black infants attending one of nine center-based child care programs. Children between the ages of 6 and 12 months were enrolled in a longitudinal study during a 20-month period. To be included in the present study, children had to be enrolled in the study between 6 and 9 months of age (mean age at entry was 7.2 months). Infants were enrolled in the nine child care programs at a mean age of 4 months. Twenty-eight children were boys and 33 were girls. Forty-nine of the children were born at full gestational age (>37 weeks); of the others, six children were born at 37 weeks, five at 36 weeks, and one at 30 weeks. On study entry, 62.3% of the children were from low income families according to the federally defined poverty level. A majority of the mothers were single (59%), and about half (54.2%) had completed high school (mean maternal educational level was 12.6 years); mean maternal age at the time of the child's birth was 24.7 years, and mean IQ was 87.9. The research protocol was reviewed and approved each year by the university's institutional research review board.

Documentation of otitis media. Children's ears were examined by a pediatric nurse practitioner under the supervision of a pediatrician. A period of 32 months elapsed from the recruitment of the first infant until the last infant's 1-year assessment. For the first 15 months of the study, ear observations were done weekly, and then biweekly for the last 17 months. The justification for changing from weekly to biweekly ear examinations was based on the difficulty (i.e., fussiness) for some infants during the weekly ear examinations and the finding of no significant differences in the incidence of OME between weekly and biweekly observations on two independent data sets (data in the current study and in our previous work[15]). In the present study, children who left participating child care centers were seen every 4 weeks at home or at their new child care site.

Ear status was determined by pneumatic otoscopy and tympanometry. The diagnosis of OME was based on otoscopic observation; tympanometry was used to corroborate the diagnosis. When otoscopic examination was not successful, tympanometric results were used as the primary diagnosis. OME was classified as purulent (acute) when the fluid in the middle ear was opaque and yellowish white. OME was classified as serous when the fluid in the middle ear was clear or straw colored in appearance. Fluid was presumed to be present when the tympanic membrane was immobile or fluid levels were observed in the middle ear. Using a portable tympanometer (Earscan, model ES-T; Micro Audiometrics Corp., Port Orange, Fla.), we classified tympanograms as flat (abnormally low mobility) when acoustic admittance was $\leq$0.2 siemens (millimhos).

Agreement between judgments of mobility on pneumatic otoscopy and tympanometry, based on 1281 observations, was 94% (κ = 0.78). Interobserver agreement between the project PNP and the pediatrician was 89% (κ = 0.65) for mobility and 91% for diagnosis (κ = 0.68), based on 70 ear observations. Interobserver agreement between the PNP and a reference otologist, whose otoscopy skills were validated against myringotomy, was 89% (κ = 0.66) for mobility and 89% (κ = 0.64) for diagnosis, based on 76 ear observations.

Children were seen for ear examinations an average of 15.2 times between study entry and 1 year of age (range, 8 to 27 times). The time interval between ear observations was weekly for 33.9% of the ear examinations, biweekly for 55.4%, and monthly for 10.3%. Treatment for acute otitis media was with antibiotics; decongestants were not prescribed.

The percentage of observation time with and without OME (unilateral, bilateral, total OME—unilateral or bilateral OME) from study entry until 1 year of age was computed for each child. Because individual children's ear status was assessed for different lengths of time (depending on age at study entry), the percentage of time that the children had OME was calculated by subtracting the date at onset of OME from the date of the resolution of the OME. The date at onset of OME was calculated as midway between the last day that the ears were normal and the first day that OME was present. Resolution of OME was calculated as midway between the last day that OME was present and the first day that the ears were normal. Next, the percentage of days with unilateral, bilateral, and total OME were totaled for each child. Finally, to compute the percentage of observation time with OME (unilateral, bilateral, and total), we divided the number of days that each child was in the study into the number of days that a child had unilateral OME, bilateral OME, and total OME.

Hearing assessment. Hearing sensitivity was evaluated behaviorally with visual reinforcement audiometry. Test stimuli consisted of frequency-modulated pure tones (500, 2000, 4000 Hz) presented through a loudspeaker in a calibrated sound field. The visual reinforcers consisted of three different sets of animated toys mounted in separate smoked-glass enclosures, with random presentation of each. Two examiners participated in each test session: an experienced pediatric audiologist who controlled the test stimuli, and a trained graduate student who remained in the test room with the subject. To activate the reinforcer, both examiners were required to "vote" affirmatively by depressing a switch. The second examiner also assisted by returning the child's attention to midline between presentations. A response was defined as a head turn or an eye-gaze shift toward the loudspeaker or visual reinforcer. Stimuli were initially presented at 60 dB HL, along with visual reinforcement. When the examiner established that the child was conditioned (two consecutive responses), the intensity level was decreased in 20 dB steps until no response was observed. Subsequent increases and decreases in intensity used a 10 dB step size. Threshold was defined as the lowest level at which the child responded at least two of four times for each frequency.

The overall validity of each session was ranked by the audiologist on a scale of 1 to 5, on the basis of the child's state (ease of conditioning, activity level, interest in reinforcer, noise level, cooperativeness) with "1" representing poor validity and "5" excellent validity. Interobserver agreement between the audiologist and the research assistant, computed for presence or absence of a response (head turn by child) during visual reinforcement audiometry for 231 sessions (63% of the sessions), was 97.4%.

Children's hearing was tested (1) routinely on study entry and every 3 months, (2) during weeks 1, 4, 7, and 13 after a diagnosis of OME, and (3) after a change in ear status (e.g., bilateral to unilateral OME, bilateral OME to normal). Hearing testing was conducted in a mobile testing unit that housed a single wall sound suite. Testing was done at each child's care center. Sound level measurements were taken periodically at the test site. Although transient or intermittent noises in the environment could necessitate a temporary suspension of testing, mean ambient noise levels during audiologic assessment were consistently within 2 dB of American National Standards Institute[16] allowable levels. To keep the audiologist and research assistant masked to children's ear status, the PNP gave the audiologist a weekly testing schedule that listed children's names but no information about ear status.

Children were seen for hearing tests an average of six times between study entry and 1 year of age (range, 4 to 12 times). Sessions judged to have a validity ranking of "1" were dropped from the data analysis, as were sessions with results from fewer than two frequencies. These accounted for only 9% of the test sessions (all sessions with a validity of "1" also had fewer than two thresholds). The thresholds for sessions in which two thresholds were obtained and in which the session validity was rated "2" or more were used to compute a hearing level for each session.

To provide a summary index of hearing loss, we considered response levels of 25 dB HL or greater, on at least half of the thresholds tested (1/2 or 2/3) in a session, indicative of significant hearing loss. Because individual children's hearing was assessed for different lengths of time (depending on age of entry), the percentage of time that children had hearing loss was then calculated by subtracting the date at onset of a hearing loss from the date at resolution of hearing loss. The date at onset of a hearing loss was calculated as midway between the last day of normal hearing and the first day that hearing loss was present. Resolution of hearing loss was calculated as midway between the last day the hearing loss was present and the first day it was within the normal range. Next, the percentage of days with significant hearing loss was totaled for each child. Finally, to compute the percentage of observation time with hearing loss, we divided the number of days that each child was in the study into the number of days that a child had a hearing loss.

Language and cognitive measures. Children's communication skills were assessed at 1 year of age with two standardized measures: the Sequenced Inventory of Communication Development—Revised[17] and the Communication and Symbolic Behavior Scales—Research Edition.[18] The SICD-R provides an overall measure of children's receptive and expressive communication skills for children aged 4 months to 4 years. A receptive communication age and an expressive communication age were derived for each scale. For the standardization sample, high interexaminer reliability and stability are reported.[17]

The CSBS is a new standardized measure designed to examine the communicative, social, and symbolic abilities of children between 8 months and 2 years of developmental age. Cluster scores (communication functions, communication means gestural, communication means vocal, communication means verbal, reciprocity, and social-affective signaling) are computed from 18 scales measuring functional communication. One cluster score (symbolic) is derived from four scales measuring symbolic development. A communication composite score (CSBS-Total) is computed by summing the scaled scores for the 18 communication scales. High levels of reliability and validity are reported in the normed edition.

Children's cognitive skills were assessed with the Bayley Scales of Infant Development.[19] Overall cognitive level is represented by the Mental Development Index. The reliability and validity of the Bayley Scales have been well documented.[19]

The standard scores on the MDI of the Bayley Scales and CSBS-Total scores were corrected for gestational age for children 37 weeks or less at birth. The SICD-R and CSBS were administered by one of two speech-language pathologists, who also administered the Bayley Scales under the supervision of a clinical psychologist. Testing was done in the sound room of a mobile test van. The speech-language pathologists and the psychologist were masked to children's OME and hearing experiences during infancy.

Child-rearing environment. The quality of the home and child care environments was assessed with the use of several instruments. The Home Observation for Measurement of the Environment—Inventory for Infants[20] examined maternal responsiveness and the overall quality and responsiveness of the home environment. Each child and family were visited at home by one of three trained observers when the child reached 9 months of age, or on study entry if the child entered the study between 9 and 11 months of age. The HOME is a 45-item semistructured observation-interview instrument composed of six subscales: emotional and verbal responsivity of the parent, acceptance of the child's behavior, organization of the environment, provision of appropriate play materials, and maternal involvement with the child. The HOME total, computed by summing the items, was used in the analyses. Moderate internal-consistency reliability, acceptable levels of test-retest reliability, and high levels of content validity have been reported for both white families and black families.[21]

The quality of the mother's teaching style was assessed with the Nursing Child Assessment Teaching Scales.[22] The teaching task, one component of the NCATS, assesses mother-child interactions in a structured situation. Parents were instructed to teach their child a block-building task. The session took place after the cognitive measurement at 1 year of age, and was videotaped. The interactions are then coded in six subscales: sensitivity to cues, response to distress, social-emotional growth fostering, cognitive growth fostering, clarity of cues, and child's responsiveness to parent. A total score also is computed by adding the subscales' scores. Interrater reliability between two trained coders based on 20 children was $r = 0.75$ (range, 0.61 to 0.83), with a weighted kappa.

The Infant/Toddler Environment Rating Scale[23] was used to assess the quality of caregiving and physical environment in the infant classes at the child care centers. The ITERS is a 35-item rating scale divided into seven sections: furnishings and display for children, personal care routines, listening and talking, learning activities, interaction, program structure, and adult needs. High reliability and validity have been reported. Each of the 35 items is rated on a 7-point scale ranging from inadequate to excellent. An average item score (ITERS-Total) was computed by dividing the sum of the items scored by the number of items scored. A trained examiner completed the ITERS during a 2- to 3-hour observation in each classroom during the spring of each child's first year in child care.

Data analysis. Data analysis involved both a descriptive and an inferential analysis to test the associations among OME, hearing loss, quality of care, and infant outcomes. The descriptive analyses involved correlating the otitis media, hearing, quality of child rearing, and child outcomes to examine the simple linear relations among them. The child outcomes were Bayley Scales MDI, SICD-R RCA, SICD-R ECA, and CSBS-Total, and were chosen because they are well accepted measures of children's communication and cognitive skills. Spearman rank-order correlations were estimated because OME and hearing loss have very skewed distributions in this sample. The inferential analysis involved fitting structural equation models[24] to the infant communication and cognitive outcomes. These models examined (1) the direct association of hearing loss with the child outcomes (proportion of time with hearing loss), quality of home environment, quality of the child care environment, maternal IQ, child gender, and whether the family's income was low and (2) the indirect association with the child outcome of maternal IQ and hearing loss through their influence on the quality of the home environment. The home environment was represented as a composite variable represented by the HOME total score (HOME-Total) and the NCATS teaching task total score (NCATS-Total). Structural equation model analyses[24] tested the direct and indirect associations between infant outcomes and hearing loss, quality of care at home, quality of care in the child care center, maternal IQ, gender of the infant, and poverty status of the family.

Structural equation model analyses[24] represent a generalization of regression model analyses. As for regression models, it is assumed that the dependent (outcome) variable can be represented as the weighted sum of the independent (predictor) variables. Structural equation models generalize regression models in two ways: the estimation of both indirect and direct associations between predictor and outcome variables, and the estimation of latent variables. Whereas regression analyses can test only the degree to which a variable is related to the outcome after adjustment for common covariance with the outcome variable that is shared between the variable and other predictors in the model (a direct effect), structural equation models permit the analysis of relations between a predictor and outcome in terms of the variable's direct effect and in terms of the variable's covariance with another variable (an indirect effect). In our analysis, we examined the extent to which hearing loss and maternal IQ covary with the quality of the home environment, resulting in indirect relations with infant development. In addition, structural equation models allow the inclusion of latent variables to represent general constructs that are not easily measured by a single indicator variable. These latent variables are estimated as a composite from several variables. In our analyses, two distinct measures of the quality of the home environment (HOME-Total and NCATS-Total) were used to create a latent variable.

Table I. Means of developmental outcomes, environmental variables, and correlations with OME and hearing (N = 61)

	Mean (SD)	Correlations with bilateral OME	Correlations with hearing >25 dB
CSBS			
Communication composite	100.6 (10.2)	−0.16	−0.10
SICD-R			
RCA (mo)	13.2 (2.1)	−0.38†	−0.42‡
ECA (mo)	14.3 (2.5)	0.05	−0.04
Bayley Scales			
MDI	115.1 (12.5)	−0.03	−0.11
HOME			
Total	34.5 (4.7)	−0.46‡	−0.49§
NCATS			
Total	60.0 (7.2)	−0.28*	−0.17
ITERS			
Total	3.0 (0.8)	−0.18	−0.21

*p <0.05.
†p <0.01.
‡p <0.001.
§p <0.0001.

RESULTS

Descriptive analyses. Descriptive analysis examined the OME experience of the children and the correlations among OME, hearing loss, quality of care, and infant outcomes. Table I presents the means and standard deviations of language, cognitive, and environmental measures.

Otitis media experience. Children who had had more bilateral OME also had less unilateral OME (r −0.82; p 0.0001) and more total OME (r 0.82; p 0.0001). Children had bilateral OME during 74.9% (SD 26.2%) of the observation time, unilateral OME in 13.6% (SD 14.1%) of the observation time, and no OME in 11.5% (SD 19.0%) of the observation period. Total OME occurred in 88.5% (SD 19.0%) of the observation time.

Hearing sensitivity. During 49% of the sessions, children had a threshold 25 dB HL or greater for 500 Hz, during 47.9% of the sessions for 2000 Hz, and during 63.3% of the sessions for 4000 Hz. When we applied the criterion for hearing loss as having at least half of the thresholds in a session at 25 dB HL or greater, children had a hearing loss in 35.3% of the test sessions. However, the percentage of time with hearing loss varied greatly. Four children never had a hearing loss, 11 had hearing loss between 1% and 19% of the observation time, 17 had hearing loss 20% to 49% of the time, 7 had hearing loss 50% to 69%, 13 had hearing loss 70% to 99%, and 9 children had hearing loss 100% of the observation period (Figure). Children who had more bilateral OME with time had more hearing loss (r 0.75; p 0.0001), and they also had higher mean thresholds (indicative of poorer hearing (r 0.67; p 0.0001). Similarly, children who had more total OME had more hearing loss with time (r 0.57; p 0.0001) and had higher mean hearing thresholds (r 0.51; p 0.0001).

Otitis media, hearing, and quality of child rearing. There were significant relationships between HOME scores and bilateral OME (r −0.46; p 0.0002), total OME (r −0.32; p

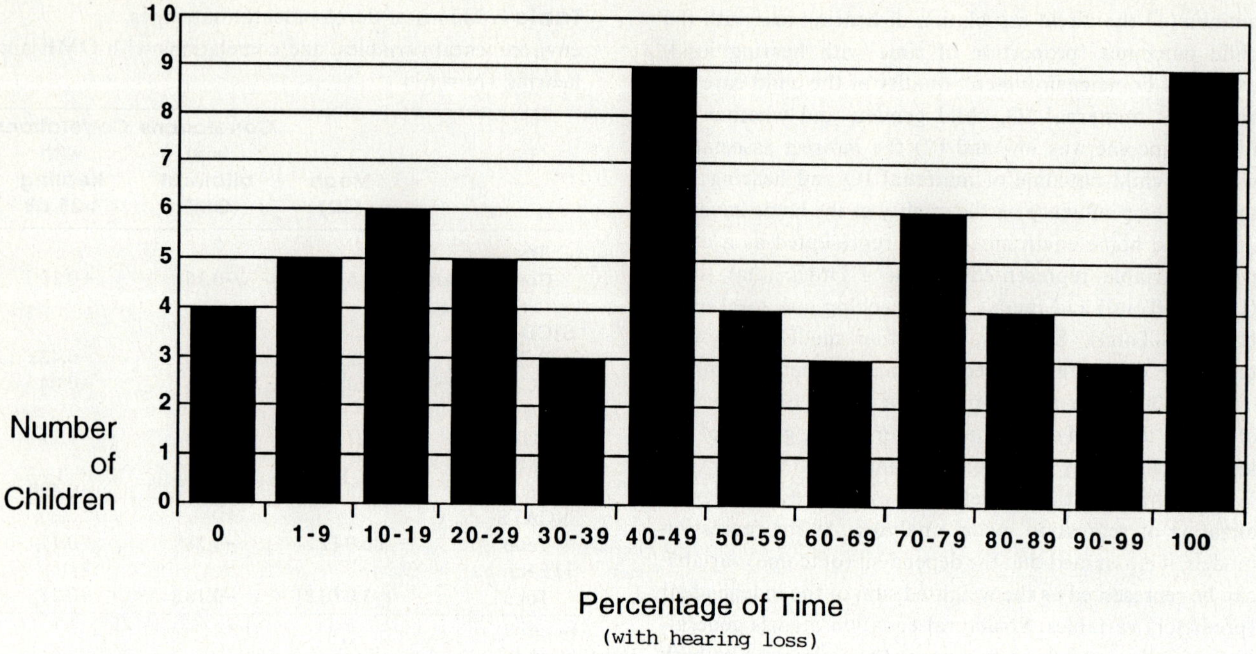

Figure. Distribution of percentage of time that children had hearing loss (hearing levels of 25 dB or greater).

0.0113), and hearing loss (r −0.49; p 0.0001). Children with more bilateral OME had had lower NCATS scores (r −0.28; p 0.0289), whereas children with more total OME had lower ITERS scores (r −0.28; p 0.0296) (Table II).

Otitis media, hearing, and child outcomes. The RCA was significantly lower for children with more bilateral OME (r −0.38; p 0.0023), more total OME (r −0.31; p 0.015), and more frequent hearing loss (r −0.42; p 0.0007) (Table I).

Structural equation model analyses. Structural equation model analyses[24] tested the direct and indirect associations between infant outcomes and hearing loss, quality of care at home, quality of care in the child care center, maternal IQ, gender of the infant, and poverty status of the family. In addition, age was included in analyses of the SICD RCA and ECA because the outcome measures were developmental ages rather than standard scores. Tests of the overall fit of the model using a goodness-of-fit index indicated that the indirect terms were needed for adequate fit of the data to the model (GFI values >0.90 are considered to provide good evidence of significant fit of data to model[24]). Analysis of the models that included an indirect association for hearing loss through quality of the home environment indicated that these models provided a good fit to all four outcome measures: the Bayley Scales MDI (GFI 0.98), the SICD-R RCA (GFI 0.98), the SICD-R ECA (GFI 0.97), and the CSBS-Total score (GFI 0.98). Analyses that excluded that indirect association resulted in poorly fitting models.

Both direct and indirect associations were obtained, as illustrated in Table II. Examination of the models indicated that direct associations between the quality of the home environment and infant outcomes were obtained for the Bayley Scales MDI ($t[54] = 8.21$; $p < 0.001$), the SICD-R RCA ($t[52] = 7.48$; $p < 0.001$), the SICD-R ECA ($t[52] = 2.34$; $p < 0.05$), and the CSBS-Total ($t[54] = 4.61$; $p < 0.001$). Indirect negative relations of OME-related hearing loss were observed with child outcomes through its association with the quality of the home care environment for the Bayley Scales MDI ($t[54] = -2.25$; $p < 0.05$), the SICD-R RCA ($t[52] = -2.51$; $p < 0.01$), the SICD-R ECA ($t[52] = -2.00$; $p < 0.05$), and the CSBS-Total ($t[54] = -2.35$; $p < 0.05$). Thus the hearing loss outcome relation was mediated by the quality of the home environment, such that OME-related hearing loss was negatively related to the home environment and the home environment was positively related to child outcomes. Finally, the indirect positive associations of child outcomes with the mother's IQ through its association with the quality of the home care environment were detected for the MDI ($t[54] = 1.77$; $p < 0.05$), the SICD-R RCA ($t[52] = 1.89$; $p < 0.05$), and the CSBS ($t[54] = 1.82$; $p < 0.05$).

DISCUSSION

This study provides further evidence documenting the high prevalence of OME among infants in group child

Table II. Testing for direct and indirect effects of hearing loss in analyses of infant development

	Regression coefficients from structural equation models			
	Bayley MDI	SICD-R RCA	SICD-R ECA	CSBS-Total
Direct effects				
Hearing loss	−0.03 (0.13)	−0.14 (0.13)	0.15 (0.15)	0.16 (0.14)
HOME	0.45‡ (0.05)	1.00 (0.13)	0.58† (0.25)	0.70‡ (0.15)
ITERS	0.16 (0.13)	−0.06 (0.11)	0.16 (0.13)	0.10 (0.13)
Poverty	0.22 (0.14)	−0.03 (0.13)	0.00 (0.14)	−0.14 (0.14)
Mother's IQ	−0.06 (0.14)	0.08 (0.12)	0.07 (0.15)	0.09 (0.14)
Sex (male)	0.06 (0.13)	−0.10 (0.11)	−0.17 (0.13)	−0.10 (0.12)
Indirect effects—through quality of home environment				
Hearing loss	−0.24* (0.11)	−0.25† (0.10)	−0.22† (0.11)	−0.25* (0.11)
Mother's IQ	0.13* (0.07)	0.13* (0.07)	0.11 (0.07)	0.13* (0.07)

Values are regression coefficients β_1 and their standard errors in parentheses.
*$p < 0.05$.
†$p < 0.01$.
‡$p < 0.001$.

care, and supports a transactional model[12] postulating an indirect association between hearing loss related to OME and the early stages of children's cognitive and language development. Bilateral OME with accompanying hearing loss was commonly experienced by infants in group care. Hearing loss was significantly correlated with receptive language. However, the results of the structural equations analysis indicated that the direct association between OME-related hearing loss and the infant language and cognitive outcomes was negligible. Hearing loss during the second 6 months of life had an indirect association with receptive language, expressive language, cognitive development, and overall communication at 1 year of age as mediated by the quality of the home environment.

These results support recent multifactorial models[11, 12] of development in that the impact of multiple factors, rather than a single factor, is important for child development, and the role of the child's environment is also considered. Study results suggest that the extent to which children have hearing loss associated with OME relates to the interaction style of the mother and the quality of the home environment, and that family factors can have important consequences for a child's development. That is, the hearing loss associated with frequent OME during early childhood may affect the establishment of responsive interaction styles between the mother and child. Mild to moderate hearing losses, caused by OME, may cause the child to appear unresponsive; the mother, in turn, may not receive the cues needed to establish a more responsive interactive style. The result may be a negative effect on the development of the child's communication and cognitive skills. Considerable research[25, 26] supports the influence of a responsive parenting style on children's language development.

Although the results of the descriptive analyses indicated a significant correlation between hearing loss and receptive communication skills, a direct effect of OME-associated hearing loss on child outcomes was not found with the structural equations analysis. Only when parenting style and quality of the home child-rearing environment were included in the statistical model was a significant relationship observed. Although many studies have reported a direct relation between OME experience and language during infancy,[4] others have not.[7] Further, two studies that documented hearing loss[1, 4] reported direct associations of hearing loss with child outcomes. Thus the results of our present study point to the importance of studying the multiplicity of factors affecting children's development.

The link between hearing loss and parenting style in this study is similar to the results reported by Black et al.[27] and by Forgays et al.,[28] although they examined OME experience rather than the hearing loss associated with OME. Black et al.[27] found that among 1- to 2-year-old children with histories of OME and low-income status, the mothers were less warm and sociable in interactions with their children than were mothers of children with little or no history of OME. In a study of middle-class white children, Forgays et al.[28] reported that mothers of 2-year-old children who had recurrent OME described themselves as more depressed and less competent, and described their children as more demanding, than did mothers of children without an OME history.

The link of OME and parenting style to child development is consistent with several other studies,[29-31] but in these studies the presence of OME rather than the hearing loss associated with OME was examined. Three recent studies found that parenting styles may interact with children's OME to affect their development.[29-31] Freeark et al.[30] studied middle-class families and found that recurrent OME during the first 3 years of life was negatively associated with children's verbal abilities at 3 to 4 years of age among children receiving low parental verbal stimulation. Chase et al.[29] reported that 1-year-old predominantly middle-class white children with a significant history of OME were less responsive to their mothers during a structured interaction, and that their mothers were less effective as teachers in comparison with the interactions of children without an OME history. Wallace et al.[31] found that mothers' interaction styles when children were 2 years of age correlated with children's expressive and receptive language skills at 3 and 4 years among children with frequent OME, but not among children without a history of OME.

In this study, many of the methodologic problems that contributed to biases in previous investigations were avoided. We used a prospective design with frequent documentation of children's OME history and hearing loss from an early age. Children were not selected for this study because of their OME histories or language difficulty. Hearing loss rather than OME experience was documented and repeatedly measured, and was examined in relation to children's communication and cognitive development. Finally, we measured multiple factors influencing development (e.g., quality of child care and parenting experiences), which allowed for a thorough analysis of potentially interactive effects. Children attending group child care are at increased risk of having OME and associated hearing loss,[32] although other studies suggest that children attending high-quality child care programs are more cognitively advanced.[33]

The results of this study should be interpreted carefully for several reasons. First, the modest level of these associations likely reflects a complex myriad of factors that, along with hearing loss, contribute to development. Second, children's OME and hearing histories before 6 months of age were not measured. Third, developmental assessments at 1 year of age are often a poor predictor of later developmental outcomes. Finally, as in any observational research, causality—that hearing loss causes differences in child-rearing patterns which affect later communication abilities—cannot be inferred directly from this study. However, the research was prospective with OME, hearing loss, and the outcomes measured carefully, and possible mediating factors (e.g., quality of the home and child care environment) were documented.

We conclude that hearing loss caused by OME had an indirect association with receptive and expressive language, cognitive development, and overall communication at 1 year of age as mediated by child-rearing factors. These results should be interpreted cautiously because infant outcomes often do not predict long-term outcomes. The study children will continue to be followed longitudinally to explore the interrelationship among OME and hearing loss, family and child care environments, and communication and cognitive development in the preschool years.

We acknowledge Elizabeth Gunn for assistance with data analysis, Rhodus Riggins and Brenda Davis for their assistance in data collection, and the families and children for participating in this study.

REFERENCES

1. Friel-Patti S, Finitzo T. Language learning in a prospective study of otitis media with effusion in the first two years of life. J Speech Hear Res 1990;33:188-194.
2. Teele DW, Klein JO, Rosner BA, the Greater Boston Otitis Media Study Group. Otitis media with effusion during the first three years of life and development of speech and language. Pediatrics 1984;74:282-7.
3. Wallace IF, Gravel JS, McCarton CM, Ruben RJ. Otitis media and language development at 1 year of age. J Speech Hear Dis 1988;53:245-51.
4. Teele DW, Klein JO, Chase C, et al. Otitis media in infancy and intellectual ability, school achievement, speech, and language at age 7 years. J Infect Dis 1990;162:685-94.
5. Sak RJ, Ruben RJ. Effects of recurrent middle ear effusion in preschool years on language and learning. Developmental and Behavioral Pediatrics 1982;3:7-11.
6. Roberts JE, Burchinal MR, Davis BP, Collier AM, Henderson FW. Otitis media in early childhood and later language. J Speech Hear Res 1991;34:1158-68.
7. Wright PF, Sell SH, McConnell KB, et al. Impact of recurrent otitis media on middle ear function, hearing, and language. J Pediatr 1988;113:581-7.
8. Gravel JS, Wallace IF. Listening and language at 4 years of age: effects of early otitis media. J Speech Hear Res 1992; 35:588-95.
9. Paradise JL, Rogers KD. On otitis media, child development, and tympanostomy tubes: new answers or old questions? Pediatrics 1986;77:88-92.
10. Ruben JR, Bagger-Sjoback D, Downs MP, et al. Complications and sequelae. Ann Otol Rhinol Laryngol 1989;98(suppl 139):46-55.
11. Huston AC, McLoyd VC, Coll CG. Children and poverty: issues in contemporary research. Child Dev 1994;65:275-82.
12. Sameroff AJ. Developmental systems: contexts and evolution. In: W. Kessen, ed. History, theories, and methods; vol 1. New York: John Wiley, 1983. (PH Mussen, Ed. Handbook of child development.
13. Feagans LV, Proctor A. Effects of mild illness in infancy on later development: the sample case of the effects of otitis media (middle ear effusion). In: Applied developmental psychology. Fisher CB, Lerner RM, eds. New York: McGraw-Hill, 1994.
14. Roberts JE, Schuele CM. Otitis media and later academic performance: the linkage and implications for intervention. Topics in Language Disorders 1990;11:43-62.
15. Roberts JE, Sanyal MA, Burchinal MR, Collier AM, Ramey CT, Henderson FW. Otitis media in early childhood and its relationship to later verbal and academic performance. Pediatrics 1986;78:423-30.
16. American National Standards Institute. Criteria for permissible ambient noise during audiometric testing. (ANSI 3.1-

1977.) New York: American National Standards Institute, 1977.

17. Hedrick DL, Prather EM, Tobin AR. Sequenced Inventory of Communication Development—Revised. Seattle: University of Washington Press, 1984.
18. Wetherby AM, Prizant BM. Communication and Symbolic Behavior Scales [Research edition]. San Antonio: Special Press, 1990.
19. Bayley N. Bayley Scales of Infant Development. New York: Psychological Corp., 1969.
20. Caldwell BM, Bradley RH. Home Observation for Measurement of the Environment. Revised ed. Little Rock: University of Arkansas, 1984.
21. Bradley RH, Caldwell BM, Rock SL, et al. Home environment and cognitive development in the first 3 years of life: a collaborative study involving six sites and three ethnic groups in North America. Developmental Psychology 1989;25:217-35.
22. Barnard KE. The Nursing Child Assessment Teaching Scales. Seattle: University of Washington, 1978.
23. Harms T, Cryer D, Clifford RM. Infant/Toddler Environment Rating Scale. New York: Teachers College Press, 1990.
24. Bollen KA. Structural equations with latent variables. New York: John Wiley & Sons, 1989.
25. Garvey C. Children's talk. Cambridge: Harvard University Press, 1984.
26. Snow CE. Parent-child interaction in the development of communicative ability. In: Schiefelbusch RL, Pickar J, eds. The acquisition of communicative competence. Baltimore: University Park Press, 1984:69-107.
27. Black MM, Gerson LF, Freeland CAB, Nair P, Rubin JS, Hutcheson JJ. Language screening for infants prone to otitis media. J Pediatr Psychol 1988;13:423-33.
28. Forgays D, Hasazi J, Wasserman R. Recurrent otitis media and parenting stress in mothers of two year old children. Dev Behav Pediatr 1992;13:321-5.
29. Chase C, Teele DW, Klein JO, Rosner BA. Behavioral sequelae of otitis media for infants at one year of age and their mothers. In: Lim DJ, Bluestone CD, Klein JO, Nelson JD, eds. Recent advances in otitis media. Abstracts of the Fifth International Symposium, Fort Lauderdale, Florida, 1991.
30. Freeark K, Frank SJ, Wagner AE, Lopez M, Olmsted C, Girard R. Otitis media, language development, and parental verbal stimulation. J Pediatr Psychol 1992;17:173-85.
31. Wallace IF, Gravel JS, Ganon EC, Ruben RJ. Two year language outcomes as a function of otitis media and parental linguistic styles. In: Lim DJ, Bluestone CB, Klein JO, eds. Recent advances in otitis media: proceedings of the Fifth International Symposium. Toronto: BC Decker, 1993.
32. Haskins R, Kotch J. Day care and illness: evidence, costs, and public policy. Pediatrics 1986;77:951-82.
33. Whitebook M, Howes C, Phillips D. Who cares? Child care teachers and the quality of care in America: national child care staffing study. Oakland, California: Child Care Employee Project, 1989.

Bacteriuria in children with neurogenic bladder treated with intermittent catheterization: Natural history

Theresa A. Schlager, MD, Susan Dilks, MD, Julie Trudell, RN, Thomas S. Whittam, PhD, and J. Owen Hendley, MD

From the Department of Pediatrics, University of Virginia, Charlottesville, and the Department of Biology, Pennsylvania State University, University Park, and the Pendleton Pediatric Infectious Disease Research Laboratory, Charlottesville, Virginia

Objective: **To determine whether bacteriuria unassociated with symptoms in patients with neurogenic bladder will lead to symptomatic infection and/or deterioration of the upper urinary tract if left untreated, we examined whether bacteriuria persisted in bladder urine of children with neurogenic bladder treated with clean intermittent catheterization (CIC) and whether persistence of bacteria led to symptomatic infection or deterioration of the upper urinary tract.**
Design: **Weekly home visits were made during 6 months of surveillance of 14 children on the CIC regimen with a normal upper urinary tract and no reflux (as determined by renal ultrasonography, voiding cystourethrography, and serum creatinine measurement). During visits a sample of bladder urine was obtained by CIC, and signs and symptoms of urinary tract infection and all medications were recorded.**
Results: **Fourteen children were observed for 323 weeks. Cultures of 70% (172/244) of the urine samples collected were positive for organisms ($\geq 10^4$ colony-forming units per milliliter), 152 (88%) for the usual pathogens and 20 (12%) for commensal organisms. Bacteriuria was associated with pyuria two thirds of the time, regardless of bacterial species. Carriage of the same pathogen for 4 weeks or longer, with associated pyuria, was common during surveillance. Despite frequent episodes of bacteriuria with associated pyuria, there were only five symptomatic infections during the 323 patient-weeks. Children remained clinically well during the study period, and their upper urinary tract did not deteriorate.**
Conclusion: **Bacteriuria persists for weeks in symptom-free children being treated with CIC for neurogenic bladder associated with a normal upper urinary tract. Before attempts are made to eradicate bacteriuria, treatment should be proved to be beneficial to this population. (J PEDIATR 1995;126:490-6)**

The majority of children with neurogenic bladder have loss of control over voiding; urinary retention and bladder distention usually occur in the absence of intervention. Obstruction caused by urinary retention may lead to deterioration of the urinary tract. In addition, urinary retention may result in reflux into the upper urinary tract and subsequent renal damage.[1] Several strategies for complete emptying of the bladder on a regular basis have been tried.[2-6] Clean in-and-out, or intermittent, catheterization of the

CIC	Clean intermittent catheterization
UTI	Urinary tract infection

Supported in part by a grant from the Spinal Cord Research Foundation.

Submitted for publication Aug. 8, 1994; accepted Sept. 16, 1994.

Reprint requests: T. Schlager, MD, University of Virginia, Department of Pediatrics, Box 386, Charlottesville, VA 22908.

0022-3476/95/$3.00 + 0 **9/73/60616**

bladder several times daily is currently the preferred method of bladder emptying in patients with neurogenic bladder, but inoculation of bacteria into bladder urine is inevitable. On the other hand, complete emptying of the bladder is thought to be critical in preventing bladder infection.[3] Bacteriuria is frequently found on CIC in patients without urinary symptoms.[7] Detection of bacteriuria presents a dilemma for the physician: Is this asymptomatic bacteriuria that does not need antimicrobial treatment, or is it an infection that would be symptomatic if it were not for the patient's sensory deficits? In addition, it is not known whether bacteriuria unassociated with symptoms in patients with neurogenic bladder will lead to symptomatic infection or deterioration of the upper urinary tract, or both, if left untreated.

We investigated both the frequency and the effect of bacteriuria in children with neurogenic bladder managed with CIC who were living at home. In our first study of symptom-free children, we found that 50% of bladder urine specimens obtained with a sterile catheter contained $\geq 10^4$ colony-forming units of bacterial pathogen(s) per milliliter.[8] Pyuria was present in half of the urine specimens with positive culture results. In the current study we investigated whether bacteriuria persisted in bladder urine and whether persistence of bacteria led to subsequent symptomatic infection or deterioration of the upper urinary tract.

METHODS

Population. The Kluge Children's Rehabilitation Center Myelomeningocele Clinic, University of Virginia, provides multidisciplinary care (neurosurgical, urologic, orthopedic, pediatrics) for more than 200 children with neurogenic bladder. Eighty percent of these children have a myelomeningocele and 20% have a traumatic spinal cord injury. Children (1 to 18 years of age) with neurogenic bladder who were on the CIC regimen were recruited for the study during a routine clinic visit. Children were enrolled if they were not receiving antimicrobial prophylaxis, had a normal serum creatinine concentration for age, had a structurally normal upper urinary tract by renal ultrasonography and a normal voiding cystourethrogram, were performing CIC four times a day, and were dry between catheterizations. If CIC did not control wetting, oxybutynin chloride was used as an adjunct.[9] An additional criterion for enrollment was geographic; patients had to live within 2 hours' driving time of the University of Virginia so that the investigator could visit the child's home weekly. The cause of the neurogenic bladder (myelomeningocele vs traumatic spinal cord lesion) and the level of the lesion (cervical, thoracic, lumbar, sacral) were recorded. Informed consent was provided by the parent (and child when appropriate) at the time of enrollment. The study was approved by the University of Virginia Human Investigation Committee. All children continued to receive medical care from their primary physicians during the study; no therapies were withheld or altered. The surveillance urine cultures were not part of the child's care, and the results were not available to either the child's physician or the investigator during the study; the results were kept on file by the research technologist in the pediatric microbiology laboratory.

Observation and surveillance cultures. Each child was visited weekly for 6 months in his or her home by an investigator (T.S.). At each visit, symptoms and signs of urinary tract infection and all medications, including antibiotics, were recorded. At each weekly visit an attempt was made to obtain a sample of bladder urine that had been collected during routine CIC on the day of the home visit. Thus information on symptoms and use of medications was available for all the weeks of observation, but a urine specimen for culture was not always obtained during each week of surveillance. Renal ultrasonography was done and serum creatinine concentration measured before study entry and after completion of surveillance to assess the effect of bacteruria on the structure and function of the urinary tract.

Catheterization was performed according to the following procedure: After hand washing, the parent or child rinsed the perineum with soap and water before inserting a sterile, soft plastic catheter into the bladder by way of the urethra. After urine flow stopped, the child performed a Valsalva maneuver (or the parent applied gentle pressure over the suprapubic area) to express the remaining urine before removal of the catheter. Urine samples were placed in a sterile urine cup and immediately refrigerated. Urine was transported on wet ice to the University of Virginia Pediatric Microbiology Laboratory, where culture inoculation and urinalysis were performed less than 10 hours after collection. Quantitative culture was done by inoculation of urine onto 5% sheep blood and MacConkey agar with a 0.001 ml calibrated loop. Urinalysis, including a dipstick reading (Multistix 10SG, Miles Inc., Diagnostic Division, Elkhart, Ind.) and a microscopic examination of the sediment from 12 ml of urine, was performed as previously described.[8]

Definitions. The appropriate definition of significant bacteriuria in terms of species and number of organisms per milliliter of urine is unclear in this population. For this study a positive urine culture result (bacteriuria) was defined as $\geq 10^4$ colony-forming units of bacteria (regardless of species) per milliliter of urine obtained by bladder catheterization.[10] Symptomatic infection (UTI) was diagnosed in accordance with guidelines developed at the Round Table Discussion of Symptoms of UTI in Neurogenic Bladder, at the October 1990 meeting of the American Academy for Cerebral Palsy and Developmental Medicine, in Orlando,

Table. Characteristics of patients and urine cultures in 14 children with neurogenic bladder during 24 weeks of surveillance

Patient No.	(Sex/age (yr)	Level of lesion	Culture results: No. positive/No. tested (%)	Culture results: No. positive for pathogens (%)
1	M/18	Cervical	19/20 (95%)	19 (100%)
2	M/5	Cervical	9/22 (41%)	8 (89%)
3	M/17	Cervical	16/19 (84%)	16 (100%)
4	F/11	Thoracic (T10)	18/22 (82%)	17 (94%)
5	M/5	Thoracic (T10)	13/18 (72%)	12 (92%)
6	M/13	Thoracic (T6)	14/15 (93%)	14 (100%)
7	M/16	Thoracic (T8)	10/20 (50%)	10 (100%)
8	M/10	Lumbar (L1)	18/18 (100%)	18 (100%)
9	M/18	Lumbar (L4)	12/18 (67%)	0 (0%)
10	F/4*	Lumbar (L4)	1/9 (11%)	1 (100%)
11	M/1†	Lumbar (L5)	10/13 (75%)	10 (100%)
12	M/14	Lumbar (L4)	15/15 (100%)	15 (100%)
13	F/2	Lumbar (L4)	4/11 (36%)	0 (0%)
14	M/4	Sacral	13/24 (54%)	12 (92%)
TOTAL			172/244 (70%)	152/172 (88%)

*Surveillance: 16 weeks only.
†Surveillance: 19 weeks only.

Fla. These guidelines defined a UTI as a positive urine culture result *with* fever, abdominal pain, change in continence pattern, or change in color or odor of urine.

The distinction between urinary tract pathogens and nonpathogens in a patient with neurogenic bladder also has not been established. For purposes of interpretation in this study, the Enterobacteriaceae, *Enterococcus* spp., *Staphylococcus aureus, Staphylococcus saprophyticus,* and group B streptococci were designated as "usual pathogens"; coagulase-negative staphylococci, α-hemolytic or nonhemolytic streptococci, and *Corynebacterium* spp. were designated as "commensal" organisms.

Bacterial carriage was defined as the number of patient-weeks during which a bacterial species was isolated from the urine. If a species was not detected in one weekly sample but was found in the sample before and the sample after the one showing negative results, the negative sample was disregarded in determination of length of carriage. For example, a species isolated on weeks 1, 2, 3, and 5 of surveillance, but not on week 4, was said to be carried for 5 patient-weeks. If a sample was not obtained for 1 or 2 weeks but the species was found in the sample before and the sample after the missing sample(s), the missing sample(s) was disregarded in determination of carriage. For example, if a species was isolated on weeks 1, 2, 3, and 6, but no sample was obtained on weeks 4 and 5, then the species was considered to be carried for 6 weeks. Finally, if administration of an antibiotic was begun during an episode of bacterial carriage, that episode of carriage was excluded from the analysis of duration of carriage (even if carriage was determined for the same organism) because the antibiotic may have spuriously terminated carriage.

Antibiotic therapy was described according to the number of patient-weeks that a patient received antibiotics. If a patient received an antibiotic for 7 days, it was described as one patient-week of therapy; if a patient received an antibiotic for 10 to 14 days, it was described as two patient-weeks of therapy.

Pyuria was defined as five or more leukocytes per high-power field on microscopy.[11] A positive leukoesterase test result was defined by dipstick reading.[12]

Statistical analysis was done with the Fisher Exact Test (two tailed).

RESULTS

Surveillance. From July 1990 to August 1992, we observed 14 children for 323 patient-weeks (Table). Twelve children completed 24 weeks of observation; two children (Nos. 10 and 11) completed 16 and 19 weeks of observation, respectively, before they moved away. There were 11 boys; six children were 1 to 5 years of age, and the remaining eight were 10 to 18 years of age. Ten children had neurogenic bladder caused by myelomeningocele; the four children (Nos. 2, 8, 9, and 10) with neurogenic bladder caused by a traumatic spinal cord injury were studied at least 6 months after the injury. Of 244 urine samples collected, 172 (70%) (range, 9 to 24 samples per child) had positive culture results—152 (88%) showing the usual pathogens with or

SURVEILLANCE WEEK

PT NO.	1	2	3	4	5	6	7	8	9	10	11	12	13	14	15	16	17	18	19	20	21	22	23	24
1	0	0	+	0	0	+	0	+	+	+	+	+	+	+	+	0	+	+	0	0	0	0	+	0
2	+	+	+	+	0	+	+	+	+	+	+	+	+	+	+	+			+	+		+		+
3	0		+	0	+	+	+	+	+	+	+	+	+		+	+	+	+	+	+	+	+	0	0
4	+	+	+	+			+	+	+	0	0	0	⊕	0	0	+	+	+		+		+		
5	+	+	+	+	+	+	+	+	+	+	+			+	+	+			+	+	+			+
6	+			+	+	+	+	+	0		+			+	⊕	+		+	+	+	+			
7	0		+	+	+	+	+	+	+	+	0	0	+		0	0		+		+		0		+
8	0		0	+	0	0	0	+	+	0	+	+	0	+	0	+	0	0	+	0	0	0	+	
9	+	+	+		+		+	+	0	0		+	+	+		+	+	+	+	+		+	+	0
10	0		0	0	+	⊕		0	+	+	+	+	+	0	0	+	⊕	0	0	+			0	0
11	0		0		0		0		0	0		+	0			0								
12	0		+	0	+	+	+	+		+			+	0		+	+		+					
13	+	+	+	+	+	+	+	⊕			+	+	+		+		+	+		+				
14	+	+	+	0		0		0		0		+					0		0	0				

Figure. Urine culture results, antibiotic use, and occurrence of symptomatic urinary tract infection in children with neurogenic bladder. *Symbols* (shown for each week): *blank* = culture not done; 0 = culture showed $<10^4$ colony-forming units of bacteria per milliliter; + = culture grew $\geq 10^4$ colony-forming units of bacteria per milliliter; *plus sign within circle* = symptomatic UTI; *shading* = antibiotic use during this week.

without commensal organisms, and 20 (12%) showing commensal organisms alone. *Escherichia coli* and *Klebsiella* spp. were the most common pathogens isolated; coagulase-negative staphylococci and *Corynebacterium* spp. were the predominant commensal organisms. There were five symptomatic infections during the 323 patient-weeks; pathogens were isolated from urine in all five infections.

The culture results, antibiotic use, and symptomatic infections by surveillance week for each of 14 children are displayed in the Figure.

Bacterial carriage. Typically two species of the usual pathogens (range, up to four per child) and one species of a commensal organism (range, up to three per child) were detected in cultures of urine specimens from each child during surveillance. Once acquired, *E. coli* and *Klebsiella* spp. often remained in bladder urine for several weeks in the absence of antibiotic therapy. Overall, carriage of pathogens was more common than carriage of commensal organisms. There were 31 episodes of carriage of a pathogen; in 15 (48%) the pathogen was carried for 4 weeks or longer (range, 1 to 24 weeks; mean, 4 weeks; median, 2 weeks). In contrast, there were 18 episodes of carriage of a commensal organism; in two episodes (18%) the commensal species was carried for 4 weeks or longer (range, 1 to 11 weeks; mean, 2 weeks; median, 1 week). Carriage of a pathogen for 4 weeks or longer occurred in 11 children, and carriage of a commensal organism for 4 weeks or longer occurred in two children. Carriage of a species of bacteria for several weeks rarely led to development of symptomatic infection because of that organism. In only one infection was the infecting species present before symptoms developed. The bacterial species responsible for four of the five infections had not previously been detected in the patient's urine before symptomatic illness.

The use of an antibiotic was frequently associated with a negative urine culture result, but the effect was only transient (Figure). During 22 of 323 patient-weeks, seven children received an antibiotic. Four courses (8 weeks) were given for symptomatic UTI and nine courses (14 weeks) for other indications (otitis media, bronchitis, pneumonia). In 1 of 13 courses of antibiotic, results of surveillance urine cultures were negative before and during therapy; in three courses the surveillance culture results remained positive; in 9 of 13 courses, results of surveillance cultures became negative. By the third surveillance week after completion of these nine courses of antibiotic therapy, all cultures were positive for a pathogen.

Pyuria. Urinalysis in addition to culture was done on all urine samples from 10 of the 14 children. The 132 samples obtained while the children were not receiving antibiotics were analyzed; the findings were not remarkable except for pyuria.

Pyuria was present in 64 (69%) of 93 samples with positive results and in 2 (5%) of 39 samples with negative culture results ($p < 0.001$). Pyuria did not differentiate asymptomatic bacteriuria from symptomatic infection because only 4 (5%) of the 64 samples with both positive culture results and pyuria were associated with symptoms of infection (urinalysis was not done during one infection). Furthermore, pyuria did not predict incipient symptomatic illness; pyuria in association with carriage of a species of bacteria commonly went on for weeks without development of symptoms. Asymptomatic pyuria was as common in urine specimens with cultures positive for commensal organisms as in those with cultures positive for pathogens. Pyuria was present in 46 (67%) of 68 cultures positive for pathogens, and in 14 (67%) of 21 positive for commensal organisms only ($p = 1.0$). The magnitude of pyuria varied but was similar for pathogens and commensal organisms. More than 20 leukocytes/mm^3 were present in 27 (59%) of 46 cultures positive for traditional pathogens, and in 9 (64%) of 14 cultures positive for commensal organisms alone ($p = 0.7$).[13]

Leukoesterase was present in 61 of 64 cultures with positive results in association with pyuria. Leukoesterase without pyuria was present in an additional seven urine samples, four of which showed negative culture results.

Effect of persistent bacteriuria on the upper urinary tract. All 14 children had a renal ultrasound study and a serum creatinine measurement within 6 to 8 months of completion of surveillance. All remained normal. Seven children who are 2 years beyond surveillance have had a second renal sonogram, and all results were unchanged.

DISCUSSION

This 6-month longitudinal observation of children with neurogenic bladder on a CIC regimen and living at home has demonstrated that bacteriuria was present three fourths of the time and that more than 80% of the bacteriuria samples contained the usual pathogens. Pyuria was associated with bacteriuria two thirds of the time regardless of bacterial species. Carriage of a species associated with pyuria did not predict symptomatic infection. Symptomatic UTI was uncommon and usually occurred at the time of acquisition of a new bacterial species. Deterioration of the upper urinary tract did not occur despite frequent bacteriuria and pyuria.

Our definition of UTI as a positive urine culture result plus "fever, abdominal pain, change in continence pattern, or change in color or odor of urine" is untested against the standard definition in children with a normal bladder and normal sensation. One could argue whether bacteriuria and change of urine color denote infection.

The findings in our patients with neurogenic bladder who were stable and had normal structure of the upper urinary tract and a normal serum creatinine concentration may not be applicable to patients with structural damage or abnormal renal function. Our 14 patients were preselected because they had a normal serum creatinine value and a normal upper urinary tract by ultrasound examination after being followed at a university center for a mean of 9.8 years (range, 1 to 18 years).[14] Thus the risk of deterioration of the upper urinary tract in this population during 6 months of observation was low. Serum creatinine values and renal ultrasonography results were followed to verify that there was no deterioration of the upper tract during the 6 months when bacteriuria was not treated.

The clinical implications of bacteriuria and pyuria are based on studies of patients with UTI and noninstrumented urinary tracts. The presence of bacteriuria is to be expected when the urinary tract is frequently instrumented.[7] However, the presence of pyuria accompanying bacteriuria is not easily explained in our symptom-free patients if one accepts the concept that pyuria denotes infection of the urinary tract. The lack of symptomatic infection despite persistent bacteriuria and pyuria in the majority of children may be due to the child's sensory deficits; if the child had sensation, we might have observed dysuria, urgency, or abdominal pain. An alternative explanation that we find more compelling is given by Andersson et al.,[15] who hypothesized that certain bacterial strains persist in the urinary tract of patients with a history of UTI and are capable of activating an inflammatory response without causing systemic disease. Andersson et al. instilled a nonvirulent *E. coli* strain (i.e., it lacked expressed adherence factors) that was isolated from a patient with stable bacteriuria and two adhering strains of *E. coli* into the bladders of women with chronic UTI. The nonvirulent strain caused stable bacteriuria for more than 30 days, but the adhering strains were eliminated from the urine within 48 hours after instillation. Bacteriuria was associated with pyuria in all cases, and the urinary leukocytes persisted for as long as bacteriuria persisted. None of the patients colonized with the nonvirulent strain had evidence of a systemic host response representing disease (fever, elevation of serum leukocytes, C-reactive protein, or erythrocyte sedimentation rate), and all maintained normal renal function without antibiotic therapy. Symptomatic disease of the urinary tract may require bacterial adherence and/or invasion of the uroepithelium so that cytokines are produced and a systemic host response is initiated.[16-20]

Several investigators[15, 16] have proposed that growth of avirulent bacteria in the urinary tract may protect against invasion by other, possibly more virulent, bacteria. Hansson et al.[16] analyzed *E. coli* strains from girls with asymptomatic bacteriuria and normal urinary tracts; he found that change in O type or electrophoretic type was uncommon during 2 to 5 years of observation. After antibiotic therapy, symptomatic urinary tract infection developed in six girls. All symptomatic infections were caused by strains of *E. coli* that were different (O type, electrophoretic type) from the pretreatment strains. They concluded that treatment of asymptomatic bacteriuria may lead to a change in urinary bacteria and increase the risk of symptomatic infection. Our study extends the findings of Andersson et al.[15] and Hansson et al.[16] to children with neurogenic bladder. Although bacteriuria and pyuria were frequent in our population, symptomatic illness was rare. Four of the five infections were due to new bacterial species, and one infection was preceded by a course of antibiotic therapy.

One reason for varying numbers of leukocytes in the urine of patients with neurogenic bladder is given by Gribble et al.[21] They observed in a study of patients with spinal cord injury who were on a CIC regimen that leukocyte counts were higher in aliquots of terminal-catheter urine (819 leukocytes/mm^3) than in midstream urine (199 leukocytes/mm^3) or in urine obtained by suprapubic aspiration (151 leukocytes/mm^3). They suggested that this difference in leukocyte numbers in terminal-catheter versus suprapubic urine was due to sedimentation of cellular elements in the neurogenic bladder. They concluded that random samples of catheter urine cannot reliably be used to quantitae pyuria in this patient population.

The sequence of events leading to a UTI is thought to begin with colonization of the periurethral area with "motile" bacteria from the stool.[22, 23] By some undefined mechanism a bacterial species then ascends into the bladder and may infect the urine or bladder mucosa or both. Long-term catheterization may facilitate movement of bacteria into the bladder urine, and bacteriuria may be the norm for patients undergoing the procedure several times a day. Attempts at eradication of bacteriuria have been largely unsuccessful.[7] Our study expands on previous work[24] that the effect of a course of antibiotic therapy on eradication of bacteria in bladder urine is brief. The concern is that use of antibiotics may result in selection of organisms that are capable of causing symptomatic infection.[25] Whether antimicrobial prophylaxis will benefit children with recurrent symptomatic infection remains to be studied. Johnson et al.[26] found that children receiving nitrofurantoin for 12 weeks had fewer episodes of bacteriuria and pyuria than those receiving placebo.

The effect of bacteriuria that continues for the lifetime of a child with a neurogenic bladder is unknown; long-term studies are needed. Our work provides an observation for 6 months and suggests that bacteriuria is to be expected in the child on a CIC regimen. Attempts to eradicate bacteriuria should be deferred until proved beneficial to this population.

We thank C. M. Kunin for his review of this manuscript.

REFERENCES

1. McGuire EJ. Clinical evaluation and treatment of neurogenic vesical dysfunction. Baltimore: Williams & Wilkins, 1984:84-98.
2. Guttman L, Frankel H. The value of intermittent catheterization in the early management of traumatic paraplegia and tetraplegia. Paraplegia 1966;4:63-85.
3. Lapides J, Kiokno AC, Silber SJ, Lowe BS. Clean, intermittent self-catheterization in the treatment of urinary tract disease. J Urol 1972;107:458-61.
4. Cass AS, Luxenberg M, Johnson CF, Gleich P. Management of the neurogenic bladder in 413 children. J Urol 1984; 132:521-5.
5. Ehrlich O, Brem AS. A prospective comparison of urinary tract infections in patients treated with either clean intermittent catheterization or urinary diversion. Pediatrics 1982; 70:665-9.
6. McGuire EJ, Savastano JA. Long-term follow-up of spinal cord injury patients managed by intermittent catheterization. J Urol 1982;129:775-6.
7. Stover SL, Lloyd LK, Waites KB, Jackson AB. Neurogenic urinary tract infection. In: Woolsey RM, Young RR, eds. Neurological clinics: disorders of the spinal cord. Philadelphia: Harcourt Brace Jovanovich, 1991:741-55.
8. Schlager TA, Dilks SA, Lohr JA, Hayden GF, Kopco JA, Hendley JW. Periurethral colonization and urinary leukocytes as markers for bacteriuria in children with neurogenic bladder. Urol Res 1992;20:361-3.
9. Abdel-Azim M, Sullivan M, Yalla SV. Disorders of bladder function in spinal cord disease. In: Woolsey RM, Young RR, eds. Neurological clinics: disorders of the spinal cord. Philadelphia: Harcourt Brace Jovanovich, 1991:727-740.
10. Hellerstein S. Recurrent urinary tract infections in children. Pediatr Infect Dis J 1982;1:271-81.
11. Kass EH. Asymptomatic infections of the urinary tract. In: Trans Assoc Am Physicians [Sixty-ninth Session] 1956;69:56-63.
12. Kusumi RK, Grover PJ, Kunin CM. Rapid detection of pyuria by leukocyte esterase activity. JAMA 1981;245:1653-5.
13. Kunin CM, White LV, Hua TH. A reassessment of the importance of "low-count" bacteriuria in young women with acute urinary symptoms. Ann Intern Med 1993;119:454-60.
14. Fernandes ET, Reinberg Y, Vernier R, Gonzalez R. Neurogenic bladder dysfunction in children: review of pathophysiology and current management. J PEDIATR 1994;124:1-7.
15. Andersson P, Engberg I, Lidin-Janson G, et al. Persistence of *Escherichia coli* bacteriuria is not determined by bacterial adherence. Infect Immun 1991;59:2915-21.
16. Hansson S, Caugant D, Jodal U, Svanborg-Eden C. Untreated asymptomatic bacteriuria in girls. I. Stability of urinary isolates. BMJ 1989;298:853-5.
17. Ko Y, Mukaida N, Ishiyama S, et al. Elevated interleukin-8 levels in the urine of patients with urinary tract infections. Infect Immun 1993;61:1307-14.
18. Agace WW, Hedges SR, Ceska M, Svanborg C. Interleukin-8

and the neutrophil response to mucosal gram-negative infection. J Clin Invest 1993;92:780-5.
19. Man P, Jodal U, Svanborg C. Dependence among host response parameters used to diagnose urinary tract infection. J Infect Dis 1991;163:331-5.
20. Hedges S, Agace W, Svensson M, Sjorgre A, Ceska M, Svanborg C. Uroepithelial cells are part of a mucosal cytokine network. Infect Immun 1994;62:2315-21.
21. Gribble MJ, Puterman ML, McCallum NM. Pyuria: its relabntionship in spinal cord injured patients on intermittent catheterization. Arch Phys Med Rehabil 1989;70:376-9.
22. Stamey TA, Sexton CC. The role of vaginal colonization with Enterobacteriaceae in recurrent urinary tract infections. J Urol 1975;113:214-7.
23. Moloney PJ, Doyle AA, Robinson BL, Fenster RH, McLoughlin MG. Pathogenesis of urinary infection in patients with acute spinal cord injury in intermittent catheterization. J Urol 1981;125:672-3.
24. Waites KB, Canupp KC, DeVivo MJ. Eradication of urinary tract infection following spinal cord injury. Paraplegia 1993; 31:645-52.
25. Mohler JL, Cowen DL, Flanigan RC. Suppression and treatment of urinary tract infection in patients with an intermittently catheterized neurogenic bladder. J Urol 1987;138:336-40.
26. Johnson HW, Anderson JD, Chambers GK, et al. A short-term study of nitrofurantoin prophylaxis in children managed with clean intermittent catheterization. Pediatrics 1994;93:752-5.

Clinical and laboratory observations

Neurodevelopmental outcome of infants with hypoplastic left heart syndrome

B. T. Rogers, MD, M. E. Msall, MD, G. M. Buck, PhD, N. R. Lyon, PNP, M. K. Norris, NP, J.-M. A. Roland, MD, R. L. Gingell, MD, D. C. Cleveland, MD, and D. R. Pieroni, MD

From the Departments of Pediatrics, Surgery, and Social and Preventive Medicine, State University of New York at Buffalo, School of Medicine and Biomedical Sciences, and Children's Hospital of Buffalo

The neurodevelopmental outcome of hypoplastic left heart syndrome in infants remains unclear. All 11 survivors of staged surgical repair of hypoplastic left heart syndrome received standardized neurodevelopmental assessments at one regional children's hospital. Seven children (64%) had major developmental disabilities. Quality-of-life outcomes must be considered when management options for children with hypoplastic left heart syndrome are evaluated. (J Pediatr 1995;126:496-8)

More than 95% of infants with hypoplastic left heart syndrome who do not receive surgical intervention will die within the first month.[1] Management options include surgical staged repair, heart transplantation, and passive euthanasia.[2] However, data on the quality of life, including neurodevelopmental outcome, are not available to compare the value of these management options.[2] The purpose of this study was to assess the growth and neurodevelopmental status of infants who underwent physiologic repair of HLHS.

GCI	General Cognitive Index
HLHS	Hypoplastic left heart syndrome
MDI	Mental Development Index
WeeFIM	Functional independence measure for children

Supported in part by Children's Guild of Buffalo, New York, and the New York State Office of Mental Retardation and Developmental Disabilities (RF150-6619D).

Submitted for publication Aug. 4, 1994; accepted Oct. 11, 1994.

Reprint requests: Brian T. Rogers, MD, Robert Warner Rehabilitation Center of, the Children's Hospital of Buffalo, 936 Delaware Ave., Buffalo, NY 14209.

0022-3476/95/$3.00 + 0 **9/22/61303**

Table. Description of patients by type of surgery and developmental outcome

Patient No.	Anomaly of the right side of the heart	Completed surgery stage	Cognition	Motor	Functional disability
1	Severe dysfunction	II	Moderate MR	Delayed*	Substantial‡
2	None	I	Suspect	Normal	None
3	None	II	Normal	Normal	Substantial
4	Moderate tricuspid regurgitation	I	Suspect	Delayed	None
5	None	III	Moderate MR	Delayed	Substantial
6	Moderate tricuspid insufficiency	Modified Fontan	Severe to profound MR	Delayed	Substantial
7	None	III	Moderate MR	Normal	Substantial
8	Mild tricuspid regurgitation	III	Severe to profound MR	CP (quadriplegia)	Substantial
9	None	III	Moderate MR	Normal	Substantial
10	Mild tricuspid regurgitation	III	Severe to profound MR	CP (extrapyramidal)	Substantial
11	Mild tricuspid regurgitation	III	Normal	Delayed	Mild†

CP, Cerebral palsy; *MR*, mental retardation.
*Motor delay: motor quotients less than 70.
†Mild functional disability: total WeeFIM scores 1 to 2 SD below the mean.
‡Substantial functional disability: total WeeFIM scores >2 SD below the mean.

METHODS

Population/sample. Institutional review board approval was obtained before this study was done. Twenty-seven consecutive infants with HLHS were born at or referred to Children's Hospital of Buffalo from September 1986 to August 1991. Twenty infants (74%) had staged surgical repair. Parents of three infants chose no surgical treatment, and four other infants died before any surgical intervention. Staged surgical repairs were performed at Children's Hospital of Philadelphia (N = 16), Children's Hospital of Buffalo (N = 3), or Children's Hospital of Boston (N = 1). The unavailability of a surgical team experienced in Norwood procedures at Children's Hospital of Buffalo was the sole reason for referral of 17 infants.

The 11 surviving infants underwent stage I repair at a mean age of 6 days. The Fontan procedure was completed on seven infants at a mean age of 25 months (range, 13 to 38 months). Additional procedures performed on the subjects in the study included atrial septectomy (n = 2), Blalock-Taussig shunt (n = 1), pulmonary artery augmentation (n = 1), and balloon aortic dilation (n = 1). Five infants (45%) had various degrees of tricuspid regurgitation, and one had right ventricular dysfunction after stage I palliation.

Neurodevelopmental assessment. Standardized neurodevelopmental assessments and physical examinations were performed on all surviving infants (N = 11; 100%) at a mean age of 38 ± 20 months (range, 11 to 67 months). The Clinical Adaptive Test–Clinical Linguistic Auditory Milestone Scale (CAT-CLAMS), Bayley Scales of Infant Development, and McCarthy Scales of Children's Abilities were used for cognitive assessments.[3-5] The WeeFIM instrument, a *f*unctional *i*ndependence *m*easure for children, was used to assess self-care, sphincter control, transfer, locomotion, communication, and social cognition.[6] Motor quotients were used to assess motor skill achievement.[7] In children with McCarthy General Cognitive Index scores <50 and Bayley Mental Development Index scores <50, mental age equivalents were used in conjunction with chronologic ages to calculate cognitive quotients (mental age/chronologic age ×100). The Clinical Adaptive Test–Clinical Linguistic Auditory Milestone Scale was used to obtain a general cognitive quotient in children with cerebral palsy. Delayed or suspect scores included McCarthy GCI scores of 69 to 89 and Bayley MDI scores of 70 to 89. McCarthy GCI scores of 50 to 68 or Bayley MDI scores of 50 to 69 were classified as indicating mild mental retardation. Moderate mental retardation represented McCarthy GCI <50, Bayley MDI <50, and cognitive quotients of 40 to 49. Children with McCarthy GCI <50 or Bayley MDI <50 and cognitive quotients <40 were classified as having severe to profound mental retardation.

Children were classified as underweight and short if their weight and length, respectively, were at less than the 5th percentile for age. Children whose head circumference was at ≥10th percentile at birth and at less than the 5th percentile for age at follow-up examination were described as having acquired microcephaly.

RESULTS

The study sample (N = 11) comprised singleton, predominantly white infants (74%). Ninety-one percent had been carried to term. Approximately half the subjects were boys (54%) and were of low socioeconomic status (50% in Hollingshead class 4 or 5). Median 1- and 5-minute Apgar scores were 7 and 9, respectively. Mean birth sizes included weight (2952 ± 724 gm), length (48.6 ± 4.1 cm), and head circumference (33.0 ± 1.7 cm). Only one infant was small for gestational age (birth weight <10%), and none had microcephaly (head circumference <10%).

At follow-up examination, five children (45%) were underweight; however, only one child had a weight/height ratio at less than the 5th percentile. Eight children (73%) had acquired microcephaly. No major or minor malformations were consistent with known genetic syndromes.

The Table outlines the cardiac and developmental status of the surviving infants. Two children (18%) had suspect cognitive development. Seven children (64%) had varying degrees of mental retardation (four moderate and three severe to profound). Two children (18%) had severe cerebral palsy. Eight children (73%) had total WeeFIM scores consistent with a substantial functional disability (>2 SD less than the mean for age). Gross motor delays occurred in five children (45%). The prevalence of mental retardation was greater in children surviving the Fontan procedure than in those undergoing stage 1 or 2, respectively. Head growth was closely associated with cognitive development. Eight (89%) of nine children with cognitive delays or mental retardation had acquired microcephaly.

Neuroimaging was performed in four children (36%). Two children had normal computed tomography scans, and one had diffuse cerebral atrophy. One child had normal findings on cranial ultrasonography at 1 week of age.

DISCUSSION

Recently an editorial review emphasized the current lack of valid data concerning the quality of life of infants with HLHS after either staged repair or transplantation.[2] To our knowledge this is the first report documenting significant neurodevelopmental disabilities in children who have had staged surgical repair of HLHS.[8, 9]

The cause of the high prevalence of developmental disabilities in our study sample remains unclear. The fact that most of our patients were transferred to other regional centers for treatment seriously compromised our ability to examine operative and postoperative factors related to outcome. However, our subjects were treated by well-trained pediatric surgical teams, and the timing of surgical repairs conformed to current accepted standards. The high prevalence of acquired microcephaly and poor growth in our patients highlights the need for more detailed analysis of potential causes of postnatal brain injury in larger prospective studies. Furthermore future neuroimaging studies may help clarify the prevalence of congenital brain anomalies or other abnormalities in survivors without extracardiac anomalies or genetic syndromes.

The quality of life of infants with HLHS surviving heart transplantation also requires clarification. A recent pilot study revealed neurodevelopmental abnormalities in three of six infants surviving heart transplantation for HLHS.[10] Large, multicenter, prospective neurodevelopmental outcome studies of infants with HLHS who receive staged surgical repair or transplantation are needed.

We thank Maryann Kihl and Mary Jane Hall for assistance in the preparation of this manuscript, and William Zorn, PhD, for performing some of the developmental assessments. Finally, we are indebted to Linda Rogers, RN, for her support and inspiration.

REFERENCES

1. Pigott JD, Murphy JD, Barber G, Norwood WI. Palliative reconstructive surgery for hypoplastic left heart syndrome. Ann Thorac Surg 1988;45:122-8.
2. Storch TG. Passive euthanasia for hypoplastic left heart syndrome. Am J Dis Child 1992;146:1426.
3. Hoon AH, Pulsifer MB, Gopalan R, Palmer FB, Capute AJ. Clinical Linguistic Auditory Milestone Scale in early cognitive assessment. J Pediatr 1993;123:S1-S8.
4. Bayley N. Bayley Scales of Infant Development. New York: Psychological Corporation, 1969.
5. McCarthy DA. Manual for the McCarthy Scales of Children's Abilities. New York: Psychological Corp, 1972.
6. Msall ME, DiGaudio K, Duffy LC, LaForest S, Granger CV. WeeFIM: normative sample of an instrument for tracking functional independence in children. Clinical Pediatr (Phila) 1994;33:431-8.
7. Capute AJ, Shapiro BK. The motor quotient: a method for the early detection of motor delay. Am J Dis Child 1985;139:940-2.
8. Jonas RA, Lang P, Hansen D, Hickey P, Castaneda AR. First-stage palliation of hypoplastic left heart syndrome: the importance of coarctation and shunt size. J Thorac Cardiovasc Surg 1986;92:6-13.
9. Starnes VA, Griffin ML, Pitlick PT, Bernstein D, Baun D, Ivens K, Shumway NE. Current approach to hypoplastic left heart syndrome: palliation, transplantation, or both? J Thorac Cardiovasc Surg 1992;104:189-95.
10. Lynch BJ, Glauser TA, Canter C, Spray T. Neurologic complications of pediatric heart transplantation. Arch Pediatr Adolesc Med 1994;148:973-9.

CURRENT LITERATURE AND CLINICAL ISSUES

Abstracts from the literature

Randomized trial of SPf66 vaccine against *Plasmodium falciparum* malaria in children in southern Tanzania

Alonso PL, Smith T, Armstrong Schellenberg JRM, et al. Lancet 1994;334:1175-81.

Objective: To determine whether three doses of SPf66 malaria vaccine in African children living in an area of intense perennial malaria transmission protects children against malaria.
Design: Randomized, double-blind, placebo-controlled trial.
Setting: A village in the Kilombero valley of southern Tanzania.
Patients: 586 children aged 1 to 5 years.
Intervention: Three doses of SPf66 malaria vaccine or placebo given at baseline and at 4 and 26 weeks.
Main outcome measures: Episodes of clinical malaria, incidence and density of parasitemia, anemia, and antibody levels to vaccine for the 1-year period after vaccination.
Results: The incidence of clinical malaria was 0.25 in the vaccine group and 0.35 in the placebo group; the incidence and density of parasitemia were similar in the two groups. After three doses, all vaccine recipients had detectable antibody; the geometric mean index was 8.3 in the vaccine group and 0.7 in the control group. Six study participants died of malaria: one in the vaccine group and five in the placebo group. Mild side effects were seen in fewer than 6%, and there were no severe side effects.
Conclusions: This study confirms that SPf66 is safe and immunogenic, and reduces the risk of clinical malaria among children exposed to intense *P. falciparum* transmission.

Comment: Severe malaria (cerebral malaria, profound anemia) kills between one and three million African children each year. The journey toward an effective vaccine against malaria has been long, hard, and expensive, and it has been made more difficult by the lack of a good in vitro correlate of immunity. This trial of the SPf66 vaccine, discovered originally in Columbia, is the first outside South America. This was a difficult test for the vaccine because malaria transmission in the Kilombero valley in Tanzania is intense compared with that at the South American trial sites. Severe disease (mainly severe anemia) occurs in the first few years of life, but by adulthood immunity has gradually developed and nearly all malaria infections are symptomless (premunition). The design and execution of this vaccine trial were good. The SPf66 vaccine was well tolerated and immunogenic, but the main outcome of the trial is tantalizing: a 31% protective efficacy with a 95% confidence interval that reaches zero is a borderline result. The lack of effect on anemia is disappointing because malaria is an important cause of anemia in malaria-endemic areas. A vaccine protective efficacy of 31% would be low for most infectious diseases, but a 31% reduction in malarial morbidity, especially if mortality rates were reduced as well, would certainly be worth achieving. In another year we will have the results of other ongoing trials with this vaccine and a clearer idea of the overall efficacy of SPf66. Will the vaccine select for resistant strains, or will it destabilize malaria and cause an increase in mortality rates in areas of intense stable transmission? Other, possibly improved, vaccines are also in development. We have not reached the end of the journey toward an ideal vaccine against falciparum malaria, but the SPf66 vaccine has held up well so far, and we are still on track.

Nicholas J. White, BSc, MD, FRCP
Director, Wellcome–Mahidol University, Oxford
Tropical Medicine Research Programme
Mahidol University
Bangkok, Thailand

School-age outcomes in children with birth weights under 750 g

Hack M, Taylor HG, Klein N, Eiben R, Schatschneider C, Mercuri-Minich N. N Engl J Med 1994;331:753-9.

Objective: To determine the developmental outcomes of children with birth weights less than 750 gm.
Design: Inception cohort with matched control subjects.
Setting: Three regional tertiary care centers in Ohio.
Patients: We matched a regional cohort of 68 surviving children born from 1982 through 1986 with birth weights less than 750 gm (mean, 670 gm; gestational age, 25.7 weeks) with 65 children weighing 750 to 1499 gm at birth and 61 children born at term.
Main outcome measures: Growth, neurosensory status, and functioning at school age in the three groups were compared. Associations of biologic and social risk factors with major developmental outcomes were examined by means of logistic-regression analyses.
Results: Children with birth weights less than 750 gm were

inferior to both comparison groups in cognitive ability, psychomotor skills, and academic achievement. They had poorer social skills and adaptive behavior, and more behavioral and attention problems. The mean (±SD) Mental Processing Composite score for the cohort was 87 ± 15, in comparison with 93 ± 14 for children with birth weights of 750 to 1499 gm and 100 ± 13 for children born at term (p <0.001). The rates of mental retardation (IQ <70) in the three groups were 21%, 8%, and 2%, respectively; the rates of cerebral palsy were 9%, 6%, and 0%; and the rates of severe visual disability were 25%, 5%, and 2%. Major cerebral ultrasonographic abnormalities were associated with mental retardation (odds ratio, 5.4; 95% confidence interval (CI), 1.8 to 15.8) and cerebral palsy (odds ratio, 15.2; 95% CI, 3.0 to 77.4). Oxygen dependence at 36 weeks of corrected age was associated with mental retardation (odds ratio, 4.5; 95% CI, 1.2 to 10.7) and severe visual disability (odds ratio, 4.3; 95% CI, 1.3 to 14.2). Social disadvantage, though associated with several adverse neuropsychologic outcomes, was not associated with major developmental impairment.
Conclusions: Children with birth weights less than 750 gm who survive represent a subgroup of very low birth weight children who are at high risk of having neurobehavioral dysfunction and poor school performance.

Comment: This report provides important information on the usefulness of applying our technologic expertise to neonates at the edge of extreme prematurity. The data may not be as sobering as a first glance might suggest. Many children with mild hearing or visual loss, or with specific language or visual-motor deficits, function relatively well if they are given appropriate support and educational interventions. The number of children enrolled in special education may reflect timely parental requests for services rather than specific adverse outcomes. Generalizability may be limited by time (given ongoing advances in neonatal intensive care) and place (the particular neonatal intensive care units where these data were collected). The authors matched their subjects with regard to age, sex, and race, and because race is so highly correlated with socioeconomic status, it may not be possible to detect an effect of the latter, independent of birth weight, on cognitive development. Although the details of any report such as this can be criticized, the general conclusion that it would be better not to be born very prematurely is well supported here and in extensive earlier literature. We need more sophisticated, quantitative approaches to predict which babies will respond to our advancing techniques; we also need to commit ourselves to prevention of extreme prematurity, which will require that we address the issue of poverty and its connection to prematurity and poor outcomes. Until then, we must continue to refine the approach in our neonatal intensive care units.

Marie C. McCormick, MD, ScD
Harvard Medical School
Boston, MA 02115

Nebulized budesonide for children with mild-to-moderate croup

Klassen TP, Feldman ME, Watters LK, Sutcliffe T, Rowe PC. N Engl J Med 1994;331:285-9.

Objective: To compare a nebulized glucocorticoid, budesonide, with placebo in outpatients with mild-to-moderate croup.
Design: Randomized, double-blind, placebo-controlled trial.
Setting: Emergency department of a children's hospital.
Patients: Children 3 months to 5 years of age were eligible for the study if their croup scores fell in the mild-to-moderate range (scores of 2 to 7 out of a possible 17).
Intervention: The patients were randomly assigned to receive either 2 mg (4 ml) of nebulized budesonide (27 children) or 4 ml of nebulized isotonic saline solution (27 children).
Main outcome measures: Subjects were assessed hourly for up to 4 hours for croup score, respiratory rate, heart rate, parental assessment of improvement, and other medical interventions by treating physicians not involved in the study.
Results: The median croup score at entry into the study was 4 in both groups. At the final study assessment, the median score was significantly lower in the budesonide group than in the placebo group (1 vs 3; p = 0.005). The patients in the budesonide group were discharged from the emergency department significantly earlier than those in the placebo group (p = 0.002). One week after enrollment, 21 patients assigned to receive placebo had received dexamethasone, in comparison with 15 patients assigned to receive budesonide (p = 0.10), and 7 patients assigned to the placebo group had been admitted to the hospital, in comparison with 1 patient assigned to the budesonide group (p = 0.05).
Conclusions: Nebulized budesonide leads to a prompt and significant clinical improvement in children with mild-to-moderate croup who come to the emergency department.

Comment: There is now consistent evidence that corticosteroids can be beneficial in the treatment of children with croup. Kairys et al.[1] reported benefit from metaanalysis of studies up to 1989. Husby et al.[2] demonstrated a prompt symptom response to inhaled budesonide, and Klassen et al.[3] showed a more rapid clinical improvement with a shorter hospital stay and a reduced rate of subsequent admission in children with mild-to-moderate croup who come to the emergency department. Geelhoed and Macdonald[4] reported an equally rapid and clinically useful response to oral and to inhaled corticosteroids. Inhaled corticosteroids have the advantage of small dose and a possible role when parenteral administration is contraindicated. Orally administered dexamethasone does, however, work as fast as budesonide, is cheaper, and is usually easier to administer. The disease may vary from sudden-onset spasmodic croup to the slower, more progressive pattern of viral croup. Most cases resolve within 2 or 3 days but many patients show improvement spontaneously within 24 hours, a finding that demonstrates the need for blinded, controlled trials with clearly defined cohorts to assess the efficacy of new interventions. It is not clear whether these varying cases of croup are separate entities that may respond differently to corticosteroids, whether some cases are allergic and others are not, whether it is possible to identify those patients who will respond to corticosteroids, at what severity these drugs should be used, what the optimal route and the lowest safe dose are, and whether the drugs do any harm. Until these questions are answered, there is evidence to suggest that corticosteroids can be used in the treatment of croup, in modest doses, for those patients whose condition fails to improve rapidly.

Louis I. Landau, MD, FRACP
Gary C. Geelhoed, MBBS, FRACP
University of Western Australia
Princess Margaret Hospital for Children
Perth, Western Australia, Australia

REFERENCES

1. Kairys SW, Olmstead EM, O'Connor GT. Steroid treatment of laryngotracheobronchitis: a meta-analysis of the evidence from randomized trials. Pediatrics 1989;83:683-93.
2. Husby S, Agertoft L, Mortensen S, Pedersen S. Treatment of croup with nebulized steroid (budesonide): a double-blind, placebo-controlled study. Arch Dis Child 1993;68:352-5.
3. Klassen TP, Feldman ME, Watters LK, Sutcliffe T, Rowe PC. Nebulized budesonide for children with mild to moderate croup. N Engl J Med 1994;331:285-9.
4. Geelhoed GC, Macdonald WBG. Comparison of oral and inhaled steroids in the treatment of croup. [Abstract] Am Rev Respir Dis 1994;149:A375.

ALSO NOTED

Effect of aerosolized recombinant human DNase on exacerbations of respiratory symptoms and on pulmonary function in patients with cystic fibrosis

Fuchs HJ, Borowitz DS, Christiansen DH, et al. N Engl J Med 1994;331:637-42.

In this trial, 968 patients were randomly assigned to receive recombinant human deoxyribonuclease (rhDNase) once daily or twice daily, or to receive placebo, for 6 months. The rhDNase regimens decreased the age-adjusted risk of pulmonary exacerbation by 28% to 37% and resulted in a slight improvement in forced expiratory volume in 1 second, with few side effects.

The effect of a recent previous visit to a physician on outcome after childhood bacterial meningitis

Kallio MJT, Kilpi T, Anttila M, Peltola H. JAMA 1994;272:787-91.

Of 325 consecutive patients aged 3 months to 15 years with bacterial meningitis, 25% had seen a physician in the 1 to 4 days before diagnosis. There was no difference in outcome between children seen first at the time of diagnosis and children who had a recent previous physician encounter.

Placebo-controlled trail of midazolam sedation in mechanically ventilated newborn babies

Jacqz-Aigrain E, Daoud P, Burtin P, Desplanques L, Beaufils F. Lancet 1994;344:646-50.

Continuously infused midazolam produced effective sedation without adverse effects on hemodynamic variables. There was no effect on the course of respiratory distress syndrome.

Isolation of *Ureaplasma urealyticum* from low birth weight infants

To the Editor:

The conclusions of Heggie et al. (J PEDIATR 1994;124:956-61) are not completely justified by the data reported or by the methods utilized. Cultures for *Ureaplasma urealyticum* were performed by inoculating undiluted clinical specimens directly onto agar, in some cases, after refrigeration without transport media. This method is likely to yield false-negative results because some especially fastidious strains may initially grow only in liquid media and must be diluted and subcultured before colonies develop on agar. Growth may be impaired by antibodies, antibiotics, bacteria, and other inhibitors present in the original specimen. If only a single tube of broth is inoculated without serial dilutions, the organism may multiply rapidly and die before the specimen can be subcultured to agar for determination of the morphologic features of the colonies. Some strains may not produce color change indicative of growth in any dilution.

We recently reviewed 1415 unselected neonatal endotracheal aspirate (ETA) cultures submitted to the University of Alabama at Birmingham Diagnostic Mycoplasma Laboratory during a 7-year period. Specimens were processed as previously described,[1] with the broth-to-agar technique, including inoculation of culture media at bedside in most instances. Without appropriate transport medium, storage of body fluids, even if refrigerated, can adversely affect organism recovery. A total of 248 ETA cultures (18%) grew *U. urealyticum*. If results had depended solely on growth of the primary inoculum on agar without benefit of broth dilutions, 65 cases (26%) would have been missed. If results had depended solely on growth of the original specimens in a single tube of broth without dilutions or inoculation of agar, 22 cases (9%) would have been missed. If results had depended solely on growth in broth or dilutions without primary inoculation onto agar, 4 cases (2%) would have been missed. The implication is that positive culture results in some neonates may not have been detected. Among six cerebrospinal fluid culture specimens in which *U. urealyticum* was isolated in addition to the ETAs, four specimens (67%) had no growth of the primary inoculum on agar and required subculture of broth, showing color change to agar before colonies could be observed. Other investigators[2, 3] have found *U. urealyticum*, *Mycoplasma hominis*, or both in cerebrospinal fluid in frequencies similar to those in our experience.

It is difficult to appreciate these negative findings because of the uncontrolled, retrospective nature of the investigation and analysis. The authors did not state how long after birth the neonates had cultures, or the criteria for collection of ETAs. The presence of other outcome variables, such as respiratory distress and pneumonia, was determined by chart review, but no information was provided regarding how they were defined or whether there was any attempt to standardize definitions across the study population. In an analysis of the relation between *U. urealyticum* isolation and rates of chronic lung disease, it is preferable to use birth weight rather than gestational age as the grouping variable, with particular emphasis on neonates weighing <1250 gm.

Neonatal infections caused by *U. urealyticum* may be acquired in utero. Thus starting treatment several days after birth would not be expected to have much effect on development of chronic lung disease, if related to *U. urealyticum*, when the organism may have been present for weeks. Therefore the value of the treatment data is questionable. No criteria for administration of erythromycin were described, nor was there any information on the duration of endotracheal intubation in those who were treated or whether there was evidence of microbiologic efficacy.

The clinical significance of *U. urealyticum* as a pathogen in cerebrospinal fluid and other sites must be studied further. We endorse the recommendation to perform a rigorously controlled erythromycin treatment trial for further assessment of the role of *U. urealyticum* as a neonatal respiratory pathogen.

Ken B. Waites, MD
Gail H. Cassell, PhD
Lynn B. Duffy, MT (ASCP)
Karen B. Searcey, MSPH
Departments of Pathology and Microbiology
University of Alabama at Birmingham
Birmingham, AL 35233
9/35/61757

REFERENCES

1. Cassell GH, Waites KB, Crouse DT, et al. Association of *Ureaplasma urealyticum* infection of the lower respiratory tract with chronic lung disease and death in very-low-birth-weight infants. Lancet 1988;2:240-5.
2. Ollikainen J, Heikkaniemi H, Korppi M, Sarkkinen H, Heinonen K. *Ureaplasma urealyticum* infection associated with acute respiratory insufficiency and death in premature infants. J PEDIATR 1993;122:756-60.
3. Valencia GB, Banzon F, Cummings M, McCormack WM, Glass L, Hammerschlag MR. *Mycoplasma hominis* and *Ureaplasma urealyticum* in neonates with suspected infection. Pediatr Infect Dis J 1993;12:571-3.

To the Editor:

The article by Heggie et al.[1] reports the isolation of genital mycoplasmas from cerebrospinal fluid and tracheal aspirates obtained from preterm infants. The authors' conclusion that isolation of ureaplasmas from the tracheas of premature infants "... do[es] not appear to be related to the presence or subsequent development of respiratory disease" is not supported by their data. Use of tracheal aspirate specimens obtained from infants supported by mechanical ventilation for several days selects infants who are more likely to have severe respiratory disease, as evidenced by the baseline prevalence of bronchopulmonary dysplasia (BPD) of 58% in this study. Fifty-six percent of the infants whose birth weights were <1500 gm had *Ureaplasma urealyticum (UU)* in their tracheal cultures. This isolation rate is two to three times the rate reported elsewhere and strongly suggests a selection bias.[2]

The microbiologic techniques used in this study were inadequate and would likely underestimate the true isolation rate. Inhibitors in body fluids, especially cerebrospinal fluid, commonly prevent the growth of ureaplasmas in the "neat" sample, necessitating serial dilutions.

In this study the lack of statistical power easily explains the lack of statistical significance.[3] For babies with birth weights <1500 gm, if an alpha of 0.05 and a one-tailed test are used and if it is assumed that the observed difference in proportions is a "true" difference, then the power (1 − beta) of this test is 0.54. With a two-tailed test, the power is 0.41. To obtain a power of 0.80 and alpha of 0.05, the investigators would need 54 infants in each group. Thus the chance of finding a difference when, in fact, one exists is about 50/50. The power of the test for infants born at 25 to 29 weeks of gestation is much less. The lack of statistical power in this study is demonstrated in the finding that a clinically significant 38% increase in the incidence of BPD ([80% *UU* positive −58% *UU* negative]/58% *UU* negative) in infants with positive culture results is not statistically significant.[4]

The authors also report that treatment of infants with *UU* colonies with erythromycin did not alter the clinical course. This finding is not unexpected. It is optimistic to expect erythromycin treatment to arrest the progression of injury and "cure" the pulmonary disease before the twenty-eighth postnatal day, when therapy was initiated after 2 or more weeks of aggressive respiratory care.[5] In one case, erythromycin therapy was started on the twenty-seventh postnatal day and the diagnosis of BPD was made on the following day. Erythromycin is bacteriostatic and would not prevent continued *UU*-antigenic challenge of the lower respiratory tract; thus inflammation would persist until the phagocytic cells of the lungs have disposed of these organisms. In a hyperoxic environment, the clearance of these organisms is delayed and the duration of inflammation is prolonged.[6]

The conclusions of the authors are difficult to endorse because of selection biases, inadequate statistical power, improper culture methods, and failure to interpret the results of erythromycin therapy in the context of normal bronchopulmonary dysplasia progression.

Dennis T. Crouse, MD, PhD
Associate Professor of Pediatrics, and Obstetrics and Gynecology
University of Tennessee at Memphis
Memphis, TN 38163

Judith M. Reese
J. Reese Consulting
Memphis, TN

9/35/61758

REFERENCES

1. Heggie AD, Jacobs MR, Butler VT, Baley JE, Boxerbaum B. Frequency and significance of isolation of *Ureaplasma urealyticum* and *Mycoplasma hominis* from cerebrospinal fluid and tracheal aspirate specimens from low birth weight infants. J PEDIATR 1994;124:956-61.
2. Cassell GH, Crouse DT, Waites, et al. Does *Ureaplasma urealyticum* cause respiratory disease in newborns? Pediatr Infect Dis J 1988;7:535-41.
3. Romano PE. The insignificance of a probability value of p < 0.05 in the evaluation of medical scientific studies. J Lab Clin Med 1988;111:501-3.
4. Detsky AS, Sackett DL. When was a "negative" clinical trial big enough? Arch Intern Med 1985;145:709-12.
5. Crouse DT, Odrezin GT, Cutter GR, et al. Radiographic changes associated with tracheal isolation of *Ureaplasma urealyticum* from neonates. Clin Infect Dis 1993;17(suppl 1):S122-30.
6. Crouse DT, Cassell GH, Waites KB, Foster JM, Cassady G. Hyperoxia potentiates *Ureaplasma urealyticum* pneumonia in mice. Infect Immun 1990;58:3487-93.

Reply

To the Editor:

Both letters, one from Waites et al. and the other from Crouse and Reese, state that dilution of specimens before inoculation of cultures results in an increased yield of *Ureaplasma* isolates, but neither provides a reference that quantifies the effect of dilution on yields from different types of specimens. Two of the three reports from which we derived our culture methods concluded that direct inoculation of specimens onto A-7 agar was more effective for isolation of *Ureaplasma* than inoculation, and thereby dilution, of specimens into liquid medium.[1,2] Furthermore, Kenny[3] did not discuss dilution of specimens, although dilution occurs when the culture method selected involves inoculation into liquid media. However, the concern of Waites et al. that growth of *Ureaplasma* may be impaired by the presence of inhibitory substances in the original specimen is valid, and the quantitative data that they present suggest that dilution may be important. Their analysis included only six cerebrospinal fluid specimens in which *Ureaplasma* was detected but 248 endotracheal aspirates (ETA) in which the organism was detected. The degree to which these specimens were diluted was not stated. On the basis of their estimate that dilution of CSF specimens would have increased our yield by 67%, our isolation rate would have increased from 0.2% to 0.6%. This difference would not have altered our conclusion that isolation of this organism from CSF specimens obtained from preterm infants as part of the evaluation for sepsis is infrequent. Their data indicate that dilution may be less important in cultures of ETA; it resulted in a lower (26%) increase in isolates. Their isolation rate from ETA specimens (17%) was the same as ours, but we recognize the possibility that dilution of ETA specimens from our population might have resulted in a somewhat higher isolation rate. More detailed data on the quantitative effects of dilution on the yield of isolates from different types of specimens would be helpful. Regarding the comments by Waites et al. that refrigeration of specimens may cause false-negative results, most of our specimens were inoculated promptly after collection and were not refrigerated.

Crouse and Reese cite the low statistical power of our study. We agree and stated clearly in our discussion, although less precisely than in the comment by Crouse and Reese, that resolution of the role of *Ureaplasma urealyticum* as a respiratory pathogen in preterm infants requires study of a larger number of infants. Low statistical power has been a problem in most studies in this area and is probably one of the reasons that several investigators in the field published a metaanalysis that combined four studies of the relation between respiratory colonization with *U. urealyticum* and chronic lung disease of prematurity.[4] The conclusion derived from this metaanalysis was that there is strong but not definitive evidence that *U. urealyticum* causes chronic lung disease of prematurity.

Crouse and Reese are incorrect in stating that 56% of infants with birth weights <1500 gm in our study had ETA specimens in which *Ureaplasma* was detected. The control subjects did not include all infants with negative culture results. As explained in our article, control subjects included all infants (birth weights <1500 gm) who had no colonization in at least two ETA specimens and who had received no antibiotics active against *Ureaplasma*. Negative results on two ETA cultures were required because we found that infants sometimes had negative culture results initially but that *Ureaplasma* was detected in subsequent cultures. In this respect, we do not agree with Waites et al. that our study was uncontrolled.

Waites et al. were also concerned about the criteria for selection of infants for culture and our use of diagnostic terms. As we explained in our article, we were not involved in determining which infants would have specimens obtained for culture or in making decisions regarding medical care. All CSF and ETA specimens from preterm infants submitted to our laboratory for bacterial culture during a 2-year period were tested for *U. urealyticum* and *Mycoplasma hominis*, and medical records were reviewed to determine frequency of outcome variables in infants with positive results and in control subjects with birth weights <1500 gm. Approximately 85% of infants in our neonatal intensive care unit require some period of endotracheal intubation for ventilation, and ETA specimens were obtained for bacterial culture from most of these infants. We defined bronchopulmonary dysplasia (BPD) very specifically because it was the outcome variable of greatest interest. For other outcome variables, the diagnosis recorded in the medical records by the attending neonatologists in our level III neonatal intensive care unit was accepted. Although the frequency of BPD by the strict definition (70%) was lower than the frequency obtained by record review (82%), the decreases were proportional in infants with *U. urealyticum* colonization and control infants. Gestational age was a factor in the definition of BPD but, contrary to the impression of Waites et al., was not used as a grouping variable.

We agree with the authors of both letters and commented in our article that delay in initiation of erythromycin therapy until 1 to 3 weeks of age may have accounted for the lack of therapeutic effect in infants with *U. urealyticum* colonization. Although we stated that a therapeutic trial of erythromycin would aid in delineation of the role of *U. urealyticum* as a pathogen in neonatal respiratory disease, we did not recommend a trial because of concern about the potential cardiotoxicity of intravenously administered erythromycin in preterm infants.[5] Two additional cases of erythromycin-related cardiotoxic effects have been reported since the reference cited in our article.[6] In a recent review to which three of the authors of these letters to the editor contributed, it was concluded that demonstration of the efficacy of an antibiotic in preventing chronic lung disease in infants with *U. urealyticum* colonization would not prove causality because another factor, presumably another pathogen susceptible to the antibiotic being used, might be causally involved.[7] We favor a rigorously controlled prospective study of respiratory disease in a sufficiently large number of preterm infants with and without *U. urealyticum* colonization to provide the statistical power necessary to prove or disprove a causal relation between *U. urealyticum* and BPD.

Alfred D. Heggie, MD
Michael R. Jacobs, MD, PhD
Verleria T. Butler, BA, MASCP
Jill E. Baley, MD
Bernard Boxerbaum, MD
Departments of Pediatrics and Pathology
Rainbow Babies and Childrens Hospital
Cleveland, OH 44106
9/35/61759

REFERENCES

1. Fiacco V, Miller MJ, Carney E, Martin WJ. Comparison of media for isolation of *Ureaplasma urealyticum* and genital *Mycoplasma* species. J Clin Microbiol 1984;20:862-5.
2. Phillips LE, Goodrich KH, Turner RM, Faro S. Isolation of *Mycoplasma* species and *Ureaplasma urealyticum* from obstetrical and gynecological patients by using commercially avaialble medium formulations. J Clin Microbiol 1986; 24:377-9.
3. Kenny GE. Mycoplasmas. In: Balows A, Hausler WJ, Herrmann KL, Isenberg HD, Shadomy HJ, eds. Manual of clinical microbiology. 5th ed. Washington, D.C.: American Society for Microbiology, 1991:478-82.
4. Wang EL, Cassell GH, Sanchez PJ, Regan JA, Payne NR, Liu P. *Ureaplasma urealyticum* and chronic lung disease of prematurity: critical appraisal of the literature on causation. Clin Infect Dis 1993;17(suppl 1):S112-6.
5. Farrar HC, Walsh-Sukys MC, Kyllonen K, Blumer JL. Cardiac toxicity with intravenous erythromycin lactobionate: two case reports and a review of the literature. Pediatr Infect Dis J 1993;12:688-91.
6. Gouyon JB, Benoit A, Betremieux P, et al. Cardiac toxicity of intravenous erythromycin lactobionate in preterm infants [Letter]. Pediatr Infect Dis J 1994;13:840-1.
7. Cassell GH, Waites KB, Crouse DT, Harasawa E. *Ureaplasma urealyticum* intrauterine infection: role in prematurity and disease in newborns. Clin Microbiol Rev 1993;6:69-87.

Band neutrophil counts in neonates

To the Editor:

The article by Schelonka et al.[1] regarding the peripheral leukocyte count and leukocyte indexes continues the ongoing challenge to find a "best" method or test that will permit an accurate diagnosis of neonatal sepsis. The authors present *no* data regarding sepsis but, instead, examine several leukocyte values at a single time in a "healthy" population of term neonates. They then compare their data with those of Manroe et al.[2] and Rodwell et al.,[3] referring to them as "neonatal sepsis-scoring systems," and conclude that these data are too restrictive. First, the Manroe data are dynamic reference ranges (i.e., ranges that are changing throughout the first 60 to 72 hours of life). Further, the authors have used the data of Manroe et al. from approximately 12 hours after birth and not 4 hours. Second, Manroe et al. never reported or suggested a "sepsis-scoring system." This is an apparent independent modification that has occurred since 1979. We have suggested on numerous occasions that the neutrophil indexes provide "supplemental" information and that a single complete blood cell count (i.e., a screening complete blood cell count) is of limited value, if any, irrespective of the method chosen. Thus one should obtain serial complete blood cell counts for at-risk neonates (up to three determinations at 12-hour intervals) and, if the clinical course is consistent with sepsis, continue treatment. On the other hand, if the clinical course is unremarkable, culture results are negative at 48 hours, and the neutrophil indexes have remained within the reference ranges,[2] discontinue administration of antibiotics. In our institution this has decreased the duration of antibiotic exposure for our term (and preterm) neonates, as well as the duration of hospitalization, with no known morbidity. It may not have improved our diagnosis of neonatal sepsis.

If the reference ranges of Manroe et al.[2] are too restrictive or neonates are now different, the ranges should be revised; however, examining neutrophil indexes as means ± SD at a single time point is not state of the art.[4] Why not reestablish the reference ranges for the first 72 hours?

Charles R. Rosenfeld, MD
Professor of Pediatrics and of Obstetrics/Gynecology
Director, Division of Neonatal-Perinatal Medicine
University of Texas Southwestern Medical Center
Dallas, TX 75235-9063
9/35/61935

REFERENCES

1. Schelonka RL, Yoder BA, desJardins SE, Hall RB, Butler TJ. Peripheral leukocyte count and leukocyte indexes in healthy newborn term infants. J PEDIATR 1994;125:603-6.
2. Manroe BL, Weinberg AG, Rosenfeld CR, Brown R. The neonatal blood count in health and disease. I. Reference values for neutrophilic cells. J PEDIATR 1979;95:89-98.
3. Rodwell RL, Leslie AL, Tudehope DI. Early diagnosis of neonatal sepsis using a hematologic scoring system. J PEDIATR 1988;112:761-6.
4. Galen RS. The normal range: a concept in transition. Arch Pathol Lab Med 1977;101:561-5.

Reply

To the Editor:

The article by Manroe et al. [see reference 2, above], of which Dr. Rosenfeld was a coauthor, was a well-designed, well-executed study and has withstood the test of time. However, we were perplexed by the observation that many healthy neonates had leukocyte values and immature/total neutrophil ratios that exceeded "normal" ranges as elucidated by Manroe et al. The proportions of immature and segmented neutrophils at our institution, most consistently followed the normative data of premature and term neonates set forth by Xanthou[1] in 1970. Xanthou stated that "in the first 2-3 days of postnatal life, a varying proportion of neutrophils, sometimes half of them, presented as band forms." Because of these conflicting observations we initiated our prospective study. Unless we misinterpreted Fig. 5 in the article by Manroe et al., a scattergram of point values for the immature/total neutrophil proportion *by hour* for the first 60 hours of life, we believe that we made time-appropriate comparisons.

We agree with Dr. Rosenfeld that serial complete blood cell counts are more sensitive predictors of sepsis in the first 24 hours of life.[2] The complete blood cell count should serve as "supplemental" information. He suggests that antibiotic exposure and duration of hospitalization may be shortened if the patient's clinical course is unremarkable, culture results are negative at 48 hours, and neutrophil values have remained within the reference ranges. Unfortunately, the reference ranges of Manroe et al. did not apply to our population in the early neonatal period.

Leukocyte reference values for the first 72 hours of life should be reexamined. However, the difficulty lies in identifying a "gold standard" to distinguish segmented and band neutrophils. We[3] and others have found that wide interreader differences exist in the interpretation of the peripheral blood smear.[4-6] Because segmented and band neutrophils exist on a continuum of cellular maturation, the establishment of discrete boundaries is artificial and subject to observer bias. Dr. Rosenfeld is well aware of the difficulties in accurate cell identification. In an earlier article of which he was a coauthor, 7% of the manual differential counts first performed by a hematology technician had to be "revised" by one of the authors because of marked discrepancies.[7] In 1993 the College of American Pathologists surveyed 6600 hematology technicians in a band neutrophil identification exercise. Because of poor reproducibility of band neutrophil identification in this large sample, the College no longer tests laboratory proficiency in the differentiation of segmented and band neutrophils. For these reasons we have discontinued a project to identify leukocyte reference ranges and neutrophil indexes for the first 48 hours of life in healthy and ill neonates.

Robert L. Schelonka, MD
Bradley A. Yoder, MD
Department of Pediatrics
Robert B. Hall, MD
Department of Pathology
Wilford Hall USAF Medical Center
2200 Bergquist Drive, Suite 1
Lackland Air Force Base, TX 78236-5300
9/35/61934

REFERENCES

1. Xanthou M. Leukocyte blood picture in healthy full-term and premature babies during neonatal period. Arch Dis Child 1970;45:242-9.

2. Greenberg DN, Yoder BA. Changes in the differential white blood cell count in screening for group B streptococcal sepsis. Pediatr Infect Dis J 1990;9:886-89.
3. Schelonka RL, Yoder BA, Hall RB, Trippett TM. Inter-reader variability of the manual differential leukocyte count in newborns [Abstract]. Pediatr Res 1994;35(4):169A.
4. Cornbleet J. 1993 CAP surveys set HG-C (band neutrophil identification exercise). Northfield, Illinois: College of American Pathologists, 1994.
5. Bacus JW. The observer error in peripheral blood cell classification. Am J Clin Pathol 1973;59:223-31.
6. Christensen RD, Rothstein G. Pitfalls in the interpretation of leukocyte counts of newborn infants. Am J Clin Pathol 1979;72:608-11.
7. Manroe BL, Rosenfeld CR, Weinberg AG, Browne R. The differential leukocyte count in the assessment and outcome of early-onset neonatal group B streptococcal disease. J PEDIATR 1977;91:632-7.

Electrocardiographic findings in Rett syndrome

To the Editor:

In 1992 we described a 14-year-old girl with Rett syndrome whose electrocardiogram showed corrected QT interval prolongation and T-wave abnormalities.[1] The QTc value was 477 msec. The T-waves were negative in leads DIII, aVF, and V_1 to V_4, and were of low amplitude in the remaining leads. The patient received no medication. Serum ion levels, including magnesium, were normal. Results of M-mode and two-dimensional echocardiography were normal. The electrocardiographic findings for two additional patients, aged 2 and 7 years, were normal.

At that time we suggested that an electrocardiographic study be done in every case of Rett syndrome, with careful measurement of the QTc interval and overall analysis of the repolarization to determine whether our observation was a casual one or may have clinical utility.

We read with interest the excellent article by Sekul et al.[2] showing that girls with Rett syndrome had significantly longer corrected QT intervals and more T-wave abnormalities than were found in age-matched healthy girls. We are pleased that Sekul et al. proved with their well-done study that we were not in error in our initial observations and suggestions. These authors are correct in pointing out that the real issue is to define the possible role of cardiac dysfunction in the sudden death associated with Rett syndrome.

Manuel Fuster-Siebert, PhD
Manual Castro-Gago, PhD
Sections of Pediatric Cardiology and Pediatric Neurology
Department of Pediatrics
Hospital General de Galicia
Santiago de Compostela, Spain

9/35/61581

REFERENCES

1. Fuster-Siebert M, Castro-Gago M. Síndrome de Rett e intervalo QT largo [Letter]. Med Clín (Barc) 1992;98:157.
2. Sekul EA, Moak JP, Schultz RJ, Glaze DG, Dunn JK, Percy AK. Electrocardiographic findings in Rett syndrome: an explanation for sudden death? J PEDIATR 1994;125:80-2.

THE JOURNAL OF
PEDIATRICS

APRIL 1995 *Volume 126* *Number 4*

SPECIAL ARTICLE

Impact of attitudes on maternal decisions regarding infant feeding

Mary Losch, PhD, Claibourne I. Dungy, MD, MPH, Daniel Russell, PhD, and Lois B. Dusdieker, MD, MS

From the Iowa Social Science Institute, the Department of Pediatrics, University of Iowa, Iowa City, and the Department of Psychology, Iowa State University, Ames

Since the early 1970s, when the proportion of new mothers who initiated breast-feeding fell to 22%,[1] there has been an increase in the amount of information provided to health professionals and women of childbearing age about the many health advantages of breast-feeding. By 1979 the rate of initiation of breast-feeding had risen to 51%[2] and reached a modern high of 62% in 1984.[3] However, the rates for initiation of breast-feeding and duration have again fallen despite continued efforts to inform health professionals and the public of the physiologic and cognitive benefits.[3-6] In light of the goals of Healthy People 2000,[7] new initiatives must be developed to reverse the current downward trend if we are to reach the goals of 75% initiation of breast-feeding at birth and 50% feeding at least some human milk until the age of 6 months. Ascertaining the factors important to a mother's decision about how to feed her infant is central to this effort. On the basis of a review of more than 200 articles in the breast-feeding and decision-making literature, this article summarizes the key findings regarding the role of attitudes in infant-feeding decisions. Only articles demonstrating the most rigorous sampling and design methods were included. In some cases, studies involving small sample sizes were included because they provided unique information. Studies reviewed were limited to investigations of Western industrialized populations, primarily in the United States, Canada, and Great Britain.

Reprint requests: Claibourne I. Dungy, MD, MPH, University of Iowa Hospitals and Clinics, Department of Pediatrics, 2569 JCP, 200 Hawkins Dr., Iowa City, IA 52242-1083.

THE JOURNAL OF PEDIATRICS 1995;126:507-14

0022-3476/95/$3.00 + 0 **9/19/61762**

For the past quarter century there have been increased efforts by researchers to identify the variables that determine how a woman will feed her infant and, if she chooses to breast-feed, how long nursing will continue. Despite methodologic limitations,[8] several associations between psychosocial factors and choices of infant feeding have consistently emerged as important in a woman's decision to breast-feed her infant. Extensive analyses of demographic variables such as age, education, income, religion, race, and parity have also been conducted. With the exception of very young mothers, who have a low rate of initiation and short duration, age has not been consistently shown to be related to initiation or duration of breast-feeding.[3, 9, 10] In the United States and England, education and social class have a direct, positive relation to the initiation and duration of breast-feeding among white populations.[3, 10-14] Related to social class (though not invariant across ethnic groups), income has also been shown to be positively correlated with breast-feeding.[15]

Racial variation has been documented as a factor associated with breast-feeding rates; in the United States, white mothers breast-feed at the highest rates and black mothers at the lowest[3, 16]; the rate for Hispanic mothers falls in between.[3] Other ethnic groups have not been sufficiently studied to determine feeding rate reliably. Data on parity tend to support the initiation of breast-feeding by higher proportions of first-time mothers,[11, 15, 17, 18] although this relationship does not always hold.[12, 19, 20]

Studies of demographic variables appear more frequently than do studies of more complex psychosocial variables,[8] even though attitudes may in fact be more important determinants of infant feeding behaviors than demographic characteristics.[21-25] Moreover, in the development of policy initiatives aimed at increasing the initiation rates and duration of breast-feeding, demographic variables are typically difficult (e.g., income, education) if not impossible (e.g., age, parity) to modify. Hence, if variables such as knowledge and attitudes are strong predictors of infant-feeding decisions, they provide much greater potential as intervention targets than more static demographic factors.

RELATION BETWEEN ATTITUDES AND BEHAVIOR

Attitudes have been studied as factors in mothers' decision making because of the assumed link with behavior. Although some early investigations questioned the ability of attitudes to predict behavior,[26, 27] current data indicate that when attitudes and behaviors are measured at the same level of specificity, the ability of attitudes to predict behavior is strong.[28, 29] In contrast, if a general attitude is measured in an attempt to predict a specific behavior, the relationship breaks down.[30] One theory[30] that has garnered a great deal of support argues that behavioral intentions are the most important predictors of behavior. Other factors such as demographic variables are viewed as indirect determinants. Several studies have found support for this theory, including its successful application to infant-feeding decisions.[31, 32]

Numerous studies have found that behavioral intentions assessed before the birth of a child are very closely linked to mothers' actual feeding practices.[9, 15, 20, 31-34] Correlations as high as 0.97 have been reported between assessments of prenatal intention and postnatal behavior.[33, 36] Other reports of correspondence between prenatal intentions and feeding choice range from 77%[33, 37] to 97%.[38] Moreover, using structural equation modeling of variables such as birth experience, early postpartum experience, feeding regimen, and timing of solid food introduction, Entwisle et al.[34] found that prenatal intentions were the strongest predictor of first-month breast-feeding behavior. Coreil and Murphy[39] reported that prenatal intended duration of breast-feeding was the strongest predictor of long-term feeding duration. Hence, a mother's intentions are closely associated with her subsequent choice of infant feeding.

WHEN ARE FEEDING DECISIONS MADE?

If the behavioral intention or the decision to feed a child in a certain way is closely linked to actual behavior, it is important to determine when mothers decide how they will feed their babies. This is a critical question in the planning of educational or attitudinal interventions aimed at increasing the rate of breast-feeding. In almost all cases, data indicate that a mother's feeding decision is made early in pregnancy or in many cases, before she becomes pregnant. Most reports indicate that nearly half[12, 38, 40] to more than three fourths[10, 20, 41] of women made feeding decisions before pregnancy. By the end of pregnancy, almost all reports indicate that at least three fourths of women have decided how they will feed their baby.[9] The large majority of adolescent mothers, who are less likely than older mothers to make feeding decisions before pregnancy, also have decided before birth how they will feed their child.[42, 43] The earlier the decision to breast-feed was made, the longer its duration.[17, 44]

Modification of breast-feeding decisions through educational or support programs provided during a mother's postpartum hospital stay may be an important method of increasing the duration of breast-feeding, but it is not likely to have a significant impact on initiation rates. In addition, the trend toward 24-hour hospital stays after uncomplicated deliveries will decrease the opportunities to provide information and support to new mothers.

FACTORS INFLUENCING ATTITUDES TOWARD INFANT FEEDING

Early attitudes. Few studies have examined the attitudes of children and adolescents toward infant-feeding issues. The limited data from this population are similar to data from studies of adult women and mothers. For example, in a group of adolescent girls, more positive attitudes toward and increased knowledge about breast-feeding have been associated with a higher likelihood of considering breast-feeding.[45] In addition, more positive attitudes toward breast-feeding were associated with greater exposure to breast-feeding mothers.[45-47] Investigations have also determined that high school students lack information and hold numerous misconceptions about breast-feeding.[48, 49] Pascoe and Berger[50] found that Israeli girls' attitudes toward breast-feeding were significantly more positive than those of U.S. girls, and a higher proportion of Israeli girls reported plans to breast-feed.

Social support and personal networks. Attitudes and information provided by various individuals in a woman's social and/or kinship network have been hypothesized to exert an influence on her decision regarding infant feeding. Husbands or partners, siblings, mothers, friends, co-workers, and health care providers have been identified as important sources of positive informational and emotional support for breast-feeding women.[51-75]

One of the most consistent findings is that sources of influence vary as a function of ethnicity. For white women, the most influential member of the social network appears to be the husband or partner. For Hispanic women, their mothers tend to exert the most influence, and for black women, close friends are most important.[52-54] In contrast, McLorg and Bryant[55] found no ethnic differences in specific social network members' influence on infant-feeding practices. In their study of white and black participants in the Supplemental Food Program for Women, Infants, and Children, the women's mothers were the most important advisers on infant-feeding issues for both racial groups; male partners were second in terms of their influence. The lack of racial differences in this study may have resulted from a lack of statistical power to detect any such effect because of the small number of women studied ($n \approx 20$ per group).

At least one recent investigation determined that in terms of risk factors for bottle feeding, "the most significant variable was lack of support from a significant other (husband, mother, other relative or friend)."[56] In this study of more than 300 indigent pregnant women, those who intended to give bottle feedngs viewed their significant others as having a negative attitude toward breast-feeding. Unfortunately, the design of the study did not allow the identification of the specific member of the social network who was most influential.

In addition to identifying important members of a woman's social support network, investigators have also begun to examine the types of support that seem to be associated with infant-feeding decisions. For example, Matich and Sims[57] measured perceived tangible (e.g., money, time, services), emotional (e.g., affection, empathy, love), and informational (e.g., facts, knowledge, advice) support in a group of pregnant women. Analyzing the relationships among sources and types of support and the intention to breast-feed, they found that informational support was higher for those intending to breast-feed. Tangible support and emotional support were not significantly associated with feeding intention. The baby's father appeared to play the largest role in providing all types of support for these women.

Fathers' attitudes. Although earlier commentaries and investigations occasionally mentioned the importance of the fathers' attitudes and their role in breast-feeding decisions,[32, 58-60] only recently have fathers' views become the primary focus of infant feeding investigations. Jordan and Wall[61] interviewed fathers on multiple occasions during their partner's pregnancy and after the birth of their child. Before the birth of the baby, most fathers were very positive toward breast-feeding and the important maternal bonding that they thought would accompany it. After the birth of the baby, however, the same men voiced concerns about feelings of inadequacy, separation from the baby, and separation from their partners because of the baby's feeding needs. Freed et al.[62] found that several attitudinal differences existed between those fathers who expressed plans to have their child breast-fed and those who planned to feed their child formula. Mirroring the relation between mothers' attitudes and feeding decisions, fathers planning to have their child breast-fed were significantly more likely to believe that breast-feeding was healthier for the baby. Those in the formula group were more likely to believe that breast-feeding is bad for the breasts and interferes with sex.

Both of these studies point to the importance of increasing the knowledge of the father when breast-feeding interventions are developed. Before the birth of a baby and even as early as childhood and adolescence, educational forums on infant feeding should include males. General information concerning the benefits of breast-feeding and its real effects (or lack of detrimental effects) should be emphasized in interventions geared toward males before they are expecting their first child. In preparation for the birth of a new baby, the information given to fathers should be candid, including a discussion of the possibilities for feelings of isolation and envy. As Jordan and Wall[61] stated, "These facts are not meant to divert couples from this infant feeding choice, but rather to help them anticipate and manage the challenges, thereby promoting greater satisfaction and success with breast-feeding"(p. 213).

Health providers' attitudes and influence. For more than two decades, the role of physicians and other health care providers in decisions on infant feeding has been debated. As Weichert[63] noted in 1975, physicians must do more than simply ask how the mother intends to feed her baby. Women must be given information concerning the potential advantages of breast-feeding. However, despite health care providers' perceptions that they are important sources of influence on mothers' infant-feeding decisions,[64] and their reports that they usually recommend breast-feeding for most pregnant patients,[65] few women (8% to 24%), report having received any feeding advice from their health care providers.[11, 13, 66, 67] Moreover, physicians, nurses, or midwives are only rarely cited by mothers as important influences in feeding decisions.[19, 67-70] When health care providers are mentioned, they are seen as giving conflicting information.[17, 66, 71] This does not mean, however, that when physicians and other health care providers actively promote breast-feeding, they have no effect. On the contrary, a woman's attitude and her physician's attitude toward breast-feeding have been shown to correspond closely. Mothers who are given positive advice about breast-feeding are much more likely to breast-feed.[11] In addition, physician-led group discussions have been shown to increase initiation rates of breast-feeding fourfold.[73] In one longitudinal study of more than 500 women, twice as many mothers were still breast-feeding at 6 weeks postpartum if they had spoken to a health care professional about feeding during a prenatal class.[74]

Although obstetricians have the greatest opportunity to provide information about the advantages of breast-feeding and hence influence patients' attitudes and subsequent behavior, they appear to be its least enthusiastic promoters.[64, 65] In the most comprehensive national survey of physician attitudes and practices, Lawrence[64] found that pediatricians, family practitioners, and nurses were more likely than obstetricians to view nutritional value, mother-infant closeness, and provision of immunity as important reasons for breast-feeding. Similarly, in a statewide survey of Louisiana physicians, only 44% of obstetricians considered breast-feeding to be very important, compared with 74% of pediatricians, 66% of general practitioners, and 65% of family practitioners.[65] Concerns about the low rates of initiation and short duration of breast-feeding have prompted some physicians to encourage their colleagues to play a more active role in influencing their patients to choose breast-feeding.[75-77] In a recent commentary, obstetricians were encouraged to refrain from supplying women in their care with formula samples and proformula advertising. The authors suggested that if obstetricians are not comfortable discussing breast-feeding issues with their patients, it may be appropriate to refer to a pediatrician before the birth of the baby.[75]

Maternity ward policies. In addition to the verbal influence that health care providers can exert, nonverbal factors such as hospital discharge packages and rooming-in policies can also play an important role in infant-feeding decisions. Using metaanalytic techniques, Dewey et al.[78] recently concluded that there was good evidence that commercial discharge packs have a negative impact on successful breast-feeding, and that breast-feeding on demand and early maternal-infant contact may have beneficial effects. They caution, however, that further investigation with rigorous methods must be completed before these relationships can be confirmed. Mixed messages are given to mothers when physicians, nursing staff, and lactation consultants devote time and effort to educating new mothers and supporting their efforts to breast-feed, only to have the new mother sent home with a package of formula and formula coupons.

PROFILES OF WOMEN WHO BREAST-FEED VERSUS THOSE WHO GIVE FORMULA

The attitudes of mothers who choose to breast-feed their infants differ from those who choose to feed their infants formula. The seminal work of Newton and Newton[24, 79] is credited with focusing interest on the important role of attitudes in "successful" breast-feeding. They found positive attitudes to be associated with more successful breast-feeding outcomes. A recent study indicates that positive attitudes are more important predictors of initiation of breast-feeding than knowledge about breast-feeding.[60] Numerous subsequent investigations have been conducted to provide a clearer picture of the specific attitudes related to choosing breast-feeding over using formula. One of the most consistent findings is that women who choose to use formula are not so much embracing this method of infant feeding as they are rejecting breast-feeding. Women who choose formula report that they dislike the thought of breast-feeding, although many acknowledge that human milk is healthier for infants.[11, 14, 70, 80-83] The most frequently cited reasons for rejecting breast-feeding are embarrassment,[84-86] fear of pain or discomfort,[70, 87] limitations on freedom and social life,[20, 85-89] and concerns that the father would not be involved in the feeding process.[68] One of the only positive attitudes expressed regarding formula feeding is the mother's view that it is the more convenient choice.[12, 38, 88-91] However, convenience is also viewed as one of the positive aspects by those who choose to breast-feed.[10, 81, 92]

In contrast to women who use formula, those who choose to breast-feed generally hold positive attitudes toward human milk and breast-feeding. Overwhelmingly, women choosing to breast-feed consider human milk to be healthier or "better" for infants than formula.[38, 92-94] These women are also more likely to believe that breast-feeding is more natural[70, 86] and results in better "bonding" or closeness with the baby.

Several investigators have noted that the reasons given for choosing either breast-feeding or formula feeding may be viewed as either "infant centered" or "mother centered."[14, 88] Mothers choosing to give formula tend to hold mother-centered views. They seem to be motivated primarily by concerns about the impact of the feeding process (e.g., convenience, comfort, assistance with feeding responsibilities). On the other hand, mothers selecting breast-feeding tend to be motivated more by concerns about the baby and his or her welfare (e.g., providing the healthiest nutrients and promoting a strong bond with the infant). Because large proportions of formula-feeding mothers acknowledge the health benefits of human milk,[37, 74] it appears that the perceived barriers associated with breast-feeding are significant motivating factors for users of formula.

The influence of the mother's attitudes on the duration of breast-feeding has not been as widely investigated as that on the initiation of breast-feeding. However, analysis of factors influencing duration have found a positive relation between duration of breast-feeding and mothers' beliefs that breast-feeding is better than formula feeding.[17, 95] In addition, mothers' confidence in their ability to breast-feed has been linked to longer duration of breast-feeding.[39, 95] In a longitudinal study, Morse[96] found that mothers' attitudes toward the problem of "leaking" of milk from their breasts were associated with duration of breast-feeding. Mothers who reported more negative feelings about leaking were more likely to breast-feed for shorter periods.

SUMMARY

It is essential that physicians and other health care professionals seeking to increase the rate of initiation and duration of breast-feeding build on the body of information concerning factors that influence a woman's attitudes about breast-feeding. The relation between positive attitudes concerning breast-feeding and its initiation is important to the development of programs targeting women before they become pregnant, and to the provision of active support for breast-feeding throughout the pregnancy, perinatal, and postnatal period. However, it is not sufficient for these programs to target only the mother or potential mother; members of a woman's social network must be considered as information targets. Educational programs must also be directed to the appropriate racial or ethnic group to develop programs that reach the individuals (father, female relative, or friend) most likely to influence the mother's breast-feeding decision.

Physicians may be very knowledgeable about the nutritional and immune properties of human milk and yet not be supportive of the act of breast-feeding. This lack of support may be manifested by the lack of verbal support for women who intend to or are in the process of breast-feeding, the provision of infant formula before or at the time of birth of the baby, or encouragement to terminate breast-feeding should the mother encounter any difficulties with lactation. To increase physician awareness of the process of breast-feeding and the properties of human milk, information about the benefits should be integrated in both the basic science and the clinical curricula of medical schools. Primary care training programs, including obstetrics, should actively involve trainees in the management of breast-feeding women so that trainees become aware of the spectrum of circumstances that confront women seeking to establish and maintain successful breast-feeding. This type of involvement would provide a contextual base for physicians' understanding the attitudes and behaviors supportive of breast-feeding.

Attitudes and behaviors of women, although more complex than demographic factors, provide a powerful tool for meeting the Healthy People 2000 goals for the initiation and duration of breast-feeding. It is important to build on the base of research reviewed here to develop new and more powerful interventions. Thus the emphasis on the known health advantages of human milk or the discovery of additional health benefits of breast-feeding should continue to be discussed because they may tip the balance in favor of breast-feeding for some women. Nevertheless, it may ultimately be more important to increase the amount of information provided to women (and girls and boys) about the practical aspects of the breast-feeding process (e.g., ease of night feeding, fathers' ability to feed mother's milk by bottle, lower cost, strategies to control leaking) than to rely solely on the positive health outcomes related to breast-feeding.

REFERENCES

1. Eckhart KW, Hendershot HE. Analysis of the reversal in breast feeding trends in the early 1970s. Public Health Rep 1984;99:410-5.
2. Martinez GA, Nalezienski JP. 1980 update: the recent trend in breast-feeding. Pediatrics 1981;64:260-3.
3. Ryan AS, Rush D, Krieger FW, Lewandoswki GE. Recent declines in breast-feeding in the United States, 1984 through 1989. Pediatrics 1991;88:719-27.

4. Bauer G, Dubanoski R, Ewald LS, Hoffman J. Breastfeeding and cognitive development of three-year-old children. Psychol Rep 1991;68:1218-22.
5. Lucas A, Morley R, Cole TJ, Lister G, Leeson-Payne C. Breast milk and subsequent intelligence quotient in children born preterm. Lancet 1992;339:261-4.
6. Rogan WJ, Gladen BC. Breast-feeding and cognitive development. Early Hum Dev 1993;31:181-93.
7. U.S. Department of Health and Human Services. Healthy People 2000: national health promotion and disease prevention objectives—full report, with commentary. Washington, D.C.: U.S. Government Printing Office, 1990:379.
8. Simopoulos AP, Grave GD. Factors associated with the choice and duration of infant-feeding practice. Pediatrics 1984; 74:603-14.
9. Holt HH, Wolkind SN. Early abandonment of breast feeding: causes and effects. Child Care Health Dev 1983;9:349-55.
10. Rousseau EH, Lescop JN, Fontaine S, Lambert J, Roy CC. Influence of cultural and environmental factors on breast-feeding. Can Med Assoc J 1982;127:701-4.
11. Jones RAD, Belsey EM. Breast feeding in an inner London borough: a study of cultural factors. Soc Sci Med 1977; 11: 175-9.
12. LeFevre M, Kruse J, Zweig S. Selection of infant feeding method: a population-based study in a rural area. J Fam Pract 1987;24:487-91.
13. Sacks SH, Brada M, Hill AM, Parton P, Harland P. To breast feed or not to breast feed. Practitioner 1976;216:183-91.
14. Switzky LT, Vietze P, Switzky HN. Attitudinal and demographic predictors of breast-feeding and bottle-feeding behavior by mothers of six-week-old infants. Psychol Rep 1979;45:3-14.
15. Stein A, Cooper PJ, Day A, Bond A. Social and psychiatric factors associated with the intention to breastfeed. Journal of Reproductive and Infant Psychology 1987;5:165-71.
16. Kistin N, Benton D, Rao S, Sullivan M. Breast-feeding rates among black urban low-income women: effect of prenatal education. Pediatrics 1990;86:741-6.
17. Jones DA, West RR. Effect of a lactation nurse on the success of breast-feeding: a randomised controlled trial. J Epidemiol Community Health 1986;40:45-9.
18. Weller SC, Dungy CI. Personal preferences and ethnic variations among Anglo and Hispanic breast and bottle feeders. Soc Sci Med 23;6:539-48.
19. Aberman S, Kirchhoff KT. Infant-feeding practices, mothers' decision making. J Obstet Gynecol Neonatal Nurs 1985; 14:394-8.
20. Mackey S, Fried PA. Infant breast and bottle feeding practices: some related factors and attitudes. Can J Public Health 1981;72:312-8.
21. Dungy CI, Losch M, Russell D, Christensen-Szalanski J. Effect of discharge samples on duration of breast-feeding. Pediatrics 1992;90:233-7.
22. Jones DA. Attitudes of breast-feeding mothers: a survey of 649 mothers. Soc Sci Med 1986;23:1151-6.
23. Dusdieker LB, Booth BM, Seals BF, Ekwo E. Investigation of a model for the initiation of breastfeeding in primigravida women. Soc Sci Med 1985;20:695-703.
24. Newton NR, Newton M. Relationship of ability to breast feed and maternal attitudes toward breast feeding. Pediatrics 1950;5:869-75.
25. Newton N, Newton M. Psychological aspects of lactation. N Engl J Med 1967;277:1179-88.
26. LaPiere RT. Attitudes versus action. Social Forces 1934; 13:230-7.
27. Wicker AW. An examination of the "other variables" explanation of attitude-behavior inconsistency. J Pers Soc Psychol 1971;19:18-30.
28. Abelson RP. Computers, polls, and public opinion: some puzzles and paradoxes. Transactions 1968;5:20-7.
29. Fishbein M, Ajzen I, eds. Belief, attitude, intention and behavior: an introduction to theory and research. Reading, Massachusetts: Addison-Wesley, 1975.
30. Ajzen I, Fishbein M. Attitude-behavior relations: a theoretical analysis and review of empirical research. Psychol Bull 1977; 84:888-918.
31. Manstead AS, Proffitt C, Smart JL. Predicting and understanding mothers' infant-feeding intentions and behavior: testing the theory of reasoned action. J Pers Soc Psychol 1983; 44:657-71.
32. Manstead AS, Plevin CE, Smart JL. Predicting mothers' choice of infant feeding method. Br J Soc Psychol 1984;23:223-31.
33. Baisch MJ, Fox RA, Goldberg BD. Breast-feeding attitudes and practices among adolescents. J Adolesc Health Care 1989;10:41-5.
34. Entwisle DR, Doering SG, Reilly TW. Sociopsychological determinants of women's breast-feeding behavior: a replication and extension. Am J Orthopsychiatry 1982;52:244-60.
35. Joffe A, Radius SM. Breast versus bottle: correlates of adolescent mothers' infant-feeding practices. Pediatrics 1987;79:689-95.
36. Radius SM, Joffee A. Understanding adolescent mothers' feelings about breast-feeding. J Adolesc Health Care 1988; 9:156-60.
37. Lyon ML, Chilver G, White DG, Woollett A. Current maternal attitudes to infant feeding methods. Child Care Health Dev 1981;7:145-51.
38. Sarett HP, Bain KR, O'Leary JC. Decisions on breast-feeding or formula feeding and trends in infant-feeding practices. Am J Dis Child 1983;137:719-25.
39. Coreil J, Murphy JE. Maternal commitment, lactation, practices, and breastfeeding duration. J Obstet Gynecol Neonatal Nurs 1988;17:237-78.
40. Eastham E, Smith D, Poole D, Neligan G. Further decline of breast-feeding. BMJ 1976;1:305-7.
41. Ekwo EE, Dusdieker LB, Booth BM. Factors influencing initiation of breast-feeding. Am J Dis Child 1983;137: 375-7.
42. Neifert M, Gray J, Gary N, Camp B. Effect of two types of hospital feeding gift packs on duration of breast-feeding among adolescent mothers. J Adolesc Health Care 1988;9: 411-3.
43. Maehr JC, Lizarraga MJL, Wingard DL, Felice ME. A comparative study of adolescent and adult mothers who intend to breastfeed. J Adolesc Health 1993;14:453-7.
44. Goodine LA, Fried PA. Infant feeding practices: pre- and

postnatal factors affecting choice of method and the duration of breastfeeding. Can J Public Health 1984;75:439-44.
45. Cusson RM. Attitudes toward breast-feeding among female high-school students. Pediatr Nurs 1985;11:189-91.
46. Banoub S, Friel JK, Hudson NI, Ross A. The effect of a promotion campaign on attitudes of adolescent females towards breastfeeding. Can J Public Health 1989;80:195-9.
47. Smith ME. Attitudes to breast-feeding. Sa Mediese Tydskrif 1984;65:234.
48. Berger A, Winter ST. Attitudes and knowledge of secondary school girls concerning breast feeding. Clin Pediatr 1980; 19:825-6.
49. Ellis DJ. Secondary school students' attitudes and beliefs about breastfeeding. J Sch Health 1983;53:600-4.
50. Pascoe JM, Berger A. Attitudes of high school girls in Israel and the United States toward breast feeding. J Adolesc Health Care 1985;6:28-30.
51. Grossman LK, Fitzsimmons SM, Larsen-Alexander JB, Sachs L, Harter C. The infant feeding decision in low and upper income women. Clin Pediatr 1990;29:30-7.
52. Baranowski T, Bee DE, Rassin DK, et al. Social support, social influence, ethnicity and the breastfeeding decision. Soc Sci Med 1983;7:367-72.
53. Bryant CA. The impact of kin, friend and neighbor networks on infant feeding practices. Soc Sci Med 1982;16:1757-65.
54. Auerbach KG, Guss E. Maternal employment and breastfeeding. Am J Dis Child 1984;138:958-60.
55. McLorg PA, Bryant CA. Influence of social network members and health care professional on infant feeding practices of econimically disadvantaged mothers. Med Anthropol 1989; 10:265-78.
56. Freed GL, Jones TM, Schandler RJ. Prenatal determination of demographic and attitudinal factors regarding feeding practice in an indigent population. Am J Perinatol 1992; 9:420-4.
57. Matich JR, Sims LS. A comparison of social support variables between women who intend to breast or bottle feed. Soc Sci Med 1992;34:919-27.
58. American Academy of Pediatrics, Nutrition Committee of the Canadian Paediatric Society, and Committee on Nutrition of the American Academy of Pediatrics. Breast-feeding: a commentary in celebration of the International Year of the Child, 1979. Pediatrics 1978;62:591-601.
59. Neville MC, Neifert MR, eds. Lactation: physiology, nutrition and breast-feeding. New York: Plenum Press, 1983.
60. Black R, Blair J, Jones VN, DuRant RH. Infant feeding decisions among pregnant women from a WIC population in Georgia. J Am Diet Assoc 1990;90:255-9.
61. Jordan PL, Wall VR. Breastfeeding and fathers: illuminating the darker side. Birth 1990;17:210-3.
62. Fraley K, Freed GL, Schanler RJ. Attitudes of expectant fathers regarding breast-feeding. Pediatrics 1992;90:224-7.
63. Weichert C. Breast-feeding: first thoughts. Pediatrics 1975; 56:987-90.
64. Lawrence RA. Practices and attitudes toward breast-feeding among medical professionals. Pediatrics 1982;70:912-20.
65. Reames ES. Opinions of physicians and hospitals of current breast-feeding recommendations. J Am Diet Assoc 1985;85:79-80.
66. Kurtz Z. Attitudes to breast feeding. Midwife Health Visit Community Nurse 1981;17:418-21.
67. Reif MI, Essock-Vitale SM. Hospital influences on early infant-feeding practices. Pediatrics 1985;76:872-9.
68. Adair LS. Feeding babies: mothers' decisions in an urban U.S. setting. Med Anthropol 1983;7:1-19.
69. Labbok MH, Simon SR. A community study of a decade of in-hospital breast-feeding: implications for breast-feeding promotion. Am J Prev Med 1988;4:62-7.
70. Dix Dustine N. Why women decide not to breastfeed. Birth 1991;18:222-5.
71. Bruce NG, Khan Z, Olsen NDL. Hospital and other influences on the uptake and maintenance of breast feeding: the development of infant feeding policy in a district. Public Health 1991;105:357-68.
72. Counsilman JJ, Mackay EV, Copeland RM. Bivariate analyses of attitudes towards breast-feeding. Aust NZ J Obstet Gynaecol 1983;23:208-15.
73. Haider SA. Encouragement of breast-feeding [Letter]. BMJ 1976; 1:650.
74. Hally MR, Bond J, Crawley J, Gregson B, Philips P, Russell I. Factors influencing the feeding of first-born infants. Acta Paediatr Scand 1984;73:33-9.
75. Howard CR, Fred M, Weitzman M. The physician as advertiser: the unintentional discouragement of breastfeeding. Obstet Gynecol 1993;81:1048-51.
76. Winikoff B, Baer E. The obstetrician's opportunity: translating "breast is best" from theory to practice. Am J Obstet Gynecol 1980;138:105-17.
77. Freed GL. Time to teach what we preach. JAMA 1993; 269:243-5.
78. Dewey KG, Lonnerdal B, Perez-Escamilla R, Pollitt E. Infant feeding policies in maternity wards and their effect on breastfeeding success: an analytical overview. Am J Public Health 1994;84:89-97.
79. Newton N, ed. Maternal emotions: a study of women's feelings toward menstruation, pregnancy, childbirth, breast feeding, infant care, and other aspects of their femininity. New York: PB Hoeber, 1955.
80. Leeper JD, Milo T, Collins TR. Infant feeding and maternal attitudes among mothers of low income. Psychol Rep 1983; 53:259-65.
81. Yeung DL, Pennell MD, Leung M, Hall J. Breastfeeding: prevalence and influencing factors. Can J Public Health 1981; 72:323-30.
82. Connolly JA, MacDonald D, Cullen JH. Breast feeding practice and factors related to choice of feeding method. Ir Med J 1981;74:166-8.
83. Fenton SJ. Factors influencing breastfeeding in a WIC population [Unpublished master's degree thesis]. University of Illinois at Chicago, 1991.
84. Mohrer J. Breast and bottle feeding in an inner-city community: an assessment of perceptions and practices. Med Anthropol 1979;3:125-45.
85. Bacon CJ, Wylie JM. Mothers' attitudes to infant feeding at Newcastle General Hospital in summer 1975. BMJ 1976; 7:308-9.
86. Gielen-Carlson A, Faden RR, O'Campo P, Paige DM. Determinants of breastfeeding in a rural WIC population. Journal of Human Lactation 1992;8:11-5.
87. Bevan ML, Mosley D, Loback KS, Solimano GR. Factors influencing breast feeding in an urban WIC program. J Am Diet Assoc 1984;84:563-7.

88. Yoos L. Developmental issues and the choice of feeding method of adolescent mothers. J Obstet Gynecol Neonatal Nurs 1985;14:68-72.
89. Brown F, Lieberman J, Winston I, Pleshette N. Studies in choice of infant feeding by primiparas: attitudinal factors and extraneous influences. Psychosom Med 1960;22:421-9.
90. Golub S. The decision to breast-feed: personality and experiential influences. Psychology 1978;15:17-27.
91. Arafat I, Allen DE, Fox JE. Maternal practice and attitudes toward breastfeeding. J Obstet Gynecol Neonatal Nurs 1981; 10:91-5.
92. Collins TR, Leeper JD, Milo T, DeMellier S. Perceptions and knowledge of breast-feeding among WIC and non-WIC pregnant women in Alabama. Ala J Med Sci 1984;21: 145-8.
93. Jeffs J. Why do mothers breast feed? Nurs Times 1977;73: 911-4.
94. Gunn TR. The incidence of breast feeding and reasons for weaning. NZ Med J 1984;97:360-3.
95. Hill PD. Predictors of breast-feeding duration among WIC and non-WIC mothers. Public Health Nurs 1991;8:46-52.
96. Morse JM. "Euch', those are for your husband!" examination of cultural values and assumptions associated with breast-feeding. Health Care for Women International 1989;11:223-32.

ORIGINAL ARTICLES

A multicenter study of alternate-day prednisone therapy in patients with cystic fibrosis

Howard Eigen, MD, Beryl J. Rosenstein, MD, Stacey FitzSimmons, PhD, Daniel V. Schidlow, MD, and the Cystic Fibrosis Foundation Prednisone Trial Group

From the Section of Pediatric Pulmonology and Critical Care, Indiana University School of Medicine, Indianapolis; the Eudowood Division of Pediatric Respiratory Sciences, Johns Hopkins University School of Medicine, Baltimore, Maryland; the Section of Pediatric Pulmonology, Department of Pediatrics, Temple University School of Medicine, St. Christopher's Hospital for Children, Philadelphia, Pennsylvania; and the Cystic Fibrosis Foundation, Bethesda, Maryland

The purpose of this study was to evaluate the efficacy and safety of alternate-day prednisone therapy in treating patients with mild-to-moderate cystic fibrosis during a 4-year period. In 15 North American cystic fibrosis centers, we screened 320 patients and enrolled 285 patients from April 1986 to December 1987. Patients were randomly assigned to take prednisone, 1 mg/kg per dose or 2 mg/kg per dose, or a matching placebo given on alternate days. Lung function, clinical status, hospitalizations, growth, and steroid side effects were monitored. During the first 24 months the percentage of the predicted forced vital capacity was greater in the 1 mg/kg group ($p < 0.0001$) and the 2 mg/kg group ($p < 0.01$) when each was compared with placebo. Patients in the 1 mg/kg group had a higher percentage of predicted forced vital capacity than placebo patients during the entire 48 months ($p < 0.0025$), but only in the group of patients who were colonized with *Pseudomonas aeruginosa* at baseline. For 48 months, the 1 mg/kg group had a higher percentage of predicted forced expiratory volume in 1 second than patients given placebo ($p < 0.02$). The prednisone-treated groups had a reduction in serum IgG concentrations (1 mg/kg vs placebo, $p < 0.007$; 2 mg/kg vs placebo, $p < 0.003$). From 6 months onward, height *z* scores fell in the 2 mg/kg group compared with those given placebo ($p < 0.001$). For the 1 mg/kg group, height *z* scores were lower from 24 months. An excess of abnormalities in glucose metabolism was seen in the 2 mg/kg group compared with the placebo group ($p < 0.005$). Our findings suggest a role for alternate-day prednisone therapy at a dose of 1 mg/kg in patients with mild to moderate cystic fibrosis. The benefit of improved lung function appears to outweigh the potential for adverse effects when the treatment period is less than 24 months. (J Pediatr 1995;126:515-23)

Presented at the meeting of the American Pediatric Society, Washington, D.C., May 1993.

Submitted for publication April 18, 1994; accepted Oct. 6, 1994.

Reprint reqeusts: Howard Eigen, MD, 702 Barnhill Drive, Room 2750, Indianapolis, IN 46202-5225

0022-3476/95/$3.00 + 0 **9/20/61098**

Glucocorticoids are administered to patients with cystic fibrosis for a variety of acute indications such as bronchiolitic syndrome of infancy,[1] refractory airways obstruction,[2] and allergic bronchopulmonary aspergillosis.[3] However, the role of long-term systemic glucocorticoid therapy in the treatment of mild-to-moderate respiratory disease is not well established. There is increasing evidence that immune-

ANOVA	Analysis of variance
CF	Cystic fibrosis
FEV_1	Forced expiratory volume in 1 second
FVC	Forced vital capacity

mediated inflammation contributes significantly to the progressive lung damage seen in patients with CF.[4] This is based on the observations that (1) patients with persistent hypogammaglobulinemia G have significantly better lung function and weight for age, and fewer hospitalizations than age-matched control subjects with normal or high concentrations of IgG,[5] (2) progression of lung disease in patients with CF is associated with rising IgG levels,[6] (3) there is a large influx of neutrophils into the airways of patients with CF,[4] (4) circulating immune complexes are present in a high percentage of the patients,[7] and (5) there is a correlation between high levels of immune complexes and disease severity.[8]

The long-term use of glucocorticoids has been evaluated in only a small number of patients with CF. In a placebo-controlled crossover trial, Pantin et al.,[9] studied the effect of a 3-week course of oral prednisolone therapy (average dose, 0.48 mg/kg) in 20 clinically stable adult patients with severe airflow obstruction. They observed no beneficial effect of prednisolone on pulmonary function, breathlessness, general well-being, or sputum production. Pneumothoraces developed in two patients and glycosuria in three during prednisolone therapy. In a 4-year placebo-controlled trial in which 45 patients with mild-to-moderate disease took prednisone at a dose of 2 mg/kg on alternate days, Auerbach et al.,[10] found that the prednisone-treated group had significant advantages over the placebo group for height, weight, forced vital capacity, forced expiratory flow in 1 second, peak expiratory flow rate, and serum IgG concentrations. The prednisone-treated group required significantly fewer admissions to the hospital for CF-related pulmonary disease than did patients in the placebo group. The investigators did not observe any steroid-related complications among the 34 patients who completed the trial.

Our study was carried out to evaluate the efficacy and safety of alternate-day prednisone therapy, in 1 mg/kg and 2 mg/kg doses given for a 4-year period to a large group of patients with CF and stable, mild-to-moderate pulmonary disease.

METHODS

We conducted a 4-year double-blind, placebo-controlled, parallel-group multicenter trial of two different doses of prednisone therapy in patients with mild-to-moderate CF. A total of 285 patients were enrolled at 15 participating CF centers in the United States and Canada. Cystic fibrosis was diagnosed on the basis of clinical signs and symptoms and two elevated sweat chloride (or sweat sodium) values according to published standards.[11] Inclusion criteria were as follows: age 6 to 14 years; clinical stability without a hospitalization for CF-related problems within 2 months of entry; serum IgG concentration within 2 SD of normal for center, or hypogammaglobulinemia; reliable performance of pulmonary function tests for at least 6 months before participation in the trial; FEV_1 more than 60% of the predicted value, and FEV_1/FVC ratio more than 60% of the predicted value. Exclusion criteria included previous therapy with oral, inhaled, or nasal corticosteroids for more than 2 weeks within 6 months of entry or any form of corticosteroid therapy in the previous month; evidence of hepatic disease, elevated fasting blood glucose concentrations, positive tuberculin skin test result, allergic bronchopulmonary aspergillosis (by clinical history and previously positive culture), or a sputum culture positive for *Pseudomonas cepacia*. Patients taking nonsteroidal antiinflammatory drugs were also excluded. Patient enrollment took place from April 1986 through December 1987. Of 320 patients screened, 285 met the study criteria and were enrolled.

Written informed consent was obtained from each patient and a parent or guardian. The study protocol and informed consent form were approved by the institutional review board at each study center.

Patients were randomly assigned to receive either prednisone, 2 mg/kg; prednisone, 1 mg/kg; or placebo. Randomization took place within each center by means of a computer-generated random number sequence in blocks of six. The study drug was given on alternate days as a single morning dose. The maximal daily dose of prednisone was 60 mg. Each patient's dosage was adjusted as they gained or lost weight. The protocol established five weight groups (average weight, 15, 20, 25, 30, and >33 kg), and the same number of tablets was given to all patients in a given weight group for all three regimens. Unused study drug was returned at each visit, and pills were counted as a measure of compliance. Patients who missed 30% or more of the total prescribed study medication were labeled as noncompliant but were included in all analyses along with the compliant patients. Patients continued all other standard therapy as prescribed at the center, including antibiotics, bronchodilators, chest physical therapy, and pancreatic enzymes.

Primary outcome measures were pulmonary function, serum IgG concentrations, growth, and hospitalization rates. Spirometry was performed by an FVC maneuver, with the results plotted as a flow volume curve. Lung volumes were measured by whole-body plethysmography. Lung function was measured with testing equipment available at each participating center. All equipment and methods of procedure for pulmonary function testing met American Thoracic Society standards.[12] All values were expressed as a percentage of the predicted value compared with the reference population reported by Knudson et al.[13] Pulmonary function was assessed at baseline and at 6, 12, 18, 24, 36, and 48 months. Patients were examined at entry and every 3 months afterward by staff physicians at each CF center. Medical management other than the study medication was prescribed by staff physicians on the basis of the center's usual clinical practices. An ophthalmology evaluation, including slit-lamp examination, evaluation of visual fields and visual acuity, and fundoscopy, was performed at baseline and then yearly. At each study visit, a modified Shwachman clinical score[14] was calculated. This scoring system assigns a maximum of 25 points for each of four clinical categories and allows comparison of clinical status among patient groups. A chest radiograph was obtained yearly. A Brasfield radiograph score,[15] which rates the chest radiograph on a 25-point scale, was assigned to all radiographs by one of the principal investigators (H.E. or B.J.R.), who were masked to the patient's treatment assignment. A serum IgG concentration was obtained during the baseline visit and then at months 3, 6, 12, 24, 36, 42, and 48. Hemoglobin A_{1c} was measured at baseline, every 3 months from months 3 to 12, and then every 6 months through month 48. A respiratory tract culture, of either a sputum or a throat swab sample, was obtained at the baseline visit and then every 6 months. A serum chemistry panel, a complete blood cell count, and a urinalysis were performed at 6-month intervals. A morning serum cortisol concentration was obtained at baseline and at 6 months. Patients who did not complete the full 48-month study had all laboratory studies repeated at the termination visit.

Adverse events were monitored at each visit, with emphasis on hyperglycemia, cataracts, liver enzyme elevation, and respiratory infections with unusual pathogens. Height and weight were measured by techniques standardized across all participating centers, and height *z* scores were calculated on the basis of age-stratified normal populations. Height *z* scores for normal populations will have a mean of zero, and an SD of 1; a child with a *z* score of −0.5, for example, will have a height that is 0.5 SD less than the mean for his age group. This was done to adjust for age differences among subjects. An interim analysis of mortality rates, hospitalization rates, pulmonary function, height and weight, and reported adverse events was carried out every 6 months by a data safety monitoring committee (DSMC). In August 1990 the DSMC recommended that the use of the study drug be discontinued for the high-dose (2 mg/kg) prednisone group. After discontinuation of use of the study drug, these patients were monitored at 3-month intervals until the completion of the study. In August 1991 the DSMC recommended discontinuance of study medication in the low-dose (1 mg/kg) group, and the trial was terminated. In both cases the DSMC recommended discontinuance of study drug dosing because of an excess number of adverse events. Monitoring of all patients at 3-month intervals continued until December 1991. Data on height, weight, cataracts, and glucose abnormalities were collected until January 1993 on those patients who had adverse events.

The study analysis was designed as an intent to treat model with all patients being carried through to completion and analysis even if they were taken off the study drug regimen. Thus no patients were lost to follow-up for the purposes of analysis. If the analysis had been performed on all patients at the end of the trial, we would have included measurements on patients in the 2 mg/kg group who had not received study drug for as long as 24 months. Therefore we elected to perform two separate analyses. The first analysis included all three treatment groups from baseline to 24 months; the second compared the 1 mg/kg per dose group with the placebo group for 48 months. All patients were included in each analysis even if they were not receiving study medication during the entire period being analyzed.

Treatment differences at baseline were tested by ANOVA, with treatment, center, and treatment by center in the model. Individual differences at baseline were accounted and adjusted for by performance of any ongoing analyses of the change from baseline. We analyzed the long-term effect of prednisone on lung function, growth, and serum IgG concentration with a repeated measures ANOVA, accounting for treatment, center, time (repeated), and all interactions. Because this interaction was not significant for any of the measurements, we then tested for the effect of treatment. A significant treatment effect indicated that there were differences among the treatments, and that these treatment differences were consistent across all time points. All pairwise comparisons for the first analysis looking at all three treatments were performed with the appropriate combination mean square error and the Satterthwaite degrees-of-freedom approximation, and were calculated only if the ANOVA yielded a significant overall treatment effect. Declines in lung function from baseline to each time point were tested for significance for each treatment group. We set $p < 0.05$ as the threshold for significance.

RESULTS

There were no significant differences among the treatment groups at the beginning of the study with the exception that the *Pseudomonas aeruginosa* colonization rate was higher in the 2 mg/kg group than in the other two groups (Table I). The patients were characterized clinically as having mild-to-moderate disease on the basis of their modified Shwachman clinical score, Brasfield radiologic

Table I. Patient characteristics at baseline

	Prednisone		
	1 mg/kg (n = 95)	2 mg/kg (n = 95)	Placebo (n = 95)
Mean age (yr)	8.9	8.9	9.3
Brasfield chest x-ray score	19.1	19.6	19.5
Shwachman clinical score	83.2	82.3	83.4
Height (cm)	130.0	130.2	132.8
Weight (kg)	27.2	26.8	29.1
Serum IgG (mg/dl)	1070.9	1087.6	1055.4
P. aeruginosa	41 (43%)	59 (62%)	53 (56%)
FVC (% predicted)	92.1	89.9	88.8
FEV_1 (% predicted)	84.0	81.4	79.2
Male (No.)	56	57	47
Female (No.)	39	38	48

score, and lung function measurements. Pulmonary function values were similar in all three groups (Table I). At baseline, there were no differences among the study groups in medical complications, history of atopy, serum immunoglobulin E concentrations, vital signs, or abnormal physical findings. The changes from baseline in the percentage of predicted FVC when the three groups were compared for 24 months are seen in Fig. 1. At all time points, the increase from baseline of the percentage of predicted FVC was greater in the patients receiving 1 mg/kg than in the placebo-treated patients ($p < 0.0001$). At all time points, the change in the percentage of predicted FVC was greater in the 2 mg/kg group than in the placebo group ($p < 0.01$). There was no significant difference in effect between the two prednisone-treated groups ($p > 0.21$).

Additionally, at 24 months, 70.4% of patients treated with prednisone, 1 mg/kg, had an increase in the percentage of predicted FVC compared with 54.9% of patients treated with 2 mg/kg and 41.6% of patients treated with placebo. During the first 2 years and for 4 years, patients in the 1 mg/kg group had a significantly better change from baseline in the percentage of predicted FEV_1 than did the placebo group ($p < 0.02$) (Fig. 2). During the first 2 years, the 2 mg/kg group was not different from the placebo group. There were no significant differences among the groups for other measures of lung function. In a comparison of patients who were colonized with *P. aeruginosa* at baseline with those who were not, only the colonized patients had a significant change in the percentage of predicted FVC on either dose of prednisone (Fig. 3, *A* and *B*).

When the group treated with prednisone, 1 mg/kg, and the placebo-treated group were compared for 48 months, the patients treated with the 1 mg/kg dose of prednisone had a greater change in the percentage of predicted FVC that was sustained for the entire term of the study ($p < 0.0025$) (Fig. 1). The mean percentage of predicted FEV_1 in the placebo group declined from 79.21% at baseline to 73.84% at 48 months ($p < 0.0015$). The percentage of predicted FEV_1 in the 1 mg/kg group did not decline significantly (83.99% at baseline and 82.70% at 48 months, $p > 0.42$). Thus, at 48 months, the 1 mg/kg group had a significantly better change in the mean percentage of predicted FEV_1 than those given placebo ($p < 0.02$).

Both of the prednisone-treated groups had a significantly greater reduction in serum IgG levels than the placebo group (1 mg/kg vs placebo, $p < 0.01$; 2 mg/kg vs placebo, $p < 0.01$; Fig. 4). Calculating the Pearson correlation coefficient for FVC against serum IgG, we were unable to identify a significant correlation with any of the treatment groups. More individual patients had a fall in serum IgG levels in the 1 mg/kg group (72.8%) and in the 2 mg/kg group (84.5%) than in the placebo group (36.4%). These differences were highly significant when the placebo group was compared with the 1 mg/kg group ($p < 0.001$) and the 2 mg/kg group ($p < 0.0001$) by chi-square analysis. Patients were stratified by whether they had been colonized with *P. aeruginosa* at baseline and the response of IgG to treatment as assessed by ANOVA. The treatment effect did not differ between the groups.

Hospitalization rates were similar in all groups, being 53%, 59%, and 59% for the 1 mg/kg, 2 mg/kg, and placebo groups, respectively. Hospital days per patient (about 19 days) were similar among the groups. Hospitalizations per patient were also not significantly different, being 1.73, 1.82, and 1.86 for the 1 mg/kg, 2 mg/kg, and placebo groups, respectively. The Shwachman score, Brasfield score, and peak expiratory flow rate were not significantly different among the prednisone-treated groups and the placebo group.

In the placebo group the majority of terminations were for noncompliance and intercurrent illness, whereas in the prednisone 2 mg/kg group the majority were for adverse events (Table II). In the prednisone 1 mg/kg group, indications for termination were equally divided among adverse events, intercurrent problems, and noncompliance.

During the first 24 months, there were 68 adverse events in the 2 mg/kg group, 39 adverse events in the 1 mg/kg group, and 25 adverse events in the placebo group (Table II). Abnormalities in glucose metabolism—either elevated hemoglobin A_{1c}, elevated fasting blood glucose concentration, or glycosuria—were encountered more frequently in the patients treated with prednisone, 2 mg/kg, than in those given 1 mg/kg ($p < 0.05$); there was no significant difference between the 1 mg/kg and placebo groups. Cataracts were seen more often in patients given prednisone, 2 mg/kg, than

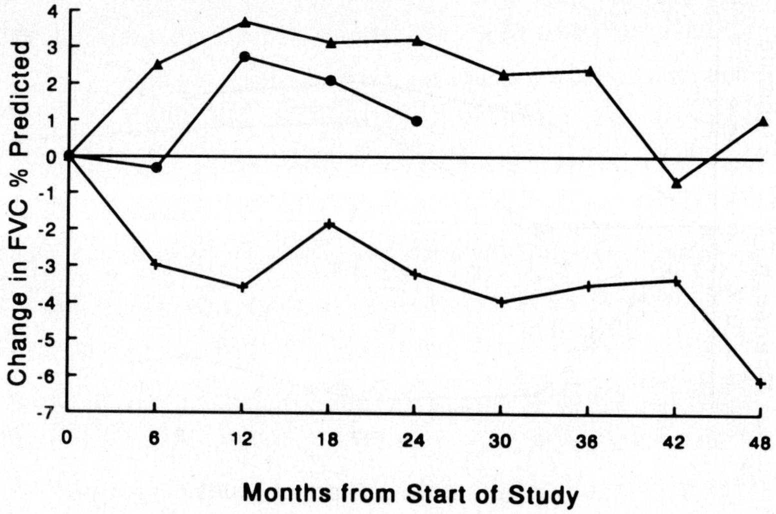

Fig. 1. Change from baseline in percentage of predicted FVC for all three groups during the first 48 months of the trial. Compared with placebo patients (+) the change in percentage of predicted FVC was greater in the 1 mg/kg group (▲) ($p < 0.0001$) and the 2 mg/kg group (●) ($p < 0.01$) at all time points during the first 24-month period. There was no difference between the 1 mg/kg and the 2 mg/kg groups ($p > 0.2$) at 24 months, but for the entire 48-month period the percentage of predicted FVC was higher in the 1 mg/kg group than in the placebo group at all time points ($p < 0.0025$).

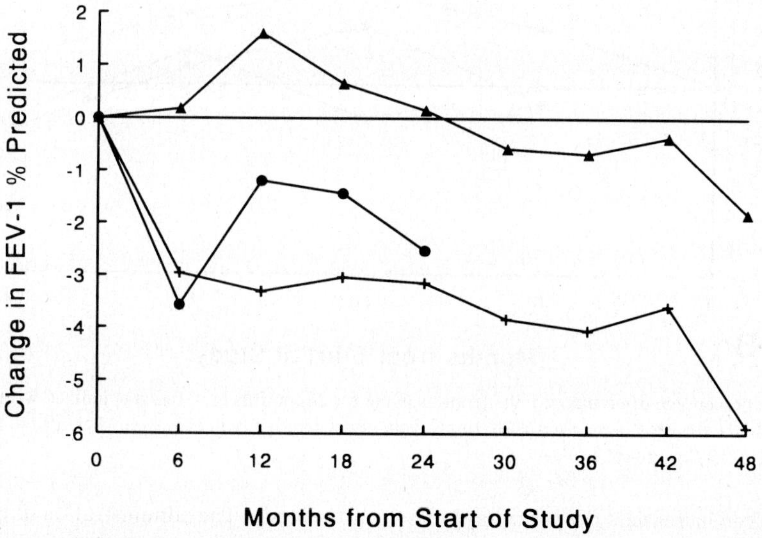

Fig. 2. Change from baseline in percentage of predicted FEV_1 for all three groups. Data for the 2 mg/kg group (●) are shown for the 24 months that this group received active drug. Data on the 1 mg/kg group (▲) and the placebo group (+) are shown for 48 months. Patients in the 1 mg/kg group had a significantly better percentage of predicted FEV_1 than did the placebo group ($p < 0.02$). During the first 24 months, the 2 mg/kg group was not significantly different from the placebo group.

in those given 1 mg/kg, but not more often than in the placebo group (Table II).

Linear growth retardation, as defined by a decrease of 1 *z* score, occurred more often in the prednisone-treated patients, either the 2 mg/kg or the 1 mg/kg group, than in those treated with placebo ($p < 0.05$). The 2 mg/kg group had a significantly greater reduction in height *z* score than the placebo-treated group from the 6-month visit onward ($p < 0.001$) (Fig. 5). For the 1 mg/kg group the reductions in height *z* scores were significant at 24, 36, and 48 months ($p < 0.001$). Placebo-treated patients who were colonized with *P. aeruginosa* grew more slowly during the course of the study and had greater decreases in height *z* scores ($p < 0.05$) than patients who were not colonized (Fig. 6). The difference in height *z* scores between colonized and noncolonized patients at baseline was not significant.

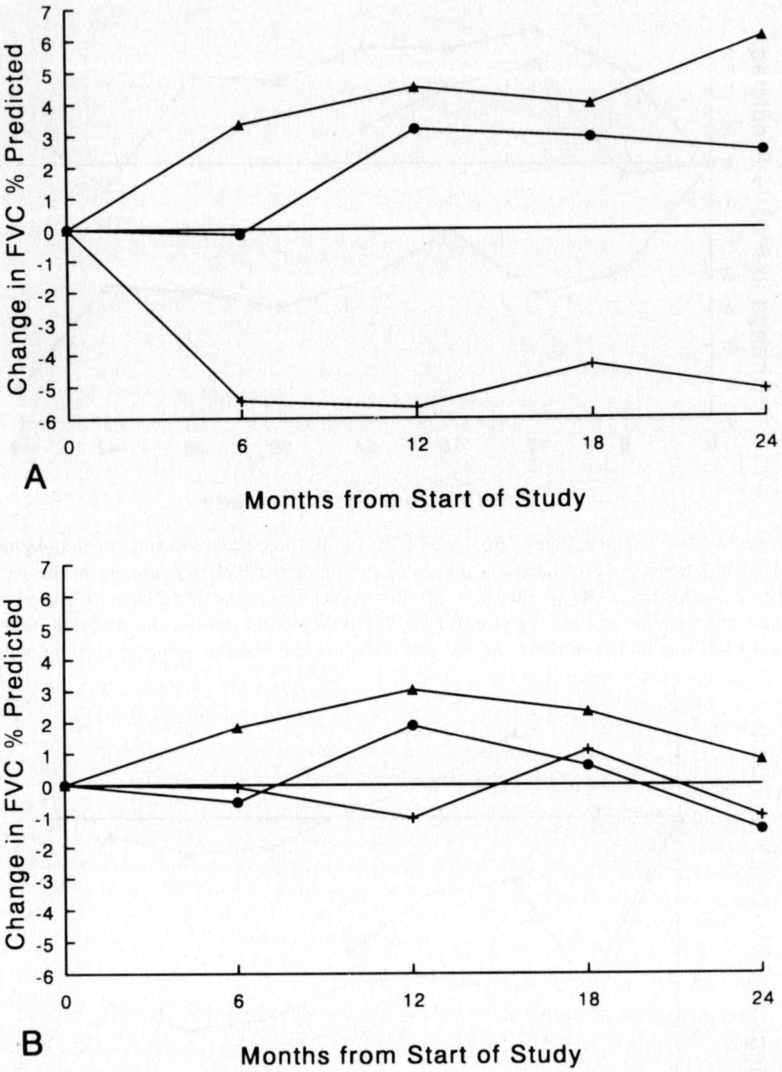

Fig. 3. Change in percentage of predicted FVC from baseline for 24 months in patients colonized with *P. aeruginosa* (**A**) and patients not colonized with *P. aeruginosa* (**B**). Improvement occurred only in colonized patients. +, Placebo group; ▲, 1 mg/kg group; ●, 2 mg/kg group.

The 2 mg/kg group had an increase in the percentage of patients colonized with *P. aeruginosa* from 62% (59/95) to 80% (43/54) ($p < 0.05$). Patients in the 1 mg/kg group had an increase in the colonization rate from 43% (41/95) to 70% (50/71) ($p < 0.01$). The colonization rate for the placebo group was not significantly changed: 53 of 95 at baseline and 42 of 71 at 48 months ($p > 0.42$).

DISCUSSION

Our findings suggest a role for alternate-day prednisone therapy, 1 mg/kg, in the treatment of patients with CF who were aged 6 to 14 years and had mild-to-moderate clinical status and *P. aeruginosa* colonization. In this group of patients, there was significant improvement in FVC, first evident at 6 months and persisting throughout the 4 years of the study. The administration of prednisone yielded no significant clinical benefit in patients who were not colonized with *P. aeruginosa*. The higher dose of prednisone did not provide additional benefit.

In previous longitudinal studies of CF patients, the percentage of predicted FVC has been noted to decline by 2% to 3% per year.[16] Given that the placebo group in our study had an 8% lower FVC at the end of 4 years than did the prednisone-treated group, it appears that prednisone therapy may have prevented the equivalent of 3 to 4 years of lung function decline. Patients with *P. aeruginosa* colonization have a more rapid decline in lung function than those not colonized,[17] and the former were the patients in our study who benefited most from prednisone therapy. The finding that the FVC did not continue to improve may be

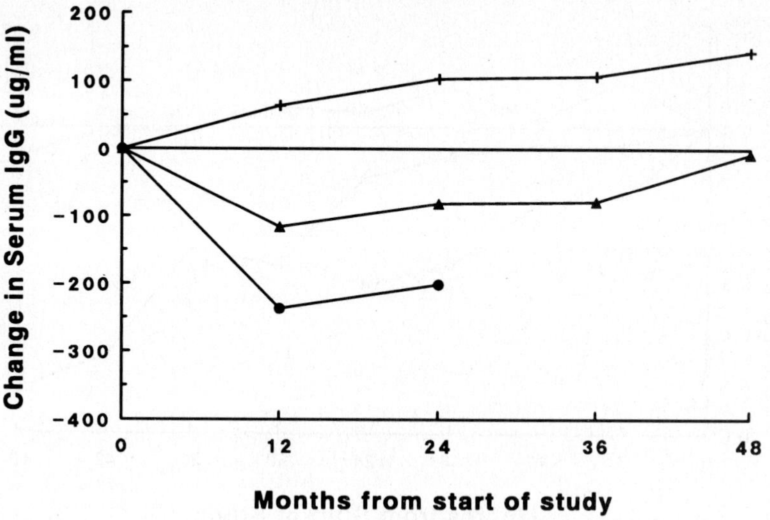

Fig. 4. Change from baseline of serum IgG concentrations. During the first 24 months IgG serum concentrations in the 2 mg/kg group (●) were significantly lower than in the placebo group (+ (p <0.01). For 4 years the IgG serum concentrations in the 1 mg/kg group (▲) were lower than in the placebo group (p <0.01).

related to the ability of prednisone to reduce active inflammation in the airways but the inability to reverse the fibrosis that results from a long-standing inflammatory process. Other than FVC and FEV_1, lung function measurements were similar in the placebo and prednisone-treated groups. Our inability to detect small differences in lung volumes is consistent with the large variability of these measurements in normal children and especially in those with CF.[18] Analysis of the data comparing the three treatment groups during the first 24 months was made necessary by the early termination of the 2 mg/kg group because of a high incidence of side effects. Had we used the intent-to-treat model and included all three groups for the entire 4-year period, the resulting analysis would have examined drug treatment effect in patients who had not been treated with active medication for as long as 2 years. This could be considered clinically invalid and may have masked a beneficial and real treatment effect of the drug. Instead, we analyzed the data in two blocks to preserve the intent-to-treat model and to obtain the greatest amount of information during the entire 4-year trial.

The mechanisms by which corticosteroids affect lung inflammation in CF are not clearly understood.[19] In patients with CF the cytokines interleukin-1β, interleukin-8, and tumor necrosis factor-α participate in pulmonary inflammation, acting as neutrophil chemoattractants.[4] Corticosteroids suppress interleukin-1 and tumor necrosis factor-α production by monocytes,[20] which may in turn reduce the inflammatory response to bacterial antigens. Patients colonized with *P. aeruginosa* had a greater response to prednisone therapy than those who were not colonized, which raises the possibility that prednisone had a greater effect in patients with more active inflammation. These data indicate that patients with *Pseudomonas* colonization are the best candidates for prednisone therapy.

Table II. Adverse events and early terminations

	Prednisone		
	1 mg/kg	2 mg/kg	Placebo
Adverse events			
Glucose abnormalities	12	26*, †	7
Diabetes	3	6	1
Intermittent hyperglycemia	3	10*	2
Intermittent glucosuria	6	10	4
Cataracts	3	11†	7
Growth retardation	24*	31*	11
Early terminations			
Intercurrent problems	13	10	12
Noncompliance/ parent request	12	4	14
Other	—	1	3

*p <0.05 compared with placebo.
†p <0.05 compared with 1 mg/kg.

Prednisone absorption in patients with CF appears to be complete.[21] Prednisolone (the active form of prednisone) is cleared more rapidly than normal in patients with CF, but it is unlikely that this rapid clearance reduced the effectiveness of the therapy in our treatment groups. However, it is possible that the effectiveness of oral prednisone therapy may have been reduced in individual patients who had rapid prednisone clearance.

Prednisone therapy also was associated with a lower serum concentration of IgG, indicating that prednisone ther-

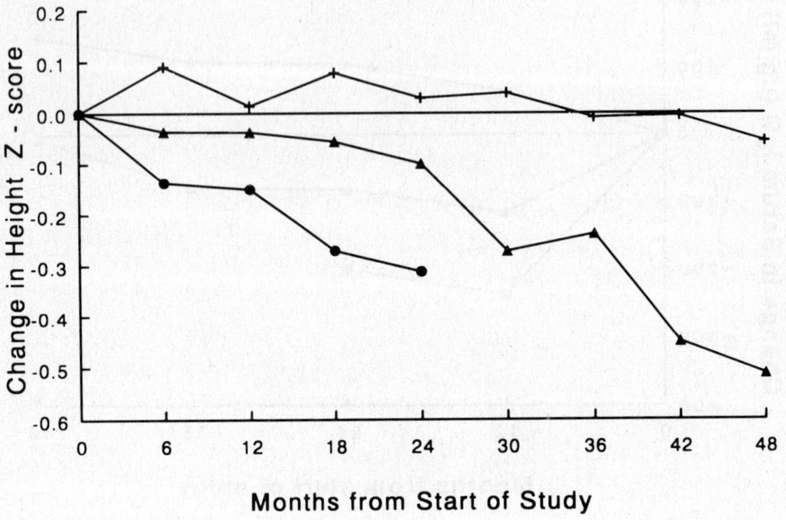

Fig. 5. Change from baseline in height z score for 48 months of the trial. The 2 mg/kg group (●) had a significantly lower height z score than in the placebo group (+) from 6 months onward ($p < 0.001$). The height z score for the 1 mg/kg group (▲) remained lower than that for the placebo group from 24 to 48 months ($p < 0.001$).

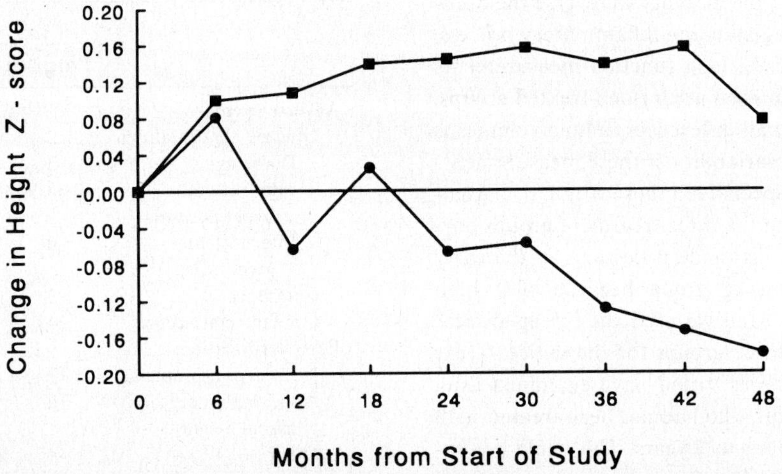

Fig. 6. Placebo-treated patients who were colonized with *P. aeruginosa* (●) grew more slowly during the course of the study and had lower height z scores ($p < 0.02$) than patients who were not colonized (■).

apy had modified the immune response. However, there was no direct correlation between decrease in serum IgG concentration and improvement in FVC.

There was a significant incidence of adverse effects, especially in the group treated with prednisone, 2 mg/kg. Auerbach et al.[10] observed no steroid-related complications in a similar but smaller trial; only 21 patients received prednisone, compared with the 190 patients who received prednisone in our trial. The adverse events seen most often were reduced linear growth and abnormalities of glucose metabolism. These are expected side effects of steroid treatment in children and should be monitored in patients treated with steroids on a long-term basis, even on an alternate-day schedule. Risk factors for the development of subcapsular cataracts in patients with CF treated with corticosteroids have been described, but in a small study these did not include duration of therapy or high dose.[22] A survey of ocular findings in patients with CF,[23] which included slit-lamp examination, did not note cataract formation. However, in our study, 7 (7%) of 95 patients in the placebo group were found to have cataracts. Whether this is a manifestation of the disease or related to other medical therapy is not known.

Height was affected from the sixth month onward in the

high-dose prednisone group, whereas patients taking the lower dose of prednisone, 1 mg/kg, had growth retardation only after 24 months of treatment. The beneficial effect of prednisone in the 1 mg/kg group was seen at 6 months and did not increase after that time. Therefore it seems prudent to discontinue prednisone therapy if there is no significant improvement in pulmonary function 6 months after therapy is initiated. Use of this dose should be limited to less than 24 months to reduce the chance of growth retardation. Growth should be monitored carefully and use of the drug discontinued at the first sign of growth retardation. The total duration of therapy must be determined individually on the basis of clinical considerations.

Our study design does not allow a more precise recommendation as to whether any subset of patients might benefit more from treatment with alternate-day prednisone. This will, of necessity, remain an individualized recommendation based on the patient's clinical course, response to standard therapy, and response to prednisone.

The participating investigators and centers were as follows: Robert Beckerman, MD, Tulane University, New Orleans, La.; Gerard Canny, MD, University of Toronto, Toronto, Ontario, Canada; Daniel Caplan, MD, Emory University, Atlanta, Ga.; Howard Eigen, MD, Indiana University, Indianapolis; Robert Fink, MD, George Washington University, Washington, D.C.; Loren Glasser, MD, Baylor College of Medicine, Houston, Tex.; Frances Harley, MD, Children's Hospital, Edmonton, Alberta, Canada; Julie Hsu, MD, Wayne State University, Detroit, Mich.; Allen Lapey, MD, Massachusetts General Hospital, Boston; Norman Lewiston, MD,† and Judy Palmer, MD, Stanford University, Palo Alto, Calif.; Raymond Lyrene, MD, and Dana Brasfield, MD, University of Alabama, Birmingham; Dennis Nielson, MD, University of Utah, Salt Lake City; Claude Prestidge, MD, University of Texas Southwestern Medical Center, Dallas; Beryl Rosenstein, MD, Johns Hopkins University, Baltimore, Maryland; and Daniel Schidlow, MD, Temple University, Philadelphia, Pa.

We are greatful to Robert Beall, PhD, for his foresight, support, and leadership during this study. We thank Lynn M. Tausig, MD, for his excellent leadership as chairman of the Cystic Fibrosis Foundation Prednisone Trial Group Data Safety Monitoring Committee. Prednisone tablets and matching placebo were supplied by Upjohn Pharmaceuticals. We especially thank Terry Reister for her help with data analysis.

REFERENCES

1. Lloyd-Still JD, Khaw KT, Shawchman H. Severe respiratory disease in infants with cystic fibrosis. Pediatrics 1974;53:678-82.
2. Mitchell IM, Corey M, Woenne R, Krastins IR, Levison H. Bronchial hyperreactivity in cystic fibrosis and asthma. J PEDIATR 1978;93:744-8.
3. Greenberger PA, Patterson R. Diagnosis and management of allergic bronchopulmonary aspergillosis. Ann Allergy 1986; 56:444-8.
4. Berger M. Inflammation in the lung in cystic fibrosis. Clin Rev Allergy 1991;9(1-2):119-42.
5. Matthews WJ, Williams M, Oliphint B, et al. Hypogammaglobulinemia in patients with cystic fibrosis. N Engl J Med 1980;302:245-9.
6. Wheeler WB, Williams M, Matthews WJ, Colten HR. Progression of cystic fibrosis lung disease as a function of serum immunoglobulin G levels: a 5-year longitudinal study. J PEDIATR 1984;104:695-9.
7. Moss RB, Lewiston NJ. Immune complexes and humoral response to *Pseudomonas aeruginosa* in cystic fibrosis. Am Rev Respir Dis 1980;121:23-9.
8. Wisnieski JJ, Todd EW, Fuller RK, et al. Immune complexes and complement abnormalities in patients with cystic fibrosis. Am Rev Respir Dis 1985;132:770-6.
9. Pantin CFA, Stead RJ, Hodson ME, Batten JC. Prednisolone in the treatment of airflow obstruction in adults with cystic fibrosis. Thorax 1986;41:34-8.
10. Auerbach HS, Williams M, Kirkpatrick JA, Colten HR. Alternate-day prednisone reduces morbidity and improves pulmonary function in cystic fibrosis. Lancet 1985;2: 686-8.
11. Shawchman H, Mahmoodian A. Pilocarpine iontophoresis sweat testing: results of seven years experience. Modern Problems in Pediatrics 1967;10:148-82.
12. American Thoracic Society. ATS Statement: Snowbird Workshop on Standardization of Spirometry. Am Rev Respir Dis 1979;119:831.
13. Knudson RJ, Lebowitz MD, Holberg CJ, Burrows B. Changes in the normal maximal expiratory flow-volume curve with growth and aging. Am Rev Respir Dis 1983;127:725-34.
14. Doerschuk CF, Matthews LW, Tucker AS, et al. A 5-year clinical evaluation of a therapeutic program for patients with cystic fibrosis. J PEDIATR 1964;65:677-9.
15. Brasfield D, Hick G, Soong S, Tiller RE. The chest roentgenogram in cystic fibrosis: a new scoring system. Pediatrics 1979; 63:24-9.
16. Corey M, Levison H, Crozier D. Five- to seven-year course of pulmonary function in cystic fibrosis. Am Rev Respir Dis 1976;114:1085-92.
17. Kerem E, Corey M, Gold R, Levison H. Pulmonary function and clinical course in patients with cystic fibrosis after pulmonary colonization with *Pseudomonas aeruginosa*. J PEDIATR 1990;116:714-9.
18. Nickerson B, Lemen RJ, Geroes CB, Wegmann MJ, Robertson G. Within-subject variability and percent change for significance of spirometry in normal subjects and in patients with cystic fibrosis. Am Rev Respir Dis 1980;122:859-66.
19. Price JF, Greatly P. Corticosteroid treatment in cystic fibrosis. Arch Dis Child 1993;68:719-21.
20. Scheimler RP. Effects of glucocorticoids on inflammatory cells relevant to their therapeutic applications in asthma. Am Rev Respir Dis 1990;141:559-69.
21. Dove AM, Szefler SJ, Hill MR, Jusko WJ, Larsen GL, Accurso FJ. Altered prednisolone pharmacokinetics in patients with cystic fibrosis. J PEDIATR 1992;120:789-94.
22. Majur M, Mroueh S, Spock A. Risk factors for the development of subcapsular cataracts in patients with cystic fibrosis and allergic bronchopulmonary aspergillosis treated with corticosteroids. Pediatr Pulmonol 1989;6:260-2.
23. Spaide RF, Diamond G, D'Amico RA, Gaerlan PF, Bisberg DS. Ocular findings in cystic fibrosis. Am J Ophthalmol 1987;103:204-10.

†Deceased.

Kawasaki disease in infants less than one year of age

Elaine A. Rosenfeld, MD, Kathleen E. Corydon, RN, and Stanford T. Shulman, MD

From the Department of Pediatrics, Northwestern University Medical School, Division of Infectious Diseases, Children's Memorial Hospital, Chicago, Illinois

Objective: **To identify risk factors for severe sequelae, analyze disease characteristics, and assess efficacy of intravenously administered immune globulin (IVGG) therapy in infants less than 12 months of age with Kawasaki disease.**
Design: **Retrospective chart review of children less than 12 months of age with Kawasaki disease between 1980 and 1993.**
Results: **Of 443 patients with Kawasaki disease, 57 (13%) were less than 1 year of age, including 14 (3%) less than 6 months. Age at onset was a predictor of the development of coronary artery aneurysms (CAA) and of giant (>8 mm) aneurysms: 11 (79%) of 14 children <6 months and 17 (44%) of 39 children 6 to 12 months of age acquired CAA (*p* = 0.06), and 5 (37%) of 14 children <6 months and 2 (5%) of 39 children 6 to 12 months of age acquired giant CAA (*p* <0.01). No specific clinical or laboratory features predicted the development of CAA, which was found in 7 (29%) of 24 patients treated with IVGG by illness day 10 and in 21 (73%) of 29 patients treated after day 10 or never treated with IVGG (*p* <0.01). Only 1 (4%) of 24 patients treated by day 10 but 6 (21%) of 29 children treated after day 10 or never treated with IVGG acquired giant CAA (*p* = 0.01). Persistent (>1 year) CAA were present in 4 (17%) of 24 IVGG-treated children by day 10 and in 14 (48%) of 29 children not treated by day 10 or never treated with IVGG (*p* <0.025). There was no difference in outcome if IVGG was given by illness day 7 or on illness days 8 to 10.**
Conclusions: **Patients with Kawasaki disease less than 6 months of age are at particularly increased risk of having CAA and giant CAA. Therapy with IVGG, given by illness day 10, is associated with substantial reduction in the frequency of CAA and giant CAA in this high-risk population. (J Pediatr 1995;126:524-9)**

Kawasaki disease is an acute febrile illness of infants and children characterized by fever for at least 5 days, with bilateral nonpurulent conjunctival injection, a polymorphous exanthem, erythema and swelling of the hands and feet, inflammatory changes of the lips and oral cavity, and acute nonpurulent cervical adenopathy.[1] In up to 25% of patients, coronary artery aneurysms develop.[2] Limited information suggests that the relatively few infants who have KD in the first year of life also have a higher incidence of cardiac sequelae with associated morbidity than do older children.[3] The goal of this study of infants less than 12 months of age at onset of KD was to assess the frequency of CAA, with emphasis on identification of risk factors for the development of CAA and on assessment of the efficacy of intravenously administered γ-globulin in the prevention of CAA.

CAA	Coronary artery aneurysms
CSF	Cerebrospinal fluid
IVGG	Intravenously administered γ-globulin
KD	Kawasaki disease

Submitted for publication May 24, 1994; accepted Oct. 24, 1994.

Reprint requests: Elaine A. Rosenfeld, MD, Children's Memorial Hospital, Division of Infectious Diseases, 2300 Children's Plaza, Box No. 20, Chicago, IL 60614.

0022-3476/95/$3.00 + 0 **9/20/61437**

METHODS

We performed a retrospective chart review of patients less than 1 year of age at the onset of KD diagnosed at Children's Memorial Hospital (CMH), Chicago, from 1980 to 1993 inclusive. Demographic, clinical, laboratory, echocardiographic, therapeutic, and follow-up data were extracted from each medical record. Typical KD was diagnosed by the presence of fever for 5 or more days with at least four of five criteria,[1] or fever plus three major criteria if CAA were recognized by echocardiography.[4]

Fever was defined as ≥38.0° C measured rectally. Day of illness was counted from the onset of fever. The first posttreatment day was defined as the 24-hour period beginning with the initiation of aspirin therapy or aspirin-plus-IVGG therapy. By echocardiography, a coronary artery was defined as abnormal if the diameter of the internal lumen was at least 3 mm; if the internal diameter of a segment was at least one and one-half times that of an adjacent segment; or if the lumen was clearly irregular.[5] Patients whose echocardiogram showed an internal coronary diameter ≥8 mm were considered to have giant CAA.[6] Normal hemoglobin values were defined as >95 gm/L (9.5 gm/dl) for infants less than 6 months of age and >105 gm/L for those 6 to 12 months. Erythrocyte sedimentation rates were determined by the Wintrobe method; other laboratory tests were performed by standard methods in the clinical laboratory.

Categorical data were analyzed statistically by chi-square analysis with the Yates correction for small numbers. Continuous data were analyzed by Student *t* test. Significance was defined as the 5% confidence level; 95% confidence intervals for difference in proportions were calculated by the method of Fleiss.[7]

RESULTS

Fifty-seven patients less than 1 year of age at the onset of KD were identified by medical record search and review of records of the division of infectious diseases. Three patients were lost to follow-up shortly after their acute illness, and one medical record was unavailable; data from the remaining 53 patients were analyzed. The 57 patients represent 13% of the total number of 443 patients with KD who were cared for at CMH during this period. No patients with known cardiac complications were referred.

Demographic features and risk of having CAA. The median age of the patients was 7 months (range, 2.25 to 11.75 months). Fourteen patients (26%) were less than 6 months of age at onset of KD; 39 were 6 to 12 months of age. Age at onset of KD strongly predicted the development of CAA, particularly of giant CAA, as assessed by echocardiography (Table I). Overall, 28 (53%) of 53 infants <12 months of age had CAA, and 7 (13%) had giant CAA; smaller coronary artery abnormalities developed in about 40% of each age group.

Table I. Relation between age at onset of Kawasaki disease and development of coronary artery aneurysms, including giant coronary artery aneurysms

	Age at onset of KD	
	Age <6 mo (n = 14)	Age 6-12 mo (n = 39)
No CAA	3 (21%)*	22 (56%)*
CAA	11 (79%)	17 (44%)
Giant CAA	5 (37%)†	2 (5%)†
Nongiant CAA	6 (42%)	15 (39%)

*p = 0.06.
†p <0.01.

The male/female ratio of patients with KD was 1.8:1. Although more boys than girls had CAA, 4 of the 8 girls and 3 of the 20 boys with CAA had giant CAA (p = 0.06), the manifestation that accounts for the large majority of KD deaths. The racial distribution of patients with KD paralleled that of CMH patients. There were no significant racial differences in CAA rates. A significant seasonal pattern for either onset of illness or the development of CAA was not demonstrated. Economic status of patients as examined by mode of payment approximated that of patients at CMH during the study. The distribution of payment status of patients in whom CAA developed did not differ from that of the patients who did not have CAA.

Clinical features and risk of CAA. The criteria for diagnosis of KD fulfilled by patients are listed in Table II. Five patients were considered to have atypical or incomplete KD, as previously described.[4] Four of these were included because of the presence of signs of KD with the subsequent development of CAA; in three of the four, giant CAA developed. The single patient considered to have atypical KD without CAA had fever, bilateral conjunctival injection, and a polymorphous exanthem; severe peripheral extremity cyanosis with subsequent severe desquamation developed later.

The frequency of specific signs and symptoms of KD was similar among patients in whom CAA developed, the subset with giant CAA, and those without CAA. Conjunctival injection and acute mucosal changes were somewhat less common in those in whom giant CAA developed than in the other groups. Peripheral extremity desquamation was more common in those in whom CAA did not develop (data not shown).

Laboratory features and risk of CAA (Table III). There were no significant differences in mean initial leukocyte counts among those who had CAA, those who had giant

Table II. Criteria for diagnosis of Kawasaki disease

	Total	Nongiant CAA (n = 21)	Giant CAA (n = 7)
Patients with CAA (n = 28)			
Fever plus 5 criteria	9	7	2
Fever plus 4 criteria	9	9	0
Fever plus 3 criteria	6	4	2
Fever plus 2 criteria*	2	1	1
Fever plus 1 criterion*	2	0	2
Patients without CAA (n = 25)			
Fever plus 5 criteria	13	—	—
Fever plus 4 criteria	11	—	—
Fever plus 3 criteria*	1	—	—

*Incomplete, or atypical, Kawasaki disease.

CAA, and those without CAA. More than half (15/28) of the patients in whom CAA developed had an initial leukocyte count of less than 20×10^9/L (20,000/mm^3). However, the initial leukocyte count exceeded 20×10^9/L in a significantly greater percentage of those in whom giant CAA developed. No significant differences in mean initial platelet counts were found among those with nongiant CAA, those with giant CAA, and those in whom CAA did not develop. The initial platelet count was normal in a comparable percentage of those who had CAA and those who did not. On the other hand, the initial platelet count exceeded 700×10^9/L (700,000/mm^3) in a significantly greater percentage of patients in whom nongiant CAA developed than in those who had none. The mean day of illness on which the initial platelet value was measured did not differ between the children who eventually had CAA and those who did not. The median peak platelet counts were significantly higher in those who had giant CAA than in those who did not have CAA.

The median initial uncorrected erythrocyte sedimentation rate was elevated comparably in all three groups of patients. The mean initial hemoglobin concentrations were significantly lower in patients who later had CAA than in those who did not. Significantly more patients in whom giant CAA developed had an initial subnormal hemoglobin value than did those who never had CAA. The mean day of illness on which the initial hemoglobin concentration was measured did not differ between the children who were anemic and those who were not. Thus neither anemia nor thrombocytosis in those who subsequently had CAA was related to a later initial evaluation.

The number of leukocytes per high-power field of initial centrifuged urine specimens varied widely in all patient groups, and no significant differences in pyuria were demonstrated. Similarly, there were no significant differences in initial alanine aminotransferase levels; 19% of patients with CAA or giant CAA had initially elevated alanine aminotransferase levels. Nineteen infants underwent lumbar puncture as part of their initial evaluation for fever. Median cerebrospinal fluid leukocyte counts, protein concentrations, or glucose concentrations were not significantly different in those with and those without CAA.

Treatment and risk of CAA. Of 53 patients, 32 (60%) were treated with IVGG and aspirin, 10 receiving IVGG, 1.6 gm/kg in four doses, and 22 receiving IVGG, 2 gm/kg in a single infusion. In 24 (75%) of 32 patients, treatment with IVGG and aspirin was instituted by the tenth illness day. All 21 patients not treated with IVGG received high doses of aspirin (80 to 100 mg/kg per day) before 1986. The mean age at onset was 7.97 months in those who were treated with IVGG and 7.25 months in those who were not. One patient received a second four-dose course of IVGG because of persistent fever and recrudescence of symptoms. CAA developed in 16 (76%) of 21 patients who did not receive IVGG, in 5 (29%) of 17 treated with IVGG and aspirin by illness day 7 ($p < 0.025$), and in 7 (29%) of 24 treated by illness day 10 ($p < 0.01$). CAA developed in 21 (73%) of 29 patients treated after day 10 or never treated with IVGG ($p < 0.01$ compared with those treated by day 10). Thus the efficacy of IVGG and aspirin given by illness day 10 to prevent CAA in this population can be estimated to be 59% (95% confidence interval, 26% to 93%). Similarly, giant CAA developed in 1 (4%) of 24 patients treated with IVGG by illness day 10, and in 6 (21%) of 29 treated after day 10 (2/8) or never treated (4/21) with IVGG ($p = 0.10$). Thus the efficacy of IVGG by illness day 10 in preventing giant CAA was estimated to be 80%, but the confidence interval is very wide (95% confidence interval, 0% to 100%). No significant difference in rates of CAA and giant CAA incidence in patients treated by illness day 7 or on illness days 8, 9, or 10 was observed. At follow-up at least 1 year after the acute illness, 4 (17%) of 24 patients treated with IVGG by illness day 10 and 14 (48%) of 29 either not treated by illness day 10 or never treated with IVGG had persistent CAA ($p < 0.025$). Thus IVGG treatment by day 10 of illness resulted in an estimated 65% reduction in long-term CAA (95% confidence interval, 17% to 100%).

The duration of pretreatment fever did not differ significantly between those treated with aspirin alone and those treated with aspirin and IVGG (mean = 9.0 and 9.2 days, respectively) (Figure). Patients who subsequently had CAA after treatment with aspirin alone tended to have more prolonged fever after institution of treatment. In patients treated with aspirin and IVGG, the proportions of febrile patients on any given posttreatment day were comparable whether or not CAA developed.

The median age at diagnosis of KD of patients in whom persistent (>1 year) CAA developed was 6.25 months

Table III. Laboratory features and risk of CAA development in Kawasaki disease

	NO CAA (n = 25)	Nongiant CAA (n = 21)	Giant CAA (n = 7)
Peripheral leukocytes			
Initial, mean (mm^3)	17,200	20,100	23,100
Initial, range (mm^3)	9,700-29,400	9,100-42,800	16,200-32,000
Initial >20,000/mm^3	6/25 (24%)‡	8/21 (38%)	5/7 (71%)‡
Platelet count			
Initial 150,000-450,000/mm^3	4/25 (16%)	7/21 (33%)	2/7 (29%)
Initial >700,000/mm^3	2/25 (8%)†	9/21 (43%)†	3/7 (43%)
Peak count, mean (mm^3)	783,7838*/†	992,071*	1,082,000†
Peak count, range (mm^3)	448,000-1,103,000	478,000-1,425,000	338,000-1,480,000
ESR >20 mm/hr	23/25 (92%)	20/21 (95%)	7/7 (100%)
Hemoglobin level			
Subnormal§	11/25 (44%)‡	15/21 (71%)	7/7 (100%)‡
Initial, mean (gm/L), (gm/dl)	103* (10.3)	88* (8.8)	81* (8.1)
Initial, range (gm/L), (gm/dl)	86-120 (8.6-12.0)	66-109 (6.6-10.9)	65-91 (6.5-9.1)
CSF leukocytes			
Initial, median (mm^3)	24 (n = 4)	6 (n = 9)	3 (n = 6)
Initial, range (mm^3)	8-190	1-153	1-97
>20/mm^3	3/4 (75%)	2/9 (22%)	1/6 (17%)

ESR, Erythrocyte sedimentation rate.
*$p < 0.001$.
†$p < 0.01$.
‡$p < 0.025$.
§<9.5 gm/dl in patients less than 6 months of age; <10.5 gm/dl in patients 6 to 12 months of age.

compared with 9.0 months for those in whom CAA did not develop ($p < 0.01$). There were no significant differences in gender, race, socioeconomic status, clinical signs or symptoms, or laboratory values between those with and those without persistent CAA. The mean day of initial evaluation of patients who later had persistent CAA was the eleventh illness day, compared with day 8 in those who never had CAA ($p < 0.02$) and day 7 in those who had CAA that did not persist ($p < 0.10$). One patient required an internal mammary coronary bypass graft at 5 years of age for persistence of giant CAA with development of significant stenosis of the left anterior descending artery and resultant compromised ventricular function. Another 6½-month-old infant with giant CAA had left anterior wall myocardial infarcts related to a massive thrombus in the left anterior descending artery at 3 and 6 weeks after onset of KD, and also had intracerebral and subdural hemorrhages as a consequence of thrombolysis and anticoagulation. She has done well neurologically and has normal cardiac function 7 years later. Another infant with giant CAA had peripheral gangrene of several fingertips, and was described recently.[8]

DISCUSSION

This retrospective review of KD in infants less than 1 year of age extends information reported in non-age-restricted reports[9] and in the few articles limited to this particular age group.[3, 10, 11] We arbitrarily divided our patients into those <6 months and those >6 months of age to be consistant with previous reports.[3, 10, 11] We failed to identify risk factors that predicted development of CAA in this population. Young age at the onset of KD, however, predicted the development of CAA in that a significantly greater proportion of children less than 6 months of age eventually had CAA and giant CAA; the latter are most strongly associated with early and late morbidity and death. Nakamura et al.[12] reported that a higher proportion of Japanese patients less than 1 year of age had CAA and substantially greater long-term survival than those older than 1 year. Shulman et al.[13] described 36 patients with KD who were less than 1 year of age during the pre-IVGG era and found that CAA developed in 31% compared with 18% in those who were 1 to 2 years of age and 10% who were more than 2 years of age. Also in the pre-IVGG era, Burns et al.[3] reported that CAA developed in 6 of 8 patients with KD who were less than 6 months of age, and Takahashi et al.[14] reported a higher prevalence of CAA in children less than 1 year of age (39%) than in older children (13%).

The male/female ratio of our population and the higher CAA risk in boys with KD are both consistent with previous epidemiologic studies of KD[9] and result in a 2.5:1 ratio of boys to girls with KD-related CAA. In this series, however, girls had fewer CAA but often had more serious CAA. In infants, KD is frequently subtle in manifestations, with a paucity of classic signs and symptoms.[3, 11] Hsiao et al.[11]

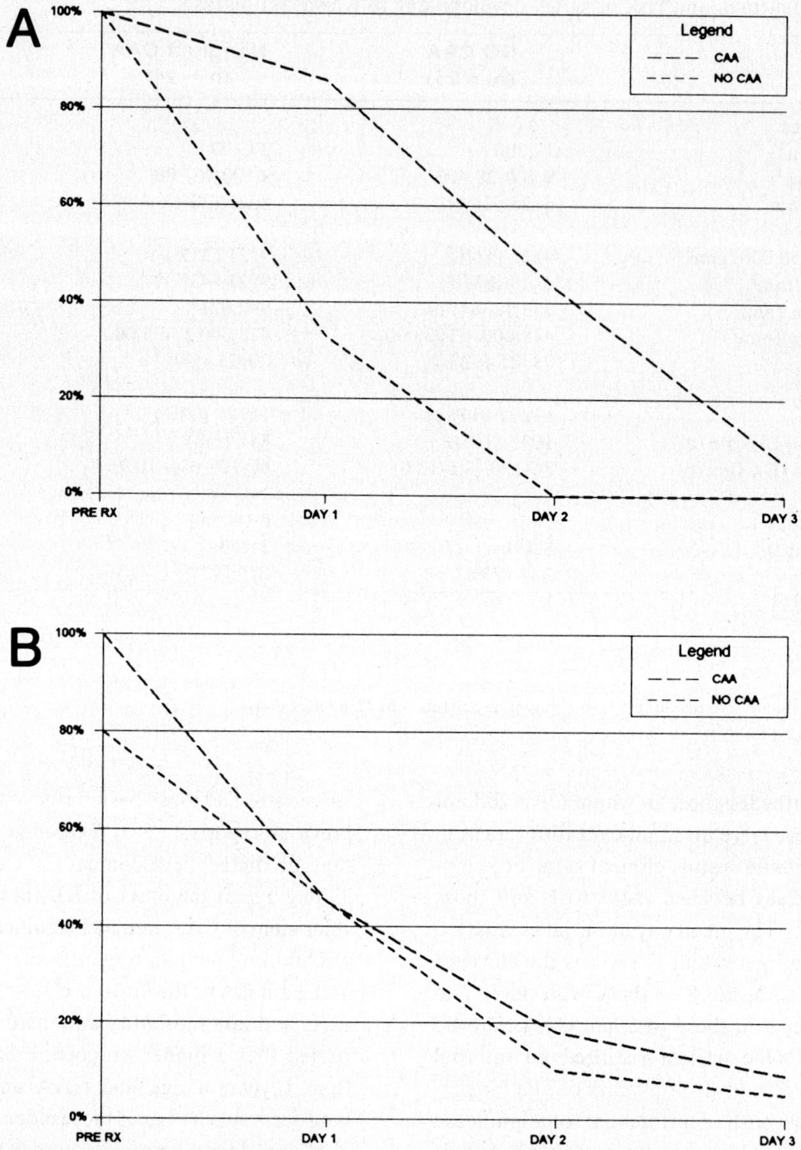

Figure. Persistence of fever after treatment with aspirin (**A**) or with aspirin and IVGG (**B**) for Kawasaki disease in patients in whom CAA did or did not later develop.

found a lower incidence of strawberry tongue and indurative edema of palms and soles in patients less than 6 months of age compared with older patients. Limbach and Lindinger[10] found that typical mucosal and lymph node changes were lacking in those less than 6 months of age. That 14% of our patients with CAA, including 43% who had giant CAA, did not fulfill classic criteria for KD emphasizes the need for a high degree of awareness of KD in the evaluation of febrile young children.

As in earlier studies, laboratory findings in our patients were nonspecific and nondiagnostic, and generally did not predict CAA development. Mild to moderate anemia without hemolysis occurred more often in those who had CAA than in those who did not, was present in all seven patients who had giant CAA, and appeared to be unrelated to duration of illness. Moderate to marked leukocytosis was particularly frequent in our patients in whom giant CAA developed. However, lack of leukocytosis did not predict an uncomplicated course of illness. Although a similar proportion of patients who later did or did not have CAA had initially normal platelet counts, an initial platelet count $>700 \times 10^9/L$ predicted the development of CAA.

We found no difference in the frequency of sterile pyuria[3, 10] in those who did and those who did not have CAA. Similarly, we did not demonstrate a predictive value of CSF pleocytosis for development of CAA. Previous reports noted CSF pleocytosis in three of seven patients less than 6 months of age (CAA developed in all three),[3] and in two of three patients less than 6 months of age.[10] Although no single clinical or laboratory finding confirms the diagnosis of KD or predicts the development of CAA, clinicians should consider KD in febrile infants who lack a source of infection and who manifest laboratory findings that support the diagnosis of KD. These include normocytic anemia, leukocytosis or thrombocytosis or both, highly elevated erythrocyte sedimentation rate, CSF pleocytosis, and sterile pyuria.

The benefit of IVGG in the treatment of KD is well documented in those more than 1 year of age,[5, 12, 15] but its efficacy in young infants has been less well studied. Newberger et al.[15] reported CAA at 7 weeks after the onset of KD in a substantially higher proportion of those less than 1 year of age who were treated with aspirin alone than in those treated with IVGG plus aspirin.[15] In a large Japanese epidemiologic study, Nakamura et al.[12] reported little difference in the prevalence of CAA among IVGG-treated patients and those given aspirin, including those less than 1 year of age. They hypothesized that this finding showed that more seriously ill patients were more likely to be treated with IVGG, often late in the course of their disease. In our retrospective study the frequency of CAA was lower in patients treated with IVGG plus aspirin by the tenth day of illness. We also observed a reduction in CAA that persisted at least 1 year in our IVGG-treated group. Takahashi et al.[14] reported more frequent and more rapid resolution of CAA in non-IVGG-treated patients less than 1 year of age than in older patients.

No fatalities occurred in our patients during either acute KD or long-term follow-up of up to 15 years. Although early studies indicated a mortality rate of about 2%, more recent data suggest a rate of about 0.08%, primarily because of acute myocarditis or late ischemic events.[2] Burns et al.[3] reported, in two of eight patients less than 6 months of age, fatalities related to ischemic cardiomyopathy and irreversible cardiogenic shock. Both our patient with two infarctions and the one who required coronary artery bypass surgery had giant CAA; neither had received IVGG by the tenth day of illness. The long-term consequences of KD were emphasized by the report of Kato et al.[16] on 21 adult Japanese survivors of apparent childhood KD who acquired serious ischemic heart disease, including myocardial infarction, angina pectoris, and dilated cardiomyopathy; three died.

Our findings indicate that infants who have KD in the first year of life, and particularly in the first 6 months, have more frequent cardiac sequelae and greater morbidity than older children.[12-14] The diagnosis of KD in these infants is often difficult because they do not have classic signs and symptoms, and individual manifestations may be subtle. Physicians evaluating fever in infants should maintain the proverbial "high index of suspicion" for the possible diagnosis of KD. Timely diagnosis and institution of treatment with IVGG and aspirin is required to minimize cardiac sequelae and long-term morbidity.

REFERENCES

1. Centers for Disease Control. Kawasaki disease—New York. MMWR 1980;29:61-3.
2. Rowley AH, Gonzalez-Crussi F, Shulman ST. Kawasaki syndrome. Curr Probl Pediatr 1991;21:387-405.
3. Burns JC, Wiggens JW, Toews WH, et al. Clinical spectrum of Kawasaki disease in infants younger than 6 months of age. J PEDIATR 1986;109:759-63.
4. Rowley AH, Shulman ST. The recognition of atypical Kawasaki disease. Report on Pediatric Infectious Diseases 1993; 3:1-2.
5. Newberger JW, Takahashi M, Beiser AS, et al. A single intravenous infusion of gamma globulin as compared with four infusions in the treatment of acute Kawasaki syndrome. N Engl J Med 1991;324:1633-9.
6. Nakano H, Ueda K, Saito A, et al. Repeated quantitative angiograms in coronary artery aneurysm in Kawasaki disease. Am J Cardiol 1985;56:846-51.
7. Fleiss JL. Statistical method for rates and proportions. 2nd ed. New York: Wiley & Sons, 1981:29-30, 64-75.
8. Tomita S, Chung K, Mas M, Gidding S, Shulman ST. Peripheral gangrene associated with Kawasaki disease. Clin Infect Dis 1992;14:121-6.
9. Mason WH, Schneider T, Takahashi M. The epidemiology and etiology of Kawasaki disease. Cardiology in the Young 1991;1:196-205.
10. Limbach HG, Lindinger A. Das Kawasaki-Syndrom bei Sauglingen im ersten Lebanshalbjahr. Klin Padiatr 1991; 203:133-6.
11. Hsiao JY, Chen MR, Huang FU, Kao HA, Sung TC. Clinical analysis of Kawasaki disease in infants below 6 months of age. Acta Paediatr Sin 1998;29:318-23.
12. Nakamura Y, Fujita Y, Nagai M, et al. Cardiac sequelae of Kawasaki disease in Japan: statistical analysis. Pediatrics 1991; 88:1144-7.
13. Shulman ST, McAuley JB, Pachman LM, Miller ML, Ruschhaupt DG. Risk of coronary abnormalities due to Kawasaki disease in urban area with small Asian population. Am J Dis Child 1987;141:420-5.
14. Takahashi M, Mason W, Lewis AB. Regression of coronary aneurysms in patients with Kawasaki syndrome. Circulation 1987;75:387-94.
15. Newberger JW, Takahashi M, Burns JC, et al. The treatment of Kawasaki syndrome with intravenous gamma globulin. N Engl J Med 1986;315:341-7.
16. Kato H, Inoue O, Kawasaki T, et al. Adult coronary artery disease probably due to childhood Kawasaki disease. Lancet 1992;340:1127-8.

Cell-mediated immune status of children with recurrent infection

Henry G. Herrod, MD, Michael S. Blaiss, MD, William R. Valenski, BS, and Sharon Gross, BS

From the Crippled Children's Foundation Research Center at Le Bonheur Children's Medical Center and Department of Pediatrics, University of Tennessee, Memphis

Objective: **To evaluate the cell-mediated immune status of children with recurrent respiratory tract infections.**
Design: **We evaluated the cell-mediated immune status of 76 patients referred because of recurrent infection. Patients were divided into those with serologic abnormalities and those without such findings. Twenty-three healthy children served as control subjects. Studies of lymphocyte phenotype included $CD4^+$ $CD29^+$ cells (an immunologically mature phenotype), lymphocyte proliferation studies, cytokine production including interleukin-2 (IL-2), IL-4, IL-6, and interferon γ), and measurement of in vitro IgM and IgG synthesis.**
Results: **Lymphocyte proliferation and T-cell phenotype were similar in both patient groups as well as in control subjects. The proportions of $CD4^+$ $CD29^+$ cells at different ages were similar in all groups. Patients with serologic abnormalities (e.g., partial IgA deficiency, partial IgG subclass deficiency) produced more IL-2 and IL-4 than did other patients. The control population had greater spontaneous IgM and IgG synthesis than the patient groups.**
Conclusion: **Routine studies of T-cell function of patients with recurrent infection provide little information useful in making clinical decisions. (J PEDIATR 1995;126: 530-6)**

Recurrent infections are common among children. The development of new diagnostic tests in recent years has raised the issue of which studies are indicated for evaluating this patient population. Evaluation of immune function in these children has focused on the humoral immune system because the clinical features (e.g., sinusitis, otitis media) found in most of these patients are consistent with bacterial infections. A relatively high proportion of children with recurrent infection have one or more serologic abnormalities.[1-5] The most frequent of these abnormalities are partial deficiency of IgA or partial deficiency in one or more of the IgG subclasses.

As more is learned about the interactions among T cells, T-cell products, and B cells, the issue of whether an abnormality in T-cell subtypes or cytokine production contributes to the pathogenesis of recurrent infections in children becomes more significant. We hypothesized that children with recurrent infection would likely have mild abnormalities in T-cell immunity. Specifically, we were interested in the proportion of $CD29^+$ $CD4^+$ cells in patients with recurrent infections. This phenotype represents a more mature immunologic phenotype of helper T cells.[6-9] We expected to find a reduction in the $CD29^+$ $CD4^+$ cell subpopulation relative to age-matched control subjects and that this reduction would be most evident in older children (>60 months) with recurrent infection. We further sought to determine whether there were differences in production of selective cytokines known to influence B-cell differentiation or in T-cell dependent in vitro immunoglobulin synthesis.

IFN	Interferon
IL	Interleukin

Submitted for publication June 28, 1994; accepted Oct. 4, 1994.
Reprint requests: Henry G. Herrod, MD, University of Tennessee, Memphis, Crippled Children's Foundation Research Center, 50 N. Dunlap—Rm. 301, Memphis, TN 38163.

0022-3476/95/$3.00 + 0 **9/20/61030**

METHODS

Study subjects. The study population consisted of 76 patients referred to the immunology clinic at Le Bonheur Children's Medical Center with a history of recurrent infection. No patient with a recognized immunodeficiency was included in the study. All patients had been treated by their primary care physicians and more than 80% had been evaluated by an allergist, otolaryngologist, or both. Infections typically involved the upper respiratory tract; symptoms of sinusitis and otitis media were most common. Some of the patients had chronic sinus symptoms, but none was acutely infected at the time of evaluation. The patient population was divided into two groups: 37 patients (mean age, 54.6 ± 29.4 months) had recurrent infections and serologic abnormalities, and 39 patients (mean age, 55.6 ± 26.9 months) had recurrent infections but no serologic abnormalities. The serologic abnormalities included partial deficiency in a major immunoglobulin isotype, partial deficiency in an IgG subclass, or various combinations of these deficiencies. Partial deficiency in major immunoglobulin isotypes and in IgG subclasses was defined as a value more than 2 SD below the geometric mean for age. We evaluated antibody production in some children older than 2 years of age after vaccination with polyvalent pneumococcal vaccine (Pneumovax).

Control subjects consisted of 23 well children ranging in age from 1 year to 18 years (mean, 67.2 ± 33.7 months). Twenty of these subjects were the children of hospital employees and three were children who were scheduled to have elective surgery. Previous studies from this laboratory and others have shown little difference in the proportion of cells bearing CD3, CD4, or CD8 phenotype or in mitogen responses in children older than 1 year of age.[10-12] For purposes of phenotypic analysis, patients and control subjects of different ages were pooled except when there were obvious age-related changes (e.g., $CD45RA^+$, $CD29^+$, $CD4^+$, $CD20^+$ cells). All studies were approved by the institutional review board of the University of Tennessee, and verbal consent to participate was obtained from the patients' parents.

Serologic studies. Quantitative immunoglobulin determinations were performed by the hospital laboratory with nephelometry; normal age-appropriate values were obtained from a local control population of more than 200 children. The IgG subclasses and pneumococcal polysaccharide studies were performed at Specialty Laboratories, (Santa Monica, Calif.) and the results were compared with that laboratory's normal values;[4] postvaccination titers of >200 ng antibody per milliliter are considered "protective."

Lymphocyte phenotype and culture studies. Lymphocyte phenotype was determined with an EPICS Profile II flow cytometer (Coulter Corp., Hialeah, Fla.) and direct conjugate two-color labeled monoclonal antibodies. The expression of the following antigens was evaluated: CD3 (T cells), CD4 (T helper cells), CD8 (cytotoxic T cells), CD20 (B cells), CD29, and CD45RA. The CD45 phenotype is a family of cell surface molecules found on nucleated hematopoietic cells.[13] Different isoforms are expressed at different times on T cells; those T cells bearing CD45RA are considered to be more immunologically naive. The CD29 molecule (β_1 integrin) is expressed on more immunologically mature $CD4^+$ cells.[14] All of these had phenotypic findings similar to those observed on initial testing. For lymphocyte transformation responses, peripheral blood mononuclear cells obtained after Ficoll-Hypaque centrifugation were cultured in the presence or absence of varying doses of phytohemagglutinin, concanavalin A, and pokeweed mitogen. The cells were pulsed with tritiated thymidine 18 hours before harvesting. In vitro cytokine production was evaluated after 72 hours of culture in either medium alone or in medium with the addition of phytohemagglutinin and phorbol myristate acetate. Supernatants from cultures were tested for individual cytokine production with the following commercially available kits: interferon γ (Genzyme Corp.), IL-2, IL-4, and IL-6 (R & D Laboratories). No manipulation of the supernatants was performed before testing.

In vitro immunoglobulin studies. The peripheral blood mononuclear cells were cultured in vitro at a concentration of 10^5 cells/ml in medium with or without pokeweed mitogen. Cultured supernatants were harvested after 7 days, and IgG and IgM concentrations were determined with an enzyme-linked immunosorbent assay as previously described.[15]

Data analysis. When appropriate, data were log-transformed before analysis. Data also were examined with nonparametric analysis including the Mann-Whitney test. Differences between the groups were considered significant when a corrected Bonferroni-Dunn test revealed a value of $p < 0.0167$.

RESULTS

Serologic studies. Of 76 patients, 37 (48%) had a partial deficiency of one or more immunoglobulin isotypes. None of the patients was totally deficient in any isotype or IgG subclass. The most common abnormality was an isolated partial IgA deficiency (18% of total cases). An isolated partial IgG subclass deficiency was found in 10% of patients; half of these had IgG2 deficiencies, and an additional 8% of patients had a combination of IgG subclass deficiencies.

Response to polysaccharide antigen. Prevaccination antibody concentrations to four pneumococcal polysaccharide serotypes (3, 7, 9, and 14) were measured in 19 of the con-

Table I. Pneumococcal polysaccharide antibody concentration

	Serotype			
	3	7	9	14
Prevaccination				
Control subjects	376 ± 161	79 ± 22	89 ± 28	162 ± 529
Recurrent infections, no serologic abnormality	440 ± 227	68 ± 42	76 ± 40	101 ± 34
Recurrent infections with serologic abnormality	134 ± 118	43 ± 9	62 ± 15	78 ± 15*
Postvaccination				
Control subjects	ND	ND	ND	ND
Recurrent infections, no serologic abnormality	1912 ± 144	171 ± 268	484 ± 243	217 ± 246
Recurrent infections with serologic abnormality	1198 ± 142	180 ± 83	221 ± 57	107 ± 22†

ND, Not done.
Data presented as the mean (±SE) concentration (in nanograms) of antibody per milliliter.
*p <0.0167 versus control group.
†p <0.0167 versus group with no serologic abnormalities.

trol patients and 33 patients older than 2 years of age (Table I). None of the differences in mean antibody titer was statistically significant except for a lower prevaccination antibody concentration to serotype 14 in patients with serologic abnormalities. Twenty-six of the patients were immunized with pneumococcal polysaccharide vaccine. The response to serotype 3 produced antibody concentrations >200 ng antibody per milliliter in all but two of the immunized patients; 75% of immunized patients had postimmunization titers of less than 200 ng antibody per milliliter to serotype 14. Patients with serologic abnormalities had a poorer response to serotype 14 than did those without serologic abnormalities. Two of the patients with normal responses to all four serotypes had a partial deficiency of an immunoglobulin isotype. Control subjects were not immunized.

Lymphocyte phenotype and mitogen responses. Table II compares the lymphocyte phenotypes found in the control population and the patients with recurrent infection. The only difference among these groups was the slightly increased proportion of $CD8^+$ cells in patients with recurrent infections with serologic abnormalities. No differences between control subjects and patients were seen in any age group for CD20 and CD45RA. There were no significant differences among the three study groups for the $CD29^+$ $CD4^+$ phenotype (Fig. 1). Responses to the mitogens phytohemagglutinin, concanavalin A, and pokeweed mitogen were similar in each study group and in control subjects (Fig. 2).

Table II. Comparison of proportion of lymphocyte phenotypes

	Group		
	Control subjects	Recurrent infection, no abnormalities	Recurrent infection with serologic abnormalities
Phenotype			
CD3	72 ± 7.4	70.5 ± 8.6	69.0 ± 8.8
CD4	45.8 ± 6.9	44.1 ± 8.3	42.8 ± 9.0
CD8	21.3 ± 9.0	23.3 ± 6.2	24.9 ± 6.2*

Data presented as the mean (±SD) percent expression of the phenotype.
*p <0.0167 compared with control subjects.

Cytokine production. In vitro cytokine production was measured in 21 patients and 14 control subjects older than 24 months of age. Fourteen subjects who had evaluations for cytokines in both the patient and control populations were older than 60 months of age. There were no significant differences in cytokine production on the basis of age; therefore data from each age group were pooled before comparison with other groups. The only difference among groups was greater spontaneous synthesis of both IL-2 and IL-4 by cells from patients with recurrent infection who had demonstrable serotype abnormalities and greater spontaneous IL-4 production by the cells of patients with no serologic abnormalities compared with values for control subjects (Fig. 3).

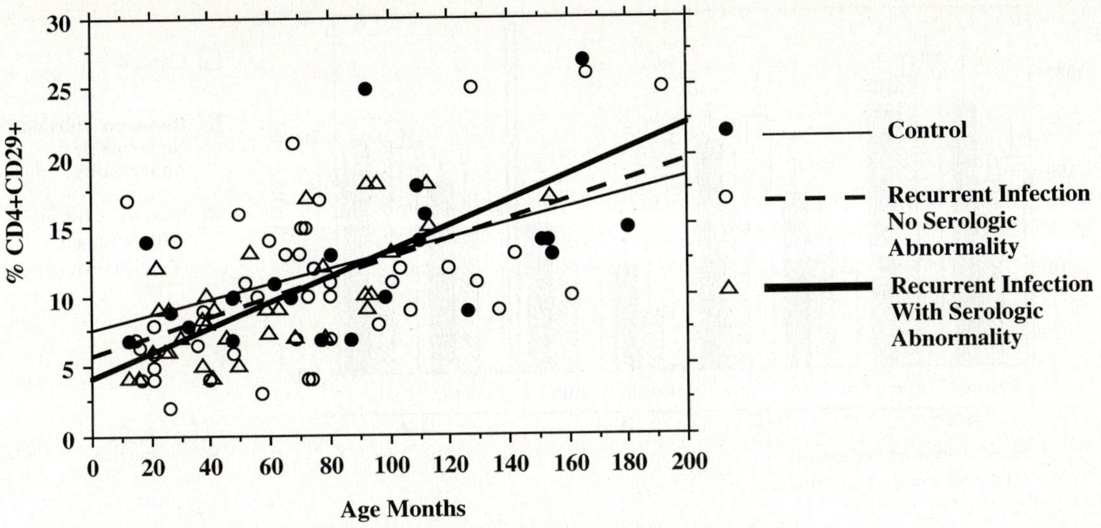

Fig. 1. Comparison of CD29$^+$ CD4$^+$ expression in subjects in the three study groups. There was no significant difference among the three groups at any age point.

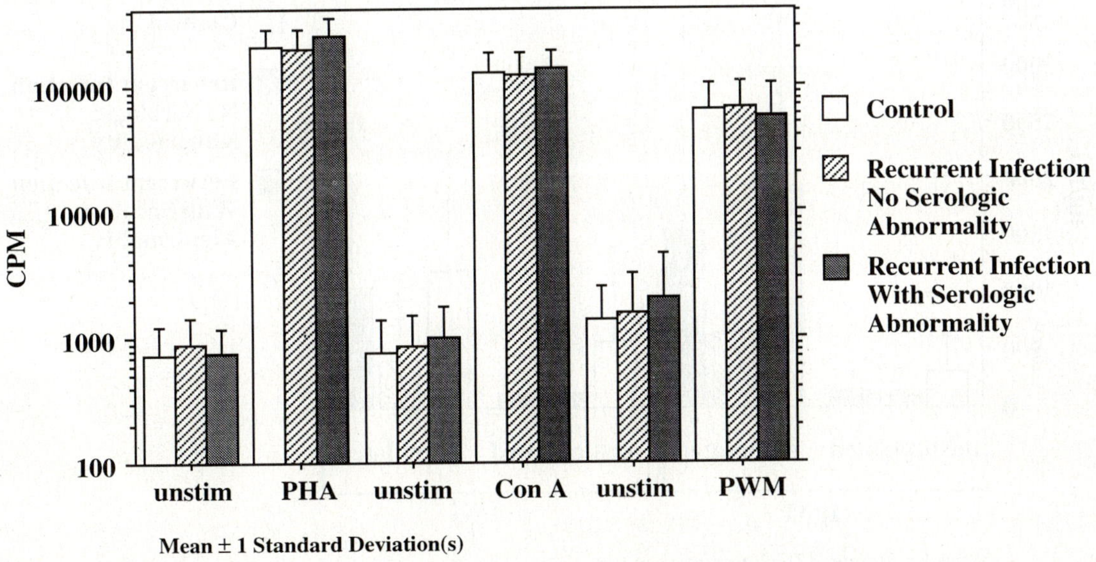

Fig. 2. Lymphocyte response to mitogen stimulation. No differences among the three study groups were noted. *PHA*, Phytohemagglutinin; *unstim*, Unstimulated; *Con A*, concanavalin A, *PWM*, pokeweed mitogen.

In vitro IgM and IgG production. There was no difference between in vitro immunoglobulin synthesis for control subjects older than 60 months of age and those less than 60 months. Therefore data from all ages were pooled for each study group. Unstimulated IgM and IgG concentrations were greater in normal subjects than in either patient group (data not shown). The IgM synthesis was greater in normal subjects after pokeweed mitogen stimulation compared with values in patients with recurrent infection without serologic abnormalities (Fig. 4). The IgG synthesis after stimulation was lower in patients without serologic abnormalities than in control subjects or in patients with serologic abnormalities.

DISCUSSION

Patients seen in a primary care setting for recurrent infection are unlikely to have any immunologic abnormalities. However, among those whose clinical problems are signif-

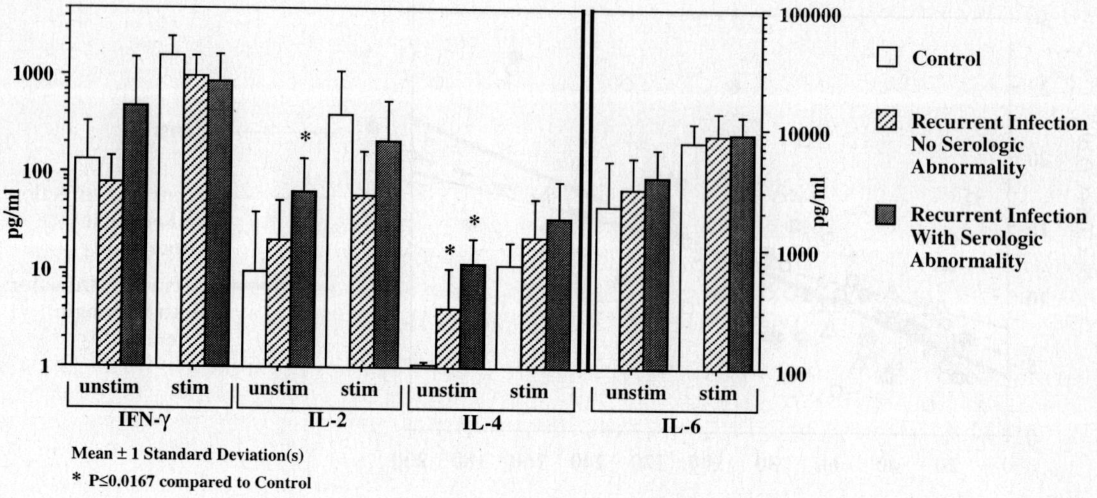

Fig. 3. Cytokine production in the three study groups.

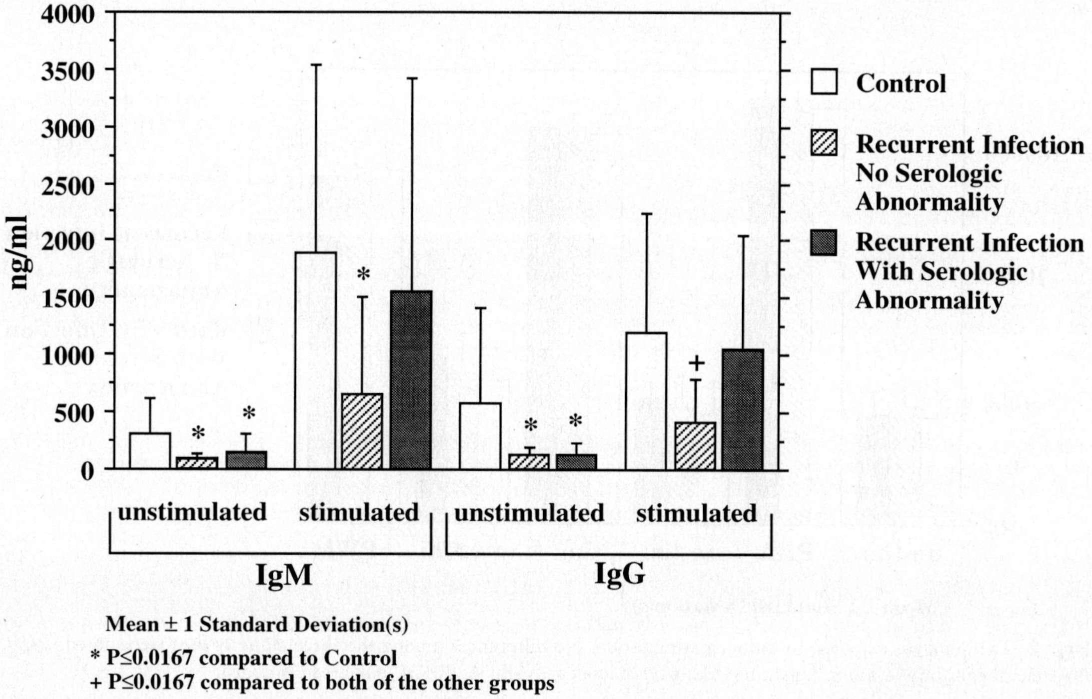

Fig. 4. In vitro IgM and IgG synthesis after stimulation with pokeweed mitogen. Spontaneous IgM and IgG production were both greater in control subjects than in either patient group ($p < 0.02$). Stimulation of IgM was greater in control subjects than in patients with no serologic abnormalities ($p < 0.02$). Stimulated IgG production by both control subjects and patients with serologic abnormalities was greater than IgG production by cells from patients with no abnormalities ($p < 0.02$).

icant enough to warrant referral for immunologic evaluation, there is a relatively high proportion of serologic abnormalities. Previous data from our center indicated that the most common serologic abnormality was a partial IgA deficiency, which was present in one third of patients.[4] Other recent studies have demonstrated that IgG subclass deficiency is also a common finding.[1, 3, 5] Almost 50% of the patients in the present study had humoral abnormalities; partial IgA and IgG subclass deficiencies were most commonly observed. A high proportion of our unvaccinated normal subjects, as well as those with recurrent infections, had low antibody concentrations to pneumococcal polysaccharides. This is in contrast to previously reported findings that most children at least 2 years of age have readily detectable antibody to most pneumococcal serotypes.[16, 17]

We hypothesized that children with recurrent infections probably had a subtle delay in "immunologic development" that might be reflected in T-cell phenotype or cytokine production. The $CD29^+$ $CD4^+$ phenotype represents a more immunologically mature cell, and we expected to find a decrease in this population of cells in children with recurrent infection. However, there was little difference in lymphocyte phenotype or lymphocyte proliferation between control subjects and patients.

There was relatively greater spontaneous production of IL-2 and IL-4 by patients who had serologic abnormalities. The basis for this is unclear, but it may be a reflection of a greater infection load in such patients, resulting in greater T-cell stimulation. Because IL-2 is produced by T helper 1 cells and IL-4 is produced by T helper 2 cells, it appears that both subpopulations might be affected.[18] Alternatively, the T helper 0 cell, which produces both IL-2 and IL-4, could be responsible for this observation. Interferon-γ, which also is produced by the T helper 1 cell subpopulation, was not different among the groups, suggesting that there may be a relatively unique trigger or response to selective stimuli that results in IL-2 and perhaps IL-4 production, but not interferon-γ production. The in vitro immunoglobulin studies were of interest in that normal subjects had higher spontaneous IgM and IgG synthesis than in either patient group. Patients without serologic abnormalities produced lower concentrations of both immunogloblins after stimulation than did the control group or the other patient group. Additional studies would be necessary to determine the basis of this decreased production of immunoglobulin in patients with recurrent infections but without serologic abnormalities.

In the past the array of tests of cell-mediated immunity were unavailable to the clinician. There was greater reliance on screening for T-cell immunity by use of delayed hypersensitivity skin tests. A positive test result indicates the following: (1) that antigen is recognized, (2) that cytokines (including chemoattractants) are released, (3) that inflammatory cells can migrate, and (4) that the inflammatory response is intact. Such tests largely measure the T-helper-1 cell response. These tests are probably not used as often in the ambulatory setting as might be indicated because of the requirement for patients to return at 48 hours for interpretation of the skin test and the relatively high proportion of poor responders even among normal young children. We believe that a multitest-type device for cell-mediated immunity is a useful screening test and should be performed, when indicated, by the primary care provider. A positive test result indicates that further evaluation of cell-mediated immunity is generally not indicated. A history compatible with T-cell dysfunction and a negative result from a battery of delayed-type hypersensitivity skin tests are indications to perform more extensive in vitro tests of T-cell function.

Overall the results of this study demonstrate that routine studies of cell-mediated immunity are of little benefit in patients with recurrent upper airway tract infections. The potential importance of enhanced IL-2 and IL-4 spontaneous production needs further evaluation.

REFERENCES

1. Shackelford PG, Polmar SH, Mayus JL, Johnson WL, Corry JM, Nahm MH. Spectrum of IgG2 subclass deficiency in children with recurrent infections: prospective study. J PEDIATR 1986;108:647-53.
2. Shapiro GG, Virant FS, Furukawa CT, Pierson WE, Bierman CW. Immunologic defects in patients with refractory sinusitis. Pediatrics 1991;87:311-6.
3. Moss RB, Carmack MA, Esrig S. Deficiency of IgG4 in children: association of isolated IgG4 deficiency with recurrent respiratory tract infection. J PEDIATR 1992;120:16-21.
4. Gross S, Blaiss M, Herrod HG. Role of immunoglobulin subclasses and specific antibody determination in the evaluation of recurrent infection in children. J PEDIATR 1992;121: 516-22.
5. Gandhi A, Brodsky L, Ballow M. Benefits of antibiotic prophylaxis in children with chronic sinusitis: assessment of outcome predictors. Allergy Proc 1993;14:37-43.
6. Morimoto C, Letvin NL, Boyd AW, et al. The isolation and characterization of the human helper inducer T cell subset. J Immunol 1985;134:3762-9.
7. Sanders ME, Makgoba MW, Sharroo SO, et al. Human memory T lymphocytes express increased levels of three cell adhesion molecules (LFA-3, CD2, and LFA-1) and three other molecules (UCHL-1, CDw29, and Pgp-1) and have enhanced IFN-γ production. J Immunol 1988;140:1401-7.
8. Akbar AN, Terry L, Tinin A, Beverly PCL, Janosy G. Loss of CD45R and gain of UCHL-1 reactivity is a feature of primed T cells. J Immunol 1988;140:2171-8.
9. Hirohata S, Lipsky PE. T cell regulation of human B cell proliferation and differentiation. Regulatory influences of CD45R+ and CD45R- T4 cell subsets. J Immunol 1989; 142: 2597-2607.
10. Herrod HG, Cooke RJ, Valenski WR, Hermann J, Dockter ME. Evaluation of lymphocyte phenotype and phytohemagglutinin response in healthy very low birthweight infants. Clin Immunol Immunopathol 1991;60:268-77.
11. Denny T, Yoger R, Gelman R. Lymphocyte subsets in healthy children during the first five years of life. JAMA 1992; 267:1484-8.

12. Hannet I, Erkelter-Yuksel F, Lydyard P, Deneys V, De Buujere M. Developmental and maturational changes in human blood lymphocyte subpopulations. Immunol Today 1992;13:215-8.
13. Koretzky GA. Role of the CD45 tyrosine phosphatase in signal transduction in the immune system. FASEB J 1993;7:420-6.
14. Pilarski LM, Yacyshun BR, Jensen GS, Pruski E, Pabst HF. Beta 1 integrin (CD29) expression on human post natal T cell subsets defined by selective CD45 isoform expression. J Immunol 1991;147:830-7.
15. Wyatt RJ, Valenski WR, Stapleton FB, et al. Immunoregulatory studies in patients with IgA nephropathy. J Clin Lab Immunol 1988;25:109-14.
16. Lawrence EM, Edwards KM, Schiffman G, Thompson JM, Vaughn WK, Wright PF. Pneumococcal vaccine in normal children. Am J Dis Child 1983;137:846-50.
17. Douglas RM, Paton JC, Duncan SJ, Hansman DJ. Antibody response to pneumococcal vaccination in children younger than 5 years of age. J Infect Dis 1983;148:131-7.
18. Salgam P, Abrams JS, Clayberger C, et al. Differing lymphokine profiles of functional subsets of CD4 and CD8 T-cell clones. Sciences 1991;254:279-82.

Supplementary sensorimotor area seizures in children and adolescents

Nancy Bass, MD, Elaine Wyllie, MD, Youssef Comair, MD, Prakash Kotagal, MD, Paul Ruggieri, MD, and Hans Holthausen, MD[a]

From the Departments of Neurology, Neurosurgery, and Radiology, Cleveland Clinic Foundation, Cleveland, Ohio.

Rationale: Some types of seizures in children may be difficult to recognize; the diagnosis of seizures arising near the mesial posterior frontal supplementary sensorimotor area (SSMA) may be especially challenging. Such seizures have been well described in adults, but few pediatric cases have been reported even though onset is typically in childhood.
Methods: We studied 11 children and adolescents with SSMA seizures diagnosed by prolonged video electroencephalography (EEG).
Results: Mean age at onset was 5.8 years, and diagnosis by video EEG was made at a mean age of 12 years. Children had at least borderline intelligence and few abnormal findings on neurologic examination. Seizures were typically brief, frequent, and predominantly nocturnal, with bilateral tonic posturing, gross proximal limb movements, and preserved consciousness. Magnetic resonance imaging showed normal findings or a superior or mesial posterior frontal tumor or cortical dysplasia. Routine EEG findings were usually normal, but prolonged EEG showed epileptiform discharges over the vertex. Seizure onset in the region of the SSMA was confirmed by subdural EEG in six patients who were studied for epilepsy surgery. Five patients had seizure-free outcome or worthwhile improvement after operation. Two nonoperated patients are seizure-free on antiepileptic medication, and three are undergoing surgical evaluation.
Conclusions: Diagnosis of SSMA seizures in children may be challenging because of unusual symptoms (bilateral tonic limb involvement with preserved consciousness) and frequently normal routine EEG findings. Video EEG may be necessary for diagnosis, and magnetic resonance imaging may reveal a focal lesion. Increased recognition of this seizure type in pediatric patients should lead to earlier diagnosis for optimal medical or surgical treatment. (J PEDIATR 1995;126:537-44)

Some seizure types in children may be difficult to recognize, especially if the routine electroencephalogram is normal, leading to confusion with nonepileptic events such as episodes of parasomnia or behavioral aberration. One particularly challenging diagnosis involves seizures arising near the supplementary sensorimotor area of the brain. The SSMA is located in the mesial posterior frontal region of each hemisphere.[1-10] Motor representation within the SSMA in each hemisphere is bilateral, with complex afferent and efferent connections with the striatum, cerebellum, and spinal cord.[11] The SSMA appears to be involved in the

EEG	Electroencephalography
FDG	Fluorodeoxyglucose
MRI	Magnetic reonance imaging
PET	Positron emission tomography
SSMA	Supplementary sensorimotor area

Submitted for publication Aug. 23, 1994; accepted Oct. 13, 1994.
Reprint requests: Elaine Wyllie, MD, Head, Pediatric Epilepsy Program, Cleveland Clinic Foundation, Desk S51, 9500 Euclid Ave., Cleveland, OH 44195-5221.

[a]Now with the Bethel Epilepsy Center, Bielefeld, Germany.

0022-3476/95/$3.00 + 0 **9/20/61269**

Table. Patient characteristics, neuroimaging, and EEG findings

Patient No.	Age at seizure onset	Age at video EEG evaluation	Intellect	Neurology examination	Seizures per day: average/maximal
1	3 yr	16 yr	Normal	Normal	2/80
2	8 yr	13 yr	FSIQ 89	Normal	4/15
3	7 yr	17 yr	FSIQ 105	Normal	1/3
4	9 yr	13 yr	Normal	Normal	4/10
5	4 yr	6 yr	Normal	Decreased fine motor RUE	3/35
6	7 yr	19 yr	FSIQ 74	Normal	5/30
7	1 yr	7 yr	Normal	Normal	3/35
8	9 mo	1 yr 2 mo	Normal	Normal	8/30
9	13 yr	16 yr	Mild difficulties: Coffin-Lowry syndrome	Normal	1/5
10	6 yr	6 yr	Normal	Normal	5/20
11	5 yr	18 yr	Mild LD	Decreased fine motor RUE	0-1/1

RUE, right upper extremity; *FSIQ*, Full Scale Intelligence Quotient; *LD*, learning disability; *ND*, not done.
*Ictal single photon emission computed tomography showed hyperperfusion in the left frontal lobe.

coordination, initiation, and integration of sequential movements.[11] Movements elicited from electrical stimulation of this area are tonic, gross, and proximal.[1, 11]

The SSMA may be the main region activated during seizures in patients with an epileptogenic zone in the posterior mesial or superior frontal area of one hemisphere. The clinical features of SSMA seizures have been characterized in older patients. In adults the events are typically frequent, brief, and predominantly nocturnal with bilateral tonic posturing of the extremities, gross proximal limb movements, and preserved awareness.[12-15] However, recognition of these seizures may be delayed because of the unusual behavior during events, almost exclusive nocturnal expression, and normal routine EEG.[13] Although SSMA seizures typically begin in childhood,[13] referral to an epilepsy center most often occurs during adulthood.

Previous reports of SSMA seizures have drawn predominantly on the adult experience. Data regarding children have been largely historical. In an effort to achieve better characterization of SSMA seizures during childhood or adolescence, we examined pediatric patients studied with video EEG.

METHODS

Eleven children and adolescents with SSMA seizures diagnosed by video EEG at the Cleveland Clinic Foundation between 1990 and 1994 were identified retrospectively from medical records. Each child was under the care of a pediatric epileptologist at the Foundation.

Video EEG. Continuous video EEG recording for 3 to 7 (mean 5.3) days was performed after decrease or discontinuation of antiepileptic drugs. Prolonged interictal EEG samples were reviewed by an electroencephalographer for slowing and epileptiform discharges, videotapes of all recorded seizures were studied for clinical symptoms, and EEGs during seizures were analyzed for location of onset.

Magnetic resonance imaging. All patients had magnetic resonance imaging with a 1.5-tesla superconducting system with a circularly polarized head coil. Sequences included a sagittal T1-weighted scout image, an axial double-echo T2-weighted sequence, and a coronal MPRAGE or 3DFast GRASS sequence.

Positron emission tomography. Four patients had interictal 18-fluorodeoxyglucose positron emission tomography performed with the Posicam system (Positron Corp., Houston, Tex.) within 40 minutes after intravenous injection of 5 to 10 mCi FDG. Patients had EEG monitoring during the FDG-PET scan to detect any seizures. A hypometabolic zone was defined by visual assessment of axial, coronal, and sagittal reconstructions and was considered present if it was apparent on two or more adjacent slices.

Ictal single photon emission computed tomography. One

MRI	PET	Interictal EEG	EEG seizures
Normal	Normal	Sharp waves: vertex and R parasagittal	R frontocentral
Normal	Hypometabolism: L frontoparietal and L temporal	Normal	L frontocentral
Ganglioglioma: L frontoparietal	ND	Sharp waves: vertex	Vertex
Low-grade astrocytoma: R cingulate gyrus	ND	Sharp waves: vertex and R parasagittal	Vertex and to the R
Normal	Hypometabolism: L centroparietal	Sharp waves: vertex	Vertex
Cortical dysplasia: L mesial frontal	ND	Sharp waves: vertex and L parasagittal	Vertex and L lateral frontal
Cortical dysplasia: L posterior frontal	Hypometabolism: L frontoparietal	Sharp waves: vertex and R parasagittal	L frontocentral
Cortical dysplasia: R superior frontal	ND	Sharp waves: R frontocentral	R frontocentral
Normal	Normal*	Sharp waves: vertex	Vertex
Normal	ND	Sharp waves: vertex	Vertex
Normal	ND	Sharp waves: vertex	Vertex

patient (No. 9) had single photon emission computed tomography on 2 separate days after intravenous injection of 10 mCi of technetium Tc 99m HMPAO (hexamethyl propylene amine oxime) performed 15 and 17 seconds after seizure onset as determined by video EEG. The scanning was performed in the nuclear medicine department within 3 hours after injection, by means of a three-headed camera system with high-resolution, low-energy collimators (Trionix, Cleveland, Ohio). A hypermetabolic zone was defined by visual assessment of axial, coronal, and saggital reconstructions and was considered present if it was apparent on two or more adjacent slices.

Subdural electrode studies. Six patients were studied with subdural electrode arrays during an evaluation for epilepsy surgery. Subdural electrode arrays included stainless steel electrodes embedded in silicone rubber (Silastic) with 1 cm distance between electrode centers. Arrays were inserted after craniotomy with the patient under general anesthesia, and then left in place for 1 to 2 weeks of recording and localization studies in the epilepsy monitoring unit. In this series, each patient had 10 electrodes over the mesial frontoparietal region suspected to be epileptogenic, and 8 to 68 electrodes over the frontoparietal convexity on that side. Video EEG was performed with subdural electrodes to localize the area of seizure onset. Cortical stimulation was performed for mapping of eloquent cortical areas.[1, 16] Electrodes were stimulated individually starting with a current intensity of 1 mA, gradually increasing in subsequent trials to clinical symptoms, EEG afterdischarges, or a maximum of 15 mA. The presence of motor signs, sensory symptoms, and afterdischarges was documented in writing, and elicited responses were videotaped. When no positive motor phenomena were noted, voluntary movements in the limbs were routinely tested to identify any negative motor responses[17] caused by motor inhibition. Patients also had median and posterior tibial evoked potential studies recorded with the subdural electrodes,[18] for localization of arm and leg somatosensory regions.

Methods of analysis. Medical records, MRIs, video EEG reports, and samples of video EEG material were retrospectively reviewed. Outcome data were augmented by telephone follow-up when needed.

RESULTS

Results for each patient are detailed in the Table. Mean age at seizure onset was 5.8 years. Mean age at definitive diagnosis with video EEG monitoring was 12 years. There was a male predominance (8 boys, 3 girls). Most patients had normal intellect. Three patients were assessed by parents and teachers to have mild intellectual difficulties requiring attendance at learning disabilities classes.

Neurologic examination. Nine patients had normal neurologic findings. Two patients had subtle motor abnormalities involving the hand contralateral to the epileptogenic focus, with decreased fine motor control.

Seizures. All patients had daily seizures. Eight patients had seizures predominantly during sleep. Four patients reported an aura before the motor phase of their seizures. Auras included crawling, tingling, or heavy sensations of the limbs in five patients and epigastric discomfort in one patient. Five patients also had rare secondarily generalized tonic-clonic seizures. By history, falling with injury was common during tonic seizures that occurred during wakefulness, but this was not observed on videotape because patients were lying on bed or seated on a chair throughout the recording period.

Recorded seizures were brief (15 to 45 seconds) and typically occurred out of sleep. Attacks were characterized by sudden sustained tonic posturing of the limbs, often with unintelligible fearful vocalization. The tonic stiffening typically affected the proximal limbs most strongly with gross involuntary limb movements. The tonic posturing affected the arms in 10 patients and the legs only in one patient. Five patients had tonic stiffening of arms and legs. It is likely that the frequency of leg stiffening was underestimated on videotape analysis, because the legs were sometimes obscured from camera view by bedcovers. Tonic limb involvement was bilateral in 10 patients.

Two patients had unusual features. Patient 2 was the only one with unilateral motor involvement during seizures; she had a "dead" or "heavy" feeling in her right arm, followed by stiffening and tonic posturing of that limb. Patient 10 was the only one who was not seen initially for tonic seizures. His complaint was that he felt "a crawling or tingling sensation in both legs" followed by "buckling of the knees and falling" eight times a day; the EEG showed runs of rhythmic vertex sharp waves during typical events. It was only after sleep deprivation during the video EEG evaluation that he had a tonic seizure with bilateral stiffening of legs and arms with preserved awareness, followed by a generalized tonic-clonic convulsion.

Although none of the patients was able to speak during seizures, all but one remained fully conscious with partial responsiveness during attacks and intact memory of ictal events. Some patients were able to stick out the tongue or squeeze an examiner's hand on command during an attack. Three patients (Nos. 1, 4, and 6) had recorded bilateral tonic seizures followed by forced turning of the head and eyes toward one side during secondary generalization. In each case the version was contralateral to the hemisphere of seizure onset.

Response to antiepileptic drugs. At the time of video EEG evaluation, trials of an average of 4 antiepileptic drugs in single- or multiple-drug regimens had failed. Most patients had experienced dose-related side effects of medication.

Special studies. The MRI findings were normal for six patients and revealed a low-grade tumor or focal cortical dysplasia in five patients. Four patients had interictal FDG-PET scan. Three patients had hypometabolism in the frontoparietal area on the side identified as epileptogenic by video EEG or MRI. The remaining patient (No. 9) had a normal FDG-PET scan, but ictal single photon emission computed tomography showed left frontal hypermetabolism.

Electroencephalography. Prolonged interictal EEG during a reduced antiepileptic medication regimen showed normal findings in one child, and focal sharp waves were increased or appeared exclusively during sleep in the remaining 10 patients. Interictal sharp waves were over the vertex (Fig. 1) in nine patients and over the right frontocentral region in one patient. Vertex sharp waves were asymmetric with greater distribution over the parasaggital region on one side in four patients, in each case ipsilateral to the hemisphere presumed to be epileptogenic on the basis of ictal EEG, MRI, or FDG-PET. When vertex sharp waves appeared only during sleep, it was difficult to distinguish them from the physiologic sharp transient waves in that area seen normally during stage I and II non-rapid-eye-movement sleep. In some cases, it was only when rare vertex sharp waves were seen during wakefulness that they were seen to be clearly epileptiform. The distinction between epileptic and physiologic sharp transient waves was often not possible on a single routine 20-minute EEG, requiring prolonged EEG recording during wakefulness and sleep with reduced doses of antiepileptic medication.

Ictal recording showed an EEG seizure pattern in every case (Fig. 2), although changes were often subtle, with low-voltage paroxysmal fast activity, or were obscured by electromyography during the tonic posturing. The EEG seizure patterns were maximal over the midline or lateral frontocentral regions. Studies with subdural electrodes (six patients) during clinical seizures showed EEG seizures over the mesial and superior lateral frontocentral region on one side in each case. The epileptogenic zone consistently overlapped with the supplementary sensorimotor area mapped by cortical stimulation and evoked potential studies.

Surgical resection. Six patients had cortical resection. Three patients had resection of mesial and superior lateral frontal cortex, and two had mesial frontal resection only. Five patients had removal of the entire zone judged to be epileptogenic on the basis of subdural EEG, and one (patient 6) had partial resection of the epileptogenic zone because of overlap with primary sensorimotor cortex.

Histopathologic analysis. Focal cortical dysplasia was confirmed histopathologically in the two operated patients with dysgenetic findings on MRI. The two resected tumors were a ganglioglioma and a low-grade astrocytoma. Two patients had only nonspecific changes, including gliosis and heterotopic neurons in the white matter.

Seizure outcome. Among the nonoperated patients, two (Nos. 8 and 10) are seizure-free with carbamazepine or valproate therapy after brief follow-up (11 and 4 months,

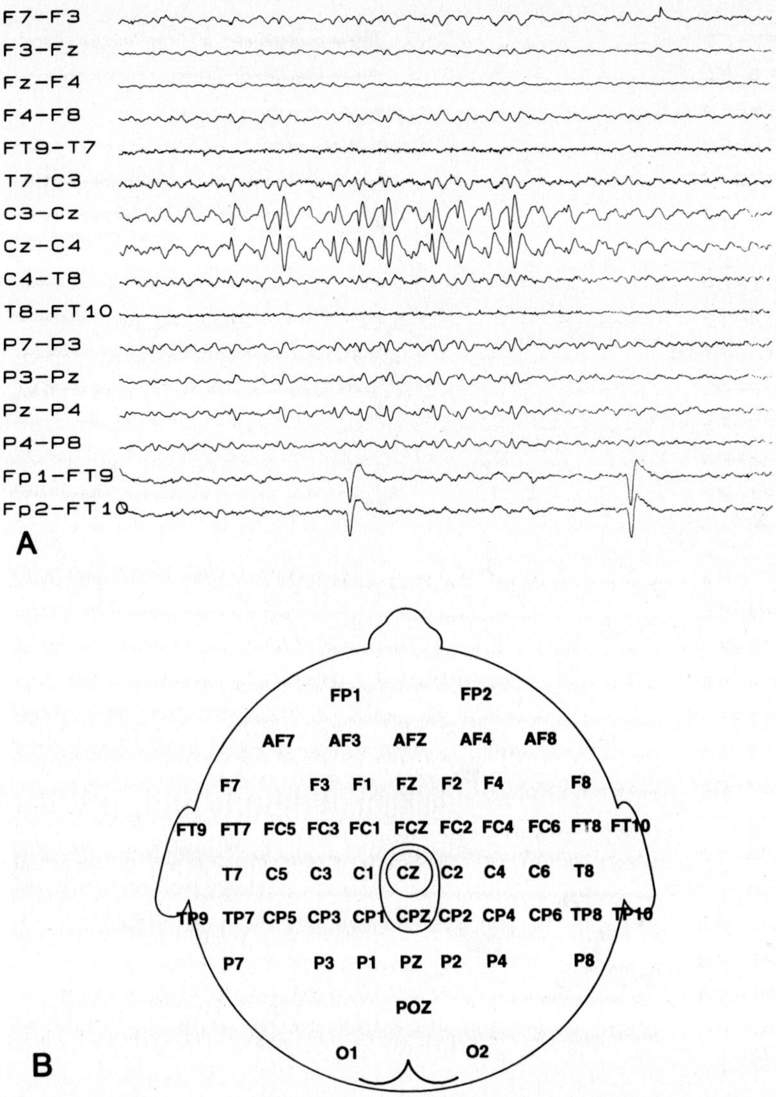

Fig. 1. A, Ten-second sample EEG from patient 9, showing a run of interictal sharp waves over the vertex during wakefulness. The sharp waves are maximal at the Cz electrode, seen best in channels C3-Cz and Cz-C4. Notice the rapid eye movements in the last two channels, indicating the awake state and eliminating the possibility that the sharp waves could be normal vertex transients of stage II sleep. **B,** Diagram showing the distribution of the sharp waves in **panel A.** On referential recording from closely spaced electrodes,[33] the sharp waves had maximal amplitude at vertex electrodes Cz and CPz over the top of the head.

respectively), and three are in the process of surgical evaluation. Of the six patients who had cortical resection, five have had marked improvement in their quality of life as a result of surgery, 2 to 31 (mean 18) months after operation. Four patients were seizure-free, and one (patient 1) had persistent seizures but worthwhile improvement. Preoperatively patient 1 had occasional daytime seizures plus seizures every night with violent motor activity that awoke him repeatedly. Postoperatively patient 1 had no daytime seizures, and nighttime seizures were so mild and infrequent that they were detectable only with video EEG.

In two patients with cortical dysplasia (Nos. 5 and 6) the epileptogenic zone overlapped with primary motor leg cortex, with EEG seizures recorded from this region with subdural electrodes. In one case (No. 6) it was decided to spare the epileptogenic region in the primary motor leg area. This patient had no postoperative leg weakness, but seizures persisted after the partial resection. In the other case (No. 5) it was decided to resect the entire epileptogenic zone as determined by ictal subdural EEG. The child was left with mild right leg weakness after resection but remains seizure-free more than 2 years after operation; he is active and fully ambulatory.

Operative complications. One patient (No. 2) had a bone

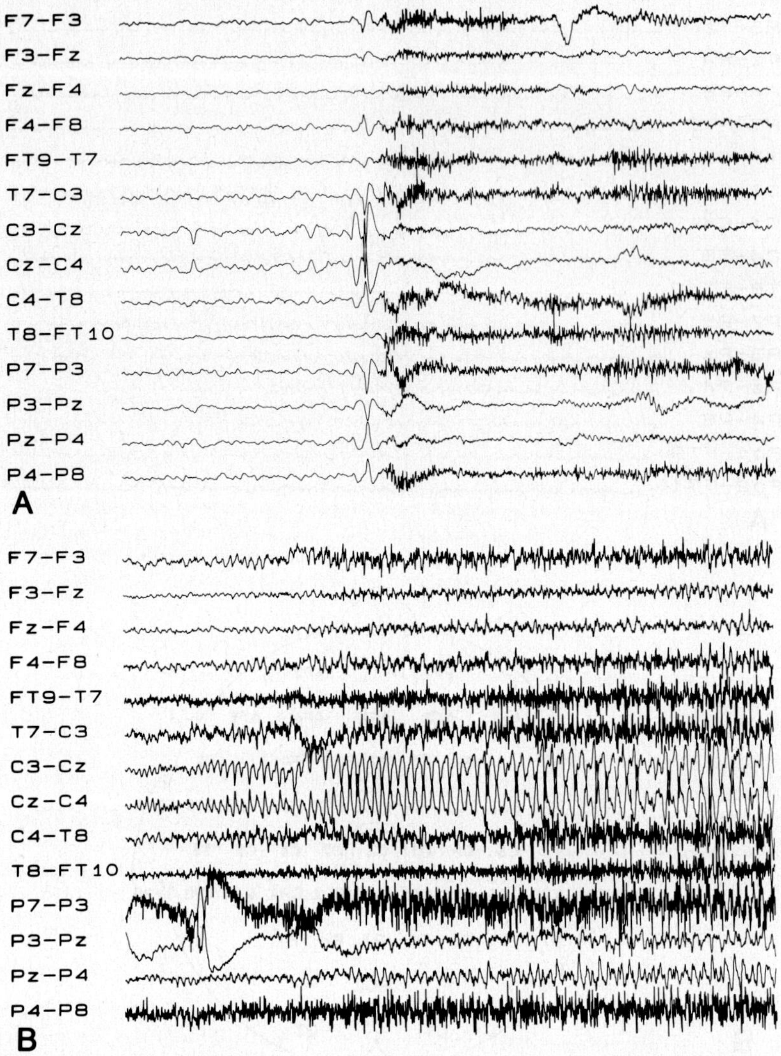

Fig. 2. A, Ten-second sample of EEG at onset of a nocturnal tonic seizure from patient 9. The initial sharp wave was maximal at the vertex, in the same region as the interictal sharp waves shown in Fig. 1. The sharp wave was followed by a generalized electrodecrement with superimposed tonic muscle artifact. **B,** Six seconds after seizure onset, the EEG showed rhythmic spiking over the vertex during evolution to a generalized tonic-clonic convulsion.

flap infection that resolved after cranioplasty. The same patient had transient mild right arm weakness for a few weeks after left mesial frontocentral resection, followed by full recovery. Patient 3 had transient problems with bimanual coordination after operation. Patient 5 had the only persistent postoperative deficit, with mild leg weakness as described above.

DISCUSSION

The diagnosis of SSMA seizures in children can be challenging. Key features in this series included brevity, nocturnal predominance, and bilateral tonic limb posturing with preserved consciousness. The posturing predominantly affected proximal musculature with stiffening and gross flailing movements. Patients usually could not speak during seizures but were able to respond to commands, afterward retaining memory for the ictal events.

The gross bilateral limb movements with preserved consciousness distinguish these SSMA seizures from more common seizure types. Focal motor seizures arising from perirolandic regions may involve preserved consciousness, but the motor activity is different, with unilateral rhythmic clonic jerking of the face or distal arm or leg, often with Jacksonian spread.[19, 20] The bilateral motor activity of SSMA seizures distinguishes them from the perirolandic motor seizures typical of benign focal epilepsy of childhood.[21] Generalized tonic-clonic seizures involve bilateral stiffening and jerking of the limbs, but consciousness is not preserved.[22] SSMA seizures are characterized by the bilaterality of generalized tonic-clonic seizures and the preserved awareness of perirolandic focal motor seizures, but they have a quality and distribution of motor activity that differ from both. Because of these distinct features, SSMA seizures have been recognized as a separate type within the frontal lobe epilepsies.[23]

Video EEG provided critical diagnostic information for our patients with SSMA seizures. As in adults,[13] a routine EEG was often normal. Prolonged recording while on a reduced regimen of antiepileptic medication was often necessary to reveal the interictal sharp waves over the vertex, or to distinguish the epileptiform discharges from the normal vertex sharp transients of stages I and II of non-rapid-eye-movement sleep. Analysis of EEG seizures was often difficult because the intense motor activity during seizures resulted in muscle and movement artifact, which obscured cortical rhythms. A clear EEG seizure was not identifiable in every event, but each patient had at least some seizures with identifiable cortical signs.

Another contribution of prolonged recording was to provide high-quality videotapes demonstrating repeated stereotyped events with clinical features typical of the SSMA seizure type. For physicians experienced in the interpretation of seizure semiology, home videotapes of the SSMA seizures may be clarifying. For three patients the videotape also provided lateralizing clues such as version of the head and eyes[24] during secondary generalization. For patients under consideration for epilepsy surgery, these lateralizing clinical features contributed to surgical planning.

Magnetic resonance imaging was another important diagnostic test in this series, revealing a low-grade tumor or focal cortical dysplasia in five patients. We believe that MRI is indicated in every case in which SSMA seizures are suspected. For patients undergoing surgical evaluation, interictal PET may give additional localizing information.

The SSMA seizures may be confused with psychogenic seizures because of the gross bilateral motor activity with preserved consciousness and the typically normal routine EEG. Several parents reported that previous physicians had recommended psychologic evaluation. In some patients the epileptic nature of the episodes was first appreciated when a typical event evolved into a secondarily generalized tonic-clonic convulsion. Kanner et al.[25] highlighted other features that may help distinguish between SSMA seizures and pseudoseizures, noting that pseudoseizures are typically longer and less stereotyped, and usually occur out of wakefulness. The age at onset may also be helpful, because psychogenic seizures rarely start before age 8 or 9 years.[26, 27]

The SSMA seizures in children may also be confused with parasomnias such as night terrors or confusional arousals. If typical events also occasionally occur during wakefulness, a diagnosis of night terrors or confusional arousals can be set aside. If episodes occur only during sleep, home videotape may clarify the diagnosis by revealing the characteristic stereotyped bilateral tonic posturing and proximal limb movements of SSMA seizures.

Lugaresi et al.[28, 29] described patients with episodes identical to SSMA seizures and attributed the events to a nonepileptic parasomnia (paroxysmal nocturnal dystonia). Several times each night, patients sat up abruptly out of sleep and had dystonic posturing of extremities with preserved consciousness. Patients were divided into two clinical groups on the basis of success or failure of treatment with carbamazepine. Some of the patients described by Lugaresi et al.[28, 29] were not studied by video EEG. It is now thought that paroxysmal nocturnal dystonic attacks are epileptic seizures arising from the frontal lobe,[15] with manifestations caused by ictal activation of the SSMA. An autosomal dominant form has been described in six families.[30]

Usual drug choices for SSMA seizures include those medications effective against partial seizures, such as carbamazepine, phenytoin, valproate, phenobarbital, primidone, or some of the newer agents. In this series, only two patients achieved good seizure control with antiepileptic medication; nine patients had refractory daily seizures. The low frequency of a benign course in our series may be due to referral bias, with patients having refractory seizures more likely to seek treatment at an epilepsy center.

The uncontrolled SSMA seizures in nine of our patients caused significant disability. Although daytime attacks were less frequent than nocturnal events for most patients, the daytime seizures typically caused abrupt, unprotected falls with injury. The nocturnal events less often caused physical injury but typically occurred several times each night and were exhausting and frightening. Because consciousness was preserved during the unpredictable episodes of uncontrollable gross motor activity, the episodes were universally perceived by patients as unpleasant. In each case, quality of life was adversely affected by the seizures, and limited independent activity.

The disability associated with refractory SSMA seizures led to consideration of surgery in nine of our patients. Six have undergone operation, and five had good results with improvement in quality of life. The patient with a poor operative outcome had only partial resection of the epileptogenic zone because of concerns about overlap with the primary motor leg area. Better results were obtained in the child who had complete resection of the epileptogenic region of cortical dysplasia, despite involvement of the primary motor leg area. Epilepsy surgery may be an effective treatment for selected pediatric patients with disabling, refractory SSMA seizures,[31] but detailed study with subdural electrodes may be important for clarification of the extent of the epileptogenic zone in relation to eloquent cortex. Careful testing has revealed subtle incoordination of bimanual movement in some older patients after resection of the SSMA,[32] but few pediatric patients have been tested with detailed paradigms.

Increased recognition of SSMA seizures in children should lead to earlier diagnosis, more effective treatment with antiepileptic medication, and earlier referral of refractory patients for surgical consideration.

REFERENCES

1. Lim SH, Dinner DS, Pillay PK, et al. Functional anatomy of the human supplementary sensorimotor area: results of extraoperative electrical stimulation. Electroencephalogr Clin Neurophysiol 1994;91:179-93.
2. Lim SH, Dinner D, Lüders HO. Cortical stimulation of the supplementary sensorimotor area. In: Lüders HO, ed. The supplementary sensorimotor area. New York: Raven Press (in press).
3. Fried I, Katz A, McCathy G, et al. Functional organization of human supplementary motor cortex studied by electrical stimulation. J Neurosurg 1991;11:3656-66.
4. Macpherson JM, Marangoz C, Miles TS, Wiesendanger M. Microstimulation of the supplementary motor area in the awake monkey. Exp Brain Res 1982;45:410-6.
5. Mitz AR, Wise SP. The somatotopic organization of the supplementary motor area: intracortical microstimulation mapping. J Neurosci 1987;7:1010-21.
6. Penfield W, Welch K. The supplementary motor area of the cerebral cortex. AMA Arch Neurol Psychiatry 1951;66:289-317.
7. Penfield W, Boldrey E. Somatic motor and sensory representation in the cerebral cortex of man as studied by electrical stimulation. Brain 1937;60:389-443.
8. Roland PE, Larsen B, Lassen NA, Skinhoj E. Supplementary motor area and other cortical areas in organization of voluntary movements in man. J Neurophysiol 1980;43:118-36.
9. Wiesendanger M. Recent developments in studies of the supplementary motor area of primates. Rev Physiol Biochem Pharmacol 1986;103:1-59.
10. Woolsey CN, Erickson TC, Gilson WE. Localization in somatic sensory and motor areas of human cerebral cortex as determined by direct recording of evoked potentials and electrical stimulation. J Neurosurg 1979;51:476-506.
11. Goldberg G. Supplementary motor area structure and function: review and hypotheses. Behav Brain Sci 1985;8:567-616.
12. Morris HH, Dinner DS, Lüders H, Wyllie E, Kramer R. Supplementary motor seizures: clinical and electroencephalographic findings. Neurology 1988;38:1075-82.
13. Morris HH. Supplementary motor seizures. In: Wyllie E, ed. The treatment of epilepsy: principles and practice. Philadelphia: Lea & Febiger, 1993:541-6.
14. Waterman K, Purves SJ, Kosaka B, Strauss E, Wada JA. An epileptic syndrome caused by mesial frontal lobe seizure foci. Neurology 1987;37:577-82.
15. Tinuper P, Cerullo A, Cirignotta F, Cortelli P, Lugaresi E, Montagna P. Nocturnal paroxysmal dystonia with short-lasting attacks: three cases with evidence for an epileptic frontal lobe origin of seizures. Epilepsia 1990;31:549-56.
16. Lüders H, Lesser RP, Dinner DS, et al. Chronic intracranial recording and stimulation with subdural electrodes. In: Engel J, ed. Surgical treatment of the epilepsies. New York: Raven Press, 1987:297-321.
17. Lüders H, Lesser RP, Morris HH, Dinner DS, Hahn J. Negative motor responses elicited by stimulation of the human cortex. In: Wolf P, Dam M, Janz D, eds. Advances in epileptology: the XVIth Epilepsy International Symposium. New York: Raven Press, 1987:229-31.
18. Lüders H, Lesser RP, Morris HH. Evoked potentials in cortical localization. J Clin Neurophysiol 1986;3:75-84.
19. Commission on Classification and Terminology of the International League Against Epilepsy. Proposal for revised clinical and electrographic classification of epileptic seizures. Epilepsia 1981;22:489-501.
20. Blume WT. Focal motor seizures and epilesia partialis continua. In: Wyllie E, ed. The treatment of epilepsy: principles and practice. Philadelphia: Lea & Febiger, 1993:393-400.
21. Loiseau P. Benign focal epilepsies of childhood. In: Wyllie E, ed. The treatment of epilepsy: principles and practice. Philadelphia: Lea & Febiger, 1993:503-12.
22. Fisch BJ. Generalized tonic-clonic seizures. In: Wyllie E, ed. The treatment of epilepsy: principles and practice. Philadelphia: Lea & Febiger, 1993:425-42.
23. Commission on Classification and Terminology of the International League Against Epilepsy. Proposal for revised classification of epilepsies and epileptic syndromes. Epilepsia 1989;30:389-99.
24. Wyllie E, Lüders H, Morris HH, Lesser RP, Dinner DS. The lateralizing significance of head and eye movements during epileptic seizures. Neurology 1986;36:606-11.
25. Kanner AM, Morris HH, Lüders H, et al. Supplementary motor seizures mimicking pseudoseizures: some clinical differences. Neurology 1990;40:1404-14.
26. Wyllie E, Friedman D, Rothner AD, et al. Psychogenic seizures in children and adolescents: outcome after diagnosis by ictal video and electroencephalographic recording. Pediatrics 1990;85:480-4.
27. Wyllie E, Friedman D, Lüders H, Morris H, Rothner D, Turnbull J. Outcome of psychogenic seizures in children and adolescents compared with adults. Neurology 1991;41:742-4.
28. Lugaresi E, Cirignotta F. Nocturnal paroxysmal dystonia: epileptic seizures or a new syndrome? Sleep 1981;4:129-38.
29. Lugaresi E, Cirignotta F, Montagna P. Nocturnal paroxysmal dystonia. J Neurol Neurosurg Psychiatry 1986;49:375-80.
30. Scheffer IE, Bhatia KP, Lopes-Cendes I, et al. Autosomal dominant frontal epilepsy misdiagnosed as sleep disorder. Lancet 1994;343:515-7.
31. Comair YG. Surgical strategies for patients with SSMA epilepsy: the Cleveland Clinic experience. In: Lüders HO, ed. The supplementary sensorimotor area. New York: Raven Press (in press).
32. Bleasel A, Lüders HO. Ablation studies in humans. In: Lüders HO, ed. The supplementary sensorimotor area. New York: Raven Press (in press).
33. Sharbrough F, Chatrian GE, Lesser RP, Lüders H, Nuwer M, Picton TW. American Electroencephalographic Society guidelines for standard electrode position nomenclature. J Clin Neurophysiol 1991;8:200-2.

Predictive factors in the determination of final height in boys with constitutional delay of growth and puberty

A. Albanese, MD, and R. Stanhope, MD, FRCP

From the Medical Unit, Institute of Child Health, London, England

Seventy-eight patients who had constitutional delay of growth and puberty were included in a retrospective study to determine whether, at the time of first evaluation, any predictive features could suggest final height outcome. Mean chronologic age was 14.3 years (range, 12 to 18 years), and all were either prepubertal or in an early stage of pubertal maturation (4 ml testicular volume). Initial mean (±SD) height standard deviation score was −2.74 (±0.71); 85% had a relatively short spine compared with subischial leg length. Mean (±SD) growth rate was 4.8 (±1.6) cm/year, and epiphyseal maturation was delayed by 2.4 (±1) years. Sixteen boys were treated with a sustained-action preparation of testosterone (50 mg monthly for 3 to 4 months), six with oxandrolone (1.25 mg daily for a mean of 4 months), and one with both drugs in sequence. At final height attainment, 58% of the boys failed to achieve their full genetic potential; among the remaining 42%, only 0.7% attained a final height above corrected mid-parental height. The relative disproportion between the segments had no significant change at final height attainment. Regression analysis showed that final height impairment (the difference between mid-parental height and final height) was negatively influenced by standing height and growth velocity when initially evaluated and positively by the degree of segmental body proportion; that is, patients who were taller, were growing at a faster rate, and who had a major degree of segmental body disproportion with a short spine and long leg length attained a final height closer to their mid-parental height, irrespective of the degree of delayed epiphyseal maturation. Neither testosterone nor oxandrolone administered during early puberty modified final height attainment or segmental proportion. We conclude that a late onset in the timing of puberty seems to be deleterious to spinal growth and consequently to final height attainment. An alternative diagnosis should be sought among patients with features of constitutional delay of growth and puberty who do not have a significant degree of body disproportion. In these patients, as well as in those who are extremely short, who have a poor growth rate, or who have an unfavorable genetic potential, an alternative therapeutic approach may be required. (J Pediatr 1995;126:545-50)

Supported in part by The Growth Child Foundation and Novo Nordisk.

Submitted for publication Oct. 19, 1993; accepted Oct. 25, 1994.

Reprint requests: R. Stanhope, MD, FRCP, Medical Unit, Institute of Child Health, 30 Guilford St., London WC1N 1EH, England.

0022-3476/95/$3.00 + 0 **9/20/61575**

Constitutional delay of growth and puberty affects mainly boys. The clinical features are relative short stature for chronologic age, delayed puberty, and delayed epiphyseal maturation. It is generally believed that height prognosis is appropriate to genetic potential, even though some authors have published contradictory data.[1-4] Presumptive diagnosis is made on clinical and anthropometric grounds and is later confirmed by the appearance or progression of spon-

CDGP	Constitutional delay of growth and puberty
GH	Growth hormone
SDS	Standard deviation score
SH	Sitting height
SLL	Subischial leg length

taneous sexual development associated with an appropriate growth acceleration. Treatment is usually offered when patients have psychologic distress associated with short stature or pubertal delay, even though they have been reassured about eventual "normal" height and sexual maturation. A 3- to 6-month course of testosterone enanthate or low doses of oxandrolone can accelerate the pubertal growth spurt without altering final height attainment.[5,6] Growth hormone can also be used to improve short-term growth rate,[7] but considering cost, the requirement for daily injections and the lack of improvement in final height,[8] it does not appear to be advantageous. One of the common features of severely delayed puberty is body disproportion at final stature, the upper segment being relatively shorter than subischial leg length.[1,2,4]

We hypothesized that CDGP may be a heterogeneous condition with different degrees of final height impairment. Our aim in this study was to identify predictive factors of final height outcome to select patients who may need further investigations or benefit from alternative therapeutic approaches.

METHODS

We analyzed the growth patterns of 78 boys with CDGP who were followed in our growth clinic until they attained final height (Table). We considered a patient as having attained final height when his growth rate was less than 2 cm/year, epiphyses were fused, and secondary sexual characteristics were adult.[1] None of our patients had low birth weight, dysmorphic syndromes, skeletal dysplasia, or chronic diseases, or had received treatment with corticosteroids. The diagnosis of CDGP was made on clinical grounds when no pubertal signs were present at chronologic age 13 years, and bone age was delayed more than 1½ years. However, when the differential diagnosis between CDGP and GH insufficiency was in doubt, pharmacologic tests of pituitary function were performed, after priming with sex steroids.[9] The results were considered normal (GH response to insulin-induced hypoglycemia or glucagon >20 mU/L, equivalent to 10 ng/ml) in all patients tested. A skeletal survey was performed when differences more than 2 standard deviation scores between the upper and lower segments were present (see below). Sixteen boys were treated with a sustained-action preparation of testosterone (50 mg monthly for 3 to 4 months), six with oxandrolone (1.25 mg daily for a mean of 4 months), and one with both drugs in sequence.

Growth, pubertal stage, epiphyseal maturation, and height prediction were assessed by standard anthropometric techniques,[10] the Tanner standards,[11,12] and the Tanner-Whitehouse method.[13] Sitting height was measured with an anthropometer (Holtain Ltd., Crymmych, Pembs, United Kingdom); SLL was estimated as standing height minus SH. Parental heights were measured, and the target height was defined according to the Tanner criteria: ([father's height (cm) + mother's height (cm) + 12.5 cm]/2 ± 8.5 cm).[14] Ninety-five percent of a couple's offspring are expected to have final height within the target height, with values normally distributed around corrected mid-parental height ([father's height (cm) + mother's height (cm) + 12.5 cm]/2). All data were expressed as SDS in comparison with the normal data of Marshall and Tanner.[11] The SDS is calculated by subtracting the population mean for a patient's peers from the patient's observed measurement and dividing by the standard deviation for that population. Therefore, when the height SDS is considered, a short patient has a negative SDS value and a tall one has a positive value. The leg length SDS was subtracted from the SH SDS to obtain a disproportion score; a normally proportioned child is expected to have a disproportion score of 0, a child with a short spine in comparison with leg length a negative score, and a child with a long spine a positive score. A disproportion score $\geq \pm 2$ represents a significant disproportion. Final height impairment was defined as the difference between corrected mid-parental height minus the patient's final height, both expressed in SDS.

Statistical analysis was by paired-sample t test. The Pearson test was used to determine significant correlation between final height on the one hand and standing height, difference between SH and SLL, chronologic age, growth velocity, and delayed bone maturation on first evaluation on the other, in addition to a stepwise multiple regression. Treatment was not entered as a variable because it is widely recognized that either testosterone or oxandrolone therapy at the above doses does not influence final height. However, one-way analysis of variance followed by the Duncan procedure was used to verify that final height and segmental body proportion did not differ in treated and untreated patients. Results are expressed as the mean (±SD).

RESULTS

The initial height SDS was −2.7 (0.7) (140.6 [8.6] cm), which increased to −2.0 (0.9) (160.5 [6.7] cm) at final height. Final height was significantly less than either corrected mid-parental height (p <0.0001) or predicted height (p <0.0001). Figure 1 shows mean value ± 2 SD of final height, mid-parental height, and predicted height SDS. When we considered the genetic target instead of mid-parental height, 58% of patients failed to achieve their full genetic potential; among the remaining 42%, only 0.7% attained a final height above mid-parental corrected height (Fig. 1). There was a significant difference between SH and SLL both initially (p <0.0001) and at final height (p <0.0001). The mean difference between the SDS values of SH and SLL was −1.2 (±1.1) at presentation (Fig. 2) and remained unmodified at a value of −1.3 (±1.0) at final height attainment (Fig. 3). In 19 patients (24%), the initial difference between SH and SLL was > −2 SDS, and in 9 (47%) of these this significant disproportion score was still present at final height attainment. In addition, 11 (14%) more patients had an initial disproportion score < −SD, but it decreased to < −2 SDS at final height. Hence, at final height, 20 (26%) patients had a severe eunuchoid habitus. All patients attained full sexual maturation, with testicular volume ≥15 ml, indicating normal gonadotrophin secretion. A significant negative correlation ($r = -0.6$; p <0.0001) was found between initial chronologic age and degree of segmental body disproportion (Fig. 2).

Multiple regression analysis, used to find most suitable predictors of final height impairment, showed that among the factors included in the analysis, only standing height, growth velocity, and degree of segmental proportion (difference between SH and SLL) were significantly associated with final height. Therefore patients who were taller, who were growing initially at a faster rate, and who had a major degree of segmental body disproportion, had less height impairment. The other variables included in the analysis were delayed bone maturation (chronologic age − bone age, expressed in years) and chronologic age at first evaluation. The relationship was described by the following regression equation:

Corrected mid-parental height SDS
− Final height SDS
= −0.39 (Initial height SDS)
−0.12 (Initial growth velocity)
+0.22 (SH SDS − SLL SDS when first seen)
+1.26
($R = 0.49$, $R^2 = 0.24$, adjusted $R^2 = 0.21$; $F = 7.8$, $p = 0.0001$)

When we classified the patients according to the treatment received (no therapy, oxandrolone or testosterone, or both oxandrolone and testosterone), the oldest patients were those treated with testosterone (p <0.05). Consequently, because they were the oldest, they also had the more pronounced body disproportion (p <0.05), with relatively long legs and short spine. However, at final height, height impairment and body proportion were similar among groups (p not significant), and the only significant difference among the boys in the four treatment options was in chronologic age (p <0.01); the patients who received testosterone were the eldest.

Table. Initial clinical data from 78 patients with CDGP

Chronologic age (yr)	14.3 (12-18)
Bone age (yr)	11.9 (7-15)
Chronologic age − bone age (yr)	2.4 ± 1.3
Height (SDS)	−2.7 ± 0.7
Height (cm)	140.6 ± 8.6
SH (SDS)	−3.5 ± 0.9
SH (cm)	73.6 ± 3.6
SLL (SDS)	−2.3 ± 0.8
SLL (cm)	67.0 ± 5.5
SH − SLL (SDS)	−1.2 ± 1.1
Growth rate (cm/yr)	4.8 ± 1.6
Height prediction (SDS)	−1.4 ± 0.8
Mid-parental height (SDS)	−0.5 ± 0.6
Father height (cm)	172.1 ± 5.7
Mother height (cm)	160.5 ± 6.7
Testicular volume (ml)	3.3 (2-8)
No. of patients	78
% of patients treated	29.5%

Values are expressed as mean ± 1 SD or mean (range).

DISCUSSION

Our data confirm that CDGP is a heterogeneous condition in which final height may be compromised; 58% of our patients failed to achieve their genetic target height, and only 4% were able to reach a final height greater than their mid-parental percentiles. The absence of correlation between final height and degree of delayed bone maturation indicates that final height prediction is not reliable in this condition. The initial standing height and growth velocity seem to be much more important than the degree of delayed bone maturation. Consequently, slow-growing patients who are extremely short in comparison with their parents need special attention despite their final height prognosis. Other therapeutic approaches, such as GH treatment, should be considered.

When the pubertal growth spurt occurs in patients with CDGP, its duration, peak height velocity and, consequently, the total pubertal height gain are reduced. If this were counterbalanced by the increased prepubertal height gain,[15] final height should not be compromised. However, during late prepuberty or early puberty, height gain is mainly the result of growth in the lower segment; spinal growth is relatively delayed compared with leg length. As a result, if puberty is delayed, spinal growth is more compromised so that, when pubertal growth acceleration occurs, a body disproportion with short SH and long SLL is already recognizable. Our results emphasize that a relatively short upper segment, compared with the lower segment, is one of the most important signs of CDGP, and that it increases when puberty is severely delayed. Its presence should always be sought and can be considered an indicator of an inadequate final height outcome. The absence of a relatively short SH in a boy older than 14 years, even in the presence of all other

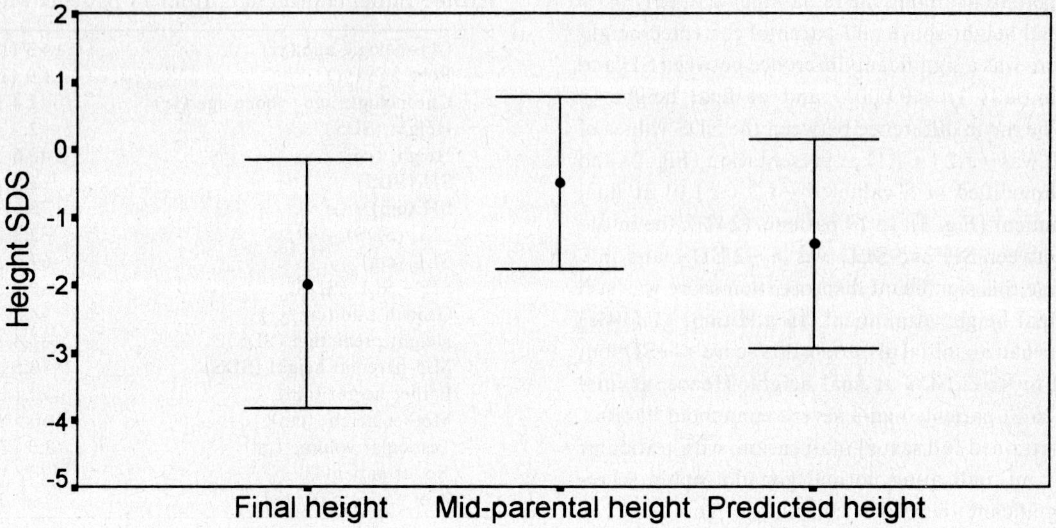

Fig. 1. Height (expressed as SDS) in 78 boys with CDGP at final stature, as well as predicted and corrected mid-parental heights.

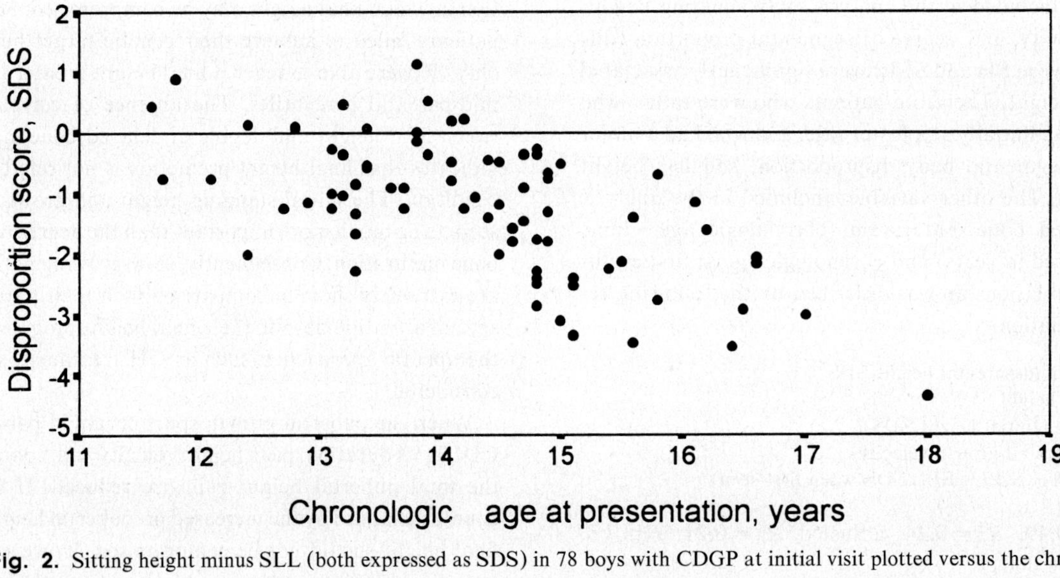

Fig. 2. Sitting height minus SLL (both expressed as SDS) in 78 boys with CDGP at initial visit plotted versus the chronologic age.

clinical signs of CDGP, should point to a different diagnosis. Recent studies have shown that during the pubertal growth spurt, spinal growth does not seem to compensate for the previous deficit[1, 2, 4]; at final height attainment an eunuchoid body disproportion is still present in most patients with CDGP. Their final height is below that expected from their corrected parental heights, partly because of their short spine. In our study short spine was also found in most patients at final height, and some of these had a disproportion score greater than −2 SD. Thus spinal growth failure was in part responsible for the failure to attain a final height appropriate to mid-parental percentiles. Because reduced mineral density has been found in the lumbar spine of adult men with CDGP,[16] vertebral mineralization also may be compromised if puberty is delayed.

We are unable to explain the failure to achieve target height in 58% of our patients other than suggesting that this

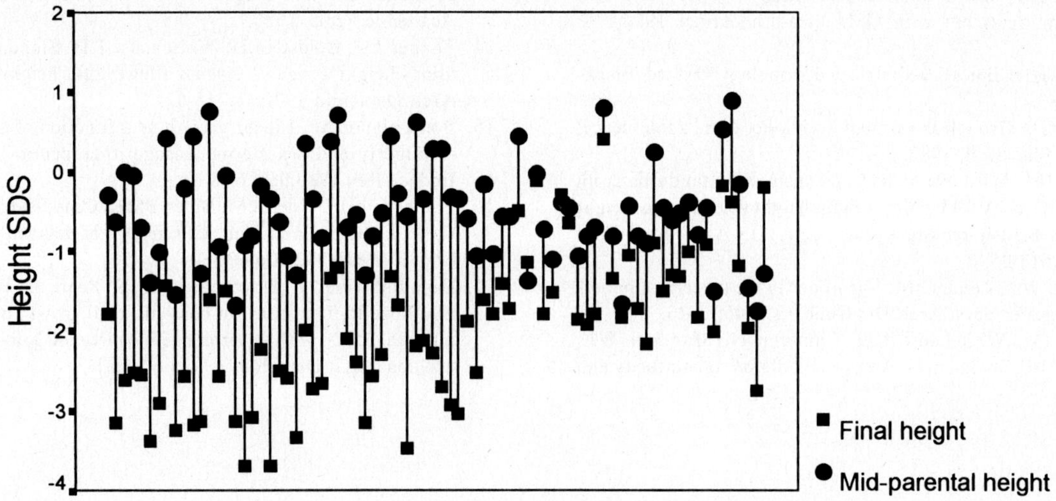

Fig. 3. Final height *(squares)* and corrected mid-parental height *(circles)* (expressed as SDS) in the 78 boys with CDGP.

may be a variant of CDGP, in association with GH insufficiency not revealed by pharmacologic tests of GH secretion or an unclassified skeletal dysplasia. We also recognize that the generally unsatisfactory final height in our patients was partly related to an artefact in the selection of patients, who were referred to our specialized growth center. It is likely that only those who had extremely short stature or a poor genetic potential came to our attention. A further selection was also undertaken by us as long-term follow-up was offered mainly to those in whom height was more compromised.

The traditional therapeutic approach in boys with CDGP is the induction of a pubertal growth spurt with either testosterone or an anabolic steroid when this is required for psychologic reasons. Treatment is therefore generally commenced at a late stage, when the patient has already had prolonged growth deceleration and, therefore, spinal growth failure. This approach does not improve final height but only accelerates the growth spurt. In our study as well, such treatment did not improve final height or body proportion attainment, presumably because of the late timing at which therapy was started (i.e., in early puberty). Because reduced spinal growth seems to be related to delayed puberty, treatment of growth delay in the prepubertal age range (11 to 12 years in boys)[17] with low doses of oxandrolone may prevent reduced spinal growth, and consequently improve final height.

We conclude that short SH compared with SLL is an important early sign of CDGP, especially when puberty is severely delayed. Its absence or minor appearance is an indicator of inadequate final height outcome; in these patients an alternative diagnosis should be carefully sought. In addition, subjects with the best final height attainment did not attain their full genetic potential, mainly because of the inadequate spinal growth. A late onset in the timing of puberty seems to be deleterious to vertebral mineralization, spinal growth, and probably to final height attainment. Thus treatment of growth delay in late prepuberty may be an effective approach for other reasons than just psychologic distress.

REFERENCES

1. Crowne EC, Shalet SM, Wallace WHB, Eminson DM, Price DA. Final height in boys with untreated constitutional delay of growth and puberty. Arch Dis Child 1990;65:1109-12.
2. Crowne EC, Shalet SM, Wallace WHB, Eminson DM, Price DA. Final height in girls with untreated constitutional delay of growth and puberty. Eur J Pediatr 1990;150:708-12.
3. Willing RP, Mahnke K, Stahnke N, Commentz JC, Sinnecker G, Winkler P. Height predictions and final height in boys with constitutional delay of growth and puberty. Horm Res 1990;33(suppl 3):34.
4. Albanese A, Stanhope R. Does constitutional delayed puberty cause segmental disproportion and short stature? Eur J Pediatr 1993;152:293-6.
5. Wilson DM, Kei J, Hintz RL, Rosenfeld GG. Effects of testosterone therapy for pubertal delay. Am J Dis Child 1988; 142:96-9.
6. Joss EE, Schmidt HA, Zuppinger ZA. Oxandrolone in constitutionally delayed growth, a longitudinal study up to final height. J Clin Endocrinol Metab 1989;69:1109-15.
7. Buyukgebiz A, Hindmarsh PC, Brook CGD. Treatment of constitutional delay of growth and puberty with oxandrolone compared with growth hormone. Arch Dis Child 1990;65:448-52.
8. Bierich JR, Nolte K, Drews K, Brugmann G. Constitutional

delay of growth and adolescence. Result of short-term and long-term treatment with GH. Acta Endocrinol 1992;127:392-6.
9. Brook CGD. Clinical paediatric endocrinology. Oxford: Blackwell, 1989.
10. Brook CGD. Growth assessment in childhood and adolescence. Oxford: Blackwell, 1982.
11. Tanner JM, Whitehouse RH, Takaishi M. Standards from birth to maturity for height, weight, height velocity and weight velocity: British children 1965. Part II. Arch Dis Child 1966;41:613-35.
12. Marshall WA, Tanner JM. Variations in the pattern of pubertal changes in boys. Arch Dis Child 1970;45:13-23.
13. Tanner JM, Whitehouse RH, Cameron N, Marshall WA, Healy MJR, Goldstein H. Assessment of skeletal maturity and prediction of adult height (TW2 method). 2nd ed. London: Academic Press, 1983.
14. Tanner JM, Goldstein H, Whitehouse RH. Standard for children's height at ages 2-9 years allowing for height of parents. Arch Dis Child 1970;45:755-62.
15. Bourguignon JP. Linear growth as a function of age at onset of puberty and sex steroid dosage: therapeutic implication. Endocr Rev 1988;9:467-88.
16. Finkelstein JS, Neer RM, Biller BMK, Crawford JD, Klibanski A. Osteopenia in men with history of delayed puberty. N Engl J Med 1992;326:600-4.
17. Papadimitriou A, Wacharasindhu S, Pearl K, Preece MA, Stanhope R. Treatment of constitutional growth delay in prepubertal boys with a prolonged course of low-dose oxandrolone. Arch Dis Child 1991;66:841-3.

Effects of dairy products on bone and body composition in pubertal girls

Gary M. Chan, MD, Karen Hoffman, and Martha McMurry, MS

From the Department of Pediatrics and the Clinical Research Center, University of Utah, Salt Lake City

Objective: To study the effect of calcium supplementation with dairy products on the bone and body composition of pubertal girls.
Design: Randomized control study with 12-month follow-up.
Setting: General community.
Subjects: Forty-eight white girls whose mean age was 11 years and sexual development at Tanner stage 2.
Intervention: One group's diet was supplemented with dairy products to the recommended dietary allowance of 1200 mg calcium daily. The other group ate their usual diet.
Main outcome measures: Bone mineral content and density were measured at the radius, femoral neck, lumbar spine, and total body bone mineral by single-photon and dual-energy x-ray absorptiometry at the start of the study and after 3, 6, 9, and 12 months. Body composition (lean body mass and body fat) was measured by dual-energy x-ray absorptiometry at the same intervals. Serum calcium, phosphate, 25-hydroxyvitamin D, 1,25-dihydroxyvitamin D, alkaline phosphatase, magnesium, and albumin concentrations were determined at the start and end of the study. The urinary calcium/creatinine ratio and hydroxyproline concentration were also determined.
Results: The dairy group had higher intakes of calcium, phosphate, vitamin D, and protein than control subjects. The dairy group had significantly greater increases during the 1-year study in bone mineral density at the lumbar spine bones (22.8% ± 6.9% vs 12.9% ± 8.3%) and in total body bone mineral (14.2% ± 7.0% vs 7.6% ± 6.0%) than control subjects. Dietary calcium, phosphate, vitamin D, and protein intakes were associated with the lumbar bone density and total body bone calcium. There were no differences in serum or urinary biochemical values between the two groups at the start or end of the study.
Conclusions: Young girls whose dietary calcium intake was provided primarily by dairy products at or above the recommended dietary allowances had an increased rate of bone mineralization. Increased intake of dairy foods did not increase overall total or saturated fat intake and was not associated with excessive weight gain or increased body fat. (J PEDIATR 1995;126:551-6)

Supported in part by grants from the National Dairy Council and by Clinical Research Center grant M01-RR0064.

Submitted for publication July 15, 1994; accepted Nov. 4, 1994.

Reprint requests: Gary M. Chan, MD, Department of Pediatrics, 50 North Medical Dr., Salt Lake City, UT 84132.

0022-3476/95/$3.00 + 0 **9/20/61905**

In the United States, dairy product consumption has declined,[1] especially during the adolescent period and in girls and women. Dairy products, especially milk, are a major source not only of calcium but also of other important nutrients such as protein and vitamins. It appears that nu-

DEXA	Dual-energy x-ray absorptiometry

Table I. Age, weight, and height

	Control group	Dairy group
Baseline		
Age (yrs)	11.2 ± 1.0	11.1 ± 0.9
Weight (kg)	37.3 ± 3.9	36.4 ± 7.3
Height (cm)	148.0 ± 4.6	145.6 ± 7.6
At 12 mo		
Weight	44.5 ± 6.3	42.8 ± 8.6
%Gain in weight	19.2 ± 6.6	17.4 ± 9.3
Height	155.4 ± 4.2	153.4 ± 7.2
%Gain in height	5.3 ± 1.2	5.2 ± 1.6

Values are expressed as mean ± SD.

trition from dairy products could be important for adolescents during their critical growth phase.[2]

Bone mass accretion during adolescence appears to be important in the development of peak bone mass, which is believed to be a major determinant of osteoporosis.[3-5] Although genetic factors may be the primary determinant of peak bone mass, calcium intake significantly affects bone mass.[3, 6, 7] The present recommended dietary allowance for calcium is highest during adolescence (1200 mg daily).[8] Unfortunately, the eating habits of many adolescents place them at risk of having calcium deficiency and of failing to achieve an optimal peak bone mass. Carbonated beverages have replaced milk in the diets of adolescents and are considered their favorite beverage.[9, 10] Low dietary calcium intake has been shown to lead to low bone density in adolescents and possibly to osteoporosis later in life.[11] We evaluated the effects of dairy products on bone and body composition of pubertal girls.

METHODS

Subjects. Forty-eight healthy white girls, aged 9 to 13 years, participated in this 12-month study. All girls were at the same sexual staging of 2, which is defined as the beginning of pubic hair and breast bud development. Sexual maturation was evaluated by examination and questionnaire. All girls were healthy and free of any chronic diseases that would affect their growth or calcium metabolism. All girls were between the 10th and 90th percentiles for both weight and height, as determined by the National Center for Health Statistics.[12] Girls who participated in school team sports were excluded. The girls in our study were randomly assigned to one of two groups: control or dairy. The control group consumed their usual diet. The dairy group's diet was supplemented weekly with dairy products to at least 1200 mg calcium daily. Dairy products included milk, cheese, and yogurt. This study was approved by our institutional review board. Informed consent was obtained from the girl's parents, and assent from each girl.

Protocol. All girls were examined at the beginning of the study and then every 3 months for 1 year. Weight and height measurements were recorded at each visit. Routine activity was assessed by questionnaire at each visit. Blood was drawn by venipuncture at the start and end of the study for determinations of serum levels of calcium, phosphate, 25-hydroxyvitamin D, 1,25-dihydroxyvitamin D, alkaline phosphatase, magnesium, and albumin. At each clinic visit, the first morning urine specimen was also collected, after 12 hours of fasting, for calcium, creatinine, and hydroxyproline determinations. Bone mineral status was determined by single-photon and dual-energy x-ray absorptiometry methods.

Dietary compliance. The dairy group received dairy products weekly. Each girl selected dairy products under the guidance of the clinical research center dietary staff to meet the minimal requirement of 1200 mg calcium daily. After each girl was given a list of dairy products of varied calcium and fat content, she chose which product she wanted. Any girl who failed to meet two consecutive weekly dietary calcium intakes of 1200 mg daily was dropped from the study. Each product was specially labeled to deter other family members from using the subject's supplements. Known amounts of dairy foods were delivered weekly, and all unused products were removed and counted. All subjects were required to record a 3-day dietary history and food frequency at the beginning and after 3, 6, 9, and 12 months of study.

Procedures. Dietary records were analyzed for total calories, calcium, phosphate, protein, fats, and vitamin D by computer software dietary programs based on U.S. Department of Agriculture handbooks and tables (MacDiet Professional, Philadelphia, Pa.). Biochemical analyses were performed as previously described.[13] Bone mineral status was determined by single-beam photon absorptiometry (SP-2 scanner; Lunar Radiation Corp., Madison, Wis.) and dual-energy x-ray absorptiometry (DEXA, XR-26 system; Norland Corp., Fort Atkinson, Wis.). With the single-beam method, the bone mineral content of the distal third of the subject's nondominant radius was measured. The accuracy error for bone mineral analyses is 2% to 4%.[14] The day-to-day error rate in infants and adults is 2.5% with the single-beam method. With the DEXA method, the subject's lean body mass, body fat, total body mineral content, and femoral neck and lumbar bone densities were measured. The DEXA method accuracy error for calcium, fat, and lean body mass averages 4.5%. The coefficient of variation for repeated scans of the lumbar spine is 1.8%. The long-term precision error for this method is 1%.[15]

Statistical analyses. Differences in weight, height, bone, and body composition between the control and dairy groups were tested by repeated measures of analyses of variance,

Table II. Daily dietary intakes

	Control group	Dairy group	p
Total calories	1403 ± 396	1464 ± 244	NS
Protein (gm)	52 ± 16	70 ± 16	0.0003
Fat (gm)	48 ± 17	51 ± 12	NS
%Total calories	31 ± 11	31 ± 7	NS
Saturated fats (gm)	14 ± 7	18 ± 8	NS
Vitamin D (IU)	128 ± 68	288 ± 95	0.0001
Calcium (mg)	728 ± 321	1437 ± 366	0.0001
Phosphorus (mg)	875 ± 318	1417 ± 340	0.0001

Values (except *p* values) are expressed as mean ± SD.
NS, Not significant.

and *t* tests with the Bonferroni corrections were used to compare categorical differences between the two groups. The correlations between variables were analyzed with regression analyses. All *p* values were two tailed.

RESULTS

Subjects. Mean ages (±SD) in the two groups were similar at the start of the study. Weights and heights were also similar at the start and end of the study. The percentages of gains in weight and height were not different between the groups (Table I). There were no differences in activity between the groups during the study. Only two girls from the dairy group failed to complete the study, and their data were not used in the final analyses.

Dietary intakes. At the start of the study, there were no differences in dietary intakes of calories, protein, fat, calcium, phosphate, and vitamin D between the groups. Daily average total calories and fat intake were similar between the two groups, but the protein, vitamin D, calcium, and phosphorus intakes were different (Table II). The experimental group received a significantly higher intake of calories (40% ± 10% vs 17% ± 9%), protein (51% ± 10% vs 27% ± 14%), phosphorus (68% ± 8% vs 41% ± 15%), fat (42% ± 14% vs 25% ± 16%), and saturated fats (60% ± 16% vs 43% ± 22%) from dairy products than the control subjects received. The most frequent dairy products selected were 2% milk, skim milk, American cheese, and then 2% chocolate milk, followed by regular fruit yogurt.

Bone mineral status, lean body mass, and percentage of body fat (Table III). There were no differences between the two groups during the study in bone mineral values, lean body mass, or percentage of body fat. The gains or increases in bone mineral density of the radius and femoral neck and in lean body mass were similar between the two groups. However, the dairy group had higher gains in lumbar bone density and total body bone mineral content (Figs. 1 and 2). The average dietary calcium ($r = 0.42$; $p < 0.01$), phosphate ($r = 0.39$; $p < 0.01$), vitamin D ($r = 0.32$; $p < 0.01$), and protein ($r = 0.36$; $p < 0.01$) intakes, but not those of fat or calories, were associated with the gains in total body bone mineral at the end of the study. The gain in the lumbar bone density was associated only with the averages of dietary calcium and vitamin D intakes ($r = 0.37$ for dietary calcium, $r = 0.41$ for vitamin D; $p < 0.01$). The girls' lean body mass was not associated with any of the dietary nutrients.

Table III. Bone mineral status, lean body mass, and percentage of body fat

	Control group	Dairy group
Baseline		
Total body bone mineral (gm)	1508 ± 167	1490 ± 291
Lumbar spine bone density (gm/cm^2)	0.665 ± 0.077	0.633 ± 0.096
Lean body mass (kg)	26.2 ± 3.3	24.7 ± 3.9
%Body fat	28.9 ± 6.4	29.7 ± 8.9
At 12 mo		
Total body bone mineral (gm)	1617 ± 152	1695 ± 317
Lumbar spine bone density (gm/cm^2)	0.748 ± 0.084	0.772 ± 0.086
Lean body mass (kg)	30.0 ± 3.3	29.0 ± 4.1
%Body fat	30.1 ± 6.0	31.3 ± 9.3

Values are expressed as mean ± SD.

Biochemical analyses. There were no differences in serum or urinary biochemical values between the two groups at the start or end of the study. The two groups did not differ in serum calcium, magnesium, phosphate, alkaline phosphatase, 25-hydroxyvitamin D, 1,25-dihydroxyvitamin D, and albumin levels. The urinary calcium/creatinine ratios and hydroxyproline values were similar. All values were within the normal range.

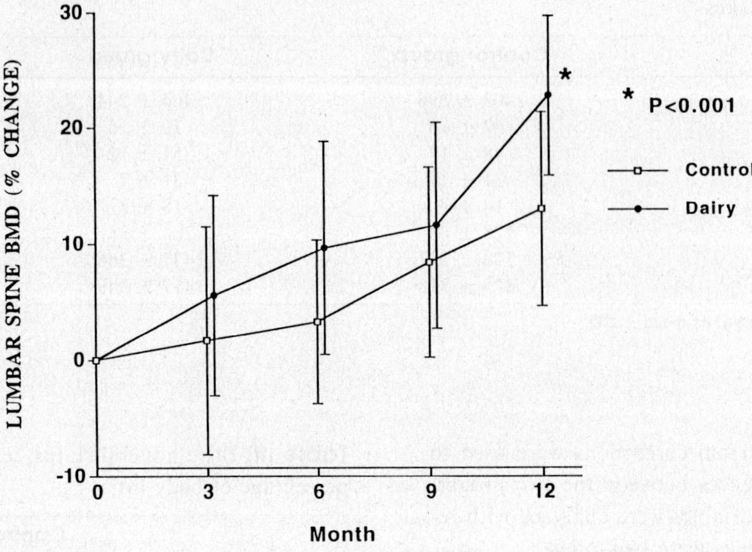

Fig. 1. Lumbar spine bone density change in the two groups. The dairy group had a higher percentage of change than the control group. Means and standard deviations are presented.

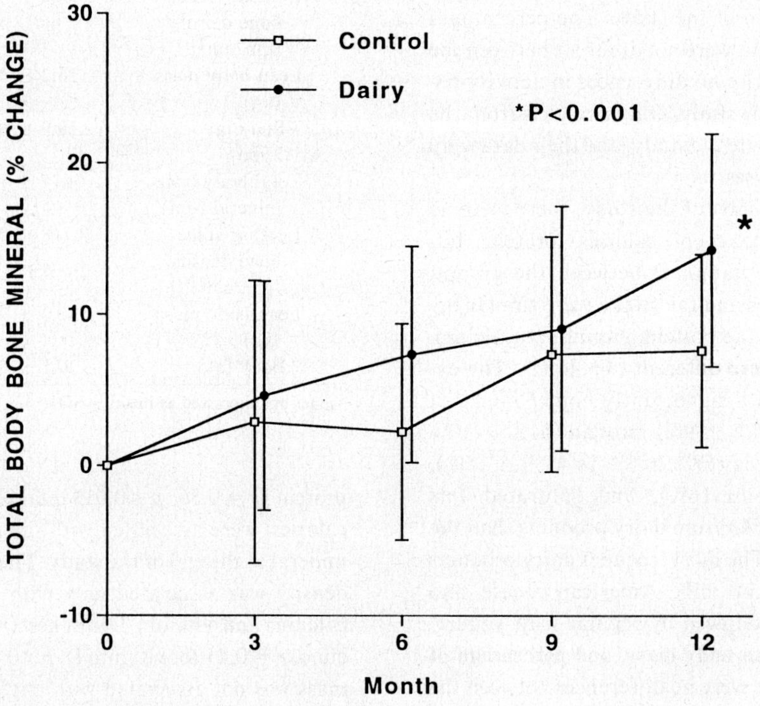

Fig. 2. Total body bone mineral change in the two groups. The dairy group had a higher percentage of change than the control group. Means and standard deviations are shown.

DISCUSSION

Our study shows that when pubertal girls supplement their diet with dairy products to the recommended dietary allowance for calcium of 1200 mg daily, the calcium, phosphorus, vitamin D, and protein intakes increase over those of control girls. However, there is concern that dairy products may contribute to a higher fat intake.[16, 17] In this study, fat intake was similar in both groups and represented approximately 30% of total calories, as currently recommended,[18] even when the girls were free to choose dairy products with different fat content. Body fat of the girls from both groups was also the same during this study. The saturated fat intake was not different in both groups, though dairy products contributed 60% to the dairy group's saturated fats in comparison with 43% to those of the control girls.

It is difficult to determine which nutrient or combination of nutrients was responsible for the gain in bone density in these girls. Dietary calcium, phosphorus, vitamin D, and protein intakes were associated with lumbar bone density and total body bone mineral. Dairy products supplied the majority of these nutrients. Several studies have indicated the relationship of calcium intake to bone mineral status in children.[3, 5, 19, 20] Two reports of studies using calcium supplementation in the form of tablets showed improvement in bone mineralization in children.[3, 20] In a clinical trial of monozygotic prepubertal male and female twins, supplementation of the diet of one group of twins with calcium citrate malate to an average of 1612 mg/day significantly increased bone mineral density of the radius (5.1%), spine (2.8%), and proximal portion of the femur (3.2%) over the values for control twins, who averaged 900 mg/day after 3 years.[3] The differences in response to calcium in this study compared with our study are that the majority of the twins were younger (average age, 9 years) and more immature (Tanner stage 1), and included both girls and boys.

Phosphate intake was associated with improved bone mineralization in this study. Excess phosphorus in nonprimates has accelerated bone resorption, leading to osteoporosis.[21] In human studies, supplemental phosphorus has been shown to have little effect on bone mineralization.[22, 23] It appears that calcium intake is a more important factor in bone mineralization than phosphate intake in a normal diet.[22, 24]

In our study, vitamin D intake was associated with bone mineralization. Adequate vitamin D status is necessary for calcium intestinal absorption and bone formation. Most of the dietary vitamin D was derived from dairy sources in both of our groups. Despite the higher intake in the dairy group, the vitamin D status of the girls, as reflected by the similar 25-hydroxyvitamin D levels, was the same.

In this study, dietary protein intake also was associated with bone mineral status. The mean protein intake from both groups was above the recommended dietary allowance of 46 gm protein daily. High protein intake has produced negative calcium balance from increased urinary calcium excretion if phosphate intake is kept low, but if the phosphate intake increases with the protein intake, the effect of a high protein intake on calcium metabolism is minimized.[25, 26] In adults, dietary protein intake has little effect on calcium absorption and metabolism.[27] The dietary calcium/protein ratio may be important in achieving a positive calcium balance; the suggested ratio is at least 16:1.[28, 29] In our study the dairy group had a ratio of 21:1, which favored calcium retention, whereas the ratio for the control group was 14:1, which may not be adequate. Dairy foods favor calcium retention because of their abundance of calcium relative to protein (36:1).[29]

We conclude that young girls who increased their dairy consumption had improved calcium, phosphorus, vitamin D, and protein intakes. For 1 year, these girls had significant gains in their total body bone mineral and lumbar bone density. Increased dairy consumption did not increase total or saturated fat intake and was not associated with weight gain or increased body fat. We believe that increased dairy consumption by young girls should be encouraged for improved bone mineralization and for better bone health to prevent adult osteoporosis.

REFERENCES

1. Science and Health Administration. Food and nutrition intakes of individuals in 1 day in the United States. Washington, D.C.: U.S. Department of Agriculture, 1980.
2. Barger-Lux M, Heaney R, Packard P, Lappe J, Recker R. Nutritional correlates of low calcium intake. Clin Appl Nutr 1992;2:39-44.
3. Johnston CJ, Miller JZ, Slemenda CW, et al. Calcium supplementation and increases in bone mineral density in children [see comments]. N Engl J Med 1992;327:82-7.
4. Matkovic V, Ilich J. Calcium requirements for growth: are current recommendations adequate? Nutr Rev 1993;51:171-80.
5. Matkovic V, Fontana D, Tominac C, Goel P, Chesnut CH. Factors that influence peak bone mass information: a study of calcium balance and the inheritance of bone mass in adolescent females. Am J Clin Nutr 1990;52:878-88.
6. Matkovic V. Calcium metabolism and calcium requirements during skeletal modeling and consolidation of bone mass. Am J Clin Nutr 1991;54:245S-60S.
7. Matkovic V, Heaney RP. Calcium balance during human growth: evidence for threshold behavior. Am J Clin Nutr 1992;55:992-6.
8. Food and Nutrition Board. Recommended dietary allowances; vol 284. 10th ed. Washington, D.C.: National Academy Press, 1989.
9. Khan MA. Observations on beverage preferences of college students at specific times. J Am Diet Assoc 1980;77:56.
10. Massey LK, Strang MM. Soft drink consumption, phosphorus intake, and osteoporosis. Perspectives in Practice 1982; 80:581-3.
11. Sandler RB, Slemenda CW, LaPorte RE, et al. Postmenopausal bone density and milk consumption in childhood and adolescence. Am J Clin Nutr 1985;42:270-4.
12. Hamill P, Drizd T, Johnson C, Reed R, Roche A, Moore W. Physical growth: National Center for Health Statistics percentiles. Am J Clin Nutr 1979;32:607-29.
13. Chan G, McMurry M, Westover K, Engelbert-Fenton K, Thomas R. The effects of increased dietary calcium intake upon

the calcium and bone mineral status of lactating adolescent and adult women. Am J Clin Nutr 1987;46:319-23.
14. Cameron J, Mazess R, Sorenson J. Precision and accuracy of bone mineral determination by direct photon absorptiometry. Invest Radiol 1968;3:141-50.
15. Chan GM. Performance of dual-energy x-ray absorptiometry in evaluating bone, lean body mass, and fat in pediatric subjects. J Bone Miner Res 1992;7:369-74.
16. American Academy of Pediatrics, Committee on Nutrition. Prudent lifestyle for children: dietary fat and cholesterol. Pediatrics 1986;78:521-5.
17. Health Nutrition Information Service. Nationwide food consumption survey: continuing survey of food intakes by individuals, women 19-50 years and their children 1-5 years, 4 days, 1986. Washington, D.C.: U.S. Department of Agriculture, 1988.
18. Nutrition Research Council. Implications for reducing chronic disease risk: report of the Committee on Diet and Health, Food and Nutrition Board; vol 750. Washington, D.C.: National Academy Press, 1989.
19. Chan G. Calcium and bone mineral status in infant's and children's nutrition. In: Lebenthal E, ed. Textbook of gastroenterology and nutrition in infancy. 2nd ed. New York: Raven Press, 1989:403-12.
20. Lloyd T, Andon M, Rollings N, et al. Calcium supplementation and bone mineral density in adolescent girls. JAMA 1993;270:841-4.
21. Draper H, Bell R. In: Draper H, ed. Advances in nutrition research; vol 2. New York: Plenum Press, 1977:23-37.
22. Wical K, Burssee P. Effects of a calcium and vitamin D supplement on alveolar ridge resorption in immediate denture patients. J Prosthet Dent 1979;41:4-8.
23. Rasmussen H, Bordier P, Marie P, et al. Effect of combined therapy with phosphate and calcitonin on bone volume in osteoporosis. Metabolic Bone Disease and Related Research 1980;2:107-12.
24. Spencer H, Kramer L, Rubio N, Osis D. The effect of phosphorus on endogenous fecal calcium excretion in man. Am J Clin Nutr 1986;43:844-51.
25. Hegsted D, Schuette S, Zemel M, Linkswiler H. Urinary calcium and calcium balance in young men as affected by level of protein and phosphorus intake. J Nutr 1981;111:553-62.
26. Schuette S, Linkswiler H. Effects on Ca and P metabolism in humans by adding meat, meat plus milk, or purified proteins plus Ca and P to a low protein diet. J Nutr 1982;112:338-49.
27. Spencer H, Kramer L, Osis D, Morris C. Effect of a high protein (meat) intake on calcium metabolism in man. Am J Clin Nutr 1978;31:2167-72.
28. Heaney R. Nutritional factors in osteoporosis. Ann Rev Nutr 1993;13:287-316.
29. Heaney R. Protein intake and the calcium economy. J Am Diet Assoc 1993;93:1259-60.

Mineral homeostasis and bone mass at diagnosis in children with acute lymphoblastic leukemia

Jacqueline M. Halton, MD, Stephanie A. Atkinson, PhD, Laurence Fraher, PhD, Colin E. Webber, PhD, W. Peter Cockshott, MB,ChB, MD,† Cherk Tam, MD, and Ronald D. Barr, MB,ChB, MD

From the Departments of Pediatrics, Radiology, and Nuclear Medicine, McMaster University, Hamilton, Ontario; Research Institute, St. Joseph's Hospital, University of Western Ontario, London; and Queen Elizabeth Hospital, University of Toronto, Toronto, Ontario, Canada

Objective: **To determine whether the osteopenia and unusual fractures observed in children with acute lymphoblastic leukemia (ALL) were related to the disease rather than to its treatment.**
Design: **Prospective analysis of the bone and mineral status in 40 consecutive children with ALL seen in a pediatric tertiary-care referral center.**
Methods: **Biochemical indicators of mineral, endocrine, and vitamin D status were measured before initiation of therapy. Bone mass was determined radiographically and by dual-photon absorptiometry of the lumbar region of the spine (L2-L4). Correlations between clinical observations, leukemia variables, bone mass, and biochemical assessment were determined.**
Results: **At the time of diagnosis musculoskeletal pain was present in 36% of patients and was more common in children with CD10-positive leukemia and leukocyte counts less than 20 $\times$ 10^9 cells/L. Radiographic evidence of osteopenia and fractures was observed in 13% and 10% of children, respectively. The mean bone mineral content was normal. Bone mass measurement *z* scores correlated with plasma 1,25-dihydroxyvitamin D_3 concentrations ($r = 0.43$, $p < 0.05$). Plasma calcium, magnesium, phosphorus, and 25-hydroxyvitamin D_3 levels were normal. Low plasma osteocalcin (mean $\pm$ SD, 1.6 $\pm$ 1.6 nmol/L) and 1,25-dihydroxyvitamin D_3 (33.4 $\pm$ 26.4 pmol/L) values were observed. Parathyroid hormone levels were low in 14% of children. Hypercalciuria was detected in 64% of children. Urinary deoxypyridinoline was lower ($p < 0.01$) than in age-matched control subjects. Histomorphometric measurements of iliac bone showed abnormalities in mineralization in the biopsy specimens from three of nine children.**
Conclusion: **Most children with ALL have alterations in bone metabolism and bone mass when first examined. These data suggest defective mineralization as the mechanism for decreased bone mass and implicate the leukemic process as causative. (J PEDIATR 1995;126:557-64)**

Supported by a grant from the Hospital for Sick Children Foundation, Toronto, Ontario, Canada. Dr. Halton held a Fellowship from the National Institute of Nutrition (Canada). Dr. Atkinson received a Career Scientist Award at McMaster University from the Ontario Ministry of Health. Dr. Fraher received a University Scholar's Award from the National Institute of Nutrition (Canada).

Submitted for publication Jan. 10, 1994; accepted Nov. 28, 1994.

Reprint requests: Stephanie Atkinson, PhD, Department of Pediatrics, McMaster University, 1200 Main St. West, Room 3V42, Hamilton, Ontario, Canada L8N 3Z5.

†Deceased.

0022-3476/95/$3.00 + 0 **9/20/62346**

We reported previously on abnormalities of mineral homeostasis and bone mass in children during treatment for acute lymphoblastic leukemia.[1] These observations were associated with clinical symptoms of musculoskeletal pain, disturbances of gait, and unusual fractures. Some children were in a debilitated state requiring confinement to a wheelchair. The cause of the observed abnormalities in bone structure in children with ALL is not known. We hypothesized that changes in bone mineral mass were associated with disturbances in mineral and vitamin D metabolism, and that both the disease state and the intensive chemotherapy contributed to the pathologic findings.

To determine whether the described abnormalities were present at diagnosis and related to the leukemic process rather than to its treatment, we prospectively assessed children seen consecutively at the time of diagnosis of ALL for alterations in biochemical mineral status and bone mass.

METHODS

Patients. Forty consecutive children (27 boys, 13 girls; aged, 0.3 to 17 years; median age, 3.9 years) with newly diagnosed ALL who were attending the hematology/oncology service in the Children's Hospital at Chedoke-McMaster, Hamilton, Ontario, were assigned a risk for relapse according to the Dana-Farber Cancer Institute criteria[2]: 18 were at standard risk, 16 at high risk, and 6 at very high risk. Children with B-cell leukemia (French-American-British classification L_3 morphologic features) were excluded. Informed consent was obtained from the children's parents for collection of blood and urine, for bone biopsy, and for bone densitometry. The study protocol was approved by the McMaster University Faculty of Health Sciences Research Ethics and Project Review Board.

ALL	Acute lymphoblastic leukemia
BMC	Bone mineral content
BMD	Bone mineral density
CALLA	Common acute lymphoblastic leukemia antigen
25-OHD$_3$	25-Hydroxyvitamin D$_3$
1,25(OH)$_2$D$_3$	1,25-Dihydroxyvitamin D$_3$
PTH	Parathyroid hormone

Clinical assessment. Physical examination, with special attention to height, weight, musculoskeletal symptoms, and gait abnormalities, was performed on admission. In addition, parents completed a pain questionnaire to determine the location and severity of musculoskeletal symptoms. Descriptive data included age at diagnosis, leukocyte count, morphologic and immunologic type of leukemia, risk category, and duration of symptoms before diagnosis.

Radiography. Anteroposterior views of the hips, knees, and ankles were reviewed by one of us (P. C.) without prior knowledge of the patients.

Bone mineral mass. Bone mineral content and bone mineral density of the lumbar vertebrae (L2 to L4) were measured with a model 2600 dichromatic densitometer with a gadolinium 153 radioisotope source (Norland Inc., Fort Atkinson, Wisc.). The BMC and BMD of the subjects were compared with normative standards established by our group for children in southwestern Ontario[3]; this comparison was computed as a proportion of the reference SD or *z* score to allow comparison across genders and at all ages.

Biochemistry. Mineral status was assessed by measurements of blood and urine before any therapy. Children with an excoriated perineum who were still in diapers were excluded from urine collections. Plasma and urine levels of calcium and magnesium were determined after dilution by standard atomic absorption spectrophotometry,[4] blood ionized calcium and pH by ion-selective electrodes (ICal; Radiometer, Copenhagen, Denmark), phosphorus by a modification of the method of Fiske and Subbarow,[5] alkaline phosphatase by a modification of the method of Bowers and McComb,[6] and creatinine by the double-slide method with the Ektakem 700 instrument (Eastman Kodak Co., Rochester, N.Y.). Parathyroid hormone was measured in the laboratory of one of us (L. F.) by a two-site immunoradiometric assay (N-tact PTH IRMA Kit, Incstar Corp., Stillwater, Minn.). Plasma 25-hydroxyvitamin D$_3$ and 1,25-dihydroxyvitamin D$_3$ were analyzed by high-pressure liquid chromatography and radiochemical assays.[7] Osteocalcin was measured by radioimmunoassay in the laboratory of Dr. Caren Gundberg.[8] Deoxypyridinoline in urine was measured according to the procedure of Black et al.[9] Aliquots of 24-hour urine collections were hydrolyzed with 11.1 mol/L hydrochloric acid at high temperatures and then prefractionated by reverse phase–column chromatography. Appropriate fractions were lyophilized and subjected to high-pressure liquid chromatography before fluorometric analysis of the deoxypyridinoline crosslinks.

Histomorphometry. Bone biopsy was performed during anesthesia at the time of bone marrow biopsy for diagnostic purposes in the final nine consecutive patients recruited for the study. A 3.3 mm core posterior iliac bone biopsy was performed with a Vilaghy-Zellerman bone biopsy needle.[10] Biopsy samples were fixed in 10% formalin, with pH adjusted to 7.4. Sections were cut and stained with Masson trichrome stain. Five morphologic measurements were done: the relative bone volume (the percentage of bone sectional area occupied by bone matrix), unmineralized bone matrix (osteoid) as percentage of total matrix volume, the thickness of osteoid tissue on the bone trabecula (osteoid width), and the formation surface (surface covered by osteoid tissue and the resorption surface as percentage of total trabecular surface). All histomorphometry findings were assessed by one of us (C. T.).

Statistics. Data are expressed as mean ± SD. Twenty-four-hour urinary excretion of mineral/creatinine ratios is expressed as median and range. Pearson correlation coefficients were used for statistical analysis, and p values less than 0.05 were considered statistically significant. Correlations between clinical observations, bone mass, and biochemical assessments were analyzed by Blossom Stat-Pack, version 2.0A (Bethesda, Md.).

RESULTS

Clinical assessment. At diagnosis all 40 children were within normal percentiles for height and weight for age (mean height, 111.3 cm; range, 67.5 to 174 cm; mean weight, 20.58 kg, range, 6.37 to 59 kg).[11] Of the 40 children, 14 had musculoskeletal pain. Lower extremity pain occurred in all children and was more frequent than pain in the upper extremity (three subjects) and spinal locations (one subject). Children with musculoskeletal symptoms had a longer duration from onset of illness to diagnosis (mean, 6.5 weeks) compared with those without (mean, 2.5 weeks; $r = 0.46, p < 0.05$). Most children (9/11) with musculoskeletal pain involving more than two sites had leukocyte counts less than 20×10^9 cells/L (20,000/mm^3), and all had expression of CD10 (CALLA). No musculoskeletal symptoms were observed in the five children with leukocyte counts greater than 100×10^9 cells/L (100,000/mm^3) (T cell type, n = 3; null cell type, n = 2).

Gait abnormalities were present in 13 children. Five children were not examined because they were unable to perform weight-bearing activities because of pain or fracture, and one child was less than 1 year of age.

Radiography. Skeletal abnormalities were present in 21 of 40 children; the most common was metaphyseal lucencies (Table I).

Bone mineral mass. Bone density measurements were not obtained in 12 children because of movement artifact (n = 4), critical illness (n = 3), or receipt of corticosteroids for more than 2 weeks before baseline assessment (n = 5). Five of our patients with ALL had significant reductions in BMD; yet only two of these five had radiographic evidence of osteopenia (Figure). The mean z scores for BMC and BMD, respectively, were −0.28 and −0.16 in boys and −0.03 and −0.76 in girls, before the initiation of chemotherapy. Two children with spontaneous fractures (vertebral and bilateral femoral compression fractures) had reduced BMD ($z = -1.06, -0.4$), but only one had osteopenia. Two children with fractures after trauma had normal bone mass (z for BMD = 0.09, 0.05).

Biochemistry. The biochemical measurements of mineral status are summarized in Table II. One child had hypercalcemia (ionic calcium, 1.41 mmol/L); he had severe osteopenia and two vertebral compression fractures. Osteocalcin values were less than the normal range for age in 87% (27/33) of prepubertal children (<9 years) and in two of seven adolescents. The children had normal vitamin D status indicated by circulating 25-OHD_3 concentrations. In contrast, the majority of children had low circulating 1,25$(OH)_2D_3$ levels. In eight children 1,25$(OH)_2D_3$ was in the low normal range (48 to 62.4 pmol/L [20 to 26 pg/ml]) and only two children had normal 1,25$(OH)_2D_3$ concentrations (91.2 and 139 pmol/L [38 and 58 pg/ml]). In 64% of patients (21/33) calcium excretion exceeded the upper limit of normal on the basis of urinary calcium/creatinine ratio, and 34% (11/32) of patients had excessive magnesium excretion (Table III). Deoxypyridinoline excretion was reduced significantly when compared with that in 20 age-matched control subjects.

Table I. Radiologic examination: Skeletal abnormalities at diagnosis*

	Patients	
Skeletal abnormality	No.	% Total
Metaphyseal lucency	11/40	28
Dense bands	7/40	18
Periosteal reaction	1/40	3
Sclerotic lesion	1/40	3
Osteopenia	5/40	13
Fracture†	4/40	10

*Present in 21 of 40 children.
†Includes vertebral compression fracture, femoral impaction fracture (two patients), and tibial fracture.

There was no significant correlation between classifications of leukemia, leukemic burden (leukocyte count), or time to diagnosis, and altered bone mass and bone minerals (Table IV). Osteocalcin values correlated positively with age. We observed a negative correlation between BMC and age.

There was no significant correlation between bone mass and bone formation measurement (osteocalcin) or bone resorption measurement (urinary deoxypyridinoline) (Table V). Bone mass measurements of the metabolically active trabecular lumbar vertebrae correlated directly with plasma 1,25$(OH_2)D_3$ level. There was a negative correlation of BMD and urinary calcium excretion.

Serum magnesium correlated positively with PTH and 1,25$(OH)_2D_3$ and negatively with urinary calcium excretion (Table VI).

Histomorphometry. The relative bone volume ranged between 6% and 18.5% (SD = 3.9), the osteoid tissue between less than 0.5% and 23% (SD = 8.5), the osteoid width between 1 and 6.5 μm (SD = 2.0), the bone formation surface

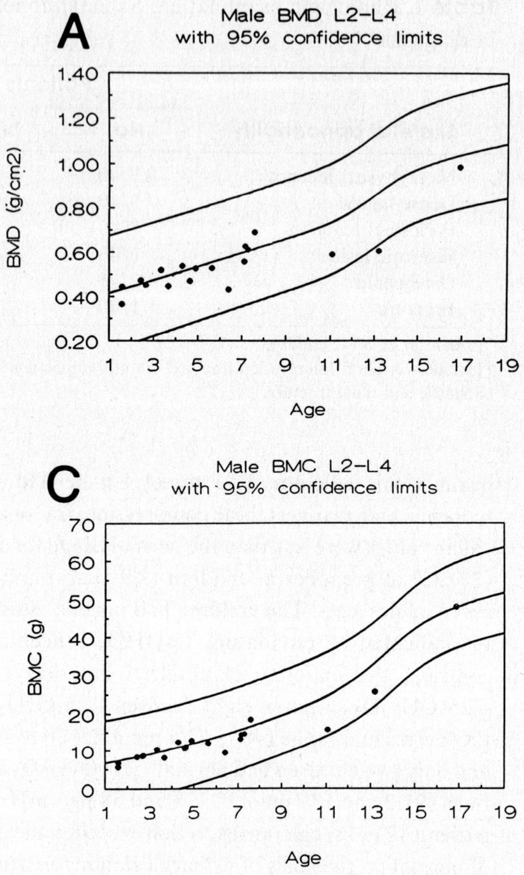

Figure. BMD for boys (**A**) and girls (**B**), and BMC for boys (**C**) and girls (**D**) at diagnosis of ALL. Normative bone mass measurements have been established at our institution for children more than 3 years of age.[13] Mean with 95% confidence intervals of these data are represented by *solid lines.*

between 2.9% and 55.5% (SD = 18.4), and the resorptive surface between less than 0.5% and 5.7% (SD = 1.7). Although there were no age-matched control subjects for comparison, four children had obviously low relative bone volume (6%, 10%, 12.2%, and 13%). Three children had a high percentage of trabecular surface covered by osteoid tissue (34.4%, 44.0%, and 55.5%) with corresponding high percentage of bone matrix not mineralized (11.3%, 23%, and 20%, respectively).

DISCUSSION

The present study establishes that the disease process contributes causally to the abnormalities observed in bone, vitamin D, and mineral metabolism in children with ALL. The observation that musculoskeletal pain was more common in the children with longer duration of symptoms, with low leukocyte counts and with CALLA-positive immunologic phenotype remains unexplained.

The metabolically active sites of bone in children are at the ends of bones close to the metaphysis, where radiographic changes in ALL are observed commonly. The incidence of radiographic osteopenia in this series was 13%, consistent with previous reports.[15] However, radiography is a subjective and rather crude method of detecting bone loss. Dual-photon absorptiometry permits measurement of bone mass (BMC and BMD) at sites that consist predominantly of trabecular bone.[3, 16-19] In our study bone mass appeared to be negatively affected by reduced concentrations of circulating $1,25(OH)_2D_3$ and an elevated urinary excretion of calcium.

Although seven children had somewhat reduced spinal BMD at diagnosis, the association between the BMD and radiographic evidence of osteopenia and fractures was inconsistent. This may reflect regional differences in bone loss in growing children. Reduced bone mass is a major concern because evidence is good that fractures result from low bone mass,[20] and studies in women suggest that bone mass predicts the probability of future fracture.[21] In addi-

Table II. Biochemical measures of mineral, endocrine, and vitamin D status

Plasma and serum measurements	Value at diagnosis*	Normal reference range
Total Ca		
(mmol/L)	2.3 ± 0.2 (2.04-2.85)	2.2-2.5 (Meites[12])
(mg/dL)	9.2 ± 0.8	8.8-10
Ionic Ca		
(mmol/L)	1.23 ± 0.08 (1.10-1.41)	1.19-1.28†
(mg/dl)	2.46 ± 0.16	2.38-2.24
Mg		
(mmol/L)	0.84 ± 0.09 (0.68-1.03)	0.77-0.93†
(mEq/L)	1.68 ± 0.18	1.54-1.86
P		
(mmol/L)	1.5 ± 0.4 (0.74-2.69)	1.0-1.5 (Meites[12])
(mg/dl)	4.6 ± 1.2	3.1-4.6
Alkaline phosphatase (U/L)	156 ± 62 (73-355)	146-362 (Meites[12])
Osteocalcin		
(nmol/L)	1.6 ± 1.6 (<0.2-6.8)	1.7-7.0
(ng/ml)	9.3 ± 9.2	10-40 (Cole et al.[13])
PTH		
(pmol/L)	2.0 ± 1.9 (0.1-7.4)	0.5-5.0
(pg/ml)	20.1 ± 19.6	3-50
25-OHD		
(nmol/L)	42.5 ± 38.0 (0-132)	12.5-125.0
(ng/ml)	17.0 ± 15.2	5-50 (Fraher et al.[7])
$1,25(OH)_2D$		
(pmol/L)	33.4 ± 26.4 (2.64-139.2)	48-156
(pg/ml)	13.9 ± 11.0	20-65 (Fraher et al.[7])

*Data are expressed as mean ± SD (range).
†Reference values for ionic calcium and magnesium are derived from an age-matched population of 19 children attending outpatient clinics for minor elective surgery at the Children's Hospital at Chedoke-McMaster.

tion, most protocols for treatment of ALL incorporate large doses of corticosteroids, which could reduce bone mass further and increase the risk for fractures.[22]

The histomorphometric evaluation of iliac crest biopsy specimens in a subset of the children suggests that there is undermineralization of bone in some children at the time of diagnosis. The high percentage of osteoid surface most likely reflects a delay in matrix mineralization. Tetracycline labeling will clarify this. The morphometric data do not reflect any acceleration in the bone resorptive process.

The reduced bone mass at the time of diagnosis may be the result of defective mineralization. We reported previously that during treatment for ALL in children hypomagnesemia, mild ionic hypocalcemia, and hypercalciuria occurred.[1] We speculated that these abnormalities in mineral metabolism were induced by one or more of the chemotherapeutic agents. In the present study, conducted at the time of diagnosis, plasma magnesium and calcium levels were normal in the group as a whole, but 18% had hypomagnesemia. For this subset it appears that low magnesium concentrations may be responsible for the low PTH levels (14%) and reduced production of $1,25(OH)_2D_3$.

Table III. Twenty-four–hour urinary excretion of mineral or deoxypyridinoline/creatinine ratio (in millimoles)

Ratio	Initial study	Normal reference range
Ca/creatinine	0.05-3.36 (0.62)*	0.26-0.48 (ref. 14)
Mg/creatinine	0.02-1.44 (0.81)*	0.52-0.94 (ref. 14)
Deoxypyridinoline/creatinine (mean ± SD)	33.7 ± 17.7†	49.8 ± 16.7‡

*Data expressed as range (median).
†$p < 0.01$; t test between values for children with ALL and age-matched control subjects.
‡Urinary deoxypyridinoline level in 20 age-matched control subjects.

Despite the normocalcemia overall, 69% of the children had excessive excretion of urinary calcium. The cause of the hypercalciuria may reflect calcium losses through bone resorption, defective kidney reabsorption, or recent immobilization. Hypercalciuria, hypermagnesiuria, and reduced $1,25(OH)_2D_3$ level suggest a possible kidney defect. However, subsequent studies by our group have shown no

Table IV. Correlation coefficients *(r)* and significance values *(p)* for leukemia variables and age versus *z* scores for bone mass, $1,25(OH)_2D_3$, and osteocalcin

	z Scores							
	BMC (n = 28)		BMD (n = 28)		$1,25(OH)_2D_3$ (n = 40)		Osteocalcin (n = 40)	
Variable	*r*	*p*	*r*	*p*	*r*	*p*	*r*	*p*
Leukocytes	−0.140	NS	−0.120	NS	−0.014	NS	0.085	NS
Immunologic phenotype (T, null, pre-B, CALLA)	−0.128	NS	0.013	NS	−0.026	NS	−0.070	NS
Risk category (standard, high, very high)	−0.126	NS	−0.080	NS	−0.112	NS	0.022	NS
Age (yr)	−0.425	<0.05	−0.100	NS	−0.150	NS	0.401	<0.01

NS, Not significant.

Table V. Correlation coefficients *(r)* and and significance values *(p)* for *z* scores for BMC and BMD versus osteocalcin, $1,25(OH)_2D_3$, urinary deoxypyridinoline/creatinine ratio, and urinary calcium/creatinine ratio

	z Score			
	BMC		BMD	
Variable (n)	*r*	*p*	*r*	*p*
Osteocalcin (28)	−0.118	NS	0.001	NS
$1,25(OH)_2D_3$ (28)	0.434	<0.05	0.383	<0.05
Urinary deoxypyridinoline/creatinine ratio (22)	0.280	NS	−0.130	NS
Urinary Ca^{++}/creatinine ratio (21)	−0.360	NS	−0.690	<0.01

NS, Not significant.

Table VI. Correlation coefficient *(r)* and significance values *(p)* for mineral and endocrine status

	Ca^{++}		Mg^{++}		PTH		$1,25(OH)_2D_3$		Urinary Ca^{++}/creatinine ratio	
Variable (n)	*r*	*p*	*r*	*p*	*r*	*p*	*r*	*p*	*r*	*p*
Ca^{++} (40)										
Mg^{++} (40)	−0.160	NS								
PTH (40)	−0.010	NS	0.516	<0.01						
$1,25(OH)_2D_3$ (40)	0.103	NS	0.519	<0.01	0.120	NS				
Urinary Ca^{++}/creatinine ratio (33)	0.200	NS	−0.340	<0.05	−0.370	NS	−0.220	NS		
Osteocalcin (40)	0.306	NS	0.020	NS	−0.040	NS	0.060	NS	−0.010	NS

NS, Not significant.

evidence of tubular dysfunction in children during treatment according to Dana-Farber Cancer Institute protocols, even during aminoglycoside therapy.[23]

The major metabolic abnormalities at onset were the strikingly low concentration of the active metabolite $1,25(OH)_2D_3$ and the low plasma osteocalcin level. As the major endocrine regulator of calcium and phosphorus, $1,25(OH)_2D_3$ acts as a hormone to stimulate intestinal absorption of calcium and phosphorus, bone resorption, and renal tubular reabsorption of calcium.[24] The active hormone $1,25(OH)_2D_3$ is also responsible for the synthesis of osteocalcin.[25] Thus in the present study the low plasma $1,25(OH)_2D_3$ level may be responsible for the low plasma osteocalcin values. Osteocalcin, a protein synthesized by osteoblasts, is an indicator of bone formation.[26] In bone resorptive states there is an increased urinary excretion of deoxypyridinoline, a breakdown product of type I collagen that is specific for bone and dentin.[27] Children with ALL at diagnosis do not have an excessive amount of bone resorption; the majority have abnormally low levels of deoxypyridinoline in the urine. However, 10 children had normal deoxypyridinoline values in the presence of low osteocalcin values. If normal bone resorption continues in the presence of decreased bone formation, the result would be an overall decrease in bone mass.

Why circulating $1,25(OH)_2D_3$ is selectively reduced in children with ALL is not known. Recent findings on the immunobiologic functions of vitamin D[28] and the binding of $1,25(OH)_2D_3$ to lymphoblasts[29] may be of some relevance to our observation of depressed concentrations of this active metabolite. Monocytes and macrophages are potential sites of synthesis of $1,25(OH)_2D_3$, but this may be curtailed in immunosuppressed patients.[28] Receptor-mediated binding of $1,25(OH)_2D_3$ to the leukemic lymphoblasts[29] may deplete circulating concentration of the active hormone further, resulting in the alterations in bone mineral status. However, we found no correlation between levels of $1,25(OH)_2D_3$ in the plasma and the leukocyte count at diagnosis (as a reflection of leukemic cell mass). Other possible mechanisms are down-regulation of the 1α-hydroxylation step, to produce the active metabolite from $25\text{-}OHD_3$, or up-regulation of metabolism to inactive products. Further studies are required, to determine the role of the reduced concentrations of $1,25(OH)_2D_3$ in the alteration of bone mass observed in children with ALL.

Receptors for $1,25(OH)_2D_3$ have been shown on immature lymphoid leukemic cells irrespective of morphologic classification.[29] Binding of $1,25(OH)_2D_3$ to receptors on immature lymphoid leukemic cells is significantly higher than that of normal mature lymphocytes.[29] We found no difference in plasma $1,25(OH)_2D_3$ among the various morphologic (L1, L2) or immunologic (T, null, pre-B, CALLA) types of leukemia. Eighty percent of childhood ALL develops as a result of monoclonal proliferation of B-cell precursors with B-lymphocyte lineage antigens being expressed sequentially (CD34 Ia, CD19, CD10, CD20, $C\mu$, Slg). In our study plasma $1,25(OH)_2D_3$ concentrations were uniformly low and did not reflect a particular maturational arrest in the B-lymphocyte lineage.

We conclude that most children with ALL have alterations in bone metabolism and bone mass when first seen. Abnormally low circulating $1,25(OH)_2D_3$ levels associated with hypercalciuria, may result in calcium and phosphate depletion, limiting bone mineralization. Serial assessments are ongoing to determine whether these initial abnormalities are prognostic indicators for the debilitating bone disease that has been observed in some children during treatment-maintained remission in ALL.[1]

REFERENCES

1. Atkinson SA, Fraher L, Gundberg CM, Andrew M, Pai M, Barr RD. Mineral homeostasis and diminished bone mass in children treated for acute lymphoblastic leukemia. J PEDIATR 1989;114:793-800.
2. Clavell LA, Gelber RD, Cohen HJ, et al. Four agent induction and intensive asparaginase therapy for treatment of childhood acute lymphoblastic leukemia. N Engl J Med 1986;315:657-63.
3. Atkinson SA, Halton JM, Hay J, Gordon C, Webber CE. Normative values for lumbar spine bone mass in children in relation to age, gender, dietary intake and physical activity [Abstract]. J Bone Miner Res 1991;6:A196, S132.
4. MacIntyre I. Flame photometry. Adv Clin Chem 1961;4:1-28.
5. Fiske CH, Subbarow Y. The colorimetric determination of phosphorus. J Biol Chem 1925;66:375-400.
6. Bowers GN, McComb RD. Measurement of total alkaline phosphatase activity in human serum. Clin Chem 1975; 21:1988-95.
7. Fraher LJ, Adami S, Clemens TL, Jones G, O'Riordan JLH. Radioimmunoassay of 1,25-dihydroxyvitamin D_2: studies on the metabolism of vitamin D_2 in man. Clin Endocrinol (Oxf) 1983;19:151-65.
8. Gundberg CM, Hauscka PV, Lian JB, Gallop PM. Osteocalcin: isolation, characterization and detection. Methods Enzymol 1972;107:516-44.
9. Black D, Duncan A, Robins SP. Quantitative analysis of the pyridinium crosslinks of collagen in urine using ion-paired reversed-phase high-performance liquid chromatography. Anal Biochem 1988;169:197-203.
10. Vilaghy MI. A bone biopsy instrument of new design. In: Fram R, Parfitt AM, Duncan H, eds. Clinical aspects of metabolic bone disease. Amsterdam: Excerpta Medica, 1973:152-3.
11. Hamill PVV, Drizd TA, Johnson CL, Reed RB, Roche AF, Moore WM. Physical growth: National Center for Health Statistics percentiles. Am J Clin Nutr 1979;32:607-29.
12. Meites S, ed. Pediatric clinical chemistry: a survey of reference (normal) values, methods and instrumentation, with commentary. 2nd ed. Washington, D.C.: American Association for Clinical Chemistry, 1981:69.
13. Cole DEC, Carpenter TO, Gundberg CM. Serum osteocalcin concentrations in children with metabolic bone disease. J PEDIATR 1985;106:770-6.
14. Ghazali S, Barratt TM. Urinary excretion of calcium and magnesium in children. Arch Dis Child 1974;49:97-101.
15. Rogalsky RJ, Black GB, Reed MH. Orthopaedic manifestations of leukemia in children. J Bone Joint Surg Am 1986;68A:494-501.
16. Glastre C, Braillon P, David L, Cochat P, Meunier PJ, Delmas PD. Measurement of bone mineral content of the lumbar spine by dual energy x-ray absorptiometry in normal children: correlations with growth parameters. J Clin Endocrinol Metab 1990;70:1330-3.
17. DeSchepper J, Derde MP, Van den Broeck M, Piepsz A, Jonckheer MH. Normative data for lumbar spine bone mineral content in children: influence of age, height, weight, and pubertal stage. J Nucl Med 1991;32:216-20.
18. Ponder SW, McCormick DP, Fawcett HD, Palmer JL, McKernan MG, Brouhard BH. Spinal bone mineral density in children aged 5.00 through 11.99 years. Am J Dis Child 1990; 144:1346-8.
19. Issenman RM, Atkinson SA, Radoja C, Fraher L. Longitudinal assessment of growth, mineral metabolism and bone mass in pediatric Crohn's disease. J Pediatr Gastro Nutr 1993; 17:401-6.

20. Seeley DG, Browner WS, Nevitt MC, and the Study of Osteoporotic Fractures Research Group. Which fractures are associated with low appendicular bone mass in elderly women? Ann Intern Med 1991;115:837-42.
21. Black DM, Cummings SR, Genant HK, et al. Axial and appendicular bone density predict fractures in older women. J Bone Miner Res 1992;7:633-8.
22. Lukert BP, Raisz LG. Glucocorticoid-induced osteoporosis: pathogenesis and management. Ann Intern Med 1990;112:352-64.
23. Wu B, Atkinson SA, Halton J, Barr RD. Nephrotoxicity by aminoglycosides is not a causative factor of hypomagnesemia in children with acute lymphoblastic leukemia [A287]. Ottawa: Canadian Federation of Biological Sciences, 1993;36:96.
24. Norman AW, Henry HL. Vitamin D: metabolism and mechanism of action. In: Favus MJ, ed. Primer on the metabolic bone diseases and disorders of mineral metabolism. New York: Raven Press, 1993:63-70.
25. Beresford JN, Gallagher JA, Poser JW, Russell RG. Production of osteocalcin by bone cells in vitro: effect of 1,25$(OH)_2D_3$, 24,25$(OH)_2D_3$ parathyroid hormone and glucocorticoids. Metab Bone Dis Relat Res 1984;5:229-34.
26. Price PA, Parthemore JG, Deftos LJ. New biochemical marker for bone metabolism: measurement by radioimmunoassay of bone GLA protein in the plasma of normal subjects and patients with bone disease. J Clin Invest 1980;66:878-83.
27. Uebelhart D, Gineyts E, Chapuy MC, Delmas PD. Urinary excretion of pyridinium crosslinks: a new marker of bone resorption in metabolic bone disease. Bone Miner 1990;8:87-96.
28. Reichel H, Koeffler HP, Norman AW. The role of vitamin D endocrine system in health and disease. N Engl J Med 1989; 320:980-91.
29. Feldman J, Federico MHH, Sonohara S, et al. Vitamin D_3 binding activity during leukemic cell differentiation. Leukemia Res 1993;17:97-101.

Pulmonary function abnormalities in Prader-Willi syndrome

Hákon Hákonarson, MD, Jay Moskovitz, MS, Karen L. Daigle, MD, Suzanne B. Cassidy, MD, and Michelle M. Cloutier, MD

From the Pediatric Pulmonary and Genetics Divisions, University of Connecticut, School of Medicine, Farmington, and the Department of Genetics, Case Western Reserve University and University Hospitals of Cleveland, Cleveland, Ohio

Objective: **To determine whether individuals with Prader-Willi syndrome (PWS) have abnormalities in pulmonary function as a result of thoracic muscle weakness.**
Design: **Testing of spirometry, flow-volume curves, lung volumes, and static respiratory pressures was performed in patients with PWS who are followed at the University of Connecticut. All tests were performed in triplicate on two or more occasions. Only reproducible tests were accepted. Established normative data were applied for all test results.**
Results: **A total of 18 male subjects (age, 17.9 ± 10.2 years (mean ± SD); range, 5-39 years) and 17 female subjects (age, 23.5 ± 13.0 years; range, 5-54 years) completed the tests. Forced vital capacity and forced expiratory volume in 1 second were reduced; the forced expiratory volume in 1 second/forced vital capacity ratio was normal, total lung capacity was in the low normal range, and residual volume was elevated. Maximum inspiratory (PI_{max}) and expiratory (PE_{max}) pressures were markedly reduced in 32 subjects tested. Fifteen subjects had PE_{max} values and 20 subjects had PI_{max} values <60 cm H_2O, respectively. There was a linear correlation between forced expiratory volume in 1 second and both PI_{max} and PE_{max} ($r = 0.71$; $r = 0.62$, respectively), and between forced vital capacity and both PE_{max} and PI_{max} ($r = 0.62$ and $r = 0.74$, respectively). There was an inverse relationship between both PI_{max} and PE_{max}, and residual volume ($r = 0.47$ and $r = 0.72$, respectively).**
Conclusion: **Children and adults with PWS have restrictive ventilatory impairment primarily as a result of respiratory muscle weakness. Efforts to improve thoracic muscle strength may be useful in improving pulmonary function in individuals with PWS. (J PEDIATR 1995;126:565-70)**

Prader-Willi syndrome is a genetic disorder characterized by infantile hypotonia, early childhood obesity, characteristic facial appearance, and various central nervous system abnormalities, including mental deficiency, hypogonadism, short stature, and behavioral disorders.[1-6] All clinically typical patients with PWS have either paternal deletion of 15q11 to q13 or maternal disomy for chromosome 15.[2, 7]

FEV_1	Forced expiratory volume in one second
FVC	Forced vital capacity
PE_{max}	Maximum expiratory pressure
PI_{max}	Maximum inspiratory pressure
PWS	Prader-Willi syndrome
RV	Residual volume
TLC	Total lung capacity
TMW	Thoracic muscle weakness

Musculoskeletal abnormalities, including a higher prevalence of scoliosis than in the general population, are common in these individuals.[8, 9]

Supported in part by a grant from the Prader-Willi Association (United States).

Submitted for publication July 6, 1994; accepted Oct. 4, 1994.

Reprint requests: Michelle M. Cloutier, MD, Pediatric Pulmonary Division MC 1827, University of Connecticut Health Center, Farmington, CT 06030.

0022-3476/95/$3.00 + 0 **9/20/61031**

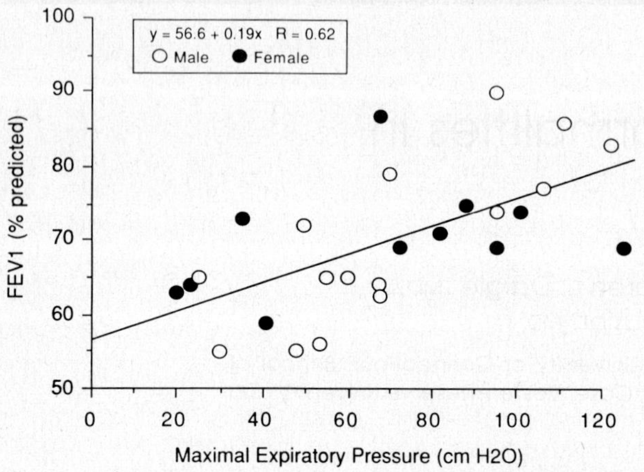

Fig. 1. The FEV_1 expressed as a function of PE_{max} in 15 male subjects *(clear circles)* and 11 female subjects *(dark circles)* with PWS, by simple regression analysis (p <0.001). The y-intercept (56.6) and slope of the line (0.19) are shown. Mean 95% confidence intervals overlapped for both groups (66.9 to 73.18).

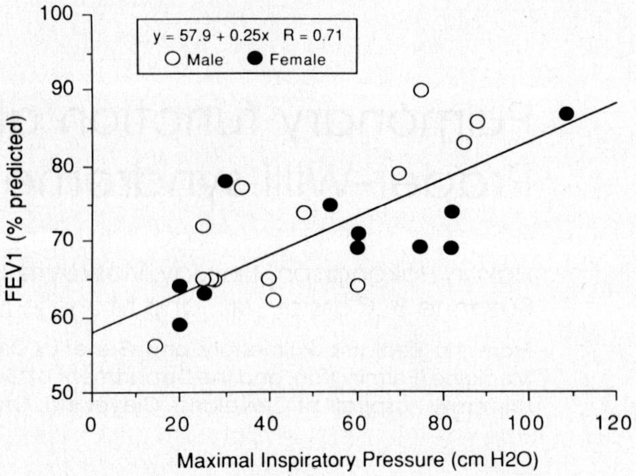

Fig. 2. The FEV_1 expressed as a function of PI_{max} in 14 male subjects *(clear circles)* and 11 female subjects *(dark circles)* with PWS, by simple regression analysis (p <0.001). The y-intercept (57.9) and slope of the line (0.75) are shown. Mean 95% confidence intervals overlapped for both groups (67.90 to 75.33).

Table I. Demographic data of the study population

	Male subjects (n = 18)	Female subjects (n = 17)
Age (yr)*	17.9 ± 10.2 (5-39)	23.5 ± 13.0 (5-54)
Weight (kg)*	59.2 ± 24.7 (29-112)	67.5 ± 29.6 (21.3-132)
Height (cm)*	144.6 ± 19.6 (108-168)	138.4 ± 12.7 (101-153)
Scoliosis	5	7
Asthma	3	3
Pneumonia	2	2
Chest surgery	0	1

*Data expressed as mean ± SD (range).

Little is known about pulmonary function in individuals with PWS. As a result of their obesity, small chest size, and scoliosis, they are at risk of having restrictive ventilatory impairment. The only study of lung function demonstrated reduced lung volumes in subjects with PWS compared with normal or obese individuals without PWS.[10] However, no study has been performed to assess thoracic muscle strength in this population, and the development of chronic lung disease has not been investigated. Hypotonia is another risk factor for the development of lung function abnormalities, and the long-term consequences and natural history of the hypotonia in PWS remain unclear. The purpose of this study was to evaluate pulmonary function in people with PWS to determine whether they have abnormal lung function and evidence of restrictive pulmonary disease as a result of thoracic muscle weakness.

METHODS

Our protocol was approved by the institutional review board at the University of Connecticut. All patients with typical features of PWS who were followed at the University of Connecticut Health Center were approached to participate.[5,6] After informed consent was obtained, a health questionnaire was completed by the subject's guardian or parent. Information obtained by questionnaire was verified by the available record. This questionnaire detailed current and previous medical history, with special emphasis on pulmonary symptoms, pulmonary disease, and previous surgery. Pulmonary function tests, consisting of spirometry, flow-volume curves, lung volumes, and static respiratory pressures, were measured with a model 6200 body plethysmograph (SensorMedics Corp., Yorba Linda, Calif.) and a mass flow sensor. Spirometry was performed with the box open and with all subjects standing. Lung volumes were obtained according to standard methods, as previously described.[11,12]

Thoracic muscle strength was assessed by measuring maximum static respiratory pressures with a mouthpiece attached to a pressure gauge. Both maximum inspiratory and maximum expiratory pressures were measured. The PI_{max} was measured by having the patient exhale to residual volume and then forcefully inhale to total lung capacity, as previously described.[11] The PE_{max} was measured by having the patient inhale to TLC and then forcefully exhale to RV.[11] Precautions were taken to avoid erroneously high or low pressures by having the subjects perform three or more measurements on two or more occasions, and the re-

Table II. Pulmonary function test results

	Male subjects	Female subjects
FVC*	64.3 ± 3.4	67.5 ± 3.4
FEV_1*	71.6 ± 2.8	71.6 ± 3.8
FEV_1/FVC	0.95 ± 0.02	0.94 ± 0.02
FEF_{25-75}*	89.0 ± 7.0	89.3 ± 7.0
RV*	188.6 ± 36.4	153.6 ± 28.3
TLC*	96.6 ± 6.8	90.4 ± 7.3
RV/TLC	0.42 ± 0.05	0.38 ± 0.05
sGAW*	87.6 ± 13.4	74.9 ± 9.5
PI_{max}	46.8 ± 5.8	48.5 ± 6.8
PE_{max}	68.2 ± 6.8	56.8 ± 9.2

FEF_{25-75}, Forced expiratory flow at 25% to 75% of forced vital capacity; *sGAW*, specific airway conductance.
Data reflect findings from 18 male subjects and 17 female subjects with PWS who completed the study.
*Data expressed as mean percentage of predicted value ± SEM. Data for PI_{max} and PE_{max} expressed as centimeters of water.

quirement that each subject sustain the maximal effort for a minimum of 3 seconds. All pulmonary function tests reported were performed in triplicate on two or more occasions. Tests were acceptable and considered reproducible if the variability in forced vital capacity, PE_{max}, and PI_{max} for individual measurements was less than 10%. Normative data used for PE_{max} and PI_{max} measurements are positive and negative pressure >60 cm H_2O, respectively, and are independent of age, size, and sex. Normative data for all other test results were based on age, sex, height, weight, and ethnic origin and were compared with those for the general population.[13, 14] All test results (except the forced expiratory volume in 1 second/forced vital capacity ratio and the RV/TLC ratio) are presented as the percentage of the predicted value. Correlation data (FEV_1 and RV as a function of thoracic muscle strength) were analyzed with simple linear regression analysis and correlation coefficient (*r*), and respective *p* values were expressed for each correlation.[15] The bronchodilator response to a β_2-agonist (Proventil MDI, Glaxo Inc., Research Trinagle Park, N.C.; two puffs) was assessed in nine subjects who had evidence of airway obstruction on initial testing, as reflected by either reduced specific airway conductance or reduced midexpiratory flow rates.

RESULTS

Study population. Thirty-nine subjects with typical features of PWS were invited to participate; 35 subjects completed the study (Table I), 1 patient refused, and 3 individuals were unable to perform reproducible tests and were excluded. Six subjects (17%) had a remote history of asthma, and four subjects (11%) had a history of recurrent pneumonia. Twelve subjects (34%) had either scoliosis, kyphoscoliosis, or a combination of the two. One female subject had undergone anterior spinal fusion for scoliosis. There was no history of active or recent smoking in the 35 subjects who completed the study.

Pulmonary function test results. Spirometry data demonstrated a decrease in FVC and FEV_1 with a normal FEV_1/FVC ratio (Table II). Lung volume measurements revealed TLC in the low normal range, elevated RV, and an increased RV/TLC ratio (Table II). Results of thoracic muscle strength measurements, as reflected by static respiratory pressures, demonstrated a significant reduction in both PE_{max} and PI_{max} in both sexes (Table II). Of 32 subjects tested, 15 (9 male subjects) had PE_{max} values <60 cm H_2O, and of these 15, 7 (5 female subjects) had PE_{max} values <40 cm H_2O. Twenty subjects (10 male subjects) had PI_{max} values <60 cm H_2O, and of these 20, 14 (7 female subjects) had PI_{max} values <40 cm H_2O. Of 10 subjects with thoracic wall abnormalities, 5 (2 male subjects) had PE_{max} values <60 cm H_2O and 7 (4 female subjects) had PI_{max} values <60 cm H_2O. The mean (±SEM) PE_{max} and PI_{max} values were 64.0 ± 16.2 cm H_2O versus 69.6 ± 7.8 cm H_2O (male subjects) and 52.8 ± 17.4 cm H_2O versus 55.8 ± 10.8 cm H_2O for PE_{max}, and 39.8 ± 10.3 cm H_2O versus 49.2 ± 7.1 (male subjects) and 46.4 ± 10.2 cm H_2O versus 49.0 ± 9.2 cm H_2O for PI_{max}, in subjects with and without thoracic wall abnormalities, respectively.

Correlations. There was a linear relationship between PE_{max} and FEV_1 (Fig. 1) and between PI_{max} and FEV_1 (Fig. 2) in both sexes. A similar relationship for PE_{max} and PI_{max} as a function of FVC was observed ($r = 0.62$ and $r = 0.74$, respectively) in both sexes with corresponding *p* values of $p < 0.005$ and $p < 0.001$, respectively. An inverse relationship was observed between PE_{max} and RV and PI_{max} as a function of RV for both sexes (Figs. 3 and 4). There was no difference in any of the relationships described above between male and female patients except for RV as a function of PI_{max}, which showed a significantly better correla-

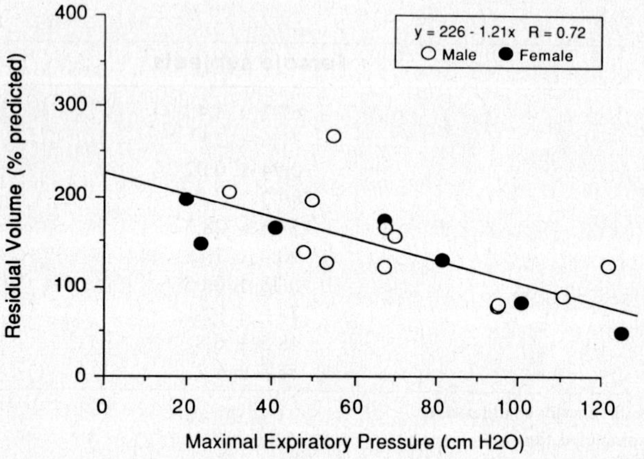

Fig. 3. Residual volume expressed as a function of PE_{max} in 12 male subjects *(clear circles)* and 7 female subjects *(dark circles)* with PWS, by simple regression analysis ($p < 0.005$). The *y*-intercept (226) and slope of the line (−1.21) are shown. Mean 95% confidence intervals overlapped for both groups (122.91 to 159.94).

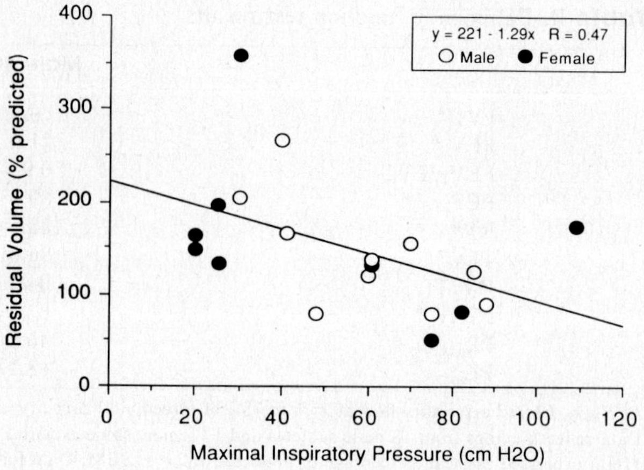

Fig. 4. Residual volume expressed as a function of PI_{max} in 10 male subjects *(clear circles)* and 9 female subjects *(dark circles)* with PWS, by simple regression analysis ($p < 0.05$). The *y*-intercept (221) and slope of the line (−1.29) are shown. Mean 95% confidence intervals were 107.10 to 177.52 for male subjects and 91.00 to 227.45 for female subjects.

tion in male subjects ($r = 0.64$) than in female subjects ($r = 0.38$) with corresponding p values of $p = 0.04$ and $p = 0.3$, respectively. There was no relationship between FVC or FEV_1 and weight expressed as a percentage of ideal body weight (data not shown).

Bronchodilator response. Nine subjects had evidence of mild obstructive airway disease on initial testing as reflected by reduced specific airway conductance or midexpiratory flows. In those nine subjects the response to an inhaled bronchodilator was examined. A 20% improvement in either specific airway conductance or expiratory flow rates at moderate to low lung volumes was demonstrated in six subjects. Restrictive ventilatory impairment was still present after bronchodilator inhalation in all subjects.

DISCUSSION

These data demonstrate that individuals of all ages with PWS have evidence of restrictive ventilatory impairment, which appears to be the result of TMW because there was no difference in the severity of restrictive ventilatory impairment in individuals who were obese, who had chest wall abnormalities, or who had a history of previous surgery. The number of subjects with such abnormalities, however, was too small to allow for statistical comparison.

Several possible reasons exist for the restrictive ventilatory impairment in patients with PWS. One of the major reasons is hypotonia. Anecdotal experience indicates that the hypotonia present at birth improves with time in these individuals,[16, 17] but no studies support this conclusion. Hypotonia can be accompanied by muscular weakness and reduced muscle mass. Restrictive ventilatory impairment has been described in patients with muscular weakness resulting from neuromuscular disorders such as Duchenne muscular dystrophy and myotonic dystrophy.[18, 19] Measurements of maximum respiratory pressures (PE_{max}, PI_{max}) provide a useful way to quantify the respiratory muscle weakness that occurs in neuromuscular diseases and to correlate these values with reductions in vital capacity.[20-22]

Our measurements demonstrate that individuals with PWS have decreased thoracic muscle strength, which could account for their restricted pulmonary function (as suggested by the relationship between static respiratory pressures and both FEV_1 and RV). The consequences of reduced thoracic muscle strength in these individuals could be severe. When the PE_{max} is reduced to <40 cm H_2O, patients can no longer breathe deeply or cough effectively, and they are unable to clear secretions from the upper airway.[18] Fifteen participants in our study had reduced PE_{max} values, and seven subjects had severely reduced values (PE_{max} <40 cm H_2O). These individuals are at substantial risk of having airway obstruction and chronic endobronchial infection as a result of a decreased ability to clear airway secretions. Increased pulmonary infection rates in people with PWS have not been reported, however, and these individuals have otherwise normal mucociliary function. Thus an additional risk factor, such as a severe upper respiratory tract infection, may be necessary for this to occur.

The cause of TMW in PWS remains unknown and may be multifactorial. Real-time ultrasound imaging is a technique that evaluates muscle size and function, and results are normal in people with PWS.[23] Results of neuromuscular studies, including muscle biopsy histologic and histochemical studies, muscle enzyme studies, and electromyography, are normal in patients with PWS.[17] However, many individuals with PWS have sleep-related problems, which may be accompanied by hypoxemia, carbon dioxide retention, or both, and could further compromise neuromuscular function.[24, 25]

Pulmonary function tests of obese but otherwise healthy individuals demonstrate both mild restrictive and obstructive pulmonary disease.[26, 27] However, there is no evidence of decreased thoracic muscle strength in obese individuals. Some of the patients in our study population were moderately obese, and obesity may have contributed to the restrictive pulmonary function. However, the correlation between static respiratory pressures and both FEV_1 and RV supports our hypothesis of TMW as the major cause of the restrictive ventilatory impairment in PWS. The stronger inverse relationship between PI_{max} and RV in male subjects may be accounted for by the relatively few subjects who were able to complete this part of the study. Total lung capacity was normal in most of our subjects, which is consistent with mild to moderate weakness of the respiratory muscles.[12]

Kyphoscoliosis is another common cause of restrictive ventilatory impairment; the degree of the scoliosis angle does not correlate with the severity of restrictive ventilatory impairment.[28] Twelve of our study subjects had mild to moderate scoliosis. However, there was no difference in the severity of restrictive pulmonary function or severity of TMW in individuals with scoliosis or other chest wall abnormalities compared with individuals without such abnormalities. The latter finding suggests that scoliosis is an unlikely cause of the restrictive pulmonary function in these patients. The number of patients, however, was small and may have masked a small contribution of scoliosis to the restrictive lung disease pattern.

Although most of the pulmonary function tests performed by our study patients are effort-dependent tests and our study subjects have mild mental deficiency, we tried to ensure full effort by performing all tests in triplicate and at different times. Only reproducible tests with a variability of less than 10% between individual measurements were accepted. Moreover, previous studies indicate that individuals with PWS have intellectual function and behavioral levels comparable with those of 7- or 8-year-old children, which is adequate to perform pulmonary function tests with consistency.

We conclude that individuals with PWS have restrictive ventilatory impairment that appears to be primarily the result of TMW. We speculate that TMW could result in decreased exercise tolerance and in a decreased ability to clear airway secretions, predisposing patients to pulmonary infections, airway obstruction, hypoxemia, and the eventual development of cor pulmonale. These are the major causes of morbidity and death in PWS.[6] Efforts to improve thoracic muscle strength may be useful in improving pulmonary function in people with PWS. Accordingly, a structured exercise program may improve thoracic muscle strength and reduce the risk of pulmonary compromise in individuals with PWS.

We thank Dr. Craig M. Schramm for his suggestions and assistance in making tables and graphs. We also thank Mary Turley, RRT, and Nancy McLellan, RRT, for their invaluable technical support and effort in obtaining test results.

REFERENCES

1. Aughton DJ, Cassidy SB. Physical features of Prader-Willi syndrome in neonates. Am J Dis Child 1990;144:1251-4.
2. Cassidy SB, Ledbetter DH. Prader-Willi syndrome. Neurol Clin 1989;7:37-54.
3. Dykens EM, Hodapp RM, Walsh K, Nach LJ. Adaptive and maladaptive behavior in Prader-Willi syndrome. J Am Acad Child Adolesc Psychiatry 1992;31:1131-6.
4. Hall BD, Smith DW. Prader-Willi syndrome. J PEDIATR 1972;81:286-93.
5. Holm VA, Cassidy SB, Butler MG, et al. Prader-Willi syndrome: consensus diagnostic criteria. Pediatrics 1993;91: 398-402.
6. Cassidy SB. Prader-Willi syndrome. Curr Probl Pediatr 1984; 14:1-55.
7. Nicholls RD. Genomic imprinting and uniparental disomy in Angelman and Prader-Willi syndromes: a review. Am J Med Genet 1993;46:16-25.
8. Soriano RM, Weisz I, Houghton GR. Scoliosis in the Prader-Willi syndrome. Spine 1988;13:209-11.
9. Rees D, Jones MW, Owen R, Dorgan JC. Scoliosis surgery in the Prader-Willi syndrome. J Bone Joint Surg Br 1989;71: 685-8.
10. Bray GA, Dahms WT, Swerdloff RS, Fiser RH, Atkinson RL, Carrel RE. The Prader-Willi Syndrome: a Study of 40 patients and a review of the literature. Medicine 1983;62:59-80.
11. Ruppel G. Lung volume tests: pulmonary mechanics. In: Mangold C, Reilly CF, eds. Manual of pulmonary function testing. 5th ed. St. Louis: Mosby–Year Book, 1991:1-72.
12. Lemen RJ. Pulmonary function testing in the office, clinic and at home. In: Kendig's disorders of the respiratory tract in children. 5th ed. Philadelphia: WB Saunders, 1990:147-54.
13. Polgar G, Promadhat V. Techniques and standards. In: Pulmonary function testing in children. Techniques and standards. Philadelphia: WB Saunders, 1971:12-256.
14. Morris JF. Spirometry in the evaluation of pulmonary function. West J Med 1976;125:110-8.
15. Ingelfinger JA, Mosteller F, Thibodeau LA, Ware JH. Regression: an overview. In: Biostatistics in clinical medicine. 2nd ed. New York: MacMillan Publishing, 1987:182-231.
16. Airede KI. Prader-Willi syndrome. East Afr Med J 1991; 68:831-8.
17. Dubowitz V. The floppy infant. In: Clinics in developmental medicine. 2nd ed. London: Heinemann Medical Books, 1980: 126-31.

18. O'Donohue WJ, Baker JP, Bell GM, et al. Respiratory failure in neuromuscular disease. JAMA 1976;235:733-6.
19. Begin R, Bureau MA, Lupien L, et al. Pathogenesis of respiratory insufficiency in myotonic dystrophy. Am Rev Respir Dis 1982;125:312-8.
20. Rochester DF. Tests of respiratory muscle function. Clin Chest Med 1988;9:249-61.
21. Rahn H, Otis AB, Chadwick LE, et al. The pressure-volume diagram of the thorax and lung. Am J Physiol 1946;46:161-78.
22. Ringquist T. The ventilatory capacity in healthy subjects: an analysis of causal factors with special references to the respiratory forces. Scand J Clin Lab Invest 1966;18(suppl 88):5-179.
23. Heckmatt JZ, Pier N, Dubovitz V. Real-time ultrasound imaging of muscles. Muscle Nerve 1988;11:56-65.
24. Kaplan J, Fredrickson PA, Richardson JW. Sleep and breathing in patients with the Prader-Willi syndrome. Mayo Clin Proc 1991;66:1124-6.
25. Clarke DJ, Waters J, Corbett JA. Adults with Prader-Willi syndrome: abnormalities of sleep and behavior. J R Soc Med 1989;82:21-4.
26. Cherniack RM. Evaluation of pulmonary function in health and disease. Dis Mon 1992;38:505-76.
27. Rubenstein I, Zanel N, Dubarry L, Hoffstein V. Airflow limitation in morbidly obese non-smoking men. Ann Intern Med 1990;112:828-32.
28. Kearon C, Viviani GR, Kirkley A, Killian KJ. Factors determining pulmonary function in adolescent idiopathic scoliosis. Am Rev Respir Dis 1993;148:288-94.

Pulmonary arteriovenous shunting in children with liver disease

Thierry Barbé, MD, Jean Losay, MD, Gilles Grimon, MD, Denis Devictor, MD, Anne Sardet, MD, Frédéric Gauthier, MD, Didier Houssin, MD, and Olivier Bernard, MD

From Hépatologie, Réanimation, and Chirurgie pédiatriques, Département de Pédiatrie, and Laboratoire de Médecine nucléaire, Hôpital de Bicêtre; Cardiologie pédiatrique, Hôpital Marie-Lannelongue; Pneumologie pédiatrique, Hôpital Trousseau; and Clinique Chirurgicale, Hôpital Cochin, Paris, France

Pulmonary arteriovenous shunting (PAVS) with hypoxemia is a severe complication of cirrhosis that may regress after liver transplantation. We report PAVS in 25 children with cirrhosis and in 1 with portal vein obstruction; proof of shunting was obtained by technetium Tc 99m microaggregated albumin pulmonary scanning or a high alveoloarterial O_2 gradient or both. Cyanosis or dyspnea or both occurred at ages ranging from 6 months to 14 years, earlier in children with biliary atresia and polysplenia syndrome (*p* <0.01). Mean arterial oxygen tension (Pao_2) was 57 mm Hg (range, 42 to 81 mm Hg) during breathing of 21% O_2 and 367 mm Hg (range, 179 to 535 mm Hg) in 100% O_2. Cardiac index was always raised, significantly more in children with biliary atresia and polysplenia syndrome (*p* <0.01). Seven untreated children died 3 months to 8 years after the diagnosis of PAVS. Eleven underwent liver transplantation: seven are alive (follow-up, 1 to 4 years) and have no signs of PAVS. The Pao_2 value during breathing of 100% O_2 was >300 mm Hg in the survivors and <200 mm Hg in the four nonsurvivors (*p* <0.01). These results indicate (1) that PAVS can occur at any age in children with portal hypertension, and that the risk is highest and earliest in children with biliary atresia and polysplenia syndrome, (2) that early liver transplantation allows regression of PAVS, and (3) that the prognosis may in part be related to the level of Pao_2 while the patient is breathing 100% O_2. The results indicate that systematic screening for PAVS should be part of the examination of these children. (J Pediatr 1995;126:571-9)

Arterial hypoxemia is present in up to 30% of adults with cirrhosis.[1] The mechanisms include hypoventilation caused by ascites, pleural effusion, and diaphragmatic dysfunction, but the most severe hypoxemia is secondary to the occurrence of intrapulmonary arteriovenous shunting, which is supposed to be related to intrapulmonary vascular dilation at the precapillary or capillary level, or to direct arteriovenous communications.[2, 3] The outcome of the hypoxemia is poor and includes permanent cyanosis, multiple organ failure, and death.[4] Until recently, severe hypoxemia was considered a contraindication to liver transplantation.[5] A few reports, however, have shown that pulmonary arteriovenous shunting can be reversed after liver transplantation in adults and older children,[6-8] but this favorable outcome has not been obtained in all cases.[9, 10] To define better the natural history and outcome of this complication in children with liver disease, with and without liver transplantation, we

$Paco_2$	Arterial carbon dioxide tension
Pao_2	Arterial oxygen tension
Po_2	Oxygen tension

Submitted for publication Jan. 25, 1994; accepted Sept. 26, 1994.

Reprint requests: O. Bernard, MD, Hépatologie pédiatrique, Hôpital de Bicêtre, 94275 Le Kremlin Bicetre, France.

0022-3476/95/$3.00 + 0 **9/20/60905**

reviewed retrospectively the records of 26 children with liver disease and pulmonary arteriovenous shunting who were investigated between 1975 and 1993.

METHODS

Patients. We studied 12 girls and 14 boys. The liver disease was cirrhosis in 25 children and portal vein obstruction in 1. The causes of cirrhosis are indicated in the Table. Gastrointestinal bleeding caused by portal hypertension had occurred in 8 of the 26 children; five were treated with endoscopic sclerotherapy. Six children underwent a surgical portosystemic shunt, for gastrointestinal bleeding in three, for Budd-Chiari syndrome in two, and for idiopathic cirrhosis (shunt carried out prophylactically elsewhere) in one. Splenectomy had been carried out during portosystemic shunts in two cases. All portosystemic shunts were later proved to be patent.

Liver function tests included serum bilirubin concentration, prothrombin time, and serum albumin concentration. Signs of portal hypertension were investigated with clinical (splenomegaly), ultrasonographic, and upper gastrointestinal tract endoscopic criteria.

During the same period, the following numbers of patients were investigated and followed in this unit: 594 children with biliary atresia, including 34 with the polysplenia syndrome; 93 children with α_1-antitrypsin deficiency and liver disease, including 54 with proven cirrhosis; 28 children with Budd-Chiari syndrome; 40 with cystic fibrosis and cirrhosis; 62 with autoimmune hepatitis and cirrhosis; and 211 with portal vein obstruction.

Diagnosis of pulmonary arteriovenous shunting. Arterial blood gases were measured with the patient in the supine position and breathing 21% oxygen, and after the patient had been breathing 100% oxygen for 15 minutes. Technetium Tc 99m macroaggregated albumin pulmonary scanning was performed in 24 children. In 2 children the degree of pulmonary shunting was not quantified by this method; in the 22 remaining children, the degree of shunting was quantified with a newly described brain/lung ratio of isotope fixation[11] (normal, <1%). Plain x-ray studies of the lungs were performed in all children. Lung function tests were carried out in 8 children, including measurement of the alveoloarterial oxygen-tension gradient in the 2 children investigated in the years 1975 to 1980, when pulmonary scanning was not yet used. Thus proof of shunting was obtained by an abnormal extrapulmonary isotope fixation on the pulmonary scintiscan in 24 children and by a high alveoloarterial PO_2 gradient in the remaining 2.

Right cardiac catheterization was carried out in 24 children, including measurement of pulmonary capillary wedge pressure and pulmonary artery pressure in all, and of cardiac index by thermodilution in 22; the latter results were compared with the results of cardiac index measured in 93 children with cirrhosis and no polysplenia syndrome who were investigated before liver transplantation and who did not have signs of pulmonary arteriovenous shunting. Pulmonary artery occlusion PO_2 was measured during cardiac catheterization in 10 children while they were breathing 21% O_2 and then 100% O_2. Pulmonary capillary angiography was carried out in 20 children during cardiac catheterization. Seventeen children underwent echocardiography. Monitoring of the pulmonary status was performed with the use of clinical data (degree of cyanosis, intensity of dyspnea) in all children, additional arterial blood gas measurements during breathing of room air in 10 children and during breathing of 100% O_2 in 9 children, and a second pulmonary scintiscan in 5.

Therapeutic methods. Early in our experience, treatment included nasal O_2 in children with permanent cyanosis, a trial of somatostatin in five children and of propranolol in one, and surgical reduction of the diameter of a splenorenal shunt in the child with portal vein obstruction; combination liver-heart-lung transplantation was performed in two children. Later, orthotopic liver transplantation was carried out in 11 children with cyclosporine and prednisone used as immunosuppressive therapy. The features of some of these children have been reported in part.[12]

Statistical analysis. Clinical data are given as medians, means, and ranges. An unpaired Student *t* test was performed to compare patients with shunting with those without shunting. Group comparisons in the population studied were performed using the Fisher, Yates, and Perry tests. We considered p values less than 0.05 significant for all analyses.

RESULTS

Diagnosis of pulmonary arteriovenous shunting. The age at which the first symptoms of pulmonary arteriovenous shunting were detected ranged from 6 months to 14 years (median, 8 years). The ages at the time of the first symptoms were significantly lower in children with biliary atresia and the polysplenia syndrome (6 months to 8 years; median, 12 months) than in the other children (3 to 14 years; median, 9 years; $p < 0.01$). The first symptoms were cyanosis during crying or on exertion and/or dyspnea on exertion in 21 children, repeated episodes of bronchopulmonary infections in 1 child, and a fortuitous abnormal finding on pulmonary scanning, blood gas measurement, or blood cell count (blood hemoglobin level, 160 gm/L at age 3½ years) in the remaining 4 children. Mean age at the time of diagnosis was 8 years (range, 6 months to 16 years). At that time cyanosis was present in 24 children, dyspnea in 19, digital clubbing in 21, numerous spider nevi in 9, and increased thoracic anteroposterior diameter in 4.

PaO_2 during inhalation of 21% O_2 ranged from 42 to 81

mm Hg (mean, 58 mm Hg); Pa_{O_2} with 100% O_2 ranged from 179 to 535 mm Hg (mean, 353 mm Hg). Mean Pa_{CO_2} was 28 mm Hg (range, 20 to 42 mm Hg). Brain/lung index of scintigraphic shunting ranged from 2.2% to 28.6% (mean, 8.4%) (Fig. 1) and was correlated with Pa_{O_2} during inhalation of room air ($r = 0.61$; $p < 0.01$) and of 100% O_2 ($r = 0.55$; $p < 0.01$). In patients 17 and 23, who did not undergo pulmonary scanning, proof of the shunting was provided by the existence of an alveoloarterial P_{O_2} gradient of 81 mm Hg in 21% O_2 in one and of 414 mm Hg in 100% O_2 in the other. Altogether, in the 13 other children studied during lung function tests or cardiac catheterization, mean alveoloarterial P_{O_2} gradients in 21% O_2 and 100% O_2 were 44 mm Hg (range, 8 to 78 mm Hg) and 126 mm Hg (range, up to 348 mm Hg), respectively.

Plain lung x-ray studies showed bilateral increased interstitial markings in each child. Lung function tests, except in the child with cystic fibrosis, did not reveal significant abnormalities except for low dynamic compliance in six of the eight children tested, and low diffusing capacity for carbon monoxide in four of five tested. Blood hemoglobin concentration was greater than the upper limit of normal for age in five children.

Echocardiography or cardiac catheterization or both ruled out a right-to-left shunt at the cardiac level in all children. Echocardiography showed normal results in 12 children and mild four-chamber enlargement in 4. Cardiac indexes ranged from 3.6 to 12.5 L/min per square meter (mean, 7 L/min); it was significantly higher in children with biliary atresia and polysplenia syndrome (median, 9.7 L/min per square meter; range, 7.1 to 12.6) than in the remaining children (median, 6.1; range, 3.6 to 7.9; $p < 0.01$). There was a slight correlation between the scintigraphic brain-lung index and the cardiac index ($r = 0.51$; $p < 0.05$). However, the median cardiac index of the 15 children with pulmonary shunting and no polysplenia syndrome was not significantly different from that of 93 other children with cirrhosis but without signs of pulmonary arteriovenous shunt (median, 5.6 L/min per square meter; range, 3 to 9.2). Pulmonary capillary wedge pressure was above normal (>12 mm Hg) in four children, and mean pulmonary artery pressure was above normal (>20 mm Hg) in three children. All children with raised mean pulmonary artery pressure also had raised pulmonary capillary wedge pressure. Pulmonary capillary angiograms showed a spongy appearance with decrease in the capillary blush in nine children and arteriovenous anastomosis with early venous filling in four.

Relation to liver condition. At the time of diagnosis, the liver and spleen were enlarged in 19 and 22 children, respectively; serum bilirubin concentration ranged from 12 to 366 μmol/L (median, 44 μmol/L), prothrombin time from 38% to 100% (median, 66%), and serum albumin concentration from 16 to 46 gm/L (median, 35 gm/L). The child with portal vein obstruction had normal liver function and did not have histologic evidence of cirrhosis. Abdominal ultrasonography displayed signs of portal hypertension in 15 of the 18 children studied. Endoscopy of the upper gastrointestinal tract showed varices in 13 of the 17 children studied. Altogether a sign of portal hypertension was present or had been present previously in all children.

Follow-up and treatment. Follow-up ranged from 1 month to 8 years, the end point being death, liver transplantation, or the time of this writing. One child was lost to follow-up, and early liver transplantation carried out within 2 months of diagnosis precluded any significant study of follow-up in three children. In 20 of the 22 remaining children, signs of hypoxemia worsened, and in two others they remained stable for a 1-year period. Worsening of shunting and hypoxemia was variable in speed but sometimes was extremely rapid (Figs. 2 and 3); cyanosis and dyspnea sometimes impaired physical activities within a few months. Three children died within 3 months, and four died within 3 to 8 years.

Somatostatin or propranolol, as well as the attempt at reducing the diameter of a surgical portosystemic shunt, did not result in any improvement in arterial blood gas values. Liver transplantation alone was undertaken in 13 children, 1 month to 3 years after the diagnosis of pulmonary arteriovenous shunting. In two instances, transplantation was carried out successfully in another institution[13] because we thought, at that time, that the extent of hypoxemia precluded liver transplantation alone. Of the 11 children who underwent transplantation of the liver in our institution, four died 4 days to 1 month after transplantation. Seven children are alive after a follow-up period ranging from 1 to 4 years; cyanosis, digital clubbing, and spider nevi have disappeared, and arterial oxygen saturation and tension during breathing of room air and/or results of pulmonary scanning returned to normal within 28 to 210 days after transplantation. Preoperative Pa_{O_2} in 100% O_2 was significantly lower in children who died after transplantation than in survivors ($p < 0.01$); preoperative Pa_{O_2} in room air was also lower in children who died than in survivors, but the significance was borderline ($p = 0.052$). Brain-lung scintiscan indexes measured in the 6 months preceding transplantation did not differ significantly between the children who died and the survivors.

Two other children underwent combination lung-heart-liver transplantation, one child at a time when severe hypoxemia was still considered a contraindication to liver transplantation alone; this patient died 2 days after surgery because of pleural hemorrhage. The other, the one with cystic fibrosis, had the combination procedure because it was deemed that the underlying lung condition would not

Text continued on p. 576

Table. Clinical features in 26 children with liver disease and pulmonary arteriovenous shunting

Patient No.	Liver disease	First symptoms		Investigations		
		Age	Type	Age	Symptoms	PaO_2 (t) (FIO_2: 0.21)
1	Biliary atresia, PSS, Kasai	6 mo	Cyanosis, dyspnea	7 mo	C + D	46
2	Biliary atresia, PSS, Kasai	9 mo	Cyanosis	9 mo	C	56
3	Biliary atresia, PSS, Kasai	12 mo	Relapsing bronchitis	17 mo	C	47
4	Biliary atresia, PSS, Kasai	14 mo	Dyspnea	17 mo	C + D	61
5	Biliary atresia, PSS, no Kasai	18 mo	Cyanosis	18 mo	C + D	44
6	Biliary atresia, PSS, Kasai, endoscopic sclerotherapy	2 yr	Cyanosis	2 yr	C	48
7	Biliary atresia, Kasai, endoscopic sclerotherapy	3 yr	Cyanosis	3 yr	C	81
8	Budd-Chiari, portacaval shunt (age 2 yr)	3 yr	Cyanosis	6 yr	C + ED	54
9	Tyrosinemia	3 yr 6 mo	Hb: 160 gm/L	4 yr	C	59
10	Cirrhosis (HCV^+), phenylketonuria	6 yr	Cyanosis, dyspnea	9 yr	C + ED	66
11	CF, portosystemic shunt (age 4 yr)	7 yr	PaO_2: 65 t (FIO_2:0.21)	9 yr	C + D	50
12	Budd-Chiari, portosystemic shunt (age 2 yr)	7 yr	Cyanosis, dyspnea	12 yr	C + D	56
13	Biliary atresia, PSS, Kasai	8 yr	Cyanosis	8 yr	C + D	44
14	Biliary atresia, Kasai	8 yr	Dyspnea	9 yr	C + D	50
15	Biliary atresia, Kasai, endoscopic sclerotherapy	9 yr	Dyspnea, cyanosis	9 yr 6 mo	C	66
16	Biliary atresia, Kasai	9 yr	Cyanosis	9 yr	C	62
17	Biliary cirrhosis (unknown cause)	9 yr 6 mo	Dyspnea	10 yr 6 mo	C + ED	61
18	Biliary atresia, Kasai	10 yr	Cyanosis, dyspnea	10 yr 6 mo	C + ED	56
19	Cirrhosis (unknown cause)	10 yr	Dyspnea	11 yr	D	70
20	*PV*, obstruction, splenorenal shunt (age 9 yr)	10 yr 6 mo	Cyanosis, dyspnea	11 yr	C + D	64
21	Biliary atresia, Kasai, endoscopic sclerotherapy	11 yr 6 mo	Cyanosis, dyspnea	11 yr 6 mo	C + D	76
22	α_1-Antitrypsin deficiency	12 yr 10 mo	Screening scintiscan	13 yr	ED	79
23	α_1-Antitrypsin deficiency; portacaval shunt (age 11 yr)	12 yr	Exertional dyspnea	15 yr 8 mo	C + ED	42
24	Biliary atresia, Kasai, endoscopic sclerotherapy	13 yr	Screening scintiscan	13 yr 6 mo	C + ED	80
25	Cirrhosis (unknown cause); splenorenal shunt (age 12 yr)	14 yr	Dyspnea	16 yr 6 mo	C + D	50
26	Autoimmune hepatitis	14 yr	Cyanosis, dyspnea	15 yr	C + ED	49

t, Torr (mm Hg); *CI*, cardiac index; *PSS*, polysplenia syndrome; *Kasai*, hepatic portoenterostomy or cholecystostomy for correction of biliary atresia; *HCV*$^+$, hepatitis C virus; *C*, cyanosis; *D*, dyspnea; *CF*, cystic fibrosis; *PV*, portal vein; *ED*, exertional dyspnea; *CF*, cystic fibrosis; *PV*, portal vein; *B/L*, brain/lung scintigraphic index of shunting (expressed as percentage); *B*, serum bilirubin concentration (expressed as micromoles per liter); *PT*, prothrombin time (expressed as percentage); *FV*, coagulation factor five (expressed as percentage); *EV*, esophageal varices; *FU*, follow-up during natural progression of the disease; *MOF*, multiple organ failure; *PAVS*, pulmonary arteriovenous shunting; *ND*, not done; *CMV*, cytomegalovirus; *FIO*$_2$, fraction of inspired oxygen.

Investigations—cont'd

PaO_2 (t) (FIO_2: 1)	Scintiscan (B/L index)	CI (L/mn/m^2)	Liver condition	Outcome
287	24.8	9.8	B: 20; PT: 86	FU: 2 mo; somatostatin: no effect; death from respiratory failure
477	4.9	7.1	B: 10; PT: 96	FU: 2 yr; scintiscan B/L: 13.7; PaO_2 (FIO_2: 1): 108 mm Hg; awaiting liver transplantation
312	24	8.1	B: 277; PT: 100	FU: 3 yr; death from respiratory failure
437	5.7	10	B: 31; PT: 100	FU: 8 mo; PaO_2 (FIO_2: 0.21): 53 mm Hg; PaO_2 (FIO_2: 1): 186 mm Hg; liver transplantation (elsewhere)
405	20	12.6	B: 338; PT: 85	FU: 1 mo; liver transplantation; alive 2 yr later; normal scintiscan: day 210
196	28.6	7.7	B: 25; PT: 100	FU: 2 mo; liver transplantation; death, day 4, MOF
418	5.9	ND	B: 73; PT: 83	FU: 5 mo; liver transplantation; alive 1 yr later; normal scintiscan: day 110
330	5.9	7.8	B: 12; FV: 100	FU: 5 yr; death, hepatic, cardiac, renal, and respiratory failure; intracranial hemorrhage
167	12	8.8	B: 46; PT: 47; grade I EV	FU: 1 mo; liver transplantation; death 20 days later, MOF
401	8.4	6.2	B: 44; PT: 56; grade I EV	FU: 12 mo; B/L: 12; PaO_2 (FIO_2: 0.21): 61 mm Hg; PaO_2 (FIO_2: 1): 386 mm Hg; liver transplantation; alive 4 yr later; normal scintiscan: day 120
270	8.7	ND	B: 16; PT: 66	FU: 1 yr; PaO_2 (FIO_2: 0.21): 44 mm Hg; combined heart-lung-liver transplantation; alive 18 mo later
290	14	ND	B: 70; PT: 51	FU: 3 mo; somatostatin: no effect; PaO_2 (FIO_2: 0.21): 41 mm Hg; B/L: 19; liver transplantation; death 1 mo later, CMV infection, MOF
449	10.4	9.7	B: 366; PT: 87	FU: 3 mo; death, MOF
179	9.9	6.2	B: 44; PT: 49; grade I EV	FU: 10 mo; somatostatin: no effect; PaO_2 (FIO_2: 0.21): 40 mm Hg; PaO_2 (FIO_2: 1): 77 mm Hg; liver transplantation (elsewhere)
437	3.3	7	B: 16; PT: 65	FU: 3 mo; liver transplantation; alive 4 yr later; normal scintiscan: day 28
268	9.4	7.9	B: 242; PT: 45; no EV	FU: 3 mo; death after superinfection
278	ND	ND	B: 65; PT: 56; grade I EV	FU: 8 yr; PaO_2 (FIO_2: 0.21): 44 mm Hg; death; superinfection, liver failure
310	7.3	6.8	B: 58; PT: 47	FU: 2 mo; liver transplantation; alive after 2 yr; normal scintiscan: day 90
530	4.7	6	B: 101; PT: 46	FU: 3 yr alive, then lost to follow-up
535	7.6	5.8	B: 35; PT: 66	FU: 6 yr; somatostatin: no effect; PaO_2 (FIO_2: 0.21): 59 mm Hg; PaO_2 (FIO_2: 1): 335 mm Hg; B/L: 10
510	3.8	6.6	B: 29; PT: 49; gastric varices	FU: 8 mo; PaO_2 (FIO_2: 0.21): 63 mm Hg; PaO_2 (FIO_2: 1): 350 mm Hg; B/L: 12.3; liver transplantation; alive after 18 mo; normal scintiscan: day 110
525	2.5	6.6	B: 13; PT: 50; grade I EV	FU: 1 yr; PaO_2 (FIO_2: 0.21): 76 mm Hg; PaO_2 (FIO_2: 1): 530 mm Hg; liver transplantation; alive 18 mo later; normal scintiscan: day 67
279	ND	5.5	B: 50; PT: 60	FU: 5 yr; death, liver failure, intracranial hemorrhage
585	2.2	6.1	B: 29; PT: 53	FU: 9 mo; PaO_2 (FIO_2: 1): 456 mm Hg; awaiting liver transplantation
250	PAVS (not quantified)	3.6	B: 57; PT: 38	FU: 12 mo; generalized cyanosis, major dyspnea; combined heart-lung-liver transplantation; death from pulmonary hemorrhage, day 2
339	PAVS (not quantified)	4.4	B: 41; PT: 60; grade II EV	FU: 2 yr; somatostatin: no effect; PaO_2 (FIO_2: 0.21): 35 mm Hg; PaO_2 (FIO_2: 1): 89 mm Hg; liver transplantation; death day 10, rejection, PV thrombosis, MOF

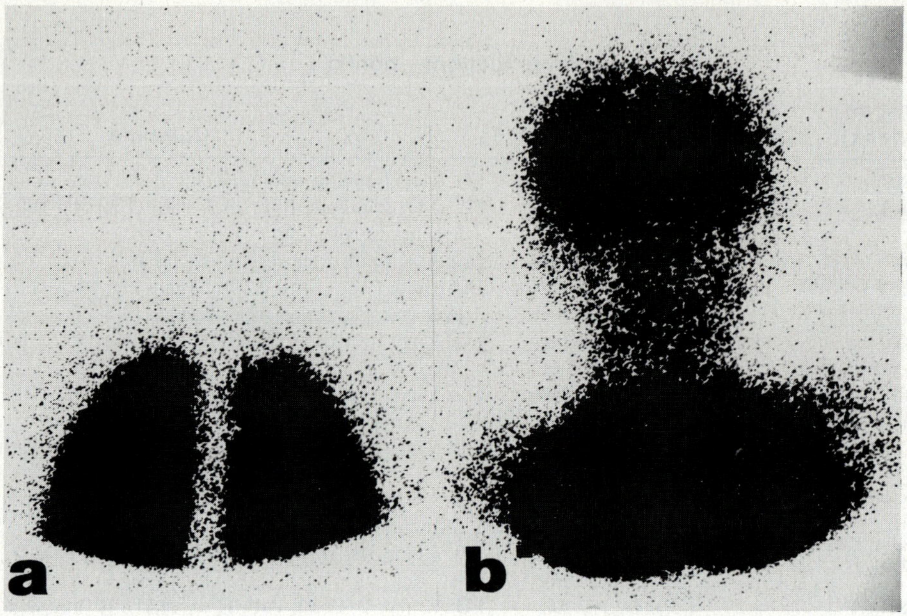

Fig. 1. Pulmonary scanning by means of technetium Tc 99m macroaggregated albumin in two children with liver disease. **a,** Scan of 6-year-old child with biliary atresia and no signs of pulmonary arteriovenous shunting. **b,** Scan of 10-year-old child with cirrhosis and pulmonary arteriovenous shunting. Note extrapulmonary isotope fixation on the brain in 10-year-old patient **b.**

allow easy recovery after liver transplantation alone. This child is alive and well 1½ years after surgery.

Outcome. Of the 26 children studied, one has been lost to follow-up, 12 have died, 3 are awaiting liver transplantation at the time of this writing, and 10 are alive after transplantation.

DISCUSSION

Our results indicate that hypoxemia associated with pulmonary arteriovenous shunting can occur in children with many types of liver diseases and at any age. Although cirrhosis was present in most of these patients, one child had portal vein obstruction with no signs of cirrhosis. Pulmonary arteriovenous shunting also has been reported in children with congenital hepatic fibrosis and noncirrhotic portal hypertension.[14, 15] Even in children with cirrhosis there did not seem to be any relationship between pulmonary arteriovenous shunting and the degree of liver cell failure. Portal hypertension thus seems to be the common etiologic factor, and the development of portosystemic circulation may play a part; such collateral vessels would allow potential vasoactive substances of digestive origin to bypass the liver and act on the pulmonary vessels.[5] The prevalence of this complication in children with liver disease may range from 0.5% in children with portal vein obstruction up to 20% in children with biliary atresia and the polysplenia syndrome; in children with other types of cirrhosis the prevalence may be close to 2% to 4%. Because of the retrospective nature of this study, these estimates are probably imprecise; for instance, the 1% prevalence in children with biliary atresia but no polysplenia syndrome is underestimated because many children died or had transplants before the age when this complication occurs, and because the search for and the interpretation of symptoms of pulmonary shunting have been more careful in recent years.

Cyanosis and exertional dyspnea were the usual initial symptoms of arteriovenous shunting. Cyanosis is alarming but is not always easy to detect in a severely jaundiced child; any kind of dyspnea should alert the physician to the possibility of pulmonary arteriovenous shunting in a child with liver disease. In two of our patients, dyspnea was initially thought to be due to asthma; in one case, this delayed proper investigations for 1 year. High blood hemoglobin or low Pa_{CO_2} values, even with nearly normal Pa_{O_2}, should also suggest the possibility of pulmonary shunting.

Early diagnosis of pulmonary arteriovenous shunting is vital in children with liver diseases because liver transplantation may allow complete regression of shunting. Pulmonary scintiscan using macroaggregated albumin particles labeled with technetium Tc 99m is a reliable diagnostic test.[16] These particles, having a diameter greater than 20 μm, normally are trapped in the pulmonary capillaries. In the presence of pulmonary arteriovenous shunting, widening of these capillaries to greater than their normal 8 to 15

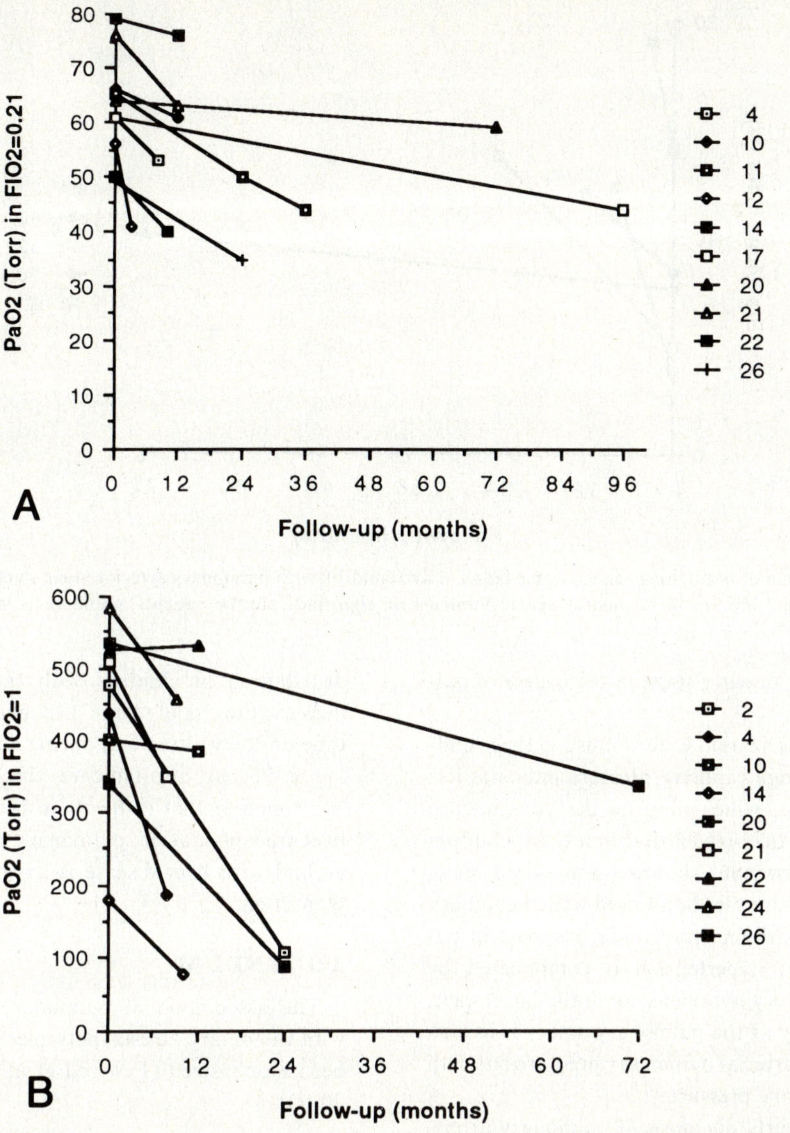

Fig. 2. Evolution of PaO_2, with time, in children with liver diseases and pulmonary arteriovenous shunting. **A,** Data on 10 children who had at least two measurements while breathing room air 3 months to 8 years apart. **B,** Data on 9 children who had at least two measurements while they were breathing 100% oxygen 8 months to 6 years apart. *Numbers on right* (panels **A** and **B**) indicate the patients' numbers as listed in the Table.

μm diameter, or opening of precapillary arteriovenous communications, allows the particles to be detected in significant amounts outside the lung.[2] A convenient means of expressing the results in children with liver diseases is to calculate the brain/lung ratio of isotope fixation.[11] This ratio, expressed as a percentage, is normally less than 1; if greater than 2, it is virtually certain to be associated with pulmonary arteriovenous shunting. A result between 1 and 2 is indeterminate, and the test should be repeated after 2 to 3 months. Because the irradiation caused by the procedure is extremely low, the test can be repeated safely, and it could be a useful screening tool in children with portal hypertension. Arterial blood gas measurements while the patient is inhaling room air and 100% O_2 are important to evaluate the severity of shunting and the prognosis. Ideally they should be carried out with a small arterial catheter. Our results suggest that PaO_2 in 100% O_2 >300 mm Hg is associated with the highest rate of survival after liver transplantation. Although liver transplantation can allow full regression of pulmonary arteriovenous shunting even when PaO_2 in 100% O_2 is very low,[7, 13] it is likely that the postoperative period will be less complicated if liver transplan-

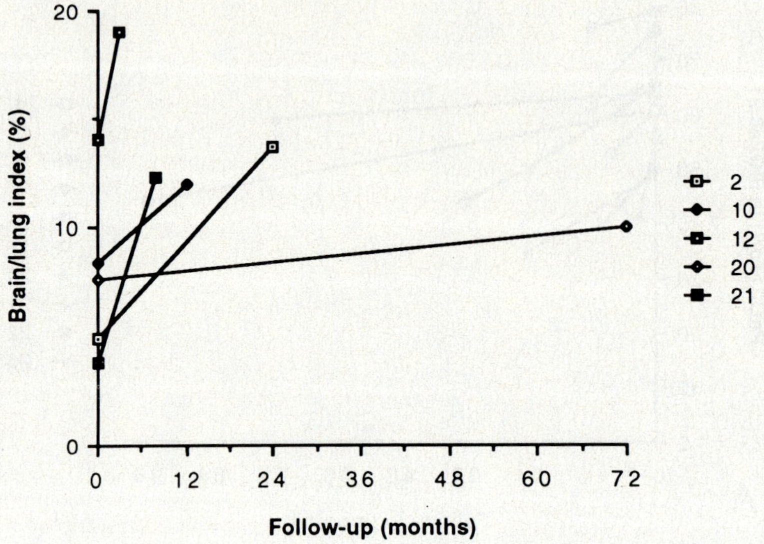

Fig. 3. Evolution of brain/lung scintigraphic index in five children with pulmonary arteriovenous shunting who were investigated twice, 3 months to 72 months apart. *Numbers on right* indicate the patients' numbers as listed in the Table.

tation is carried out at an early stage in the course of pulmonary shunting.

Right cardiac catheterization is also of use in these children. An increased wedge capillary pressure indicates left ventricular dysfunction, which may be the consequence both of hypoxia and of the high cardiac index. All children with pulmonary arteriovenous shunting and raised mean pulmonary artery pressure also had raised wedge capillary pressure. These results differ from those observed in patients in whom portal hypertension is complicated by primary pulmonary artery hypertension; in the latter case, plexogenic arteriopathy of the pulmonary artery is associated with raised mean arterial pulmonary pressure but with a normal wedge capillary pressure.[17]

The importance of early diagnosis of pulmonary arteriovenous shunting in children with liver disease is highlighted by the rapid progression of hypoxia, which was observed in many cases, and by the complete reversal of shunting after early liver transplantation. We thus emphasize the need for regular screening for pulmonary arteriovenous shunting in all children with portal hypertension, regardless of its cause. Special attention should be paid to every suggestive clinical symptom; pulmonary scintiscan or contrast-enhanced echocardiography[5] should be carried out and repeated in case of doubt. Scintiscans could even become part of a systematic screening program, so that pulmonary arteriovenous shunting could be detected as early as possible and the child provided with the best possible chances of success of liver transplantation. In many of these children, malnutrition, abdominal adhesions caused by prior surgery for biliary atresia, and atypical vascular distribution in children with the polysplenia syndrome increase the risk of severe postoperative complications. The time on the waiting list, during which worsening of shunting will occur, also indicates the need for early detection. We conclude that rather than being a contraindication to liver transplantation, pulmonary arteriovenous shunting in a child with liver disease is an indication for liver transplantation.

ADDENDUM

The association of pulmonary arteriovenous shunting with the biliary atresia–polysplenia syndrome has recently been emphasized (Fewtrell et al. Arch Dis Childh 1994; 70:501-4).

We thank Prof. Garre for follow-up data on patient 17 and Prof. J. B. Otte for follow-up data on patients 4 and 14.

REFERENCES

1. Sherlock S. Diseases of the liver and biliary system. Oxford: Blackwell, 1989:82-6.
2. Krowka MJ, Cortese DA. Pulmonary aspects of liver diseases and liver transplantation. Clin Chest Med 1989;10:593-616.
3. Rodriguez-Roisin R, Agusti AGN, Roca J. The hepatopulmonary syndrome: new name, old complexities. Thorax 1992; 47:897-902.
4. Kravath RE, Scarpelli E, Bernstein J. Hepatogenic cyanosis: arteriovenous shunts in chronic active hepatitis. J PEDIATR 1971;78:238-45.
5. Krowka MJ, Cortese DA. Hepatopulmonary syndrome: an evolving perspective in the era of liver transplantation. Hepatology 1990;11:138-42.
6. Stoller JK, Moodie D, Schiavone WA, et al. Reduction of in-

trapulmonary shunt and resolution of digital clubbing associated with primary biliary cirrhosis after liver transplantation. Hepatology 1990;11:54-8.
7. McCloskey JJ, Schleien C, Schwarz K, Klein A, Colombani P. Severe hypoxemia and intrapulmonary shunting resulting from cirrhosis reversed by liver transplantation in a pediatric patient. J PEDIATR 1991;118:902-4.
8. Laberge JM, Brandt ML, Lebecque P, et al. Reversal of cirrhosis-related pulmonary shunting in two children by orthotopic liver transplantation. Transplantation 1992;53:1135-8.
9. Mews CF, Dorney SF, Sheil AG, Forbes DA, Hill RE. Failure of liver transplantation in Wilson's disease with pulmonary arteriovenous shunting. J Pediatr Gastroenterol Nut 1990; 10:230-3.
10. Ibarguen E, Gross CR, Savik SK, Sharp HL. Liver disease in alpha-1-antitrypsin deficiency: prognostic indicators. J PEDIATR 1990;117:864-70.
11. Grimon G, Andre L, Bernard O, Raffestin B, Desgrez A. Early radionuclide detection of intrapulmonary shunts in children with liver diseases. J Nucl Med 1994;35:1328-32.
12. Hobeika J, Houssin D, Bernard O, et al. Orthotopic liver transplantation in children with chronic liver disease and severe hypoxemia. Transplantation 1994;57:224-8.
13. Van Obbergh L, Carlier M, Clement de Clety S, et al. Liver transplantation and pulmonary gas exchanges in hypoxemic children. Am Rev Respir Dis 1993;148:1408-10.
14. Maggiore G, Borgna-Pignatti C, Marni E, Abbati G, Magrini U. Pulmonary arteriovenous fistula: an unusual complication of congenital hepatic fibrosis. J Pediatr Gastroenterol Nut 1983;2:183-6.
15. Babbs C, Warnes TW, Haboubi NY. Noncirrhotic portal hypertension with hypoxaemia. Gut 1988;29:129-31.
16. Stanley NN, Ackrill P, Wood J. Lung perfusion scanning in hepatic cirrhosis. BMJ 1972;4:639-43.
17. Lockhart A. Pulmonary arterial hypertension in portal hypertension. Clin Gastroenterol 1985;14:123-38.

Book review

Epilepsy in children. 2nd ed.

Aicardi J. New York: Raven Press Books, 1994. 555 pages. $95.

Dr. Aicardi has done it again. This long-awaited update of his textbook on epilepsy in children is everything that we have come to expect. His clear, narrative style is highly accessible, even to those with limited experience in epilepsy. He tempers an exhaustive review of the literature (2552 references) with his extensive clinical experience. He has a remarkable ability to place an often bewildering group of disorders within a coherent, logical framework.

The book begins with a superlative comparison of epileptic versus nonepileptic seizures, accompanied by a helpful discussion of the various factors that influence and provoke clinical expression of seizures. The next chapter reviews the classification of seizures and contains an excellent discussion of the different classification schemes. Dr. Aicardi is clearly not invested in one scheme or another but has a superb ability to place them all in perspective and elucidate the strengths and weaknesses of each.

The next section of the book describes individual seizure types. Within each chapter, the author discusses the clinical manifestations, typical and atypical electroencephalographic patterns, causes, differential diagnosis, and management of the particular type of seizure. Excellent discussions of the controversies in nosology help clarify the literature and bring order to this otherwise confusing field.

The last several chapters cover the prognosis and management of epilepsy. These reflect the author's wealth of clinical experience and offer many helpful suggestions for working with children and their parents. The principles of management are well delineated and offer an abundance of information, even for experienced clinicians.

The references for the entire textbook are grouped in alphabetic order in the back of the book. Placing them at the end of each chapter or section would facilitate the search for references pertaining to a particular topic.

The figures are clear and well captioned and illustrate key points within the text. The prose is an easy, narrative style and eminently readable. The book is well indexed and easy to use as a reference. This book is essential reading for all pediatric neurologists and epileptologists. It would also be a helpful addition to the library of anyone who treats children with epilepsy.

Phillip S. Riback, MD
Section of Child Neurology, Department of Neurology
Albany Medical College
Albany, NY 12208

CLINICAL AND LABORATORY OBSERVATIONS

Life-threatening infection in two children with hemoglobin S–beta-thalassemia

Amy Lynch, MD, and Joseph D. Tobias, MD

From the Division of Pediatric Critical Care and Anesthesia, Vanderbilt University, Nashville, Tennessee

Life-threatening infections with *Streptococcus pneumoniae* and parvovirus occurred in two patients with hemoglobin S–β-thalassemia. We recommend that acute febrile illnesses in the presence of any hemoglobinopathy be considered potentially life threatening, and managed accordingly. (J PEDIATR 1995;126:581-2)

Although overwhelming infections have been described in patients with homozygous hemoglobin abnormalities, the heterozygote state of sickle cell disease is relatively benign and characterized by an expected symptom-free existence and normal longevity. However, when one Hgb S gene is paired with a second abnormal hemoglobin, such as hemoglobin C, hemoglobin D, or β-thalassemia, the resultant disorder can vary in severity.

The combination of a sickle gene and a β-thalassemia gene occurs in 0.06% of black persons.[1] We report two cases of life-threatening infections in patients with heterozygous sickle–β-thalassemia to remind clinicians that such children should have early detection of infectious illnesses to prevent severe complications similar to those seen in their homozygous counterparts.

CASE REPORTS

Patient 1. A previously healthy black 6-year-old boy with sickle trait awoke the morning of admission with vomiting, diarrhea, cough, and fever. The symptoms worsened progressively and he was found unresponsive by his father. In the emergency department, initial findings were as follows: temperature, 40.6° C; pulse, 156 beats/min; respirations, 52 breaths/min; and blood pressure, 80 mm Hg by palpation. Physical examination showed extreme lethargy, dry mucous membranes, and decreased peripheral pulses. Results of laboratory studies included the following: hematocrit, 0.15; leukocyte count, $20.9 \times 10^9/L$ ($20{,}900/mm^3$); platelet count, $90 \times 10^9/L$ ($90{,}000/mm^3$); prothrombin time, 23 seconds; and partial thromboplastin time, 84 seconds. The initial mean corpuscular volume was 94.6 μm^3 with an erythrocyte distribution width index of 17.7%; many sickle cells were seen on the peripheral smear. The patient received intravenously administered fluids and antibiotics, and was transferred to the pediatric intensive care unit where his course was characterized by progressive respiratory failure, hemodynamic instability, renal failure, and disseminated intravascular coagulation. The initial blood culture grew *Streptococcus pneumoniae*, and the patient was found to have osteomyelitis of the left tibia. Hemoglobin electrophoresis from admission revealed 91% hemoglobin S, 7% hemoglobin A, and 2% hemoglobin F. His condition gradually improved and he was discharged from the pediatric intensive care unit to complete the antibiotic course. Mild renal dysfunction was noted as a result of acute tubular necrosis.

Patient 2. A 14-year-old black girl had a 2-day history of headache, backache, and abdominal discomfort that was thought to be of viral origin. A blood count revealed a leukocyte count of $12 \times 10^9/L$ ($12{,}000/mm^3$), hematocrit 0.27 (27%), and a positive sickle cell test result. The day of admission, the patient became progressively more agitated and was in an obtunded state when seen in the emergency department. On arrival, finding were as follows: temperature, 38.7° C; pulse, 168 beats/min; respirations, 32 breaths/min; and blood pressure, 128/80 mm Hg. Physical examination showed an obtunded state and marked respiratory distress. Laboratory studies revealed hematocrit of 0.17, platelet count $79 \times 10^9/L$ ($79{,}000/mm^3$), and leukocyte count $5.1 \times 10^9/L$ ($5100/mm^3$) with 28% neutrophils, 67% lymphocytes, 2% monocytes, 1% eosinophils, and 2% metamyelocytes. The mean corpuscular volume was 66 μm^3 with an erythrocyte distribution width index of 14.7%. The reticulocyte count was 0.2%, and results of coagulation studies were normal. A computed tomographic scan of the head showed normal findings, and analysis of cerebrospinal fluid revealed 2 leukocytes per high-power field, no erythrocytes; glucose 6.2 mmol/L (111 mg/dl), and protein concentration 190 mg/dl. Blood, urine, and cerebrospinal fluid samples were obtained for culture, and intravenous antibiotic therapy was started. Her course was characterized by progressive respiratory failure, hemodynamic instability, and massive blood product requirements. He-

Submitted for publication June 21, 1994; accepted Oct. 25, 1994.

Reprint requests: Amy Lynch, MD, Vanderbilt University, Medical Center North T-0118, Nashville, TN 37232.

0022-3476/95/$3.00 + 0 **9/22/61574**

moglobin electrophoresis at the time of admission revealed 68.9% hemoglobin S, 26.8% hemoglobin A, and 4.3% hemoglobin F. The patient died of cardiorespiratory failure 4 days after the onset of symptoms. Postmortem examination revealed diffuse bone marrow infarction with fat embolism syndrome. Polymerase chain reaction on serum DNA obtained at autopsy revealed human parvovirus B19. Her spleen was massively enlarged with evidence of recent massive infarction. This girl had an 8-year-old brother who had been seen in another emergency department in cardiopulmonary arrest the week before her admission. He had sickle cell trait and had had a preceding viral illness. Resuscitation efforts were unsuccessful; a postmortem examination was not performed.

DISCUSSION

Patients with abnormal heterozygous hemoglobinopathies are generally thought to have milder disease with fewer complications than those with homozygous defects. Sickle cell and β-thalassemia genes have been described in the same individual.[2-4] Patients with sickle thalassemia syndromes often have nearly normal hemoglobin levels with little evidence of sickling on peripheral smear. Hemoglobin A concentration has been considered to have prognostic value in patients with sickle cell–β-thalassemia, but this is controversial.[2, 5, 6]

The pathogen *S. pneumoniae* is the most common cause of serious bacterial infection in patients with sickle cell disease.[7] We are unaware of previously reported cases of overwhelming infections in patients with sickle cell–β-thalassemia. There has been a report of a 9-year-old child with hemoglobin SC disease who died of pneumococcal sepsis.[8] In addition, a recent review described seven cases of fatal pneumococcal septicemia in children with hemoglobin SC disease.[9]

Reports of life-threatening infections in a group previously not thought to be at increased risk promote consideration of prophylaxis, vaccination, or both interventions. The routine use of polyvalent pneumococcal vaccine in functionally asplenic hosts is effective,[10] but does not afford complete protection.

Patients with chronic anemia as a result of a hemolytic condition usually can compensate for decreased erythrocyte survival by increasing bone marrow activity. Parvovirus infection causes aplastic crises in patients with hemolytic anemias; apparent outbreaks among siblings or "cluster groups" have been reported.[11] Even temporary cessation of bone marrow activity results in a 10% to 15% drop in hematocrit per day. In the sibling of the second child, a rapidly fatal aplastic crisis ensued without prior history of hemolytic anemia or any clinical conditions that would have prompted medical attention.

These two case histories suggest that children with sickle cell–β-thalassemia may be at risk of having a life-threatening infection and should be managed accordingly.

REFERENCES

1. Motulsky AG. Frequency of sickling disorders in U.S. blacks. N Engl J Med 1973;288:31-3.
2. Sergeant GR, Ashcroft MT, Sergeant BE, Milner PF. The clinical features of sickle cell/beta-thalassemia in Jamaica. Br J Haematol 1973;24:19-30.
3. El-Hazmi MAF, Al-Swailem AR. Sickle cell-$\beta 0$ thalassaemia in Saudi Arabia. Hum Hered 1987;37:211-6.
4. Schiliro G, Samperi P, Testa R, et al. Clinical, hematological and molecular features in Sicilians with Hb S–β-thalassemia. Am J Hematol 1992;41:264-9.
5. Atweh GF, Forget BG. Clinical and molecular correlations in the sickle/β^+-thalassemia syndrome. Am J Hematol 1987;24: 31-6.
6. Stevens MCG, Maude GH, Beckford M, et al. Haematological change in sickle cell–haemoglobin C disease and in sickle cell–beta-thalassemia: a cohort study from birth. Br J Haematol 1985;60:279-92.
7. Barrett-Conner E. Bacterial infection and sickle cell anemia. Medicine 1971;50:97-112.
8. Chilcote RR, Dampier C. Overwhelming pneumococcal septicemia in a patient with HbSC disease and splenic dysfunction. J Pediatr 1984;104:734-6.
9. Lane PA, Rogers ZR, Woods GM, et al. Fatal pneumococcal septicemia in hemoglobin SC disease. J Pediatr 1994;124: 859-62.
10. Amman AJ, Addiego JE, Wara DW, et al. Polyvalent pneumococcal polysaccharide immunization of patients with sickle cell anemia and patients with splenectomy. N Engl J Med 1977;297:897-900.
11. Sergeant GR, Topley JM, Mason K, et al. Outbreak of aplastic crisis in sickle cell anemia associated with parvovirus-like agent. Lancet 1981;2:595-7.

Development of a vaccine tracking system to improve the rate of age-appropriate primary immunization in children of lower socioeconomic status

Jon S. Abramson, MD, T. Michael O'Shea, MD, MPH, D. Lee Ratledge, BS, Michael R. Lawless, MD, and Laurence B. Givner, MD

From the Department of Pediatrics, Bowman Gray School of Medicine of Wake Forest University, Winston-Salem, North Carolina

We conducted a randomized, controlled trial to determine the effectiveness of an immunization tracking system designed to increase the number of infants of lower socioeconomic status who receive their primary series of vaccinations at age-appropriate times. By 7 months of age, 91% (274/301) of the infants in the intervention group were up-to-date on their primary series of vaccinations versus 72% (214/296) of the infants in the control group (*p* <0.0001). The estimated cost of follow-up for each infant in the intervention group was $18.05. (J Pediatr 1995; 126:583-6)

Although immunization rates have increased during the past decade, less than 70% of 2-year-old children in the United States are fully vaccinated.[1] An important factor in predicting which children will be delayed with their immunizations is low socioeconomic status. The main goal of the Childhood Immunization Initiative is completion of the recommended vaccinations for at least 90% of children by their second birthday (an exception of at least 70% is made for hepatitis B vaccine).[2]

One method of increasing appropriate vaccination rates is improved follow-up systems. All states are now developing tracking systems, but there are few prospective, controlled studies of their effectiveness. This article describes the effectiveness of a newly developed tracking system for increasing the number of children of lower socioeconomic status who receive their primary vaccination series on schedule.

METHODS

Patients and study design. More than 98% of the approximately 5600 infants born in Forsyth County, North Carolina, each year are delivered at Forsyth Memorial Hospital. Most infants of families of lower socioeconomic status receive their health care either at Reynolds Health Center, which is the Forsyth County public health center, or at Brenner Childrens' Hospital continuity clinic. These facilities are staffed by physicians at the Bowman Gray School of Medicine.

Infants born at Forsyth Memorial Hospital were eligible for inclusion if their mother indicated that the infant's primary care would be at the Reynolds Health Center or Brenner Childrens' Hospital clinics. Study enrollment took place on weekdays; infants born and discharged over the weekend were not enrolled. The project coordinator obtained the names, birth dates, addresses, and telephone numbers of mother and child; in addition to the home telephone number, other telephone numbers (i.e., work, relatives, or friends) were also obtained and the mother was asked the best times to phone her. These data were entered into a relational database (DATAEASE, DataEase International, Trumbull, Conn.) adapted for this project, and were maintained on a portable personal computer. Data collected from tracking immunizations were added as they became available. The database allowed for generation of automated lists of individuals who were due to receive reminder cards or phone calls.

All eligible children were randomly assigned to the inter-

Hib	*Haemophilus influenzae* type be conjugate vaccine
DTP	Diphtheria-tetanus-pertussis vaccine
OPV	Oral poliomyelitis vaccine

Supported by Merck Sharpe & Dohme.

Presented at the meetings of the Infectious Disease Society of America in New Orleans, La., Oct. 16-17, 1993, and the Society for Pediatric Research, Seattle, Wash., May 4, 1994.

Submitted for publication Sept. 2, 1994; accepted Oct. 24, 1994.

Reprint requests: Jon S. Abramson, MD, Department of Pediatrics, Bowman Gray School of Medicine, Medical Center Blvd., Winston-Salem, NC 27157.

0022-3476/95/$3.00 + 0 **9/22/61438**

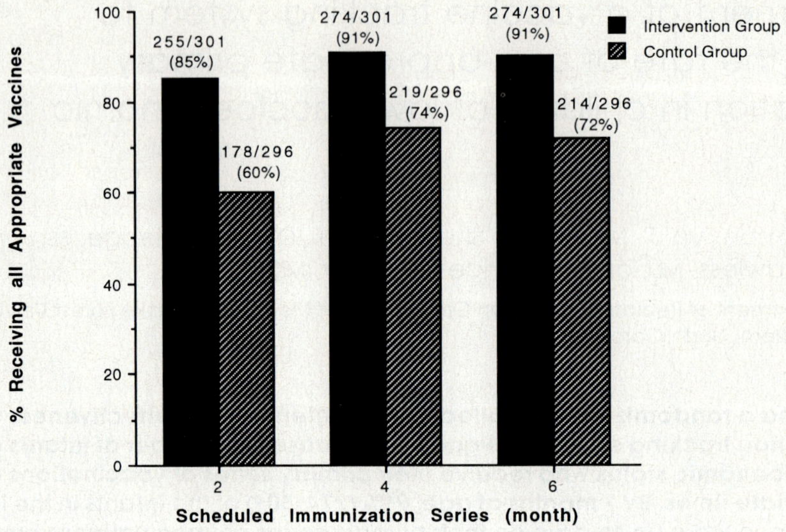

Figure. The percentage of infants in the intervention and control groups who received their primary series of vaccines at age-appropriate times ($p < 0.00001$ at each scheduled immunization).

vention or to the control group. The project coordinator met with each mother in the intervention group during the hospitalization. Informed consent was obtained only from mothers of children randomly assigned to the intervention group, with the rationale that control infants would be vaccinated and followed using procedures identical to current standard community practice. The study was approved by the clinical research practices committee of the Bowman Gray School of Medicine.

Parents of infants in the intervention group were sent reminder postcards 1 week before the target vaccination dates. Immunization records were extracted from manual entries into logbooks kept by personnel at both clinics. Records were examined weekly by the project coordinator, and the information was entered into the database. For infants in the intervention group who did not receive a scheduled vaccination, the parents were reminded again of scheduled vaccinations by a single postcard. At the same time, phone calls to the family were made once a week until (1) the infant received the vaccinations, (2) a family member indicated that the primary health care provider had changed, or (3) the infant was more than 1 month behind on scheduled immunizations. Most phone contacts were with mothers, but contact with any family member was considered acceptable. Infants in the control group received no intervention except the public health department's routine policy of sending a single postcard to families of infants who did not keep their scheduled appointments; control infants whose families did not make an initial appointment received no reminders.

The primary outcome was the proportion of infants in each group who received their primary series of immunizations at age-appropriate times. This end point is of interest because children who do not complete their primary series of vaccinations on schedule are at high risk of remaining behind on their immunizations.[3] During the study period, the vaccine schedule at the Reynolds Health Center and Brenner Childrens' Hospital clinics was as follows: diphtheria-tetanus-pertussis vaccine at 2, 4, and 6 months; oral polio myelitis vaccine at 2 and 4 months; *Haemophilus influenzae* type b conjugate vaccine at 2, 4, and 6 months; and hepatitis B vaccine at 1, 2, and 6 months. Infants were considered vaccinated at age-appropriate times if they received the appropriate immunizations within 1 month of this schedule. All infants were followed until they completed their primary series of immunizations or they reached 7 months of age. Routine use of hepatitis B vaccine was begun 3 months after the study was initiated. Therefore infants enrolled before this time were considered fully immunized if they received all other scheduled vaccines.

The cost of the tracking system for each infant in the intervention group was determined as follows: Total cost including computer, personnel, and supplies/Number of infants in the intervention group.

Statistics. The chi-square test was used to examine differences in proportions. The 95% confidence limits for risk differences were determined as described by Simon.[4]

RESULTS

From Jan. 7 through Oct. 15, 1993, 601 infants were enrolled in this study (302 and 299 infants in the intervention and control groups, respectively). By study design, all infants were from families of lower socioeconomic status. The two groups were also similar for race, number of siblings, maternal age, and marital status. One parent of an infant in the intervention group refused to participate. One infant in the intervention group and three control infants moved out of state and were lost to follow-up. The parents of four infants in the intervention group and seven control infants changed health care providers within the state during the follow-up period; vaccination status was determined at 7 months of age for these 11 children, and all but one in each group were up-to-date on their immunizations (these children were included in the analysis on an intention-to-treat basis). Thus the study analysis included 301 infants in the intervention group and 296 control infants.

The percentages of children receiving their primary vaccinations at age-appropriate times are shown in the Figure. At 7 months of age, 91% (274/301) of infants in the intervention group versus 72% (214/296) of control infants were up-to-date on vaccinations, a 19% difference in the risk of being delayed at 7 months of age (95% confidence limits, 13%, 25%; chi-square, 35.1; $p = 3 \times 10^{-9}$). The corresponding risk differences at 2 and 4 months were, respectively, 25% (confidence limits, 18%, 31%) and 17% (confidence limits, 11%, 23%). Routine immunization with hepatitis B vaccine began 3 months after study initiation. Subsequently each child who had received the 2- and 6-month hepatitis B vaccines also received all other scheduled vaccines.

Of those children fully immunized by 7 months of age, 28% (78/274) in the intervention versus 44% (95/214) in the control group missed their first scheduled appointment (chi-square value, 13.3; $p = 0.0002$), and therefore received postcard or telephone reminders or both. Most infants in both groups who did not complete their primary immunization series by 7 months of age were delayed in receiving some or all of their immunizations (DTP, OPV, Hib, and hepatitis B) at 2 months of age (62% [18/29] and 78% [68/86] of infants in the intervention and control groups, respectively [chi-square value, 3.3; $p = 0.07$]). Of those infants in the intervention group who missed one scheduled vaccination, 35% (106/301) required one or more reminder phone calls (Table). For those infants who missed two or more scheduled vaccinations, phone calls were made to an additional 14% (43/301) of families.

The total cost of following each infant in the intervention group through 7 months of age was $18.05. This figure was corrected for time spent by the project coordinator in following control group infants. The costs included the following: (1) coordinator's salary and fringe benefits: 18 hours a week at $10.63/hour; cost per infant, $12.77, (2) ongoing supplies (postage and telephone), $1.11 per infant, and (3) startup items (computer, software, and printer), $4.17 per infant; the cost of this tracking system minus the startup costs was $13.78 per infant.

Table. Families in the intervention group to whom phone calls were made

No. requiring phone calls	Intervention group No. %
For only one vaccination series	106/301 (35)
1 Phone call	84/106 (79)
≥2 Phone calls	22/106 (21)
For multiple vaccination series	43/301 (14)
1 Phone call/vaccination series	28/43 (65)
≥2 Phone calls/vaccination series	15/43 (35)
Place family was contacted: total calls made*	188
Home	134/188 (71)
Work	17/188 (9)†
Other (e.g., relative)	37/188 (20)†

Data represent the number (percentage) of families in the intervention group to whom telephone calls were made because their infant missed a scheduled vaccination.

*Of 301 families, 35 (12%) did not have home telephones.

†Of the total number of contacts made at work or at other places, 21% and 79%, respectively, were with families that did not have a home telephone.

DISCUSSION

Prior studies have indicated that reminder postcards increase age-appropriate vaccination rates.[5-7] However, these studies have been limited in the strength of their conclusion because they either did not follow the children for all indicated vaccines or they evaluated vaccine status at a single time point. Our study demonstrates that an immunization tracking system that follows infants from birth and utilizes both mail and telephone reminders can substantially increase the rate of timely vaccination. The methods used to ensure vaccination compliance in the children assigned to the interventional tracking system differed from the method in the control group in several ways: (1) the importance of receiving scheduled vaccinations was discussed soon after birth only with intervention group mothers, (2) only intervention group families were sent a postcard reminder before each scheduled vaccination, and (3) only intervention group families were contacted by telephone.

Several factors appear to have contributed to the success of our tracking system. Our data, showing that a greater percentage in the control group than in the intervention group missed their first scheduled appointment, indicate that one or both tracking system components that occurred before the first scheduled vaccination (i.e., project coordinator's interaction with mothers at birth, the preappointment postcard reminder) helped increase the mothers' compliance with the scheduled appointments. Enrollment of infants at birth also avoids the problem that infants who have not been scheduled for an initial appointment are unknown to immunization providers.

Components of the tracking system instituted after a missed vaccine appointment were also needed; 35% of infants in the intervention group missed a vaccination appointment and required postcard and telephone reminders. Further studies are needed to evaluate the relative contributions of each of the components of this tracking system to its overall success, as well as the effectiveness of this type of program in other settings (e.g., locales with large inner-city populations).

The immunization tracking program cost $18.05 per child. This figure will vary for other sites, because it is dependent on multiple factors including location, number of infants tracked, baseline age-appropriate vaccination rates, and the duration of tracking. Additionally, potentially cost-effective measures could be incorporated into this tracking system (e.g., telephone calls by trained volunteers). Although any tracking system will require expenditures, such programs will prevent diseases and ultimately reduce health care costs. For each dollar invested in measles-mumps-rubella, DTP, and OPV vaccines, it is estimated that $16.30, $6.20, and $3.40, respectively, is saved (personal communication, Dr. Stephen Hadler, Centers for Disease Control and Prevention, May 12, 1994).

The nationwide use of effective vaccination-tracking systems is an important component for achieving and maintaining high vaccination rates in preschool-age children. The tracking system described herein effectively increased the level of up-to-date primary vaccination in our community, and potentially could accomplish the Childhood Immunization Initiative goal of up-to-date immunization of 90% of 2-year-old children.[2] The effectiveness of other types of tracking systems used in various locales also needs to be prospectively evaluated.

REFERENCES

1. Centers for Disease Control and Prevention. Vaccination coverage of 2-year-old children—United States, 1993. MMWR Morb Mortal Wkly Rep 1994;43:705-9.
2. Centers for Disease Control and Prevention. Reported vaccine-preventable diseases—United States, 1993, and the Childhood Immunization Initiative. MMWR Morb Mortal Wkly Rep 1994;43:57-60.
3. Centers for Disease Control and Prevention. Retrospective assessment of vaccination coverage among school-aged children—selected U.S. cities. MMWR Morb Mortal Wkly Rep 1992;41:103-7.
4. Simon R. Confidence intervals for reporting results of clinical trials. Ann Intern Med 1986;105:429-35.
5. Byrne EB, Schaffner W, Dini EF, Case GE. Infant immunization surveillance: cost vs effect. A prospective, controlled evaluation of a large-scale program in Rhode Island. JAMA 1970;212:770-3.
6. Young SA, Halpin TJ, Johnson DA, Irvin JJ, Marks JS. Effectiveness of a mailed reminder on the immunization levels of infants at high risk of failure to complete immunizations. Am J Public Health 1980;70:422-4.
7. Tollestrup K, Bubbard BB. Evaluation of a follow-up system in a county health department's immunization clinic. Am J Prev Med 1991;7:24-8.

Portal vein thrombosis caused by protein C and protein S deficiency associated with cytomegalovirus infection

Ravit Arav-Boger, MD, Shimon Reif, MD, and Yoram Bujanover, MD
From the Department of Pediatrics and the Division of Pediatric Gastroenterology, Dana Children's Hospital, Tel Aviv Medical Center, Tel Aviv, Israel

A 4-month-old girl who was examined because of splenomegaly had portal vein thrombosis, which apparently resulted from a combination of cytomegalovirus infection and deficiency of both protein S and protein C. The cytomegalovirus infection, by damaging endothelial cells, may have triggered a cascade of events that was ultimately expressed as portal vein thrombosis resulting from deficiency of proteins S and C. (J PEDIATR 1995;126:586-8)

Submitted for publication July 25, 1994; accepted Oct. 25, 1994.

Reprint requests: Yoram Bujanover, MD, Division of Pediatric Gastroenterology, Dana Children's Hospital, Tel Aviv Medical Center, 6 Weizman St., Tel Aviv 64239, Israel.

0022-3476/95/$3.00 + 0 9/22/61573

Portal vein thrombosis in early childhood may be a result of perinatal events such as omphalitis, umbilical vein cannulation, intraabdominal sepsis, dehydration, or hypercoagulability states.[1] In more than 50% of cases, the cause of prehepatic portal vein thrombosis is unknown.[1]

We describe a 4-month-old girl with portal vein thrombosis associated with both cytomegalovirus infection and deficiency of proteins C and S.

CASE REPORT

The patient was born at term after an uneventful pregnancy to apparently healthy parents. Birth weight was 3200 gm, and the perinatal history was unremarkable. A 2-year-old sister was healthy. At the age of 4 months, the patient was evaluated because of splenomegaly. On physical examination, the spleen was palpable 8 cm and the liver 3 cm below the costal margin. Laboratory tests revealed the following: hemoglobin, 1.7 mmol/L (11 gm/dl); erythrocyte count, 6.7×10^9/L (6700/mm^3); platelet count, 163×10^9 (163,000/mm^3); erythrocyte sedimentation rate, 8 mm/hr; alkaline phosphatase, 583 U/L; total protein, 61 gm/L; albumin, 40 gm/L; aspartate aminotransferase, 125 U/L; alanine aminotransferase, 145 U/L; prothrombin time, 16 seconds; and partial thromboplastin time, 29 seconds. Results of serologic studies for hepatitis A, B, and C were negative, as was testing of IgM for Epstein-Barr virus. The serum IgG concentration was 20.48 gm/L. Test results of IgM and IgM for cytomegalovirus (assessed with an enzyme-linked immunosorbent assay kit, Sorin, France) were highly positive. Toxoplasmosis, VDRL, and rubella serologic test results were negative; cytomegalovirus was isolated from the urine.

Eye examination revealed no gross abnormality, and there was no evidence of chorioretinitis. Skull x-ray studies showed no calcifications, and brain-stem evoked response auditory potential, chest x-ray study, and electrocardiographic findings were normal. Doppler ultrasound examination of the abdomen revealed an enlarged spleen, mild ascitic fluid, narrowing of the portal vein, and multiple collateral vessels in the portal area.

At the age of 8 months, the patient was referred to our hospital for further evaluation. On physical examination, she appeared to be well developed, and psychomotor assessment scores were appropriate for age. The spleen was palpated 8 cm and the liver 3 cm below the costal margin. Laboratory test results were as follows: hemoglobin, 1.7 mmol/L (11 gm/dl) with normal indexes; leukocyte count, 11×10^9 cells/L (11,000/mm^3); hemoglobin electrophoresis results were appropriate for age; total protein, 55 gm/L; albumin, 34 gm/L; globulin, 21 gm/L; aspartate aminotransferase, 52 U/L; alanine aminotransferase, 76 U/L; alkaline phosphatase, 162 U/L; triglycerides, 1.54 mmol/L (136 mg/dl); prothrombin time, 14.3 seconds; partial thromboplastin time, 25.3 seconds; IgM, 1400 mg/L; IgG, 8.8 gm/L; IgA, 1.86 gm/L; α-fetoprotein, 61 μg/L (61 ng/ml); α_1-antitrypsin, 2.5 gm/L; ceruloplasmin, 429 mg/L. Results of the sweat test were negative. Serologic cytomegalovirus test results were negative for IgM; the IgG level was 1:1000.

Doppler ultrasonography revealed splenomegaly, mild ascites, and typical changes of portal vein thrombosis with cavernous malformation. Blood flow in the portal vein was hepatopetal. Computed tomography confirmed the ultrasound finding of classic cavernous malformation with multiple collateral vessels in the portal area.

Gastro esophageal endoscopy demonstrated grade III esophageal varices, with normal gastric and duodenal mucosa. Liver biopsy specimens revealed normal architecture with no inflammation or inclusion bodies.

Further investigations were performed to determine the cause of portal vein thrombosis. Immunoassay of proteins S and C and activity assays (performed according to the manufacturers' instructions with the Protein S Activity Assay kit [Behringwerke AG, Marburg, Germany] and Dade Protein C Chromogenic Assay [Baxter Diagnostics AG, Duedinger, Switzerland] showed deficiency of both proteins (Table). Antithrombin III activity was 83% (normal, 74% to 126%). The mother had a decreased level of protein S antigen (64%). The father's respective levels were normal; the sister's protein S antigen level was 42%.

Table. Protein S and protein C levels in serum of the patient

Age (mo)	Protein S antigen* (%)‡	Protein C antigen† (%)§
9	32	35
11	42	37
14	19	31
20	29	36
26	33	38

*Free protein S (activity) was 58%.
†Free protein C (activity) was 36%.
‡Normal, 70% to 140%.
§Normal, 70% to 140%.

Treatment for portal hypertension was initiated with the administration of propranolol at a dose of 2 mg/kg twice a day. At 17 months of age, the patient was readmitted to the hospital with massive hematemesis, the result of active variceal bleeding. Because of the severe blood loss (hemoglobin level, 5 gm/dl), she required two blood transfusions. She then underwent sequential sclerotherapy. Splenomegaly and portal hypertension are still present, but the patient's condition is currently stable and she is doing well. She is being treated with propranolol, and there is no hematologic evidence of hypersplenism.

DISCUSSION

One of the few inherited abnormalities that causes a hypercoagulable state in children is protein S deficiency.[2] Protein S is a vitamin K–dependent cofactor of protein C, which is a vitamin K–dependent serine proteinase. When protein C is activated by thrombin, it inactivates factors Va and VIIIa, acting as a potent anticoagulant. Heterozygous individuals with protein S and C deficiency have a tendency for development of venous thrombosis. Their protein S and C levels are approximately one half those of normal values, and they rarely have symptoms before adolescence. Cases of childhood stroke, arterial thrombosis, deep vein thrombosis, and other related conditions have been reported.[3-5]

The prevalence and the clinical importance of these vitamin K–dependent anticoagulants have not been clearly defined. In one large series, protein S deficiency was found in approximately one of 300 individuals, but most had no history of thrombotic episodes. Thus deficiencies of protein S, protein C, or both contribute to thrombosis, but they are seldom the sole cause. Damaged endothelium or vascular injury may also act as contributing factors.[6] In several reports, total protein S levels, but not the free protein, were correlated with thrombotic events,[7] but other studies suggested that the free protein S is relevant to its activity as a cofactor.[3]

Of neonates with congenital cytomegalovirus infection, 90% to 95% have no symptoms in the neonatal period; splenomegaly may be the sole manifestation.[8] The virus can initiate endothelial inflammation and vasculitis, especially in patients with acquired immunodeficiency syndrome. Infection of endothelial cells can produce occlusive vascular ischemia.[9] The exposure of our patient to cytomegalovirus could have occurred in utero or perinatally.

Because it damages endothelial cells, cytomegalovirus infection could have triggered a cascade of events that finally led to the development of portal vein thrombosis.

This patient had heterozygous deficiency of protein S and low protein C levels. Her mother had moderately reduced levels of protein S antigen, and her sister had low levels of protein S antigen. Neither of them had any thromboembolic phenomena. Further tests revealed that free protein S was also reduced. The protein C level was normal in the other members of the family. Few reports describe such combined deficiencies, and it has been recommended that they be sought in families already known to be lacking one antithrombotic protein.[10, 11] Perhaps the deficiency of proteins C and S was the result of cytomegalovirus-related hepatitis. Previous reports of such low protein C levels have associated them with severe liver damage.[12] However, in our patient there was no substantial evidence of liver damage, although a slight elevation of liver enzyme activity had been present, and the normal liver histologic findings may not support this hypothesis. Moreover, the detection of abnormal levels of protein S in other members of the family strengthens the argument that a genetic defect, associated with the cytomegalovirus infection, was important in the development of portal vein thrombosis in this infant.

Anticoagulants are the preferred treatment in protein S deficiency, but because of the esophageal varices, we were reluctant to use them to treat this child, and therefore administered only propranolol. Liver transplantation could correct the protein S deficiency, but in light of the preserved liver function and the possibility of cure as a result of recanalization in the thrombus, this option was deferred.

Reports of portal vein thrombosis associated with proteins S and C deficiency are rare.[13] This case report demonstrates the possible interaction between cytomegalovirus infection, with its endothelial cell–damaging effect, and a genetic hypercoagulable state resulting in portal vein thrombosis in early infancy.

REFERENCES

1. Bernard O, Alvarez, Brunelle F, Hadchouel P, Alagille D. Portal hypertension in children. Clin Gastroenterol 1985;14:33-54.
2. Lusher JM. Diseases in coagulation: the fluid phase. In: Nathan DG, Oski FA, eds. Hematology of infancy and childhood. Philadelphia: WB Saunders, 1987:1293-342.
3. Comp PC, Esmon CT. Recurrent venous thromboembolism in patients with a partial deficiency of protein S. N Engl J Med 1984;311:1525-8.
4. Horowitz IN, Galvis AG, Gompers ED. Arterial thrombosis and protein S deficiency. J Pediatr 1992;121:934-7.
5. Devilat M, Toso M, Morales M. Childhood stroke associated with protein C or S deficiency and primary antiphospholipid syndrome. Pediatr Neurol 1993;9:67-70.
6. Rick ME. Protein C and protein S. Vitamin K–dependent inhibitors of blood coagulation. JAMA 1990;263:701-3.
7. Engesser L, Broekmans AW, Briet E, et al. Hereditary protein S deficiency: clinical manifestations. Ann Intern Med 1987; 106:677-82.
8. Demmler GJ. Acquired cytomegalovirus infections. In: Feigin RD, Cherry JD, eds. Textbook of pediatric infectious diseases. 3rd ed. Philadelphia: WB Saunders, 1992;2:1532-47.
9. Koskinen P, Lemstrom K, Bruggeman C, Lautenschlager I, Hayry P. Acute cytomegalovirus infection induces a subendothelial inflammation (endothelialitis) in the allograft vascular wall. A possible linkage with enhanced allograft arteriosclerosis. Am J Pathol 1994;144:41-50.
10. Jobin F, Vu L, Lessard M. Two cases of inherited triple deficiency in a large kindred with thrombotic diathesis and deficiency of antithrombin III, heparin cofactor II, protein C and protein S. Thromb Haemost 1991;66:295-9.
11. Brenner B, Tavori S, Zivelin A, et al. Hereditary deficiency of all vitamin K-dependent procoagulants and anticoagulants. Br J Haematol 1990;75:537-42.
12. Shulman HM, Hinterberger W. Hepatic veno-occlusive disease–liver toxicity syndrome after bone marrow transplantation. Bone Marrow Transplant 1992;10:197-214.
13. Sas G, Blaski G, Petro I, et al. A protein S deficient family with portal vein thrombosis. Thromb Haemost 1985;54:724.

Absence of infection in breast-fed infants born to hepatitis C virus–infected mothers

Ho-Hsiung Lin, MD, PhD, Jia-Horng Kao, MD, Hong-Yuan Hsu, MD, PhD, Yen-Hsuan Ni, MD, Mei-Hwei Chang MD, Su-Cheng Huang, MD, Lih-Hwa Hwang, PhD, Pei-Jer Chen, MD, PhD, and Ding-Shinn Chen, MD

From the Departments of Obstetrics and Gynecology, and Pediatrics, Graduate Institute of Clinical Medicine and Hepatitis Research Center, College of Medicine, National Taiwan University, Taipei, Taiwan, Republic of China

The role of breast-feeding in perinatal transmission of hepatitis C virus (HCV) was explored in 15 HCV-infected mothers and their infants. The 15 carrier mothers had anti-HCV titers ranging from 1:80 to 1:40,000 and also had HCV–ribonucleic acid with concentrations ranging from 10^4 to 2.5×10^8 copies/ml. Both anti-HCV antibody and HCV–ribonucleic acid were present in colostral samples in much lower levels, but none of the 11 breast-fed infants had evidence of HCV infection for up to 1 year of age. Thus breast-feeding seems safe for these infants. (J PEDIATR 1995;126:589-91)

Many body fluids and secretions, including saliva, semen, urine, and stool, have been examined for the presence of hepatitis C virus–ribonucleic acid; the results have been conflicting.[1-4] Data from human milk are also limited.[2, 3] This prompted us to study the status of HCV-RNA in the colostrum of HCV carrier mothers, and to explore the possibility of transmission of HCV to their infants by breast-feeding.

Approval for the collection and analysis of human samples in the study was obtained from the health and ethics committee. The project conformed to the requirements of the human research committee.

METHODS

Subjects. Between April 1992 and January 1993, we recruited 15 carrier mothers with anti-HCV antibody from among 40 pregnant HCV carriers described in our previous studies,[5, 6] and 3 healthy mothers as control subjects. Maternal blood, 10 ml, and colostrum, 10 ml, were taken from each subject within 5 days post partum. For colostral samples, the yellowish fat in the top layer was removed after centrifugation at 1000*g* and 4° C for 30 minutes, and the supernatant was collected.[7] The precipitate was washed twice with phosphate-buffered saline solution and finally restored to its original volume with the same solution. All the supernatants and precipitates of colostrum and maternal sera were stored at −40° C until analysis. Blood samples were collected from the infants at 1, 3, 6, 9, and 12 months of age.

cDNA	Complementary DNA
HCV	Hepatitis C virus
HIV	Human immunodeficiency virus
PCR	Polymerase chain reaction
RNA	Ribonucleic acid

Serologic assays and quantitation of HCV genome. In serum and colostrum (supernatant and precipitate) samples, the anti-HCV titer was determined by a second-generation enzyme immunoassay kit (Abbott Laboratories, North Chicago, Ill.) with serial tenfold and then twofold dilutions, and HCV-RNA by reverse transcription–polymerase chain reaction.[5] Each of the serial blood samples of the 15 neonates was tested for anti-HCV and HCV-RNA. The detailed procedures of the reverse transcription–PCR were described previously.[5, 8]

The HCV–complementary DNA concentration of each sample was quantified by a competitive PCR assay.[9] Extraction of RNA and synthesis of cDNA were the same as described previously. One tenth of the cDNA was mixed with serial dilutions of competitor DNA that differed from the cDNA of interest by a small insertion (56 base pairs).

Supported by the National Science Council (NSC82-0419-B-002-394-MC), Executive Yuan, Republic of China.

Submitted for publication Oct. 11, 1994; accepted Nov. 28, 1994.

Reprint requests: Ding-Shinn Chen, MD, Hepatitis Research Center, National Taiwan University Hospital, No. 7, Chung-Shan South Road, Taipei, Taiwan 100, Republic of China.

0022-3476/95/$3.00 + 0 **9/22/62352**

Table. Hepatitis C virus in the sera and colostra of HCV carrier mothers

	Maternal serum		Colostral supernant		Colostral precipitate	
Patient No.	Anti-HCV titer	HCV-cDNA* (copies/ml)	Anti-HCV titer	HCV-cDNA (copies/ml)	Anti-HCV titer	HCV-cDNA (copies/ml)
1	1:10,000	2.5×10^8	1:4	1.25×10^2	1:1	<250
2	1:40,000	1.25×10^8	1:20	1.25×10^4	1:2	<250
3	1:40,000	2.5×10^7	1:20	<250	1:2	<250
4	1:1,000	1.25×10^7	1:10	1.25×10^4	1:1	<250
5	1:80	5×10^6	1:1	1.25×10^3	—	<250
6	1:2,000	2.5×10^6	1:10	<250	—	<250
7	1:800	2.5×10^6	1:1	1.25×10^3	—	<250
8	1:200	10^6	1:2	<250	—	<250
9	1:800	10^5	1:10	1.25×10^2	—	<250
10	1:800	2×10^4	1:2	<250	—	<250
11	1:400	4×10^4	1:1	<250	—	<250
12	1:800	2×10^4	1:4	<250	—	<250
13	1:200	2×10^4	1:2	<250	—	<250
14	1:80	10^4	1:1	<250	—	<250
15	1:100	10^4	1:1	<250	—	<250

*HCV-cDNA is detected by the competitive PCR.

The mixtures were coamplified by nested PCR with two sets of primers. For both PCRs, 35 cycles were performed as follows: denaturation at 95° C for 1 minute, primer annealing at 55° C for 1 minute, and extension at 72° C for 1 minute. Both PCR assays were done in 25 μl of mixture, and 1 μl of the first PCR product was transferred to the second PCR mixture. The preparation of competitor DNA and determination of HCV-cDNA concentrations have been described previously.[9] The sensitivity of our competitive assay is approximately 250 copies/ml in each specimen.

All 18 maternal sera were evaluated for human immunodeficiency virus by Enzygnost–Anti-HIV microanalysis kit (Behringwerke AG, Marburg, Germany).

RESULTS

All 15 mothers with, and the three mothers without, anti-HCV antibody had no anti-HIV antibody. The anti-HCV and HCV-RNA titers for maternal serum and colostrum are shown in the Table. The reciprocal anti-HCV titers of the 15 carrier mothers ranged from 1:80 to 1:40,000, and serum HCV-RNA was present in all; the three healthy mothers had negative results. By the competitive PCR assay, HCV-cDNA concentrations in the 15 maternal sera ranged from 10^4 to 2.5×10^8 copies/ml. Comparing anti-HCV titer to HCV-cDNA concentration, we found that extremely high titers of anti-HCV (> 1:10,000) in the serum usually correlated with a high HCV-cDNA concentration (>10^8 copies/ml), whereas titers of 1:80 to 1:2000 in the serum had no such correlation. In colostral samples, although both anti-HCV antibody and HCV-RNA were present in all, the titers were much lower; anti-HCV titers ranged from 1:1 to 1:20, and HCV-cDNA from <250 to 1.25×10^4 copies/ml. The precipitates of colostrum had the lowest anti-HCV titer and HCV-cDNA concentration. Anti-HCV titer of the colostrum correlated with that of the corresponding maternal serum, but a similar correlation did not seem to be present for HCV-RNA. Thus the blood-to-colostrum gradient of HCV was estimated to be from 10^{-3} to 10^{-7}.

Of 15 infants, 11 (except infants 4, 7, 8, and 13) were breast fed for 3 weeks to 4 months, with a mean duration of 2 months. All infants had no anti-HCV antibody and no HCV-RNA at the end of follow-up, and thus apparently were not infected by HCV.

DISCUSSION

In contrast to previous studies indicating that HCV-RNA cannot be detected in the milk of HCV carrier mothers,[2, 3] our data show that both anti-HCV antibodies and HCV-RNA were present in the colostrum of HCV carrier mothers without HIV coinfection. Although the exact causes of this discrepancy remain unclear, it might be explained by the difference in primer pairs used[3] or by the higher HCV-cDNA concentrations (10^4 to 10^8 copies/ml) in our carrier mothers.[2]

Concerning the amount of virus in both the serum and body secretions, Hsu et al.[3] proposed that the blood-to-secretion gradient of HCV would be 10^{-6} to 10^{-7}, in contrast to 10^{-3} to 10^{-4} for hepatitis B virus. However, our data showed that the blood-to-colostrum gradient of HCV ranged from 10^{-3} to 10^{-7}, and no evident correlation was found between paired maternal serum and colostrum samples. These discrepant results may be caused by the use of different primer pairs and quantitation methods; we employed competitive PCR for quantitation in our study, whereas Hsu et al. used serial dilutions to quantify serum HCV-RNA. Although the blood-to-secretion gradient exists for both hepatitis B virus and HCV, the origin of the hepatitis viruses in the body fluids might be due to occult hemorrhage (unpublished data), especially in the colostrum, because skin abrasion of the nipple is easily induced by suckling. Nonetheless, although HCV can be found in the milk, infection through breast-feeding apparently is infrequent. In our study, none of the infants fed human milk for up to 4 months had HCV infection by 1 year of age. The observation suggests that breast-feeding need not be discouraged for infants born to HCV carrier mothers. This conclusion may be explained by several factors. First, the HCV amount in the colostrum may be so low as to be unable to infect the newborn infant; infants had already encountered HCV by mucocutaneous exposure to maternal blood during delivery,[9, 10] which may be a more efficient method of infection than breast-feeding. Second, the tiny amount of HCV present in the colostrum may be easily inactivated in the gastrointestinal tract.[7] Finally, the integrity of the oral and gastrointestinal mucosa may effectively preclude HCV infection via the oral route.

We conclude that although anti-HCV antibody and HCV-RNA are present in the colostrum of HCV carrier mothers without HIV coinfection, breast-feeding usually does not cause HCV transmission in their infants and thus should not be discouraged.

We thank Mrs. Mei-Chen Lo for her skillful technical assistance.

REFERENCES

1. Wang JT, Wang TH, Lin JT, Sheu JC, Lin SM, Chen DS. Hepatitis C virus RNA in saliva of patients with posttransfusion hepatitis C infection [Letter]. Lancet 1991;337:48.
2. Ogasawara S, Kage M, Kosai K, Shimamatsu K, Kojiro M. Hepatitis C virus RNA in saliva and breast milk of hepatitis C carrier mothers [Letter]. Lancet 1993;341:561.
3. Hsu HH, Wright TL, Luba D, et al. Failure to detect hepatitis C virus genome in human secretions with the polymerase chain reaction. Hepatology 1991;14:763-7.
4. Fried MW, Shindo M, Fong TL, Fox PC, Hoofnagle JH, Di Bisceglie AM. Absence of hepatitis C viral RNA from saliva and semen of patients with chronic hepatitis C. Gastroenterology 1992;102:1306-8.
5. Lin HH, Kao JH, Leu JH, et al. Comparison of three different immunoassays and PCR for the detection of hepatitis C virus infection in pregnant women in Taiwan. Vox Sang 1993;65:117-21.
6. Lin HH, Hsu HY, Chang MH, et al. Low prevalence of hepatitis C virus and infrequent perinatal or spouse infections in pregnant women in Taiwan. J Med Virol 1991;35:237-40.
7. Lin HH, Hsu HY, Chang MH, Chen PJ, Chen DS. Hepatitis B virus in the colostra of HBeAg-positive carrier mothers. J Pediatr Gastroenterol Nutr 1993;17:207-10.
8. Okamoto H, Okada S, Sugiyama Y, et al. Detection of hepatitis C virus RNA by a two-stage polymerase chain reaction with two pairs of primers deduced from 5′-noncoding region. Jpn J Exp Med 1990;60:215-22.
9. Lin HH, Kao JH, Hsu HY, et al. Possible role of high-titer maternal viremia in perinatal transmission of hepatitis C virus. J Infect Dis 1994;169:638-41.
10. Ohto H, Terazawa S, Sasaki N, et al. Transmission of hepatitis C virus from mothers to infants. N Engl J Med 1994; 330:744-50.

Viral measurement by polymerase chain reaction–based assays in human immunodeficiency virus–infected infants

Paul E. Palumbo, MD, Shirley Kwok, BA, Sharon Waters, BS, Yvonne Wesley, RN, Dan Lewis, MS, Nancy McKinney, MS, Arlene Bardeguez, MD, Edward M. Connor, MD, and James M. Oleske, MD, MPH

From the Departments of Pediatrics and of Obstetrics and Gynecology, University of Medicine and Dentistry of New Jersey–New Jersey Medical School, and Children's Hospital of New Jersey, Newark, and Roche Molecular Systems, Alameda, California

Serial samples from human immunodeficiency virus–infected infants in the first year of life were analyzed by quantitative human immunodeficiency virus polymerase chain reaction assays. Very high, persistent levels of plasma RNA and proviral DNA were detected throughout the study period, suggesting the absence of an effective immune response. Most patients had normal CD4 lymphocyte counts and were symptom free for the first 3 to 6 months despite high levels of viral replication. These findings support the evaluation of early intervention (before symptoms develop) and efforts to establish the predictive value of these assays. (J Pediatr 1995;126:592-5)

The vertical transmission of human immunodeficiency virus from mother to infant presents many diagnostic and therapeutic challenges. Our understanding of the pathophysiology of primary infection is limited and is derived mainly from studies in symptomatic adults.[1-8] A transient burst of circulating HIV is detectable by both culture and molecular amplification methods in such adults but is quickly suppressed in most cases by an effective immune response. Similar details concerning mechanism(s) of transmission and early viral replication in the young infant are needed to guide intervention strategies. This study was undertaken to measure virus levels in early pediatric HIV infection by means of polymerase chain reaction analysis of both plasma and peripheral blood mononuclear cells.

Supported in part by grants from the Centers for Disease Control and Prevention (No. U64/CCU202219-08), the National Institutes of Health (No. IUO1 AI 25883-01), and the Foundation of the University of Medicine and Dentistry of New Jersey (No. 8-90). Dr. Connor is now with MedImmune Inc., Gaithersburg, Md.

Presented at the Annual Meeting of the American Pediatric Society and the Society for Pediatric Research, Seattle, Wash., May 1994.

Submitted for publication Aug. 10, 1994; accepted Nov. 14, 1994.

Reprint requests: Paul E. Palumbo, MD, Division of Infectious Diseases, MSB F578, Department of Pediatrics, University of Medicine and Dentistry of New Jersey–New Jersey Medical School, 185 S. Orange Ave., Newark, NJ 07103.

0022-3476/95/$3.00 + 0 **9/22/62072**

METHODS

Study population. Fourteen HIV-infected infants from a prospectively examined HIV transmission cohort were selected on the basis of specimen availability. Single plasma samples from nine uninfected neonates (1 to 10 days of age) born to HIV-infected mothers were also included. All

AIDS	Acquired immunodeficiency syndrome
HIV	Human immunodeficiency virus
MNC	Blood mononuclear cells
PCR	Polymerase chain reaction

infants were born between January 1991 and April 1993, providing a minimum observation period of 1 year. HIV infection was established within the first 3 months of life by means of positive results on two viral detection assays (PCR or viral culture or both) performed at two separate times.

Serial blood samples from the first year of life were analyzed; all had at least one data point within 30 days of age. Antiretroviral therapy was not administered to any infant during the period of the PCR analyses. One infant died as a result of *Pneumocystis carinii* pneumonia at 4 months of

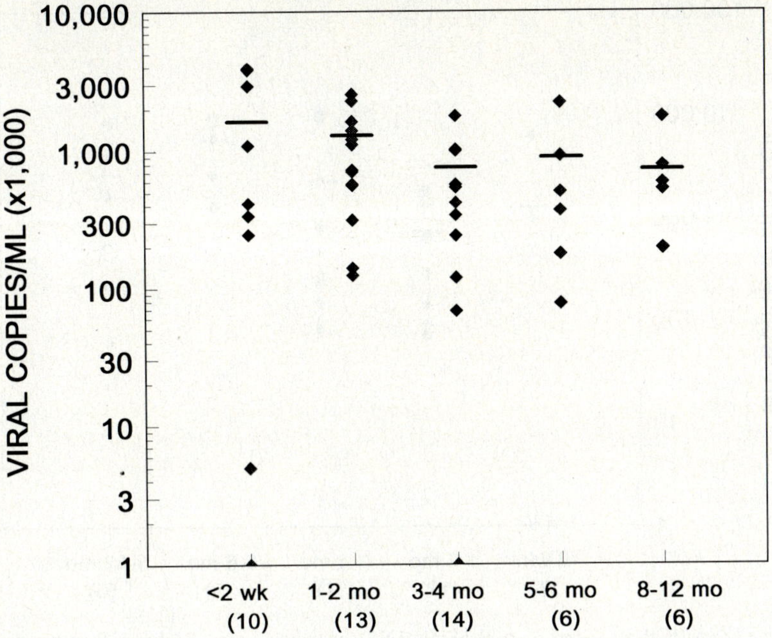

Fig. 1. Quantitative RNA PCR results from 49 plasma specimens from 14 infants. Results are reported as number of HIV RNA copies per milliliter of plasma. *Bars* represent age group means, and *numbers in parentheses* represent number of specimens analyzed.

age. The Centers for Disease Control and Prevention classification at 12 months of age was P-2–symptomatic disease for nine infants (one with an AIDS-defining condition) and P-1–asymptomatic disease for four infants. In two infants from the group with P-2 classification AIDS-defining illnesses developed by 14 months of age. Among the entire group of 14 infants, six had age-appropriate CD4 lymphocyte counts for the first 12 months of life and 10 had normal values through 4 months. In addition, 7 of the 14 infants were asymptomatic through 6 months of life.

Sample processing. Whole blood was collected in tubes containing anticoagulant (heparin or acid-citrate-dextrose) and processed within 4 hours. We extracted RNA from 200 μl of plasma either by the guanidinium isothiocyanate-isopropanol method[9] (acid-citrate-dextrose samples) or by the silica particle carrier method[10] (heparinized samples). Recovery of RNA from the same specimen with the use of either method is equivalent (S. Kwok: unpublished data).

Quantitative PCR. Blood mononuclear cells were assayed at two concentrations (2.5×10^4 and 10×10^4) in triplicate by 28-cycle PCR with a modification of the Amplicor kit (Roche Diagnostic Systems, Nutley, N.J.). Fivefold serial dilutions (from 6250 to 10 cells) of 8E5 cells infected with a single copy of HIV per cell were amplified in a background of 1×10^5 uninfected cells to create a standard curve. Twenty-eight cycles of PCR have been demonstrated to produce a consistent linear relationship between 10 and 1000 8E5 cells (P. E. Palumbo: unpublished data).

Plasma HIV RNA was quantified by reverse-transcription PCR[9, 11] with a single enzyme, recombinant *Thermus thermophilus* DNA polymerase, an internal standard RNA, as well as deoxyuridine triphosphate and uracil-*N*-glycosylase for DNA carryover prevention.

RESULTS

Quantitative RNA PCR. Quantitative RNA PCR was performed on 49 plasma specimens from 14 infants (Fig. 1). Viral RNA was undetectable in three specimens: two at 3 and 10 days of age, and one at 3 months. Of the remaining 46 specimens, 43 had values greater than 10^5 viral copies/ml, including 17 with more than 10^6 copies/ml. The highest mean value of 12.8 ($\pm$16.3) $\times 10^5$ viral copies/ml occurred among specimens obtained in the first 2 weeks of life; the lowest group mean was 5.9 ($\pm$5.1) $\times 10^5$ viral copies/ml in the 3- to 4-month age category. Viral RNA was not detected in single plasma samples collected from nine uninfected infants between 1 and 10 days of age.

Ten infants had plasma specimens collected within the first 12 days of life. Six of these neonates, classified as "early positives" (i.e., detectable proviral DNA and/or virus by cultivation), had a mean plasma RNA level of $1.708 \times 10^6 \pm 1.603 \times 10^6$ copies/ml (range, 0.246×10^6 to $3.85 \times$

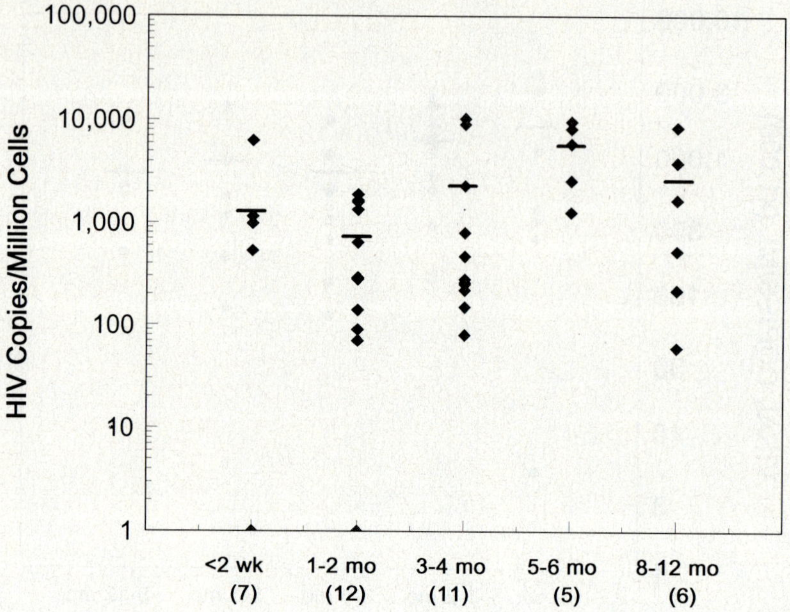

Fig. 2. Quantitative DNA PCR results on 41 peripheral MNC specimens from 11 infants. Results are reported as number of HIV DNA copies per 10^6 MNCs tested. *Bars* represent age group means, and *numbers in parentheses* represent number of specimens analyzed.

10^6) that was about 10 times higher than the mean of $0.085 \pm 0.168 \times 10^6$ copies/ml (range, negative to 0.337×10^6) for four neonates who were negative by DNA PCR and culture during this period. In three of six infants in the early-positive group AIDS-defining illnesses have developed compared with none of four in the initially negative group.

Three infants within the first 30 days of life had detectable plasma RNA levels (5×10^5, 314×10^5, and 337×10^5 copies/ml) in the face of negative assays for proviral DNA within circulating MNCs.

Quantitative DNA PCR. Forty-one MNC samples from 11 infants were available, and in four cases the initial MNC sample was negative by qualitative DNA PCR. The results for the remaining 37 samples are depicted in Fig. 2. Four samples had fewer than 100 DNA copies per 10^6 MNCs, 16 resulted in values between 100 and 1000 DNA copies per 10^6 MNCs, and 17 ranged between 10^3 to 10^4 copies.

DISCUSSION

Measurement of circulating viral load in primary HIV infection has been difficult because of assay limitations and obstacles identifying persons with acute disease. Four groups have reported HIV measurement studies with the use of culture and PCR-based techniques in a small group of adults.[1-5] Peak plasma viral levels as measured by culture detected a median tissue culture infective dose ($TCID_{50}$ per milliliter) of 10 to 10^4 per milliliter and 10^5 to 10^7 viral copies per milliliter as measured by RNA PCR. Culture of MNCs detected a tissue culture infective dose of 10^2 to 10^4 per 10^6 cells in the acute phase, and 7×10^3 to 13×10^3 copies per 10^6 MNCs were detected by DNA PCR. Viral levels declined rapidly during the ensuing 2 to 10 weeks in conjunction with an effective immune response. In the case of six patients examined serially with RNA PCR, plasma viral RNA levels decreased by a factor of 20 to 235 from peak values during a 1- to 4-month period but were always detectable at between 10^3 to 3×10^5 copies per milliliter during the early convalescent phase.[2, 3]

The levels of plasma viremia detected in this study of 14 infants are comparable to those reported in acutely infected adults with symptomatic disease. Seven of 12 infants tested in the first month of life had more than 10^6 copies/ml of plasma; and 10 of 12 had more than 10^5 copies/ml. Mean values for all age groups through 1 year were greater than 5×10^5 copies per milliter and only three infants past neonatal age had time points with viral copies at values less than 10^5 copies per milliliter. When viral levels declined from initial time points, the decrease was only in the range of twofold to tenfold. This is in contrast with findings in adults, who have a more pronounced decline in circulating viral RNA. In addition, plasma and MNC culture-based assays in both adults with primary infection and the few studied newborn infants peak abruptly and fall to very low or undetectable levels within weeks to a few months, in contrast to the more persistent viral RNA levels observed in this study.[1-4, 7, 8] Persistence of high plasma RNA levels through the first year of life, as detected by PCR, supports the concept of an immature immune system incapable of suppressing viral replication and dissemination.[12]

Generally high and persistent levels of proviral DNA within circulating MNCs were also seen in the first year of life within this cohort. If each infected MNC harbors a single provirus, the average infected cell ratio was 1 in 400 circulating MNCs, with peak ratios of 1 in 100 cells. There were four examples of either negative qualitative or low-level quantitative DNA PCR in the first month of life together with an elevated plasma RNA (3×10^5 to 3.8×10^6 viral copies per milliliter). In addition, one infant with negative DNA PCR findings and culture at 1 day of age had detectable viral RNA in plasma (5000 copies per milliliter). These findings are suggestive of either significant viral replication within the noncirculating cellular compartment in the early phase of infection (e.g., lymph node and spleen) or robust viral replication in a small number of infected circulating lymphocytes. Recent studies have reported extensive viral replication in lymphoid organs during the latent period after primary infection in adults.[13, 14]

Determination of the clinical predictive value of plasma or cellular viral measurement was not possible in this study because of the small sample size. Examples of both rapid progression to AIDS and asymptomatic clinical courses were observed in infants with persistently high levels of virus in this cohort. This is a critical issue that requires further investigation in large-scale, prospective studies. Additional variables such as virus phenotype, host genotype, and individual immune response also need to be systematically investigated.

The majority of infants were symptom free and had age-appropriate CD4 lymphocyte counts for the first 3 to 6 months, despite early and persistent high-level viremia and substantial viral burden in circulating MNC. These findings strongly support the evaluation of early intervention strategies before symptoms develop.

We thank R. J. Simonds and J. Sninsky for reviewing the manuscript, and the families whose participation made this study possible. The 8E5 cell line was obtained from Dr. Thomas Folks through the National Institutes of Health AIDS Research and Reference Reagent Program.

REFERENCES

1. Clark SJ, Saag MS, Decker WD, et al. High titers of cytopathic virus in plasma of patients with symptomatic primary HIV-1 infection. N Engl J Med 1991;324:954-60.
2. Piatak M, Luk KC, Saag MS, et al. Viral dynamics in primary HIV-1 infection [Letter]. Lancet 1993;341:1099.
3. Piatak M, Saag MS, Yang LC, et al. High levels of HIV-1 in plasma during all stages of infection determined by competitive PCR. Science 1993;259:1749-54.
4. Daar ES, Moudgil T, Meyer RD, and Ho DD. Transient high levels of viremia in patients with primary HIV-1 infection. N Engl J Med 1991;324:961-4.
5. Graziosi C, Pantaleo G, Butini L, et al. Kinetics of HIV-1 DNA and RNA synthesis during primary HIV-1 infection. Proc Natl Acad Sci U S A 1993;90:6405-9.
6. Niu MT, Stein DS, Schnittman SM. Primary HIV-1 infection: review of pathogenesis and early treatment intervention in humans and animal retrovirus infections. J Infect Dis 1993;168:1490-501.
7. Alimenti A, Luzuriaga K, Stechenberg B, Sullivan JL. Quantitation of HIV in vertically infected infants and children. J Pediatr 1991;119:225-9.
8. Luzuriaga K, McQuilken P, Alimenti A, Somasundaran M, Hesselton R, Sullivan JL. Early viremia and immune responses in vertical HIV-1 infection. J Infect Dis 1993;167:1008-13.
9. Mulder J, McKinney N, Christopherson C, et al. Rapid and simple PCR assay for quantitation of HIV-1 RNA in plasma: application to acute retroviral infection. J Clin Microbiol 1994;32:292-300.
10. Boom R, Sol CJ, Salimans MM, et al. Rapid and simple method for purification of nucleic acids. J Clin Microbiol 1990;28:495-503.
11. Myers TW, Sigua CL, Gelfand DH. High temperature reverse transcription and PCR with *Thermus thermophilus* DNA polymerase. Miami Short Rep 1994;4:87.
12. Luzuriaga K, Koup RA, Pikora CA, Brettler DB, Sullivan JL. Deficient human deficiency type 1–specific cytotoxic T cell responses in vertically infected children. J Pediatr 1991;119:230-6.
13. Pantaleo G, Graziosi C, Demarest JF, et al. HIV infection is active and progressive in lymphoid tissue during the clinically latent stage of disease. Nature 1993;362:355-8.
14. Embretson J, Zupancic M, Ribas JL, et al. Massive covert infection of helper T lymphocytes and macrophages by HIV during the incubation period of AIDS. Nature 1993;362:359-62.

Outcome of partial splenectomy for type I Gaucher disease

A. Zimran, MD, D. Elstein, PhD, R. Schiffmann, MD, A. Abrahamov, MD, M. Goldberg, MD, J. A. Bar-Maor, MD, R. O. Brady, MD, P. C. Guzzetta, MD, and N. W. Barton, MD, PhD

From the Gaucher Clinic and Department of Surgery A, Shaare Zedek Medical Center, Jerusalem, and the Department of Pediatric Surgery, Rambam Medical Center, Haifa, Israel; the Developmental and Metabolic Neurology Branch, National Institutes of Health, Bethesda, Maryland; and the Division of Pediatric Surgery, University of Texas, Southwestern Medical Center, Dallas

Partial splenectomy was introduced to achieve the benefits of splenectomy and to avoid the risk of overwhelming infection in patients with symptomatic Gaucher disease. We observed regrowth of the splenic remnant, reemergence of preoperative symptoms, and new bone involvement among most of our patients who had undergone partial splenectomy. Enzyme replacement therapy has markedly limited indications for splenectomy, partial or total, for Gaucher disease. (J Pediatr 1995;126:596-7)

The majority of patients with symptomatic Gaucher disease have splenic enlargement, which may be enormous, causing thrombocytopenia, anemia, abdominal discomfort with early satiety, severe abdominal pain associated with infarcts, and mechanical interference with adjoining organs.[1] Until the recent introduction of enzyme replacement therapy,[2] surgical removal of the spleen was a common therapeutic procedure to correct the hematologic abnormalities and to relieve the symptoms of mechanical compression.[1] Partial splenectomy was suggested as a means of reversing the hematologic and mechanical complications of splenomegaly while reducing the risk of overwhelming infection.[3] Recent reports have noted fewer secondary complications in patients who had undergone partial splenectomy relative to those in patients who had had total splenectomy.[4-6] We describe our experience with long-term clinical outcome in 24 patients with type I Gaucher disease who have undergone partial splenectomy.

METHODS

All our patients with Gaucher disease who had undergone partial splenectomy were included; 16 were from Israel and 8 from Washington, D.C. Indications for partial splenectomy included severe hypersplenism and mechanical complications resulting from massive enlargement of the spleen. There were 17 female and 7 male patients. Age at partial splenectomy ranged between 6 and 48 years; 17 patients were less than 18 years of age. The patients have been followed for up to 13 years after partial splenectomy (mean follow-up, 7.3 years). Seven other patients were not included in the current survey because they required emergency total splenectomy because of bleeding within 24 hours of partial splenectomy.

RESULTS

In 21 (87.5%) of the 24 patients significant regrowth of the splenic remnant developed with reemergence of all presurgical symptoms, and total splenectomy or enzyme replacement therapy was required after partial splenectomy. Mild to moderate bone involvement was present in seven patients (29%) preoperatively. During postsurgical follow-up (often <3 years), new bone-related complications, including avascular necrosis of the hip joints in nine patients (37.5%), developed in 12 patients (50%). The severity of the previous skeletal involvement progressed in six of seven patients; in two of these patients, avascular necrosis developed. Progression occurred in both children and adults. Six patients (25%) were free of bone-related symptoms during their follow-up period.

DISCUSSION

Partial splenectomy was associated with a higher risk of postoperative bleeding complications relative to total splenectomy and with eventual regrowth of the residual spleen and reestablishment of all original symptoms in our patients with Gaucher disease. Seven patients required emergency

Submitted for publication July 1, 1994; accepted Nov. 8, 1994.
Reprint requests: Ari Zimran, MD, Gaucher Clinic, Shaare-Zedek Medical Center, P.O. Box 3235, Jerusalem 91031, Israel.
9/22/61902

total splenectomy and multiple blood transfusions. Regrowth of the splenic remnant occurred in 21 of our 24 patients and in all seven patients described by Cohen et al.[6] Fleshner et al.[5] described an 18-month-old girl in whom rapid regrowth of the splenic remnant developed; she required splenectomy and then bone marrow transplantation but died 21 months later.

Enzyme replacement therapy may decrease spleen volume by 50% to 75% within the first 2 years of treatment; thus the rationale for splenectomy should be reevaluated. In addition, Pastores et al.[7] and Zimran et al.[8] reported comparable responses to enzymatic treatment in patients with or without a spleen; consequently, there appears to be no role for splenectomy, either total or partial, as a preparatory procedure to enhance the clinical response to enzyme replacement therapy. Our suggestions for the indications for splenectomy in the era of enzyme replacement therapy are limited to the following very specific situations: (1) when enzyme replacement is not a suitable option (e.g., where the cost is prohibitive), (2) life-threatening thrombocytopenia or a critical need for surgery (such as coronary bypass) in a patient with a very low platelet count, (3) inferior vena cava syndrome, (4) unremitting abdominal pain resulting from recurrent splenic infarction, and (5) severe restrictive pulmonary disease with incipient respiratory failure. Under these circumstances we prefer total splenectomy in adults or adolescents but may consider partial splenectomy in children less than 6 years of age.

REFERENCES

1. Zimran A, Kay A, Gelbart T et al. Gaucher disease: clinical, laboratory, radiologic and genetic features of 53 patients. Medicine 1992;71:337-53.
2. Barton NW, Brady RO, Dambrosia JM, et al. Replacement therapy for inherited enzyme deficiency: macrophage-targeted glucocerebrosidase for Gaucher's disease. N Engl J Med 1991; 325:1464-70.
3. Beutler E. Newer aspects of some interesting lipid storage diseases: Tay-Sachs and Gaucher disease. West J Med 1977; 126:46-54.
4. Guzzetta PC, Riley EJ, Merrick HFW, Verderese C, Barton N. Elective sub-total splenectomy: indications and results in 33 patients. Ann Surg 1990;211:34-42.
5. Fleshner PR, Aufsus AH Jr, Grabowski GA. A 27 year experience with splenectomy for Gaucher's disease. Am J Surg 1991; 161:69-75.
6. Cohen IJ, Katz K, Freud E, Zer M, Zaizov R. Long-term follow-up of partial splenectomy in Gaucher's disease. Am J Surg 1992;164:345-7.
7. Pastores GM, Sibille AR, Grabowski GA. Enzyme therapy in Gaucher disease type I: dosage, efficacy and adverse effects in 33 patients treated for 6 to 24 months. Blood 1993;82:408-16.
8. Zimran A, Elstein D, Kannai R, et al. Low-dose enzyme replacement therapy for Gaucher's disease: effects of age, sex, genotype and clinical features on response to treatment. Am J Med 1194;97:3-13.

Deletion of mitochondrial DNA in patient with chronic tubulointerstitial nephritis

Agnès Rötig, PhD, Françoise Goutières, MD, Patrick Niaudet, MD, Pierre Rustin, PhD, Dominique Chretien, PhD, Geneviève Guest, MD, Jacqueline Mikol, MD, Marie-Claire Gubler, MD, and Arnold Munnich, MD, PhD

From the Unité de Recherches sur les Handicaps Génétiques de l'Enfant INSERM U393, Unité de Recherches de Néphrologie Pédiatrique, INSERM U192 and Département de Pédiatrie, Hôpital des Enfants-Malades, Paris, France, and the Service d'Anatomopathologie, Hôpital Lariboisière, Paris, France

We report a mitochondrial DNA deletion (2.6 kb) in a boy with tubulointerstitial nephritis in whom chronic renal failure and leukodystrophy subsequently developed. Elevated lactate values in plasma and cerebrospinal fluid were

Submitted for publication July 26, 1994; accepted Oct. 24, 1994.
Reprint requests: Arnold Munnich, MD, INSERM U393, Hôpital des Enfants Malades, 149 rue de Sèvres, 75743 Paris-Cedex 15, France.

0022-3476/95/$3.00 + 0 9/22/61435

suggestive of a defect in the mitochondrial respiratory chain. High amounts of deleted mitochondrial DNA were present in muscle and cerebral white matter. On the basis of this observation, we suggest giving consideration to genetic defects of oxidative phosphorylation in any attempt to determine the origin of unexplained chronic tubulointerstitial nephritis, especially when seemingly unrelated organs are involved. (J PEDIATR 1995;126:597-601)

Respiratory chain deficiency can be manifested in infancy by a range of initial findings, including pancytopenia, hepatic failure, diabetes mellitus, deafness, hypertrophic cardiomyopathy, muscle weakness, dwarfism, villous atrophy, or proximal tubulopathy.[1] Tubulointerstitial nephritis has not been regarded as an initial manifestation of respiratory chain deficiency. We report here a mitochondrial DNA deletion in a male patient with tubulointerstitial nephritis and chronic renal failure with clinical onset as nephronophthisis.

CASE REPORT

A boy born to unrelated healthy parents (birth weight 3 kg) did well during the first years of life except for persistent intestinal obstruction after appendectomy at 5 years of age. At 11 years of age he had anemia and polyuria (height 131 cm [−2 SD], weight 27 kg [−2 SD]). Blood pressure was 130/60 mm Hg. Moderate proteinuria (0.5 gm/day) with no sign of proximal tubulopathy or renal failure was noted; the serum creatinine concentration was 206 μmol/L (2.3 mg/dl), and creatinine clearance was 30 ml/min per 1.73 m^2. Ultrasonography revealed highly echogenic kidneys with no evidence of obstruction. The patient had end-stage renal failure within 1 year. Hemodialysis was started when he reached 13 years of age, and he received a cadaveric kidney transplant 1 year later. Immunosuppressive therapy consisted of antilymphocyte globulin for 2 weeks, prednisone, and azathioprine. Cyclosporine therapy was started 2 weeks later, and graft function remained normal during the next 5 years. However, the patient had severe growth retardation (−6 SD at the age of 16 years), and despite an absence of growth hormone deficiency, he was given recombinant growth hormone therapy. At 17 years of age, difficulties at school became obvious and he had to repeat his first year of professional school. At the age of 19 years, he was referred to a neurologist because of dizziness and vertigo during the preceding 6 months. Neurologic findings were normal, but nonspecific signs of demyelination were observed on magnetic resonance imaging (disseminated patchy areas of increased signal on T2-weighted sequences in the white matter of the cerebral hemispheres). His neurologic status rapidly worsened and he became severely mentally disabled with cerebellar ataxia and bilateral pyramidal track signs; magnetic resonance imaging showed marked extension of the cerebral lesions, with diffuse hypersignal on T2, hyposignal of the whole white matter on T1, and cavitation suggesting necrosis in the frontal lobes. This profile suggested a leukodystrophic process, and an unrelated degenerative disorder was first considered. Late-onset metachromatic leukodystrophy, Krabbe disease, and adrenoleukodystrophy were ruled out (not shown), and a subacute multifocal leukoencephalitis caused by immunosuppressive therapy was considered. A stereotactic brain biopsy specimen of the frontal white matter ruled out papovavirus infection and showed evidence of marked spongiosis with demyelination gliosis and marked thickening of the arterial walls. He now uses a wheelchair and is mentally retarded, and he has severe retinitis pigmentosa and mild sensorineural deafness.

METHODS

Plasma lactate-pyruvate and ketone body molar ratios (3-hydroxybutyrate/acetoacetate) were determined in the patient and in control subjects as indexes of the oxidation-reduction status in cytoplasm and mitochondria, respectively.[2] A needle biopsy of the kidney and an open biopsy of the deltoid were performed with local anesthesia and the specimens were processed for histologic studies and for spectrophotometric and polarographic analyses of mitochondrial respiratory enzymes. Enzyme activities were also measured in cerebral white matter homogenates, lymphocytes, and cultured skin fibroblasts.[3]

mtDNA	Mitochondrial DNA
NADH	Nicotinamide adenine dinucleotide, reduced form

For Southern blotting, total DNA (5 μg) derived from muscle or lymphocytes was digested, separated by agarose gel (0.7%) electrophoresis, and transferred onto nylon filters (Hybond N^+; Amersham Corp., Arlington Heights, Ill.). The filters were hybridized with [^{32}P] deoxycytidine triphosphate–labeled mtDNA probes (2×10^6 cpm/ml). For characterization of the nucleotide sequence at the boundaries of the deletion, 1 μg of total DNA was submitted to polymerase chain reaction amplification (30 cycles) with two oligonucleotide primers (primer A: nt 10390–nt 10409; primer B: nt 13496–nt 13476). DNA was amplified by mixing 100 pmol of each primer with 2.5 U Taq polymerase (Perkin Elmer Cetus, Norwalk, Conn.). Amplified DNA was purified on a 2% low melting point agarose gel and recovered by heating for 5 minutes at 65° C. Direct sequencing was performed on an automatic DNA sequencer (model 373A; Applied Biosystems, Foster City, Calif.) with 3.2 pmol of primer A, 100 ng of DNA, and 9.5 μl of sequencing reaction mixture (Applied Biosystems) and compared with the wild type of sequence.[4]

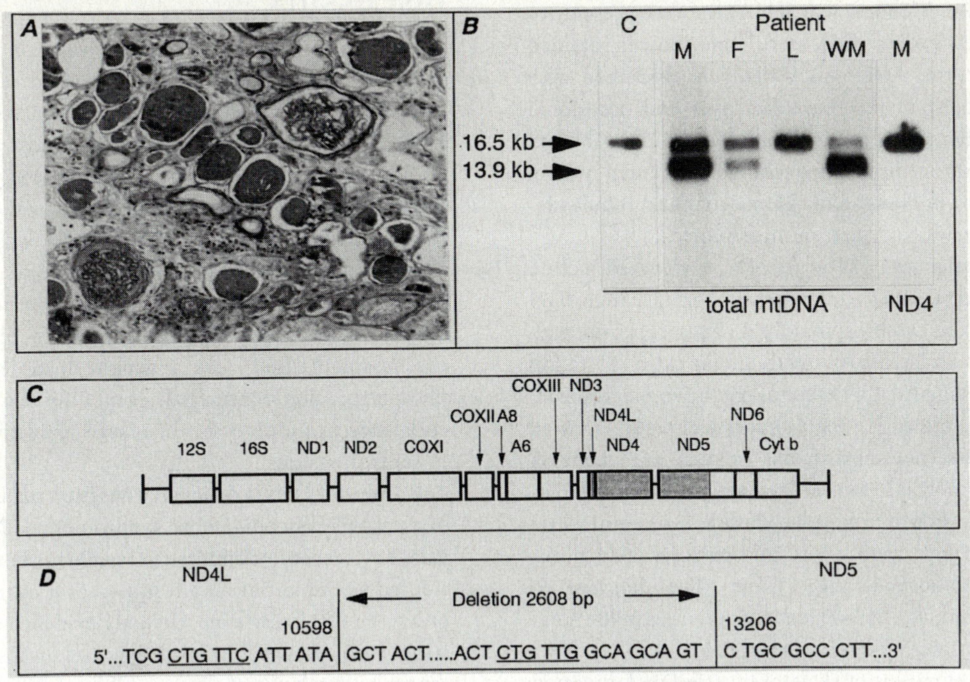

Figure. **A,** Periodic acid–Schiff stain of renal biopsy. Note the severe tubulointerstitial nephropathy with obstruction of the tubular lumen by hyaline casts, the focal thickening of the tubular basement membrane, the interstitial fibrosis, and the glomerular sclerosis. **B,** Southern blot analysis of total DNA extracted from the patient's muscle *(M)*, cerebral white matter *(WM)*, skin fibroblasts *(F)*, and circulating lymphocytes *(L)*, and of control DNA *(C)* digested with the restriction enzyme *Pvu II*. **C,** Map of human mtDNA, showing the extent of the deletion in the patient. **D,** Characterization of the nucleotide sequence at the boundaries of the mtDNA deletion. *COX*, Cytochrome *c* oxidase; *Cyt b*, cytochrome *b*.

Table. Respiratory chain enzyme activities in muscle, cerebral white matter, cultured skin fibroblasts, and circulating lymphocytes of the patient

	Enzyme activities (nmol/min/mg protein)				Ratios		
	NCCR	SCCR	QCCR	COX	COX/NCCR	COX/SCCR	COX/QCCR
Muscle mitochondria	283 (36-1288)	283 (63-803)	455 (354-897)	817 (194-2655)	2.9 (3.4 ± 0.8)	2.9 (3.1 ± 0.5)	1.8 (1.5 ± 0.2)
White matter	—	22 (11-72)	42 (41-214)	75 (37-253)	—	3.4 (3.4 ± 0.4)	1.8 (1.6 ± 0.4)
Fibroblasts	—	36 (15-73)	88 (58-136)	105 (37-213)	—	2.9 (2.9 ± 0.4)	1.2 (1.2 ± 0.2)
Lymphocytes	—	167 (23-98)	—	509 (65-240)	—	3.04 (3.1 ± 0.4)	—

Control ranges (enzyme activities) and means ± SD (ratios) are in parentheses.
NCCR, NADH cytochrome *c* reductase; *SCCR*, succinate cytochrome *c* reductase; *QCCR*, quinol cytochrome *c* reductase; *COX*, cytochrome *c* oxidase; *SQDR*, succinate quinone DCPIP reductase (*DCPIP*, dichlorophenol indophenol).

RESULTS

Histopathologic examination of the kidney showed prominent tubulointerstitial changes characterized by marked, and nearly diffuse, interstitial fibrosis with tubular lesions consisting of obstructions of the tubular lumen by hyaline casts. Moderate thickening of the tubular basement membrane around atrophic tubules was seen focally. Within these areas, glomeruli were totally sclerosed or had irregular thickening and wrinkling of the basement membrane and retraction of the tuft within thickened Bowman capsules (Figure, *A*). Mononuclear infiltrates were present focally. Only a few groups of glomeruli and tubules retained a normal structure. Arteriolar walls were thickened with major hypertrophy of the muscular layer and occasional pericellular sclerosis. Immunofluorescent studies showed granular deposits of third component of complement within sclerotic glomeruli. Nonspecific glomerular and tubular lesions were observed by electron microscopy.

When the patient was 19 years of age, elevated lactate concentration in plasma (>2.7 mmol/L; normal range, 0.63 to 2.44) and in the cerebrospinal fluid (7 mmol/L; normal, <2.4), with a high lactate/pyruvate molar ratio (15 to 20; normal, <12), suggested a defect of oxidative metabolism.

The muscle, stained by the Gomori technique, showed ragged-red fibers (not shown), but isolated mitochondria had apparently normal respiratory enzyme activities (Table). Similarly, oxidative phosphorylation in cerebral white matter, circulating lymphocytes, and cultured skin fibroblasts was in the normal range (Table). The high level of rotenone-resistant, NADH-dependent activities made measurement of complex I activity impossible.

Southern blot analysis of skeletal muscle DNA digested with restriction enzyme *Pvu* II (cleavage at nt 2652) and hybridization using a full-length mtDNA probe detected two populations of mtDNA, one normal (16.5 kb, 35%) and one partly deleted (13.9 kb, 62%; Figure). Subsequent hybridization with an NADH dehydrogenase-4 (ND4) probe revealed only one normal *Pvu* II fragment (Figure). The same pattern was observed in cerebral white matter and skin fibroblasts (Figure, *B*). Deleted mtDNA molecules were also found in cerebral white matter (86%) and in skin fibroblasts (36%). No deleted mtDNA molecules were observed by Southern blot analysis of leukocyte DNA (Figure, *B*).

The polymerase chain reaction amplification and sequence analysis, carried out to characterize the end points of the deletion, showed that the abnormal junction was located between the ND4L and ND5 genes and resulted in an ND4L-ND5 chimeric gene (Figure, *C*). The deletion spanned 2608 bp (nt 10598 to nt 13206) and skipped part of the gene for ND4L, the genes for ND4, ND5, and three tRNA genes ($tRNA^{His}$, $tRNA^{Ser}$, $tRNA^{Leu}$). Sequence analysis also showed that directly repeated sequences (6 bp) were present in the wild type of genome close to the boundaries of the deletion (Figure, *D*). Because the 5′ repeat was located six nucleotides away from the end point of the deletion, the retention of the 5′ repeat in the rearrangement is likely. Finally, PCR amplification using specific oligonucleotide primers detected the abnormal junction in the proband's lymphocyte DNA but not in his mother (not shown). Neither the needle biopsy specimen of the kidney nor the kidney transplant was available for investigation.

DISCUSSION

We report here an mtDNA deletion in a patient with tubulointerstitial nephritis that resulted in a concentrating defect and chronic renal failure. Nephronophthisis was initially considered because it is the most frequent cause of tubulointerstitial nephritis in childhood, but this diagnosis remained questionable because specific thickening of the basement membrane in the tubules was not observed. The disease remained unexplained, and only when it progressed to involvement of the central nervous system, with elevated lactate concentrations in plasma and the cerebrospinal fluid, was a genetic disorder of oxidative phosphorylation considered; eventually the diagnosis was confirmed by the detection of a large-scale mtDNA deletion in several tissues.

Respiratory chain deficiency has been regarded as a cause of de Toni–Fanconi–Debré syndrome in infancy.[5,6] Hitherto, however, tubulointerstitial nephritis has not been considered as the initial manifestation of a mitochondrial disorder. To our knowledge, the only evidence of tubulointerstitial involvement in a mitochondrial disease is the recent report by Szabolcs et al.[7] describing tubular atrophy and interstitial fibrosis in an 8-year-old girl with megaloblastic anemia and growth retardation; a chronic tubulointerstitial nephropathy developed in the course of the disease. Why our patient had no proximal tubulopathy is intriguing, especially inasmuch as the reabsorption of electrolytes and amino acids by the proximal tubule is energy dependent. Similarly, it is surprising that no enzyme deficiency was detected in skeletal muscle because two thirds of mtDNA molecules were deleted in this tissue. One can speculate that the proportion of the wild type of mtDNA in muscle was sufficient to achieve normal respiratory activity in both the skeletal muscle and the proximal tubule. Alternatively, intramitochondrial heteroplasmy might allow complementation between normal and deleted molecules and result in normal respiratory enzyme activity. By contrast, brain involvement gradually became obvious and may have been related to an increased proportion of deleted mtDNA molecules in the white matter, although the high level of rotenone-resistant, NADH-dependent activity precluded a reliable measurement of complex I activity in this tissue. Whatever the mechanism, we suggest that respiratory enzyme deficiency be considered when one is elucidating the origin of tubulointerstitial nephritis of unknown origin, especially in association with seemingly unrelated early-onset symptoms and a progressive course.

REFERENCES

1. Munnich A, Rustin P, Rötig A, et al. Clinical aspects of mitochondrial disorders. J Inher Metab Dis 1992;15:448-55.
2. Robinson BH. Lactic acidemia. In: Scriver CR, Beaudet AL,

Sly WS, Valle D, eds. The metabolic bases of inherited disease. New York: McGraw-Hill, 1989:869-88.
3. Rustin P, Chretien D, Gérard B, et al. Biochemical and molecular investigations in respiratory chain deficiencies. Clin Chim Acta 1994;228:35-51.
4. Anderson S, Bankier AT, Barrell BG, et al. Sequence and organization of the human mitochondrial genome. Nature 1981; 290:457-65.
5. Ogier H, Lombes A, Scholte HR, et al. De Toni–Fanconi–Debré syndrome with Leigh disease revealing severe muscle cytochrome *c* oxidase deficiency. J PEDIATR 1987;112:734-9.
6. Niaudet P, Heidet L, Munnich A, et al. Deletion of the mitochondrial DNA in a case of De Toni–Debré–Fanconi syndrome and Pearson syndrome. Pediatr Nephrol 1994;8:164-8.
7. Szabolcs MT, Seige R, Shanske S, Bonilla E, DiMauro S, D'Agati V. Mitochondrial DNA deletion: a cause of chronic tubulointerstitial nephropathy. Kidney Int 1994;45:1388-96.

Plasma erythropoietin reference ranges in children

Brian Krafte-Jacobs, MD, Jacqueline Williams, MD, and Steven J. Soldin, PhD

From the Departments of Critical Care and Laboratory Medicine, Children's National Medical Center, and the Departments of Pediatrics and Pathology, George Washington University School of Medicine, Washington, D.C.

Plasma erythropoietin values were determined in 1122 hospitalized and outpatient children aged 1 to 18 years with a commercially available enzyme-linked immunosorbent assay. A computerized approach based on the Hoffman technique was used to establish erythropoietin reference ranges. Plasma erythropoietin values ranged from 1.0 to 21.9 mIU/ml in male subjects, and from 1.1 to 20.5 mIU/ml in female subjects (2.5th to 97.5th percentiles). (J PEDIATR 1995;126:601-3)

Erythropoietin is a glycoprotein produced in renal peritubular interstitial cells that is responsible for maturation and proliferation of the erythroid cell line in human beings. Increased plasma erythropoietin values are seen in conditions that result in decreased oxygen flow to the kidneys, such as anemia and hypoxia.[2] Decreased erythropoietin concentrations have been noted in a variety of neoplastic, inflammatory, and infectious conditions, as well as in renal failure, burns, and acute anemia or acute hypoxia associated with critical illness.[3] Anemia resulting from diminished endogenous erythropoietin production in these disease states has led to an increasing therapeutic use of recombinant erythropoietin. Measurement of erythropoietin concentrations has been found to be useful in monitoring prereplacement and postreplacement therapy in these patients.[4] In addition, erythropoietin values are useful in differentiating several categories of anemia[5] and polycythemia.[6] Interpretation of erythropoietin concentrations has been hindered by an absence of gender- and age-adjusted reference ranges in children. Given the difficulty in obtaining blood specimens from large numbers of children, we used readily available residual specimens from both outpatient and hospitalized children for the determination of erythropoietin concentrations. Statistical methods were then applied to the data to establish reference ranges for plasma erythropoietin in children.

Supported in part by a research grant from R&D Systems, Inc.
Submitted for publication Aug. 30, 1994; accepted Oct. 24, 1994.
Reprint requests: Brian Krafte-Jacobs, MD, Division of Critical Care Medicine, Children's Hospital Medical Center, 3333 Burnet Ave., Cincinnati, OH 45229-3039

0022-3476/95/$3.00 + 0 **9/22/61436**

METHODS

Patients and sample collection. Excess plasma samples were obtained from a population of outpatient and hospitalized children after routine clinical chemistry testing was performed. The population included male and female patients aged 1 to 18 years. Visibly hemolyzed samples were excluded. Samples were identified only by age and gender. Samples were kept refrigerated for less than 24 hours at 2° to 4° C and then frozen at −70° C. The study used excess plasma that otherwise would have been discarded; therefore no informed consent was required. No effort was made to exclude children with diseases known to affect erythropoietin values because the analytic procedure used effectively excludes outlier values resulting from these conditions.

Table. Plasma erythropoietin concentrations in hospitalized children

	Male subjects			Female subjects		
Age (yr)	No.	2.5% (mIU/ml)	97.5% (mIU/ml)	No.	≤2.5% (mIU/ml)	≤97.5% (mIU/ml)
1-3	122	1.7	17.9	97	2.1	15.9
4-6	89	3.5	21.9	76	2.9	8.5
7-9	79	1.0	13.5	80	2.1	8.2
10-12	98	1.0	14.0	90	1.1	9.1
13-15	100	2.2	14.4	148	3.8	20.5
16-18	66	1.5	15.2	77	2.0	14.2

Erythropoietin assay. Erythropoietin concentrations were determined in duplicate on 100 μl plasma samples with an enzyme-linked immunosorbent assay (Quantikine IVD, R&D Systems, Minneapolis, Minn.). The assay is based on a spectrophotometric double-antibody sandwich method that can detect erythropoietin concentrations as low as 0.25 mIU/ml with high specificity.[7] Appropriate control samples were run in each assay with a mean of 10.8 ± 1.7 SD mIU/ml (range, 6.9 to 14.2 mIU/ml) and coefficient of variation of 15.5%.

Statistical analysis. Patient age and gender, and plasma erythropoietin values were entered into a spreadsheet program. Outlier values were removed according to the criterion method of Chauvenet and Crymble.[8] Briefly, after calculating a mean and SD for each data set, the Chauvenet method rejects a value if the probability of obtaining the value is less than ½*n*, where *n* equals the number of values in the data set. After these values are excluded, a new mean and SD are calculated, and the Chauvenet method is applied to the new data set. This process is repeated until no additional outlier values can be excluded. Each data set remaining after applying the Chauvenet method was further truncated with the Hoffman method[9] to ensure that abnormal results were eliminated. The method was modified to allow for computerized handling of the data. Generally, the top 10% and the bottom 10% of the data were discarded, and the 2.5th to 97.5th percentiles were calculated on the remaining 80% of the data, assuming a normal distribution. The 2.5th to 97.5th percentiles were used as the final reported reference ranges.

RESULTS

The results are displayed in the Table. Plasma erythropoietin values ranged from 1.0 to 21.9 mIU/mL in male subjects, and from 1.1 to 20.5 mIU/mL in female subjects (2.5th to 97.5th percentiles). With the exception of 13- to 15-year-old female subjects, upper limits of erythropoietin values in each age group tended to be higher in male subjects.

DISCUSSION

Determination of plasma erythropoietin values is important in characterizing a variety of conditions in which erythropoietin production may be either deficient or excessive. In addition, decisions regarding initiation or continuation of recombinant erythropoietin replacement therapy can be facilitated by knowledge of endogenous erythropoietin values. Reliable erythropoietin reference ranges in children are essential in the interpretation of these values.

Beckman et al.[10], who used a radioimmunoassay, reported normal pediatric erythropoietin concentrations of 0.4 to 52.0 mU/ml (2.5% to 97.5%). Unfortunately, samples were obtained from only 29 children of unreported gender, and the results were not delineated by age. In their review of seven studies in normal adults, Goldberg et al.[11] noted serum erythropoietin values ranging from 1.2 to 15.0 mU/ml (2.5%) to 16.5 to 38.8 mU/ml (97.5%) by radioimmunoassay. The results of these adult studies with radioimmunoassay are consistent with our results with an enzyme-linked immunosorbent assay technique.

Plasma samples obtained from male patients had somewhat higher erythropoietin values than those obtained from female patients. This finding is consistent with previous studies showing that adult men have higher erythropoietin values and higher erythroid cell counts than women, most likely a result of higher androgen levels.[12] Male subjects have higher testosterone concentrations than female subjects in all age categories.[13] In addition, estrogens decrease erythropoietin production, which may further explain the male-female differences noted in the study.[12] Female subjects in the 13- to 15-year age group were an exception to the above; their erythropoietin values were higher than those of their male counterparts. We speculate that increased blood loss after menarche may be responsible for upregulating erythropoietin values in these patients.

The erythropoietin reference ranges established in this study should help in the delineation of conditions associated with erythropoietin deficiency or excess. In addition, recombinant erythropoietin therapy can be initiated after comparison of an individual patient's erythropoietin value with a reference range of children of the same age and gender.

REFERENCES

1. Christensen RD. Recombinant erythropoietin. Pediatr Rev 1991;12:244-8.
2. Erslev AJ. Erythropoietin. N Engl J Med 1991;324:1339-44.
3. Krafte-Jacobs B, Levetown ML, Bray GL, Ruttimann UE, Pollack MM. Erythropoietin response to critical illness. Crit Care Med 1994;22:821-6.
4. Chandra M, McVicar M, Clemmons G, et al. Role of erythropoietin in the reversal of anemia of renal failure with continuous ambulatory peritoneal dialysis. Nephron 1987;46:312-5.
5. Bray GL, Taylor B, O'Donnell R. Comparison of the erythropoietin response in children with aplastic anemia, transient erythroblastopenia, and iron deficiency. J PEDIATR 1992;120: 528-32.
6. Koeffler HP, Goldwasser E. Erythropoietin radioimmunoassay in evaluating patients with polycythemia. Ann Intern Med 1981;94:44.
7. Quantikine IVD human EPO immunoassay handbook. Minneapolis, Minn: R & D Systems, 1994.
8. Chauvenet W, Crymble GG. Quality control service notes. East Scarborough, Ontario: Warner Chilcott Diagnostics, 1973:26-7.
9. Hoffman RG. Statistics in the practice of medicine. JAMA 1963;185:864-73.
10. Beckman BS, Brookins JW, Garcia MM, Fisher JW. Measurement of erythropoietin in anephric children. Pediatr Nephrol 1989;3:75-9.
11. Goldberg MA, Schneider TJ, Khan S, Petersen JR. Clinical validation of an RIA for natural and recombinant erythropoietin in serum and plasma. Clin Biochem 1993;26:183-9.
12. Fried W. Erythropoietin and the kidney. Nephron 1975;15:327-49.
13. Pediatric endocrine testing. San Juan Capistrano, California: Nichols Institute Diagnostics, 1993:38.

THE BOOK SHELF **André D. Lascari,** *Editor*

Book review

Perinatal and pediatric pathophysiology: a clinical perspective

Gluckman PD, Heyman MA, eds. Boston: Little, Brown, 1993. 760 pages. $125.

The editors sought to develop a text that would bridge the gap between clinical and basic science as they relate to pediatrics. Although there are numerous texts in pediatrics and the basic sciences (such as biochemistry, cell physiology, and molecular biology), there are very few that relate the scientific basis with the clinical or developmental perspective. A major difficulty in developing such a text is to choose a group of contributors who can integrate the basic and clinical sciences in an easy-to-understand style. The majority of the authors work in clinical departments but have exceptionally strong reputations in basic science research. It is to the editors' credit that the contributors selected for their position on the "cutting edge" of research are also aware of the needs of the clinician in understanding the tools of modern biology. This text has the resources to serve as a companion to any pediatrician involved in clinical research.

The book is divided into two parts: a basic science review of cell biology, biochemistry, and physiology as they relate to growth and development (covering five chapters); and a systems approach to pathophysiology (covering 10 chapters). Each system chapter begins with a review of basic science concepts and developmental aspects, and ends with a description of clinically relevant disease processes. The chapters are written in a style that is easy to read and understand. The references are not extensive, but they are current and excellent sources of further reading and information. Tables and figures are used effectively to illustrate a concept described in the text. The index is organized in a manner that allows easy access to the topic in question.

This textbook is a good compilation of a large amount of developmental biology as it relates to molecular and cellular processes. The rapidity of the explosion of knowledge in cellular and molecular physiology makes texts such as this an important source of information for the pediatrician-in-training as well as the "practicing" pediatrician.

Michael J. Horgan, MD
Section of Neonatal/Perinatal Medicine
Department of Pediatrics
Albany Medical College
Albany, NY 12208

Changing trends in the epidemiology and pathogenesis of neonatal chronic lung disease

Mario A. Rojas, MD, Alvaro Gonzalez, MD, Eduardo Bancalari, MD, Nelson Claure, MS, Catherine Poole, MD, and Galdino Silva-Neto, MD

From the Department of Pediatrics, Division of Neonatology, University of Miami School of Medicine, Miami, Florida

Objective: **To assess the role of specific risk factors that may predispose preterm infants with mild or no initial respiratory distress syndrome to the development of chronic lung disease (CLD).**
Study design: **Clinical data were collected prospectively from 119 ventilator-supported preterm infants with birth weights between 500 and 1000 gm, who survived more than 28 days and required fewer than 3 days of treatment with fraction of inspired oxygen >25% during the first 5 days of life. Logistic regression analysis was used in a multivariate assessment of risk factors for CLD.**
Results: **Chronic lung disease occurred in 44 of the patients (37%). The analysis showed that low birth weight, patent ductus arteriosus (PDA), and sepsis were significant risk factors for CLD. The corresponding odds ratios for CLD and their 95% confidence intervals (CI) were as follows: 2.9 per 100 gm birth weight decrement (CI, 1.7 to 4.8); 6.2 (CI, 2.1 to 18.4) for PDA; and 4.4 (CI, 1.3 to 14.5) for sepsis. When sepsis and PDA occurred simultaneously, the odds ratio for CLD increased to 48.3 (CI, 6.3 to >100) in comparison with infants without these conditions. Episodes of PDA were categorized as either early (occurring during the first week of life) or late (after the first week), and the respective odds ratios for CLD were 2.8 (CI, 0.8 to 9.4) and 21.1 (CI, 5.6 to 80) in comparison with infants without PDA. For the duration of symptomatic PDA, the odds ratio for CLD was 3.5 per week that the PDA remained open (CI, 1.9 to 6.5).**
Conclusion: **CLD is a frequent sequela in very low birth weight infants with mild or no respiratory distress syndrome. In this population, the development of late episodes of PDA, usually in association with a nosocomial infection, seems to play a primary role in the pathogenesis of CLD. (J PEDIATR 1995;126:605-10)**

Originally, chronic lung disease was observed primarily in preterm infants with severe respiratory distress syndrome who were exposed to high oxygen concentrations and positive airway pressures.[1] In recent years, however, less severe forms of CLD have been observed frequently in infants with mild or no initial RDS.[2-4] This change in clinical pattern suggests that risk factors different from those associated with the severity of the initial respiratory course are responsible for the development of CLD in these infants.

CI	Confidence interval
CLD	Chronic lung disease
FIO_2	Fraction of inspired oxygen
PDA	Patent ductus arteriosus
RDS	Respiratory distress syndrome

The objective of this study was to assess the role of spe-

Supported by University of Miami Project: New Born.
Submitted for publication Oct. 26, 1993; accepted Oct. 24, 1994.
Reprint requests: Eduardo Bancalari, MD, University of Miami School of Medicine, Division of Neonatology, Department of Pediatrics (R-131), PO BOX 016960, Miami, FL 33101.

0022-3476/95/$3.00 + 0 **9/23/61439**

cific risk factors that may result in a predisposition to CLD in a large population of premature infants with birth weight <1000 gm, and with mild or no initial RDS. The risk factors considered were birth weight, gender, race, Apgar scores, mean airway pressure during the first 3 days, presence of pneumothorax, pulmonary interstitial emphysema, intracranial hemorrhage, sepsis, and episodes of clinically symptomatic patent ductus arteriosus.

METHODS

We prospectively examined all consecutively born preterm infants with birth weights between 500 and 1000 gm who were delivered at the University of Miami/Jackson Memorial Medical Center during a 2-year period beginning in March 1989. Only infants who required mechanical ventilation were included in the study. Infants with symptomatic congenital infections or major congenital anomalies were excluded. Detailed perinatal and neonatal information was abstracted on a daily basis by means of specific data forms. Respiratory data included the median daily fraction of inspired oxygen administered during the first 2 months of life (data obtained from the hourly recorded F_{IO_2} values during each 24-hour period), total duration of oxygen therapy, and duration and characteristics of ventilatory support. Because the effect of the severity of initial respiratory failure on the development of CLD is well established, we selected only those infants with minimal or no respiratory failure who required fewer than 3 days in an F_{IO_2} >0.25 during the first 5 days of life.

Infants were examined at least daily for clinical signs of PDA, which was diagnosed when a compatible murmur or two-dimensional color Doppler echocardiographic evidence of left-to-right ductal shunting was associated with one or more of the following clinical signs: hyperactive precordium, bounding pulses or wide pulse pressure (>25 mm Hg), or radiographic evidence of pulmonary edema or cardiomegaly or both. Medical therapy for a suspected PDA remained at the discretion of the attending physician; because of unstable clinical status, some infants were treated for PDA before echocardiographic confirmation. However, echocardiographic evaluation was performed before surgical ligation in all infants whose PDA failed to close with indomethacin therapy or in those for whom this therapy was contraindicated. All symptomatic PDAs were managed according to the neonatal intensive care unit's guidelines, which included intravenous indomethacin administration at a starting dose of 0.2 mg/kg, followed by two doses of 0.1 mg/kg every 12 hours if the infant was younger than 48 hours, 0.2 mg/kg if between 3 and 7 days of life, or 0.25 mg/kg if older than 7 days. Contraindications for indomethacin administration were a serum creatinine concentration >160 μmol/L (1.8 mg/dl), oliguria (urine output <0.5 ml/kg per hour), evidence of bleeding diathesis, and platelet count $<75 \times 10^9$/L (<75,000/mm^3). Surgical ligation was performed when indomethacin therapy failed or was contraindicated.

The patients were also examined closely for signs of sepsis, and appropriate cultures and blood cell counts were done when infection was suspected. Sepsis was defined as the presence of at least one positive blood culture result in association with (1) one or more of five clinical signs (lethargy, arterial hypotension, poor skin perfusion, hypothermia, and apnea) and/or (2) abnormal leukocyte count with an increase in the proportion of immature forms (immature/mature granulocyte ratio >0.3). An effort was made to document more than one positive blood culture result, especially if a coagulase-negative staphylococcus was identified in the culture. Infants with an isolated positive blood culture result who were free of symptoms were not considered to have sepsis. Infants with two or more consecutive blood cultures positive for the same microorganism were considered to have sepsis regardless of their symptoms.

Chronic lung disease was defined as the need for supplemental oxygen for 28 days or longer during the first 2 months of life, in association with chest radiographic findings compatible with CLD (persistent hazy opacification or cystlike pattern of density and lucency). Radiographs were evaluated by a pediatric radiologist (C.P.) who had no knowledge of the patients' initial respiratory diagnosis or clinical outcome.

Neonatal management, including nutritional support, fluid intake, the use of diuretics, indomethacin, sedation, oxygen supplementation, and ventilatory support, was provided uniformly for all infants according to the neonatal intensive care unit's guidelines. The goal of the ventilatory management was to use the lowest mean airway pressure and F_{IO_2} necessary to maintain appropriate blood gas values (pH, 7.30 to 7.45; arterial oxygen tension, 50 to 80 mm Hg; arterial carbon dioxide tension, 40 to 50 mm Hg; base excess, ±5 mEq/L). Pulse oximetry was used continuously to monitor oxygen saturation and maintain it, as closely as possible, between 88% and 95%. All information was stored in a computerized database for subsequent analysis.

Statistical analysis. Categorical variables were analyzed by the chi-square test, the Mann-Whitney (Wilcoxon) rank-sum test, and the Mantel-Haenszel test when adjustment for birth weight was necessary. Differences in continuous variables were assessed by the Student *t* test and analysis of variance. Statistical significance was considered as a *p* value <0.05. In an attempt to define the role of different risk factors associated with the development of CLD, we performed univariate analyses to compare infants with and those without CLD for the following variables: birth weight, gender, race, gestational age, Apgar scores, presence of pneumothorax, pulmonary interstitial emphysema, intracranial hemorrhage, sepsis, and episodes of PDA during the first 2 months of life.

The univariate analysis was followed by a multivariate analysis to assess the independent relationship of a particular variable with the presence of CLD after adjustment for the remaining variables in the model. For this step of the analysis we used backward stepwise logistic regression analysis[5] (BMDP Statistical Software, University of California, Los Angeles) applied to a model that did not include interactions. The initial model included the following variables: birth weight, gender, race, Apgar scores, mean airway pressure during the first 3 days, presence of pneumothorax, pulmonary interstitial emphysema, intracranial hemorrhage, sepsis, and episodes of PDA. The analytic method evaluates the contribution of each variable to the model, eliminates, in a stepwise fashion, those variables whose contribution is not significant, and selects the ones whose contribution is significant independently of the effect of the other variables in the model.

The next analytic strategy was to perform new logistic regression analyses with models that included the variables selected in the previous step and their interactions and the duration of a symptomatic PDA, together with indicator variables corresponding both to the time that the ductus was recognized and to the temporal interaction between PDA and sepsis. To assess the importance of time of occurrence of PDA as a risk factor for CLD, we categorized the infants into three groups: those with early PDA (infants with PDA occurring during the first 7 days of life and without recurrence); those with late PDA (infants with either new or recurrent episodes of PDA that occurred after the first 7 days of life); and those with no PDA. A temporal relationship between sepsis and PDA was considered when sepsis preceded PDA or developed while the ductus remained open, with a time interval no longer than 5 days between both diagnoses. The logistic model used to analyze the temporal interaction between sepsis and PDA and the development of CLD included the following four categories: no PDA or sepsis, PDA temporally related to sepsis, PDA not temporally related to sepsis, and sepsis alone.

RESULTS

A total of 258 preterm infants with birth weights between 500 and 1000 gm were born at the University of Miami/Jackson Memorial Medical Center during the 2 years of the study. Of these, 93 infants (36%) died during the first 28 days of postnatal life and were excluded from the analysis. Of the 165 survivors, 46 infants met one of the following exclusion criteria: 16 did not require mechanical ventilation; 28 had severe RDS with high oxygen requirements during the first 5 days of life; 1 had a symptomatic congenital infection; and 1 had congenital heart disease.

A total of 119 ventilator-supported infants with low initial oxygen requirements who survived more than 28 days were included in the final analysis. Their demographic and clinical characteristics are shown in Table I. Only 52 infants (44%) had mild RDS; 23 of them were treated with exogenous surfactant (surfactant was available for the treatment of RDS only during the second year of the study). Most of the remaining infants underwent intubation because of the presence of apnea or poor respiratory effort or both. More than half of these infants had at least one episode of sepsis (64 [54%]). Of all blood cultures with positive results, 46% grew *Staphylococcus epidermidis*, 32% *Candida albicans*, and 22% other microorganisms. An additional blood culture positive for *S. epidermidis* was documented in 56% of the infants with sepsis. The incidence of PDA was also high (69 infants [58%]), being confirmed by echocardiogram in 51 (74%). Most of them had symptoms during the first week of life and were treated successfully with indomethacin. Thirty-four infants had late episodes of PDA (32 confirmed by echocardiogram [94%]); 26 of these episodes were recurrences of a previous episode in which the ductus had closed with indomethacin therapy. Of all the PDA episodes, 24 (35%) failed to respond to medical treatment, and the infants required surgical ligation. Twenty-four infants had an episode of PDA temporally related to an episode of infection.

Of the 119 study infants, 44 (37%) met the criteria for the diagnosis of CLD. The diagnoses of sepsis and PDA were associated with a marked increase in the incidence of CLD. Of 69 infants with PDA, 37 (54%) eventually had CLD compared with 7 (14%) of 50 infants without PDA (*p*

Table I. Demographic and clinical characteristics of the 119 infants included in the study

Birth weight (gm)*	802 ± 111
Gestational age (wk)*	26.8 ± 1.7
MAP first 3 days (cm H_2O)*	5.6 ± 1.4
IMV first 3 days (breaths/min)*	19.6 ± 9.9
FIO_2 first 3 days (%O_2)*	25.1 ± 7.1
Apgar score	
At 1 min†	4 (1-9)
At 5 min†	6 (1-9)
Days in oxygen†	13 (0-138)
Days in IPPV†	30 (1-119)
Gender (%male)	47
Race (%black)	65
RDS (%)	44
Sepsis (%)	54
PDA (%)	58
ICH (%)	47
PIE (%)	6
PTX (%)	11

MAP, Mean airway pressure; *IMV*, intermittent mandatory ventilation; *IPPV*, intermittent positive-pressure ventilation; *ICH*, intracranial hemorrhage; *PIE*, pulmonary interstitial emphysema; *PTX*, pneumothorax.
*Results are mean ± SD.
†Results are median (range).

Table II. Univariate analysis of clinical characteristics according to the presence of CLD

	CLD (n = 44)	No CLD (n = 75)	p
Birth weight (gm)*	730 ± 90	845 ± 100	<0.001
Gestational age (wk)*	25.8 ± 1.4	27.4 ± 1.5	<0.001
Apgar score			
At 1 min†	4 (1-9)	4 (1-8)	NS
At 5 min†	6 (2-9)	6 (1-9)	NS
Gender (%male)	55	43	NS
Race (%black)	61	68	NS
PDA (%)	84	43	<0.001
Sepsis, first month (%)	79	39	<0.001
ICH (%)	55	43	NS
PTX (%)	18	7	NS
PIE (%)	9	4	NS

NS, Not significant; *ICH*, intracranial hemorrhage; *PTX*, pneumothorax; *PIE*, pulmonary interstitial emphysema.
*Results are mean ± SD.
†Results are median (range).

<0.01, Mantel-Haenzsel test, with adjustment for birth weight). Among the 64 infants with sepsis, CLD was diagnosed in 35 (55%) compared with 9 (16%) of 55 infants without sepsis ($p < 0.05$, Mantel-Haenzsel test). As seen in Table II, univariate analyses for the comparison of infants with and those without CLD showed statistically significant differences ($p < 0.001$) in four variables: birth weight, gestational age, incidence of PDA, and incidence of sepsis.

As shown in the Figure, in a multiple logistic regression analysis of a model with no interaction terms, the variables birth weight, PDA, and sepsis were statistically significant predictors of CLD, after adjustment for all remaining variables in the model. The corresponding odds ratios for CLD and their 95% confidence intervals were as follows: 2.9 (CI, 1.7 to 4.8) per 100 gm birth weight decrement; 6.2 (CI, 2.1 to 18.4) for PDA; and 4.4 (CI, 1.3 to 14.5) for sepsis. On the other hand, other previously reported risk factors for CLD, such as gender, race, low Apgar score, and mean airway pressure, did not reach significance. Results of subsequent logistic regression analyses are presented in Table III. As indicated in model A, the odds ratio for CLD comparing late PDA with no PDA was statistically significant (odds ratio, 21.1; $p < 0.001$; 95% CI, 5.6 to 79.9). Model B shows that, in comparison with infants in whom PDA or sepsis did not develop, infants with a PDA temporally related to sepsis were at a significantly higher risk of having CLD (odds ratio, 48.3; $p < 0.001$; 95% CI, 6.3 to >100). This result suggests a synergistic interaction between PDA and sepsis in the pathogenesis of CLD. Model C, analysis of duration of symptomatic PDA and development of CLD, demonstrates an odds ratio for CLD of 3.5 for each week that the infant had a symptomatic PDA ($p < 0.001$; 95% CI, 1.9 to 3.5). Among the 16 infants in whom the PDA remained symptomatic for more than 2 weeks, in 15 (94%) the PDA was temporally associated with sepsis; CLD subsequently developed in all of them.

Table III. Odds ratios for development of CLD: Results of logistic regression analyses with adjustment for birth weight (models A, B, and C) and sepsis (models A and C)

Condition	Odds ratio	95% CI	p
Model A: PDA time of presentation*			
Early PDA	2.8	0.8-9.4	0.08
Late PDA	21.1	5.6-79.9	<0.001
Model B: temporal relation between PDA and sepsis†			
Sepsis alone	1.5	0.2-10.1	0.67
PDA not related to sepsis	4.5	0.8-24.7	0.06
PDA related to sepsis	48.3	6.3->100	<0.001
Model C: duration of symptomatic PDA (per wk increment)	3.5	1.9-6.5	<0.001

*Reference group: infants without PDA.
†Reference group: infants without PDA or sepsis.

DISCUSSION

With the introduction of surfactant therapy and new strategies for mechanical ventilation in infants with RDS, it was anticipated that the incidence of CLD would decrease; however, most clinical trials have failed to confirm this expectation.[6-8] On the contrary, investigators have reported an increasing incidence of CLD in preterm infants with mild or no RDS.[3, 4, 9] During the 2-year period of our study, CLD developed in 66 (45%) of 147 surviving ventilator-supported infants with birth weights between 500 and 1000 gm. This incidence is close to reported figures for this complication in this birth weight range.[2, 10-13] The majority of infants in whom CLD developed came from this subgroup of "low risk" infants (i.e., those infants who had only mild or no RDS and therefore were not exposed to established risk factors for CLD, such as high inspired oxygen concentrations and airway pressures). This observation supports a changing epidemiology of CLD, and strongly suggests that factors other than those associated with the severity of the initial respiratory failure play a role in the pathogenesis of chronic lung damage.

The results of this study showed that after birth weight, which is a recognized risk factor for CLD, sepsis, and PDA were the variables most significantly associated with an increased risk of CLD in these infants. Furthermore, when they occur simultaneously, the higher odds ratio for CLD indicates an interaction between the two. The fact that other previously reported risk factors for CLD such as male gender, race, and low Apgar scores were not associated with

CLD in these "low risk" infants suggests that these factors increase the risk of CLD by affecting the severity of the initial respiratory failure.

The presence of a PDA has a negative effect on lung function, thus increasing the risk of chronic pulmonary damage,[14-16] but these effects can be reversed by prompt intervention to close the ductus.[17, 18] The role of infection in the development of CLD is less clear; however, there is accumulating evidence to support the hypothesis that inflammation plays an important role in the pathogenesis of CLD. Evaluation of lung lavage from ventilator-supported premature infants has shown that prolonged neutrophil influx[19] and increased cytokine activity[20] are associated with development of CLD. Colonization with specific microorganisms such as cytomegalovirus and *Ureaplasma urealyticum* also has been associated with increased risk of CLD.[21-23] Although both PDA and infection have independently been associated with CLD, the possible interaction between these two factors has not been assessed. There is evidence that sepsis may adversely influence the outcome of a PDA. Salzer et al.[24] described indomethacin closure failure in six of seven infants with a PDA associated with sepsis. Infections may also delay the effective medical or surgical closure of the PDA. Thus sepsis can prolong the duration of an open ductus, and by this mechanism explain the synergistic association between sepsis and PDA that increases the risk of CLD. Such an association is supported by our finding that episodes of PDA limited to the first week of life did not significantly increase the risk of CLD. On the other hand, late episodes of PDA, frequently temporally related to sepsis and lasting for longer periods, were associated with a significant increase in the risk of CLD.

A limitation of our study is that our protocol of surveillance for PDA was based on clinical observation, and in some of the patients with clinically symptomatic PDA we could not obtain a confirmatory echocardiographic evaluation before treatment. This may have resulted in some false-positive results or missed diagnoses of PDA. However, it is unlikely that our conclusions were affected, because the majority of unconfirmed episodes of PDA occurred early and were of short duration. On the other side, most "silent" PDAs develop symptoms later, and the clinical significance of those which never produce symptoms is questionable.[25] Ninety-four percent of the late episodes of PDA and 100% of those which failed to close with indomethacin were evaluated by echocardiogram before surgical closure. In terms of the diagnosis of sepsis, our criteria were based on clinical symptoms and laboratory confirmation, but routine surveillance cultures were not performed. We do not believe that this would affect the conclusions significantly because we used strict diagnostic criteria for the analysis. Although *S. epidermidis* could be considered a skin contaminant, all the

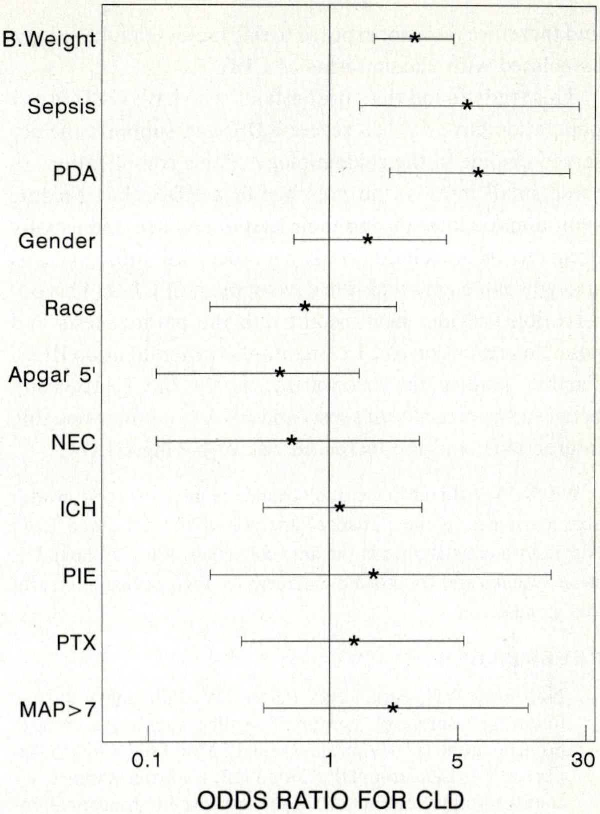

Figure. Odds ratios (*) and their 95% CIs for the development of CLD—logistic regression analysis of the 119 infants. We analyzed birth weight per 100-gram decrement; gender, comparing male versus female infant; race, comparing black versus nonblack infant; Apgar score ≤5 at 5 minutes; and *(MAP)* ≥7 cm H_2O during the first 3 days of life. *NEC*, Necrotizing enterocolitis; *ICH*, intracranial hemorrhage; *PIE*, pulmonary interstitial emphysema; *PTX*, pneumothorax.

infants had symptoms and most of them had more than one documented positive blood culture result. It can be argued that infants with CLD were more likely examined for murmurs and, similarly, more likely to have blood culture specimens taken. However, most infants in this study who had PDA or sepsis, or both, had no significant respiratory disease before the episode, and the symptoms and increased oxygen requirements developed in association with the diagnosis of sepsis or PDA.

Only infants with birth weights less than 1000 gm were included in this study because in our institution the incidence of CLD in larger infants is very low. We elected to use birth weight rather than gestational age as an inclusion criterion because of the difficulty of accurately assessing gestational age in extremely premature infants. Although the selection of infants according to their initial respiratory course was arbitrary, our intention was to define a group of infants who initially had mild respiratory failure and therefore were not exposed to risk factors that have been associated with classic forms of CLD.

This study found that most infants who have CLD in our population have not had severe RDS, and supports the observed change in the epidemiology of this complication. In these small infants, the presence of a PDA that became symptomatic later during their hospital course and usually occurred in association with a nosocomial infection was strongly associated with the development of CLD. This observation provides new insight into the pathogenesis and possible prevention of CLD in infants with mild or no RDS. Further studies are needed to clarify the relationship between the presence of sepsis and PDA (and their possible interaction), and the increased risk of having CLD.

We thank William Feuer and Orlando Gomez for their invaluable assistance in the statistical analysis of the data, and Rosa Nuñez for her assistance in the data collection. We also thank Dr. Ilene Sosenko and Dr. Ronald Goldberg for their critical review of this manuscript.

REFERENCES

1. Northway WH, Rosan RC, Porter DY. Pulmonary disease following respiratory therapy of hyaline membrane disease: bronchopulmonary dysplasia. N Engl J Med 1967;276:357-68.
2. Parker RA, Lindstrom DP, Cotton RB. Improved survival accounts for most, but not all, of the increase in bronchopulmonary dysplasia. Pediatrics 1992;90:663-8.
3. Wung JT, Koons AH, Driscoll JM, James LS. Changing incidence of bronchopulmonary dysplasia. J PEDIATR 1979; 95:845-7.
4. Heneghan MA, Sosulski R, Baquero JM. Persistent pulmonary abnormalities in newborns: the changing picture of bronchopulmonary dysplasia. Pediatr Radiol 1986;16:180-4.
5. Dixon WJ, Brown MB, Engelman L, Jennrich RI, eds. BMDP statistical software manual; vol 1, 1990 revision. Berkeley: University of California Press.
6. Horbar JD, Soll RF, Sutherland JM, et al. A multicenter randomized, placebo-controlled trial of surfactant therapy for respiratory distress syndrome. N Engl J Med 1989;320:959-65.
7. Truog WE, Prueitt JL, Woodrum DE. Unchanged incidence of bronchopulmonary dysplasia in survivors of hyaline membrane disease. J PEDIATR 1978;92:261-4.
8. Long W, Thompson T, Sundell H, et al. Effects of two rescue doses of a synthetic surfactant on mortality rate and survival without bronchopulmonary dysplasia in 700- to 1350-gram infants with respiratory distress syndrome. J PEDIATR 1991; 118:595-605.
9. O'Brodovich HM, Mellins RB: Bronchopulmonary dysplasia: unresolved neonatal acute lung injury. Am Rev Respir Dis 1985; 132:694-709.
10. Avery ME, Tooley WH, Keller JB, et al. Is chronic lung disease in low birth weight infants preventable? a survey of eight centers. Pediatrics 1987;79:26-30.
11. Palta M, Gabbert D, Weinstein MR, et al. Multivariate assessment of traditional risk factors for chronic lung disease in very low birth weight neonates. J PEDIATR 1991;119:285-92.
12. Van Marter LJ, Pagano M, Allred EN, et al. Rate of bronchopulmonary dysplasia as a function of neonatal intensive care practices. J PEDIATR 1992;120:938-46.
13. Horbar JD, McAuliffe TL, Adler SM, et al. Variability in 28-day outcomes for very low birth weight infants: an analysis of 11 neonatal intensive care units. Pediatrics 1988;82:554-9.
14. Cotton RB, Stahlman MT, Bender HW, et al. Randomized trial of early closure of symptomatic patent ductus arteriosus in small preterm infants. J PEDIATR 1978;93:647-51.
15. Merritt TA, Harris JP, Roghmann K, et al. Early closure of patent ductus arteriosus in very-low-birth-weight infants: a controlled trial. J PEDIATR 1981;99:281-6.
16. Brown ER. Increased risk of bronchopulmonary dysplasia in infant with patent ductus arteriosus. J PEDIATR 1979;95:865-6.
17. Gerhardt T, Bancalari E. Lung compliance in newborns with patent ductus arteriosus before and after surgical ligation. Biol Neonate 1980;38:96-105.
18. Stefano JL, Abbasi S, Pearlman SA, et al. Closure of the ductus arteriosus with indomethacin in ventilated neonates with respiratory distress syndrome: effects on pulmonary compliance and ventilation. Am Rev Respir Dis 1991;143:236-9.
19. Ogden BE, Murphy S, Saunders GC, Johnson JD. Lung lavage of newborns with respiratory distress syndrome: prolonged neutrophil influx is associated with bronchopulmonary dysplasia. Chest 1983;83:31-3s.
20. Bagghi A, Viscardi RM, Taciak V, et al. Increased activity of interleukin-6 but not tumor necrosis factor-α in lung lavage of premature infants is associated with the development of bronchopulmonary dysplasia. Pediatr Res 1994;36:244-52.
21. Sawyer MH, Edwards DK, Spector SA. Cytomegalovirus infection and bronchopulmonary dysplasia in premature infants. Am J Dis Child 1987;141:303-5.
22. Cassell GH, Crouse DT, Cannup KC, et al. Association of *Ureaplasma urealyticum* infection of the lower respiratory tract with chronic lung disease and death in very low birth weight infants. Lancet 1988;2:240-4.
23. Fujimura M, Takeuchi T, Ando M, et al. Elevated immunoglobulin M levels in low birth weight neonates with chronic respiratory insufficiency. Early Hum Dev 1983;9:27-32.
24. Salzer HR, Salzer-Muhar U, Pollak A, Weninger M. Sepsis and indomethacin failure in premature infants with symptomatic ductus arteriosus [Letter]. Lancet 1987;1:977.
25. Hammerman C, Strates E, Valaitis S. The silent ductus: its precursors and its aftermath. Pediatr Cardiol 1986;7:121-7.

Long-chain polyunsaturated fatty acids in preterm infants: Status at birth and its influence on postnatal levels

Magritha M. H. P. Foreman–van Drongelen, MD,
Adriana C. van Houwelingen, MD, PhD, Arnold D. M. Kester, PhD,
Tom H. M. Hasaart, MD, PhD, Carlos E. Blanco, MD, PhD, and
Gerard Hornstra, PhD

From the Departments of Human Biology and of Methodology and Statistics, University of Limburg, Maastricht, The Netherlands, and the Departments of Obstetrics and Gynecology and of Neonatology, University Hospital Maastricht, Maastricht, The Netherlands

To determine the influence of the prenatal long-chain polyunsaturated fatty acid (LCP) supply on prenatal growth and on postnatal LCP levels, we studied 52 preterm infants and assessed the relations between the LCP status at birth (reflecting the prenatal LCP supply), gestational age and prenatal growth, and the relation between the LCP status at birth and at 37 to 42 weeks of gestational age. After a correction for gestational age at birth, significant relations ($p \leq 0.05$) were observed between anthropometric measurements at birth (weight, head circumference, and length) and LCP levels in the umbilical artery wall, the LCP content of which reflects the long-term fetal LCP status. Independent of the neonatal diet (human milk or formula), LCP levels in erythrocyte phospholipids at term were positively related to levels in the umbilical artery wall (docosahexaenoic acid (22:6*n*-3): $p \leq 0.0003$; arachidonic acid (20:4*n*-6): $p = 0.02$). Postnatal diet significantly influenced LCP levels in plasma phospholipids at term (docosahexaenoic acid: $p \leq 0.004$; arachidonic acid: $p = 0.02$); formula-fed infants had lower values. We conclude that the LCP status of preterm infants at birth is related to prenatal growth. Moreover, next to the postnatal enteral diet, the LCP status at birth significantly affects LCP levels at term postconceptional age. This finding may warrant further studies of the effects of essential fatty acid–enriched maternal diets during pregnancy on the neonatal LCP status at birth. (J Pediatr 1995;126:611-8)

Long-chain polyunsaturated fatty acids (chain length of 20 carbon atoms or more and at least one double bond more than the parent essential fatty acids, linoleic acid [18:2*n*-6] or α-linolenic acid [18:3*n*-3]; Fig. 1) are of major importance in fetal and infant development. The LCPs docosahexaenoic acid (22:6*n*-3) and arachidonic acid (20:4*n*-6) are the predominant polyunsaturated fatty acids in the structural lipids of the human brain[1-3] and retina.[4] In addition, considerable amounts of AA are found in membrane

AA	Arachidonic acid (20:4*n*-6)
DHA	Docosahexaenoic acid (22:6*n*-3)
EFA	Essential fatty acid
GA	Gestational age
HC	Head circumference
LCP	Long-chain polyunsaturated fatty acid
PL	Phospholipid

Supported by a grant from Nutricia, Zoetermeer, The Netherlands.

Submitted for publication June 30, 1994; accepted Oct. 6, 1994.

Reprint requests: Magritha M. H. P. Foreman–van Drongelen, MD, Department of Human Biology, University of Limburg, PO Box 616, 6200 MD Maastricht, The Netherlands.

0022-3476/95/$3.00 + 0 **9/23/61096**

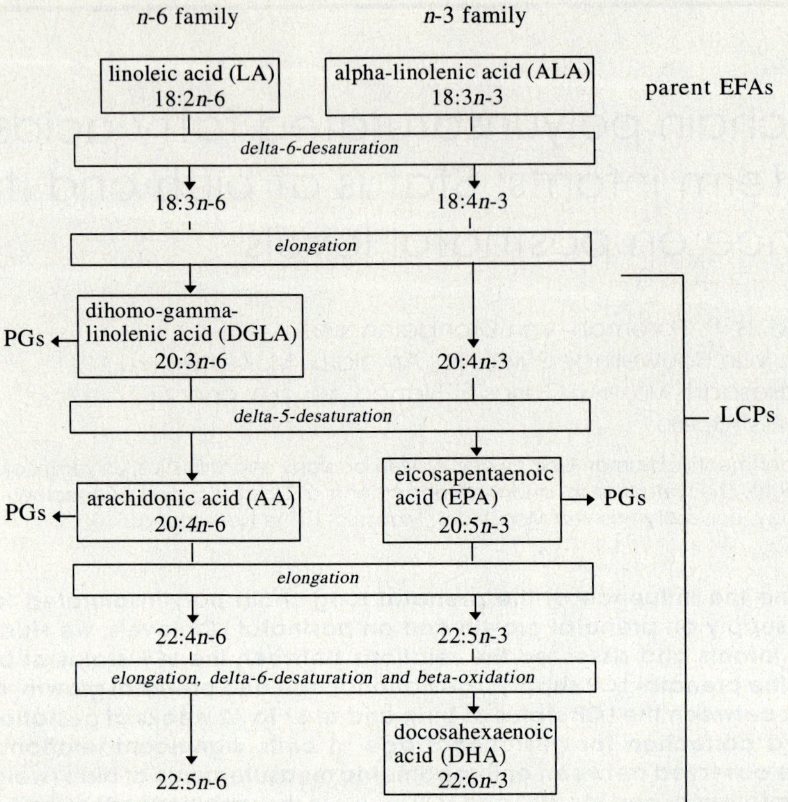

Fig. 1. Main pathways of *n*-6 and *n*-3 fatty acid conversion. *PGs*, Prostaglandins (and other eicosanoids).

phospholipids throughout the body. Furthermore, AA, dihomo-γ-linolenic acid (20:3*n*-6), and eicosapentaenoic acid (20:5*n*-3) are precursors of prostaglandins and other eicosanoids (Fig. 1) that have important bioregulatory functions.

Dietary studies have demonstrated that preterm infants who receive a conventional artificial formula as their main source of dietary lipids have a poorer LCP status than infants fed their own mother's milk.[5-9] This discrepancy has been attributed to the presence of small but significant amounts of DHA, AA, and other LCPs in human milk, and to their absence in the majority of the commercially available artificial formulas.[10-12] These formulas usually contain substantial amounts of the parent essential fatty acids, linoleic acid and α-linolenic acid, which can be converted to *n*-6 and *n*-3 LCPs in the human body (Fig. 1). However, the desaturase capacity of premature newborn infants is probably too limited to guarantee an adequate supply of LCPs solely through metabolic conversion of these two fatty acids.[13, 14] Adding LCPs to artificial formulas reduces the differences in the LCP status of formula-fed and breast-fed preterm infants.[7, 8, 15-17] The LCP status has also been related to anthropometric measurements, both at birth[18, 19] and thereafter.[20]

Leaf et al.[21] recently observed a positive correlation between plasma LCP levels at birth (reflecting the prenatal LCP supply) and those at term postconceptional age (40 weeks of gestational age). This relation was independent of the type of postnatal diet, indicating that the intrauterine experience of the fetus may set the pattern for postnatal LCP levels.[22] However, the study was confined to plasma PLs and lacked information on the erythrocyte fraction of the blood, the LCP content of which may be a more accurate reflection of LCP levels in the brain.[23]

The aim of our study was to explore the nature of the relation between the LCP status at birth and that in the term period (37 to 42 weeks of GA) in a group of preterm infants. To this end, the LCP levels in PLs extracted from plasma, from erythrocytes, and from the umbilical artery walls were studied; the last is considered to reflect the long-term fetal LCP status.[24, 25] In addition, the potential relations among LCP status at birth, GA at birth, and weight, head circumference, and length at birth were studied.

METHODS

Infants. The population studied comprised 52 preterm infants (GA, 26 to 36 weeks; birth weight, 650 to 1860 gm). The infants had no metabolic disease or congenital malformations. A 3 ml sample of venous cord blood and approximately 15 cm of umbilical cord were collected immediately after delivery to provide information on the LCP status at birth. This material was collected as part of a dietary study of preterm infants,[9] which was approved by the medical ethics committee of the University Hospital of Maastricht; written informed consent was obtained from one or both parents.

All infants were admitted to the neonatal care unit, where their birth weights were assessed on a calibrated infant scale and recorded to the nearest 5 gm. Head circumference and crown-heel length were measured, to the nearest millimeter, with a tape on the third day of life. Crown-heel length was measured with the infants in the supine position.

Subsequently, between 1½ and 2 hours after a feeding, 0.5 ml blood samples were taken by venous puncture or heel prick, in conjunction with a diagnostic puncture, and collected in tubes containing ethylene diaminetetraacetic acid. For 28 infants, blood samples collected at 37 to 42 weeks of GA were available. The fatty acid data on these latter infants were used to assess the influence of the LCP status at birth on postnatal LCP levels.

The study populations are described in Table I. Of the infants followed until the term period, 10 received their own mother's milk and 18 received a commercially available artificial formula as their main source of dietary lipids. The preterm human milk contained, on average, 0.34% (wt/wt) of DHA and 0.58% (wt/wt) of AA. No detectable amounts of DHA, AA, and other LCPs were present in the artificial formulas; their linoleic acid and α-linolenic acid contents ranged from 10.8% to 18.1% (wt/wt) and from 0.34% to 1.47% (wt/wt), respectively.[9] In the group of infants fed human milk, only two infants received less than 90% (vol/vol) human milk during the study period; their human milk intakes were 50.2% and 68.4% (vol/vol). Infants raised on artificial formulas consumed no human milk.

Until the infants were receiving full enteral feedings, they received parenteral nutrition according to current standards. Up to 22.5 kcal (per kilogram per day) of intravenous lipids (Intralipid 10% and 20%, and Vitalipid, which contain up to 0.2% and 0.3% [wt/wt] of DHA and AA, respectively[9]) was given as a source of fat. The majority of the infants received their first enteral intake during the first week of life, and they were receiving full enteral feedings of 100 to 120 kcal/kg per day at, on average, the fourteenth day of life. Some infants also received intravenous erythrocyte and plasma infusions as part of the treatment.

Laboratory analysis. Plasma and erythrocyte samples were prepared as described previously.[9] A 15 μm umbilical cord sample was obtained, cut into three segments of 5 μm each, and rinsed with saline solution (sodium chloride, 0.9% [wt/vol]). One segment was used for further analysis, including isolation of the arterial vessel walls from the surrounding tissue. The vessel walls were frozen in liquid nitrogen and pulverized in an aluminum mortar with a stainless steel pestle, which were cooled in liquid nitrogen. The pulverized samples were freeze dried for 16 hours, followed by immediate fatty acid analysis.

Table I. Characteristics of study population

	Infants involved in correlations at birth (*n* = 44)	Infants followed until term period* (*n* = 28)
Maternal age (yr)	28.6 ± 4.9	29.1 ± 4.7
Gestational age (wk)	30.6 ± 2.6	32.3 ± 2.9
Birth weight (gm)	1355 ± 344	1380 ± 330
Head circumference (cm)	27.6 ± 2.8	28.1 ± 3.0
Length (cm)	40.5 ± 3.4	40.6 ± 3.7
SGA (*P* <2.3)	0	8 (29%)
pH of umbilical artery blood	7.18 ± 0.12	7.16 ± 0.12
Follow-up after birth (wk)		6.4 ± 2.6
Age at first enteral intake (days)		6 ± 3
Age at full enteral intake (days)		14 ± 8
Intravenous lipids (kcal/kg/day)†		5.4 ± 4.5
Intravenous plasma (ml)†		17.4 ± 27.6
Intravenous erythrocytes (ml)†		28.4 ± 44.3
Human milk: formula		10:18

Values expressed as mean ± SD, except for number (%) of SGA subjects and number of subjects who were fed human milk/number who were fed infant formula.
SGA, Small for gestational age (birth weight percentile <2.3).
*Term period: 37 to 42 weeks of gestational age.
†Value represents average amount received per day during entire follow-up period.

At the start of the fatty acid analysis, 1,2-dinonadecanoyl phosphatidylcholine (19:0 PC) was added to every sample as an internal standard. Samples were analyzed as described previously,[9] with modification by the use of the method of Bligh and Dyer[26] for the extraction of total lipids from 10 to 30 mg freeze-dried vessel-wall tissue and by the use of a CP-Sil 88 column (Chrompack, Middelburg, The Netherlands) for the separation and quantification of the fatty acid methylesters in the vessel wall samples.

Fatty acid amounts present in the PL fraction were quantified on the basis of the amount of 19:0 internal standard fatty acid methylester recovered. Absolute fatty acid levels were expressed as milligrams per liter of plasma or erythrocyte suspension, or as milligrams per kilogram of dry weight of cord vessel wall tissue. Relative fatty acid levels were expressed as a percentage (weight/weight) of total fatty acid methylesters.

Data analysis. The p values $\leq$0.05 were considered sig-

Table II. Fatty acid composition (% [wt/wt],* mean ± SD) of phospholipids in umbilical artery vessel walls and in plasma and erythrocytes at birth and at term postconceptional age (37 to 42 weeks of gestational age)

Fatty acid	Umbilical artery (n = 38)	Plasma at birth (n = 39)	Plasma at term (n = 27)	Erythrocytes at birth (n = 39)	Erythrocytes at term (n = 28)
20:3*n*-6 (DGLA)	0.89 ± 0.26	3.99 ± 0.88	2.81 ± 0.70	1.68 ± 0.54	1.22 ± 0.47
20:4*n*-6 (AA)	11.06 ± 2.23	16.97 ± 1.96	7.71 ± 1.68	11.73 ± 4.42	7.32 ± 2.86
Σ*n*-6 (LCP)†	17.78 ± 3.25	22.07 ± 1.78	11.38 ± 1.99	16.21 ± 5.97	10.60 ± 4.16
20:5*n*-3 (EPA)‡		0.27 ± 0.16	0.17 ± 0.11	0.12 ± 0.10	0.10 ± 0.09
22:6*n*-3 (DHA)	4.20 ± 0.97	3.84 ± 0.88	1.85 ± 0.79	2.71 ± 1.39	1.28 ± 0.77
Σ*n*-3 (LCP)†,‡		4.42 ± 0.99	2.39 ± 1.03	3.19 ± 1.65	1.85 ± 1.05
Σ*n*-3 + *n*-6 (LCP)†	21.99 ± 3.90	26.49 ± 2.27	13.77 ± 2.88	19.41 ± 7.47	12.45 ± 5.14
Total*	15533 ± 4478.8	659.89 ± 149.68	1060.0 ± 174.7	1027.4 ± 267.1	924.7 ± 262.9

Detailed results, containing all fatty acids separately, are available on request.
DGLA, Dihomo-γ-linolenic acid (20:3*n*-6); *EPA*, eicosapentaenoic acid.
*Total amount of PL-associated fatty acids expressed as milligrams per kilogram dry weight for umbilical artery vessel walls and as milligrams per liter for plasma and for erythrocyte suspension. Fatty acid concentrations can be calculated from the relative fatty acid levels and the total amounts of PL-associated fatty acids.
†Σ*n*-6 LCP = sum of *n*-6 long-chain polyunsaturated fatty acids (20:3*n*-6, 20:4*n*-6, 22:4*n*-6, and 22:5*n*-6); Σ*n*-3 LCP = sum of *n*-3 long-chain polyunsaturated fatty acids (20:4*n*-3, 20:5*n*-3, 22:5*n*-3 and 22:6*n*-3); and Σ*n*-3 + *n*-6 LCP = sum of all (*n*-3 and *n*-6) long-chain polyunsaturated fatty acids.
‡No *n*-3 fatty acids other than DHA (22:6*n*-3) were detectable in the vessel walls of the umbilical artery.

nificant. Relations between *n*-3 and *n*-6 LCP levels at birth, GA at birth, and anthropometric measurements at birth were explored by linear regression (Pearson correlation coefficients). Significant correlations between the LCP status and anthropometric measures were corrected for GA at birth, by multiple regression analysis.

The influence of the LCP status at birth on postnatal LCP levels was evaluated for the two LCPs of primary interest, DHA and AA, by means of multiple regression analysis. The regression equation formulated was as follows: LCPs in blood at term = A + B_1 * LCPs in cord blood + B_2 * LCPs in umbilical artery wall + B_3 * Diet + B_4 * Follow-up (days). The dependent variable was the DHA or AA status in the term period. As indicators of the DHA or AA status at birth, the levels of these fatty acids in the PL fraction of venous cord blood (plasma or erythrocytes) and the umbilical artery walls were entered as potential explanatory variables. The potential relation between LCP status at birth and postnatal LCP levels was corrected for the type of postnatal enteral diet, which was entered as a dummy variable with zero for human milk and one for artificial formula. Moreover, the period (days) between birth and the blood sampling in the term period (follow-up) was entered as a continuous variable. Separate equations were calculated for DHA and AA, for the plasma and the erythrocyte component of the blood, and for the absolute and relative fatty acid data. Using an F test, we tested the overall relation between the LCP status at term and both indicators of the LCP status at birth, correcting for diet and follow-up. To guard against spurious correlations, we present separate *p* values for the two LCP indicators only when the F test result was significant.

RESULTS

Relation between LCP status at birth and GA at birth. In Table II, mean values for the fatty acids studied (percentage [wt/wt] and total amounts of PL-associated fatty acids) are listed. Birth weights of eight infants were at less than the 2.3rd percentile of the Amsterdam growth charts.[27] These small-for-gestational-age infants were not included in the analyses of the relations among LCP status, GA, and anthropometric measurements at birth. No umbilical cord sample was available from 6 of the remaining 44 infants, and no acceptable blood sample could be obtained from the cords of five other infants.

In cord plasma PLs, significant positive relations were found between GA at birth and the relative levels of DHA, the sum of all *n*-3 LCPs, and the sum of all LCPs ($p < 0.01$). In the arterial cord vessel walls, significant positive correlations were observed between GA at birth and relative levels of AA, the sum of all *n*-6 LCPs, the sum of all LCPs ($p < 0.001$ for all), and DHA ($p < 0.05$). No significant relations were found between GA and plasma or cord artery wall levels of dihomo-γ-linolenic acid or eicosapentaenoic acid, nor between GA and absolute LCP levels in plasma or umbilical artery walls, nor between GA and LCP levels in erythrocyte PLs.

Relation between LCP status at birth and prenatal growth. No significant correlations were observed for any of the anthropometric measurements with the LCP status measured in cord plasma or erythrocyte PLs. The relations of LCP levels in the umbilical artery wall with birth weight are based on 38 infants, with HC on 31 infants, and with length on 29 infants, because of missing values for the latter two growth measures. All significant correlations between anthropometric measurements and LCP levels in umbilical artery wall PLs could at least partly be attributed to the significant positive correlation between the anthropometric measurement and GA at birth ($p < 0.0005$).

After correction for GA at birth, only absolute and relative DHA levels remained significantly related to birth weight ($p = 0.03$ for both). Absolute levels of AA, the sum of all *n*-6 LCPs ($p = 0.05$ for both), the sum of all LCPs ($p = 0.03$) and DHA ($p = 0.01$), and the relative level of DHA ($p = 0.05$) remained significantly related to HC at birth. The absolute level of DHA remained significantly related to length at birth ($p = 0.02$). Cord artery wall levels of dihomo-γ-linolenic acid were not significantly related to any of the measures of prenatal growth.

Relation between LCP status at birth and at term. From three of the 28 infants followed until the term period, no cord blood sample was available; from two infants, the umbilical vessel wall sample was missing. As a result, 23 complete sets of data were available for the regression analyses concerning erythrocytes. From one infant, the plasma sample collected at term was lost during fatty acid analysis, so for the regression analyses of the plasma data, 22 complete sets were used.

The postnatal diet was the only explanatory variable for absolute ($p = 0.004$) and relative ($p = 0.0004$) plasma levels of DHA and relative plasma levels of AA ($p = 0.02$) at term postconceptional age; postnatal levels in the infants raised on formula were lower than in those fed their own mother's milk. The absolute AA level in plasma PLs at birth was the only explanatory variable (positive correlation, $p = 0.02$) for the absolute AA level at term (Fig. 2, *A*).

Absolute ($p = 0.0003$) and relative ($p < 0.0001$) DHA levels and the absolute AA level ($p = 0.02$) in the umbilical artery wall were positively related to the corresponding LCP levels in erythrocyte PLs at term (Fig. 2, *B*). No significant explanatory variables were found for the relative level of AA in erythrocytes in the term period.

Detailed information on the results described (e.g., correlation coefficients) is available on request.

DISCUSSION

One of the objectives of this study was to enhance the knowledge of the relations between the LCP status at birth, GA at birth, and anthropometric measurements. The GA was positively correlated with relative *n*-3 LCP amounts in cord plasma PLs and with relative *n*-6 and *n*-3 LCP amounts in the umbilical artery walls. We consider the higher *n*-6 and *n*-3 levels observed with advancing GA to be an indication of an adequate response to the increasing demand for *n*-6 and *n*-3 LCPs, which are necessary for fetal brain and body growth, in the third trimester of pregnancy.

Increasing plasma *n*-3 levels with increasing GA have also been observed by others.[19, 28, 29] Plasma *n*-6 levels have been reported to increase[28] or to decrease[29] with advancing GA, or, as in this study, no significant relation was observed.[18, 19] Fatty acid levels in plasma PLs are affected by relatively short-term (dietary) influences. Therefore we also studied umbilical artery walls, because their LCP composition can be looked on as a long-term reflection of the fetal LCP status.[24, 25] They are regarded as such because human umbilical vessels have no vasa vasorum, and human tissue cannot synthesize EFAs, so their walls have no other way to obtain EFAs than from the blood flowing through them. As a consequence, the LCP composition of the umbilical artery walls represents the EFA and LCP content of the backflow from the fetus to the mother and thereby indicates the lowest estimate of the fetal LCP status.

After correction for GA at birth, anthropometric measurements at birth were significantly related to LCP levels in the umbilical artery wall only. Because LCP levels in cord plasma and erythrocyte PLs are considered to be relatively short-term indicators of the fetal LCP status, their correlation with measures of a long-term process such as fetal growth can be expected to be less distinct. The levels of DHA in the arterial cord vessel walls were significantly related to weight and HC, as well as to length at birth, and absolute *n*-6 LCP levels correlated with HC. Others have observed a positive relation of both *n*-3 and *n*-6 LCPs to birth weight and HC, in premature[19] and term[24, 30] newborn infants. Koletzko and Braun[18] reported a positive relation between birth weight and relative levels of AA and the sum of all *n*-6 LCPs in plasma triglycerides of newborn preterm infants. No such relation was observed for *n*-3 LCPs, so they concluded that LCPs of the *n*-6 series specifically seem to be associated with tissue growth in utero. However, the correlations observed in the above-mentioned studies were not always corrected for GA. In our population, significant correlations for percentage levels of AA and the sum of all *n*-6 LCPs to both birth weight and HC were completely attributable to GA at birth.

In the current study, we observed a striking relation between prenatal growth and DHA status; this fatty acid was significantly related to all three anthropometric measures, independent of the GA at which the infant was born. DHA has a highly specific distribution in the human body, being present in high concentrations in brain, retina, spermatozoa, and mitochondria.[31] Perhaps an explanation for the consistent relation between DHA status and prenatal growth may be sought in the high DHA concentration in mitochondrial membrane phospholipids and its potential influence on mitochondrial metabolic functions.[32]

We also demonstrated that the LCP status at term is determined, not only by the postnatal diet, but also by the LCP status at birth. The observed relations did not change when

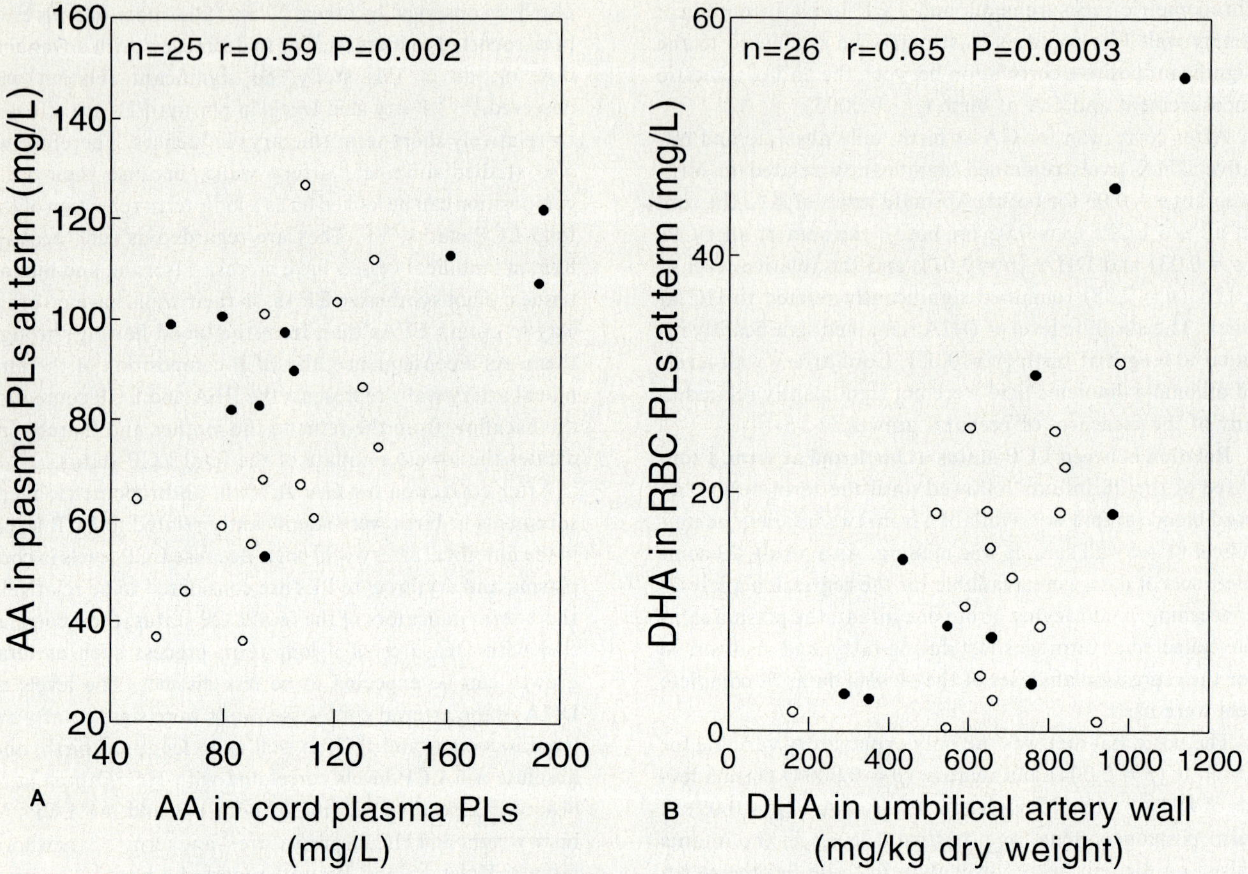

Fig. 2. A, Influence of AA (20:4*n*-6) status at birth, measured in cord plasma PLs, on the absolute AA status in plasma PLs in the term period (at term, 37 to 42 weeks of GA). Type of postnatal enteral diet: ● = human milk, ○ = artificial formula. **B,** Influence of DHA (22:6*n*-3) status at birth, measured in walls of umbilical arteries, on the absolute DHA status in erythrocyte PLs in the term period. Type of postnatal enteral diet: ● = human milk; ○ = artificial formula. **A** and **B,** *Scatterplots* contain all available information, including data on the infants from whom incomplete data sets were obtained. The given Pearson correlation coefficients and significance levels result from linear regression between the two variables in each of the scatterplots.

the data on SGA infants were not included in the statistical analysis. The DHA and AA levels in the walls of the umbilical arteries of preterm infants were positively related to the DHA and AA content of erythrocyte PLs collected at the time when these infants were expected to be born. Recent studies in preterm populations have demonstrated the importance of both the *n*-6 and the *n*-3 LCP status for several functional[33-36] and anthropometric measures.[20, 37] These studies pointed out the importance of an adequate LCP content of the early enteral diet of premature infants. However, our observation that higher LCP levels at birth result in higher postnatal levels stresses the significance of an appropriate prenatal LCP supply, because this is a major determinant of the LCP status at birth. The only potential way to achieve a change in this prenatal LCP supply is through an adaptation of the fatty acid content of the maternal diet during pregnancy (e.g., through an enhanced maternal EFA intake). The results of an earlier study support the feasibility of such an intervention.[38]

Besides the observed relation between the LCP status at birth and LCP levels at term postconceptional age, the type of postnatal diet was demonstrated to be the major determinant of postnatal LCP levels in plasma PLs, indicating that conventional artificial formulas (containing no *n*-6 and *n*-3 LCPs) are unable to maintain the postnatal LCP status of preterm infants at levels that can be obtained with preterm human milk. Our observation that the type of oral nutrition received by an infant influences the postnatal LCP status when measured in plasma PLs, but not when measured in erythrocyte PLs, is in agreement with the findings of recent studies.[8, 16]

We conclude that in preterm infants, there are significant

relations between the LCP status at birth, GA at birth, and indicators of prenatal growth. Moreover, both the postnatal dietary LCP supply and the prenatal LCP supply, which is reflected in the LCP status at birth, were found to affect postnatal LCP levels in preterm infants. Considering the importance of LCPs for normal brain and retinal function, the latter observation may warrant further studies of the effects of EFA-enriched maternal diets during pregnancy on the neonatal LCP status at birth.

We express our appreciation for the skilled assistance obtained from the Analytical Biochemical Laboratory, in Assen, The Netherlands (fatty acid analyses of blood samples), and from Mrs. M. M. G. Simonis (fatty acid analyses of umbilical artery wall samples).

REFERENCES

1. Svennerholm L. Distribution and fatty acid composition of phosphoglycerides in normal human brain. J Lipid Res 1968; 9:570-9.
2. Crawford MA, Casperd NM, Sinclair AJ. The long-chain metabolites of linoleic and linolenic acids in liver and brain in herbivores and carnivores. Comp Biochem Physiol 1976; 54B:395-401.
3. Sastry PS. Lipids of nervous tissue: composition and metabolism. Prog Lipid Res 1985;24:69-176.
4. Fliesler SJ, Anderson RE. Chemistry and metabolism of lipids in the vertebrate retina. Prog Lipid Res 1983;22:79-131.
5. Carlson SE, Rhodes PG, Ferguson MG. Docosahexaenoic acid status of preterm infants at birth and following feeding with human milk or formula. Am J Clin Nutr 1986;44:798-804.
6. Pita ML, Fernández MR, De-Lucchi C, et al. Changes in the fatty acids pattern of red blood cell phospholipids induced by type of milk, dietary nucleotide supplementation, and postnatal age in preterm infants. J Pediatr Gastroenterol Nutr 1988; 5:740-7.
7. Koletzko B, Schmidt E, Bremer HJ, Haug M, Harzer G. Effects of dietary long-chain polyunsaturated fatty acids on the essential fatty acid status of premature infants. Eur J Pediatr 1989;148:669-75.
8. Clandinin MT, Parrott A, Van Aerde JE, Hervada AR, Lien E. Feeding preterm infants a formula containing C_{20} and C_{22} fatty acids simulates plasma phospholipid fatty acid composition of infants fed human milk. Early Hum Dev 1992;31:41-51.
9. Foreman–van Drongelen MMHP, van Houwelingen AC, Kester ADM, et al. Long-chain polyene status of preterm infants with regard to the fatty acid composition of their diet: comparison between absolute and relative fatty acid amounts in plasma and red blood cell phospholipids. Br J Nutr 1995;73:405-22.
10. Jensen RG, Hagerty MM, McMahon KE. Lipids of human milk and infant formulas: a review. Am J Clin Nutr 1978; 31:990-1016.
11. Lammi-Keefe CJ, Jensen GJ. Lipids in human milk: a review. II. Composition and fat-soluble vitamins. J Pediatr Gastroenterol Nutr 1984;3:172-98.
12. Jensen RG, Ferris AM, Lammi-Keefe CJ. Lipids in human milk and infant formulas. Ann Rev Nutr 1992;12:417-41.
13. Clandinin MT, Chappell JE, Leong S, Heim T, Swyer PR, Chance GW. Extrauterine fatty acid accretion in infant brain: implications for fatty acid requirements. Early Hum Dev 1980;4:131-8.
14. Chambaz J, Ravel D, Manier M-C, Pepin D, Mulliez N, Bereziat G. Essential fatty acid interconversion in the human fetal liver. Biol Neonate 1985;47:136-40.
15. Carlson SE, Rhodes PG, Rao VS, Goldgar DE. Effect of fish-oil supplementation on the *n*-3 fatty acid content of red blood cell membranes in preterm infants. Pediatr Res 1987; 21:507-10.
16. Carlson SE, Cooke RJ, Rhodes PG, Peeples JM, Werkman SH, Tolley EA. Long-term feeding of formulas high in linolenic acid and marine oil to very low birth weight infants: phospholipid fatty acids. Pediatr Res 1991;30:404-12.
17. Carlson SE, Cooke RJ, Rhodes PG, Peeples JM, Werkman SH. Effect of vegetable and marine oils in preterm infant formulas on blood arachidonic and docosahexaenoic acids. J PEDIATR 1992;120:159-67.
18. Koletzko B, Braun M. Arachidonic acid and early human growth: is there a relation? Ann Nutr Metab 1991;35:128-31.
19. Leaf AA, Leighfield MJ, Costeloe KL, Crawford MA. Long-chain polyunsaturated fatty acids and fetal growth. Early Hum Dev 1992;30:183-91.
20. Carlson SE, Werkman SH, Peeples JM, Cooke RJ, Tolley EA. Arachidonic acid status correlates with first year growth in preterm infants. Proc Natl Ac Sci USA 1993;90:1073-7.
21. Leaf AA, Leighfield MJ, Ghebremeskel K, Costeloe KL, Crawford MA. Polyunsaturated fatty acids in plasma choline phosphoglycerides of preterm infants [Abstract]. Third International Congress on Essential Fatty Acids and Eicosanoids, Adelaide, Australia, 1992:77.
22. Hornstra G. Essential fatty acids, pregnancy and pregnancy complications: a round table discussion. In: Sinclair A, Gibson R, eds. Essential fatty acids and eicosanoids. Invited papers from the Third International Congress, Champaign, Illinois: American Oil Chemist's Society, 1993:177-82.
23. Carlson SE, Carver JD, House SA. High fat diets varying in ratios of polyunsaturated to saturated fatty acid and linoleic and linolenic acid: a comparison of rat neural and red cell membrane phospholipids. J Nutr 1986;116:718-25.
24. Crawford MA, Doyle W, Drury P, Lennon A, Costleloe K, Leighfield M. n-6 and n-3 fatty acids during early human development. J Intern Med 1989;225:159-69S1.
25. Hornstra G, Houwelingen AC van, Simonis M, Gerrard JM. Fatty acid composition of umbilical arteries and veins: possible implications for the fetal EFA-status. Lipids 1989;24:511-7.
26. Bligh EG, Dyer WJ. A rapid method for total lipid extraction and purification. Can J Biochem Physiol 1959;37:911-7.
27. Kloosterman GJ. Ontwikkeling van embryo tot foetus [in Dutch]. In: Kloosterman GJ, chief ed. De Voortplanting van de Mens. Bussum, The Netherlands: Uitgeversmaatschappij Centen, 1983:71-5.
28. Friedman Z, Danon A, Lamberth EL, Mann WJ. Cord blood fatty acid composition in infants and in their mothers during the third trimester. J PEDIATR 1978;92:461-6.
29. Houwelingen AC van, Foreman–van Drongelen MMHP, Al MDM, Hornstra G, Nicolini U. Fetal essential fatty acid status during gestation [Abstract]. Am J Clin Nutr 1993;57:815S.
30. Felton CV, Chang TC, Crook D, Marsh M, Robson SC, Spencer JAD. Umbilical vessel wall fatty acids after normal and retarded fetal growth. Arch Dis Child 1994;70:F36-9.

31. Salem N, Kim H-Y, Yergey JA. Docosahexaenoic acid: membrane function and metabolism. In: Simopoulos AP, Kifer RR, Martin RE, eds. Health effects of polyunsaturated fatty acids in seafood. Orlando: Academic Press, 1986:263-317.
32. Houtsmuller UMT. Specific biological effects of polyunsaturated fatty acids. In: Vergroesen AJ, ed. The role of fats in human nutrition. London: Academic Press, 1975:331-51.
33. Uauy RD, Birch DG, Birch EE, Tyson JE, Hoffman DR. Effect of dietary omega-3 fatty acids on retinal function of very-low-birth-weight neonates. Pediatr Res 1990;28:485-92.
34. Carlson SE, Werkman SH, Rhodes PG, Tolley EA. Visual-acuity development in healthy preterm infants: effect of marine-oil supplementation. Am J Clin Nutr 1993;58:35-42.
35. Birch E, Birch D, Hoffman D, Hale L, Everett M, Uauy R. Breast-feeding and optimal visual development. J Pediatr Ophthalmol Strabismus 1993;30:33-8.
36. Bjerve KS, Brubakk AM, Fougner KJ, Johnsen H, Midthjell K, Torstein V. Omega-3 fatty acids: essential fatty acids with important biological effects, and serum phospholipid fatty acids as markers of dietary omega-3 fatty acid intake. Am J Clin Nutr 1993;57:801-6S.
37. Carlson SE, Cooke RJ, Werkman SH, Tolley EA. First year growth of preterm infants fed standard compared to marine oil *n*-3 supplemented formula. Lipids 1992;27:901-7.
38. Houwelingen AC van, Hornstra G, Simonis M, et al. Essential fatty acid composition of umbilical arteries and veins after fish oil supplementation during pregnancy. In: Drevon CA, Baksaas I, Krokan HE, eds. Omega-3 fatty acids: metabolism and biological effects. Basel, Switzerland: Birkhauser, 1993:125-9.

FELLOWSHIPS

Fellowships available in pediatric subspecialties and those for general academic pediatric training are listed once a year, in **January,** in THE JOURNAL OF PEDIATRICS. Each **June,** forms for listing fellowships available for the academic year beginning 18 months after publication are sent to the Chairman of the Department of Pediatrics at major hospitals in the United States and Canada. In addition, **a copy of the application form appears in the July, August, and September issues** of THE JOURNAL (please use the current form). Should you desire to list fellowships, a separate application must be made *each* year for *each* position. All applications must be returned to Mosby–Year Book, Inc., by **October 15** preceding the listing year to ensure publication. Additional forms will be supplied on request from the Journal Editing Department, Mosby–Year Book, Inc., 11830 Westline Industrial Drive, St. Louis, MO 63146-3318/800-325-4177, ext. 4317, or 314-453-4317.

Influence of energy substrates on respiratory gas exchange during conventional mechanical ventilation of preterm infants

Philippe Chessex, MD, Sylvie Bélanger, MD,[a] Bruno Piedboeuf, MD,[a] and Marjolain Pineault, PhD

From the Perinatal Service, Pharmacy and Research Center, Hôpital Sainte Justine, and the Department of Pediatrics, University of Montreal, Montreal, Quebec, Canada

Objective: **The purpose of this study was to determine the optimal parenteral feeding regimen for infants with compromised respiratory function.**
Methods: **We studied the influence of varying the source of energy on respiratory gas exchange in 10 infants who were supported by mechanical ventilation and who received intravenous feedings. Two isoenergetic parenteral regimens were infused consecutively; the level of fat intake was varied inversely with that of glucose. Under similar ventilator settings, transcutaneous partial pressures of oxygen and carbon dioxide, as well as indirect calorimetry were measured during each regimen.**
Results: **Despite the higher carbon dioxide production during the glucose-rich regimen (8.9 ± 0.7 vs 7.9 ± 0.4 ml/kg per minute, $p < 0.05$ by analysis of variance), transcutaneous partial pressure of carbon dioxide remained unaffected, suggesting ventilatory compensation as documented by the increased ($p < 0.002$) alveolar ventilation. This was not associated with a detectable rise in oxygen consumption, but with a significant change in partial pressure of oxygen (77 ± 5 vs 66 ± 3 mm Hg, $p < 0.05$).**
Conclusions: **Ventilator-dependent infants with early and mild bronchopulmonary dysplasia, who receive intravenous feedings of a moderate load of glucose-based energy, can compensate for enhanced carbon dioxide production by increasing their respiratory drive, with a beneficial effect on oxygenation compared with that observed when energy is derived from lipid-based solutions. (J PEDIATR 1995;126:619-24)**

Supported by a grant from Clintec Technologies, Inc., by the Medical Research Council of Canada, and by the Foundation of Hôpital Sainte Justine.

Submitted for publication July 29, 1994; accepted Nov. 11, 1994.

Reprint requests: Philippe Chessex, MD, Research Center, Sainte Justine Hospital 3175 Côte Sainte Catherine Montreal Québec, H3T 1C5, Canada.

[a]Now at the Centre de recherche, Centre hospitalier universitaire de l'Université Laval, Sainte Foy, Québec G1V 4G2, Canada.

0022-3476/95/$3.00 + 0 **9/23/61933**

Several groups have studied the effect of varying the source of energy on respiratory gas exchange.[1-5] However, the appropriate ratio of glucose and lipid-based energy remains to be defined for parenterally fed newborn infants with chronic lung disease who are supported by mechanical ventilation. Infants with bronchopulmonary dysplasia are hypermetabolic[6-10] and therefore have increased carbon dioxide production. Because alveolar ventilation is proportional to $\dot{V}CO_2$,[11] there is a theoretical advantage in diminishing $\dot{V}CO_2$ to avoid further compromising the respiratory system of those with abnormal lung function. We hypothesized that

BPD	Bronchopulmonary dysplasia
CHO	Glucose-rich regimen
LIP	Lipid-rich regimen
$TcPco_2$	Transcutaneous partial pressure of carbon dioxide
$TcPo_2$	Transcutaneous partial pressure of oxygen
$\dot{V}A$	Alveolar ventilation
$\dot{V}E$	Minute ventilation
$\dot{V}co_2$	Carbon dioxide production
$\dot{V}o_2$	Oxygen consumption

the source of energy could influence the respiratory gas exchange in infants who are supported by mechanical ventilation for compromised lung function, because of the specific effects of the combustion of glucose and lipids on $\dot{V}co_2$.

From the comparison of the stoichiometric equations for the oxidation of glucose and palmitate,[12] it appears that for the same amount of energy provided by both substrates, and in the event of their complete oxidation, fat would produce 25% less carbon dioxide. A comparable metabolic response can be observed in vivo in newborn infants with normal lung function when 35% of glucose energy is replaced by a lipid emulsion providing the same amount of energy.[3] Furthermore, glucose loading could stimulate glucose utilization for lipogenesis, which in turn would contribute to increased $\dot{V}co_2$ as well as oxygen consumption.[1] The clinical consequences of these metabolic adaptations remain questionable in patients who can provide adequate ventilatory compensation. However, in patients with compromised lung function, glucose-based energy might cause an increase in ventilatory demand, leading to respiratory distress,[13, 14] especially in premature infants who have a higher metabolic rate and hence a higher $\dot{V}co_2$ per unit body mass. Therefore in newborn infants with pulmonary dysfunction, a high glucose load might aggravate preexisting carbon dioxide retention, which in turn could lead to further diaphragmatic fatigue.[15]

On the other hand, recent reports suggest that lipid emulsions might be contaminated by hydroperoxides.[16-18] The immaturity of the antioxidant systems puts the newborn infant at risk of morbidity related to cellular lesions caused by oxidants, such as the peroxides found in lipid emulsions. This could explain the discrepancies between reports in adults suggesting beneficial effects of intravenously administered lipids during ventilation[19] versus publications in neonates warning about its hazards.[17, 20] These warnings are supported by clinical correlates suggesting that lipid emulsions cause decreased oxygenation[21] and have deleterious effects on morbidity and mortality rates.[22, 23]

Therefore the aim of this study was to assess the effect on respiratory gas exchange of varying glucose and lipid intakes isoenergetically in newborn infants who received mechanical ventilation for respiratory distress.

METHODS

Measurements were to be performed in a paired fashion, in parenterally fed infants whose ventilator settings were stable. This prerequisite was established from previous experience in infants who received mechanical ventilation for BPD,[9] which showed a large interindividual variation in respiratory gas exchange linearly related to the need for ventilatory support. Approval by the human ethics committee of Sainte-Justine Hospital and informed parental consent were obtained before the investigation.

The study population consisted of parenterally fed newborn infants who were receiving prolonged conventional ventilatory support. To be assigned to the investigation, the infants' respiratory condition had to be stable (i.e., the ventilator settings had to remain similar for 2 days before assignment and presumably for 4 to 6 days thereafter, representing the duration of the protocol). The ventilation was managed by the attending physician in an attempt to maintain oxygen saturation between 90% and 95%, and partial pressure of carbon dioxide between 45 and 65 mm Hg. Measurements were performed only when air leaks around the endotracheal tube were clinically undetectable.[24] The infants were housed in convective incubators, with their abdominal skin temperature regulated by a servocontrol mechanism at 36.4° to 36.5° C. Total parenteral nutrition was initiated independently by the infants' physicians, based on feeding intolerance. The study was performed when parenteral intakes were being gradually increased, as in the case of intermittent and unsuccessful attempts at enteral alimentation.

The experimental protocol consisted of a paired crossover design, in which each infant served as his or her own control subject. Each patient received two 2- to 3-day periods (P1 and P2) of isoenergetic (300 kJ/kg per day, or 70 kcal/kg per day) and isonitrogenous (420 mg/kg per day) parenteral regimens infused consecutively, during which the level of fat intake (low fat [0.5 to 1.0 gm/kg per day] versus high fat [2.0 to 2.5 gm/kg per day]) varied inversely with that of glucose (high glucose [14 to 16 gm/kg per day] versus low glucose [8 to 10 gm/kg per day]). Half of the patients were initially given the glucose-rich regimen (high glucose and low fat) and the other half the lipid-rich regimen (high fat and low glucose). Measurements were performed on the last day of each period. The crossover was limited to a period of 2 to 3 days in an attempt to ensure similar ventilatory conditions during both periods. Total parenteral nutrition was delivered through peripheral lines as previously reported.[3] The lipid emulsion (Intralipid 10%; KabiVitrum AB, Stockholm, Sweden) was administered in a piggyback fashion with the amino acid dextrose solution (Travasol 10% Blend C; Clintec Canada, Mississauga, Ontario, Canada). All solutions were supplemented with electrolytes, trace elements (Micro + 6 Pediatric; Sabex International Montreal, Quebec, Canada), and a multivitamin preparation (MVI Pediatric; Rhône Poulenc Rorer, Montreal, Quebec, Canada).

Respiratory gas exchange variables, $\dot{V}O_2$ (in milliliters per kilogram per minute at standard temperature and pressure that contains no water vapor), carbon dioxide production (in milliliters per kilogram per minute at standard temperature and pressure that contains no water vapor), and minute ventilation (in milliliters per kilogram per minute) were measured with a previously validated[25, 26] indirect calorimeter (MGM/Jr; Utah Medical Products, Inc., Midvale, Utah) that can be used as an open-circuit system with a head hood[3, 27] or as a closed-circuit system[9, 28] in newborn infants supported by mechanical ventilation. This metabolic cart consists of a pneumotachometer, a zirconium oxygen sensor, and an infrared photometry carbon dioxide analyzer, integrated with a microprocessor that records data read every 20 seconds. A two-way nonrebreathing valve allowed for connection of the indirect calorimeter to the ventilator circuit with the addition of less than 1 ml of dead space. Before each measurement, calibrations were performed with known gas mixtures. Three-hour measurements were recorded, and physical activity[29] was continuously monitored by an experienced observer. A resting state (0 on the Freymond activity scale[29]) corresponded to the condition in which an infant had no body or limb movement, eyes open or closed. Periods of at least 30 minutes spent under resting conditions were used for data analysis. Resting energy expenditure was calculated from $\dot{V}O_2$ and respiratory quotient ($\dot{V}CO_2/\dot{V}O_2$) with classic equations of indirect calorimetry.[25] Paired measurements were conducted at approximately the same time of the day.

Concomitantly, transcutaneous partial pressures of oxygen and carbon dioxide (model 7690 Microgas analyzer with Combi Sensor, Kontron Electronic AG, Zurich, Switzerland) were continuously recorded every 10 seconds with a desktop computer.[3] The electrode was heated at 44° C and calibrated before each measurement. After installation, the sensor was allowed to stabilize for more than 20 minutes, before 3-hour data collection. The ventilatory index[30] (mean airway pressure × fraction of inspired oxygen × $100/TcPO_2$) was used to follow the severity of the respiratory condition. Alveolar ventilation was calculated as $\dot{V}A = \dot{V}CO_2 \times 863/TcPCO_2$ (in milliliters per kilogram per minute at body temperature, ambient pressure, and saturated with water vapor),[11] assuming that the $TcPCO_2$ value was similar enough to alveolar partial pressure of carbon dioxide for paired comparisons. Routine biochemical monitoring was performed and determinations were carried out according to standard analytical techniques (Parallel; American Monitor Corp., Indianapolis, Ind.).

Table I. Nutrient intakes in 10 parenterally fed newborn infants who received mechanical ventilation for chronic lung disease

	CHO	LIP
Energy		
(kcal/kg/day)	69 ± 2	68 ± 2
(kJ/kg/day)	288 ± 17	284 ± 17
Glucose (gm/kg/day)	14.1 ± 0.5	9.9 ± 0.2
Nonprotein energy intake as glucose (%)	86 ± 2	60 ± 1
Lipids (gm/kg/day)	0.8 ± 0.1	2.0 ± 0.1
Nonprotein energy intake as lipids (%)	14 ± 2	40 ± 1
Nitrogen (mg/kg/day)	417 ± 16	417 ± 16
Fluids (ml/kg/day)	167 ± 14	163 ± 10

Data are expressed as mean ± SEM.
For the sake of clarity, the table does not show the crossover in which half of the studies started with LIP.

Statistics. The paired crossover design[31] allowed us to evaluate separately by analysis of variance for repeated measures the effects of treatment (LIP vs CHO), time or evolution of the clinical condition (P1 vs P2), and sequence of administration or carryover (starting either LIP or CHO). The level of significance was set at $p < 0.05$.

RESULTS

Of the 14 patients who were initially enrolled in the study, four were excluded because they did not complete the protocol for the following reasons: noncompliance with the nutritional protocol (n = 1), important modifications in the ventilator settings, clinical condition, or both (one after CHO, and one after LIP), and audible leak around the endotracheal tube in the second period of the protocol (n = 1). The clinical characteristics of the 10 patients who completed the paired observations, and who therefore represent the study population, were as follows: birth weight (mean ± SEM), 1.13 ± 0.15 kg (range, 0.65 to 2.3 kg); gestational age, 28 ± 1 weeks (range, 26 to 30 weeks); age at study, 22 ± 3 days (range, 9 to 42 days); and study weight, 1.13 ± 0.07 kg (range, 0.95 to 1.64 kg). During the initial stage of ventilation, the patients had radiologic and clinical features of respiratory distress syndrome. All subjects eventually had chronic lung disease of prematurity as defined by oxygen dependency after 30 days of life. Eight infants had received surfactant as a rescue treatment within the first 24 hours of life. One infant (birth weight, 2.3 kg; gestational age, 30 weeks) born with nonimmune hydrops fetalis was studied at 23 days of age with a weight of 1.64 kg. The following medications were given during both pe-

Table II. Respiratory gas exchange data in 10 parenterally fed newborn infants who received mechanical ventilation for chronic lung disease

	CHO	LIP
$\dot{V}O_2$ (ml/kg/min)	8.6 ± 0.6	8.1 ± 0.4
$\dot{V}CO_2$ (ml/kg/min)	8.9 ± 0.7	7.9 ± 0.4*
$TcPO_2$ (mm Hg)	77 ± 5	66 ± 3*
$TcPCO_2$ (mm Hg)	51 ± 4	53 ± 4
$\dot{V}_A$ (ml/kg/min)	153 ± 7	132 ± 6*
$\dot{V}_E$ (ml/kg/min)	315 ± 27	276 ± 18

Data are expressed as mean ± SEM.
For the sake of clarity, the table does not show the crossover in which half of the studies started with LIP.
*p <0.05.

riods of the protocol: diuretics (n = 2), xanthines (n = 6), and antibiotics (n = 3); none of the subjects received dexamethasone. No infant had laboratory-proved septicemia. Before the study, five infants had received indomethacin for treatment of a patent ductus arteriosus, which was not hemodynamically active during the protocol.

By design, CHO and LIP differed only in the source of energy (Table I). Because the study was performed during the phase in which parenteral nutrient intakes are gradually increased, the infused energy had not reached target intakes of 80 to 90 kcal/kg per day, which are attained by combining the maximum intakes in both studied regimens. Most infants in our institution are fed through peripheral lines to minimize the risk of infections; thus the upper limit of osmolality (750 to 800 mOsm/L) was reached with CHO.[32] There was no change in the need for ventilatory support, because mean airway pressure (CHO 5.8 ± 0.7 vs LIP 5.7 ± 0.6 cm H_2O) as well as fraction of inspired oxygen (CHO 0.33 ± 0.03 vs LIP 0.35 ± 0.03) remained stable during the protocol; hence the ventilatory index (CHO 29 ± 7 vs LIP 33 ± 5) was not statistically affected by treatment ($F_{(1,8)}$ = 2.6) or time ($F_{(1,8)}$ = 5.2).

For the sake of clarity, and because there was no effect of time or carryover, the respiratory gas exchange data are presented in Table II without the crossover. The $\dot{V}CO_2$ value was higher (p <0.05) during CHO ($F_{(1,8)}$ = 9.2). However, no significant difference ($1 - \beta > 80\%$) in $\dot{V}O_2$ was detected between CHO and LIP ($F_{(1,8)}$ = 1.3). There was a significant change in respiratory quotient between CHO and LIP (1.05 ± 0.02 vs 0.96 ± 0.01; p <0.02). During both regimens the respiratory quotient was different from 1 (p <0.05). Under resting conditions the mean energy expenditure (CHO 62 ± 5 kcal/kg per day [259 ± 21 kJ/kg per day] vs LIP 58 ± 3 kcal/kg per day [243 kJ/kg per day]) approximated the mean energy intake, which explains the poor growth of these infants at the time of study.

Despite the higher $\dot{V}CO_2$ during CHO, $TcPCO_2$ remained unchanged ($F_{(1,8)}$ = 1.3), but there was a significant difference in $TcPO_2$ ($F_{(1,8)}$ = 9.0). Although the change in $\dot{V}_E$ was not significant ($F_{(1,8)}$ = 3.87), it was linearly related (r = 0.82, p <0.01) to the change in $\dot{V}_A$, which was higher (p <0.002) during the CHO phase of the study ($F_{(1,8)}$ = 25.9).

Routine blood monitoring showed similar results in both regimens (CHO vs LIP: pH 7.31 ± 0.01 vs 7.32 ± 0.01; glucose 4.5 ± 0.4 [n = 6] vs 5.2 ± 1.1 [n = 6] mmol/L; chloride 100 ± 3 [n = 10] vs 101 ± 3 [n = 7] mmol/L; sodium 136 ± 2 [n = 10] vs 137 ± 1 [n = 8] mmol/L; potassium 4.6 ± 0.2 [n = 10] vs 4.6 ± 0.4 [n = 7] mmol/L; and calcium 2.6 ± 0.3 [n = 7] vs 2.6 ± 0.4 [n = 7] mmol/L). During LIP, plasma triglyceride and cholesterol levels were 0.78 ± 0.2 (n = 6) and 3.5 ± 0.2 (n = 6) mmol/L, respectively. No glycosuria was detected.

DISCUSSION

To provide the elevated energy required to sustain growth in infants with BPD, high parenteral glucose intakes are often given by central access lines.[8] This might be associated with a respiratory quotient >1, indicating that glucose not directly oxidized is used for de novo synthesis of fat from glucose. In adults, lipogenesis from glucose does not seem to contribute substantially to fat reserves[33]; in newborn infants, because the energy intake must exceed expenditure to sustain adequate growth, fat synthesis from glucose is an active metabolic pathway.[34] Depending on the extent of fat synthesis from glucose, lipogenesis might be associated with an increase in $\dot{V}O_2$. Under those circumstances, the extra energy provided by glucose could be offset by the increase in metabolic rate.[8] On the other hand, with a well-balanced diet, such extremes of metabolic adaptation do not seem to occur, even in infants with BPD.[10] In this study, which provided only a moderate energy intake, CHO did not produce deleterious effects on the respiratory gas exchange even if it was associated with a respiratory quotient >1.

The $\dot{V}O_2$ of the study population was 30% higher than that of parenterally fed infants with normal respiratory function[3, 5] and 25% higher than in infants in the acute stage (<24 hours of life) of relatively severe respiratory distress syndrome.[28] This hypermetabolism of infants with chronic lung disease confirms previous observations.[6, 7, 9, 10] However, in infants supported by mechanical ventilation, respiratory gas exchange data could be underestimated if there were leaks around the endotracheal tube.[24] However, the fact that our subjects had $\dot{V}O_2$ similar to that of enterally fed infants with BPD[10] strengthens the validity of our measurements. It could be argued, however, that the opposing effects of several factors influencing energy expenditure[9, 35] may explain why our subjects and those enterally fed infants[10] had similar metabolic rates, despite such diverse clinical characteristics. In the same way, opposing effects might explain the absence of changes in $\dot{V}O_2$ during CHO and LIP.

It was initially debatable whether differences in respiratory gas exchange would be detectable in infants receiving ventilatory support by a conventional respirator, because the intermittent mandatory ventilation might conceal small spontaneous ventilatory adaptations by the infants. However, despite the increased $\dot{V}CO_2$ during CHO, $TcPCO_2$ remained unaffected, suggesting a ventilatory compensation as documented by the increased $\dot{V}A$. The significantly higher $TcPO_2$ observed during CHO, which was also reported in other studies under similar nutritional conditions,[3,4] could be further evidence of increased $\dot{V}A$ disproportionate to the change in $\dot{V}O_2$. This hypothesis is supported by similar findings in a group of healthy adults breathing spontaneously, in whom the metabolism of carbohydrate was shown to increase $\dot{V}E$ sufficiently to raise arterial partial pressure of oxygen significantly.[36]

Because the experimental design did not enable us to separate the effects of CHO from those of LIP, an opposite point of view would be that $TcPO_2$ was significantly lower during LIP. By stimulating cyclooxygenase production and inhibiting prostacyclin synthase,[37] the hydroperoxides contaminating the lipid emulsion could produce an overall vasoconstriction[17] and a decrease in lung perfusion, and hence affect respiratory gas exchange and oxygenation. This possibilitiy is supported by the presence of diet-induced modifications in $\dot{V}A$, an index for both ventilation and perfusion, while $\dot{V}E$ remained unchanged, suggesting a mismatch between ventilation and perfusion. Similarly, Peirera et al.[10] did not detect changes in $\dot{V}E$ in patients with BPD, despite an increased $\dot{V}CO_2$ during enteral feeding with a high-carbohydrate formula compared with a high-fat formula.

We conclude that ventilator-dependent infants fed parenterally with a moderate glucose-based energy intake can compensate for the enhanced $\dot{V}CO_2$ by increasing their respiratory drive. However, caution is necessary in extrapolating these conclusions to those infants receiving a more positive energy balance or those with a greater degree of lung compromise and ventilator dependency.

We thank Jocelyne Vallée, RN, for her assistance in this study.

REFERENCES

1. Van Aerde JE, Sauer PJ, Pencharz PB, Smith JM, Swyer PR. Effect of replacing glucose with lipid on the energy metabolism of newborn infants. Clin Sci 1989;76:581-8.
2. Nose O, Tipton J, Ament M, Yabuchi H. Effect of the energy source on changes in energy expenditure, respiratory quotient, and nitrogen balance during total parenteral nutrition in children. Pediatr Res 1987;21:538-41.
3. Piedboeuf B, Chessex P, Hazan J, Pineault M, Lavoie JC. Total parenteral nutrition in the newborn infant: energy substrates and respiratory gas exchange. J PEDIATR 1991;118:97-102.
4. Salas-Salvado J, Molina J, Figueras J, Masso J, Marti-Henneberg C, Jimenez R. Effect of the quality of infused energy on substrate utilization in the newborn receiving total parenteral nutrition. Pediatr Res 1993;33:112-7.
5. Van Aerde JE, Sauer P, Pencharz PB, Smith JM, Heim T, Swyer P. Metabolic consequences of increasing energy intake by adding lipid to parenteral nutrition in full-term infants. Am J Clin Nutr 1994;59:659-62.
6. Kao LC, Durand DJ, Nickerson BG. Improving pulmonary function does not decrease oxygen consumption in infants with bronchopulmonary dysplasia. J PEDIATR 1988;112:616-21.
7. Kurzner SI, Garg M, Bautista DB, Sargent CW, Bowman M, Keens TG. Growth failure in bronchopulmonary dysplasia: elevated metabolic rates and pulmonary mechanics. J PEDIATR 1988;112:73-80.
8. Yunis KA, Oh W. Effects of intravenous glucose loading on oxygen consumption, carbon dioxide production, and resting energy expenditure in infants with bronchopulmonary dysplasia. J PEDIATR 1989;115:127-32.
9. Billeaud C, Piedboeuf B, Chessex P. Energy expenditure and severity of respiratory disease in very low birth weight infants receiving long-term ventilatory support. J PEDIATR 1992; 120:461-4.
10. Peirera GR, Baumgart S, Bennett MJ, et al. Use of high-fat formula for premature infants with bronchopulmonary dysplasia: metabolic, pulmonary and nutritional studies. J PEDIATR 1994;124:605-11.
11. McCann E, Goldman S, Brady J. Pulmonary function in the sick newborn infant. Pediatr Res 1987;21:313-25.
12. Flatt JP. Energetics of intermediary metabolism. In: Kinney JM, ed. Assessment of energy metabolism in health and disease. (Ross Conference on Medical Research.) Columbus, Ohio: Ross Laboratories, 1980:77-87.
13. Covelli HD, Black WJ, Olsen SM, Beekman J. Respiratory failure precipitated by high carbohydrate loads. Ann Intern Med 1981;95:579-81.
14. Askanazi J, Elwyn DH, Silverberg PA, Rosenbaum SH, Kinney JM. Respiratory distress secondary to a high carbohydrate load: a case report. Surgery 1980;87:596-8.
15. Juan G, Calverley P, Talamo C, Schnader J, Roussos C. Effect of carbon dioxide on diaphragmatic function in human beings. N Engl J Med 1984;310:874-9.
16. Bélanger S, Lavoie JC, Pineault M, Chessex P. Bound-iron admixture tp parenteral nutrition (TPN) causes peroxidation of the lipid emulsion [Abstract]. Pediatr Res 1994;35: 307.
17. Helbock HJ, Motchnik PA, Ames BN. Toxic hydroperoxides in intravenous lipid emulsions used in preterm infants. Pediatrics 1993;91:83-8.
18. Pitkänen O, Hallman M, Anderson S. Generation of free radicals in lipid emulsion used in parenteral nutrition. Pediatr Res 1991;29:56-9.
19. Skeie B, Askanazi J, Rothkopf MM, Goldstein S, Rosenbaum SH. The beneficial effects of fat on ventilation and pulmonary function. Nutrition 1987;3:149-54.
20. Pitkänen OM. Peroxidation of lipid emulsions: A hazard for the premature infant receiving parenteral nutrition? Free Radic Biol Med 1993;13:239-45.
21. Peirera G, Fox W, Stanley C, Baker L, Schwartz J. Decreased

oxygenation and hyperlipemia during intravenous fat infusions in premature infants. Pediatrics 1980;66:26-30.
22. Pitkänen O, Hallman M, Andersson SM. Correlation of free oxygen radical-induced lipid peroxidation with outcome in very low birth weight infants. J PEDIATR 1990;116:760-4.
23. Hammerman C, Aramburo MJ. Decreased lipid intake reduces morbidity in sick premature neonates. J PEDIATR 1988;113:1083-8.
24. Dietrich KA, Romero MD, Conrad SA. Effects of gas leak around endotracheal tubes on indirect calorimetry measurements. JPEN J Parenter Enteral Nutr 1990;14:408-13.
25. Mayfield SR. Technical and clinical testing of a computerized indirect calorimeter for use in mechanically ventilated neonates. Am J Clin Nutr 1991;54:30-4.
26. Alverson DC, Isken VH, Cohen RS. Effect of booster blood transfusions on oxygen utilization in infants with bronchopulmonary dysplasia. J PEDIATR 1988;113:722-6.
27. Billeaud C, Piedboeuf B, Jéquier JC, Chessex P. Relative contribution of physical activity to neonatal oxygen consumption. Early Hum Dev 1993;32:113-20.
28. Hazan J, Chessex P, Piedboeuf B, Bourgeois M, Bard H, Long W. Energy expenditure during synthetic surfactant replacement therapy for neonatal respiratory distress syndrome. J PEDIATR 1992;120:S29-33.
29. Freymond D, Schutz Y, Decombaz J, Micheli JL, Jéquier E. Energy balance, physical activity, and thermogenic effect of feeding premature infants. Pediatr Res 1986;20:638-45.
30. Merritt AT, Hallman M, Bloom BT, et al. Prophylactic treatment of very premature infants with human surfactant. N Engl J Med 1986;315:785-90.
31. Hills M, Armitage PL. The two-period cross-over clinical trial. Br J Clin Pharmacol 1979;8:7-20.
32. Pineault M, Chessex P, Piedboeuf B, Bisaillon S. Beneficial effect of coinfusing a lipid emulsion on venous patency. JPEN J Parenter Enteral Nutr 1989;13:637-40.
33. Acheson KJ, Schutz Y, Bessard T, Ravussin E, Jéquier E, Flatt JP. Nutritional influences on lipogenesis and thermogenesis after a carbohydrate meal. Am J Physiol 1984;246:E62-E70.
34. Van Aerde J, Sauer P, Pencharz P, Heim T, Smith J, Swyer P. Glucose and fat requirements in the intravenously fed newborn infant. In: Stern L, Orzalesi M, Friis-Hansen B, eds. Physiologic foundations of perinatal care III. New York: Elsevier, 1989:60-74.
35. Chessex P, Reichman B, Verellen G, et al. Influence of postnatal age, energy intake, and weight gain on energy metabolism in the very low-birth-weight infant. J PEDIATR 1981;99:761-6.
36. Saltzman HA, Salzano JV. Effects of carbohydrate metabolism upon respiratory gas exchange in normal men. J Appl Physiol 1971;30:228-31.
37. Lavoie JC, Chessex P. The increase in vasomotor tone induced by a parenteral lipid emulsion is linked to an inhibition of prostacyclin production. Free Radic Biol Med 1994;16: 795-9.

Birth order, delivery route, and concordance in the transmission of human immunodeficiency virus type 1 from mothers to twins

Anne-Marie Duliège, MD, MS, Christopher I. Amos, PhD, Susanne Felton, MA, Robert J. Biggar, MD, the International Registry of HIV-Exposed Twins,[a] and James J. Goedert, MD

From the Biocine Company, Emeryville, California; the Department of Epidemiology, M. D. Anderson Cancer Center, Houston, Texas; the Research Triangle Institute, Washington, D.C.; and the Viral Epidemiology Branch, National Cancer Institute, Rockville, Maryland

***Background*: We evaluated data from prospectively identified twins to understand better the mechanisms and covariates of mother-to-infant transmission of human immunodeficiency virus (HIV).**

***Methods*: Using data obtained from an international collaboration and multivariate quasilikelihood modeling, we assessed concordance, birth order, route of delivery, and other factors for HIV infection in 115 prospectively studied twin pairs born to HIV-infected women. Actuarial methods were used to evaluate overall survival and survival free of acquired immunodeficiency syndrome for HIV-infected twins.**

***Results*: Infection with HIV occurred in 35% of vaginally delivered firstborn (A) twins, 16% of cesarean-delivered A twins, 15% of vaginally delivered secondborn (B) twins, and 8% of cesarean-delivered B twins. In a multivariate model, the adjusted odds ratios for HIV infection were 11.8 (confidence interval: 3.1 to 45.3) for concordance of infection with the co-twin, 2.8 (confidence interval: 1.6 to 5.0) for A versus B twins, and 2.7 (confidence interval: 1.1 to 6.6) for vaginally delivered versus cesarean-delivered twins. Among A twins, 52% (lower confidence limit: 6%) of the transmission risk was related to vaginal delivery. Comparing vaginally delivered A twins (infants most exposed to vaginal mucus and blood) to cesarean-delivered B twins (infants least exposed), 76% (lower confidence limit: 48%) of the transmission risk was related to vaginal exposure. Infected B twins had slightly reduced Quetelet indexes and more rapid development of illnesses related to acquired immunodeficiency syndrome.**

***Conclusions*: These results indicate that HIV infection of B twins occurs predominantly in utero, whereas infection of A twins (and, by implication, singletons) occurs predominantly intrapartum. We propose that intrapartum transmission is responsible for the majority of pediatric HIV infections and that reducing exposure to HIV in the birth canal may reduce transmission of the virus from mother to infant. (J PEDIATR 1995;126:625-32)**

Supported in part by contract NO1-CP-95612 from the National Cancer Institute.

Submitted for publication Aug. 8, 1994; accepted Oct. 26, 1994.

Reprint requests: Anne-Marie Duliège, MD, MS, Biocine-Chiron, 4560 Horton St., Emeryville, CA 94608-2916.

[a]Contributors to the International Registry of HIV-Exposed Twins are listed before the reference list. Address inquiries about the Registry to Dr. Goedert at 6130 Executive Blvd., Suite 434, Rockville, MD 20852.

9/23/61577

In industrialized countries, the overall transmission rate of fhuman immunodeficiency virus type 1 from mother to child is currently estimated to be approximately 15% to 25%.[1-6] Risk of transmission is higher with more advanced disease in the mother, whether ascertained by the duration of HIV infection, clinical status, or degree of immunodeficiency.[5, 7] The roles of maternal humoral and cellular immunity in protecting against transmission are not yet clear.[8] Transmission probably occurs both in utero and intrapartum, but clinical and molecular virologic studies of mothers and children have not yet clarified the mechanisms or proportions of transmission by each route.[9-12]

In a previously published study of twin pairs born to 66 mothers who were infected with HIV-1,[13] we found that HIV-1 infection was more common in firstborn than in second-born twins. We suggested that a substantial proportion of transmission occurred during labor or delivery and that contact with the birth canal may be particularly important in the transmission process. We have now collected information on 148 sets of twins with known infection status. The three primary goals of the current study were to confirm our initial findings, to evaluate intrauterine and intrapartum factors that may affect the risk of HIV-1 transmission among the subset of sets of twins that came to medical attention through prospective follow-up of infants born to HIV-1–infected mothers, and to compare the progression of HIV-1–related disease in firstborn and second-born HIV-1–infected twins.

AIDS	Acquired immunodeficiency syndrome
CI	Confidence interval
HIV	Human immunodeficiency virus
HIV-1	Human immunodeficiency virus type 1

METHODS

Data for the International Registry of HIV-Exposed Twins were abstracted from clinical records and submitted on standardized forms by collaborators, mainly pediatricians, obstetricians, infectious disease specialists, and nurse practitioners, in 14 countries. Follow-up forms were sent to all participants to update information about the infection status of twins, to obtain additional details related to birth conditions, and to enroll new sets of twins. For most sets, zygosity was assessed by clinical criteria (including gender, placentation, and physical appearance). Firstborn twins were designated as A twins, second-born twins as B twins. HIV-1 status (infected, uninfected, or indeterminate) included clinical and laboratory criteria as previously reported.[13]

The risk of infection in the twin pairs was assessed by quasilikelihood modeling.[14] This approach estimated the marginal probability of infection for each twin from predictors with adjusted odds ratios (and 95% confidence intervals) rather than relative risks, thereby allowing for the within-twin correlation of infection. Similar results (not presented) were obtained with the McNemar test for the matched twin pairs and with log-linear models of each twin's risk adjusted for the co-twin's infection status. Twin sets with mixed deliveries (that is, the A twin delivered vaginally, the B twin by cesarean section) were excluded when the effect of route of delivery on the risk of HIV-1 infection was evaluated. To assess effects of continuous covariates, specifically birth weight (in grams), birth length (in centimeters), Quetelet index (weight/length^2), and head circumference (in centimeters), we performed logistic regression with HIV-1 infection in one twin as the outcome, with and without adjustment for the co-twin's infection status.[15] As in the previous study,[13] co-twins were considered to have equal birth weights if their weights did not differ by more than 10%. To compare concordance of infection for monozygous and dizygous pairs, the kappa (κ) coefficient $\pm$ one standard error was used.[16] The proportions of maternal acquired immunodeficiency syndrome by continent and of vaginal deliveries by AIDS status were compared by the chi-square test.

The proportions of transmission that could be attributed to (1) method of delivery and (2) exposure to birth canal products were estimated as the fractions of exposed twins who were infected, minus the fractions of nonexposed twins who were infected, divided by the fractions of exposed twins who were infected.[17] Among the A twins, the attributable proportion from vaginal delivery was obtained by comparing the infected fraction delivered vaginally with the infected fraction delivered by cesarean section. We also calculated a proportion attributable to birth-canal exposure by comparing vaginally delivered A twins (the infants most exposed to birth canal products) and cesarean-delivered B twins (the infants least exposed to birth canal products). The lower 95% confidence limits for the attributable proportions were determined by the percentile method applied to 5000 paramedic bootstrap replications.[18] One-tailed estimates were justified because we focused on the minimal proportions of infection that could be prevented by avoiding the exposure. Kaplan-Meier actuarial survival curves were compared by log-rank tests.

RESULTS

Data from 203 sets of twins and two sets of triplets born to HIV-1–infected women had been recorded in the Registry by Dec. 1, 1993. Complete data on HIV-1 infection status were available for 148 sets, including 115 sets of twins

Table. Factors for mother-to-infant transmission of HIV-1 infection in 115 prospectively identified twin sets*

		No. of sets by HIV-1 infection status				% HIV-1 infected		
	Total No. of sets	Neither infected	Both infected	A twin infected	B twin infected	Overall	A twins	B twins
All sets	115	81	11	19	4	20	26	13
Delivery								
Both vaginal	65	41	9	14	1	25	35	15
Both cesarean	38	30	1	5	2	13	16	8
Zygosity								
Monozygotic	24	17	3	4	0	21	29	13
Dizygotic	73	49	7	13	4	21	27	15
Birth weight concordance								
Twin A heavier	22	17	3	1	1	18	18	18
Same (±10%)	55	39	5	11	0	19	29	9
Twin A lighter	28	17	2	6	3	23	29	18
Gestational age (wk)								
<34	27	20	3	3	1	19	22	15
34-37	55	39	3	11	2	17	25	9
>37	23	13	5	5	0	33	43	22
Mother's race								
Black	72	51	9	9	3	21	25	17
White	22	14	2	6	0	23	36	9
Other/unknown	21	16	0	4	1	12	19	5
Mother's route of infection								
Intravenous drug abuse	57	45	4	6	2	14	18	11
Sexual/other	53	36	4	11	2	20	28	11
Mother with AIDS								
Yes	11	6	1	3	1	27	36	18
No	54	42	4	7	1	15	20	9
HIV infected sibling								
Yes	13	10	0	3	0	12	23	0
No	57	39	5	10	3	20	26	14
Continent								
North America	72	54	8	8	2	18	22	14
Europe	26	19	1	5	1	15	23	8
Africa	16	8	2	5	1	31	44	19
Breast fed								
Both	12	8	0	3	1	17	25	8
Neither	63	45	7	10	1	20	27	13

*Numbers may not sum to 115 due to missing values.

ascertained by the collaborators prospectively (by follow-up of infants born to HIV-infected mothers), 28 sets ascertained by clinical signs or symptoms of HIV-1 infection in one or both twins, and five sets with uncertain modes of ascertainment. Both sets of triplets were excluded from the analysis of HIV-1 risk factors, one set because of uncertain HIV-1 infection status and the other because infection status was not ascertained prospectively. The 115 prospectively ascertained sets were predominately from North America (63%) and Europe (23%) but included 16 sets (14%) from Africa and one from Australia. These 115 sets include 32 sets that were previously reported.[13]

Major risk factors. The crude prevalence of HIV-1 infection among 115 prospectively followed twin sets (230 infants) was 20%—26% for A twins and 13% for B twins (Table). In 80% of the sets, both twins had similar infection status (neither infected 70%, both infected 10%). Concordance of infection status was 83% in monozygotic and 77% in dizygotic twin pairs. Thus the kappa coefficients were not significantly higher in monozygotic ($\kappa = 0.52 \pm 0.19$) than in dizygotic twins ($\kappa = 0.32 \pm 0.12$). Adjusted for concordance within pairs, the odds ratio of HIV-1 infection for A twins compared with B twins was 2.4 (Cl: 1.4 to 4.0). Excluding sets of twins previously reported,[13] the A twins were still significantly more likely to become infected than B twins (odds ratio: 2.9; Cl: 1.3 to 6.6).

Vaginal delivery was associated with an approximately twofold greater risk of transmission than cesarean delivery:

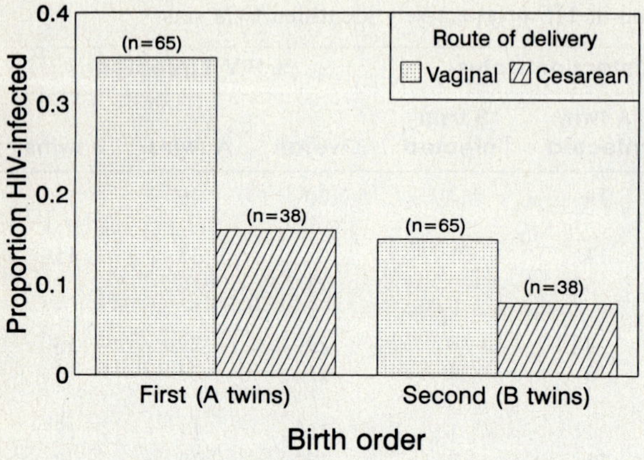

Fig. 1. Proportions of infants infected with HIV-1 from 103 sets of twins born to HIV-1–infected women, by order of birth (first is A twin, second is B twin) and route of delivery (vaginal or cesarean). Rate of infection was increased approximately twofold for A twins compared with B twins and for vaginal compared with cesarean delivery.

35% of A twins delivered vaginally compared with 16% of A twins delivered by cesarean section; for B twins, 15% were infected with vaginal delivery and 8% with cesarean delivery (Fig. 1). By quasilikelihood modeling, the adjusted odds ratios of infection were 11.8 (Cl: 3.1 to 45.3) for concordance, 2.8 (Cl: 1.6 to 5.0) for first birth, and 2.7 (Cl: 1.1 to 6.6) for vaginal delivery.

Attributable proportions. We estimated the proportion of infection attributable to route of delivery and the proportion attributable to birth canal exposure. For these analyses we excluded the African twins, all of whom were born vaginally. Among A twins, 52% of HIV-1 transmission was related to vaginal delivery (lower confidence limit, 6%). When A twins delivered vaginally were compared with B twins delivered by cesarean section, 76% of the transmission risk was related to vaginal exposure (lower confidence limit, 48%).

Secondary risk factors. Transmission of HIV-1 was 31% in Africa, 18% in North America, and 15% in Europe (Table); the differences were not statistically significant. All twins from Africa were delivered vaginally and were breast fed. By comparison, 56% of non-African twins were vaginally delivered, and only 3% were breast fed. In addition, the prevalence of AIDS was 38% in African and 10% in non-African mothers ($p = 0.16$). Thus it was not possible to dissect the risks associated with geography, breast-feeding, and AIDS illness. Despite universal breast-feeding and a higher prevalence of maternal AIDS, the excess risk of HIV-1 infection for A twins (44%) compared with B twins (19%) was evident in the African sets (adjusted odds ratio, 3.4; Cl, 0.8 to 14.0).

Transmission of HIV-1 also appeared to be more frequent when the mother had AIDS, and the rate of infection was twice as high for A twins as for B twins whether or not AIDS had developed in the mother (Table). Mothers with AIDS were more likely than mothers without AIDS to deliver vaginally (91% vs 50%; $p = 0.01$). In a four-variable quasilikelihood model including concordance and birth order, odds ratios of HIV-1 transmission were 3.7 (Cl, 0.9 to 15.4) for vaginal delivery and 1.4 (Cl, 0.4 to 5.00) for mothers with AIDS.

In three of the twin sets, only one infant was reported to have been breast fed and infected with HIV-1. In a fourth set, scalp electrodes were used only on the A twin, who also became infected. Excluding these four sets and two others with uncertain breast-feeding histories, the odds ratios for HIV-1 infection were 2.2 (Cl, 1.0 to 4.9) for first birth, 2.4 (Cl, 0.6 to 9.3) for vaginal delivery, 1.4 (Cl, 0.4 to 5.4) for mothers with AIDS, and 11.1 (Cl, 1.7 to 71.3) for concordance in the 53 non-African sets with complete data.

Other factors. In univariate analyses, HIV-1 infection of the B twin, but not of the A twin, was associated with longer body length (odds ratio, 1.04 per cm; Cl, 1.01 to 1.07 per cm), lower Quetelet index (odds ratio, 14.3 per gm/cm^2; Cl, 1.8 to 112.7 per gm/cm^2), and larger head circumference (odds ratio, 1.0 per cm; Cl, 1.0 to 1.1 per cm). However, these associations were not significant in models that included concordance of infection with the A twin.

In 50 of the 105 sets with adequate data, birth weights differed between co-twins by at least 10% (Table). In multivariate quasilikelihood models, difference in birth weight was not associated with HIV-1 infection ($p > 0.1$) and did not reduce the associations of HIV-1 infection with the co-twin's HIV-1 status (odds ratio, 23.8), first birth (odds ratio, 2.9), or vaginal delivery (odds ratio, 2.6).

Risk of HIV-1 did not appear to be associated with gestational age, zygosity, having an older sibling with HIV-1 infection, or mother's source of HIV-1 infection (Table). The male/female sex ratio was 1:1, and there was no evidence of a sex difference in risk of HIV-1 infection or of an interaction between sex and birth order (data not shown).

Survival analysis. Including all 148 sets that had complete HIV-1 infection data, 84 children were infected, including 54 A twins, 27 B twins, and one set of triplets.[13] Including the first two triplets as twins, information on survival was available for 52 A twins and 27 B twins, and on the incidence of AIDS for 51 A twins and 26 B twins. The median duration of follow-up for the group was 25 months (mean, 35 months) and was similar for A twins and B twins. Of the 52 infected A twins, 16 (31%) have died, compared with seven (26%) of the 27 infected B twins. The 3-year actuarial survival rate was 69% for A twins and 75% for B twins

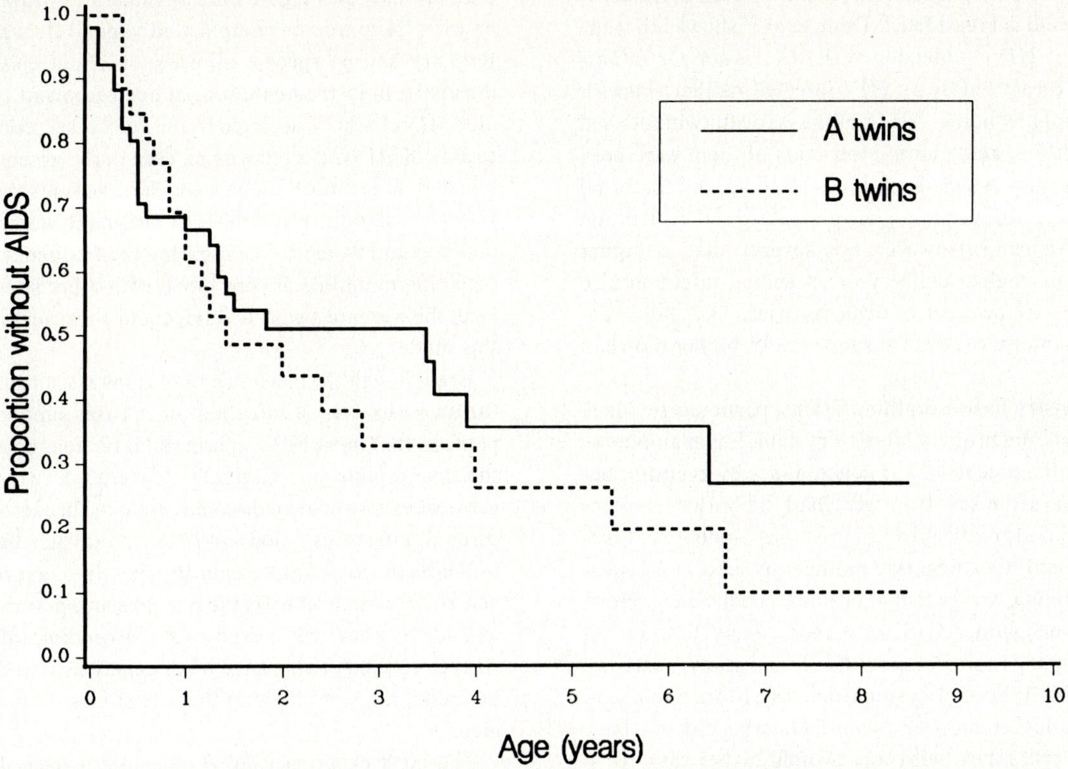

Fig. 2. AIDS-free actuarial survival estimated by the Kaplan-Meier method for twins who were infected with HIV. AIDS-free survival was slightly but not significantly better for firstborn *(A)* compared with second-born *(B)* twins ($p = 0.54$).

($p = 0.94$). Twenty-seven (53%) of the 51 A twins and 19 (73%) of the 26 B twins have AIDS. Median actuarial AIDS-free survival time was 42 months for A twins and 17 months for B twins ($p = 0.54$; Fig. 2).

DISCUSSION

Twins born to HIV-infected women provide a unique perspective on the epidemiology and natural history of HIV-1 infection and AIDS. Infection with HIV-1 was concordant in 80% of our 115 prospectively followed twin pairs, a level similar to that previously reported for 18 twin sets not included in this Registry.[19] With such high concordance, which presumably reflects the mother's level of infectiousness during the twin pregnancy and at the time of delivery, the strongest risk factor for an infant in our study was infection of the co-twin. Among the 20% of HIV-discordant twin sets, the A twin was more likely to be infected than the B twin, even among newly ascertained twin sets, which confirms our previous results.[13]

In both univariate and multivariate analysis, there was a significant, twofold lower risk of HIV-1 infection with cesarean delivery. With the acknowledgment that the Registry approach is an observational study and not a clinical trial, the magnitude of the effect of cesarean delivery, as well as the lack of attenuation after adjustment for birth order, concordance with the co-twin, maternal AIDS, and birth weights, all argue that the protective effect of cesarean delivery is real and clinically meaningful. We had hoped to evaluate the indications for cesarean delivery and the duration of rupture of membranes, but the available data were too sparse. We suggest that twin pregnancies represent high-risk obstetric conditions in which cesarean deliveries are more often elective and more likely to occur before or sooner after the rupture of membranes than for singletons, thus reducing the risk of ascending infections. No randomized clinical trial to reduce perinatal transmission of HIV-1 with elective cesarean delivery before or shortly after rupture of membranes has been reported. However, some reduction in risk with cesarean delivery has been found in most observational studies of singletons, an effect that was statistically significant in a recent metaanalysis.[20]

Mother-to-infant transmission of HIV-1 can occur during gestation, during labor or delivery, or even after delivery if the child is breast fed.[21] Dunn et al.[22] showed that the incidence of HIV-1 infection was 14% higher for infants who were breast fed by an HIV-infected mother than for those fed only by bottle. All 16 of the African twin sets had been breast fed, and a large proportion of them were born to mothers with AIDS. Both breast-feeding and maternal AIDS may contribute to higher perinatal HIV-1 infection rates in African.[5] However, we suspect that a higher frequency of vaginal delivery or ascending infection also contributes,[7, 23] because African A twins, like their non-African counterparts, were at substantially higher risk than B twins.

The Registry has several limitations, particularly a lack of specimens and primary laboratory data. For example, we found no difference in HIV-1 concordance by zygosity, but few of our same-sex twin sets had laboratory studies performed to support clinical impressions of identity. Likewise, we could not categorize mothers by laboratory measures of viremia, antigenemia, or immunodeficiency. However, mothers with AIDS were more likely to transmit HIV-1, as noted in singleton births.[5] In our study, nearly all mothers with AIDS had a vaginal delivery. More important, among the larger number of mothers who did not have AIDS, the risk for A twins was twofold higher than for B twins, a finding that points to a significant rate of intrapartum transmission among women who did not have overt disease.

The mechanisms of intrapartum HIV-1 infection remain unclear. Three hypotheses can be suggested. First, infection might occur with mixing of maternal and fetal blood during the contractions. This hypothesis seems unlikely because B twins are exposed to uterine contractions for a longer period and should be at higher risk than A twins.

Second, breaks in the skin could become contaminated by infected maternal blood or secretions. Fetal scalp monitoring does cause a wound, and this procedure was associated with higher HIV-1 transmission in at least some European centers.[5] In this model, ready access to the A twin's but not the B twin's scalp would lead to a higher risk for the A twin. However, scalp electrodes and other traumatic procedures were reported so rarely to the Registry that they could not account for the observed effect of birth order. They also would not have occurred in deliveries to African women, among whom the birth order effect was apparent.

Third, the infant might be infected through mucous membranes or by swallowing maternal blood or secretions before or during passage through the birth canal. Episiotomy and tears of the cervix or vagina introduce blood into the birth canal, and some centers in the European Collaborative Study had higher transmission rates with episiotomy or with traumatic or complicated vaginal deliveries.[5] The Registry had no specific information about episiotomy or intrapartum instrumentation, but cell-free and cell-associated HIV-1 can be detected in the genital secretions of 12% to 50% of HIV-infected women even in the absence of gross blood.[24] One study suggested that genital shedding of HIV-1 is significantly higher in pregnant women than in nonpregnant women.[25] Comparing the frequency of HIV-1 detection in umbilical cord blood with other sites, particularly the neonate's gastric fluid, could shed further light on this model.

Even though the mechanisms of transmission are unclear, the increased risk of infection for A twins supports the hypothesis that most HIV-1 perinatal infections occur around the time of delivery. Vaginally delivered A twins have the greatest exposure to birth-canal products, because they pass through infectious mucus and blood, and because they are in the birth canal longer than B twins. In a cesarean delivery, the A twin usually is the one presenting at the cervical os and thus has ready exposure to ascending infections.[23] Therefore the A twins have birth experiences and, not surprisingly, rates of infection that are similar to those of singletons.

The birth experiences of B twins differ from those of A twins. Although vaginally delivered B twins are exposed to the birth canal, the duration of exposure usually is relatively short. In addition, the A twin will have dilated and, to some extent, mechanically cleansed the canal. We found that infected B twins tended to be smaller than uninfected B twins. This suggests that some growth retardation with in utero infection may occur but would be difficult to detect in A twins and singletons, among whom most infections probably occur in the intrapartum period. Cesarean section–delivered B twins never enter the birth canal and have only remote exposure to blood and mucus that ascends into the uterus. Except for their exposure to blood during cesarean delivery, B twins have a relatively minimal exposure that might be close to the baseline rate of HIV-1 infection in utero. We used this baseline rate of in utero transmission to estimate that at least half of mother-to-infant transmissions of HIV-1 occurred by exposure to the birth canal. This frequency corroborates studies of the prevalence of HIV-1 infection that can be detected during the first few days of life.[26-29]

We conclude that three factors were strongly associated with HIV-1 infection of twins: HIV-1 status of the co-twin, birth order, and vaginal delivery. These results are consistent with the hypothesis that exposure to HIV-1–contaminated blood and mucus in the birth canal accounts for the majority of subsequent infection in infants. Although we base this conclusion on a study of twins, it likely applies to both single and multiple births.

Our data indicate that elective cesarean section may be a useful method of avoiding exposure to HIV-1 in the birth canal. However, cesarean delivery may not be as effective as zidovudine in reducing mother-to-infant transmission. We found that the mother-to-infant HIV-1 transmission rate may be halved with cesarean delivery, whereas zidovudine reduced the rate by two thirds.[30] Unfortunately, in many developing countries that have a high prevalence of HIV-1 among pregnant women, zidovudine is not available and cesarean delivery cannot be a routine intervention. To investigate a potential alternative, we have initiated a clinical trial of vaginal cleansing during labor, using a soap that neutralizes HIV-1 in vitro, to reduce infants' birth-canal exposure to HIV-1 and other infections.[31] If such a simple, sustainable intervention proves to be safe and effective, it could be used to reduce HIV-1 perinatal transmission everywhere.

We are indebted to Dr. Frances Yellin, Atlantic Research Corporation, for assistance with computer programming, and to Sally Canchola for technical assistance.

Contributors to the International Registry of HIV-Exposed Twins are as follows: University of New South Wales, Randwick, Australia: J. Ziegler and M. Cruikshank; Hospital St. Pierre, Brussels, Belgium: J. Levy; Royal Free Hospital, London: M. A. Meates; Great Ormond Street Hospital, London: D. Gibb; HIV in Newborn French Collaborative Group, France: M. J. Mayaux, J. P. Teglas, C. Laurent, S. Blanche, and C. Rouzioux; Frauenklinik Finkenau, Hamburg, Germany*: G. Helling-Giese, U. Mattner, and P. H. Hoeger; Coombe Lying-In Hospital, Dublin, Ireland: T. Conlon and E. Griffin; Hospital S. Martino, University of Genoa, Italy: A. De Maria; S. Camillo Hospital, Rome, Italy: A. Benedetto; University of Milan, Italy: N. Principi; University of Padova, Italy: C. Giaquinto and A. Giancomelli; City Hospital, Edinburgh, Scotland: J. Mok; Catalan Registry of Seropositive Children, Generalitat de Catalunya, Barcelona, Spain: J. Casabona, C. Fortuny, S. Uriz, and J. M. Pérez; General and University Hospital, Valencia, Spain: M. C. Tuset-Ruiz, P. Leon, and J. F. Y. Elorza; La Fe Children's Hospital, Valencia, Spain: C. Canosa; Kinderspital Zurich, Zurich, Switzerland: B. Brandle, R. Seger, and D. Nadal; University Hospital, Geneva, Switzerland: O. Irion and C. A. Wyler; Llandough Hospital, Cardiff, Wales: P. Davis; ORSTOM-Congo-France/Harvard School of Public Health, Boston, Mass.: M. Lallemant and S. Lallemant-Le Coeur; Center Hospital of Kigali, Rwanda: D. G. Hitimana, P. Le Page, P. Van de Perre, and F. Dabis; Uganda/Case Western Reserve University Collaboration, Kampala, Uganda: L. Marum, C. Ndugwa, D. Tindyebwa, E. Aceng, F. Mmiro, T. Sutongas, and K. Olness; Project SIDA, Kinshasa, Zaire/Centers for Disease Control and Prevention, Atlanta, Ga.: M. St. Louis; Hospital Sainte-Justine, Montreal, Quebec, Canada: N. La Pointe; Albert Einstein College of Medicine, Bronx, N.Y.: A. Rubinstein and D. Burge; Bay State Medical Center, Springfield, Mass.: B. W. Stechenberg; Boston City Hospital, Boston, Mass.: E. Cooper and A. M. Regan; Bridgeport Hospital, Bridgeport, Conn.: S. Shipkowitz; Bronx Lebanon Hospital Center, Bronx, N.Y.: A. Wiznia; Cedars-Sinai of Los Angeles, Los Angeles, Calif.: P. A. Brunell and T. Courville; Children's Hospital of Philadelphia, Philadelphia, Pa.: R. Rutstein; Children's Hospital, Boston, Mass.: K. McIntosh; Children's Hospital of Northern California, Oakland, Calif.: A. Petru and M. O'Leary; Children's Hospital of Los Angeles, Los Angeles, Calif.: J. Church and S. Taylor; Children's Medical Center, Dallas, Tex.: J. Squires and M. Mallory; Children's Memorial Hospital, Chicago, Ill.: R. Yogev and B. Klauke; Children's National Medical Center, Washington, D.C.: T. Rakusan and S. Plumley; Cook–Fort Worth Children's Medical Center, Fort Worth, Tex.: M. M. Shelton; Duke University Medical Center, Durham, N.C.: C. Wilfert and B. Lane; Harlem Hospital Center, New York, N.Y.: E. J. Abrams; Howard University Hospital, Washington, D.C.: S. Rana; Jersey City Medical Center, Jersey City, N.J.: O. Chandavasu and S. Puvabanditsin; Lincoln Hospital Center, Bronx, N.Y.: J. H. Chow, K. Shah, S. Nachman, and R. O'Neill; Montefiore Medical Center, Bronx N.Y.: P. Selwyn and E. Shoenbaum; Mount Sinai, New York, N.Y.: A. Barzilai and R. Warford; New York Medical College, Valhalla: A. Gupta and L. Ahern; North Shore University Hospital, Manhasset, N.Y.: S. Pahwa and N. Pnugoti; Ramon Ruiz Arnau University Hospital, Bayamon, Puerto Rico: D. E. Garcia-Trias; St. Luke's/Roosevelt Hospital Center, Bayside, N.Y.: S. Bakshi; State University of New York Health Sciences Center at Brooklyn: S. Landesman, H. Mendez, and G. Moroso; State University of New York, Brooklyn, N.Y.: R. D. Mendez-Bautista and S. Fikrig; Children's Medical Center, State University of New York at Stonybrook: S. Nachman and A. Belman; Texas Children's Hospital, Baylor College of Medicine, Houston: M. W. Kline and C. Hanson; New York Hospital–Cornell Medical Center, New York, N.Y.: P. Edelson and G. Hinds; Tulane School of Medicine, New Orleans, La.: R. Van Dyke and R. Clark; University of California, San Francisco, Calif.: D. W. Wara and E. B. Manio; University of Connecticut Health Center, Farmington: G. Johnson and L. Wells; University of Illinois, Chicago: C. L. Park; University of Maryland, Baltimore: J. P. Johnson and L. Alger; University of Massachusetts, Worcester: K. Luzuriaga; University of Miami, Miami, Fla.: T. Mastrucci, M. R. Sunkutu, and Z. Rodriguez; University of Texas Medical School, Houston: M. Doyle and J. Reuben; University of California at Los Angeles Medical Center: Y. Bryson and M. Dillon; Yale–New Haven Hospital, New Haven, Conn.: B. J. Simpson and W. Andiman; University of Chile, Santiago*: P. Uribe.

REFERENCES

1. Chin J, Sankaran G, Mann J. Mother-to-infant transmission of HIV: an increasing global problem. In: Kessel E, Awan AK,

*Not included in current analysis.

*Not included in current analysis.

eds. Maternal and child health care in developing countries. Thun, Switzerland: Ott Publishers, 1989:299-306.
2. Dabis F, Msellati P, Dunn D, et al. Estimating the rate of mother-to-child transmission of HIV. Report of a workshop on methodological issues. Ghent (Belgium), 17-20 February 1992. AIDS 1993;7:1139-48.
3. Italian Multicenter Study. Epidemiology, clinical features, and prognostic factors of pediatric HIV infection. Lancet 1988;2:1043-5.
4. Andiman WA, Simpson J, Olson B. Rate of transmission of HIV type 1 infection from mother to child and short-term outcome of neonatal infection. Am J Dis Child 1990;144: 758-66.
5. European Collaborative Study. Risk factors for mother-to-child transmission of HIV-1. Lancet 1992;339:1007-12.
6. Blanche S, Rouzioux C, Moscato ML, et al. A prospective study of infants born to women seropositive for human immunodeficiency virus type 1. N Engl J Med 1989;320: 1643-8.
7. St. Louis ME, Kamenga M, Brown C, et al. Risk of perinatal HIV-1 transmission according to maternal immunologic, virologic, and placental factors. JAMA 1993;269:2853-9.
8. Ljunggren K. Moschese V, Broliden PA. Antibodies mediating cellular cytotoxicity and neutralizing correlate with a better clinical stage in children born to HIV-infected mothers. J Infect Dis 1990;161:198-202.
9. Courgnaud V, Laure F, Brossard A, et al. Frequent and early in utero HIV-1 infection. AIDS Res Hum Retroviruses 1991; 7:337-41.
10. Ehrnst A, Lindgren S, Dictor M. HIV in pregnant women and their offspring: evidence for late transmission. Lancet 1991; 338:203-7.
11. Lindgren S, Anzen B, Bohlin AB, et al. HIV and child-bearing: clinical outcome and aspects of mother-to-infant transmission. AIDS 1991;5:1111-6.
12. Wolinsky SM, Wike CM, Korber BTM, et al. Selective transmission of human immunodeficiency virus type-1 variants from mothers to infants. Science 1992;255:1134-7.
13. Goedert JJ, Duliège AM, Amos CI, Felton S, Biggar RJ, International Registry of HIV-Exposed Twins. High risk of HIV-1 infection for first born twins. Lancet 1991;338: 1471-5.
14. Qaquish BF, Liang K-Y. Marginal models for correlated binary responses with multiple classes and multiple levels of nesting. Biometrics 1992;48:939-50.
15. Bonney GE. Logistic regression for dependent binary observations. Biometrics 1987;43:951-73.
16. Bishop YMM, Fienberg SE, Holland PW. Discrete multivariate analysis. Cambridge: Massachusetts Institute of Technology Press, 1975:395-6.
17. Benichou J. Methods of adjustment for estimating the attributable risk in case-control studies: a review. Stat Med 1991; 10:1753-73.
18. Hinkley DV. Bootstrap methods. J Royal Stat Soc B 1988; 50:321-37.
19. De Martino D, Tovo P-A, Galli L, et al. HIV-1 infection in perinatally exposed siblings and twins. Arch Dis Child 1991; 66:1235-8.
20. Villari P, Spino C, Chalmers TC, Lau J, Sacks HS. Cesarean section to reduce perinatal transmission of human immunodeficiency virus: a metaanalysis. Online Journal of Current Clinical Trials 1993 (Jul 8) (document No. 74).
21. Van de Perre P, Simonon A, Deo-Gratias H, et al. Infective and anti-infective properties of breastmilk from HIV-1–infected women. Lancet 1993;341:914-8.
22. Dunn DT, Newell ML, Ades AE, Peckham CS. Risk of human immunodeficiency virus type 1 transmission through breast-feeding. Lancet 1992;340:585-8.
23. Romero R, Shamma F, Avila C, et al. Infection and labor. VI. Prevalence, microbiology, and clinical significance of intraamniotic infection in twin gestations with preterm labor. Am J Obstet Gynecol 1990;163:757-61.
24. Wofsy CB, Cohen JB, Hauer LB, et al. Isolation of AIDS-associated retrovirus from genital secretions of women with antibodies to the virus. Lancet 1986;1:527-9.
25. Henin Y, Mandelbrot L, Henrion R, Pradinaud R, Coulaud JP, Montagnier L. Virus excretion in the cervicovaginal secretions of pregnant and non-pregnant HIV-infected women. J Acquir Immune Defic Syndr 1993;6:72-5.
26. Krivine A, Yakudima A, Le May M, et al. A comparative study of virus isolation, polymerase chain reaction, and antigen detection in children of mothers infected with human immunodeficiency virus. J PEDIATR 1990;116:372-6.
27. Rogers MF, Ou C-Y, Kilbourne B, et al. Advances and problems in the diagnosis of human immunodeficiency virus infection in infants. Pediatr Infect Dis J 1991;10:523-31.
28. Borkowsky W, Krasinski K, Pollack H, Hoover W, Kaul A, Ilmet-Moore T. Early diagnosis of human immunodeficiency virus infection in children <6 months of age: comparison of polymerase chain reaction, culture, and plasma antigen capture techniques. J Infect Dis 1992;166:616-9.
29. Luzuriaga K, McQuilken P, Alimenti A, Somasundaran M, Hesselton R, Sullivan JL. Early viremia and immune responses in vertical human immunodeficiency virus type 1 infection. J Infect Dis 1993;167:1008-13.
30. Centers for Disease Control and Prevention. Zidovudine for the prevention of HIV transmission from mother to infant. MMWR Morb Mortal Wkly Rep 1994;43:285-7.
31. Burman LG, Christensen P, Christensen K, et al. Prevention of excess mortality associated with group B streptococcus by vaginal chlorhexidine disinfection during labor. Lancet 1992; 340:65-9.

Clinical and laboratory observations

Placement of umbilical venous catheters with use of bedside real-time ultrasonography

Mark Greenberg, MD, Hamid Movahed, MD, Beverly Peterson, and Raul Bejar, MD

From the Departments of Neonatology and Pediatrics, University of California–San Diego, San Diego, California

Real-time ultrasonography was used to assess the position of umbilical venous catheters tips in 79 newborn infants (birth weight range, 400 to 4200 gm). The position of the umbilical venous catheters determined by ultrasonography was compared with the projection of the catheter tip on the closest vertebral body shown on a standard chest radiograph. Of the catheters initially placed with radiographic guidance, 56% were repositioned because of unsatisfactory location. Ultrasonography is more precise than radiography because it allows direct visualization of the catheter tips in relation to internal vascular structures. When ultrasonography is unavailable, placement at the ninth thoracic vertebral body ensures safe positioning. (J Pediatr 1995;126:633-5)

Radiography has been the method of choice to estimate the position of umbilical venous catheters,[1, 2] but the drawbacks of this method include ionizing radiation, variability of the right atrium–inferior vena cava junction position in relation to bony landmarks, and the need for multiple studies. Ultrasonography has been shown to be useful in determining position of catheters in relation to cardiac chambers, but a comparison with bony radiographic landmarks has not been done.[3] We assessed the utility of ultrasonography to visualize UVCs, and describe the relationship between the body locations of the catheters tips and the closest vertebral bodies seen on chest radiographs.

METHODS

Seventy-nine infants (median birth weight, 1600 gm; range, 480 to 4200 gm) admitted to the infant special care unit at the University of California–San Diego Medical Center who required UVC insertion for clinical care were enrolled in the study between June 1992 and December 1993. The protocol was approved by the institutional review board, and parental written consent was obtained. Heparin-bonded polyurethane catheters (5F and 3.5F) were inserted by the clinical team to a distance determined by shoulder-to-umbilicus-length curves with the intention of positioning the UVC tip at the level of the RA-IVC junction.[4] Indications for UVC placement included vascular access for administration of fluids and vasoactive medications, exchange transfusion, and monitoring of central venous pressure. The position of the catheters was determined by concurrent ultrasound and radiography examinations. The position shown by ultrasonography was compared with the nearest vertebral body obtained on the radiographs. Ultrasound studies were performed with a model 128XP color Doppler scanner equipped with a 7 Mhz transducer (Acuson, Mountain View, Calif.). Apical four-chamber, parasternal short-axis, and subcostal views were used to image the catheter (Fig. 1). A small volume of saline solution (0.5 ml) was injected

RA-IVC	Right atrium–inferior vena cava
UVC	Umbilical venous catheter

Submitted for publication June 14, 1994; accepted Oct. 4, 1994.

Reprint requests: Mark Greenberg, MD, 2220 River Run Dr., No. 113, San Diego, CA 92108.

0022-3476/95/$3.00 + 0 **9/24/61032**

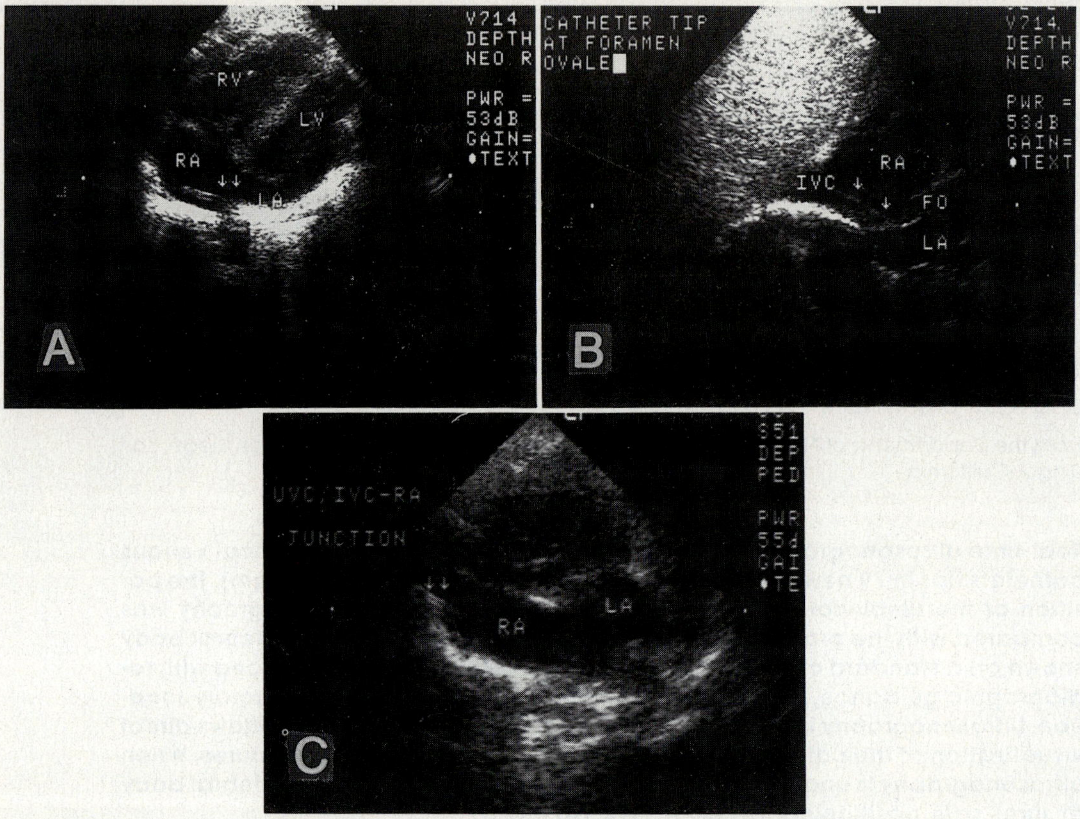

Fig. 1. Ultrasound study of UVC. **A,** Apical four-chamber view of a catheter lying in the left atrium. **B,** Subcostal view of the same catheter shows the catheter holding open the foramen ovale. Saline solution injection revealed flow to both the right atrium and left atrium. **C,** Parasternal short-axis view shows the catheter at the RA-IVC junction, after repositioning.

as a contrast medium to determine the exact position of the catheter tip.

A standard chest radiograph was obtained each time the catheter position was changed. After the initial radiograph, the catheter tip was repositioned to the RA-IVC junction with ultrasound guidance. After expertise with ultrasonography was achieved, the catheters in 35 patients were positioned with ultrasound guidance during the insertion procedure, followed by a radiograph.

Oxygen saturation and temperature were monitored during the ultrasound procedure. The fraction of inspired oxygen and heat sources were adjusted to maintain normal oxygen saturation and normothermia. Patients also had monitoring for catheter-related sepsis, thrombosis, and necrotizing enterocolitis for the duration of catheter use.

RESULTS

We compared 95 radiographs and ultrasound studies for 79 patients. In all patients the catheters were easily seen (Fig. 1). Initial placement of 60 UVCs was done with radiographs and ultrasonography was used in placement of the remaining 35 UVCs. Of the 60 catheters placed with radiographic guidance, 34 (56%) were repositioned because of unsatisfactory location, requiring more than one radiograph.

Figure 2 shows the relationship between the anatomic location of the catheters visualized by ultrasonography and the projection of the catheter tips on the thoracic vertebral bodies. All catheters at T6 and above were in the heart; 18 (58%) of 31 catheters were located in the left atrium. At T7, 14 (82%) of 17 catheters were incorrectly positioned with the tip in the right atrium. At T8-T9, 34 (90%) of 38 catheters were correctly positioned at the RA-IVC junction (100% at T9; $n = 17$). Catheters at T11 and below were all in the liver proximal to the ductus venosus.

The ultrasound procedures were tolerated by all infants, and there were no adverse effects. A transient increase in oxy-

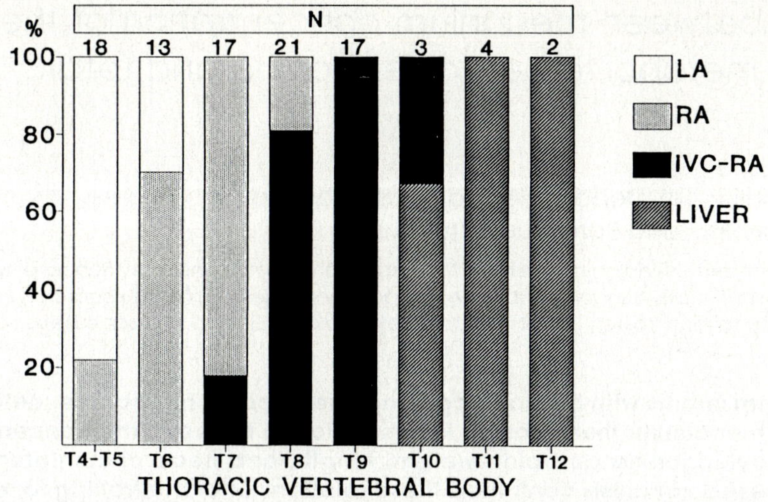

Fig. 2. Comparison between the UVC body locations determined by ultrasonography and the thoracic vertebral bodies projected in radiographs. *LA*, Left atrium; *RA*, right atrium.

gen requirement, which reversed on completion of the study, was common during both ultrasonography and radiography.

There was no apparent catheter-related sepsis or necrotizing entercolitis in any of the study infants while the catheter was in place. All catheters were functional at the time of removal. One infant had an atrial dysrhythmia that resolved with ultrasound-guided repositioning of the catheter.

DISCUSSION

Our data indicate that real-time ultrasonography at the bedside can be used to determine the position of UVCs in critically ill term and preterm infants. Although the catheters were visualized in all patients, fluid injection was helpful to image the exact position of the tip. Real-time ultrasonography was more effective than radiography because the location of the UVC in the body could be determined, and the catheters could be positioned at the RA-IVC junction during the initial insertion procedure. Furthermore, real-time ultrasound scanning during insertion avoids false passage to the portal sinus or advancement to the left atrium, reducing the risk of complications.

This study also shows that proper placement of UVCs can be estimated by use of radiography to position the catheter tips between the top of T8 to the bottom of T9. However, multiple studies are usually required when radiography alone is used to position the catheters. Ultrasound scanning can be expensive and is not routinely available on a 24-hour basis in most units. Catheter positioning can be accomplished with radiography when ultrasonography is not available.

Although the incidence of complications in this study was low, thrombosis, vascular injury and portal hypertension may occur. Emboli and damage to the foramen ovale also may occur with malpositioned catheters. Thus care should be taken with insertion and positioning of catheters, and UVCs should be used only when clinically indicated.

We conclude that the use of ultrasonography at the bedside for proper placement of UVCs is feasible and safe, and offers advantages over radiography. When ultrasonography is not available, we advocate placement of lines at T8-T9; the majority of catheters placed at this location will lie at the RA-IVC junction.

REFERENCES

1. Rosen S, Reich S. Umbilical venous catheterization in the newborn: identification of correct positioning. Radiology 1970; 95:335-40.
2. Baker D, Berdon W, James S. Proper localization of umbilical arterial catheters and venous catheters by lateral roentgenogram. Pediatrics 1969;43:34-9.
3. Oppenhiemer D, Carroll B. Ultrasonic localization of neonatal umbilical catheters. Radiology 1982;142:281-2.
4. George L, Waldman J, Cohen ML, et al. Umbilical vascular catheters: localization by two dimensional echocardio/aortography. Pediatr Cardiol 1982;2:237-43.
5. Dunn P. Localization of the umbilical catheter by post mortem measurement. Arch Dis Child 1966;41:69-75.

Relation between meconium concentration of the cocaine metabolite benzoylecgonine and fetal growth

Mark Mirochnick, MD, Deborah A. Frank, MD, Howard Cabral, MPH, Adrian Turner, BSc, and Barry Zuckerman, MD

From the Department of Pediatrics, Boston City Hospital and Boston University School of Medicine, the Boston University School of Public Health, and the General Clinical Research Center, Boston City Hospital and Boston University School of Medicine, Boston, Massachusetts

Among 95 term infants with benzoylecgonine, the cocaine metabolite, detectable in their meconium, there was an inverse relation between the concentration of benzoylecgonine and birth weight, length, and head circumference. Multiple regression analysis confirmed these relations after controlling for gestational age and maternal use of marijuana, cigarettes, and alcohol. These data suggest a dose-response relation between the magnitude of prenatal cocaine exposure and impaired fetal growth. (J PEDIATR 1995;126:636-8)

The impact of maternal cocaine dose on the fetus remains unknown, in large part because of the difficulty in quantifying maternal drug use.[1] Qualitative meconium drug analysis is more sensitive than urine drug testing in identifying cocaine-exposed neonates.[2-4] We hypothesized that there is a dose-response relation between prenatal cocaine exposure and impaired fetal growth, and that meconium benzoylecgonine concentration, serving as a biologic marker for the amount of prenatal cocaine exposure, would correlate with fetal growth impairment.[5-8]

METHODS

We studied infants participating in a large prospective study of the neonatal and long-term effects of prenatal cocaine exposure. After informed consent was obtained, infants were enrolled within 2 days of delivery if they met enrollment criteria including gestational age more than 36 weeks; absence of serious illness, congenital malformations, or fetal alcohol syndrome; and no known maternal use of illicit drugs except cocaine and marijuana. The study protocol included collection of infant meconium and maternal urine samples for drug testing; maternal interview for prenatal drug, alcohol, and cigarette use; and neonatal physical examination with Dubowitz gestational age assessment.

A single meconium sample from one diaper was collected from each study infant before 72 hours of age. Infant meconium and maternal urine samples were frozen at −30° C until analysis by radioimmunoassay (Abuscreen RIA, Roche Diagnostics Systems, Inc., Montclair, N.J.) for benzoylecgonine, opiates, amphetamines, benzodiazepines, and cannabinoids. Meconium analysis was performed according to a modification of the method of Ostrea.[2, 9] Radiolabeled spiking experiments demonstrated 95% to 99.5% recovery of spiked radiolabeled drug metabolites from meconium. Benzoylecgonine concentrations in the original meconium samples were calculated with the assumption of complete extraction.

Statistical analysis was performed with simple and multiple linear regression analyses, with log transformation of meconium benzoylecgonine concentration and self-reported days of cocaine, cigarette, and alcohol use. Mean substitution was used for missing covariate data points.

RESULTS

Adequate meconium samples were collected from 217 infants. Ninety-five (44%) of the infants had meconium assay results that were positive for benzoylecgonine. Of the 111 infants known by maternal self-report, urine screen, or both, to be exposed to cocaine meconium assay results were positive for benzoylecgonine in 86 (77%). Of the 106 infants classified as unexposed to cocaine after maternal interview, urine screen, or both, results of meconium benzoylecgonine

Supported by grant No. DAO6532-03 from the National Institute on Drug Abuse and grant No. MO1RR00533-25 from the National Centers for Research Resources, General Clinical Research Centers, National Institutes of Health.

Submitted for publication June 27, 1994; accepted Nov. 9, 1994.

Reprint requests: Mark Mirochnick, MD, Boston City Hospital, Maternity 2, 818 Harrison Ave., Boston, MA 02118.

0022-3476/95/$3.00 + 0 **9/24/61931**

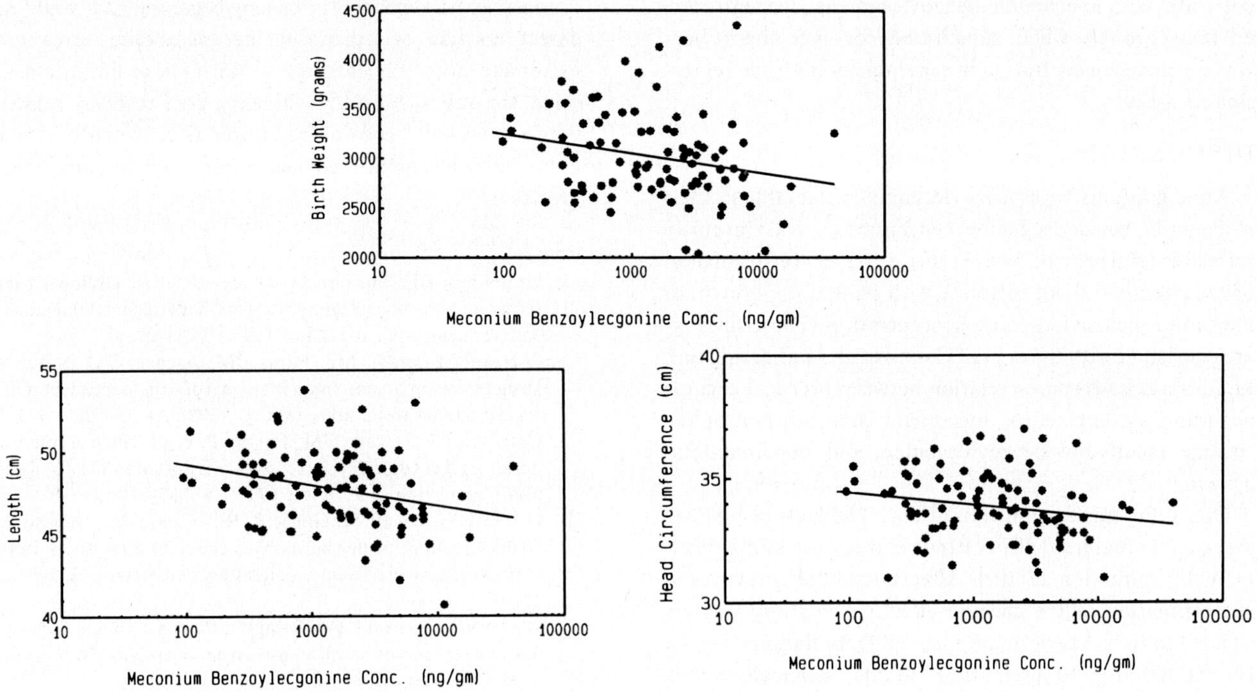

Figure: Relation between meconium benzoylecgonine concentration and birth weight ($r = -0.23$; $p = 0.02$), length ($r = -0.29$; $p = 0.005$), and head circumference ($r = -0.20$; $p = 0.05$).

Table. Results of multiple regression analysis of meconium benzoylecgonine concentration, gestational age, and maternal alcohol, cigarette, and marijuana use versus growth measurements

	Birth weight (gm) (n = 95)		Length (cm) (n = 93)		Head circumference (cm) (n = 93)	
Independent variable	**Regression coefficient**	***p***	**Regression coefficient**	***p***	**Regression coefficient**	***p***
Meconium benzoylecgonine concentration (log)	−0.22	0.02	−0.28	0.004	−0.20	0.04
Gestational age	0.32	0.002	0.22	0.02	0.31	0.002
Alcohol use (log of average daily use + 1)	−0.22	0.03	−0.26	0.01	−0.24	0.02
Cigarette use (log of average daily use + 1)	−0.27	0.49	−0.26	0.51	−0.24	0.51
Marijuana use (1 = yes, 0 = no)	0.12	0.23	0.12	0.84	0.06	0.56

To assess the relative importance of each independent variable in the model, we calculated standardized regression coefficients after transformation of each independent variable to a *z* scale. These coefficients allow the comparison of the relative impact of each independent variable on outcome variables after adjustment for the effects of the other independent variables in the model. Length and head circumference measurements were not available for two infants.

assays were positive in 9 (8%). Benzoylecgonine meconium concentrations ranged from 94 to 40,000 ng/gm, with a mean of 3020 ng/gm and a median of 1673 ng/gm. Among the 95 infants with benzoylecgonine detectable in their meconium, there were significant negative correlations between meconium benzoylecgonine concentration and birth weight ($r = -0.23$; $p = 0.02$), length ($r = -0.29$; $p = 0.005$), and head circumference ($r = -0.20$; $p = 0.05$) (Figure). After controlling for gestational age and maternal use of marijuana, cigarettes, and alcohol, meconium benzoylecgonine concentration was still independently associated with decreased fetal growth (Table). Maternal self-reported days of cocaine use did not significantly correlate with meconium benzoylecgonine concentration or fetal growth when substituted for meconium benzoylecgonine concentration in the single or multiple regression analysis.

DISCUSSION

Among infants with benzoylecgonine detectable in their meconium, benzoylecgonine concentration was inversely related to fetal growth, whereas maternal self-report of days of cocaine use did not correlate with either fetal growth or meconium benzoylecgonine concentration. These findings are consistent with the data of Ostrea et al.,[4] indicating that there is a dose-response relation between prenatal cocaine exposure, as reflected by meconium concentration of the cocaine metabolite benzoylecgonine, and impaired fetal growth.

Our study has several limitations. The lack of biologic markers for maternal alcohol and cigarette use might result in underestimation of their effects on fetal growth and overestimation of the cocaine effect.[5] The study was restricted to term newborn infants, and these findings cannot be extrapolated to premature infants. Benzoylecgonine was detectable in the meconium of only 77% of infants born to mothers identified as using cocaine by history, urine drug screening, or both. Our sensitivity is comparable with that reported in studies comparing maternal hair and infant meconium assays (74% to 92%).[3, 10] There are several possible explanations for false-negative results of meconium drug assays. Meconium drug assays are unable to detect drug use before the start of meconium formation late in the fourth month of gestation. The drug or metabolite being assayed may not be evenly distributed throughout an infant's meconium and may be missed by assay of a single aliquot taken from one stool sample. Our radioimmunoassay was specific for benzoylecgonine and would not detect cocaine or other cocaine metabolites except at extremely high concentrations. With these limitations in mind, the data suggest that there is a dose-response relation between prenatal cocaine exposure, as reflected by meconium benzoylecgonine concentration, and impaired fetal growth.

REFERENCES

1. Hutchings, DE. The puzzle of cocaine's effects following maternal use during pregnancy: Are there reconcilable differences? Neurotoxicol Teratol 1993;15:281-6.
2. Ostrea EM, Brady MJ, Parks PM, Asensio DC, Naluz A. Drug screening of meconium in infants of drug-dependent mothers: an alternative to urine testing. J Pediatr 1989;115:474-7.
3. Callahan CM, Grant TM, Phipps P, et al. Measurement of gestational cocaine exposure: sensitivity of infants' hair, meconium, and urine. J Pediatr 1992;120:763-8.
4. Ostrea EM, Brady M, Gause S, Raymundo AL, Stevens M. Drug screening of newborns by meconium analysis: a large-scale prospective, epidemiologic study. Pediatrics 1992;89:107-13.
5. Zuckerman B, Frank DA, Hingson R, et al. Effects of maternal marijuana and cocaine use on fetal growth. New Engl J Med 1989;320:762-8.
6. Bingol N, Fuchs M, Diaz V, et al. Teratogenicity of cocaine in humans. J Pediatr 1987;110:93-6.
7. Oro AS, Dixon SD. Perinatal cocaine and methamphetamine exposure: maternal and neonatal correlates. J Pediatr 1987; 111:571-8.
8. Chasnoff IJ. Cocaine and pregnancy: clinical and methodologic issues. Clin Perinatol 1991;18:113-23.
9. Mirochnick M, Rehm K, Brown E, Frank D, Perez A, Turner A. Revised and expanded method for meconium drug analysis. Pediatr Res 1992;31:63A.
10. Ostrea EM, Welch RA. Detection of prenatal drug exposure in the pregnant woman and her newborn infant. Clin Perinatol 1991;18:629-45.

Efficacy of frequent nebulized ipratropium bromide added to frequent high-dose albuterol therapy in severe childhood asthma

Suzanne Schuh, MD, David W. Johnson, MD, Sheilagh Callahan, RN, Gerald Canny, MD, and Henry Levison, MD

From the Divisions of Emergency, Clinical Pharmacology, and Chest, the Department of Pediatrics, Hospital for Sick Children, Toronto, Ontario, Canada

Objective: **The objective of this trial was to determine the efficacy of frequent nebulized ipratropium added to high-dose albuterol therapy in children with severe asthma.**
Methods: **One hundred twenty children (5 to 17 years) of age) with severe acute asthma (forced expiratory volume in 1 second (FEV_1), <50% of the predicted value) were enrolled into a randomized double-blind three-arm placebo-controlled trial comparing three groups: group 1, three doses of nebulized ipratropium bromide within 60 minutes (250 μg/dose); group 2, one dose of ipratropium; group 3, no ipratropium. All patients were also treated with three doses of nebulized albuterol within 60 minutes (0.15 mg/kg per dose). Pulmonary function and clinical measures were assessed every 20 minutes for up to 120 minutes.**
Results: **The groups were comparable at baseline. At 120 minutes, the mean percentage of predicted FEV_1 improved from 33.4% to 56.7% in group 1, from 34.2% to 52.3% in group 2, and from 35.4% to 48.4% in group 3 ($p = 0.0001$). The differences between groups were larger in those children with a baseline $FEV_1 \leq 30\%$ of the predicted value: FEV_1 increased from 24.5% to 50.9% in group 1, from 25.0% to 39.8% in group 2, and from 25.9% to 36.5% in group 3 ($p = 0.0001$). In group 1, 38% of the patients were hospitalized after the study, 44% in group 2, and 46% in group 3 (p value not significant). However, in patients with $FEV_1 \leq 30\%$, the hospitalization rates were 27% in group 1, 56% in group 2, and 83% in group 3 ($p = 0.027$). There were no toxic effects attributable to ipratropium.**
Conclusion: **The addition of repeated doses of nebulized ipratropium to frequent high-dose albuterol therapy in patients with acute severe asthma is both safe and more effective than albuterol alone; its use in patients with very severe asthma may reduce hospitalizations. (J PEDIATR 1995;126:639-45)**

Supported by the Ontario Ministry of Health (Emergency Medical Services) and Boehringer Ingelheim.

Presented in part at the Society for Pediatric Research meeting in Seattle, Wash., May 2, 1994.

Submitted for publication Sept. 28, 1994; accepted Dec. 15, 1994.

Reprint requests: Suzanne Schuh, MD, Emergency Department, Hospital for Sick Children, 555 University Ave., Toronto, Ontario M5G 1X8, Canada.

0022-3476/95/$3.00 + 0 **9/25/62808**

Frequent administration of nebulized β_2 agonists and of corticosteroids at the time of onset has been shown to be more effective than less aggressive therapy for acute exacerbations of asthma.[1-5] However, many children do not respond adequately to this regimen and require prolonged treatment and hospitalization. Nebulized ipratropium bromide, an acetylcholine antagonist, has been used as an adjunct to therapy for asthma in Europe and in Canada for almost a decade. Well-executed studies have demonstrated,

ANOVA	Analysis of variance
ED	Emergency department
FEV_1	Forced expiratory volume in 1 second

in both adults and children, that the combination of ipratropium and a β_2 agonist is superior to the use of a β_2 agent alone.[6-12] However, all these studies have used either low-dose or infrequent albuterol therapy, potentially resulting in a submaximal response to this drug. Because of the current widespread use of frequent, high-dose β_2 agonist therapy in severe asthma, we thought it important to establish whether the addition of ipratropium bromide to this already aggressive treatment provides additional benefit. Further, the relative efficacy of administering a single dose versus multiple doses of nebulized ipratropium has not been established.

The objective of this trial was to study the efficacy and safety of the addition of three doses versus one dose of nebulized ipratropium bromide to frequent administration of albuterol, in comparison with albuterol alone in the emergency department treatment of severe childhood asthma.

METHODS

The study design was a double-blind, randomized, placebo-controlled trial with three study groups: all patients received three nebulizations of albuterol in combination with either no ipratropium, one dose of ipratropium, or three doses of ipratropium. The study took place in the emergency department of the Hospital for Sick Children, Toronto, between October 1991 and December 1993. Included in the study were children with an acute asthma attack who were 5 through 17 years of age and were able to perform the pulmonary function testing reliably; baseline forced expiratory volume in 1 second was less than 50% of the predicted value. Excluded were children who had had their first wheezing episode only, those who had used ipratropium within 4 hours of this ED visit, those with a previous admission to the intensive care unit, children with concurrent cardiopulmonary disease, those near death and therefore requiring immediate intervention, and patients with known or suspected hypersensitivity to the study drugs. Informed consent was obtained for all the patients, and the study was approved by the ethics committee of this hospital. An experienced research nurse (S.C.) enrolled all patients and performed all observations. The randomization code was generated by the hospital pharmacy department from a standard table of random numbers in blocks, so that after each nine patients there would be three subjects allocated to each group. A log of all patients screened for this trial listed reasons for those excluded.

After arrival of the patient in the ED and initial assessment by the ED staff, the research nurse evaluated each child for study eligibility, and obtained written consent. She also completed a questionnaire detailing demographics, history of present condition, and current medications. The pharmacy department provided three vials that contained either ipratropium or placebo (0.9% saline solution) labeled Nos. 1, 2, and 3. Albuterol-ipratropium and albuterol-saline mixtures are indistinguishable in both the liquid and the nebulized states. The patient, the research nurse, and the investigator were masked to the group assignment.

All patients received three standard doses of nebulized albuterol (Allen & Hanbury Canada), 0.15 mg/kg per dose, 20 minutes apart. Those in group 1 also got three doses of ipratropium bromide (Boehringer Ingelheim), 250 μg/dose (1 ml = 1 dose) mixed with the albuterol; those in group 2 received only one dose of ipratropium, and those in group 3 received no ipratropium. The nurse thus mixed the weight-appropriate albuterol dose from the ED stock with 1 ml of the content of vials marked Nos. 1, 2, and 3 (ipratropium or placebo). The inhalations were given by nebulizer (Whisper Jet; Intec Medical, Inc. [Marquest Medical Products, Inc.], Engelwood, Colo.) with 2 ml of 0.9% saline solution at an O_2 flow of 6 to 7 L/min. A tight-fitting plastic face mask was used, and each inhalation lasted about 15 minutes. To avoid a potential confounder, we administered neither corticosteroids nor other bronchodilators during the study.

The primary outcome measure was the difference (between groups) in the change of the percentage of predicted FEV_1. The FEV_1 was measured by a portable, battery-operated hand spirometer (P. K. Morgan Ltd., Kent, United Kingdom). After the initial demonstration and teaching, the pulmonary function tests were performed in sets of six (to ensure maximal effort and to allow for a learning curve) and expressed as a percentage of that predicted for height and sex.[13] The highest FEV_1 from each set was used in the analysis.[14, 15] Secondary outcomes included the changes in the accessory muscle score, wheeze score, dyspnea score, overall score (Table I), respiratory rate, heart rate, and oxygen saturation (Nellcor Inc., Hayward, Calif.).

All outcome measures were taken at baseline (time 0), at 20, 40, and 60 minutes (i.e., after each treatment), and at 80 and 120 minutes. Side effects (as reported by the patient or observed by the research nurse) were monitored. Disposition and additional therapy (after the study) in the ED were also noted. Children with respiratory distress at the end of the study were admitted. The decision to hospitalize the patients was made by the ED staff pediatrician not involved in the trial and unaware of the outcome measure changes (except for the oxygen saturation). The research nurse also followed all patients (by telephone) 72 hours af-

Table I. Clinical scores

Severity	Accessory muscle score	Wheeze score	Dyspnea score
0	No retractions	No wheeze and well	Absent dyspnea
1	Intercostal retractions	End-expiratory wheeze	Normal activity and speech; minimal dyspnea
2	Intercostal and suprasternal retractions	Pan-expiratory ± inspiratory wheeze	Decreased activity; 5- to 8-word sentences; moderate dyspnea
3	Nasal flaring	Wheeze audible without stethoscope	Concentrates on breathing; <5-word sentences; severe dyspnea

Table II. Baseline characteristics of study groups: Clinical demographics

	Group 1 (n = 40)	Group 2 (n = 39)	Group 3 (n = 41)
Age (yr)*	9.2 ± 2	9.3 ± 3	9.4 ± 3
Duration of symptoms (hr)*	22 ± 21	31 ± 24	30 ± 18
ED visits for asthma (total within past 2 years—as reported by the parents)	86	67	61
URI (within past 7 days)	34	28	29
Fever (within 48 hr)	2	3	5
Atopy (personal and/or family history): asthma, eczema, hay fever	38	35	39
FEV_1 (% predicted)*	33.4 ± 7	34.2 ± 9	35.4 ± 8
Respiratory rate (breaths/min)*	30.6 ± 7	30.8 ± 8	28.3 ± 7
Heart rate (beats/min)*	120.4 ± 19	123.6 ± 19	121.0 ± 19
Oxygen saturation % (room air)*	94.4 ± 3	94.2 ± 3	93.2 ± 8
Accessory muscle score	2.3	2.4	2.1
Wheeze score	2.2	2.5	2.1
Dyspnea score	1.8	2.1	1.7

URI, Upper respiratory tract infection.
*Values are expressed as mean ± SD.

ter discharge regarding repeated visits to the ED or hospitalizations for asthma at this or other institutions.

Before the study, we estimated that the minimal requirement for a "positive" result was the difference between groups in the mean improvement of the percentage of predicted FEV_1 of at least 8. In addition, each patient was defined as an "excellent responder" if the percentage of predicted FEV_1 improved by ≥ 30 from baseline to 120 minutes (e.g., from 30% to 60% of the predicted value) and as a "poor responder" if it improved by <5. It was also decided to stop the study if the patient had (1) cardiac tachyarrhythmia (except sinus tachycardia), (2) severe clinical deterioration (as judged by the nonstudy ED supervisor) requiring immediate additional intervention or precluding reliable pulmonary function measurement, and (3) severe eye pain or visual acuity changes.

During the 3 weeks before the start of the study, the research nurse was trained to measure pulmonary function and the various scoring measurements by the principal investigator and the chief technician of the pulmonary function laboratory. Furthermore, a videotape of 23 children of various ages and with asthma of varying severity was produced during this period, to obtain interobserver reliability ratings on the accessory muscle and the dyspnea scores between the research nurse and the principal investigator for the quality assurance measurement.

The primary analysis was the repeated measures analysis of variance on the difference between groups in the changes in the percentage of predicted FEV_1 with time. Several secondary analyses were also performed, including ANOVA on the differences in the respiratory rate, heart rate, and O_2 saturation. The changes in the various scores were analyzed by repeated measures ANOVA. The score differences between baseline and 120 minutes among the three groups were compared by using the Kruskal-Wallis test (nonparametric equivalent of ANOVA). The proportions of excellent and poor responders and the hospitalization rates were examined by the chi-square and the Fisher Exact tests. The required number of subjects was calculated according to the following: clinically significant difference in improvement between groups in the percentage of predicted $FEV_1 \geq 8$, standard deviation in the control group of 13.7[1] ($\alpha = 0.05$; $\beta = 0.01$). The appropriate formula yields the total number of 120.[16]

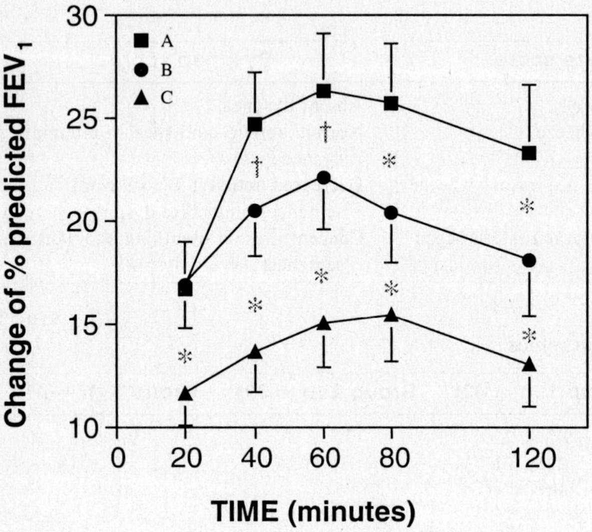

Fig. 1. Mean difference (±SEM) from baseline of percentage of predicted FEV_1 with time in group 1 (three ipratropium doses), group 2 (one ipratropium dose), and group 3 (no ipratropium). Repeated measures ANOVA: $p = 0.0001$. $^*p < 0.01$. $^\dagger p < 0.05$.

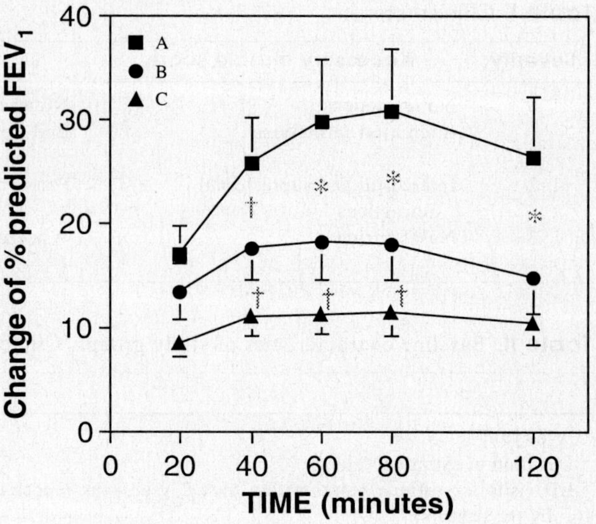

Fig. 2. Mean difference (±SEM) from baseline of the percentage of the predicted FEV_1 with time in groups 1 (three ipratropium doses), 2 (one ipratropium dose), and 3 (no ipratropium); very severe group). Repeated measures ANOVA, $p = 0.0001$. $^*p < 0.01$. $^\dagger p < 0.05$.

RESULTS

During the study period (Oct. 15, 1991, to Dec. 12, 1993) 1586 children more than 5 years of age with asthma were seen in our ED; 435 of these arrived while the nurse was on duty (usually between 2 and 10 PM). The exclusions comprised 204 patients with baseline FEV_1 50% of the predicted value or greater, 33 patients previously enrolled in this study, 21 with coexistent medical problems, 32 children who did not perform the pulmonary function test satisfactorily, 15 whose condition was unstable and required immediate intervention, 11 who had no history of wheezing or asthma or of bronchodilator therapy, 6 who had received ipratropium within 4 hours of arrival, and 2 who arrived without a parent. One patient was 19 years of age and thus went to another institution, and 16 patients were missed. Eight families refused to participate.

A total of 121 children were originally enrolled (64 boys), but one parent changed his mind and demanded withdrawal before the start of the experimental therapy. This left 120 patients for analysis. Group 1 consisted of 40 patients, group 2 of 39, and group 3 of 41. Randomization produced equivalent groups with respect to contributory variables such as demographics, duration of present illness, baseline severity measures, and medications before arrival (Table II).

Repeated measures ANOVA showed significant differences in improvement among the three groups ($p = 0.0001$) (Fig. 1) and even larger differences in patients with FEV_1 less than 30% of the predicted value ($p = 0.0001$) (Fig. 2). Seven patients had to stop the trial prematurely at either 60 or 80 minutes; three children (one each in groups 1, 2, and 3) stopped cooperating before the 120-minute measurement, and three children in group 2 and one child in group 3 were too ill to continue. Two patients had missing data at 80 minutes (because of vomiting), but both had recovered by 120 minutes. Separate analyses—with and without the nine subjects with missing data—were carried out. In this former analysis the missing data were substituted by the data from the preceding observation (Fig. 1). These nine patients were omitted in the latter analysis, with similar results (ANOVA: $F = 3.31$, $p = 0.0003$). Post hoc analysis showed that most of the differences between improvements in group 1 versus group 2 and improvements in group 2 versus group 3 were statistically significant (Figs. 1 and 2). To compare the mean changes with time in the secondary variables, we used the repeated measures ANOVA (Table III). The differences between groups in the dyspnea score were also significant when the Kruskal-Wallis test was performed ($p = 0.014$). The differences for the other scores were not significant by this test.

There were 23 "excellent" responders in the trial (% $FEV_1 \uparrow \geq 30$ at 120 minutes): 10 of 40 children in group 1, 11 of 30 in group 2, and 2 of 41 in group 3 (Fisher Exact Test, $p = 0.009$). A total of 22 children responded "poorly" (% $FEV_1 \uparrow < 5$ at 120 minutes): 4 of 40 children in group 1, 8 of 39 in group 2, and 10 of 41 in group 3 (Fisher Exact Test, $p = 0.225$).

Fifteen patients (38%) in group 1 were hospitalized after the study, 17 (44%) in group 2, and 19 (46%) in group 3 (p value not significant). However, when the severe cases were examined (baseline $FEV_1 \leq 30\%$), the differences were larger: 27% were hospitalized in group 1, 56% in group 2, and 83% in group 3 (chi-square test, $p = 0.027$). According to the telephone follow-up, four children had to come back to the ED for further treatment within 72 hours after discharge home (1 in group 1, 3 in group 3), of whom 1 had to be hospitalized (group 3). After the study was completed, 21 (53%) of 40 children in group 1 needed further inhaled bronchodilators in the ED before disposition, 31 (79%) of 39 needed them in group 2, and 30 (73%) of 41 in group 3 ($p = 0.029$). Of the patients with severe symptoms, 27% needed further inhaled bronchodilator therapy after the study in group 1, 75% in group 2, and 100% in group 3 ($p = 0.00045$). Before disposition, the patients received oral or intravenous corticosteroid therapy.

Side effects were not significantly different in the three groups. None caused termination or significant delay in the experimental therapy, and all had resolved by the end of the trial despite continued treatment. One child (group 1) had red and slightly painful conjuctivitis 3 to 5 minutes after the start of the first treatment; both the visual acuity and the pupillary size were normal. The conjunctivitis abated about 40 minutes later and did not recur despite continued experimental treatment. One child (group 3) had a sudden decrease of O_2 saturation into the 60% range while having a coughing spasm followed by a 10-second syncope. He subsequently coughed up large amounts of mucus, after which the O_2 saturation rose to a nearly normal level.

During the training period there was a 100% interobserver agreement in the dyspnea score between the nurse (S.C.) and the principal investigator, and a 91.5% interobserver agreement in the accessory muscle score (a difference of 1 point in two patients).

DISCUSSION

Our study shows a significant benefit of the addition of repeated doses of nebulized ipratropium to frequent high-dose albuterol therapy in children with severe acute asthma. This benefit seems especially marked in children with very severe baseline status, in whom this regimen also resulted in lower hospitalization rates.

Ipratropium is an acetylcholine antagonist. Although parasympathetic fibers occur primarily in the larger airways,[17] ipratropium may have a generalized action throughout the lung.[18] In contrast, β-adrenergic receptors are more peripherally distributed.[19] This property of differential action, as well as the different pharmacologic mechanisms,

Table III. Secondary outcome measures: Mean changes from baseline to 120 minutes

	Group 1	Group 2	Group 3	p*
Accessory muscle score	−1.4	−1.2	−0.9	0.014
Wheeze score	−1.4	−1.6	−1.0	0.011
Dyspnea score	−1.1	−1.3	−0.8	0.018
Respiratory rate (breaths/min)	−3.0	−5.0	−3.1	NS
Heart rate (beats/min)	+15.3	+9.9	+15.1	NS
O_2 saturation (%)	+1.3	+1.4	+0.1	NS

NS, Not significant.
*By ANOVA.

provides a rationale for using these drugs together. Several studies of adults have demonstrated their synergy.[6-9] Several pediatric studies also show the benefit of this combination, albeit not all. Both Beck et al.[10] and Reisman and Galdes-Sebalt[11] showed differences in pulmonary function improvement in children with acute asthma who were receiving the ipratropium-albuterol mixture, in comparison with albuterol alone. Watson et al.[12] found the ipratropium-fenoterol combination to be beneficial, although the statistical difference from fenoterol alone was marginal (possibly because of small patient numbers). Several other studies showed no added benefit from the anticholinergic drugs,[20-22] but these projects had methodologic problems, such as nonuniform frequency of administration of the study drugs,[20] enrollment of subjects with mild disease,[21] or lack of objective measurement of pulmonary function in many subjects.[22] To date, all the authors dealing with the subject have used submaximal β-agonist therapy—that is, either low or infrequent doses. Given the efficacy of frequent high doses of albuterol,[2] any further benefit of the addition of anticholinergics was in question before this trial.

The ideal dosage and the ideal dosing frequency of ipratropium are unknown. Davis et al.[23] found the optimal dose to be between 75 and 250 μg in stable patients with nonacute disease—a scenario not fully comparable to severe, acute disease. The present recommendation in Canada is to use this drug at 4- to 6-hour intervals.[5] Reisman et al.[11] showed that the additional benefit of ipratropium can be maintained by further doses at 40 and 80 minutes, with no toxic effects. Our trial demonstrates that the addition of one ipratropium dose to frequent high-dose albuterol therapy results in a small clinical benefit and that frequent administration is necessary to produce a clinically significant difference from albuterol alone. This benefit was most obvious in the sickest children. A significant vagal component to bronchospasm must be present in many of these children with asthma, a view previously expressed by others.[10, 11]

This benefit is further supported by the differences in the various scores. These scores have been partially validated and have been shown to correlate with the objective "gold standard" measurement of the FEV_1.[24] These scores are much more crude measures than the FEV_1 and thus do not identify changes in group 1 versus group 2. The credibility of the various measurements is markedly enhanced by the single-observer design of this trial, which eliminated the interobserver reliability issue. Lack of changes in the respiratory rate and the oxygen saturation likely represents poor responsiveness of these outcome measures to therapy in the older children. The relative insensitivity of oxygen saturation is due in part to the curvilinear oxygen-hemoglobin dissociation curve, which accounts for minimal saturation changes when the oxygen tension is greater than 60 mm Hg.

Ipratropium is of low lipid solubility, and thus is poorly absorbed systemically.[25] Toxic effects of this drug are therefore negligible, even at very high doses.[6] Both transient anisocoria and angle-closure glaucoma have been reported in adults.[26, 27] Our trial did not show any atropine-attributable side effects, nor any differences in toxic effects between the groups. Paradoxical bronchoconstriction had been reported in infants treated with isoosmolar, preservative-free ipratropium solution.[28] However, the lack of masking and randomization casts some doubt on the validity of the data of that study.

Acute asthma exacerbations often result from suboptimal initial therapy. Only three children had had corticosteroids prescribed before the study. This undertreatment had probably contributed to the severity of the disease in many patients.

This study has some limitations. Systemic corticosteroids were not administered during the study. This design eliminates their possible confounding effect, but current management of severe asthma calls for early steroid therapy. However, it is very likely that the responses would have been similar because the study was of only 2 hours' duration (insufficient time for steroids to act). Although our trial shows a benefit of repeated doses of ipratropium in children with a baseline FEV_1 17% to 49% of the predicted value and even greater improvement in more severe cases, it was not the goal of this experiment to find the FEV_1 above which this regimen ceases to have significant benefit. Infrequent doses of ipratropium may be sufficient in many children with a baseline FEV_1 greater than 30% of the predicted value. The results of this study are not generalizable to patients with milder asthma, who usually respond readily to albuterol alone.

We conclude that this trial demonstrates the benefit and safety of the addition of frequent nebulized doses of ipratropium to frequent albuterol therapy in severe childhood asthma, with a decrease in hospitalizations in the very severe cases.

We thank all medical and nursing staff for their support and Dr. David Jaffe for his encouragement.

REFERENCES

1. Schuh S, Parkin P, Rajan A, et al. High versus low dose, frequently administered nebulized albuterol in children with severe, acute asthma. Pediatrics 1989;83:513-8.
2. Tal A, Levy N, Bearman JE. Methylprednisolone therapy for acute asthma in infants and toddlers. Pediatrics 1990;86:350-6.
3. Littenberg B, Gluck EH. A controlled trial of methylprednisolone in the emergency treatment of acute asthma. N Engl J Med 1986;314:150-2.
4. Scarfone RJ, Fuchs S, Nager AL, Shane SA. Controlled trial of oral prednisone in the emergency department treatment of children with acute asthma. Pediatrics 1993;92:513-8.
5. Canadian Pharmaceutical Association. Compendium of pharmaceutical and specialties. 20th ed. Ottawa: CK Productions, 1994.
6. Rebuck AS, Chapman KR, Brande AC. Anticholinergic therapy of asthma. Chest 1982;82(suppl 1):55S-7S.
7. Rebuck AS, Chapman KR, Abbound R, et al. Nebulized anticholinergic and sympathamimetic treatment of asthma and chronic obstructive airways disease in the emergency room. Am J Med 1987;82:59-64.
8. O'Driscoll BF, Taylor RJ, Horsley M, Chambers DK, Bernstein A. Nebulized salbutamol with and without ipratropium bromide in acute airflow obstruction. Lancet 1989;1:1418-20.
9. Higgins RM, Stradling RJ, Lane DM. Should ipratropium bromide be added to β-agonists in treatment of severe acute asthma? Chest 1988;94:718-22.
10. Beck R, Robertson C, Galdes-Sebaldt M, Levison H. Combined salbutamol and ipratropium bromide by inhalation in the treatment of severe acute asthma. J PEDIATR 1985;107:605-8.
11. Reisman J, Galdes-Sebaldt M, Kazim F, et al. Frequent administration by inhalation of salbutamol and ipratropium bromide in the initial management of severe acute asthma in children. J Allergy Clin Immunol 1988;82:1012-8.
12. Watson WTA, Becker AB, Simons FER. Comparison of ipratropium solution, fenoterol solution, and their combination administered by nebulizer and face mask to children with acute asthma. J Allergy Clin Immunol 1988;82:1012-8.
13. Weng T, Levison H. Standards of pulmonary function in children. Am Rev Respir Dis 1969;99:879-92.
14. American Thoracic Society. Snowbird workshop on standardization of spirometry. Am Rev Respir Dis 1979;119:831-8.
15. American Thoracic Society. Standardization of spirometry—1987 update. Am Rev Respir Dis 1987;136:1255-98.
16. Fleiss J. The design and analysis of clinical experiments [Appendix A-2]. New York: John Wiley & Sons, 1986.
17. Reisman J, Canny G, Levison H. The role of anticholinergic drugs in paediatric airways disease. In: Gross N. Anticholinergic therapy in obstructive airways disease. London: Franklin Scientific Publications, 1993:169-70.
18. Partridge M, Saunders K. Site of action of ipratropium

bromide and clinical and physiological determinants of response in patients with asthma. Thorax 1981;36:530-3.
19. Barnes PJ, Basbaum CB, Nael JA. Autoradiographic localization of autonomic receptors in airway smooth muscle. Am Rev Respir Dis 1983;127:758-62.
20. Storr J, Lenney W. Nebulized ipratropium and salbutamol in asthma. Am J Dis Child 1986;61:602-3.
21. Boner AL, De Stefano G, Niero E, Vallone G, Gaburro D. Salbutamol and ipratropium bromide solution in the treatment of bronchospasm in asthmatic children. Ann Allergy 1987; 58:54-8.
22. Cook JJ, Fergusson DM, Dawson KP. Ipratropium and fenoterol in the treatment of acute asthma. Pharmatherapeutics 1985;4:383-6.
23. Davis A, Vickerson F, Worsley G, et al. Determination of dose-response relationship for ipratropium in asthmatic children. J PEDIATR 1984;105:1002-5.
24. Kerem E, Canny G, Tibshirani R, et al. Clinical-physiological correlations in acute asthma. Pediatrics 1991;87:481.
25. Lichterfeld A. Safety of Atrovent Scand J Respir Dis 1979; 60(suppl 103):143-7.
26. Jannum DR, Mickel SF. Anisocoria and aerosolized anticholinergics. Chest 1986;90:148-9.
27. Shah P, Dhurjon L, Metcalfe T, Gibson J. Acute angle closure glaucoma associated with nebulized ipratropium bromide and salbutamol. BMJ 1992;304:40-1.
28. O'Callahan C, Milner AD, Swarbrick A. Paradoxical bronchoconstriction in wheezing infants after nebulized preservative-free, iso-osmolar ipratropium bromide. BMJ 1989; 299: 1433-4.

Treatment of purpura fulminans in meningococcemia with protein C concentrate

Georges E. Rivard, MD, Michèle David, MD, Catherine Farrell, MD, and Hans Peter Schwarz, MD

From the Division of Hematology-Oncology and the Department of Pediatrics, Hôpital Sainte-Justine, Université de Montréal, Montréal, Québec, Canada, and Immuno AG, Vienna, Austria

Objective: **To evaluate the clinical and laboratory effects of protein C concentrate as an adjunct to conventional therapy in the treatment of meningococcemia with purpura fulminans.**
Design: **Case series (pilot study).**
Setting: **Intensive care unit in a tertiary care pediatric hospital.**
Patients: **Four children (aged 3 months to 15 years) requiring intensive treatment for meningococcemia with shock, disseminated intravascular coagulation, and purpura fulminans.**
Intervention: **Intravenous administration of a protein C concentrate (100 IU/kg every 6 hours).**
Main outcome measures: **Plasma protein C amidolytic activity, fibrinogen, and D-dimers; evolution of skin and limb lesions.**
Results: **Treatment with protein C concentrate led to a rise in plasma protein C activity levels to within normal limits in all patients, associated with an increase in plasma fibrinogen and a bimodal decrease in D-dimers. No adverse effects were noted. All patients had reversal of organ dysfunction despite the severity of the initial illness. Two patients recovered completely with no sequelae; two required amputations.**
Conclusions: **These encouraging clinical and laboratory results and the absence of side effects warrant the initiation of a double-blind, randomized controlled multicenter trial to determine the role of protein C replacement in the treatment of meningococcemia-associated purpura fulminans. (J PEDIATR 1995; 126:646-52)**

Despite recent advances in the management of septic shock,[1] meningococcemia with purpura fulminans still carries a high risk of death[2, 3] and of mutilating complications.[4] In a recently published study of children with meningococcemia, of 20 patients who were in shock and had disseminated intravascular coagulation, seven died and extremity amputation was necessary in three.[5] Meningococcemia is associated with clinical and laboratory evidence of DIC,[6] which is frequently combined with severe protein C deficiency.[7, 8] Protein C levels are reduced in patients with septic shock, especially with meningococcemia and purpura fulminans.[2, 5, 9-14] Moreover, nonsurviving patients have lower protein C levels than surviving patients.[2, 11, 15]

APC	Activated protein C
DIC	Disseminated intravascular coagulation
PAI-1	Plasminogen activator inhibitor type 1

Submitted for publication July 18, 1994; accepted Oct. 11, 1994.
Reprint requests: Georges E. Rivard, MD, Division of Hematology-Oncology, Hôpital Sainte-Justine, 3175 Chemin Côte Sainte-Catherine, Montréal, Québec H3T 1C5, Canada.

0022-3476/95/$3.00 + 0 **9/25/61302**

Table. Clinical and biochemical characteristics at time of admission of patients with purpura fulminans caused by meningococcemia

	Normal range	Patient 1*	Patient 2	Patient 3†	Patient 4
Age	—	15 yr	13 yr	11 yr	3 mo
Sex	—	F	M	F	M
Time from onset of skin lesions to PC infusion (hr)	—	20	7	14	8
Severity of skin lesions‡	—	++++	+	++	+
Mental status	—	IRR	LET	IRR	LET
N. meningitidis type	—	C	C	C	B
Leukocytes (10^9/L)	4-10	10.6	16.5	18.4	12.3
Platelets (10^9/L)	150-440	93	121	22	138
PT (INR)	0.8-1.35	4.4	1.6	3.9	4.5
APTT (sec)	25-36	109	38	114	117
Fibrinogen (g/L)	2-4	0.35	1.4	1.0	0.78
D-Dimers (μg/ml)	<0.25	8	8	16	2
Factor V (IU/ml)	0.5-1.5	0.05	0.57	0.21	0.09
Factor VIII (IU/ml)	0.5-1.5	0.08	1.6	0.36	0.12
Protein C (IU/ml)	0.7-1.2	0.10	0.47	0.14	<0.1
Protein S (IU/ml)	0.7-1.4	0.41	0.5	0.4	0.3
α_2-Antiplasmin (IU/ml)	0.8-1.3	0.13	0.72	0.27	0.32
PAI-1 (U/ml)	<10	180	35	94	228
Interleukin-6 (pg/ml)	<10	3100	370	2800	1625

PC, Protein C concentrate; *IRR*, irritable; *LET*, lethargic; *PT*, prothrombin time; *INR*, international normalized ratio; *APTT*, activated partial thromboplastin time.
*Required bilateral mid-thigh and right mid-forearm amputations
†Required bilateral submalleoar amputations.
‡Graded from + to ++++.

The acquired deficiency of protein C in sepsis may contribute to the pathogenesis of purpura fulminans,[2, 13] and early replacement of protein C may limit hemostatic system activation, interrupt DIC, and ultimately result in normalization of the microcirculation and improvement in organ function. Administration of purified human activated protein C decreases the incidence and severity of endotoxin-induced septic shock in an animal model.[16] Furthermore, administration of purified protein C concentrate was associated with correction of acquired protein C deficiency, reversal of biochemical evidence of DIC, and arrest of clinical signs of development of septic shock–related purpura fulminans in a child who was not responding to aggressive conventional treatment.[14]

We report our experience with the use of a purified protein C concentrate as an adjunct to aggressive conventional therapy in the management of four children with meningococcemia and purpura fulminans. This prospective pilot study was initiated to explore the feasibility of conducting a larger randomized, controlled study.

METHODS

Patients. Children with a clinical presentation suggestive of meningococcemia, cutaneous lesions compatible with purpura fulminans, and laboratory evidence of DIC were eligible for the study. Two girls and two boys, ranging in age from 3 months to 15 years, were treated.

Materials. Protein C Concentrate (Human) Vapor Heated was supplied by Immuno AG (Vienna, Austria). This product is a monoclonal antibody–purified, virus-inactivated concentrate of protein C for intravenous use and was described previously.[17] It is manufactured from pooled human plasma and contains protein C in a sterile lyophilized form. One international unit is defined as the protein C activity in 1 ml of a normal human plasma pool, based on a snake venom (Protac) activity assay calibrated against the first international standard of protein C.[18]

Study procedures. The study was approved by the ethics committee of Sainte-Justine Hospital of Montreal, and informed consent was given by parents of all patients before administration of the protein C concentrate. Patients were admitted to the intensive care unit of the hospital, and aggressive conventional antibiotic treatment and supportive care were initiated, including fluid resuscitation, vasoactive amines, and mechanical ventilation when indicated. Protein C concentrate was administered after stabilization of ventilation and hemodynamic functions. Blood specimens for laboratory studies were obtained immediately before and at

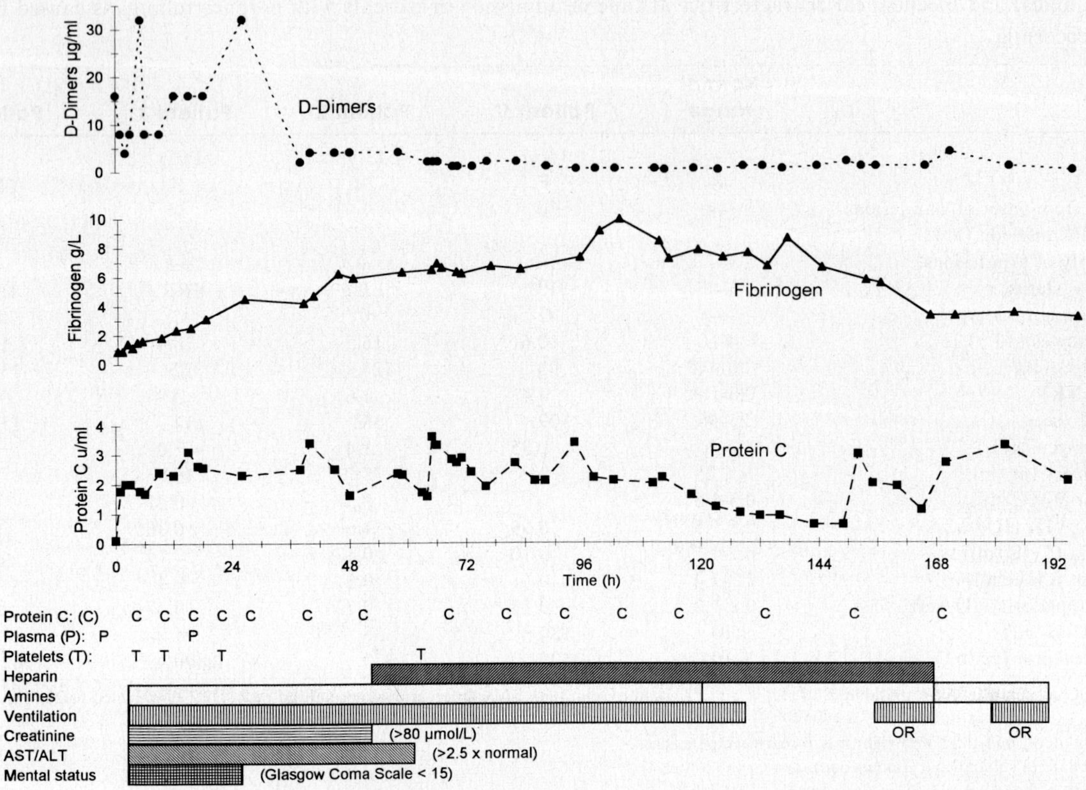

Fig. 1. Course of clinical and laboratory observations in patient 1. *AST*, Aspartate aminotransferase; *ALT*, alanine aminotransferase; *OR*, reintubation.

the following intervals after the initial dose of protein C: 30 minutes and 1, 4, and 6 hours. During the subsequent 72 hours, specimens were obtained immediately before and 30 minutes after the administration of protein C. Protein C was administered intravenously at a dose of 100 IU/kg during a 15- to 20-minute period. Identical doses of the same lot of the protein C concentrate were given every 6 hours during the acute phase. Patient 1 received further doses once or twice daily, for a total of 9 days.

Laboratory and clinical tests. Complete blood cell counts, including platelet counts, were obtained by standard techniques with an automated instrument. Blood specimens for coagulation studies and other specialized tests were drawn through arterial or venous catheters with a double-syringe technique and put in siliconized Vacutainer glass tubes containing buffered citrate solution (Becton Dickinson & Co., Rutherford, N.J.). Each specimen was submitted to double centrifugation at 12,000*g* for 10 minutes at 4° C and tested immediately, or snap-frozen in a methanol–dry ice mixture and stored at −80° C until use.

Routine coagulation tests were performed by standard methods. The following measurements were performed with commercial kits (Diagnostica-Stago, Asnières, France): D-dimers, protein C amidolytic activity, functional protein S activity, plasminogen activator inhibitor type 1 amidolytic activity, and α_2-antiplasmin amidolytic activity. Interleukin-6 was measured with an immunoassay kit (BioSources International Inc., Camarillo, Calif.). Results are expressed in appropriate units and compared with normal ranges as recommended for each commercial kit. Where applicable, results are expressed in international units; 1 IU is defined as the activity of the respective substance in 1 ml of a normal human plasma pool. A normal plasma pool was constructed by mixing equal volumes of plasma from 23 normal adult male subjects. Normal ranges given in the Table are based on results from this pool.

Neurologic status was assessed by the Glasgow Coma Scale.

RESULTS

Clinical and laboratory observations at the time of admission are given in the Table. The severity of the skin lesions varied from mild (+) to severe (+ +++). Two patients were irritable and two were lethargic. No patient had leukopenia, and all had laboratory evidence of DIC. Blood cultures grew *Neisseria meningitidis* type C in three of the patients and type B in one patient. The time from onset of skin lesions to initiation of treatment with protein C concentrate varied from 7 to 20 hours, depending on time of referral of patients. All patients had low levels of protein C and protein S activity. The PAI-1 activity was moderately to markedly increased in all patients, whereas α_2-antiplasmin was decreased in the three patients with the clinically most severe disease. The interleukin-6 value was increased in all patients, with higher levels in the patients who had more extensive skin lesions.

Figures 1 to 4 summarize the course of laboratory and clinical observations in the four patients. The initial dose of protein C concentrate was sufficient to raise plasma protein C activity levels to within normal limits for each patient, and subsequent doses maintained protein C values within normal limits. After the first dose of protein C concentrate, the plasma level of D-dimers fell abruptly in each patient, only to rise again rapidly and very transiently before progressively falling toward normal values during the subsequent days of treatment. Meanwhile, fibrinogen rose progressively and steadily during the first days of treatment to reach higher-than-normal levels for each patient. No adverse effects were observed with any of the protein C concentrate infusions.

For patient 1 the attending physician elected to give a 5-day infusion of heparin at a therapeutic dosage. This patient, who was transferred to us from another hospital at a relatively advanced stage of the disease, required vasoactive agents on days 1 to 5 and again on days 7 to 14. In the other patients, vasoactive agents were required for only 24 to 48 hours.

Assisted ventilation was necessary for only a relatively short time in patients 2, 3, and 4; assisted ventilation became acutely necessary immediately after platelet transfusion for low platelet counts in patients 3 and 4. It is impossible to know whether platelet transfusions contributed to the need for prolonged respiratory support in patient 1 because assisted ventilation was already in use when they were given.

In none of the patients did we observe deterioration of kidney or liver function as assessed on the basis of the course of creatinine and transaminase levels during hospitalization. Overall, abnormal levels of laboratory values quickly returned to normal limits. Brain function returned to normal within 24 hours in all four patients. Patients 2 and 4 recovered completely with no sequelae. Patient 1 required bilateral mid-thigh and right mid-forearm amputations, and skin grafts on her left breast. In patient 3, bilateral submalleolar amputations were necessary.

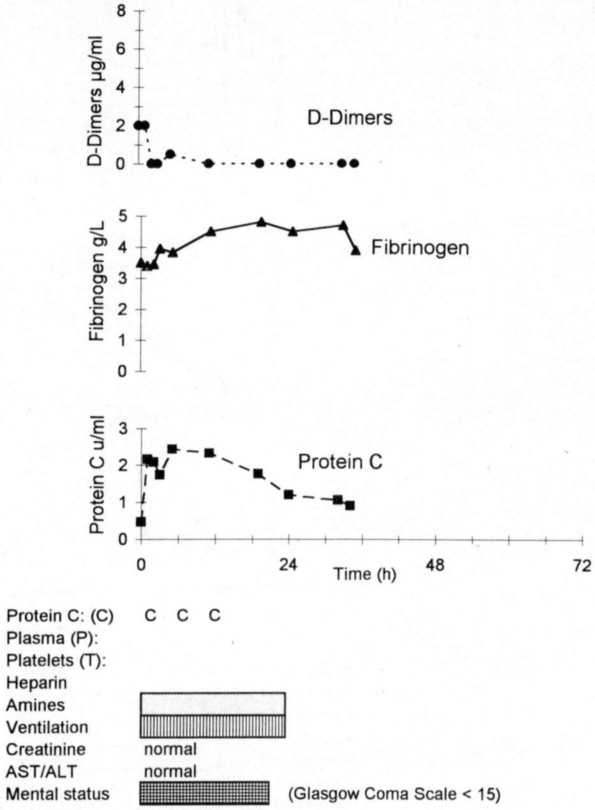

Fig. 2. Course of clinical and laboratory observations in patient 2. *AST*, Aspartate aminotransferase; *ALT*, alanine aminotransferase.

DISCUSSION

The administration of a highly purified protein C concentrate resulted in normalization of circulating protein C levels in plasma in these patients, in association with a rise in fibrinogen, which indicates that the protein C zymogen infused was converted to APC in vivo, thus limiting thrombin generation and interrupting DIC.[19] The decrease in D-dimers, a marker of cross-linked fibrin, immediately after the administration of protein C is consistent with previous observations made in patients with severe congenital protein C deficiency, in whom substitution of protein C resulted in normalization of D-dimer levels, and circulating protein C levels less than 25% were associated with an increase in D-dimers, indicating coagulation system activation and recurrence of DIC and purpura fulminans.[17]

In our patients, we observed a secondary rise in D-dimers that was associated with a decrease in PAI-1 levels (data not shown). In vitro studies have demonstrated the ability of APC to form a complex with and neutralize PAI-1.[20] By allowing in situ generation of plasmin, this or other mech-

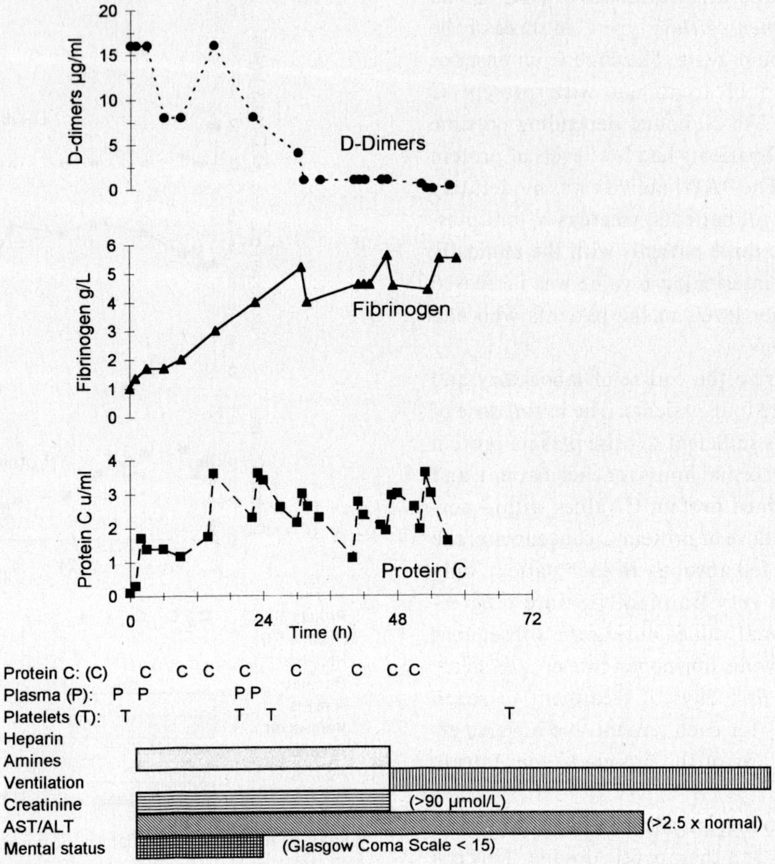

Fig. 3. Course of clinical and laboratory observations in patient 3. *AST*, Aspartate aminotransferase; *ALT*, alanine aminotransferase.

anisms of APC-induced fibrinolysis might have been responsible for the removal of fibrin deposits from organs, resulting in a rise in D-dimers and thus possibly preserving organ function. On the other hand, the secondary rise in D-dimers might also be attributable to the mobilization of cross-linked fibrin from the necrotic skin lesions on improvement of the microcirculation. It has been suggested that APC has antiinflammatory properties; infusion of APC prevents the coagulopathic, hepatotoxic, and lethal effects of *Escherichia coli* infusion in baboons.[16] In addition, the observation that the protein C concentrate used in this study attenuated the hemorrhagic necroticizing lesions of the localized Shwartzman reaction in rabbits serves as a rationale for its use in meningococcemia-associated purpura.[21] A role for APC in inflammatory responses is also suggested by interactions that have been observed in vitro between APC and monocytes[22]: (1) APC significantly decreases lipopolysaccharide-induced cytokine production by cultured human monocytes; (2) APC inhibits CD14 down-regulation induced by interferon gamma; and (3) APC inhibits CD11 down-regulation induced by lipopolysaccharides. The in vivo relevance of these observations remains to be determined.

A further rationale for the beneficial effects of APC in sepsis might be based on the ability of APC to act as a natural anticoagulant in destroying the activated forms of factors V and VIII,[23] which would lead to decreased generation of thrombin. The limitation of thrombin formation may be crucial in modulating the outcome of the systemic inflammatory response syndrome if one considers the cellular humoral responses to minuscule concentrations of thrombin.[24] Inhibition of thrombin formation by APC may abort the progression of the inflammatory cascade that contributes to the pathophysiologic events in sepsis and may prevent such consequences of (local) thrombin generation as activation, adhesion, and aggregation of platelets; release of vasoactive and proinflammatory material; increase in endothelial permeability; expression of platelet activating

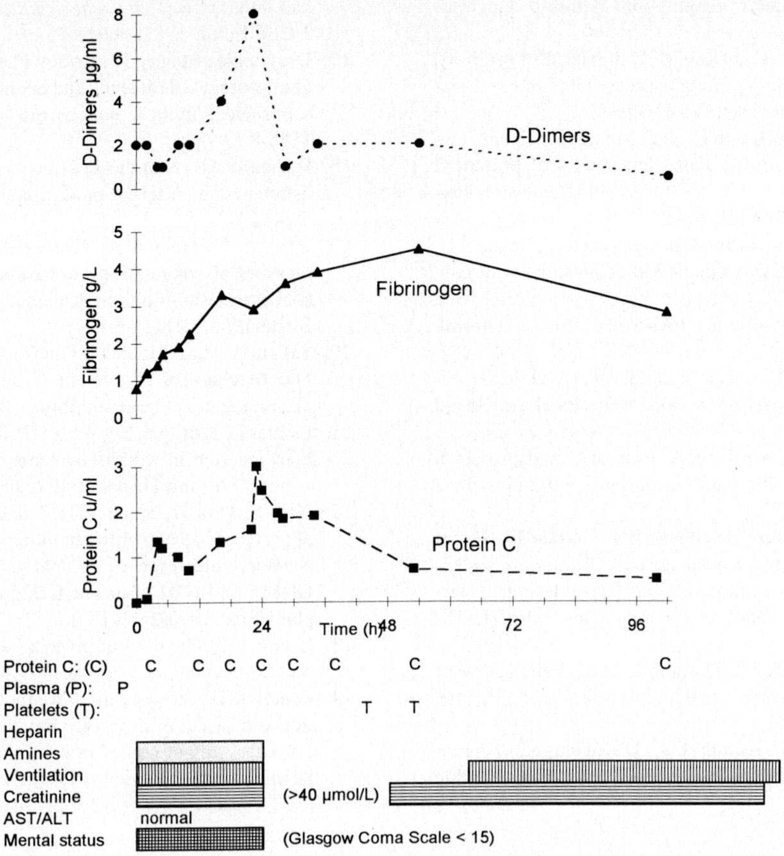

Fig. 4. Course of clinical and laboratory observations in patient 4. *AST*, Aspartate aminotransferase; *ALT*, alanine aminotransferase.

factor and granule membrane protein-140 on endothelial cells (which results in adhesion of polymorphonuclear neutrophil leukocytes); and inhibition of nitric oxide synthesis.

The progression of skin lesions in meningococcemia-associated purpura fulminans is very rapid. The fact that amputation was necessary only in the two patients who received the protein C concentrate at a relatively late stage leads us to conclude that the early initiation of treatment is crucial. The prompt reversal of organ dysfunction and the rapid normalization of measures of hemostasis, even in our patients with late irreversible skin damage, suggest that correction of plasma protein C levels could contribute to a decrease in morbidity and mortality rates for patients with this condition. However, evidence of the efficacy and safety of this therapeutic modality should be obtained in a double-blind, randomized, controlled multicenter trial.

We thank Kathryn Nelson for valuable suggestions and linguistic supervision.

REFERENCES

1. Parrillo JE. Pathogenetic mechanism of septic shock. N Engl J Med 1993;328:1471-7.
2. Powars DR, Rogers ZR, Patch MJ, McGehee WG, Francis RB. Purpura fulminans in meningococcemia: association with acquired deficiencies of proteins C and S [Letter]. N Engl J Med 1987;317:571-4.
3. Tesoro LJ, Selbst SM. Factors affecting outcome in meningococcal infections. Am J Dis Child 1991;145:218-20.
4. Genoff MC, Hoffer MM, Achauer B, Formosa P. Extremity amputations in meningococcemia-induced purpura fulminans. Plast Reconstr Surg 1992;89:878-81.
5. Leclerc F, Hazelzet J, Jude B, et al. Protein C and S deficiency in severe infectious purpura of children: a collaborative study of 40 cases. Intensive Care Med 1992;18:1-4.
6. Spicer TE, Rau JM. Purpura fulminans. Am J Med 1976; 61:566-70.
7. Marlar RA, Endres-Brooks J, Miller C. Serial studies of protein C and its plasma inhibitor in patients with disseminated intravascular coagulation. Blood 1985;66:59-63.
8. Scully MF, Toh CH, Hoogendoorn H, et al. Activation of protein C and its distribution between its inhibitors, protein C inhibitor, α_1-antitrypsin and α_2-macroglobulin in patients with

disseminated intravascular coagulation. Thromb Haemost 1993;69:448-53.
9. Hesselvik JF, Malm J, Blombäck M, Dahlbäck B. Protein C, protein S and C4b-binding protein in severe infection and septic shock. Thromb Haemost 1991;65:126-9.
10. Fourrier F, Lestavel P, Chopin C, et al. Meningococcemia and purpura fulminans in adults: acute deficiencies of protein C and S and early treatment with antithrombin III concentrates. Intensive Care Med 1990;16:121-4.
11. Brandtzaeg P, Sandset PM, Joo GB, Ovstebo R, Abilgaard U, Kierulf P. The quantitative association of plasma endotoxin, antithrombin, protein C, extrinsic pathway inhibitor and fibrinopeptide A in systemic meningococcal disease. Thromb Res 1989;55:459-70.
12. Blanco A, Guisasola JA, Solis P, Bachiller R, Gonzalez H. Fibronectin in mengingococcal sepsis. Acta Paediatr Scand 1990;79:73-6.
13. Madden RM, Gill JC, Marlar RA. Protein C and protein S levels in two patients with acquired purpura fulminans. Br J Haematol 1990;75:112-7.
14. Gerson WT, Dickermann JD, Bovill EG, Golden E. Severe acquired protein C deficiency in purpura fulminans associated with disseminated intravascular coagulation: treatment with protein C concentrate. Pediatrics 1993;91:418-22.
15. Lorente JA, García-Frade LJ, Landin L, et al. Time course of hemostatic abnormalities in sepsis and its relation to outcome. Chest 1993;103:1536-42.
16. Taylor FB, Chang A, Esmon CT, D'Angelo A, Vigano-D'Angelo S, Blick KE. Protein C prevents the coagulopathic and lethal effects of *Escherichia coli* infusions in the baboon. J Clin Invest 1987;79:918-25.
17. Dreyfus M, Magny JF, Bridey F, et al. Treatment of homozygous protein C deficiency and neonatal purpura fulminans with a purified protein C concentrate. N Engl J Med 1991; 325: 1565-8.
18. Hubbard AR. Standardization of protein C in plasma: establishment of an international standard. Thromb Haemost 1988; 59:464-7.
19. Conard J, Bauer KA, Gruber A, et al. Normalization of markers of coagulation activation with a purified protein C concentrate in adults with homozygous protein C deficiency. Blood 1993;82:1159-64.
20. Sakata Y, Loskutoff DJ, Gladson CL, Hekman CM, Griffin JH. Mechanism of protein C–dependent clot lysis: role of plasminogen activator inhibitor. Blood 1986;68:1218-23.
21. Pichler L, Hruby E, Schwarz HP. Attenuation of the Shwartzman reaction in rabbits by human activated protein C [Abstract]. Thromb Haemost 1991;65:1205.
22. Grey S, Hau H, Salem HH, Hancock WW. Selective effects of protein C on activation of human monocytes by lipopolysaccharide, interferon-γ, or PMA: modulation of effects on CD11b and CD14 but not CD25 or CD54 induction. Transplant Proc 1993;25:2913-4.
23. Esmon CT. The roles of protein C and thrombomodulin in the regulation of blood coagulation. J Biol Chem 1989;264:4743-6.
24. Esmon CT. Cell-mediated events that control blood coagulation and vascular injury. In: Palade GE, Alberts BM, Spudich JA, eds. Annual review of cell biology; vol 9. Palo Alto, California: Annual Reviews, 1993:1-25.

Control of severe pain in children with terminal malignancy

John J. Collins, MBBS, FRACP, Holcombe E. Grier, MD, Hannah C. Kinney, MD, and Charles B. Berde, MD, PhD

From the Pain Treatment Service, Division of Hematology/Oncology, and Departments of Anesthesia, Medicine, and Pathology, Children's Hospital, Boston; the Department of Pediatric Oncology, Dana-Farber Cancer Institute, Boston; and the Departments of Anesthesia, Pediatrics, and Pathology, Harvard Medical School, Boston, Massachusetts

Objective: To identify the characteristics of the subset of children with malignancy in whom massive opioid infusions are needed during the terminal phase.
Design: Retrospective review of the records of the 199 patients who died of malignancy after treatment at Children's Hospital, Boston, from March 1989 to July 1993, identifying characteristics of patients who required massive opioid infusions (operationally defined as infusion of >3 mg/kg per hour of morphine dose equivalent) during the terminal phase.
Results: Twelve patients (6%) required massive opioid infusions, and eight of these patients required extraordinary measures (epidural or subarachnoid infusion and/or sedation) to achieve adequate analgesia. The duration of epidural or subarachnoid infusions in three patients ranged from 3 to 9 days, and minimal complications occurred. The duration of sedation ranged from 1 to 15 days. Maximal intravenous opioid dosing ranged from 3.8 to 518 mg/kg per hour of morphine equivalent. The maximal infusion rate (exceeding all previous published reports) occurred in an infant with an isolated metastasis in the periaqueductal gray matter, a brain-stem site linked to mediating analgesia and defense reactions. The need for massive opioid dosing in 11 of 12 patients was associated with tumor spread to the spinal nerve roots, nerve plexus, large peripheral nerve, or spinal cord compression.
Conclusions: Standard dosing of opioids adequately treats most cancer pain in children; however, a significant group requires more extensive management. These problems occur more commonly among patients with solid tumors metastatic to spine and major nerves. (J PEDIATR 1995;126:653-7)

The fear of pain is one of the overriding concerns of children with cancer and of their parents.[1] The World Health Organization (WHO) analgesic ladder is a program for pain control in patients with cancer. It involves stepwise prescription of analgesics according to pain severity, ranging from acetaminophen and nonsteroidal antiinflammatory drugs for mild pain to strong opioids for severe pain. This approach is effective for children, as well as adults, with cancer.[2-4]

The Maunuksela study[5] of children with terminal malignancy at the Children's Hospital, University of Helsinki, showed that approximately half of their subjects required analgesics, and one patient required epidural analgesia. In our practice a small subset of children with terminal malignancy require massive doses of opioids (operationally defined as >3 mg/kg per hour of intravenous morphine dose equivalent, or approximately 100-fold greater than standard starting infusion rates) and/or extraordinary mea-

Supported by grants from the Department of Oncology, Children's Hospital, Sydney, New South Wales, Australia, and the Department of Anesthesia, Children's Hospital, Boston, Massachusetts (Dr. Collins), and by the Anesthesia Patient Safety Foundation, Christopher Coakley Memorial Fund, and Mayday Fund (Dr. Berde).

Submitted for publication July 25, 1994; accepted Nov. 2, 1994.

Reprint requests: Charles B. Berde MD, PhD, Director, Pain Treatment Service, Farley 306, Children's Hospital, 300 Longwood Ave., Boston, MA 02115.

0022-3476/95/$3.00 + 0 **9/25/61755**

sures (epidural or subarachnoid infusion, or deep sedation) to achieve adequate analgesia. To better understand the characteristics of patients with massive opioid requirements and to gain potential insight into the cause(s) of massive opioid need, we retrospectively reviewed 199 charts of children dying of cancer at the Children's Hospital, Boston, and the Dana-Farber Cancer Institute, Boston, Mass.

METHODS

The study protocol was approved by the clinical investigation committee at the Dana-Farber Cancer Institute and Children's Hospital, Boston. A retrospective chart analysis was made of the inpatient and outpatient records of the Dana-Farber Cancer Institute and Children's Hospital, Boston, and the hospice agency records (if appropriate) of the 199 patients who died of malignancy after treatment at Children's Hospital, Boston, from March 1989 to July 1993. During this time the WHO algorithm[2] was systematically applied. Eligibility for inclusion in the chart review required that the age of the patient at the time of initial diagnosis was less than 18 years. Patients were divided into two groups: (1) required massive opioid infusions (operationally defined as >3 mg/kg per hour of intravenous morphine dose equivalent) during the terminal phase of their illness and (2) did not require massive opioid infusions. Morphine equivalent doses were calculated with standard opioid conversion tables.[6]

Patient records were analyzed to obtain the following information: patient demographics; tumor type, location, treatment, and metastatic spread during the terminal phase; opioid dose range, duration, adequacy, and limiting side effects of opioid analgesia; requirement for sedative-hypnotics; success or failure of other analgesic modalities; character and treatment of nonpainful, distressing symptoms (e.g., seizures, air hunger, myoclonic jerks); and autopsy data when available. Pain assessment at Children's Hospital, Boston, is routinely performed by nurses using a 0 to 10 numeric self-report scale for children aged 6 to 7 years or older, and a behavioral-physiologic measure, the Objective Pain Scale,[7] for younger children or for older children who cannot do self-report measures. Adequacy of analgesia for the purposes of the study represents a composite of impressions by patients, parents, nurses, and physicians.

The Fisher Exact Test and the unpaired t tests were used to test for significant differences ($p < 0.05$) in selected demographic, tumor, and analgesic features between the two groups of patients.

RESULTS

Patient characteristics. The 199 patients ranged in age at the time of death from 5 months to 20½ years. Forty-four percent had leukemia-lymphoma, 33% solid tumors, and 23% central nervous system tumors. Of the 199 patients, 12 (6%: 7 female, 5 male) required massive opioid infusion. An additional six patients, not described here, received relatively low-dose opioid infusions (<3 mg/kg per hour of intravenous morphine dose equivalent) but required epidural or spinal infusions, or celiac plexus blockade, primarily for limiting the side effects of the opioids (e.g., nausea, clouded sensorium, respiratory depression).

Pain management strategies before massive opioid infusions. As the severity of the pain increased, escalation of opioid doses was made initially by the oral route. If orally administered opioids were not tolerated, they were replaced with either intermittent intravenous infusions of opioids administered by the nursing staff or by patient-controlled analgesia; the latter (three patients) used continuous infusions with a "rescue" option. Continuous infusions of opioids were commenced in the intermittent-infusion group or continued in the group with patient-controlled analgesia, and were increased incrementally to massive doses as the severity of the pain necessitated. Although other delivery routes (subcutaneous infusion, transdermal administration of fentanyl) were used by other patients among the larger population, all patients in the massive opioid subgroup received high doses only via the intravenous route. Adjuvant analgesic agents (corticosteroids, tricyclic antidepressants, psychostimulants) were used in the treatment of eight patients before escalation to massive opioid requirements.

Massive opioid infusions. The duration of opioid use for the 12 patients requiring high doses ranged from 6 to 240 days; the maximal dosage range was 3.8 to 518 mg/kg per hour of intravenous morphine dose equivalent. The logarithmic escalation of the intravenous morphine dose equivalent in the 12 patients indicates that rapid dose escalation occurred in the last 2 weeks of life in the majority of patients (Fig. 1). Of the 12 patients requiring massive infusions of opioids, 4 patients obtained satisfactory analgesia with opioids alone (Fig. 2). The opioids used as massive intravenous infusions during the terminal phase were hydromorphone (7 patients) and morphine sulfate (5 patients).

Predictors of massive opioid use. Patients who required massive opioid infusions did not vary in age from those who did not require such infusions (unpaired t test, $p < 0.05$). Solid tumors (10 patients), however, were overrepresented in patients requiring massive doses of opioids (Fisher Exact Test, $p < 0.01$). Among patients with solid tumors (66 patients in the total group), spread to the spinal nerve roots, nerve plexus, large peripheral nerve, or spinal cord compression, based on clinical and/or autopsy data, increased the likelihood of massive opioid infusion requirement (Fisher Exact Test, $p < 0.01$).

Extraordinary measures. Five patients who required rapid acceleration in opioid infusions in the last few days of life required the addition of continuous sedation (benzodiazepines, propofol, barbiturates, nitrous oxide) to achieve

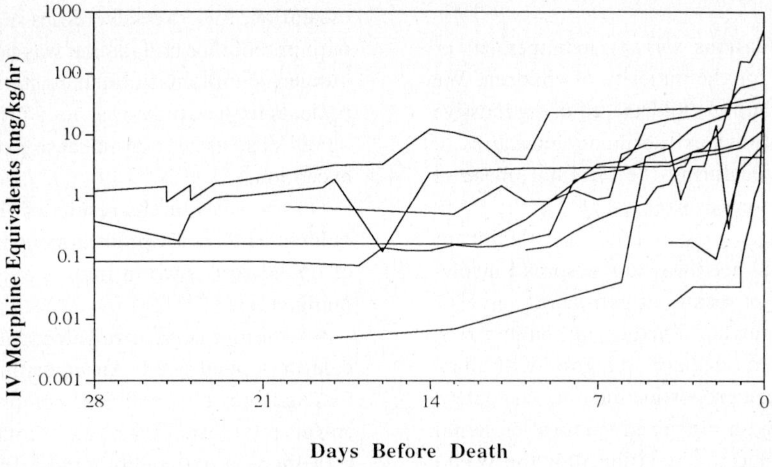

Fig. 1. Logarithmic escalation of opioid dose in patients requiring massive doses of opioid in terminal pediatric malignancy.

adequate analgesia. Another three patients required the addition of sedatives during the terminal phase because of anxiety or agitation (two patients) or air hunger (one). Duration of the use of sedatives ranged from 1 to 15 days; all patients continued to receive opioid analgesia while receiving sedatives. Infusion rates for pentobarbital ranged from 0.2 to 28 mg/kg per hour. The most extreme cases have been reported previously.[8]

Three patients required supplementary analgesia with epidural or spinal infusions. One patient had effective spinal analgesia until a delay occurred in changing syringes containing the spinal infusion. This patient subsequently required deep sedation.[8] Duration of regional anesthetic administration in these three patients ranged from 3 to 9 days; all died in the hospital. Each required the addition of local anesthetic to epidural or spinal opioids to achieve an adequate ratio of analgesia to side effects. Apart from a post-lumbar-puncture headache, effectively treated with an epidural blood patch (an injection of autologous blood in the epidural space), there were no major complications resulting from epidural or spinal infusions.

Tumor type, metastatic spread, and autopsy findings. Of the 12 patients receiving massive opioid infusions, 10 had solid tumors, one a central nervous system tumor, and one an acute lymphoblastic leukemia. On the basis of imaging studies, clinical history and examination, or autopsy data, 11 of the 12 patients had evidence of involvement of spinal nerve roots, nerve plexus, large peripheral nerve, or spinal cord compression by tumor.

One infant had an axillary rhabdoid tumor with localized brain-stem metastases in the periaqueductal gray matter of the mesencephalon; the brachial plexus was not examined at autopsy. This infant had massive opioid resistance, receiving 518 mg/kg per hour of intravenous morphine dose equivalent before death, a dose exceeding all previously published reports.[9] This infant eventually required deep sedation to achieve adequate analgesia.

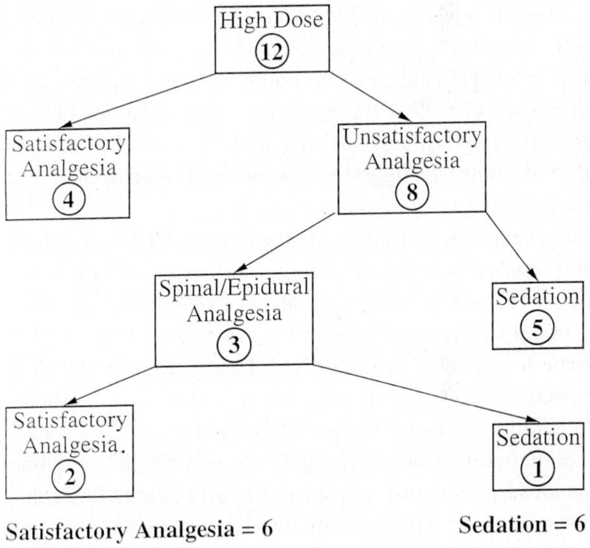

Fig. 2. Algorithm representing management of patients requiring high-dose opioid therapy in terminal pediatric malignancy.

Nonpainful symptoms. All patients had nonpainful symptoms. Air hunger occurred in seven patients and was managed with opioids or sedation or both. Myoclonic jerks, thought to be a side effect of massive opioid doses, were described in two patients and continued despite an infusion of the general anesthetic agent propofol in one patient and an infusion of a sedative anxiolytic agent, midazolam, in another. One patient had muscle spasms of the legs, which continued despite the use of a skeletal muscle relaxant agent, baclofen, and a sedative anxiolytic agent, lorazepam.

DISCUSSION

The WHO recommendations for the management of cancer pain are effective for the majority of children. We have identified a small group of children requiring massive opioid dosing with or without extraordinary measures to achieve adequate analgesia during the terminal phase of their illness. Solid tumors were overrepresented in the group requiring massive opioid infusions, and the most significant predictor of massive opioid need was tumor spread involving spinal nerve roots, major plexus, or peripheral nerve, or causing spinal cord compression. Further, although a proportion of patients received adequate analgesia with massive opioid infusions alone, a proportion did not. To achieve adequate analgesia, this group required epidural or spinal infusions, or sedation beyond that envisioned by the WHO analgesic ladder. The need for massive opioid dosing usually is a nearly terminal event; the majority of our patients began to require massive opioid infusions during the last 2 weeks of life.

There is ongoing debate regarding the degree of opioid responsiveness of neuropathic pain.[10] Arner and Meyerson[11] provided evidence that adults with neuropathic pain do not achieve adequate analgesia with a fixed opioid dose as well as do patients with nociceptive pain. Portenoy et al.,[12] in contrast, suggested that opioid responsiveness is a matter of degree, and that many patients with neuropathic pain can achieve adequate analgesia with opioids, although they may require higher dosing, rational use of adjuvants, and/or more aggressive treatment of opioid side effects.

In our study, neuropathic pain was associated with resistance to standard opioid dosing. However, sufficient dose escalation provided adequate analgesia for some patients. This supports the contention of Portenoy et al.[12] that neuropathic pain is not necessarily opioid resistant and that opioid response must be explored in all patients through a range of doses. However, many of our patients could not achieve acceptable analgesia even with more than 100-fold escalation of starting infusion rates, suggesting that opioid resistance and failure of the usual progression of the WHO algorithm may occur more frequently in this subpopulation.

An unexpected autopsy finding was the metastatic involvement of the periaqueductal gray matter in the midbrain in an infant who was receiving the intravenous morphine dose equivalent of 518.5 mg/kg per hour at the time of death. Electrical stimulation of the periaqueductal gray matter has produced analgesia in human subjects and is thought to be an important part of the descending endogenous inhibitory pain control system, and a key region involved in the mediation of defense reactions.[13]

Myoclonic jerks were witnessed in two patients receiving high intravenous doses of morphine. The role of morphine in producing myoclonus is controversial and may be more related to the use of concomitant medications,[14] the rate of escalation, and excessive doses of morphine.[15] Treatment with propofol or midazolam was not effective. Terminal air hunger, symptomatic of metastatic lung disease in seven patients in this study, was not a primary reason for massive opioid dose escalation in these patients, with one possible exception.

On the basis of the results of this study, we offer some guidelines to assist practitioners managing the emergency of opioid resistance in infants and children with terminal malignancy:

1. Consider nerve involvement as the cause of rapidly escalating opioid need. An algorithm for the diagnosis and management of spinal cord compression caused by cancer is well established for adults[16] and includes high-dose steroid therapy and radiotherapy. In selected cases, decompressive surgery may be indicated and may be palliative.[17]

2. Consider the use of regional anesthetic infusions if appropriate escalation of intravenous opioid infusions do not provide adequate analgesia despite optimal use of adjunctive therapies. Three patients in this study received epidural or subarachnoid infusions for 3 to 9 days, with an acceptable rate of complications and with generally satisfactory analgesia. A regimen for the conversion of intravenous to equianalgesic epidural or intrathecal administration of opioid and a schedule for the subsequent reduction in the intravenous opioid dose has been published by Krames.[18] These guidelines are approximate and must be modified by clinical circumstances. The use of a local anesthetic may significantly alter spinal and epidural opioid requirements.

3. The choice of deep sedation generally assumes that there is no acceptable means of providing analgesia with preservation of alertness. We strongly recommend continuing high-dose opioid infusions along with sedative-hypnotic use in these circumstances, to avoid situations in which the patient has unrelieved pain but inadequate clarity of sensorium to communicate regarding the pain.

4. Communicating with the dying child and the family is a difficult issue for which practitioners have few guidelines. When a child requires regional anesthesia for analgesia during the terminal phase of a malignancy, discussion should be age appropriate and should anticipate potential causes of distress for the child, including the side effects of motor blockade and numbness of the lower extremities, and potential loss of bladder function. The issue of prolonged sedation raises many ethical issues that have been discussed elsewhere.[8] The trade-off between sedation and inadequate pain relief requires consideration of the wishes of the patient and family.

Dr. R. T. Wilder and Dr. M. Levine provided assistance with statistical analysis. Dr. R. T. Wilder and Ms D. Hu assisted with graphics.

REFERENCES

1. Lansky SB, Ritter-Sterr C, List MA, Hart MJ. Psychiatric and psychological support of the child and adolescent with cancer. In: Pizzo PA, Poplack DG, eds. Pediatric oncology. Philadelphia: JB Lippincott, 1989:1127-39.
2. Berde C, Ablin A, Glazer J, et al. Report of the Subcommittee on Disease-related Pain in Childhood Cancer. Pediatrics 1990; 86:818-25.
3. Miser AW. Management of pain associated with childhood cancer. In: Schecter NL, Berde CB, Yaster M, eds. Pain in infants, children and adolescents. Baltimore: Williams & Wilkins, 1993:411-24.
4. McGrath PA. Pain control. In: Doyle D, Hanks GWC, MacDonald N, eds. Oxford textbook of palliative medicine. London: Oxford University Press, 1993:685-9.
5. Maunuksela E, Saarinen UM, Lähteenoja KM. Prevalence and management of terminal pain in children with cancer: five-year experience in Helsinki, Finland. In: Tyler DC, Krane EJ, eds. Advances in pain research therapy. New York: Raven Press, 1990:383-90.
6. Portenoy RK. Practical aspects of pain control in the patient with cancer. Cancer Journal for Clinicians 1988;38:327-52.
7. Broadman LM, Rice LJ, Hannallah RS. Testing the validity of an objective pain scale for infants and children [Abstract]. Anesthesiology 1988;69:A770.
8. Truog RD, Berde CB, Mitchell C, Grier HE. Barbiturates in the care of the terminally ill. N Engl J Med 1992;327:1678-82.
9. Coyle N, Adelhardt J, Foley KM, Portenoy RK. Character of terminal illness in the advanced cancer patient: pain and other symptoms in the last four weeks of life. Journal of Pain and Symptom Management 1990;5:83-93.
10. Wall PD. Neuropathic pain. Pain 1990;43:267-8.
11. Arner S, Meyerson BA. Lack of analgesic effect of opioids on neuropathic and idiopathic forms of pain. Pain 1988;33:11-23.
12. Portenoy RK, Foley KM, Inturrisi CE. The nature of opioid responsiveness and its implications for neuropathic pain: new hypotheses derived from studies of opioid infusions. Pain 1990; 43:273-86.
13. Hosobuchi Y, Adams JE, Linchitz R. Pain relief by electrical stimulation of the central gray matter in humans and its reversal by naloxone. Science 1977;197:183-6.
14. Potter JM, Reid DB, Shaw RJ, Hackett P, Hickman PE. Myoclonus associated with treatment with high doses of morphine: the role of supplemental drugs. BMJ 1989;299:150-3.
15. McQuay HJ, Gorman DJ, Hanks GW [Letter]. BMJ 1989; 299:684.
16. Portenoy RK, Lipton RB, Foley KM. Back pain in the cancer patient: an algorithm for evaluation and management. Neurology 1989;37:134-8.
17. Rossitch E, Madsen JR. Neurosurgical procedures for the relief of pain in children and adolescents. In: Schecter NL, Berde CB, Yaster M, eds. Pain in infants, children, and adolescents. Baltimore: Williams & Wilkins, 1993:237-44.
18. Krames ES. Intrathecal infusional therapies for intractable pain: patient management guidelines. Journal of Pain and Symptom Management 1993;8:36-46.

Clinical and laboratory observations

Diarrhea associated with enteral benzodiazepine solutions

J. D. Marshall, MD, H. C. Farrar, MD, and G. L. Kearns, PharmD

From the Division of Critical Care Medicine and the Section on Clinical Pharmacology, Department of Pediatrics, University of Arkansas for Medical Science, Little Rock, and the Pediatric Pharmacology Research Unit, Arkansas Children's Hospital, Little Rock

Diarrhea occurred in an infant given large enteral doses of benzodiazepine solutions that contained the carriers propylene glycol and polyethylene glycol. This adverse drug effect may be avoided by prescribing the tablet formulations appropriately prepared for enteral administration. (J Pediatr 1995;126:657-9)

Supported in part by National Institute of Child Health and Human Development grant No. 1 U10 HD31324-01.

Submitted for publication Aug. 26, 1994; accepted Oct. 14, 1994.

Reprint requests: J. D. Marshall, MD, Arkansas Children's Hospital, Division of Critical Care Medicine, 800 Marshall St., Little Rock, AR 72202.

0022-3476/95/$3.00 + 0 **9/26/61270**

Continuous high-dose infusions of short-acting benzodiazepines such as midazolam are frequently administered for extended sedation and anxiolysis in the pediatric intensive care unit. Dependence and tolerance may occur after long-term exposure to benzodiazepines, and rapid withdrawal may precipitate symptoms ranging from restlessness to generalized seizure activity.[1-3] It is our practice to discontinue CHDI as soon as the noxious stimuli of the intensive care environment are diminished. To prevent withdrawal symptoms, we substitute a longer-acting enteral preparation such as lorazepam. The enteral dose may then be decreased slowly while close clinical observation for withdrawal symptoms is maintained. The individual benzodiazepine doses may be extraordinarily high, depending on the tolerance of the individual. Recently we encountered an unusual adverse effect of high-dose therapy with an enteral lorazepam solution.

CASE REPORT

The patient, an 11 kg, 9-month-old girl with tracheobronchial malacia and bronchopulmonary dysplasia, had pneumonitis requiring brief neuromuscular blockade and prolonged midazolam CHDI for optimal mechanical ventilation; her maximal dose of midazolam was 0.3 mg/kg per hour plus occasional parenteral doses of lorazepam, 2 mg/kg, for a total benzodiazepine dose of 168 mg/24 hr. When her acute lung disease had sufficiently resolved, the midazolam CHDI and parenteral lorazepam therapy were converted to enteral lorazepam administration at 30 mg every 4 hours for a total dose of 180 mg/24 hr. This high dose did not completely sedate the infant but did control her agitation. A 10% decrease in the total dose each day was ordered, and the patient was transferred to an intermediate care unit.

CHDI	Continuous high-dose infusion
PEG	Polyethylene glycol
PG	Propylene glycol

Three days after conversion to enteral lorazepam therapy, the patient had intractable, frequent watery stools and was unable to gain weight despite elemental formula changes. Results of an extensive evaluation for enteral inflammation, infectious agents, and toxins were negative. None of the patient's concomitant medications (e.g., phenobarbital, prednisone, furosemide, captopril) was suspected of being the cause of her diarrhea because all of them had been tolerated for at least 2 weeks without apparent adverse effects. Review of her medication list showed that she was receiving 14 ml (28 mg) of lorazepam oral solution (Intensol) every 4 hours. This preparation contains propylene glycol at 40% weight per volume and polyethylene glycol 400 at 60% weight per volume. Thus the patient was receiving PG, 34 gm/24 hr, and PEG, 50 gm/24 hr, both osmotically active, nonabsorbed substances. Assuming that such a large daily enteral osmotic load could be responsible for her diarrhea, we converted the lorazepam formulation to crushed tablets; the diarrhea resolved completely within 2 days.

Administration of crushed lorazepam tablets through the patient's gastrostomy tube became difficult, and mild symptoms consistent with benzodiazepine withdrawal (e.g., irritability, restlessness) were noted. Consequently, midazolam CHDI at 0.3 mg/kg per hour was reinstated, and enteral diazepam, 0.5 mg/kg per day, divided every 8 hours as crushed tablets (i.e., 2 mg/dose) was given through the gastrostomy tube in 30 ml of water. Escalation of the diazepam dose to 2.5 mg every 6 hours (approximately 1 mg/kg per day) on the third day of enteral therapy was required to control agitation. On the fifth day of enteral treatment, a substitution of diazepam oral solution (Roxane Laboratories Inc., Columbus, Ohio) was made and not communicated to the physicians caring for the patient. Within 2 days, frequent watery stools (approximately 14 gm/kg per day) reappeared, prompting the discovery of the formulation change. The diazepam enteral solution contained PG at 50% wt/vol and PEG 1000 at 15% wt/vol. We subsequently prescribed diazepam crushed tablets at 4 mg every 6 hours, and the diarrhea resolved within 36 hours. Midazolam CHDI was successfully discontinued and the patient was adequately sedated with enteral diazepam therapy alone, which permitted effective, long-term ventilatory management. The patient's diarrhea remained fully resolved.

DISCUSSION

The inclusion of PG and PEG in these oral preparations of benzodiazepines is required to enhance solubility and to preserve and stabilize the formulations.[4] Because the amount of PG and PEG in these preparations is low, the administration of currently recommended therapeutic doses of each drug[5] is generally not associated with diarrhea or other adverse gastrointestinal effects.

The requirement for high-dose benzodiazepine therapy in our patient resulted in doses of PG and PEG capable of producing osmotic diarrhea. We believe that our patient's diarrhea was drug induced because the problem occurred only when oral solutions of lorazepam and diazepam containing PG and PEG were administered, and promptly remitted when tablet formulations of these same benzodiazepines were prescribed. Cardiac arrhythmias, central nervous system depression, and seizures also have been reported with overdoses of PG but were not observed in our patient.[6]

We conclude that drug-induced diarrhea is a previously unrecognized iatrogenic complication associated with the use of high-dose oral benzodiazepine solutions that contain PG and PEG. This adverse effect can be avoided by substituting the tablet formulations of these drugs.

REFERENCES

1. Boisse N, Quaglietta N, Samoriski G, Guarino J. Tolerance and physical dependence to a short-acting benzodiazepine, midazolam. J Pharm Exp Ther 1990;252:1125-33.
2. Fialip J, Aumitre O, Eschalier A, Maradeix B, Dordain G, Lavarenne J. Benzodiazepine withdrawal seizures: analysis of 48 case reports. Clin Neuropharmacol 1987;10:538-44.

3. Sury M, Billingham I, Russel G, Hopkins C, Thorington R, Viviori E. Acute benzodiazepine withdrawal syndrome after midazolam infusions in children [Letter]. Crit Care Med 1989;17:301-2.
4. Gennaro A, ed. Remington's pharmaceutical sciences. 18th ed. Easton, Pennsylvania: Mack Publishing, 1990:219, 1317.
5. Benitz W, Tatro D. The pediatric drug handbook. 2nd ed. Chicago: Year Book Medical Publishers, 1988:85-6, 108-9.
6. American Academy of Pediatrics Committee on Drugs. "Inactive" ingredients in pharmaceutical products. Pediatrics 1985;76:635-43.

Prepubertal gynecomastia during growth hormone therapy

Saul Malozowski, MD, PhD, and Bruce V. Stadel, MD, MPH

From the Division of Metabolism and Endocrine Drug Products, Center for Drug Evaluation and Research, U.S. Food and Drug Administration, Rockville, Maryland

We report 22 cases of prepubertal gynecomastia diagnosed during growth hormone (GH) treatment. The age and dose range were 2 to 12 years and 1.8 to 0.3 mg/kg per week, respectively. In most of the patients, gynecomastia appeared between 0.5 and 7 months after GH was started. Three boys were using drugs other than GH. This condition appears to be self-limited and benign. (J Pediatr 1995;126:659-61)

Gynecomastia occurs in about 70% of boys during puberty,[1] but prepubertal gynecomastia is rare.[2] When gynecomastia does occur before puberty, there is usually evidence of endogenous or exogenous estrogenic stimulation.[3-7] To our knowledge, drugs other than sex steroids have not been associated with prepubertal gynecomastia, although many drugs have been related to its occurrence in adults.[8] In this report, we describe 22 cases of gynecomastia that developed before puberty in boys treated with growth hormone.

METHODS

Cases of gynecomastia diagnosed during GH treatment of prepubertal boys were identified by reviewing "adverse drug experience" reports to the U.S. Food and Drug Administration. We defined "prepubertal" as a reported age of ≤12 years and, if recorded, Tanner stage I or testicular volume ≤2 ml or both. Neonatal gynecomastia was excluded by requiring that the age be ≥2 years. The first six cases meeting these criteria were found by searching the existing adverse drug experience database of the Food and Drug Administration. Subsequent inquiries to pharmaceutical companies that market GH domestically and abroad led to the reporting of 16 additional cases.

RESULTS

We identified 22 cases of prepubertal gynecomastia that were diagnosed during GH treatment. All boys were 2 to 12 years of age at diagnosis, with a median age of 7 years. Five were described as in Tanner stage I with testicular volume ≤2 ml, five as being in Tanner stage I with no data on testicular volume, and two as having a testicular volume ≤2 ml with no data on Tanner stage. Ten cases were reported with no data on Tanner stage or testicular volume; the age range for this subgroup was 2 to 12 years (median, 7 years). The cases were reported from the United States and Europe, with no evidence of geographic clustering.

GH	Growth hormone

The diagnosis leading to GH treatment was reported to be GH deficiency in 18 cases; the other four were cases of short stature—one with intrauterine growth retardation, one with Noonan syndrome, one with Aarskog syndrome, and one with a GH neurosecretory disorder. One boy with GH deficiency also had asthma and allergic rhinitis, one had

The contents of this manuscript represent the views of the authors and do not constitute an official position of the U.S. Food and Drug Administration.

Submitted for publication Aug. 12, 1994; accepted Oct. 6, 1994.

Reprint requests: Saul Malozowski, MD, PhD, U.S. Food and Drug Administration, HFD-510, Room 14B-03, Rockville, MD 20857.

9/26/61102

cryptorchidism (age 7 years, Tanner stage and testicular volume unreported), one had rickets, and one had undergone bone marrow transplantation at 2½ years of age for acute lymphoblastic leukemia, with complications of host-versus-graft disease and scleroderma. No current medications other than GH were reported except for three patients—one taking ketotifen (a histamine receptor antagonist), theophylline, and cromolyn sodium for asthma; one taking vitamin D for rickets; and one taking thyroid hormone.

The GH dose ranged from approximately 1.8 to 0.3 mg/kg per week, by subcutaneous injection, for the 16 cases with dosages reported. The time from the start of GH therapy to diagnosis of gynecomastia ranged from 0.5 to 7 months for 13 cases and from 1 to 8 years for eight; the interval was not stated for one. The gynecomastia was unilateral in nine boys and bilateral in seven; laterality was not stated for six. Mammary size was reported for three patients—as 1, 2, and 5 cm. One boy was described as having increased areolar pigmentation, but none was reported to have spontaneous or induced mammary discharge.

Hormonal determinations were available in eight cases. Serum estrogen, testosterone, and prolactin concentrations were determined in most of these cases; all results were within normal limits for age and sex. No other laboratory abnormalities were reported, except for liver enzyme elevations in the one patient with Aarskog syndrome.

In one boy the gynecomastia resolved within 3 months after GH therapy was stopped, but it reappeared when GH therapy was restarted. In another, the gynecomastia also resolved after treatment with GH was stopped, but no information was given about whether treatment was restarted. In five patients the gynecomastia regressed spontaneously while administration of GH was continued. No information is available about the clinical evolution of the other cases.

DISCUSSION

Our findings are in accordance with those of Rudman et al.,[9] who reported the occurrence of gynecomastia in 4 of 26 elderly men treated with GH in a clinical trial. Their four cases all appeared between 2 and 7 months after GH therapy was started; three resolved after treatment was stopped, and one resolved spontaneously while GH therapy was continued. In addition, regression of breast symptoms after the administration of GH-inhibiting drugs has been described in a patient with gynecomastia and lung cancer, who had elevated GH levels.[10] Thus the role of GH in the development of gynecomastia appears well substantiated in adult men.

Tanner staging or testicular volume, or both, in 12 of our patients indicated their prepubertal status, and one boy without this information was reported as having cryptorchidism. Although data on sexual maturity were not available for the remaining nine patients, we believe that they were also prepubertal because their age range was 2 to 12 years, and puberty tends to be delayed in GH-deficient children.[11] Pubertal gynecomastia usually appears when puberty has advanced to Tanner stage III-IV (ages 14 and 15 years).[12]

The mechanism underlying stimulation of gynecomastia by GH has not been established. However, GH receptors have been identified in human breast cell lines,[13] and GH could be stimulating growth directly through these, or through lactogenic receptors,[14] or indirectly through the production of insulin-like growth factor.[15] In this study, plasma levels of estradiol were within normal limits in all eight patients with levels reported.

We cannot estimate the incidence of prepubertal gynecomastia during GH treatment, because we do not have data on the number of boys $\leq$12 years of age who have been treated with GH in the countries from which our adverse drug experience reports came, and because substantial underreporting is likely even with our efforts to solicit data on known cases. However, in 1983 Haibach et al.[2] were able to identify only 43 published case reports of prepubertal gynecomastia, and in 1985 Descamps et al.[16] reported only 16 additional cases, of which 13 were described as "idiopathic." Our finding of 22 cases associated specifically with GH therapy seems large in this context. In addition, gynecomastia was first detected in 63% of the cases in the first 6 months of therapy; the lack of an even time distribution suggests that this association is drug related and that it is more commonly seen soon after GH is initially given. We have not identified any reports of premature thelarche in prepubertal girls treated with GH.

Although our findings indicate that the course of GH-induced gynecomastia in prepubertal boys is time limited and benign, breast examinations should be performed routinely in patients receiving GH.

REFERENCES

1. Nydick M, Bustos J, Dale J, Rawson RW. Gynecomastia in adolescent boys. JAMA 1961;178:449-54.
2. Haibach H, Rosebholtz MJ. Prepubertal gynecomastia with lobules and acini: a case report and review of the literature. Am J Clin Pathol 1983;80:252-5.
3. Hemsell DL, Edman CD, Marks JF, Siiteri PK, MacDonald PC. Massive extraglandular aromatization of plasma androstenedione resulting in feminization of a prepubertal boy. J Clin Invest 1977;60:455-64.
4. Payne AH, Perkins LM, Giorgiou M, Quinn PG. Intratesticular aromatase site of activity and possible function of testicular estradiol. Steroids 1987;50:435-48.
5. Brodie A, Inkster S. Aromatase in the human testis. J Steroid Biochem Mol Biol 1993;44:549-55.

6. Bhettay E, Bonnici F. Pure oestrogen-secreting feminizing adrenocortical adenoma. Arch Dis Child 1977;52:241-3.
7. Edidin DV. Prepubertal gynecomastia associated with estrogen-containing hair cream. Am J Dis Child 1982;136:587-8.
8. Braunstein GD. Gynecomastia. N Engl J Med 1993;328:490-505.
9. Rudman D, Feller AG, Cohn L, Shetty KR, Rudman IW, Draper MW. Effects of human growth hormone in body composition in elderly men. Horm Res 1991;36(suppl 1):73-81.
10. Matucci Cerinic M. Response of hypertrophic osteoarthropathy to drugs inhibiting growth hormone [Letter]. J Reumathol 1984; 11:865-6.
11. Goodman HG, Grumbach MM, Kaplan SL. Growth and growth hormone. II. A comparison of isolated growth hormone deficiency and multiple pituitary-hormone deficiency in 35 patients with idiopathic pituitary dwarfism. N Engl J Med 1968; 278:57-68.
12. Biro FM, Lucky AW, Huster GA, Morrison JA. Hormonal studies and physical maturation in adolescent gynecomastia. J Pediatr 1990;116:450-5.
13. Murphy LJ, Murphy LC, Stead B, Sutherland RL, Lazarus L. Modulation of lactogenic receptors by progestins in cultured human breast cancer cells. J Clin Endocrinol Metab 1986;62:280-7.
14. Fradkin JE, Eastman RC, Lesniak MA, Roth J. Specificity spillover at the hormone receptor: exploring its role in human disease. N Engl J Med 1989;320:640-5.
15. Rosen N, Yee D, Lippman ME, Paik S, Cullen KJ. Insulin-like growth factors in human breast cancer. Breast Cancer Res Treat 1991;18:S55-62.
16. Descamps H, Chaussain JL, Job JC. Les gynecomasties du garcon avant la puberte. Arch Fr Pediatr 1985;42:87-9.

New books received

Toxicologic emergencies. 5th ed.
Goldfrank LR et al. Norwalk, Connecticut: Appleton & Lange, 1994. 1589 pages. $175.

Down syndrome: successful parenting of children with Down syndrome
Unruh JF. Eugene, Oregon: Fern Ridge Press, 1994. 120 pages. $13.95.

Viral infections of the gastrointestinal tract. 2nd ed.
Kapikian AZ, ed. New York: Marcel Dekker, 1994. 785 pages. $195.

Exercise and children's health
Rowland TW. Champaign, Illinois: Human Kinetics, 1990. 368 pages. $29.50.

Pediatric telephone medicine. 2nd ed.
Brown J. Philadelphia: JB Lippincott, 1994. 320 pages. $29.95.

Neonatology: management, procedures, on-call problems, diseases and drugs. 3rd ed.
Gomella TC, ed. Norwalk, Connecticut: Appleton & Lange, 1994. 620 pages. $24.95.

Pediatric psychooncology
Bearison DJ, Mulhern RK, eds. New York: Oxford University Press, 1994. 247 pages. $45.

Practitioner's guide to developmental and psychological testing
Aylward GP. New York: Plenum, 1994. 258 pages. $37.50.

Sickle cell disease: basic principles and clinical practice
Embury SH, Hebbel RP, Mohandas N, Steinberg MH, eds. New York: Raven Press, 1994. 928 pages. $145.

Respiratory illness in children. 4th ed.
Phelan P. Boston: Blackwell, 1994. 414 pages. $125.

Learning and memory
Anderson JR. New York: John Wiley & Sons, 1995. 488 pages. $39.95.

Fever in paediatric practice
El-Radhi AS. Boston: Blackwell, 1994. 258 pages. $49.95.

Pediatric trauma: initial assessment and management
Ford EG, Andrassy RJ. Philadelphia: WB Saunders, 1994. 416 pages. $59.

Clinical biochemistry and the sick child. 2nd ed.
Clayton BE, Round JM, eds. Boston: Blackwell, 1994. 555 pages. $160.

Coping in young children
Zeitlin S, Williamson GG. Baltimore: Paul H. Brookes, 1994. 309 pages. $36.

Maternal-fetal toxicology. 2nd ed.
Koren G, ed. New York: Marcel Dekker, 1994. 821 pages. $175.

Leukocyte-depleted blood products
Lane TA, Myllyla G, eds. Basel: Karger, 1994. 150 pages. $137.75.

Pediatric nephrology
Drukker A, Gruskin AB. Basel: Karger, 1994. 242 pages. $219.25.

Child abuse and neglect: a clinician's handbook
Hobbs CJ, Hanks HGI, Wynne JM. Edinburgh, Scotland: Churchill Livingstone, 1993. 325 pages. $79.95.

Otoendoscopically guided surgery
Thomassin J. Paris: Springer-Verlag France, 1994. 128 pages. $77.

Your child and health care
Rosenfeld LR. Baltimore: Paul H. Brookes, 1994. 576 pages. $25.

A three-month-old girl with fever and hepatomegaly

V. Faye Jones, MD, and John J. Buchino, MD

From the Departments of Pediatrics and Pathology, University of Louisville School of Medicine and Kosair Children's Hospital, Louisville, Kentucky

CASE PRESENTATION

A 3-month-old black girl was admitted to Kosair Children's Hospital with a 3-day history of fever and "congestion." Diarrhea developed and she became increasingly irritable. She had been treated by her physician initially for bilateral otitis media with amoxicillin. On the evening of admission she became lethargic, and her temperature spiked to 40.9° C. She was taken to Kosair Children's Hospital Emergency Department for evaluation.

Further history obtained on admission revealed the infant to be the product of an uncomplicated term pregnancy, labor, and delivery. Transient hyperbilirubinemia developed during the neonatal period and resolved without treatment. There was no history of serious illness or hospitalization. The family history was unremarkable except for an upper respiratory infection in a sibling 2 weeks before the patient's admission to the hospital. The patient had five normal siblings.

Physical examination on admission to the hospital revealed a 3-month-old black girl who was arousable and active but in mild to moderate respiratory distress. Vital signs were as follows: temperature 40.9° C; heart rate 184 beats/min; respirations 46 breaths/min; blood pressure 136/78 mm Hg; and weight 6 kg. The skin was slightly dry but had no rashes or discoloration. Findings of examination of the head, eyes, nose, throat, and neck were within normal limits. The tympanic membranes were erythematous with decreased mobility. Auscultation of the chest revealed scattered basilar rhonchi. The heart had a normal sinus rhythm. The abdomen was distended. The liver was palpable 2 cm below the right costal margin. A large, reducible umbilical hernia was present. Genital and neurologic findings were normal.

Submitted for publication Nov. 28, 1994; accepted Nov. 28, 1994.

Reprint requests: John J. Buchino, MD, Chief of Pathology, Kosair Children's Hospital, PO Box 35070, Louisville, KY 40232.

THE JOURNAL OF PEDIATRICS 1995;126:663-8

0022-3476/95/$3.00 + 0 **9/32/62355**

Results of laboratory studies included a hemoglobin concentration of 93 gm/L; hematocrit value 0.27; and leukocyte count 10.3×10^9/L, with 0.06 neutrophils, 0.24 band forms, 0.60 lymphocytes, 0.01 monocytes, and 0.09 atypical lymphocytes. The platelet count was 35×10^9/L. Serum chemical values included the following: sodium 130 mmol/L; potassium 5.3 mmol/L; chloride 112 mmol/L; bicarbonate 11 mmol/L; blood urea nitrogen 6.43 mmol urea/L (18 mg/dl); and glucose 3.89 mmol/L (70 mg/dl). Arterial blood gas studies while the patient was breathing room air revealed the pH to be 7.3; partial pressure of oxygen 106 mm Hg; partial pressure of carbon dioxide 15 mm Hg; and bicarbonate 7 mmol/L, with a base excess of −17.9 mmol/L. Prothrombin time was 17 seconds, and partial thromboplastin time was 82.5 seconds. Protamine sulfate test results were negative. Fibrin split products were >10 mg/L. Cerebrospinal fluid examination showed 0.1×10^6/L (10 leukocytes/mm^3), (0.4 monocytes, 0.6 neutrophils), with a protein concentration of 300 mg/L (30 mg/dl) and glucose 3.11 mmol/L (56 mg/dl). A chest roentgenogram was interpreted as normal. Results of blood, urine, and cerebrospinal fluid cultures were negative. The impression of the patient's condition on admission was (1) probable sepsis with diffuse intravascular coagulation, (2) possible pneumonia with respiratory insufficiency, and (3) metabolic acidosis.

CD	Cluster designation
CMV	Cytomegalovirus
EBV	Epstein-Barr virus
HSV	Herpes simplex virus

The infant was admitted to the pediatric intensive care unit. Antibiotic therapy with ampicillin and chloramphenicol was begun. She was also given 2 units of random donor platelets and fresh-frozen plasma at 10 ml/kg per dose. On the next morning, the physical examination showed increasing hepatomegaly to 9 cm below the right costal margin, and splenomegaly of 7.5 cm below the left costal margin. Another complete blood cell count revealed a leukocyte count of $19.2 \times 10^9/L$, with 0.03 juvenile forms, 0.29 band forms, 0.11 neutrophils, 0.40 lymphocytes, 0.08 monocytes, and 0.09 atypical lymphocytes. Hemoglobin concentration and hematocrit values were 66 gm/L and 0.17, respectively. The platelet count was $99 \times 10^9/L$. The bicarbonate level was 11 mmol/L and the glucose level was 1.1 mmol/L (20 mg/dl). Other test results included the following: alanine aminotransferase 988 U/L; aspartate aminotransferase 270 U/L; total bilirubin 73.5 μmol/L (4.3 mg/dl); conjugated bilirubin 27.4 μmol/L (1.6 mg/dl); total protein 43 gm/L; albumin 31 gm/L; ammonia 301.3 μmol/L (422 μg/L); and fibrin split products >40 mg/L. Protamine sulfate test results were positive. Results of a spot urine test for vanillylmandelic acid were within normal limits. Serum lactic acid was 3.27 mmol/L (29.5 mg/dl) with a cerebrospinal fluid level of 4.9 mmol/L (44.1 mg/dl). Bone marrow aspirate had no neuroblastoma or leukemic infiltrate. Arterial blood gas studies revealed pH 7.11; partial pressure of oxygen 39 mm Hg; partial pressure of carbon dioxide 31 mm Hg; and bicarbonate 9 mmol/L. An additional chest roentgenogram showed mild perihilar infiltrates in the right lung. Ultrasound examination of the abdomen revealed marked hepatomegaly and splenomegaly without focal abnormalities.

The patient's condition continued to deteriorate, requiring tracheal intubation. Gentamicin and 20% dextrose were added to her therapy. She continued to require fresh frozen plasma; in addition, she was given packed erythrocytes. Despite therapy, pulmonary and gastrointestinal bleeding developed. Continuing hypoglycemia required frequent glucose infusions. On the afternoon of the second hospital day, the patient became hypotensive, and inotropic therapy with dopamine and dobutamine was provided. Later that evening a total exchange transfusion was performed. Ten minutes later the patient had a cardiopulmonary arrest. Efforts to revive her were unsuccessful.

CLINICAL FINDINGS AND DISCUSSION

DR. JONES: In summary, our patient, a 3-month-old black girl, was seen in the emergency department with fever and congestion. She was noted to be arousable and active but in moderate respiratory distress. She was admitted to the hospital; her course was marked by progressive hepatosplenomegaly, liver failure, coagulopathy, and hypoglycemia. She died within 24 hours. The differential diagnosis of this child's condition can be divided into four general categories: infectious, inflammatory, metabolic, and neoplastic disorders.

In a 3-month-old child, infectious disease is a primary consideration. The duration and severity of her illness suggest overwhelming sepsis with a bacterial infection. However, we are given no information about other predisposing factors such as sickle cell anemia or an inherited immunodeficiency. The three most common pathogens for this age group are *Streptococcus pneumoniae*, *Neisseria meningitidis*, and *Haemophilus influenzae*.[1-3] Each has its peak occurrence in children less than 2 years of age. Although these organisms can cause respiratory symptoms and progressive liver failure, splenomegaly would be unusual. It would also be unusual to have negative results on blood, urine, and cerebrospinal fluid cultures with the degree of illness that our patient exhibited.

One must also consider endemic organisms as a cause of acute infection. In Kentucky, histoplasmosis is an endemic organism affecting 90% of the population by age 20 years.[4] It is caused by *Histoplasma capsulatum* and can occur in three forms. Asymptomatic primary infection is the most common, occurring in about 50% of persons infected. Symptomatic, acute pulmonary histoplasmosis typically is manifested as an influenza-like illness of abrupt onset of fever, myalgia, headache, and mild hepatosplenomegaly. The most serious type is disseminated histoplasmosis, which typically affects infants, young children, and persons with immunosuppression. It begins as an acute pulmonary infection with fever, cough, and dyspnea, and then quickly progresses to involve multiple organ systems. Physical examination may reveal rales, diffuse lymphadenopathy, and hepatosplenomegaly; a roentgenogram of the chest may show abnormalities—typically, diffuse interstitial pneumonia. Patients eventually have disseminated intravascular coagulopathy and gastrointestinal bleeding.[5] This child's lack of exposure, absence of lymphadenopathy, and inconsistent chest roentgenogram speak against disseminated histoplasmosis as a cause of death. Further, histiocytes containing the organism are usually evident on bone marrow examination.

Hepatosplenomegaly can also be caused by viral infections. Acquired infection with cytomegalovirus is usually asymptomatic. However, pneumonia, hepatitis with mild hepatic enlargement, protracted mild diarrhea, and petechial rashes may occur when CMV infection is acquired in infancy or childhood. Splenomegaly more typically occurs in older children and adults.[6] The course of illness is not as fulminant as this case.

Infection with Epstein-Barr virus can cause some of the problems found in our patient. Liver enlargement occurs in approximately one third of the patients infected; elevation of enzyme activities occurs in up to 80%. Splenomegaly is found in about half of the patients, though extension to 2 to 3 cm below the costal margin, rather than massive enlargement, is the rule. Other findings common in children include neutropenia, thrombocytopenia, and nonspecific respiratory disease. However, the majority of patients acutely infected with EBV have pharyngitis and lymphadenopathy, posterior cervical most often, but other nodal groups can be affected.[7] Therefore I would eliminate both CMV and EBV infection from further consideration.

Disseminated herpes simplex virus infection must be considered in the differential diagnosis of this patient's condition. It typically causes fever and mucocutaneous involvement, though skin lesions are not a prerequisite of infection. Generally, there is involvement of the liver, lungs, spleen, adrenal glands, kidneys, marrow, and usually the brain. This ultimately leads to hepatitis, pneumonitis, shock, disseminated intravascular coagulopathy, and bleeding, with death occurring within days or weeks. Laboratory data can show pancytopenia, elevation of liver function values, hypoglycemia, and cerebral spinal fluid pleocytosis. This potentially lethal form of disease usually occurs in patients who are in the first 3 to 4 weeks of life, malnourished, or immunosuppressed. There was no history of exposure to HSV.[8] Thus HSV infection would be an unlikely cause of infection.

Reye syndrome must be considered in a child who has a change in consciousness, elevated aminotransferase values, metabolic acidosis, and hypoglycemia. The typical history is of a child with a preceding viral infection treated with aspirin who appears to be recovering, and then has the sudden onset of emesis, followed by confusion and deterioration of liver function, which results in elevation of alanine and aspartate aminotransferases to twice normal concentrations and elevation of ammonia levels. Although Reye syndrome can affect all ages, it is rare in children less than 2 years of age. Splenomegaly and pneumonia are not the typical findings for this illness, and our patient had no history of aspirin ingestion.[9]

Because an obvious infectious cause cannot be well fitted with the clinical findings, a noninfectious cause should be explored. Collagen vascular diseases such as systemic lupus erythematosus and systemic juvenile rheumatoid arthritis can produce hepatosplenomegaly, pneumonia, and anemia. However, the incidence of these diseases is extremely low before 5 years of age, and they usually have an insidious onset. In addition, rash and arthritis are common findings for each disease process, and they were not present in our patient.[10, 11]

Metabolic disorders frequently have their clinical onset in infancy. Glycogen storage disease type IV usually becomes symptomatic in the first year of life, with failure to thrive and hepatosplenomegaly. The hepatic disease is progressive, with the development of cirrhosis and ascites; death occurs during early childhood.[12] Other metabolic diseases include fructose-1,6-diphosphatase deficiency and disorders of amino acid metabolism. Hypoglycemia, acidosis, and hepatomegaly are the principal hallmarks of these disorders, but splenomegaly and hematopoietic disorders are not typical.[13] A recently described constellation of abnormalities are the fatty acid oxidation defects. Children with these defects can have a Reye-like syndrome with hepatomegaly, acidosis, elevated serum ammonia values, and increased aminotransferase activity.[14] Again, splenomegaly and blood dyscrasias are not typical. Although metabolic disorders can mimic almost any pediatric disease, the absence of any prior nutritional difficulties and the child's overall health status make metabolic disorders seem less likely.

Anemia, thrombocytopenia, and hepatosplenomegaly could be caused by a neoplastic process. In this age group, congenital leukemia, neuroblastoma, lymphoma, and histiocytoses should be considered. Congenital leukemia accounts for fewer than 1% of childhood cancers. The disease usually is characterized by cutaneous infiltration, hemorrhage, and a high leukocyte count, and is often associated with a chromosome abnormality. The most common are Down syndrome, Turner syndrome, mosaic trisomy 9, and mosaic monosomy 7.[15] Our patient had none of these characteristics, and results of bone marrow aspiration were negative. Neuroblastoma is one of the most common tumors found in childhood; approximately 50% of patients are less than 2 years of age at the time of diagnosis.[16] Increased amounts of vanillylmandelic acid are found in about 90% of patients. Bone marrow involvement is expected, with extensive disease, as in our patient.

Lymphoma is the third most common cancer in children in the United States. It is divided into two broad categories: Hodgkin disease and non-Hodgkin lymphoma. Hodgkin disease is more common in older children and adolescents. The most common initial finding is the presence of enlarged, asymptomatic cervical or supraclavicular lymph nodes. Usually the lymph node has a "rubbery" consistency. Approximately 30% of patients will have systemic symptoms including fever, night sweats, and weight loss. Hepatosplenomegaly may be present. Bone marrow involvement results in neutropenia, thrombocytopenia, and anemia.[17, 18] Although this girl had some features of this disease, her age and lack of lymphadenopathy make Hodgkin disease unlikely.

Non-Hodgkin lymphoma is more common in younger children. Erythrophagocytic T-gamma lymphoma has been reported to cause fever, hepatosplenomegaly, anemia, thrombocytopenia, and hyperbilirubinemia, but lymphadenopathy is a common feature.[18, 19] In this category of lymphoma, a solid tumor mass is generally found. It was not apparent in our patient.

We are left with an unusual type of disease—the histiocytic syndromes, which result from the proliferation of cells

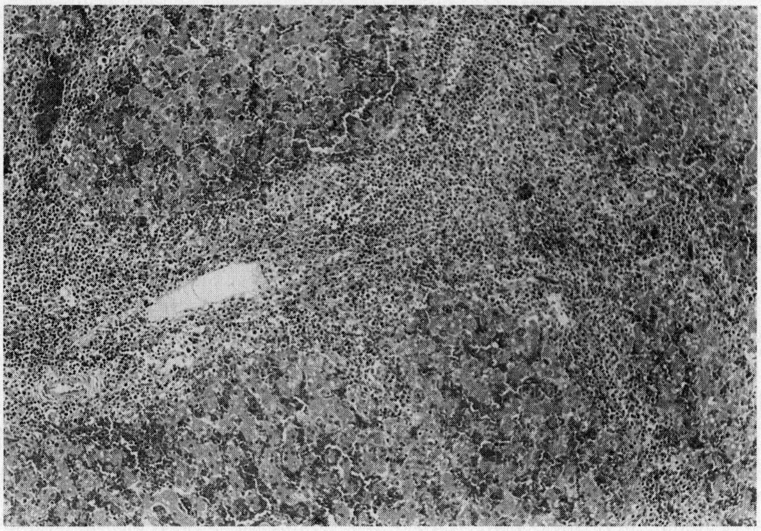

Fig. 1. Low-power photomicrograph of liver, showing marked periportal cellular infiltrate. (Hematoxylin-eosin stain; ×100.)

of the mononuclear phagocytic system. As pediatricians, we are familiar with class I histiocytosis—histiocytosis X, or Langerhans cell histiocytosis. Historically, it has been divided into three subgroups on the basis of the location of the lesions: eosinophilic granuloma, Hand-Schüller-Christian disease, and Letterer-Siwe syndrome. Recently Willman et al.[20] presented evidence that Langerhans cell histiocytosis is a clonal neoplastic disorder with highly variable biologic behavior. The disseminated form of Langerhans cell histiocytosis mainly affects infants and is rapidly progressive. It primarily affects soft tissues with only minimal or no bone involvement. Skin involvement is common, seborrheic dermatitis predominating. Lymphadenopathy occurs in 50% of affected individuals. Chest roentgenograms typically have the appearance of miliary tuberculosis. Anemia, thrombocytopenia, and hepatosplenomegaly are common features of disseminated disease.[21] The lack of skin involvement, absence of lymphadenopathy, and a normal chest roentgenogram, in light of the severity of our patient's illness, makes disseminated Langerhans cell histiocytosis unlikely.

The class II histiocytoses involve the antigen-processing type of mononuclear phagocyte. Familial erythrophagocytic lymphohistiocytosis, an inherited autosomal-recessive disease, and infection-associated hemophagocytic syndrome are the most common entities in this category. Each of them is characterized by a striking erythrophagocytosis, not identified in our patient.[22]

Malignant histiocytosis (class III histiocytosis) is a nonhereditary process of the histiocytic line. It occurs in all decades of life, though rarely before 1 year of age. It can produce a fulminant systemic disease, or it can be localized in a lymph node or an extranodal site. In 96% of patients, fever is the initial symptom. The majority of patients also have hepatosplenomegaly and respiratory symptoms. Chest roentgenograms may demonstrate a bilateral reticulonodular interstitial pneumonitis.[23]

Laboratory data typically reveal anemia, granulocytopenia, and thrombocytopenia. Bone marrow involvement has been reported in only approximately 25% of patients at initial diagnosis. Hyperbilirubinemia and elevated aminotransferase activities are common. Usually there is increasing liver dysfunction with elevation in the prothrombin and partial thrompoplastin times and in serum ammonia levels. Hypoglycemia and disseminated intravascular coagulopathy occur as the liver continues to fail.[23, 24] There is a high fatality rate in untreated cases. I conclude that this girl's clinical findings, laboratory data, and radiographic findings are most consistent with an infiltrative neoplastic process, malignant histiocytosis being the most likely clinical diagnosis.

Clinical diagnosis: *Malignant histiocytosis*

PATHOLOGIC FINDINGS AND DISCUSSION

Dr. Adams: This child's initial antibiotic therapy included ampicillin and chloramphenicol. Use of this antibiotic combination in this hospital allows us to estimate that this patient was probably seen sometime before the use of third-generation cephalosporins became common in the 1980s.

Dr. Buchino: Dr. Adams is correct. This is an old case, dating back to early 1984. So I will tell you what we thought then and how things have evolved during the past 10 years.

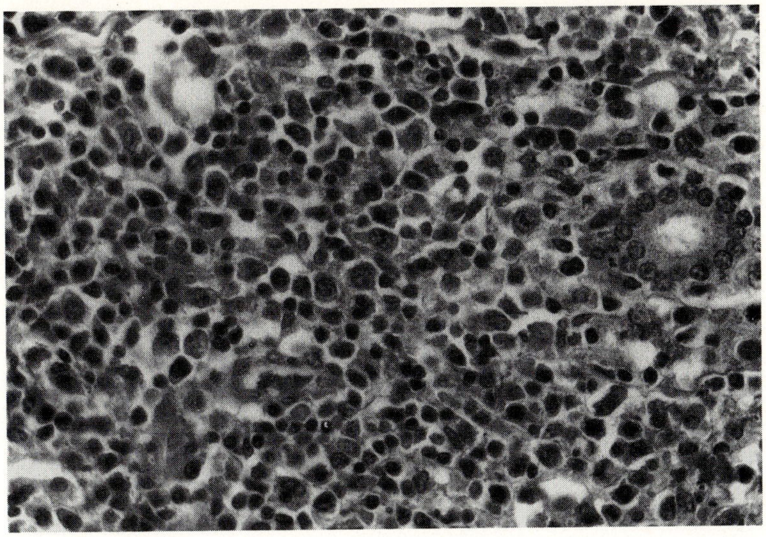

Fig. 2. High magnification of hepatic cellular infiltrate. Cells are characterized by large but variable-sized nuclei, which were generally hyperchromatic. Immunoperoxidase staining characterized them as T cell in origin. (Hematoxylin-eosin stain; ×400.)

A complete autopsy was performed. Significant findings at the time of gross examination included a markedly enlarged liver and spleen, each of which was approximately three times the expected weight for a child of this age. Additionally, the kidneys and lungs were significantly heavier than expected. Focal lesions were not present in any of these organs.

Microscopic examination revealed a distinct cellular infiltrate in the liver, spleen, kidneys, and lymph nodes. The infiltrate in the liver was perhaps most striking in that it predominantly involved the portal regions, but scattered foci were present in mid-zonal and central lobular areas as well (Fig. 1). These infiltrates were characterized by cells having moderately pleomorphic, hyperchromatic nuclei ranging from approximately half the size to slightly larger than a hepatic cell nucleus (Fig. 2). Nuclear infolding was common. The larger cells had abundant eosinophilic cytoplasm that was occasionally vacuolated. Immunoperoxidase staining at that time was positive for lysozyme. Similar findings characterized the infiltrates noted in the spleen, kidneys, and lymph nodes.

Microscopic examination of the lungs failed to reveal the presence of infiltrative disease. Rather, marked, diffuse alveolar damage was present with hyaline membrane formation. Moderate pulmonary congestion was noted as well. I interpret these pulmonary findings as being a result of this patient's shock.

Bone marrow sections contained a few scattered clusters of abnormal cells amid normal hematopoietic elements. On the basis of the patient's clinical course and morphologic findings, we originally concluded that a diagnosis of malignant histiocytosis was warranted.

However, since that time, several advances have taken place that allow us to define entities such as this more precisely. One important advance was the advent of immunophenotyping of leukocytes based on cell-surface antigens characteristic of mature leukocytes and their various precursors. The process of defining monoclonal antibodies for leukocytes was initially confusing because independent laboratories were producing new monoclonal antibodies, each with its own nomenclature and no uniform method of confirming specificity. Fortunately, after four international workshops, some 2000 monoclonal antibodies have been categorized according to their specificity for human leukocyte surface antigens. Approximately 80 monoclonal antibody categories, or cluster designations (CDs), have resulted.[25]

Using immunohistochemistry techniques, I recently tested liver tissue from this case for a battery of CD antigens. The infiltrative cells were negative for CD68 (a histiocyte-macrophage marker), CD30 (a Reed-Sternberg cell–associated marker), CD20 (a B-cell marker), and peanut agglutinin (a Langerhans cell marker). In contrast, there was marked positive staining for common leukocyte antigen and CD45RO (a T-cell marker). On the basis of these findings, I conclude that the cell of origin in the infiltrative process was not a histiocyte but, rather, a T cell. This finding is similar to that of others who have retrospectively evaluated cases initially diagnosed as malignant histiocytosis.[26] Several such cases have been reclassified, often, but not exclusively, as T cell in origin. It now appears that true malignant histiocytosis is extremely rare.

A reasonable question that arises is whether this disease should be called a leukemia or a lymphoma. The former implies a bone marrow origin, so the designation of leukemia does not seem appropriate. On the other hand the term *lymphoma* typically implies a tumoral mass and does not quite fit, either. Therefore I prefer the term *T-cell disease*.

Another question that can be raised is whether or not this disease was a true malignancy. Certainly from a clinical standpoint it behaved in a malignant fashion, but the possibility remains that the patient's condition resulted from an exaggerated immune response. Gene rearrangement techniques might help to answer this question by proving a monoclonal cell origin. Unfortunately, we are not able to perform those tests at this time.

"Final" anatomic diagnosis: *Malignant T-cell disease*

REFERENCES

1. Davidson M, Schrader CD, Parkinson AJ, Campbell JF, Facklam RR, Wainwright RB. Invasive pneumococcal disease in an Alaska native population, 1980 through 1986. JAMA 1989;261:715-8.
2. Wong VK, Hitchcock W, Mason WH. Meningococcal infections in children: a review of 100 cases. Pediatr Infect Dis J 1989;8:224-7.
3. Dajani AS, Asmar BI, Thirumoorthi MC. Systemic *Haemophilus influenzae* disease: an overview. J PEDIATR 1979; G4:355-64.
4. Medoff G, Kobayashi GS. Histoplasmosis. In: Feigin RO, Cherry JD, eds. Textbook of pediatric infectious diseases; vol 2. 2nd ed. Philadelphia: WB Saunders, 1987:1974-6.
5. Weinberg GA, Kleiman MB, Grosfeld JL, Weber TR, Wheat LJ. Unusual manifestations in histoplasmosis in childhood. Pediatrics 1983;72:99-105.
6. Starr SE. Cytomegalovirus. Pediatr Clin North Am 1979;26: 283-93.
7. Sumaya CV, Ench Y. Epstein-Barr virus infectious mononucleosis in children. I. Clinical and general laboratory findings. Pediatrics 1985;75:1003-10.
8. Kohl S. Postnatal herpes simplex virus. In: Oski F, De Angelis CD, Feigin RD, McMillan JA, Warshaw JB, eds. Principles and practice of pediatrics. 2nd ed. Philadelphia: JB Lippincott, 1994: 1319-30.
9. Berman S. Reye's syndrome/metabolic disorders. In: Berman S, ed. Pediatric decision making. 2nd ed. Philadelphia: BC Decker, 1991:340-1.
10. Ramirez-Seijas F, Cepero-Akselrad A. Systemic lupus erythematosus in children. Int Pediatr 1993;8:334-43.
11. Ostrov BE, Goldsmith DP, Athreya BH. Differentiation of systemic juvenile rheumatoid arthritis from acute leukemia near the onset of disease. J PEDIATR 1993;122:595-8.
12. Ward JC. Inborn errors of metabolism of acute onset in infancy. Pediatr Rev 1990;11:205-16.
13. Gruppuso PA, Schwartz R. Hypoglycemia in children. Pediatr Rev 1989;11:117-24.
14. Hale DE, Bennett MJ. Fatty acid oxidation disorders: a new class of metabolic disease. J PEDIATR 1992;121:1-11.
15. Lanzkowsky P, ed. Manual of pediatric hematology and oncology. New York: Churchill Livingstone, 1989:217-50, 303-14.
16. Lopez-Ibor B, Schwartz AD. Neuroblastoma. Pediatr Clin North Am 1985;32:755-78.
17. Windebank KP, Gilchrist GS. Hodgkin disease. Pediatr Ann 1988;17:204-23.
18. Link MP, Donaldson SS. The lymphomas and lymphadenopathy. In: Nathan DG, Osk FF, eds. Hematology of infancy and childhood; vol 2. 4th ed. Philadelphia: WB Saunders, 1992: 1319-53.
19. Kadin ME, Kamoun M, Lamberg J. Erythrophagocytic T-gamma lymphoma: a clinicopathologic entity resembling malignant histiocytosis. N Engl J Med 1981;304:648-53.
20. Willman CL, Busque L, Griffith BB, et al. Langerhans' cell histiocytosis (histiocytosis X): a clonal proliferative disease. N Engl J Med 1994;331:154-60.
21. Osband ME, Pochedly C. Histiocytosis X: an overview. Hematol Oncol Clin North Am 1987;1(1):1-7.
22. Perry MC, Harrison EG, Burgert EO, Gilchrist GS. Familial erythrophagocytic lymphohistiocytosis. Cancer 1976;38:209-18.
23. Zucker JM, Caillaut JM, Vanel D, Gerard-Marchant R. Malignant histiocytosis in childhood. Cancer 1980;45:315-26.
24. Jurco S, Starling K, Hawkins EP. Malignant histiocytosis in childhood. Hum Pathol 1983;14:1059-65.
25. Jasani B, Schmid KW. Immunocytochemistry in diagnostic histopathology. New York: Churchill Livingstone, 1993:36.
26. Schnitzer B, Roth MS, Hyder DM, Ginsburg D. Ki-1 lymphomas in children. Cancer 1988;61:1213-21.

Reacting to a suggestion, the Editorial Board of THE JOURNAL made a decision in 1992 to publish a series of "profiles" of American pediatricians whose careers began in the 1920s and 1930s, whose contributions had been seminal, and who were no longer alive. The profiles were to be written by a colleague or student who knew the subject well. These publications replicated an initiative of THE JOURNAL in the 1950s, when 30 such men (all selected from that era were men) were profiled, covering the origins of American pediatrics.* The new series was initially limited to 14 individuals, 12 men and 2 women, selected through ballot by a group of senior pediatricians.

The response to this series has been positive. We have therefore extended the list to another 14 pediatricians: 10 men and 4 women. It is safe to predict that should there be another series some years from now, the proportion of women will be 50% or more. As before, the judgment of the seven senior pediatricians who served as the newest selection committee may differ from that of at least some readers, whose preferences have equal standing. All will surely agree, however, that each of those selected played an important role in bringing American pediatrics to its present eminent stature—some by serving as departmental leaders, some by elegant, innovative research, and some by founding a subspecialty within pediatrics.

We hope that all our readers will enjoy reading these offerings, which have been generously and enthusiastically submitted for publication. Some of you will be first learning of the origins of our present knowledge and development; others will be reveling in pleasant nostalgia. We would appreciate knowing your reaction to the whole series. After these profiles, the next group probably should not be chosen for another 15 to 20 years.—*Laurence Finberg, MD, Guest Editor*

We are very grateful to Dr. Finberg for continuing to organize and direct this effort to record the contributions of the leaders of American pediatrics. The willingness of the authors to undertake the task has been heartwarming, and we will continue to publish the profiles in the order in which they are received, at approximately bimonthly intervals.—*Joseph M. Garfunkel, MD, Editor*

Josef Warkany

Josef Warkany and I first met in 1956, when I had the misfortune to speak after he did to a group of social workers at the Children's Bureau (U.S. Department of Health, Education, and Welfare). His presentation sparkled with humor and interest, enhanced by his Viennese accent. We spoke on environmental causes of birth defects—5 years before the epidemic of thalidomide embryopathy occurred and at the same time that cerebral palsy was being caused by maternal ingestion, during pregnancy, of fish contaminated with methylmercury dumped as factory waste into Minamata Bay, Japan.

Josef Warkany (1902–1992) had to make his own way in teratology. Although congenital malformations had been described since ancient times, scientific study of their environmental causes was thought to be unpromising; the prevailing belief was that nothing beyond inheritance need be considered. He came to this subject by chance. After he received his medical degree from the University of Vienna in 1926, he had a 1-year residency at the Children's University Clinic, under Professor Clemens von Pirquet, the pioneer in immunology. He spent several years as an assistant at another children's hospital, where his laboratory research was on conventional subjects—vitamin D, calcium, and phosphorus. Next, he sought but did not find an academic position that combined clinical pediatrics with experimental research in Europe. When he learned of a 1-year research scholarship under Dr. A. Graeme Mitchell at the new Children's Hospital Research Foundation in Cincinnati, Ohio, he applied and was accepted. He arrived there in 1932. At the end of the year, during which he did more research on vitamin D, he was asked to become a permanent member of the staff. He was put in charge of an outpatient

*Veeder BS, ed. Pediatric profiles. St. Louis: CV Mosby, 1957.

THE JOURNAL OF PEDIATRICS 1995;126:669-72
9/20/60615

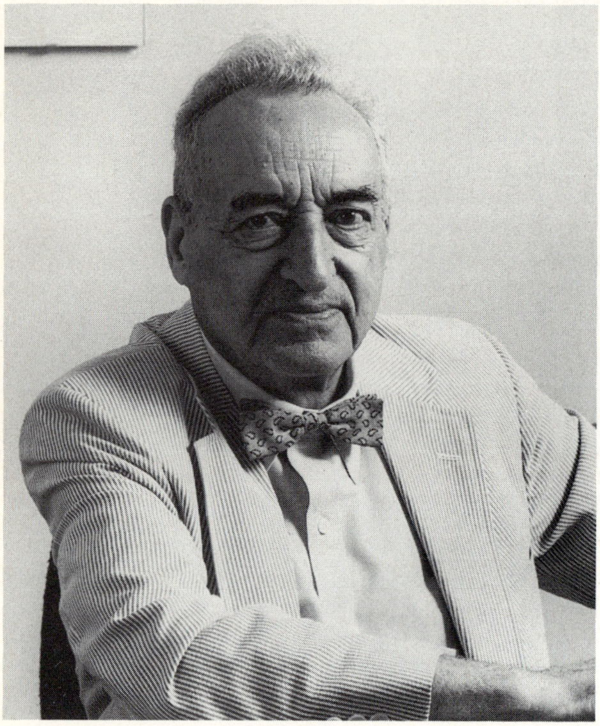

Josef Warkany

endocrine clinic, to which children with a variety of congenital malformations were referred. His curiosity about the cause of their malformations led him into this unexplored field of clinical and laboratory research.[1]

During World War I, he had gone as a teenager into remote valleys in Austria to buy food not available in Viennese shops. There he saw some strange dwarfs—endemic cretins who were children of goitrous mothers. Later, in Cincinnati, he began his experimental work in teratology with Rose Nelson[2] by trying to breed goitrous rats, using a goitrogenic diet that also caused rickets; to prevent rickets, vitamin D was added. The offspring were retarded in growth and maturation. After clearing the tissues of the young by immersing them in a solution that stains and shows the ossified skeleton (Schultz-Dawson method), Warkany and Nelson found that 43% had a specific array of bony malformations. When the experiment was repeated with the addition of dried pig liver to improve growth and maturation, the skeletal malformations did not occur. In place of the pig liver, various synthetic nutritional factors were added individually and in combination, until riboflavin was found to be the ingredient in pig liver that prevented the malformations.[3] Here was key evidence that congenital malformations could be caused by altering the environment. At about the same time, Norman Gregg showed that rubella infection during pregnancy was related to a malformation syndrome in the child.

Serendipity also led Warkany to the cause of acrodynia, sometimes called pink disease because of the color of the rash, which was accompanied by red hands and feet, signs of infection, and, at times, loss of hair, teeth, and jawbone. It was particularly prevalent in the southern United States, Australia, Switzerland, and England, but not in Cincinnati. On seeing such a patient in 1945, Warkany thought of poisoning by arsenic or thallium as a possible cause. The Kettering Laboratory of Applied Physiology was in a building next door, so he asked that the patient's urine be tested there for metals. The results were negative for arsenic and thallium but positive for mercury. It had come from calomel, teething powders, or ointments used to treat diaper rash or the mother's nipples.

In Great Britain doubts were raised about the new-found cause because a case-control study there showed no significant difference in mercury exposure in the groups with versus those without acrodynia. The authors referred to Warkany's claim as transatlantic madness, until it was pointed out that in Britain such exposure was so common that case subjects and control subjects had similar histories. Dose or diminished susceptibility apparently explained why the disease did not develop in some exposed children. British antilewisite (BAL) promoted elimination of mercury, the disappearance of disease, and the belief that mercury was the cause of the disease. Prevention followed, when mercury was eliminated in medications.

Warkany published a wonderful article, "Acrodynia: Postmortem of a Disease,"[4] a copy of which was sent by a friend to Berton Rouché, who wrote on medical mysteries for *The New Yorker*. In response to the suggestion that he adapt it for the magazine, Rouché wrote, "I might have tried if Dr. Warkany had not done it so well."

Until 1961, infants with birth weights less than 2500 gm were labeled as premature. In that year Warkany et al.[5] called attention to intrauterine growth retardation as a cause of smallness for gestational age, an observation so obvious that it is a wonder it was not made long before. His interest in growth-retarded children stimulated him to determine whether stunting existed before birth.

Warkany continued his experimental studies of congenital malformations throughout his career. Clinically his special interest was in the cause of mental retardation. He published material on anatomic abnormalities and on syndromes caused by cytogenetic abnormalities after techniques were developed for such studies. He wrote overviews for volumes of reports on mental retardation and developmental disabilities, and otherwise sowed seeds for others to cultivate.[6] As with any truly creative person, versatility was his hallmark.

In 1945, Year Book Medical Publishers invited him to write a book on congenital malformations within the next 2 years. He meticulously summarized his voluminous notes from index cards, added comments for each section, and submitted them for publication 25 years later. The 1309-page volume, *Congenital Malformations: Notes and Comments*,[7] covers the literature from the earliest history through 1970. Interest in the cause of congenital malformations was promoted when Warkany and Kalter[8, 9] published two-part reviews in *The New England Journal of Medicine* in 1961 and again in 1983.

Warkany was also a leader of four ad hoc conferences on congenital malformations held in 1956 to 1960. These conferences were forerunners of the Teratology Society, now in its thirty-fourth year, which he helped found and served as its first president. He and Virginia Apgar provided a special luster to its annual meetings.

When the question of drug safety arose in 1961 because of the epidemic of thalidomide-induced phocomelia abroad, he was a constant consultant to various health agencies, where he characteristically spoke with a voice of reason. In the mood of the times, he saw an opportunity to promote further interest in teratology through a series of workshops sponsored by drug manufacturers and other organizations. Four were held in the United States, one in Europe, and one in the Far East. All were fully subscribed and very successful.

In 1965 he was instrumental in procuring federal funds to establish the Institute for Developmental Research in its own new building as part of the (Cincinnati) Children's Hospital Research Foundation. The laboratories are devoted to research on mental retardation, brain malformations, and metabolic disorders associated with brain malfunction.

In the early 1960s Warkany brightened the institute's study section on human embryology and development. At a coffee break during a meeting in the Stone House at the National Institutes of Health, a group emerged from a neighboring meeting room. They had beards when beards were not yet in fashion. "Psychiatrists?" Joe was asked. "No", he said, "they spend a lot of time on each application, and I can tell you, they did not have beards when they went in there." At meetings, he improvised in response to questions: at a symposium on neurofibromatosis he was asked what he thought of the designation "neurocristopathy." He replied: "I don't know. I'm a 'neo-neurocristian.' "

He was often asked to keynote a meeting or to be the after-dinner speaker, and he excelled at this.[10] He kept improving on the theme "research then and now." In a favorite story he told how, when he started in Vienna, he was given one rabbit to study. In time the veins of the ear were destroyed by repeated venipunctures, and when he said, "Herr Professor, I need a rabbit," the professor's encouraging attitude changed to indignation as he said, "But you already have one."[11] Occasionally Joe referred to himself as a one-rabbit investigator. He cringed when people quoted *The New York Times* in describing him as the father of modern teratology.

On both his trips to Japan he grew quickly in the eyes of his hosts from a scientist known to them only by his works to the popular superstar of teratology. Once again it was the warmth of his personality and his quick wit that unified the group—he created a camaraderie between East and West far beyond the ordinary. In this situation, new to him and of short duration, his excellent qualities, scientific and personal, ignited enthusiasm for a previously neglected but important area of pediatrics.

Since childhood, Warkany had enjoyed drawing, etching, and painting. In Cincinnati, Dr. Mitchell, his chief, shared this hobby and introduced Joe to the local art club. The two men found etchers to teach them how to make drypoints and aquatints, which Joe produced throughout his life. His work, in the style of the Aschan school of American art,[12-15] was exhibited in one-man shows (where it often sold out) and in group shows that traveled nationally and abroad. His style of speech and writing live on in his 79-page autobiography.[1] Other short biographic sketches have been published,[6, 12-16] including one with Japanese perception and charm by Yasuko Nishimura,[15] daughter of the founder of modern teratology in Japan.

Joe Warkany received awards from the March of Dimes, from *Modern Medicine* (for distinguished achievement), and from societies for mental retardation, cerebral palsy, cleft palate, and hydrocephalus. He also received two honorary degrees (University of Illinois and Thomas Jefferson Medical College, Philadelphia). In pediatrics he was a triple-crown winner. He received all three major awards: Borden, Mead-Johnson, and Howland. The Howland Award must have been particularly gratifying because he was so atypical—he had been neither a department head nor a leader of mainstream pediatric research. It was a stirring sight to see him rise to accept the award.

Robert W. Miller, MD
National Cancer Institute, EPN-400
Bethesda, MD 20892-7360

Thanks to Steve Warkany for providing the photograph.

REFERENCES

1. Warkany J. Story of a teratologist. Issues Rev Teratol 1988; 4:1-79.
2. Warkany J, Nelson RC. Appearance of skeletal abnormalities in the offspring of rats reared on a deficient diet. Science 1940;92:383-4.
3. Warkany J, Schraffenberger E. Congenital malformations induced in rats by maternal nutritional deficiency. V. Effects of purified diet lacking riboflavin. Proc Soc Exp Biol Med 1943; 54:92-4.
4. Warkany J. Acrodynia: postmortem of a disease. Am J Dis Child 1966;112:147-56.
5. Warkany J, Monroe BB, Sutherland BS. Intrauterine growth retardation. Am J Dis Child 1961;102:249-79. [Citation classic: Current Contents, No. 49, December 3, 1979.]
6. Brent RL. Biography of Josef Warkany [with curriculum vitae]. Teratology 1982;25:137-51.
7. Warkany J. Congenital malformations: notes and comments. Chicago: Year Book Medical, 1971.
8. Warkany J, Kalter H. Congenital malformations. N Engl J Med 1961;265:993-1001, 1046-52.
9. Kalter H, Warkany J. Congenital malformations: etiologic factors and their role in prevention. N Engl J Med 1983; 308:424-31, 491-7.
10. Warkany J. Research then and now. In: Mulvihill JJ, Miller RW, Fraumeni JF Jr, eds. Genetics of human cancer. New York: Raven Press, 1977:483-8.
11. Warkany J. Acceptance of the Howland Award. Pediatr Res 1970;4:431-4.
12. Wertelecki W. Of dreaming on solid grounds and silent triumphs of one man: a story about Josef Warkany. Am J Med Genet 1989;33:522-36.
13. Cohen MM. Josef Warkany, 1902–1992: a personal remembrance. J Craniofac Genet Dev Biol 1994;14:1-6.
14. Wilson JG. Presentation of the Howland Award to Josef Warkany. Pediatr Res 1970;4:427-30.
15. Nishimura Y. Dr. Josef Warkany in Scarlet Oaks. Congenital Anomalies (Jpn) 1988;28:127-9.
16. Kalter H. Josef Warkany, 1902–1992. Teratology 1993;48:1-3.

ADDITIONAL PUBLICATIONS OF NOTE BY JOSEF WARKANY

Warkany J. Congenital malformations induced by maternal nutritional deficiency. J PEDIATR 1944;25:476-80.

Warkany J, Schraffenberger E. Congenital malformations induced by rats by roentgen rays. AJR Am J Roentgenol 1974;57:455-63.

Warkany J. Etiology of congenital malformations. Adv Pediatr 1947;2:1-63.

Warkany J, Hubbard DM. Mercury in the urine of children with acrodynia. Lancet 1948;1:829-30.

Warkany J. Congenital malformations induced by maternal dietary deficiency: experiments and their interpretation. The Harvey Lectures 1952–1953;48:89-109.

Kalter H, Warkany J. Experimental production of congenital malformations in mammals by metabolic procedure. Physiol Rev 1959;39:69-115.

Warkany J, Weinstein ED, Soukup SW, Rubinstein JH, Curless MC. Chromosome analysis in a children's hospital. Pediatrics 1964;33:290-305.

Warkany J. Syndromes. Am J Dis Child 1971;121:365-70.

Warkany J. History of teratology. In: Wilson JG, Fraser FC, eds. Handbook of teratology; vol 1. New York: Plenum, 1977:3-45.

Warkany J. Terathanasia. Teratology 1978;17:187-92.

Warkany J, Lemire R, Cohen MM Jr. Mental retardation and congenital malformations of the central nervous system. Chicago: Year Book Medical, 1981.

Warkany J. Prevention of congenital malformations. Curr Probl Pediatr 1983;13:1-26.

EDITORIAL CORRESPONDENCE

Motor and cognitive development in children with congenital hypothyroidism

To the Editor:

We appreciate the difficulty in conducting a long-term follow-up study of children with congenital hypothyroidism such as the one reported by Kooistra et al. (J PEDIATR 1994;124:903-9). The article concludes that hypothyroid children with low screening thyroxine (T_4) concentrations (<50 nmol/L), despite early treatment, are likely to have borderline intelligence and motor problems. If taken at face value, this implies that families with athyreotic children should be resigned to a less-than-optimal outcome. This is also disheartening news for the physician, especially if he or she is convinced that nothing can be done to prevent the cognitive and motor problems. However, before such a pessimistic (and self-defeating) attitude is allowed to overtake us, it is crucial to ask whether the children in the study were treated adequately.

A careful reading of the article shows that no data confirm the authors' statement of adequate T_4 replacement therapy. With the exception of the screening mean T_4 values, we can find no figures relative to T_4 and thyrotropin concentrations during the first year of life, when inadequate levels of circulating T_4 correlate significantly with poor developmental outcome.[1] Another disturbing issue was that the patients were examined only four times during the first year of life. Thus prolonged intervals of inadequate treatment might not have been detected for several months between examinations. Under such circumstances, it is not surprising that an athyreotic infant (deprived of any endogenous T_4) would fare considerably worse than the infant with a functioning ectopic thyroid gland. A single blood specimen obtained 1 week before testing of a 7½- or 9½-year-old child is an unreliable marker for adequacy of treatment during the first year of life.

We contend, on the basis of several studies,[2-4] that early and adequate treatment, including frequent monitoring, will ensure optimal outcome in all children with hypothyroidism, regardless of type.

We quote an earlier statement: "Physicians must be dissatisfied with less than normal performances by patients whose hypothyroidism was treated early as a result of neonatal screening."[5] To think otherwise could instill an air of futility in the management of such patients and thus result in a self-fulfilling prophecy.

Marvin L. Mitchell, MD
New England Regional Newborn Screening Program
State Laboratory Institute
Jamaica Plain, MA 02130

Robert Z. Klein, MD
Department of Pediatrics
Dartmouth Medical School
Lebanon, NH
9/35/62073

REFERENCES

1. New England Congenital Hypothyroidism Collaborative. Effects of neonatal screening for hypothyroidism: prevention of mental retardation by treatment before clinical manifestations. Lancet 1981;2:1095-8.
2. Illicki A, Larsson A. Psychomotor development of children with congenital hypothyroidism diagnosed by neonatal screening. Acta Paediatr Scand 1988;77:142-7.
3. Heyerdahl S. Follow-up study of hypothyroidism in Norway. In: Delange F, ed. Research in congenital hypothyroidism. New York: Plenum Press, 1989;298-9.
4. Dubuis JM, Richer F, Glorieux J, et al. Should all patients with congenital hypothyroidism (CH) be treated with 10-15 μg/kg/day of levothyroxine (T4)? [Abstract]. Pediatr Res 1994;572:98A.
5. New England Congenital Hypothyroidism Collaborative. Elementary school performance of children with congenital hypothyroidism. J PEDIATR 1990;116:27-32.

Reply

To the Editor:

Drs. Mitchell and Klein contend that early and adequate treatment will ensure optimal outcome in all children with hypothyroidism. Our observation that some patients with congenital hypothyroidism (CH) detected by neonatal screening have a less favorable cognitive and motor outcome is interpreted as disheartening news for physicians. Drs. Mitchell and Klein seem to have just one explanation: it cannot be the patient, so it must be the doctor, and they demand proof that our patients with CH were treated adequately.

We consider it a blessing that in the 1970s a group of North American investigators, among them Drs. Mitchell and Klein, showed that the devastating effects of CH are preventable by introducing neonatal mass screening. In those days it was thought that fetal hypothyroidism had little or no impact on cerebral development, because early-treated patients had such favorable outcomes. Moreover, it was thought that there was no significant maternal-fetal transfer of thyroid hormone, and it was argued that a fetus could develop properly even in the absence of any thyroid hormone. Now we know that thyroxine (T_4) passes the placenta, and we are aware of the devastating effects of maternal hypothyroidism on the developing central nervous system. The fetal brain needs thyroid hormone, although the questions of when and how much remain to be answered. It is hard to believe that the limited maternal supply of T_4 is sufficient in all cases of severe CH; we have demonstrated that T_4 levels in cord blood from infants with a complete inability to produce T_4 show considerable variation,[1] and that especially in severe CH, plasma T_4 concentrations decrease during the first few weeks after birth. In our opinion, one can hardly expect all children with CH to have completely normal motor skills and intelligence even when they are treated early and adequately.

In the Netherlands the neonatal thyroid screening was set up according to the American methods. Treatment criteria also fit well with the guidelines published by the New England Congenital Hypothyroidism Collaborative.[2] The Dutch health care system guarantees that every patient has access to the same quality of treatment and follow-up. There is no reason to believe that Dutch pediatricians provide less adequate care than their colleagues abroad.

The criteria that we used for scoring treatment compliance are provided in our article.[3] Hormone levels were measured frequently, with the interval increasing gradually from at least once a week to about once every 3 months after 1 year of age. On the basis of the hormone level readings, almost all patients received adequate long-term treatment. Some irregularities in the administration of T_4 may have occurred, but it is highly unlikely that such irregularities coincided preferentially with cases of severe CH.

The only way to determine the cerebral damage caused by fetal and neonatal hypothyroidism is to correlate the individual cognitive and motor outcome with data concerning severity and duration of the hypothyroid phase, and with other complicating factors. This requires etiologic classification of the study population. Many studies, in particular those of the New England Congenital Hypothyroidism Collaborative,[2, 4-6] have presented data only on the CH population as a whole. By including milder cases, such studies risk "diluting" the effects of the severe cases. Mitchell and Klein refer to three smaller studies to illustrate their contention that "early and adequate treatment, including frequent monitoring, will ensure optimal outcome in all children with hypothyroidism, regardless of type." One of these studies reports that at 6 years of age, 13 children with athyrosis had a mean IQ of 84, whereas 22 children with ectopic or hypoplastic glands had a mean IQ of 100.[7]

Two recent publications from the United Kingdom support our (unfortunate) results.[8, 9] Simons et al.[8] tested the IQs of patients with CH at about the same age as we did. Their subgroup of patients with very low pretreatment plasma T_4 concentrations (defined as $\leq$40 nmol/L) had a mean full-scale IQ 10 points below that of matched control subjects, and their subgroup of patients with moderately decreased pretreatment plasma T_4 levels (>40 nmol/L) had a mean full-scale IQ similar to that of the control group. Timing of the T_4 replacement therapy (23 ± 9 days [mean ± SD] for the Dutch patients with low neonatal T_4 levels,[3] 26 days [range, 10 to 40 days] for the British patients with low neonatal T_4 levels,[8] and 25 ± 15 days [mean ± SD] for the whole group of patients from New England [presumably slightly earlier for patients with severe CH])[5] cannot explain the differences in cognitive outcome. Although the Finnish screening program may be unique, enabling treatment to start at a median age of only 6 days, Virtanen et al.[10] concluded that some damage is inevitable and that its degree correlates with the severity of the [intrauterine] CH. Tillotson et al.[9] concluded that the severity of CH has a threshold effect on brain development, probably determined prenatally.

Physicians must accept the fact that some patients with CH already have some cerebral damage at the time of referral, because of exposure to very low T_4 levels prenatally or during the short interval between birth and referral. It is misleading to promise all parents beforehand a completely normal cognitive and motor development for their children. On the other hand, screening organizations should never rest in their attempts to reduce the time interval between birth and administration of the first dose of T_4 as much as possible.

Thomas Vulsma, MD, PhD
Department of Pediatric Endocrinology, G8-220
Academic Medical Center of the University of Amsterdam
Meibergdreef 9
1105 AZ Amsterdam, The Netherlands

Libbe Kooistra, MSc
Laboratory of Experimental Clinical Psychology
University of Groningen
Grote Kruisstraat 2/1
9712 TS Groningen, The Netherlands
9/35/62074

REFERENCES

1. Vulsma T, Gons MH, de Vijlder JJM. Maternal-fetal transfer of thyroxine in congenital hypothyroidism due to a total organification defect or thyroid agenesis. N Engl J Med 1989; 321:13-6.
2. New England Congenital Hypothyroidism Collaborative. Correlation of cognitive test scores and adequacy of treatment in adolescents with congenital hypothyroidism. J PEDIATR 1994; 124:383-7.
3. Kooistra L, Laane C, Vulsma T, Schellekens JMH, van der Meere JJ, Kalverboer AF. Motor and cognitive development in children with congenital hypothyroidism: a long-term evaluation of the effects of neonatal treatment. J PEDIATR 1994;124:903-9.
4. New England Congenital Hypothyroidism Collaborative. Neonatal hypothyroidism screening: status of patients at 6 years of age. J PEDIATR 1985;107:915-9.
5. New England Congenital Hypothyroidism Collaborative. Effects of neonatal screening for hypothyroidism: prevention of mental retardation by treatment before clinical manifestations. Lancet 1981;2:1095-8.
6. New England Congenital Hypothyroidism Collaborative. Elementary school performance of children with congenital hypothyroidism. J PEDIATR 1990;116:27-32.
7. Heyerdahl S. Intellectual development of children with congenital hypothyroidism in Norway. In: Delange F, Fisher DA, Glinoer D, eds. Research in congenital hypothyroidism. New York: Plenum Press, 1989:298-9.
8. Simons WF, Fuggle PW, Grant DB, Smith I. Intellectual development at 10 years in early treated congenital hypothyroidism. Arch Dis Child 1994;71:232-4.
9. Tillotson SL, Fuggle PW, Smith I, Grant DB. Relation between biochemical severity and intelligence in early treated congenital hypothyroidism: a threshold effect. Br Med J 1994; 309:440-5.
10. Virtanen M, Santavuori P, Hirvonen E, Perheentupa J. Multivariate analysis of psychomotor development in congenital hypothyroidism. Acta Paediatr Scand 1989;78:405-11.

Opsoclonus-myoclonus, ataxia, and coincident neuroblastoma

To the Editor:

Koh et al.[1] describe 10 children with neuroblastoma and the paraneoplastic opsoclonus-myoclonus syndrome. The long survival of children so affected appeared to be a consequence of the following factors: (1) favorable histologic characteristics according to the Shimada classification, (2) tumors with a single copy of the N-*myc* oncogene, (3) localized tumor, and (4) a high percentage of extraabdominal tumors. Several points regarding this article are instructive.

First, paraneoplastic neurologic syndromes are most often associated with long survival in children and adults. This phenomenon has been explained by the findings in patients with neurologic paraneoplastic syndromes, limited disease, and favorable tumor biology. The authors elegantly expand on this thesis by demonstration of a single copy of N-*myc*, an oncogene which, when amplified, independently predicts unfavorable prognosis.

Second, paraneoplastic syndromes are clinically defined, and the definition is augmented by laboratory demonstration of syndrome-specific autoantibodies. This laboratory tool is frequently used in diagnosing paraneoplastic disorders in adults; however, I know of no similar pediatric experience. An autoantibody associated with the opsoclonus-myoclonus syndrome in women with breast cancer is termed anti-Ri.[2] Anti-Ri appears to be a specific marker of the opsoclonus-myoclonus syndrome and warrants investigation in children with neuroblastoma both with and without the paraneoplastic disorder.

Finally, common themes in neurologic paraneoplastic disorders are the presence of fixed neurologic deficits notwithstanding early diagnosis and, often, curative treatment of the underlying cancer. No effective therapies for neurologic paraneoplastic syndromes have been identified. The data supporting the presence of adrenocorticotropic hormone in children with opsoclonus-myoclonus are not compelling, given the poor outcome reflected by the high incidence of encephalopathy and variable response time to treatment. Edmondson et al.[3] suggested intravenous immune globulin therapy, but no long-term follow-up was available; this therapy may warrant further study.

Marc C. Chamberlain, MD
Department of Neurosciences
Division of Neurology/Oncology
University of California, San Diego
La Jolla, CA 92093-0812
9/35/62447

REFERENCES

1. Koh PS, Raffensperger JG, Berry S, et al. Long-term outcome in children with opsoclonus-myoclonus and ataxia and coincident neuroblastoma. J PEDIATR 1994;125:712-6.
2. Luque FA, Furneaux HM, Ferziger R, et al. Anti-Ri: an antibody associated with paraneoplastic opsoclonus and breast cancer. Ann Neurol 1991;29:241-51.
3. Edmondson JC, Nichter CA, Selman JE, DeVivo DC, Gold AP. Use of intravenous gamma globulin therapy for postinfectious acute cerebellar ataxia/opsoclonus of childhood [Abstract]. Ann Neurol 1992;32:440.

Blood flow velocities and neonatal asphyxia

To the Editor:

The report by Akinbi et al. (J PEDIATR 1994;125:625-7) claims that blood flow velocity profiles correlate with birth asphyxia. To meet the authors' diagnostic criteria for birth asphyxia, infants had to have a cord blood pH <7.20 *or* a 5-minute Apgar score ≤7. The literature is replete with evidence that neither of these is diagnostic of asphyxia. In 1986 the American Academy of Pediatrics Committee on the Fetus and Newborn noted that Apgar scores at 1 and 5 minutes correlate poorly with either cause or outcome, that scores alone should not be considered evidence of asphyxia, and that a score of 7 is normal.[1]

Similar problems exist when cord pH values are misused as singular indicators of asphyxia. In the study by Ruth and Raivio,[2] positive predictive value and sensitivity of cord pH values <7.16 (i.e., more than 2 SD below the mean) for adverse outcomes linked to asphyxia were 8% and 21%, respectively. This is not surprising because nearly 15% of all live-born singletons delivered at term have cord arterial pH values <7.20, the value used by Akinbi et al. to diagnose birth asphyxia.[3] Furthermore, the correlation between Apgar score and cord pH is poor. Only 19% of low Apgar scores are associated with significant acidosis, and only 27% of infants with acidosis have low Apgar scores.[4]

A joint statement by the American Academy of Pediatrics and the American College of Obstetricians and Gynecologists noted that the term *asphyxia* should be reserved for clinical situations characterized by "damaging acidemia, hypoxia and metabolic acidosis."[5] Most causes of asphyxia predate parturition and have little to do with intrapartum events. In this regard, the term *birth asphyxia* is imprecise and should not be used.[5] It is a label that implies causality, has substantial medicolegal implications, and belies the scientific investigations that have been performed during the last 25 years.

Stephen J. Elliott, MD
Department of Pediatrics
Baylor College of Medicine
Houston, TX 77030
9/35/62449

REFERENCES

1. American Academy of Pediatrics. Use and abuse of the Apgar score. Pediatrics 1986;78:1148-9.
2. Ruth VJ, Raivio KO. Perinatal brain damage: predictive value of metabolic acidosis and the Apgar score. Br Med J 1988; 297:24-7.
3. Gilstrap LC, Leveno KJ, Burris J, Williams ML, Little BB. Diagnosis of birth asphyxia on the basis of fetal pH, Apgar score, and newborn cerebral dysfunction. Am J Obstet Gynecol 1989;161:825-30.

4. Sykes GS, Molloy PM, Johnson P. Do Apgar scores indicate asphyxia? Lancet 1982;1:494-6.
5. American Academy of Pediatrics, and American College of Obstetricians and Gynecologists. Guidelines for perinatal care. 3rd ed. Elk Grove Village, Illinois: American Academy of Pediatrics, 1992:221-4.

Reply

To the Editor:

We appreciate Dr. Elliott's comment about the stringency of our diagnostic criteria for diagnosis of birth asphyxia. Although the joint statement by the American Academy of Pediatrics and the American College of Obstetricians and Gynecologists relates specifically to neurologic outcome, his point is well taken. Our study was not intended as a validation of either the Apgar score or umbilical cord blood pH. Neither of these two measurements, singly or in combination, accurately predicts morbidity. The cutoff point for the 5-minute Apgar score used in our study was actually <7. Many studies have used the same criteria that we used[1-4]; two of the studies cited by Dr. Elliott used a 5-minute Apgar score of 7 as one of their criteria.[5, 6] However, this was neither our rationale nor a justification. The fact that only 0.6% of live births will meet the criterion of pH $\leq$7.00,[7] as Dr. Elliott would have preferred for us to use, would preclude most studies that attempt to correlate clinical conditions that engender anxiety in caretakers of newborn infants (in this case, timing of enteral feedings) with established means of assessing neonatal physiologic status. The point in our report—that the two indexes we examined, peak systolic blood flow and pulsatility index, were worse with worsening cord blood pH and lower Apgar scores—should not be obfuscated by this distinction of the American Academy of Pediatrics definition of birth asphyxia from acidemia at birth.

H. Akinbi, MD
V. Bhutani, MD
S. Abbasi, MD
Section on Newborn Pediatrics
Pennsylvania Hospital
Philadelphia, PA 19107
9/35/62448

REFERENCES

1. Thilaganathan B, Athanasiou S, Ozmen S, Creighton S, Watson NR, Nicholaides KH. Umbilical cord blood erythroblast count as an index of intrauterine hypoxia. Arch Dis Child 1994;70:F192-4.
2. Samueloff A, Langer O, Berkus M, Field N, Xenakis E, Ridgway L. Is fetal heart variability a good predictor of fetal outcome? Acta Obstet Gynecol Scand 1994;73:39-44.
3. Bruner JB, Levy DW, Arger PH. Doppler ultrasonography of the umbilical cord in complicated pregnancies. South Med J 1993;86:418-22.
4. Fraser WD, Marcoux S, Moutquin JM, Christen A, Canadian Early Amniotomy Study Group. Effect of early amniotomy on the risk of dystocia in nulliparous women. N Engl J Med 1993;328:1145-9.
5. Sykes GS, Molloy PM, Johnson P, et al. Do Apgar score indicate asphyxia? Lancet 1982;1:494-6.
6. Ruth VJ, Raivio KO. Perinatal brain damage: predictive value of metabolic acidosis and Apgar score. BMJ 1988;297: 24-7.
7. Gilstrap LC, Leveno KJ, Burris J, Williams LM, Little BB. Diagnosis of birth asphyxia on the basis of fetal pH, Apgar score, and newborn cerebral dysfunction. Am J Obstet Gyncol 1989;161:825-30.

A new defect in vitamin D metabolism

To the Editor:

We read with interest the article by Casella et al.[1] and the Editor's Column[2] on a possible new defect in vitamin D metabolism. The importance of a singular observation is enforced if more patients with similar findings are disclosed. Thus we describe two Turkish sisters with similar findings (i.e., rickets at the age of 3 years and reappearance of the rickets after successful treatment with vitamin D).

The initial observations included difficulties in walking, low 25-hydroxyvitamin D concentration and low calcium and phosphate levels in serum, elevated alkaline phosphatase activity, and signs of rickets by x-ray examination. After treatment with vitamin D, normalization of all described abnormal findings occurred 6 to 12 months later. Between the ages of 8 to 13 years, after discontinuation of vitamin D therapy, both patients several times had mild to severe symptoms of active rickets (difficulties in walking, pain in the knees, typical x-ray findings, elevated alkaline phosphatase activity, and low serum values for 25-hydroxyvitamin D). Treatment with orally administered vitamin D (5000 to 10,000 U daily) led each time to the disappearance of clinical symptoms and the abnormal laboratory findings.

There is no consanguinity and no evidence of metabolic bone disease in the parents or the five siblings. The patients both received vitamin D supplementation (500 U daily) during the first year of life. Nutritional intake and outdoor activity were comparable with those of other children, and there was no treatment with anticonvulsive drugs. Growth and weight gain were normal, as were results of liver and kidney function tests and examinations for malabsorption.

The patients of Casella et al. and ours have in common late-onset rickets that can be treated successfully with vitamin D but reappears without further vitamin D supplementation, and there is evidence that they require the supplementation for an extended period or even for life. They do not fulfill the diagnostic criteria of vitamin D–dependent rickets type I or II.[3] The early symptoms and the first response to vitamin D treatment resemble the condition of late-onset vitamin D deficiency, but reappearance and familial occurrence distinguish it from a simple form of vitamin D deficiency.

The cause of the enhanced vitamin D requirement remains obscure; the proposed defect in 25-hydroxylation is possible but still hypothetical.[1] The supplementation of vitamin D in all these patients led to an increase in the 25-hydroxycholecalciferol levels, which indicates that at least some hydroxylation occurred. Other conceivable defects are an impairment of either the endogenous formation or the degradation of vitamin D.[4] More biochemical observations are required to establish the molecular defect in this type of "familial recurrent vitamin D–dependent rickets."

Walter Nützenadel, MD
Otto Mehls, MD
Günter Klaus, MD
University Hospital of Heidelberg
Department of Pediatrics
Im Neuenheimer Feld 150
D-69120 Heidelberg, Germany
9/35/62349

REFERENCES

1. Casella SJ, Reiner BJ, Chen TC, Holick MF, Harrison HE. A possible genetic defect in 25-hydroxylation as a cause of rickets. J PEDIATR 1994;124:929-32.
2. Finberg L. Rickets: another genetic cause [Editorial]. J PEDIATR 1994;124:927.
3. Marx SJ. Vitamin D and other calciferols. In: Scriver CR, Beaudet AL, Sly WS, Volle D, eds. The metabolic basis of inherited disease. 6th ed. New York: McGraw-Hill, 1989: 2029-45.
4. Webb AR, Decosta B, Holick MF. Sunlight degradation of vitamin D_3. In: Norman AW, Schaefer K, Grigoleit HG, von Herrath D, eds. Vitamin D: molecular, cellular and clinical endocrinology. New York: Walter de Gruyter, 1988:656-7.

Reply

To the Editor:

The clinical findings reported by Drs. Nützenadel, Mehls, and Klaus are similar to those of the siblings described in our article and accompanying commentary. If these children have a defect in 25-hydroxyvitamin D hydroxylase, then we predict that they will sustain normal levels of calcidiol (25-hydroxyvitamin D) when given physiologic doses of that prehormone. Such a response would make it unlikely that the rickets resulted from an accelerated degradation of 25-hydroxyvitamin D, and would provide further evidence that these two kindreds have the same malady. We believe that the probable defect is a primary deficiency of the 25-hydroxylase enzyme, so one should not name it "recurrent."

Samuel J. Casella, MD
Johns Hopkins Children's Center
CMSC-3-110
600 N. Wolfe St.
Baltimore, MD 21287-3311

Laurence Finberg, MD
Children's Medical Center of Brooklyn
Brooklyn, NY 11203-2098
9/35/62348

Criteria for studies of antibiotic therapy for acute otitis media

To the Editor:

Aspin et al.[1] report the results of a collaborative comparative study of clarithromycin versus amoxicillin-clavulanate in the treatment of acute otitis media in children. The purpose of this letter is not to comment in detail on the work of Aspin et al. but to propose three measures that would ensure uniform criteria for physical signs of acute disease and a more reliable basis for the interpretation of studies of antibiotic efficacy in the treatment of acute otitis media.

First, we recommend the development of precise diagnostic criteria for acute otitis media. Currently each pharmaceutical manufacturer defines the condition differently in its study protocols. Thus Aspin et al. required minimal criteria (i.e., abnormal color and decreased mobility of the tympanic membrane). These criteria provide no means for reliably distinguishing secretory otitis media (otitis media with effusion) from acute otitis media. Both conditions can produce fussiness, irritability, sleep disturbance, and petulance. Pneumatic otoscopy reveals opacification and limited mobility of the eardrum in patients with either condition. We recommend that three well-defined criteria be used for diagnosis in future clinical studies of acute otitis media: (1) limitation of lateral and medial mobility of the eardrum when air pressure in the ear canal is alternately reduced and amplified, (2) opacification of the pearly luster of reflected light on the surface of the eardrum, and (3) bulging or fullness of the eardrum. The findings that the eardrums are abnormal in color and poorly mobile, but are in the neutral position or retracted (as in secretory otitis media or otitis media with effusion), are insufficient for use as minimal criteria for acute otitis media. Bulging or fullness of the tympanic membrane is an absolute requirement.

Second, a minimum of 80% recovery of accepted middle-ear pathogens should be required of all collaborative sites. We have reported that more than 90% recovery of such pathogens is possible, provided that appropriate protocols are followed before the tympanocentesis needle is introduced into the middle ear.[2]

We also suggest that the U.S. Food and Drug Administration and the pharmaceutical company sponsors insist that a subset of sites participating in collaborative studies perform a second tympanocentesis after 3 to 5 days of antibiotic treatment. Only then will we learn whether some agents are less effective than others in sterilizing the middle ear.

Third, we urge those responsible for setting criteria for determining antimicrobial susceptibility testing procedures to update the design of cephalosporin testing. We believe that the 30 μg cephalothin disk should no longer be the standard for cephalosporin testing. Specific disks, including cefprozil, cefpodoxime, cefaclor, cefixime, and loracarbef, should be widely available with concentrations of 1 to 3 μg.

Finally, the U.S. National Committee for Clinical Laboratory Standards (NCCLS) proposed that disk susceptibility testing for *Haemophilus influenzae* be done on *Haemophilus* test media and not on chocolate Mueller-Hinton agar; that a 0.5 McFarland standard, preferably determined by a photometric device, be used to standardize inoculum of colony-forming units of bacteria; and that minimal inhibitory concentration determinations be used to confirm antibiotic resistance.[3]

Our ability to interpret antibiotic efficacy studies in children with acute otitis media rests on precise diagnostic criteria, a minimally acceptable yield of bacterial pathogens, and appropriate laboratory procedures. Development and use of standardized measures will require the collaborative efforts of investigators, the pharmaceutical industry, and the U.S. Food and Drug Administration.

Richard H. Schwartz, MD
William J. Rodriguez, MD
Children's Hospital National Medical Center
111 Michigan Ave., NW
Washington, DC 10010
9/35/62531

REFERENCES

1. Aspin MM, Hoberman A, McCarty J, et al. Comparative study of the safety and efficacy of clarithromycin and amoxicillin-clavulanate in the treatment of acute otitis media in children. J PEDIATR 1994;125:136-41.
2. Nelson JD, McCracken GH Jr, eds. Susceptibilities of middle ear pathogens [report of communication from RH Schwartz, Vienna, Va.]. Pediatr Infect Dis J Newsletter 1994;20(7):14.
3. Scriver SR, Hoban DJ, McGeer A, et al. Surveillance of susceptibility testing methodologies for *Haemophilus influenzae* om Canada, including evaluation of disk diffusion test. J Clin Microbiol 1994;32:2013-15.

Adult respiratory distress syndrome in children, associated with miliary tuberculosis

To the Editor:

We read with interest the article by Davis et al.,[1] who examined the incidence, clinical course, predictors of death, and associated acute disease with the adult respiratory distress syndrome (ARDS) in children. Infectious pneumonia was one of the most common acute diseases from which ARDS developed by a direct mechanism, but miliary tuberculosis (MT) was not present as a cause of ARDS.[2] We describe a 4-year-old boy who had ARDS as a result of MT. He was admitted to the pediatric intensive care unit because of serious respiratory distress caused by interstitial pneumonia. Fifteen days before admission, the boy began to have fever, cough, and loss of weight. He had no previous infection or family history of immunodeficiency. He required tracheal intubation and mechanical ventilation at admission. He had leukocytosis and neutrophilia, and the chest radiograph showed bilateral diffuse interstitial infiltrates. Antibiotic and antiviral empiric treatment were started; results of studies for viruses, bacteria, fungi, *Pneumocystis carinii*, and mycobacteria were negative. On the fifth day of admission the lungs had not improved and fever persisted. The boy also had hepatosplenomegaly, hypertriglyceridemia, and hypofibrinogenemia. Biopsy of a bone marrow aspirate was done to rule out hemophagocytic syndrome. *Mycobacterium tuberculosis* bacilli and a small number of reactive hemophagocytic histiocytes were found. Antituberculosis chemotherapy was started.

The ARDS evolved in the first hours; high respiratory assistance (maximal fraction of inspired oxygen, 1; maximal positive end-expiratory pressure, 12 cm H_2O; maximal peak inspiratory pressure, 47 cm H_2O) with an alveolar-arterial oxygen tension difference >450 mm Hg was needed throughout the clinical course. As a complication of the mechanical ventilation, pneumothorax and pneumomediastinum developed on the second day. Because the child's condition did not improve with the conventional therapy, arteriovenous hemofiltration was initiated on the fifth day but was ineffective. The patient died on the nineteenth day of refractory hypoxemia. A nosocomial infection contributed to his death. Pathologic findings from autopsy confirmed the diagnosis of ARDS, MT, and hemophagocytic syndrome.

The ARDS associated with MT has not been described in children and only exceptionally in adults.[2] This case allows its inclusion as a cause of ARDS in children. This is important because the incidence of tuberculosis is increasing, and we will probably see more new cases of ARDS in the near future.[3] Miliary tuberculosis is a treatable cause of ARDS; early diagnosis and treatment are very important to improve the outcome.

Amelia Martinez-Azagra, MD
Ana Serrano, MD
Juan Casado-Flores, MD
Pediatric Intensive Care Unit
Hospital Niño Jesús
University Autónoma de Madrid
Avda. Menéndez Pelayo, 65
28009, Madrid, Spain
9/35/62351

REFERENCES

1. Davis SL, Furman DO, Costarino AT Jr. Adult respiratory distress syndrome in children: associated disease, clinical course and predictors of death. J PEDIATR 1993;123:35-45.
2. Dyer RA, Chapel WA, Potgieter PD. Adult respiratory distress syndrome associated with miliary tuberculosis. Crit Care Med 1985;13:12-5.
3. Starke JR, Jacobs RF, Jereb J. Resurgence of tuberculosis in children. J PEDIATR 1992;120:839-55.

Reply

To the Editor:

Martinez-Azagra et al. call attention to a point of controversy relating to the adult respiratory distress syndrome: When does an infectious pneumonia become ARDS? Indeed, can an infectious pneumonia ever be considered the cause of ARDS? In our study,[1] we used the clinical criteria of Murray et al.[2] (diffuse radiodensities on chest roentgenogram, hypoxemia in the presence of therapeutic positive end-expiratory pressure, and abnormal respiratory system compliance) to define ARDS. Although it may be argued that this definition is too broad and that lung biopsy is necessary to differentiate an infectious pneumonia from ARDS, we found a similar clinical course and outcome regardless of cause. Moreover, most clinical studies of ARDS use similar "noninvasive" criteria for case identification.

Some investigators have sought a defining change in chemistry or other marker to identify patients with ARDS; however, there is no acceptable sine qua non for the syndrome. Many clinicians and investigators hope that future work will demonstrate an inflammatory mediator or other compound, the presence or absence of which will define ARDS.

Our view is that ARDS is at times the result of, or is caused by, an infectious pneumonia. We agree that tuberculosis, particularly when the inflammation is systemic, as in miliary tuberculosis, may trigger a reaction in the lung, causing ARDS.

Susan L. Davis, MD
Department of Pediatrics
Texas Children's Hospital
Houston, TX 77030-2399
9/35/62350

REFERENCES

1. Davis SL, Furman DP, Costarino AT. Adult respiratory distress syndrome in children: associated disease, clinical course, and predictors of death. J PEDIATR 1993;123:35-45.
2. Murray JF, Matthay MA, Luce JM, Flick MR. An expanded definition of the adult respiratory distress syndrome. Am Rev Respir Dis 1988;138:720-3.

Techniques for measurement of resting energy expenditure in children

To the Editor:

We read with interest the article by Goran et al.[1] Having completed a study of energy expenditure in prepubescent children,[2] we can appreciate the work involved. However, we have reservations concerning the method used for measurement of resting energy expenditure (REE) and the impact of this method on the conclusions.

The authors' definition of REE included both the thermogenic effect of food and any spontaneous movement by the subjects. The lack of control inherent in this definition introduces additional variance and makes it difficult to compare this study with others. For example, the "usual" breakfasts consumed by the subjects were of unknown size and composition, and may have increased REE by 0% to 20%. We found that nondisabled children between the ages of 4 and 7 years further increase REE by 2% to 15% because of movement made while watching television or videotapes.[2] When we adjusted for observed spontaneous movement, the correlation between REE and fat-free mass in our control subjects increased from $r = 0.86$ to 0.91.[2]

The authors make a number of conclusions without acknowledging that these also are probably in error. With no attempt to quantify the subjects' movement, gender differences in spontaneous activity cannot be determined, and it cannot be determined whether the gender differences in REE are related to differences in true REE or to differences in movement. The finding that fat mass is a predictor of REE also may be an artifact; movement requires more energy in the obese subject because of greater limb weight. Griffiths and Payne[3] and Weinsier et al.[4] used completely different definitions of REE and different measurement methods. Finally, because thermogenesis and movement are likely to inflate the variation in REE, any apparent r value is reduced, and thus a significant relationship may have been missed during the regression analysis.

Although we recognize the difficulty of measuring REE in this age group, we do not believe that it is impossible. The authors' idea that this is "normal" REE and that the results and conclusions are therefore generalizable is difficult to accept, especially when some individuals' REE under these "normal" conditions exceeded the child's total daily energy expenditure.[5]

Dale A. Schoeller, PhD
Department of Medicine
University of Chicago
Chicago, IL 60637

Amy Luke, PhD
Department of Preventive Medicine & Epidemiology
Loyola University
Maywood, IL 60153
9/35/62654

REFERENCES

1. Goran MI, Kaskoun M, Johnson R. Determinants of resting energy expenditure. J PEDIATR 1994;125:362-7.
2. Luke A, Roizen NJ, Sutton M, Schoeller DA. Energy expenditure in children with Down syndrome: correcting metabolic rate for movement. J PEDIATR 1994;125:829-38.
3. Griffiths M, Payne PR. Energy expenditure in small children of obese and non-obese parents. Nature 1976;260:698-700.
4. Weinsier RL, Schutz Y, Bracco D. Reexamination of the relationship of resting metabolic rate to fat-free mass and to the metabolically active components of fat-free mass in humans. Am J Clin Nutr 1992;55:790-4.
5. Goran MI, Carpenter WH, Poehlman ET. Total energy expenditure in 4- to 6-year-old children. Am J Physiol 1993;264:E706-11.

Reply

To the Editor:

Schoeller and Luke emphasize that our article should be interpreted with caution because resting energy expenditure (REE) was measured under conditions that were less than optimal. In our experience with hundreds of measurements, the key to obtaining reliable measures of REE in children is to minimize stress. We therefore allowed the children to watch videotaped cartoons and to eat their normal breakfast at home before reporting to the laboratory. This protocol ensures that young children maintain a relaxed and cooperative mood during testing, thus leading to excellent measurement reliability (the test-retest reliability is ~5%).

We have completed studies (unpublished observations) in which we compared the postprandial protocol with the more typical "basal" conditions used in adults. Metabolic rate was ~11% higher when measured under postprandial conditions. This finding is consistent with measurements of postprandial REE by Maffeis et al.,[1] suggesting that the elevation in metabolic rate with the postprandial protocol is explained by the additional energy cost of meal consumption. In addition, we found that the correlation between REE and fat-free mass was stronger when measurements were performed under postprandial (r = 0.88) versus "basal" conditions (r = 0.64), but the regression slope was similar. These findings suggest that the postprandial protocol reduces measurement noise without compromising the nature of the relationship between REE and fat-free mass.

We believe that allowing children to watch television is another factor that contributes to more reliable and less "fidgety" measurement of REE. This is supported by data from two other laboratories. Dietz et al.[2] showed that children move less when they watch television, in comparison with asking them to sit still, and Klesges et al.[3] showed that energy expenditure was reduced during television viewing in obese and nonobese girls.

A final advantage of the postprandial protocol is that the measurements are performed under conditions that are physiologically representative (a 12-hour fasted state is not natural for a young child). Schoeller and Luke challenge this idea because we published data in which REE exceeded total energy expenditure in several children.[4] In 100 studies we have noted a higher REE in four cases (by 20 to 50 kcal/day). Our interpretation of REE being higher than total energy expenditure is that the relevant techniques are subject to measurement error.

Although we do not advocate the use of the alternative protocol in all situations, it does offer several advantages: (1) it is reproducible, (2) children may move less during measurement, (3) it is practical and can be applied to large numbers of children or in a clinical setting, and (4) the measurement is performed under conditions that would be encountered during the course of a typical day. As pointed out by Schoeller and Luke, the limitations to such a protocol are that metabolic rate cannot be resolved into its basal and postprandial components and that it may be difficult to compare data with other studies.

Michael I. Goran, PhD
Associate Professor
Director, Energy Metabolism Research Unit
Department of Nutrition Sciences
University of Alabama at Birmingham
Birmingham, AL 35294

Rachel Johnson, RD, PhD
Assistant Professor
Department of Nutrition Sciences
University of Vermont
Burlington, VT 05404
9/35/62655

REFERENCES

1. Maffeis C, Schutz Y, Zoccante L, Micciolo R, Pinelli L. Meal-induced thermogenesis in lean and obese prepubertal children. Am J Clin Nutr 1993;57:481-5.
2. Dietz WH, Bandini LG, Morelli JA, Peers KF, Ching PLYH. Effect of sedentary activities on resting metabolic rate. Am J Clin Nutr 1994;59:556-9.
3. Klesges RC, Shelton ML, Klesges LM. The effects of television on metabolic rate: potential implications for childhood obesity. Pediatrics 1993;91:281-6.
4. Goran MI, Carpenter WH, Poehlman ET. Total energy expenditure in 4 to 6 year old children. Am J Physiol 1993;264:E706-E711.

Placebo-controlled versus comparative studies of drug effects

To the Editor:

The Fluticasone Propionate Collaborative Pediatric Working Group administered two doses of the inhaled steroid, fluticasone propionate, in a double-blind, crossover study with placebo to children with seasonal allergic rhinitis.[1] They demonstrated that this new corticosteroid was significantly better than a placebo, although there appeared to be no significant dose-response effect. After reading this article, my major question relates to the rationale for performing it. It is well documented that topical nasal steroids provide benefit for noninfectious inflammatory nasal disease, allergic or nonallergic. Therefore it is virtually a foregone conclusion that a topical nasal steroid sprayed into the noses of children with seasonal allergic rhinitis will be better than nothing. The relevant issue for the clinician, however, is not whether something is better than nothing but whether something is better than something else. The study provides no guidance regarding the potential advantage, if any, of intranasal fluticasone therapy over other inhaled corticosteroids or maintenance antihistamine therapy. Is fluticasone more or less effective and more or less well tolerated than other inhaled corticosteroids or twice-daily treatment with antihistamines, either hydroxyzine[2, 3] or even the least expensive antihistamine, chlorpheniramine.[3]

The medical community, and medical journals in particular, need to demand more of companies that market new drugs than simply demonstrating that the new product is better than nothing, especially because the new drug is generally more expensive. "Better-than-nothing" studies may meet minimal FDA standards, but clinical decision making requires more information than that. The studies referenced above for hydroxyzine and chlorpheniramine therapy suggest degrees of clinical benefit that appear greater than that apparent in this study, and with equally good tolerance during sustained maintenance therapy. I encourage journal editors and reviewers to be on the frontline in encouraging clinical trials that actually aid clinical decision making.

Miles M. Weinberger, MD
Professor of Pediatrics
Director, Allergy and Pulmonary Division
University of Iowa Hospitals and Clinics
Iowa City, IA 52242-1083
9/35/62806

REFERENCES

1. Fluticasone Propionate Collaborative Pediatric Working Group. Treatment of seasonal allergic rhinitis with once-daily intranasal fluticasone propionate therapy in children. J PEDIATR 1994;125:628-34.

2. Schaaf L, Hendeles L, Weinberger M. Suppression of seasonal allergic rhinitis symptoms with daily hydroxyzine. J Allergy Clin Immunol 1979;63:129-33.
3. Wong L, Hendeles L, Weinberger MM. Pharmacological prophylaxis of allergic rhinitis: relative efficacy of hydroxyzine and chlorpheniramine. J Allergy Clin Immunol 1980;67:223-8.

Reply

To the Editor:

I agree that clinical studies comparing the efficacy and safety of a new drug with those of an alternative therapy provide the clinician with the most useful information. The U.S. Food and Drug Administration requires data from two well-controlled (i.e., randomized, double-blind, and placebo-controlled) clinical studies to establish efficacy and safety of a new drug. Our study and a 2-week study[1] comparing fluticasone therapy with use of placebo in children with seasonal allergic rhinitis were conducted to meet these requirements. We included children between the ages of 4 and 11 years in our studies. Because of U.S. Food and Drug Administration regulations, we could not compare an investigational corticosteroid agent with a currently marketed, second-generation antihistamine (e.g., terfenadine) or a currently marketed intranasal corticosteroid agent (e.g., beclomethasone dipropionate), because terfenadine is not indicated for use in children <12 years of age and beclomethasone is not indicated for use in children <6 years of age. However, fluticasone has been compared with terfenadine,[2,3] astemizole,[4,5] and beclomethasone[6,7] in adolescents and adults with seasonal allergic rhinitis.

Finally, in our study, chlorpheniramine maleate was allowed as a rescue antihistamine for relief of symptoms of rhinitis uncontrolled by study treatment. During the screening period, all three groups of patients used similar amounts of the rescue antihistamine. However, during the treatment period, significantly fewer children receiving either dosage of fluticasone used rescue antihistamine. Although more children receiving placebo used rescue antihistamine, nasal symptoms did not improve.

Comparative clinical studies in children are necessary. This population, especially children as young as 4 years, has been ignored to some extent by pharmaceutical manufacturers because of the stringent regulatory constraints surrounding studies in this population. I hope that the results of our study provide clinically relevant information regarding the efficacy and safety of an intranasal corticosteroid in children with allergic rhinitis.

Stanley P. Galant, MD
Fluticasone Propionate Collaborative
Pediatric Working Group
Orange, CA 92668
9/35/62805

REFERENCES

1. Grossman J, Banov C, Bronsky EA, et al. Fluticasone propionate aqueous nasal spray is safe and effective for children with seasonal allergic rhinitis. Pediatrics 1993;92:594-9.
2. Meltzer E, Orgel H, Backhaus J, et al. Intranasal fluticasone propionate once daily is more effective than terfenadine twice daily in relieving symptoms of seasonal allergic rhinitis [Abstract]. J Allergy Clin Immunol 1992;89:302.
3. Bronsky E, Dockhorn R, Meltzer E, et al. Intranasal fluticasone propionate is more effective than terfenadine for treatment of seasonal rhinitis. [Abstract]. Ann Allergy 1994;72:86.
4. Stricker WE, Klimas IT, Mendelson L, et al. Intranasal fluticasone is more effective than astemizole for seasonal allergic [Abstract]. Ann Allergy 1994;72:86.
5. Lemanske R, Dunn K, Galant S, et al. Fluticasone propionate aqueous nasal spray is more effective than astemizole in the treatment of seasonal allergic rhinitis [Abstract 15]. J Allergy Clin Immunol 1994; 93:165.
6. Ratner P, Paul BR, Findlay SR, Hampel F, Martin B, Kral K, Rogenes PR. Fluticasone propionate given once daily is as effective for seasonal allergic rhinitis as beclomethasone dipropionate given twice daily. J Allergy Clin Immunol 1992;90:285-91.
7. LaForce CF, Dockhorn RJ, Findlay SR, et al. Fluticasone propionate: an effective alternative treatment for seasonal allergic rhinitis in adults and adolescents. J Fam Pract 1994; 38:145-52.

Reply

In general, we agree with the principles set forth by Dr. Weinberger. We accept for publication the best of the papers that we receive. Given a choice between a placebo-controlled trial and a comparative trial of the same drug, we almost certainly would choose the latter.

Joseph M. Garfunkel, MD
Editor
9/35/62804

Standards for home care of sick children

To the Editor:

We read with great interest the contribution of Goldberg et al.[1] to the growing literature on pediatric home care. We commend them for their leadership of home care issues.

Although the authors argue eloquently that skilled pediatricians need to be involved with all aspects of pediatric home care, they neglect the role of the nurse-caregiver in developing care plans, managing resources, and delivering care within the home. Pediatric home care requires a commitment by a team of providers, of which the pediatrician is one member. Currently the physician role in home care tends to be limited; patient care and administrative duties are assumed by individuals trained in nursing, business, and health care administration.

The growth of the pediatric home care market has attracted the attention of home care providers who have dedicated their services to adults and the elderly with the support of Medicare dollars. As market competition has increased, providers have looked to pediatrics and other niche markets to increase market share. Consequently, pediatric home care services are being provided by individuals with managerial, organizational, and nursing expertise oriented toward adult care but with little or no experience in caring for medically fragile children.

Pediatricians should make certain that their patients are cared for by competent home care agencies staffed with pediatric nurses and ancillary staff. Home health agencies may offer pediatric services without making a complete commitment to children through pediatric-specific policies and procedures, agency organization, and the hiring of competent pediatric nursing and other ancillary staff. Pediatricians cannot rely solely on accreditation by governmental and nongovernmental agencies to ensure good care because these bodies do not have standards specific for pediatric home care.

As Goldberg et al. state, the validation of pediatric-specific home care services ultimately will be established by outcome data. Home care providers who specialize in pediatrics should be able to demonstrate better cost and clinical outcomes for children compared with other providers. With the assistance of academic programs such as the authors', further outcomes research will lay the scientific foundation to ensure that this vital area of health care delivery remains the purview of dedicated pediatric specialists. Furthermore, such research can serve as the basis for development of independent standards for pediatric home care, preferably under the auspices of organizations such as the American Academy of Pediatrics and the American Academy of Home Care Physicians.

Mark S. McConnell, MD
Departments of Pediatrics and Anesthesia
Lucille Salter Packard Children's Hospital
Stanford University School of Medicine
Stanford, CA 94305

Ronald M. Perkin, MD
Professor of Pediatrics
Loma Linda University Children's Hospital
Loma Linda University School of Medicine
Loma Linda, CA 92354
9/35/62890

REFERENCE

1. Goldberg AI, Gardner HG, Gibson LE. Home care: the next frontier of pediatric practice. J PEDIATR 1994;125:686-90.

Reply

To the Editor:

We did not intend to neglect the role of nurses or the importance of understanding that the physician is part of a multidisciplinary team. Our concern is that home care has evolved with limited physician input in its design, and with limited direct participation of physicians in discharge planning and care in the home. Physicians must understand home care to be able to assume their appropriate roles and responsibilities. They must understand that the home care plan is a medical prescription for which they are medically and legally responsible. If physicians would get more involved, more acute, subacute, and long-term care could be transferred into the home. Greater physician involvement is one of the key issues of the current Home Care Initiative being convened by the Health Care Financing Administration. As a result, new Current Procedural Terminology codes have been approved for 1995 for physician care oversight (case management) in the home.

Pediatric home care is family centered. The family is in charge; all professionals are guests in their home. Successful home care requires an interdisciplinary team of which the physician is only one member. All members of the team—nurses, social workers, therapists, and others—have significant roles and responsibilities that must be defined and predetermined. Because physicians must learn and value the importance of roles and responsibilities of the other team members, an "experience-based" curriculum is justified.

We applaud Drs. McConnel and Perkin for their emphasis on provision of pediatric home care by organizations and professionals with knowledge and insight about the special needs of children and their families. They justify the physician oversight responsibility when they describe the need to ensure quality pediatric care because we do not have standards specific for pediatric home care. We need to create these pediatric "standards" on the basis of outcome data. Home care may not be the appropriate choice for all families or all situations. Rigorous selection criteria are needed regarding medical, psychosocial, environmental, technologic, organizational, and financial aspects. Unless home care is designed with an integrated management approach, it may not be cost saving. The future growth of home care can be justified only by rigorous outcomes research. We agree that these efforts are major responsibilities of academic programs and professional associations dedicated to the advancement of home care.

Allen I. Goldberg, MD
M. Harry Gardner, MD
Lewis E. Gibson, MD
Sections of Home Health and Pulmonary Medicine
Department of Pediatrics
Loyola University Medical Center
Maywood, IL 60153
9/35/62891

CORRECTION

In the January 1995 listing of fellowships in pediatric subspecialties and general academic training (volume 126, pages 25A to 70A), the following fellowship was listed under **adolescent medicine** (p. 25A) but should have been listed under **allergy**: Iowa (Iowa City), University of Iowa Hospitals and Clinics, Miles M. Weinberger, MD, Director.

THE JOURNAL OF
PEDIATRICS

MAY 1995 *Volume 126* *Number 5, Part 1*

MEDICAL PROGRESS

Bone mineralization, hypothalamic amenorrhea, and sex steroid therapy in female adolescents and young adults

Albert C. Hergenroeder, MD

From the Department of Pediatrics, Adolescent Medicine and Sports Medicine Section, Baylor College of Medicine, Texas Children's Hospital, Houston

Osteoporosis is a disease manifested primarily in postmenopausal women. Reduced bone mass in adulthood is a risk factor for osteoporosis; for some women the disease has its onset in the second decade, when peak bone mass should be achieved. Women who have reached age 20 years and have missed 50% of their expected menstrual periods, such as women with hypothalamic amenorrhea, are likely to have reduced bone mineral density and will be at greater risk for osteoporosis.[1] Because peak bone mass is a major determinant of osteoporosis and the second decade is a critical time in the achievement of peak bone mass, providers of health care for adolescents need to understand the factors that optimize bone mineralization during the second decade.

DISCUSSION

Influences on bone mineralization

Puberty. The vast majority of bone mass is acquired by the end of the second decade,[2-4] and most of the increase in bone size and density occurs relatively early in puberty. Puberty is associated with accelerated bone mineralization, especially trabecular bone (lumbar spine and femoral neck). Minimal increase of BMD occurs after 2 years postmenarche.[4] Body weight and pubertal stage are positively associated with BMD in adolescent girls.[5-9] The effect of weight as a determinant of BMD may be tempered in mid to late puberty compared with early puberty.[8-10] The total increase in whole body bone mineral and half the increase in spine mineral during puberty is related to changes in bone size rather than to an increase in bone mineral per unit volume.[9] A small but potentially important fraction of bone mass accretion occurs in the third decade.[11] Girls have greater BMD than boys up to the late teens, at which time BMD becomes and remains greater in men.[12] Black girls have greater BMD than white girls at all ages, although this difference may not appear until mid to late puberty.[13-16]

BMD	Bone mineral density
DEXA	Dual-energy x-ray absorptiometry
DMPA	Depot medroxyprogesterone acetate
OCP	Oral contraceptive pills

Calcium intake. Adequate calcium intake is important in achieving peak bone mass. Whether calcium supplementation in puberty increases peak BMD or simply allows peak BMD to be achieved earlier remains a question.[17-19] The current recommended daily allowance of calcium is 1200 mg. An increase of calcium intake to 1500 mg/day has been proposed for adolescents and young adults.[5, 18, 20, 21] However, in adolescent girls with anorexia nervosa, increased calcium intake alone may not improve BMD because of in-

Supported by National Institutes of Health grant M01RR-00188, General Clinical Research Center.

Reprint requests: Albert C. Hergenroeder, MD, Texas Children's Hospital, 6621 Fannin St., 3-3340, Houston, TX 77030-2399.

THE JOURNAL OF PEDIATRICS 1995;126:683-9

0022-3476/95/$3.00 + 0 **9/18/63479**

creased excretion and decreased absorption of calcium.[22] Increasing calcium intake above the recommended daily allowance may have the long-term benefit of increasing BMD, but only if the regimen is continued through childhood and adolescence.[17,21] Normal bone mineralization requires optimal calcium intake through childhood, adolescence, and adulthood. Most adolescent girls consume much less than the RDA for calcium.[21]

Exercise and bone mineralization. New bone formation occurs when strain is applied across that bone,[23] whereas the absence of strain, such as that occurring with bed rest, is associated with rapid and significant bone demineralization.[24] The degree of BMD increase is related to the strain of the exercise across the bone. The magnitude of the stress appears to be more important than the number of repetitions[25, 26]; BMD is remarkably increased in weight lifters.[27, 28] The relationship between exercise and BMD is complex and incompletely understood. BMD changes at the hip and lumbar spine differ depending on the type of exercise program in premenopausal women[29-33]; this emphasizes the importance of measuring BMD at more than one site when ongoing change in BMD is assessed. The increased BMD associated with exercise is not limited to weight-bearing activities: non-weight-bearing exercise also favors bone formation.[34] Not all athletes have increased BMD; swimmers have been shown to have reduced BMD.[35-37] The beneficial effect of exercise on BMD can be lost and significant bone loss can result if women exercise to the point of low body weight, amenorrhea, anovulation, or luteal-phase inadequacy.[30, 38-41] Runners and dancers with normal menses have increased BMD compared with that of amenorrheic runners and dancers.[3, 39, 40] Weight is a cofactor possibly mediating the effects of amenorrhea on BMD.[3, 41] Young adult runners with anovulatory or short-luteal-phase eumenorrhea may lose bone rapidly.[38]

In summary, exercise promotes bone mineralization in most women and is to be encouraged. In the minority of girls and women who exercise to the point of excessive weight loss and amenorrhea or oligomenorrhea, exercise is part of a lifestyle that promotes bone demineralization.

Measurement of bone mineral density. There are two types of bone: cortical and trabecular. Both types are present throughout the skeleton; the largest percentage overall, especially in the appendicular skeleton, is cortical bone. Early studies of BMD used single-photon absorptiometry, in which a beam of monoenergetic radiation was passed across a limb and the decrease in the intensity of the beam was a function of the amount of mineral in the bone. Single photon absorptiometry is limited to measuring BMD of the appendicular skeleton and cannot measure BMD in areas where the highest bone turnover and the earliest bone loss might occur, notably the spine and hip. Dual-energy x-ray absorptiometry measures BMD at two energies (frequencies), eliminating the need for a constant thickness of soft tissue around the bone.[42] DEXA can be used to measure BMD at any site and is the current standard of BMD measurement. DEXA measures BMD without distinguishing between cortical and trabecular bone. Trabecular bone is present in a higher percentage in bones that are common sites of fracture in postmenopausal women (e.g., femoral neck and lumbar spine). These sites are of particular interest and are usually reported separately in studies of BMD. To assess a patient's bone mineralization, the physician should order a DEXA scan of the hip and lumbar spine, because osteopenia can be present at one site but not necessarily both.

Women at risk for premature bone loss. Young women at risk of having hypothalamic amenorrhea and oligomenorrhea include athletes, ballet dancers, and those with eating disorders. Many factors may predispose young women who diet or exercise, or both, to amenorrhea and oligomenorrhea. The reader is referred to previous publications for further review.[43-46] There is a higher incidence of delayed menarche and menstrual dysfunction in girls who started intensive athletic training before menarche.[47] However, menarche may occur at a later age in these athletes anyway; that is, they may have been destined to have delayed menarche even without intense athletic training.[48] Menstrual cycles may be more vulnerable to disruption by exercise and dieting during the early postmenarchal period.[49, 50] Related to hypothalamic-pituitary-ovarian axis maturation, previous pregnancy appears to be associated with a protective effect against exercise-induced amenorrhea, and girls and women in whom amenorrhea develops during exercise training are more likely to have abnormal menstrual function before beginning training.[51, 52]

The amenorrhea associated with athletics and eating disorders is characterized by a disruption of the pulsatile release of gonadotropin-releasing hormone, resulting in low levels of gonadotropins and secondarily reduced levels of estrogen and progesterone. The mechanism by which intense athletic training predisposes women to menstrual disorders is unknown. The concept of "energy drain" (i.e., the failure to supplement the energy cost of exercise with increased caloric intake) has been implicated.[45, 47, 53] Some female athletes maintain body weight despite surprisingly low energy intakes.[39, 49, 54, 55] In these studies, energy intake was significantly lower among amenorrheic than eumenorrheic athletes. In contrast, Wilmore et al.[56] reported no differences in energy intake between amenorrheic and eumenorrheic runners. Although systematic underestimation of true energy intake cannot be ruled out, weight-conscious athletes may be prone to erratic eating habits and periods of negative energy balance. A direct effect of negative energy balance on menstrual status has been demonstrated in a controlled feeding study in which short-term energy deprivation (60% reduction in usual intake) inhibited ovulation and menstruation in susceptible thin women.[57] The controlling influence of energy availability (rather than body weight or composition) on gonadotropin release is evident from the initiation of luteinizing hormone pulsatility within a few hours and ovulation within 3 or 4 days after the start of ad libitum feeding in severely growth-restricted female rats, long before significant changes in body size and body composition could occur.[45, 58] Lower percentages of body fat, greater weight loss since the onset of training, and lower initial body weight at the onset of training are more common in runners with amenorrhea than in runners with normal menses. The mechanism by which body fat affects menstrual function is not completely understood. Frisch and McArthur[50] hypothesized that menarche occurs at a minimum percentage of body fat of 17% and that maintenance of regular menstruation requires a minimum 22% body fat. This critical body fat hypothesis has been challenged, and the consensus is that there are no specific body fat levels at which menarche and normal menstruation occur.[59-61]

Depending on the definition of secondary amenorrhea, the method used to gather and interpret information, the intensity of exercise, and age of the subjects, the prevalence of secondary amenorrhea in female athletes and dancers ranges from 3% to 66%.[47, 59, 62] It has been estimated that 5% to 33% of athletes and dancers have eating disorders.[63, 64] The prevalence of anorexia nervosa among adolescent girls ranges from 0.1% to 1%. A present or past history of eating disorders has been reported in 2% to 5% of female college students.[65] The majority of patients with bulimia report a history of secondary amenorrhea, and nearly half currently report irregular menses.[66]

In summary, young women at risk of having premature bone loss include those with hypothalamic amenorrhea and oligomenorrhea. The cause of the hypothalamic amenorrhea is not established, but inadequate caloric intake relative to the activity level is important. Some girls and women are predisposed to athletics-related menstrual problems, especially those with delayed menarche and oligomenorrhea before training.

Bone mineral density in women with hypothalamic amenorrhea. Osteopenia and osteoporotic fractures are recognized complications of anorexia nervosa.[67-71] Improvements in BMD can occur as women recover from anorexia nervosa, but the longer the duration of the illness, the more likely that osteopenia will result. Likewise, those who do not recover from anorexia nervosa will have poorer recovery of BMD.[70, 72-74] It appears that recovery of BMD can precede the return of spontaneous menstruation; this suggests an independent effect of weight gain on BMD accretion and that recovery of BMD can occur in the absence of estrogen supplementation. Amenorrheic subjects can achieve significant increases in BMD even during the third decade and before regular menses resume; the gains are associated with weight increase and increased caloric intake.[75-77]

Effect of treatment with estrogen or progestin or both on BMD in young women with hypothalamic amenorrhea. Long-term estrogen replacement therapy is associated with a reduced risk of osteoporotic fractures and increased BMD in postmenopausal women.[78] The beneficial effect of estrogen therapy on BMD in young adult women with hypothalamic amenorrhea or oligomenorrhea remains to be established by a prospective, randomized, clinical trial.[11, 79-81] One randomized clinical trial found no difference in the change of BMD of the spine, wrist, and foot for 2 years in amenorrheic subjects treated with conjugated estrogen, 0.625 mg per day for 21 days per month, and medroxyprogesterone, 10 mg per day for 10 days per month, compared with a placebo group.[82] All subjects received 1200 mg of calcium per day. Weight was suggested as a cofactor mitigating the effects of estrogen deficiency on BMD, as others have suggested.[3, 36, 77] In a nonrandomized clinical trial, no improvement in wrist BMD was noted for 2 years in 20-year-old estrogen-deficient women treated with the same conjugated estrogen-progestin protocol mentioned above,[83] but hip and spine BMD were not assessed. Thus treatment with conjugated estrogen (0.625 mg daily, 21 days per month) has not been associated with improved BMD in adolescent and young adult women with estrogen deficiency associated with hypothalamic amenorrhea, in contrast to improvements in BMD in postmenopausal women treated with the same dose of estrogen.[84, 85] In one observational, prospective study of a convenience sample and a second nonrandomized, retrospective study of patients with anorexia nervosa, oral contraceptive use was associated with an increase in total body bone mass and lumbar spine BMD.[11, 70] That orally administered contraceptive pills have a beneficial effect on BMD in premenopausal women remains to be established by means of a double-masked, randomized, placebo-controlled trial.

Progesterone deficiency may play an important role in bone loss.[38] Treatment with medroxyprogesterone (10 mg/day for 10 days per month for 12 months) has been associated with an increase in lumbar spine BMD in comparison with a decrease in an untreated group of 21- to 45- year-old women in a randomized, double-masked, placebo-controlled clinical trial.[86] It is not clear why treatment with progestin alone was associated with improved BMD and no increase in BMD was associated with progestin plus estrogen treatment; possibly the body weights and weight changes of the groups in the studies were different. Lending evidence to the role of progesterone as a bone trophic hormone[87] is a study showing that serum progesterone concentration was significantly related to lumbar spine BMD in eumenorrheic runners, but the progesterone concentration and lumbar spine BMD were not related in oligomenorrheic runners or sedentary control subjects.[88] Treatment with progestin alone represents a deviation from the current standard of replacement with estrogen and progestin for young women with risk of premature bone loss, but medroxyprogesterone therapy has been as effective as conjugated estrogen and medroxyprogesterone in combination in preventing loss of appendicular but not spinal BMD in postmenopausal women.[84, 89] Cundy et al.[90] raised the concern that long-term depot medroxyprogesterone acetate treatment could be associated with loss of BMD; the proposed mechanism is hypoestrogenemia caused by suppression of the release of luteinizing hormone and follicle-stimulating hormone by the continuous release of progestin. Progestin-only therapy may improve bone mineralization in adult women with hypothalamic amenorrhea or oligomenorrhea related to athletics or eating disorders, but to date there are no data on the effect of progestin treatment alone on BMD in amenorrheic or oligomenorrheic teenage girls. There is also no evidence that oral progestin therapy, 10 days per month, is associated with BMD loss in young girls with hypothalamic amenorrhea or oligomenorrhea.

Treatment of young girls at risk of having bone demineralization. The treatment of amenorrhea in the athlete or patient with an eating disorder should include correction of any primary cause for the amenorrhea. If the subject has hypothalamic amenorrhea, she needs education about the proposed cause of hypothalamic amenorrhea and the potential complications, including osteopenia. Reduction in training to levels at which normal menstrual cycles resume is encouraged. However, reduced training may not be an option for a female athlete. In athletes with amenorrhea for more than 6 months, BMD should be measured, and if the patient has osteopenia at the hip or spine, then hormonal treatment should be considered. However, the criteria for initiating estrogen replacement therapy, the dose, and the beneficial effect of estrogen-progestin therapy on BMD in adolescents and young adults with hypothalamic amenorrhea or oligomenorrhea are not established. It appears that replacement doses of conjugated estrogen, which are appropriate for postmenopausal women, are not adequate to improve BMD in teenagers and young adults. Whether higher doses of estrogen (i.e., oral contraceptive pills) for longer periods of time would improve BMD in teenage girls and young adult women is not yet established. Likewise, there are no data to support the use of progestin therapy alone in teenage girls. Optimal calcium intake is to be encouraged; for amenorrheic 12- to 25-year-old women, the daily recommended dose is 1200 to 1500 mg calcium. Increased calcium intake alone will not necessarily improve calcium balance and will probably have no effect on bone mineralization in women with hypothalamic amenorrhea who do not increase their caloric intake, reduce their training, and possibly take hormone replacement.[22]

SUMMARY AND CONCLUSIONS

1. The vast majority of bone mineralization in girls occurs by the middle of the second decade.
2. Premature bone demineralization occurs in women with hypothalamic dysfunction manifest as amenorrhea and oligomenorrhea, associated with athletics, dancing, and eating disorders.
3. In young women with amenorrhea associated with weight loss, BMD loss will be occurring soon after the amenorrhea develops. Treatment to prevent BMD loss or promote BMD accretion should begin soon, probably within 6 months after amenorrhea occurs.
4. Women who recover from anorexia nervosa at a young age (<15 years of age) can have normal total body BMD, but regional (lumbar spine and femoral neck) BMD may remain low. The longer the anorexia nervosa persists, the less likely it is that the BMD will return to normal. Girls and women with anorexia nervosa need to be rehabilitated early in the disease to maximize BMD accretion.
5. Conjugated estrogen, in doses that improve bone mineralization in postmenopausal women and in combination with medroxyprogesterone, has not been shown to improve BMD in young women with hypothalamic amenorrhea. The role of orally administered medroxyprogesterone at a dose of 10 mg per day, 10 days per month, in improving BMD in teenage girls with hypothalamic amenorrhea or oligomenorrhea remains to be established.
6. Treatment with OCP may have a beneficial effect on BMD in young women with hypothalamic amenorrhea, but this has not been established in a double-masked, randomized, controlled trial. Doing a double-masked trial using OCP will be difficult because estrogen-deficient subjects treated with OCP will be likely to have menstrual bleeding, whereas those treated with placebo will not. In addition, the risk of pregnancy in a sexually active subject, who does not know whether she is receiving OCP, is too great for some subjects.
7. Osteoporosis is a major cause of morbidity and death. Peak bone mass is a major determinant of the risk of osteoporosis, and the second decade is the critical period of peak bone mass acquisition; thus providers of health care for adolescents need to understand the factors that affect bone mineralization during this period, and advise patients accordingly.

REFERENCES

1. Lloyd T, Meyers C, Buchanan JR, Demers LM. Collegiate women athletes with irregular menses during adolescence have decreased bone density. Obstet Gynecol 1988;72:639-42.
2. Gilsanz V, Gibbens DT, Roe TF, et al. Vertebral bone density in children: effect of puberty. Radiology 1988;166:847-50.
3. White CM, Hergenroeder AC, Klish WJ. Bone mineral density in eumenorrheic and amenorrheic, 15-21 year old females. Am J Dis Child 1992;146:31-5.
4. Theintz G, Buchs D, Rizzoli R, et al. Longitudinal monitoring of bone mass accumulation in healthy adolescents: evidence for marked reduction after 16 years of age at the levels of lumbar spine and femoral neck in female subjects. J Clin Endocrinol Metab 1992;75:1060-5.
5. Slemenda CW, Reister TK, Hui SL, Miller JZ, Christian JC, Johnston CC. Influences on skeletal mineralization in children and adolescents evidence for varying effects of sexual maturation and physical activity. J Pediatr 1994;125:201-7.
6. Ponder SW, McCormick DP, Fawcett HD, Palmer JL, McKernan MG, Brouhard BH. Spinal bone mineral density in children aged 5.00 through 11.99 years. Am J Dis Child 1990; 144:1346-8.
7. Chan GM. Dietary calcium and bone mineral status of children and adolescents. Am J Dis Child 1991;145:631-4.
8. Lloyd T, Rollings N, Andon MB, et al. Determinants of bone density in young women. I. Relationships among pubertal development, total body bone mass and total body bone density in premenarchal females. J Clin Endocrinol Metab 1992; 75:383-7.
9. Katzman DK, Bachrach LK, Carter DR. Clinical and anthropometric correlates of bone mineral acquisition in healthy adolescent girls. J Clin Endocrinol Metab 1991;73:1332-9.
10. Rubin K, Schirduan V, Gendreau P, Sarfarazi M, Mendola R, Dalsky G. Predictors of axial and peripheral bone mineral density in healthy children, with special attention to the role of puberty. J Pediatr 1993;123:863-70.
11. Recker RR, Davies KM, Hinders SM, Heaney RP, Stegman MR, Kimmel DB. Bone gain in young adult women. JAMA 1992;268:2403-8.
12. McCormick DP, Ponder SW, Fawcett HD, Palmer JL. Spinal bone mineral density in 335 normal and obese children and adolescents: Evidence for ethnic and sex differences. J Bone Miner Res 1991;6:507-13.
13. Trotter M, Broman GE, Peterson RR. Densities of bones of white and Negro skeletons. J Bone Joint Surg 1960;42:50-8.
14. Li JU, Specker BL, Ho Ml. Bone mineral content in black and white children. Am J Dis Child 1989;143:1346-9.
15. Gilsanz V, Roe T, Mora S, Costin G, Goodman WG. Changes in vertebral bone density in black girls and white girls during childhood and puberty. N Engl J Med 1991;325:1597-600.
16. Garn SM, Solomon MA, Friedl J. Calcium intake and bone quality in the elderly. Ecol Food Nutr 1981;10:131-3.
17. Lloyd T, Andon MB, Rollings N, et al. Calcium supplementation and bone mineral density in adolescent girls. JAMA 1993;270:841-4.
18. Johnston CC, Miller JZ, Slemenda CW, et al. Calcium supplementation and increases in bone mineral density in children. N Engl J Med 1992;327:82-7.
19. Slemenda CW, Reister TK, Peacock M, Johnston CC. Bone growth in children following the cessation of calcium supplementation. J Bone Miner Res 1993;8:S154.
20. Shangold M, Rebar RW, Wentz AC, Schiff I. Evaluation and management of menstrual dysfunction in athletes. JAMA 1990;263:165-9.
21. Matkovic V, Ilich J. Calcium requirements for growth: are current requirements adequate? Nutr Rev 1993;51:171-80.
22. Abrams SA, Silber TJ, Esteban NV, et al. Mineral balance and bone turnover in adolescents with anorexia nervosa. J PEDIATR 1993;123:326-31.
23. Lanyon LE, Goodship AE, Pye CJ, MacFie JH. Mechanically adaptive bone remodeling. J Biomech 1982;15:141-54.
24. Donaldson CL, Hulley SB, Vogel JM, Hattner RS, Bayers JH, McMillan DE. Effect of prolonged bed rest on bone mineral. Metabolism 1970;19:1071-84.
25. Carter DR. Mechanical loading history and skeletal biology. J Biomech 1987a;20:1095-109.
26. Carter DR, Fryhrie DP, Whalen RT. Trabecular bone density and loading history regulation of connective tissue biology by mechanical energy. J Biomech 1987b;20:785-94.
27. Pocock NA, Eisman J, Gwinn T, et al. Muscle strength, physical fitness, and weight, but not age, predict femoral neck bone mass. J Bone Miner Res 1989;4:441-8.
28. Virvidakis K, Georgiou E, Korkotsidis A, Ntalleb K, Proukakis C. Bone mineral content of junior competitive weight lifters. Int J Sports Med 1990;11:244-6.
29. Gleeson PB, Protas EJ, LeBlanc AD, Schneider VS, Evans HL. Effects of weight lifting on bone mineral density in premenopausal women. J Bone Miner Res 1990;5:153-8.
30. Rockwell JC, Sorensen AM, et al. Weight training decreases vertebral bone denisty in premenopausal women: a prospective study. J Clin Endocrinol Metab 1990;71:988-93.
31. Snow-Harter C, Bouxsein ML, Lewis BT, Carter Dr, Marcus R. Effects of resistance and endurance exercise on bone mineral status of young women: a randomized exercise intervention trial. J Bone Miner Res 1992;7:761-9.32.
32. Robinson TL, Snow-Harter C, Taaffe DR, Gillis D, Shaw J, Marcus R. Gymnasts exhibit higher bone mass than runners despite similar prevalence of amenorrhea and oligomenorrhea. J Bone Miner Res 1995;10:26-35.
33. Nilsson BE, Westlin NE. Bone density in athletes. Clin Orthop 1971;77:179-82.
34. Aloia JF, Cohn SM, Ostuni JA, Cane R, Ellis K. Prevention of involutional bone loss by exercise. Ann Intern Med 1978; 89:356-8.
35. Risser WL, Lee EJ, LeBlanc A, Poindexter HBW, Riser JMH, Schneider V. Bone density in eumenorrheic female college athletes. Med Sci Sports Exerc 1990;22:570-4.
36. McCullough RG, Bailey DA, Whalen RL, Houston CS, Faulkner RA, Craven BR. Bone density and bone mineral content of adolescent soccer athletes and competitive swimmers. Pediatr Exerc Sci 1992;4:319-30.
37. Grimston SK, Willows ND, Hanley DA. Mechanical loading regime and its relationship to bone mineral density in children. Med Sci Sports Exerc 1993;25:1203-10.
38. Prior JC, Vigna YM, Schechter MT, Burgess AE. Spinal bone loss and ovulatory disturbances. N Engl J Med 1990;323; 1221-7.
39. Drinkwater BL, Nelson K, Chestnut CH, Bremner WJ, Shainholtz S, Southworth MD. Bone mineral content of amenorrheic and eumenorrheic athletes. N Engl J Med 1984; 311:277-81.
40. Cann CE, Martin MC, Genant HK, Jaffe RB. Decreased spi-

nal mineral content in amenorrheic women. JAMA 1984; 251:626-9.
41. Warren MP, Brooks-Gunn J, Fox RP, Lancelot C, Newman D, Hamilton WG. Lack of bone accretion and amenorrhea: evidence for a relative osteopenia in weight-bearing bones. J Clin Endocrinol Metab 1991;72:847-53.
42. Davis MR. Screening for postmenopausal osteoporosis. Am J Obstet Gynecol 1987;156:1-5.
43. DeSouza MJ, Metzger DA. Reproductive dysfunction in amenorrheic athletes and anorexic patients: a review. Med Sci Sports Exerc 1991;23:995-1007.
44. Loucks AB, Vaitukaitis J, Cameron JL, et al. The reproductive system and exercise in women. Med Sci Sports Exerc 1992;24:S288-93.
45. Loucks AB. Physical activity, fitness and female reproductive morbidity. In: Bouchard C, Shepard RJ, Stephens T, eds. Physical activity, fitness and health. Champaign, Illinois Human Kinetics Publishers, 1994.
46. Golden NH, Shenker IR. Amenorrhea in anorexia nervosa: etiology and implications. Adolescent Medicine, State of the Art Reviews 1992;3:503-17.
47. Warren WP. The effect of exercise on pubertal progression and reproductive function in girls. J Clin Endocrinol Metab 1980;51:1150-7.
48. Stager JM, Wigglesworth JK, Hatler LK. Interpreting the relationship between age of menarche and prepubertal training. Med Sci Sports Exerc 1990;22:54-8.
49. Marcus R, Cann R, Madvig P, et al. Menstrual function and bone mass in elite women distance runners: endocrine and metabolic features. Ann Intern Med 1985;102:158-63.
50. Frisch RE, McArthur JW. Menstrual cycles: fatness as a determinant of minimum weight for height necessary for their maintenance or onset. Science 1974;185:949-51.
51. Baker ER. Menstrual dysfunction and hormonal status in athletic women. Fertil Steril 1981;36:691-6.
52. Schwartz B, Cumming DC, Riordan E, Selye M, Yen SSC, Rebar RW. Exercise-associated amenorrhea: a distinct entity? Am J Obstet Gynecol 1981;141:662-70.
53. Loucks AB, Heath EM, Law T, Verdun M, Watts JR. Dietary restriction reduces luteinizing hormone (LH) pulse frequency during waking hours and increases LH pulse amplitude during sleep in young menstruating women. J Clin Endocrinol Metab 1994;78:910-5.
54. Kaiserauer S, Snyder AC, Sleeper M, Zierath J. Nutritional, physiologic, and menstrual status of distance runners. Med Sci Sports Exerc 1989;21:120-5.
55. Nelson ME, Fisher EC, Catsos PD, Meredith CN, Turksoy RN, Evan WJ. Diet and bone status in amenorrheic runners. Am J Clin Nutr 1986;43:910-6.56.
56. Wilmore JH, Wambsgans KC, Brenner M. Is there energy conservation in amenorrheic compared with eumenorrheic distance runners? J Appl Physiol 1992;72(1):15-22.
57. Kurzer MS, Calloway DH. Effects of energy deprivation on sex hormone patterns in healthy menstruating women. Am Physiol Soc 1986;251:E483-8.
58. Bronson FH. Food-restricted, prepubertal rats: rapid recovery of luteinizing hormone pulsing with excess food, and full recovery of pubertal development with gonadotropin-releasing hormone. Endocrinology 1986;118:2483-7.
59. Hergenroeder AC, Fiorotto ML, Klish WJ. Body composition in ballet dancers measured by total body electrical conductivity. Med Sci Sports Exerc 1991;23:528-33.
60. Sanborn CF, Albrecht BH, Wagner WW. Athletic amenorrhea lack of association with body fat. Med Sci Sports Exerc 1987;19:207-12.
61. de Ridder CM, Thijssen JHH, Bruning PF, Van den Brande JL, Zonderland ML, Erich WBM. Body fat mass, body fat distribution, and pubertal development a longitudinal study of physical and hormonal sexual maturation of girls. J Clin Endocrinol Metab 1992;75:442-6.
62. Lutter JM. Prevalence of menstrual change in athletes and active women. In: Puhl J, Brown C, eds. The menstrual cycle and physical activity. Champaign, Illinois: Human Kinetics Publishers, 1986:29.
63. Garner DM, Garfinkel PE. Socio-cultural factors in the development of anorexia nervosa. Psychol Med 1980;10:647-56.
64. Brooks-Gunn J, Warren MP, Hamilton LH. The relation of eating problems and amenorrhea in ballet dancers. Med Sci Sports Exerc 1987;19:41-4.
65. Kurtzman FD, Yager J, Landvesk J, Wiesmeier E, Bodurka DC. Eating disorders among selected female student populations at UCLA. J Am Diet Assoc 1989;89:45-53.
66. Weltman EA, Stein RC, Doershuk CF, Moir RN, Palmer K, Jaffe AC. Weight and menstrual function in patients with eating disorders and cystic fibrosis. Pediatrics 1990;85:282-7.
67. Rigotti NA, Nussbaum SR, Herzog DB, Neer RM. Osteoporosis in women with anorexia nervosa. N Engl J Med 1984;311:1601-6.
68. Brotman AW, Stern TA. Osteoporosis and pathologic fractures in anorexia nervosa. Am J Psychiatry 1985;142:495-6.
69. Dugowson CE, Drinkwater BL, Clark JM. Nontraumatic femur fracture in an oligomenorrheic athlete. Med Sci Sports Exerc 1991;23:1323-5.
70. Seeman E, Szmukler GI, Formica C, Tsalamandris C, Mestrovic R. Osteoporosis in anorexia nervosa: the influence of peak bone density, bone loss, oral contraceptive use, and exercise. J Bone Miner Res 1992;7:1467-74.
71. Bachrach IK, Guido D, Katzman MD, Litt IF, Marcus R. Decreased bone mineral density in adolescent girls with anorexia nervosa. Pediatrics 1990;86:440-7.
72. Herzog W, Minne H, Deter C, et al. Outcome of bone mineral density in anorexia nervosa patients 11.7 years after first admission. J Bone Miner Res 1993;8:597-605.
73. Bachrach LK, Katzman DK, Litt IF, Guido D, Marcus R. Recovery from osteopenia in adolescent girls with anorexia nervosa. J Clin Endocrinol Metab 1991;72:602-6.
74. Rigotti NA, Neer RM, Skates SJ, Herzog DB, Nussbaum SR. The clinical course of osteoporosis in anorexia nervosa: a longitudinal study of cortical bone mass. JAMA 1991;265: 1133-8
75. Biller BMK, Coughlin JF, Saxe V, Schoenfeld D, Spratt DI, Klibanski A. Osteopenia in women with hypothalamic amenorrhea: a prospective study. Obstet Gynecol 1991;78:996-1001.
76. Jonnavithula S, Warren MP, Fox RP, Lazaro MI. Bone density is compromised in amenorrheic women despite return of menses a 2-year study. Obstet Gynecol 1993;81:669-74.
77. Drinkwater BL, Nilson K, Ott S, Chestnut CH. Bone mineral density after resumption of menses in amenorrheic athletes. JAMA 1986;256:380-2.
78. Ettinger B, Genant HK, Cann CE. Long-term estrogen replacement therapy prevents bone loss and fractures. Ann Intern Med 1985;102:319-24.
79. Lindsay R, Rohme J, Kandus B. The effect of oral contracep-

tive use on vertebral bone mass in pre- and postmenopausal women. Contraception 1986;34:333-40.
80. Kleerekoper M, Brienza RS, Schultz LR, Johnson CC. Oral contraceptive use may protect against low bone mass. Arch Intern Med 1991;151:1971-6.
81. Kritz-Silverstein D, Barrett-Connor E. Bone mineral density in postmenopausal women as determined by prior oral contraceptive use. Am J Public Health 1993;83:100-2.
82. Warren MP, Fox RP, DeRogatis AJ, Hamilton WG. Osteopenia in hypothalamic amenorrhea a 3-year longitudinal study Abstract . Program of the Endocrine Society Annual Meeting, Anaheim, California, 1994.
83. Emans SJ, Grace E, Hoffer FA, Gundberg C, Ravnikar V, Woods ER. Estrogen deficiency in adolescents and young adults impact on bone mineral content and effects of estrogen replacement therapy. Obstet Gynecol 1990;76:585-92.
84. Gallagher JC, Kable WT. Goldgar D. Effect of progestin therapy on cortical and trabecular bone: comparison with estrogen. Am J Med 1991;90:171-8.
85. Prince RL, Smith M, Dick IM, et al. Prevention of postmenopausal osteoporosis. a comparative study of exercise, calcium supplementation, and hormone replacement. N Engl J Med 1991;325:1189-95.
86. Prior JC, Vigna YM, Barr SI, Rexworthy C, Lentle BC. Cyclic medroxyprogesterone treatment increases bone density. Am J Med 1994;96:521-30.
87. Prior JC. Progesterone as a bone-trophic hormone. Endocrine Reviews 1990;11;386-98.
88. Snead DB, Weltman A, Weltman JY, et al. Reproductive hormones and bone mineral density in women runners. J Appl Physiol 1992;72;2149-56.
89. McNeely SG, Schinfeld JS, Stovall TG, Ling FW, Buxton BH. Prevention of osteoporosis by medroxyprogesterone acetate in postmenopausal women. Int J Gynaecol Obstet 1991;34: 253-6.
90. Cundy T, Evans M, Roberts H, Wattie D, Ames R, Reid IR. Bone density in women receiving depot medroxyprogesterone acetate for contraception. BMJ 1991;303:13-6.

Relationship between insulin resistance and abnormal lipid profile in obese adolescents

Julia Steinberger, MD, Catherene Moorehead, MS, Victor Katch, EdD, and Albert P. Rocchini, MD

From the Division of Pediatric Cardiology, University of Minnesota, Minneapolis, and the Division of Pediatric Cardiology and the Department of Kinesiology, Division of Physical Education, University of Michigan, Ann Arbor

Objective: **To determine whether the lipid abnormalities observed in obese adolescents are associated with insulin resistance.**
Methods: **We evaluated the relationship between lipid levels and insulin resistance in 82 obese adolescents. Insulin resistance was assessed by fasting insulin level and sum of the insulin values after an oral glucose tolerance test in all 82, and were compared with data from 40 nonobese adolescents. Whole-body glucose uptake during euglycemic hyperinsulinemia (M value) was performed in 19 of the obese adolescents and compared with that of 24 nonobese young adults.**
Results: **The obese adolescents had significantly elevated low-density lipoprotein cholesterol (LDL-C) (3.09 ± 0.73 mmol/L; 119 ± 28.2 mg/dl) and triglycerides (1.22 ± 0.62 mmol/L; 108 ± 54.6 mg/dl) and low high-density lipoprotein cholesterol (HDL-C) levels (0.94 ± 0.24 mmol/L; 36 ± 9.1 mg/dl) when compared with values in the nonobese subjects. M values were significantly depressed in the obese compared with the nonobese subjects. Adiposity significantly correlated with low HDL-C and elevated triglyceride values. From the variables representing insulin resistance, the strongest correlation with the abnormal lipid profile was found for the M value. A stepwise multiple regression analysis revealed that the M value was the only step entered into the relationship for triglycerides and LDL-C, and both M value and fasting insulin were entered for HDL-C.**
Conclusion: **In obese adolescents the degree of insulin resistance explains a significant portion of the variance in the levels of triglycerides, LDL-C, and HDL-C. (J PEDIATR 1995;126:690-5)**

In young persons obesity, non-insulin-dependent diabetes mellitus, hypertension, and atherosclerotic cardiovascular disease are uncommon. However, by 70 years of age, the incidence of these metabolic disorders reaches epidemic proportions. The link between these conditions is believed by some investigators to be insulin resistance.[1-4] It is not clear, however, whether the link is causal and, if so, which is the cause and which the effect. Recent studies with the use of the euglycemic insulin clamp technique in normoglycemic persons have suggested that insulin resistance can be linked with lipid and lipoprotein abnormalities.[5] Insulin resistance has been associated with elevated fasting and postprandial insulin levels, and has been hypothesized to play a major role in dyslipidemia in persons with normal glucose tolerance and in those with impaired glucose tolerance and non-insulin-dependent diabetes. Lipid abnormalities have also been reported in obese adults, who have elevated trig-

Supported in part by granst (Nos. Ro1-AM-20572, M01-RP-00042, 2R01-HL-35743, and 2P60 AM-20572 from the National Institutes of Health.

Submitted for publication July 22, 1994; accepted Nov. 28, 1994.

Reprint requests: Julia Steinberger, MD, Division of Pediatric Cardiology, University of Minnesota Hospital and Clinic, Box 94, 420 Delaware St. SE, Minneapolis, MN 55455.

0022-3476/95/$3.00 + 0 **9/20/62345**

lyceride and low-density lipoprotein cholesterol levels and low levels of high-density lipoprotein cholesterol.[7-11]

The purpose of this study was to determine whether similar lipid abnormalities occur in normoglycermic obese adolescents and whether these lipid abnormalities are associated with insulin resistance.

METHODS

The patient population is described in Table I. None of the subjects was taking any medications or had any medical illness, including kidney, liver, endocrine, or cardiovascular disease. Obesity was defined as weight-for-height greater than the 75th percentile for age and sex, and triceps and subscapular skin-fold thicknesses greater than the 80th percentile for age and sex.[12] Four of the 82 obese adolescents (5%) had a family history for hypertension and 41 of 82 (50%) had one or more first-degree relatives who were obese. There was no significant difference between obese and nonobese adolescents regarding a family history of dyslipidemia; we did not perform lipid profile studies in family members. The study protocol was approved by the institutional review board, and the parents of all the subjects gave informed consent before the study began.

HDL-C	High-density lipoprotein cholesterol
LDL-C	Low-density lipoprotein cholesterol
M value	Whole-body glucose uptake during euglycemic hyperinsulinemia

Experimental protocol. All children were recruited from a consecutive group of patients seen in an obesity clinic. The majority had been referred by a family physician, although some were self-referred. Forty-five of the obese and 26 of the nonobese children were included in previous studies.[13, 14] The adolescents were studied as outpatients at the Clinical Research Center. After an overnight fast of 12 hours, all adolescents reported for the study before 8 AM; a heparin lock was inserted in an antecubital vein, and blood was drawn for insulin, glucose, lipids, and lipoprotein determinations. For the majority of subjects the lipid profiles were performed on one occasion. An oral glucose tolerance test with a glucose load of 1.75 gm/kg (maximum load, 75 gm) was performed in all obese and nonobese adolescents. Blood was sampled for glucose and insulin at baseline and 15, 30, 45, 60, 90, and 120 minutes after the glucose load. The sum of the insulin values at these time points was used as an estimate of insulin resistance. After lunch, all adolescents had body composition measured by hydrostatic weighing as described by Katch et al.[15]

On a separate day 19 of the obese adolescents returned for a euglycemic insulin clamp procedure; they did not significantly differ in any measured variable from the other 63 adolescents. With the adolescents in a semisupine position, polyethylene cannulas were inserted into an antecubital vein in one arm and into a warmed dorsal hand vein in the other arm. After 30 minutes a primed constant infusion of insulin was administered, beginning at a dose of 800 mU/m^2 and exponentially decreasing for 10 minutes. A constant dosage of 40 mU/m^2 per minute was then given. Concomitantly with the insulin, an intravenous infusion of 20% glucose was administered by a variable infusion syringe pump (Harvard Apparatus, Mills, Mass.). Blood samples were obtained at 5-minute intervals for determination of blood glucose concentration. The glucose infusion rate was varied every 5 minutes to keep glucose concentration constant at baseline values. The amount of glucose required to maintain euglycemia was used as an estimate of whole-body glucose disposal.

Table I. Demographic data of the patient population

	Obese (n = 82)	Nonobese (n = 40)	*p*
Mean age ± SD (yr)	12.6 ± 1.2	13.3 ± 0.6	NS
Sex: No. (%)			
M	34 (41)	18 (45)	NS
F	48 (59)	22 (55)	NS
Ethnic background: No. (%)			
White	54 (66)	28 (70)	NS
Black	12 (15)	8 (20)	NS
Hispanic	6 (7)	4 (10)	NS
Family history: No. (%)			
Hypertension	4 (5)	0	
Obesity	41 (50)	0	

NS, Not significant.

Laboratory procedures. Lipid and lipoprotein values were determined from fresh serum samples drawn after a 12-hour overnight fast. Lipoprotein fractionation was performed with ultracentrifugation and selective precipitation. Cholesterol and triglycerides from the whole serum and from lipoprotein fractions were assayed by automated enzymatic methods. LDL-C values were derived from the triglyceride and HDL-C levels. Blood glucose was measured by the glucose oxidase method. Plasma insulin was determined by a radioimmunoassay.

Statistical analysis. All values are reported as means ± SD. Analysis of variance was used to compare differences between obese and nonobese adolescents. Lipid and lipoprotein values were adjusted for age, race, and sex by use of the SD score *(z)*, calculated according to the formula $z = x - x'/\text{SD}$, where x is measured lipid value, x' is mean of the expected lipid for age, race, and sex,[16] and the SD is of the expected lipid value for age, race, and sex. The rela-

Table II. Fasting plasma lipid level, fasting plasma insulin level, and sum of the insulin levels after oral glucose tolerance test in 82 obese and 40 nonobese adolescents

	Obese (N = 82)	Nonobese (N = 40)
Triglycerides: mmol/L (mg/dl)	2.80 ± 1.4 (108 ± 54.6)*	1.4 ± 0.5 (54 ± 19.5)
LDL cholesterol: mmol/L (mg/dl)	3.09 ± 0.7 (119 ± 28.2)*	1.7 ± 0.5 (69 ± 20.2)
Total cholesterol: mmol/L (mg/dl)	4.5 ± 0.7 (173 ± 27.3)*	3.5 ± 0.8 (137 ± 29)
HDL cholesterol: mmol/L (mg/dl)	0.9 ± 0.2 (36 ± 9.1)*	1.4 ± 0.4 (54 ± 13.9)
Fasting insulin: 10^{-2}IU/L (μU/ml)	22.7 ± 17.3*	9 ± 12.6
Σ Insulin, 10^{-2} IU/L (μU/ml)†	540 ± 391.3*	245 ± 163.8

Values are expressed as mean ± SD. Conversion factors: 1 mg/dl = 0.0258 mmol/L; 1 μU/ml = 10^{-2} IU/L.
*p <0.001, obese versus nonobese subject.
‡After an oral glucose tolerance test.

Table III. Simple and partial correlations between HDL-C, LDL-C, and triglyceride levels versus percent body fat, fasting insulin level, sum of the insulins after oral glucose tolerance test, and M value

	Simple correlation *(R)*			Partial correlation *(R)**		
Variable	HDL-C	LDL-C	Triglycerides	HDL-C	LDL-C	Triglycerides
Body fat (%)	−0.54†	0.24	0.34‡	−0.43†	0.1	0.1
Fasting insulin	−0.60†	0.18	0.38‡	−0.36‡	0.01	0.04
Σ Insulin	−0.64†	0.30†	0.52†	−0.62†	0.29*	0.51†
M value	0.77†	−0.55†	−0.60†	0.70†	−0.49†	−0.59†

Σ *Ins*, Sum of insulin values after oral glucose tolerance test.
*Calculated for Σ Insulin, and body fat (n = 82) and did not take into account the effect that M value had on the relationships because only 19 of the subjects had M value measured. The partial correlation for M value took into account all the other variables.
†p <0.001.
‡p <0.01.

tionships between lipid and lipoprotein determinations and fasting insulin, sum of the insulin values after an oral glucose tolerance test, and whole-body glucose uptake were assessed with Pearson product-moment correlations, partial correlations, and regression models. Because lipid values are affected in childhood by age, sex, and race, to compare our group of obese adolescents with the adolescent population in general, a z-score distribution was calculated for each of the lipid values with data from *The Lipid Research Clinics Population Studies Data Book*.[16]

RESULTS

Obese adolescents and nonobese adolescents were not significantly different with regard to age, sex, and race (Table I). When compared with the nonobese group, the obese adolescents were both significantly heavier (mean body weight, 69.9 ± 2.5 kg vs 44.3 ± 2.9 kg, p <0.001) and significantly more adipose (mean percent body fat, 37.4% ± 1.1% vs 20.1% ± 10%, p <0.001). Body mass index was significantly greater in the obese (mean, 21.6) compared with the nonobese subjects (mean, 14.2; p <0.001). Similar differences were noted between the groups regarding blood pressure, which was significantly higher in the obese compared with the nonobese adolescents (mean, 126 ± 3/79 ± 3 mm Hg vs 108 ± 4/63 ± 3 mm Hg, p <0.01). The obese adolescents had significantly higher triglyceride, total cholesterol, and LDL-C levels (p <0.01) and significantly lower HDL-C values (p <0.01) (Table II). The obese adolescents had LDL-C and triglyceride distributions that were significantly skewed to the right (LDL-C mean z = 0.97 ± 0.13, p <0.01; triglyceride mean z = 1.4 ± 0.19, p <0.01). The HDL-C distribution of the obese adolescents was significantly skewed to the left (HDL-C mean z = −1.5 ± 0.09, p <0.01).

When compared with the nonobese adolescents, the obese adolescents had significantly higher (p <0.001) fasting plasma insulin levels and sums of the insulin values during the oral glucose tolerance test (Table II). Although we have not performed euglycemic insulin clamps on nonobese adolescents, we have performed insulin clamps on 24 nonobese young adults 18 to 24 years old (mean, 22.3 years).[13, 17] Compared with these nonobese young adults, the obese adolescents had significantly reduced M values both when related to body surface area (342 ± 14 vs 164.9 ± 13 mg [glucose]/m^2 per minute, p <0.001) and weight (8.7 ± 0.6 vs 4.1 ± 0.3 mg [glucose]/kg per minute, p <0.001). Table III summarizes the simple and partial correlations of LDL-C, HDL-C, and triglyceride with percent body fat,

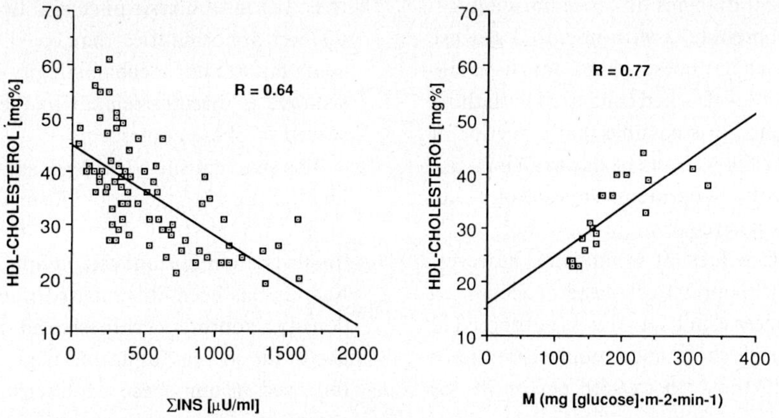

Fig. 1. Linear correlation between low HDL-C and insulin resistance. Insulin resistance is measured by sum of insulin values during oral glucose tolerance test *(ΣINS) (left panel)* and M value *(right panel)*. Significant linear relationship was observed between two estimates of insulin resistance and HDL-C level (Σ INS vs HDL-C, $r = -0.64$, $p < 0.001$; M value vs HDL-C, $r = 0.77$, $p < 0.001$).

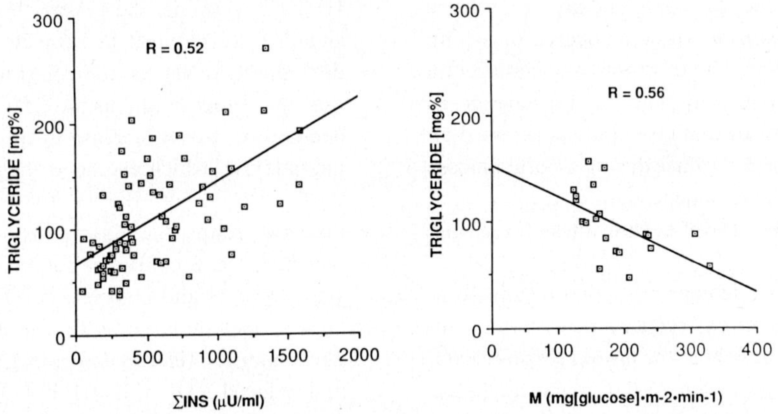

Fig. 2. Linear correlation between triglyceride level and insulin resistance. Insulin resistance is measured by sum of insulin values during oral glucose tolerance test *(ΣINS) (left panel)* and M value *(right panel)*. Significant linear relationship was observed between two estimates of insulin resistance and triglyceride level (ΣINS vs triglycerides, $r = 0.052$, $p < 0.001$; M value vs triglycerides, $r = -0.56$, $p < 0.001$).

fasting insulin, sums of the insulin values during the oral glucose tolerance test, and M value. HDL-C and triglycerides were the two lipid variables that had the highest correlation with the degree of insulin resistance as assessed by sums of the insulin values during an oral glucose tolerance test and M value (Figs. 1 and 2). In all 82 obese adolescents with these measurements we performed stepwise multiple regression analysis. The sum of the insulin values was the only variable significantly related to triglycerides ($F = 32$) and LDL-C ($F = 12.5$); both the sum of the insulin values ($F = 34$) and percent body fat ($F = 9.6$) were significantly related to HDL-C when controlled for age, sex, race, and weight. Similarly, in the 19 obese adolescents in whom M value was also measured, stepwise multiple regression analysis revealed that M value was the only significant predictive variable for triglycerides ($F = 36.1$) and LDL-C ($F = 10.3$), and both M value ($F = 52$) and fasting insulin value ($F = 5.1$) were significantly associated with HDL-C levels.

DISCUSSION

The current study reports that when compared with either our nonobese control subjects or the adolescent population included in *The Lipid Research Clinics Population Studies Data Book*, obese adolescents have an abnormal "atherogenic" lipid profile consisting of elevated LDL-C and triglycerides levels, and low HDL-C levels. Similar lipid profiles have been reported in obese and nonobese adults with non-insulin-dependent diabetes, in obese normoglycemic adults, and in nonobese adults with impaired glucose tolerance.[4, 5, 18-20] Although our obese adolescents have significantly elevated LDL-C levels when compared with those of the nonobese adolescents, it is possible that a portion of the apparent elevation in LDL-C could be due to an increase in the intermediate-density lipoprotein cholesterol,[21] because LDL-C values were derived from the total cholesterol, triglyceride, and HDL-C values. It is unlikely, however, that intermediate-density lipoprotein cholesterol accounted for the majority of the increase in LDL-C value observed in our obese subjects, because these obese adolescents have triglyceride values within the 75th to 95th percentile for age, sex, and race.

Many investigators have speculated that the link between these metabolic disorders is insulin resistance. In the current study we have documented not only that obese adolescents have insulin resistance (as documented by fasting hyperinsulinemia, a hyperinsulinemia response to an oral glucose load, and reduced M value but also that there is a significant relationship between the degree of insulin resistance and the abnormal lipid profile associated with obesity. With multiple regression analysis we have documented that the degree of insulin resistance as assessed either by the sum of the insulin values during an oral glucose tolerance test or by M value, independent of the degree of adiposity, is the best predictor of each of these three lipid abnormalities.

Amiel et al.[22] previously demonstrated that insulin-stimulated glucose metabolism was reduced in pubertal children, and it is possible that part of the insulin resistance observed in the obese group was due to their pubertal status. However, the insulin-stimulated glucose uptake in our obese adolescents was still significantly lower (164.9 ± 13 mg/m^2 per minute) than that reported by Amiel et al. for pubertal boys and girls (199 ± 16 and 203 ± 21 mg/m^2 per minute). We also showed that for obese subjects the abnormal glucose uptake correlated with an abnormal lipid profile. We were unable to perform insulin clamps in nonobese adolescents for comparison with the obese adolescents, because this was judged to be unethical by the committee on the use of human subjects in research at our institution. Without data from nonobese control subjects, the insulin values in obese adolescents may be functions, in unknown proportions, of insulin resistance and decreased clearance of insulin. The comparison with nonobese young adults was used to define a normal range of insulin-mediated glucose uptake. Although we have demonstrated a relationship between insulin resistance and the lipid abnormalities of obese adolescents, we have not proven that this relationship is causal. There are at least two explainations for the observed association between insulin resistance and lipid abnormalities: (1) insulin resistance and lipid abnormalities are two distinct abnormalities that coexist in many obese adolescents but are not mechanistically related; or (2) insulin resistance is directly related to the lipid abnormalities observed in obese adolescents.

The mechanism whereby insulin resistance could cause an alteration in lipid metabolism was not directly examined in the current study. However, there is evidence that insulin plays an important role in lipid metabolism. Hyperinsulinemia has been documented to enhance hepatic very low density lipoprotein synthesis and thus may directly contribute to the increased plasma triglyceride and LDL-C levels observed in our obese adolescents.[23, 24] Resistance to the action of insulin on lipoprotein lipase in peripheral tissues may also contribute to elevated triglyceride and LDL-C levels.[25, 26] Golay et al.[27] suggested that insulin resistance may be responsible for the reduced levels of HDL-C observed in patients with non-insulin-dependent diabetes. These investigators have shown that despite enhanced HDL-C synthesis, the plasma HDL-C concentration was significantly reduced in subjects with non-insulin-dependent diabetes versus control subjects. They documented that the decrease in plasma HDL-C level was entirely accounted for by an increase in the rate of apo-A1/HDL-C degradation, which exceeded the enhanced rate of its synthesis. Within both the control and non-insulin-dependent diabetic groups, the plasma insulin concentration and the plasma HDL-C concentration (and apo-A1 clearance rate) were strongly and inversely correlated.

We conclude not only that obese adolescents have lipid abnormalities (elevated serum LDL-C and triglycerides, and reduced HDL-C levels) but also that these lipid abnormalities correlate with the degree of insulin resistance. Further studies are necessary to determine whether these lipid abnormalities are directly caused by insulin resistance. Weight reduction is known to improve insulin resistance and lipid profile in obese subjects, and we may expect this to have the same effect in the obese children of this study. A number of these obese adolescents had been enrolled in a weight loss program, but compliance was variable, and repeated studies are to be performed.

REFERENCES

1. Kissebah AH, Adams PW, Wynn V. Inter-relationship between insulin secretion and plasma free fatty acid and triglyceride transport kinetics in maturity onset diabetes and the effect of phenethylbiguanide (Phenformin). Diabetologia 1974; 10:119-30.
2. Laakso M, Barrett-Connor E. Asymptomatic hyperglycemia is associated with lipid and lipoprotein changes favoring atherosclerosis. Arteriosclerosis 1989;9:665-72.
3. Reaven GM, Greenfield MS. Diabetic hypertriglyceridemia: evidence of three clinical syndromes. Diabetes 1981;30:66-75.

4. Tobey TA, Greenfield M, Kraemer F, Reaven GM. Relationship between insulin resistance, insulin secretion, very low density lipoprotein kinetics and plasma triglyceride levels in normotriglyceridemic man. Metabolism 1981;30:165-71.
5. Abbott WGH, Lillioja S, Young AA. Relationships between plasma lipoprotein concentrations and insulin action in an obese hyperinsulinemic population. Diabetes 1987;36:897-904.
6. Garg A, Helderman JH, Koffler M, Ayuso R, Rosenstock J, Raskin P. Relationship between lipoprotein levels and in vivo insulin action in normal young white men. Metabolism 1988; 37:982-7.
7. Evans DH, Hoffman RG, Kalkhoff RK, et al. Relationship of body fat topography to insulin sensitivity and metabolic profiles in premenopausal women. Metabolism 1984;33:68-75.
8. Haffner SM, Stern MP, Hazuda HP, et al. Do upper body and centralization adiposity measure different aspects of regional body fat distribution: relationship to non-insulin-dependent diabetes mellitus, lipids and lipoproteins. Diabetes 1987;36:43-51.
9. Haffner SM, Fong D, Hazuda HP, Pugh PA, Patterson JK. Hyperinsulinemia, upper body adiposity, and cardiovascular risk factors in non-diabetics. Metabolism 1988;37:338-45.
10. Kissebah AH, Vydelingum N, Murray R, et al. Relationship of body fat distribution to metabolic complications of obesity. J Clin Endocrinol Metab 1982;54:254-60.
11. Krotkiewski M, Bjorntop P, Sjostrom C, et al. Impact of obesity on metabolism in men and women: importance of regional adipose distribution. J Clin Invest 1983;72:1150-62.
12. Rocchini AP, Katch V, Anderson J, et al. Blood pressure in obese adolescents: effects of weight loss. Pediatrics 1988;82:16-23.
13. Rocchini AP, Katch V, Kveselis D, et al. Insulin and renal retention in obese adolescents. Hypertension 1989;14:367-74.
14. Rocchini AP, Morehead C, Katch V, Key J, Finta KM. Forearm resistance vessel abnormalities and insulin resistance in obese adolescents. Hypertension 1992;19:615-20.
15. Katch FI, Michael ED, Hovath SM. Estimation of blood volume by underwater weighing: description of a simple method. J Appl Physiol 1967;23:811-3.
16. Lipid Metabolism Branch. The lipid research clinics population studies data book; vol 1: The prevalence study. National Institutes of Health publication No. 80-1527, July 1980.
17. Rocchini AP, Moorehead C, London M, Antishin J. Salt sensitivity and insulin resistance. Circulation 1990;82(suppl III-):III-87.
18. Olefsky JM, Farquhar JW, Reaven GM. Reappraisal of the role of insulin in hypertriglyceridemia. Am J Med 1974;57:551-60.
19. Reaven GM, Lerner RL, Stern MP, Farquhar JW. Role of insulin in endogenous hypertriglyceridemia. J Clin Invest 1967; 46:1756-67.
20. Zavaroni I, Dall'Aglio E, Alpi O, et al. Evidence for an independent relationship between plasma insulin and concentration of high density lipoprotein cholesterol and triglyceride. Atherosclerosis 1985;55:259-66.
21. Steiner G. Hypertriglyceridemia and carbohydrate intolerance: interrelations and therapeutic implications. Am J Cardiol 1986;57:27G-30G.
22. Amiel SA, Sherwin RS, Simonson DC, Lauritano AA, Tamborlane WV. Impaired insulin action in puberty. N Engl J Med 1986;315:215-9.
23. Orchard TJ, Becker DJ, Bates M, Kuller LH, Drash AL. Plasma insulin and lipoprotein concentrations: an atherogenic association? Am J Epidemiol 1983;118:326-37.
24. Stalder M, Pometta D, Suenram A. Relationship between plasma insulin levels and high density lipoprotein cholesterol levels in healthy men. Diabetologia 1981;21:554-8.
25. Pykallsto OJ, Smith PH, Brunzell JD. Determinants of human adipose tissue lipoprotein lipase: effect of diabetes and obesity on basal and diet induced activity. J Clin Invest 1975;56:1108-17.
26. Sadur CN, Yost TJ, Eckel RH. Insulin responsiveness of adipose tissue lipoprotein lipase is delayed but preserved in obesity. J Clin Endocrinol Metab 1984;59:1176-82.
27. Golay A, Zech L, Shi MZ, Chiou Y-AM, Reaven GM, Chen Y-DI. High density lipoprotein (HDL) metabolism in noninsulin-dependent diabetes mellitus: measurement of HDL turnover using tritiated HDL. J Clin Endocrinol Metab 1987; 65:512-8.

Differences in morbidity between breast-fed and formula-fed infants

Kathryn G. Dewey, PhD, M. Jane Heinig, PhD, and
Laurie A. Nommsen-Rivers, MS, RD

From the Department of Nutrition and Program in International Nutrition, University of California, Davis

To determine whether breast-feeding is protective against infection in relatively affluent populations, morbidity data were collected by weekly monitoring during the first 2 years of life from matched cohorts of infants who were either breast fed (BF) (N = 46) or formula fed (FF) (N = 41) until at least 12 months of age. Cohorts were matched for characteristics such as birth weight and parental socioeconomic status, and we controlled for use of day care in data analysis. Mean maternal educational level was high (16 years) in both groups. In the first year of life the incidence of diarrheal illness among BF infants was half that of FF infants; the percentage with any otitis media was 19% lower and with prolonged episodes (>10 days) was 80% lower in BF compared with FF infants. There were no significant differences in rates of respiratory illness; nearly all cases were mild upper respiratory infections. Morbidity rates did not differ significantly between groups in the second year of life, but the mean duration of episodes of otitis media was longer in FF than BF infants (8.8 ± 5.3 vs 5.9 ± 3.5 days, respectively; *p* = 0.01). These results indicate that the reduction in morbidity associated with breast-feeding is of sufficient magnitude to be of public health significance. (J Pediatr 1995;126:696-702)

Despite numerous studies demonstrating the protective effect of breast-feeding against infection, particularly in disadvantaged populations,[1-4] debate still continues as to whether the magnitude of this effect in affluent populations has public health significance.[5] In industrialized countries comparisons of morbidity rates between breast-fed and formula-fed infants must usually take into account confounding factors such as parental socioeconomic status, maternal education, access to health care, parental smoking, and use of day care, in addition to issues regarding reporting biases and reverse causality. In such studies reduced diarrheal morbidity of BF relative to FF infants has been reported by many[6-16] but not all[17-19] researchers. Likewise, the evidence regarding protection against otitis media[10, 19-27] and respiratory illnesses[9, 14, 19, 28-34] has been mixed. Conflicting results may be due to inadequate study design, lack of control of confounding variables, differences in the definition or duration of breast-feeding, or insufficient sample size.

Short of random assignment of infants to be breast fed or formula fed, which is not ethically or practically feasible, the optimal study design to evaluate morbidity differences is one in which infants are either fully breast fed or formula fed throughout the first year of life, the groups are matched for as many potentially confounding variables as possible, and morbidity data are collected longitudinally by continuous, frequent monitoring. The Davis Area Research on Lactation, Infant Nutrition, and Growth (DARLING) study[35-40] was designed to meet these criteria. We present the comparisons of morbidity rates between BF and FF infants during the first 2 years of life.

BF	Breast-fed
FF	Formula-fed

Supported by U.S. Department of Agriculture grants 86 CRCR 1-1968 and 89-37200-4450, and by a gift from the Mead-Johnson Nutritional Group, Evansville, Ind.

Submitted for publication July 29, 1994; accepted Nov. 28, 1994.

Reprint requests: Kathryn G. Dewey, PhD, Department of Nutrition, University of California, Davis, CA 95616-8669.

0022-3476/95/$3.00 + 0 **9/20/62344**

Table I. Characteristics of study groups

	BF (n = 45)	FF (n = 41)
Birth weight (gm)*	3653 ± 536	3602 ± 452
Infant sex (% male)	53	49
Maternal age (yr)*	30.8 ± 4.7	30.5 ± 5.6
Maternal education (yr)*	16.4 ± 1.9	15.6 ± 2.4
Parity (% primiparas)	40	37
Pregnancy weight gain (kg)*	15.1 ± 4.8	16.2 ± 5.5
Parental height (cm)*	173 ± 5	171 ± 7
Race/ethnicity (% white non-Hispanic)	89	85
Income (% >$30,000/yr)	49	68
Parental smoking (No.)		
Households	4	4
Mothers	2	3
Fathers	3	3
Day care use		
In first yr (%)	42	76†
Hr/wk*		
Age 0-6 mo	(n = 15) 7.3 ± 5.3	(n = 28) 13.8 ± 8.8†
Age 6-12 mo	(n = 19) 15.8 ± 10.4	(n = 29) 27.7 ± 14.3†
Age 12-18 mo	(n = 25) 14.0 ± 9.7	(n = 30) 26.3 ± 16.4†
No. of siblings*	1.02 ± 1.27	0.80 ± 0.75

*Mean ± SD.
†$p < 0.05$.

METHODS

Study design. The objective of the DARLING study was to compare growth, nutrient intake, morbidity, and activity levels during the first 2 years of life between matched cohorts of infants who were either breast fed (n = 46) or formula fed (n = 41) until at least 12 months of age. Selection criteria and details regarding recruitment and attrition are described elsewhere.[35] Briefly, 92 mothers were recruited into the BF group, of whom 19 dropped out before 3 months (primarily because they were too busy to complete the intake measurements) and another 27 dropped out between 3 and 12 months (primarily because their infants weaned themselves before 12 months [n = 12] or because the mothers became too busy). Two infants in the BF group dropped out because of illness (infant botulism, pneumonia). Average morbidity rates from 0 to 3 and from 3 to 6 months for infants who dropped out did not differ significantly from those of the 46 infants who remained in the study for the full 12 months. In the FF group 52 mothers were recruited, of whom six dropped out before 3 months and five did so between 3 and 12 months (none dropped out because of infant illness). Human milk was the major form of milk for BF infants throughout the first year, except for occasional bottles of cow milk or formula (<120 ml/day). Eighteen infants breast fed for 12 to 14 months, 10 for 15 to 17 months, 5 for 18 to 23 months, and 13 for 24 months or longer. Mothers in the FF group had decided prenatally not to breast-feed at all (n = 11) or to terminate breast-feeding by 3 months (n = 30); all used an iron-fortified cow milk–based formula, and nearly all introduced formula within the first 4 weeks. Neither BF nor FF infants received solid foods before they attained 4 months of age. Stratified matching was used to ensure that the groups were similar in parental socioeconomic status, education, ethnicity, and anthropometric characteristics, and in infant sex and birth weight. In these analyses one BF infant was excluded because of incomplete morbidity data.

Table I shows the characteristics of the two cohorts. Average birth weight and maternal educational level were high in both groups. Mothers in the FF group were more likely to be employed full time than those in the BF group. It was not possible to match for employment because the choice of infant-feeding method was strongly related to the mother's expected work schedule. As a result, there were significant differences between groups in the percentage who used day care and in the amount of time infants spent in day care (Table I). Parental smoking was very uncommon in both groups.

Morbidity. All mothers were contacted once a week to record the nature and duration (in days) of all symptoms of infant illness. In addition, any diagnoses made by personal physicians were recorded. Mothers were given a calendar on which to record symptoms daily. Morbidity data were subsequently grouped into four categories:

- *Respiratory symptoms* were defined as any upper or lower respiratory tract symptoms other than a clear nasal discharge.
- *Diarrhea* was defined as two or more runny stools per

day that differed from the child's usual stool consistency

- *Acute otitis media* was diagnosed by a physician, with duration defined on the basis of symptoms of fever or continued discomfort. Prolonged otitis media was defined as an episode lasting more than 10 days, as determined by a physician on reexamination.
- *Other symptoms or disorders* included unexplained fevers, vomiting, chickenpox, and other nonrespiratory viral exanthems.

For these analyses the prevalence and incidence of each category of illness for each child were calculated in both 6-month (0 to 6, 6 to 12, 12 to 18, and 18 to 24 months) and 12-month (0 to 12 and 12 to 24 months) intervals, but statistical comparisons between groups were made only for 12-month intervals, to eliminate the problem of seasonal variability. Prevalence was calculated as the number of days the child was ill during each interval (defined as "episodic prevalence" by Kleinbaum et al.[41]). When data analysis required categorization of the outcome variable, period prevalence was calculated, either as the percentage of children with or without illness during the interval, or the percentage falling into each of three categories on the basis of the number of days the child was ill during the interval (e.g., 0, 1 to 20, or >20 days of otitis media). Incidence was calculated as the number of episodes per 100 days at risk (i.e., not including days when that illness was already present) but is also presented as the crude rate of episodes per year. When data analysis required categorization of the outcome variable, the percentage of infants with zero, one, or two or more episodes of illness during the interval was calculated.

Data analysis. Data were analyzed with the Statistical Package for the Social Sciences, SPSS Inc., Chicago, Ill.[42] Only those infants with complete data for a given interval were included in the analyses for that interval. Each infant was considered as the unit of analysis (rather than each day of observation) to avoid autocorrelation, and mean values were compared between groups. One FF infant left the country for 2 months when he was 10 months old and was therefore excluded from the analyses during intervals that included that time period. During the second year four BF and six FF infants left the study, primarily because their families relocated out of the area.

Several methods were used to assess group differences in morbidity outcomes. The distribution of each outcome variable was examined to determine whether the assumption of normality was valid. Except for respiratory illness, the majority of the morbidity variables were highly skewed and the distributions were not improved by transforming the data. In bivariate analyses Student *t* tests were used when the data were normally distributed; otherwise, nonparametric methods (Mann-Whitney U tests, chi-square tests) were used to compare groups.

To control for potentially confounding variables, we examined differences between groups, using multiple regression analysis for respiratory illness outcome variables. Potential confounders included day care use and number of siblings. Two alternative indices of day care use were used in the regression models: (1) number of hours per week, or (2) day care "score," the number of hours per week multiplied by the usual number of children at the day care site.

For diarrhea, otitis media, and other illnesses logistic regression or hierarchic log linear models had to be used for multivariate analyses. In logistic regression analyses the outcome variable was presence or absence of illness in a given interval (period prevalence). For log-linear models the outcome variable included three categories of incidence or prevalence, as described previously. In both the logistic regression and log-linear models, day care use was categorized as none versus some, and number of siblings was categorized as zero or one or more (relatively few infants had more than one sibling). The dichotomous categorization of day care use was chosen because there was no evidence that the amount of time spent in day care (other than use vs nonuse) was associated with a further increased risk of morbidity (except for respiratory illness). Log-linear models were determined by backward elimination of terms. Likelihood ratio chi-square tests were used to test whether the simplified models differed significantly from the model with all variables included; significance values of $p > 0.10$ indicate that the simplified model was a good fit. (To avoid confusion with the usual convention of $p < 0.05$ for other tests, the significance levels of the log-linear results reported in the next section are not listed; all were >0.10.)

RESULTS

Respiratory illness. On average, infants had symptoms of respiratory illness about 11% of the time during the first 6 months and 16% to 20% of the time from 6 to 24 months. Nearly all these illnesses were mild upper respiratory illnesses; in both groups together there were only 10 episodes of physician-diagnosed lower respiratory illnesses during the first two years of life (three BF, seven FF infants). Six infants (three BF, three FF) were hospitalized because of illness during the 2-year period, all for pneumonia.

Before the multivariate analyses were completed, the relationships of day care use and number of siblings to the morbidity outcome variables in the first year of life were examined. The incidence of respiratory illness was positively related to day care use (whether expressed as hours per week or as day care score) in the FF group (for day care score, $r = 0.43$, $p < 0.05$) but not in the BF group ($r = 0.17$,

Table II. Incidence and prevalence of respiratory illnesses, diarrhea, otitis media, and other illnesses

	Age 0-12 mo					Age 12-24 mo				
	BF		FF		Statistical significance‡	BF		FF		Statistical significance‡
	Unadjusted*	Adjusted†	Unadjusted*	Adjusted†		Unadjusted*	Adjusted†	Unadjusted*	Adjusted†	
Respiratory illnesses										
Incidence§	1.9 ± 1.1	2.1	1.8 ± 0.8	1.7	NS	1.9 ± 1.0	2.0	2.3 ± 1.5	2.0	NS
No. of episodes/yr	5.5 ± 2.8	5.9	5.3 ± 2.3	4.9	NS	5.6 ± 2.2	5.8	6.0 ± 3.0	5.6	NS
Prevalence (ill days/yr)	55.5 ± 31.1	62.3	59.4 ± 28.2	59.6	NS	59.9 ± 30.6	61.9	72.9 ± 43.1	66.4	NS
Diarrhea										
Incidence§	0.16 ± 0.16	0.14	0.33 ± 0.38	0.31	Significant; log-linear	0.50 ± 0.50	0.50	0.45 ± 0.46	0.44	NS
No. of episodes/yr	0.56 ± 0.59	0.49	1.18 ± 1.34	1.07	Significant; log-linear	1.71 ± 1.65	1.71	1.56 ± 1.54	1.49	NS
Prevalence (ill days/yr)	3.0 ± 5.3	2.6	6.5 ± 7.1	6.3	NS	9.9 ± 11.1	10.7	11.1 ± 12.6	11.2	NS
Otitis media										
Incidence§	0.35 ± 0.44	0.45	0.55 ± 0.46	0.53	Significant; log-linear	0.39 ± 0.53	0.43	0.48 ± 0.52	0.45	NS
No. of episodes/yr	1.22 ± 1.5	1.53	1.85 ± 1.5	1.78	Significant; log-linear	1.32 ± 1.62	1.41	1.53 ± 1.46	1.43	NS
Prevalence (ill days/yr)	7.2 ± 10.5	10.0	17.2 ± 17.9	15.8	Significant; log-linear	9.3 ± 14.1	11.1	18.0 ± 26.6	17.3	NS
Other										
Incidence§	0.18 ± 0.25	0.24	0.15 ± 0.18	0.14	NS	0.29 ± 0.26	0.29	0.23 ± 0.19	0.25	NS
No. of episodes/yr	0.64 ± 0.88	0.86	0.53 ± 0.64	0.49	NS	1.05 ± 0.92	1.05	0.81 ± 0.67	0.88	NS
Prevalence (ill days/yr)	2.9 ± 3.7	3.4	2.0 ± 3.3	1.8	NS	4.9 ± 4.3	5.2	3.8 ± 4.9	4.5	NS

NS, Not significant.
*Values expressed as mean ± SD.
†Adjusted for day care score and number of siblings, with analysis of covariance techniques.[43]
‡Multivariate analyses, controlled for day care use and number of siblings, were used. Multiple regression was used for respiratory illness; logistic regression and log-linear analyses were used for all other categories of morbidity, as explained in Methods.
§Episodes per 100 days at risk.

$p > 0.05$). Number of siblings was positively related to incidence of respiratory illness in the BF group ($r = 0.32$, $p < 0.05$) but not in the FF group.

Controlling for day care use and number of siblings, we found no significant differences in incidence or prevalence of respiratory illness between BF and FF infants up to 12 months or from 12 to 24 months of age (Table II).

Diarrheal illness. Diarrheal illness was relatively uncommon, ranging from 0.2% of days among BF infants in the first 6 months to 3.3% of days among FF infants at 12 to 18 months (Fig. 1). The percentage of infants with diarrheal illness was positively associated with day care use (categorized as none vs some use) in the FF group (20% [2/10] vs 68% [21/31], respectively; chi-square value = 7.0, $p < 0.01$) but not in the BF group (54% [14/26] vs 47% [9/19], respectively; chi-square value = 0.2). Diarrheal illness was not significantly associated with number of siblings in either group.

Table II shows that the incidence of diarrheal illness among FF infants was approximately twice that of BF infants during the first year of life. The percentage of infants with zero, one, or two or more episodes of diarrheal illness in the first year was 49%, 47%, and 4% among BF infants versus 45%, 30%, and 35% among FF infants, respectively; this difference was significant by log-linear analysis even when controlled for day care use and number of siblings. Diarrheal morbidity during the second year of life did not differ significantly between groups.

Otitis media. The prevalence of otitis media (Fig. 2) in the first 6 months was low (0.9% of days among BF infants, 2.1% of days among FF infants); thereafter the prevalence ranged from 2.2% to 3.1% of days among BF infants and from 4.2% to 7.2% of days among FF infants. The percentage of infants with otitis media was not significantly associated with day care use; it was associated with number of

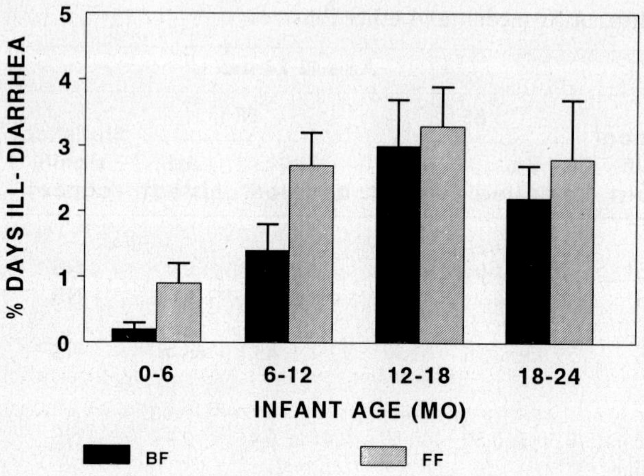

Fig. 1. Prevalence (unadjusted) of diarrheal illness among BF versus FF infants (mean ± SEM).

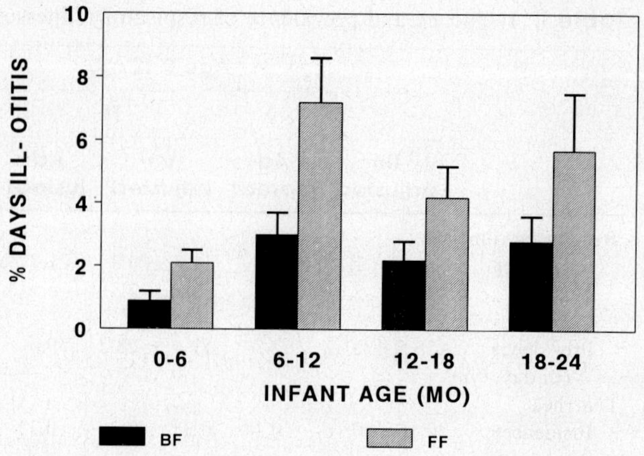

Fig. 2. Prevalence (unadjusted) of otitis media among BF versus FF infants (mean ± SEM).

siblings only among FF infants (53% [8/15] vs 92% [24/26] for FF infants with zero or one or more siblings, respectively, $\chi^2 = 8.4$, $p < 0.01$; among BF infants these percentages were 56% [10/18] vs 59% [16/27], respectively).

Incidence of otitis media differed significantly between BF and FF infants during the first year of life (Table II): the percentage of infants with zero, one, or two or more episodes was 42%, 24%, and 34% among BF infants versus 18%, 25%, and 57% among FF infants, respectively (statistically significant by log-linear analysis, when controlled for day care use and number of siblings). The mean age at onset of the first episode was 43 ± 24 weeks versus 31 ± 20 weeks in the BF and FF groups, respectively ($p < 0.05$). Period prevalence of otitis media also differed between groups up to 12 months of age: the percentage of infants with 0, 1 to 20, or more than 20 days of illness was 42%, 49%, and 9% among BF infants versus 18%, 45%, and 37% among FF infants, respectively (significant by log-linear analysis, controlled for day care use and number of siblings). Average duration of episodes of otitis media was significantly greater among FF infants than among BF infants in both the first year (8.7 ± 6.3 days vs 5.6 ± 2.2 days, respectively; $p = 0.01$) and second year (8.8 ± 5.3 days vs 5.9 ± 3.5 days, respectively; $p = 0.01$) of life. When compared with the percentage in the BF group, the percentage of FF infants with prolonged ear infections (one or more ear infections that lasted >10 days) was five times higher in the first year (34% [14/41] vs 7% [3/45] in FF and BF groups, respectively; $p < 0.05$) and 3.6 times higher in the second year of life (36% [13/36] vs 10% [4/41], respectively, $p < 0.05$). There were relatively few cases of recurrent otitis media (defined as four or more episodes in a 12-month period): in children up to 12 months of age, zero cases in the BF group and four in the FF group were reported, and from 12 to 24 months four cases in the BF group and five in the FF group were reported.

Other illnesses. Symptoms of other illnesses were present only 0.1% to 0.2% of days in the first 6 months and 0.9% to 1.4% of days from 6 to 24 months. Incidence and prevalence of other illnesses were not significantly related to day care use or number of siblings. There were no significant differences between BF and FF infants with regard to these illnesses (Table II).

DISCUSSION

These results indicate that breast-feeding during the first year of life is protective against diarrheal illness and otitis media, even in a relatively affluent, highly educated population. The findings are consistent with those of most previous reports[6-16, 20-23, 26, 27] but add to the evidence because the groups were carefully matched for many potentially confounding variables. Because mothers who breast-feed generally tend to be of higher income and educational level and smoke less than those who formula-feed, most other studies have required extensive statistical adjustment for these differences. The only significant difference in characteristics between our study groups was use of day care, which was controlled for in the analyses. In addition, we chose the most conservative method for analyzing the data, that is, considering each child, rather than each day of observation, as the unit of analysis. Nevertheless, the differences in rates of diarrhea and otitis media between BF and FF infants were statistically significant.

Our data indicate that the incidence of diarrhea is about 50% lower in BF than in FF infants during the first year of life. Among other recent studies, Howie et al.[14] found a similar or greater reduction in gastrointestinal illness associated with breast-feeding in a large prospective study in

Scotland. In contrast, Rubin et al.[19] found no significant relationship between type of feeding and the incidence of gastroenteritis in Denmark. However, the latter study was based on monthly questionnaires mailed to parents, to which the response rate declined with infant age to only 44% at 12 months. In addition, the two main comparison groups in the Danish study both included mixed-fed infants, because the investigators defined BF infants as those whose mothers reported providing more human milk than formula and FF infants as those who were provided more formula than human milk. When breast-feeding is more strictly defined and morbidity surveillance is complete, breast-feeding has been linked to reductions in both the incidence and severity of gastrointestinal illness.[13, 14] Numerous components have been identified in human milk that likely contribute to these protective effects.[4]

The percentage of BF infants in our study with one or more episodes of otitis media during the first year of life was 19% lower, and that of infants with prolonged episodes (>10 days) was 80% lower compared with FF infants. Even in the second year of life infants who had been breast-fed were less likely to have prolonged episodes of otitis media. Similar results were found in a large prospective study in Arizona, in which there was an 18% reduction in the percentage of infants with otitis media during the first year in those exclusively breast fed for at least 4 months, and a 51% reduction in the percentage of infants with recurrent otitis media who were exclusively breast fed for more than 6 months.[26] Although feeding position may explain part of this difference, it is likely that secretory IgA and prostaglandins in human milk reduce otitis by affecting the ability of pathogens to attach or to cause an inflammatory response.[44-47]

We did not observe any significant differences in the incidence or prevalence of respiratory illnesses between BF and FF infants. However, the vast majority of episodes were mild upper respiratory illnesses. Previous studies have indicated that the protective effect of breast-feeding is greatest for lower respiratory illnesses.[14, 28-31] The sample size in our study was not large enough to detect differences in more severe respiratory illnesses.

Taken as a whole, the results of this and other studies indicate that the protective effect of breast-feeding against illness is of public health significance even in relatively affluent populations. This study evaluated differences in morbidity associated with breast-feeding during the first 12 months of life. Although nursing for this duration is at present uncommon in the United States, other studies have shown a substantial protective effect even with breast-feeding of shorter duration.[14, 26] In addition to reducing morbidity, the evidence suggests that the cost savings in health care from promoting breast-feeding could be large, given that more than $1 billion is spent each year on diagnosis and treatment of otitis media alone,[48] and that gastrointestinal illnesses are a major reason for hospitalization during the first year of life.[49]

We are grateful for the assistance of Linda Stuart and Wendy Kristy, the cooperation of the study participants, the help of our team of student assistants, the statistical advice of Janet M. Peerson, and comments on the manuscript by Kenneth H. Brown.

REFERENCES

1. Feachem RG, Koblinsky MA. Interventions for the control of diarrheal diseases in young children: promotion of breastfeeding. Bull World Health Organ 1984;62:271-91.
2. Cunningham AS, Jelliffe DB, Jelliffe EFP. Breastfeeding and health in the 1980s: a global epidemiologic review. J PEDIATR 1991;118:659-66.
3. Huffman SL, Combest C. Role of breastfeeding in the prevention and treatment of diarrhea. Diarr Dis Res 1990;8:68-81.
4. Institute of Medicine. Nutrition during lactation. Washington, DC: National Academy Press, 1991.
5. Bauchner H, Leventhal JM, Shapiro ED. Studies of breastfeeding and infections: how good is the evidence? JAMA 1986;256:887-92.
6. Cunningham AS. Morbidity in breastfed and artificially fed infants II. J PEDIATR 1979;95:685-9.
7. Paine R, Coble RJ. Breastfeeding and infant health in a rural US community. Am J Dis Child 1982;136:36-8.
8. Lo CW. Chronic diarrhea. Pediatrics 1983;72:786-800.
9. Forman MR, Graubard BI, Hoffman HJ, Beren R, Harley EE, Bennett P. The Pima infant feeding study: breastfeeding and respiratory infections during the first year of life. Int J Epidemiol 1984;13:447-53.
10. Myers MG, Fomon SJ, Koontz FP, McGuinness GA, Lachenbuch PA, Hollingshead R. Respiratory and gastrointestinal illnesses in breast and formula-fed infants. Am J Dis Child 1984;138:629-32.
11. McFarlane PI, Miller V. Human milk in the management of protracted diarrhea of infancy. Arch Dis Child 1984;59:260-5.
12. Koopman JS, Turkish VJ, Monto AS. Infant formulas and gastrointestinal illness. Am J Public Health 1985;75:477-80.
13. Duffy LC, Byers TE, Riepenhoff-Talty M, La Scolea LJ, Zielezny M, Ogra PL. The effects of infant feeding on rotavirus-induced gastroenteritis: a prospective study. Am J Public Health 1986;76:259-63.
14. Howie PW, Forsyth JS, Ogston SA, Clark A, du V Florey C. Protective effect of breastfeeding against infection. Br Med J 1990;300:11-6.
15. van den Bogaard C, van den Hoogen HJM, Huygen FJA, van Weel C. The relationship between breastfeeding and early childhood morbidity in a general population. Fam Med 1991;23:510-5.
16. Ruuska T. Occurrence of acute diarrhea in atopic and nonatopic infants: the role of prolonged breastfeeding. J Pediatr Gastroenterol Nutr 1992;14:27-33.
17. Adebonojo FO. Artificial vs breastfeeding: relation to infant health in a middle class American community. Clin Pediatr 1972;11:25-9.
18. Cushing AH, Anderson L. Diarrhea in breastfed and nonbreastfed infants. Pediatrics 1982;70:921-5.
19. Rubin DH, Leventhal JM, Krasilnikoff PA, et al. Relationship

between infant feeding and infectious illness: a prospective study of infants during the first year of life. Pediatrics 1990;85:464-71.
20. Teele DW, Klein JO, Rosner B. Epidemiology of otitis media during the first seven years of life in children in greater Boston: a prospective cohort study. J Infect Dis 1989;160:83-94.
21. Kero P, Piekkala P. Factors affecting the occurrence of acute otitis media during the first year of life. Acta Paediatr Scand 1987;76:618-23.
22. Saarinen UM. Prolonged breastfeeding as prophylaxis for recurrent otitis media. Acta Paediatr Scand 1982;71:567-71.
23. Sipila M, Karma P, Pukander J, Timonen M, Kataja M. The Bayesian approach to the evaluation of risk factors in acute and recurrent acute otitis media. Acta Otolaryngol (Stockh) 1988;106:94-101.
24. Tainio VM, Savlahti E, Salmenpera L, Arjomaa P, Siimes MA, Perheentupa J. Risk factors for infantile recurrent otitis media: atopy but not type of feeding. Pediatr Res 1988;23:509-12.
25. Harsten G, Prellner K, Heldrup J, Kalm O, Kornfalt R. Recurrent acute otitis media. Acta Otolaryngol (Stockh) 1989;107:111-9.
26. Duncan B, Ey J, Holberg CJ, Wright AL, Martinez FD, Taussig LM. Exclusive breastfeeding for at least 4 months protects against otitis media. Pediatrics 1993;91:867-72.
27. Owen MJ, Baldwin CD, Swank PR, Pannu AK, Johnson DL, Howie VM. Relation of infant feeding practices, cigarette smoke exposure, and group child care to the onset and duration of otitis media with effusion in the first two years of life. J Pediatr 1993;123:702-11.
28. Pullan CR, Toms GL, Martin AJ, Gardner PS, Webb JKG, Appleton DR. Breastfeeding and respiratory syncytial virus infection. Br Med J 1980;281:1034-6.
29. Watkins CJ, Leeder SR, Corkhill RT. The relationship between breast and bottle feeding and respiratory illness in the first year of life. J Epidemiol Community Health 1979;33:180-2.
30. Woodward A, Douglas RM, Graham NMH, Miles H. Acute respiratory illness in Adelaide children: breastfeeding modifies the effect of passive smoking. J Epidemiol Community Health 1990;44:224-30.
31. Wright AL, Holberg CJ, Martinez FD, Morgan WJ, Taussig LM. Breastfeeding and lower respiratory tract illness in the first year of life. Br Med J 1989;299:945-9.
32. Frank AL, Taber LH, Glezen WP, Kasel GL, Wells CR, Paredes A. Breastfeeding and respiratory virus infection. Pediatrics 1982;70:239-45.
33. Anderson LJ, Parker RA, Strikas RA, et al. Day-care attendance and hospitalization for lower respiratory tract illness. Pediatrics 1988;82:300-8.
34. Margolis PA, Greenberg RA, Keyes LL, et al. Lower respiratory illness in infants and low socioeconomic status. Am J Public Health 1992;82:1119-26.
35. Dewey KG, Heinig MJ, Nommsen LA, Peerson JM, Lonnerdal B. Growth of breast-fed and formula-fed infants from 0 to 18 months: the DARLING study. Pediatrics 1992;89:1035-41.
36. Dewey KG, Heinig MJ, Nommsen LA, Peerson J, Lonnerdal B. Breastfed infants are leaner than formula-fed infants at 1 year of age: the DARLING study. Am J Clin Nutr 1993;57:140-5.
37. Dewey KG, Heinig MJ, Nommsen LA, Lonnerdal B. Maternal vs infant factors related to breast milk intake and residual milk volume: the DARLING study. Pediatrics 1991;87:829-37.
38. Dewey KG, Heinig MJ, Nommsen LA, Lonnerdal B. Adequacy of energy intake among breastfed infants in the DARLING study: relationships to growth velocity, morbidity and activity levels. J Pediatr 1991;119:538-47.
39. Heinig MJ, Nommsen LA, Peerson JM, Lonnerdal B, Dewey KG. Energy and protein intakes of breastfed and formula-fed infants during the first year of life and their association with growth velocity: the DARLING study. Am J Clin Nutr 1993;58:152-61.
40. Heinig MJ, Nommsen LA, Peerson JM, Lonnerdal B, Dewey KG. Intake and growth of breastfed and formula-fed infants in relation to the timing to introduction of complementary foods: the DARLING study. Acta Paediatr 1993;82:999-1006.
41. Kleinbaum DG, Kupper LL, Morgenstern H. Epidemiologic research. Belmont, Calif: Lifetime Learning Publications, 1982.
42. Norusis MJ. Statistical Package for the Social Sciences: SPSS users guide. New York: McGraw-Hill, 1983.
43. Neter J, Wasserman W, Kutner MH. Applied linear statistical models. 2nd ed. Homewood, Ill: Richard D Irwin, 1985:871-3.
44. Hanson LA, Ahlstedt S, Andersson B, et al. Protective factors in milk and the development of the immune system. Pediatrics 1985;75(suppl):172-6.
45. Backon J. Prolonged breastfeeding as a prophylaxis for recurrent otitis media: relevance of prostaglandins. Med Hypotheses 1984;13:161.
46. Fantone JC, Kunkel SL, Ward PA, Zurier RB. Suppression by prostaglandin E_1 of vascular permeability induced by vasoactive inflammatory mediators. J Immunol 1980;125:2591-6.
47. Fantone JC, Kunkel SL, Ward PA, Zurier RB. Suppression of human polymorphonuclear function after intravenous infusions of prostaglandin E_1. Prostaglandins Med 1981;7:195-8.
48. Schappert SM. Office visits for otitis media: United States, 1975-90. Adv Data 1992;8:1-19.
49. Leventhal JM, Shapiro ED, Aten CB, Berg AT, Egerter SA. Does breastfeeding protect against infections in infants less than 3 months of age? Pediatrics 1986;78:896-903.

Use of polymerase chain reaction for improved diagnosis of tuberculosis in children

Christophe Delacourt, MD, Jean-Dominique Poveda, MD, Corinne Chureau, Nicole Beydon, MD, Bruno Mahut, MD, Jacques de Blic, MD, Pierre Scheinmann, MD, and Guy Garrigue, MD

From the Service de Pneumologie et Allergologie Pédiatriques, Hôpital des Enfants Malades, the Service de Pédiatrie Générale, Hôpital Robert Debré, and the Centre de Biologie Médicale Spécialisée, Institut Pasteur, Paris, France

Objective: **To study the value of a rapid diagnostic method based on the amplification by polymerase chain reaction (PCR) of a fragment of the IS*6110* insertion element for the detection of *Mycobacterium tuberculosis* in children.**
Design: **We tested 199 specimens obtained from 68 children referred for evaluation of suspected tuberculosis.**
Results: **In 83.3% of children with active disease and 38.9% with tuberculous infection but no evidence of disease, at least one positive PCR result was observed. No child without tuberculosis had positive PCR results (100% specificity). The sensitivity of the PCR was increased by testing of multiple samples from the same child and use of Chelex particles (Bio-Rad Laboratories, Ivry, France) rather than guanidine isothiocyanate–silica particles for DNA extraction. Bronchoalveolar lavage samples were no more useful than gastric aspirates.**
Conclusions: **If appropriate laboratory methods are used, DNA amplification is a reliable method for the early diagnosis of tuberculosis in children and appears to be very helpful in clinical pediatric practice when the diagnosis of active tuberculosis is difficult or needs to be rapidly confirmed. (J PEDIATR 1995; 126:703-9)**

Despite the numerous efforts to control tuberculosis in developed countries, the disease remains a major health problem, especially in urban areas. Its incidence increased in the 1980s both in the United States[1] and in Europe.[2] The influx of high-risk persons and the prevalence of HIV infection may largely account for this increase.[3] Early detection is of major importance in the control of tuberculosis, but many cases of tuberculous disease in children may be unrecognized because of the poor sensitivity of currently available diagnostic methods.[4] The diagnosis of tuberculosis in children is often supported only by epidemiologic, clinical, and radiographic findings. Fiber-optic bronchoscopy also may be helpful for the initial diagnosis.[5] The recovery of tubercle bacilli, which establishes the diagnosis with certainty, is difficult in children.[6] Other laboratory analyses are thus required to improve the early diagnosis of tuberculosis in children. We have recently shown that serodiagnosis may be useful in children with active disease,[7] but this approach is limited by the need to establish locally the normal values, thus making generalized use difficult.

BAL	Bronchoalveolar lavage
BCG	Bacille Calmette-Guérin
HIV	Human immunodeficiency virus
PCR	Polymerase chain reaction

A DNA amplification for *Mycobacterium tuberculosis* is a potentially valuable technique. In principle it offers the possibility of a rapid, sensitive, and specific test for tuber-

Submitted for publication July 5, 1994; accepted Dec. 13, 1994.
Reprint requests: Christophe Delacourt, MD, Service de Pneumo-Pédiatrie, Hôpital des Enfants Malades, 149 rue de Sèvres, 75015 Paris, France.

0022-3476/95/$3.00 + 0 **9/20/62803**

Table I. Study population

	Clinically active disease	Infection without disease	Suspicion of infection	No tuberculosis	Total
No. of children	24	18	11	15	68
Age (yr), mean ± SD	4.5 ± 4.4	4.8 ± 4.0	5.5 ± 4.8	6.1 ± 4.0	5.1 ± 4.2
Sex ratio (M/F)	9:15	10:8	8:3	5:10	32:36
BCG vaccination (%)	65.2	66.7	72.7	80	70.5
Ethnic origin					
European	9	11	2	8	30
African	13	6	7	6	32
Asian	1	1	2	1	5
South American	1	0	0	0	1

culosis. Many studies in adults have reported a high degree of sensitivity in detecting *M. tuberculosis* in clinical samples by means of DNA amplification.[8, 9] However, in practice the reliability of the method may be limited by the generation of false-positive reactions because of the amplification of contaminating DNA. Using an appropriate amplification technique, including suitable controls during the complete procedure, and retesting doubtful positive samples appear to be necessary, to minimize the number of false-positive results.[10] We evaluated the usefulness of DNA amplification for the diagnosis of tuberculosis in children and assessed the technical requirements for this approach.

METHODS

Patients. Specimens were obtained from 68 children 1 month to 16.4 years of age who were being investigated at our pediatric department for suspected tuberculosis. Tuberculosis was suspected on the basis of a history of close contact with active tuberculosis, the clinical and roentgenographic findings, and the results of tuberculin skin tests. The diagnosis was established according to the recommendations of the American Thoracic Society.[11] Twenty-four patients were thus considered as having tuberculous infection with clinically active disease because they had clinical or radiographic evidence of tuberculosis with a positive reaction to the tuberculin skin test. Three of these 24 children were HIV seropositive, one received immunosuppressive therapy after kidney transplantation, and one had cystic fibrosis. Clinical symptoms and chest radiographic abnormalities improved in all patients after appropriate treatment.

Eighteen patients were considered to have tuberculous infection without disease because they had a positive reaction to the tuberculin skin test without clinical or radiographic abnormalities; 11 of them had been recently and massively exposed to active pulmonary disease and had an increase of at least 10 mm in their intradermal skin test response. The other seven patients had no known contact with pulmonary disease but had an increase in induration of their intradermal skin test response of more than 15 mm.

In 11 other children the diagnosis of tuberculous infection without disease was classified as "suspected," on the basis of (1) strong tuberculin skin test reactions (>15 mm) in children who had received the bacille Calmette-Guérin vaccine for whom no previous test results were available for comparison, or (2) no modification of tuberculin test results despite extensive contact with active tuberculosis. Nevertheless, all these 11 children received preventive therapy.

Finally, 15 children had diagnoses other than tuberculous infection. Eleven of these children had bacterial or viral bronchopulmonary infection with negative tuberculin skin test results and completely recovered after appropriate treatment. The four remaining children had the following diagnoses: immunodeficiency with pulmonary aspergillosis, allergic alveolitis, bronchiectasis, and cat scratch disease.

Mean age, sex ratio, ethnic origin, and BCG vaccination history of all children are reported in Table I.

Clinical specimens. One hundred ninety-nine specimens were collected from the 68 children (Table II). Two or more specimens collected on consecutive days were obtained from 52 children; 80% of the samples were gastric aspirates. Sixty-four of the 199 specimens were obtained from the 24 children with clinically active tuberculosis, 51 from the 18 children with tuberculous infection without disease, 30 from the 11 children with suspected tuberculous infection, and 54 from the 15 children without tuberculosis, who were considered control subjects.

Gastric aspirates. Gastric content was aspirated early in the morning after the child had fasted for at least 8 to 10 hours and while he or she was still in bed. Samples of 2 to 5 ml were obtained without lavage.

Microscopic examination and cultivation of mycobacteria. Fresh samples were first decontaminated with 4% sodium hydroxide NaOH (vol/vol). After 45 minutes of incubation (37° C) the reaction was neutralized with 15%

Table II. Total number of samples collected from 68 children and percentage of samples culture positive or PCR positive among the 42 children with tuberculosis (24 children with active disease and 18 infected children without disease)

	Total No. of samples	Children with tuberculosis: No. of samples	Culture positive samples (%)	PCR-positive samples* (%)
Gastric aspirates	160	86	4	31
BAL	22	20	20	50
Urine	7	1	0	100
CSF	6	4	0	50
Lymph node biopsy	3	3	33	100
Pleural fluid	1	1	0	0
TOTAL	199	115	7	37

*Definitive PCR results were those obtained after false-positive detection procedure and controls with the Chelex 100 extraction technique.

sulfuric acid (vol/vol). The samples were then centrifuged at 3000*g* for 20 minutes. The pellet was stained for acid-fast bacilli with auramine stain and cultured both on Löwenstein-Jensen and on Coletsos media. Bronchoalveolar lavage specimens were directly centrifuged. The pellet was incubated for 30 minutes at room temperature with 15% sulfuric acid (vol/vol) and the reaction was stopped with 20% NaOH (vol/vol).

DNA amplification

Sample preparation and DNA extraction. Gastric aspirates and BAL samples were subjected to the N-acetylcysteine–NaOH procedure and then concentrated by centrifugation; cerebrospinal fluid, urine, and pleural fluid samples were directly centrifuged. Biopsy specimens were first digested with proteinase K and then centrifuged. All pellets were resuspended in 100 μl of distilled water. DNA was extracted with either guanidine isothiocyanate and silica particles[12] or Chelex 100 particles[13] (Bio-Rad Laboratories, Ivry-sur-Seine, France) as indicated elsewhere. Five microliters and 10 μl of the guanidine isothiocyanate–silica extraction or 10 μl of the Chelex 100 extraction were used for DNA amplification of the IS*6110* sequence as previously described.[8] Briefly, PCR amplification was performed in a 100 μl mixture containing 50 mmol/L potassium chloride, 10 mol/L, tris(hydroxymethyl) aminomethane HCl (pH 8.3), 1.5 mmol/L magnesium chloride, 125 μmol/L each deoxyadenosine triphosphate, deoxycytidine triphosphate, deoxyguanosine triphosphate, and deoxythymidine triphosphate, 250 nmol/L each primer and 2.5 U of Taq polymerase (Perkin-Elmer, St. Quentin en Yvelines, France). Amplified DNA was isolated by electrophoresis in agarose gel, transfer onto a nylon membrane, and hybridization with a horseradish peroxidase–labeled probe (kindly provided by Sanofi-Diagnostics Pasteur, Marnes la Coquette, France), and detected with a chemiluminescent substrate (ECL-Amersham, Les Vlis, France).

Prevention of false-positive results. Carryover contamination was prevented by following the usual recommendations[14]; performing pre-PCR, PCR, and post-PCR steps of the procedure in three separate rooms with appropriate positive and negative air pressure regulation; and forbidding any turn back from a post-PCR to a pre-PCR area on the same day. Appropriate negative and positive controls were included at each step. No result was recorded if any controls gave discrepant results. To detect cross-contamination between positive and negative samples, we treated all samples in the same order throughout DNA extraction and PCR preparation. Positive results given by consecutive samples in the sequence and taken from different patients were considered as doubtful, and samples were retested.

Statistical analysis. Results are expressed as means ± SD. The chi-square test was used for statistical comparisons. Sensitivity (the fraction of children with tuberculosis who had a positive PCR result), specificity (the fraction of children without the disease and having a negative PCR result), positive predictive value (the fraction of children having a positive PCR result who had the disease), and negative predictive value (the fraction of children with a negative PCR result who did not have the disease) were calculated by standard methods.[15]

RESULTS

Overall results. Ten children with active disease had a bacteriologic confirmation of tuberculosis (five with positive smears), including five children with positive culture obtained from specimens other than those tested by PCR (one with positive smear). The PCR technique was much more sensitive than smears or culture for the diagnosis of both clinically active tuberculosis and tuberculous infection without disease (Table III). The procedure for prevention of false-positive PCR results, as defined in Methods, allowed false positives for four children to be corrected and

Table III. Bacteriologic and *M. tuberculosis* DNA amplification results in children divided into four groups according to their tuberculous status

Tuberculous status	Children with positive result (%)		
	Smears	Culture	PCR
Active disease	20.8	41.7	83.3
Infection without disease	0	0	38.9
Suspected infection	0	0	0
No tuberculosis	0	0	0

Results are expressed as the percentage of children with positive smears or culture, or at least one PCR-positive sample.

thus to achieve a specificity of 100% for the diagnosis of tuberculosis, instead of 86.7% before correction. Positive and negative predictive values of PCR were 74.1% and 90.2%, respectively, for identifying children with active disease, and 25.9% and 73.2%, respectively, for identifying children with tuberculous infection without active disease.

Analysis of samples

Bacteriologic data. Smears were obtained for 198 of the 199 specimens tested by PCR and were positive in only four cases. Cultures on Löwenstein-Jensen for 196 of these specimens gave positive results in eight specimens (including all four that gave positive smears) (Table II).

Results of PCR. All samples were analyzed by PCR with a blind protocol; doubtful positive results, defined as positive results for consecutive samples taken from different patients, were systematically retested. PCR results were then compared with bacteriologic and clinical data.

Initial blind analysis of all specimens. Initial DNA amplification gave positive results in 44 of the 199 specimens tested after guanidine isothiocyanate–silica extraction. According to the criteria defined previously, and although all negative controls had negative results in the corresponding PCR series, 11 positive results were considered as doubtful in series involving 33 samples. Cross-contamination between samples was suspected, and all samples from these series were retested with the same extraction procedure, when enough material remained available. Twenty-eight samples of 33 were available for retesting (19/22 negative, 9/11 positive): 19 were confirmed negative; two were confirmed positive; and seven initially positive samples were found repeatedly negative, and the initial results were therefore considered as false positive. The two initially positive samples that could not be retested were from two children with other repeatedly positive samples and were considered as true-positive samples. After correction of false-positive results, findings of 37 of the 199 specimens were considered as positive.

Comparison of PCR results with bacteriologic data. The four specimens with positive smear results also had positive results by PCR. After the initial corrections for false-positive results, DNA amplification and culture had the same results in 166 of the 196 specimens, either positive for tuberculosis complex (n = 7) or negative (n = 159). Discrepancies were found for 30 specimens; 29 were culture negative and PCR positive, and one was PCR negative and culture positive (but smear negative).

Table IV. Number of PCR-positive samples according to the chronologic order of collection for the 17 tuberculous children from whom two or more samples were collected and having at least one positive PCR result

No. of samples from each child (No. of children)	No. of positive samples according to chronologic order of collection					
	1st	2nd	3rd	4th	5th	6th
2 (2)	2	1	—	—	—	—
3 (6)	2	4	2	—	—	—
4 (5)	1	2	1	4	—	—
5 (2)	0	2	2	0	1	—
6 (2)	1	2	1	1	2	2
TOTAL	6/17	11/17	6/15	5/9	3/4	2/2

Control procedure: Comparison of two DNA extraction methods. Because false-positive results had been attributed to cross-contamination with confirmed positive samples, other undetected cross-contaminations between positive and negative samples were possible. We therefore tested all the samples that remained available with another DNA extraction technique, to compare the feasibility and sensitivity of the two techniques. Ninety-six samples were thus retested with the Chelex 100 extraction procedure. No false-positive result was observed. Guanidine isothiocyanate–silica and Chelex 100 extractions gave the same results in 89 of the 96 specimens tested with both techniques. Twelve were positive for tuberculosis complex and 77 were negative. Discrepancies were found for seven specimens, six of which were negative after guanidine isothiocyanate–silica extraction and positive after Chelex 100 extraction, and one of which was Chelex 100 negative and guanidine isothiocyanate–silica positive. The only sample that was culture positive and PCR negative after guanidine isothiocyanate–silica extraction had a positive result after Chelex 100 treatment.

Thus the results obtained with the Chelex 100 extraction procedure confirmed the specificity of those obtained after guanidine isothiocyanate–silica extraction. DNA extraction with Chelex particles significantly improved the sensitivity of the PCR technique both for patients with active disease ($p = 0.0002$) and for patients with tuberculous infection without disease ($p = 0.0003$) (Table II).

Comparison of definitive PCR results with clinical data. False-positive PCR results detected by the systematic prevention procedure were obtained for two children with suspected tuberculous infection and for two patients without tuberculosis. After correction, positive PCR results were obtained in 20 children with clinically active disease, including three children whose results were recognized as positive only after the Chelex 100 extraction procedure, and in seven children with tuberculous infection but no disease. None of the children with suspected tuberculosis or without tuberculosis had positive PCR results. All 10 children with active disease and bacteriologic confirmation of tuberculosis had at least one positive PCR result. Among the three HIV-positive children with active disease, all had at least one positive PCR result but only one had a positive culture result. Similarly, the child with cystic fibrosis and active tuberculosis (revealed by strong tuberculin test positivity, rapid lung function degradation, and hilar adenopathies) was PCR positive and culture negative.

Some children had both positive and negative specimens, suggesting that testing numerous samples taken on consecutive days improves the detection of *M. tuberculosis*. Overall, only 16 children with either active tuberculosis or infection without disease had a positive PCR result with the first sample collected; analysis of several samples was required to recognize another seven children with active disease and four children with infection without disease as having positive PCR results. In 12 children with tuberculosis PCR results remained negative despite two or more samples collected. We further examined the proportion of positive PCR results according to the chronologic order of collection in the 17 children with tuberculosis from whom two or more samples were collected and at least one positive PCR result (Table IV) was found. The proportion of positive PCR results among the first samples collected from these 17 children was 41% as compared with 65% for the second samples, 40% for the third samples, and 64% for the fourth and subsequent samples. Furthermore, in children with only one positive PCR result and one or more negative results (n = 8), the positive sample was obtained in 50% of cases by the third (n = 2) or fourth sample (n = 2) tested by PCR.

Value of gastric aspirates and BAL. We investigated whether analysis of BAL samples would be better than the analysis of gastric aspirates for detection of *M. tuberculosis*. Sixteen children with tuberculosis had both BAL (16 specimens) and gastric aspirates (38 specimens) collected. Positive culture results were obtained for two BAL and for three gastric aspirate samples. Analysis by PCR of these samples showed that six BAL specimens (37.5%) from six children and 15 gastric aspirates (39.5%) from 11 children yielded positive findings; the difference was not significant. Five children had positive results in both gastric aspirate and BAL samples. We also investigated whether the probability that a gastric aspirate would be PCR positive correlated with its time of collection after BAL. Eight children had gastric aspirates collected both on the morning after BAL collection and on other days. Four of the eight gastric aspirates (50%) collected on the morning after lavage collection had positive results as compared with four of the 13 gastric aspirates (30.8%) collected on other days; the difference was not significant.

DISCUSSION

The diagnosis of tuberculosis in children can be difficult and is often delayed. Bacterial proof of the infection, and especially positive smears, are rarely obtained. Amplification of *M. tuberculosis*–specific DNA sequences in clinical samples is the most sensitive method of detection available.[16] However, the usefulness of this approach to the diagnosis of tuberculosis in children has not been well evaluated. Only one recent study reported encouraging results: 60% of children with primary tuberculosis had a positive PCR result.[17] We detected mycobacterial DNA after amplification by PCR in clinical samples from most of the children with active disease. Surprisingly, we also found that 40% of children with tuberculous infection without disease had at least one positive PCR result. Sensitivity was improved by testing several samples from each child. Finally, the risk of sporadic false-positive results can be considerably reduced by retesting doubtful positive results and by increasing the number of negative control samples.

Our study confirmed the difficulty in obtaining bacterial proof of tuberculous infection in children. Only 21% of children with active disease had positive smears and 42% had positive cultures. DNA amplification by PCR identified *M. tuberculosis* in clinical samples from more than 80% of the children with active tuberculosis. Moreover, more than 70% of children with active disease but no bacterial proof of the infection, had a positive PCR result. The difference between PCR and bacteriologic data was mostly related to the small number of organisms in samples from children. Polymerase chain reaction technique is more sensitive than microscopy for the detection of *M. tuberculosis*. DNA amplification can detect 500 *M. tuberculosis* cells per milliliter of sputum, whereas microscopy has a sensitivity of 10^4 to 10^5 organisms/ml.[10]

M. tuberculosis was also detected in 40% of children with tuberculous infection without disease. It is very unlikely that these positive results were false positives, because a rigorous protocol was followed to prevent carryover contamination and negative control samples yielded consistently negative results. Positive specimens from these children were never considered as doubtful (i.e., no association in their series to positive samples from other children), and results were repeatedly positive when retesting was possible. Furthermore, only children with a certain diagnosis of tuberculous infection had positive results. None of the children with either contact with tuberculosis and a negative tuberculin test result, or an unclear history of increased tuberculin reactivity, had a positive PCR result. Recognition of infected patients without symptoms is difficult in pediatric practice. Given a history of exposure to active pulmonary disease and a positive tuberculin skin test result, the absence of radiographic evidence of tuberculosis usually leads to the conclusion that there is no disease. However, we previously demonstrated that more than half these infected children had enlarged lymph nodes as assessed by computed tomography.[18] Our present study shows that *M. tuberculosis* was present at a sufficient density to be detected in gastric aspirates from 40% of these infected children; these results highlight the artificial character of the clinical distinction between infection and disease. In clinical practice the pathophysiologic significance of this remains unknown, and we did not address the question of whether infected children without disease but with positive PCR results should be treated differently from those with negative PCR results. Guidelines for treatment of infected children, as defined by current clinical and radiographic criteria, recommend either a one-drug regimen with isoniazid[19] or a two-drug regimen combining isoniazid and rifampicin[20]; beneficial effects have been demonstrated for both regimens. Thus, according to these established criteria, PCR is not a good test to distinguish between tuberculous infection and disease, and therefore to determine how a child should be treated. We therefore consider it unjustified to collect gastric aspirates for PCR routinely in children with suspected tuberculous infection without disease.

The high sensitivity of the PCR technique in children with tuberculosis was achieved largely by testing several samples from each child. In agreement with a previous report,[17] our results showed that most children with positive PCR results also had some negative specimens. The first sample collected was PCR positive in only 60% of children who later were recognized as PCR positive after two or more specimens were tested. However, the ideal number of samples to be collected from each child for maximal sensitivity cannot be stated from our study; the third or fourth specimen collected was the sole positive PCR result for four children, and only one child with repeatedly negative results had more than four samples analyzed by PCR.

The extraction technique also had an effect on the sensitivity of the PCR test. DNA purification with Chelex 100 particles was better than extraction with guanidine isothiocyanate and silica particles. The guanidine isothiocyanate–silica method has been reported to eliminate inhibitors[8] but has also been described as being less sensitive than other methods.[21] In our hands the Chelex 100 procedure proved better at eliminating inhibitors than the silica technique and was more reproducible (data not shown).

The sensitivity was not influenced by the site from which the specimens were collected; PCR tests of BAL samples and gastric aspirates from the same patients gave similar results in terms of sensitivity. Previous studies reported that cultures of BAL were no more likely to recover tubercle bacilli than cultures of gastric aspirates.[22]

False positivity is a constant problem with the PCR technique. A recent masked comparison among several laboratories showed the importance of appropriate precautions and of including negative controls for both DNA purification and amplification procedures.[10] Despite these precautions false-positive results were present in our study. Although the BCG genome is amplified by IS*6110* PCR, it is very unlikely that prior BCG vaccination accounted for these false-positive results in samples from the respiratory tract. Previous evaluation in our laboratory showed that the BCG genome was not detectable by PCR in blood samples shortly after BCG vaccination (data not shown). However, cross-contamination was easily suspected with our false-positive detection procedure because of the presence of several other positive results in the same series. The routine approach in our laboratory is to consider as doubtful and to retest all samples appearing positive among other positive results in the same series, even when all negative control samples yield negative results. Retesting positive samples reduces the number of false-positive results to less than 25 per 10,000 samples.[10] Our control procedures eliminated false-positive results, and positive results in children with tuberculosis were highly reproducible. Only one sample from a child with active disease had a negative PCR result in a control test with Chelex 100, despite an initial positive result. That the initial result for this sample was a false positive was unlikely because no other sample in its series was positive and the negative control samples had negative results. Bacterial heterogeneity of the sample or the presence of undetected inhibitors could explain this discrepancy. Finally, we observed false-positive results despite negative water controls giving negative results, underlining the need to increase the number of negative control samples for each procedure.

We conclude that DNA amplification is a sensitive method for the detection of *M. tuberculosis* in clinical samples from children with tuberculosis. However, technical considerations, including the DNA purification procedure, the use of suitable control samples, and the retesting of doubtful positive samples, considerably influence sensitivity and specificity. When suitable precautions are taken, DNA amplification for *M. tuberculosis* appears to be very valuable in pediatric clinical practice, although its high cost limits its indications. We believe that PCR for children is best used when the diagnosis of active tuberculosis is difficult and needs to be confirmed rapidly to exclude other diagnoses, especially in cases with a potentially false-negative tuberculin skin test result (for example, in immunosuppressed children or in neonates). In our study positive PCR results obtained in HIV-infected children or in the child with cystic fibrosis highlight the potential usefulness of the PCR technique in patients in whom the diagnosis of tuberculosis is difficult.

REFERENCES

1. Nemir RL, Krasinski K. Tuberculosis in children and adolescents in the 1980s. Pediatr Infect Dis J 1988;7:375-9.
2. Huret B, Haury B, Moyse C. Les cas de tuberculose déclarés en France en 1992. Bull Epidemiol Hebdomadaire 1993;52: 243-5.
3. Starke JR. Modern approach of the diagnosis and treatment of tuberculosis in children. Pediatr Clin North Am 1988; 35:441-64.
4. Starke JR. Childhood tuberculosis: a diagnostic dilemma. Chest 1993;104:329-30.
5. de Blic J, Azevedo I, Burren CP, Le Bourgeois M, Scheinmann P. The value of fiberoptic bronchoscopy in childhood pulmonary tuberculosis. Chest 1991;100:688-92.
6. Inselman LS, Kendig EL. Tuberculosis. In: Chernick V, Kendig EL, eds. Disorders of the respiratory tract in children. Philadelphia: WB Saunders, 1990:730-69.
7. Delacourt C, Gobin J, Gaillard JL, de Blic J, Veron M, Scheinmann P. Value of ELISA using antigen 60 for the diagnosis of tuberculosis in children. Chest 1993;104:393-8.
8. Brisson-Noel A, Aznar C, Chureau C, et al. Diagnosis of tuberculosis by DNA amplification in clinical practice evaluation. Lancet 1991;338:364-6.
9. Eisenach KD, Sifford MD, Cave MD, Bates JH, Crawford JT. Detection of *Mycobacterium tuberculosis* in sputum samples using a polymerase chain reaction. Am Rev Respir Dis 1991; 144:1160-3.
10. Noordhoek GT, Kolk AHJ, Bjune G, et al. Sensitivity and specificity of PCR for detection of *Mycobacterium tuberculosis*: a blind comparison study among seven laboratories. J Clin Microbiol 1994;32:277-84.
11. American Thoracic Society. Diagnostic standards and classification of tuberculosis. Am Rev Respir Dis 1990;142:725-35.
12. Boom R, Sol CJA, Salimans MMM, Jansen CL, Wertheim-van Dillen PME, van der Noordaa J. Rapid and simple method for purification of nucleic acids. J Clin Microbiol 1990;28:495-503.
13. De Lamballerie X, Zandotti C, Vignoli C, Bollet C, De Micco P. A one step microbial DNA extraction method using "Chelex 100" suitable for gene amplification. Res Microbiol 1992; 143:785-90.
14. Kwok S, Higuchi R. Avoiding false positives with PCR. Nature 1989;339:237-8.
15. Toman K. Sensitivity, specificity and predictive value of diagnostic tests. Bull Int Union Tuberc 1981;56:18-28.
16. Hermans PWM, Schuitema ARJ, Van Soolingen D, et al. Specific detection of Mycobacterium tuberculosis complex strains by polymerase chain reaction. J Clin Microbiol 1990; 28:1204-13.
17. Pierre C, Olivier C, Lecossier D, Boussougant Y, Yeni P, Hance AJ. Diagnosis of primary tuberculosis in children by amplification and detection of mycobacterial DNA. Am Rev Respir Dis 1993;147:420-4.
18. Delacourt C, Mamou Mani T, Bonnerot V, et al. Computed tomography with normal chest radiograph in tuberculous infection. Arch Dis Child 1993;69:430-2.
19. American Thoracic Society. Treatment of tuberculosis and tuberculosis infection in adults and children. Am J Respir Crit Care Med 1994;149:1359-74.
20. Ormerod LP. Chemotherapy and management of tuberculosis in the United Kingdom: recommendations of the Joint Committee of the British Thoracic Society. Thorax 1990;45:403-8.
21. Wilson SM, McNerney R, Nye PM, Godfrey-Faussett PD, Stoker NG, Voller A. Progress toward a simplified PCR and its application to diagnosis of tuberculosis. J Clin Microbiol 1993;31:776-82.
22. Abadco DL, Steiner P. Gastric lavage is better than bronchoalveolar lavage for isolation of *Mycobacterium tuberculosis* in childhood pulmonary tuberculosis. Pediatr Infect Dis J 1992; 11:735-8.

Encephalopathy in children with perinatally acquired human immunodeficiency virus infection

Mark N. Lobato, MD, M. Blake Caldwell, MD, MPH, Paulus Ng, MPH, Margaret J. Oxtoby, MD, and the Pediatric Spectrum of Disease Clinical Consortium

From the Pediatric and Family Studies Section, Epidemiology Branch, Division of HIV/AIDS, National Center for Infectious Diseases, Centers for Disease Control and Prevention, Public Health Service, U.S. Department of Health and Human Services, Atlanta, Georgia

***Objective*: To define the incidence, characteristics, and survival of children with perinatally acquired human immunodeficiency virus (HIV) infection and encephalopathy.**
***Design*: Cross-sectional and longitudinal data collected from 1811 HIV-infected children in a multicenter active surveillance study.**
***Setting*: Health departments and medical centers in six areas of the United States.**
***Results*: HIV encephalopathy was diagnosed in 178 (23%) of 766 children with perinatally acquired immunodeficiency syndrome (AIDS). The median age at diagnosis of encephalopathy was 19 months. Among infected children, the estimated risk of having HIV encephalopathy by age 12 months was 4.0% (95% confidence interval, 2.6% to 6.0%). Children with HIV encephalopathy had more hospitalizations (median, 4) than children with other AIDS-defining conditions (median, 2; $p = 0.002$) and lower $CD4^+$ T-lymphocyte counts in the first year of life (median, 444 cells/mm^3). Estimated median survival after diagnosis was 22 months, similar to the 20 months for children with *Pneumocystis carinii* pneumonia.**
***Conclusion*: HIV encephalopathy in chidren with perinatally acquired AIDS is a common condition and is associated with severe morbidity evidenced by frequent hospitalizations, severe immunodeficiency, and short survival. (J Pediatr 1995;126:710-5)**

The human immunodeficiency virus is the primary agent associated with progressive encephalopathy in persons with the acquired immunodeficiency syndrome.[1] The exact timing of HIV infection of the central nervous system is unknown; however, early neurologic signs may precede detectable immunologic defects.[2] Early in the HIV epidemic, encephalopathy was a recognized feature of HIV infection in infants and children.[3, 4] Developmental delays, loss of previously acquired milestones, cognitive impairment, microcephaly, weakness, spastic paresis, and hyperreflexia are the most common manifestations of HIV encephalopathy in

ADC	AIDS-defining condition
AIDS	Acquired immunodeficiency syndrome
CI	Confidence interval
HIV	Human immunodeficiency virus
LIP	Lymphoid interstitial pneumonia
PCP	*Pneumocystis carinii* pneumonia

Presented in part at the First National Conference on Human Retroviruses and Related Infections, Washington, D.C., Dec. 12-16, 1993.

Submitted for publication Sept. 21, 1994; accepted Dec. 2, 1994.

Reprint requests: M. Blake Caldwell, MD, MPH, Division of HIV/AIDS, Centers for Disease Control and Prevention, 1600 Clifton Rd., MS E-45, Atlanta, GA 30333.

9/20/62446

children.[5] Treatment with zidovudine or dideoxyinosine improves IQ scores in children with symptomatic HIV infection, including encephalopathy.[6-9]

This study describes the epidemiologic features and survival of children with HIV encephalopathy, and examines possible predictors of the development of encephalopathy and associated clinical findings among children with perinatally acquired HIV infection.

METHODS

Patient population. We used data collected through the Pediatric Spectrum of Disease Project in six sites in the United States. This project conducts active surveillance of HIV-exposed children by methods previously described.[10] Briefly, the Centers for Disease Control and Prevention, several state and local health departments, and several clinical centers initiated the project in 1988. Participating hospitals reported about one fifth of the reported perinatal AIDS cases in the United States in 1992. The medical records of children who are less than 13 years of age, who are HIV infected or whose mothers are infected, and whose infection status is indeterminate infection (classification E) were reviewed in the six study sites (Los Angeles County, 9 hospitals in New York City, the Commonwealth of Massachusetts, 3 cities in Texas, Washington, D.C., and 12 counties in the San Francisco Bay area). Data were abstracted anonymously from all available medical records at the time of enrollment and subsequently at 6-month intervals. Data collected on each child included age, sex, race or ethnicity, mode of HIV transmission, maternal HIV risk factors, date of birth, birth weight, gestational age at birth, results of urine toxicology screening at birth, date of conditions indicative of AIDS, other HIV-related illnesses, $CD4^+$ T-lymphocyte measurements, use of antiretroviral therapy or prophylaxis for opportunistic infections, dates of hospital admissions, and cause and date of death. No personal identifiers were collected.

Case definitions. The 1987 AIDS surveillance case definition defines HIV encephalopathy in infected children as the presence of one or more of the following: progressive neurologic deterioration, loss of developmental milestones, or symmetric motor dysfunction.[11] Brain imaging and analysis of the cerebrospinal fluid or autopsy should be used to exclude other possible conditions that may explain these findings. Individual clinicians use different exclusion criteria because neuroimaging may be nonspecific[12]; HIV encephalopathy may be diagnosed presumptively. Therefore the project collects information that allows a definitive or presumptive diagnosis of HIV encephalopathy and defines presumptive encephalopathy as clinically diagnosed disease in the absence of neuroimaging or other laboratory studies.

Because children with the presumptive diagnosis of HIV encephalopathy were not different from those with definitive diagnoses in their demographic features, characteristics at birth, or survival, we included in the definition of HIV encephalopathy a presumptive diagnosis (32% of children with HIV encephalopathy) as well as a definitive diagnosis. For this analysis, all children with HIV encephalopathy (definitive or presumptive) were considered to have AIDS.

We examined correlates between HIV encephalopathy and HIV-related diseases, including other AIDS-defining conditions, and also the reported association of encephalopathy with HIV-related cardiomyopathy. For this analysis, any diagnosis noted in the medical record of cardiomyopathy or cytomegalovirus disease of an organ other than liver, spleen, or lymph nodes in a child more than 1 month of age was accepted.

Statistical analysis. We analyzed data collected from 1988 through 1992 on children with perinatally acquired HIV infection. Analysis of demographic and clinical features compared children who had HIV encephalopathy as an initial or subsequent diagnosis with all other children who had severe HIV infection. Analysis of clinical outcomes, $CD4^+$ T-lymphocyte counts, and survival compared children by means of the diagnosis date of the specific condition when it was the initial diagnosis (i.e., the date of AIDS diagnosis). Categoric data were compared by using the Yates-corrected chi-square test and nonparametric data by the Kruskal-Wallis test. Statistical significance was evaluated at the level of $p < 0.05$. We used the product-limit method to estimate the incidence of HIV encephalopathy for children followed prospectively from age 3 months or less. Hospitalization rates were computed per 100 person-years from birth to the date of the last clinical contact. Children were censored at the time of diagnosis of HIV encephalopathy, death, or last contact. We compared $CD4^+$ T-lymphocyte counts measured within a month before or after the date of diagnosis of HIV encephalopathy, *Pneumocystis carinii* pneumonia, lymphoid interstitial pneumonia, and other ADCs. Because $CD4^+$ T-lymphocyte counts in children decline physiologically during the first few years of life, the $CD4^+$ cell counts for children by diagnosis were stratified into age groups from birth to 11 months and from 12 to 71 months. After being stratified for the age of the children, the median $CD4^+$ T-lymphocyte counts of children with different diagnoses were compared by using the SAS NPAR1WAY procedure.[13] When the median $CD4^+$ cell counts among all groups were significantly different, the median $CD4^+$ cell counts in the four diagnostic groups were compared for each age stratum by using this procedure with a level of significance of $p < 0.0125$. Time to death after the diagnosis of specific ADCs was estimated by using the product-limit method. Confidence intervals for survival times were calculated by the Brookmeyer-Crowley meth-

Table. Demographic and birth characteristics of children with HIV encephalopathy compared with other children with perinatally acquired AIDS

Characteristic	Encephalopathy No.	Encephalopathy %	Other AIDS No.	Other AIDS %	p
Diagnosis at <12 months	31/95*	33	268/671	40	NS†
Male	92/176	52	299/590	51	NS
White race	40/172	23	70/581	12	<0.001‡
Birth weight <2500 gm	46/135	34	135/448	30	NS
Gestational age <37 wk	35/136	26	121/453	27	NS
Vaginal delivery	93/120	78	336/417	81	NS
Nursery stay >7 days	40/97	41	115/305	38	NS
Positive results on urine toxicology screen	12/38	32	42/121	35	NS
Maternal injection drug use	70/123	57	243/411	59	NS

NS, Not significant.
*Diagnosis denotes first AIDS diagnosis.
†NS = $p > 0.05$.
‡Was not significant when controlled for study site.

od,[14] and survival curves were compared by the Breslow statistic.[15] Because the survival relationships did not change when children with both HIV encephalopathy and either PCP or LIP were excluded from the analysis, these children were included in the survival analysis.

RESULTS

Children with HIV encephalopathy. Of 1811 perinatally infected children, 766 (42.3%) had AIDS; their median age at the last medical evaluation was 37 months. HIV encephalopathy, the fourth most common ADC reported, was diagnosed in 178 (23.2%) children with perinatally acquired AIDS and 9.8% of all children with perinatally acquired HIV infection. At the time of AIDS diagnosis, 95 children (12.4%) had HIV encephalopathy: 76 had only encephalopathy and 19 had more than one ADC. Eighty-three children (10.8%) had HIV encephalopathy diagnosed after an initial diagnosis of AIDS. In all, 81% of children with HIV encephalopathy received treatment with zidovudine at some time.

Of the 178 children with HIV encephalopathy, 133 (74.7%) had the diagnosis before age 36 months, and 15 (8.4%) after 60 months of age. The median age at the diagnosis of HIV encephalopathy was 19 months (range, 1 to 141 months). In comparison, the median age at diagnosis was 6 months for children with PCP and 24 months for those with LIP. The age at the diagnosis of HIV encephalopathy did not differ significantly by race or ethnicity.

The characteristics of children with HIV encephalopathy were not different from the characteristics of all other children with AIDS, except for race (Table). Overall, white children (23.3%) were more likely to have HIV encephalopathy than black (16.9%) but not Hispanic (24.2%) children. However, analysis stratified by study site found no significant difference for HIV encephalopathy between white children and black children. No other demographic or birth characteristic differentiated children in whom HIV encephalopathy developed from those who had other ADCs.

To estimate the incidence of HIV encephalopathy, we analyzed data from 503 HIV-infected children followed prospectively from age 3 months or younger. The median follow-up time was 19 months (range, 1 to 128 months). HIV encephalopathy was diagnosed in 15 children by age 1 year and in 31 by age 4 years. The estimated risk of HIV encephalopathy by age 12 months was 4.0% (95% confidence interval, 2.6% to 6.0%), and by age 48 months was 13.9% (95% CI, 9.3% to 18.5%).

Clinical outcomes associated with HIV encephalopathy. Children with HIV encephalopathy were more likely than children with other ADCs to have cardiomyopathy (41% vs 18%) (risk ratio, 3.15; 95% CI, 1.96 to 5.03; $p < 0.001$). No other correlations with HIV-related conditions were found.

Hospitalizations after birth were more frequent among children with HIV encephalopathy (median, 4; range, 0 to 25) than among children with all other ADCs (median, 2; range, 0 to 34; $p = 0.002$), PCP (median, 2), or LIP (median, 2). Hospitalization rates were highest for children with encephalopathy, who had 0.837 hospitalization per person-year (520 hospitalizations per 621.5 person-years), compared with 0.785 hospitalization per person-year (613/781.3) in children with PCP, and significantly higher ($p < 0.001$) than in children with LIP, who had 0.401 hospitalization per person-year (617/1540.3).

The $CD4^+$ T-lymphocyte counts were performed within a month of diagnosis for 41 children with HIV encephalopathy, 75 with PCP, 69 with LIP, and 52 with AIDS excluding encephalopathy, PCP, or LIP, when the condition represented the initial AIDS diagnosis. The median $CD4^+$

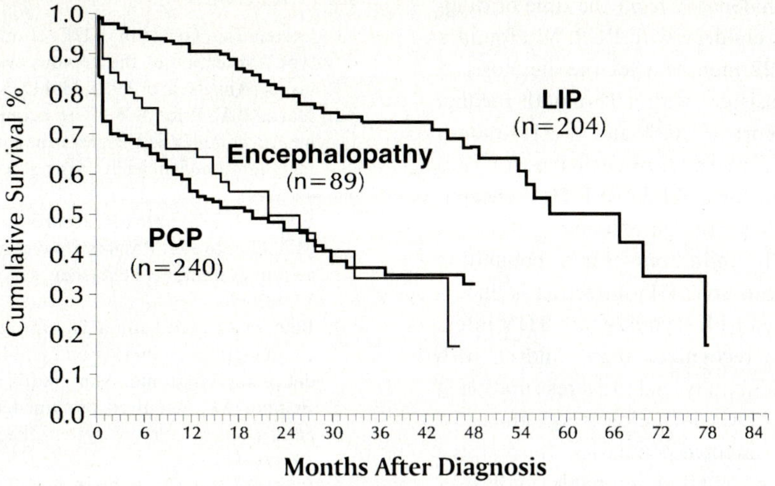

Figure. Cumulative survival from time of diagnosis to death for perinatally HIV-infected children diagnosed with HIV encephalopathy, PCP, and LIP.

T-lymphocyte count among children from birth to 11 months of age at diagnosis of HIV encephalopathy was 444 cells/mm^3, not statistically different from the median counts for children with PCP, LIP, or other ADCs. The median count for children from 12 to 71 months with HIV encephalopathy was 281 cells/mm^3—similar to the median count for children with other ADCs, and significantly lower than the median count for children with LIP ($p = 0.01$).

Survival times (Figure) from the diagnosis of HIV encephalopathy, PCP, LIP, and other ACDs as the initial AIDS condition were estimated. Median survival time after the diagnosis of HIV encephalopathy was 22 months (95% CI, 15 months to 33 months), slightly longer than the 20 months' (95% CI, 12 to 28; $p = 0.043$) median survival time after the diagnosis of PCP. In contrast, the median survival time of children with LIP was 67 months (95% CI, 54 to 70; $p < 0.001$) and of children with other ADCs, 36 months (95% CI, 26 to 48; $p = 0.019$).

DISCUSSION

Encephalopathy caused by HIV infection is common among children with perinatally acquired HIV. In our study, about 10% of HIV-infected children and 23% of children with AIDS had HIV encephalopathy. The finding that HIV encephalopathy represents 12% of initial AIDS diagnoses is similar to the proportion (13%) with encephalopathy among pediatric AIDS cases reported to the British Pediatric Surveillance System, which includes HIV encephalopathy diagnosed on the basis of clinical critieria without supporting laboratory evidence.[16] In contrast to earlier studies that found the rate of HIV encephalopathy after an AIDS diagnosis to be less than 5%,[17-19] we found a 12% rate, probably because of the longer follow-up time of this study. Other studies have shown that the proportion of HIV encephalopathy in children younger than 14 years is higher than that for older age-groups except in persons older than 70 years.[20]

Although the age range at the diagnosis of HIV encephalopathy was broad, most cases of encephalopathy were diagnosed by 3 years of age; the highest risk occurred in the first year of life. In the future, the median age at diagnosis may increase as more children are followed for a longer time. Increasing numbers of children with HIV encephalopathy will reach school age and have special needs.

We found no demographic or birth characteristics that would help predict the development of encephalopathy among children with perinatally acquired HIV infection. With control for the study site, there was no significant association between race and HIV encephalopathy. It is possible that the differences in race represent differences in site-specific diagnostic practices.

This analysis and a previous study have correlated HIV encephalopathy with cardiomyopathy.[21] HIV can have multiple direct and indirect effects on both the central nervous system and the heart, especially on the autonomic nervous system.[22] However, further investigation is necessary to establish common causes and to explain the observed association in our study and others. We were unable to confirm the findings of several investigators of an association between HIV encephalopathy and cytomegalovirus disease.[23, 24]

Our analysis and that of Duliege et al.[25] suggest that children with HIV encephalopathy often are severely immunodeficient, and that survival time for children with HIV encephalopathy is poor. Morbidity is also high, as evidenced by the number of hospitalizations. The survival of children with HIV encephalopathy from the time of diagnosis is similar to that of children with PCP. We found a median survival time of 22 months after the diagnosis of HIV encephalopathy, consistent with a 15-month median survival time in New York State[26] and a 31.4-month median survival time in a recent European report,[27] but longer than the 11 months for children with HIV encephalopathy found in an earlier study in Miami.[17]

This study has several limitations. First, population studies have shown that pediatric HIV infection is underdiagnosed and that children with asymptomatic HIV infection are less likely to be recognized than children with symptomatic infection.[28] This may lead to overestimation of the prevalence of specific ADCs, including encephalopathy, among the pediatric HIV-infected population. Second, the HIV encephalopathy case definition probably underestimates the incidence of central nervous system dysfunction caused by HIV, because subtle manifestations of dysfunction may not be included. Third, the data collected are abstracted from charts and reflect only diagnoses and information recorded in the medical record. These data may be incomplete or delayed, although periodic record review improves completeness.

Encephalopathy represents a common and serious manifestation of HIV infection, as measured by the proportion of children affected, the number of hospitalizations, the associated severe immunodeficiency, and short survival time. For HIV-infected children, regular neurologic and developmental evaluations should be part of their routine care.[29] Antiretroviral therapy is recommended for any child with HIV encephalopathy.[30]

The following are investigators with the Pediatric Spectrum of Disease Clinical Consortium: in Massachusetts, Ho-Wen Hsu, MD (Principal Investigator), Barbara Stechenberg, MD, Kenneth McIntosh, MD, Stephen Pelton, MD, Cody Meissner, MD, Suzanne Tobin, RN, Mark Pasternack, MD, and John Sullivan, MD; in Los Angeles, California, Laurene Mascola, MD (Principal Investigator), Philip Brunell, MD, Carol Berkowitz, MD, Nadia Ewing, MD, Andrea Kovacs, MD, Joseph Church, MD, Steve Taylor, MD, Audra Deveikis, MD, and Yvonne Bryson, MD; in San Francisco, California, Yvonne Maldonado, MD (Principal Investigator), Ann Petru, MD, Catherine Albin, MD, Charles Prober, MD, and Diane Wara, MD; in New York City, Pauline Thomas, MD (Principal Investigator), Arye Rubinstein, MD, Geniveve Lambert, MD, Ruth Stein, MD, Susan Champion, MD, Herman Mendez, MD, Nathan Litman, MD, Donna Futterman, MD, Senih Fikrig, MD, Joseph Servia, MD, and Margaret Hilgartner, MD; in Washington, D.C., Robert Parrott, MD (Principal Investigator), Tamara Rakusan, MD, Yvette Reid, MD, and Antoine Fomafod, MD; and in Texas, Karl Shaner, DrPH (Principal Investigator), Mark Kline, MD, Janet Squires, MD, and Terence Doran, MD, PhD.

REFERENCES

1. Epstein LG, Gendelman HE. Human immunodeficiency virus type 1 infection of the nervous system: pathogenetic mechanisms. Ann Neurol 1993;33:429-36.
2. Navia BA, Price RW. The acquired immunodeficiency dementia complex as the presenting or sole manifestation of human immunodeficiency virus infection. Arch Neurol 1987; 44:65-9.
3. Epstein LG, Sharer LR, Joshi VV, Fojas MM, Koenigsberger MR, Oleske JM. Progressive encephalopathy in children with acquired immune deficiency syndrome. Ann Neurol 1985; 17:488-96.
4. Belman AL, Ultmann MH, Horoupian D, et al. Neurological complications in infants and children with acquired immune deficiency syndrome. Ann Neurol 1985;18:560-6.
5. Belman AL. Acquired immunodeficiency syndrome and the child's central nervous system. Pediatr Clin North Am 1992; 39:691-714.
6. Pizzo PA, Eddy J, Falloon J, et al. Effect of continuous intravenous infusion of zidovudine (AZT) in children with symptomatic HIV infection. N Engl J Med 1988;319:889-96.
7. Brouwers P, Moss H, Wolters P, et al. Effect of continuous-infusion zidovudine therapy on neuropsychologic functioning in children with symptomatic human immunodeficiency virus infection. J Pediatr 1990;117:980-5.
8. McKinney RE, Maha MA, Connor EM, et al. A multicenter trial of oral zidovudine in children with advanced human immunodeficiency virus disease. N Engl J Med 1991;324:1018-25.
9. Butler KM, Husson RN, Balis FM, et al. Dideoxyinosine in children with symptomatic human immunodeficiency virus infection. N Engl J Med 1991;324:137-44.
10. Caldwell MB, Mascola L, Smith W, et al. Biologic, foster, and adoptive parents: care givers of children exposed perinatally to human immunodeficiency virus in the United States. Pediatrics 1992;90:603-7.
11. Centers for Disease Control. Revision of the CDC surveillance case definition for acquired immunodeficiency syndrome. MMWR 1987;36(suppl 1):1S-15S.
12. DeCarli C, Civitello LA, Brouwers P, Pizzo PA. The prevalence of computed tomographic abnormalities of the cerebrum in 100 consecutive children symptomatic with the human immune deficiency virus. Ann Neurol 1993;34:198-205.
13. SAS/STAT user's guide: version 6, vol 2. 4th ed. Cary, North Carolina: SAS Institute, 1990.
14. Brookmeyer R, Crowley J. A confidence interval for the median survival time. Biometrics 1982;38:29-41.
15. Breslow NE. A generalized Kruskal-Wallis test for comparing K samples subject to unequal patterns of censorship. Biometrika 1970;57:579-94.
16. Ades AE, Davison CF, Holland FJ, et al. Vertically transmitted HIV infection in the British Isles. BMJ 1993;306:1296-9.
17. Scott GB, Hutto C, Makuch RW, et al. Survival in children with perinatally acquired human immunodeficiency virus type 1 infection. N Engl J Med 1989;321:1791-6.
18. Blanche S, Tardieu M, Duliege AM, et al. Longitudinal study of 94 symptomatic infants with perinatally acquired human immunodeficiency virus infection. Am J Dis Child 1990;144: 1210-5.
19. European Collaborative Study. Neurologic signs in young children with human immunodeficiency virus infection. Pediatr Infect Dis J 1990;9:402-6.

20. Janssen RS, Nwanyanwu OC, Selik RM, Stehr-Green JK. Epidemiology of human immunodeficiency virus encephalopathy in the United States. Neurology 1992;42:1472-6.
21. Luginbuhl LM, Orav EJ, McIntosh K, Lipschultz SE. Cardiac morbidity and related mortality in children with HIV infection. JAMA 1993;269:2869-75.
22. Freeman R, Roberts MS, Friedman LS, Broadbridge C. Autonomic function and human immunodeficiency virus infection. Neurology 1990;40:575-80.
23. Cooper ER, Schwartz T, Brena A, Regan AM, Pelton SI. Cytomegalovirus as a cofactor in transmission and progression of perinatal HIV infection. Pediatric AIDS and HIV Infection: Fetus to Adolescence 1992;3:302-7.
24. Fiala M, Singer EJ, Graves MC, et al. AIDS dementia complex complicated by cytomegalovirus encephalopathy. J Neurol 1993;240:223-31.
25. Duliege AM, Messiah A, Blanche S, Tardieu M, Griscelli C, Spira A. Natural history of human immunodeficiency virus type 1 infection in children: prognostic value of laboratory tests on the bimodal progression of disease. Pediatr Infect Dis J 1992;11:630-5.
26. Turner BJ, Denison M, Eppes SC, Houchens R, Fanning T, Markson LE. Survival experience of 789 children with the acquired immunodeficiency syndrome. Pediatr Infect Dis J 1993:12:310-20.
27. Salamina G, Ancelle-Park RA, Downs AM, de Vincenzi I, Brunet JB. Vertically acquired AIDS cases in Europe [Abstract PoC 4242]. Eighth International Conference on AIDS, Amsterdam, the Netherlands, July 1992.
28. Hsu HW, Moye J Jr, Kunches L, et al. Perinatally acquired human immunodeficiency virus infection: extent of clinical recognition in a population-based cohort. Pediatr Infect Dis J 1992;11:941-5.
29. El-Sadr W, Oleske JM. Evaluation and management of early HIV infection. (Publication No. AHCPR 94-0572-90-3.) Rockville, Maryland: U.S. Department of Health and Human Services, 1994 (Jan).
30. Working Group on Antiretroviral Therapy, National Pediatric HIV Resource Center. Antiretroviral therapy and medical management of the human immunodeficiency virus–infected child. Pediatr Infect Dis J 1993;12:513-22.

Long-term efficacy of recombinant hepatitis B vaccine and risk of natural infection in infants born to mothers with hepatitis B e antigen

Ping-Ing Lee, MD, Chin-Yun Lee, MD, Li-Min Huang, MD, PhD, and Mei-Hwei Chang, MD

From the Department of Pediatrics, National Taiwan University Hospital, Taipei, Taiwan, Republic of China

To evaluate the long-term protection afforded by the vaccine, recombinant hepatitis B (HB) vaccine was given to 171 infants born to hepatitis B e antigen–positive carrier mothers. Group A (53 infants) and group B (57 infants) received four doses of HB vaccine at birth and at 1, 2, and 12 months of age, with a dose of 20 μg in group A and 10 μg in group B. Group C (61 infants) received three 20 μg doses of HB vaccine at birth and at 1 and 6 months of age. These children were followed up annually up to 5 years of age. Six children (4%) became HB carriers before 1 year of age, and the carrier state persisted to the end of follow-up. The overall seropositive rate of HB surface antibody (anti-HBs) dropped from 99% at 1 year of age to 83% at 5 years of age. Among 548 serum pairs taken at 1-year intervals from children negative for HB surface antigen (HBsAg), a fourfold rise of anti-HBs titer was noted in 58 (11%) and a 10-fold rise of anti-HBs was noted in 17 (3%). Maternal HB core antibody disappeared in most children (151/152, 99%) before 2 years of age. Natural infections, as judged by persistence or reappearance of HB core antibody, occurred in 19 of 163 (12%) HBsAg-negative children. None of these episodes was associated with HBsAg positivity. We conclude that the long-term protection afforded by recombinant HB vaccine is satisfactory and that a further booster dose before 5 years of age is not necessary. (J Pediatr 1995;126:716-21)

The carrier rate for hepatitis B in the Taiwanese general population has been 15% to 20%, and perinatal hepatitis B virus transmission has accounted for 40% to 50% of the carrier pool.[1-3] Although long-term carriage of HBV in children is usually asymptomatic,[4, 5] it may lead to chronic hepatitis, liver cirrhosis, and hepatocellular carcinoma in later life.[6] Many studies have demonstrated the efficacy of HB vaccine in reducing the incidence of long-term carriage in neonates at high risk.[7-12] Most studies have shown that both the plasma-derived vaccines and the recombinant vaccines are equivalent in immunogenicity, protective efficacy, and safety.[8, 13, 14]

Anti-HBc	Hepatitis B core antibody
Anti-HBs	Hepatitis B surface antibody
HB	Hepatitis B
HBeAg	Hepatitis B e antigen
HBsAg	Hepatitis B surface antigen
HBV	Hepatitis B virus

A potential problem with HB vaccination is that vaccine-induced antibody levels might decline with age. Accordingly, a booster dose in later life has been recommend-

Supported by National Science Council grants NSC 79-0419-B002-180, NSC 80-0419-B002-207, and NSC 81-0419-B002-608.

Submitted for publication Sept. 14, 1994; accepted Dec. 12, 1994.

Reprint requests: Chin-Yun Lee, MD, Department of Pediatrics, National Taiwan University Hospital, 7 Chung-Shan South Rd., Taipei, Taiwan, Republic of China.

0022-3476/95/$3.00 + 0 **9/20/62710**

ed.[11, 15-18] Follow-up studies of vaccinated persons have identified rare HBV infections in those who had responded to HB vaccine.[8, 12, 19-24] The vast majority of these infections, however, have been manifest only by hepatitis B core antibody positivity. Most of the follow-up data available have come from studies of plasma-derived vaccine. There are even fewer follow-up data of vaccinated infants born to hepatitis B e antigen–positive carrier mothers. Such data are of prime importance because these infants are at sustained risk of contracting HBV infection through contact with the carrier mother and other family members.[1]

We have followed until 5 years of age 171 infants born to HBeAg-positive carrier mothers and given recombinant HB vaccine.[7] This report describes the pattern of blood HB markers in these children, to evaluate the long-term protection afforded by recombinant HB vaccines.

METHODS

Subjects. High-risk infants for HBV infection were identified by screening pregnant women for hepatitis B surface antigen and HBeAg. Those born to HBeAg-positive carrier mothers were recruited into the study with written consent from parents. Blood samples were obtained from the mothers after delivery to confirm the presence of HBeAg. A total of 171 infants was recruited and completed the vaccination schedule from 1988 to 1989.

Vaccination schedules. All infants received 0.5 ml (145 IU) of HB immune globulin within 24 hours of birth. The recombinant HB vaccine (Engerix-B) was provided by SmithKline Beecham Biologicals, Rixensart, Belgium. Three protocols were adopted. Group A (53 infants) and group B (57 infants) received four doses of HB vaccine at birth and at 1, 2, and 12 months of age. The dose of HB vaccine was 20 μg in group A and 10 μg in group B. Group C (61 infants) received three doses of 20 μg HB vaccine at birth and at 1 and 6 months of age. All infants were subjected to blood sampling at birth and at 6 months and 1 year of age. An additional blood sample was collected at 14 months of age in group A and group B. These children were then followed up annually up to 5 years of age. A blood sample was collected at each visit.

Laboratory studies. Hepatitis B surface antibody, anti-HBc, and HBsAg were tested by radioimmunoassay (Abbott Laboratories, North Chicago, Ill.). Serum alanine aminotransferase levels were assayed by an autoanalyzer. Anti-HBs was considered positive when its value exceeded 10 mIU/ml. A carrier was defined as a person with persistently positive HBsAg for more than 6 months.

Definitions and statistics. In children negative for HBsAg, a natural infection of HBV was defined as a persistence of anti-HBc beyond 3 years of age or reappearance of anti-HBc after it had become negative. Only samples negative for HBsAg were included in the calculation of geometric mean titer of anti-HBs. Analysis of variance was used to compare geometric mean titers of anti-HBs among groups. Differences in frequency between groups were examined by chi-square test. Linear regression for the anti-HBs levels in HBsAg-negative children was computed by the following model: $\log_e$ (anti-HBs) = A + $B_1 \times \log_e$ (peak anti-HBs after vaccination) + $B_2 \times \log_e$ (days since booster).[15]

RESULTS

Hepatitis B surface antigen and anti-HBs. After completion of initial vaccination schedules, six infants (4%) were seropositive for HBsAg and remained so throughout the follow-up period (Table I). The overall protective efficacy of HB vaccine was 96%, assuming that 88% of the unvaccinated infants born to HBeAg-positive mothers would become carriers.[25] One carrier child was lost to follow-up at 3 years of age. All the other 165 infants remained HBsAg negative during the follow-up period.

The percentage of children with anti-HBs decreased with age. Only one HBsAg-negative infant (1%) was seronegative for anti-HBs at 1 year of age; the rate increased to 23 of 135 (17%) at the end of follow-up (Table I). The percentage of children at 5 years of age with anti-HBs was highest in group A and lowest in group C ($p < 0.05$). The mean anti-HBs level also decreased with age. During the follow-up period the geometric mean titer of anti-HBs in group A tended to be the highest and that in group C tended to be the lowest (analysis of variance, $p < 0.05$ except for 4-year group) (Table I). Levels of anti-HBs were not affected by gender in any age interval or in any vaccination group.

Titers of anti-HBs in HBsAg-negative children were analyzed by the regression model proposed by Coursaget et al.[15] to compare our results with those of other studies. At any age anti-HBs titer may thus be estimated by the following equation: $\log_e$ (anti-HBs) = 7.4 + 0.67 $\times \log_e$ (peak anti-HBs after vaccination) − 1.0 $\times \log_e$ (days since booster) ($r = 0.48$, SD = 1.8).

Maternal anti-HBc. All infants were anti-HBc positive at birth. All six carrier children were positive for anti-HBc throughout the follow-up period. Among the 165 noncarrier children, two remained anti-HBc positive before they were lost to follow-up at 2 years of age and five who had been followed up for at least 3 years were persistently positive for anti-HBc throughout the follow-up period. The other 158 noncarrier children lost anti-HBc by the age of 3 years. The timing of anti-HBc disappearance could not be determined in six cases because of irregular visits. Among the remaining 152 children, two thirds of them lost anti-HBc before 12 months, and all but one child lost anti-HBc before 2 years of age (Table II). The timing of disappearance of maternal

Table I. Hepatitis B surface antigen and anti-HBs in 171 children vaccinated with recombinant HB vaccines

Vaccination group	Age (yr) 1*	2	3	4	5
Group A					
No.	53	48	44	44	46
HBsAg+	3 (6%)	3 (6%)	3 (7%)	3 (7%)	3 (7%)
HBsAg−					
Anti-HBs−	0	1 (2%)	1 (2%)	2 (5%)	3 (7%)
Anti-HBs+	50 (94%)	44 (92%)	40 (91%)	39 (89%)	40 (87%)
GMT (mIU/ml)	371	307	223	108	106
Group B					
No.	57	56	51	47	45
HBsAg+	1 (2%)	1 (2%)	1 (2%)	1 (2%)	1 (2%)
HBsAg−					
Anti-HBs−	0	1 (2%)	4 (8%)	4 (9%)	6 (13%)
Anti-HBs+	56 (98%)	54 (96%)	46 (90%)	42 (89%)	38 (84%)
GMT (mIU/ml)	250	187	118	57	51
Group C					
No.	61	54	56	52	49
HBsAg+	2 (3%)	2 (4%)	1 (2%)	1 (2%)	1 (2%)
HBsAg−					
Anti-HBs−	1 (2%)	4 (7%)	6 (11%)	6 (12%)	14 (29%)
Anti-HBs+	58 (95%)	48 (89%)	49 (88%)	45 (87%)	34 (69%)
GMT (mIU/ml)	158	92	66	56	30

+, Positive; −, negative; *GMT*, geometric mean titer of anti-HBs.
*Blood samples were taken at 14 months of age in groups A and B, and at 12 months of age in group C.

Table II. Timing of disappearance of maternal anti-HBc in 152 children

Vaccination group	Age at disappearance of anti-HBc <6 mo	6-12 mo	12 mo-2 yr	2 yr-3 yr
Group A (n = 45)	5 (11)	24 (53)	16 (36)	0
Group B (n = 53)	12 (23)	28 (53)	13 (25)	0
Group C (n = 54)	9 (17)	24 (44)	20 (37)	1 (2)
TOTAL (n = 152)	26 (17)	76 (50)	49 (32)	1 (1)

Values represent number (percentage) of cases that disappeared.

Table III. Reappearance of anti-HBc in HBsAg-negative children

Vaccination group	Age (yr) at reappearance of anti-HBc 1	2	3	4	5	Total
Group A (n = 46)	0	0	1	0	2	3 (7%)
Group B (n = 55)	2	0	0	3	2	7 (13%)
Group C (n = 57)	1	1	2	0	0	4 (7%)
TOTAL (n = 158)	3	1	3	3	4	14 (9%)

Values represent number of cases that reappeared.

anti-HBc did not correlate with either different vaccination schedules or peak anti-HBs levels after vaccination.

Natural infections in HBsAg-negative children. Five HBsAg-negative children, three in group A and two in group C, were persistently positive for anti-HBc beyond 3 years of age. They were regarded as having had a natural HBV infection before 3 years of age, although the precise age at infection could not be determined. Among 158 HBsAg-negative children who had lost their anti-HBc at some time during follow-up, 14 of them (9%, or 2.0 per 100 person-years) had a reemergence of anti-HBc positivity (Table III). Acquisition of anti-HBc was distributed evenly during the 5-year follow-up period. The rate of anti-HBc reappearance was similar in the three vaccination groups (*p*

>0.05). When all cases with persistence or reappearance of anti-HBc are considered, 19 (12%) episodes of natural infection were found among 163 assessable HBsAg-negative children. All the serum alanine aminotransferase levels were within the normal range (<35 IU/L) during the study period.

Fluctuations of anti-HBs level. Some anti-HBs levels fluctuated during follow-up, to an extent that they did not conform to the general tendency of the anti-HBs titer to decline. Among 548 serum pairs taken at 1-year intervals from HBsAg-negative children, a fourfold rise of anti-HBs titer was noted in 58 (11%) and a 10-fold rise of anti-HBs was noted in 17 (3%). A rise of anti-HBs titer was to be expected in children with reappearance of anti-HBc. However, only two significant increases of anti-HBs titer were seen among 11 children who had had reappearance of anti-HBc beyond 1 year of age. One had a fourfold rise and the other had a 12-fold rise of anti-HBs. Data from three children with reappearance of anti-HBc before 1 year of age could not be analyzed because a dose of HB vaccine was given when the anti-HBc status changed.

DISCUSSION

This report demonstrates that recombinant HB vaccine is effective in protecting high-risk infants from HBV infection, both in the perinatal period and during follow-up for 5 years. Although the rate of seropositivity and the mean level of anti-HBs tended to be higher in those receiving higher doses of HB vaccine, protective efficacy within the 5-year study period was essentially the same among different vaccination groups. All the carrier children acquired HBV infection before 1 year of age, a finding similar to those of other studies.[9, 12]

In our study the prevalence of anti-HBs in HBsAg-negative children dropped from 99% to 83% during a 4-year period. The long-term anti-HBs positivity rate in vaccinated children has varied markedly among different reports, ranging from 58% to 100% in studies with a follow-up of 4 to 6 years.[10-13, 16, 17, 19-22, 26] Many factors, such as type of vaccine, vaccination schedule, ethnic group, age, and infection risk of study subjects may contribute to the differences.

It is generally agreed that the persistence of anti-HBs correlates with the initial peak antibody level,[8, 17, 20, 22, 26] which in turn correlates with the dose of vaccine administered.[8] On the other hand, the rate of decrease in anti-HBs level was independent of peak antibody level, vaccine dose, and age.[15, 19, 22] It is therefore likely that the most important factor producing different rates of persistent anti-HBs is a different peak anti-HBs level attained after vaccination. This fact may also be reflected in our results: among three vaccination groups, a higher mean titer of peak anti-HBs was associated with a higher rate of seropositivity at the end of follow-up. Coursaget et al.[15] proposed the following regression model to describe the changes of anti-HBs titer over time: $\log_e$ (anti-HBs) $= A + B_1 \times \log_e$ (peak anti-HBs after vaccination) $+ B_2 \times \log_e$ (days since booster). They demonstrated that all the values of B_2 in different studies were equal to -1. With the same regression model our data yielded the same value for B_2. These results indicate that the rate of decrease in anti-HBs titer is similar among studies and that putting peak anti-HBs levels into a regression model may make different study results comparable.

All infants were positive for anti-HBc at birth. This antibody was thought to have been acquired from their mothers, because it has been shown that injection of HB immune globulin did not affect the status of anti-HBc in subsequent follow-up.[27] Almost all maternal anti-HBc disappeared before children reached 2 years of age. Therefore a positive anti-HBc beyond 2 years of age may be regarded as evidence of a previous HBV infection. Thus 12% of the episodes of presumed natural infection were identified among HBsAg-negative children in this study. None of these episodes was accompanied by a positive HBsAg. This fact indicated that the risk of becoming a carrier after HBV infection is contracted in later life is minimal, although a few instances of new carrier status had been reported in some long-term follow-up studies.[19, 20, 22-24]

Whether these HBV infections in successfully vaccinated children of HBeAg-positive mothers were due to a breakthrough of latent perinatal infection or were acquired after infancy remains unknown. In a previous study we demonstrated that almost all children with hepatocellular carcinoma in Taiwan were seropositive for HBsAg and most such HBV infections were acquired from their carrier mothers.[28] If latent infection exists in these anti-HBc–positive vaccinated children, there will be a risk of hepatocellular carcinoma in later life. Further follow-up and application of sensitive methods to detect HBV, such as polymerase chain reaction, will be helpful to elucidate this issue.

The annual rate of HBV infection acquired in HBsAg-negative vaccinated children was 2.0%, as judged by reappearance of anti-HBc. Such an infection risk is lower than that in a previous study in Taiwan, which showed the annual incidence of HBV infection to be 5.0% in unvaccinated preschool children.[1] The latter study involved a general population, including both low-risk and high-risk children. Hepatitis B vaccination may thus prevent not only the risk of becoming a carrier but also infections manifested by anti-HBc positivity. Consistent with this finding is a report from Senegal[18] demonstrating a higher annual rate of HBV infection in unvaccinated (11.5%) than in vaccinated children (1.5%). A serologic survey done recently in Taiwan showed that the risk of HBV infection decreased among both the vaccinated and the unvaccinated children after a mass HB vaccination program.[2] This observation indicates that the risk of horizontal HBV infection may be reduced by a decrease in the number of infected persons.

These observations indicate that HB vaccination may lower the overall risk of natural infection not only because of the immunity elicited by the vaccine but also because of a reduced risk of horizontal transmission after a mass vaccination program. After infection by HBV the risk of becoming a carrier is minimal, as shown by our results and by the fact that those infected by horizontal transmission of HBV at older ages are at lower risk of becoming carriers.[1] We therefore conclude that a further booster dose of HB vaccine is not necessary before 5 years of age. On the other hand, a further decline of anti-HBs level is to be expected after 5 years of age and sexual contact is a potential route of HBV transmission.[29] If further follow-up data indicate a significant risk of HBV infection after puberty, a booster dose of HB vaccine is necessary before these children begin sexual activity.

As in other studies, some anti-HBs levels did not decrease steadily in time. In HBsAg-negative children a fourfold rise of anti-HBs titer was noted in 11% and a 10-fold rise of anti-HBs in 3%. In previous reports, such increases of anti-HBs were regarded as evidence of natural infection. However, criteria for such a "natural booster" have differed among studies.[13, 18, 20] In other instances[10, 12, 20, 27] this term was used casually, without a clear definition.

It is impossible to define a natural booster without a control group that is completely devoid of risk of HBV infection. With the present data we can state only that some natural boosters apparently did occur during follow-up. Although the exact frequency of such events could not be determined, it seemed likely that they took place in a small group of vaccinated children. Other factors might also contribute to the fluctuations of anti-HBs level, such as the natural occurrence of mild fluctuation, technical errors in assays, and nonspecific increase due to concurrent illness.[13] We agree with Coursaget et al.[15] that such a booster effect during the first 5 years may not be significant in maintaining immunity, because the rates of decrease of anti-HBs were similar in nonendemic and endemic areas.

REFERENCES

1. Beasley RP, Hwang LY, Lin CC, et al. Incidence of hepatitis B virus infections in preschool children in Taiwan. J Infect Dis 1982;146:198-204.
2. Tsen YJ, Chang MH, Hsu HY, Lee CY, Sung JL, Chen DS. Seroprevalence of hepatitis B virus infection in children in Taipei, 1989: five years after a mass hepatitis B vaccination program. J Med Virol 1991;34:96-9.
3. Stevens CF, Beasley RP, Tsui JJ, Lee WC. Vertical transmission of hepatitis B antigen in Taiwan. N Engl J Med 1975; 292:771-4.
4. Chang MH, Sung JL, Lee CY, et al. Factors affecting clearance of hepatitis B e antigen in hepatitis B surface antigen carrier children. J PEDIATR 1989;115:385-90.
5. Lee PI, Chang MH, Lee CY, et al. Changes of serum hepatitis B virus DNA and aminotransferase levels during the course of chronic hepatitis B virus infection in children. Hepatology 1990;12:657-60.
6. Beasley RP, Hwang LY, Lin CC, Chien SC. Hepatocellular carcinoma and hepatitis B virus: a prospective study of 22707 men in Taiwan. Lancet 1981;2:1129-33.
7. Lee CY, Huang LM, Chang MH, et al. The protective efficacy of recombinant hepatitis B vaccine in newborn infants of hepatitis B e antigen-positive-hepatitis B surface antigen carrier mothers. Pediatr Infect Dis J 1991;10:299-303.
8. Stevens CE, Toy PT, Taylor PE, Lee T, Yip HY. Prospects for control of hepatitis B virus infection: implications of childhood vaccination and long-term protection. Pediatrics 1992;90: 170-3.
9. Poovorawan Y, Sanpavat S, Pongpunglert W, et al. Long term efficacy of hepatitis B vaccine in infants born to hepatitis B e antigen-positive mothers. Pediatr Infect Dis J 1992;11:816-21.
10. Resti M, Azzari C, Rossi ME, Lami CA, Tucci F, Vierucci A. Five-year follow-up of vaccination against hepatitis B virus in newborns vaccinated with a reduced number of doses. Vaccine 1991;9:15-8.
11. Gonzalez ML, Gonzalez JB, Salva F, Lardinois R. A 7-year follow-up of newborns vaccinated against hepatitis B. Vaccine 1993;11:1033-6.
12. Ding L, Zhang M, Wang Y, Zhou S, Kong W, Smego RA Jr. A 9-year follow-up study of the immunogenicity and long-term efficacy of plasma-derived hepatitis B vaccine in high-risk Chinese neonates. Clin Infect Dis 1993;17:475-9.
13. Lai CL, Wong BCY, Yeoh EK, Lim WL, Chang WK, Lin HJ. Five-year follow-up of a prospective randomized trial of hepatitis B recombinant DNA yeast vaccine vs. plasma-derived vaccine in children: immunogenicity and anamnestic responses. Hepatology 1993;18:763-7.
14. Greenberg DP. Pediatric experience with recombinant hepatitis B vaccines and relevant safety and immunogenicity studies. Pediatr Infect Dis J 1993;12:438-45.
15. Coursaget P, Yvonnet B, Gilks WR, et al. Scheduling of revaccination against hepatitis B virus. Lancet 1991;337: 1180-3.
16. Moyes CD, Milne A, Waldon J. Very low dose hepatitis B vaccination in the newborn: anamnestic response to booster at four years. J Med Virol 1990;30:216-8.
17. Yvonnet B, Coursaget P, Chotard J, et al. Hepatitis B vaccine in infants from an endemic area: long-term anti-HBs persistence and revaccination. J Med Virol 1987;22:315-21.
18. Coursaget P, Yvonnet B, Chotard J, et al. Seven-year study of hepatitis B vaccine efficacy in infants from an endemic area (Senegal). Lancet 1986;2:1143-5.
19. Whittle HC, Inskip H, Hall AJ, Mendy M, Downes R, Hoare S. Vaccination against hepatitis B and protection against chronic viral carriage in the Gambia. Lancet 1991;337:747-50.
20. Hadler SC, Francis DP, Maynard JE, et al. Long-term immunogenicity and efficacy of hepatitis B vaccine in homosexual men. N Engl J Med 1986;315:209-14.
21. Delage G, Rémy-Prince S, Montplaisir S. Combined active-passive immunization against the hepatitis B virus: five-year follow-up of children born to hepatitis B surface antigen-positive mothers. Pediatr Infect Dis J 1993;12:126-30.

22. Jilg W, Schmidt M, Deinhardt F. Persistence of specific antibodies after hepatitis B vaccination. J Hepatol 1988;6:201-7.
23. Hsu NHM, Chen DS, Chuang CH, et al. Studies on the efficacy of a mass immunization program against hepatitis B in Taiwan: a three-year follow-up. In: Coursaget P, Tong MJ, eds. Progress in hepatitis B immunization. Paris: John Libby Eurotext, 1990:509-17.
24. Hwang LY, Lee CY, Beasley RP. Five-year follow-up of HBV vaccination with plasma-derived vaccine in neonates: evaluation of immunogenicity and efficacy against perinatal transmission. In: Hollinger FB, Lemon SM, Margolis HS, eds. Viral hepatitis and liver disease. Baltimore: Williams & Wilkins, 1991:759-61.
25. Beasley RP, Hwang LY, Lee GCY, et al. Prevention of perinatally transmitted hepatitis B virus infection with hepatitis B immune globulin and hepatitis B vaccine. Lancet 1983; 2:1099-102.
26. Goh KT, Tan KL, Kong KH, Oon CJ, Chan SH. Comparison of the immune response of four different dosages of a yeast-recombinant hepatitis B vaccine in Singapore children: a four-year follow-up study. Bull WHO 1992;70:233-9.
27. Heijtink RA, Weber YAM, Mazel JA. Hepatitis B vaccination in newborn babies [Letter]. Lancet 1988;1:1226.
28. Chang MH, Chen DS, Hsu HC, Hsu HY, Lee CY. Maternal transmission of hepatitis B virus in childhood hepatocellular carcinoma. Cancer 1989;64:2377-80.
29. Hou MC, Wu JC, Kuo BIT, et al. Heterosexual transmission as the most common route of acute hepatitis B virus infection among adults in Taiwan: the importance of extending vaccination to susceptible adults. J Infect Dis 1993;167:938-41.

Cerebral vein thrombosis in childhood systemic lupus erythematosus

Yosef Uziel, MD, MSc, Ronald M. Laxer, MD, FRCPC, Susan Blaser, MD, FRCPC, Maureen Andrew, MD, FRCPC, Rayfel Schneider, MBBCh, FRCPC, and Earl D. Silverman, MD, FRCPC

From the Divisions of Rheumatology, Department of Pediatrics, the Department of Diagnostic Imaging, Hospital for Sick Children and Hospital for Sick Children Research Institute, University of Toronto, Toronto, Canada, and the Department of Pediatrics, Children's Hospital, McMaster University, Hamilton, Canada

We describe three cases of cerebral vein thrombosis (CVT) in girls with systemic lupus erythematosus. Severe, persistent, unremitting headache was a common manifestation. In the first patient, although the clinical features were suggestive of CVT, the diagnosis was delayed and she had a significant cerebral infarct. In the other two patients the diagnosis was made earlier and led to more rapid treatment; the institution of early therapy may have prevented further sequelae. The CVT was diagnosed in all patients with a combination of computed tomography and magnetic resonance imaging studies without the need for angiography. All patients were treated for their underlying systemic lupus erythematosus and with anticoagulation. All are receiving long-term low doses of warfarin and have not had any recurrences. (J PEDIATR 1995;126:722-7)

Systemic lupus erythematosus is a complex multisystem autoimmune disease with multiple clinical manifestations; neuropsychiatric involvement occurs in up to 50% of children with SLE. The common clinical symptoms include seizures, organic brain syndrome, headache, functional psychosis, cranial nerve palsies, and peripheral neuropathies.[1-3] Cerebral vein thrombosis is a rare manifestation of SLE. The thrombosis may be caused by neuropsychiatric SLE or a result of antiphospholipid antibodies. Only a few cases of CVT in SLE have been described, and only two of them were in children.[4-7]

We describe three young girls with SLE who had headache and were found to have CVT. We emphasize the need for increased awareness of this entity and the importance of early diagnosis, to prevent or reduce the morbidity associated with CVT.

Supported in part from a grant from the Ontario Lupus Association and a grant from The Hospital for Sick Children Foundation.

Submitted for publication July 5, 1994; accepted Dec. 5, 1994.

Reprint requests: E. D. Silverman, MD, Division of Rheumatology, The Hospital for Sick Children, 555 University Ave., Toronto, Ontario, Canada M5G 1X8.

0022-3476/95/$3.00 + 0 **9/20/62530**

METHODS

The presence of antinuclear antibodies was assessed by indirect immunofluorescence on HEp-2 human cell lines. Anti–double-stranded DNA antibodies and anti–extractable nuclear antigen antibodies were tested by enzyme-linked immunosorbent assay and by immunoblotting.

ANA	Antinuclear antibodies
CT	Computerized tomography
CVT	Cerebral vein thrombosis
dsDNA	Double-stranded-DNA
MR	Magnetic resonance
SLE	Systemic lupus erythematosus

The dilute one-stage prothrombin time was carried out with a 1:500 dilution of thromboplastin. Results of more than 55 seconds undiluted and 57 seconds in the 1:1 mix with plasma were considered abnormal (>2 SD greater than the mean values). The dilute activated partial thromboplastin time was performed with a commercially available

Table I. Laboratory findings at time of diagnosis of CVT

	Patient 1	Patient 2	Patient 3	Normal values
Hemoglobin (gm/L)	111	83	119	
WBC (×10^9 cells/L)	9	8.3	4	
Platelet (×10^9 cells/L)	125→5	153	229	
Coombs test	–	+	–	
C3 (gm/L)	0.21	0.28	0.5	0.51-0.95
C4 (gm/L)	0.06	<0.03	0.13	0.08-0.44
ANA	1:1280	1:1280	1:640	1:40
PT (sec)	11	13.4	11.5	10.5-13.5
PTT (sec)	26	26.3	28.2	25-40
Syphilis test	UD	–	–	

PT, Prothrombin time; *PTT*, partial thromboplastin time; *UD*, unrecorded data.

reagent (Dade Actin FSL, Baxter, Miami, Fla.). Results of more than 40 seconds undiluted and 37 seconds in the 1:1 mix were considered abnormal (>2 SD greater than the mean values). The dilute viper venom time kit (American Diagnostica Inc., Wellmark Diagnostics Ltd., Guelph, Ontario, Canada) was used in the detection of the lupus anticoagulant by combining Russel viper venom, plant phospholipids, and calcium in a single reagent. The assay was run with an automated coagulation machine (ACL, Milan, Italy). Samples with positive responses were run again to confirm the findings. The detection and measurement of IgG and/or IgM anticardiolipin antibodies was performed with a commercially available enzyme-linked immunosorbent assay (Advanced Biologic Products Inc., Brampton, Ontario, Canada). Patients were considered to have positive findings only if the IgG and/or IgM assays were positive on two separate occasions.

CASE REPORTS

Case 1. A 17-year-old girl was seen because of fatigue, malar rash, mouth ulcers, pleuritic chest pain, and headache. The diagnosis of SLE was confirmed by the presence of ANA and anti-ds-DNA antibodies. Despite treatment with hydroxychloroquine and prednisone (30 mg/day), her headache persisted and was severe enough to necessitate treatment with ketorolac. Six weeks later she became confused, disoriented, and aphasic, and had generalized tonic-clonic seizures. She was transferred to the Hospital for Sick Children, Toronto. Computed tomography and magnetic resonance imaging of the brain revealed a left temporal lobe infarct with a central hemorrhage and a lateral transverse sigmoid sinus thrombosis (Fig. 1). Magnetic resonance venography confirmed sinus thrombosis but inadequately demonstrated the acute hemorrhage (Fig. 1). Laboratory findings (Table I) were consistent with active SLE. The lupus anticoagulant was present, but anticardiolipin antibodies were absent (Table II).

The patient was treated intravenously with heparin and phenobarbital, and pulse doses of methylprednisolone, 1 gm/day for 3 consecutive days, followed by high daily doses of methylprednisolone. Her course was complicated by severe thrombocytopenia (platelet count, <5 × 10^9 cells/L) that was unresponsive to intravenous immune globulin and platelet transfusions. On hospital day 6 a new intracerebral hemorrhage developed and a craniotomy was required, to evacuate a hematoma. After surgery the patient was treated intravenously with cyclophosphamide and plasmapheresis, and after a prolonged, complicated course in the hospital she was discharged with minimal neurologic deficits. She completed a 1½-year course of cyclophosphamide intravenously and daily prednisone in tapering doses. She received anticoagulation with warfarin and has had no new thrombotic events.

Case 2. An 11-year-old girl had constitutional symptoms including fever and malaise; a positive Coombs test result with a hemolytic anemia and thrombocytopenia; and the presence of ANA, anti-dsDNA antibodies, and of lupus erythematosus cells. She had relatively mild disease that was easily controlled until 2 years later, when increased fatigue, pleuritic chest pain, fever, and headache developed in association with a decrease in serum complement levels. The headache was intense and accompanied by photophobia and meningeal signs. Central nervous system infection was excluded. Unenhanced and enhanced CT of her brain revealed incomplete sagittal sinus thrombosis with congestion of the transverse sinuses. This was confirmed on MR images that also showed some focal periventricular signal abnormalities, thought to be related to small-vessel disease; no evidence of venous thrombosis–related infarction or edema was present (Fig. 2). Laboratory findings were consistent with active SLE (Table I) and documented the presence of the lupus anticoagulant and anticardiolipin antibodies (Table II). After treatment with heparin and intravenously administered methylprednisolone the headache resolved and no further thrombosis was found during a follow-up of 10 months. She has continued treatment with warfarin and tapering doses of prednisone.

Case 3. A 14-year-old girl was seen because of persistent choreiform movements of her right hand and leg, diffuse arthralgia, and secondary amenorrhea but no headache. Her medical and family histories were negative. Results of the physical examination were normal except for right-sided choreiform movements. Laboratory examinations revealed ANA at a titer of 1:320 and the presence of antiphospholipid antibodies. Findings of a brain CT scan were normal. A cerebral single-photon emission CT scan revealed minor

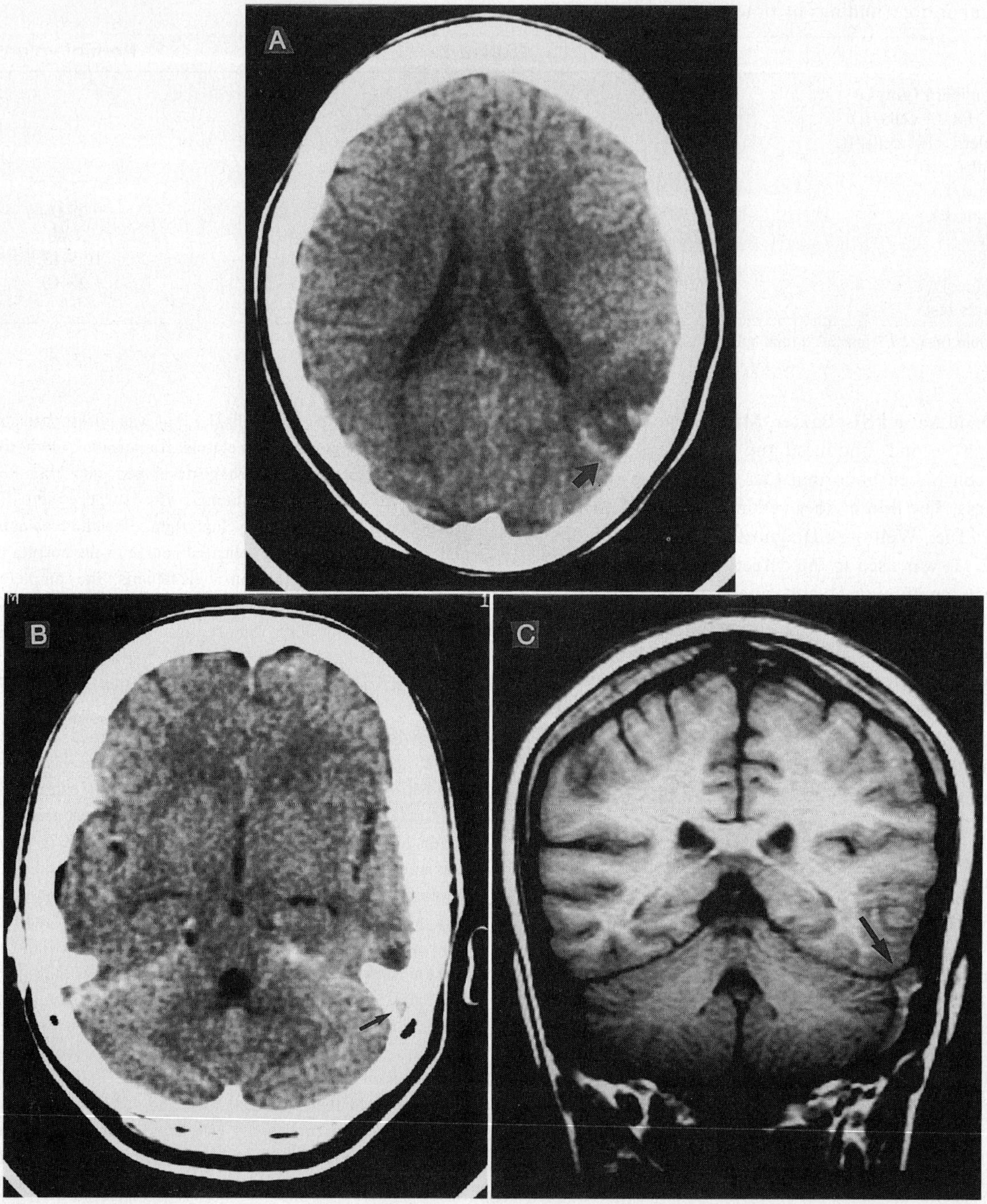

Fig. 1. A, Unenhanced axial CT scan demonstrates left temporal parenchymal hemorrhage *(arrow)*. **B,** Enhanced axial CT scan demonstrates delta sign *(arrow)* involving left sigmoid sinus. **C,** Coronal T1-weighted (600/20) MR image demonstrates isointense signal *(arrow)* of acutely thrombosed sigmoid sinus.

uptake defects in the anterior parietal lobes bilaterally, consistent with vasculitis. Low-dose aspirin therapy was commenced. Six months later her chorea worsened and was accompanied by arthralgia. Laboratory investigation now revealed the presence of anti-Sm antibodies. She had started therapy with 60 mg/day prednisone with good response of her chorea and arthralgia. After the dose of prednisone was tapered, the symptoms recurred.

She was readmitted to the hospital 3 months later because of arthralgia, myalgia, swallowing difficulties, auditory hallucinations, decreased concentration, chest pain, abdominal pain, and head-

Table II. Laboratory tests for the determination of the lupus anticoagulant and anticardiolipin antibodies

Patient No.	dPT (sec) Neat	dPT (sec) Dilute (1:1)	dAPTT (sec) Neat	dAPTT (sec) Dilute (1:1)	dVVT (sec)	dVVT (ratio of control)	ACLA (gm/L)
1	79.1	76.1	41.5	40.2	50.2	1.6	11
2	97.1	91.4	35.7	40.2	58.4	1.88	24
3	76.6	66	37.6	34.8	26.3	0.87	2.5
Control	43-55	43-57	28-40	29-37	31	1.3	0-13

ACLA, IgG anticardiolipin antibodies; *dAPTT*, dilute activated partial thromboplastin time; *dPT*, prothrombin time; *dVVT*, dilute viper venom time.

ache. The headache was daily, throbbing, and persistent. Results of the physical examination were normal. Laboratory findings were consistent with SLE (Table I) and the presence of the lupus anticoagulant. However, anticardiolipin antibodies were not detected (Table II). The cerebrospinal fluid examination yielded normal findings. Somatosensory evoked potentials, nerve conduction velocity, and electroencephalographic findings were all normal. Holter monitoring revealed sinus bradycardia (range, 36 to 56 beats/min). Contrast-enhanced CT and MR scans of the brain revealed small, nonobstructing, focal-filling defects within the left sigmoid sinus. These findings were consistent with small, nonobstructing thrombi. Cerebral angiogram revealed flow defects in the superior sagittal sinus but no definite evidence of thrombosis. She was treated with intravenous pulse doses of methylprednisone, 1 gm/day for 3 consecutive days, and heparin initially and then warfarin. After 20 months of follow-up she did not have any further thrombotic episodes and was receiving tapering doses of prednisone and daily warfarin.

DISCUSSION

Neuropsychologic involvement occurs in approximately 50% of children with SLE. Arterial and venous thrombosis may occur as a result of active CNS vasculitis, or as the result of the lupus anticoagulant or antiphospholipid antibodies. Cerebral vein thrombosis, although rare, should be considered in patients with SLE and CNS involvement, severe or unremitting headache, and/or antiphospholipid antibodies. Our first patient had a headache for several weeks before examination. Our two other patients had early radiologic evaluation because of their clinical symptoms and were found to have early, incomplete CVT before neurologic deficits developed. For maintenance all patients have received low-dose oral anticoagulation and treatment of their SLE and have had no further thrombotic events during follow-up periods of 10 to 18 months.

Tension or vascular headaches occur in 25% of patients with SLE and are the most common type of headache in these patients.[8] Migraine headache may also occur and may be a sign of central nervous system involvement. These headaches are usually severe and may require an increase in treatment, but each episode lasts only hours.[9] The clinical signs and symptoms of CVT may be variable. Headache is the main early symptom, but increased intracranial pressure, papilledema, seizures, focal neurologic deficits such as hemiparesis, and altered mental status leading to coma and death are reported. The clinical findings vary depending on the veins or sinuses obstructed, and the presence or absence of alternative drainage pathways. Associated seizures, papilledema, and hemiparesis are supportive of the diagnosis of CVT, but severe headache alone may be the earliest feature. Severe, persistent, throbbing, unremitting headache, unresponsive to analgesic drugs, should raise the index of suspicion to the possibility of CVT and in our opinion is an indication for radiologic evaluation.

The pathogenesis of CVT in SLE is likely related to the presence of antiphospholipid antibodies, which increase the risk of thrombosis.[10] The anti-phospholipid antibody syndrome is associated with arterial or venous thrombotic events, thrombocytopenia, and the presence of anti-phospholipid antibodies. It may occur as an isolated event and cause CVT,[11] but in children it is more commonly caused by SLE. Platelets, tissue factors, protein C, thrombomodulin, and endothelial cell antigens are all potential targets for anti-phospholipid antibodies. Thrombotic events, arterial or venous, occurred in 9% of children with SLE in one series[12] and may be the initial sign. It is possible that multiple vascular injuries and active SLE are risk factors in addition to the presence of antiphospholipid antibodies for the development of a thrombotic event.[13]

The confirmation of CVT is by radiologic studies; CT scanning is the usual initial investigation for patients with severe, unremitting, acute headache because acute cerebral hemorrhage may be missed by MR imaging.[14] Small ventricles associated with diffuse swelling may be seen, although the parenchymal attenuation may be normal and the ventricles normally sized or large. Findings suggestive of CVT include the "cord" or "dense triangle" signs, which refer to the dense cortical veins or thrombosed sinuses seen on unenhanced CT in the presence of acutely congealed blood.[15-17] The "delta" or "empty triangle" signs may be seen and refer to the opacification of collateral veins in the wall of the sinus contrasting with the nonopacified thrombus within the sinus.[17, 18] A normal CT scan finding does not exclude CVT, particularly if coronal imaging or wide windows of the enhanced study have not been obtained. These

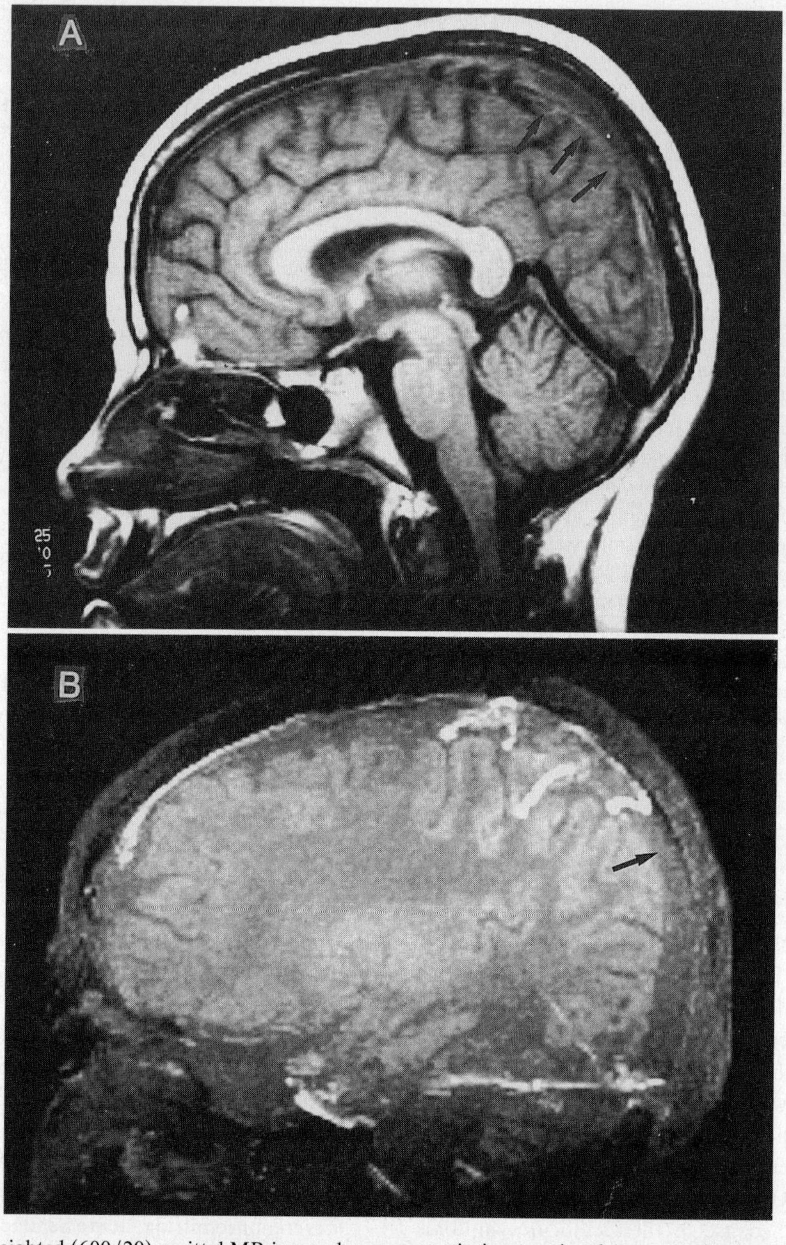

Fig. 2. A, T1-weighted (600/20) sagittal MR image demonstrates isointense signal *(arrows)* of acutely thrombosed portion of superior sagittal sinus. **B,** Sagittal MR venogram confirms finding in **A.** Note dilated and congealed cortical veins.

views are not routinely obtained unless the diagnosis of CVT has been considered before the study. Cerebral angiography was formerly considered to be the standard in the diagnosis of CVT and may still be required in some cases.[19] However, MR imaging and MR venogram are now considered to be the preferred diagnostic evaluations because of their ability to visualize the thrombus directly and because of their noninvasive nature.[20]

A normal prothrombin time, partial thromboplastin time, negative syphilis test result, and absence of anticardiolipin antibodies as screening test results do not exclude the presence of anti-phospholipid antibodies, as demonstrated in our patients. When the problem is suspected, special tests for the lupus anti-coagulant should be done.[21] All three of our patients had the lupus anticoagulant, but anticardiolipin antibodies were present in only one. Published evidence favors anticoagulation therapy with heparin for the acute stage of CVT, even when intracerebral hemorrhage is present.[22] In a prospective study patients who were treated with heparin had better neurologic outcome than in the control patients.[22] Rarely, local fibrinolytic therapy has been used.[23] The long-term management of CVT is unclear. However, we favor long-term anticoagulation therapy with warfarin to keep the international normalized ratio between 2 and 3 in the acute phase (first 3 months), followed by lower doses of warfarin to keep the international normalized ratio between 1.5 and 2.0, in the hope of preventing further thrombotic events. In addition, we advocate therapy for the underlying SLE with corticosteroids and immunosuppressive therapy as necessary.

Although intracranial sinus thrombosis is rare as compared with other thrombotic events in SLE, it may occur and progress to the cerebral veins, leading to significant neurologic morbidity or death. Increase in the suspicion index for the unusual "lupus headache" should lead to radiologic investigations. Early diagnosis and more intensive therapy for SLE, and particularly anticoagulation therapy, may prevent associated complications of CVT.

REFERENCES

1. Lang BA, Silverman ED. A clinical overview of systemic lupus erythematosus in childhood. Pediatr Rev 1993;14:194-201.
2. Bluestein HG. Neuropsychiatric manifestations of systemic lupus erythematosus. N Engl J Med 1987;317:309-10.
3. Yancey CL, Doughty RA, Arthreya BA. Central nervous system involvement in childhood systemic lupus erythematosus. Arthritis Rheum 1981;24:1385-95.
4. Vidailket M, Piette JC, Wechsler B, Bousser MG, Brunet P. Cerebral venous thrombosis in systemic lupus erythematosus. Stroke 1990;21:1226-31.
5. Kaplan RE, Springate JE, Feld LG, Cohen MF. Pseudo tumor cerebri associated with cerebral venous sinus thrombosis, internal jugular vein thrombosis, and SLE. J PEDIATR 1985;107:266-8.
6. Parnass SM, Goodwin JA, Patel DV, Levinson DJ, Rheinhard JD. Dural sinus thrombosis: a mechanism for pseudotumor cerebri in systemic lupus erythematosus. J Rheumatol 1987;14:152-5.
7. Li EK, Kay RL, Cohen MG. Cerebral venous thrombosis in systemic lupus erythematosus. Stroke 1991;22:281-3.
8. Atkinson RA, Affenzeller O. Headache in small vessel disease of the brain: a study of patients with systemic lupus erythematosus. Headache 1975;15:198-201.
9. Brandt KD, Lessell S. Migrainous phenomena in systemic lupus erythematosus. Arthritis Rheum 1978;21:7-16.
10. Petri M, Hochberg M, Hellman D, et al. Incidence of and predictors of thrombonic events in systemic lupus erythemotous (SLE): a five year prospective study [Abstract]. Arthritis Rheum 1991;34:S44.
11. Levine SR, Kieran S, Puzio K, Feit H, Patel SC, Welch KM. Cerebral venous thrombosis with lupus anticoagulants: report of two cases. Stroke 1987;18:801-4.
12. Montes de Oca MA, Babron MC, Bletry O, et al. Thrombosis in systemic lupus erythematosus: a French collaborative study. Arch Dis Child 1991;66:713-7.
13. Petri M. The clinical syndrome associated with antiphospholipid antibodies. J Rheumatol 1992;19:505-7.
14. Justich E, Lammer J, Fritsch G, Beitzke A, Walter GF. CT diagnosis of thrombosis of dural sinuses in childhood. Eur J Radiol 1984;4:294-5.
15. Rao KCVG, Knipp HC, Wagner EJ. CT findings in cerebral sinus and venous thrombosis. Radiology 1981;140:391-8.
16. Patronas NJ, Duda EE, Mirfakhraee M, Wollmann RL. Superior sagittal sinus thrombosis diagnosed by computed tomography. Surg Neurol 1981;15:11-4.
17. Buonanno F, Moody DM, Ball MR, Laster DW. Computed cranial tomographic findings in cerebral sino-venous occlusion. J Comput Assist Tomogr 1978;2:281-90.
18. Virapongse C, Cazenave C, Quisling R, Sarwar M, Hunter S. The empty delta sign: frequency and significance in 76 cases of dural sinus thrombosis. Radiology 1987;162:779-85.
19. Vines FS, Davis DO. Clinical radiological correlation in cerebral venous occlusive disease. Radiology 1971;98:9-22.
20. Hulcelle PJ, Dooms GC, Mathurin P, Cornelis G. MRI assessment of unsuspected dural sinus thrombosis. Neuroradiology 1989;31:217-21.
21. NcNeil HP, Chesterman CN, Krillis SA. Anticardiolipin antibodies and lupus anticoagulants comprise separate antibody subgroups with different phospholipid binding characteristics. Br J Haematol 1989;73:506-13.
22. Einhäupl KM, Villringer A, Meister W, et al. Heparin treatment in sinus venous thrombosis. Lancet 1991;338:597-600.
23. Persson L, Lilja A. Extensive dural sinus thrombosis treated by surgical removal and local streptokinase infusion. Neurosurgery 1990;26:117-21.

Low-density lipoprotein apheresis as long-term treatment for children with homozygous familial hypercholesterolemia

R. Jeff Zwiener, MD, Ricardo Uauy, MD, PhD,[a] Mary L. Petruska, RN, and Beverley A. Huet, MS

From the Department of Pediatrics and The General Clinical Research Center, The University of Texas Southwestern Medical Center, and Children's Medical Center of Dallas

***Objective*: To determine the safety and efficacy of long-term dextran sulfate–affinity column low-density lipoprotein (LDL) apheresis for the treatment of children with receptor-negative homozygous familial hypercholesterolemia (HFH).**
***Study design:* Two children with HFH (pretreatment cholesterol levels 22.1 to 24.7 mmol/L (ranges 850 to 950 mg/dl) began LDL apheresis treatments at ages 7 and 10 years, respectively. The LDL apheresis treatment interval was generally either 7 or 14 days; for the last 2 years of the study the treatment interval was 7 days. The patients had 167 and 188 LDL apheresis procedures during 64 and 70 months, respectively.**
***Results*: Individual procedures decreased total blood cholesterol levels by 63% to 68%. When the treatment interval was 7 days, the patients' time-averaged mean total cholesterol levels decreased to 7.3 ± 0.65 mmol/L (280 ± 25 mg/dl) and 6.4 ± 0.55 mmol/L (247 ± 22 mg/dl), respectively. Both children remained clinically well with normal growth and development. There was significant regression of xanthomas in both patients. The older patient required heart surgery for preexisting aortic stenosis and coronary ostial stenosis, but neither patient had progression of hypercholesterolemia-related cardiovascular disease. With the exception of iron (deficiency in patient 1), there was no evidence of depletion of serum components. Adverse reactions to LDL apheresis were rare and never severe.**
***Conclusions*: Dextran sulfate–affinity column LDL apheresis is effective long-term treatment for children with receptor-negative HFH. (J PEDIATR 1995;126:728-35)**

Supported by U.S. Public Health Service grant M01-RR00633 and Kaneka Corp., Osaka, Japan.

Submitted for publication May 4, 1994; accepted Dec. 5, 1994.

Reprint requests: R. Jeff Zwiener, MD, Division of Pediatric Gastroenterology and Nutrition, Department of Pediatrics, University of Texas Southwestern Medical Center, 5323 Harry Hines Blvd., Dallas, TX 75235-9063.

[a]Now Professor of Pediatrics, Instituto de Nutricion y Tecnologia de los Alimentos, Universidad de Chile, Santiago.

0022-3476/95/$3.00 + 0 **9/20/62528**

Children with homozygous familial hypercholesterolemia have extreme hypercholesterolemia caused principally by the accumulation of low-density lipoprotein in blood. This rare autosomal recessive disease stems from a variety of

HDL	High-density lipoprotein
HFH	Homozygous familial hypercholesterolemia
LDL	Low-density lipoprotein
VLDL	Very low density lipoprotein

mutations in the LDL-receptor gene, resulting in a marked decrease or absence of receptor activity. Early in the patient's childhood prominent xanthomas and symptomatic coronary heart disease develop. Death from premature myocardial infarction usually occurs before age 20 years.[1] The receptor-negative form of HFH is unresponsive or minimally responsive to cholesterol-lowering therapies such as a low-fat diet, drugs,[2] ileal bypass surgery, biliary diversion, and portacaval shunting. Serial plasma exchange (plasmapheresis) has been used successfully in prolonging the lives of patients with HFH, but the frequency of treatment and therefore the effectiveness are limited because of the nonspecific depletion of all plasma components.[3, 4] Liver-heart transplantation has effected the long-term survival of one child, but eventually long-term transplant-related complications led to death.[5]

LDL apheresis selectively removes the predominant cholesterol-containing particles from blood. The patient's plasma is filtered through an affinity column loaded with dextran sulfate covalently bound to a cellulose matrix.[6] This material has a high affinity and binding capacity for apolipoprotein B–containing lipoproteins and therefore selectively removes LDL and very low density lipoprotein from the plasma.[7] We have previously reported the safety and efficacy of this technique in a pilot study for acutely lowering blood cholesterol levels.[8] We now report its long-term use as the primary therapy for two children with severe HFH.

METHODS

Subjects. Two children, a sister and brother (patients 1 and 2, respectively) with severe HFH, were studied in the Pediatric Clinical Research Center at Children's Medical Center of Dallas. At the time of entry into the study the children were 7 and 10 years old, respectively. Both children had extreme hypercholesterolemia; the average total cholesterol level was 24.7 mmol/L (950 mg/dl) for patient 1 and 22.1 mmol/L (850 mg/dL) for patient 2. The LDL-receptor activity in skin fibroblasts and blood lymphocytes was less than 1% of normal values. The parents and a younger sibling had cholesterol levels consistent with heterozygous familial hypercholesterolemia. Both children had manifestations of systemic cholesterol deposition; there were multiple large cutaneous xanthomas and advanced atherosclerotic disease as evidenced by aortic ejection murmurs and carotid bruits. Patient 2 had decreased carotid artery blood flow as measured by Doppler ultrasound blood flow studies. Both patients had normal cardiac perfusion by thallium stress test function, and neither patient had signs or symptoms of myocardial ischemia. They both failed to respond to dietary therapy and to the 3-hydroxy-3-methylglutaryl coenzyme A reductase inhibitor lovastatin.[2] Neither child required pharmacologic agents for heart disease.

Low-density lipoprotein apheresis. Two LDL apheresis systems were used: a single-column system (Liposorber LA-40, Kaneka Corp., Osaka, Japan) and a more sophisticated regenerating dual-column system (Liposorber LA-15, Kaneka Corp.). The clinical use of both systems has been previously described in detail.[8, 9] The recently developed dual-column system replaced the single-column system early in the study because of two major advantages: (1) the extracorporeal volume is smaller (the column volume is 150 ml vs 400 ml) and (2) column saturation does not limit cholesterol removal because the dual columns alternate as the adsorption column and the regenerating column. The goal for each procedure was to treat 1½ to 2 blood volumes as determined by the following equation: Weight in Kilograms ×80 ml/kg × 2. The columns were discarded after each treatment. The duration of most procedures was 2 to 3 hours.

Low-density lipoprotein–receptor activity determinations. The assays for skin fibroblast and blood lymphocyte LDL-receptor activity were done by previously described methods.[10, 11]

Laboratory determinations. With standard techniques, all lipid and lipoprotein determinations were performed by Medical Research Laboratories, Cincinnati, Ohio, which maintained Centers for Disease Control–National Heart, Lung, and Blood Institute part III standardization.[12-15] Apolipoproteins A1, AII, B, and E, and lipoprotein (a), were quantified with enzyme-linked immunosorbent assays.[16] All other laboratory measurements were also performed by Medical Research Laboratories with standard techniques.

Experimental design. The study was approved by the institutional review board of the University of Texas Southwestern Medical Center. Informed written consent was obtained from the parents and children. The Liposorber LA-40 and LA-15 systems were granted investigational device exemption status by the Food and Drug Administration. The regular home diet was maintained throughout the study period. A multivitamin preparation and iron supplement were provided empirically to replace losses resulting from blood drawing and lipid removal.

The LDL apheresis treatment interval with the dual-column system (LA-15) varied from 1 to 4 weeks. When the asymptomatic perfusion abnormalities were seen on thallium scan in patient 2 (the older patient), the interval was shortened to 1 week so that for the last 24 months of the data collection period, LDL apheresis was consistently done weekly.

Blood lipids (total cholesterol; LDL, high-density lipoprotein, and VLDL cholesterol; and triglycerides) were measured before and after LDL apheresis with every procedure. Complete blood cell count and blood chemistry studies (sodium, potassium, chloride, calcium, phosphorus, total protein, albumin, total bilirubin, alanine aminotransferase, aspartate aminotransferase, alkaline phosphatase, creatine phosphokinase, urea nitrogen, creatinine, uric acid, and glucose) were measured before and after LDL apheresis with the first few LDL apheresis procedures. However, when it became apparent that no clinically relevant short-term changes in these values occurred with LDL apheresis, only measurements before LDL apheresis were done and the measurement interval was increased to 6 weeks and then later to 12 weeks. Laboratory studies before and after LDL apheresis were obtained 5 minutes before the start of apheresis and 5 minutes after completion of the procedure. Levels of apolipoproteins (AI, AII, B, E), lipoprotein (a), immunoglobulins (IgA, IgG, IgM), vitamin E, vitamin A, and folate were measured before LDL apheresis at intervals ranging from 4 to 16 weeks. Complement (C3a, C4a, and C5a) was measured before and after LDL apheresis for the first three LA-15 LDL apheresis procedures. Exercise thallium scans, Doppler carotid ultrasound studies, and echocardiograms were done at the outset of the study and then prospectively throughout the study.

Statistical methods. The time-averaged mean lipid value was defined as the mean of the means of the post–LDL apheresis values and the subsequent pre–LDL apheresis values. The 7- and 14-day treatment interval periods were defined when LDL apheresis was performed every 6 to 8 days or every 13 to 15 days, respectively. Lipid values were compared between the 7- and 14-day treatment interval periods for each patient, with the Wilcoxon rank-sum test. The Wilcoxon signed-rank test was used to compare the apolipoprotein and lipoprotein (a) levels before and after LDL apheresis. Linear regression models were constructed to assess the rebound of blood lipid levels after LDL apheresis. Pearson or Spearman correlation coefficients were used to assess the trend over time with regard to serum chemistry and vitamin levels. For all analyses a two-tailed p value of 0.05 was considered statistically significant. No adjustment for multiple testing was used. A change of 20% or greater was considered biologically significant. Clinically relevant changes were those outside the accepted normal laboratory values for age and sex. Data management and statistical analysis were performed with CLINFO and BMDP software.

RESULTS

The LDL apheresis treatments began for patient 1 on Feb. 1, 1988 (at age 7.5 years), and for patient 2 on Aug. 19, 1987 (at age 10.2 years). The data in this report were collected from these dates through June 15, 1993, when the children were 12.8 and 16 years of age, respectively. At the time of this evaluation, patient 1 had undergone 167 LDL apheresis procedures in 64 months (26 LA-40 procedures and 141 LA-15 procedures) and patient 2 had undergone 188 LDL apheresis procedures in 70 months (38 LA-40 procedures and 150 LA-15 procedures).

Lipids and apolipoproteins. Table I summarizes the changes in blood lipid levels with LDL apheresis. Only data obtained with the dual-column system (LA-15) are shown. To demonstrate the effect of varying the interval between LDL apheresis treatments, the data are partitioned into two periods: the 14-day treatment interval period and the 7-day treatment interval period. In the short term LDL apheresis markedly reduced total blood cholesterol levels; the mean decrease with each treatment was 63% to 68%. Although the treatment interval (7 vs 14 days) did not affect the percentage magnitude of this short-term decrease, the 7-day interval achieved significantly lower mean pre–LDL apheresis levels (36% lower) and mean post–LDL apheresis levels (38% to 43% lower) and hence a significantly lower (36% to 38% lower) time-averaged mean total cholesterol level. Total cholesterol levels, when the mean untreated baseline value was compared with the time-averaged means, decreased by 53.5% during the 14-day treatment interval period and by 71% during the 7-day treatment interval period. The reduction in total cholesterol levels was due mainly to the removal of LDL; the mean decrease in LDL levels with each treatment was 69% to 77%. As for the changes in total cholesterol level, the 7-day interval achieved a 41% lower time-averaged mean LDL for both patients. As expected, the apolipoprotein B–containing VLDL decreased in parallel with the LDL. In contrast, HDL decreased by only 15% to 24% on average. Triglyceride values decreased with LDL apheresis by 17% to 42% in the short term.

The long-term effect of LDL apheresis on total cholesterol levels is graphically depicted in Fig. 1. The time-averaged mean total cholesterol decreased more during the 7-day treatment interval period than during the 14-day treatment interval period.

The changes in apolipoproteins and lipoprotein (a) are shown in Table II. Low-density lipoprotein apheresis caused a 60% to 70% decrease in apolipoprotein B, apolipoprotein E, and lipoprotein (a), and only a 25% to 28% decrease in apolipoprotein A-I and apolipoprotein A-II.

Cholesterol reaccumulated in serum after LDL apheresis. The instantaneous rates of increase of the serum total cholesterol levels ranged from 1.8 mmol/L/day (69.5 mg/dl per day) at baseline to 0.15 mmol/L per day (6.1 mg/dl per day) on day 7. Low-density lipoprotein cholesterol reaccumulated at a similar rate.

Vitamin levels. Blood levels of vitamins E and A decreased in the short term by 70% to 82% with LDL apheresis, and these levels returned to baseline levels within 24 hours (data not shown). Despite the passive removal of these fat-soluble vitamins as components of the LDL particle, there was no laboratory or physical evidence for vitamin E or A de-

Table I. Changes in blood lipid levels with LDL apheresis in two children with receptor-negative HFH

	LDL apheresis treatment interval				7-day vs 14-day interval			
	7 days		14 days		Change (%)		p*	
Variable	Patient 1	Patient 2	Patient 1	Patient 2	Patient 1	Patient 2	Patient 1	Patient 2
Total cholesterol (mg/dl)	n = 68	n = 88	n = 27	n = 27				
Before LDL apheresis	420 ± 34	370 ± 29	661 ± 48	580 ± 33	−36	−36	<0.001	<0.001
After LDL apheresis	133 ± 13	121 ± 16	216 ± 54	214 ± 34	−38	−43	<0.001	<0.001
Time-averaged mean†	280 ± 25	247 ± 22	439 ± 40	396 ± 27	−36	−38	<0.001	<0.001
LDL cholesterol (mg/dl)	n = 68	n = 88	n = 27	n = 27				
Before LDL apheresis	352 ± 28	308 ± 27	586 ± 46	499 ± 33	−40	−38	<0.001	<0.001
After LDL apheresis	81 ± 13	72 ± 12	163 ± 52	156 ± 31	−50	−54	<0.001	<0.001
Time-averaged mean	221 ± 23	192 ± 20	376 ± 38	328 ± 27	−41	−41	<0.001	<0.001
VLDL cholesterol (mg/dl)	n = 5	n = 5	n = 10	n = 9				
Before LDL apheresis	17 ± 8	28 ± 13	32 ± 16	43 ± 21	−47	−35	0.031	0.205
After LDL apheresis	7 ± 1	9 ± 5	10 ± 8	11 ± 5	−30	−18	0.616	0.316
HDL cholesterol (mg/dl)	n = 68	n = 88	n = 27	n = 28				
Before LDL apheresis	48 ± 9	39 ± 6	53 ± 6	42 ± 5	−9	−7	0.055	0.036
After LDL apheresis	36 ± 8	32 ± 6	41 ± 4	35 ± 3	−12	−9	0.027	0.015
Time-averaged mean	42 ± 8	35 ± 5	46 ± 5	38 ± 3	−9	−8	0.009	0.034
Triglycerides (mg/dl)	n = 68	n = 88	n = 27	n = 28				
Before LDL apheresis	96 ± 39	116 ± 44	112 ± 49	207 ± 81	−14	−44	0.118	<0.001
After LDL apheresis	76 ± 33	84 ± 39	61 ± 28	117 ± 58	25	−28	0.023	0.002
Time-averaged mean	86 ± 27	100 ± 30	84 ± 30	158 ± 46	2	−37	0.575	<0.001

Blood lipid values expressed as mean ± SD. To convert total, LDL, VLDL, and HDL cholesterol to millimoles per liter, multiply by 0.02586. To convert triglycerides to millimoles per liter, multiply by 0.01129.
*Difference between 7-day and 14-day treatment interval by Wilcoxon rank-sum test.
†Mean of the means of the post–LDL apheresis and the subsequent pre–LDL-apheresis values.

Table II. Changes in blood apolipoprotein and lipoprotein (a) levels with LDL apheresis in two children

	Before LDL-apheresis		After LDL apheresis			
	No. of measurements	Mean ± SD (mg/dl)	No. of measurements	Mean ± SD (mg/dl)	Change (%)	p*
Patient 1						
Apolipoprotein A-1	21	119.8 ± 14.1	21	86.4 ± 12.5	−27.9	<0.001
Apolipoprotein A-II	21	58.2 ± 8.9	21	40.0 ± 6.4	−31.3	<0.001
Apolipoprotein B	21	330.9 ± 85.0	21	101.8 ± 47.5	−69.2	<0.001
Apolipoprotein E	21	14.2 ± 4.1	21	5.5 ± 2.6	−61.3	<0.001
Lipoprotein (a)	21	7.3 ± 2.6	20	2.5 ± 1.0	−65.8	<0.001
Patient 2						
Apolipoprotein A-I	21	98.9 ± 14.4	20	76.9 ± 13.8	−22.2	<0.01
Apolipoprotein A-II	21	50.0 ± 5.5	20	37.4 ± 6.2	−25.2	<0.001
Apolipoprotein B	21	304.2 ± 68.7	20	92.2 ± 30.4	−69.7	<0.001
Apolipoprotein E	21	14.0 ± 3.4	20	5.2 ± 2.0	−62.9	<0.001
Lipoprotein (a)	21	2.8 ± 0.5	18	1.1 ± 0.2	−60.7	<0.001

The data are from both patients 1 and 2 with the dual-column (LA-15) system. Data from the 7-day and 14-day treatment intervals are combined.
*Wilcoxon signed-rank test.

ficiency for the study period. When data from both patients were combined, the mean pre–LDL apheresis blood level of vitamin E (n = 26) was 28.8 ± 8.8 μmol/L (12.4 ± 3.8 mg/L; normal, 5 to 20 mg/L) and of vitamin A (n = 26) was 1.65 ± 0.4 μmol/L was (47.1 ± 11.5 μg/dl; normal, 25 to 48 μg/dl). No values were less than the lower limits of normal, and there was no decline in vitamin E and A blood levels before LDL apheresis over time. At the end of the study period vitamin E status as gauged by the ratio of vitamin E to total lipid was normal (1.0 to 1.2 mg vitamin E per gram of total lipids before LDL apheresis).[17] Vitamin D levels were not monitored, but there was no evidence of

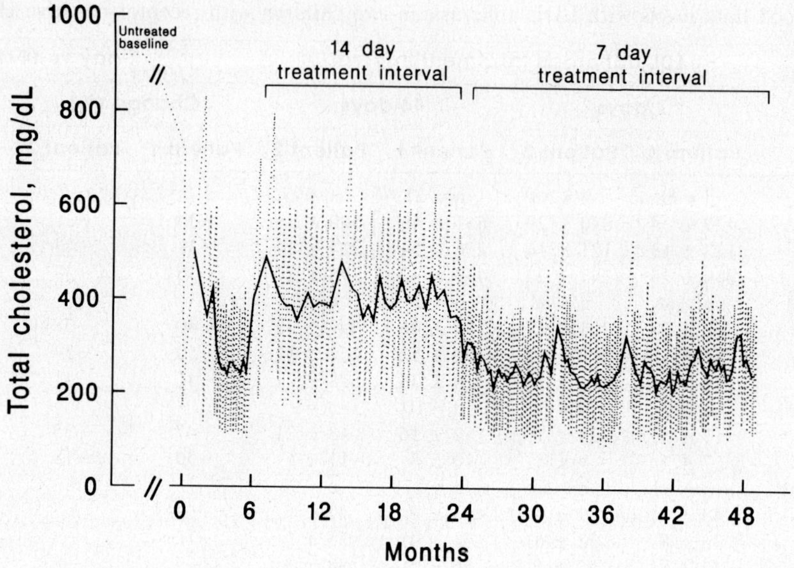

Fig. 1. Long-term effects of LDL apheresis on total cholesterol levels. Peaks are levels before LDL apheresis, and troughs are levels after LDL apheresis. Line is drawn through points on rebound curves halfway between post–LDL apheresis value and subsequent pre–LDL apheresis value. Seven-day treatment interval period (88 treatments in 27 months; mean treatment interval, 7.0 ± 0.3 days), when compared with 14-day treatment interval period (28 treatments for 17 months; mean treatment interval, 14 ± 0.6 days), markedly decreases levels before and after LDL apheresis, and time-averaged mean cholesterol level. Data shown are from patient 2, with use of dual-column system (LA-15). Patient 1 (data not shown) responded in similar fashion.

vitamin D deficiency, no physical or radiologic evidence of rickets, and no alteration in calcium or phosphorus metabolism.

The water-soluble vitamins folate and vitamin B_{12} were not removed by LDL apheresis (data not shown) For the study period there was no decrease in blood folate or vitamin B_{12} levels, before LDL apheresis, indicating that depletion did not occur over time.*

Hematologic and coagulation studies. There were transient statistically significant but clinically irrelevant changes in the hematologic indices (hematocrit, platelet count, prothrombin time, and partial thromboplastin time) before and after LDL apheresis.* For the most part, all short-term changes in the hematologic indices corrected to baseline by the time of the next LDL apheresis treatment. Iron deficiency anemia eventually occurred in patient 1, who required oral iron supplementation throughout the study period.

Chemistry and immunoglobulin values. There were transient but clinically irrelevant changes in the serum chemistry values with LDL apheresis. For the duration of the study no depletion or accumulation of any of the serum chemistry or immunoglobulin values occurred. Renal or hepatic dysfunction was never evident.*

Complement activity. There was evidence for C3 activation during five of six procedures as indicated by a marked increase (300% to 2700%) in post–LDL apheresis C3a levels. In contrast, C4a levels decreased 20% to 100% with LDL apheresis. For C5a levels no consistent pattern was noted; some levels decreased and others increased.* No adverse effects were noted in relation to these observed short-term changes in complement induced by LDL apheresis.

Cardiovascular disease. The children never had signs or symptoms suggestive of myocardial ischemia. In patient 2, however, a possible inferolateral perfusion defect developed on thallium stress test at age 12.5 years. By age 13.8 years, although still asymptomatic, he had a definite inferoposterior perfusion abnormality during exercise. Cardiac catheterization showed severe aortic stenosis with a peak-to-peak gradient of 63 mm Hg. There was also 90% stenosis of the right coronary ostium and 50% stenosis of the left coronary ostium. Despite these lesions the coronary arteries had normal caliber with no evidence of atheroma distal to the ostia. At age 14 years he had a pericardial patch aortoplasty to relieve supravalvular aortic stenosis and right coronary artery ostial stenosis. Intraoperative palpation of the coronary arteries distal to the ostia confirmed the lack of atheroma. The aortic biopsy showed marked intimal thickening caused by myointimal hyperplasia and dense fibroplasia. This intimal plaque had a necrotic center with atheromatous material and dystrophic calcification. After surgery the

*Exact values available on request from the authors.

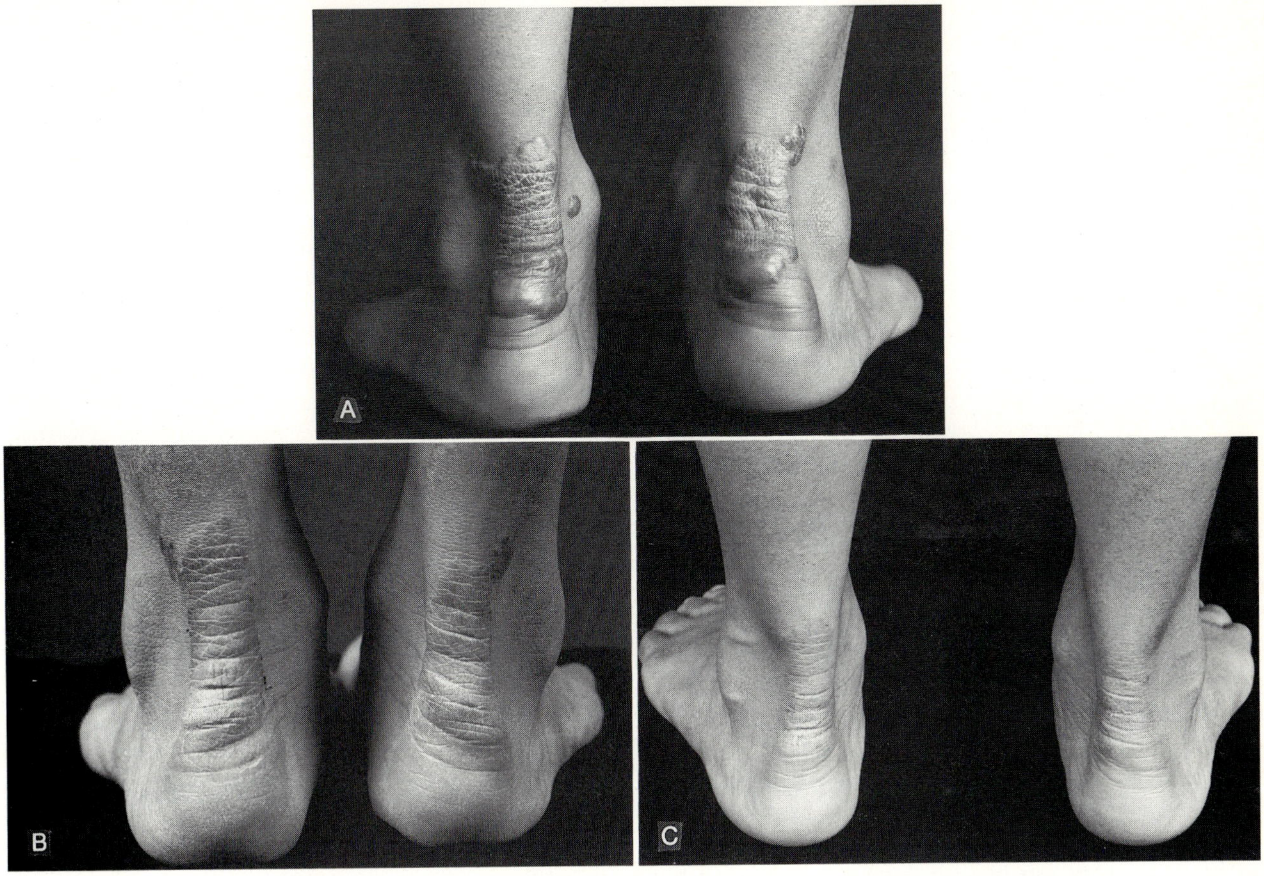

Fig. 2. Patient 1. Regression of xanthomas in HFH treated with LDL apheresis. There was marked regression of xanthomas with serial LDL apheresis during study. Patient before start of LDL apheresis treatments (age 7 years) (**A**), after 1 year of LDL apheresis treatments (age 8 years) (**B**), and after 3 years of LDL apheresis treatments (age 10 years) (**C**). Patient 2 had similar response.

results of the thallium stress test normalized. Patient 1 continued to have a normal thallium stress test result.

Serial echocardiograms showed gradually worsening aortic stenosis in both patients. In patient 2 the estimated peak-to-peak aortic valve gradient increased from 17 to 65 mm Hg during the course of the study. Both patients had gradually worsening left ventricular hypertrophy (mild to moderate by end of study) and aortic insufficiency (mild for patient 1, moderate for patient 2). Nevertheless, both children continued to have normal ventricular size and function.

There was no progression in either patient of carotid stenosis as measured by blood flow velocity with Doppler ultrasonography; loss of diameter was never more than 20%.

Xanthomas. The children had marked regression of xanthomas, as shown in Fig. 2. After 3 years of LDL apheresis, only residual hyperpigmented cutaneous scars were present at the previous locations of the xanthomas.

Growth and development. Growth and development during the study period were normal. Both children progressed normally through puberty to Tanner stage 4 or 5. Patient 1, the 13-year-old girl, had regular menses during the last year of the study. Bone age, as determined radiographically at the end of the study period, was appropriate for chronologic age.

Adverse reactions and complications. Adverse reactions to LDL apheresis included occasional mild abdominal cramps. Patient 1 had urticaria during three procedures in the first year; there has been no recurrence of the rash. Of the 355 LDL apheresis procedures started, only 12 were discontinued; the rest were completed successfully. Patient 1 had three vasovagal reactions with bradycardia, hypotension, and diaphoresis, which responded to cessation of LDL apheresis and infusions of fluid. Future problems were avoided by priming the system with 5% albumin. Six procedures were discontinued for problems with intravenous access, one because of an uncooperative patient, one because of a minor system malfunction, and one because of a temporary electrical power interruption. We consistently achieved, with the exceptions noted previously, adequate intravenous access from the antecubital veins.

Cost. We estimate the cost of weekly LDL apheresis treatments to be $25,000 to $50,000 per year.

DISCUSSION

This study establishes dextran sulfate–affinity column LDL apheresis as a safe and effective long-term treatment of receptor-negative HFH in children as young as 7 years. Other investigators have used this therapy for children, but no study has documented successful treatment for such a prolonged period.[3, 6, 9, 18, 19] Most patients of this age with receptor-negative HFH have either died, have severe symptomatic coronary artery disease, or have undergone liver transplantation.[20] Additional objective observations that support the efficacy of LDL apheresis include the regression of xanthomas, the lack of coronary atherosclerosis distal to the coronary ostia, and the lack of progression of carotid arterial stenosis.

Both children had progression of their cardiovascular disease, but we believe that this does not indicate failure of long-term LDL apheresis treatment. Rather, preexisting cardiovascular lesions progressed independent of hypercholesterolemia. Supravalvular aortic stenosis and coronary artery ostial stenosis have been described in HFH.[21-25] We speculate that the atheromas in the thoracic aorta become fibrosed and calcified; thus, despite lipid depletion with serial LDL apheresis, the potential for normal aortic root growth is impaired by these static restrictive lesions. Worsening of the aortic pressure gradient occurs in time, with normal growth and increasing cardiac output, whereas coronary artery ostial stenosis develops as a result of local aortic fibrosis. In addition, atheroma formation on the leaflets results in scarring and abnormal valve growth; this lesion is also irreversible, and progression of valve damage occurs as a result of trauma caused by high-velocity blood flow across the damaged valve. The echocardiogram data suggest that patient 1 (now 13 years old) will also require corrective surgery, as did patient 2, and that both patients will possibly require additional surgery, including aortic valve replacement. Thus we believe that LDL apheresis treatment should begin early in life, before cardiovascular disease becomes established, and that the minimum practical treatment interval should be used. For these children the 7-day treatment interval achieved a time-average mean cholesterol concentration between 5.2 and 7.8 mmol/L (200 and 300 mg/dl).

The LDL apheresis takes advantage of the intrinsic charge affinity of dextran sulfate to cysteine-rich apolipoprotein B, allowing for the selective removal of apolipoprotein B–containing LDL and VLDL.[7] The dextran sulfate–apolipoprotein B bond can be readily dissociated by hypertonic saline solution, thus restoring the material's affinity and binding capacity for apoprotein B. Other methods of specific extracorporeal removal of cholesterol being used by other investigators are immunoadsorption by anti–apolipoprotein B antibodies,[26-28] double-membrane filtration,[6, 29-31] and heparin-induced LDL precipitation.[32, 33] Although some of these procedures have been used long term for the treatment of severe HFH, none has been reported to be an effective and practical long-term therapy for HFH.

Reduction in serum LDL cholesterol level may induce regression of atheromas and improvement in clinical status.[34-36] Coronary angiography was not done before LDL apheresis was begun, so regression cannot be documented in these patients. However, progression of atherosclerosis was prevented and, although not proved, regression of atheroma probably occurred. The preservation of normal HDL levels in conjunction with marked lowering of LDL may cause atheromatous lesions to regress. Additional studies with patients with less severe but nevertheless refractory forms of hypercholesterolemia may serve to expand the therapeutic possibilities of this treatment.

We conclude that dextran sulfate–affinity column LDL apheresis is the current treatment of choice for children with receptor-negative HFH. It may be administered safely and practically for many years while patients maintain an excellent quality of life.

We thank Dr. Sarah Blumenschein and Dr. Thomas Zellers of the Division of Pediatric Cardiology for their contribution to the clinical care of the patients.

REFERENCES

1. Goldstein JL, Brown MS. Familial hypercholesterolemia. In: Scriver CR, Beaudet AL, Sly WS, Valle D, eds. The metabolic basis of inherited disease. 6th ed. New York: McGraw-Hill, 1989:1215-50.
2. Uauy R, Vega GL, Grundy SM, Bilheimer DM. Lovastatin therapy in receptor-negative homozygous familial hypercholesterolemia: lack of effect on low-density lipoprotein concentrations or turnover. J PEDIATR 1988;113:387-92.
3. Berger GM, Firth JC, Jacobs P, Wood L, Marais AD, Horak A. Three different schedules of low-density lipoprotein apheresis compared with plasmapheresis in patients with homozygous familial hypercholesterolemia. Am J Med 1990;88:94-100.
4. Thompson GR, Miller JP, Breslow JL. Improved survival of patients with homozygous familial hypercholesterolemia treated with plasma exchange. Br Med J 1985;291:1671-3.
5. Bilheimer DW, Goldstein JL, Grundy SM, Starzl TE, Brown MS. Liver transplantation to provide low-density-lipoprotein receptors and lower plasma cholesterol in a child with homozygous familial hypercholesterolemia. N Engl J Med 1984; 311:1658-64.
6. Yokoyama S, Yamamoto A, Hayashi R, Satani M. LDL-aph-

eresis: potential procedure for prevention and regression of atheromatous vascular lesion. Jpn Circ J 1987;51:1116-22.
7. Yokoyama S, Hayashi R, Kikkawa T, et al. Specific sorbent of apolipoprotein B-containing lipoproteins for plasmapheresis: characterization and experimental use in hypercholesterolemic rabbits. Arteriosclerosis 1984;4:276-82.
8. Uauy R, Zwiener RJ, Phillips MJ, Petruska ML, Bilheimer DW. Treatment of children with homozygous familial hypercholesterolemia: safety and efficacy of low-density lipoprotein apheresis. J PEDIATR 1992;120:892-8.
9. Gordon BR, Kelsey SF, Bilheimer DW, et al. Treatment of refractory familial hypercholesterolemia by low-density lipoprotein apheresis using an automated dextran sulfate cellulose adsorption system: The Liposorber Study Group. Am J Cardiol 1992;70:1010-6.
10. Brown MS, Goldstein JL. A receptor-mediated pathway for cholesterol homeostasis. Science 1986;232:34-47.
11. Cuthbert JA, Lipsky PE. Identification of low density lipoprotein receptor abnormalities by assaying functional receptors on proliferating lymphocytes. Arteriosclerosis 1989;9:I43-9.
12. Steiner PM, Freidel J, Bremner WF, Stein EA. Standardization of micromethods for plasma cholesterol, triglyceride and HDL-cholesterol with the Lipid Clinics' methodology [Abstract]. J Clin Chem Clin Biochem 1981;19:850.
13. Warnick GR, Albers JJ. A comprehensive evaluation of the heparin manganese precipitation procedure for estimating high-density lipoprotein cholesterol. J Lipid Res 1978;19:65-76.
14. Friedewald WT, Levy RI, Fredrickson DS. Estimation of the concentration of low-density lipoprotein cholesterol in plasma, without use of the preparative ultracentrifuge. Clin Chem 1972;18:499-502.
15. Myers GL, Cooper GR, Winn CL, Smith SJ. The Centers for Disease Control–National Heart, Lung, and Blood Institute Lipid Standardization Program: an approach to accurate and precise lipid measurements. Clin Lab Med 1989;9:105-35.
16. Stein EA, DiPersio L, Pesce AJ, et al. Enzyme-linked immunoabsorbent assay of apolipoprotein AII in plasma, with use of a monoclonal antibody. Clin Chem 1986;32:967-71.
17. Sokol RJ, Heubi JE, Iannaccone ST, Bove KE, Balistreri WF. Vitamin E deficiency with normal serum vitamin E concentrations in children with chronic cholestasis. N Engl J Med 1984; 310:1209-12.
18. Thiery J, Walli AK, Janning G, Seidel D. Low-density lipoprotein plasmaphaeresis with and without lovastatin in the treatment of the homozygous form of familial hypercholesterolaemia. Eur J Pediatr 1990;149:716-21.
19. Mol MJ, Stalenhoef AF. Homozygous familial hypercholesterolaemia: metabolic studies and treatment with LDL apheresis. Neth J Med 1990;36:279-87.
20. Goldstein JL, Brown MS. The LDL receptor defect in familial hypercholesterolemia: implications for pathogenesis and therapy. Med Clin North Am 1982;66:335-62.
21. Rose V, Wilson G, Steiner G. Familial hypercholesterolemia: report of coronary death at age 3 in a homozygous child and prenatal diagnosis in a heterozygous sibling. J PEDIATR 1982; 100:757-9.
22. Stanley P, Chartrand C, Davignon A. Acquired aortic stenosis in a twelve-year-old girl with xanthomatosis. N Engl J Med 1965;273:1378-80.
23. Hendry WG, Seed M. Homozygous familial hypercholesterolaemia with supravalvar aortic stenosis treated by surgery. J R Soc Med 1985;78:334-5.
24. Beppu S, Minura Y, Sakakibara H, et al. Supravalvular aortic stenosis and coronary ostial stenosis in familial hypercholesterolemia: two-dimensional echocardiographic assessment. Circulation 1983;67:878-84.
25. Sprecher DL, Schaefer EJ, Kent KM, et al. Cardiovascular features of homozygous familial hypercholesterolemia: analysis of 16 patients. Am J Cardiol 1984;54:20-30.
26. Riesen WF. Experience with low-density lipoprotein apheresis by polyclonal and monoclonal anti-apolipoprotein B antibodies and by dextran sulfate cellulose. Curr Stud Hematol Blood Transfus 1990;57:208-19.
27. Richter WO, Jacob BG, Ritter MM, Suhler K, Vierneisel K, Schwandt P. Three-year treatment of familial heterozygous hypercholesterolemia by extracorporeal low-density lipoprotein immunoadsorption with polyclonal apolipoprotein B antibodies. Metabolism 1993;42:888-94.
28. Borberg H, Gaczkowski A, Hombach V, Oette K, Stoffel W. Treatment of familial hypercholesterolemia by means of specific immunoadsorption. J Clin Apheresis 1988;4:59-65.
29. Mabuchi H, Michishita I, Sakai T, et al. Treatment of homozygous patients with familial hypercholesterolemia by double-filtration plasmapheresis. Atherosclerosis 1986;61:135-40.
30. Homma Y, Mikami Y, Tamachi H, et al. Comparison of selectivity of LDL removal by double filtration and dextran-sulfate cellulose column plasmapheresis. Atherosclerosis 1986; 60:23-7.
31. Franceschini G, Busnach G, Vaccarino V, Calabresi L, Gianfranceschi G, Sirtori CR. Apheretic treatment of severe familial hypercholesterolemia: comparison of dextran sulfate cellulose and double membrane filtration methods for low density lipoprotein removal. Atherosclerosis 1988;73:197-202.
32. Seidel D, Armstrong VW, Schuff-Werner P. The HELP-LDL-apheresis multicentre study, an angiographically assessed trial on the role of LDL-apheresis in the secondary prevention of coronary heart disease. I. Evaluation of safety and cholesterol-lowering effects during the first 12 months: HELP Study Group. Eur J Clin Invest 1991;21:375-83.
33. Eisenhauer T, Schuff-Werner P, Armstrong VW, Talartschik J, Scheler F, Seidel D. Long-term experience with the HELP system for treatment of severe familial hypercholesterolemia. Asaio Trans 1987;33:395-7.
34. Cashin-Hemphill L, Mack WJ, Pogoda JM, Sanmarco ME, Azen SP, Blankenhorn DH. Beneficial effects of colestipol-niacin on coronary atherosclerosis: a four-year follow-up. JAMA 1990;264:3013-7.
35. Brown G, Albers JJ, Fisher LD, et al. Regression of coronary artery disease as a result of intensive lipid-lowering therapy in men with high levels of apolipoprotein B. N Engl J Med 1990; 323:1289-98.
36. Kane JP, Malloy MJ, Ports TA, Phillips NR, Diehl JC, Havel RJ. Regression of coronary atherosclerosis during treatment of familial hypercholesterolemia with combined drug regimens. JAMA 1990;264:3007-12.

Pathophysiology of calcium metabolism in children with vitamin D–deficiency rickets

Klaus Kruse, MD

From the Department of Pediatrics, Medical University of Luebeck, Luebeck, Germany

Objective: **To improve understanding of the biochemical events in vitamin D–deficiency rickets (VDR).**
Methods: **We investigated 51 untreated patients, 2 to 36 months of age, during three stages of VDR. Nineteen of these patients were also studied during therapy with 5000 to 10,000 U vitamin D_3 (cholecalciferol) and 0.5 to 1 gm calcium. Together with calcium and inorganic phosphate in serum and urine, we measured (1) parathyroid hormone (PTH) secretion (intact serum PTH) and action on the kidney (urinary adenosine 3′,5′-cyclic monophosphate (cAMP)/creatinine ratio; (2) serum alkaline phosphatase level; (3) urinary hydroxyproline/creatinine ratio; and (4) serum 1,25-dihydroxyvitamin D (1,25$(OH)_2$D) level.**
Results: **The untreated patients had secondary hyperparathyroidism (high serum PTH and urinary cAMP/creatinine ratio), low calcium and phosphate concentrations in serum, and increased bone turnover (elevated serum alkaline phosphatase and OHP/creatinine ratio), whereas serum 1,25$(OH)_2$D was low, normal, or even slightly elevated. Serum calcium level was positively correlated to serum 1,25$(OH)_2$D and to OHP/creatinine ratio, indicating that normocalcemia in untreated rickets (stage 2) is at least partially maintained by 1,25$(OH)_2$D–induced calcium mobilization from bone. There was no correlation between serum calcium and serum PTH, or between serum PTH and urinary cAMP/creatinine ratio or serum phosphate, indicating disturbed regulation and action of PTH. During vitamin D treatment, serum 1,25$(OH)_2$D values increased to supranormal concentrations in association with the restoration of the physiologic relationship of PTH to serum calcium and phosphate concentrations and urinary cAMP/creatinine ratio.**
Conclusion: **Circulating 1,25$(OH)_2$D has an important role in the pathophysiology of VDR before and during treatment, mainly by influencing the bone and kidney response to endogenous PTH. (J Pediatr 1995;126:736-41)**

Vitamin D–deficiency rickets occurs as a result of low vitamin D intake in association with decreased exposure to sunlight. The disorder is biochemically characterized by elevated serum alkaline phosphatase activity, normal or decreased serum levels of calcium and inorganic phosphate, secondary hyperparathyroidism, and decreased 25-hydroxyvitamin D serum concentrations.

Fraser et al.[1] described three stages of VDR on the basis of laboratory and clinical data: stage 1 arises from impaired intestinal Ca absorption and Ca resorption from bone, resulting in hypocalcemia; hyperaminoaciduria and hyperphosphaturia are absent, and serum P is normal. Hypophosphatemia develops in stages 2 and 3; serum Ca is normal in stage 2 and hypocalcemia returns in stage 3, in which the clinical and radiologic findings of rickets are severe. Hyperaminoaciduria and hyperphosphaturia occur in these two later stages as indirect evidence of secondary hyper-

Submitted for publication May 10, 1994; accepted Dec. 1, 1994.

Reprint requests: Klaus Kruse, MD, Klinik fuer Paediatrie der Medizinischen Universitaet zu Luebeck, Kahlhorststrasse 31-35, D-23538 Luebeck, Germany.

0022-3476/95/$3.00 + 0 **9/20/62438**

parathyroidism. This concept of three successive stages appears somewhat theoretic and does not account for several pathophysiologic interrelations among parathyroid activity, P, Ca, and vitamin D, and bone metabolism.[2] The weakness of the study of Fraser et al. is the lack of measurements of serum parathyroid hormone and vitamin D metabolites.

During the last several years we investigated untreated vitamin D–deficient children with the aim to gain insight into the pathophysiologic events of the disorder, with special reference to the interactions of the most important Ca-regulating hormones, PTH and 1,25-dihydroxyvitamin D.

AP	Alkaline phosphatase
cAMP	Adenosine 3′,5′-cyclic phosphate
$1,25(OH)_2D$	1,25-Dihydroxyvitamin D
25(OH)D	25-Hydroxyvitamin D
OHP	Urinary hydroxyproline
PTH	Parathyroid hormone
TmP/GFR	Maximal tubular phosphate reabsorption rate in relation to glomerular filtration rate
VDR	Vitamin D–deficiency rickets

METHODS

We studied 51 children (33 boys) with VDR, 2 to 36 months of age (median, 16 months). The patients were not selected and attended several pediatric clinics, mainly from the northern part of Germany, from 1989 to 1994. All children had a history of deficient vitamin D intake.

The diagnosis of VDR was based on radiologic signs of rickets and laboratory findings such as elevated AP activity, low 25(OH)D concentration (<12.5 nmol/L; 5 ng/ml), and low or normal Ca and P levels in serum. None of the patients received anticonvulsant drugs or had evidence of renal, hepatic, or intestinal disease.

After an overnight fast, 2-hour morning urine specimens and blood were obtained at about 9 AM for the determination of Ca, P, and creatinine levels; AP activity; PTH, 25(OH)D, and $1,25(OH)_2D$ levels in serum; and P, creatinine, cAMP, and hydroxyproline in urine. The urine was collected by having the children spontaneous void into an attached urine bag.

In 19 of these patients Ca metabolism was also investigated 1 to 3 weeks after initiation of oral treatment with 5000 to 10,000 U vitamin D_3 and 0.5 to 1 gm Ca. The 51 untreated patients were divided into three groups reflecting the three stages of VDR. The stage 1 (n = 8) group had low serum Ca (<2.1 mmol/L; 8.4 mg/dl) and normal serum P; the stage 2 group (n = 31), had normal serum Ca and serum P level less than 1.68 mmol/L (5.2 mg/dl) (−1 SD or more less than the age-dependent mean value); and the stage 3 group (n = 12) had low levels of both serum a C and P. The clinical and radiologic signs of rickets were mild in stage 1 and moderate to severe in stages 2 and 3. The age at the time of admission ranged from 2 to 26 months (median, 4 months) in stage 1 VDR, 6 to 36 months (median, 20 months) in stage 2, and 4 to 36 months (median, 16 months) in stage 3.

Urinary Ca, OHP, and cAMP levels were related to creatinine excretion. The maximal rate of tubular P reabsorption in relation to the glomerular filtration rate was determined according to the method of Walton and Bijvoet.[3, 4] Urinary hydroxyproline,[5] cAMP,[6] and intact PTH[7] were assayed as previously described. The normal range of serum PTH in children is 1.1 to 5.8 pmol/L (range, 10 to 55 ng/L). Calcium, P, creatinine, and AP levels were measured with standard automatic analyzer techniques. Serum 25(OH)D was determined with a competitive protein-binding assay (normal range, 24 to 120 nmol/L [10 to 50 ng/ml]). Serum $1,25(OH)_2D$ was assayed with a test kit (Nichols Institute Diagnostics, San Juan Capristano, Calif.). The detection limit is 7 pmol/L; the intraassay and interassay variances at a concentration of 96 pmol/L are about 10% and 14%, respectively. The normal range in children less than 3 years of age in our laboratory is 48 to 144 pmol/L (20 to 60 pg/ml). To eliminate the influence of age, we calculated the OHP/creatinine ratio, which is age dependent during the first 3 years,[5] as SD score by the equation $(X_i - X)/SD$, where X_i is the actual individual value, X is the mean value for age, and SD is the standard deviation at that age. The other measured variables are not age dependent during the ages of 2 to 36 months.[5-7]

Most of the individual values in the patients were not distributed normally. Therefore the median and range were calculated, and the Mann-Whitney U test was used for statistical comparison. Differences were considered to be significant at a level of $p < 0.05$. Correlations between variables of interest were examined by linear regression analysis.

RESULTS

Calcium metabolism in different stages of VDR. Table I summarizes the median values and ranges of several biochemical variables in the untreated patients, who were divided into three groups according to the stage of VDR. As previously defined, serum Ca level was low in stages 1 and 3 but normal in stage 2, whereas serum P level was normal in stage 1 but low in stages 2 and 3.

The median value of serum AP activity was elevated in stage 1, with a significant further increase in stage 2 and a decrement thereafter. The index of bone degradation, OHP/creatinine ratio, was in the upper normal range in stage 1, increased significantly in stage 2, and decreased slightly in stage 3.

Serum PTH and urinary cAMP/creatinine ratio were

Table I. Calcium metabolism in three stages of VDR

Values (units)	Normal range	n	Stage 1 Median (range)	n	Stage 2 Median (range)	n	Stage 3 Median (range)	p Stage 1 vs Stage 2	p Stage 2 vs Stage 3	p Stage 1 vs Stage 3
Serum										
Ca (mmol/L)	(2.1-2.65)	8	1.69 (1.35-1.93)	31	2.38 (2.10-2.60)	12	1.85 (1.43-2.03)	<0.001	<0.01	NS
P (mmol/L)	(1.45-2.37)	8	2.06 (1.74-2.74)	31	1.13 (0.42-1.65)	12	1.28 (0.58-1.52)	<0.001	NS	<0.01
AP (U/L)	(200-600)	8	1221 (800-1926)	31	1637 (896-5096)	12	1297 (758-4835)	<0.05	NS	NS
PTH (ng/L)	(10-55)	8	149 (90-271)	31	199 (85-1056)	12	260 (56-729)	NS	NS	<0.05
$1,25(OH)_2D$ (pmol/L)	(48-144)	3	73 (15-83)	16	217 (81-439)	7	76 (60-146)	<0.001	<0.001	NS
Urine										
TmP/GFR (mmol/L)	(1.3-2.6)	6	1.75 (1.39-2.35)	21	1.19 (0.42-1.77)	10	1.13 (0.35-2.13)	<0.001	NS	<0.05
cAMP/creatinine ratio (nmol/mg)	(4.7-11.5)	6	20.5 (12-32)	20	26.5 (8-43)	10	31 (17-45)	NS	NS	<0.05
OHP/creatinine ratio (SD score)	(−2 to +2)	6	1.6 (−2.3 to +12)	20	8.3 (2-20)	10	5 (0.7-16)	<0.01	NS	NS

NS, Not significant.

Table II. Relationship between PTH and $1,25(OH)_2D$ and indices of Ca and bone metabolism in patients with VDR before and 1 to 3 weeks after treatment with vitamin D

	Serum Ca	Serum P	TmP/GFR	Serum AP	OHP/creatinine ratio	cAMP/creatinine ratio	25(OH)D	$1,25(OH)_2D$
Pretreatment (n = 51)								
PTH	NS	NS	NS	$r = 0.46$, n = 51, $p <0.001$	NS	NS	NS	NS
$1,25(OH)_2D$	$r = 0.55$, n = 26, $p <0.01$	NS	NS	NS	$r = 0.43$, n = 22, $p <0.05$	NS	$r = 0.55$, n = 26, $p <0.01$	
1-3 wk treatment (n = 19)								
PTH	$r = -0.59$, n = 19, $p <0.01$	$r = -0.56$, n = 19, $p <0.05$	$r = -0.57$, n = 18, $p <0.05$	NS	NS	$r = 0.78$, n = 14, $p <0.001$	NS	NS
$1,25(OH)_2D$	NS	NS	NS	$r = 0.69$, n = 13, $p <0.01$	$r = 0.68$, n = 12, $p <0.05$	NS	NS	

NS, Not significant.

elevated in stage 1; there was a further increase in the later stages and significantly higher values in stage 3 in comparison with stage 1.

The median value of serum $1,25(OH)_2D_3$ was normal in stages 1 and 3, and significantly elevated in stage 2 (Fig. 1), thus showing a pattern resembling that of serum Ca and OHP/creatinine ratio (Table I).

Parathyroid hormone and $1,25(OH)_2D$ before and during vitamin D treatment. The relationship of the Ca-regulating hormones PTH and $1,25(OH)_2D$ in all patients before and during vitamin D treatment is depicted in Table II. The intact serum PTH level was elevated in all 51 untreated patients. The PTH level was correlated only with serum AP. Vitamin D_3 treatment resulted in normalization of the physiologic relationships of PTH to serum Ca and serum P levels, TmP/GFR, and urinary cAMP level.

The serum levels of $1,25(OH)_2D$ were measured in only 26 untreated and 19 treated patients. As depicted in Fig. 1, the levels were decreased in only one patient but were normal (n = 12) or even elevated (n = 13) in the other untreated patients, and were markedly increased during vitamin D therapy. In the untreated patients the $1,25(OH)_2D$ concentrations were positively correlated with serum Ca (Fig. 2) and 25(OH)D levels. Serum Ca level was significantly higher (mean ± SD: 2.28 ± 0.23 vs 2.03 ± 0.28 mmol/L, $p <0.02$) in patients with elevated $1,25(OH)_2D$

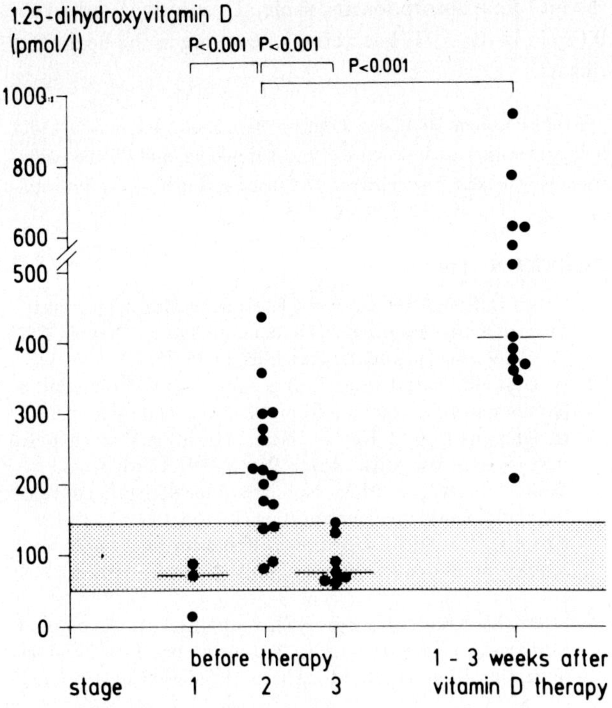

Fig. 1. Individual and median serum concentrations of $1,25(OH)_2D$ in children with VDR during its three stages and during vitamin D_3 therapy.

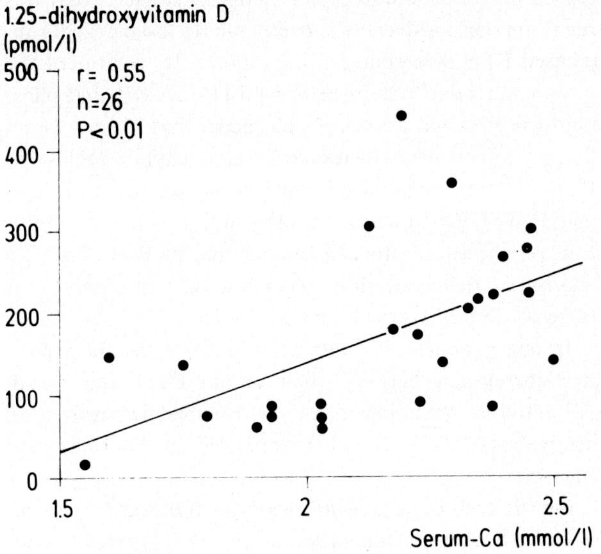

Fig. 2. Relationship between $1,25(OH)_2D$ and serum Ca concentrations in untreated vitamin D–deficient children.

levels (>144 pmol/L, n = 13) than in those with normal values (<144 pmol/L, n = 13). There was a positive correlation of $1,25(OH)_2D$ with the OHP/creatinine ratio in the untreated patients and with OHP/creatinine ratio and serum AP during vitamin D treatment.

There was a negative correlation between the urinary cAMP excretion and serum P level ($r = -0.52$, n = 36, $p < 0.01$) and TmP/GFR ($r = -0.58$, n = 36, $p < 0.001$), in the untreated but not in the treated patients (data not shown). Concentrations of PTH, serum Ca, and P; TmP/GFR; and urinary cAMP/creatinine ratio normalized 2 to 3 weeks after initiation of vitamin D therapy, although both serum AP level and OHP/creatinine ratio remained elevated.

DISCUSSION

The present study confirms that vitamin D depletion (low serum 25(OH)D levels), secondary hyperparathyroidism, and high bone turnover are the hallmarks of VDR in children. The serum levels of Ca, P, and $1,25(OH)_2D$ are of minor diagnostic relevance; these values may be normal, and $1,25(OH)_2D$ may even be increased in VDR. The latter observation confirms investigations in other vitamin D–deficient children[8, 9] and adults.[10, 11] In the face of secondary hyperparathyroidism, hypocalcemia, and hypophosphatemia (i.e., in conditions of maximal stimulation of renal $1,25[OH]_2D$ synthesis) the $1,25(OH)_2D$ serum levels in these patients seem to be inadequately low.[8, 9]

Our findings of a positive correlation between 25(OH)D and $1,25(OH)_2D$ serum concentrations before vitamin D_3 treatment, and the marked increase of $1,25(OH)_2D$ concentration during vitamin D_3 administration, confirm the observations of other authors[8, 10, 12-14] and indicate that there is a limitation to the synthesis of $1,25(OH)_2D$, which is probably due to the deficiency of the substrate 25(OH)D. The circulating $1,25(OH)_2D$ levels seem to have important effects in the pathophysiology of VDR, especially in the defense against hypocalcemia. Thus our finding of a positive relationship between $1,25(OH)_2D$ and serum Ca concentration, and between $1,25(OH)_2D$ and the index of bone degradation, OHP, provides evidence that the normocalcemia in untreated vitamin D–deficient children is maintained at least partially by $1,25(OH)_2D$-induced mobilization of Ca from bone.

In untreated patients we could not find the physiologic inverse relation between PTH and serum Ca level, the main regulator of PTH secretion. In addition, there also seemed to be a disturbance of PTH action on its main target organ, the kidney. This is reflected by a lack of correlation between PTH serum levels, and urinary cAMP excretion, TmP/GFR, and, consequently, serum P concentrations. In the first stage of VDR, in the face of elevated PTH and urinary cAMP levels but normal serum P level and TmP/GFR, one may postulate a block beyond the step of cAMP production. In stages 2 and 3 of VDR, the presence of elevated urinary cAMP excretion and hypophosphatemia suggests that this renal hyporesponsiveness is overcome by the markedly increased PTH secretion. During vitamin D_3 treatment the physiologic relationships between PTH, cAMP, and phosphaturia returned, favoring the concept that vitamin D deficiency affects the activation of renal adenylate cyclase by PTH.[15-18] The negative correlation between serum P level and TmP/GFR to urinary cAMP indicates that a significant renal postreceptor defect, reported by Rao et al.[19] in vitamin D–deficient adults, does not exist in children, at least not during stages 2 and 3 of VDR.

In our patients with untreated VDR we found a positive correlation between their serum PTH and serum AP activity, indicating that their osteoblastic response to endogenous PTH was not as impaired as the kidney response.

On the basis of our results and those of others,[2, 8] the following pathophysiologic mechanisms are suggested in children with VDR. In the first stage impaired intestinal Ca absorption and Ca resorption from bone lead to hypocalcemia with secondary hyperparathyroidism that in turn stimulates the osteoblastic activity, reflected by elevated serum AP activity. Usually stage 1 proceeds to stage 2 in a short time; the secondary hyperparathyroidism and the associated increase in serum $1,25(OH)_2D$ level normalize serum Ca concentration by mobilizing it from bone (as reflected by the marked increase of the index of osteoclastic bone degradation, OHP/creatinine ratio).

It is unclear why the hypersecretion of PTH continues despite the normocalcemia. It may be related to the circulating $1,25(OH)_2D$ levels, which are not appropriately elevated to suppress the parathyroid glands and restore the disturbed Ca homeostasis.[2, 8] The fact that the patients do not have hypercalcemia despite elevated $1,25(OH)_2D$ and PTH concentrations may be explained by the inadequate influx of Ca from gut, kidney, and bone. During this second stage of VDR, hypophosphatemia and the PTH- and $1,25(OH)_2D$-induced bone degradation lead to manifest rickets.

In stage 3 hypocalcemia develops again, mainly because of the absolute or relative deficiency of $1,25(OH)_2D$ caused by a further depletion of its substrate, 25(OH)D. The disturbed secretion of $1,25(OH)_2D$ leads to a further decrease in intestinal Ca absorption and to insufficient Ca mobilization from bone despite continuous hyperparathyroidism, because $1,25(OH)_2D$ is required for PTH to resorb bone.[20, 21] The combination of hypocalcemia and hypophosphatemia causes a marked reduction of the product of Ca and P (Ca × P), with severe clinical and radiologic signs of rickets.

Vitamin D_3 treatment leads to a marked rise of $1,25(OH)_2D$ with a consecutive normalization of serum Ca (by intestinal absorption and skeletal resorption) and serum P (by inhibiting PTH secretion), resulting in the healing of rickets.

I thank Sabine Tiemann, Gudrun Pauch, and Ritva Schroeder for performing the biochemical measurements, and all the pediatricians who sent frozen serum and urine specimens, and information regarding several patients.

REFERENCES

1. Fraser D, Koogh SW, Scriver CR. Hyperparathyroidism as the cause of hyperaminoaciduria and phosphaturia in human vitamin D deficiency. Pediatr Res 1967;1:425-35.
2. Arnaud CD. Parathyroid hormone and its role in the pathophysiology of the common forms of rickets and osteomalacia. In: Glorieux FH, ed. Rickets. Nestlé Nutrition Workshop Series; vol 21. New York: Raven Press, 1991:47-61.
3. Walton RJ, Bijvoet OLM. Nomogram for derivation of renal threshold phosphate concentration. Lancet 1975;2:309-10.
4. Kruse K, Kracht U, Göpfert G. Renal threshold phosphate concentration ($TmPO_4$/GFR). Arch Dis Child 1982;57:217-23.
5. Kruse K, Kracht U. Die Hydroxyprolin-Ausscheidung im Morgen-Urin: ein geeigneter Parameter des Knochen-Umsatzes im Kindesalter. Monatsschr Kinderheilkd 1983;131:797-803.
6. Kruse K, Kracht U. Urinary adenosine-3′-5′-monophosphate excretion in childhood. J Clin Endocrinol Metab 1981;53:1251-5.
7. Kruse K, Pankau R, Gosch A, Wohlfart K. Calcium metabolism in Williams-Beuren syndrome. J PEDIATR 1992; 121:902-7.
8. Markestad T, Halvorsen S, Seeger Halvorsen K, Aksnes L, Aarskog D. Plasma concentrations of vitamin D metabolites before and during treatment of vitamin D deficiency rickets in children. Acta Paediatr Scand 1984;73:225-31.
9. Chesney RW, Zimmermann J, Hamstra A, DeLuca HF, Mazess RB. Vitamin D metabolite concentrations in vitamin D deficiency: are calcitriol levels normal? Am J Dis Child 1981;135:1025-8.
10. Papapoulos SE, Fraher LJ, Clemens TL, Gleed J, O'Riordan JLH. Metabolites of vitamin D in human vitamin D deficiency: effect of vitamin D_3 or 1,25-dihydroxycholecalciferol. Lancet 1980;2:612-6.
11. Eastwood JR, de Wardener ME, Gray RW, et al. Normal plasma $1,25\text{-}(OH)_2$ vitamin D concentrations in nutritional osteomalacia. Lancet 1979;1:1377-9.
12. Rasmussen H, Baron R, Broadus A, et al. $1,25(OH)_2D_3$ is not the only D metabolite involved in the pathogenesis of osteomalacia. Am J Med 1980;69:360-7.
13. Mallet E, Nguyen T, Garabedian M, Bassuyau JP. Circulating parathyroid hormone and dihydroxylated vitamin D metabolites after oral 25 hydroxycholecalciferol in infantile rickets. Horm Metab Res 1982;14:503-4.
14. Stanbury SW, Taylor CM, Lumb GA, et al. Formation of vitamin D metabolites following correction of human vitamin D deficiency. Miner Electrolyte Metab 1981;5:212-27.
15. Forte LR, Nickols GA, Anast CS. Renal adenylate cyclase and the interrelationship between parathyroid hormone and vitamin D in the regulation of urinary phosphate and adenosine cyclic 3′5′-monophosphate excretion. J Clin Invest 1976;57:559-68.

16. Kruse K, Bartels H, Kracht U. Parathyroid function in different stages of vitamin D deficiency rickets. Eur J Pediatr 1984; 141:158-62.
17. Lewin IG, Papapoulos SE, Hendy G, Tomlinson S, O'Riordan JLH. Reversible resistance to the renal action of parathyroid hormone in human vitamin D deficiency. Clin Sci 1982; 62:381-7.
18. Marguet C, Basuyou JP, Leroy M, Brunelle Ph, Mallet E. Gs-unit activity in vitamin D deficiency rickets [Abstract]. Pediatr Res 1994;36:27.
19. Rao DS, Parfitt AM, Kleerekoper M, Pumo BS, Frame B. Dissociation between the effects of endogenous parathyroid hormone on adenosine 3′,5′-monophosphate generation and phosphate reabsorption in hypocalcemia due to vitamin D depletion: an acquired disorder resembling pseudohypoparathyroidism type II. J Clin Endocrinol Metab 1985;61:285-90.
20. Rasmussen H, DeLuca H, Arnaud CD, Hawker C, v Stedingk M. The relationship between vitamin D and parathyroid hormone. J Clin Invest 1963;42:1940-6.
21. Arnaud CD, Rasmussen H, Anast C. Further studies on the relationship between parathyroid hormone and vitamin D. J Clin Invest 1966;45:1955-64.

Use of peritoneal dialysis, continuous arteriovenous hemofiltration, and continuous arteriovenous hemodiafiltration for removal of ammonium chloride and glutamine in rabbits

Denis S. Semama, MD, Frédéric Huet, MD, Jean-Bernard Gouyon, MD, Christian Lallemant, MD, and Jean Desgres, PhD

From the Service de Pédiatrie 2 et laboratoire de Néphrologie-Hémaphérèse-Transplantation, and the laboratoire de Biochimie, CHUR du Bocage, Dijon, France

Objective: **We compared the ability of peritoneal dialysis, hemofiltration, and continuous hemodiafiltration to remove infused ammonium chloride.**
Study design: **Anesthetized adult rabbits received an intravenous infusion of ammonium chloride. Two methods of removal of ammonium chloride were performed in each animal and compared. In group 1 (n = 6), peritoneal dialysis (dialysate = 75 ml · kg^{-1}) and continuous arteriovenous hemofiltration (CAVH) with a polysulfone 800 cm^2 hemofilter (Minifilter Plus; Amicon Division, W. R. Grace & Co., Danvers, Mass.) were simultaneously performed for 40 minutes. In group 2 (n = 6), peritoneal dialysis and continuous arteriovenous hemodiafiltration (CAVHD) (dialysate flow = 1000 ml · hr^{-1}) were simultaneous performed for 40 minutes. In group 3 (n = 6), CAVH and CAVHD were performed successively in random order for 30 minutes each.**
Results: **Animals had high and stable ammonium chloride and glutamine plasma levels during the experimental procedure. No significant difference in ammonium chloride clearance was observed between PD and CAVH (group 1). In comparison with PD or CAVH, CAVHD resulted in significantly higher clearances of ammonium chloride (40% ± 10% vs 96% ± 34%, respectively) and of glutamine (195% ± 17% vs 77% ± 25%, respectively).**
Conclusion: **The overall results indicate that CAVHD should be considered for hyperammonemia when peritoneal dialysis is indicated but unfeasible or inefficient. (J Pediatr 1995;126:742-6)**

Hyperammonemia is encountered in various inborn errors of urea synthesis, including deficiencies of carbamoyl phosphate synthetase, ornithine transcarbamylase, argininosuccinate synthetase, argininosuccinate lyase, and argininase.[1] The accumulation of ammonia can lead to vomiting, lethargy, seizures, and coma. Hyperammonemia results in a rise in intracranial pressure by causing a breakdown of cerebral autoregulation, astrocytic swelling, and changes in cerebral metabolism; another possibility is the accumulation of intra-

Presented in part at the 4th International Meeting of the European Society for Developmental Pharmacology, May 1994, York, England.

Submitted for publication July 27, 1994; accepted Nov. 4, 1994.

Reprint requests: Jean-Bernard Gouyon, MD, Service de Pédiatrie 2, CHUR du Bocage, 2 bd Mal. de Lattre de Tassigny, 21034 Dijon Cedex, France.

0022-3476/95/$3.00 + 0 **9/20/61796**

cellular glutamine, a major end product of ammonia detoxification in cerebral tissue.[2]

When hyperammonemia is symptomatic, exchange transfusions or peritoneal dialysis may be required. However, failures with these therapies have been described.[3,4] Continuous venovenous and arteriovenous hemofiltration have rapidly reduced ammonium blood levels in neonates with inborn errors of metabolism.[5-7] Hemofiltration removes non-protein-bound low weight molecules by an ultrafiltration mechanism, and has been used as a simple, safe, and effective treatment in fluid-overloaded infants and neonates with acute renal failure.[8] The basic hemofiltration procedure has been modified recently by instilling dialysate in the ultrafiltrate compartment, thus leading to a marked improvement in removal of solutes such as urea[9] and branched-chain amino acids.[10] This "continuous hemodiafiltration" combines the convective transport of hemofiltration with the diffusive transport of hemodialysis.

CAVH	Continuous arteriovenous hemofiltration
CAVHD	Continuous arteriovenous hemodiafiltration
PD	Peritoneal dialysis

The overall data suggest that continuous arteriovenous hemodiafiltration could improve removal of ammonium (molecular weight: 17.03 daltons) and glutamine (molecular weight: 146.15 daltons) as compared with hemofiltration and PD. The scarcity of data on ammonium removal by CAVHD[11] has led us to use an experimental animal model to compare PD, hemofiltration, and continuous hemodiafiltration clearances simultaneously.[10]

METHODS

Animal preparation. Experiments were performed in 18 male New Zealand white rabbits weighing 2.88 ± 0.04 kg and maintained on a standard diet. Food was withheld approximately 24 hours before the study. Animals were anesthetized with an intravenous injection of 30 mg · kg^{-1} of sodium pentobarbital; anesthesia was maintained by small intravenous doses of the same drug, as required. The trachea was cannulated to allow mechanical ventilation (respirator, model 662; Harvard Apparatus Inc., Natick, Mass.). Respiratory rate was 40 min^{-1}, tidal volume was 17 ml · kg^{-1}, and fraction of inspired oxygen was 1 throughout the experiment. The body temperature was maintained at 38° C by using a warming operating table. The left carotid artery was catheterized with a 4F 110 mm catheter (Seldicath, 1.3 mm; Plastimed, St.-Leu-la-Forêt, France) for blood sampling and continuous mean blood pressure monitoring (Hewlett-Packard Pressure Recorder, model 78205D, Hewlett-Packard Co., Palo Alto, Calif.). The right jugular vein was catheterized (4F 110 mm catheter) for drug infusion. The right femoral vein was catheterized (22-G 25 mm catheter; Critikon, Chatenay Malabry, France) for intravenous solute infusion. After completion of this initial surgical procedure, a priming dose of ammonium chloride (125 mg · kg^{-1}) was administered through the jugular vein and ammonium serum concentration was maintained by infusing 125 mg · kg^{-1} · h^{-1}. After the beginning of the infusion of ammonium chloride, a polyethylene catheter (Trocar catheter, Argyle, Morangis, France) was surgically inserted in the peritoneal cavity to allow PD in some animals (see below). Approximately 60 minutes was spent for animal preparation and 60 minutes was then allowed for subsequent equilibration.

Experimental procedures. The experimental protocol started 60 minutes after the start of ammonium chloride infusion in each group.

Group 1 (n = 6). Hemofiltration and PD were simultaneously performed for a 40-minute period to obtain similar experimental conditions (systemic hemodynamics, hematocrit, oncotic pressure, and ammonium blood levels) for these two procedures.

The dialysate solution used for PD contained per liter: 83 mmol of glucose, 145 mmol of sodium, 45 mmol of bicarbonate, and 102 mmol of chloride. This solution was warmed to 37° C and dose of a 75 ml · kg^{-1} was peritoneally infused after the equilibration period. Dialysate was left in the peritoneal cavity for 40 minutes. Instillation and dialysate return took approximately 3 and 5 minutes, respectively. Drainage fluid never showed macroscopic blood contamination.

Continuous arteriovenous hemofiltration started at the end of dialysate instillation and lasted for 40 minutes. CAVH was performed with an 800 cm^2 polysulfone hemofilter (Minifilter Plus; Amicon Division, W. R. Grace & Co., Danvers, Mass.). Lines connected the hemofilter with the cervical arterial and venous catheters; the extracorporeal volume was 15 ml. The arterial line allowed prefilter blood samplings, and the venous line allowed postfilter blood samplings. According to the manufacturer's recommendations, hemofilters were filled with heparinized (5000 IU · L^{-1}) isotonic saline solution. Heparin (loading dose: 200 IU · kg^{-1}; maintenance dose: 20 IU · kg^{-1} · h^{-1}) was used to prevent hemofilter clotting. Ultrafiltrate was drained through a 105 cm tube to a preweighed bag. Ultrafiltrate was totally replaced by infusing, through the femoral vein, a substitute fluid that contained per liter: 123 mmol of sodium chloride, 4 mmol of potassium chloride, 30 mmol of sodium bicarbonate, and 8.3 mmol of glucose.

Arterial blood samplings were performed at the first, twentieth, and fortieth minute and venous blood samplings at the twentieth minute. Ammonium chloride and glutamine concentrations were determined in each arterial blood sample and in peritoneal dialysate and ultrafiltrate. Oncotic pressure, oxygen saturation, and pH were measured in the arterial blood samples. Hematocrit was measured in arterial and venous blood samples to calculate the filter blood flow.

Group 2 (n = 6). CAVHD and PD were simultaneously performed for a 40-minute period. During CAVHD, a dialysate flow of 1000 ml · hr^{-1} was obtained with a peristaltic pump (VM 8000m; Vial Medical, St.-Martin-Le-Vinoux, France). The dialysate composition was similar to that of the substitute fluid, and the ultrafiltrate and dialysate fluids were collected together in the collecting bag. The experimental procedure of this group was similar to that described in group 1.

Group 3 (n = 6). Rabbits were successively submitted to CAVH and CAVHD in random order. Each period lasted 30 minutes. CAVH was performed as in group 1 and CAVHD as in group 2. Arterial blood sampling was performed at the first and thirtieth minute of each period. Ammonium chloride and glutamine concentrations were determined in each arterial blood sample and in collected solutes. Oncotic pressure, oxygen saturation, and pH were also measured in the arterial blood samples.

Analytic methods. During CAVH, the ultrafiltrate was calculated from the change in weight of preweighed bags without correction for specific gravity. During CAVHD, the ultrafiltrate volume was calculated by subtracting the infused dialysate from the collected fluid. During PD, the dialysate volume was assumed to be the infused volume (75 ml · kg^{-1}).

Ammonium was analyzed by an enzymatic method (Cobas Fara, Roche, Neuilly-Sur-Seine, France) and glutamine by column chromatography on an amino acid analyzer (system 6300 high-performance analyzer, Beckman Instruments, Spinco Division, Palo Alto, Calif.). Oncotic pressure and arterial gas values were measured with an oncometer (Osmomat 050; Gonatec, Berlin, Germany) and pH/blood gas analyzer 168 (Ciba Corning Diagnostics Corp., Medfield, Mass.), respectively.

Data analysis. Blood flow (Qb), plasma flow (Qp), and clearance rate (C) were derived from the following equations[8]:

$$Qb = \frac{Qf \times HCT_o}{Hct_o - Hct_i}$$

where Qf = ultrafiltrate rate, and Hct_i and Hct_o = hematocrit at the inlet and the outlet.

$$Qp = Qb \times (1 - Hct_i)$$

$$C_{PD} = \frac{\text{Concentration of solute in PD fluid}}{\text{Mean concentration of solute in arterial plasma}} \times \frac{\text{Dialysate volume}}{\text{PD duration}}$$

$$C_{CAVH} = \frac{\text{Concentration of solute in ultra filtrate fluid}}{\text{Mean concentration of solute in arterial plasma}} \times Qf$$

$$C_{CAVHD} = \frac{U \times V}{P}$$

where U = solute concentration in fluid drained in the collecting apparatus, V = rate (ml·kg^{-1}·min^{-1}) of fluid drained in the collecting apparatus, and P = mean plasma solute concentration during the CAVHD period.

Comparisons of the efficiencies of PD, CAVH, and CAVHD within each group were assessed statistically by the Wilcoxon signed-rank test. Comparisons between group 1 and group 2 were performed with the Mann-Whitney test. We considered *p* values <0.05 statistically significant. All data were expressed as means ± SE.

RESULTS

Basal plasma ammonium chloride and glutamine levels determined in the 18 rabbits were 73.6 ± 11.9 μmol · L^{-1} and 307.9 ± 16.4 μmol · L^{-1}, respectively. Infusion of ammonium chloride always induced a significant increase in plasma ammonium chloride and glutamine concentrations reaching 575.3 ± 44.5 μmol · L^{-1} and 474.6 ± 25.6 μmol · L^{-1}, respectively. No hemofilter showed fiber clotting at the end of the experiment.

Comparison between PD and CAVH (group 1). Mean values for blood and plasma flow and ultrafiltrate rate during CAVH were 12.50 ± 0.99 ml · kg^{-1} · min^{-1}, 8.47 ± 0.63 ml · kg^{-1} · min^{-1}, and 0.97 ± 0.07 ml · kg^{-1} · min^{-1}, respectively. No significant differences for ammonium chloride and glutamine clearances were found between PD and CAVH (Table I).

Comparison between PD and CAVHD (group 2). Mean values for blood and plasma flow and ultrafiltrate rate during CAVHD were 9.77 ± 1.20 ml · kg^{-1} · min^{-1}, 7.03 ± 0.82 ml · kg^{-1} · min^{-1}, and 0.74 ± 0.09 ml · kg^{-1} · min^{-1}, respectively. In comparison with PD, CAVHD resulted in significantly and consistently higher clearances for ammonium chloride (40% ± 10%) and glutamine (195% ± 17%) (Table I).

Comparison between groups 1 and 2. We found no significant difference between groups 1 and 2 for operational parameters, ultrafiltrate rate, and ammonium clearance for PD (Table II). In comparison with CAVH in group 1, CAVHD in group 2 resulted in significantly higher clearances for ammonium chloride and glutamine (Table I). To verify that this difference could not be ascribed to any intergroup difference, we compared CAVH and CAVHD in the same group of animals (group 3).

Comparison between CAVH and CAVHD (group 3). Mean blood pressure, arterial pH, arterial oxygen saturation, hematocrit, oncotic pressure, body temperature, and ammonium chloride levels were similar during CAVH and CAVHD (Table III). Mean values for ultrafiltrate rate

Table I. Values of ammonium and glutamine clearances in the three groups during the PD, CAVH, and CAVHD periods

	Group 1		Group 2		Group 3	
	PD	CAVH	PD	CAVHD	CAVH	CAVHD
C_{NH_4Cl} (ml · kg^{-1} · min^{-1})	1.75 ± 0.11	1.77 ± 0.24	1.83 ± 0.17	2.61 ± 0.40*,†	1.16 ± 0.25	1.96 ± 0.26*
$C_{glutamine}$ (ml · kg^{-1} · min^{-1})	0.57 ± 0.05	0.82 ± 0.10	0.38 ± 0.02	1.12 ± 0.10*,†	0.78 ± 0.04	1.35 ± 0.16*

Values are expressed as mean ± SE.
C_{NH_4cl}, Ammonium clearance; $C_{glutamine}$, glutamine clearance.
*p <0.05 significant difference when clearance values are compared between the two procedures performed in the same group.
†p <0.05 significant difference when clearance values of CAVH in group 1 are compared with those of CAVHD in group 2.

Table II. Comparison of the operational parameters, ultrafiltrate rate, and ammonium clearance for PD between group 1 and group 2

	Group 1	Group 2
pH	7.53 ± 0.06	7.49 ± 0.03
Arterial oxygen saturation (%)	99.8 ± 0.02	99.8 ± 0.04
Protein plasma levels (gm · L^{-1})	36.8 ± 2.7	32.9 ± 1.4
Oncotic pressure (mm Hg)	14.3 ± 1.2	11.8 ± 0.7
Hematocrit (L)	0.32 ± 0.02	0.28 ± 0.02
Heart rate (beats · min^{-1})	215 ± 17	195 ± 7
Mean blood pressure (mm Hg)	78 ± 4	71 ± 3
Body temperature (° C)	38.6 ± 0.2	38.3 ± 0.3
Blood flow in the hemofilter (ml · kg^{-1} · min^{-1})	12.50 ± 0.99	9.77 ± 1.20
Ultrafiltrate rate (ml · kg^{-1} · min^{-1})	0.97 ± 0.07	0.74 ± 0.09
Ammonium clearance for PD (ml · kg^{-1} · min^{-1})	1.75 ± 0.11	1.83 ± 0.17

No significant difference was found. Values are expressed as mean ± SE.

Table III. Comparison of the experimental parameters influencing the efficiency of CAVH and CAVHD in group 3

	CAVH	CAVHD
NH_4Cl (mmol · L^{-1})	651.8 ± 95.9	692.5 ± 75.2
Mean blood pressure (mm Hg)	79.8 ± 3.9	80.6 ± 6.8
Ultrafiltrate rate (ml · kg^{-1} · min^{-1})	0.97 ± 0.08	0.94 ± 0.15
pH	7.58 ± 0.01	7.57 ± 0.04
Arterial oxygen saturation (%)	99.9 ± 0.02	99.8 ± 0.02
Hematocrit (L)	0.29 ± 0.01	0.29 ± 0.01
Oncotic pressure (mm Hg)	13.7 ± 0.8	13.9 ± 0.9
Body temperature (° C)	38.5 ± 0.27	38.4 ± 0.27

No significant difference was found. Values are expressed as mean ± SE.

during CAVH and CAVHD were similar (Table III). In comparison with CAVH, CAVHD allowed significantly and consistently higher clearances for ammonium chloride (96% ± 34%) and glutamine (77% ± 25%) (Table I).

DISCUSSION

We recently demonstrated that this experimental model was valuable for the comparison of efficiency of PD, CAVH, and CAVHD because hemofiltration or continuous hemodiafiltration could be simultaneously performed with PD to obtain similar experimental conditions (systemic hemodynamics, hematocrit, oncotic pressure, and solute blood levels) during the experiments.[10] This study shows that this model is valuable for the comparison of these three procedures for the treatment of hyperammonemia in the neonatal period. The ammonium blood levels in this study were close to those requiring extracorporeal removal in neonates with congenital urea cycle enzymopathies. Lettgen et al.[5] and Thompson et al.[6] described the use of PD or continuous venovenous hemofiltration in neonates with ammonium blood levels of 600 to 700 μmol · L^{-1}. Moreover, as previously described by Ballard et al.[12] in neonates, the induction of hyperammonemia in our model induced a significant rise in glutamine plasma concentrations.

Besides these similarities with the neonatal hyperammonemia, our model allowed the assessment of hemofilters with a filtration surface already used in human neonates with acute renal failure.[13-15] Hemofilters were used with blood flow, plasma flow, and ultrafiltration rates that were comparable with values recorded in neonates treated for acute renal failure by continuous venovenous hemofiltration or CAVH.[6,16] The values for blood flow and ammonium clearances obtained in our study were close to those obtained with CAVH in a neonate with ornithine transcarbamylase deficiency.[17]

The use of CAVHD produced a constant and significant increase in ammonium clearance in comparison with PD; the clearance of ammonium obtained with PD was slightly better than that observed in human neonates.[3, 18] The ammonium clearance obtained with CAVHD in group 2 was significantly higher than that observed with CAVH in group 1, and this result was confirmed when the two procedures were performed in the same animals (group 3); CAVHD allowed a 96% increase in ammonium clearance in comparison with CAVH. This result could be explained by the mechanism of continuous hemodiafiltration, which combines the convective transport of hemofiltration with the diffusive transport of hemodialysis, thus leading to a marked improvement in the removal of solutes with low molecular weight and unbound to plasma proteins.[19]

These data indicate that CAVHD, which has been used safely in children and neonates,[20, 21] was the more efficient method of removing ammonium in our study. This result is important because CAVHD was also the more efficient in clearing glutamine, which has been involved in the mechanisms by which hyperammonemia causes its cerebral toxic effects.[2] Moreover, intermittent hemodialysis, which has been shown to be rapidly effective in neonates with an inborn error of metabolism,[18, 22, 23] frequently induces hypotension[4] and may aggravate brain hypoperfusion, in opposition to CAVHD.

We conclude that continuous hemodiafiltration should be considered in hyperammonemia when peritoneal dialysis is indicated but unfeasible or inefficient. Further studies will be needed to define the benefits of continuous hemodiafiltration for hyperammonemia in infants.

We thank Ms. N. Wittig for valuable technical assistance.

REFERENCES

1. Maestri NE, Hauser ER, Bartholomew D, Brusilow SW. Prospective treatment of urea cycle disorders. J PEDIATR 1991; 119:923-8.
2. Watson AJ, Karp JE, Walker WG, Chambers T, Risch VR, Brusilow SW. Transient idiopathic hyperammonemia in adults. Lancet 1985;2:1271-74.
3. Siegel NJ, Brown RS. Peritoneal clearance of ammonia and creatinine in a neonate. J PEDIATR 1973;82:1044-6.
4. Donn SM, Swartz RD, Thoene JG. Comparison of exchange transfusion, peritoneal dialysis, and hemodialysis for the treatment of hyperammonemia in an anuric newborn infant. J PEDIATR 1979;95:67-70.
5. Lettgen B, Bonzel KE, Colombo JP, et al. Therapy of hyperammonaemia caused by carbamyl-phosphate synthetase deficiency with peritoneal dialysis and haemofiltration. Monatsschr Kinderheilkd 1991;139:612-7.
6. Thompson GN, Butt WW, Shann FA, et al. Continuous venovenous hemofiltration in the management of acute decompensation in inborn errors of metabolism. J PEDIATR 1991; 118:879-84.
7. Sperl W, Geiger R, Maurer H, et al. Continuous arteriovenous hemofiltration in a neonate with hyperammonaemic coma due to citrullinaemia. J Inher Metab Dis 1992;15:158-9.
8. Lieberman KV. Continuous arteriovenous hemofiltration in children. Pediatr Nephrol 1987;1:330-8.
9. Gouyon JB, Petion AM, Huet F, Lallemant C. Urea removal by hemofiltration and hemodiafiltration. Biol Neonate 1994; 65:36-40.
10. Gouyon JB, Desgres J, Mousson C. Removal of branched-chain amino acids by peritoneal dialysis, continuous arteriovenous hemofiltration, and continuous arteriovenous hemodialysis in rabbits: implications for maple syrup urine disease treatment. Pediatr Res 1994;35:357-61.
11. Falk MC, Knight JF, Roy LP, et al. Continuous venovenous haemofiltration in the acute treatment of inborn errors of metabolism. Pediatr Nephrol 1994;8:330-3.
12. Ballard RA, Vinocur B, Reynolds JW, et al. Transient hyperammonemia of the preterm infant. N Engl J Med 1978; 299:920-5.
13. Lopez-herce J, Dorao P, Delgado MA, Espinosa L, Ruza F, Martinez MC. Continuous arteriovenous haemofiltration in children. Intensive Care Med 1989;15:224-7.
14. Bambauer R, Jutzler GA, Philippi H, et al. Hemofiltration and plasmapheresis in premature infants and newborns. Artif Organs 1988;12:20-6.
15. Zobel G, Ring E, Müller W. Continuous arteriovenous hemofiltration in premature infants. Crit Care Med 1989;17: 534-6.
16. Ronco C, Brendolan A, Bragantini L, et al. Treatment of acute renal failure in newborns by continuous arterio-venous hemofiltration. Kidney Int 1986;29:908-15.
17. Ring E, Zobel G, Stöckler S. Clearance of toxic metabolites during therapy for inborn errors of metabolism. J PEDIATR 1990;117:349-50.
18. Wiegand C, Thompson T, Bock GH, Mathis RK, Kjellstrand CM, Mauer SM. The management of life-threatening hyperammonemia: a comparison of several therapeutic modalities. J PEDIATR 1980;96:142-4.
19. Geronemus R, Schneider N. Continuous arteriovenous hemodialysis: a new modality for treatment of acute renal failure. Transactions of the American Society for Artificial Internal Organs 1984;30:610-4.
20. Assadi FK. Treatment of renal failure in an infant by continuous arteriovenous hemodialysis. Pediatr Nephrol 1988;2: 320-2.
21. Bishof NA, Welch TR, Strife F, Ryckman FC. Continuous hemodiafiltration in children. Pediatrics 1990;85:819-23.
22. Rutledge SL, Havens PL, Haymond MW, McLean RH, Kan JS, Brusilow SW. Neonatal hemodialysis: effective therapy for the encephalopathy of inborn errors of metabolism. J PEDIATR 1990;116:125-8.
23. Brewer ED. Rapid removal of blood ammonia by hemodialysis in newborns: successful treatment of 5 infants <4 kg [Abstract]. J Am Soc Nephrol 1990;1:349.

EDITOR'S COLUMN

Use of intravenous lipids in neonates

Reports concluding that lipid emulsions are safe and effective[1, 2] when administered to ill newborn infants contrast sharply with work suggesting that various hazards may be associated with lipid infusion.[3-8] More recent laboratory efforts have been directed to determining the possible sources of undesirable metabolic and pulmonary effects. In a study of lipid peroxidation, different bottles from four batches of a 20% lipid emulsion (Intralipid) marketed in the western United States were found to contain between 214 and 655 μmol lipid hydroperoxide per liter.[7] In this issue of THE JOURNAL, Neužil et al.[8] further document the propensity of lipid emulsions to undergo peroxidation, and show that light accelerates this reaction. Because of variation in LOOH content, the authors selected low LOOH (<16 μmol/L) samples and then investigated the effect of light exposure. Exposure to ambient light increased the LOOH content of the samples from 7 to 10 μmol/L to 60 μmol/L. Phototherapy lights produced significant effects, increasing LOOH content to more than 90 μmol/L in the clinical setting and 600 μmol/L in the more controlled laboratory environment. Protecting the emulsions from light by using aluminum foil or by adding the antioxidant ascorbic acid directly to the bottles eliminated the phototherapy effect.

Physiologic studies in adults have demonstrated deterioration of pulmonary function, including a fall in arterial oxygen saturation, during the infusion of lipid emulsions.[9] These findings have been duplicated in infants.[3] In addition, a nearly tenfold increase in the mortality rate was reported in 4- to 28-day-old infants weighing 600 to 800 gm at birth who were randomly selected to receive 20% Intralipid beginning on the first day of life.[5] Other clinical studies, however, have not demonstrated adverse effects despite apparently adequate sample size.[2] Lipid hydroperoxides or their breakdown products are capable of producing a wide range of biologic injury and are therefore plausible mediators of the toxic effects associated with lipid emulsions.[7, 10] The concentrations of LOOH reported for different bottles and batches of emulsion, even from the same manufacturer, range from 7 to 655 μmol/L.[7, 8] Brand, batch, and bottle differences in LOOH content are therefore a confounding variable and may account for the disparate findings in clinical studies. Until we account for the content of toxic by-products in the preparations studied, it will be impossible to compare studies, predict clinical outcomes, or apply metaanalysis to published clinical trials.

There are several mechanisms by which LOOH could cause lung injury: (1) the aldehydic breakdown products of LOOH bind and inactivate cysteine sulfhydryl groups, which are critical for the action of surfactant protein C[10]; (2) LOOH combines with neutrophil superoxide to produce a potent lipid peroxidation initiator, peroxyl radical, which is also capable of attacking the methionine residue at the active site of α_1-antitrypsin[11]; (3) LOOH produces aberrations in prostanoid and leukotriene synthesis[7]; and (4) LOOH at nanomolar concentrations increases the binding of monocytes to endothelial cells and increases the production of monocyte chemotactic factor, thereby potentially stimulating inflammation.[12] The ability of phototherapy to produce LOOH in lipid emulsions during infusion,[8] combined with the ability of LOOH to modify the production of vasoactive prostanoids,[7] may explain the increased incidence of patent ductus arteriosus and the changes in mesenteric blood flow that have been noted in infants being treated with phototherapy.[13, 14] Lipid emulsions have also been associated with retinopathy of prematurity.[6] That LOOH could induce a cascade of lipid peroxidation in the retina is not surprising given the exquisite sensitivity of docosahexaenoic acid to peroxidation; this fatty acid makes up 30% of retinal lipid. Although all these mechanisms are of interest in understanding the biologic issues involved and also provide fertile areas for research, the practical solution is to take the toxins out of the emulsions.

See related article, p. 785.

LOOH	Lipid hydroperoxide

Clinicians need a lipid preparation free of toxic by-products. Neužil et al.[8] suggest that the addition of ascorbic acid to the emulsions may reduce the formation of LOOH. This proposal could represent an inexpensive and effective option if safety can be demonstrated, but current guidelines of the U.S. Food and Drug Administration might require extensive testing before a reformulated emulsion could be placed on the market, and the addition of ascorbate at the bedside will not remove LOOH produced during manufacture,

THE JOURNAL OF PEDIATRICS 1995;126:747-8

0022-3476/95/$3.00 + 0 **9/21/64031**

storage, and distribution. In our view, one should also consider a manufacturing process that eliminates one of the reactants necessary for the formation of LOOH, namely oxygen. Currently, the production process uses nitrogen in an attempt to remove air. However, nitrogen, being lighter than air, may allow reentry of air into the system. The use of argon, a much heavier inert gas, to degas the emulsion and fill the bottle head space may circumvent this problem and sharply limit the formation of LOOH.

Adequate nutrition for extremely low birth weight infants remains an elusive goal despite extensive research and the development of improved enteral and parenteral formulations. The critically ill neonate is at the greatest disadvantage. Lipids provide essential fatty acids and calories, and improve nitrogen use without an increase in carbon dioxide production that can be associated with high rates of glucose infusion.[15] On the negative side are studies that find an increase in retinopathy of prematurity,[6] bronchopulmonary dysplasia,[4] and mortality rates[5] when infants are given lipid preparations, particularly in the first few days of life. These complications are plausibly related to the content of lipid peroxidation products. The conflicts inherent in this situation are not easily resolved. It may be desirable to protect emulsions from light, particularly phototherapy light, and it is known that lipids should be infused at the slowest possible rate, but most questions remain unanswered. When should lipids be started? Beginning on the first day of life is associated with increased mortality rates for the most fragile infants,[5] beginning on the second or third day is associated with an increase in retinopathy of prematurity,[6] and starting at 7 days of age or later invites nutritional deficiencies. How much lipid should we administer? The need for essential fatty acids can be met with 0.5 gm/kg per day, but this has little effect on caloric needs. Because of the problem with peroxidation products in the emulsions, should we limit the maximum dose to 2.0 or 2.5 gm/kg per day? The clinician is left with questions but no clear answers, and this quandary is unlikely to be resolved without improved emulsions and further clinical trials.

Harold J. Helbock, MD
Department of Molecular and Cell Biology
University of California
Berkeley, CA 94720
Division of Neonatology
Children's Hospital—Oakland
Oakland, CA 94609

Bruce N. Ames, PhD
Department of Molecular and Cell Biology
University of California
Berkeley, CA 94720

REFERENCES

1. Sosenko I, Frank L. Nutritional influences on lung development and protection against chronic lung disease. Semin Perinatol 1991;15:462-8.
2. Gilbertson N, Kovar I, Cox D, Crowe L, Palmer N. Introduction of intravenous lipid administration on the first day of life in the very low birth weight neonate. J PEDIATR 1991;119:615-23.
3. Pereira G, Fox W, Stanley C, Baker L, Schwartz J. Decreased oxygenation and hyperlipidemia during intravenous fat infusions in premature infants. Pediatrics 1980;66:26-30.
4. Cook R. Factors associated with chronic lung disease in preterm infants. Arch Dis Child 1991;66:776-9.
5. Sosenko I, Rodriguez-Pierce M, Bancalari E. Effect of early initiation of intravenous lipid administration on the incidence and severity of chronic lung disease in premature infants. J PEDIATR 1993;123:975-82.
6. Hammerman C, Aramburo M. Decreased lipid intake reduces morbidity in sick premature neonates. J PEDIATR 1988;113:1083-8.
7. Helbock H, Motchnik P, Ames B. Toxic hydroperoxides in intravenous lipid emulsions used in preterm infants. Pediatrics 1993;91:83-8.
8. Neužil J, Darlow B, Inder T, Sluis K, Winterbourn C, Stocker R. Oxidation of parenteral lipid emulsion by ambient and phototherapy lights: potential toxicity of routine parenteral feedings. J PEDIATR 1995;126:785-90.
9. Venus B, Prager R, Patel C, Sandoval E, Sloan P, Smith R. Cardiopulmonary effects of Intralipid infusion in critically ill patients. Crit Care Med 1988;16:587-90.
10. Esterbauer H, Schaur R, Zollner H. Chemistry and biochemistry of 4-hydroxynonenal, malonaldehyde and related aldehydes. Free Radic Biol Med 1991;11:81-128.
11. Chamulitrat W, Cohen M, Mason R. Free radical formation from organic hydroperoxides in isolated human polymorphonuclear neutrophils. Free Radic Biol Med 1991;11:439-45.
12. Chin J, Azhar S, Hoffman B. Inactivation of endothelial derived relaxing factor by oxidized lipoproteins. J Clin Invest 1992;89:10-8.
13. Barefield E, Dwyer M, Cassady G. Association of patent ductus arteriosus and phototherapy in infants weighing less than 1000 grams. J Perinatol 1993;13:376-80.
14. Yao A, Martinussen M, Johansen O, Brubakk A. Phototherapy-associated changes in mesenteric blood flow response to feeding in term neonates. J PEDIATR 1994;124:309-11.
15. Van Aerde J, Sauer P, Pencharz P, Smith J, Heim T, Swyer P. Metabolic consequences of increasing energy intake by adding lipid to parenteral nutrition in full-term infants. Am J Clin Nutr 1994;59:659-62.

CLINICAL AND LABORATORY OBSERVATIONS

Disseminated intravascular coagulation associated with granulocyte colony-stimulating factor therapy in a child with human immunodeficiency virus infection

Brigitta U. Mueller, MD, Richard Burt, MD, Leslie Gulick, MD, Freda Jacobsen, RN, Philip A. Pizzo, MD, and McDonald Horne, MD

From the Pediatric Branch, Clinical Oncology Program, National Cancer Institute, Bethesda, Maryland; the Hematology Service, Department of Clinical Pathology, Warren Grant Magnuson Clinical Center, Bethesda, Maryland; and the Department of Pediatrics, Children's Medical Center of Brooklyn, Brooklyn, New York

We report a case of disseminated intravascular coagulopathy, apparently caused by exposure to granulocyte colony-stimulating factor (G-CSF). The medical records of patients treated for more than 30 consecutive days with subcutaneously administered G-CSF were reviewed for the occurrence of thrombocytopenia or coagulation abnormalities. New-onset thrombocytopenia with a platelet count less than 100 × 10^9 cells/L (<100,000 cells/mm^3) developed in 9 of 23 patients (39%) after a median of 11 weeks of treatment with G-CSF at dosages between 1 and 10 μg/kg per day. (J PEDIATR 1995;126:749-52)

Zidovudine causes neutropenia in 48% of children and adults infected with HIV-1.[1] Recombinant granulocyte colony-stimulating factor is being used successfully in HIV-infected patients with intractable neutropenia who have no other treatment options.[2] However, experience with the long-term use of G-CSF is limited, and new and unexpected side effects may occur. We report a case of disseminated intravascular coagulation, apparently caused by exposure to this growth factor.

CASE REPORT

A boy with vertically acquired HIV infection was initially treated with zidovudine when he was 5½ years of age. However, it had to be discontinued 18 months later because of neutropenia, and he was then treated for a few weeks with zalcitabine, but he continued to have neutropenia.

When first examined at 7 years of age at the Pediatric Branch, National Cancer Institute, the patient was free of symptoms and active infection but had a leukocyte count of 2.0 × 10^9 cells/L (2000 cells/mm^3), with an absolute neutrophil count of 0.28 × 10^9 cells/L (280 cells/mm^3) and an absolute monocyte count of 0.32 × 10^9 cells/L (320 cells/mm^3). His platelet count was 325 × 10^9 cells/L (325,000 cells/mm^3), hemoglobin level 7.5 mmol/L (12.1 gm/dl), absolute $CD4^+$ cell count 0.013 × 10^9 cells/L (13/mm^3; 1%), and serum p24 antigen level 47 pg/ml (limit of detection, 30 pg/ml). He was receiving acyclovir, 200 mg four times a day, as prophylaxis against herpes simplex virus stomatitis and trimethoprim-sulfamethoxazole (60 mg/300 mg) twice daily three times a week as prophylaxis against *Pneumocystis carinii* pneumonia.

The patient was enrolled in a protocol for the treatment of HIV-infected children who have had hematologic toxic effects during zidovudine treatment. Therapy was initiated with G-CSF (provided by Amgen Inc., Thousand Oaks, Calif.) at a dose of 1 μg/kg body weight given as a daily subcutaneous injection, and zidovudine at an oral dose of 180 mg/m^2 every 6 hours.[2] The prophylactic antibiotic therapy was continued. To maintain his ANC between 1.5 × 10^9 and 5.0 × 10^9 cells/L (1500 to 5000 cells/mm^3), the dosage of G-CSF was increased during a period of 6 weeks to 5 μg/kg per day. While receiving this dosage, the patient underwent

ANC	Absolute neutrophil count
APTT	Activated partial thromboplastin time
DIC	Disseminated intravascular coagulation
G-CSF	Granulocyte colony-stimulating factor
HIV	Human immunodeficiency virus
PT	Prothrombin time

Submitted for publication Aug. 18, 1994; accepted Nov. 18, 1994.

Reprint requests: Brigitta U. Mueller, MD, Pediatric Branch, National Cancer Institute, Bldg. 10, Room 13N240, Bethesda, MD 20892.

9/22/62138

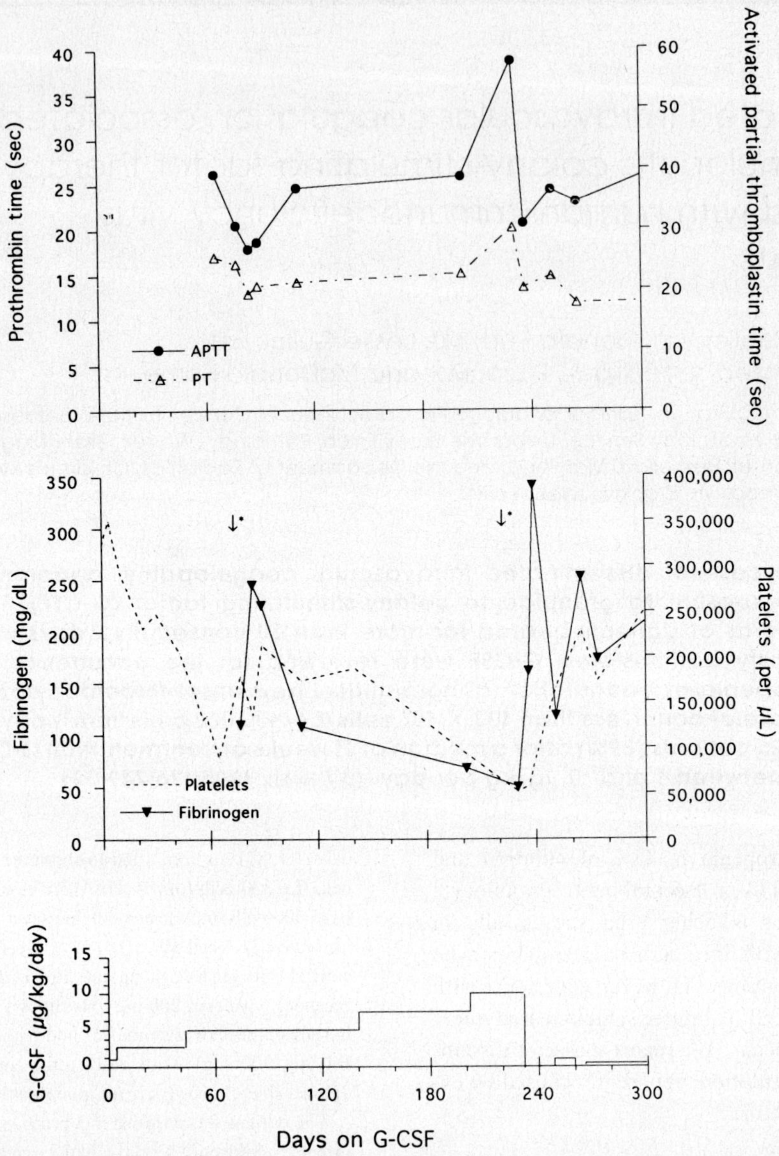

Figure. Platelet count and coagulation values of index patient during therapy with G-CSF. Dosage of G-CSF was between 1 and 10 μg/kg per day, given subcutaneously; after day 260 it was 1 μg/kg every other day. Patient was treated on two occasions with fresh-frozen plasma, cryoprecipitate, and platelet transfusions (↓*).

colonoscopy (Figure; day 77) and a bowel biopsy at another hospital because of chronic diarrhea. He subsequently had bleeding of the lower gastrointestinal tract and received fresh-frozen plasma, cryoprecipitate, and platelet and erythrocyte transfusions. Coagulation tests at that time revealed a prothrombin time of 16.2 seconds (normal, 9.4 to 13.7 seconds), an activated partial thromboplastin time of 30.7 seconds (normal, 22.5 to 34.8 seconds), and a plasma fibrinogen concentration of 3.23 μmol/L (110 mg/dl) (normal, 4.7 to 10.17 μmol/L [160 to 346 mg/dl]).

On day 111 the patient was found to have a plasma fibrinogen level of 3.17 μmol/L (108 mg/dl) with a PT of 14.2 seconds, an APTT of 36.8 seconds, and a platelet count of 174 × 10^9 cells/L (174,000 cells/mm^3), still receiving 5 μg/kg per day of G-CSF. On day 141 the dosage of G-CSF was increased to 7.5 μg/kg per day because of persistent neutropenia, and on day 200 the patient's plasma fibrinogen level was 1.99 μmol/L (68 mg/dl) with a PT of 15.1 seconds, an APTT of 38.7 seconds, and a platelet count of 93 × 10^9/L (93,000 cells/mm^3). Because of an ANC of 0.86 × 10^9 cells/L (860 cells/mm^3), the G-CSF dosage was further increased to 10 μg/kg per day. Throughout this time zidovudine was continued at 180 mg/m^2 every 6 hours.

On day 230 the patient underwent a bone marrow aspiration and biopsy, which showed marked hypercellularity with a left shift in granulocytic maturation. The procedure led to protracted oozing from the puncture site. The patient's fibrinogen level and platelet count had decreased further, and he had multiple coagulation ab-

Table. Coagulation values on day 230 of G-CSF therapy, before blood was given for profuse and protracted bleeding from bone marrow biopsy site

	Patient's value	Normal value
PT (sec)	20.1	9.4-13.7
APTT (sec)	57.8	22.5-34.8
Platelet count (cells/L; cells/mm^3)	52×10^9; 52×10^3	150×10^9-350×10^9; 150×10^3-350×10^3
Plasma fibrinogen (μmol/L; mg/dl)	1.47; 50	4.7-10.1; 160-346
Thrombin time (sec)	37	25-35
Fibrin(ogen) degradation products* (mg/L; μg/ml)	80-160; 80-160	<2; <2
D-Dimer† (mg/L; μg/ml)	16-32; 16-32	<0.5; <0.5
Fibrinogen antigen‡ (gm/L; mg/dl)	0.64; 64	1.8-3.5; 180-350
Thrombin-antithrombin complexes§ (μg/L; ng/ml)	111; 111	1.3-4.0; 1.3-4.0
Plasmin-antiplasmin complexes‖ (μg/L)	3570	120-790
Factor VIII (kU/L)	31	50-150
Prothrombin (kU/L)	51	50-150

*Spli-Prest, Diagnostica Stago, Asnières-sur-Seine, France.
†D-Di Test, Diagnostica Stago.
‡NOR-Partigen Fibrinogen Kit, Behringwerke AG, Marburg, Germany.
§Enzygnost TAT, Behringwerke AG.
‖EIA APP, Behringwerke AG.

normalities (Table). The prolonged PT was only partially corrected by 1:1 mixing with pooled normal plasma, but levels of factors V, VII, IX, X, XI, and XII, and results of liver function tests, were within normal limits. Administration of G-CSF was discontinued on day 232. The zidovudine was replaced with didanosine, 120 mg/m^2 every 8 hours.

On day 237 the patient's PT was 13.5 seconds, APTT was 30.9 seconds, fibrinogen level was 4.73 μmol/L (161 mg/dl), fibrin(ogen) degradation products was 20 to 40 mg/L (20 to 40 μg/ml), and D-dimer was 4 to 8 mg/L (4 to 8 μg/ml), but the platelet count remained low at 58×10^9 cells/L (58,000 cells/mm^3). Because of an ANC of 0.19×10^9 cells/L (190 cells/mm^3), G-CSF was started again at 1 μg/kg per day. However, on day 252 the fibrinogen level had again decreased to 3.47 μmol/L (118 mg/dl), and the PT had risen to 14.8 seconds. The concentration of thrombin-antithrombin complexes was 27 μg/L (27 ng/ml), and that of plasmin-antiplasmin complexes was 2439 μg/L. The platelet count, however, had increased to 165×10^9/L (165,000 cells/mm^3). The therapy with G-CSF was again discontinued. Within 10 days the PT decreased to 11.8 seconds, the fibrinogen rose to 7.41 μmol/L (252 mg/dl) and the concentration of D-dimer was less than 0.5 mg/L (<0.5 μg/ml). The G-CSF was restarted at a dose of 1 μg/kg every other day. At this dose the patient's PT, APTT, and fibrinogen level remained normal; D-dimer level was less than 0.5 μg/ml; and the ANC was maintained greater than 1.0×10^9 cells/L (1000/mm^3).

METHODS

The medical records of all other HIV-infected patients who were treated at our institution for more than 30 consecutive days with subcutaneously administered G-CSF were reviewed for the occurrence of thrombocytopenia or coagulation abnormalities. Patients received G-CSF at a dose of 1 to 20 μg/kg per day administered subcutaneously with the goal of maintaining the ANC between 1.5×10^9 to 5.0×10^9 cells/L (1.5×10^3 to 5.0×10^3/mm^3). The leukocyte and platelet counts were monitored on a regular basis, but because coagulation abnormalities were initially not known to occur, baseline values were not available for all the patients.

RESULTS

Twenty-eight patients were assessable (20 male, 8 female; median age, 9.6 years; range, 0.4 to 20.5 years), and each had been treated according to a protocol for children with previous hematologic toxic effects from zidovudine.[2] Eleven boys had hemophilia A, and several patients had advanced HIV disease. Five patients had preexisting thrombocytopenia, and seven patients had preexisting coagulation abnormalities (other than hemophilia). The patients were treated with G-CSF for a median of 32 weeks (range, 4 to 138 weeks) with individualized doses. Twenty-five treatment regimens included zidovudine, five didanosine, and two lamivudine; three patients continued to receive G-CSF during more than one antiretroviral regimen.

Thrombocytopenia developed in nine patients (39%) after a median of 11 weeks (range, 2 to 28 weeks) of treatment with G-CSF at doses between 1 and 10 μg/kg per day. In five patients a new coagulopathy developed during treatment with G-CSF (increased PT in three; increased APTT in five; increased FDP in two; decreased fibrinogen level in two). Four of the five patients had recurrent chronic pancreatitis or liver dysfunction, which could also have contributed to the coagulation abnormalities. The fifth patient had an unexplained elevation of the APTT (47.9 seconds) and a slightly elevated D-dimer level (1 mg/L, 1 μg/ml). The presence of a lupus anticoagulant was ruled out in all these patients.

DISCUSSION

Therapy with G-CSF for a prolonged period of time has been limited to a small number of patients with aplastic anemia or severe chronic neutropenia.[3, 4] Side effects have been few and include bone pain, elevation of alkaline phosphatase and lactic dehydrogenase levels, acute febrile neutrophilic dermatosis (Sweet syndrome), and one case of acute anaphylaxis.[3-5] Mild thrombocytopenia has been noted occasionally,[2, 3] even in healthy granulocyte donors undergoing leukopheresis after stimulation with G-CSF.[6]

Our patient appears to have had an additional adverse effect of G-CSF, DIC. Because no other possible cause for the coagulopathy (e.g., liver disease, infection, autoimmune phenomena, malignancy, trauma, or pancreatitis) could be identified, the patient's therapy with zidovudine and G-CSF were both discontinued and didanosine therapy was begun. Within a week the coagulopathy had been corrected except for the thrombocytopenia. Within 2 weeks after G-CSF was restarted, the fibrinogen had decreased and thrombin-antithrombin and plasmin-antiplasmin complex, fibrinogen degradation product, and D-dimer levels were again elevated. No other medications had been changed and the patient's general clinical status was otherwise stable. Therefore G-CSF was discontinued for the second time, and the evidence of DIC once more disappeared within 2 weeks.

Thrombocytopenia occurs in 10% to 20% of HIV-infected children and adults,[7] and mild coagulation abnormalities (e.g., prolonged APTT) are seen in patients who have a lupuslike anticoagulant.[8] In our initial analysis of the treatment with G-CSF and zidovudine we attributed the thrombocytopenia to prolonged exposure to a myelosuppressive drug and to progressive HIV disease.[2] On review of the records of 28 other patients who had been treated with G-CSF and various antiretroviral drugs, five more cases of coagulopathy and nine cases of thrombocytopenia were identified. In most instances the abnormalities could have been due to other causes such as pancreatitis, liver dysfunction, opportunistic infections, or HIV infection. In one case, however, no cause was apparent for a prolonged APTT and minimally elevated D-dimer concentration, indicating that mild DIC could have been present.

The bone marrow of patients treated with G-CSF often shows a high percentage of blasts and excessive granules in the immature myeloid cells. Our index patient's bone marrow showed immature myeloid hyperplasia at the height of his DIC. If granulopoiesis is stimulated on a long-term basis by G-CSF, it is conceivable that the disturbed maturation of these cells might lead them to disintegrate in the marrow, thereby releasing thromboplastins, in a manner similar to the mechanism of DIC that commonly occurs with acute promyelocytic leukemia. However, further studies are needed to test this hypothesis.

Our experience with a small number of HIV-infected children treated for a prolonged time with G-CSF underlines the need for continued careful observation to detect previously unknown side effects and to define the optimal dose for the individual patient. Until more is known about the long-term effects, the use of growth factors should be restricted to the patient with no other treatment options who can be followed up regularly.

REFERENCES

1. McKinney RE, Maha MA, Connor EM, et al. A multicenter trial of oral zidovudine in children with advanced human immunodeficiency virus disease. N Engl J Med 1991;324:1018-25.
2. Mueller BU, Jacobsen F, Butler KM, Husson RN, Lewis LL, Pizzo PA. Combination treatment with azidothymidine and granulocyte colony-stimulating factor in children with human immunodeficiency virus infection. J PEDIATR 1992;121:797-802.
3. Dale DC, Bonilla MA, Davis MW, et al. A randomized controlled phase III trial of recombinant human granulocyte colony-stimulating factor (Filgrastim) for treatment of severe chronic neutropenia. Blood 1993;81:2496-502.
4. Bonilla MA, Gillio AP, Ruggeiro M, et al. Effects of recombinant granulocyte colony-stimulating factor on neutropenia in patients with congenital agranulocytosis. N Engl J Med 1989;320:1574-80.
5. Park JW, Mehrotra B, Barnett BO, Baron AD, Venook AP. The Sweet syndrome during therapy with granulocyte colony-stimulating factor. Ann Intern Med 1992;116:996-8.
6. Bensinger WI, Price TH, Dale DC, et al. The effects of daily recombinant human granulocyte colony-stimulating factor administration on normal granulocyte donors undergoing leukapheresis. Blood 1993;81:1883-8.
7. Rigaud M, Leibovitz E, Sin Quee C, et al. Thrombocytopenia in children infected with human immunodeficiency virus: long-term follow-up and therapeutic considerations. J Acquir Immune Defic Syndr 1992;5:450-5.
8. Cohen AJ, Philips TM, Kessler CM. Circulating coagulation inhibitors in the acquired immunodeficiency syndrome. Ann Intern Med 1986;104:175-80.

Association of symptoms with *Helicobacter pylori* infection in children

Siobhan M. Gormally, MD, Nan Prakash, MRCP, Marie T. Durnin, SRN, Leslie E. Daly, PhD, Marguerite Clyne, PhD, Barry M. Kierce, MB, and Brendan Drumm, MD

From the Department of Paediatrics and the Department of Public Health Medicine and Epidemiology, University College Dublin, and Children's Research Centre, Our Lady's Hospital for Sick Children, Dublin, Ireland

The aim of this study was to determine prospectively whether *Helicobacter pylori*–associated gastritis is associated with specific symptoms by evaluating whether these symptoms are relieved by treatment of the infection. Symptoms resolved after the eradication of *H. pylori* in only three of eight children with *H. pylori*–associated gastritis alone, in comparison with all six children with duodenal ulcer disease. (J Pediatr 1995;126:753-6)

Helicobacter pylori is the major cause of chronic gastritis in children.[1-3] Furthermore, *H. pylori* infection of the gastric mucosa determines the natural history of duodenal ulcer disease in children and adults.[4] The relationship of chronic *H. pylori*–associated gastritis to symptoms is controversial.[5] Although several studies have attempted to demonstrate an association between *H. pylori* gastritis in adults and dyspepsia not caused by an ulcer, the relationship is unclear. The high incidence of infection among adult patients makes it difficult to study symptoms in infected as compared with noninfected persons.[6]

Children represent an excellent group in whom to evaluate whether *H. pylori*–associated gastritis is a symptomatic condition. Children in developed countries have a low incidence of infection and fewer confounding causes of gastrointestinal symptoms, thereby making it easier to identify specificity of symptoms.[2] In this study we prospectively evaluated symptoms in children with *H. pylori*–associated gastritis and determined whether these gastrointestinal symptoms were modified by treatment of the infection.

METHODS

Two hundred fifty-six patients underwent upper gastrointestinal endoscopy between May 1991 and March 1993. During each examination two biopsy specimens were obtained from the first part of the duodenum. In addition, two biopsy specimens were taken from the antral mucosa; one was used for a rapid urease test (Clo, Delta West, Bentley, Western Australia), and the second was sent for histologic assessment. If the rapid urease test result was positive (up to 24 hours), the patient was entered into the study. In some of the children a third gastric biopsy specimen was obtained for culture. Children were considered to be infected by *H. pylori* if both the rapid urease test result was positive and the cresyl violet stain demonstrated spiral organisms on the gastric mucosa. After treatment, resolution of infection was confirmed if both test results were negative.

A previously used detailed questionnaire[7] to determine the presence of symptoms was completed by one of us (S. M. G.) for each patient with *H. pylori* infection. The symptoms assessed included the presence of abdominal pain, nocturnal awakening, and vomiting. The presence or absence of epigastric tenderness was also noted. No attempt was made to score the severity of symptoms. A score of 1 point was given for each factor. A maximum score of 4 was therefore attainable.

Histologic examination of biopsy specimens. Gastric and duodenal biopsy specimens were fixed in 10% neutral formalin, embedded in paraffin wax, and cut at 5 μm. The sections were stained with hematoxylin and eosin for light microscopy.

Gastritis was defined according to established histologic criteria with the Sydney classification. Gastritis was classified as acute or chronic or as a special form (e.g., granulomas, eosinophilic infiltration).

Formalin-fixed specimens were stained with cresyl violet to identify *H. pylori*. The organisms were easily identified because of their spiral or curved shape and their unique location beneath and within the layer of mucus on the surface of the gastric mucosa.

Submitted for publication June 28, 1994; accepted Nov. 28, 1994.

Reprint requests: B. Drumm, MD, Children's Research Centre, Our Lady's Hospital for Sick Children, Crumlin, Dublin 12, Ireland.

0022-3476/95/$3.00 + 0 **9/22/62347**

Table. Symptoms and abdominal findings present in children with and those without ulcers

	No. (%) of patients		
	No ulcer (n = 12)	Duodenal ulcer (n = 7)	*p* v
Total with symptoms	10 (83)	7 (100)	NS
Abdominal pain	10 (83)	7 (100)	NS
Nocturnal awakening	3 (25)	5 (71)	<0.05
Epigastric tenderness	5 (42)	4 (57)	NS
Vomiting	6 (50)	4 (57)	NS

NS, Not significant.

Chronic nonspecific duodenitis was defined according to Hasan et al.[8] Duodenitis was characterized by the presence of neutrophils in the lamina propria, crypts, or surface epithelium, and by an increase in the number of mononuclear cells.

All the biopsy specimens were examined by a pathologist who was unaware of the clinical history, endoscopic findings, or the urease test result. Gastric biopsy specimens were cultured as previously described.[9]

Treatment. Treatment for *H. pylori* infection included a combination of colloidal bismuth subcitrate (Denol), one tablet (120 mg) four times a day for 4 weeks, and metronidazole, 20 mg/kg per day (to a maximum of 200 mg three times daily) for 2 weeks. At least 1 month after the completion of treatment, symptoms were reassessed with the same questionnaire. The patients were then immediately reexamined by endoscopy.

Statistical analysis. Results are expressed as mean ± SD or as medians for the symptom scores. Differences between groups were compared by the Wilcoxon rank-sum test or chi-square test as appropriate. Significance of changes within groups were assessed with the sign test.

The study was approved by the ethics committee at Our Lady's Hospital for Sick Children, Dublin. Fully informed parental consent was obtained.

RESULTS

Nineteen children had *H. pylori* infection of the gastric mucosa. The children ranged in age from 6.1 to 14.7 years (mean age ± SD, 11.7 ± 2.5 years). The male/female ratio was 1.4:1. None of these children had a history of alcohol consumption, smoking, or use of nonsteroidal antiinflammatory medication.

Endoscopic features. The gastric mucosa did not appear red or inflamed in any of the children. Nodularity of the antral mucosa was present in 11 (58%) of 19 children with *H. pylori* gastritis. Seven children had duodenal ulcers at endoscopy.

Histology. Histologic evidence of gastritis was present in all 19 children. All the children had chronic gastritis, and acute gastritis was never present. Furthermore, gastric atrophy and intestinal metaplasia did not occur in these children. Nine of the children in the group without ulcers had moderate gastritis, two had mild gastritis, and one had severe gastritis. This was not significantly different from the seven children with ulcers, 6 of whom had moderate gastritis and one mild gastritis. Duodenitis was present in 7 of the 19 children, including 6 of the 7 patients with duodenal ulcer disease, as shown by biopsy specimens of their duodenal mucosa.

Symptoms. The major indication for endoscopy was vomiting in 10 patients, abdominal pain in 7, and possible malabsorption in 2. The prevalence of abdominal pain, vomiting, and epigastric tenderness was similar in both the group with ulcers and the group without ulcers (Table). Nocturnal awakening was the only symptom that helped to distinguish between the two groups ($p < 0.05$) (Table).

Response to treatment. Of the 19 children studied, *H. pylori* was eradicated in 16 of 19 (84%). *H. pylori* was cleared in 10 of 12 (83%) patients with gastritis alone and similarly in 6 (86%) of 7 with gastritis and duodenal ulceration.

Ulcer-free group. In the ulcer-free group, 10 children had symptoms (Table). The two children without symptoms underwent endoscopy to rule out malabsorption.

In 10 of these 12 children, *H. pylori* was cleared from the gastric mucosa after treatment with bismuth and metronidazole. In 8 of the 10 children who had symptoms before treatment *H. pylori* cleared from the gastric mucosa. Of these eight children, 3 (38%) became free of symptoms, which was not statistically significant. One of the children whose *H. pylori* infection failed to clear became free of symptoms despite persistent infection.

The median symptom score before treatment among the 10 children whose *H. pylori* infection subsequently cleared was 1.5. After eradication of *H. pylori* the mean symptom score (0.5) did not differ.

Group with ulcers. In the group with ulcers, the mean age and male/female ratio did not differ from those of the ulcer-free group.

All children had symptoms before treatment. In six of the seven children (88%) *H. pylori* cleared after treatment. In each of these six children, duodenal ulceration had healed at the time of follow-up endoscopy. The median symptom score of these six children was 3.5 before treatment. Symptoms resolved completely in all six patients ($p < 0.05$). The one patient whose *H. pylori* infection failed to clear from the gastric mucosa after treatment continued to have duodenal ulceration and symptoms. The response of symptoms to clearing of *H. pylori* in the group with ulcers (n = 6), in comparison with the ulcer-free group (n = 10), was highly significant ($p < 0.01$).

DISCUSSION

In our study, *H. pylori* gastritis, in the absence of duodenal ulcer disease, did not cause symptoms. After eradication of *H. pylori*, symptoms consistently resolved only in those patients who had duodenal ulcer disease associated with *H. pylori* gastritis. *H. pylori* infection is uncommon among children in developed countries, and therefore specific symptoms are easier to identify. Furthermore, smoking, alcohol use, and nonsteroidal antiinflammatory drug ingestion are usually not confounding variables in children. Some previous studies have suggested that abdominal pain is associated with *H. pylori* infection of the gastric mucosa.[10, 11] This study was specifically designed to determine whether symptoms were cleared when *H. pylori* was eradicated.

There is no validated system for scoring symptoms in children or adults with dyspepsia not caused by ulcers.[12] In a major review of studies of non-ulcer-related dyspepsia in adults, Talley[12] suggested that the duration of symptom-free periods is a better measure than a symptom score. He further notes that this system allows for comparisons between results from different groups. We made no attempt to score the severity of symptoms. We simply assessed the presence or absence of a symptom or clinical finding. We believe that the use of this system strengthens our ability to draw conclusions from the results. We reevaluated the presence or absence of symptoms and epigastric tenderness before reassessment of the children's *H. pylori* status to remove possible observer bias. Our finding that eradication of *H. pylori* infection was associated with clearance of symptoms only if duodenal ulceration was present is similar to the finding of Katelaris et al.[13] in adults. They found an association between symptoms and the presence of peptic ulcer disease, but there was no association between symptoms and *H. pylori* colonization of the gastric mucosa or gastritis. Our findings are also in agreement with an earlier study carried out with our colleagues in Toronto.[7] In that study, symptoms of children who were infected with *H. pylori* could not be differentiated from those of children who were not infected before endoscopy.

Some epidemiologic studies have indicated that *H. pylori* is not a cause of symptoms in children. Serologic studies from the United States and Europe have shown up to 30% of symptom-free children are infected.[5, 14] Furthermore the prevalence of *H. pylori*–specific antibodies in children with recurrent abdominal pain is similar to that in symptom-free children.[14] Infection as assessed by the urea breath test is very uncommon in North American children with recurrent abdominal pain.[10]

Other studies have suggested that *H. pylori* infection may be more common among children with gastrointestinal symptoms.[5, 11] Ashorn et al.[14] found that 22% of children with recurrent abdominal pain were infected with *H. pylori*. However, such studies are impossible to interpret if the prevalence of infection among children in the general population is not included.

Studies in adults also suggest that *H. pylori* gastritis in the absence of ulcer disease is an asymptomatic condition. The prevalence of infection in symptom-free adults is high.[6] In a population-based study in Norway, 36% of a group of symptom-free adults had *H. pylori* colonization of the gastric mucosa.[15] In India 97% of subjects had *H. pylori* colonization in a population-based study.[13] It is not possible to differentiate adult patients with non-ulcer-related dyspepsia who are infected with *H. pylori* from those who are not infected.[5] Abdominal pain occurs with equal frequency in those who have *H. pylori* colonization and those do not.[16] Although treatment of *H. pylori* infection has been reported to provide relief of symptoms in adults with dyspepsia, similar relief was obtained in patients treated identically or with placebo in whom the infection was not cleared.[17]

All the infected children in this study had chronic gastritis. This is a consistent finding in studies of children with *H. pylori* infection. In contrast, adult patients usually have an acute gastritis.

This study suggests that *H. pylori* gastritis in the absence of duodenal ulcer disease is not a cause of symptoms in children. Attention needs to be focused on the possible association between early colonization by *H. pylori* and the subsequent development of gastric cancer.[18] Presently the eradication of *H. pylori* in children without duodenal ulcer disease may not be necessary and should possibly be confined to patients entered into treatment trials. Eradication of *H. pylori* has now to be considered as a major part of the treatment of duodenal ulcer disease in children and in adults.[4]

REFERENCES

1. Drumm B, Sherman P, Cutz E, Karmali M. Association of *Campylobacter pylori* on the gastric mucosa with antral gastritis in children. N Engl J Med 1987;316:1557-61.
2. Drumm B, Perez-Perez GI, Blaser MJ, et al. Intrafamilial clustering of *Helicobacter pylori* infection. N Engl J Med 1990;322:359-63.
3. Drumm B. *Helicobacter pylori* and the pediatric patient. Gastroenterol Clin North Am 1993;22:169-82.
4. Israel D, Hassall E. Treatment and long-term follow-up of *Helicobacter pylori*–associated duodenal ulcer disease in children. J Pediatr 1993;123:53-8.

5. Gormally SM, Drumm B. *Helicobacter pylori* and gastrointestinal symptoms. Arch Dis Child 1994;70:165-6.
6. Dooley CP, Cohen H, Fitzgibbons PL, et al. Prevelance of *Helicobacter pylori* infection and histologic gastritis in asymptomatic persons. N Engl J Med 1989;321:1562-6.
7. Reifen R, Rasooly I, Drumm B, Millson ME, Murphy K, Sherman PM. *Helicobacter pylori* infection in children: is there specific symptomatology? Dig Dis Sci 1994;39:1488-92.
8. Hasan M, Sircus W, Ferguson A. Duodenal mucosal architecture in nonspecific and ulcer-associated duodenitis. Gut 1983;22:637-41.
9. Clyne M, Drumm B. Adherence of *Helicobacter pylori* to primary human gastrointestinal cells. Infect Immun 1993; 61:4051-7.
10. Fiedorek SC, Casteel HB, Pumphrey CL, et al. The role of *Helicobacter pylori* in recurrent, functional abdominal pain in children. Am J Gastroenterol 1992;87:347-9.
11. Ashorn M, Maki M, Ruuska T, et al. Upper gastrointestinal endoscopy in recurrent abdominal pain of childhood. J Pediatr Gastroenterol Nutr 1993;16:273-7.
12. Talley NJ. A critique of therapeutic trials in *Helicobacter pylori*–positive functional dyspepsia. Gastroenterology 1994; 106:1174-83.
13. Katelaris PH, Tippett GHK, Norbu P, Lowe DG, Brennan R, Farthing MJG. Dyspepsia, *Helicobacter pylori* and peptic ulcer in a randomly selected population in India. Gut 1992; 33:1462-6.
14. van der Meer SB, Forget PP, Loffeld RJLF, Stobberingh E, Kuijten RH, Arends JW. The prevalence of *Helicobacter pylori* serum antibodies in children with recurrent abdominal pain. Eur J Pediatr 1992;151:799-801.
15. Bernersen B, Johnsen R, Bostad L, Straume B, Sommer A, Burhol PG. Is *Helicobacter pylori* the cause of dyspepia? BMJ 1992;304:1276-9.
16. Parsonnet J, Blaser MJ, Perez-Perez GI, Hargrett-Bean N, Tauxe RV. Symptoms and risk factors of *Helicobacter pylori* infection in a cohort of epidemiologists. Gastroenterology 1992;102:41-6.
17. Patchett S, Beattie S, Leen E, Keane C, O'Morain C. Eradicating *Helicobacter pylori* and symptoms of non-ulcer dyspepsia. BMJ 1991;303:1238-40.
18. The Eurogast Study Group. An international association between *Helicobacter pylori* and gastric cancer. Lancet 1993; 341:1359-62.

Use of the gonadotropin-releasing hormone agonist triptorelin in the diagnosis of delayed puberty in boys

Giorgio Zamboni, MD, Franco Antoniazzi, MD, and Luciano Tatò, MD

From the Department of Pediatrics, Endocrine Unit, University of Verona, Italy

To differentiate gonadotropin deficiency from delayed puberty in teenage boys, 0.1 mg/m² of triptorelin, a gonadotropin-releasing hormone agonist, was administered subcutaneously at 4 AM. Serum gonadotropins and testosterone levels were determined at baseline and 4 hours after the injection. The increase in blood gonadotropin and testosterone levels was significantly greater in patients with delayed puberty than in those with gonadotropin deficiency. (J PEDIATR 1995;126:756-8)

Distinguishing between constitutional delayed puberty and gonadotropin deficiency is difficult in teenage boys.[1,2] Evaluation of the gonadotropin and testosterone response to a single test dose of nafarelin, a gonadotropin-releasing hormone agonist, can distinguish delayed puberty from gonadotropin deficiency in teenage years.[2] We propose use of a modified test with triptorelin, a synthetic GnRH analog, that differs from natural GnRH in that it has D-tryptophan in place of L-glycine in position 6 in the peptide chain (D-trp[6]–luteinizing hormone–releasing hormone).

FSH	Follicle-stimulating hormone
GnRH	Gonadotropin-releasing hormone
LH	Luteinizing hormone

Submitted for publication Oct. 20, 1994; accepted Nov. 28, 1994.
Reprint requests: Giorgio Zamboni, MD, Clinica Pediatrica dell'Università, Policlinico Borgo Roma, 37134 Verona, Italy.

0022-3476/95/$3.00 + 0 **9/22/62353**

METHODS

Eighteen male subjects with constitutional delayed puberty were examined. They showed absence of pubertal de-

Table I. Clinical characteristics of study patients and control subjects

	Patients		Control subjects	
	Delayed puberty (n = 18)	Gonadotropin deficiency (n = 10)	Prepubertal (n = 16)	Pubertal (n = 15)
Chronologic age (yr)	15.8 ± 0.6 (15.0-17.0)	16.8 ± 1.1 (15.2-18.9)	9.3 ± 0.9 (6.9-11.0)	17.5 ± 0.4 (16.8-18.0)
Bone age (yr)	13.0 ± 0.7 (11.5-14.1)	14.6 ± 1.1 (13.8-17.0)	9.1 ± 1.2 (6.7-10.5)	17.3 ± 0.3 (16.5-18.0)
Height (cm)	151.6 ± 7.6 (140.8-169.2)	158.2 ± 7.0 (145.0-170.6)	132.6 ± 5.7 (118.7-140.0)	173.6 ± 4.4 (170.0-182.0)
Target height (cm)	171.4 ± 5.1 (163.0-182.0)	170.2 ± 4.6 (164.0-177.0)	172.9 ± 5.8 (160.0-185.0)	174.2 ± 4.0 (170.0-182.0)
Testicular volume (ml)	3.1 ± 0.8 (2-4)	2.8 ± 0.7 (2-4)	2.2 ± 0.4 (2-3)	20.9 ± 2.9 (16-25)
Penis length (cm)	5.8 ± 1.2 (4-8)	5.2 ± 1.5 (2.5-7.5)	5.1 ± 0.8 (4-7)	12.7 ± 0.8 (11-14)

Data are means ± SD (range).

Table II. Gonadotropin and testosterone levels before and after triptorelin treatment in study patients and control subjects

	Patients		Control subjects	
	Delayed puberty (n = 18)	Gonadotropin deficiency (n = 10)	Prepubertal (n = 16)	Pubertal (n = 15)
LH (IU/L)				
Pretreatment	1.6 ± 0.7 (0.1-2.6)	0.5 ± 0.6 (0.05-1.7)	0.8 ± 0.7 (0.05-2.9)	5.0 ± 0.8 (3.5-6.8)
Posttreatment	22.8 ± 7.8* (13.5-38.1)	4.0 ± 2.6 (0.1-8.6)	3.8 ± 2.2 (0.1-8.8)	21.3 ± 1.6 (19.1-23.9)
FSH (IU/L)				
Pretreatment	2.2 ± 1.0 (0.8-4.5)	1.2 ± 1.1 (0.05-3.0)	1.7 ± 0.6 (0.7-2.9)	3.7 ± 0.7 (2.3-5.2)
Posttreatment	11.6 ± 4.6† (2.9 ± 18.2)	3.5 ± 1.8 (0.5-5.8)	13.4 ± 2.9† (9.1-18.8)	16.5 ± 0.9 (15.0-18.0)
Testosterone (nmol/L)				
Pretreatment	1.0 ± 0.6 (0.3-3.1)	0.7 ± 0.3 (0.17-1.7)	0.3 ± 0.17 (0.13-0.7)	20.8 ± 3.1 (12.1-26.0)
Posttreatment	3.4 ± 1.7*,‡ (1.0-9.0)	0.7 ± 0.7 (0.17-2.4)	0.7 ± 0.3 (0.17-1.3)	26.3 ± 1.3 (22.5-27.7)

Data are means ± SD (range).
*Significant (p <0.01) versus patients with gonadotropin deficiency and prepubertal control subjects.
†Significant (p <0.01) versus patients with gonadotropin deficiency.
‡Significant (p <0.01) versus pretreatment value.

velopment at a chronologic age of 15.0 years or older, but clear pubertal signs developed within 12 months from the start of the study, clinically confirming the diagnosis of delayed puberty. Ten patients with gonadotropin deficiency were studied, including four with panhypopituitarism, two who had undergone surgically removal of craniopharyngioma, and four with Kallmann syndrome. Sixteen normal prepubertal children examined for supposed micropenia or small testicles and 15 normal pubertal volunteers served as control subjects. Informed consent was obtained from the patients or their guardians.

The basal blood levels of luteinizing hormone, follicle-stimulating hormone, and testosterone were determined at 8 AM, on day 1. On day 2, at 4 AM, 0.1 mg/m^2 of triptorelin (Decapeptyl, Ipsen-Biotech, Paris, France) was administered subcutaneously and blood samples for LH, FSH, and testosterone were collected 4 hours after injection. The timing of the injection and blood sampling was chosen on the basis of a previous study with five normal adult volunteers, showing gonadotropin peaks 4 hours after triptorelin administration. The blood samples were kept frozen at −30° C until simultaneously assayed in duplicate.

Serum LH and FSH concentrations were determined by an immunoenzymefluorometric assay, with the Stratus II fluorometric analyzer. The commercial kits were obtained from Baxter Diagnostics Inc., Deerfield, Ill. The mean intraassay and interassay coefficients of variation were 2.8% and 5.3%, respectively, for LH and 2.6% and 4.3%, respectively, for FSH. Serum testosterone level was determined by radioimmunoassay with a commercially available kit obtained from Diagnostic Systems Laboratories, Webster, Tex. Statistical analysis was performed with unpaired and paired two-tailed Student t test; the significance of changes was determined by analysis of variance.

RESULTS

There were no differences in clinical characteristics between subjects affected by delayed puberty and those with gonadotropin deficiency (Table I). After triptorelin administration serum LH, FSH, and testosterone levels increased in subjects with delayed puberty and this increase was greater than in patients with gonadotropin deficiency ($p < 0.01$ for all values) (Table II). Blood LH increase in boys with delayed puberty was comparable to that of pubertal control subjects, whereas in patients with gonadotropin deficiency it was comparable to that of prepubertal control subjects.

Serum FSH level increase in boys with delayed puberty was comparable to that of prepubertal control subjects, and in both groups of subjects, it was much greater than that found in patients with gonadotropin deficiency ($p < 0.01$). Serum testosterone levels rose significantly only in boys with delayed puberty ($p < 0.01$, before vs after treatment).

DISCUSSION

The majority of children with delayed puberty are boys with constitutional delay of growth and puberty. It is difficult to distinguish this common and benign condition from true gonadotropin deficiency[1, 2] despite the variety of endocrine tests developed for this purpose.[3-8] There is evidence that gonadotropin synthesis is greater in teenaged boys with delayed puberty than in those with gonadotropin deficiency,[2] but virtually all previous tests show overlap between the two groups.

Normally, pituitary gonadotropic cells undergo a priming by endogenous GnRH. In gonadotropin deficiency, such a priming is insufficient[9, 10] and the gonadotropic cells need additional pharmacologic priming before a response to GnRH can be elicited. Teenaged boys with delayed puberty were distinguished from those with gonadotropin deficiency by stimulating gonadotropin secretion with a single injection of nafarelin. Prepubertal control subjects were not included in that original study[2]; in addition, the test lasted 24 hours and included frequent blood sampling. Our modifications make the test simpler because only two blood samples are required. For practical purposes the triptorelin injection could be made at 8 AM and blood drawn at noon.

The results of our study confirm that GnRH agonists can stimulate gonadotropin secretion and can differentiate delayed puberty from gonadotropin deficiency. After triptorelin injection, the patients with gonadotropin deficiency showed blood gonadotropins and testosterone significantly lower than those reached by subjects with delayed puberty. There was overlap in the FSH and testosterone responses between the two groups. Only LH values did not overlap among patients in either group.

In conclusion, persons with constitutional delayed puberty, with a bone age greater than 11½ years, show an increase in LH level after triptorelin stimulation, which distinguishes them from patients with gonadotropin deficiency. The triptorelin test could be an important screening tool to exclude gonadotropin deficiency in boys with delayed puberty; it appears to be simple, effective, relatively inexpensive, and well tolerated.

REFERENCES

1. Ibanez L, Potau N, Zampolli M, et al. Use of leuprolide acetate response patterns in the early diagnosis of pubertal disorders: comparison with the gonadotropin-releasing hormone test. J Clin Endocrinol Metab 1994;78:30-5.
2. Ehrmann DA, Rosenfield RL, Cuttler L, Burstein S, Cara JF, Levitsky LL. A new test of combined pituitary-testicular function using the gonadotropin-releasing hormone agonist nafarelin in the differentiation of gonadotropin deficiency from delayed puberty: pilot studies. J Clin Endocrinol Metab 1989; 69:963-7.
3. Cohen HN, Wallace AM, Beastall GH, Fogelman I, Thomson JA. Clinical value of adrenal androgen measurement in the diagnosis of delayed puberty. Lancet 1981;1:689-92.
4. Dunkel L, Pertheentupa J, Sorva R. Single versus repeated dose human chorionic gonadotropin stimulation in the differential diagnosis of hypogonadotropic hypogonadism. J Clin Endocrinol Metb 1985;60:333-7.
5. Moshang JrT, Marx BS, Cara JF, Snyder P. The prolactin response to thyrotropin-releasing hormone does not distinguish teenaged males with hypogonadotropic hypogonadism from those with constitutional delay of growth and development. J Clin Endocrinol Metab 1985;61:1211-3.
6. Santen RJ, Kulin HE, Loriaux DL, Friend J. Spironolactone stimulation of gonadotropin secretion in boys with delayed adolescence. J Clin Endocrinol Metab 1976;43:1386-90.
7. Savage MO, Preece MA, Cameron N, et al. Gonadotropin response to LHRH in boys with delayed growth and adolescence. Arch Dis Child 1981;56:552-6.
8. Wagner TOF, Brabant F, Warsch F, Hesch RD, Van Zur Muhlen A. Pulsatile gonadotropin-releasing hormone treatment in idiopathic delayed puberty. J Clin Endocrinol Metab 1986;62:95-101.
9. Crowley JrWF, Beitins IZ, Vale W, et al. The biologic activity of a potent analogue of gonadotropin-releasing hormone in normal and hypogonadotropic men. N Engl J Med 1980; 302:1052-7.
10. Partsch CJ, Hermanussen M, Sippell WG. Differentiation of male hypogonadotropic hypogonadism and constitutional delay of puberty by pulsatile administration of gonadotropin-releasing hormone. J Clin Endocrinol Metab 1985;60:1196-203.

Relationship of growth hormone deficiency and leukemia

Robert Rapaport, MD, Sharon E. Oberfield, MD, Leslie Robison, PhD, Sonia Salisbury, MD, Raphael David, MD, Jayashree Rao, MD, and Geoffrey P. Redmond, MD

From the University of Medicine and Dentistry—New Jersey Medical School and Children's Hospital of New Jersey, Newark; New York University School of Medicine, New York; University of Minnesota, Minneapolis; Dalhousie University, Halifax, Nova Scotia, Canada; Louisiana State University, New Orleans; and The Department of Pediatrics, Foundation for Developmental Endocrinology, Beachwood, Ohio

The use of growth hormone (GH) has been implicated as a possible risk factor for leukemia. We present data from six patients that support a working hypothesis that an increased risk of leukemia may exist in patients with GH deficiency not related to exogenous use of GH. (J Pediatr 1995;126:759-61)

Although treatment with growth hormone has generally been considered safe, there has been concern regarding a possible increased risk of leukemia in patients who have received GH therapy.[1, 2] In a recent summary report the relative risk of leukemia in pituitary GH recipients compared with the general population was 2.5.[1] One of us[3] has previously reported cases of leukemia in two children with GH deficiency who were never treated with GH. We now report the occurrence of leukemia without exposure to exogenous GH in a total of six patients: three patients with classic GH deficiency, one with partial GH deficiency, and two with panhypopituitarism.

METHODS

The clinical and hormonal data of the six patients described in this report are presented in the Table. None received GH treatment. Three of the six patients had classic GH deficiency, as defined as a peak stimulated GH level of less than 7 ng/ml. One patient (No. 6) had partial GH deficiency (peak GH, between 7 and 10 ng/ml); her subsequent growth rate was normal without GH treatment. In two patients (Nos. 3 and 4) with panhypopituitarism, formal GH testing was not performed. Both had multiple pituitary deficits indicating a degree of pituitary damage, which, in view of their primary tumors and therapy, would almost certainly have caused GH deficiency. In one of them (patient 4) a somatomedin C level was 0.19 μg/ml, which was compatible with GH deficiency. Four of our patients (Nos. 1, 3, 4, and 5) had CNS tumors, which were treated with radiation. Of these four, one (patient 3) had a craniopharyngioma. The time of onset of leukemia ranged from 1½ to 5½ years after initial diagnosis. Four of the six patients had acute lymphocytic leukemia; one each had nonlymphocytic leukemia or acute myelogenous leukemia.

The absence of data regarding the number of children with untreated GH deficiency in the population from which the reported cases were derived does not allow us to quantify how our findings compare with the occurrence of leukemia in the general population. To obtain a general idea of the size of a nontreated population with GH deficiency required to observe the number of cases of leukemia reported, we used the age-, sex-, and race-specific leukemia incidence rates from the National Cancer Institute's Surveillance, Epidemiology and End Results Program[4] and the characteristics of the population of GH-treated children from the National Collaborative Growth Study (Genentech Inc., South San Francisco, Calif.). Assuming that the population with GH deficiency has the same incidence of leukemia as the general population, we estimated that approximately 55,000 person-years of follow-up (i.e., 5500 nontreated children with GH deficiency followed up for an average of 10 years) would be required, to expect to observe one case of leukemia. This expected figure can be used as a reference point for the observed cases presented in this report.

ALL	Acute lymphocytic leukemia
AML	Acute myelogenous leukemia
GH	Growth hormone
IGF-1	Insulin-like growth factor–1

Submitted for publication Oct. 10, 1994; accepted Dec. 21, 1994.
Reprint requests: Sharon E. Oberfield, MD, New York University Medical Center, 550 First Ave., New York, NY 10016.

0022-3476/95/$3.00 + 0 9/22/62893

Table. Clinical and hormonal data

Patient No.	Sex	Race	Age (yr) Primary diagnosis	Age (yr) Leukemia Dx	Radiation dose (cGy)	Type of leukemia	Primary diagnosis	GH* (ng/ml)
1	M	White	0.8	4	4960	ALL	Astrocytoma	4.6
2	F	White	1.2	6	None	ALL	Optic nerve hypoplasia	2.8
3	F	White	12.5	15.5	5000	NLL	Craniopharyngioma	†
4	F	White	13.3	19	3000	ALL	Germinoma	†
5	M	White	19.5	21	5040	AML	Meningioma	3.5
6	F	Black	1.0	3.0	None	ALL	Idiopathic GH deficiency	8.7

NLL, Nonlymphocytic leukemia.
*Peak GH to provocative stimulation tests (including arginine HCl, L-dopa, insulin, and clonidine).
†Formal test for GH was not done but patient had adrenocorticotropic hormone, thyroid stimulating hormone, and gonadotropin deficiencies.

DISCUSSION

In addition to these six patients, we are aware of three other patients with leukemia who had GH deficiency but who had not received any hormone treatment.[2] These findings raise the possibility that GH deficiency rather than treatment with GH may be related to the development of leukemia.

The effects of GH on the hemopoietic and immune systems have recently been reviewed.[5] Blatt et al.[6] reported that only supraphysiologic doses of GH resulted in increased human leukemic lymphoblast colony formation. Most other authors have demonstrated increased leukemic cell proliferation in response to exposure to GH.[7] Human marrow granulopoiesis in vitro was enhanced by GH but inhibited by anti–insulin-like growth factor–1 receptor antibodies, suggesting that paracrine effects of IGF-1 mediated the GH effect.[8] Zadik et al.[9] studied the effects of GH and IGF-1 on bone marrow cells derived from five children with ALL and four children with AML, and on peripheral blood cells of three patients with chronic myelogenous leukemia during remission with use of a blast colony formation assay. Both GH and IGF-1 increased blast colony numbers in a dose-dependent fashion in eight of nine patients with ALL and AML. Growth hormone and IGF-1 did not increase peripheral blood blast colony formation in the patients with chronic myelogenous leukemia.

One of us[10] has suggested that the proliferative responses to GH may depend on the GH status of the subjects tested. The responses to phytohemagglutanin of peripheral blood lymphocytes derived from most normal children were decreased by the addition of GH, whereas peripheral blood lymphocytes derived from children with GH deficiency during treatment with GH had greater spontaneous and phytohemagglutinin-stimulated proliferation than did the cells of the normal children.

Forty occurrences of leukemia in children undergoing GH therapy have been reported since 1987 (reference 11; D. Frasier: personal communication).[11] Fradkin et al.[1] suggested that a 2.5-fold increase in risk of leukemia occurred in patients with GH deficiency who were treated with GH. However, there also seemed to be an increased association of leukemia in patients who had the primary diagnosis of craniopharyngioma. Further, the role of other risk factors, such as radiation exposure, could not be discounted. Recently the suggestion was made that growth failure may be an initial sign of Fanconi anemia. In children with early Fanconi anemia the development of leukemia may be related to the unrecognized underlying disease state rather than the treatment with GH.[12]

The prevalence of GH deficiency in the general population is not known, although Lindsay et al.[13] suggested that the prevalence in Utah is at least one in 3480 persons. The number of untreated children with GH deficiency in the general population is also unknown. Although we believe that the number of persons in the population who have GH deficiency and do not receive treatment is not large, it is not possible to determine with any level of precision how the cases of leukemia described here compare with the expected occurrence in the general population.

We estimated that approximately 5500 untreated children with GH deficiency followed up for an average of 10 years would be required, to expect to observe one case of leukemia (see Methods). Accordingly, for the six observed cases the population at risk would need to consist of a cohort providing approximately 330,000 person-years of follow-up. If we restrict the number of cases to four patients with documented GH deficiency, then 220,000 person-years would be needed. If we excluded patient 6, who, although found to have partial GH deficiency subsequently grew at a normal velocity without treatment, then 165,000 persons per year would be needed. We believe, however, that patient 6 should be included, because it is not unlikely that patients with similar GH profiles would have been treated with GH before long-term follow-up may have revealed a normal growth rate. The cause of leukemia risk is confounded by the four patients who had treatment-induced GH deficiency as a result of their previous malignancy and who had received radiation therapy. Children treated for cancer have an increased risk of having a second malignant neoplasm.[14] Moreover, children treated for CNS tumors are at an increased risk of acute leukemia.[15] Because of the small number of reported cases and the high correlation between treatment of CNS tumors, treatment-induced GH deficiency, and risk of secondary leukemia, it is not possible to determine the contribution of the initial cancer and its treatment independent of GH deficiency. However, if we consider the two cases of non-malignancy-associated GH deficiency, the estimates indicate that the population at risk would need to include approximately 110,000 person-years, or 11,000 untreated children with GH deficiency followed up for an average of 10 years, to expect to observe two cases of leukemia (assuming general population rates). Because of the small expected number (i.e., two cases), this estimate is associated with a large range of potential error, and the population at risk could be as small as 9500 person-years before reaching a 95% level of confidence that the excess risk is not greater than 1.

These crude estimates assume that the characteristics (age, sex, race) of untreated children with GH deficiency are similar to those of treated children with GH deficiency. It could be argued that this is not the case and that untreated children with GH deficiency include a higher proportion of nonwhite children with GH deficiency. Use of the incidence rates for treated children, however, represents a conservative approach because black children in the general population have a lower incidence of leukemia.[4]

There is increasing evidence that the endocrine system, and GH in particular, is linked with the hematopoietic and immune systems. Further, the use of GH has been implicated as a possible risk factor for leukemia. Although confounding factors are present and data are limited, our cases support a working hypothesis that there may be an increased risk of leukemia in patients with GH deficiency that is not related to exogenous use of GH.

REFERENCES

1. Fradkin JE, Mills JL, Schonberger LB, et al. Risk of leukemia after treatment with pituitary growth hormone. JAMA 1993; 270:2829-32.
2. Watanabe S, Mizuno S, Oshima L, Tsunematsu Y, Fujimkoto J, Komkiyama A. Leukemia and other malignancies among GH users. J Pediatr Endocrinol 1993;6:99-109.
3. Redman GP, Shu S, Norris D. Leukemia and growth hormone. Lancet 1988;1:1335.
4. Ries LAG, Hankey BF, Mioller BA, Hartman AM, Edwards BK. Cancer statistics review: 1973-88. Bethesda, Md: National Cancer Institute, 1991, National Institutes of Health publication 91-2789.
5. Rapaport R. Effect of growth hormone on immune functions. In: Gupta D, Wollman HA, Fedor-Freybergh, eds. Pathophysiology of immune-neuroendocrine communication circuit. Heidelberg: Springer-Verlag, 1994;91-131.
6. Blatt J, Wenger S, Stitely S, Lee P. Lack of mitogenic effects of growth hormone on human leukemic lymphoblasts. Eur J Pediatr 1987;146:257-60.
7. Estrov Z, Meir R, Barak Y, Zaizov R, Zadik Z. Human growth hormone and insulin-like growth factor-1 enhance the proliferation of human leukemic blasts. J Clin Oncol 1991;9:394-9.
8. Mercha S, Tatarsky J, Hochberg Z. Enhancement of human granulopoiesis in-vitro by biosynthetic insulin-like growth factor 1/somatomedin C and human growth hormone. J Clin Invest 1988;81:791-7.
9. Zadik Z, Estrov Z, Karov Y, Hahn T, Barak Y. The effect of growth hormone and IGF-1 on clonogenic growth of hematopoietic cells in leukemic patients during active disease and during remission: a preliminary report. J Pediatr Endocrinol 1993;6:79-83.
10. Rapaport R, Oleske J, Ahdieh H, et al. Effects of human growth hormone on immune function: in-vitro studies in cells of normal and growth hormone deficient children. Life Sci 1987;41:2319-24.
11. Shalet SM. Leukemia in children treated with growth hormone. J Pediatr Endocrinol 1993;6:109-11.
12. Butturini A, Bernasconi S, Izzi G, Gertner JM, Bale RP. Short stature, Fanconi's anaemia and risk of leukemia after growth hormone therapy. Lancet 1994;34:1576.
13. Lindsay RM, Feldkamp M, Harris D, Robertson J, Rallison M. Utah Growth Study: growth standards and the prevalence of growth hormone deficiency. J PEDIATR 1994;125:29-35.
14. Meadows AT, Baum E, Fossati-Bellani F, et al. Second malignant neoplasms in children: an update of the Late Effects Study Group. J Clin Oncol 1985;3:532-8.
15. Tucker MA, Meadows AT, Boice JD, Hoover RN, Fraumeni JF. Cancer risk following treatment of childhood cancer. In: Fraumeni JF, Boice JD, eds. Radiation carcinogenesis: epidemiological and biological significance. New York: Raven Press, 1983:211-24.

Permanent heterotopic ossification at the injection site after diphtheria-tetanus-pertussis immunizations in children who have fibrodysplasia ossificans progressiva

Thomas F. Lanchoney, BS, Randolph B. Cohen, MD, David M. Rocke, PhD, Michael A. Zasloff, MD, PhD, and Frederick S. Kaplan, MD

From the Departments of Orthopedic Surgery, Pediatrics, and Genetics, University of Pennsylvania School of Medicine, Philadelphia, and the Graduate School of Management, University of California, Davis

In patients who have fibrodysplasia ossificans progressiva, routine childhood diphtheria-tetanus-pertussis immunizations administered by intramuscular injection caused a significant risk of permanent heterotopic ossification at the site of injection ($p < 10^{-8}$), whereas measles-mumps-rubella immunizations administered by subcutaneous injection posed no significant risk. Intramuscular injections should be avoided, if possible, once a diagnosis of fibrodysplasia ossificans progressiva has been established. (J PEDIATR 1995;126:762-4)

Fibrodysplasia ossificans progressiva is an extremely rare, disabling, heritable disorder of connective tissue characterized by congenital malformation of the great toes[1, 2] and by progressive heterotopic ossification of tendons, ligaments, fasciae, and skeletal muscle,[3, 4] which begin during childhood.[2, 5-7] Fibrous nodules appear in soft connective tissues[7] and herald impending ossification at an anatomic site. Nodules mature through an endochondral process to form permanent foci of heterotopic bone that bridge and immobilize adjacent joints. Heterotopic ossification may be exacerbated by soft tissue injury, surgical trauma, intramuscular injections, or dental therapy.[2] Autosomal dominant transmission has been documented,[3] but the genetic defect remains unknown.

We surveyed and examined the patient-members of the International Fibrodysplasia Ossificans Progressiva Association (IFOPA) who were 21 years of age or younger, to determine the risk of heterotopic bone formation that resulted from childhood immunizations.

Supported in part by grants from the International Fibrodysplasia Ossificans Progressiva Association and the National Institutes of Health.

Submitted for publication Oct. 25, 1994; accepted Dec. 13, 1994.

Reprint requests: Frederick Kaplan, MD, Department of Orthopedics, Hospital of the University of Pennsylvania, Silverstein Two, 3400 Spruce St., Philadelphia, PA 19104.

0022-3476/95/$3.00 + 0 **9/22/62713**

METHODS

A survey requesting information about patients' immunization histories was mailed to the 32 patient-members of the IFOPA 21 years of age or younger. These 32 patients comprised more than 40% of all patients in the United States known to have FOP and more than 90% of all patients in the United States who were 21 years of age or younger.[5] The survey asked for information concerning the administration of childhood immunizations, whether any FOP disease flare-ups resulted from the immunizations, the type(s) of immunization and route of administration that were temporally associated with the flare-up, and a detailed description of the flare-up. The patients were requested to verify information with pediatricians, parents, family members, or caretakers. Detailed medical records were available regarding the times and anatomic locations of new heterotopic ossification events dating back to early childhood in all patients. Follow-up was attempted in person or by telephone with all surveyed members. Members who did not return the form could not be contacted, and no follow-up was possible. The study was designed to determine the incidence of heterotopic ossification events resulting directly from immunizations in patients who had FOP, and the type of vaccine or route of administration that may have been associated with an ossification event.

DTP	Diphtheria-tetanus-pertussis
FOP	Fibrodysplasia ossificans progressiva

The survey was sent to FOP patients who were 21 years of age or younger because this subgroup of all FOP patients would be expected to have considerably better recall and more accurate records of their immunization history than the older patient-members of the IFOPA. Patient confidentiality was guaranteed in public reporting of all results.

Two of us (M. A. Z. and F. S. K.) conducted personal follow-up interviews with 19 of the 23 children who responded to the survey, including all six of the children in whom ossification developed after the immunization and 12 of the 16 children who were fully immunized but who did not have a flare-up as a result of the diphtheria-tetanus-pertussis immunization.

Exact hazard rates for ossification of the elbow-arm and knee-thigh regions were calculated from the results of the joint survival data of Rocke et al.[1] on the basis of the hypothesis that the reactions to immunization leading to ossification would have occurred within x days of injection. The annual rate of ossification for the elbow-arm region is 0.042 (joint with constant hazard), and for the knee-thigh region at age 2 years is 0.005 (joint with increasing hazard).[1] The chance of ossification of one or the other or both is less than or equal to the sum of these, or 0.047. Because the event initiating ossification occurred within 1 day of the immunization in all cases, one may use the daily hazard rate: $0.047 \div 365 = 0.0001$. The chance of three or more such events in 22 is (under the null hypothesis that the ossification had no causal relationship to the immunization that preceded it) less than 10^{-8}.

RESULTS

The postal survey was returned by 23 of the 32 patients (72%). Seven male (30%) and 16 female patients, ranging in age from 15 months to 21 years (mean age, 11 years) participated. Twenty-two of the 23 patients (96%) had received intramuscular childhood immunizations with the DTP vaccine. Sixteen of the 22 patients (73%) reported no complications after the injections; six patients (27%), all female, reported flare-ups of the FOP at the injection site within 6 hours of having received the immunization (expected occurrences, 0.0001; $p < 10^{-8}$).

In all six patients reporting flare-ups, new bone formation developed at the injection site within 6 weeks of the immunization, as verified by detailed medical records and roentgenograms. Three of the six patients reported no loss of joint mobility as a result of the heterotopic ossification; the other three patients reported permanent loss of joint motion. In one patient restrictive ossification developed about the elbow after an immunization in the arm, and in two patients restrictive ossification developed about the knee after an immunization in the thigh. All six patients implicated the DTP immunization as the cause of the flare-up. None of the 22 immunized patients reported an ossification event as a result of a subcutaneous measles-mumps-rubella immunization (expected occurrences, 0.0001; not significant).

DISCUSSION

Minor injection site reactions occur commonly after DTP immunizations,[8] but clinically significant ossification at the injection site in the 80.1 million children immunized from 1978 to 1990 has not been reported.[9] Our study indicates that routine intramuscular administration of DTP vaccines to children who have FOP poses significant risk of inciting heterotopic ossification at the site of injection. The postal survey may have introduced methodologic biases. The nine patient-members who did not return the questionnaire might have been involved in litigation involving alleged vaccine injuries and failed to respond on legal advice, may not have had sufficient technical help by family or caretakers to respond, did not wish to respond, or never received the survey. Reliance on the memory of patients and family members, and use of old immunization records, may have also introduced bias into the data, but detailed medical records and roentgenograms were available for confirmation in all cases. Additionally, recall bias may have involved events that were forgotten, although it is unlikely that a patient would have forgotten a complication such as permanent heterotopic ossification. We believe that the young patients in this study were representative of young patients who have the disease and that determination of heterotopic ossification events was accurate.

The diagnosis of FOP can be established readily by the presence of congenital malformation of the great toes together with roentgenographic evidence of progressive heterotopic ossification in characteristic locations.[2, 5, 7] The appearance of subfascial nodules in a child who has bilateral malformation of the great toes, even before the roentgenographic appearance of heterotopic ossification, strongly suggests the diagnosis of FOP and underscores the need for restraint in the administration of intramuscular injections.[4]

Although all states mandate immunizations for children entering school, exemptions from state immunization requirements exist. According to the Centers for Disease Control and Prevention, all 50 states, the District of Columbia, and Puerto Rico permit medical exemption from vaccination.[10, 11] Therefore legal requirements for immunization can be avoided in children who have FOP.

Presently, three vaccines, DTP, *Haemophilus influenzae* type b, and hepatitis B vaccine, are recommended for intramuscular use only.[12] However, a modified subcutaneous administration could be considered. Hepatitis B vaccine, for example, produces lower titers when given subcutaneously.

No other risk from this route of administration is apparent, and extra doses might overcome any problem with lower titers. Tetanus toxoid is recommended for administration with diphtheria toxoid and pertussis but can be administered subcutaneously.[13] The surveyed 27% prevalence (95% confidence interval, 8% to 44%) of heterotopic ossification developing after intramuscular DTP immunizations in children who have FOP must be balanced against the unknown risk of not immunizing these children and leaving them vulnerable to infectious disease.[11, 14] Intramuscular immunization of children who have FOP presents a unique dilemma to parents, pediatricians, and family practitioners; the risk of disabling heterotopic ossification must be balanced against the risk of life-threatening infectious disease in the nonimmunized child.

We recommend avoiding intramuscular immunizations in patients who have FOP until safe alternate routes of administration become available. The risk/benefit ratio of routine intramuscular immunizations must be considered in the context of the family and community setting for each child who has FOP.

REFERENCES

1. Rocke DM, Zasloff M, Peeper J, Cohen RB, Kaplan FS. Age and joint specific risk of initial heterotopic ossification in patients who have fibrodysplasia ossificans progressiva. Clin Orthop Rel Res 1994;301:243-8.
2. Connor JM, Evans DAP. Fibrodysplasia ossificans progressiva: the clinical features and natural history of thirty-four patients. J Bone Joint Surg 1982;64-B:76-83.
3. Kaplan FS, McCluskey W, Hahn G, Tabas JA, Muenke M, Zasloff M. Genetic transmission of fibrodysplasia ossificans progressiva: a report of a family. J Bone Joint Surg 1993;75-A:1214-20.
4. Kaplan FS, Tabas JA, Gannon FH, Finkel G, Hahn GV, Zasloff MA. The histopathology of fibrodysplasia ossificans progressiva: an endochondral process. J Bone Joint Surg 1993; 75-A:220-9.
5. Cohen RB, Hahn GV, Tabas JA, et al. The natural history of fibrodysplasia ossificans progressiva: a study of forty-four patients. J Bone Joint Surg 1993;75-A:215-9.
6. Kaplan FS, Tabas JA, Zasloff MA. Fibrodysplasia ossificans progressiva: a clue from the fly? Calcif Tiss Int 1990;47:117-25.
7. Rogers JG, Geho WB. Fibrodysplasia ossificans progressiva: a survey of forty-two cases. J Bone Joint Surg 1979;61-A:909-14.
8. Cody CL, Baraff LJ, Cherry JD, Marcy SM, Manclark CR. Nature and rates of adverse reactions associated with DTP and DT immunizations in infants and children. Pediatrics 1981; 86:650-60.
9. Howson CP, Howe HJ, Fineberg HV, eds. Adverse effects of pertussis and rubella vaccines. Washington, DC: National Academy Press; 1991:193.
10. Department of Health and Human Services. State immunization requirements 1991-1992. Atlanta: Public Health Service, Centers for Disease Control and Prevention, 1992.
11. Peter G. Current concepts: childhood immunizations. N Engl J Med 1992;327:1794-800.
12. Centers for Disease Control and Prevention. General recommendations on immunization: guidelines from the Immunization Practices Advisory Committee. Ann Intern Med 1989; 111:133-42.
13. Plotkin SA, Mortimer EA. Vaccines. Philadelphia: WB Saunders; 1988:58.
14. Gardner P, Schaffner W. Current concepts: immunization of adults. N Engl J Med 1993;328:1252-8.

Dysmorphic features in patients with complex glycerol kinase deficiency

Angela Scheuerle, MD, Frank Greenberg, MD, and Edward R. B. McCabe, MD, PhD

From the Department of Molecular and Human Genetics and the Department of Pediatrics, Baylor College of Medicine, Houston, Texas

Complex glycerol kinase deficiency is a contiguous gene syndrome consisting of a deletion of the glycerol kinase locus, together with the genes for adrenal hypoplasia congenita or Duchenne muscular dystrophy or both. We describe an

Supported by National Institutes of Health training grant 5 T32 GM07526-16 and by the Baylor Mental Retardation Research Center, Houston, Tex.

Submitted for publication Aug. 30, 1994; accepted Nov. 15, 1994.

Reprint requests: Angela Scheuerle, MD, Division of Medical Genetics, Department of Pediatrics, University of Texas Medical School, Houston, 6431 Fannin St., Room 3144, Houston, TX 77030.

0022-3476/95/$3.00 + 0 **9/22/62075**

infant with complex glycerol kinase deficiency and mildly dysmorphic features similar to those seen in other patients, including an "hourglass" appearance of the middle of the face; hypertelorism; rounded palpebral fissures; esotropia; wide, flattened earlobes; and a downturned mouth. The combination of medical history and characteristic facies should prompt the request for specific laboratory tests diagnostic for this potentially treatable condition. (J PEDIATR 1995; 126:764-7)

Complex glycerol kinase deficiency results from the contiguous deletion on Xp21 of all or part of the gene for glycerol kinase together with that for adrenal hypoplasia congenita and/or Duchenne muscular dystrophy.[1] The patients typically have historical, physical, and laboratory findings consistent with each of these diseases. DMD adversely affects motor development and longevity but does not cause severe, life-threatening problems in infancy.[2] Isolated GKD can lead to reversible electroencephalographic and intellectual impairment, particularly in the face of a high fat intake or prolonged fasting.[3] The condition may be managed with relative ease by reducing the fat (and therefore glycerol intake) in the diet.[1, 3] All patients with DMD and GKD have had significant developmental delays. The component of complex GKD that requires emergent treatment is the adrenal hypoplasia and insufficiency.[4] Reported deaths in these patients have all occurred as a result of addisonian crisis.[1]

AHC	Adrenal hypoplasia congenita
DMD	Duchenne muscular dystrophy
GK	Glycerol kinase
GKD	Glycerol kinase deficiency

To date, more than 30 cases of complex GKD have been reported.[1] The clinical findings in 20 of these cases have been reviewed.[5, 6] Abnormalities include delays in growth and development, abnormal genitalia, and osteoporosis. Unusual facial features such as strabismus, hypertelorism, and "drooping mouth" are mentioned in some of the patients, but the reports are not consistent. We describe an infant with newly diagnosed complex GKD who had a striking facial similarity to other patients. The recognition of the typical facial features may aid in early diagnosis and treatment of complex GKD.

CASE REPORT

A white boy was born at term after an uneventful pregnancy to a 32-year-old woman (gravida 3, para 2, aborta 1) who received good prenatal care. Delivery was induced because of late heartbeat decelerations. Apgar scores were 6 and 8 at 1 and 5 minutes, respectively. He was taken to the neonatal nursery but was transferred later to the neonatal intensive care unit because of apnea, cyanosis, and feeding problems. He was noted persistently to be very pale. The mother and her siblings were all noted to have glucosuria, but none had had diabetes diagnosed. The parents' older child was a healthy 4-year-old girl. The mother's serum cholesterol concentration was reported to be 6.5 mmol/L (250 mg/dl), and the father's was 5.6 mmol/L (215 mg/dl).

Birth weight was 3.040 kg (50th percentile), length was 48.9 cm (50th percentile), and head circumference was 35.6 cm (90th percentile). Other facial measurements included the following: inner canthal distance, 17.5 mm (20th percentile); outer canthal distance, 57.5 mm (20th percentile); ears, 3.5 cm (40th percentile); and philtrum, 1 cm. Examination revealed a pale male infant with slightly upslanting palpebral fissures, a straight nose, and a triangular face (Figure). Results of heart and lung examinations were normal. There was no abdominal organomegaly, and male genitalia were normal, with testes descended bilaterally. Muscle tone was decreased, but the normal neonatal reflexes were present. The skin had no birthmarks or unusual pigmentation.

Feeding problems continued. Tracheoesophageal fistula and palatal cleft were ruled out. Computed tomographic scan of the brain revealed no structural deformity or mass lesion.

Findings of routine electrolyte analyses of the patient at 2 days of age were normal. After parenteral nutrition with lipid emulsion was begun, triglyceride levels were 7.22 gm/L (722 mg/dl) (normal, .02 to 1.5 gm/L). After lipid administration was discontinued, plasma triglyceride levels remained greater than normal and ranged from 3.8 to 5.4 gm/L. Measurements of other plasma levels were as follows: cholesterol, 4.6 mmol/L (178 mg/dl) (normal, 1.3 to 3.1 mmol/L); high-density lipoprotein 1.29 mmol/L (50 mg/dl) (normal, 1 to 1.9 mmol/L); aspartate aminotransferase, 565 IU/L (normal, 35 to 140 U/L); alarine aminotransferase, 328 IU/L (normal, 6 to 50 IU/L); and γ-glutanyl transferase, 152 IU/L (normal, 10 to 160 IU/L).

At 13 days of age, the patient's body became limp, apnea developed, and his heart monitor revealed ventricular tachycardia. Electrolyte analysis showed metabolic acidosis (bicarbonate, 8 mmol/L) with sodium level, 124 mmol/L; potassium level, 10 mmol/L; and chloride level, 101 mmol/L. Venous lactate and ammonia values were normal. Resuscitation included administration of bicarbonate, calcium, glucose, and insulin, and resulted in some normalization of electrolyte values.

Urine organic acid analysis revealed a high urine glycerol level (normally undetectable). Serum creatine kinase level was 13,500 IU/L (normal, 60 to 305 IU/L). Routine peripheral blood lymphocyte chromosome analysis showed a 46,XY normal male karyotype at the 550-band level. Fluorescence–in situ hybridization analysis revealed a deletion of the GK gene in the patient and his mother but not in his sister. Results of molecular genetic studies

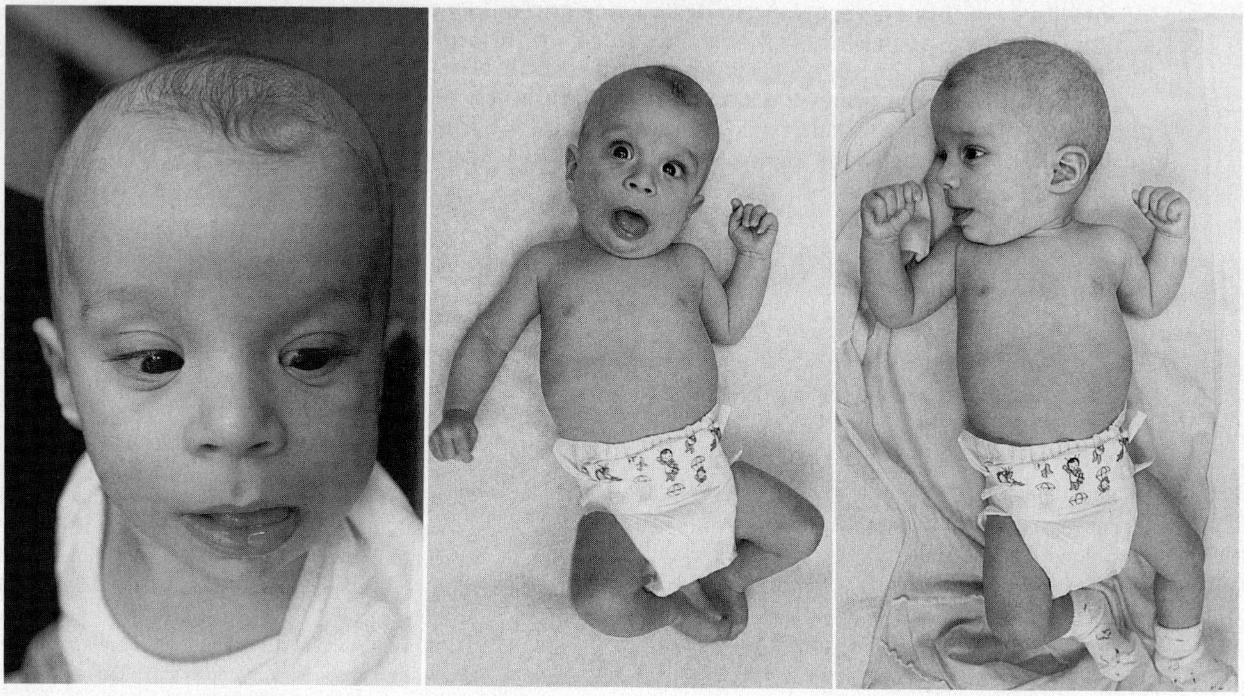

Figure. Three views of patient at 4 months of age. Note hourglass appearance of midfacial region; wide, flat earlobes; and general hypotonia.

were consistent with a deletion involving the adrenal hypoplasia congenita, GK, and DMD loci.

The patient remained in the hospital a total of 6 weeks; discharge was delayed by feeding difficulty. At home he received daily oral glucocorticoid (hydrocortisone) and mineralocorticoid (fludrocortisone) replacements and sodium chloride supplementation for maintenance. His parents were instructed in manipulation of his steroid doses in response to illness or other stress. When he was reexamined at 4 months of age, his height and weight were at the 10th percentile for age and his head circumference was at the 50th percentile. His diet consisted of a standard infant formula, and his interim health had been good except for one afebrile upper respiratory infection. Developmentally he was already showing signs of delay, because he had only poor head control and was not yet rolling over, pushing up when prone, or sitting with support. He was noted to have mildly dysmorphic facial features reminiscent of previously described patients with complex GKD. He did not have any pigmentation changes.

DISCUSSION

Patients with complex GKD have features of each of the individual genes involved in the contiguous gene deletion syndrome. By definition, all patients have loss of the GK locus together with one or more closely flanking genes, most frequently AHC and DMD. Much larger deletions, extending to include the ornithine transcarbamylase locus, have also been described.[7] The clinical manifestations in patients with complex GKD can be nonspecific, as evidenced by the apnea and feeding problems during the first day of life in our patient; however, life-threatening adrenal insufficiency may develop as a result of deletion of AHC gene. This condition is manifested as hyperkalemia and hyponatremia, but the loss of glucocorticoid function may also lead to hypoglycemia. Therefore prompt clinical recognition and management of complex GKD would benefit these patients.

Recognition of the distinct dysmorphic facies associated with complex GKD is one way of facilitating the clinical diagnosis of this disorder. The most prominent facial features are the forehead and eyebrows, and the root and bridge of the nose, which combine to give an "hourglass" appearance to the midfacial region. Other facial characteristics are hypertelorism; rounded palpebral fissures; esotropia; wide, flattened ear lobes; and a downturned mouth. The observation that all the patients with complex GKD, even those in different ethnic groups, have similar facies leads us to conclude that this combination of features is characteristic of complex GKD; however, they are subtle and might not be easily recognizable as a distinct dysmorphic syndrome.

Other historic and clinical features of complex GKD should assist in the recognition of the syndrome. This is an X-linked disorder, and nearly all the patients have been male.[8] Many of the patients with complex GKD have had failure to thrive and short stature.[5] Abnormal genitalia, including anorchia and cryptorchidism, are frequently seen.[5, 9] Neurologic abnormalities include spasticity with weakness and a peculiar, repetitive "handwashing" motion similar to that demonstrated by girls with Rett syndrome (unpublished observation by one of us [E.R.B.M.]). Pathologic fractures have been observed in association with radiologic findings of osteoporosis. Patients with AHC deletions may have addisonian pigmentation and features of hypogonadotrophic hypogonadism.[9, 10] All the patients with involvement of the GK and DMD loci have had significant psychomotor retardation.[11] Female carriers may also have mild to moderate mental retardation.[6] Duchenne muscular dystrophy and the milder Becker muscular dystrophy each has been reported in persons with complex GKD whose deletions included the DMD locus. Abnormalities in the ocular expression of the DMD gene product, dystrophin, are associated with vision impairment, protanomalous color blindness, and an abnormal electroretinogram, a combination of findings referred to as Oregon eye disease,[12] which is a condition similar to but with a different cause from that of Åland Island eye disease.[13]

Adrenal hypoplasia congenita, suggested by electrolyte imbalances, may be diagnosed by subnormal response of serum cortisol levels to exogenous administration of adrenocornotropic hormone and by decreased levels of gonadotropins. A deficiency in GK results in glyceroluria and hyperglycerolemia. Direct analysis of glycerol levels is available, but an increased serum glycerol level may be suspected in the face of extraordinarily high triglyceride levels. This phenomenon of "pseudodypertriglyceridemia" is an artifact of the test for triglycerides, which is based on the measurement of free glycerol.[1] Initial laboratory evaluation for Duchenne muscular dystrophy should include measurement of serum creatine kinase.

Routine chromosome analysis may reveal a large deletion. Direct DNA analysis of the DMD gene can evaluate the presence or absence of each of the known exons. Fluorescence–in situ hybridization studies can be used to demonstrate deletions of the GK gene in both affected male patients and female carriers. Specific probes for the flanking genes, AHC and DMD, are being developed. All these molecular genetic tests can be used for prenatal diagnosis with chorionic villus sampling or amniocentesis.

We conclude that the diagnosis of complex GKD may be delayed because the most prominent clinical findings (developmental delay, short stature, and osteoporosis) may not become apparent until later. We describe what may be a characteristic facies associated with complex GKD that should aid in early diagnosis and prophylactic treatment.

We thank Dr. Lisa Shaffer for the cytogenetic analyses, Drs. Antonio Baldini and Elizabeth Lindsay for the fluorescence–in situ hybridization assays, and the patients, their families, and their physicians for their helpfulness.

REFERENCES

1. McCabe ERB. Disorders of glycerol metabolism. In: Scriver CR, Beaudet AL, Sly WS, Valle D, eds. The metabolic and basis of inherited disease 5th ed. New York: McGraw-Hill 1994;16:1652.
2. Zellweger H, Niedermeyer E. Central nervous system manifestations in childhood muscular dystrophy (CMD) I. Ann Paediat 1965;205:25-42.
3. Ginns EI, Barranger JA, McClean SW, et al. A juvenile form of glycerol kinase deficiency with episodic vomiting, acidemia, and stupor. J Pediatr 1984;104:736-9.
4. Kohlschütter A, Willig HP, Schlamp D, et al. Infantile glycerol kinase deficiency: a condition requiring prompt identification: clinical, biochemical, and morphological findings in two cases. J Pediatr 1987;146:575-81.
5. Wise JE, Matalon R, Morgan AM, McCabe ERB. Phenotypic features of patients with congenital adrenal hypoplasia and glycerol kinase deficiency. Am J Dis Child 1987;141:744-7.
6. Fries M, Lebo R, Schonberg S, et al. Mental retardation locus in Xp21 chromosome microdeletion. Am J Med Genet 1993;46:363-8.
7. Hammond J, Howard NJ, Brookwell R, Purvis-Smith S, Wilcken B, Hoogenraad N. Proposed assignment of loci for X-linked adrenal hypoplasia and glycerol kinase genes [Letter]. Lancet 1985;1:54.
8. Bartley JA, Miller DK, Hayford JA, McCabe ERB. Concordance of X-linked glycerol kinase deficiency with X-linked congenital adrenal hypoplasia. Lancet 1982;2:733-6.
9. Zachmann M, Illig R, Prader A. Gonadotropin deficiency and cryptorchidism in three prepubertal brothers with congenital adrenal hypoplasia. J Pediatr 1980;97:255-7.
10. Goonewardena P, Dahl N, Ritzen M, van Ommen GJ, Pettersson U. Molecular Xp deletion in a male: suggestion of a locus for hypogonadotropic hypogonadism distal to the glycerol kinase and adrenal hypoplasia loci. Clin Genet 1989;35:5-12.
11. Davies KE, Patterson M, Kenwrick SM, et al. Fine mapping of glycerol kinase deficiency and adrenal hypoplasia within Xp21 on the short arm of the human X chromosome. Am J Med Genet 1988;29:557-64.
12. Davies KE, Mandel J-L, Monaco AP, Nussbaum RL, Willard HF. Report of the Committee on the Genetic Constitution of the X Chromosome. Cytogenet Cell Genet 1991;58:853-966.
13. Alitalo T, Kruse TA, Forsius H, Eriksson AW, de la Chapelle A. Localization of the Åland Island eye disease locus to the pericentromeric region of the X chromosome by linkage analysis. Am J Hum Genet 1991;48:31-8.

THE BOOK SHELF **André D. Lascari,** *Editor*

Book review

Sickle cell disease: basic principles and clinical practice

Embury S, Hebbel R, Mohandas N, Steinberg M, eds. New York: Raven Press, 1994. 902 pages. $145.

This is a very large, comprehensive, albeit expensive, treatise with 81 contributors (15 pediatric hematologists and a foreword by Linus Pauling). The 59 chapters are organized into seven sections. Two sections cover the biochemistry of sickle hemoglobin, erythrocyte membranes, and red cell metabolism. Chapters in the section on pathophysiology include vascular modulation, regulation of fetal hemoglobin, pathogenesis of vasoocclusion and hemolytic anemia, and the immune deficit.

The fourth section of the book discusses the origin and dispersion of the sickle cell gene, sickle cell trait, sickle cell disease in Africa, compound heterozygous states, and the natural history in children and adults. Clinical laboratory diagnosis, laboratory values, and prenatal diagnosis are presented in the section on diagnosis.

The largest section, clinical considerations, consists of 17 chapters individually covering all the organ systems, as well as neonatal screening, psychosocial issues, growth and development, and obstetric and gynecologic issues.

Therapeutic considerations are covered in chapters discussing health care maintenance, treatment of pain, nursing care, transfusion therapy, iron overload, and surgery and anesthesia. Pharmacologic modulation of fetal hemoglobin, bone marrow transplantation, gene therapy, and development of drug therapy are the concluding chapters.

The text is well illustrated with figures and tables and includes 16 color plates. A minor criticism is the absence of caution regarding respiratory isolation of patients admitted with aplastic crisis, and avoidance of exposure to pregnant health care personnel unless they are known to be immune to the parvovirus 19.

Overall, this is an excellent repository of the state of knowledge of the biochemical, clinical, and therapeutic aspects of sickle cell disease; controversial issues are identified and opposing opinions are presented in a dispassionate discourse. The book surpasses the several other recently published texts devoted solely to sickle cell disease and is highly recommended for all medical school, hospital, and pediatric and medicine department libraries.

André D. Lascari, MD
Children's Hospital
Albany Medical College
Albany, NY 12208

Effect of pulse dexamethasone therapy on the incidence and severity of chronic lung disease in the very low birth weight infant

Beverly S. Brozanski, MD, Judith G. Jones, BSN, RNC, Carol H. Gilmour, MD, Michael J. Balsan, MD, Roger L. Vazquez, MD,[a] Barbara A. Israel, MD,[b] Beverley Newman, MD,[c] Francis B. Mimouni, MD,[d] and Robert D. Guthrie, MD[e]

From the Divisions of Neonatology and Radiology, Department of Pediatrics, University of Pittsburgh, Pittsburgh, Pennsylvania

We conducted a prospective, randomized, double-blind trial to assess the efficacy and safety of pulse doses of dexamethasone on survival without supplemental oxygen in very low birth weight infants at high risk of having chronic lung disease. Seventy-eight infants with birth weights ≤1500 gm who were ventilator dependent at 7 days of postnatal age were randomly assigned to receive pulse doses of dexamethasone, 0.5 mg/kg per day, divided twice daily (n = 39), or an equivalent volume of saline solution placebo (n = 39), for 3 days at 10-day intervals until they no longer required supplemental oxygen or assisted ventilation, or reached 36 weeks of postmenstrual age. At study entry, the groups did not differ by birth weight, gestational age, or severity of lung disease. At 36 weeks of postmenstrual age, there was both a significant increase in survival rates without oxygen supplementation (*p* = 0.03) and a significant decrease in the incidence of chronic lung disease (*p* = 0.047) in the group that received pulse therapy. Supplemental oxygen requirements were less throughout the study period in the group that received repeated pulse doses of dexamethasone (*p* = 0.013). The total numbers of deaths and the durations of supplemental oxygen, ventilator support, and hospital stay did not differ between groups. Recorded side effects in the pulse therapy group were minimal and included an increase in the use of insulin therapy for hyperglycemia (*p* <0.05). We conclude that in this population of very low birth weight infants, treatment with pulse doses of dexamethasone resulted in improvement in pulmonary outcome without clinically significant side effects. (J Pediatr 1995;126:769-76)

Supported by grants from the Magee-Women's Health Foundation Research Fund and the GCRC/National Institutes of Health 5M01RR00084.

Presented in part at the Society for Pediatric Research, Washington, D.C., May 1993.

Submitted for publication Aug. 22, 1994; accepted Dec. 5, 1994.

Reprint requests: Beverly S. Brozanski, MD, Department of Pediatrics, Division of Neonatology, Magee-Womens Hospital, 300 Halket St., Pittsburgh, PA 15213-3180.

[a]Now at Pediatric and Neonatal Associates, Western Pennsylvania Hospital, Pittsburgh, PA 15224.

[b]Now at Department of Pediatrics, Mercy Hospital of Pittsburgh, Pittsburgh, PA 15219.

[c]Now at Department of Radiology, Children's Hospital of Pittsburgh, Pittsburgh, PA 15213.

[d]Now at Department of Pediatrics, Maimonides Medical Center, Brooklyn, NY 11219.

[e]Now at Allegheny General Hospital, Pittsburgh, PA 15212.

0022-3476/95/$3.00 + 0 **9/23/62529**

The use of dexamethasone therapy in various dosing regimens to prevent or ameliorate chronic lung disease in the very low birth weight infant is widespread in the practice of neonatology. Short-term dexamethasone therapy has been shown to decrease oxygen and ventilator requirements and improve pulmonary mechanics, but is associated with exacerbations requiring a return to pretreatment ventilator support after dexamethasone therapy has been discontinued.[1] Conventional long-term dexamethasone therapy also has resulted in improvement in both pulmonary function and gas exchange.[2, 3] However, multiple side effects have been associated with long-term steroid therapy, including hypertension,[4] growth failure,[5] left ventricular hypertrophy,[6] ischemic brain injury,[7] and an increased rate of infection.[8]

In children with steroid-responsive inflammatory disease, pulse dosing regimens have been found to be clinically effective and to be associated with fewer side effects.[9, 10] Therefore we designed a prospective, double-blind, placebo-controlled, randomized clinical trial to examine the clinical effects of repeated 3-day pulses of dexamethasone therapy in preterm infants at high risk of CLD. We hypothesized that repeated pulses of dexamethasone would increase survival without supplemental oxygen, decrease the severity of lung disease, and minimize clinical side effects.

CLD	Chronic lung disease
F_{IO_2}	Fraction of inspired oxygen
GA	Gestational age
IVH	Intraventricular hemorrhage
LVH	Left ventricular hypertrophy
VLBW	Very low birth weight

METHODS

Study design. Infants with birth weights ≤1500 gm who required ventilator support at 7 days of postnatal age were eligible for recruitment. Infants with complex congenital anomalies, pulmonary hypoplasia, or hemodynamic instability were excluded from the study. After informed consent was obtained, patients enrolled in the study were randomly assigned to receive either pulse doses of dexamethasone or saline solution placebo. Randomization, achieved by use of a random numbers table, was stratified according to sex and birth weight (<1000 gm vs ≥1000 gm). Treatment allocation was recorded on cards enclosed in sequentially numbered envelopes that were kept in the pharmacy department and were available only to the pharmacist who selected the next envelope and distributed the assigned study drug.

Beginning at 7 days of postnatal age, study infants received either pulse doses of dexamethasone (0.25 mg/kg per dose) or an equivalent volume of saline solution intravenously twice daily for 3 days. Courses of study drug were repeated every 10 days until the infant reached 36 weeks of postmenstrual age, or the infant no longer required ventilator support or supplemental oxygen. Total exposure to pulse doses of dexamethasone was dependent on gestational age and the clinical course of each infant. For example, an infant at 32 weeks of GA would be eligible for only two courses, whereas an infant at 25 weeks of GA would be eligible for a maximum of seven courses of study drug. An occasional dose of study drug was administered as an intramuscular injection when intravenous access was not possible.

This research protocol was approved by the human research review and experimentation committee at Magee-Womens Hospital.

Clinical care of infants. Clinical care was performed at the discretion of the neonatology attending physicians, who remained unaware of patient group assignment. For all infants, supplemental oxygen and mechanical ventilation were adjusted to maintain an arterial oxygen tension of 60 to 80 mm Hg or oxygen saturation within 93% to 96% (Nellcor pulse oximeter, Nellcor, Inc., Haywood, Calif.). Ventilator support was provided with a pressure-limited ventilator (Sechrist Industries, Inc., Anaheim, Calif.). Infants were given therapy with surfactant (Exosurf Neonatal, Burroughs Wellcome, Research Triangle Park, N.C.; Survanta, Ross Laboratories, Columbus, Ohio; or Infasurf, ONY, Amherst, N.Y.) in a rescue mode if they had an alveolar-arterial oxygen tension difference <0.22. Blood gas measurements and chest radiographs were obtained as clinically indicated. At 1 month of postnatal age and 36 weeks of postmenstrual age, chest radiographs of all study infants were obtained.

Nutritional and metabolic support followed our nursery routine, which included introduction of parenteral nutrition (Trophamine, Kendall McGaw Inc., Irvine, Calif., and 20% Intralipid, Kabi Pharmacia Inc., Clayton, N.C.) by day 3 of life; this regimen was then advanced according to clinical and laboratory findings. Enteral feeding was introduced by days 5 to 7 of life and advanced during 7 to 10 days as tolerated. Caloric intake was adjusted to maintain an average weight gain of 10 to 20 gm/day. Fluid intake was not restricted unless clinical signs of pulmonary edema developed. Transfusion of packed erythrocytes was used to maintain the capillary hematocrit at greater than 0.38 while the infants required mechanical ventilation. Diuretics, bronchodilators, and methylxanthines were used to improve pulmonary function as clinically indicated. Because of our experience of observing growth failure and cardiac hypertrophy with the use of long-term dexamethasone therapy,[6] routine therapy for CLD in our nursery did not include long-term, continuous steroid treatment. Glucocorticoids were not available to study infants under any other dosing regimen until after 36 weeks of postmenstrual age.

Table I. Maternal demographics

	Pulse doses of dexamethasone	Placebo
Age (yr)	24.8 ± 1	26.5 ± 1
Corticosteroids	8/39	9/39
Hypertension	6/39	6/39
Chorioamnionitis	13/39	14/39
Delivery mode (vaginal: cesarean section)	22:17	24:15
Illicit drug use	3/39	9/39

Outcome criteria. Pulmonary outcome variables included the following: (1) survival without supplemental oxygen, analyzed both at 1 month of postnatal age and 36 weeks of postmenstrual age, and (2) severity of lung disease, which was assessed by mean airway pressure, requirement for supplemental oxygen, and total duration of positive-pressure ventilation, oxygen therapy, and hospitalization. Oxygen therapy was analyzed as a continuous variable before and after each course of study drug, and as a dichotomous variable for days of oxygen supplementation with fraction of inspired oxygen ≥0.30. This value of supplemental oxygen was chosen as a point of comparison between the two groups as an indicator of readiness for discharge.

Clinical surveillance. The medical records were reviewed to obtain the following data: supplemental oxygen and ventilator requirements on the day before and the day after each 3-day treatment course; total days of assisted ventilation and supplemental oxygen; days of supplemental oxygen with FiO_2 ≥0.30; use of exogenous surfactant; air leak; mean arterial pressure; hyperglycemia (defined as serum glucose concentration of >8.3 mmol/L [150 mg/dl] or Dextrostix [Miles Laboratory, Elkhart, Ind.] >13.9 mmol/L [250 mg/dl] with glycosuria); sepsis (defined as a positive blood culture result) or pneumonia (defined by chest radiographic changes and treatment with antimicrobial therapy for 7 to 10 days); intraventricular hemorrhage; patent ductus arteriosus; pharmaceutical therapy including diuretics, methylxanthines, and bronchodilators; retinopathy of prematurity; or death. A neonatologist who was unaware of treatment group determined the cause of death by chart review and autopsy results. Echocardiograms were obtained for each patient after every other course of study drug to monitor for evidence of LVH as defined by a left ventricular free wall thickness ≥4 mm.[11] Chest radiographs at 1 month of postnatal age and 36 weeks of postmenstrual age were scored by a pediatric radiologist (B.N.) who was unaware of the treatment group assignments.[12]

Statistical analysis. The sample size was determined by review of patients at our own institution for the occurrence of a poor pulmonary outcome (dependence on mechanical ventilation or death at 1 month postnatal age). It was determined that a sample size of 38 infants in each group was required to show a 35% improvement in pulmonary outcome with an alpha error of 0.05 and a power of 80%. Minitab software package (Minitab, Inc., State College, Pa.) was used to perform a Student *t* test for continuous variables and chi-square analysis for discrete variables. The BMDP software package (Statistical Software, Inc., Los Angeles, Calif.) was used for repeated-measures analysis of variance to test for differences in mean airway pressure, mean arterial pressure, and oxygen requirements; and for the survival analysis to evaluate the effect of pulse dexamethasone therapy on duration of hospital stay and on the requirement for supplemental oxygen and mechanical ventilation. Results are expressed as the mean ± SEM, or as a percentage. Statistical significance was defined as $p < 0.05$.

Table II. Patient characteristics at study entry

	Pulse doses of dexamethasone	Placebo
GA (wk)	25.6 ± 0.3	26.0 ± 0.3
Birth weight (gm)	794 ± 27	814 ± 24
Sex (M/F)	19/20	20/19
Single/multiple birth	27/12	26/13
Race (white/nonwhite)	25/14	19/20
5-minute Apgar score (≤5)	7/38	7/38
Surfactant use	35/39	34/39
IVH (>grade 2)	0/39	2/39
Patent ductus arteriosus	35/39	33/39
FiO_2	0.43 ± 0.03	0.39 ± 0.03
Mean airway pressure	7.3 ± 0.4	6.3 ± 0.3

RESULTS

Patient population. From March 1991 to April 1993 there were 356 infant survivors at 7 days of age with birth weights ≤1500 gm in our neonatal intensive care unit. Of these, 232 infants did not require mechanical ventilation at 7 days postnatal age and were not eligible for enrollment. Of the 124 eligible infants, parents declined participation for 27 infants, and 9 infants were not enrolled because of a complex psychosocial situation or because death appeared to be imminent. Eighty-eight patients were enrolled in the study.

Contingency analysis of all randomly assigned patients (n = 88) with regard to the primary end point showed that the percentage of infants who were alive and without the need for supplemental oxygen at 36 weeks of postmenstrual age was greater in the group that received pulse doses of dexamethasone than in the placebo group (pulse therapy = 40% vs placebo = 20%; $p = 0.038$). Ten patients were

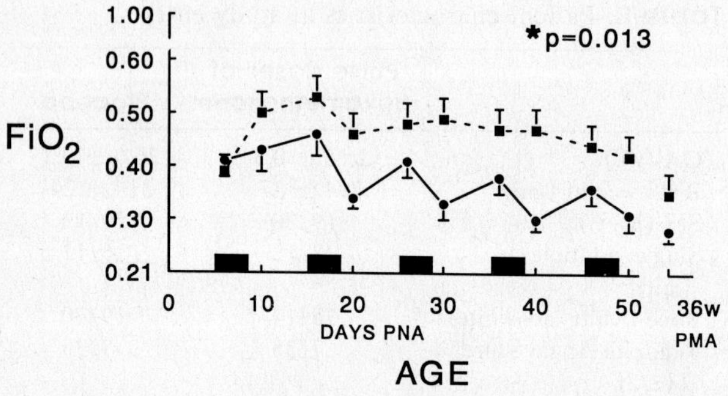

Fig. 1. Supplemental oxygen requirement (mean ± SE) before and after each dosing period (indicated on *x*-axis by black square) to 36 weeks of postmenstrual age. Treatment with pulse doses of dexamethasone is shown with *solid line*, placebo with *broken line*. Except at study entry, the data points were significantly different between groups. *PNA*, Postnatal age; *PMA*, postmenstrual age.

withdrawn during the study because of pharmacy error (dexamethasone 2 infants, placebo group 1 infant), parental choice (placebo group two infants), or attending physician request (pulse therapy group 1 infant, placebo group 4 infants). All five of the patients withdrawn from the study by the attending physician subsequently received an extended course of dexamethasone. The three patients withdrawn for pharmacy error received mixed treatment with both pulse doses of dexamethasone and placebo. However, because the study did not provide for a treatment crossover arm, inclusion of this mixed treatment of eight infants (10% of the population) in the data analysis would result in significant biases with regard to other outcomes. Therefore, the data reported here represent only the 78 infants who completed the full experimental protocol.

There were no differences between the groups for maternal demographic variables (Table I). Patient groups were not different with respect to GA, birth weight, sex distribution, race, or multiple birth (Table II). At study entry, there were no differences in severity of illness as assessed by Apgar score, surfactant therapy, prevalence of patent ductus arteriosus, or IVH more severe than grade 2. Before the first course of study drug at 7 days of postnatal age, the groups were not different with respect to supplemental oxygen requirement or mean airway pressure.

Pulmonary outcome. The requirement for supplemental oxygen (Fig. 1) was significantly less throughout the study in the pulse therapy group compared with the placebo group ($p = 0.013$). Mean airway pressure (recorded only for patients with endotracheal tubes in places) was not different between groups. Mean airway pressure was analyzed to 40 days of age because beyond that point only half of the study infants required mechanical ventilation.

Survival without supplemental oxygen at 30 days of

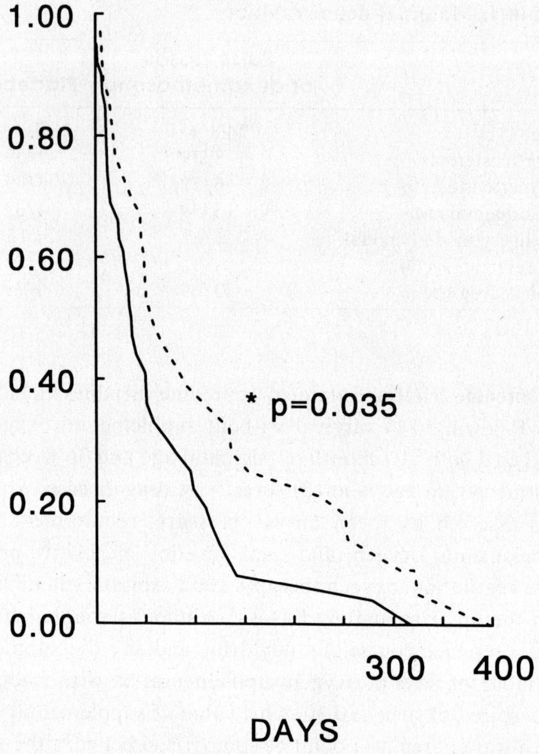

Fig. 2. Life table analysis: proportion of infants with supplemental oxygen requirement of (FIO_2 ≥0.30 as a function of postnatal age in days. Treatment with pulse doses of dexamethasone is shown with *solid line*, placebo with *broken line*.

postnatal age was not different between groups. Of the survivors at 30 days (pulse therapy group = 37, placebo = 32), 89% in the group that received pulse doses of dexamethasone and 97% in the placebo group had a persistent oxygen requirement. However, the FIO_2 required in the infants who received pulse doses of dexamethasone at 30 days of postnatal age was significantly less (pulse therapy, $FIO_2 = 0.33 \pm 0.02$; placebo, $FIO_2 = 0.49 \pm 0.04$; $p = 0.001$).

At 36 weeks of postmenstrual age, there was a greater than twofold increase in survival without the need for supplemental oxygen in the pulse therapy group compared with the placebo group (pulse therapy = 17/39 vs placebo = 7/39; $p = 0.03$). Among survivors at 36 weeks of postmenstrual age (pulse therapy = 37, placebo = 30), the percentage of infants without CLD (CLD defined as the requirement for any supplemental oxygen at 36 weeks of postmenstrual age) was greater in the group that received pulse doses of dexamethasone (pulse therapy 46% vs placebo 23%; $p = 0.047$).

Survival analysis showed a significant decrease in the number of days in supplemental oxygen with $FIO_2 \geq 0.30$ (Fig. 2) in the pulse therapy group compared with the pla-

Table III. Clinical outcome

	Pulse doses of dexamethasone	Placebo
Hyperglycemia	24/39	21/39
Insulin therapy	10/39	1/39*
Growth (gm/kg/day)	14.3 ± 0.5	15.4 ± 0.6
Hypertension	0/39	0/39
Air leak	15/39	18/39
Sepsis	13/39	13/39
Left ventricular hypertrophy	9/37	1/36†
Death	4/39	9/39
Necrotizing enterocolitis	6/39	6/39
Retinopathy of prematurity (>stage 2)	11/74	6/60
Gastrointestinal bleeding	5/39	2/39
Worsening IVH (>grade 2)	0/39	6/39‡

*$p = 0.026$.
†$p = 0.006$.
‡$p = 0.025$.

cebo group ($p < 0.035$). Mean days of ventilation required (pulse therapy 49 ± 11 days, placebo 74 ± 25 days), days in the hospital (pulse therapy 115 ± 11 days, placebo 140 ± 15 days) and total days requiring any supplemental oxygen (pulse therapy 150 ± 25 days, placebo 209 ± 32 days) were not statistically different between groups. Chest radiograph scores were not different between groups at either 30 days of postnatal age or 36 weeks of postmenstrual age.

Clinical surveillance (Table III). Hyperglycemia was no more prevalent in the group that received pulse doses of dexamethasone than in the placebo group. However, there was a significant difference in the degree of hyperglycemia as assessed by the requirement for insulin therapy. Ten infants in the pulse therapy group required insulin, which was limited to the time of pulse therapy, compared with one infant in the placebo group ($p = 0.026$). Average daily weight gain from study entry to 36 weeks postmenstrual age was not different between groups (pulse therapy 14.3 ± 0.5 gm kg per day, placebo 15.4 ± 0.6 gm/kg per day). There was also no difference in total fluid or caloric intake throughout the course of the study. Body weight at 36 weeks of postmenstrual age was similar between groups (pulse therapy 1854 ± 62 gm vs placebo 1885 ± 61 gm, $p = 0.7$). Mean arterial pressure (Fig. 3) was not different before each course of study drug. However, transient increases in mean arterial pressure occurred in the pulse therapy group during each administration of study drug ($p < 0.001$). No infant in either group could be classified as hypertensive according to the standards established by Tan,[13] and none required treatment.

Table IV. Cause of death

	Pulse doses of dexamethasone	Placebo
Lung disease	3	2
Sepsis	0	1
Necrotizing enterocolitis	1	4
IVH (>grade 2)	0	2
TOTAL	4	9

There was no difference in air leak or in suspected or documented sepsis. A diagnosis of LVH was made in 9 of the 37 infants in the pulse therapy group compared with 1 of 36 infants in the placebo group ($p = 0.006$). When these hypertrophic changes were noted during the first 6 months of the study, the protocol was altered to add an additional follow-up echocardiogram before discharge. Of the 10 infants with LVH, six had additional echocardiograms before discharge. Regression of LVH was noted in all six patients.

There were four deaths (Table IV) in the pulse therapy group and nine in the placebo group ($p = 0.022$). There were no significant differences in retinopathy of prematurity (>stage 2), necrotizing enterocolitis, or gastrointestinal hemorrhage. There was significantly more postenrollment IVH with greater severity that grade 2 in the infants receiving placebo ($p = 0.025$). Pharmacologic therapy (use of diuretics, methylxanthines, and bronchodilators) was similar in the two groups.

DISCUSSION

We have shown that treatment with pulse doses of dexamethasone leads to improved pulmonary outcome in the VLBW infant at high risk of CLD. In this population of preterm infants who were ventilator dependent at 7 days of postnatal age, pulse therapy resulted in a marked increase in survival without the need for supplemental oxygen at 36 weeks of postmenstrual age, a decrease in requirement for supplemental oxygen, and a decrease in the duration of oxygen supplementation with $F_{IO_2} \geq 0.30$. Total duration of supplemental oxygen requirement, of the need for mechanical ventilation, and of total hospital stay were not significantly different.

Our finding of improvement in pulmonary outcome associated with the use of dexamethasone is consistent with previous reports of randomized, double-blind, and placebo-controlled trials,[2-4, 14-17] but the pulse dosing regimen with dexamethasone makes this study different. Pulse steroid therapy has been used in an attempt to avoid the complications and side effects associated with long-term steroid use and, at the same time, achieve antiinflammatory effects similar to those associated with daily steroid dosing.[9] The usual side effects may occur, but are less frequent than with

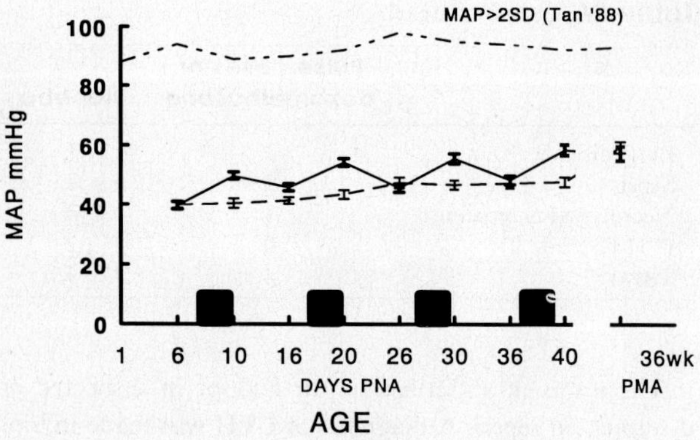

Fig. 3. Mean arterial pressure (MAP ± SE) before and after each dosing period (indicated on the *x*-axis by *black square*) during the first four courses (to 40 days postnatal age) and 36 weeks postmenstrual age. Pulse dexamethasone is shown with *solid line*, placebo with *broken line*. PNA, Postnatal age; *PMA*, postmenstrual age; *Tan '88*, see reference 13.

conventional modes of steroid therapy.[10] We chose a 3-day dosing schedule (0.5 mg/kg per day for 3 days) because this regimen has been shown to improve lung function.[1, 8] Mammel et al.[8] reported a significant decrease in intermittent mandatory ventilator rate, peak inspiratory pressure, requirement for supplemental oxygen, and alveolar-arterial oxygen gradient in infants with bronchopulmonary pulmonary dysplasia treated with 3 days of dexamethasone therapy. However, to sustain this clinical improvement, infants required continuous treatment with dexamethasone therapy for more than 30 days. Yoder et al.[1] also reported that ventilator-dependent premature infants at 14 days of postnatal age who were treated with dexamethasone for 3 days showed an improvement in respiratory system compliance and an increase in expiratory air flow at 25% vital capacity. Again, clinical deterioration occurred after dexamethasone therapy was discontinued. Our regimen of repeated pulse therapy was designed to secure and maintain the benefits reported with a single 3-day pulse. The requirement for supplemental oxygen was significantly less in the pulse therapy group throughout the study, and survival analysis demonstrated a significant decrease in days of oxygen supplementation with $FiO_2 \geq 0.30$. Although these infants were still oxygen dependent, they may qualify for earlier discharge from the neonatal intensive care unit.

We found no difference between groups in total days on artificial ventilation. Some investigators have reported a dexamethasone-associated decrease in the duration of mechanical ventilation[2, 3, 14, 15]; others have found no difference.[4, 16, 18] Direct comparisons are difficult because of differences in infant age at study entry and various durations of dexamethasone therapy. Protocols that reported a decrease in ventilator days tended to enroll infants between 2 and 6 weeks of life.[2, 3, 14, 15] Other studies that began treatment at less than 10 days of postnatal age demonstrated no difference in total time of ventilation requirement.[4, 16, 18] This observation underscores the fact that nonpulmonary factors such as apnea, infant weight, muscle mass, and nutritional state may play a role in the need for continuing mechanical ventilation.

We were able to show a significant increase in the survival rate without supplemental oxygen in the infants in the pulse therapy group at 36 weeks of postmenstrual age. With the increasing rate of survival of the VLBW infant, 36 weeks of postmenstrual age is a better point of comparison for the need for supplemental oxygen and the incidence of CLD.[18] In the study by Sanders et al.,[19] the use of two doses of intravenously administered dexamethasone within the first 24 hours of life did not affect the survival rate without supplemental oxygen at 36 weeks of postmenstrual age (dexamethasone 68%, placebo 43%, difference not significant). The difference between the two studies in long-term pulmonary outcome may be related to sustained improvement with repeated pulse therapy.

The prevalence of CLD in the placebo group as defined by the requirement for supplemental oxygen was 97% at 30 days of postnatal age and 77% at 36 weeks of postmenstrual age. In the year before the start of the study, approximately 30% of all infants with birth weights <1500 gm at our institution were discharged with a diagnosis of CLD. This rate is comparable to results reported in recent trials of surfactant replacement.[20, 21] The disparity in the rate of CLD at 30 days of postnatal age in this study, when compared with CLD in all infants of similar birth weight at our institution, underscores the fact that birth weight alone is not a sensitive indicator for development of CLD. Entry criteria for this study were designed to include the subgroup of infants with the highest likelihood of having long-term pulmonary morbidity, to avoid glucocorticoid exposure of infants who are at a lower risk of having CLD.

Multiple investigators have reported poor growth in association with the use of dexamethasone therapy. Yeh et al.[16] used a 12-day course of dexamethasone beginning at 12 hours of life and demonstrated a significant decrease in weight gain in dexamethasone-treated infants that persisted through 4 weeks of life. Although growth was slowed during the 3-day pulse therapy with dexamethasone in our study,[22] the overall growth rate was not altered by the use of this protocol. We also found a significant increase in hyperglycemia that required short-term treatment with insulin in the pulse therapy group. Close attention to glucose monitoring and subsequent intervention is important in any preterm infant exposed to exogenous glucocorticoids. Mean arterial blood pressure was transiently increased in the pulse therapy group, but the increase was not sufficient to require pharmacologic treatment. Likewise, although LVH was more prevalent in the pulse therapy group, it was clinically insignificant and regressed before discharge in all six of the infants examined. This experience is in contrast to the reports of significant left ventricular outflow tract obstruction in infants receiving long-term steroid treatment.[6, 23]

The decrease in severe IVH in the pulse therapy group may indicate that steroids play a role in stabilization of capillary membranes or alteration of cerebral blood flow. Alternatively, an improvement in the overall ventilatory status of the infants in the pulse therapy group may account for this decrease in severe IVH.

The precise mechanism by which pulse doses of dexamethasone improve pulmonary outcome in high-risk VLBW infants remains speculative. Evolving CLD has a marked inflammatory component, and known actions of corticosteroid therapy include decreasing inflammatory cell recruitment and activation, as well as diminishing production or release of mediators of inflammation, or both.[24] Serial tracheal bronchial lavage samples from infants with respiratory distress syndrome in whom CLD later develops show an initial airway infiltration by polymorphonuclear leukocytes followed by an increase in alveolar macrophages.[25] Multiple mediators of inflammation have been documented in the airways of infants with evolving CLD.[26] Glucocorticoid treatment of infants with evolving CLD has been shown to decrease the number of airway inflammatory cells[1] and alveolar macrophage hydrogen peroxide production,[27] as well as tracheobronchial lavage levels of histamine,[28] leukotrienes,[29] tumor necrosis factor,[30] platelet-derived growth factor,[31] and fibronectin.[32] The relative importance of corticosteroid-induced suppression of these and other inflammatory mediators in improving pulmonary outcomes in VLBW infants is unknown. Further research in this area may provide the groundwork for the development of mediator specific, effective, and safe pharmacologic agents for the treatment of evolving CLD in VLBW infants. In the meantime, we believe that pulse dexamethasone therapy results in optimal antiinflammatory effects with minimal side effects.

We thank David R. Brown, MD, for his original contributions to the design of this project, Giovanni G. Laneri, MD, for his help as a study patient monitor, Joan Sentipal-Walerius, MS, RD, for her assistance with calculation of fluid and caloric intake, and Deborah M. Flotta and Frederick S. Sherman, MD, who performed and interpreted all of the echocardiograms. We also thank the nurses and pharmacists of the neonatal intensive care unit at Magee-Women's Hospital for their assistance in the completion of the study. Finally, we acknowledge Elaine Harris for data entry.

REFERENCES

1. Yoder MC Jr, Chua R, Tepper R. Effect of dexamethasone on pulmonary inflammation and pulmonary function of ventilator-dependent infants with bronchopulmonary dysplasia. Am Rev Respir Dis 1991;143:1044-8.
2. Avery GB, Fletcher AB, Kaplan M, Brudno DS. Controlled trial of dexamethasone in respirator-dependent infants with bronchopulmonary dysplasia. Pediatrics 1985;75:106-11.
3. Cummings JJ, D'Eugenio DB, Gross SJ. A controlled trial of dexamethasone in preterm infants at high risk for bronchopulmonary dysplasia. N Engl J Med 1989;320:1505-10.
4. Kari MA, Heinonen K, Ikonen RS, Koivisto M, Raivio KO. Dexamethasone treatment in preterm infants at risk for bronchopulmonary dysplasia. Arch Dis Child 1993;68:566-9.
5. Ohlsson A, Calvert SA, Hosking M, Shennan AT. Randomized controlled trial of dexamethasone treatment in very-low-birth-weight infants with ventilator-dependent chronic lung disease. Acta Paediatr 1992;81:751-6.
6. Israel BA, Sherman FS, Guthrie RD. Hypertrophic cardiomyopathy associated with dexamethasone therapy for chronic lung disease in preterm infants. Am J Perinatol 1993;10:307-10.
7. Noble-Jamieson CM, Regev R, Silverman M. Dexamethasone in neonatal chronic lung disease: pulmonary effects and intracranial complications. Eur J Pediatr 1989;148:365-7.
8. Mammel MC, Green TP, Johnson DE, Thompson TR. Controlled trial of dexamethasone therapy in infants with bronchopulmonary dysplasia. Lancet 1983;1:1356-8.
9. Miller JJ III. Prolonged use of large intravenous steroid pulses in the rheumatic diseases of children. Pediatrics 1980;65:989-94.
10. Pentikäinen PJ. Pharmacological aspects of corticosteroid pulse therapy. Scand J Rheumatol Suppl 1984;54:6-9.
11. Allen LD. Manual of fetal echocardiography. Norwell, Massachusetts: MTP Press, 1986:48-55.
12. Toce SS, Farrell PM, Leavitt LA, Samuels DP, Edwards DK. Clinical and roentgenographic scoring systems for assessing bronchopulmonary dysplasia. Am J Dis Child 1984;138:581-5.
13. Tan KL. Blood pressure in very low birth weight infants in the first 70 days of life. J PEDIATR 1988;112:266-70.
14. Harkavy KL, Scanlon JW, Chowdhry PK, Grylack LJ. Dexamethasone therapy for chronic lung disease in ventilator- and oxygen-dependent infants: a controlled trial. J PEDIATR 1989; 115:979-83.
15. Kazzi NJ, Brans YW, Poland RL. Dexamethasone effects on the hospital course of infants with bronchopulmonary dysplasia who are dependent on artificial ventilation. Pediatrics 1990;86:722-7.
16. Yeh TF, Torre JA, Rastogi A, Anyebuno MA, Pildes RS. Early postnatal dexamethasone therapy in premature infants with severe respiratory distress syndrome: a double-blind, controlled study. J PEDIATR 1990;117:273-82.
17. Collaborative Dexamethasone Trial Group. Dexamethasone therapy in neonatal chronic lung disease: an international placebo-controlled trial. Pediatrics 1991;88:421-7.
18. Shennan AT, Dunn MS, Ohlsson A, Lennox K, Hoskins EM. Abnormal pulmonary outcomes in premature infants: predic-

tion from oxygen requirement in the neonatal period. Pediatrics 1988;82:527-32.
19. Sanders RJ, Cox C, Phelps DL, Sinkin RA. Two doses of early intravenous dexamethasone for the prevention of bronchopulmonary dysplasia in babies with respiratory distress syndrome. Pediatr Res 1994;36:122-8.
20. Zola EM, Overbach AM, Gunkel JH, et al. Treatment investigational new drug experience with new drug experience with Survanta (beractant). Pediatrics 1993;91:546-51.
21. Horar JD, Wright LL, Soll RF, et al. A multicenter randomized trial comparing two surfactants for the treatment of neonatal respiratory distress syndrome. J PEDIATR 1993;123:57-66.
22. Gilmour C, Sentipal-Walerius J, Jones J, Doyle J, Mimouni F. Pulse dexamethasone does not impair growth and body composition of very low birth weight infants. J Am Coll Nutr 1993;12:577A.
23. Werner JC, Sicard RE, Hanson TWR, Solomon E, Cowett RM, Oh W. Hypertrophic cardiomyopathy associated with dexamethasone therapy for bronchopulmonary dysplasia. J PEDIATR 1992;120:286-91.
24. Stenmark KR. Steroids. In: Bancalari E, Stocker JT, eds. Bronchopulmonary dysplasia. Washington, D.C.: Hemisphere Publishing, 1988:36-65.
25. Merritt TA, Stuard ID, Puccia J, et al. Newborn tracheal aspirate cytology: classification during respiratory distress syndrome and bronchopulmonary dysplasia. J PEDIATR 1981;98:949-56.
26. Groneck P, Götze-Speer B, Oppermann M, Eiffert H, Speer CP. Association of pulmonary inflammation and increased microvascular permeability during the development of bronchopulmonary dysplasia: a sequential analysis of inflammatory mediators in respiratory fluids of high-risk preterm neonates. Pediatrics 1994;93:712-8.
27. Clement A, Chadelat K, Sardet A, Grimfield A, Tournier G. Alveolar macrophage status in bronchopulmonary dysplasia. Pediatr Res 1988;23:470-3.
28. Balsan MJ, Jones JG, Brozanski BS, Fireman P, Guthrie RD. Effect of pulse dexamethasone therapy on histamine levels in tracheobronchial lavage samples (TBLS) from premature infants with evolving bronchopulmonary dysplasia. Am Rev Respir Dis 1993;147:A422.
29. Davidson D, Drafta D, Wilkens BA. Elevated urinary leukotriene E_4 in chronic lung disease of extreme prematurity: relationship to ventilatory support and dexamethasone therapy. Am Rev Respir Dis 1994;149:A544.
30. Murch SH, MacDonald TT, Wood CBS, Costeloe KL. Tumour necrosis factor in the bronchoalveolar secretions of infants with the respiratory distress syndrome and the effect of dexamethasone treatment. Thorax 1992;47:44-7.
31. Watts CL, Fanaroff, AA. Platelet-derived growth factor (PDGF) response to dexamethasone in infants with bronchopulmonary dysplasia (BPD) [Abstract]. Pediatr Res 1993;33:349.
32. Watts CL, Bruce MC. Effect of dexamethasone therapy on fibronectin and albumin levels in lung secretions of infants with bronchopulmonary dysplasia. J PEDIATR 1992;121:597-607.

Effect of the arterial oxygenation level on cardiac output, oxygen extraction, and oxygen consumption in low birth weight infants receiving mechanical ventilation

Andreas Schulze, MD, Robin K. Whyte, MBBS, R. Clifton Way, MD, and John C. Sinclair, MD

From the Department of Pediatrics, Divisions of Neonatology and Cardiology, McMaster University, Hamilton, Ontario, and the Department of Pediatrics, Dalhousie University, Halifax, Nova Scotia, Canada

Objective: **To investigate the effects on oxygenation of targeting the higher versus the lower end of the currently recommended range for pulse oximetry (Spo_2).**
Design: **Nonrandomized crossover trial with the use of within-subject comparisons (two-tailed paired *t* test).**
Setting: **Level III neonatal intensive care unit of a university hospital.**
Patients: **Twenty infants whose lungs were mechanically ventilated (mean ± SD: birth weight, 1192 ± 396 gm; gestational age, 28.7 ± 2.7 weeks; age at time of study, 42 ± 26 hours).**
Interventions: **The inspired oxygen concentration was adjusted to achieve Spo_2 readings of 93% to 96% versus 89% to 92% (Ohmeda pulse oximeter) or 95% to 98% versus 91% to 94% (Nellcor oximeter).**
Measurements: **Cardiac output was measured by echocardiography, oxygen content of arterial blood samples by cooximetry, and oxygen consumption by indirect calorimetry.**
Results: **The inspired oxygen concentrations required to achieve the Spo_2 target ranges were 39.8% ± 8.3% versus 28.7% ± 6.1% (p <0.001). The respective arterial oxygen contents were 18.0 ± 2.6 ml/dl versus 16.9 ± 2.5 ml/dl (p <0.001). Oxygen consumption was unchanged. In the lower-oxygen condition no compensatory increase in cardiac output was detected; thus the estimated mixed venous oxygen tension decreased and the oxygen extraction ratio increased. Venous admixture increased from 15% ± 6% to 31% ± 9% in the lower-oxygen condition (p <0.001).**
Conclusions: **The "low normal" Spo_2 target range allowed for less oxygen exposure. No signs of mismatch between systemic oxygen delivery and demand could be detected. (J PEDIATR 1995;126:777-84)**

Supported in part by Deutsche Forschungsgemeinschaft (A.S.).

Presented in part at the annual meetings of the Society for Pediatric Research/American Pediatric Society, Seattle, Wash., May 3, 1994, and the German-Austrian Society for Neonatology and Pediatric Intensive Care, Graz, Austria, Oct. 14, 1994.

Submitted for publication Aug. 22, 1994; accepted Nov. 18, 1994.

Reprint requests: John C. Sinclair, MD, McMaster University, Faculty of Health Sciences, Department of Pediatrics, 1200 Main St. West, Room 4G40, Hamilton, Ontario, Canada L8N 3Z5.

0022-3476/95/$3.00 + 0 **9/23/62137**

During O_2 therapy, current reference standards for arterial partial pressure of oxygen and saturation of hemoglobin in arterial blood with O_2, measured by pulse oximetry, are based essentially on physiologic normal values in healthy infants. Few data are available about the safety of extrapolating these standards to low birth weight infants undergoing intensive care. Moreover, no single measurement of arterial O_2 tension or saturation can describe the complex oxygenation system in terms of O_2 demand and reserve.[1, 2] Systemic oxygen transport (oxygen supply) depends not only on hemoglobin oxygen saturation but also on the hemoglobin concentration and on cardiac output, both of which may vary considerably. Oxygen consumption (oxygen uptake) can change within a few minutes in infants.[3] The mixed venous oxygen saturation reflects the venous oxygen content, which accounts for about half the body's oxygen store.[4]

CaO_2	Arterial blood oxygen content (milliliter per deciliter)
$Cc'O_2$	Pulmonary end-capillary blood oxygen content (milliliter per deciliter)
CO	Cardiac output (milliliters per minute per kilogram)
COHb	Carboxyhemoglobin (grams per deciliter)
$C\bar{v}O_2$	Mixed venous blood oxygen content (milliliter per deciliter)
FIO_2	Fraction of inspired oxygen
[Hb]	Hemoglobin concentration (grams per deciliter)
MetHb	Methemoglobin (grams per deciliter)
P_AO_2	Alveolar partial pressure of oxygen (millimeters of mercury)
PaO_2	Arterial partial pressure of oxygen (millimeters of mercury)
SaO_2	Functional saturation of hemoglobin in arterial blood with oxygen, measured by cooximetry (oxyhemoglobin ÷ [oxyhemoglobin + reduced hemoglobin]) (%)
SOT	Systemic oxygen transport (milliliters per kilogram per minute)
SpO_2	Saturation of hemoglobin in arterial blood with oxygen, measured by pulse oximetry (%)
$S\bar{v}O_2$	Mixed venous hemoglobin oxygen saturation (percent)
tHb	Total hemoglobin (grams per deciliter)
$\dot{V}O_2$	Oxygen consumption (milliliters per minute per kilogram)

Recommended PaO_2 levels have ranged from 40 to 100 mm Hg.[5-7] The American Academy of Pediatrics Committee on Fetus and Newborn currently recommends a PaO_2 range of 50 to 80 mm Hg during administration of supplemental O_2 to a premature neonate.[8] Depending on O_2 half-saturation pressure, a PaO_2 range of 45 to 100 mm Hg corresponds approximately to a range for SpO_2 readings of 89% to 98%.[9-11] These ranges are broad enough to allow for different policies of O_2 administration: we could choose to aim at either the upper end or the lower end of the range.

We hypothesized that targeting SpO_2 to "high normal" as opposed to "low normal" readings would affect not only PaO_2 and SaO_2 but other, potentially equally important measures of O_2 status. We designed a study to provide data about O_2 supply, demand, and reserve in low birth weight infants given intensive care in two different situations: when SpO_2 readings were targeted either to the upper limit or to the lower limit of the normal range. Our specific aims were to estimate quantitatively the effects on CO, O_2 extraction, $\dot{V}O_2$, and mixed venous O_2 content.

METHODS

Subjects. Low birth weight infants were selected for study from among all infants admitted to the neonatal intensive care unit at McMaster University Medical Center. Infants were enrolled if they met all the following inclusion criteria: (1) mechanical ventilation for respiratory distress, (2) fraction of inspired oxygen less than 0.6, (3) arterial catheter in place for clinical management, (4) stable cardiovascular condition, (5) all nutrition received parenterally, (6) nursing given under servo-controlled radiant warmer, and (7) informed parental consent. Exclusion criteria were (1) congenital malformations, (2) audible endotracheal tube leak, or (3) left-to-right ductal or atrial shunt by echocardiography. Echocardiograms were done for all infants before the study to rule out a left-to-right shunt.

Protocol. We performed a paired comparison in which each patient was studied at each of two different oxygenation levels. The FIO_2 was adjusted to achieve measurement periods with high-normal and low-normal SpO_2 readings. The target SpO_2 ranges were 93% to 96% versus 89% to 92% if the infant was monitored with an Ohmeda Biox 3700 oximeter (Ohmeda Monitoring Systems, Louisville, Colo.) and 95% to 98% versus 91% to 94% if the Nellcor N-100 oximeter (Nellcor Inc., Hayward, Calif.) was used. Different SpO_2 values were chosen for the two instrument brands because of the different ways they calculate SpO_2 (fractional vs functional hemoglobin O_2 saturation).[9] To minimize clinical disruption, we exposed the infants first to the study target range closest to the saturation level that had been chosen previously by the clinicians. Data acquisition was attempted if the SpO_2 readings had been stable for at least 30 minutes after adjustment of the FIO_2 without a further requirement to change the FIO_2 within that time period. No attempts were made to restrict the measurements to a specific behavioral state, but data acquisition was not performed if an infants had excessive body movement. The following measurements were done during each observation period: PaO_2, SaO_2, CO, and $\dot{V}O_2$. If an umbilical venous catheter was in place with its tip in the right atrium, we also measured right atrial oxygen pressure and saturation.

This protocol was approved by the McMaster University Research Advisory Group (ethics board). Informed written consent was obtained from at least one parent for each child.

Measurements. Oxygen consumption was measured by indirect calorimetry with the MGM/jr. metabolic gas monitor (Utah Medical Products Inc., Midvale, Utah) in line with the ventilator. A nonrebreathing valve (Hans Rudolph Inc., Kansas City, Mo.) was inserted between the endotracheal tube and the ventilator circuit so that the expired gas was separated for analysis from the continuous fresh gas flow of the ventilator and fed back into the expiratory part of the ventilator circuit after passing through the gas analyzer. A test to rule out an endotracheal tube leak was performed by application of gentle manual pressure externally around the larynx; if the mean expired air flow as measured by the metabolic gas monitor increased, this was taken as evidence of a leak and the infant was excluded from the study. Oxygen consumption was calculated for standard temperature and pressure conditions (0° C, 760 mm Hg) from measurements of FIO_2 and fraction of mean expired oxygen, mean expired carbon dioxide, expiratory minute volume, and barometric pressure. Oxygen consumption was measured for 20 to 30 minutes during each study period. During these periods the monitor sampled data every 20 seconds.

Arterial and right atrial blood samples were analyzed for the total hemoglobin level, oxyhemoglobin, carboxyhemoglobin, and methemoglobin with a multiwavelength hemoximeter (model OSM-3; Radiometer, Copenhagen, Denmark). One determination of the percentage of fetal hemoglobin was obtained for each infant at the beginning of the study. If the instrument returned fetal [Hb] greater than 100%, we assumed that the true concentration was 100%. The estimate of the percentage of fetal hemoglobin was then used to correct all subsequent cooximetry results for the amount of fetal hemoglobin present. Blood gases and pH values were obtained with an AVL 995 pH and blood gas analyzer (AVL Scientific Corp., Roswell, Ga.).

Cardiac output was determined by Doppler echocardiography[12] in each infant during each measurement period with an ATL Ultramark 4 system (Advanced Technology Laboratories Inc., Bothell, Wash.) with a mechanical multifrequency duplex sensor; 7.5 MHz were used for imaging. The wall filter was set at 200 Hz. Cardiac output was calculated as follows: CO = Mean systolic flow velocity × Ejection time × Aortic cross-sectional area × Heart rate. Aortic diameter was measured from the parasternal long-axis view near the base of the aortic valve leaflets with the M-mode trailing edge–to–leading edge method at end-diastole.[13] The mean of three consecutive determinations of the inner aortic diameter was used. Systolic blood flow velocity was measured from the suprasternal or a high right parasternal position with a range-gated, 5 MHz Doppler transducer. The sample volume of 1.5 mm was placed inside the ascending aorta as close to the aortic annulus as possible. Angle correction was attempted if the Doppler beam appeared to be angled more than 15 degrees in the two-dimensional image. The ejection time was obtained from the Doppler tracing. Heart rates were derived from the simultaneously recorded electrocardiogram. For each CO determination the mean of three repeated measurements was averaged. The Doppler transducer was lifted and newly placed for each measurement. All CO measurements were done by one investigator (A.S.).

Further calculations. (The format of all the following equations assumes that the parameters are used with the units given in the list of abbreviations.) The arterial hemoglobin-bound O_2 content was calculated as follows:

$$CaO_2 = SaO_2 \cdot 1.39 \cdot ([tHb]-[COHb]-[MetHb]) \quad (1)$$

Systemic oxygen transport was then given as follows:

$$SOT = \frac{CaO_2}{100} \cdot CO \quad (2)$$

"Apparent" hemoglobin-bound $C\bar{v}O_2$ was derived as follows:

$$C\bar{v}O_2 = CaO_2 - \frac{100 \cdot \dot{V}O_2}{CO} \quad (3)$$

This allowed the calculation of the O_2 extraction ratio:

$$O_2 \text{ extraction ratio} = \frac{Ca - \bar{v}O_2}{CaO_2} \quad (4)$$

Mixed venous O_2 saturation was given as follows:

$$S\bar{v}O_2 = \frac{C\bar{v}O_2}{1.39 \cdot ([tHb] - [COHb] - [MetHb])} \quad (5)$$

We derived venous admixture according to the shunt equation,[14] assuming 100% hemoglobin O_2 saturation in the pulmonary end-capillary blood:

$$\text{Percentage of venous admixture} = \frac{Cc'O_2 - CaO_2}{Cc'O_2 - C\bar{v}O_2} \times 100 \quad (6)$$

To assess the validity of the assumption that hemoglobin in pulmonary end-capillary blood was fully saturated with O_2 in both observation periods, we calculated the ideal alveolar partial pressure of O_2 from the alveolar gas equation in the following form[14]:

$$PAO_2 = (P_{barometric} - P_{H_2O}) \cdot FIO_2 - \frac{\text{Arterial } CO_2 \text{ pressure}}{\text{Respiratory quotient}} \quad (7)$$

The physically dissolved blood O_2 content was disregarded because O_2 pressure estimates for mixed venous blood

Table I. Oxygen delivery and O_2 uptake variables in 20 low birth weight infants when high-normal or low-normal Spo_2 readings were targeted

	Spo_2 target range		
	High-normal (n*)	Low-normal (n*)	p† (n‡)
Pao_2 (mm Hg)	78 ± 14 (18)	52 ± 6 (19)	<0.001 (18)
Arterial pH	7.31 ± 0.06 (18)	7.31 ± 0.06 (19)	NS (18)
Arterial CO_2 pressure (mm Hg)	47.9 ± 10 (18)	47.5 ± 10 (19)	NS (18)
Sao_2 (%)	97 ± 1.7 (20)	92 ± 3.8 (20)	<0.001 (20)
Cao_2 (ml/dl)	18.0 ± 2.56 (20)	16.9 ± 2.51 (20)	<0.001 (20)
Heart rate (beats/min)	142 ± 17 (20)	143 ± 14 (20)	NS (20)
CO (ml/min/kg)	263 ± 52 (20)	253 ± 44 (20)	NS (20)
SOT (ml/min/kg)	47.3 ± 10.6 (20)	42.4 ± 8.7 (20)	0.009 (20)
$\dot{V}o_2$ (ml/min/kg)	7.59 ± 1.5 (20)	7.64 ± 1.2 (20)	NS (20)
Right atrial O_2 pressure (mm Hg)	47 ± 8 (9)	39 ± 7 (11)	<0.001 (9)
Measured right atrial o_2 saturation (%)	87.9 ± 4.8 (13)	79.6 ± 7.5 (13)	<0.001 (11)
Calculated $S\bar{v}o_2$ (%)	79.4 ± 6.0 (20)	73.4 ± 7.3 (20)	<0.001 (20)
$C\bar{v}o_2$ (ml/dl)	15.0 ± 2.6 (20)	13.7 ± 2.7 (20)	<0.001 (20)
Arterial–mixed venous difference in O_2 content (ml/dl)	3.00 ± 0.98 (20)	3.13 ± 0.81 (20)	NS (20)
O_2 extraction ratio	0.169 ± 0.055 (20)	0.190 ± 0.060 (20)	0.005 (20)

Values are means ± SD.
*Number of patients with data available on the parameter.
†Paired two-tailed *t* test.
‡Number of pairs available for *t* test.

Table II. Precision of O_2 status measurements

	Coefficient of variation (%)	
	High-normal Spo_2 (n = 20)	Low-normal Spo_2 (n = 20)
Cao_2	1.08 ± 1.05	2.29 ± 2.55
CO	4.85 ± 3.05	6.51 ± 4.39
$\dot{V}O_2$	13.31 ± 6.48	13.12 ± 5.65

Values are means ± SD.

would require exact knowledge of the position and shape of the individual O_2 dissociation curve. Moreover, O_2 measurements were available only for a subset of the arterial and right atrial blood samples because [Hb] and saturation measurements were given priority over O_2 pressure measurements if the available blood sample volume was small. As estimated from infants who had blood gases measured, this simplification introduces less than 1% error for our data analysis.

Data analysis. Two-tailed paired *t* tests were used to test for differences between the two oxygenation conditions. A *p* value less than 0.05 was considered significant. Measurement precision was assessed by the coefficient of variation. For the Cao_2 determinations this assessment was based on up to three replicate measurements that were available for single, individual blood samples. For all CO determinations, three repeated measurements were obtained in each infant in each observation period. On average, 60 $\dot{V}o_2$ measurements were performed in each infant in each period.

RESULTS

Twenty infants were enrolled between August 1993 and April 1994. Their birth weight was 1192 ± 396 gm (mean ± SD; range, 690 to 2010 gm); the gestational age was 28.7 ± 2.7 weeks (range, 25 to 33 weeks). Infant age at the time of the study was 42 ± 26 hours (range, 11 to 96 hours). Eighteen infants had hyaline membrane disease according to clinical and radiologic criteria and had received exogenous surfactant before the study. At the time of study two infants were receiving dopamine and two others received aminophylline. All infants received continuous-flow, pressure-limited, time-cycled ventilation with the following settings (mean ± SD): peak inspiratory pressure, 18.9 ± 3.7 cm H_2O; end-expiratory pressure, 3.9 ± 0.3 cm H_2O; ventilator rate, 41.6 ± 15.1 min^{-1}; mechanical inspiratory time, 0.4 ± 0.02 seconds. The infants' core temperature was 36.8° ± 0.2° C. Their caloric intake from parenteral nutrition at the time of the study was 29.4 ± 7.4 kcal/kg per day.

The inspired O_2 concentration required to achieve the target Spo_2 levels was 39.8% ± 8.3% (mean ± SD; range, 26% to 55%) for the high-normal O_2 condition and 28.7% ± 6.1% (range, 21% to 39%) for the low-normal O_2 condition (p <0.001, n = 20). The P_{AO_2} values in the two observation periods were 236 ± 55 mm Hg and 154 ± 41 mm Hg, respectively (p <0.001, n = 18). This difference in O_2 environment yielded significant differences in the oxygenation status of the arterial blood (Table I): the Cao_2 decreased from 18.0 to 16.9 ml/dl, a relative reduction of 6.1%

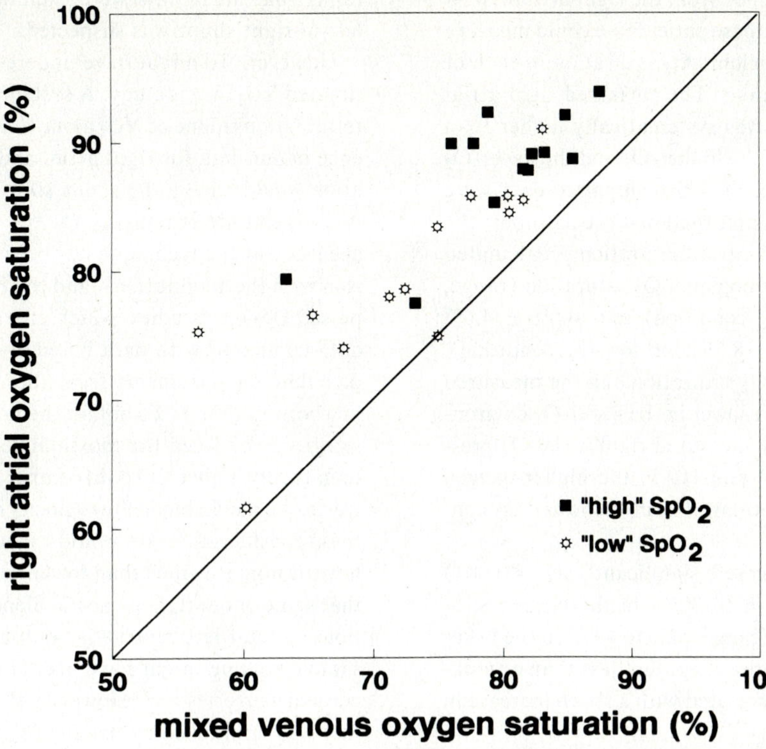

Fig. 1. Relation of measured hemoglobin O_2 saturation in samples of right atrial blood to calculated $S\bar{v}O_2$.

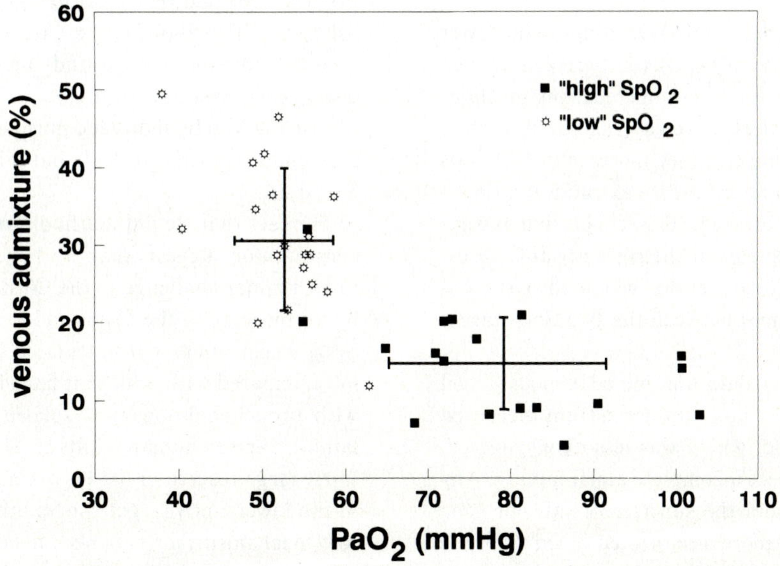

Fig. 2. Relation between venous admixture and PaO_2.

in the lower-O_2 condition. There was no compensatory increase in CO in response to this reduction. As a result, SOT decreased in the lower-O_2 environment. Oxygen consumption remained virtually identical in the two situations, and therefore the O_2 extraction ratio increased. The calculated $S\bar{v}O_2$ and $C\bar{v}O_2$ decreased. There were no detectable differences in the arterial blood pH, CO_2 pressure, base deficit, or bicarbonate concentration.

Blood samples were obtained from the right atrium in 14 of the 20 infants. In nine of these patients we could measure both blood gases and hemoglobin O_2 saturation in each of the two oxygenation conditions. The measured right atrial hemoglobin O_2 saturation was systematically higher than the calculated $S\bar{v}O_2$ in both the higher-O_2 and the lower-O_2 environments (Table I; Fig. 1). Thirteen paired data were available in both the high- and the low-O_2 conditions; the difference (measured right atrial saturation − calculated $S\bar{v}O_2$) was 8.2% ± 4.1% hemoglobin O_2 saturation (range, 3.2% to 16% for high-O_2 condition) and 6.8% ± 4.6% saturation (range, 0% to 18.7% for low-O_2 condition). The measured right atrial O_2 saturation and the measured right atrial O_2 pressure were lower in the lower-O_2 environment (Fig. 1; Table I). The measured right atrial O_2 pressure ranged from 31 to 59 mm Hg in the higher-oxygen condition and from 28 to 50 mm Hg in the lower-O_2 condition.

Venous admixture increased significantly ($p < 0.001$) from 15% ± 6% (range, 6% to 32%) in the higher SpO_2 target range to 31% ± 9% (range, 12% to 49%) in the lower target range. Arterial O_2 pressure values less than approximately 60 mm Hg were associated with a sharp increase in venous admixture (Fig. 2).

The precision of the measurements of the CaO_2, CO, and $\dot{V}O_2$ is given in Table II.

DISCUSSION

These data show that targeting SpO_2 readings to the lower as opposed to the higher end of the currently recommended normal range in low birth weight infants receiving mechanical ventilation decreased the CaO_2 on average by more than 6%. We did not find a compensatory increase in CO; $\dot{V}O_2$ remained unchanged. Therefore the O_2 extraction ratio increased and the $S\bar{v}O_2$ decreased. This conclusion is supported by direct measurements of the right atrial O_2 pressure and right atrial O_2 saturation, which also showed highly significant differences between the two SpO_2 target ranges.

Calculated oxygenation data for mixed venous blood were systematically but variably different from measured data for right atrial blood, which was less deoxygenated. The discrepancy may reflect incomplete atrial mixing. Any oversampling of blood from the superior or inferior vena cava before it mixes with more desaturated blood from the coronary sinus may cause a higher O_2 content of the sample compared with the mixed venous oxygenation level.[15] This explanation contradicts the theoretic expectation that atrial mixing should be complete in the newborn infant and that monitoring of atrial oxygenation could replace mixed venous measurements.[4, 16] We cannot rule out a minor left-to-right atrial shunt that went undetected by echocardiography, but all infants were excluded from the study if a left-to-right shunt was suspected.

However, we might have underestimated CO or overestimated $\dot{V}O_2$ in this study. A systematic error in the CO determinations alone or $\dot{V}O_2$ alone to explain the mean difference in our data for right atrial and mixed venous oxygenation would have to be about 10%. An underestimation of this magnitude is unlikely for the following reasons. The accuracy of the technique has been established in comparison with thermodilution[17] and the Fick method.[18] We used pulsed Doppler studies, which give consistently higher CO data compared with data based on continuous-wave Doppler flow measurements from the suprasternal window in newborn infants.[13] To obtain the aortic blood flow velocity integral, we traced the maximal velocity, which gives systematically higher CO data compared with a technique that traces the modal blood flow velocity of the spectrum.[19] From these considerations we would expect a bias in our CO data toward higher rather than lower data. We cannot rule out that some of our data on aortic blood flow are underestimations of total left ventricular output, because the Doppler sample volume might have been distal to the origin of the coronary arteries.[13, 20] However, the potential for this artifact was minimized by placing the sample volume as close to the aortic annulus as possible.

It is unlikely that we systematically overestimated O_2 consumption in this study. The accuracy of the instrument we used for indirect calorimetry has been well established.[21-24] Our data on $\dot{V}O_2$ are consistent with previous reports from other groups studying low birth weight infants during their first days of life.[23, 25] A major source of bias in measuring $\dot{V}O_2$ by indirect calorimetry in intubated infants is an endotracheal tube leak, but this would give falsely low $\dot{V}O_2$ data.[26]

The fact that we did not find a response in CO and $\dot{V}O_2$ consumption suggests that our lower range of CaO_2 constitutes a minor challenge to the O_2 supply system that is met by an increase in the O_2 extraction ratio. Even in the low SpO_2 target range, our calculated O_2 extraction ratios are low compared with data that have been reported in infants with bronchopulmonary dysplasia,[24] in healthy newborn lambs,[27] and in human adults.[28] According to these data, a fairly large reserve in the O_2 extraction ratio remains even in the lower SpO_2 target range; other potential compensatory mechanisms may not need to be called into play. On the other hand, the ability of newborn infants, when faced with stress, to invoke additional CO has been questioned.[2] However, CO as measured by echocardiography can change in response to circulatory challenges such as a patent ductus arteriosus in premature infants[29] or in response to changes in total body erythrocyte mass.[30] Oxygen consumption and CO_2 production may decrease during acute hypoxia within a few minutes in newborn infants[31] and animals.[32-34] Conversely, hyperoxia increases O_2 consumption in newborn infants,[3] newborn rats,[35] lambs,[36] and mice.[37] The reported magnitude of these changes in CO and metabolic rate was much higher than the intraindividual variability of our measurements. The coefficient of variation for three repeated measures of CO by a single operator in our study is almost identical with that of other ultrasound studies.[38] The intraindividual variability of our $\dot{V}O_2$ data is also close to, or lower than, that of other reports.[23, 25, 39, 40] It is unlikely that substantial effects on CO or on $\dot{V}O_2$ in our infants would have escaped detection.

The effect on venous admixture of targeting the lower as opposed to the higher SpO_2 range is obviously more profound than that on O_2 uptake. The right-to-left shunt fraction rapidly increased in the lower SpO_2 target range. However, the rise in venous admixture might be overestimated if the underlying assumption of fully oxygenated pulmonary end-capillary blood is more violated in the low-O_2 compared with the high-O_2 environment. The mean O_2 pressure required for 90% saturation of hemoglobin from a similar group of low birth weight infants at birth has been reported to be as low as 40.8 ± 3.6 mm Hg.[7] Therefore even if we make an allowance for a lower in vivo pH, the mean P_{AO_2} of 154 mm Hg in our lower O_2 target range seems to justify the assumption of fully saturated pulmonary end-capillary blood. Approximately 60 mm Hg is the inflection point less than which there is a steep rise in venous admixture with decreasing PaO_2. Systemic O_2 supply may therefore be more unstable as the PaO_2 decreases to less than 60 mm Hg. The fact that the variability of the SaO_2 was higher in the lower-O_2 environment compared with the higher-O_2 condition may reflect such increased instability, presumably because of increased pulmonary vascular resistance.

On the basis of these results, we speculate that O_2 supply becomes more stable if high-normal SpO_2 readings are targeted. This is achieved at the expense of higher O_2 tensions at all levels of the oxygenation system, with the associated increased risk of O_2 toxicity. On the other hand, during periods with low-normal SpO_2 readings, we could not find compensatory changes at the level of systemic O_2 delivery or $\dot{V}O_2$ that might indicate stress on the system. The average $C\bar{v}O_2$ suggested a well-preserved O_2 reserve capacity. However, O_2 supply might be more unstable because of larger changes in venous admixture for any given change in O_2 pressure.

Short-term measurements of O_2 status are unlikely to provide conclusive evidence in favor of either O_2 administration strategy. A formal comparison in a randomized controlled trial with long-term outcome measures is therefore necessary to decide O_2 administration policies; relevant clinical outcomes should include the death rate and the rates of eye, lung, and brain damage in survivors.[41] The fact that the currently accepted range of arterial oxygenation allowed a mean difference of 11% in the inspired O_2 concentration shows that such a trial would test the effects of a quantitatively important difference in O_2 exposure.

We thank the following workers for their assistance and support: Jim Kane, chief technologist, Cardiorespiratory Services; Joei Cannon, Rose Durocher, and Janice Robinson, echocardiography technicians; The Masters and Wardens Association of Hamilton (Masonic Foundation of Ontario) for the donation of the MGM/jr metabolic gas monitor; the nursing staff of the neonatal unit; and the babies (and their parents) who participated in this study.

REFERENCES

1. Dudell G, Cornish JD, Bartlett RH. What constitutes adequate oxygenation? Pediatrics 1990;85:39-41.
2. Lister G, Moreau G, Moss M, Talner NS. Effects of alterations of oxygen transport on the neonate. Semin Perinatol 1984; 8:192-204.
3. Mortola JP, Frappell PB, Dotta A, et al. Ventilatory and metabolic responses to acute hyperoxia in newborns. Am Rev Respir Dis 1992;146:11-5.
4. Whyte RK. Mixed venous oxygen saturation in the newborn: can we and should we measure it? Scand J Clin Lab Invest Suppl 1990;203:203-11.
5. Swyer PR, Boston RW, Murdock A, et al. Oxygen therapy in the newborn infant: statement by the Fetus and Newborn Committee of the Canadian Paediatric Society. Can Med Assoc J 1975;113:750-1.
6. American Academy of Pediatrics recommendations on oxygen use. Pediatrics 1976;57:S635-7.
7. Emond D, Lachance C, Gagnon J, Bard H. Arterial partial pressure of oxygen required to achieve 90% saturation of hemoglobin in very low birth weight newborns. Pediatrics 1993;91:602-4.
8. American Academy of Pediatrics, American College of Obstetricians and Gynecologists. Guidelines for perinatal care. 3rd ed. Washington, DC: 1992:197-203.
9. Thilo EH, Andersen D, Wasserstein ML, Schmidt J, Luckey D. Saturation by pulse oximetry: comparison of the results obtained by instruments of different brands. J PEDIATR 1993; 122:620-6.
10. Hay WW, Brockway JM, Eyzaguirre M. Neonatal pulse oximetry: accuracy and reliability. Pediatrics 1989;83:717-22.
11. Blanchette T, Dziodzio J, Harris K. Pulse oximetry and normoxemia in neonatal intensive care. Respir Care 1991;36:25-32.
12. Snider AR, Serwer GA. Methods for obtaining quantitative information from the echocardiographic examination. In: Echocardiography in pediatric heart disease. Chicago: Year Book, 1990:78-133.
13. Hudson I, Houston A, Aitchison T, Holland B, Turner T. Reproducibility of measurements of cardiac output in newborn infants by Doppler ultrasound. Arch Dis Child 1990;65:15-9.
14. Nunn JF. Applied respiratory physiology. 3rd ed. London: Butterworths, 1987.
15. Scheinman MM, Brown MA, Rapaport E. Critical assessment of use of central venous oxygen saturation as a mirror of mixed venous oxygen in severely ill patients. Circulation 1989;40:165-72.

16. Hirschl RB, Palmer P, Heiss KF, Hultquist K, Fazzalari F, Bartlett RH. Evaluation of the right atrial venous oxygen saturation as a physiologic monitor in a neonatal model. J Pediatr Surg 1993;28:901-5.
17. Mellander M, Sabel K-G, Caidahl K, Solymar L, Eriksson B. Doppler determination of cardiac output in infants and children: comparison with simultaneous thermodilution. Pediatr Cardiol 1987;8:241-6.
18. Alverson DC, Eldridge M, Dillon T, Yabek SM, Berman W. Noninvasive pulsed Doppler determination of cardiac output in neonates and children. J Pediatr 1982;101:46-50.
19. Mandelbaum-Isken VH, Linderkamp O. Cardiac output by pulsed Doppler in neonates using the apical window. Pediatr Cardiol 1991;12:13-6.
20. Gardin JM. Estimation of volume flow by Doppler echocardiography. Echocardiology 1987;4:17-28.
21. Chwals WJ, Lally KP, Woolley MM, Mahour GH. Measured energy expenditure in critically ill infants and young children. J Surg Res 1988;44:467-72.
22. Mayfield SR, Uauy R. Validation of a computerized indirect calorimeter for use in research studies of ventilated neonates [Abstract]. Pediatr Res 1986;20:414A.
23. Mayfield SR. Technical and clinical testing of a computerized indirect calorimeter for use in mechanically ventilated neonates. Am J Clin Nutr 1991;54:30-4.
24. Alverson DC, Isken VH, Cohen RS. Effect of booster blood transfusions on oxygen utilization in infants with bronchopulmonary dysplasia. J Pediatr 1988;113:722-6.
25. Richardson P, Bose CL, Bucciarelli RL, Carlstrom JR. Oxygen consumption of infants with respiratory distress syndrome. Biol Neonate 1984;46:53-6.
26. Chwals WJ, Lally KP, Woolley MM. Indirect calorimetry in mechanically ventilated infants and children: measurement accuracy with absence of audible airleak. Crit Care Med 1992;20:768-70.
27. Lister G, Walter TK, Versmold HT, Dallman PR, Rudolph AM. Oxygen delivery in lambs: cardiovascular and hematologic development. Am J Physiol 1979;237:H668-75.
28. Ronco JJ, Fenwick JC, Tweeddale MG, et al. Identification of the critical oxygen delivery for anaerobic metabolism in critically ill septic and nonseptic humans. JAMA 1993;270:1724-30.
29. Lindner W, Seidel M, Versmold HT, Döhlemann C, Riegel KP. Stroke volume and left ventricular output in preterm infants with patent ductus arteriosus. Pediatr Res 1990;27:278-81.
30. Hudson I, Cooke A, Holland B, et al. Red cell volume and cardiac output in anemic preterm infants. Arch Dis Child 1990;65:672-5.
31. Cross KW, Tizard JPM, Trythall DAH. The gaseous metabolism of the new-born infant breathing 15% oxygen. Acta Pediatr 1958;47:217-37.
32. Mortola JP, Rezzonico R. Metabolic and ventilatory rates in newborn kittens during acute hypoxia. Respir Physiol 1988;73:55-68.
33. Mortola JP, Rezzonico R, Lanthier C. Ventilation and oxygen consumption during acute hypoxia in newborn mammals: a comparative analysis. Respir Physiol 1989;78:31-43.
34. Mortola JP, Matsuoka T. Interaction between CO_2 production and ventilation in the hypoxic kitten. J Appl Physiol 1993; 74:905-10.
35. Mourek J. Oxygen consumption during ontogenesis in rats with high and low oxygen content. Physiol Bohemoslov 1959;8:106-11.
36. Alexander G, Williams D. Summit metabolism and cardiovascular function in young lambs during hyperoxia and hypoxia. J Physiol (Lond) 1970;208:85-97.
37. Mortola JP, Tenney SM. Effects of hyperoxia on ventilatory and metabolic rates in newborn mice. Respir Physiol 1986; 63:267-74.
38. Claflin KS, Alverson DC, Pathak D, Angelus P, Backstrom C, Werner S. Cardiac output determinations in the newborn: reproducibility of the pulsed Doppler velocity measurement. J Ultrasound Med 1988;7:311-5.
39. Billeaud C, Piedboeuf B, Chessex P. Energy expenditure and severity of respiratory disease in very low birth weight infants receiving long-term ventilatory support. J Pediatr 1992; 120:461-4.
40. Shortland GJ, Fleming PJ, Walter JH. Validation of a portable indirect calorimetry system for measurement of energy expenditure in sick preterm infants. Arch Dis Child 1992;67:1207-11.
41. Duc G, Sinclair JC. Oxygen administration. In: Sinclair JC, Bracken MB, eds. Effective care of the newborn infant. Oxford: Oxford University Press, 1992:178-99.

Oxidation of parenteral lipid emulsion by ambient and phototherapy lights: Potential toxicity of routine parenteral feeding

Jiří Neužil, PhD, Brian A. Darlow, MD, Terrie E. Inder, MBChB, Karl B. Sluis, BSc, Christine C. Winterbourn, PhD, and Roland Stocker, PhD

From the Biochemistry Group, The Heart Research Institute, Camperdown, Sydney, New South Wales, Australia, and the Departments of Paediatrics and Pathology, Christchurch School of Medicine, Christchurch Hospital, Christchurch, New Zealand

Vitamin E can be a prooxidant in isolated lipoprotein suspensions. Because lipid emulsions used in parenteral nutrition are lipoprotein-like suspensions rich in polyunsaturated fatty acids and vitamin E, we hypothesized that vitamin E may act as a prooxidant in lipid emulsions, as it is in lipoprotein suspensions. We therefore exposed an intravenously administered lipid emulsion (Intralipid) to a single spotlight commonly used in the treatment of neonatal jaundice, and measured the formation of triglyceride hydroperoxides by using high-performance liquid chromatography with postcolumn chemiluminescence detection. Concentrations of these hydroperoxides in different batches of fresh Intralipid were usually approximately 10 μmol/L but increased up to 60 times after exposure to phototherapy light for a period of 24 hours, even though significant amounts of vitamin E were present at the end of the exposure. Triglyceride hydroperoxides were formed during phototherapy light exposure whether the Intralipid was in plastic tubing used routinely for infusion or in glass containers. Ambient light also caused significant peroxidation of the formula lipids, although to a much lesser extent than observed with phototherapy light. For infants in the neonatal intensive care unit who were receiving Intralipid but not phototherapy, solutions being infused at the end of 24 hours contained a mean of 40 μmol/L hydroperoxides. For infants receiving phototherapy, the mean was 97 μmol/L. Phototherapy light–induced formation of triglyceride hydroperoxides was prevented by covering the Intralipid with aluminum foil or supplementation with sodium ascorbate before light exposure. We conclude that Intralipid is highly susceptible to oxidation and that elevated levels of oxidized lipids can be formed during its clinical use, especially when Intralipid infusion is combined with phototherapy. Because lipid hydroperoxides are cytotoxic and can cause adverse effects, inadvertent infusion of rancid Intralipid may add to the numerous problems encountered by premature neonates. (J PEDIATR 1995;126:785-90)

Supported by the National Health and Medical Research Council of Australia (grants No. 910284 and No. 940915 to R. S.) and the Health Research Council of New Zealand.

Presented at the Annual Meeting of the American Pediatric Society and the Society for Pediatric Research, San Diego, Calif., May 1995.

Submitted for publication Aug. 23, 1994; accepted Dec. 9, 1994.

Reprint requests: Roland Stocker, PhD, Biochemistry Group, The Heart Research Institute, 145 Missenden Road, Camperdown, Sydney, 2050 New South Wales, Australia.

0022-3476/95/$3.00 + 0 **9/23/62652**

See commentary, p. 747.

NICU	Neonatal intensive care unit

Parenteral lipid emulsions derived from either soybean or safflower oil provide essential fatty acids and are a concentrated source of calories for preterm infants. However, lipid infusions in preterm neonates are associated with problems (reviewed by Stahl et al.[1]), including inefficient plasma lipid clearance, displacement of bilirubin from albumin, and impaired pulmonary function.

Earlier reports suggested that lipid emulsions used in parenteral feeding of infants are susceptible to peroxidation, as judged indirectly by the formation of pentane and malondialdehyde.[2] More recently Helbock et al.[3] demonstrated the presence of high concentrations of oxidized lipids in stored lipid emulsions before their administration. Lipid hydroperoxides in either free form or within lipid emulsions are cytotoxic and cause marked damage to endothelial cells of the thoracic aorta when administered intravenously.[4] Lipid hydroperoxides also modulate lipoxygenase[5] and cyclooxygenase[6]; the latter enzyme is responsible for the biosynthesis of important vasoregulatory prostaglandins. Moreover, perfusion of umbilical veins with lipid emulsions causes vasoconstriction, which has been linked to an inhibition in the production of the vasodilator prostaglandin I_2 and an increase in the vasoconstrictor prostaglandin $F_{2\alpha}$.[7] These findings, together with the observation that the concentration of lipid hydroperoxides in plasma of healthy human beings is very low (i.e., measurable in nanomolar amounts),[8] suggest that intravenous infusion of oxidized Intralipid presents a potentially serious problem.

Phototherapy could potentially enhance lipid oxidation. We have exposed an intravenously administered lipid emulsion (Intralipid; Kabi Pharmacia AB, Stockholm, Sweden) to ambient room light and single spotlight under simulated and real phototherapy conditions in a neonatal intensive care unit to determine whether this produces high levels of lipid hydroperoxides.

METHODS

Exposure of Intralipid to various conditions was performed in the Christchurch Women's Hospital NICU, where the ambient temperature is 25° C. A single spotlight unit (Healthdyne Phototherapy Light, model PT 1400-2; Air-Shields, Hatboro, Pa.) was used for phototherapy. The lamps emit light of 400 to 520 nm wavelength. The light is routinely directed at the neonate's chest and abdomen, with the drip site and extension tubing containing fluids frequently exposed, whereas the syringe and infusion pump are located on one side.

Solutions of 20% Intralipid are imported by the local distributor (Baxter Healthcare Ltd., Auckland, New Zealand) in 250 ml clear glass bottles with a 2-year expiration date. The distributor prepares 50 ml aliquots in plastic syringes that have a 30-day expiration date if stored at 4° C, and these are dispensed by the hospital pharmacy. Solutions of Intralipid were exposed either to ambient room light or a single phototherapy spotlight at a distance of 32 to 46 cm. Light fluxes were quantified at baseline and at 24 hours with a model 451 Minolta Air-Shields Fluoro-Lite Meter, which measures irradiances in $\mu W/cm^2$ per nanometer within a wavelength range of 400 to 520 nm.[3] The irradiances used were as recommended for effective phototherapy.[9]

To simulate the clinical situation, the syringes were placed on the bench in the NICU in ambient lighting and connected to standard minibore plastic extension tubing of 1.8 ml capacity (catalog number BC 567, Codan Medlon, Inc., Burbank, Calif.). In the experimental system, the tubing but not the syringe was exposed to phototherapy light. In control samples, syringes and tubing remained in ambient lighting throughout. Samples of lipid (1.5 ml) were taken from the syringes and distal end of the tubing at baseline and after 24 hours.

To investigate the time course of oxidation of Intralipid in different conditions, syringes containing 20% Intralipid were exposed to phototherapy light and samples were taken at intervals up to 24 hours. The syringes were glass, plastic, plastic covered in aluminum foil, or glass to which 2 cm of plastic infusion tubing was added. In further experiments, sodium ascorbate was added to Intralipid in plastic syringes at a final concentration of 1 mmol/L and at pH 7.4. Control conditions were provided by Intralipid with ascorbate added and exposed to ambient light, and Intralipid with an equivalent volume of distilled water added in place of ascorbate and exposed to either phototherapy or ambient light for 24 hours.

Samples of direct clinical relevance were obtained from six neonates receiving Intralipid infusion. Intralipid was removed at baseline and at 24 hours from both the syringe and distal end of the infusion tubing from three infants exposed to phototherapy light and three neonates in ambient lighting.

The Intralipid samples were placed immediately on dry ice and stored at −80° C until they were transported to Sydney on dry ice for analyses; they remained frozen until analyzed. For each shipment, baseline samples that have not been exposed to ambient or phototherapy light served as control samples. Results were included only if these control samples contained <15.9 μmol/L triglyceride hydroperoxides (i.e., two SD values greater than the mean value [see below]).

Table. Levels of triglyceride hydroperoxides in Intralipid taken from the reservoir and distal end of the infusion tubing before and after a 24-hour exposure to ambient room or phototherapy light

	Triglyceride hydroperoxides (μmol/L)			
	Intralipid reservoir		Infusion tubing	
Condition	Baseline	After 24 hr	Baseline	After 24 hr
Simulated				
Ambient light	9.9 ± 1.8	27.4 ± 7.3*	7.5 ± 1.2	59.2 ± 9.7*
Phototherapy light	9.2 ± 0.5	32.4 ± 6.2*	9.6 ± 2.9	633.9 ± 82.5*
Clinical				
Ambient light	5.4	26.9 ± 18.0	5.5	39.9 ± 9.0*
Phototherapy light	6.8	77.8 ± 17.0*	7.0	92.7 ± 4.7*

The results of experiments that simulated the clinical situation (Simulated) and Intralipid samples actually used for parenteral nutrition of neonates (Clinical) are shown. The results represent mean values ± SD of three separate experiments, except for the baseline clinical values, which represent the mean of two separate experiments. All baseline values were within 2 SD of the mean value of fresh Intralipid samples.
*Values different ($\alpha < 0.0005$) from those in fresh Intralipid; Wilcoxon Rank Sum Test (two-sample).

Intralipid samples were extracted and analyzed for unoxidized lipids and triglyceride hydroperoxides by high-performance liquid chromatography with ultraviolet and postcolumn chemiluminescence detection.[10, 11] To verify chemiluminescence-positive peaks as hydroperoxides, an aliquot of the Intralipid sample was treated with sodium borohydride.[12] The amounts of triglyceride hydroperoxides in Intralipid extracts were determined by area comparison of the eluting peaks with those of a standard of cholesteryl linoleate hydroperoxide, assuming an equal response of both hydroperoxides.[13] Vitamin E isomers in the hexane layer in the Intralipid biphasic extract were analyzed by high-performance liquid chromatography with electrochemical detection.[14] For sodium ascorbate stability studies, fresh Intralipid was supplemented with sodium ascorbate (Aldrich Chemical, St. Louis, Mo.) at 100 μmol/L (final concentration) and incubated at 25° C. At various times an aliquot was removed, extracted,[10] and the aqueous methanol layer was analyzed for ascorbate.[15]

RESULTS

We initially examined extracts of Intralipid as obtained from the local pharmacy before exposure to light (i.e., "baseline" Intralipid) for their contents of lipid hydroperoxides by means of high-performance liquid chromatography with specific postcolumn chemiluminescence detection for hydroperoxides. Analyses of 59 such baseline Intralipid samples revealed concentrations of triglyceride hydroperoxides of 7.8 ± 4.0 μmol/L (mean value ± SD). One of the seven shipments contained baseline Intralipid samples with an initial content of triglyceride hydroperoxides of ≅100 μmol/L; the samples of that shipment were excluded.

Treatment of these samples with sodium borohydride, which reduces hydroperoxides to the corresponding alcohols that themselves are not chemiluminescence active,[13] largely eliminated the chemiluminescence-positive peaks detected in untreated samples and typical for triglyceride hydroperoxides. This demonstrated that the chemiluminescence-positive peaks were indeed hydroperoxides.[10, 12, 13] Analysis of a baseline Intralipid sample for its endogenous vitamin E showed ≅60 μmol/L γ-tocopherol and 20 μmol/L each of the δ- and α-isomers; α-tocopherol is biologically the most active form of vitamin E.[16]

To simulate the clinical situation in the NICU, we exposed Intralipid dispensed in standard infusion plastic tubing to either ambient or phototherapy light at irradiances recommended for effective therapy. The plastic tubing was connected to a syringe (used as the Intralipid reservoir). The syringes always remained in ambient light. As shown in the Table, levels of triglyceride hydroperoxides in all the syringes increased threefold during the 24-hour period. There was an additional doubling of the peroxide concentration in the tubing exposed to ambient light, whereas the concentration in the tubing exposed to phototherapy light increased to 65-fold that of the original Intralipid solution. Such high levels of triglyceride hydroperoxides occurred despite the presence of vitamin E, because even at the 24-hour exposure to phototherapy light, 72.5% ± 5.5% and 88% ± 2% (means ± SD, n = 3) of the original α- and γ-tocopherol, respectively, remained in the most heavily oxidized Intralipid sample.

For Intralipid samples used clinically for infusion into neonates (Table), the increases in triglyceride hydroperoxides under ambient light were similar to those seen in the simulated conditions. For infants undergoing phototherapy, hydroperoxide accumulation both in the syringes and in the tubing after 24 hours was higher than with ambient lighting. The values for the accumulated hydroperoxides in the tubing were lower than in the simulated experiments because the Intralipid solution was passing through the light beam rather than remaining static under the phototherapy light. Furthermore, in the clinical situation, with alterations

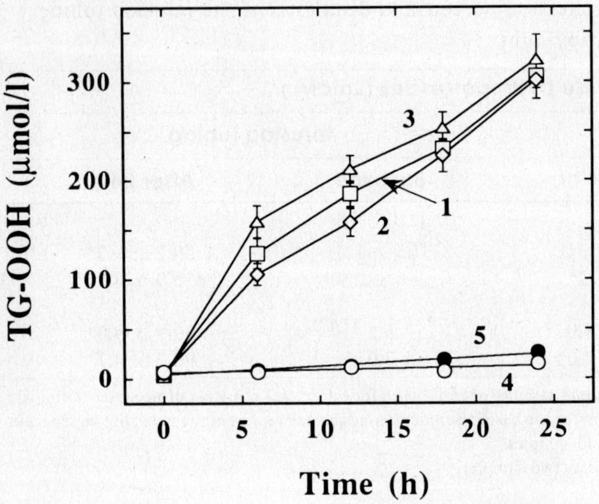

Figure. Kinetics of accumulation of triglyceride hydroperoxides in Intralipid exposed to phototherapy light under conditions that mimic the situation in an NICU. A solution of 20% Intralipid was dispensed into a glass reservoir containing plastic tubing (*line 3*), plastic *(line 1)* or glass reservoir *(line 2)*, plastic reservoir covered with aluminum foil *(line 4)*, or a plastic reservoir after supplementation with 1 mmol/L sodium ascorbate *(line 5)* and exposed to phototherapy light for up to 24 hours. For all samples the light fluxes measured were 11.7 to 25.9 $\mu W/cm^2$ per nanometer for 24 hours. At the time points indicated, aliquots were withdrawn, extracted, and their hexane extracts analyzed for the presence of triglyceride hydroperoxides and α-tocopherol as described in the Methods section.

in the neonate's position and the placement of the light, a variable length of the tubing was exposed to phototherapy for a variable proportion of the 24 hours.

To determine whether photosensitization by the plastic tubing was an important factor, we performed additional experiments, again under conditions that simulated the situation in the NICU. The time-dependent increase in triglyceride hydroperoxides on exposure to phototherapy light was similar for Intralipid in plastic or glass syringes (Figure, *lines 1 and 2*). At least 8% more triglyceride hydroperoxides accumulated in Intralipid dispensed in a glass syringe to which plastic infusion tubing was added *(line 3),* indicating some photosensitizing effect of the plastic tubing. However, these differences were small compared with those related to phototherapy versus ambient light exposure (Table), suggesting that the irradiance applied was largely responsible for hydroperoxide formation.

Oxidation of Intralipid was inhibited almost completely by covering the syringe with aluminum foil (Figure). Supplementation of Intralipid with 1 mmol/L sodium ascorbate before exposure to phototherapy light also inhibited hydroperoxide formation by ≅95%. Addition of water (as a control substance instead of ascorbate) did not affect the rate of triglyceride hydroperoxide formation, and ascorbate also inhibited peroxide formation in ambient light (data not shown). When added to Intralipid at 25° C and under ambient light, ascorbate at 100 μmol/L autooxidized linearly at a rate of 13.5 μmol/L per hour, so that significant and increasing amounts of its oxidation product(s) will be present in the Intralipid.

DISCUSSION

These data show that Intralipid is highly oxidizable under routine clinical conditions in an NICU, and this may result in high concentrations of lipid hydroperoxides being administered intravenously to large numbers of patients receiving this form of parenteral nutrition. This problem is particularly marked for neonates undergoing phototherapy, because this form of lighting is associated with greater prooxidant effect. Lipid oxidation occurs despite high concentrations of vitamin E, but appears to be preventable by the relatively simple maneuvers of wrapping the syringes and tubing in aluminum foil, or adding ascorbate to the infusate.

The high susceptibility of Intralipid to oxidation may appear surprising because it contains large amounts of endogenous vitamin E. The latter is generally regarded as the most efficient chain-breaking, lipid-soluble antioxidant.[16] However, recent reports have revealed that for vitamin E to be an efficient antioxidant in *isolated* lipoprotein emulsions, it requires a suitable "coantioxidant," such as vitamin C (ascorbate),[17, 18] ubiquinol,[19, 20] or albumin-bound bilirubin.[21] These coantioxidants eliminate the vitamin E radical that is formed from the interaction of the vitamin with initiating radical oxidants, which can have an adverse effect by *promoting* lipid peroxidation.[18, 19] Intralipid is also an emulsion of large particles, made of a triacylglycerol core surrounded by a monolayer of phospholipids.[22] Hence vitamin E is likely to act similarly in Intralipid as in lipoproteins, and in the absence of suitable coantioxidants may cause formation of triglyceride hydroperoxides during storage.[17-19] Therefore increasing the concentration of this antioxidant alone is not likely to increase the oxidation resistance of Intralipid.

Two recent reports have examined the formation of lipid hydroperoxides in infant feeding formulas. Helbock et al.,[3] who used a method similar to ours, reported values of lipid hydroperoxides as high as 650 μmol/L in 20% Intralipid taken from the samples prepared by the pharmacy of the University of California, both before and after a 20-hour exposure to ambient light. The extent to which the differences in initial lipid peroxide concentrations are related to differences in the manufactured batches, handling, the processing of Intralipid in the local pharmacy or hospital before its use, or a combination of these factors, is not clear. Another report[23] showed that the level of lipid peroxides in human milk and infant formula was very low (<0.5 μmol/L for the formula, ~1.5 μmol/L for the milk). Unlike Intralipid, the formula contained vitamin C, and human milk possesses natural antioxidant defenses. Exposure of these preparations to phototherapy light did not increase the concentration of lipid hydroperoxides.[23]

Intravenous infusion with oxidized Intralipid in preterm neonates may be a clinically significant hazard. The highest level of lipid hydroperoxides detected in infused Intralipid ($\simeq$100 μmol/L, Table) is some five orders of magnitude higher than that present in plasma of healthy adult human subjects.[8] Thus, even when the slow infusion rate, hemodilution, and rapid in vivo clearance of Intralipid (i.e., in the minute time scale) are considered, the overall plasma concentration of lipid hydroperoxides derived from the infused oxidized Intralipid may well be within or even above the concentration range of endogenous hydroperoxides; local hydroperoxide concentrations would be expected to be even higher.

In addition to a direct cytotoxic effect,[4] lipid hydroperoxides in oxidized Intralipid could conceivably cause (pulmonary) vasoconstriction through interference with the endogenous synthesis of vasoregulatory prostaglandins,[5, 6] inactivation of endothelium-derived relaxing factor, or both, as has been shown for oxidized low-density lipoprotein and the lipids extracted from it.[24] In vitro oxidation of low-density lipoprotein results in non-cyclooxygenasederived esterified prostanoids (F_2-isoprostanes),[25] some of which are potent vasoconstrictors in their free form. Therefore esterified isoprostanes may also be formed during phototherapy light–induced oxidation of Intralipid and become biologically active during infusion and hydrolysis.

Several strategies might minimize this potentially serious problem. One simple solution is to protect the Intralipid from light exposure by wrapping the tubing and syringe with aluminum foil; in the future an aluminum foil sleeve or dark tubing may be used to solve the problem identified here. Addition of ascorbate to Intralipid, although very effective and inexpensive, cannot currently be recommended, because side effects of relatively high concentrations of ascorbate, its oxidation products, or both cannot be excluded. However, combining commercial water-soluble vitamin preparations used in parenteral nutrition with Intralipid in the syringe may be beneficial because some of these preparations contain ascorbate.

We found a greater accumulation of hydroperoxides in the syringes for neonates receiving phototherapy even though they were theoretically not exposed to the spotlight. However, syringes may have been exposed while lights were redirected during periods when access to the infant was required. Thus phototherapy lights should be turned off rather than redirected during infant care procedures.

In this study, the analyses of lipids actually given to neonates were similar to the simulated conditions of light exposure described, and this will provide a useful model for further testing. Although we exclusively tested only one commonly used brand of lipid supplement, one form of phototherapy, and in only one NICU, we believe that the results are widely applicable because these variables are similar in many hospital settings.

We conclude that parenteral nutrition with Intralipid administered under standard practices in an NICU results in the formation and intravenous infusion of relatively high levels of oxidized lipids. This may present an additional source of morbidity in premature neonates, but appears preventable by minimizing the exposure of the lipid to ambient and phototherapy lights.

We thank Drs. W. Jessup, L. Krithrides, and D. Celermajer for critical reading of the manuscript.

REFERENCES

1. Stahl GE, Spear ML, Mamosh M. Intravenous administration of lipid emulsions to premature infants. Clin Perinatol 1986; 13:133-62.
2. Pitkänen O, Hallman M, Andersson S. Generation of free radicals in lipid emulsion used in parenteral nutrition. Pediatr Res 1991;29:56-9.
3. Helbock HJ, Motchnik PA, Ames BN. Toxic hydroperoxides in intravenous lipid emulsions used in preterm infants. Pediatrics 1993;91:83-7.
4. Yagi K, Ohkawa H, Ohnishi N, Yamashita M, Nakashima T. Lesions of aortic intima caused by intravenous administration of linoleic acid hydroperoxides. J Appl Biochem 1981;3:58-65.
5. Hatzelmann A, Schatz M, Ullrich V. Involvement of glutathione peroxidase activity in the stimulation of 5-lipoxygenase activity by glutathione-depleting agents in human polymorphonuclear leukocytes. Eur J Biochem 1989;180:527-33.
6. Markey CM, Alward A, Weller PE, Marnett LJ. Quantitative studies of hydroperoxide reduction by prostaglandin H synthase. J Biol Chem 1987;262:6266-79.
7. Lavoie JC, Chessex P. The increase in vasomotor tone induced by parenteral lipid emulsion is linked to an inhibition of prostacyclin production. Free Radic Biol Med 1994;16:795-9.
8. Bowry VB, Stanley KK, Stocker R. High-density lipoprotein is the major carrier of lipid hydroperoxides in human blood plasma from fasting donors. Proc Natl Acad Sci U S A 1992;89:10316-20.
9. Modi N, Keay AJ. Phototherapy for neonatal hyperbilirubinaemia: the importance of dose. Arch Dis Child 1983; 58:406-9.
10. Sattler W, Mohr D, Stocker R. Rapid isolation of lipoproteins and assessment of their peroxidation by HPLC postcolumn chemiluminescence. Methods Enzymol 1994;233:469-89.
11. Mohr D, Stocker R. Radical-mediated oxidation of isolated human very low density lipoprotein. Arterioscler Thromb 1994;14:1186-92.
12. Frei B, Yamamoto Y, Niclas D, Ames BN. Evaluation of an isoluminol chemiluminescence assay for the detection of hydroperoxides in human blood plasma. Anal Biochem 1988; 175:120-30.
13. Yamamoto Y, Brodsky MH, Baker JC, Ames BN. Detection and characterization of lipid hydroperoxides at picomole lev-

els by high-performance liquid chromatography. Anal Biochem 1987;60:7-13.
14. Pascoe GA, Duda CT, Reed DJ. Determination of α-tocopherol and α-tocopherylquinone in small biological samples by high-performance liquid chromatography with electrochemical detection. J Chromatogr 1987;414:440-8.
15. Behrens WA, Madere R. A highly sensitive high-performance liquid chromatography method for the estimation of ascorbic and dehydroascorbic acid in tissues, biological fluids, and foods. Anal Biochem 1987;165:102-7.
16. Burton GW, Ingold KU. Vitamin E: application of the principles of physical organic chemistry to the exploration of its structure and function. Acc Chem Res 1986;19:194-201.
17. Bowry VW, Ingold KU, Stocker R. Vitamin E in human low-density lipoprotein. When and how this antioxidant becomes a pro-oxidant. Biochem J 1992;288:341-4.
18. Bowry VW, Stocker R. Tocopherol-mediated peroxidation. The pro-oxidant effect of vitamin E on the radical-initiated oxidation of human low-density lipoprotein. J Am Chem Soc 1993;115:6029-40.
19. Ingold, KU, Bowry VW, Stocker R, Walling C. Autooxidation of lipids and antioxidation by α-tocopherol and ubiquinol in homogeneous solution and in aqueous dispersions of lipids. The unrecognized consequences of lipid particle size as exemplified by the oxidation of human low-density lipoprotein. Proc Natl Acad Sci U S A 1993;90:45-9.
20. Stocker R, Bowry VW, Frei B. Ubiquinol-10 protects human low-density lipoprotein more efficiently against lipid peroxidation than does α-tocopherol. Proc Natl Acad Sci U S A 1991; 88:1646-50.
21. Neužil J, Stocker R. Free and albumin-bound bilirubin are efficient co-antioxidants for α-tocopherol, inhibiting plasma and low density lipoprotein lipid peroxidation. J Biol Chem 1994; 269:16712-9.
22. Rotenberg M, Rubin M, Bor A, Meyuhas D, Talmon Y, Lichtenberg D. Physico-chemical characterization of Intralipid emulsions. Biochim Biophys Acta 1991;1086:265-72.
23. van Zoeren-Grobben D, Moison RMW, Ester WM, Berger HM. Lipid peroxidation in human milk and infant formula: effect of storage, tube feeding and exposure to phototherapy. Acta Paediatr 1993;82:645-9.
24. Chin JH, Azhar S, Hoffman BB. Inactivation of endothelial-derived relaxing factor by oxidized lipoproteins. J Clin Invest 1992;89:10-8.
25. Lynch SM, Morrow JD, Roberts LJ II, Frei B. Formation of noncyclooxygenase-derived prostanoids (F2-isoprostanes) in plasma and low-density lipoprotein exposed to oxidative stress in vitro. J Clin Invest 1994;93:998-1005.

Plasma mineral concentrations in preterm infants fed a nutrient-enriched formula after hospital discharge

Sujatha Rajaram, PhD, Susan E. Carlson, PhD, Winston W. K. Koo, MBBS, and W. Emmett Braselton, PhD

From the Department of Pediatrics and The Department of Obstetrics and Gynecology, University of Tennessee, Memphis, and the Department of Pharmacology and Toxicology, Michigan State University, East Lansing

Objective: To determine whether prolonged feeding of preterm infant formula to preterm infants can accelerate recovery to normal plasma zinc levels without affecting plasma mineral homeostasis.
Design: Part of concurrent prospective feeding trials in a university hospital–based population.
Subjects and intervention: Preterm infants (n = 33; birth weight, 1037 ± 157 gm) were fed a preterm infant formula with higher concentrations of zinc, copper, calcium, magnesium, and potassium until 2 months past expected term, then a term infant formula. Term infants (n = 38; birth weight, 3318 ± 401 gm) fed this term infant formula from birth were a reference group for comparison with study infants and with published values. Plasma mineral levels were analyzed by inductively coupled plasma atomic emission spectroscopy.
Results: Preterm infants fed a preterm infant formula after discharge from the hospital appeared to achieve normal plasma zinc concentrations by at least 2 months past term without adverse effects on mineral homeostasis. (J PEDIATR 1995;126:791-6)

Currently, nutrient-enriched formula is used routinely in the treatment of hospitalized preterm infants in the United States. Recent reports have also shown that prolonging the feeding of preterm infant formula after discharge of the infant from the hospital can improve nutritional status,[1-3] growth,[4] and bone mineralization.[5] In addition, a zinc supplement provided after patient discharge at levels found in preterm infant formula has been shown to improve Zn status, linear growth velocity, and early motor development.[6] However, data on plasma concentrations of minerals during prolonged feeding of preterm infant formula are minimal. These data may be important because there is presently no assurance that extended feeding of the nutrient-enriched preterm infant formulas does not result in supraphysiologic concentrations of plasma minerals. The goal of this study was to compare Zn, calcium, copper, magnesium, potassium, and iron concentrations of preterm infants fed a preterm infant formula until 2 months after expected term delivery. Data from a group of term infants were obtained as a basis for comparison with study infants and as a reference

ICP/AES	Inductively coupled plasma atomic emission spectroscopy
PCA	Postconceptional age
SRM	Standard reference material

Supported by grants from the National Eye Institute (R01 EY08770), the National Institute of Child Health and Human Development (R01-HD 31329), the National Center for Research Resources (M01 RR00211) and a gift from Ross Products Division, Abbott Laboratories, Columbus, Ohio.

Presented in part at the annual meeting of the Federation of American Societies for Biology and published as an abstract in FASEB J 1994;8:A460.

Submitted for publication Aug. 24, 1994; accepted Dec. 1, 1994.

Reprint requests: Susan E. Carlson, PhD, Newborn Center, Room 201, 853 Jefferson Ave., Memphis, TN 38163.

0022-3476/95/$3.00 + 0 **9/23/62437**

Table I. Neonatal and perinatal characteristics of term and preterm infants studied

Variable	Mean ± SD (range) Term (n = 38)	Preterm (n = 33)
Birth weight (gm)	3318 ± 401 (2600-4190)	1037 ± 157 (747-1275)
Gestational age (wk)	40.0 ± 1.0 (38-42)	27.8 ± 1.4 (24-30)
Black/white ratio	35:3	28:5
M/F ratio	18:20	17:16
Apgar (5 min)	9.0 ± 0.2 (8-10)	7.2 ± 1.2 (4-10)
Maternal age (yr)	22.0 ± 4.0 (17-33)	22.0 ± 5.0 (16-33)
Maternal height (cm)	162.5 ± 6.3 (150-180)	164.1 ± 5.9 (152-178)
Gravidity	2.8 ± 1.2 (1-5)	2.5 ± 1.2 (1-5)

group for term infants studied with methods other than inductively coupled plasma atomic emission spectroscopy, the multielement assay used here.

METHODS

Preterm and term infants were the subjects of separate randomized trials that ran concurrently. Each trial was designed primarily to determine whether infant development could be improved by the addition of long-chain n-3 or n-6 fatty acids to formula. Because preterm infants fed term infant formula after discharge had a high incidence of biochemical vitamin A deficiency,[2] to avoid the possibility of marginal nutritional status confounding developmental outcomes, both control and experimental preterm groups were fed a nutrient-enriched preterm infant formula until 2 months of age (this and all subsequent ages indicate age after expected term). Instead of including the type of formula fed at discharge as part of the randomization, which would have increased the time necessary for enrollment from 3 to 6 years, the decision was made to obtain information on mineral status, which could be helpful in subsequent randomized trials.

The mineral content of the control (Similac Special Care and Similac With Iron, Ross Products Div., Abbott Laboratories, Columbus, Ohio) and experimental formulas based on these products was identical. Parental consent was obtained before enrollment, according to a protocol approved by the institutional review board of the University of Tennessee, Memphis. If sufficient blood was available for mineral analysis at a planned blood draw (250 μl), a separate sample of blood was prepared for mineral analyses (see Blood Collection). Only preterm infants for whom blood was available from at least three of six planned blood draws and term infants for whom blood was available from at least two of four planned blood draws were included in the analyses. The preterm and term infants constituted subsets of 33 of 59, and 38 of 59 infants, respectively; their neonatal and perinatal characteristics are shown in Table I.

Preterm infants received a parenteral solution containing Zn (3.2 mg/L) and Cu (0.16 mg/L) from approximately 48 hours of age. The volume of parenteral solution was increased to 125 ml/kg per day for 96 hours. Preterm formula was started at approximately 72 hours of age and the volume increased gradually to 150 ml/kg per day, which provided 120 kcal/kg per day (Table II). On average, infants had a postnatal age of 3½ weeks when they achieved a formula intake of 150 ml/kg per day. Parenteral feedings were decreased gradually and stopped when enteral intakes of preterm formula reached approximately 80 kcal/kg per day.

Infants were discharged from the hospital when they weighed approximately 1800 gm but continued receiving preterm formula until 2 months past expected term. They returned for follow-up at 0, 2, 4, 6, 9, and 12 months after term. From 2 to 12 months they were provided a standard formula (Similac With Iron Ross Products Div., Abbott Laboratories; 5.1 mg/L Zn or 0.75 mg Zn per 100 kcal). Term infants were fed a formula with the same vitamin and mineral composition as Similac With Iron formula from birth through 12 months of age. All formulas were provided at no cost and as needed to parents, and the parents of study infants were encouraged to provide free access to formula as an exclusive feeding to infants to 4 months past term. In addition, parents received money for transportation. Parents were interviewed by a nutritionist at each follow-up visit and asked to describe their child's usual intake of formula. If the diet history was determined to be unreliable, the data were not included. From 4 months past term, both term and preterm infants consumed a mixed diet, which included both formula and variable amounts of other foods. Only reports of recent formula intake obtained at each visit were used to obtain an estimate of mineral intake from formula. Mean reported formula intakes up to age 1 month were 0.20 ± 0.08 L/kg per day and 0.21 ± 0.03 L/kg per day in term and preterm infants, respectively. Reported formula intake was unchanged through 4 months in term infants and then declined progressively, reaching 0.10 L/kg per day by 12 months. The formula intake of preterm infants declined progressively throughout infancy, reaching 0.08 L/kg per day by 12 months.

Blood collection. Heparinized blood samples were collected in trace element–free vials (Sarstedt, Newton, N.C.). Samples from preterm infants were collected at term (39 ± 1 week postconceptional age) and at 2 (48 ± 1 weeks PCA), 4 (57 ± 1 weeks PCA), 6 (69 ± 1 weeks PCA), 9

(79 ± 1 weeks PCA), and 12 months (92 ± 1 weeks PCA). Blood samples from term infants were obtained at 2, 4, 6, and 12 months. Samples were collected between 10 AM and 2 PM, and all infants were well and eating at 3- to 4-hour intervals on the day of sampling; the samples were not postprandial. After immediate separation from blood cells, plasma was stored in sterile polypropylene microtubes (Sarstedt) at −70° C until the mineral analyses were performed.

Instrumentation and analytic methods. An ICP/AES, a polyscan 61E simultaneous/sequential instrument (Thermo Jarrell Ash Corp., Franklin, Mass.) interfaced to a U-5000 Ultrasonic Nebulizer (Cetac Technologies Inc., Omaha, Neb.), was used for plasma mineral analyses. The validity and sensitivity of the ICP/AES technique for measuring mineral concentrations in plasma and other biologic fluids have been documented.[7-9] The small sample necessitated addition of the ultrasonic nebulization technique for additional sensitivity. The analysis involved the overnight digestion (95° C) of 0.1 ml of plasma with 0.5 ml of Baker-analyzed Ultrex II nitric acid (Baxter Diagnostics, Inc., McGaw Park, Ill.) in tetrafluoroethylene (Teflon) containers (Savillex Corp., Minnetonka, Minn.). After digestion the samples were removed from the oven, cooled to room temperature, and brought to a final volume of 10 ml by gravimetric addition of grade I water (Millipore Corp., Bedford, Mass.) to a predetermined net weight of 10.224 gm.

Mineral standards (Johnson-Matthey/Aesar, Ward Hill, Mass.) were made up in 5% nitric acid containing 30 ppm Na to matrix match with the plasma samples. The accuracy of the assay was verified by comparing the readings obtained from the standards with National Institute of Standards and Technology (NIST) multielement mix A-1 standard reference material 3171a and multielement mix B SRM 3172, diluted to 1 ppm with 5% nitric acid with 30 ppm Na. Quality control was achieved by determining the concentration of Zn in control bovine serum and/or human serum prepared in the same manner as the samples and comparing the values with that of NIST bovine serum (SRM 1598) and/or human serum 909a (NIST, Gaithersburg, Md.). The ICP/AES value for Zn in 0.1 ml (n = 40) of the control bovine serum (mean ± SD) is 0.92 ± 0.14 ppm, and the established mean in bovine serum is 0.92 ppm (range, 0.85 to 0.98 ppm). Our ICP/AES values for all minerals studied in the certified serum were within 2% to 3% of the established mean and were in the accepted range.

Statistical analysis. The General Linear Model procedure of statistical application system (SAS) version 6.0 (SAS Institute, Cary, N.C.) was employed for all statistics. After a preliminary analysis, which showed that the inclusion of long-chain n-3 or n-6 fatty acids did not influence any plasma mineral, this variable was not considered further. A repeated-measures analysis of variance, corrected for subject effects and missing data, was performed for each mineral to determine the effects of gestational age at birth (term or preterm) and time (study age) on plasma concentration. Within each analysis were 276 individual analyses. The Fisher least significant difference obtained from these analyses was used for comparisons to obtain within-group (study age) and between-group (gestational age at birth) differences. A difference with $p < 0.05$ was considered statistically significant.

Table II. Selected mineral composition of study formulas

Nutrient*	Term formula	Preterm formula
K (mg/L)	710	1047
Ca (mg/L)	493	1462
Mg (mg/L)	40.6	97.4
Zn (mg/L)	5.1	12.2
Cu (μg/L)	608	2030
Fe (mg/L)	12.2	14.62

*From Ross Laboratories Product Handbook, Ross Products Div., Abbott Laboratories, Columbus, Ohio, June 1992. The term infant formula contained 676 kcal/L, and the preterm infant formula contained 812 kcal/L.

RESULTS

Longitudinal changes in plasma concentrations of K, Ca Mg, Cu, Zn, and Fe are shown in Table III. In both term and preterm infants plasma K generally decreased with increasing age ($p < 0.0001$). The plasma K concentration obtained in preterm infants differed from that of term infants ($p < 0.009$), but this appeared to be due completely to a lower 12-month plasma K concentration in term compared with preterm infants. Mean plasma Ca and Mg concentrations remained constant throughout the study period, and the concentrations were similar in term and preterm infants.

The mean plasma Zn concentration in the preterm group at term was significantly lower than at every subsequent age (Table III). However, even at term, most preterm infants (92%) had a plasma Zn concentration greater than 65 μg/dl. In term infants the mean plasma Zn concentration increased significantly between 6 and 12 months ($p < 0.001$). Compared with term infants, preterm infants had a significantly higher plasma Zn level at 4 months ($p < 0.02$) and a lower plasma Zn level at 12 mo ($p < 0.05$) of age.

There were wide ranges in plasma Cu and Fe concentrations for both term and preterm groups at all ages (Table III). Plasma Cu concentrations also increased significantly with increasing age in both term ($p < 0.03$) and preterm ($p < 0.0001$) infants. Plasma Fe concentration decreased in time ($p < 0.05$) and was higher in preterm compared with term infants ($p < 0.004$).

DISCUSSION

Infant formulas specially designed for the nutrient needs of premature infants contain Zn concentrations of 10 to

Table III. Plasma concentrations of K, Ca, Mg, Zn, Cu, and Fe in term and preterm infants during the first year of life

Age* (mo)	K (mmol/L)		Ca (mg/dl)		Mg (mg/dl)	
	Term	Preterm	Term	Preterm	Term	Preterm
0	NA	5.0 ± 0.6[a]	NA	9.4 ± 1.0	NA	2.1 ± 0.3
2	4.8 ± 0.5[a]	4.8 ± 0.6[a, b]	9.7 ± 0.8	9.9 ± 0.9	2.0 ± 0.3	2.0 ± 0.3
4	4.4 ± 0.5[b]	4.6 ± 0.6[b, c]	9.7 ± 0.7	9.7 ± 0.9	2.0 ± 0.2	2.0 ± 0.3
6	4.3 ± 0.5[b]	4.4 ± 0.6[c, d]	9.4 ± 0.8	9.9 ± 1.0	2.0 ± 0.3	2.0 ± 0.3
9	NA	4.4 ± 0.7[c, d]	NA	9.8 ± 0.9	NA	2.1 ± 0.3
12	4.2 ± 0.6[b]	4.6 ± 0.7[b, d, †]	9.8 ± 0.7	9.6 ± 0.9	1.9 ± 0.2	2.0 ± 0.3
Repeated measures ANOVA						
Gestational age	0.009		NS		NS	
Study age	0.0001		NS		NS	

Concentration values are least-squares means ± SD from repeated-measures analysis of variance. Study ages with *different letters as superscripts* are significantly different from each other (p <0.05).
Conversion factors for SI units: Ca, mg/dl × 0.25 = mmol/L; Cu, μg/dl × 0.16 = μmol/L; Fe, μg/dl × 0.18 = μmol/L; Mg, mg/dl × 0.41 = μmol/L; Zn, μg/dl × 0.15 = μmol/L.
NA, Not available; *NS*, not significant.
*Adjusted for expected term.
†Preterm infants differ from term infants of the same age (p <0.05).

12.2 mg/L and are routinely used for in-hospital feeding of preterm infants in the United States. However, preterm formula given only during the hospital stay, with the feeding of standard formula after hospital discharge,[10-14] is not adequate to prevent a decline in plasma Zn levels.[14-16] Our data demonstrate that preterm infants fed preterm formula for 2 to 3 months after discharge from the hospital achieve a plasma Zn concentration equivalent to that of term infants on or before an adjusted age of 2 months.

The Subcommittee on Recommended Daily Allowances[17] has proposed a Zn intake of 5 mg/day for formula-fed term infants, on the basis of the Zn intake of normal breast-fed infants; this value takes into account the lower bioavailability of Zn from formulas. Assuming an absorption of 20%,[18] this would allow for Zn retention of 1 mg/day, and would meet the estimated Zn requirement of healthy term infants in the early postnatal period of 0.8 mg/day. In our term reference group the mean Zn intake exceeded 5 mg/day, and the mean plasma Zn concentration at each study age was similar to normal adult values.[19] In contrast, preterm infants who presumably retained Zn at approximately 1 mg/day for 3 weeks had declines in plasma Zn concentration.[16] The preterm infants in our study had Zn intakes of 9 mg/day from term to 2 months. If their Zn absorption was similar to that of formula-fed term infants, they should have had Zn retention of 1.5 to 2 mg/day during this interval. Judging from the fact that they rapidly achieved plasma Zn concentrations similar to those of term infants, this intake appears to have been reasonable.

Marginal Zn status has been shown to result in slower growth[20, 21] and poorer immune function,[22, 23] and to alter behavior in rats[24] and nonhuman primates.[25] In the only randomized trial to study the effects of supplementing the diet of preterm infants with Zn after discharge from the hospital, Friel et al.[6] observed higher plasma Zn concentration, linear growth velocity, and scores for motor development. Additional studies are required to determine whether other improvements in behavior (e.g., those influenced by feeding preterm formula compared with term formula[26] and human milk[27]) are associated with Zn intake from different types of feedings.

Plasma K, Ca, and Mg concentrations are normally well regulated and maintained within narrow ranges.[28] Despite intakes of Ca and Mg from preterm infant formula two times higher than those from standard formula, the preterm infants studied here had concentrations of plasma Ca and Mg comparable to those of formula-fed term infants. Higher K intakes of preterm compared with term infants did not influence plasma K concentration during the first 2 months of infancy, and both term and preterm infants had a normal decline in plasma K concentration in time.

Plasma Cu does not reflect hepatic Cu stores immediately after preterm birth, presumably because ceruloplasmin concentration is low.[29] Hence a low plasma Cu concentration does not necessarily indicate poor Cu stores. The mean Cu concentration of 61 μg/dl in preterm infants at term corrected age was lower than the normal reference range for adults (80 to 120 μg/dl) but increased to within normal limits by 2 months past term. A similar increase was reported up to 3 months of age by L'Abbe and Friel[1] in infants, regardless of dietary Cu intake. The progressive increase in plasma Cu throughout infancy in term and preterm infants was virtually identical to that reported by these authors and also did not appear to be influenced by Cu intake. Nevertheless, the group fed Cu intakes two times higher until 3 months past term had higher erythrocyte Cu,

Table III—cont'd

Zn (μg/dl)		Cu (μg/dl)		Fe (μg/dl)	
Term	Preterm	Term	Preterm	Term	Preterm
NA	80.1 ± 19.0[a]	NA	61.5 ± 41[a]	NA	92.7 ± 55
93.3 ± 18.6[a]	101.4 ± 18.5[b]	84.2 ± 39.4[a]	85.8 ± 40[b]	88.3 ± 31.4	108.4 ± 55
92.0 ± 18.1[a]	106.6 ± 19.1[b,†]	105.7 ± 38.5[b]	111.8 ± 42[c]	72.0 ± 30.2	106.2 ± 57†
97.3 ± 18.4[a]	103.2 ± 18.6[b]	112.6 ± 39.1[b]	121.1 ± 41[c,d]	70.4 ± 29.3	84.1 ± 56
NA	106.7 ± 19.1[b]	NA	139.8 ± 42[d]	NA	85.4 ± 55
112.9 ± 18.4[b]	100.9 ± 18.7[b,†]	144.0 ± 38.5[c]	147.3 ± 42[d]	81.3 ± 30.5	88.7 ± 58
NS		NS		0.004	
0.0002		0.001		0.05	

Zn–superoxide dismutase levels, suggesting there was an advantage to prolonged feeding of higher Cu intakes.[1]

Because both term and preterm infants received formulas with 1.8 mg Fe per 100 kcal, we cannot explain why plasma Fe concentration during infancy was somewhat higher in preterm compared with term infants. This may have been related to early erythrocyte transfusions received by preterm infants. There was also a small but significant decrease in plasma Fe in time in both term and preterm infants; this decrease fits with parental reports that infants gradually replaced energy from Fe-fortified formula with that from foods lower in Fe concentration. Despite these significant differences, however, the means in plasma for both term and preterm infants at all ages were well within the normal adult range of 35 to 140 μg/dl.[30]

We conclude that prolonged feeding of nutrient-enriched formula to preterm infants can accelerate achievement of normal plasma Zn values in preterm infants without adverse effects on other plasma mineral levels.

The technical assistance of Kirk Stuart is gratefully acknowledged. We appreciate the assistance of Susan Werkman and Amy Ford in conducting this study.

REFERENCES

1. L'Abbe MR, Friel JK. Copper status of very low birth weight infants during the first 12 months of infancy. Pediatr Res 1992;32:183-8.
2. Peeples JM, Carlson SE, Werkman SH, Cooke RJ. Vitamin A status of preterm infants during infancy. Am J Clin Nutr 1991;53:1455-9.
3. Carlson SE, Peeples JM, Werkman SH, Koo WWK. Plasma retinol and retinol binding protein concentrations in very preterm infants fed preterm formula in early infancy. Eur J Clin Nutr (in press).
4. Lucas A, Bishop NJ, King FJ, Cole TJ. Randomised trial of nutrition for preterm infants after discharge. Arch Dis Child 1992;67:324-7.
5. Bishop NJ, King FJ, Lucas A. Increased bone mineral content of preterm infants fed with a nutrient enriched formula after discharge from hospital. Arch Dis Child 1993;68:573-8.
6. Friel JK, Andrews WL, Matthew JD, et al. Zinc supplementation in very low birth weight infants. J Pediatr Gastroenterol Nutr 1993;17:97-104.
7. Stowe HD, Braselton WE, Slanker M, Kaneene JB. Multielement assays of canine serum, liver, and kidney by inductively coupled argon plasma emission spectroscopy. Am J Vet Res 1986;47:822-7.
8. Fassel VA. Quantitative elemental analyses by plasma emission spectroscopy. Science 1978;202:183-91.
9. Nixon DE, Moyer TP, Johnson P, et al. Routine measurement of calcium, magnesium, copper, zinc and iron in urine and serum by inductively coupled plasma emission spectroscopy. Clin Chem 1986;32:1660-5.
10. Gibson RS, Dewolfe MS. Changes in serum zinc concentrations of some Canadian full term and low birthweight infants from birth to six months. Acta Paediatr Scand 1981;70:497-500.
11. Altigani M, Murphy JF, Gray OP. Plasma zinc concentration and catch up growth in preterm infants. Acta Paediatr Scand Suppl 1989;357:20-33.
12. Friel JK, Gibson RS, Peliowski AD, Watts J. Serum zinc, copper and selenium concentrations in preterm infants receiving enteral nutrition or parenteral nutrition supplemented with zinc and copper. J PEDIATR 1984;104:763-8.
13. McMaster D, Lappin TRJ, Halliday HL, Patterson CC. Serum copper and zinc levels in the preterm infant: a longitudinal study of the first year of life. Biol Neonate 1983;44:108-13.
14. Tyrala EE, Manser JI, Brodsky NL, et al. Serum zinc concentrations in growing premature infants. Acta Paediatr Scand 1983;72:695-8.
15. Koo WW, Succop P, Hambidge KM. Serum alkaline phosphatase and serum zinc concentrations in preterm infants with rickets and fractures. Am J Dis Child 1989;143:1342-5.
16. Tyrala EE. Zinc and copper balances in preterm infants. Pediatrics 1986;77:513-7.
17. Subcommittee on the Tenth Edition of the RDAs, Food and Nutrition Board, Commission on Life Sciences, National Research Council. Recommended dietary allowances. Washington, DC: National Academy Press, 1989:205-11.
18. Hambidge KM, Krebs NF. Upper limits of zinc, copper and manganese in infant formulas. J Nutr 1989;119:1861-4.
19. Pilch SM, Senti FR, eds. Assessment of zinc nutritional status of the U.S. population based on data collected in the Second National Health and Nutrition Examination Survey, 1979.

1980. Bethesda, Md: Life Sciences Research Office, Federation of American Societies for Experimental Biology, 1984.
20. Walravens PA, Hambidge KM. Growth of infants fed a zinc supplemented formula. Am J Clin Nutr 1976;29:1114-21.
21. Walravens PA, Krebs NF, Hambidge KM. Linear growth of low income preschool children receiving a zinc supplement. Am J Clin Nutr 1983;38:195-201.
22. Chandra KP, Au B. Single nutrient deficiency and cell-mediated immune responses. I. Zinc. Am J Clin Nutr 1980;33:736-8.
23. Schlesinger L, Arevalo M, Arrendondo S, et al. Effect of a zinc-fortified formula on immunocompetence and growth of malnourished infants. Am J Clin Nutr 1992;56:491-8.
24. Halas ES, Heinrich MD, Sandstead HH. Long-term memory deficits in adult rats due to postnatal malnutrition. Physiol Behav 1979;22:991-7.
25. Golub MS, Gershwin ME, Hurley LS, Hendrickx AG, Saito WY. Studies of marginal zinc deprivation in rhesus monkeys: infant behavior. Am J Clin Nutr 1985;42:1229-39.
26. Lucas A, Morley R, Cole TJ, et al. Early diet in preterm babies and developmental status at 18 months. Lancet 1990;335:1477-81.
27. Lucas A, Morley R, Cole TJ, et al. Early diet in preterm babies and developmental status in infancy. Arch Dis Child 1989;64:1570-8.
28. Gibson RS. Principles of nutritional assessment. New York: Oxford University Press, 1990:487-510.
29. Hillman LS. Serial serum copper concentrations in premature and SGA infants during the first 3 months of life. J PEDIATR 1981;98:305-8.
30. Cook JD, Bothwell TH, Covell AM, et al. Reports of the International Nutrition Anemia Consultative Group. Washington, DC: The Nutrition Foundation, 1985.

Clinical and laboratory observations

Evidence of increased intrauterine bone resorption in term infants of mothers with insulin-dependent diabetes

Sergio Demarini, MD, Bonny L. Specker, PhD, Rosa I. Sierra, MS, Menachem Miodovnik, MD, and Reginald C. Tsang, MBBS

From the Perinatal Research Institute, Division of Neonatology, Departments of Pediatrics and of Obstetrics and Gynecology, University of Cincinnati Medical Center, Children's Hospital Medical Center, Cincinnati, Ohio

Infants of diabetic mothers (IDMs) have lower bone mineral content than control subjects at birth. We measured cord blood propeptide of type I procollagen (PICP), a marker of bone formation, and telopeptide of type I collagen (ICTP), a marker of bone resorption, in 25 term IDMs and 20 term control subjects. Concentrations of ICTP were higher in IDMs than in control subjects; there was no difference in PICP concentrations. We conclude that osteoclastic activity appears to be higher in IDMs than in control subjects in utero. (J PEDIATR 1995;126:796-8)

Supported in part by the Diabetes in Pregnancy Program Project (HICHD 11725) and by a grant from the J. Miglierina Foundation, Varese, Italy (Dr. Demarini).

Submitted for publication Aug. 5, 1994; accepted Nov. 14, 1994.

Reprint requests: Reginald C. Tsang, MBBS, Department of Pediatrics, University of Cincinnati Medical Center, 231 Bethesda Ave., ML 541, Cincinnati, OH 45267-0541.

0022-3476/95/$3.00 + 0 **9/24/62071**

Infants of diabetic mothers have decreased bone mineral content at birth in comparison with control subjects.[1] Decreased BMC in infants is correlated with poor maternal glycemic control, especially in the first trimester.[1] Possible explanations include either decreased intrauterine bone accretion rate or increased intrauterine bone resorption rate. The aim of this study was to evaluate differences in cord blood concentrations of carboxyterminal propeptide of human type I procollagen, a marker of bone formation, and of cross-linked carboxyterminal telopeptide of type I collagen, a marker of bone resorption, between IDMs and normal term newborn infants.

We tested the following hypotheses: (1) concentrations of PICP, a marker of bone formation, would be higher in IDMs than in control subjects because fetal hyperinsulinemia may have an anabolic effect on bone,[2] and (2) concentrations of ICTP, a marker of bone resorption, also would be higher in IDMs than in control subjects because high cord blood 1,25-dihydroxyvitamin D_3 concentrations have been reported in IDMs[3] and because $1,25(OH)_2D_3$ may increase bone resorption.

BMC	Bone mineral content
ICTP	Cross-linked carboxyterminal telopeptide of type I collagen
IDMs	Infants of diabetic mothers
$1,25(OH)_2D_3$	1,25-Dihydroxyvitamin D_3
PICP	Carboxyterminal propeptide of human type I procollagen

METHODS

Twenty-five term infants (gestational age, 38.8 ± 0.8 weeks; range, 38 to 41 weeks) born to women with insulin-dependent diabetes (class B-RT) from 1990 to 1993 were enrolled in the study. All women were entered prospectively during pregnancy and were followed in the diabetes clinic at the university hospital as part of a National Institutes of Health–sponsored diabetes-in-pregnancy program. The goals of glucose control were a fasting blood glucose value of less than 5.55 mmol/L (100 mg/dl) and a 90-minute postprandial blood glucose level of less than 7.77 mmol/L (140 mg/dl). Patients measured their blood glucose concentrations with a reflectance meter at least twice daily, and the patient's instruments were verified against laboratory instruments every 4 weeks. All patients were seen weekly throughout pregnancy. Details of the program have been published previously.[4] Twenty healthy term infants (gestational age, 39.9 ± 0.9 weeks; range, 38 to 41 weeks) represented the control population.

Cord blood PICP was measured by an equilibrium radioimmunoassay from Incstar Corp., (Stillwater, Minn.). Adult reference concentrations are 50 to 170 μg/L for women and 38 to 202 μg/L for men. Intraassay and interassay variations are 3.5% and 7.0%, respectively. Cord blood ICTP was measured by a radioimmunoassay obtained from Incstar. The normal adult range is 1.8 to 5.0 μg/L. Intraassay and interassay variations are 6.2% and 7.9%, respectively.

Results were expressed as means ± SD. Differences in mean serum concentrations of PICP and ICTP between IDMs and control subjects were analyzed with the Student t test. A p value <0.05 was considered significant. Analysis of covariance was used for analysis of multiple variables and their interaction.

RESULTS

As expected, IDMs had a higher mean birth weight at term than normal infants (3854 ± 816 vs 3416 ± 378 gm; $p = 0.005$) and were more likely to be delivered by cesarean section (11/25 vs 0/20; $p < 0.0001$). There was no difference in PICP serum concentrations between IDMs and control subjects: 1408 ± 489 versus 1407 ± 419 μg/L ($p = 0.99$). Concentrations of ICTP were significantly higher in IDMs than in control subjects: 76.1 ± 17.3 versus 63.7 ± 13.5 μg/L ($p = 0.01$). Both PICP and ICTP serum concentrations were considerably higher than those in normal adults. By analysis of covariance, neither birth weight ($p = 0.2$) nor mode of delivery ($p = 0.7$) had any influence on ICTP differences between groups.

DISCUSSION

Decreased BMC is a well-known complication of diabetes in children and adults,[5] and IDMs have been reported to have a decreased BMC in comparison with normal newborn infants, although the reason is not known.[1] We attempted to elucidate the mechanism for decreased BMC in IDMs by measuring cord blood concentrations of biochemical markers of bone formation and resorption. PICP is a marker of osteoblastic activity. Type I collagen represents approximately 90% of the organic matrix of bone, synthesized and deposited by osteoblasts. PICP splits off from procollagen in a 1:1 molar ratio during formation of type I collagen, and is released into extracellular fluid. The serum PICP concentration correlates with the rate of bone formation as measured histomorphometrically.[6] ICTP is a marker of bone resorption, being liberated during the degradation of type I collagen.[6,7]

We found no differences in an index of bone formation (PICP) between IDMs and control infants; however, we found biochemical evidence of increased bone resorption. Increased bone resorption in utero theoretically may occur in IDMs because serum $1,25(OH)_2D_3$ concentrations are increased at birth in such infants[3] and because this hormone stimulates bone resorption and intestinal calcium absorption.[8] Fetal rats have absent intestinal 1,25$(OH)_2D_3$ receptors[9]; it is hypothesized that, in utero, 1,25$(OH)_2D_3$ might lack intestinal effects but cause increased bone resorption.

We conclude that (1) osteoclastic activity in utero appears to be higher in IDMs than in control infants, and (2) osteoblastic activity seems to be similarly elevated in both IDMs and control infants in comparison with adults. For further clarification of the mechanism underlying the lower BMC in IDMs, more studies are needed to assess the correlation between neonatal BMC values and biochemical indexes of bone turnover.

We thank Mona Ho, MS, and Kay Ellis for their excellent technical assistance.

REFERENCES

1. Mimouni F, Steichen JJ, Tsang RC, Hertzberg V, Miodovnik M. Decreased bone mineral content in infants of diabetic mothers. Am J Perinatol 1988;5:339-43.
2. Kream BE, Smith MD, Canalis E, Raisz LG. Characterization of the effect of insulin on collagen synthesis in fetal rat bone. Endocrinology 1985;116:296-302.
3. Steichen JJ, Tsang RC, Ho M, et al. Perinatal magnesium, calcium and 1,25$(OH)_2D$ in relation to prospective randomized management of maternal diabetes [Abstract]. Calcif Tissue Int 1972;33:317A.
4. Demarini S, Mimouni F, Tsang RC, Khoury J, Hertzberg V. Impact of metabolic control of diabetes during pregnancy on neonatal hypocalcemia: a randomized study. Obstet Gynecol 1994;83:918-22.
5. Levine ME, Boisseau VC, Avioli LV. Effects of diabetes mellitus on bone mass in juvenile and adult onset diabetes. N Engl J Med 1976;294:241-5.
6. Eriksen EF, Charles P, Melsen F, Mosekilde L, Risteli L, Risteli J. Serum markers of type I collagen formation and degradation in metabolic bone disease: correlation with bone histomorphometry. J Bone Miner Res 1993;8:127-32.
7. Risteli J, Elomaa I, Niemi S, Novamo A, Risteli L. Radioimmunoassay for the pyridinoline cross-linked carboxyterminal telopeptide of type I collagen: a new serum marker of bone collagen degradation. Clin Chem 1993;39:635-40.
8. Boyle IT, Miravet L, Gray RW, et al. The response to 25-hydroxy and 1,25-dihydroxyvitamin D in nephrectomized rats. Endocrinology 1972;90:605-10.
9. Halloran BP, DeLuca HF. Appearance of the intestinal cytosolic receptor for the 1,25-dihydroxyvitamin D_3 during neonatal development in the rat. J Biol Chem 1981;256:7338-42.

Bacteriologic failure of amoxicillin-clavulanate in treatment of acute otitis media caused by nontypeable *Haemophilus influenzae*

Janak A. Patel, MD, Barbara Reisner, PhD, Negar Vizirinia, MD,* Mary Owen, MD, Tasnee Chonmaitree, MD, and Virgil Howie, MD

From Departments of Pediatrics and Clinical Microbiology, University of Texas Medical Branch, Galveston

Objective: **To evaluate the rate of bacteriologic failure of amoxicillin-clavulanate in the treatment of acute otitis media (AOM) and to identify the risk factors associated with failure.**

Methods: **Ninety-nine subjects (mean age, 21.4 months) with AOM were treated with amoxicillin-clavulanate in two prospective study trials that compared efficacy of two experimental antibiotics with amoxicillin-clavulanate. Tympanocentesis for microbiologic studies was performed in all subjects at enrollment; at 3 to 6 days, during amoxicillin-clavulanate therapy; and at other times when clinically indicated. The subjects were followed up for 1 month. Clinical, bacteriologic, and virologic characteristics of the subjects were analyzed.**

Results: **Bacteriologic failure of treatment occurred in none of 39 subjects (0%) with *Streptococcus pneumoniae*, two of 25 (8%) with *Moraxella catarrhalis*, and 11 of 29 (38%) with nontypeable *Haemophilus influenzae* (NTHi) infection. The failure rate for NTHi was higher than that for other pathogens ($p = 0.0007$) and was increased when compared with the preceding study period ($p = 0.017$). Bacteriologic failure was also associated with clinical failure ($p = 0.041$). In subjects with AOM caused by NTHi the rates of adequate drug compliance were comparable in both success and failure groups. Antimicrobial susceptibility testing by minimum inhibitory concentration and minimum bactericidal concentration (MIC/MBC) assays showed that amoxicillin-clavulanate resistance was not significantly associated with bacteriologic failure of treatment. However, in two subjects, MIC/MBC of the NTHi isolates during therapy were higher than MIC/MBC of the isolates before therapy; these strains of isolates pretherapy and during therapy were discordant as determined by outer membrane protein analysis. The bacteriologic failure rate was higher in nonwhite boys ($p = 0.026$) and in subjects with a history of three or more previous episodes of AOM ($p = 0.008$). Other factors such as age, bilaterality of disease, polymicrobial infection, and biotype pattern of NTHi were not associated with treatment failure. When children with adequate drug compliance were analyzed separately, only those with concomitant viral infection of the nasopharynx or middle ear were**

Supported in part by grants from the National Institute of Child Health and Human Development (HD-27841), The Upjohn Company, and Abbott Laboratories.

Submitted for publication Feb. 21, 1994; accepted Dec. 9, 1994.

Reprint requests: Janak Patel, MD, Division of Pediatric Infectious Diseases, Children's Hospital at the University of Texas Medical Branch, Galveston, TX 77555-0371.

*Now at the Department of Pediatrics, Univeristy of Texas Medical School, Houston.

0022-3476/95/$3.00 + 0 **9/20/62651**

found to be at an increased risk of bacteriologic failure of treatment ($p = 0.04$). *Conclusions:* The bacteriologic failure rate of amoxicillin-clavulanate therapy for AOM caused by NTHi was higher in the current study period than in the preceding period. Factors contributing to treatment failure were race, gender, proneness to otitis, and concomitant viral infection. **(J PEDIATR 1995;126:799-806)**

Acute otitis media is the most common childhood illness requiring treatment with antibiotics. Since the early 1980s, nontypeable *Haemophilus influenzae* and *Moraxella catarrhalis,* the pathogens that cause AOM, have developed an increased resistance to amoxicillin through production of β-lactamase. Consequently, β-lactamase–stable antibiotics such as amoxicillin-clavulanate are often used in the management of AOM.

Several investigators have shown a high level of efficacy of amoxicillin-clavulanate for management of AOM. However, we now describe an increased frequency of bacteriologic failure of amoxicillin-clavulanate during a 3-year study period, especially for infection with NTHi. We analyzed the clinical, bacteriologic, and virologic factors responsible for the failure. The concern for emergence of failure of amoxicillin-clavulanate is warranted because this drug is frequently used to compare the efficacy of newer antibiotics and to treat cases of AOM in which treatment with other antibiotics has failed.

AOM	Acute otitis media
MBC	Minimum bactericidal concentration
MEF	Middle ear fluid
MIC	Minimum inhibitory concentration
NTHi	Nontypeable *Haemophilus influenzae*
NW	Nasal wash
OMP	Outer membrane protein
RSV	Respiratory syncytial virus

METHODS

Study population. From October 1989 to April 1991, children 2 months to 8 years of age, seen for AOM at the pediatric clinic of the University of Texas Medical Branch at Galveston, were enrolled prospectively in two drug study trials comparing the efficacy of two experimental antibiotics (clarithromycin or cefpodoxime), with amoxicillin-clavulanate as the control drug.[1] The studies were approved by the institutional review board. The subjects were enrolled after a parental or guardian consent was obtained. Of 276 subjects enrolled, data from 99 subjects who were treated with amoxicillin-clavulanate were analyzed for this report. The diagnosis of AOM was made by pneumatic otoscopic signs of inflammation (bulging, red or yellow discoloration, and decreased motility of tympanic membrane) and symptoms (fever, irritability, or otalgia) of less than 2 weeks in duration. Subjects were excluded if they had received antibiotic therapy within the previous 3 days; were allergic to penicillin; currently had tympanostomy tubes in place or had a history of any other middle ear surgery; or had a chronic perforation of the tympanic membrane, sensorineural hearing loss, gastrointestinal disease with malabsorption, or severe cardiac, hepatic, renal, or immunologic disease. Eligible subjects received amoxicillin-clavulanate at a dose of 40 mg/kg per day of amoxicillin in three equal doses for 10 days. The parents were asked to record the dates and times that the medication was given to the subjects and to return bottles of unused medication at the end of therapy. Compliance was documented by both the parents' diary and calculation of the weight of the consumed medication (during therapy and at the end of therapy). Inadequate compliance was defined as taking less than 80% of the prescribed medication or failing to return the medication bottles or parent's diary.

Sample collection. At enrollment (visit 1) tympanocentesis was performed to collect middle ear fluid (MEF-1) for viral and bacterial studies as previously described.[1] In subjects with bilateral otitis media, tympanocentesis was performed in both ears. Nasal wash was also obtained for viral studies. The subjects than began amoxicillin-clavulanate treatment.

Follow-up visits were scheduled at 3 to 6 days after initiation of treatment (visit 2), at the end of therapy (visit 3, days 9 to 12), and approximately 1 month after initiation of therapy (visit 4). At each follow-up visit the clinical response to therapy was assessed. Repeated tympanocentesis and viral studies were routine during visit 2, except in some patients without bacterial pathogen in MEF-1. If persisting bacteria were found or patients had symptoms, the antibiotic treatment was changed. Tympanocentesis was also performed on visit 3 or 4 when judged by the investigators to be clinically indicated. All MEF from repeated tympanocentesis was labeled MEF-2. The subject was considered to have clinical improvement or cure when signs and symptoms of AOM were improved or absent, and no drainage of MEF occurred. Clinical failure was defined as the presence of persistent fever, otalgia, erythema of the tympanic membrane, or purulent drainage with or without positive bacterial culture. Bacteriologic failure was defined by the presence of pathogenic bacteria in MEF-2 with or without clinical symptoms. The clinical and

The clinical and bacteriologic responses were evaluated separately for each ear. At the end of therapy good response was considered when the resolution of AOM was uneventful. A prolonged course was considered when clinical and/or bacteriologic failure occurred at any time during the course (visit 2 or 3).

Identification and drug susceptibility of NTHi. MEF was cultured for aerobic bacteria, and the organisms were identified with standard techniques that are available in clinical microbiology laboratories. All NTHi isolates were initially tested for amoxicillin-clavulanate susceptibility by the Kirby-Bauer disk diffusion method. According to recent criteria of the National Committee on Clinical Laboratory Standards, a disk zone size of 19 mm or less was considered to indicate susceptibility. All NTHi isolates were also tested for β-lactamase production with the chromogenic cephalosporinase assay (Becton Dickinson, Cockeysville, Md.).

Additional drug susceptibility testing of NTHi was performed by determining minimum inhibitory concentration and minimum bactericidal concentration. Briefly, approximately 10,000 colony-forming units of freshly grown NTHi were placed in wells of commercial microtiter plates (Sensititer plates, Radiometer, Westlake, Ohio) containing amoxicillin-clavulanate (amoxicillin/clavulanate ratio, 1:0.5) at twofold dilutions ranging from 0.5/0.25 to 16/8 μg/ml. After overnight incubation in 5% carbon dioxide at 37° C, MIC was determined by observing the minimum concentrations of amoxicillin-clavulanate required to inhibit the turbidity caused by bacterial growth. According to the criteria of the National Committee on Clinical Laboratory Standards, MIC of 4/2 μg/ml or less is considered susceptible, whereas 8 μg/ml or greater is considered resistant. For determination of MBC 10 μl of bacterial suspensions from the wells of the MIC plate were plated on chocolate agar and incubated overnight in 5% carbon dioxide at 37° C to observe for growth of colonies of NTHi. Minimum bactericidal concentration represented the minimum concentration of amoxicillin-clavulanate required to inhibit growth of 99% of bacteria colonies. All susceptibility studies were done in duplicate.

Analysis of outer membrane protein of NTHi. The outer membrane protein fraction was isolated from NTHi as described by Murphy et al.[2] Briefly, fresh NTHi colonies grown on chocolate agar were scraped, washed twice in phosphate-buffered saline solution, and resuspended in a buffer containing 0.05 mol/L sodium phosphate, 0.15 mol/L sodium chloride, and 0.05 mol/L ethylenediaminetetraacetic acid, adjusted to pH 7.4. The suspension was incubated at 60° C for 45 minutes and subjected to mild shearing by three passages through a 25-gauge hypodermic needle attached to a 50 ml syringe. Whole organisms were separated from the suspension by centrifugation at 10,000 *g* for 20 minutes at 4° C. Ultracentrifugation of the supernatant at 80,000 *g* for 2 hours at 4° C was done to form a pellet of the OMP preparation. The pellet was resuspended in 50 mmol/L tris (hydroxymethyl) aminomethane containing 1% sodium dodecyl sulfate, and the protein concentration was determined with BCA Protein Assay Kit (Pierce, Rockford, Ill.). The OMP preparations were then analyzed by sodium dodecyl sulfate–polyacrylamide gel electrophoresis.

Biotyping of NTHi. The biotypes of isolates were determined with the Minitek system (BBL Microbiology Systems, Cockeysville, Md.) as described by Back and Oberhofer.[3] The specific substrates tested were ornithine, indole, urea, and *o*-nitrophenyl-β-D-galactopyranoside.

Virologic studies. Samples of MEF were diluted with 1 ml of phosphate-buffered saline solution and inoculated into cell cultures within 2 to 3 hours of specimen collection. Viral culture methods for MEF and NW have been previously described.[1] Rapid viral antigen detection was performed on both MEF and NW. Detection of respiratory syncytial virus in MEF was performed by enzyme immunoassay (RSV EIA Diagnostic Kit, Abbott Laboratories, North Chicago, Ill.). For NW the cell pellet from the centrifuged specimen was smeared onto microscopic slides and used for rapid antigen detection by an indirect fluorescence antibody technique, with commercially prepared antisera for RSV, influenza A and B, parainfluenza (types 1, 2, and 3), and adenovirus (Bartels Viral Respiratory Panel, Baxter Healthcare Corp., W. Sacramento, Calif.).

Statistical analysis. The incidence of bacteriologic failure in the two study periods (1988 vs 1989 to 1991) was analyzed by *z* test and chi-square analysis. The variables, such as bacteriologic and clinical response, gender, race, history of recurrent otitis media, and concurrent presence of viruses or other bacteria, were converted to indicator (dummy) variables and then analyzed by Pearson product-moment correlation test. The microbiologic studies of NTHi were analyzed by Fisher Exact Test. All power values were calculated at an alpha value of 0.05. All statistical and data manipulations were performed on a personal microcomputer with Sigmastat (Jandel Scientific, San Rafael, Calif.) statistical software package.

RESULTS

Clinical outcome. Of the 99 subjects analyzed in the study, 91 completed a follow-up of at least 10 days. The mean age of the subjects was 21.4 months; 40.8% of subjects were white, 31.8% were black, and 27.4% were Hispanic. Bacterial cultures of MEF-1 grew *Streptococcus pneumoniae*, NTHi, and *M. catarrhalis* from 39%, 30%, and 25% of subjects, respectively. Eighteen percent of subjects had more than one pathogen. Twenty-three percent of subjects

Table I. Comparison, during two study periods, of failure rates of amoxicillin-clavulanate treatment for various bacterial pathogens in subjects with AOM

Bacterial pathogens	1988 (Previous study) No. treated	1988 (Previous study) No. (%) failed	1989-1991 (Current study) No. treated	1989-1991 (Current study) No. (%) failed
S. pneumoniae	15	1 (7)	39	0 (0)[a]
NTHi	15	0 (0)[b]	29	11 (38)[c]
M. catarrhalis	5	0 (0)	25	2 (8)[d]

Significance for *c* versus *a* and *d*, $p = 0.0007$ (power = 0.95) as calculated by chi-square analysis; for *b* versus *d*, $p = 0.017$ (power = 0.70) as calculated by *z* test.

had no identifiable bacterial pathogens. The subjects who had bacteriologic failure (MEF-2 had the same bacterial species as MEF-1) are stated in Table I; these subjects are also compared with those of the preceding study year.[4] The results show that the rate of bacteriologic failure of amoxicillin-clavulanate had increased significantly in the subjects with infection caused by NTHi when compared with infections caused by other pathogens and when compared with results from the preceding study period. All subjects with AOM caused by NTHi (n = 29) were therefore analyzed in further detail.

Characteristics of NTHi subjects. Table II shows the characteristics of the subjects with AOM caused by NTHi and treated with amoxicillin-clavulanate who were bacteriologically cured or in whom treatment failed. The majority of the bacteriologic failures (64%) were detected within the first 6 days (visit 2); the remainder occurred within 14 days of diagnosis. Overall, 55% of subjects with AOM caused by NTHi had concomitant viral infection of the middle ear or the nasopharynx. This rate was not significantly different from the 58% rate of virus infection in children with other bacteria in MEF.

The bacteriologic failure rate was significantly related to clinical failure rate. Furthermore, the rate of adequate drug compliance was comparable in both success and failure groups. Because the bacteriologic failure rate was clinically important and unrelated to lack of drug compliance, we evaluated the additional risk factors that may be associated with failure. Nonwhite race was significantly associated with bacteriologic failure, although on further analysis only treatment in nonwhite boys (five black and four Hispanic) was associated with failure. History of three or more episodes of AOM (otitis proneness) was also a significant risk factor for bacteriologic failure. Additional correlation analysis showed that subjects with recurrent otitis media were also more likely to be nonwhite boys ($p = 0.008$, power = 0.76) and to have inadequate documentation of drug compliance ($p = 0.004$, power = 0.824). The mean age, bilaterality of disease, and polymicrobial infection (more than one bacterial species in the MEF) were not associated with bacteriologic failure of treatment.

When subjects with adequate drug compliance were analyzed separately (10 in success group vs 6 in failure group), only those with concomitant viral infection of the nasopharynx or middle ear were found to be at an increased risk of bacteriologic failure ($p = 0.04$, $r = -0.52$, power = 0.54). In the treatment failure group four of six subjects had viral infection: one subject each had cytomegalovirus, RSV, and influenza A virus in MEF; one subject each had cytomegalovirus and enterovirus in NW only; and one subject had enterovirus and adenovirus in NW at two different visits. In the successfully treated group, three of 10 subjects had viral infection: two subjects had RSV in MEF, and one subject had coxsackievirus group A9 in NW.

Antibiotic susceptibility to NTHi. The summary of antibiotic susceptibility testing is given in Table III. β-Lactamase production was not associated with higher failure rate. By Kirby-Bauer disk diffusion method none of the NTHi isolates was resistant to amoxicillin-clavulanate. However, further susceptibility testing by MIC and MBC assays showed that two isolates (7%), one each from a subject in the successful treatment and failed treatment groups, were resistant to amoxicillin-clavulanate. These two subjects had unilateral otitis media. Two other isolates from MEF-2 of the failure group (Figure; patients 8 and 9) had MIC values more than eight times higher than the initial isolates (MEF-1) of the same subjects, indicating the selection of a tolerant strain during therapy. Overall, the rate of antibiotic resistance was not signficantly associated with bacteriologic failure treatment.

Identification of NTHi by OMP profiles and biotyping. The pairs of NTHi strains present in MEF-1 and MEF-2 in the treatment failure group were compared by OMP analysis (Figure). The OMP profile of each MEF-1 isolate was unique for each subject. Nine MEF-1/MEF-2 pairs, including the left- and right-sided MEF-1 and MEF-2 of patient 11, were identical. However, two MEF-2 isolates of patients 8 and 9 had different OMP profiles and an eightfold increase in MIC and MBC (described earlier) when compared with MEF-1 isolates. The remainder of the pairs that had identical OMP profiles had no differences in MIC

Table II. Demographic characteristics of 29 subjects with AOM caused by NTHi whose treatment with amoxicillin-clavulanate failed or succeeded

	Bacteriologic success (n = 18)	Bacteriologic failure (n = 11)	r*
Clinical failure	8	9	0.404[a]
Age (mo)†	16.4 ± 11.0	14.2 ± 7.7	0.043
Race (white/nonwhite)	10:8	1:10	0.465[b]
Gender (M/F)	8:10	7:4	−0.186
Race and gender			
White boys	4	0	0.313
Nonwhite boys	4	7	−0.414[c]
White girls	6	1	0.275
Nonwhite girls	4	3	−0.057
History of recurrent otitis	2	6	−0.479[d]
Adequate drug compliance	10	6	0.010
Bilaterality	11	6	−0.080
Concurrent viral infection‡	10	6	0.010
Polymicrobial bacterial infection	3	4	−0.223

Significance: Values marked by superscripts *a, b, c,* and *d* are significant at $p = 0.041, 0.011, 0.026, 0.008$, respectively; power = 0.56, 0.73, 0.61, 0.76, respectively.
*Correlation coefficient calculated by Pearson product-moment correlation test; $r = 0.36$ for $p < 0.05$ at 28 degrees of freedom.
†Expressed as mean ± SD.
‡Positive viral diagnostic test results in MEF or NW.

Table III. Microbiologic studies of NTHi from subjects with AOM who were treated with amoxicillin-clavulanate

	Bacteriologic success (n = 18)	Bacteriologic failure (n = 11)	p*
β-Lactamase–producing strain	6	4	>0.999
Resistance to amoxicillin-clavulanate			
By Kirby-Bauer disk	0	0	
By MIC†	1	1	>0.999
MEF-2 strain different from MEF-1 strain	NA	2	
MIC of MEF-2 >MEF-1‡	NA	2	
Biotype MEF-1§			
Type I	9	5	>0.999
Type II	3	5	0.254
Type III	2	1	>0.999
Type IV	6	2	0.685
Type V	1	0	>0.999

NA, Not applicable.
*Calculated by Fisher Exact Test.
†MIC of each isolate was 16 μg/ml.
‡A more than fourfold difference was considered significant.
§Three subjects in successfully treated group and three in treatment failure group had different biotypes in contralateral MEF.

and MBC values. Biotype analysis showed that biotype I occurred most frequently in MEF-1.

DISCUSSION

Because of the rising incidence of β-lactamase–producing bacterial pathogens, β-lactamase–stable antibiotics are increasingly being used in the treatment of otitis media. In this regard amoxicillin-clavulanate is considered to provide ideal antibacterial coverage and is frequently used to compare efficacy of newer β-lactamase–stable antibiotics in the treatment of otitis media. However, we found a high rate of bacteriologic failure with amoxicillin-clavulanate for treatment of AOM, and the failure was specifically associated with AOM caused by NTHi. This problem was clinically important because bacteriologic failure was also associated with clinical failure requiring a change in antibiotic treatment.

In the only study to date in which bacteriologic failure of amoxicillin-clavulanate in the treatment of AOM has been described, Mendelman et al.[5] noted failure rate of 10% in children infected with NTHi, and failure rates of 33% and 9% in children infected with *S. pneumoniae* and *M. catarrhalis*, respectively. However, the sample size (n = 5) was smaller than in the current report, and only 42% of these

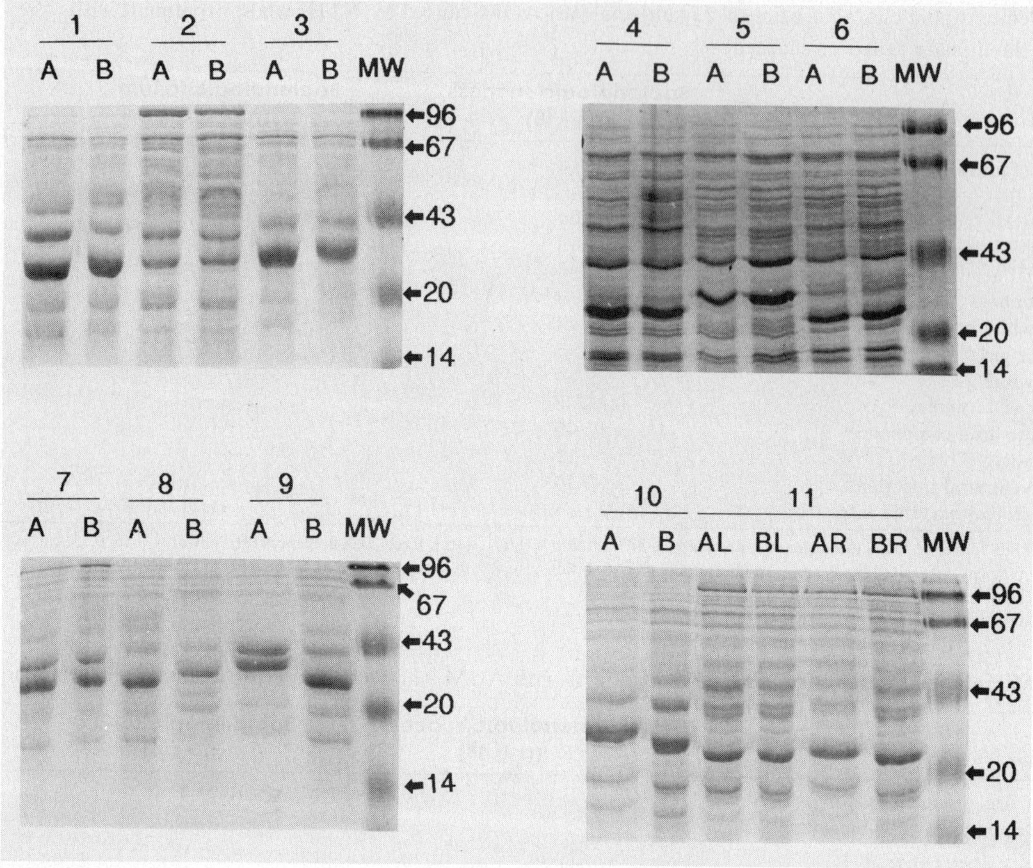

Figure. Outer membrane protein profile of NTHi from paired MEF of subjects whose treatment with amoxicillin-clavulanate failed. Numbers above lanes signify patient identification. *A*, Outer membrane protein of bacteria isolated before therapy (MEF-1); *B*, OMP of bacteria isolated during therapy (MEF-2). Patient 11 also had OMP analysis of bacterial isolates from left-sided *(AL, BL)* and right sided *(AR, BR)* MEF. *MW*, Molecular weight marker lane. Numbers at *right* of each gel are molecular weight standards expressed as kilodaltons.

subjects were examined with repeated tympanocentesis during therapy; hence the bacteriologic failure rate was not determined. Furthermore, the amoxicillin-clavulanate susceptibility was determined by Kirby-Bauer disk test only, and factors responsible for failure were not investigated. In studies of adults with chronic bronchitis,[6] amoxicillin-clavulanate–resistant strains of NTHi have been isolated from sputum, although the incidence of bacteriologic failure and the clinical progression of disease have not been well characterized.

In the present study we showed that the rate of adequate drug compliance was similar in both bacteriologic success and failure groups, and hence the possibility of antibiotic resistance as a cause of failure was explored. Resistance of NTHi to amoxicillin-clavulanate is primarily caused by the presence of altered penicillin-binding proteins on the bacterial cell wall.[6] Previous studies have shown that MIC and MBC assays are more accurate than the Kirby-Bauer disk test in the detection of such ampicillin-resistant, non-β-lactamase–producing NTHi.[7] In the present study the Kirby-Bauer disk test detected neither of the two isolates that were found to be resistant by MIC and MBC assays. The amoxicillin-clavulanate resistance rate of 7% is higher than the recently reported rates of 0.2% to 2.5% in respiratory secretions from subjects studied in the United States[6]; however, our sample size is rather small for a meaningful comparison.

Two persistent bacterial isolates from the treatment failure group had an eightfold increase in MIC and MBC levels when compared with the initial isolates of the same subjects. Further analysis of these two pairs of isolates by the OMP profile showed that the MEF-2 isolates were different from the initial isolates. These results suggest that a more tolerant strain of NTHi may have been selected during treatment with amoxicillin-clavulanate. This pattern of selection of a tolerant isolate during therapy for AOM has not previously been described. For other patients in the failure group the OMP profiles of both MEF-1 and MEF-2 isolates were identical and their MIC and MBC levels were similar. The results of the OMP profiles agree with those of Barenkamp et al.,[8] who demonstrated that the OMP profiles of the first isolates were identical to those of the second isolates obtained within 30 days.

Overall, the rate of amoxicillin-clavulanate resistance in our study was not statistically associated with bacteriologic failure. Previous studies have shown that NTHi is the most frequent pathogen associated with treatment failure despite the use of appropriate antibiotics.[9, 10] NTHi is also the most frequently found pathogen in MEF of children with recurrent or chronic otitis media during antimicrobial therapy.[11, 12] One possible explanation is that antibiotics do not achieve the optimal MIC in MEF, which is necessary to inhibit the growth of NTHi. For example, the peak concentration of amoxicillin in MEF after an oral dose of amoxicillin-clavulanate has been shown to be approximately 1 μg/ml.[13] Although antibiotic concentrations were not measured in our subjects, the MIC and MBC values of our study isolates were higher than 1 μg/ml in 40% and 55%, respectively.

Additional evaluation of risk factors showed that nonwhite boys and otitis-prone subjects were more likely to have treatment failure. An explanation for the higher failure rate in otitis-prone subjects is provided by the study of Yamanaka and Faden,[14] who showed that otitis-prone children mount an inadequate anamnestic antibody response to NTHi. However, nonwhite children were not investigated in that study. Other studies have shown that male gender and certain racial groups, such as the Eskimos, Maoris, and Pacific Islanders, have an increased susceptibility to chronic otitis media or poor antimicrobial response.[9, 15, 16] Black and Hispanic children who were included in our study have not been studied extensively for bacterial species–specific responses to antibiotics. In a study in which black infants were found to have a lower incidence of otitis media, cultures of MEF were not done.[17] Additional correlation analysis in our study showed that the otitis-prone subjects were more likely to be nonwhite boys and children with inadequate documentation of drug compliance. It is unclear how these three factors are interrelated for AOM caused by NTHi, because none contributed to bacteriologic failure in AOM caused by other pathogens.

Attempts have previously been made to characterize the biochemical properties of NTHi by the biotyping method and to correlate them with types of clinical disease. Long et al.[18] reported that 67% of NTHi strains from subjects with AOM were biotype I. Our study of AOM showed a similar pattern. DeMaria et al.[19] showed that 53% of NTHi strains from subjects with chronic bacterial otitis media with effusion were biotype II and that biotype IV was infrequent. A similar trend for biotype distribution was found among our subjects who had persistent NTHi despite drug therapy. These results suggest that the biotype II strains may have a survival advantage.

When we removed from analysis those subjects with inadequate documentation of drug compliance, to better explore the mechanisms of antimicrobial failure in subjects who were clearly compliant, we found that concomitant viral infection of either the nasopharynx or middle ear was associated with an increased risk of bacteriologic failure. This observation is in keeping with our previous observation that viral infection of the nasopharynx or middle ear was associated with treatment failure in AOM caused by a variety of pathogens.[1] The mechanisms of virus-associated bacteriologic failure to respond to antimicrobial treatment are poorly understood. Giebink[20] showed that influenza virus infection alters the distribution of antibiotic in the middle ear. Furthermore, viruses alter host immune responses to bacterial infection,[21] which may be particularly important for hosts with antibiotic diffusion into the MEF that is less than the required MIC for NTHi.

If gender, race, and concomitant viral infection are important determinants for resolution of AOM caused by NTHi, it is not clear why similar rates of failure were not detected in our previous study with amoxicillin-clavulanate. The amoxicillin-clavulanate susceptibility of NTHi in children may be decreasing gradually, undetected by MIC and MBC assays. It is also possible that NTHi is developing a survival advantage in subjects with weak immune responses, which may occur in nonwhite and otitis-prone populations.

We conclude that there is a significant incidence of failure of amoxicillin-clavulanate to eradicate NTHi in children with AOM. Although the exact cause of bacteriologic treatment failure is unknown, important contributing factors were race, gender, proneness to otitis, and concomitant viral infection. This report points to the need for continued study of mechanisms of failure of antimicrobial agents in the treatment of AOM.

We thank Catherine Rimlinger, MA, for manuscript review.

REFERENCES

1. Chonmaitree T, Owen MJ, Hedgepeth D, Horlick D, Howie VM. Effect of viral respiratory tract infection on outcome of acute otitis media. J Pediatr 1992;120:856-62.
2. Murphy TF, Dudas KC, Mylotte JM, Apicella MA. A subtyping system for nontypeable *Haemophilus influenzae* based on outer-membrane proteins. J Infect Dis 1983;147:838-46.
3. Back AE, Oberhofer TR. Use of the Minitek system for biotyping *Haemophilus* species. J Clin Microbiol 1978;7:312-3.
4. Howie VM. Otitis media. Pediatr Rev 1993;14:320-3.
5. Mendelman PM, Del Beccaro MA, McLinn SE, Todd WM.

Cefpodoxime proxetil compared with amoxicillin-clavulanate for the treatment of otitis media. J PEDIATR 1992;121:459-65.
6. Jorgensen JH. Update on mechanisms and prevalence of antimicrobial resistance in *Haemophilus influenzae.* Clin Infect Dis 1992;14:1119-23.
7. Mendelman PM, Chaffin DO, Clausen C, et al. Failure to detect ampicillin-resistant, non-β-lactamase-producing *Haemophilus influenzae* by standard disk susceptibility testing. Antimicrob Agents Chemother 1986;30:274-80.
8. Barenkamp SJ, Shurin PA, Marchant CD, et al. Do children with recurrent *Haemophilus influenzae* otitis media become infected with a new organism or reacquire the original strain? J PEDIATR 1984;105:533-7.
9. Harrison CJ, Marks MI, Welch DF. Microbiology of recently treated acute otitis media compared with previously untreated acute otitis media. Pediatr Infect Dis 1985;4:641-6.
10. Teele DW, Pelton SI, Klein JO. Bacteriology of acute otitis media unresponsive to initial antimicrobial therapy. J PEDIATR 1981;98:537-9.
11. Liston TE, Foshee WS, McClesky FK. The bacteriology of recurrent otitis media and the effect of sulfisoxazole chemoprophylaxis. Pediatr Infect Dis 1984;3:20-4.
12. Gates GA, Holt GR, Wachtendorf CA, Hearne EM, Jorgenson JH. Microbiology of medically treated chronic otitis media with effusion. In: Lim DJ, Bluestone CD, Klein JO, Nelson JD, eds. Recent advances in otitis media with effusion. Philadelphia: BC Decker, 1984: 145-6.
13. Fraschini F, Scaglione F, Falchi M, et al. Pharmacokinetics and tissue distribution of amoxicillin plus clavulanic acid after oral administration in man. J Chem 1990;2:171-7.
14. Yamanaka N, Faden H. Antibody responses to outer membrane protein of nontypeable *Haemophilus influenzae* in otitis-prone children. J PEDIATR 1993;122:212-8.
15. Teele DW, Klein JO, Rosner B. Epidemiology of otitis media during the first seven years of life in children in Greater Boston: a prospective, cohort study. J Infect Dis 1989;160:83-94.
16. Ryodhouse N. Antibiotic treatment of otitis media with effusion. N Z Med J 1991;104:380-2.
17. Marchant CD, Shurin PA, Turczyk VA, Wasikowski DE, Tutihasi MA, Kinney SE. Course and outcome of otitis media in early infancy: a prospective study. J PEDIATR 1986;104:826-31.
18. Long SS, Teter MJ, Gilligan PH. Biotype of *Haemophilus influenzae*: correlation with virulence and ampicillin resistance. J Infect Dis 1983;147:800-6.
19. DeMaria DS, Lim DJ, Barnishan J, Ayers LW, Birck HG. Biotypes of serologically nontypeable *Haemophilus influenzae* isolated from the middle ears and nasopharynges of patients with otitis media with effusion. J Clin Microbiol 1984;20:1102-4.
20. Giebink GS. Otitis media update: pathogenesis and treatment. Ann Otol Laryngol 1992;101:21-3.
21. Chonmaitree T. Viral otitis media. Pediatr Ann 1990;19:522-32.

Clinical trial of vitamin A as adjuvant treatment for lower respiratory tract infections

Chris L. Kjolhede, MD, MPH, Francisco J. Chew, MD,
Anne M. Gadomski, MD, MPH, and Diana P. Marroquin, MD

From the Department of International Health, Johns Hopkins University, Baltimore, Maryland; the Division of Nutrition and Health, Instituto de Nutricion de Centro America y Panama (INCAP), Guatemala City, Guatemala; and the Department of Pediatrics, University of Maryland, Baltimore

Objective: To test the efficacy of a high dose of vitamin A as adjuvant treatment for radiographically confirmed cases of acute lower respiratory tract infection (ALRI).
Design: Randomized, double-masked, placebo-controlled clinical trial.
Setting: Two large urban hospitals in Guatemala City.
Patients: Sequential sample of 263 children aged 3 to 48 months, identified in the emergency departments and admitted to the hospital.
Interventions: Vitamin A (100,000 IU for children less than 1 year of age, and 200,000 IU for older children) or placebo in addition to standard treatment for ALRI which included antibiotics, oxygen, bronchodilators, and intravenously administered solutions.
Measurements and main results. The children were assessed every 8 hours. There were neither statistically nor clinically significant differences by treatment group in the rate of normalization in respiratory rate, oxygen saturation, temperature, or clinical score. Duration of hospitalization was not different by treatment group. Adverse outcomes (mechanical ventilation, prolonged hospitalization, readmission or transfer, and death) were equally distributed between the two groups.
Conclusions: Treatment with high doses of vitamin A over and above standard care for infants and children with non-measles-related ALRI is not efficacious for the current episode. Additional trials among populations in which vitamin A deficiency is more prevalent and severe should be considered. (J PEDIATR 1995;126:807-12)

Supported by a grant from the Thrasher Research Fund and from Cooperative Agreement DAN-5116-A-00-8051-00 between the Department of International Health, Johns Hopkins University, and the U.S. Agency for International Development, Office of Nutrition. Additional support was received from the World Health Organization, Control of Diarrheal Diseases/Acute Respiratory Illness Program.

Submitted for publication Sept. 22, 1994; accepted Dec. 29, 1994.

Reprint requests: Chris L. Kjolhede, MD, MPH, Research Institute, Mary Imogene Bassett Hospital, 1 Atwell Rd., Cooperstown, NY 13326.

0022-3476/95/$3.00 + 0 **9/25/62982**

Several large, population-based supplementation studies have shown that vitamin A can reduce childhood mortality rates,[1-3] but few studies have reported this effect in infants less than 12 months of age, in whom the mortality rate for acute lower respiratory tract infection is very high.[4] Clinical trials of high-dose vitamin A supplementation during

ALRI	Acute lower respiratory tract infection
RR	Respiratory rate
Spo_2	Oxygen saturation (as determined by pulse oximetry)

Table I. Baseline characteristics by treatment group

	Vitamin A (n = 132)	Placebo (n = 131)
Age		
% 3-5 mo (n)	37 (49)	33 (43)
% 6-11 mo (n)	33 (43)	39 (51)
% 12+ mo (n)	30 (40)	28 (37)
% Male (n)	61 (81)	64 (84)
Ethnic group*		
% Ladino (n)	83 (110)	82 (107)
% Mayan Indian (n)	17 (22)	17 (22)
Principal diagnosis		
% Pneumonia (n)	91 (120)	90 (118)
% Bronchiolitis (n)	9 (12)	10 (13)
Median respiratory rate (breaths/min)	62	62
% Febrile (n)	31 (41)	32 (42)
% SpO_2 <90	52 (69)	44 (56)†
% Chest indrawing (n)	96 (127)	97 (127)
Median days of cough before admission	4	4
Median hematocrit	34	34
Retinol (μmol/L)		
Median	0.92	0.87
% <0.70 (n)	28 (37)	28 (37)
Median weight/length *z* score	−0.69	−0.63
Median birth weight	3.08	3.13
Hospital		
% Roosevelt (n)	66 (87)	60 (79)
% IGSS (n)	34 (45)	40 (52)
Median number of children at home	3	3

*Data missing on two subjects.
†Data missing on three subjects

measles have also demonstrated a beneficial effect.[5-7] Numerous epidemiologic studies have reported significant relationships between vitamin A deficiency and respiratory morbidity.[8-11] A community-based intervention trial in Thailand of vitamin A in children aged 3 to 5 years demonstrated that control children had nearly three times the respiratory morbidity; other subgroups of children in the same study did not have the same protective effect.[12]

The World Health Organization[13] (WHO) recommends giving high doses of vitamin A to children who have acute or prolonged diarrhea or ALRI. The presumed rationale for this recommendation is either that the vitamin A will improve the outcome of the current illness or that the contact with the health care system and resulting dose of vitamin A will improve vitamin A status. The efficacy of such supplementation as either treatment or to improve vitamin A status has not been demonstrated. One clinical trial of high-dose vitamin A supplementation during diarrhea failed to demonstrate any benefit.[14]

The current clinical trial was designed to test the efficacy of one aspect of the WHO recommendation, that is, to assess the adjuvant effect of high-dose vitamin A supplementation on the course of an episode of radiologically confirmed ALRI requiring inpatient care. Specifically, this study was designed to test the hypothesis that treatment with a high dose of vitamin A in oil (100,000 IU for those <12 months of age; 200,000 IU for those >12 months) in children hospitalized for ALRI will increase the rate of improvement as indicated by the rate of defervescence and of the return to age-appropriate respiratory rates, by the resolution of oxygen desaturation (if any), and by shorter duration of hospitalization.

METHODS

Study subjects were recruited from those infants and children with ALRI seen at the emergency services of the Hospital Roosevelt and the Instituto Guatemalteco de Seguridad Social (IGSS) Hospital in Guatemala City, Guatemala. Children between 3 and 48 months of age were considered for enrollment into the study if they had a history of cough, and/or tachypnea (respiratory rate, >40/min), and/or difficulty in drinking or eating, and/or clinical signs of difficulty in breathing (e.g., chest indrawing or subcostal retraction), and/or presence of central cyanosis. Children were individually randomly selected with balanced blocks of eight randomly ordered integers if they met the following disease definitions: (1) pneumonia, with clinical evidence of pulmonary infiltrate (e.g., rales, decreased breath sounds, dullness to percussion) and infiltrate present on chest radiograph, and/or (2) bronchiolitis, with wheezing in a child less than 18 months of age and a chest radiograph with hyperinflation or peribronchial thickening or diffuse infiltrates.

Children with asthma, tuberculosis, xerophthalmia, or pneumonia associated with measles and other exanthematous diseases, or with a history of receipt of multivitamin supplements or high-dose vitamin A supplementation within the last 4 months, were excluded. Severely malnourished children, defined as less than 70% of the median of the normal weight/height ratio according to the National Center for Health Statistics reference, were also excluded.

A study pediatrician collected the history of respiratory symptoms from the child's caretaker. This baseline evaluation included demographics, history of the present disease and prior respiratory diseases, immunization status, feeding problems, number of children in the home, and maternal education. Degree of crowding and indicators of environmental air pollution, such as mode of cooking and parents' smoking habits, were also determined. Consent for participation in the study was given by each child's caretaker, who had read or heard about the study and its risks and benefits. Complete physical and eye examinations and anthropometric measures were done after the interview. Chest radiographs (posteroanterior and lateral) were obtained to confirm clinical diagnoses for every child.

The subjects were randomly assigned to receive one dose of either vitamin A in oil (100,000 IU and 20 mg of vitamin E for children <1 year of age, or 200,000 IU and 40 mg of vitamin E if older), or a placebo containing 20 mg vitamin E for children less than 1 year of age or 40 mg if older. The placebo and treatment capsules (Banner Gelatin, Inc., Pa.) were otherwise similar and were enclosed in uniquely numbered, opaque envelopes before use. The vitamin A capsules were the same dosage and similar in appearance to the high-dose vitamin A capsules provided by United Nations Children's Fund (UNICEF) throughout the developing world. Vitamin E is included in high-dose vitamin A capsules as a preservative.

While hospitalized, the child's condition was evaluated every 8 hours by the study pediatrician or the study nurses or both. Respiratory rates were measured by observing chest wall movements for 1 minute with the use of a timer with an audible cue (Miconta, Elizabeth, N.J.; Tandy Corp., Fort Worth, Tex.). According to hospital policy, rectal temperatures were measured at Hospital Roosevelt and axillary temperatures were measured at IGSS with digital thermometers (B-D Digital Fever Thermometer; Becton Dickinson & Co., Rutherford, N.J.). Fever was defined as a temperature greater than 37.7° C at IGSS or greater than 38.3° C at Hospital Roosevelt. Oxygen saturation and heart rate were measured with a Nellcor N-10 pulse oximeter (Nellcor Inc., Hayward, Calif.). Children with an oxygen saturation less than 90% were considered to have desaturation.

A standardized scoring and evaluation form, adapted from Silverman et al.,[15] was used to assess the child's clinical status each 8 hours. The presence of grunting, nasal flaring, intercostal retractions, and chest indrawing (subcostal retractions for children older than 18 months) was each scored as 0, 1, or 2. The child's general appearance (i.e., level of interaction, attentiveness, consolability, and vigor of crying) was similarly scored. Once a child's lungs were mechanically ventilated, the last score before intubation was carried in the analysis until extubation. Pictorial illustrations were included on the evaluation form to increase face validity and to reduce interrater variability.

All study personnel were extensively trained in the determination of RR, chest indrawing, pulse oximetry, and clinical scoring before the trial and at two points during the study. Testing of interrater variability of respiratory rate measurement and clinical scoring, especially assessment of chest indrawing, was conducted before the trial. Interrater variability was also assessed monthly by having the nurses examine a child and determine the RR at the same time as the study pediatrician. When RRs were determined concurrently by the nurses and the pediatrician, more than 80% fell within a range of ±5 of the rate counted by the pediatrician; for very high rates the variability was higher. The interrater variability in the assessment of the grades of severity of chest indrawing was also determined periodically. The percentage of agreement was more than 90% for grades of "chest indrawing" and nearly 97% when the presence or absence of chest indrawing was assessed.

Table II. Primary clinical outcomes during hospitalization

	Vitamin A (n = 132)	Placebo (n = 131)
Mean RR* (breaths/min)	49.3 (8.5)	49.8 (7.8)
Mean temperature* (°F)	98.6 (0.8)	98.6 (0.8)
Mean Spo_2* (%)	91.2 (3.4)	91.1 (3.1)
Number of shifts in hospital	16.1 (15.4)	15.5 (13.0)
Number of shifts with fever	1.1 (1.5)	1.3 (2.1)
Percent of shifts with fever	8.1 (11.8)	8.6 (10.8)
Number of shifts with Spo_2 <90%	3.9 (5.1)	3.8 (4.6)
Percent of shifts with Spo_2 <90%	26.4 (27.6)	27.2 (27.5)
Number of shifts with elevated RR	7.2 (6.0)	7.7 (7.6)
Percent of shifts with elevated RR	50.8 (30.4)	51.8 (29.3)

Values are expressed as mean (SD).
*Group means (SD) of individuals' means of observations during hospitalization.

We attempted to standardize the use of antibiotics among hospital pediatricians through presentations at staff meetings and through close monitoring by the study pediatrician. The WHO acute respiratory infection manual for small hospitals[16] was used as a guide.

A standard hospital diet that met the recommended dietary allowance for vitamin A was provided to all children who could eat. Intravenous solutions and nasogastric feedings were administered as indicated by the patient's clinical condition; otherwise the diet provided in the hospital met the recommended dietary allowance.

The study subjects were discharged at the discretion of the attending pediatrician or by the decision of the parent. Transfers to other clinical services, readmissions, and deaths after discharge were recorded. Subjects were reexamined 2 weeks or more after discharge from the hospital.

Ethical approval was granted by the School of Hygiene and Public Health Committee on Human Volunteers, Johns Hopkins University, and by the Instituto de Nutricion de Centro America y Panama (INCAP) Comite de Etica.

Table III. Characteristics of study deaths

Study group	Age (mo)	Sex	Admission diagnosis	Days in hospital	Possible cause of death
Vitamin A	4	M	Pneumonia	2	Pertussis
Placebo	11	M	Bronchiolitis, malnutrition	2	Delayed treatment, supraventricular tachycardia
Placebo	14	F	Pneumonia, malnutrition	7	Hemothorax, resistant *Staphylococcus*
Vitamin A	3	M	Pneumonia	9	Aminophylline toxicity

Laboratory studies. Hematocrit, leukocyte count and differential counts, blood culture specimens, and urine specimens for antimicrobial activity were obtained at the time of admission. The disk diffusion method was used to test urine for antimicrobial activity; a drop of urine was placed on agar that was growing a lawn of very susceptible *Staphylococcus epidermidis*, and zones of inhibited growth were measured the next day. Nasopharyngeal secretions were obtained by aspiration within 24 hours of admission and evaluated for respiratory syncytial virus, influenza A and B, parainfluenza 1, 2, and 3, and adenovirus, by means of viral antigen detection kits (Respiratory Panel—IFA [immunofluorescence assay]; Chemicon International Inc., Temecula, Calif.). Blood samples for the serum retinol concentration were drawn at the time of admission and 2 weeks or more after discharge from hospital. Retinol levels were determined by the spectrophotometric method of analysis, modified from that of Bessey et al.,[17] in the biochemistry laboratory of INCAP. The International Vitamin A Consultative Group recommendations for the handling and storage of serum samples were observed.[18]

Analysis. Data were entered with the Epi Info program (version 5.0, USD Inc., Stone Mountain, Ga.) and analyzed with the SAS program (version 6.0, SAS Institute, Inc., Cary, N.C.). Analysis of variance was used to compare continuous variables and chi-square tests for dichotomous or categorical outcomes. Because each child had three observations per day and was often hospitalized for several days, we computed a treatment group mean by averaging each individual's mean value for RR, temperature, and Spo_2, respectively, using all of that subject's observations. We employed the method used by DiGiulio et al.[19] to compare the group means of slopes of improvement curves generated by means of linear regressions of RR, temperature, and Spo_2 by time (intervals of 3, 5, and 7 days). Survival analysis was used to assess the impact of treatment during the course of hospitalization.

RESULTS

We enrolled 267 children from October 1991 to March 1993. Four children were excluded from the final analysis because of age more than 48 months or evidence of asthma or both. Comparison of key variables at baseline revealed no significant differences between the vitamin A and placebo groups (Table I).

Clinical outcomes (Table II). There were no differences between the treatment groups in mean RR, temperature, or Spo_2. There were no differences in mean number of shifts or percentage of shifts with elevated RR, fever, or desaturation, or in total number of shifts in hospital by treatment group. Clinical scores revealed rapid improvement in the condition of most subjects in both groups, with no consistent differences. During hospitalization, there were also no differences in the number of changes in antibiotics or in the receipt of bronchodilators (salbutamol, theophylline-aminophylline) or steroids, by treatment group. Survival analysis of the number of observations (duration of hospitalization) by treatment group revealed no differences.

Laboratory findings. Two hundred thirteen children had nasopharyngeal aspirations sent for viral antigen detection; 204 had adequate cells present. One hundred twelve children (55%) had respiratory syncytial virus, 11 had parainfluenza 1 or 3, and 3 had adenovirus; there were no significant differences in viral etiologic findings by treatment group. Two hundred thirty-five children had blood cultures. Four cultures showed positive results in the vitamin A group and four in the placebo group. These blood cultures were positive for *Staphylococcus aureus* (4), *Streptococcus pneumoniae* (1), *Haemophilus parainfluenzae* (1), *Pseudomonas aeruginosa* (1), and *Klebsiella sp.* (1). Eight children had lung punctures; two were infected with *S. pneumoniae* and one each with *H. influenzae* and coliform species. One of these four children was in the vitamin A group and three were in the placebo group. Two hundred sixty children had their urine tested for antimicrobial activity shortly after admission; more than 85% in each group had positive test results, and there was no difference between groups.

There was no significant difference between the baseline retinol levels by group (Table I). The median number of days between initial and subsequent levels was 19.5 for the vitamin A group and 21 for the placebo group. Of those subjects hospitalized for 10 days or less and for whom the initial retinol value was low (<0.70 μmol/L), the mean change in levels in the vitamin A group was 0.67 μmol/L (n=23) and in the placebo group was 0.73 μmol/L (n=27); these levels were not significantly different.

Adverse outcomes. There was no significant difference in several adverse outcomes between the vitamin A and placebo-treated groups, even if all adverse events were grouped together. Eight children required mechanical ventilation during the study, four in each group. Thirteen children required hospitalization for more than 14 days, 8 in the vitamin A and 5 in the placebo group. There were 17 readmissions to the study hospitals for acute respiratory illnesses, 9 in the vitamin A group and 8 in the placebo group, and 3 transfers to other clinical services for infectious complications, 2 in the vitamin A group and 1 in the placebo group. There were four deaths during hospitalization, two in each of the treatment groups (Table III). Two children died after discharge from the hospital; both were in the vitamin A group.

DISCUSSION

This randomized, double-masked, placebo-controlled trial demonstrates the lack of efficacy of vitamin A as adjuvant treatment of ALRI requiring hospitalization in this population. The effect size was estimated a priori to be 1.5 days of hospitalization. With a standard deviation of 4 days and error probabilities of 0.05 (type I) and 0.2 (type II), the estimated sample size was 56 per study group. The power of this study to detect a clinically important difference varied by outcome measure. When $\alpha = 0.05$ and $n = 131$ were assumed, there was a power of 84% to detect a reduction in duration of hospitalization of 25%, a power of 80% to detect a 46% reduction in the number of 8-hour observation intervals with Spo_2 <90 mm Hg, and a power of 93% to detect a reduction by 1 day of elevated RR. Smaller, statistically significant differences cannot be detected with the sample size achieved but are probably not clinically significant. The strengths of our trial include the rigorous study design, the careful standardization of the multiple clinical assessments, and the supporting radiologic, microbiologic, and biochemical data.

There is a consensus on the benefits of vitamin A for reducing childhood mortality rates.[20] There is little agreement, however, regarding the efficacy of vitamin A for reducing childhood morbidity rates. There are several potential reasons for the lack of efficacy in our trial. First, the severity of ALRI illness in children included in this study may overwhelm any beneficial effect that vitamin A may provide. There may be an increased excretion of vitamin A during acute infection, as suggested by Stephensen et al.,[21] which may also explain the hyporetinolemia observed in other infections.[22] The increased excretion of retinol may reduce the likelihood that absorbed retinol could have the same impact as it might if there were no acute infection.

Additionally, the dose of vitamin A that we delivered may have been insufficient and the preparation may not have been the optimal form. Studies from Africa[6, 7] that reported a significant protective effect of vitamin A during measles used at least 400,000 IU vitamin A and as a water-miscible preparation. In light of our findings, the dose and preparation of retinol that WHO recommends for pneumonia (200,000 IU once, and oil based), which is what we used, may need to be reexamined.

Last, the vitamin A status in this population is relatively replete compared with populations used for the vitamin A mortality trials, and thus our subjects may not be expected to respond to treatment with vitamin A. There is a vitamin A sugar fortification program currently in place in Guatemala, though its effectiveness is unreported. Both of our treatment groups had higher mean retinol levels during convalescence. On the basis of the relatively normal baseline retinol levels (≥0.70 μmol/L being considered sufficient) and the lack of a substantially greater response in retinol levels of the vitamin A–treated group, we conclude that our population was not particularly deficient. Our findings are generalizable, nevertheless, to many populations in the developing world, including nearly all the western hemisphere. Similarly designed trials in which vitamin A deficiency is more prevalent and severe may be warranted. Prophylactic high-dose vitamin A therapy has not been addressed in this study but has not been shown to prevent ALRI in several trials in the developing world.[23, 24]

We are grateful for the contributions of our study nurses, and for the cooperation of the staff of the Hospital Roosevelt and the IGSS Hospital. We also thank Malathi Ram, Omar Dary, Humberto Mendez, Patricia Caceres, Flory Cano, and Jorge Pellecer for their important contributions to this study. We are especially indebted to Monica Grandien, of the Swedish Institute for Infectious Disease Control, for the analysis of nasopharyngeal aspirates.

REFERENCES

1. Sommer A, Tarwotjo I, Djunaedi E, et al. Impact of vitamin A supplementation on childhood mortality: a randomized controlled community trial. Lancet 1986;2:1169-73.
2. West KP, Pokhrel RP, Katz J, et al. Efficacy of vitamin A in reducing preschool child mortality in Nepal. Lancet 1991; 338:67-71.
3. Rahmathullan L, Underwood BA, Thulasiraj RD, et al. Reduced mortality among children in southern India receiving a small weekly dose of vitamin A. N Engl J Med 1990;323:929-35.
4. Selwyn BJ. The epidemiology of acute respiratory tract infection in young children: comparison of findings from several developing countries. Reviews of Infectious Diseases 1990; 12(supp 8):S870-88.
5. Barclay AJ, Foster A, Sommer A. Vitamin A supplements and mortality related to measles: a randomized clinical trail. BMJ 1987;294:294-6.
6. Hussey GD, Klein M. A randomized, controlled trial of vita-

min A in children with severe measles. N Engl J Med 1990;323:160-4.
7. Coutsoudis A, Broughton M, Coovadia HM. Vitamin A supplementation reduces measles morbidity in young African children: a randomized, placebo-controlled, double-blind trial. Am J Clin Nutr 1991;54:890-5.
8. Milton RC, Reddy V, Naidu AN. Mild vitamin A deficiency and childhood morbidity: an Indian experience. Am J Clin Nutr 1987;46:827-9.
9. Sommer A, Katz J, Tarwotjo I. Increased risk of respiratory disease and diarrhea in children with preexisting mild vitamin A deficiency. Am J Clin Nutr 1984;40:1090-5.
10. Tielsch JM, West KP, Katz J, et al. Prevalence and severity of xerophthalmia in southern Malawi. Am J Epidemiol 1986;124:561-8.
11. Solon FS, Popkin BM, Fernandez TL, Latham MC. Vitamin A deficiency in the Philippines: a study of xerophthalmia in Cebu. Am J Clin Nutr 1978;31:360-8.
12. Bloem M, Wedel M, Egger RJ, et al. Mild vitamin A deficiency and risk of respiratory tract disease and diarrhea in preschool and school children in northeastern Thailand. Am J Epidemiol 1990;131:332-9.
13. Vitamin A supplements: a guide to their use in the treatment and prevention of vitamin A deficiency and xerophthalmia. Geneva: World Health Organization, 1988.
14. Henning B, Stewart K, Zaman K, Alam AN, Brown KH, Black RE. Lack of therapeutic efficacy of vitamin A for non-cholera, watery diarrhoea in Bangladeshi children. Eur J Clin Nutr 1992;46:437-43.
15. Silverman WA, Anderson DH. A controlled trial of the effects of water mist on obstructive signs, death rate and necropsy findings among premature infants. Pediatrics 1956;17:1-10.
16. Respiratory infections in children: management in small hospitals—a manual for doctors. Geneva: World Health Organization, 1988.
17. Bessey OT, Lowry OH, Brock MJ, Lopez JA. The determination of vitamin A and carotene in small quantities of blood serum. J Biol Chem 1946;166:177-88.
18. Arroyave G, Chichester CO, Flores H, et al. Biochemical methodology for the assessment of vitamin A status. Washington, D.C.: The Nutrition Foundation, 1982.
19. DiGiulio GA, Kercsmar CM, Krug SE, Alpert SE, Marx CM. Hospital treatment of asthma: lack of benefit from theophylline given in addition to nebulized albuterol and intravenously administered corticosteroids. J PEDIATR 1993;122:464-9.
20. Beaton GH, Martorell R, L'Abbé KA, et al. Effectiveness of vitamin A supplementation in the control of young child morbidity and mortality in developing countries: final report. Toronto: International Nutrition Program, Department of Nutritional Sciences, University of Toronto, January 1993.
21. Stephensen CB, Alvarez JO, Kohatsu J, Hardmeier R. Vitamin A is excreted in the urine during acute infection. Am J Clin Nutr 1994;60:388-92.
22. Butler JC, Havens PL, Sowell AL, et al. Measles severity and serum retinol (vitamin A) concentration among children in the United States. Pediatrics 1993;91:1176-81.
23. Stansfield SK, Louis MP, Lerebours G, Augustin A. Vitamin A supplementation and increased prevalence of childhood diarrhoea and acute respiratory infections. Lancet 1993;342:578-82.
24. Bhandari N, Bhan MK, Sazawal S. Impact of massive dose of vitamin A given to preschool children with acute diarrhoea on subsequent respiratory and diarrhoeal morbidity. BMJ 1994;309:1404-7.

Clinical and laboratory observations

Fatal hemolysis induced by ceftriaxone in a child with sickle cell anemia

Juan C. Bernini, MD, Mahmoud M. Mustafa, MD, Laurie J. Sutor, MD, and George R. Buchanan, MD

From the Departments of Pediatrics and Pathology, University of Texas Southwestern Medical Center at Dallas, and the Center for Cancer and Blood Disorders, Children's Medical Center, Dallas, Texas

A 2-year-old boy with sickle cell anemia had a massive, fatal hemolytic reaction after administration of an intravenous dose of ceftriaxone. Laboratory studies demonstrated the presence of an IgM antibody against ceftriaxone, binding to and destroying the patient's erythrocytes by an immune complex mechanism. This rare complication should be considered in the differential diagnosis when hemoglobinuria develops in a child after administration of ceftriaxone or a similar agent. (J Pediatr 1995;126:813-5)

It has become standard practice to administer ceftriaxone, a third-generation cephalosporin, to infants and children with diverse febrile illnesses.[1] In particular the efficacy of ceftriaxone in the treatment of febrile patients with sickle cell disease has been well documented.[2, 3] Ceftriaxone therapy has few complications except for rare penicillin-like allergic reactions and transitory (and usually asymptomatic) biliary sludging. Immune hemolytic anemia has been reported in adults, but severe hemolytic reactions have not been reported during childhood or in patients with sickle cell disease.

CASE REPORT

A 24-month-old black male child with sickle cell anemia, diagnosed by the Texas Department of Health's newborn screening program, and reactive airway disease was followed in the hematology-oncology clinic at Children's Medical Center of Dallas. His steady-state hemoglobin value was approximately 70 gm/L, and hematocrit was 0.20 to 0.23. He began prophylactic penicillin therapy at the time of his initial visit to the clinic when he was 6 months of age. For the next 18 months his clinical course was characterized by several episodes of acute chest syndrome, fever, splenic sequestration, and vasoocclusive crises. At 13 and 20 months of age he received blood transfusions. No abnormalities were detected by pretransfusion serologic tests, and he had no untoward reactions after transfusions. At 10 months of age he began to receive ceftriaxone for febrile illness according to an institutional management protocol.[3] He received a total of 14 doses of ceftriaxone on several different occasions.

See related article, p. 816.

IHA	Immune hemolytic anemia

Beginning when the patient was 16 months of age, the clinical course was complicated by six unexplained episodes of hemoglobinuria occurring transiently during the initial hours of hospitalizations for acute illnesses. The result of a quantitative glucose-6-phosphate dehydrogenase assay was normal. No further studies were undertaken to investigate the hemoglobinuria. The patient had a decline in hemoglobin concentration during only one of these episodes; this was ascribed to hemolysis resulting from sepsis, although the blood cultures were negative.

Ten days after a routine follow-up clinic visit, during which no

Supported in part by Children's Cancer Fund of Dallas and Consejo Nacional para Investigaciones Científicas y Tecnológicas, San José, Costa Rica.

Submitted for publication Dec. 7, 1994; accepted Jan. 20, 1995.

Reprint requests: George R. Buchanan, MD, Department of Pediatrics, University of Texas Southwestern Medical Center, 5323 Harry Hines Blvd., Dallas, TX 75235-9063.

0022-3476/95/$3.00 + 0 **9/26/63482**

Table I. Laboratory results before and after intravenous administration of ceftriaxone

Test	Before ceftriaxone	After ceftriaxone (20 min)
Hemoglobin (gm/L)	70	9
Hematocrit	0.20	0.015
Leukocyte count ($\times 10^9$ cells/L)	23	6.7
Platelets ($\times 10^9$ cell/L)	399	50
Reticulocytes (%)	17	NA
Serum potassium (mmol/L)	NA	9
Serum phosphate (mmol/L)	NA	4.5

NA, Not available.

changes in findings of physical examination or in steady-state laboratory values were noted, the patient was seen in the emergency department after an acute onset of fever and vomiting. His temperature was 40.2° C, but he did not appear seriously ill. According to protocol, blood cultures and a complete blood cell count were determined and a dose of ceftriaxone (75 mg/kg) was administered intravenously. His initial laboratory results were within the steady-state values (Table I). Review of the peripheral blood smear showed some sickle and target cells, marked polychromasia, and Howell-Jolly bodies, but no erythrocyte agglutination or fragmentation. Twenty minutes after the administration of the ceftriaxone dose, he became unresponsive and had a cardiorespiratory arrest. Repeated laboratory testing showed severe anemia (Table I). Despite vigorous resuscitative efforts, including transfusion and intensive care support, he remained in shock and died 36 hours later with evidence of multiple organ failure. Permission to perform an autopsy was denied. Blood cultures obtained before the administration of the ceftriaxone were sterile.

In retrospect, review of the patient's medical record indicated that the transient episodes of hemoglobinuria noted previously had occurred immediately after the administration of ceftriaxone on five separate occasions.

METHODS AND RESULTS

The serologic evaluations, most of which were performed after the patient's death on specimens obtained shortly after the patient's cardiorespiratory arrest, included determination of blood type and crossmatch, direct antiglobulin test with polyspecific serum and with anti-IgG and anti-C3d, Donath-Landsteiner test, cold agglutinin titer, and serum complement determination; all tests were performed according to standard methods (Table II). Blood samples were also sent to the American Red Cross Blood Services (Los Angeles, Calif.) to determine whether the patient's serum or erythrocytes contained antibodies against ceftriaxone. The patient's serum was tested against ceftriaxone-coated, enzyme-treated, and untreated erythrocytes, and in the presence of ceftriaxone against uncoated erythrocytes[4] (Table II). Titration studies of the patient's serum were performed in the presence of fresh complement and ceftriaxone against enzyme-treated erythrocytes. The 37° C agglutinin reacted to a titer of 1:512, the hemolysin to a titer of 1:8, and the antiglobulin to a titer of 1:512. Dithiothreitol treatment[5] of the patient's serum reversed the agglutination seen at 37° C in the presence of ceftriaxone against enzyme-treated erythrocytes, thus indicating the antibody to be in the IgM class.

DISCUSSION

Drug-induced IHA in children is commonly associated with a congenital defect of the erythrocyte (i.e., glucose-6-phosphate dehydrogenase deficiency) and rarely is related to an immunologic reaction. Although many pediatric and hematology reference books list drugs as a cause of IHA,[6-9] cephalosporin-induced IHA has not been described in children.

Cephalosporins frequently interact nonspecifically with the erythrocyte membrane, resulting in a positive direct antiglobulin test result, but hemolysis is rare. Since the introduction of the first-generation cephalosporins, only five well-documented cases of IHA complicating the use of these agents have been reported in 25 years.[10] With the advent of second- and third-generation cephalosporins, the incidence of cephalosporin-induced IHA appears to be increasing.[10-13] To our knowledge only four episodes of IHA, one of them fatal, have been triggered by a third-generation cephalosporin,[13-16] and ours is the first report of such a complication in a child or in a patient with a sickle hemoglobinopathy. In addition, this is only the second fatality known to have resulted from IHA related to a third-generation cephalosporin agent.[13] Our patient had clinical evidence of intravascular hemolysis characterized by a striking decline in the hemoglobin concentration, reticulocytosis, increased serum phosphorus and potassium concentrations, and hemoglobinuria. The presence of IHA was confirmed by several commonly performed tests (i.e., a strongly positive direct antiglobulin test result with anticomplement reagents and a low serum complement level).

The immune mechanisms by which second- and third-generation cephalosporins induce IHA are different from those described for the first-generation agents. An IgM antibody directed against ceftriaxone, which then mediates erythrocyte destruction by an immune complex mechanism, has been at least one of the processes implicated in the five reported cases (including ours) of third-generation cephalosporin-induced IHA. On the other hand, an IgG antibody, through a drug-absorbent (penicillin-like) mechanism, has been responsible for all reported cases of first-generation cephalosporin–induced IHA.[10] It has been suggested that the immune complex (drug-antidrug complex) binds to the erythrocyte membrane, activating complement and causing intravascular hemolysis.

Table II. Laboratory findings in patient with fatal ceftriaxone-induced immune hemolytic anemia

Test	Reaction with patient's cells	Reaction with patient's serum	Reaction with plasma, complement, and ceftriaxone
Direct antiglobulin	Agglutination 3+		
IgG	Agglutination ±		
C3	Agglutination ±		
Indirect antiglobulin		–	
Cold agglutinin titer		–	
Donath-Landsteiner antibody		–	
Serum complement			
C3 (mg/dl)		69 (range 73-180)	
C4 (mg/dl)		9.9 (range 15-45)	
Patient's ceftriaxone-coated RBCs		Nonreactive	
Patient's untreated RBCs			Agglutination 3½+
Patient's enzyme-treated RBCs			Agglutination, 2½+, Hemolysis 3+

Agglutination and hemolysis are scored on scale from 0 to 4+.
–, Negative results.

In most prior cases cephalosporin-induced IHA appeared 7 to 10 days after drug exposure.[17] Our patient's immediate and massive hemolysis most likely resulted from sensitization by repeated exposure to ceftriaxone during the previous months. This notion is supported by the retrospective observation that the prior episodes of hemoglobinuria were temporally related to the administration of a cephalosporin. It is possible that our patient's underlying anemia may have exacerbated the drug-induced hemolytic event.

The incidence of drug-induced IHA caused by ceftriaxone or other third-generation cephalosporins may be underestimated; many cases have probably not been reported.[10] Physicians should be aware of the clinically severe and potentially fatal hemolytic reactions that can occur after parenteral administration of the second- and third-generation cephalosporin agents. Hemoglobinuria should be carefully evaluated, and IHA should always be considered in the differential diagnosis in a child with signs of intravascular hemolysis after the parenteral administration of cephalosporins.

We acknowledge Dr. George Garratty, American Red Cross Blood Services, Los Angeles, Calif., for performing the ceftriaxone-induced antibody assays, and Dr. William Chappell for editorial assistance.

REFERENCES

1. Bradley JS. Once-daily ceftriaxone in the treatment of pediatric infections. Chemotherapy 1991;3(suppl):3-6.
2. Wilimas JA, Flynn PM, Harris S, et al. A randomized study of outpatient treatment with ceftriaxone for selected febrile children with sickle cell disease. N Engl J Med 1993;329:472-6.
3. Rogers ZR, Morrison RA, Vedro D, Buchanan GR. Outpatient management of febrile illness in infants and young children with sickle cell anemia. J PEDIATR 1990;177:736-9.
4. Petz LD, Garratty G. Acquired immune hemolytic anemias. New York: Churchill Livingstone, 1980:267-304.
5. Walker RH, ed. Technical manual. 11th ed. Bethesda, Md: American Association of Blood Banks, 1993.
6. Stockman JA III. Diseases of the blood. In: Behrman RE, Kliegman RM, Nelson WE, Vaughan VC III, eds. In: Nelson textbook of pediatrics. 14th ed. Philadelphia: WB Saunders, 1992:1229-56.
7. Martin PL, Pearson HA. The hemolytic anemias. In: Oski FA, DeAngelis CD, Feigin RD, McMillan JA, Warshaw JB, eds. Principles and practice of pediatrics. 2nd ed. Philadelphia: JB Lippincott, 1994:1663-6.
8. Schreiber AD, Gill FM, Manno CS, eds. Autoimmune hemolytic anemia. In: Nathan DG, Oski FA, eds. Hematology of infancy and childhood; vol 1. 4th ed. Philadelphia: WB Saunders, 1993:496-510.
9. Klemperer MR. Hemolytic anemias: immune defects. In: Miller DR, Baehner RL, eds. Blood diseases of infancy and childhood. 6th ed. St Louis: CV Mosby, 1990:233-60.
10. Garratty G. Immune cytopenia associated with antibodies. Transfus Med Rev 1993;7:255-67.
11. Ehmann WC. Cephalosporin-induced hemolysis: a case report and review of the literature. Am J Hematol 1992;40:121-5.
12. Garratty G, Nance S, Lloyd M, Domen R. Fatal immune hemolytic anemia due to cefotetan. Transfusion 1992;32:269-71.
13. Garratty G, Postoway N, Schwellenbach J, McMahill PC. A fatal case of ceftriaxone (Rocephin)-induced hemolytic anemia associated with intravascular immune hemolysis. Transfusion 1991;31:176-9.
14. Shulman IA, Arndt PA, McGehee W, Garratty G. Cefotaxime-induced hemolytic anemia due to antibodies reacting in vitro by more than one mechanism. Transfusion 1990;30:263-6.
15. Chambers LA, Donovan LM, Kruskall MS. Ceftazidime-induced hemolysis in a patient with drug-dependent antibodies reactive by immune complex and drug adsorption mechanisms. Am J Clin Pathol 1991;95:393-6.
16. Salama A, Göttsche B, Schleiffer T, Mueller-Eckhardt C. "Immune complex" mediated intravascular hemolysis due to IgM cephalosporin-dependent antibody. Transfusion 1987;27:460-3.
17. Chenoweth CE, Judd WJ, Steiner EA, Kauffman CA. Cefotetan-induced immune hemolytic anemia. Clin Infect Dis 1992;15:863-5.

Fatal hemolysis caused by ceftriaxone

André D. Lascari, MD, and Kristina Amyot, MD

From the Departments of Pediatrics and Pathology, Albany Medical College, Albany, New York

After receiving ceftriaxone intravenously, a boy with leukemia died suddenly of massive hemolysis. The diagnosis was made retrospectively only after a similar case of sudden fatal immune hemolysis after intravenous administration of ceftriaxone was reported. (J Pediatr 1995;126:816-7)

Ceftriaxone is a third-generation cephalosporin antibiotic that has gained wide popularity because it provides bactericidal levels against common pediatric pathogens for more than 24 hours. In August 1994 a boy with leukemia died suddenly and unexpectedly in our clinic after intravenous administration of ceftriaxone and a platelet transfusion. Four months later the report of a similar case led retrospectively to the highly probable diagnosis of fatal immune hemolysis resulting from intravenous administration of ceftriaxone.[1]

CASE REPORT

Juvenile chronic myelocytic leukemia was diagnosed in a 5-year-old boy with neurofibromatosis. During the previous year he had received three courses of cefaclor for otitis media. The patient was initially treated with hydroxyurea, and a search was started for a bone marrow donor. Three months later he received four doses of cytosine arabinoside for 2 consecutive weeks. He was then admitted to the hospital because of fever and neutropenia, received vancomycin and ceftazidime intravenously for 4 days, and was then discharged from the hospital to receive ceftriaxone intravenously daily for 9 days because of persistent neutropenia. He had no history of dark urine at this time.

A splenectomy had been done 4 months after onset of leukemia because of its massive size and poor responses to platelet transfusions. A bone marrow donor was identified, but the patient's disease was not under control and he received a 4-day course of daunomycin, VP-16 (etoposide), 6-thioguanine, and dexamethasone. The day after discharge the patient was seen in the clinic to get a platelet transfusion before a day visit to a summer camp. The hemoglobin concentration was 62 gm/L (6.2 gm/dl), leukocyte count was 0.7×10^9 cells/L (700 cells/mm^3), and platelet count was 1×10^9 cells/L (1000 cells/mm^3). He was afebrile and did not appear sick but had an earache, and the left tympanic membrane was markedly inflamed. Amoxicillin was prescribed and ceftriaxone (50 mg/kg) was given intravenously for 30 minutes because of the neutropenia and the impending day trip to camp. A platelet transfusion was then started, and 45 minutes later he suddenly sat up and screamed with ear pain. Blood was draining from his left ear, and he then stiffened, appeared pale, and became unresponsive. Jaundice was not evident. Ten minutes later he had a cardiac arrest and could not be resuscitated. The hemoglobin level at the time of the patient's death was 14 gm/L (1.4 gm/dl) and the platelet count was 111×10^9 cells/L (111,000 cells/mm^3). Results of a erythrocyte antibody screening, performed before the ceftriaxone was administered, was negative.

Autopsy on the next day revealed generalized leukemic involvement with massive generalized lymphadenopathy, hepatomegaly, hepatic fibrosis, pleural effusions (210 ml on the left side, 170 ml on the right), and ascites (100 ml). Striking hemophagocytosis was present in the lymph nodes and in the spleen, which had been removed 1 month previously. No internal hemorrhage was found. The brain was normal. Cultures of the blood, liver, and lung grew multiple organisms (*Candida albicans*, enterococcus, *Bacillus* species, coagulase-negative staphylococci) strongly suggestive of contamination. No histologic evidence of any bacterial or fungal infection was found in any tissue.

Four months later the two blood smears done the day of death showed no erythrocyte clumping on the first blood cell count (hemoglobin, 62 gm/L [6.2 gm/dl]) but striking clumping on the second smear (hemoglobin, 14 gm/L [1.4 gm/dl]). Blood was not available for serologic studies.

See related article, p. 813.

DISCUSSION

The immediate cause of death of this patient was unexplained until a recent case report of a sudden collapse and death in a child with sickle cell anemia who also had received ceftriaxone intravenously.[1] Our patient's initial low platelet count and the precipitous drop in hemoglobin level suggested a massive internal hemorrhage. Hemolysis was never considered, and therefore appropriate serologic tests were not done. The patient did not become jaundiced; there likely was not time for the breakdown of hemoglobin to bilirubin, because death occurred within an hour of the administration of ceftriaxone.

Submitted for publication Dec. 29, 1994; accepted Jan. 25, 1995.

Reprint requests: André D. Lascari, MD, Department of Pediatrics, Hematology/Oncology, A-24, Albany Medical College, 47 New Scotland Ave., Albany, NY 12208-3478.

0022-3476/95/$3.00 + 0 **9/26/63691**

Although platelets were being given at the time of death, to our knowledge platelet transfusions have not been incriminated as a cause of such a mssive hemolytic reaction. Erythrophagocytosis was present in the spleen, which had been removed 2 weeks after the first exposure to ceftriaxone, and erythrophagocytosis was striking in the lymph nodes at autopsy. The erythrophagocytosis and an apparent increase in transfusion requirements during the last month of life point to a shortened erythrocyte survival time. No clinical evidence of an infection-associated hemophagocytic syndrome was found,[2] and the erythrophagocytosis remains unexplained.

Our patient had previously received ceftriaxone, as had the other described patient.[1] The marked erythrocyte clumping observed on the blood smear, the precipitous drop in hemoglobin level with no evidence of hemorrhage at autopsy, and the absence of erythrocyte antibodies just before the antibiotic administration point to the high probability that massive hemolysis was the terminal event and that it was caused by ceftriaxone. In the previously reported case the patient had a cardiovascular collapse within 20 minutes of an intravenous dose of ceftriaxone and had a decrease in hemoglobin level from 70 gm/L (7.0 gm/dl) to 9 gm/L (0.9 gm/dl). Despite vigorous resuscitative efforts, the child died 36 hours later. The direct antiglobulin test result was strongly positive, and the patient's serum strongly agglutinated washed erythrocytes in the presence of complement and ceftriaxone.

A similar but not as precipitous reaction has been described in an adult who had a decrease in hematocrit from 0.45 (45%) to 0.15 (15%) within 8 days after receiving intravenous ceftriaxone for the first 6 days of therapy.[3] The serum of that patient contained an antibody that also reacted strongly when the serum was added to the drug and erythrocytes. Although immune hemolysis has been reported with other cephalosporin antibiotics, the onset has usually been during the course of days.[1, 4]

Ceftriaxone is widely used, particularly because it can be administered once daily and thus may allow outpatient treatment instead of admission to the hospital. Whether intramuscular administration would minimize the risk of sudden hemolysis and death, and whether patients with a preexisting hemolytic anemia are the only ones at risk, remain to be determined.

REFERENCES

1. Bernini J, Mustafa M, Buchanan G. Fatal immune-mediated hemolysis induced by ceftriaxone in a child with sickle cell anemia [Abstract 716]. Blood 1994;84(10, suppl 1):183a.
2. Risdall R, McKenna R, Mesbit M, Krivit W. Virus associated hemophagocytic syndrome. Cancer 1979;44:993-1002.
3. Garratty G, Postoway N, Schwellenbach J, McMahill P. A fatal case of ceftriaxone (Rhocephin)-induced hemolytic anemia associated with intravascular immune hemolysis. Transfusion 1991;31:176-9.
4. Ehmann W. Cephalosporin-induced hemolysis: a case report and review of the literature. Am J Hematol 1992;40:121-5.

Furosemide-associated fever

Herbert W. Clegg, MD, and Donald A. Riopel, MD

From Eastover Pediatrics, The Sanger Clinic, and the Department of Pediatrics and Division of Pediatric Cardiology, Carolinas Medical Center, Charlotte, North Carolina

We describe a 5-month-old infant who had fever of unknown origin leading to an exhaustive evaluation during a 7-week period. Fever caused by the use of furosemide was proved; the fever resolved after discontinuation of this medication and recurred after its reintroduction. (J Pediatr 1995;126:817-8)

Most drugs can cause fever, and certain agents are particularly associated with drug fever.[1] Furosemide is not considered among these agents.

Submitted for publication Sept. 12, 1994; accepted Dec. 12, 1994.

Reprint requests: Herbert W. Clegg, MD, Eastover Pediatrics, 2711 Randolph Rd., Suite 501, Charlotte, NC 28207.

0022-3476/95/$3.00 + 0 **9/26/62711**

We recently cared for a patient with fever of unknown cause in whom drug fever was suspected early but not proved until late in her course.

CASE REPORT

A 5-month-old girl with trisomy 21 (Down syndrome) (47,XX; +21) was noted to have a complete atrioventricular canal defect shortly after birth. When she was 2 weeks old, treatment with digoxin and furosemide was begun for congestive heart failure. When she was 6 weeks old, a temperature of 37.8° to 38.4° C and cough were noted and she required hospitalization. A chest x-ray study revealed a right upper lobe infiltrate, and nasal secretions were positive by enzyme immunoassay for respiratory syncytial virus and by direct fluorescence antibody testing for *Chlamydia trachomatis*. She received ribavirin and erythromycin, and hydralazine was added to her regimen because of worsening heart failure.

Low-grade fever persisted after the respiratory symptoms were much improved. Hydralazine was discontinued without a change in the fever and was reintroduced. A fine maculopapular rash appeared on the patient's trunk, and her fever subsided for 10 days.

When the patient was 11 weeks of age, a temperature of 38.4° to 39° C recurred without other symptoms or signs except those associated with chronic heart failure. Hydralazine was again discontinued. Because of a persistent daily fever of 38.4° to 39° C for 3 weeks and negative results of an outpatient examination for a focus of infection, she was hospitalized for further examination. The results of a blood cell count, sedimentation rate, electrolyte panel, liver enzymes profile, chest x-ray study, urinalysis, echocardiogram, abdominal ultrasonography, cerebrospinal fluid and bone marrow examinations, and gallium citrate scan were normal. Skin tests with intermediate purified protein derivative and *Candida* antigen (1:100), and for antinuclear antibody, and cultures of blood (three sets), urine, cerebrospinal fluid, and bone marrow yielded negative results. Viral cultures of throat and stool grew only poliovirus type 2, consistent with a vaccine virus, because she had recently received her second dose of oral vaccine.

After 6 weeks of persistent daily fever to 39° C, digoxin was withheld for 6 days; the fever pattern was unchanged. Furosemide was then withheld, and the fever abruptly ceased. After 72 hours without fever, heart failure was considered worse, and digoxin and furosemide were again given. Fever to 39° C recurred after the first dose of furosemide. This agent was discontinued, and chlorothiazide was substituted. Fever resolved within 24 hours and did not recur.

DISCUSSION

The most common clinical toxic effects associated with furosemide are abnormalities of fluid balance and electrolytes; other side effects are rarely observed.[2-5] Anaphylaxis, marked by angioedema, urticaria, and hypotension, has been noted after intravenous furosemide,[6] as has cardiac arrest.[7] Furosemide is structurally related to sulfonamide antibiotics and thiazide diuretics. This may be important if true allergic reactions occur with one of these agents.[6, 8]

Except in a single case, furosemide oral solution has not, according to the manufacturer and our review of the literature, been reported to be a cause of fever. Fever has been described in an elderly patient who had autoimmune findings suggesting a furosemide-induced lupuslike syndrome.[9] Moreover, in three surveillance studies of more than 3500 hospitalized furosemide recipients, fever was not listed as an adverse reaction.[3-5]

The adverse drug experience files of the Food and Drug Administration contained 20 possible cases of fever associated with furosemide (J. Creamer: personal communication, Dec. 22, 1992). In these patients either other drugs were given concomitantly or the patient did not receive a rechallenge with the drug to demonstrate a relationship more conclusively.

Our experience suggests that furosemide may cause drug fever. In the differential diagnosis of persistent fever, all drugs being administered should be considered as possible causes of the fever.

REFERENCES

1. Mackowiak PA, LeMaistre CF. Drug fever: a critical appraisal of conventional concepts. Ann Intern Med 1987;106:728-33.
2. Weiner IM. Diuretics and other agents employed in the mobilization of edema fluid. In: Gilman AG, Rall TW, Nies AS, Taylor P, eds. Goodman and Gilman's the pharmacological basis of therapeutics. 8th ed. New York: Pergamon Press, 1990:723-5.
3. Greenblatt DJ, Duhme DW, Allen MD, Koch-Weser J. Clinical toxicity of furosemide in hospitalized patients: a report from the Boston Collaborative Drug Surveillance Program. Am Heart J 1977;94:6-13.
4. Naranjo CA, Busto U, Cassis L. Furosemide-induced adverse reactions during hospitalization. Am J Hosp Pharm 1978;35:794-8.
5. Lowe J, Gray J, Henry DA, Lawson DH. Adverse reactions to frusemide in hospital inpatients. Br Med J 1979;2:360-2.
6. Hansbrough JR, Wedner HJ, Chaplin DD. Anaphylaxis to intravenous furosemide. J Allergy Clin Immunol 1987;80:538-41.
7. Rance CP. Cardiac arrest after intravenous frusemide. Lancet 1969;1:1265-6.
8. Sullivan TJ. Cross-reactions among furosemide, hydrochlorothiazide, and sulfonamides. JAMA 1991;265:120-1.
9. Lin RY. Unusual autoimmune manifestations in furosemide-associated hypersensitivity angiitis. N Y State J Med 1988;88:439-40.

Rebound severe methemoglobinemia from ingestion of a nitroethane artificial-fingernail remover

Kevin C. Osterhoudt, MD, Catherine C. Wiley, MD,
Robert Dudley, MD, Sandra Sheen, BSN, and Fred M. Henretig, MD

From the Department of Pediatrics, University of Pennsylvania School of Medicine, Children's Hospital of Philadelphia, and the Poison Control Center, Philadelphia

We describe life-threatening methemoglobinemia in a child who ingested a nitroethane artificial-fingernail remover initially mistaken to be an acetone-based polish remover. Nitroethane-induced methemoglobinemia may be delayed and recurrent; patients ingesting this substance may warrant close observation for at least 24 hours. Care givers are cautioned to determine the precise substance involved in ingestions of potentially toxic fingernail products. (J PEDIATR 1995;126:819-21)

Methemoglobinemia occurs when an oxidative stress converts hemic iron from the ferrous to the ferric state, rendering it less capable of binding oxygen. Acquired cases of methemoglobinemia in children occur in approximately equal proportions from two distinctly different stressors: (1) endogenous illness, usually characterized by gastroenteritis with metabolic acidosis, and (2) acute overdose of, or therapeutic exposure to, an exogenous oxidant agent.[1] Cosmetic fingernail products include many potentially hazardous chemicals. Reported childhood poisonings have included acetone intoxication caused by nail polish remover,[2] cyanide intoxication caused by acetonitrile-containing nail glue remover,[3, 4] methemoglobinemia resulting from ingestion of N,N-dimethyl-*p*-toluidine used to make artificial fingernails,[5] and methemoglobinemia caused by nitroethane artificial-fingernail remover.[6] This report of nitroethane ingestion is unusual in that the child had delayed and recurrent severe methemoglobinemia.

CASE REPORT

A 13-month-old girl weighing 10.2 kg who had ingested a fingernail product thought to be an acetone-based fingernail polish remover was seen in the emergency department. She had previously been healthy and was receiving no medications. The symptom-free infant was discharged without specific treatment after a brief period of observation. Seven hours after ingestion the patient returned for reevaluation because of emesis and lethargy. At this time the ingested substance was identified as the Remove brand of artificial nail remover (Gena Laboratories Inc., Duncanville, Tex.), which contains 100% nitroethane. A maximum of 90 ml was missing from the previously used bottle. The infant had tachypnea (respiratory rate, 44 breaths/min) and cyanosis; yet an arterial blood gas study in room air showed a pH of 7.35, carbon dioxide pressure of 26 mm Hg, and oxygen pressure of 103 mm Hg. She remained cyanotic despite the administration of 80% supplemental oxygen. The lungs were clear with good aeration bilaterally. The infant's heart rate was 120 beats/min, and her blood pressure was 100/55 mm Hg. Heart rhythm was regular; no murmur was detected by auscultation. Examination of the abdomen showed no abnormalities, and the patient had no history of diarrheal illness. Peripheral capillary refill time was less than 2 seconds. The patient's cyanosis, refractory to supplemental oxygen, suggested methemoglobinemia, which was confirmed. Her hospital course (Table) was notable for the delayed onset (7 hours) of severe methemoglobinemia. A rebound elevation of methemoglobin to 53% occurred after methylene blue therapy and an asymptomatic period. Her total hemoglobin concentration was 107 gm/L (10.7 gm/dl). Liver enzyme levels in the serum remained within laboratory standard values for age, and glucose-6-phosphate dehydrogenase was not deficient when measured on outpatient follow-up.

DISCUSSION

The abrupt onset of cyanosis, unresponsive to oxygen administration, in a previously well child is the long recognized hallmark of methemoglobinemia.[7] Numerous oxidant agents have been associated with this phenomenon. Methemoglobinemia results in cellular hypoxic trauma by decreasing oxygen-carrying capacity and by shifting the oxyhemoglobin dissociation curve to the left with subsequent diminished oxygen release to the tissues. As levels rise greater than 10% to 15%, most patients are visibly cyanotic; at 30% to 50%, dysphoria, headache, lethargy, and vomiting ensue. Progressively higher levels are associated with

Submitted for publication Aug. 23, 1994; accepted Nov. 28, 1994.

Reprint requests: Fred M. Henretig, MD, Department of Pediatric Emergency Medicine, The Children's Hospital of Philadelphia, 34th and Civic Center Boulevard, Philadelphia, PA 19104.

0022-3476/95/$3.00 + 0 **9/26/62343**

Table. Methemoglobin level, clinical appearance, and treatment after ingestion of nitroethane

Time (hr)	Methemoglobin level (%)	Clinical findings	Methylene blue dose* (mg/kg)
7	48	Emesis, lethargy, cyanosis	3.5
17	19	No symptoms	—
23	53	No Cyanotic alert	2
35	24	No symptoms	—
42	5.5	No symptoms	—
60	0.4	No symptoms	—

*Administered by intravenous bolus infusion.

increasingly altered sensorium, and levels greater than 70% are potentially lethal. Classic therapy includes provision of supplemental oxygen and the use of the antidote methylene blue. Children with glucose-6-phosphate dehydrogenase deficiency in whom methemoglobinemia develops are resistant to therapy with methylene blue because it utilizes reduced nicotinamide adenine denucleotide phosphate, derived from the hexose monophosphate shunt pathway, as a cofactor in reducing hemic iron.[8]

Nitroethane has the chemical formula $CH_3CH_2NO_2$. It is a colorless liquid with a mild fruity odor. Now commercially available as an artificial fingernail glue remover, it has also been used as a rocket propellant, as an intermediate in pharmaceutical manufacture, and as an industrial solvent. Many standard toxicologic resources such as the text *Medical Toxicology*[9] and *The Poisindex*[10] have no discussions concerning nitroethane toxicity. Although the *Handbook of Toxic and Hazardous Chemicals and Carcinogens* (second edition) mentions the potential for toxic effects as a result of contact, inhalation, and ingestion, there is no mention of methemoglobinemia as a possible sequela.[11] Animal studies have suggested that similar compounds were low-potency methemoglobin formers.[12]

Symptomatic methemoglobinemia developed 10 hours after ingestion in one previous patient with nitroethane poisoning[6] and 7 hours after ingestion in our patient. In animal models nitroethane is not absorbed sufficiently from the skin to result in systemic injury but is rapidly absorbed through the lungs and gastrointestinal tract.[13] The delayed onset of methemoglobinemia in the human poisonings suggests biotransformation to other toxic metabolites. Nitroethane has been shown in animal studies to be metabolized to aldehyde and nitrite, with the end product being the eventual oxidation to nitrate:[14]

$$CH_3CH_2NO_2 \rightarrow CH_3CHO + HNO_2 + H_2O \xrightarrow{O} NO_3^-$$

This process results in complete clearance of nitroethane within 30 hours in rats.[14] Nitrites are acknowledged as formers of methemoglobin.[15] Organic nitrates are of themselves rather inert. However, nitrates can be metabolized back to inorganic nitrite by the liver[16] or by nitrite-producing bacteria in the gastrointestinal tract.[17] The reviewed metabolic fate likely accounts for the delayed methemoglobinemia observed in our patient and for the severe rebound elevation in methemoglobin noted several hours after apparent resolution. Methylene blue is an oxidizing agent in its own right, and doses of 5 mg/kg have been implicated in asymptomatic methemoglobinemia.[8] However, we do not believe that the rebound methemoglobinemia observed was iatrogenic because the initial dose of methylene blue administered was only 3.5 mg/kg, and subsequent treatment with methylene blue had the expected effect of again lowering the methemoglobin level. Delayed gastrointestinal absorption and/or enterohepatic recirculation of nitroethane may also have contributed to the rebound phenomenon.

The growing number of potentially toxic compounds used in the cosmetic fingernail industry led to confusion in the initial treatment of this patient. This confusion has hindered appropriate medical treatment in other published accounts, including one fatal case.[3, 4] In most cases newer products such as acetonitriles and methemoglobin-generating agents are mistaken for older, more familiar, acetone-based products. Nitroethane, which is currently sold commercially without child-resistant packaging, has been observed to cause methemoglobinemia and thus is another potentially toxic fingernail product. When confronted with ingestions of fingernail products, pediatricians and poison control centers must be diligent in correctly identifying the compound involved, because treatment varies and may be lifesaving. Our experience demonstrates that nitroethane-induced methemoglobinemia may be delayed in onset and recurrent; patients ingesting this substance may warrant close observation for at least 24 hours after ingestion.

REFERENCES

1. Avner JR, Henretig FM, McAneney CM. Acquired methemoglobinemia: the relationship of cause to course of illness. Am J Dis Child 1990;144:1229-30.

2. Gamis AS, Wasserman GS. Acute acetone intoxication in a pediatric patient. Pediatr Emerg Care 1988;4:24-6.
3. Caravati EM, Litovitz TL. Pediatric cyanide intoxication and death from an acetonitrile-containing cosmetic. JAMA 1988;260:3470-3.
4. Rainey PM, Roberts WL. Diagnosis and misdiagnosis of poisoning with the cyanide precursor acetonitrile: nail polish remover or nail glue remover? Am J Emerg Med 1993;11:104-8.
5. Potter JL, Krill CE, Neal D, Kofron WG. Methemoglobinemia due to ingestion of N,N-dimethyl-p-toluidine, a component used in the fabrication of artificial fingernails. Ann Emerg Med 1988;17:1098-100.
6. Hornfeldt CS, Rabe WH. Nitroethane poisoning from an artificial fingernail remover. J Toxicol Clin Toxicol 1994;32:321-4.
7. Henretig FM. Cyanosis unresponsive to oxygen administration in three children. Pediatr Emerg Care 1985;1:205-7.
8. Harvey JW, Keitt AS. Studies of the efficacy and potential hazards of methylene blue therapy in aniline-induced methaemoglobinemia. Br J Haematol 1983;54:29-41.
9. Ellenhorn MJ, Barceloux DG. Medical toxicology: diagnosis and treatment of human poisoning. New York: Elsevier, 1988.
10. Poisindex. Denver, Colo: Micromedex Corp., 1994.
11. Sittig M, ed. Handbook of toxic and hazardous chemicals and carcinogens. 2nd ed. Parkridge, NJ: Noyes, 1985:657-8.
12. Treon JF, Dutra FR. Physiological response of experimental animals to vapor of 2-nitropropane. Arch Ind Hyg Occup Med 1952;5:52-61.
13. Machle W, Scott EW, Treon JF. Metabolism of mononitroparaffins: recovery of nitroethane from animal organism. J Ind Hyg Toxicol 1942;24:5-9.
14. Scott EW. Metabolism of mononitroparaffins: concentration of nitroethane, nitrite, and nitrate in blood of rabbits during exposure by inhalation and oral administration. J Ind Hyg Toxicol 1943;25:20-25.
15. Curry S. Methemoglobinemia. Ann Emerg Med 1982;11:214-21.
16. Needleman P, Blehm D, Rotskoff KS. Relationship between glutathione-dependent denitration and the vasodilator effectiveness of organic nitrate. J Pharmacol Exp Ther 1969; 165:286-8.
17. Buenger JW, Mauro VF. Organic nitrate-induced methemoglobinemia. Drug Intell Clin Pharm 1989;23:283-8.

Effect of corticosteroids on survival of children with acquired immunodeficiency syndrome and *Pneumocystis carinii*–related respiratory failure

Gwenn E. McLaughlin, MD, Satranjan S. Virdee, MBBS, Charles L. Schleien, MD, Bernard H. Holzman, MD, and Gwendolyn B. Scott, MD

From the Division of Pediatric Critical Care Medicine, Division of Pediatric Infectious Disease and Immunology, Department of Pediatrics, University of Miami School of Medicine, Miami, Florida

The medical records of patients with acquired immunodeficiency syndrome were reviewed to evaluate the effect of our adoption to the pediatric population of the National Institutes of Health recommendation for adjunctive corticosteroid therapy in adults with *Pneumocystis carinii* pneumonia. In 21 episodes of P. carinii–related respiratory failure, only adjunctive corticosteroids were associated with a significant improvement in survival to successful removal of the tracheal tube, from a historical rate of 11% to 91%. (J Pediatr 1995;126:821-4)

Supported by grant AI23524 from the National Institutes of Health.

Submitted for publication July 29, 1994; accepted Dec. 8, 1994.

Reprint requests: Gwenn E. McLaughlin, MD, Department of Pediatrics, University of Miami School of Medicine, P.O. Box 016960 (R-131), Miami, FL 33101.

0022-3476/95/$3.00 + 0 **9/26/62653**

Impending respiratory failure is the most common reason for admission of pediatric patients with AIDS to an ICU, and *Pneumocystis carinii* pneumonia accounts for more than 50% of these admissions; reported mortality rates have been 50% to 85% once respiratory failure has developed.[1-6] The results of several randomized controlled trials that evaluated the efficacy of corticosteroids in adult patients with AIDS and PCP[7-10] prompted the National Institute of

Allergy and Infectious Diseases to convene a collaborative panel, which recommended *early* adjunctive therapy with corticosteroids for adults with moderate to severe respiratory failure caused by PCP.[11] No recommendations were made for treatment of children less than 12 years of age. In addition, corticosteroid administration before the development of respiratory failure was emphasized, because one report suggested that a delay in therapy did not improve survival but did increase the incidence of complications.[10]

To date there is little information about the efficacy of corticosteroids in children with AIDS and PCP-related respiratory failure. One group reported a 100% survival rate to the time of successful removal of the tracheal tube in four infants who received corticosteroids.[6] The present study was undertaken to test the hypothesis that corticosteroids alone have led to improved survival from PCP in the pediatric population even when respiratory failure has already occurred. Because children with AIDS and respiratory failure seen at our institution from 1983 to 1986 have previously been reported,[1] we reviewed the charts of all children with AIDS who subsequently required mechanical ventilation.

METHODS

A retrospective review of the records of patients admitted to the pediatric ICU at Jackson Memorial Hospital, Miami, from January 1987 to June 1993, who met criteria for AIDS, *P. carinii* infection, and acute respiratory failure was conducted. Forty-three hospitalizations were identified by the hospital's computerized records system with the code of the International Classification of Diseases, ninth revision,—Clinical Modification for HIV infection (042.1) and the current procedural terminology codes for mechanical ventilation (94656 and 94657). To assure that all appropriate patients were identified, this list was compared with the pediatric ICU admission log. The diagnosis of AIDS was made according to criteria developed by the Centers for Disease Control and Prevention.[12] The presence of HIV infection was confirmed by enzyme-linked immunosorbent assay and Western blot in all patients except for two infants with negative serologic findings, who were found to have HIV infection by culture. *P. carinii* was identified by Giemsa stain of fluid obtained by either bronchoscopy or lung lavage through the endotracheal tube after insertion of an endotracheal tube for respiratory failure. Acute respiratory failure was defined as (1) an arterial partial pressure of oxygen of less than 75 mm Hg with a fraction of inspired oxygen of 0.5 obtained just before insertion of the tracheal tube, (2) the presence of new diffuse interstitial infiltrates on chest radiograph, and (3) the exclusion of left ventricular failure or intracardiac shunting by clinical examination and a normal cardiac silhouette by chest radiograph. No patients met criteria for respiratory failure as a result of bronchoscopy.

AIDS	Acquired immunodeficiency syndrome
CMV	Cytomegalovirus
HIV	Human immunodeficiency virus
PCP	*Pneumocystis carinii* pneumonia

Antiprotozoal therapy was initiated intravenously with trimethoprim and sulfamethoxazole (20 mg/kg per day trimethoprim) in all but one case. Patients who failed to improve after 4 to 5 days were given pentamidine isethionate (4 mg/kg per day). Routine cultures for bacteria, cytomegalovirus, and mycobacteria were also obtained. All patients were initially treated with a third-generation cephalosporin until results of blood, urine, bronchoscopic, or tracheal aspirate cultures, and of cytologic studies, became available. No open lung biopsies were performed during the study period. Before October 1990 after no improvement with conventional therapy, four of 11 patients with proved PCP, who were already receiving mechanical ventilation, received corticosteroids (2 to 4 mg/kg methylprednisolone per day intravenously, divided into four doses daily) at the discretion of the attending physician. After October 1990 all patients with PCP received corticosteroids either when the Giemsa stain results became available or when mechanical ventilation was begun pending results of the Giemsa stain. Corticosteroids were continued for 14 days, and subsequently the dose was tapered for 1 week.

During the ICU stay infants received pressure-controlled, time-cycled ventilation (Sechrist, Anaheim, Calif.). Children weighing more than 10 kg received volume-controlled, time-cycled ventilation. The goal of ventilation therapy was to maintain a pH greater than 7.35 and an arterial oxygen pressure of 60 mm Hg or greater with a fraction of inspired oxygen of an FiO_2 less than 0.6.

Differences between groups for parametric data were determined by a two-tailed Student *t* test. Differences in proportions (categoric data) were determined by chi-square analysis. Differences were considered significant at $p < 0.05$.

RESULTS

Twenty-one episodes of PCP-related respiratory failure requiring mechanical ventilation were identified in 19 patients ranging in age from 3 to 156 months (median age, 6 months). Infection with HIV was acquired perinatally in 20 patients (95%). For 71% of these episodes PCP was the initial illness for AIDS and the patient was less than 10 months of age (median age, 5.5 months). Only two children were receiving PCP prophylaxis at the time of admission to the hospital. For the total study period rates of successful removal of the tracheal tube and discharge from the ICU

Table. Comparison of patients with PCP and acute respiratory failure

Variable	Before Oct. 1990 (n = 9)	After Oct 1990 (n = 11)	p
Median (range) age, in mo	6 (4-104)	5 (2-58)	NS
Antiprotozoal therapy at ICU admission*	9 (82)	9 (75)	NS
Antiretroviral therapy at ICU admission*	1 (9)	3 (25)	NS
Corticosteroids*	4 (44)	11 (100)	0.02
$CD4^+$ lymphocytes (%)	7 ± 13	6 ± 11	NS
Days from presentation to therapy for PCP†	4 ± 4	3 ± 3	NS
Alveolar-arterial gradient (mm Hg)†	435 ± 136	363 ± 199	NS
Lactate dehydrogenase (IU/ml)†	3260 ± 2302	2907 ± 1813	NS
Maximum positive end-expiratory pressure (cm H_2O)†	10 ± 2	10 ± 3	NS
Maximum peak inspiratory pressure PIP (cm H_2O)†	55 ± 13	34 ± 15	0.003
Days of mechanical ventilation†	15 ± 11	8 ± 3	NS
Survival to successful tracheal extubation*	1 (11)	10 (91)	0.002
Survival to discharge from ICU*	1 (11)	8 (72)	0.02

NS, Not significant.
*Values represent number (percentage) of patients.
†Value expressed as mean ± SD.

were 52% and 43%, respectively. These data include a child in whom PCP was neither treated nor diagnosed before death but was identified on autopsy.

Initial analysis of the 20 episodes in which PCP was identified showed a 67% survival rate (10/15) to successful removal of the tracheal tube in patients who received corticosteroids versus 20% (one of five) in those who did not (*p* not significant). All four children who received corticosteroids as salvage therapy before October 1990 died. When these children were excluded from analysis, early corticosteroid administration was associated with an improved survival rate to removal of the tracheal tube (91% [10/11] vs 20% [one of five] in those who did not receive corticosteroids, $p < 0.05$).

To look at the effect of early adjuvant corticosteroid therapy, patients with PCP seen after October 1990 who received early treatment according to the practice described were compared with all patients with documented PCP seen before October 1990. Survival rates for documented PCP-related acute respiratory failure improved from 11% before October 1990 to 91% for successful tube removal ($p < 0.01$) and to 76% for discharge from the ICU ($p < 0.05$) for patients subsequently treated early with corticosteroids. As demonstrated in the Table, there were no differences between the conventionally treated patients with PCP and those who received early corticosteroid therapy in age, sex, race, mode of HIV transmission, or percentage of CD4-positive lymphocytes. There were no differences in timing of either antiprotozoal therapy or antiretroviral therapy, to suggest earlier recognition or treatment of PCP or AIDS in the group receiving early corticosteroid treatment. There were no differences in mean alveolar-to-arterial oxygen gradient or lactate dehydrogenase level immediately before tracheal intubation, indicating no differences in severity of initial lung disease. A difference between the two treatment groups was detected only for the mean maximal peak inspiratory pressure, which was greater in the conventional treatment group. This difference likely reflects ongoing pulmonary deterioration in the nonsurvivors, because when nonsurvivors were excluded from analysis, no difference in mean maximal PIP was noted between patients in the two groups whose tubes were successfully removed. Additional potentially confounding variables such as complications of ICU care, hours of exposure to hyperoxia, and decisions regarding limitation of therapy were also evaluated and were found not to differ between groups (data not presented).

Infants less than 10 months of age, who may have had primary *P. carinii* infection and thus a potentially different pathophysiologic response to the infection, were analyzed separately (n = 15). In this age group patients who received corticosteroids at any time were more likely to survive to successful removal of the tracheal tube than infants who did not receive corticosteroids (66% [n = 12] vs no survivors [n = 3], $p < 0.05$). Among the variables listed in the Table, no differences were detected between those who received corticosteroids and those who did not. Infants who received corticosteroids early had a 100% survival rate to removal of the tracheal tube and a 75% survival rate to discharge from the ICU.

In two infants who received corticosteroids a second fatal episode of respiratory failure developed within days of successful removal of the tracheal tube. In one patient fungal sepsis was associated with adult respiratory distress syndrome. The second infant died of shock caused by disseminated CMV infection. These complications are not clearly related to corticosteroid therapy; in two infants who did not receive corticosteroids fungal sepsis also developed, and a third infant who received corticosteroids had CMV gastroenteritis that responded to ganciclovir therapy.

DISCUSSION

The present study reports a marked improvement in survival after PCP-related respiratory failure when early adjunctive corticosteroid therapy was given. Vernon et al.[1] first reported poor ICU survival rates for children with AIDS and respiratory failure. In this previous study from our institution the survival rate to discharge from the ICU for 15 children who underwent mechanical ventilation was 15%. Similarly, Notterman et al.[2] reported eight episodes of PCP-related respiratory failure with an ICU survival rate of 12%, without adjunctive corticosteroids. Sleasman et al.[6] reported a survival rate of zero in seven children with respiratory failure who received no corticosteroids and a 100% survival rate in the next four patients, who received adjunctive corticosteroids; for these four patients the survival rate to discharge from the ICU was 75%. Two other groups have reported survival rates of approximately 50% from PCP-related respiratory failure not treated with corticosteroids.[3, 4] The indications for mechanical ventilation were not described in either of these studies, and some of the data indicate that the patients had less severe disease than those in the present study. Differences in the severity of lung disease may account for the differences in reported survival rates.

A reluctance to administer corticosteroids to children with HIV infection stems from the immunosuppressive properties of these agents. Two patients in the present study had life-threatening CMV infections within 1 month after corticosteroid therapy. There have been similar reports of adult patients with AIDS who died of overwhelming CMV infection weeks after corticosteroid therapy.[13, 14] Thus we recommend surveillance for CMV infection when corticosteroids are given.

This retrospective study can be criticized for lacking a concurrent control group to rule out unidentified confounding variables that may affect outcome. Because all patients were cared for at a single institution, some of these variables may have been indirectly controlled. On the basis of data concerning adults, the practice of administering corticosteroids to children with confirmed PCP has now become widespread, potentially precluding the development of a randomized controlled trial in this patient population. Our study suggests that adjunctive corticosteroid therapy is beneficial in children even when respiratory failure has already occurred.

REFERENCES

1. Vernon DD, Holzman BH, Lewis P, Scott GB, Birriel JA, Scott MB. Respiratory failure in children with acquired immunodeficiency syndrome and acquired immunodeficiency syndrome-related complex. Pediatrics 1988;82:223-8.
2. Notterman DA, Greenwald BM, DiMaio-Hunter AD, Wilkinson JD, Krasinski K, Borkowsky W. Outcome after assisted ventilation in children with acquired immunodeficiency syndrome. Crit Care Med 1990;18:18-20.
3. Marolda J, Pace B, Bonforte RJ, Kotin NM, Rabinowitz J, Kattan M. Pulmonary manifestations of HIV infection in children. Pediatr Pulmonol 1991;10:231-5.
4. Bye MR, Bernstein MD, Glaser J, Kleid D. *Pneumocystis carinii* pneumonia in young children with AIDS. Pediatr Pulmonol 1990;9:251-3.
5. Abadco DL, Rao M, Kravath RE, Steiner P. The role of assisted ventilation in survival after respiratory failure in children with AIDS. Am J Dis Child 1992;146:1052-5.
6. Sleasman JW, Hemenway C, Klein AS, Barrett DJ. Corticosteroids improve survival of children with AIDS and *Pneumocystis carinii* pneumonia. Am J Dis Child 1993;147:30-4.
7. Montaner JSG, Lawson LM, Levitt N, Belzberg A, Schechter MT, Ruedy J. Corticosteroids prevent early deterioration in patients with moderately severe *Pneumocystis carinii* pneumonia and the acquired immunodeficiency syndrome (AIDS). Ann Intern Med 1990;113:14-20.
8. Gagnon S, Boota AM, Fischl MA, Baier H, Kirksey OW, Voie LL. Corticosteroids as adjunctive therapy for severe *Pneumocystis carinii* pneumonia in the acquired immunodeficiency syndrome. N Engl J Med 1990;323:1444-50.
9. Bozzette SA, Sattler FR, Chiu J, et al. A controlled trial of early adjunctive treatment with corticosteroids for *Pneumocystis carinii* pneumonia in the acquired immunodeficiency syndrome. N Engl J Med 1990;323:1451-7.
10. Clement M, Edison R, Turner J, et al. Corticosteroids as adjunctive therapy in severe *Pneumocystis carinii* pneumonia: a prospective placebo-controlled trial [Abstract]. Am Rev Respir Dis 1989;139(suppl):250.
11. National Institutes of Health–University of California. Consensus statement on the use of corticosteroids as adjunctive therapy for pneumocystis pneumonia in the acquired immunodeficiency syndrome. N Engl J Med 1990; 323:1500-4.
12. Centers for Disease Control. Classification system for human immunodeficiency virus infection (HIV) in children under 13 years of age. MMWR 1987;36:225-30.
13. Amundson DE, Murray KM, Brodine S, Oldfield EC. High-dose corticosteroid therapy for *Pneumocystis carinii* pneumonia in patients with acquired immunodeficiency syndrome. South Med J 1989;82:711-8.
14. Clumeck N, Hermans P. Corticosteroids as adjunctive therapy for *Pneumocystis carinii* pneumonia in patients with AIDS [Letter]. N Engl J Med 1991;324:1666-7.

Human synthetic calcitonin therapy for hypercalcemia of immobilization

Sushma Kaul, MD, and Joseph J. Sockalosky, MD

From the Departments of Pediatrics and Pediatric Endocrinology, University of Minnesota Health Center, Minneapolis, Minnesota, and Children's Health Care, St. Paul, Minnesota

We studied four children with hypercalcemia of immobilization resulting from quadriplegia. After a trial of conventional therapy, human synthetic calcitonin was given subcutaneously at 0.5 to 2.5 mg per day in divided doses. Serum calcium concentrations returned to normal levels in all patients, decreasing an average of 0.72 mmol/L (2.9 mg/dl) within 4 to 10 days. Calcitonin therapy was effective for periods varying from 3 to 10 months. In one patient a bladder stone developed without nephrocalcinosis. (J Pediatr 1995;126:825-7)

The syndrome of hypercalcemia of immobilization includes elevated serum and urinary calcium levels, increased urinary hydroxyproline excretion, and marked osteopenia.[1] The hypercalcemia develops within days to weeks of immobilization but may be unrecognized because of the nonspecific nature of the symptoms, such as lethargy, alteration in mood, nausea, vomiting, and anorexia. Hypercalcemia and hypercalciuria may result in nephrocalcinosis, nephrolithiasis, renal failure, and other systemic complications.[1] It is therefore important to recognize the subtle signs and symptoms promptly and treat the hypercalcemia immediately to prevent complications.

The most effective treatment for hypercalcemia of immobilization is remobilization.[2] However, active movement is not always possible, and passive range of motion exercises are ineffective.[3] Conventional treatment with intravenously administered saline solution and furosemide is often ineffective in controlling hypercalcemia. Other pharmacologic agents such as glucocorticoids and bisphosphonates are associated with long-term side effects.[4] Calcitonin, a product of the C cells of the thyroid gland, lowers the serum calcium concentration when given in supraphysiologic concentrations. However, calcitonin therapy has been reported to be only transiently effective because of the development of resistance to its effects after several days of therapy.[4]

Submitted for publication July 6, 1994; accepted Nov. 1, 1994.

Reprint requests: Joseph J. Sockalosky, MD, Assistant Professor of Pediatrics, Pediatric Endocrinology, Box 404 UMHC, 420 Delaware St., SE, Minneapolis, MN 55455.

0022-3476/95/$3.00 + 0 **9/26/61760**

We report the successful use of human synthetic calcitonin therapy for prolonged periods in four pediatric patients with hypercalcemia of immobilization.

METHODS

We retrospectively studied four boys with quadriplegia in whom hypercalcemia of immobilization developed and who were treated with human synthetic calcitonin at Gillette Childrens Hospital and Childrens Hospital St. Paul. Patients 1, 2, and 3 had C3-C4 spinal cord injury; patient 4 had quadriplegia caused by panmyelitis after intrathecal administration of cytosine arabinoside for the treatment of Burkitt lymphoma.

This study was not prospective, and initiation of treatment and laboratory evaluations were not standardized. Before initiation of calcitonin therapy, all four patients were well hydrated with intravenous fluids and were given furosemide. Two patients were given a course of glucocorticoids (prednisone, 2 mg/kg/per day, or hydrocortisone, 75 mg/m^2 per day) either before or during calcitonin therapy. Calcitonin was given because of poor response to conventional therapy. Human synthetic calcitonin was given subcutaneously to all four patients in doses ranging from 0.03 to 0.12 mg/kg per day, divided every 6 to 12 hours. Dietary restriction of calcium and vitamin D was strictly followed in patients 1, 3, and 4 by use of Calcilo XD, a dietary supplement containing low amounts of calcium and no vitamin D. Serum liver enzyme activity, blood urea nitrogen concentrations, and creatinine were measured periodically to monitor hepatic and renal function. Serum calcium and phosphorus levels were measured initially every 12 to 24 hours and, once normal levels were achieved, every 3 to 5

Table. Summary of patient response to human synthetic calcitonin therapy

	Patient 1	Patient 2	Patient 3	Patient 4
Age (yr)	0.92	12.5	12.5	12.5
Duration of immobilization before hypercalcemia (wk)	5	4	6	4
Duration of hypercalcemia before start of calcitonin therapy (wk)	3.5-4	1.5	4.0	10.0
Total duration of calcitonin therapy (wk)	44	12	25	29
Dose of calcitonin (mg/kg/day in divided doses, every 6 to 12 hr)	0.03-0.06	0.03-0.06	0.08-0.12	0.03-0.07
Mean serum calcium before start of calcitonin therapy (mmol/L [mg/dl])*	2.86 (11.5)	2.99 (12.0)	3.00 (12.4)	3.54 (14.2)†
Mean serum calcium during calcitonin therapy (mmol/L [mg/dl])*	2.24 (9.0)	2.27 (9.1)	2.54 (10.2)	2.51 (10.1)†
Mean urine Ca/Cr ratio before start of calcitonin therapy‡	0.85	0.4	0.44	1.7
Mean urine Ca/Cr ratio during calcitonin therapy‡	0.2	0.24	0.2	—

Ca, calcium; *Cr*, creatinine.
*Normal range, 2.12 to 2.64 mmol/L (8.5 to 10.4 mg/dl).
†Corrected for serum albumin.
‡Normal range, <0.2.

days. The urine calcium/creatinine ratio was measured randomly on morning samples in three patients. Abdominal ultrasonography was done at regular intervals to evaluate the development of nephrocalcinosis and nephrolithiasis.

RESULTS

During the first few weeks of immobilization, total serum calcium concentration was normal in all four patients (Table). Results of other laboratory tests indicative of hepatic and renal function were normal. In patient 4, corrected total serum calcium values (because of hypoalbuminemia) were monitored by adjusting the serum total calcium concentration by 0.20 mmol/L (0.8 mg/dl) for each 10 gm by which the serum albumin level was above or below 40 gm/L (each 1 gm above or below 4.0 gm/dl).[5] Patient 1 had normal serum parathyroid hormone (intact) and vitamin D (25-hydroxyvitamin D_3 and 1,25-dihydroxyvitamin D_3) levels at the beginning and at the end of calcitonin therapy.

In all patients the serum calcium concentration was >2.64 mmol/L (>10.6 mg/dl) after 4 to 6 weeks of immobilization. Typical signs and symptoms of hypercalcemia, such as anorexia, nausea, vomiting, irritability, and hypertension, were present in patients 2, 3, and 4. Isotonic saline solution infusions and furosemide were temporarily and minimally effective in all four patients. Similarly, use of hydrocortisone or prednisone in patients 3 and 4 was not effective in achieving normal serum calcium values. With institution of synthetic human calcitonin therapy, serum calcium values returned to normal within 6 to 12 days. The serum calcium concentration decreased, with an average drop of 0.72 mmol/L (2.9 mg/dl) in all four patients (Table). There was a decrease in the urine calcium/creatinine ratio to normal or near normal values in the three patients in whom it was measured. Serum phosphorus levels remained within the normal range for age in all four patients.

Side effects of calcitonin therapy were relatively mild and did not interfere with appetite or lead to any weight loss. Patient 2 had daytime nausea. Patient 3 had hot flashes, nausea, and abdominal pain; he refused injections at times because of these symptoms. Patient 4 had hot flashes and nausea. Nephrocalcinosis did not develop in any of the patients, but patient 3 had a single bladder calculus. In patients 2, 3, and 4, administration of calcitonin was stopped when the serum calcium value returned to normal, but reinstitution of therapy was required when hypercalcemia recurred. With the reinstitution of calcitonin therapy after intervals of days to weeks, the serum calcium values promptly returned to normal in all three patients.

DISCUSSION

In patients with hypercalcemia of immobilization, analysis of bone biopsy specimens has shown a loss of trabecular bone volume, increased osteoclastic resorption surface, and decreased osteoblastic bone formation.[6] Four possible pathophysiologic mechanisms have been proposed for these changes; these include lack of mechanical stress, poor vascularity, metabolic changes in bone, and denervation. Normal mechanical stress generates a piezoelectric charge with a negative charge on the concave surface of the bone, leading to bone deposition. The lack of mechanical stress results in an abnormality of electrical charge on the bone surface. Immobilization results in less bone deposition and increased bone resorption.[7] Decreased blood flow to immobilized bone also leads to decreased mineral deposition. Increased partial pressure of carbon dioxide and decreased pH associated with poor blood flow lead to an acidic environment locally in immobilized bone. Parathyroid hormone activity presumably increases in the local acidic environment, resulting in increased osteoclast cell activity, loss of bone mass, and hypercalcemia.[8] Weight-bearing bones are more likely to react to immobilization. The rate of bone loss is inversely related to age, and ranges from 15% of trabecular bone in elderly women to almost 50% in immobilized adolescents.[6]

If the patient is unable to return to an active, ambulatory state, hypercalcemia may persist for months despite aggressive conventional treatment.[2] The resulting prolonged negative calcium balance predisposes the patient to osteoporosis. In addition, more than 50% of children immobilized because of spinal cord injury who have hypercalcemia may have urolithiasis and other systemic complications of hypercalcemia.[9]

Isotonic, isometric exercises and longitudinal compressions do not alter the pathophysiologic process of hypercalcemia of immobilization.[3] Administration of glucocorticoids in relatively high doses improves hypercalcemia of immobilization but leads to bone demineralization and other well-known systemic toxic effects, making these agents far from ideal for treatment of this entity.[4] Bisphosphonates, the antiosteoclastic agents, are also inhibitors of skeletal mineralization and, if used for long periods, may lead to clinical osteomalacia, bone pain, and fractures. They are also nephrotoxic.[4]

Calcitonin lowers serum calcium by inhibiting bone resorption. It inhibits osteoclast cell activity and decreases osteoclast cell numbers if used for prolonged periods.[10] It temporarily induces proximal renal tubular calciuresis, which also lowers serum calcium values.[11] Various in vitro studies suggest that calcitonin, unlike bisphosphonates, is an osteoblast stimulator.[12] Salmon calcitonin effectively controls hypercalcemia, but the effect is sustained for only a few days because of development of anticalcitonin antibodies in 40% to 70% of patients. Antibody development to human calcitonin is rare.[11] Phosphorus balance also affects the effectiveness of calcitonin therapy. In experimental animals, phosphate loading enhances and phosphate depletion inhibits the hypocalcemic effect of calcitonin; the escape phenomenon therefore may be averted by the concomitant use of phosphate.[13]

In our study the effectiveness of human synthetic calcitonin therapy persisted for periods varying from 3 to 10 months with tolerable side effects. We postulate that use of human calcitonin does not stimulate clinically significant antibody formation, resulting in a sustained and potent effect. Another possible explanation for the prolonged effectiveness of calcitonin in our patients is that normal serum phosphorus levels were maintained. We cannot exclude the possibility that calcitonin is more effective in hypercalcemia of immobilization than in other hypercalcemic syndromes because of its direct osteoclast inhibitory effect.

REFERENCES

1. Evans RA, Bridgeman M, Hills E, Dunstan CR. Immobilization hypercalcemia. Miner Electrolyte Metab 1984;10:244-8.
2. Stewart AF, Broadus AE. In: Felig P, Baxter JD, Broadus AE, Frohman LA, eds. Endocrinology and metabolism. 2nd ed. New York: McGraw Hill, 1987:1416.
3. Hantman DA, Vogel JM, Donaldson CL, Friedman R, Goldsmith RS, Hulley SB. Attempts to prevent disuse osteoporosis by treatment with calcitonin, longitudinal compression and supplementary calcium and phosphate. J Clin Endocrinol Metab 1973;36:845-58.
4. Carey DE, Paisz LG. Calcitonin therapy in prolonged immobilization hypercalcemia. Arch Phys Med Rehabil 1985;66:640-4.
5. Shane E. Clinical manifestations and acute management of hypercalcemic states. In: Favus MJ, ed. Primer on the metabolic bone diseases and disorders of mineral metabolism. New York: American Society for Bone and Mineral Research, 1990:107-8.
6. Minaire P, Despassio J, Berard E, et al. Effects of clodronate on immobilization bone loss. Bone 1987;8(suppl 1):563-8.
7. Becker RO. Electrical osteogenesis-pro and con. Calcif Tissue Int 1978;26:93-7.
8. Karpati RM, Mark RHK, Lemley KV. Hypercalcemia, hypertension and acute renal insufficiency in an immobilized adolescent. Child Nephrol Urol 1991;11:215-9.
9. Tori JA, Kewelramani LS, Orth MS. Urolithiasis in children with spinal cord injury. Paraplegia 1978;16:357-65.
10. Chambers TJ, Moore A. The sensitivity of isolated osteoclasts to morphological transformation by calcitonin. J Clin Endocrinol Metabol 1983;57:819-24.
11. Deftos LJ, First BP. Calcitonin as a drug. Ann Intern Med 1981;95:192-7.
12. Carstens JHJ, Feinblatt JD. Future horizons for calcitonin: a U.S. perspective. Calcif Tiss Int 1991;49(suppl 2):S2-S6.
13. Brautbar N, Luboshitzky R. Combined calcitonin and oral phosphate treatment for hypercalcemia in multiple myeloma. Arch Intern Med 1974;137:914-6.

Estimation of energy requirements in persons with severe central nervous system impairment

Linda G. Bandini, RD, PhD, Heidi Puelzl-Quinn, MS, RD, Julie A. Morelli, BS, and Naomi K. Fukagawa, MD, PhD

From the Department of Pediatrics, Division of Gastroenterology and Nutrition, New England Medical Center, and the Developmental Evaluation Center, Children's Hospital Center, Boston, Massachusetts; the Clinical Research Center, Massachusetts Institute of Technology, Cambridge; and Rockefeller University, New York, New York

We measured resting metabolic rate (RMR) in 12 persons (aged 10 to 30 years) with severe impairment of the central nervous system requiring gastrostomy feedings, and compared our findings with the RMR predicted from standardized equations. The RMR was 70.6% ± 15.7% of that predicted from the Mayo Clinic nomogram, 63.7% ± 18% of that predicted from the Food and Agriculture Organization/World Health Organization/United Nations University equation, and 75.4% ± 17.3% of that predicted from the Robertson and Reid equation. Energy intake was 756 ± 225 kcal/day and RMR was 708 ± 231 kcal/day; RMR adjusted for changes in body energy stores was 729 ± 231 kcal/day. No significant differences were found between energy intake and RMR, or between energy intake and the sum of RMR and changes in body energy stores. These findings demonstrate that standardized equations overestimate energy needs of individuals with severe CNS impairment. Measures of energy intake adjusted for weight changes represent a valid method to determine energy requirements in a group of individuals with severe CNS impairment. Length was found to be significantly correlated with RMR (*r* = 0.79; *p* <0.01). When the regression equation was tested on another group of subjects from the same residential facility, the equation predicted energy needs reasonably well for those individuals with similar energy intakes but not for all patients with CNS disorders. (J PEDIATR 1995;126:828-32)

Standard equations based on height, weight, and age for healthy children and adults are used to determine metabolic rate and energy requirements of different groups of persons. However, standard equations may not be applicable to individuals with severe central nervous system disorders, who often have alterations in body composition. We have observed that children, adolescents, and young adults with severe CNS disorders who are exclusively receiving gastrostomy feedings are able to maintain their weight or grow consistently on energy intakes less than 7 kcal/cm. In absolute terms, these diets range from 500 to 1100 kcal/day, which are 16% to 50% of the recommended

See related article, p. 833.

FAO/WHO/UNU	Food and Agriculture Organization/ World Health Organization/ United Nations University
RMR	Resting metabolic rate

Supported by grant M01-RR00088 from the National Center for Research Resources, National Institute of Health, to the General Clinical Research Center (Massachusetts Institute of Technology), and by grant P30 DK476200, Boston Obesity Nutrition Research Center.

Submitted for publication June 13, 1994; accepted Nov. 11, 1994.

Reprint requests: Linda G. Bandini, RD, PhD, Department of Pediatric Gastroenterology and Nutrition, New England Medical Center, 750 Washington St., Box 213, Boston, MA 02111.

0022-3476/95/$3.00 + 0 **9/20/61936**

dietary allowance estimated for age. The extremely low energy intakes often make physicians, nurses, and dietitians hesitant to accept the adequacy of these diets. We previously reported that nonambulatory individuals with spastic cerebral palsy and myelodysplasia have low energy requirements.[1] Culley and Middleton[2] reported that energy requirements of ambulatory children with mild to moderate motor dysfunction were 13.9 kcal/cm, whereas children with severe motor dysfunction who were nonambulatory had energy requirements of 11.9 kcal/cm. Individuals with severe CNS disorders represent a different type of disability that appears to reduce energy requirements further.

The purpose of this study was to determine the energy needs of a population of individuals with severe CNS disorders. The first objective was to confirm that standardized equations used to determine metabolic rate significantly overestimate energy requirements in individuals with CNS disorders. The second objective was to demonstrate that in those individuals with CNS disorders who are exclusively receiving gastrostomy feedings, energy intake data, together with weight change, provide an accurate, practical, and useful method of determining energy requirements of individuals with severe CNS disorders. Fried and Pencharz[3] found this technique to be valid in the management of children with spastic quadriplegia who were fed through a gastrostomy.

METHODS

Subjects. Seven female and five male subjects ranging in age from 10 to 30 years participated in this study. The population included prepubertal, pubertal, and adult subjects. All individuals had severe CNS disorders (CNS malformations, n = 5; CNS infections and encephalitis, n = 3; perinatal asphyxia, n = 1; CNS impairment of unknown cause, n = 3) were nonambulatory, and were totally dependent on staff for all activities of daily living. Energy intake less than or equal to 7 to 8.2 kcal/cm was the criterion for entry into the study. This level of intake was selected because many of the patients were receiving less than 7 kcal/cm, and there was no documentation in the literature of energy needs this low.

Informed consent was obtained from either the parents or guardian of the subjects. The protocol was approved by the institutional review boards at the Massachusetts Institute of Technology (MIT), Cambridge, Mass., and Children's Hospital, Boston, Mass.

Subjects were weighed in diapers at the residential facility within a day of their visit to the MIT Clinical Research Center. During this visit, measurements of resting metabolic rate and of body length, head circumference, and triceps skin-fold thickness were made. Scoliosis and contractures in this population make body length measurement difficult and use of alternative measurements (such as arm span) to assess length impossible. Therefore we defined body length as the straightest length possible for each individual subject lying on his or her side or back. Length measured when the subjects were lying on their back was compared with the sum of the lengths of five specific segments of the body. These latter segments included the length (1) from the inferior aspect of lateral malleolus to the joint space of the knee, (2) from the joint space to the greater trochanter, (3) from the greater trochanter to the iliac crest, (4) from the sacrum to the base of the occiput, and (5) from the base of the occiput to the top of the head. The correlation between segmented length and straight length was significant ($r = 0.89$). Because of the complexity associated with obtaining the segmented length, we chose to use overall straight, unsegmented length.

Resting metabolic rate. Resting metabolic rate was measured for 30 minutes by open-circuit indirect calorimetry with a ventilated hood, as previously described.[4] With subjects lying on their side or supine, RMR was calculated from measures of oxygen consumption and carbon dioxide production according to the modified Weir formula.[5] The accuracy of this system for measuring energy expenditure is within 3%.[4] Measurements were made 2 to 4 hours after the last feeding and after a 30-minute rest period in bed. Under the conditions of this study, RMR included the thermic effect of food. Two subjects who missed their feeding before coming to MIT were measured 5 to 7 hours postprandially. The caloric content of the meal ranged from 120 to 250 kcal, and therefore the contribution of the thermic effect of food would be small (approximately 12 to 25 kcal). Because of the severe cognitive impairments, subject behavior could not be controlled. Some individuals napped; others had petit mal seizures during the measurement. The staff reported that these behaviors were typical of each individual.

Energy balance. Daily energy intakes were determined from the caloric intake of the gastrostomy feedings during a six-month period (3 months before and 3 months after the MIT visit). Because some of the subjects were children, weight changes associated with growth and consequently changes in metabolic rate would be expected after prolonged periods. Therefore a period 3 months before and 3 months after testing was selected as the period in which to assess energy needs based on energy balance. One subject was hospitalized with pneumonia for 3 weeks subsequent to his visit to MIT and therefore was not included in the energy balance analysis. Seven subjects consumed the same caloric intake for 6 months; the other four individuals had changes in energy intake during this period (mean change = 131 kcal/day). Energy intake of those who had caloric changes are reported as weighted averages of the feedings. The number of days during the 6-month period on

Table. Subject characteristics

	Study group (n = 12)	Test group A (n = 12)	Test group B (n = 8)
Sex	5M/7F	6M/6F	5M/3F
Age (yr)	18.7 ± 6.2	16.6 ± 5.9	18.6 ± 5.9
Weight (kg)	32.5 ± 6.4*	36.7 ± 7.1	41.2 ± 10.7
Length (cm)	122.0 ± 13.1†	142.7 ± 12.2	150.7 ± 13.5
BMI (kg/m^2)	26.5 ± 4.2	25.5 ± 3.3	27.0 ± 4.8
TSF (mm)	13.9 ± 5.0	N/A	N/A
Energy intake (kcal/day)	788 ± 242‡	999 ± 164‡	1530 ± 323‡

Values are expressed as mean ± SD.
BMI, Body mass index; *TSF*, triceps skin-fold thickness; *N/A*, not available.
*p <0.05: study group < test group B.
†p <0.05: study group < test group A = test group B.
‡p <0.05: study group < test group A < test group B.

each diet was used in the calculation of the average daily intake for the 6-month period.

Subjects were weighed in diapers but without clothes at the residential facility during the first week of each month. These weights, obtained during a 6-month period, were used to calculate energy balance. Changes in energy stores were also calculated for the 6-month period. Because prepubertal, pubertal, and adult subjects were included, two assumptions were made in these calculations:

1. All weight changes were assumed to be adipose tissue, with a caloric content of 7200 kcal/kg[6] in female subjects more than 15 years of age and in male subjects more than 18 years of age. Of the 12 subjects, 8 fell into this group.
2. Because the other four subjects may have been growing, we assumed that weight changes were due to changes in both fat-free mass and adipose tissue. The caloric equivalent of fat-free mass is approximately 1000 kcal/kg. The percentage contribution of fat-free mass and fat to weight gain was estimated to be 84% and 16%, respectively, with a caloric equivalent of 2280 kcal/kg.[7]

Changes in energy stores during the 6-month period were determined by dividing total caloric stores by 185 days, which represents an average to account for variation in the day that the individual was weighed and the number of days in each month. Energy intake was compared with the sum of energy expenditure and the change in energy stores to determine how well energy intake predicted energy expenditure. Because these subjects did not engage in any physical activity, RMR represented their total daily energy expenditure.

Energy intake and weight and length measurements were obtained from an additional 20 patients with CNS disorders living at the same residential facility who were in the same age range as the subjects who participated in the study. These patients were fed exclusively by gastrostomy feedings; their energy intake during a 5- to 6-month period varied less than 50 kcal/day. Data from these subjects were used to test the applicability of the regression equation for determining energy intake derived from the study subjects. The patients were divided into two groups: test group A had energy intakes similar to those of the study group (≤8.2 kcal/cm), and test group B had energy intakes higher than those of the study group (>8.2 kcal/cm). The characteristics of the study subjects and of test groups A and B are provided in the Table.

Statistics. Relationships between metabolic rate and anthropometric indexes, and estimates of body length, were obtained by Pearson product moment correlations (Statistical Analysis Systems, SAS Institute Inc., Cary, N.C.). Comparisons between energy intake and energy expenditure, and between predicted and measured metabolic rates, were made by a paired t test. The comparisons between the study group and the two test groups were done with a one-way analysis of variance followed by pairwise comparisons among sample means by means of a Student-Newman-Keuls test.

RESULTS

Resting metabolic rate was significantly lower than that predicted by standardized equations based on age, weight, height, and gender. Measured RMR was 70.6% ± 15.7% (mean ± SD; range, 47.8% to 103.5%) of that predicted from the Mayo Clinic Nomogram,[8] 63.7% ± 18% (range, 37.8% to 96.8%) of that predicted from the FAO/WHO/UNU equation,[9] and 75.4% ± 17.3% (range, 51.8% to 110.9%) of that predicted from the Robertson and Reid equation.[10] Measures of RMR would have been even lower had our subjects been studied after a 10- to 12-hour fast.

Energy intake and energy expenditure were compared in 11 of the 12 subjects. One subject was excluded from this analysis because of hospitalization. Energy intake was 756 ± 225 kcal/day (mean ± SD; range, 412 to 1090). The RMR was 708 ± 231 kcal/day (range, 365 to 1095). The sum of RMR and the change in body energy stores was 730 ± 229 kcal/day (range, 394 to 1126). The differences between energy intake and RMR or between energy intake and the sum of RMR plus the change in body energy stores were not significant.

Length was the best predictor of metabolic rate in these subjects and explained 62% of the variance in metabolic rate (Figure) ($r = 0.79$; $p < 0.01$). Body surface area was also significantly correlated with metabolic rate ($r = 0.72$; $p < 0.01$), but weight was not ($r = 0.52$; $p < 0.08$).

The regression line describing the relationship between length and RMR was used to predict energy expenditure in the test groups (A and B) from the same residential facility (Table). Although the energy intakes in the two test groups

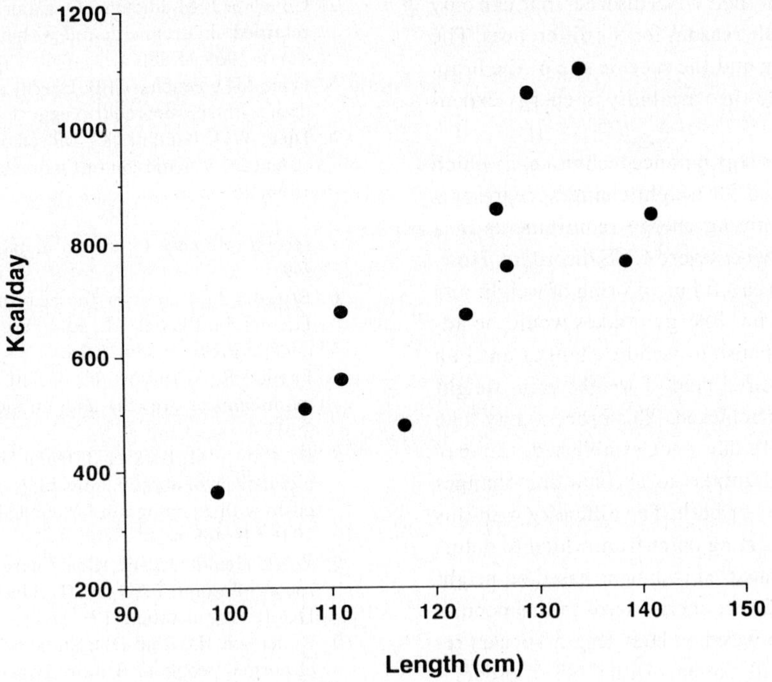

Figure. Relationship between RMR and body length: RMR = 13.4 · Length − 925.6 (r = 0.79).

were not necessarily weight-maintaining diets, the energy intakes did not differ from estimated requirements by more than ±150 kcal/day and in some instances promoted either slow weight gain or weight loss. Both test groups A and B were similar in age, weight, length, or body mass index (Table). The prediction of energy expenditure in test group A did not differ significantly from their daily energy intake; the mean difference between predicted energy expenditure and actual energy intake was 8.3 ± 131.3 kcal. However, for those with energy intakes >8.2 kcal/cm (test group B), the regression equation significantly underestimated energy needs. The mean difference in energy intake and predicted energy expenditure was 422.7 ± 197.8 kcal/day.

DISCUSSION

Studies of energy expenditure in persons with disabilities are limited. The RMR in adolescents and young adults with myelodysplasia and Prader-Willi syndrome[1, 11] was significantly lower than predicted, and was attributed to decreases in fat-free mass. In contrast, in adolescents and young adults with cerebral palsy who also had reduced fat-free mass, RMR did not differ from that predicted from age and weight.[1] These discrepancies highlight the heterogeneity of the energy requirements of the disabled population and the difficulty of selecting appropriate energy intakes for an individual.

Our study demonstrates that RMR is significantly reduced in individuals with severe CNS disorders and that the use of standardized equations will overestimate RMR and thus energy requirements. In subjects with severe CNS disorders, RMR as a percentage of predicted RMR based on the FAO/WHO/UNU equation was much lower (63%) than the RMR that we reported for a group of adolescents with cerebral palsy or myelodysplasia (97% and 88%, respectively).[1] Length but not weight was significantly correlated with metabolic rate. The lack of a significant correlation of weight and metabolic rate is in contrast to findings in unaffected children,[12] adolescents,[13] and adults,[14] and is probably due to variation in body composition among the subjects.

The observation that length explains 62% of the variance in RMR observed in this population suggests that length may be a useful predictor of RMR. When we tested this regression equation on a separate group of individuals with severe CNS disorders who had similar intakes to those in the study group, the estimated energy needs did not differ from their intakes. However, when the regression equation was used to predict energy requirements in another group of patients with severe CNS disorders with greater energy intakes, their energy requirements were underestimated. The disparity in the predictions of energy expenditure in the two test groups is not easily explained. Because of the small sample size and the heterogeneity of the subject population with respect to the cause of their CNS disorder, one can only speculate about the possible reasons for the differences. The age at onset of the disease and the specific site of the brain affected may contribute to the variability in energy expenditure.

We conclude that the energy balance technique, in which energy intakes are adjusted for weight changes, represents a valid method of determining energy requirements in a population of individuals with severe CNS disorders. However, this process requires careful monitoring of weight and intake for an extended time. Energy intakes would be adjusted periodically in response to weight changes until an optimal intake for the desired goal of weight gain, weight loss, or weight stability is achieved. This process may take several months to complete but, once established, requires only slight adjustment of intake to account for changes caused by growth or illness or both. The difficulty with this method is in choosing a starting point from which to determine caloric intake. Standardized equations based on height and weight grossly overestimate energy needs in this population. A predictive equation based on body length appears reliable for certain, but not all, patients with CNS disorders.

We thank the staff at the Children's Extended Care Center and the MIT Clinical Research Center for their assistance with the study, Dr. Ray Gleason for his help with the statistical analysis, and Dr. William Dietz for providing medical coverage and reviewing this manuscript.

REFERENCES

1. Bandini LG, Schoeller DA, Fukagawa NK, Wykes LJ, Dietz WH. Body composition and energy expenditure in adolescents with cerebral palsy or myelodysplasia. Pediatr Res 1991; 29:70-7.
2. Culley WJ, Middleton TO. Caloric requirements of mentally retarded children with and without motor dysfunction. J PEDIATR 1969;75:380-4.
3. Fried MD, Pencharz PB. Energy and nutrient intakes of children with spastic quadriplegia. J PEDIATR 1991;119:947-9.
4. Dietz WH, Bandini LG, Morell JA, Ching PLYH. Effect of sedentary activities on resting metabolic rate. Am J Clin Nutr 1994;59:556-9.
5. Weir JB. New methods for calculating metabolic rate with special reference to protein metabolism. J Physiol 1949;109: 1-9.
6. Brouwer E. Report of the Subcommittee on Constants and Factors. In: Blaxter KL, ed. Energy metabolism. London: Academic Press, 1965:425-38.
7. Payne PR, Waterlow JC. Relative energy requirements for maintenance, growth, and physical activity. Lancet 1971; 2:210-1.
8. Boothby WM, Berkson J, Dunn HL. Studies of the energy of metabolism of normal individuals: a standard for basal metabolism with a nomogram for clinical application. Am J Physiol 1936;116:468-84.
9. World Health Organization. Energy and protein requirements: report of a joint FAO/WHO/UNU meeting. Geneva: World Health Organization, 1985:71-8.
10. Robertson JD, Reid DD. Standards for the basal metabolism of normal people in Britain. Lancet 1953;1:940-3.
11. Schoeller DA, Levitsky LL, Bandini LG, Dietz WH, Walczak A. Energy expenditure and body composition in Prader-Willi syndrome. Metabolism 1988;37:115-20.
12. Fontvielle AM, Harper IT, Ferraro RT, Spraul M, Ravussin E. Daily energy expenditure by five-year-old children, measured by doubly labeled water. J PEDIATR 1993;123: 200-7.
13. Bandini LG, Schoeller DA, Dietz WH. Energy expenditure in obese and nonobese adolescents. Pediatr Res 1990;27:198-203.
14. Ravussin E, Burnand B, Schutz Y, Jequier E. Twenty-four-hour energy expenditure and in obese, moderately obese, and control subjects. Am J Clin Nutr 1982;35:566-73.

Body composition in children with spastic quadriplegic cerebral palsy

Virginia A. Stallings, MD, Christine E. Cronk, ScD, Babette S. Zemel, PhD, and Edward B. Charney, MD

From the Divisions of Gastroenterology and Nutrition, and of Child Development and Rehabilitation Medicine, Children's Hospital of Philadelphia, University of Pennsylvania School of Medicine, Philadelphia, and the Department of Anthropology, Southern Illinois University at Carbondale

Objective: To determine the pattern of body composition and nutritional status in a group of prepubertal children with spastic quadriplegic cerebral palsy (SQCP) compared with healthy control children.
Study design: Subjects were enrolled for this cross-sectional study from two tertiary care settings. One hundred thirty-six subjects with SQCP, 2 to 12 years of age, were evaluated by anthropometric measures, or by anthropometric and total body water (TBW) measures (n = 28), with 39 control subjects.
Results: Body composition and nutritional status indicators were significantly reduced in children with SQCP. Accretion of fat-free mass with age was smaller for children with SQCP. Calculation of body fat from two skin folds correlated best with measures of fat mass from TBW.
Conclusion: Malnutrition is common in children with SQCP. Clinically available, serial anthropometric measures enable the clinician to identify malnourished children with SQCP. (J PEDIATR 1995;126:833-9)

Spastic quadriplegic cerebral palsy, the most severe form of cerebral palsy, is characterized by mental and growth retardation, abnormal oral motor skills, and restricted ambulation. Although the application of medical, computer, and engineering techniques has improved many aspects of the clinical care of these children, disease-specific nutritional support has been limited. Errors in conventional measures of body size (e.g., height or recumbent length) arise from the spasticity and joint contractures in these children, making reliable evaluation of body size difficult. Recent work has documented the utility and accuracy of upper arm or lower leg lengths as replacements for unreliable measures of height.[1-3] Nutritional assessment of patients with SQCP also has been limited because information based on more directly measured body composition (e.g., total body water from deuterium oxide dilution, body cell mass from potassium-40 measurements) is lacking. Thus the accuracy of body fat and fat-free mass estimates based on clinically available anthropometry is unknown.

See related article, p. 828.

CP	Cerebral palsy
D_2O	Deuterium oxide [dilution]
FFM	Fat-free mass
FM	Fat mass
SQCP	Spastic quadriplegic cerebral palsy

An implicit assumption by some clinical caregivers of children with SQCP is that abnormalities in growth and body composition are due to unalterable aspects of the disease process. Our research group has demonstrated that a

Supported by the United Cerebral Palsy Foundation, the Children's Seashore House, the General Clinic Research Center (NIH-RR-00240), and the Nutrition Center of Children's Hospital of Philadelphia.

Submitted for publication May 31, 1994; accepted Dec. 15, 1994.

Reprint requests: Virginia A. Stallings, MD, Division of Gastroenterology and Nutrition, Children's Hospital of Philadelphia, 34th Street and Civic Center Blvd., Philadelphia, PA 19104.

0022-3476/95/$3.00 + 0 **9/73/62807**

Table I. Distributions for age, *z* scores, percentage of medians for anthropometry, and D_2O-derived variables for children with SQCP and control children

	SQCP group (n = 136, 108, or 28)*		Control group (n = 39)	
	Mean	SD	Mean	SD
Age (yr)	7.5	2.3	6.5	2.0
z Score				
Upper arm length	−1.29	1.26†	—	—
Lower leg length	−1.96	1.56†	—	—
Height	—	—	−0.39	1.05
Weight	−2.00	0.72‡	−0.09	0.87
Muscle area	−0.32	1.11‡	0.27	0.98
%Median skin-fold thickness				
Triceps	61	25‡	107	29
Subscapular	88	27‡	111	30
Slaughter[13] FM (kg)	1.6	1.0‡	3.4	1.2
Slaughter FFM (kg)	12.7	3.7‡	18.5	4.8
D_2O-derived FM (kg)	2.9	2.0‡	4.6	1.8
D_2O-derived FFM (kg)	13.5	3.2‡	17.6	4.9

*Data based on a sample size of 136 children with SQCP, except as follows: Slaughter FM and FFM, n = 108; D_2O = derived FM and FFM, n = 28.
†p <0.01 by one sample t test.
‡p <0.01 by independent t test, or by Mann-Whitney U test for percentage of median triceps and subscapular skin-fold thickness.

significant part of the abnormal growth and body composition in children with SQCP is directly attributable to poor nutritional status, independent of other factors such as disease severity, age, race, gender, pubertal status, and midparental height.[2] These findings emphasize the need for more accurate and routine nutritional status assessment in an effort to prevent nutrition-related growth failure. This report provides information on body composition of prepubescent children with SQCP in comparison with a group of normal children. The relationship of age, ethnicity, gender, and nutritional supplementation to body composition is explored, and the relationship of directly measured body composition to clinically available indicators of body composition is assessed.

SUBJECTS

Prepubertal children between 2 and 12 years of age with a diagnosis of spastic quadriplegia, and a group of healthy control children, were enrolled in this study. Children with SQCP were recruited from two university-based, tertiary care centers, the Children's Seashore House at Children's Hospital of Philadelphia, Philadelphia, Pa., and the A. I. duPont Institute, in Wilmington, Del. The diagnosis of SQCP was based on a neurologic examination by a developmental pediatrician or pediatric neurologist. SQCP was defined as severe involvement of both upper and lower extremities. Children with SQCP were excluded from the study if they had any other chronic illnesses (e.g., cardiac, renal, gastrointestinal, or congenital syndromes) or used any medication (e.g., steroids, thyroxine) known to affect growth or body composition. Children in the anthropometric measurement group were enrolled and measured during a routine office visit. All eligible subjects were asked to participate, and about 90% of the eligible children entered the study. The families who declined to participate most often stated it was because of the lack of time on that specific day. Most children who had total body water determinations were also recruited during routine office visits, with follow-up contact to schedule the overnight admission and measurements. Some children were enrolled by a telephone call from their developmental pediatrician or clinical coordinator to the parent when no convenient clinic visit was scheduled. There was no recruitment strategy based on race, gender, nutritional status, or disease severity. Control children were recruited from the general hospital community and siblings of subjects, and were selected to be comparable in fat-free body mass to children with SQCP. Informed consent was obtained from the parent or legal guardian, and the protocol was approved by the Children's Hospital of Philadelphia Institutional Review Board.

METHODS

All children had an anthropometric assessment, including weight, upper arm circumference, and skin-fold thicknesses (triceps, biceps, suprailiac, subscapular), by methods described by Cameron.[4] Skin-fold thicknesses were measured with a pair of Holtain calipers. Upper arm circumference was measured with plastic measuring tape (Inser Tape, Ross Laboratories, Columbus, Ohio), and weight was measured with a digital electronic scale. Linear growth

Table II. Regression analysis for D_2O-derived FM and FFM on age, gender (0 = male, 1 = female), black ethnicity (0 = white and other, 1 = black), and gastrostomy supplementation (0 = no supplementation, 1 = gastrostomy)

	Source							
	DF	Σ Squares	F value	Pr>F	Estimate	T for HO (variable = 0)	Pr>T	SEE
Dependent variable: D_2O-derived fat mass (kg)								
Model	4	66.558	9.57	0.0001				
Error	23	40.000						
CORRECTED TOTAL	27*	106.558						
Variable								
Intercept					4.420	4.04	0.0005	1.0954
Age					−0.085	−0.76	0.4578	0.1122
Gender					−0.895	−1.53	0.1397	0.5849
Black ethnicity					−1.791	−3.42	0.0023	0.5237
Gastrostomy					1.747	2.67	0.0138	0.6549
Dependent variable: D_2O-derived fat-free mass (kg)								
Model	4	179.295	10.26	0.0001				
Error	23	100.467						
CORRECTED TOTAL	27†	279.762						
Variable								
Intercept					4.763	2.74	0.0116	1.7360
Age					1.051	5.91	0.0001	0.1778
Gender					0.430	0.46	0.6568	0.9269
Black ethnicity					1.540	1.86	0.0764	0.8300
Gastrostomy					−0.337	−0.32	0.7487	1.0380

DF, Degrees of freedom; *SEE*, standard error of the estimate.
*R^2 = 0.625.
†R^2 = 0.641.

in children with SQCP was measured with a Holtain anthropometer for upper arm length (acromion-radial length) and lower leg length (tibial-sphyrion length) by methods previously described.[1, 4, 5] Height in control children was obtained by methods described by Cameron[4] and a Holtain stadiometer. For all measurements, two replicates were obtained and the mean value was used in analysis. Pubertal development was assessed by means of Tanner staging.[6] All measurements were conducted by one of two trained anthropometrists during an office visit.

For a subsample of the SQCP group (called the SQCP body composition subgroup) and all control children, an estimate of total body water was obtained by D_2O dilution with the use of methods described by Schoeller et al.,[7] during an overnight admission to the General Clinical Research Center. After a baseline urine collection, a D_2O dose of 0.14 gm/kg of estimated total body water was given by nasogastric tube to the SQCP subjects and orally to the control subjects. Urine was collected overnight, and the volume was noted for adjustment for isotope losses during the equilibration period. For SQCP subjects, urine samples were obtained from diapers with cotton batting pads, from which the urine was extracted. Samples from the overnight and morning voids were analyzed for D_2O at the University of Chicago Clinical Nutrition Research Center. Total body water was used to derive a value for FFM, which was in turn used in combination with body weight to estimate body fat mass. Age-appropriate FFM hydration factors were used.[8, 9] Measurements for all of these subjects were collected by a single investigator.

Information on demographic and clinical characteristics and variables associated with SQCP was collected. Ambulatory status was categorized as totally wheelchair-bound versus having some ambulation. Cognitive ability was based on educational classification and, when available, recent developmental testing. Children were classified as dyskinetic when they had choreiform or athetotic movements. Oral motor status was rated on a 5-point scale (0 = no difficulty, 5 = difficulty on all areas tested) based on the presence or absence of tongue thrust, fluid or food loss during eating, coughing or gagging during eating, excessive time required for meals, and difficulty in consuming textured foods. Nutritional supplementation was defined as the routine use of commercially available nutritional products by mouth, or by nasogastric, gastrostomy, or gastrojejunal feeding tubes.

All statistical analyses were performed with the SAS program.[10] The *z* scores for linear growth measures (standard deviation scores) were used so that age and gender groups could be combined. Reference values for height and weight were drawn from the National Center for Health Statistics data,[11] and for lower leg and upper arm lengths

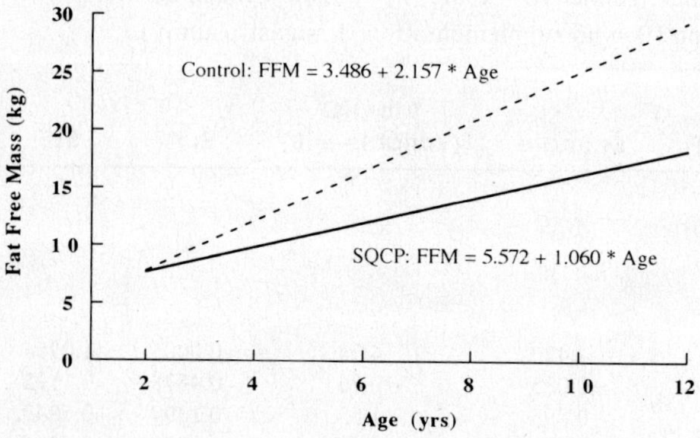

Figure Plot of regression lines for FFM (in kilograms) against age (in years) for control and SQCP children.

from Snyder et al.[5] Reference values for triceps and subscapular skin folds and upper arm muscle area (computed from upper arm circumference and triceps skin fold) from Frisancho[12] were used. Percentage medians were used instead of *z* scores for triceps and subscapular skin folds because of the skewness of the reference data, which made the use of *z* scores inappropriate for this sample of children. Estimates of FM and FFM from two skin-fold measurements were computed with the Slaughter prediction equations[13] shown below.

Equations for estimation of percentage of body fat in prepubertal children from the triceps and subscapular skin-fold measurements (in millimeters) are as follows:

All girls:

$$\% \text{ Body fat} = 1.33 (\text{Triceps} + \text{Subscapular}) - 0.013 (\text{Triceps} + \text{Subscapular})^2 - 2.5$$

White boys:

$$\% \text{ Body fat} = 1.21 (\text{Triceps} + \text{Subscapular}) - 0.008 (\text{Triceps} + \text{Subscapular})^2 - 1.7$$

Black boys:

$$\% \text{ Body fat} = 1.21 (\text{Triceps} + \text{Subscapular}) - 0.008 (\text{Triceps} + \text{Subscapular})^2 - 3.2$$

When the sum of triceps and subscapular skin folds is >35 mm, the following equations are used:

All girls: $\% \text{ Body fat} = 0.546 (\text{Triceps} + \text{Subscapular}) + 9.7$

All boys: $\% \text{ Body fat} = 0.783 (\text{Triceps} + \text{Subscapular}) + 1.6$

Regression analyses were used to explore the relationships of FFM and FM to age, gender, ethnicity, nutritional supplementation, and body size. When appropriate, interaction terms were included in the regression analyses to test for significant interaction effects. The relationship of FM derived from D_2O to anthropometric indicators of FM was assessed by correlation and regression analyses. Because of the skewness of the skin-fold thickness measures, log-transformed values were used. A *t* test was used to test for significant differences in slopes between SQCP and control groups from regression analysis.

RESULTS

A total of 136 children with SQCP participated; 58 girls and 50 boys (75 white, 33 black) enrolled in the clinical assessment protocol. The body composition subgroup included 11 girls and 17 boys (15 white, 13 black) who also completed the protocol for stable isotope determination of total body water. The approximate race and gender distributions for the Children's Hospital and duPont CP centers are, respectively, 28, 70% white; 64, 25% black; 8, 5% other; 46, 50% female, and 54, 50% male. Eighteen girls and 21 boys, all white, comprised the control group. For the two linear growth measurements (lower leg length and upper arm length), technical errors were between 1 and 2 mm, and represented less than 1% of the variability in the data. Errors for all skin-fold thicknesses were about 0.1 mm, which represented about 2% of the total variability for these measurements. These technical errors were comparable to those reported in a similar sample,[14] and to intraobserver errors reported for the national reference data used in this study.[11, 15]

About half of the SQCP group were severely or profoundly cognitively delayed, and nearly 90% used a wheelchair. Seizure disorders occurred in about 40% of these children. Ten percent had athetoid or choreiform movement as well as spasticity. Forty-five percent of the children had scores of 5 on the oral motor assessment, indicating difficulty on all items in this assessment scale. More than 60% of the children had never been prescribed a specific nutritional supplementation program. The most common types of nutritional intervention were the placement of gastrostomy feeding tubes (18%) and oral supplementation (14%).

Table I shows distributions for age, *z* scores, and percentage of the medians for anthropometry, and for FM and FFM derived from D_2O and from the two skin-fold prediction equations from Slaughter et al.[13] The *z* scores and percentage of the medians for the control children were near expectation (i.e., near 0 for height and weight *z* scores, near 100% for percentage of median triceps and subscapular values). For the SQCP sample, the proxy measures for height (upper arm and lower leg lengths) were significantly reduced below the reference means by 1 to 2 SD, and weight was reduced by 2 SD. Reduction of skin-fold thicknesses was greatest at the triceps site, about 60% of median reference value; subscapular fat was reduced to about 85%. Suitable reference data for biceps and suprailiac skin folds were not available. Arm muscle area was closer to normal values in the SQCP group than were other anthropometric measurements. All anthropometric values for SQCP children were significantly lower than those for the control children by *t* test or Mann-Whitney U test (for percentage of the medians) at $p < 0.01$. The 28 children in the SQCP body composition subgroup had anthropometric measurement values similar to those of the full SQCP group. Values for D_2O FM and FFM were significantly lower in the children with SQCP than in the control group.

The effects of age, gender, black ethnicity, and feeding supplementation on the D_2O-derived measures of FM and FFM for children with SQCP were analyzed by regression analyses (Table II). The D_2O-derived FM showed significant negative effects from black ethnicity (on average, 1.8 kg less than white subjects) and significant positive effects from gastrostomy feeding (on average, 1.7 kg more than in children without gastrostomies). Comparison of mean values of FM showed that white children had nearly twice the amount of FM (4.2 kg) as black children (2.4 kg), and children with gastrostomy feeding tubes had nearly twice as much FM (4.2 kg) as those who were not gastrostomy fed (2.4 kg). No significant interaction effects were observed. The effects of age and gender on D_2O-derived FM were not significant.

The D_2O-derived FFM showed only the expected significant positive effect from age (Table II). The Figure shows this relationship for both SQCP and control children. The FFM for age in the children with SQCP was similar to that in the control group at 2 years of age but diverged progressively through the end of the age intervals evaluated. The slopes of the two lines were both significant and positive, but the SQCP slope (1.06) was significantly smaller ($p < 0.01$) than that for control subjects (2.16).

Correlations of anthropometric and direct measures of fat mass. Correlation coefficients were used to assess the relationship of anthropometric indicators of FM and D_2O-derived FM (Table III). For SQCP, the log of the suprailiac skin fold and the two skin-fold–derived FM measures[14] had the highest correlations with D_2O-derived FM (range, $r = 0.57$ to 0.70). For control children, the level of correlation was very similar to that seen in the SQCP children, and the two skin-fold–derived FM values had the highest correlation with D_2O-derived FM. Scatter plots revealed that much of the variability for the SQCP children was related to the high body fat levels in gastrostomy-fed children. Correlation analyses excluding these children were therefore repeated; in general, correlations were lower, with only two (log suprailiac and two skin-fold–derived FM values) reaching statistical significance (Table III).

Table III. Correlations of FM for D_2O with log values for skin-fold thickness, sum of four skin-fold thicknesses, and Slaughter FM, with FM from D_2O measures for the body composition SQCP subsample and the control group

	SQCP group		
	All (n = 28)	Without gastrostomy (n = 19)	Control group (n = 39)
Triceps	0.57†	0.38	0.57†
Subscapular	0.57†	0.23	0.57†
Biceps	0.57†	0.30	0.43†
Suprailiac	0.70†	0.56†	0.52†
Four skin folds	0.67†	0.42	0.57†
Slaughter[13] FM	0.69†	0.51*	0.75†

*$p < 0.05$.
†$p < 0.01$.

DISCUSSION

Malnutrition and growth failure in children with CP have been described during the past 30 years,[16-20] including recent reports of children with diplegia or hemiplegia[21] and spastic quadriplegia.[2] Nevertheless, nutritional disorders in these children are not as frequently recognized and treated as they are in children with other chronic pediatric diseases with more easily recognized nutrition-related growth failure (e.g., cystic fibrosis, Crohn disease). The lack of nutritional treatment is due, in part, to the difficulty in identifying which child with SQCP is undernourished in a disease state that includes skeletal muscle atrophy, joint contractures, and motor disorders. We selected the prepubertal age range for evaluation to decrease the variations in the patterns of growth and the concomitant accretion of FM and FFM associated with pubertal development.

This group of children with SQCP was severely affected and is likely representative of the type of children with SQCP cared for in larger, interdisciplinary CP programs. As reported earlier in a similar sample, all measures of body size and fatness were markedly reduced in comparison with those of unaffected children and with national reference data.[2] Upper arm length was less compromised than the lower leg length. The subcutaneous fat stores at the upper extremity triceps site were more reduced than fat at the subscapular site. This pattern of retention of truncal fat has been seen in other groups of malnourished children.[22-24] The estimate of muscle area was the least reduced of all the anthropometric measures. This pattern of malnutrition also was observed in our earlier study of children with SQCP[2] and in another report of poorly nourished children.[25] However, muscle area is calculated from the mid-arm circumference and triceps skin-fold measurements, so this finding may be an artifact of the depleted fat stores at the triceps site.

Direct measures of body composition showed that the children with SQCP had a significant reduction in both FM and FFM compartments and that the reduction in FM was associated with ethnicity; the black children had lower FM than white children. Other investigators have shown that during childhood, black children have greater bone density, less body fat, and lower mean triceps skin-fold thickness than white children.[26, 27] Therefore it is possible that a portion of the ethnic difference in body composition in the group of children with SQCP was related to differences in body composition seen also in unaffected children. Alternatively, black children may have more severe growth failure because they have more severe CP, less utilization of the medical system, or less effective medical and nutritional care. Identifying racial differences was not a specific aim of the study, and the sample size and racial distribution for children with CP and for control children were not adequate to address this issue. Further work is required to determine whether black children with SQCP have a disproportionally abnormal pattern of body composition or a greater frequency of nutrition-related growth failure, and to identify the cause. Children with SQCP have worsening growth failure with age, with reductions in both FFM compartment and in limb lengths. Similar findings were seen in the previous report of children with SQCP,[2] and were related to poor nutritional status.

Body composition was estimated from anthropometric measurements and D_2O dilution. The correlation between FM from anthropometric measurements using the Slaughter two skin-fold equations and total body water measurements by D_2O was similar in both SQCP and control children. The Slaughter equations yielded a value that systematically underestimated FM from D_2O by 1.3 kg in both subjects with SQCP and control subjects.

We conclude that growth failure and abnormal body composition are common in prepubertal children with SQCP who are dependent on caregivers for their daily food supply. Undernutrition or overnutrition may be recognized in these patients by periodic examination of weight, upper arm length, lower leg length, triceps skin fold, subscapular skin fold, and upper arm circumference. Collection every 6 months of these anthropometric measurements and calculation of the appropriate interpretive information (percentile, percentage of the median, *z* score, and FM and FFM from the Slaughter skin-fold equations) will document the growth patterns and nutritional status. Growth charts for upper arm and lower leg lengths are available.[28] Undernutrition or obesity will be apparent from the semiannual growth and body composition trends, and may be readily treated with available dietary modification and feeding techniques.[29-33] The clinical goals are prevention of malnutrition throughout the life span of children with SQCP, and effective nutritional rehabilitation for children with existing malnutrition. This strategy not only will improve growth but also may improve physiologic and functional capacity, resulting in improved quality of life.

We gratefully acknowledge the participation and efforts of the children, families, and staff of the CP centers at the A. I. duPont Institute and the Children's Seashore House. In addition, we acknowledge special contributions of Jayne Chalfin-Davies, MSN, RD; Drs. Dale Schoeller, Freeman Miller, and Steven Bachrach; and Marilyn Boos, RN, Debbie Cole, Greg Maislin, Betty Leifer, Damary Vargas, and Deirdre MacLeod.

REFERENCES

1. Spender QW, Cronk CE, Charney EB, Stallings VA. Assessment of linear growth of children with cerebral palsy: use of alternative measures to height or length. Dev Med Child Neurol 1989;31:206-14.
2. Stallings VA, Charney EB, Davies JC, Cronk CE. Nutrition-related growth failure of children with quadriplegic cerebral palsy. Dev Med Child Neurol 1993;35:126-38.
3. Johnson RK, Ferrara MS. Estimating stature from knee height for persons with cerebral palsy: as evaluation of estimation equations. J Am Diet Assoc 1991;91:1283-4.
4. Cameron N. The methods of auxological anthropometry. In: Falkner F, Tanner JM, eds. Human growth; vol 2. New York: Plenum Press, 1986:1-42.
5. Snyder RG, Schneider LW, Owings CL, Golomb DH, Schork MA. Anthropometry of infants, children and youths to age 18 for product safety design. (Report No. Um-HSRI-77-17.) Bethesda, Maryland: Consumer Product Safety Commission, 1977.
6. Tanner JM, ed. Growth at adolescence. London: Blackwell Scientific, 1962.
7. Schoeller DA, Leitch C, Brown C. Doubly labeled water method: in vivo oxygen and hydrogen isotope fractionation. Am J Physiol 1986;251:R1137-43.
8. Fomon SJ, Haschke F, Ziegler EE, Nelson SE. Body composition of reference children from birth to age 10 years. Am J Clin Nutr 1982;35:1169-75.
9. Boileau R, Lohman T, Slaughter M, Ball T, et al. Hydration of the fat-free body in children during maturation. Hum Biol 1984;56:651-66.
10. SAS user's guide: statistics. Cary, North Carolina: SAS Institute, 1986.
11. Hamill PVV, Drizd TA, Johnson CL, Reed RB, Roche AF. Physical growth: National Center for Health Statistics percentiles. Am J Clin Nutr 1979;32:607-29.
12. Frisancho AR. Anthropometric standards for the assessment of growth and nutritional status. Ann Arbor: University of Michigan Press, 1990.
13. Slaughter MH, Lohman TG, Boileau RA, et al. Skinfold

equations for estimation of body fatness in children and youth. Hum Biol 1988;60:709-24.
14. Spender QW, Hediger ML, Cronk CE, Stallings VA. Fat distribution in children with cerebral palsy. Ann Hum Biol 1988; 15:191-6.
15. Johnson C, Fulwood R, Abraham S, Bryner J. Basic data on anthropometric measurements and angular measurements of the hip and knee joints for selected age groups 1-74 years of age: United States, 1971–1975. (Vital Health Statistics, series 11, No. 219; DHHS publication No. [PHS] 81-1669.) Hyattsville, Maryland: National Center for Health Statistics, 1981.
16. Sterling HM. Height and weight of children with cerebral palsy and acquired brain damage. Arch Phys Med Rehabil 1960;41:131-5.
17. Tobias JS, Saturen P, Larios G, Posniak AO. Study of growth patterns in cerebral palsy. Arch Phys Med Rehabil 1961; 41:475-81.
18. Culley WJ, Jolly DH, Mertz ET. Heights and weights of mentally retarded children. Am J Ment Defic 1963;68:203-9.
19. Hammond MI, Lewis MN, Johnson EW. A nutritional study of cerebral palsied children. J Am Diet Assoc 1966;49:196-201.
20. Thelander HE, Pryor HB. Growth deviations in handicapped children. Clinical Pediatrics 1967;6:501-12.
21. Stallings VA, Charney EB, Davies JC, Cronk CE. Nutritional status and growth of children with diplegic or hemiplegic cerebral palsy. Dev Med Child Neurol 1993;35:997-1006.
22. Cameron N, Johnston FE, Kgamphe JS, Lunz JS. Body fat patterning in rural South African black children. Am J Hum Biol 1992;4:353-64.
23. Bogin B, MacVean RB. Nutritional and biological determinants of body fat patterning in urban Guatemalan children. Hum Biol 1981;53:259-68.
24. Hammond MI, Lewis MN, Johnson EW. A nutritional study of cerebral palsied children. J Am Diet Assoc 1966;49:196-201.
25. Schumacher LB, Kretchmer N. Upper arm anthropometric characteristics of immigrant children in the newcomer schools of San Francisco. Hum Biol 1988;60:623-38.
26. Cronk CE, Roche AF. Race- and sex-specific reference data for triceps and subscapular skinfolds and weight stature.[2] Am J Clin Nutr 1982;35:347-54.
27. Bell WH, Shary J, Stevens J, Garza M, Gordon L, Edwards J. Demonstration that bone mass is greater in black than in white children. J Bone Miner Res 1991;6:719-23.
28. Stallings VA, Zemel BS. Nutritional assessment of the disabled child. In: Sullivan PB, Rosenbloom L, eds. Feeding the disabled child. Clinics in Developmental Medicine (in press).
29. Shapiro BK, Green P, Krick J, Allen D, Capute AJ. Growth of severely impaired children: neurological versus nutritional factors. Dev Med Child Neurol 1986;28:729-33.
30. Patrick J, Boland M, Stodki D, Murray GE. Rapid correction of wasting in children with cerebral palsy. Dev Med Child Neurol 1986;29:734-9.
31. Rempel GR, Colwell SO, Nelson RP. Growth in children with cerebral palsy fed via gastrostomy. Pediatrics 1988;82:857-62.
32. Sanders KD, Cox K, Cannon R, et al. Growth response to enteral feeding by children with cerebral palsy. JPEN J Paren Enteral Nutr 1990;14:23-6.
33. Fried MD, Pencharz PB. Energy and nutrient intakes of children with spastic quadriplegia. J PEDIATR 1991;119:947-9.

THE BOOK SHELF

André D. Lascari, *Editor*

Book review

Pediatric psychooncology

Bearison D, Mulhern R, eds. New York: Oxford University Press, 1994. 247 pages. $45.

It was not until the late 1960s that articles appeared by Doris Howell, Audrey Evans, Morris Green, William Easson, and Stanford Friedman, among others, offering guidance as to how to provide emotional support for terminally ill children and their families. At that time a provocative article entitled, "Who's afraid of death on a leukemia ward?" by J. Vernick and M. Karon (Am J Dis Child 1965;109:393-7) stirred the discussion of telling children with cancer about their diagnosis. One of the "fathers" of pediatric oncology adamantly proclaimed, in response to the article, that "One should never tell the child the diagnosis." We have come a long way since that time in our knowledge and ability to support such children as they and their families cope with the tragedy of childhood cancer.

This book provides an excellent review of the present state of the art and research involving the many emotional issues such patients and the families face. It was written for a broad audience with interests in psychologic research and the care of children with cancer.

There are 12 contributors, most of whom are psychologists from several major children's cancer centers. The medical overview chapter would be very helpful for the nononcologist. Other chapters discuss coping with pediatric cancer, pain and symptoms management, and medical compliance. Because more children are surviving cancer, the chapter on neuropsychologic late effects assumes even greater relevance. An individual chapter is devoted to the very important topic of sibling adaptation.

The chapter on the emotional aspects of bone marrow transplantation is most helpful because there is very little in the pediatric literature on this subject. The remaining chapters cover implications of survival, care of the dying child and the bereaved, and future directions.

This is an excellent resource for all health care workers who are involved in the care of children with cancer.

André D. Lascari, MD
Children's Hospital
Albany Medical College
Albany NY 12208

CURRENT LITERATURE AND CLINICAL ISSUES

Abstracts from the literature

Feeding of *Bifidobacterium bifidum* and *Streptococcus thermophilus* to infants in hospital for prevention of diarrhoea and shedding of rotavirus

Saavedra JM, Bauman NA, Oung I, Perman JA, Yolken RH. Lancet 1994;344:1046-9.

Objective: To determine whether the addition of *Bifidobacterium bifidum*, which constitute the predominant intestinal flora of breast-fed infants, and *Streptococcus thermophilus*, an organism that hydrolyses lactose and produces lactic acid, to infant formula will prevent nosocomial acute diarrhea.

Design: Randomized, double-blind, placebo-controlled trial.

Setting: A 46-bed inpatient unit of a facility for the long-term care of children with chronic illnesses in Baltimore, Md.

Patients: Fifty-five infants aged between 5 and 24 months admitted during an 18-month period, excluding breast-fed infants, those with a history of allergy to cow milk, and those receiving lactose-free protein hydrolysate formulas for a malabsorptive disorder.

Intervention: Infants were randomly selected to receive either supplemented formula or control formula for the duration of their hospital stay. They were stratified at enrollment by age (<12 months, >12 months) and by the proportion of energy intake from infant formula (≤50%, >50%). The formulas were casein based and contained vegetable oil, corn syrup solids, and lactose. Both formulas were isocaloric, with the same nutrient distribution. The supplemented formula contained 1.9×10^8 colony-forming units (CFU) of *B. bifidum* and 0.14×10^8 CFU of *S. thermophilus* per gram of powdered formula. The formulas were diluted with distilled water according to clinical needs as assessed by the infant's physician and nutritionist. Caloric densities varied from 0.53 to 1 kcal/ml.

Main outcome measures: Episodes of diarrhea (≥5 liquid stools per day for <7 days), duration of episodes of diarrhea, number of stools per day, stool weight, and rotavirus shedding.

Results: The groups were similar with respect to indexes of formula intake: mean number of days that each formula was fed per subject, mean volume ingested per day, daily energy intake per kilogram of body weight, and energy density of the formula. Episodes of diarrhea occurred in two infants (5.9%) fed the supplemented formula versus eight of the infants (31%) fed the control formula. The cumulative incidence of diarrhea was analyzed and displayed on a Kaplan-Meier plot, and was significantly less for infants fed the supplemented formula. Of the 10 episodes of diarrhea, 7 were associated with rotavirus shedding; 5 of these were in the group fed the control formula. No other viral or bacterial pathogens were identified in any of the episodes of diarrhea. Ten children (38%) fed the control formula shed rotavirus at some point in the study versus only three children (10%) in the supplemented group.

Conclusions: Feeding of a formula supplemented with *B. bifidum* and *S. thermophilus* substantially reduces the incidence of acute diarrheal disease in hospitalized infants.

Comment: This double-blind, placebo-controlled study is the first to confirm that the addition of acid-producing, probiotic bacteria can be used to lower the risk of hospital-acquired diarrhea in high-risk children. Many of the children in this study were malnourished and immunocompromised, and at high risk of having diarrhea. As pointed out by the authors, these or similar bacteria can be cultivated cheaply and added to other foods. The use of the Kaplan-Meier curves was effective in illustrating differences in the acquisition of nosocomial diarrhea, and seems appropriate for expressing the increase in the risk of acquiring a complication as the duration of hospitalization increases. The data on the duration of shedding of rotavirus, which are used as one of the underpinnings of the conclusion that the supplemented formula decreases rotaviral shedding, are not

The following journals are reviewed for every Abstracts section: *Lancet, Pediatric Infectious Disease Journal, New England Journal of Medicine, Journal of the American Medical Association,* and *Archives of Pediatrics*. In addition, the following were reviewed for this issue: *Biology of the Neonate, Clinical Infectious Diseases, Annals of Emergency Medicine, American Journal of Human Genetics, American Journal of Medical Genetics, Teratology,* and *Pediatric Emergency Care*.

9/34/63755

presented. The setting of the study is appropriate because it addresses the subjects at highest risk of acquiring this infection, and it allows sufficient duration of observation to see the difference between the two groups emerge.

Wallace A. (Skip) Gleason, Jr., MD
University of Texas–Houston Health Science Center
Houston, TX 77030

Reduction of maternal-infant transmission of human immunodeficiency virus type 1 with zidovudine treatment

Connor EM, Sperling RS, Gelber R, et al. N Engl J Med 1994;331:1173-80.

Objective: To assess the efficacy and safety of zidovudine in reducing the risk of maternal-infant transmission of human immunodeficiency virus (HIV).
Design: Randomized, double-blind, placebo-controlled trial.
Setting: Fifty-nine centers in the United States and Puerto Rico.
Patients: A total of 477 HIV-infected pregnant women (at 14 to 34 weeks of gestation) with $CD4^+$ T-lymphocyte counts greater than 200 cells/mm^3, who had not received antiretroviral therapy during the current pregnancy, were enrolled.
Intervention: Antepartum administration of zidovudine (100 mg orally five times daily), intrapartum administration of zidovudine (2 mg/kg body weight, given intravenously for a 1-hour period, and then 1 mg/kg per hour until delivery), and zidovudine therapy given to the newborn infant (2 mg/kg orally every 6 hours for 6 weeks).
Main outcome measures: Infection with HIV in infants (infants with at least one culture of peripheral-blood mononuclear cells positive for HIV were classified as HIV infected), adverse effects in mothers and infants, and maternal $CD4^+$ T-lymphocyte count.
Results: A total of 477 pregnant women were enrolled; during the study period, 409 women gave birth to 415 liveborn infants. HIV-infection status was known for 363 births (180 in the zidovudine group, 183 in the placebo group). Thirteen infants in the zidovudine group and 40 in the placebo group were infected with HIV. The proportions infected at 18 months, as estimated by the Kaplan-Meier method, were 8.3% (95% confidence interval [CI], 3.9%, 12.8%) in the zidovudine group and 25.5% (CI, 18.4%, 32.5%) in the placebo group. This corresponds to a 67.5% (CI, 40.7%, 82.1%) relative reduction in the risk of HIV transmission ($z = 4.03$; $p = 0.00006$). Minimal short-term toxic effects were observed. The mean hemoglobin concentration at birth in the infants in the zidovudine group was significantly lower than in the placebo group. By 12 weeks of age, hemoglobin values in the two groups were similar.
Conclusions: In pregnant women with mildly symptomatic HIV disease and no prior treatment with antiretroviral drugs during the pregnancy, a regimen consisting of zidovudine given antepartum and intrapartum to the mother, and to the neonate for 6 weeks, reduced the risk of maternal-infant HIV transmission by approximately two thirds.

Comment: There is one absolute truism associated with the epidemic of HIV infection: prevention is the ultimate goal. Treatment of those infected with HIV is limited, both in options and long-term efficacy. The hypothesis that the administration of zidovudine during the last two trimesters of pregnancy and during delivery, and to neonates for 6 weeks, decreases maternal HIV transmission has been resoundingly proved in the study results from protocol 076 of the Pediatric AIDS Clinical Trials Group, as reported in this article. The reduction of transmission from approximately 25% for placebo to 8% for zidovudine-treated maternal-infant pairs is remarkable. The earlier-than-expected results from protocol 076 were, in part, due to the sensitivity and specificity of the HIV polymerase chain reaction method in serving as an early marker of neonatal HIV infection. This technique had not been established when protocol 076 was initiated but, during the study, became accepted as an early diagnostic tool in perinatal HIV infection. A significant amount of data remains to be evaluated in the protocol 076 database, which may help define which of the treatment phases (prenatal, intrapartum, neonatal) is most responsible for the decrease in maternal-fetal HIV transmission. This analysis will be critical if the findings of the study are to be applied to the majority of HIV-infected pregnant women. The results of protocol 076 have also emphasized the need to provide prenatal care to all pregnant women, including counseling and encouraging voluntary HIV testing. Unfortunately, for economic reasons, the benefits of protocol 076 are not available to women in the developing world.

James M. Oleske, MD, MPH
University of Medicine and Dentistry
of New Jersey Medical School
Newark, NJ 07103

Early intervention in low-birth-weight premature infants: Results through age 5 years from the Infant Health and Development Program

Brooks-Gunn J, McCarton CM, Casey PH, et al. JAMA 1994;272:1257-62.

Objective: To evaluate the persistence of effects on health and development at age 5 years of the Infant Health and Development Program, an early childhood intervention that was provided to low birth weight (LBW) premature infants from neonatal discharge through age 3 years.

Design: Randomized, controlled, multicenter trial, stratified by two LBW groups: lighter (≤2000 gm) and heavier (2001 to 2500 gm).
Setting: Eight socioeconomically heterogeneous clinical sites.
Participants: Of 985 eligible infants weighing 2500 gm or less and born at 37 weeks of gestational age or earlier, 377 infants were randomly assigned to the intervention group and 608 to the follow-up–only group. About two thirds of the infants in each group were in the lighter LBW stratum, and one third were in the heavier LBW stratum.
Intervention: The intervention group received both home visits (from neonatal discharge through age 3 years) and center-based schooling (from 1 to 3 years of age). Children in both groups received pediatric surveillance.
Main outcome measures: Cognitive development, behavioral competence, and health status.
Results: At age 5 years, the intervention group had full-scale IQ scores similar to those of children in the follow-up–only group. However, in the heavier LBW stratum, children in the intervention group had higher full-scale IQ scores (3.7 points higher; $p = 0.03$) and higher verbal IQ scores (4.2 points higher; $p = 0.02$). No significant differences between the intervention and follow-up–only groups in cognitive measures at age 5 years were noted in the lighter LBW infants. The intervention and follow-up groups were similar in behavior and health measures regardless of LBW stratum.
Conclusion: The early childhood intervention provided in the first 3 years of life had effects on heavier LBW premature infants' IQ and verbal performance at age 5 years that were not observed in lighter LBW premature infants. The intervention did not affect health or behavior at age 5 years in either LBW stratum.

Comment: This study was well designed and well executed. Rather than being complacent with the success of their early childhood intervention program for children aged 3 years, the investigators rightly chose to test the relative endurance of these earlier gains 2 years after the cessation of the program. Between 4 and 5 years of age, 87% of the children in both groups had attended a community day care center. It is not surprising that earlier advantages were now diluted, with modest differences persisting only in heavier infants. However, it is debatable whether the observed 3- to 4-point IQ difference represents significant educational advantage. The investigators recognize that reliance on IQ scores alone may be misleading, and that school performance would be more relevant. It is therefore important that they continue their inquiry and also determine the cost-effectiveness of this program. One cannot help wondering, however, about the feasibility of implementing this extremely intensive and costly intervention program routinely, even if remarkable benefits were demonstrated.

Saroj Saigal, MD, FRCP(C)
McMaster University Health Sciences Center
Hamilton, Ontario L8N 3Z5, Canada

Educational attainment in long-term survivors of childhood acute lymphoblastic leukemia

Haupt R, Fears TR, Robison LL, et al. JAMA 1994; 272:1427-32.

Objective: To determine the impact of treatment on scholastic performance in the first cohort of survivors of childhood acute lymphoblastic leukemia who are old enough to have completed their educational experience.
Design: Retrospective cohort study.
Setting: Twenty-three institutions in the Childrens Cancer Group.
Subjects: A total of 593 adult survivors of childhood acute lymphoblastic leukemia and 409 sibling control subjects.
Main outcome measures: Enrollment in special programs, grades during high school, graduation from high school, college admission, and college graduation.
Results: After diagnosis, survivors were more likely than their sibling control subjects to enter a special education program (relative risk [RR] = 3.4; $p < 0.01$) or a program for learning-disabled children (RR = 3.6; $p < 0.01$), while just as likely to enter programs for gifted and talented children (RR = 1.0). The risk associated with special education and learning-disability programs increased with increasing doses of cranial radiotherapy. Despite these problems, survivors generally had the same probability as their siblings of finishing high school, entering college, and earning a bachelor's degree. However, survivors treated with 24 Gy and those whose diagnosis was made before 6 years of age were less likely to enter college (RR = 0.67 and 0.6, respectively; $p < 0.01$).
Conclusions: This large study demonstrates that survivors of childhood acute lymphoblastic leukemia have a greater likelihood of being placed in special education or learning-disability programs than their siblings, but that most are able to overcome these problems. Dose of cranial radiotherapy and age at diagnosis are the most important education-related risk factors.

Comment: Increasing survival rates after childhood leukemia have resulted in a large population of long-term survivors and prompted heightened interest in their psychologic outcome. This study, conducted within the Childrens Cancer Group, examined the impact of cancer and its treatment on scholastic attainment in 593 survivors of childhood leukemia. Control subjects consisted of 409 siblings. Factors examined included the use and dose of cranial irradiation, intrathecal methotrexate, gender, age at treatment, and time elapsed since treatment. A strength of this study was its large number of subjects (more than 1000), so it was surprising that there were instances when power was insufficient to conduct analyses on some subgroups. The results suggest that survivors can, in general, expect to attain educational levels similar to those of healthy children despite a higher enrollment in special education programs during primary and secondary school. As expected, those treated with cranial irradiation have less success. Although the study confirms what other studies have reported in a way that may be more ecologically valid than psychometric test scores, it does not add significantly to our understanding of the specific factors associated with poor academic outcome after treatment for leukemia.

Bartlett D. Moore III, PhD
University of Texas M. D. Anderson Cancer Center
Houston, TX 77030

ALSO NOTED

Surveillance of pharyngeal colonization: detection and control of serious bacterial illness in low birth weight infants

Finelli L, Livengood JR, Saiman L. Pediatr Infect Dis J 1994;13:854-9.

This study examined the common practice of routine surface culture (which is used to predict the organism involved in serious bacterial illness) by means of a prospective cohort design in a neonatal intensive care unit. Pharyngeal cultures were poor predictors of the causative organism: concordance was only 11% for bacteremia or infection present in the cerebral spinal fluid. The investigators concluded that this test has no apparent utility in the neonatal intensive care unit.

Randomized comparison of amoxicillin and erythromycin in treatment of genital chlamydial infection in pregnancy

Alary M, Joly JR, Moutquin J-M, et al. Lancet 1994; 334:1461-5.

In this double-blind, placebo-controlled trial, 1 of 100 amoxicillin-treated women versus 12 of 99 erythromycin-treated women stopped therapy because of unacceptable side effects of medication, and one remaining woman in the amoxicillin group had a culture positive for *Chlamydia* at follow-up—an overall failure rate of 12% in the erythromycin group and 2% in the amoxicillin group ($p = 0.005$).

A controlled trial of intravenous immune globulin for the prevention of serious bacterial infections in children receiving zidovudine for advanced human immunodeficiency virus infection

Spector SA, Gelber RD, McGrath N, et al. N Engl J Med 1994;331:1181-7.

Monthly intravenous doses of immune globulin decreased the rate of serious bacterial infection from 24.3% to 16.9%, but the benefit appeared to be limited to children not receiving trimethoprim-sulfamethoxazole prophylaxis; the 2-year survival rate was not affected.

Edith Potter

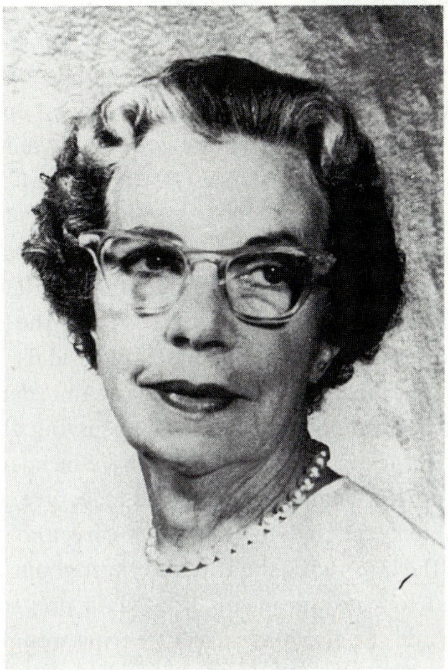

The only daughter of a locomotive engineer, Edith Potter was born in Wisconsin and during early childhood moved to Minnesota. She completed medical school at the University of Minnesota in 1925 and interned at Minneapolis Hospital, and then went to Vienna for further studies. When she returned to Minnesota in 1927, she started a medical practice and, at the same time, took pathology courses with Dr. E. T. Bell, the University of Minnesota's chairman of pathology, whom she said had the greatest influence on her professional life. Thereafter, she accepted a pathology fellowship and obtained her doctor of philosophy degree in pathology in 1934.

Dr. Potter then moved to Chicago and worked with Dr. F. L. Adair, the chief of the newly opened Chicago Lying-in Hospital. While there, she became alarmed at the high infant mortality rate and focused her interest in the study and causes of infant deaths, devoting her professional career to the study of perinatal pathology.

As a young physician in the 1930s, Edith Potter established, virtually single-handedly, the medical subspecialty of perinatal pathology. Her pioneering work at the Chicago Lying-in Hospital (the obstetrics-gynecology teaching unit for the University of Chicago School of Medicine) in the causes of deaths in newborn infants resulted in a significant decline in infant mortality rates.

Early in her career, Dr. Potter had become alarmed at the high infant mortality rate. "Up to that time," she explained, "when a baby died it was considered an act of God. There was very little known about that time of life; even the word 'perinatal' did not yet exist. What little material there was, was dispersed among many medical journals."

It was customary in those days for the health departments in many cities to bury any baby who died within the first month of life, or any stillborn baby, so that the family would not be put to any expense. To be able to do the necessary studies to determine the cause of the babies' deaths, Edith Potter made it difficult for a mortician to obtain a burial permit for any child on whom an autopsy had not been performed. Subsequently the medical examiner made autopsies mandatory for all perinatal deaths in Chicago.

Through postmortem studies of stillborn and newborn infants in Chicago, Dr. Potter showed that the two leading causes of perinatal death at that time were intracranial hemorrhage and anoxia brought about by long labors and traumatic delivery methods. She and Dr. Adair published the preliminary results of their studies in 1940 in *Fetal and Neo-Natal Death*. In 1952 the first edition of what is now *Pathology of the Fetus and Newborn Infant* was published. It was revised in 1961 and, with Dr. John Craig, the third edition was completed in 1976. This text is monumental and represents the first comprehensive presentation of perinatal pathology, including a spectacular array of malformations that Dr. Potter had personally studied.

Edith Potter spent 33 years at the University of Chicago Medical School as pathologist at the Chicago Lying-in Hospital, and rose from the rank of instructor to full professor. During this time she was director of the laboratories, including surgical pathology, and she performed autopsies on more than 10,000 fetuses and infants. She authored a total of six books and published 140 scientific papers. She was the first woman member of the American Gynecological Society. Among her scores of honors are awards from the University of Minnesota, the New York Infirmary, the National Association for Retarded Children, the American Gynecological Society, and the City of Hope. In 1983 she was inducted into the Hall of Fame of the American Col-

THE JOURNAL OF PEDIATRICS 1995;126:845-6

0022-3476/95/$3.00 + 0 **9/20/60734**

lege of Obstetricians and Gynecologists, in Washington, D.C. She received honorary degrees from the University of Brazil, the University of Pennsylvania, and the University of South Florida. She was also made an honorary member of the Society for Pediatric Pathology.

Dr. Potter was among the first to do research on the Rh factor, and her work included a number of papers and her book *Rh: Its Relation to Congenital Hemolytic Disease and to Intragroup Transfusion Reactions*, published in 1947. She was the first to discover a distinctive facial appearance in infants with urinary system defects associated with oligohydramnios, now called the "Potter facies" and the "Potter sequence."

Dr. Potter traveled extensively during her career and continued to travel after her retirement. In 1950, she spent several months in South America, studying the causes of stillbirths and infant deaths, and lectured widely in Brazil, Uruguay, and Argentina. During that same decade, she traveled to Japan and Korea, as well as serving as consultant to the Surgeon General of the Army. She spent several months in Australia and New Zealand to lecture and investigate problems related to maternity care and perinatal deaths. In the late 1950s she traveled throughout Africa to lecture and to study problems related to pregnancy and childbirth, and she also made a lecture trip through Central America. In 1960 she went on a month-long mission to the Soviet Union to investigate maternal and child healthcare services.

After retirement from the University of Chicago and the Chicago Lying-in Hospital in 1967, with her husband Alvin Meyer, an architectural sculptor whom she married in 1943, Dr. Potter moved to Fort Myers, Florida. She pursued interests in tropical horticulture and earned a reputation as a gourmet cook. While still pursuing her interests in medical research, she continued to study the effects of diethylstilbestrol (DES) on the reproductive tracts of men and women.

After the death of her first husband in 1976, Dr. Potter married a family friend, Frank Deats, who was also an architect and an accomplished water colorist. She was widowed again in 1983.

Edith Potter had a zest for life. At 87 years of age she said, "I'm busier now than I have ever been—isn't life wonderful!"

Those who knew Dr. Potter personally recall with great fondness and admiration the strength of her character, her great human qualities, and her zest for knowledge. Her life can be described as inspirational. Despite her battle against colon cancer, she pursued her life and interests to the full. In 1988, in tribute to her years of dedicated service to medical education, the annual Edith Potter Lectureship was established at the University of South Florida at Fort Myers.

Dr. Edith Potter Deats died March 22, 1993, at sea while taking a cruise in the Caribbean, at the age of 91 years.

Looking back over the nearly nine decades of an extraordinary life, Dr. Edith Potter said she had few regrets. "I only wish I had asked for more help and more money to do my work. That's really the only thing I would change."

Enid Gilbert-Barness, MD
Tampa, Florida

EDITORIAL CORRESPONDENCE

Cost of ribavirin therapy for respiratory syncytial virus infection

To the Editor:

Englund et al.[1] compared standard ribavirin therapy (6 gm administered by aerosol during an 18-hour period) with high-dose, short-duration ribavirin therapy (6 gm administered during 2-hour periods three times a day). They concluded that the high-dose, short-duration therapy improved access to patients by health care workers and allowed patient visits by family members. The drug cost for the high-dose, short-duration therapy is three times as much as standard therapy. I doubt that increasing drug costs can be justified by increased patient access. The study was supported by a grant from ICN Pharmaceuticals, the manufacturer of ribavirin.

I suggest that the authors next compare ribavirin therapy, 6 gm administered during an 18-hour period, with ribavirin, 6 gm administered during a 2-hour period once daily. Drugs costs would then be the same in both groups, and the results could determine differences in efficacy, safety, and environmental issues.

Eric D. Marquardt, PharmD
Department of Pharmacy
University of California, Davis Medical Center
2315 Stockton Blvd.
Sacramento, CA 95817
9/35/62989

REFERENCE

1. Englund JA, Piedra PA, Ahn Y-M, Gilbert BE, Hiatt P. High-dose, short duration ribavirin aerosol therapy compared with standard ribavirin therapy in children with suspected respiratory syncytial virus infection. J PEDIATR 1994;125:635-41.

Reply

To the Editor:

Dr. Marquardt stated that using high-dose, short-duration ribavirin therapy would result in a tripling of drug costs. He is mistaken. As stated in the Methods section of our article, we used either 6 gm ribavirin per 300 ml water (20 mg/ml during 18 hours) or 6 gm per 100 ml water (60 mg/ml during 6 hours; i.e., for a 2-hour period three times daily),[1] thus using the standard 6 gm vial of drug daily. With both regimens, the ribavirin solution was changed once a day, resulting in the use of a single, 6 gm vial of drug per day per patient. The drug costs were the same, with concomitant improvement in patient access, patient compliance, and reduction in environmental contamination (not merely in patient access).

This study was based on earlier animal studies in cotton rats and mice, indicating comparable efficacy between the two ribavirin regimens,[2, 3] as well as our subsequent pharmacokinetic evaluation in infected children.[4] Dr. Marquardt asked us to study ribavirin administered during one 18-hour period per day versus that administered during a 2-hour period each day because of "drug costs." Because drug costs are already the same, and there are no animal studies or pharmacokinetic models published on this schedule, such a study would be difficult for us to rationalize. However, we recognize that the cost of ribavirin therapy is exceedingly high and is a major roadblock to its widespread use. It is unfortunate that prices have recently been substantially increased, which in our opinion may result in drug being administered to fewer patients who might potentially benefit.

Janet A. Englund, MD
Pedro A. Piedra, MD
Brian E. Gilbert, PhD
Departments of Microbiology and Immunology, and Pediatrics
Baylor College of Medicine
Houston, TX 77030
9/35/62990

REFERENCES

1. Englund JA, Piedra PA, Ahn Y-M, Gilbert BE, Hiatt P. High-dose, short-duration ribavirin aerosol therapy compared with standard ribavirin therapy in children with suspected respiratory syncytial virus infection. J PEDIATR 1994;125:635-41.
2. Wyde PR, Wilson SZ, Petrella R, Gilbert BE. Efficacy of high dose-short duration ribavirin aerosol in the treatment of respiratory syncytial virus-infected cotton rats and influenza B virus-infected mice. Antiviral Res 1987;7:211-20.
3. Wyde PR, Wilson SZ, Gilbert BE, Smith RHA. Protection of mice from lethal influenza virus infection with high dose-short duration ribavirin aerosol. Antimicrob Agents Chemother 1986;30:942-4.
4. Englund JA, Pedro PA, Jefferson LS, Wilson SZ, Taber LH, Gilbert BE. High-dose, short-duration ribavirin aerosol therapy in children with suspected respiratory syncytial virus infection. J PEDIATR 1990;117:313-20.

Opsoclonus-myoclonus and recurrent neuroblastoma

To the Editor:

The article by Koh et al.[1] again brings to the forefront the value of opsoclonus-myoclonus and ataxia in heralding occult neuroblastoma. The authors note that opsoclonus and other neurologic symptoms may resolve and recur with or without treatment, but do not mention that these signs can signal recurrence of the malignancy itself—a scenario illustrated by a patient under our care who had no neurologic symptoms when first seen but who had opsoclonus and ataxia on two later recurrences of her neuroblastoma. There is no previous report of this phenomenon, and this has major implications for managing patients with this disorder.

In our patient, stage IV neuroblastoma (with elevated urinary homovanillic and vanillylmandelic acid concentrations and a normal serum ferritin level) was diagnosed at the age of 4½ years after a cervical mass was noted. She had no neurologic symptoms at the time. She was successfully treated with chemotherapy, total body irradiation, and autologous bone marrow transplant. After 18 months of remission, opsoclonus, ataxia, and dysarthria developed. There are two previously reported cases of delayed-onset opsoclonus (occurring at 7 and 15 months, respectively) after treatment for neuroblastoma.[2, 3] We initially considered that our patient might be included in this category; however, during her evaluation we found recurrent abdominal neuroblastoma. She was treated with radiation therapy for the tumor and prednisone for the opsoclonus; remission of the tumor and resolution of opsoclonus were achieved. Eight months later, she was again noted to have opsoclonus and an exacerbation of her ataxia while being weaned from steroid therapy. She was found to have recurrent neuroblastoma and was successfully treated with chemotherapy and a syngeneic bone marrow transplant from an identical twin sister. Her recurrent opsoclonus resolved after another course of steroid therapy. Our patient has had learning difficulties, both because of the time spent in treatment and bilateral hearing loss and cataracts as a result of her treatment. Although her development is within normal limits, she has multiple behavioral difficulties requiring intervention.

We believe that this unique presentation of this paraneoplastic syndrome in a readily recognized case of neuroblastoma emphasizes the need to pursue the diagnosis of neuroblastoma (or recurrent neuroblastoma) aggressively in any child who has these abnormal neurologic symptoms.

William T. Basco, Jr., MD
Miguel Abboud, MD
Department of Pediatrics
Kenton R. Holden, MD
Department of Neurology
Medical University of South Carolina
Charleston, SC 29425
9/35/62987

REFERENCES

1. Koh PS, Raffensperger JG, Berry S, et al. Long-term outcome in children with opsoclonus-myoclonus and ataxia and coincident neuroblastoma. J PEDIATR 1994;125:712-6.
2. Delalieux C, Ebinger G, Maurus R, Sliwowski H. Myoclonic encephalopathy and neuroblastoma [Letter]. N Engl J Med 1975;292:46-7.
3. Rupprecht L, Mortier W. Cerebellåre bewegungsstörung und neuroblastoma. (Cerebellar motor disturbance and neuroblastoma). Monatschr Kinderheilkd 1975;123:392-3.

Cystic fibrosis and episodic arthritis

To the Editor:

We read with interest the article by Wulffraat et al.[1] about cystic fibrosis (CF) and arthritis. The authors affirm that episodic arthritis in patients with CF resembles reactive arthritis and the arthritis of Reiter syndrome, disorders associated with the presence of HLA-B27. This statement, however, is not completely correct because reactive arthritis and Reiter syndrome, usually much more frequent in patients in whom HLA-B27 antigen is present, can also develop in patients without HLA-B27 antigen, even in the absence of its cross-reactive antigens, such as HLA-B7, HLA-B22, and HLA-B40.[2]

Wulffraat et al. also discuss the character of CF arthritis, underline the limited clearance capacity of the reticuloendothelial system in this situation, and describe the results of sputum cultures of patients, but they do not stress the importance of *Pseudomonas aeruginosa* colonization in the pathogenesis of arthritis or vasculitic lesions associated with CF episodic arthritis. Sixteen patients with purpuric rash and five of eight patients with CF arthritis described by Schidlow et al.[3, 4] had *Pseudomonas* species in their respiratory secretions. In our center, three of 125 patients (two male subjects and one female subject) have episodic arthritis. The age at onset was the second decade of life. All these patients have liver involvement, have chronical *P. aeruginosa* colonization, and have high levels of anti–*P. aeruginosa* antibodies. Arthritis is pauciarticular and asymmetric; the most commonly affected joints are the knees, ankles, and proximal interphalangeals, and in two cases purpuric rash is present on the skin of the lower extremities. Laboratory investigations reveal an increased erythrocyte sedimentation rate and elevated levels of C-reactive protein and immunoglobulins. Results of tests to detect antinuclear antibody and rheumatoid factor are negative. The third and fourth components of complement, total hemolytic complement, and uric acid values are all within normal range. Enzyme-linked immunosorbent assay to detect circulating immune complexes binding the C1q and C3d subunits of complement, detectable in 20.3% of all our patients with CF, indicates the presence of these substances in two patients with CF arthritis. No association with HLA type has been shown. Recurrence of acute arthritis had been described by the patients before antibiotic treatment was administered. The duration of episodes varied from 2 to 7 days with recurrence at intervals of several weeks. Episodic arthritis has been nondestructive, without progression to erosive arthritis. Our patients are usually treated with nonsteroidal antiinflammatory drugs, but in some episodes arthritis remitted spontaneously. The clinical pattern and the frequent association with purpuric rash may be related to circulating immune complex arthritis. In our experience,[5] routine rheumatologic studies fail to reveal any explanation for the nature of these attacks, but continuous antigenic stimulation produced by the persistence of *P. aeruginosa* may be responsible for immune stimulation, production of antibodies against *P. aeruginosa* and immune complexes. Tissue deposition of circulating immune complexes containing *P. aeruginosa* antigen and a malfunction of clearance by the mononuclear phagocyte system in the damaged liver could be responsible for acute episodic CF arthritis.

G. Taccetti, MD
S. Campana, MB
L. Marianelli, MD
Cystic Fibrosis Center
Meyer Hospital
University of Florence
Florence, Italy

S. Turchini, MD
Medical Clinic III Institut
University of Florence
Florence, Italy
9/35/63324

REFERENCES

1. Wulffraat NM, de Graeff-Meeder ER, Rijkers GT, van der Laag H, Kuis W. Prevalence of circulating immune complexes in patients with cystic fibrosis and arthritis. J PEDIATR 1994;125:374-8.
2. Ford DK. Reiter's syndrome: reactive arthritis. In: McCarty DJ, ed. Arthritis and allied conditions. Philadelphia: Lea & Febiger, 1989:944-53.
3. Schidlow DV, Goldsmith DP, Palmer J, Huang NN. Arthritis in cystic fibrosis. Arch Dis Child 1984;59:377-9.
4. Schidlow DV, Panitch HB, Zaeri N, Zenel J, Alpert BE. Purpuric rashes in cystic fibrosis. Am J Dis Child 1989;143:1030-2.
5. Taccetti G, Campana S, Ferrari R. Cystic fibrosis and acute episodic arthritis: our experience. Clin Exp Rheumatol 1994;12(suppl 10):S-134.

Reply

To the Editor:

Taccetti et al. state that the artritis seen in patients with cystic fibrosis cannot be entirely compared with the arthritis in Reiter syndrome because this arthritis occurs both in individuals with and without HLA-B27 antigen. However, the purpose of our statement was merely to describe the clinical resemblance of the arthritis with patients with Reiter syndrome, in the majority of whom HLA-B27 is present.

We fully agree with Tacetti et al. that *Pseudomonas aeruginosa* colonization should be considered as a possible cause for arthritis mediated by circulating immune complexes. However, *P. aeruginosa* is one of the bacteria most frequently found in the sputum of all patients with CF who have respiratory problems.[1, 2] *P. aeruginosa* was detected in the sputum of 6 of the 8 patients in the arthritis group and in 10 of the 14 patients in our control group. The mere presence of a *P. aeruginosa* infection cannot be an explanation for the arthritis. It is then tempting to speculate on differences in the response to the *P. aeruginosa* infection. The occurrence of circulating immune complexes in patients with CF is well known.[3] A limited clearance capacity of the circulating immune complexes containing the *P. aeruginosa* antigen may cause arthritis in some individuals, but this was not tested in our study.

The degree of liver involvement in our study was the same in both CF groups, as was the degree of pulmonary involvement, but we must stress that we studied a pediatric population.

N. M. Wulffraat, MD, PhD
E. R. de Graeff-Meeder, MD, PhD
G. T. Rijkers, PhD
H. van der Laag, MD
W. Kuis, MD, PhD
University Hospital for Children and Youth "Het Wilhelmina Kinderziekenhuis"
Utrecht, The Netherlands
9/35/63325

REFERENCES

1. Elborn JS, Shale DJ. Lung injury in cystic fibrosis. Thorax 1990;45:970-3.
2. Fegan M, Francis P, Hayward AC, Fuerst JA. Heterogeneity, persistence, and distribution of *Pseudomonas aeruginosa* genotypes in cystic fibrosis patients. J Clin Microbiol 1991;29:2151-7.
3. Wisnieski JJ, Todd EW, Fuller RK, et al. Immune complexes and complement abnormalities in patients with cystic fibrosis. Am Rev Respir Dis 1985;132:770-6.

Helicobacter pylori infection in neurologically impaired children

To the Editor:

Proujansky et al.[1] reported on the observation that the incidence of symptomatic *Helicobacter pylori* infection is increased in children with severe neurologic impairments. The authors describe a number of clinical features associated with the manifestations of this infection. We recently treated a 6-year-old boy with severe idiopathic mental retardation who had rumination and numerous other behavioral disorders. He had a history of gastroesophageal reflux as an infant that was previously successfully treated with metoclopramide. He had frequent episodes of regurgitating his food, chewing on it and swallowing, or occasionally spitting it out. A 99mTc-sulfur colloid milk scan revealed delayed gastric emptying, with no reflux or aspiration. Results of upper gastrointestinal series showed no anatomic abnormality, but delayed gastric emptying and nodularity of the distal antrum and duodenal bulb. Upper endoscopy revealed duodenal and plyloric irritation. Intraoperative gastric biopsy showed severe acute inflammation, and an acridine orange stain indicated the presence of *Helicobacter pylori*. The child was treated with amoxicillin, metronidazole, bismuth subsalicylate, and ranitidine. Clinical improvement and decreased frequency of rumination were noted, and weight remained stable. Cisapride was later added to his therapeutic regimen as a prokinetic agent.

Rumination occurs more frequently in patients with developmental disabilities. Treatable medical causes such as delayed gastric emptying or *Helicobacter* infection could facilitate development of a behavior pattern of rumination by making the gastric contents available to the mouth. In addition to the symptoms described by Proujansky et al., rumination may be a possible symptom of *Helicobacter* infection in individuals with developmental disabilities.

Joyce Elizabeth Mauk, MD
Children's Seashore House and
University of Pennsylvania School of Medicine
Philadelphia, PA, 19104
9/35/63158

REFERENCE

1. Proujansky R, Shaffer SE, Vinton NE, Bachrach SJ. Symptomatic *Helicobacter pylori* infection in young patients with severe neurologic impairment. J PEDIATR 1994;125:750-2.

Reply

To the Editor:

Our article focused on the association between *Helicobacter pylori* and a diverse group of symptoms in neurologically impaired patients; we did not devote significant attention to the variable nature of clinical presentations. One of our patients who had refusal to feed had been thought to have predominantly a behavioral disorder. Only after documentation of *H. pylori* infection and a prompt increase in appetite with effective therapy did it become clear that this was not a behavioral disorder. It is our belief that the usual symptoms of *H. pylori* infection such as nausea, vomiting, dyspeptic symptoms, or anorexia could potentially lead to a number of behavioral responses in the neurologically impaired patient. It will be interesting to observe, as this diagnosis is pursued more aggressively in this group of patients, the full spectrum of clinical manifestations. At the same time, for some of our patients *H. pylori* infection was coexistent with other gastrointestinal problems, particularly gastroesophageal reflux. Thus attributing a specific behavior or symptom to the presence of *H. pylori* infection in a specific patient requires demonstration of improvement of this symptom with effective therapy for *Helicobacter* infection, and documentation of resolution of the infectious process.

Roy Proujansky, MD
Stephen Shaffer, MD
Nancy Vinton, MD
Steven Bachrach, MD
Alfred I. duPont Institute
Wilmington, DE 19899
9/35/63157

Promotion of healthy eating habits in children

To the Editor:

I enjoyed the article by Whitaker et al.,[1] but was disappointed that the results were only modest. During the study intervention, the selection of low-fat food items by students in the school cafeterias increased by 4% compared with baseline. The intervention involved modifying elementary school lunch menus to emphasize the low-fat entrees. The parents of the students were mailed a package that included a modified menu, an educational pamphlet on healthy diets, and a letter explaining the availability of low-fat diets in the menu. No component of the intervention directly educated the children on the significance of low-fat diets in disease prevention. This specific component is essential for promoting positive behavior change.

Behavior change can result from the modification of three types of factors that influence health behaviors—predisposing factors, enabling factors, and reinforcing factors.[2] Predisposing factors include individuals' knowledge, attitudes, and beliefs surrounding a particular health issue. Enabling factors provide access to resources or teach particular skills to assist in the modification of the behavior. Reinforcing factors either positively or negatively influence a particular behavior to encourage and maintain behavior change. In this study, the predisposing factors were not specifically addressed.

Encouraging changes in the dietary habits of children for health promotion and disease prevention can be a challenging and difficult task. Effective change can be achieved by multiple and integrative strategies that target all three types of factors that influence the behavior.

Sherry R. Crump, MD
Morehouse School of Medicine
Department of Community Health and
Preventive Medicine
720 Westview Dr. S.W.
Atlanta, GA 30310
9/35/63154

REFERENCES

1. Whitaker RC, Wright JA, Koepsell TD, Finch AJ, Psaty BM. Randomized intervention to increase children's selection of low-fat foods in school lunches. J PEDIATR 1994;125:535-40.
2. Green LW. Prevention and health education. In: Last JM, Wallace RB, eds. Public health and preventive medicine. 13th edt. Norwalk, Connecticut: Appleton & Lange, 1992:787-802.

Reply

To the Editor:

We agree, in principle, with an approach to dietary interventions that integrates different strategies for behavior change,[1] but we deliberately omitted a direct educational component targeting the students. In choosing among intervention strategies, we considered their potential efficacy, cost, ease of implementation, and generalizability. Failure to consider these factors may lead to designing interventions that cannot be maintained in the study setting after the formal research has ended, or cannot be transferred to other settings where resources are more modest. Our approach, therefore, was to find a minimal, rather than maximal, intervention that would result in changing a specific observed dietary behavior—selection of low-fat foods in school lunches.

Unfortunately, there is little evidence that changes in nutrition knowledge, attitudes, or beliefs in children (predisposing factors) are related to changes in observed (as distinct from reported) dietary behavior.[2] The beneficial effects, if any, of classroom nutrition education on eating behavior have been hard to detect. Nutrition education curricula are difficult to implement evenly across units of intervention (schools, classes, or students). School food-service departments may not have adequate resources, and teachers may already be burdened by competing curriculum demands (e.g., drug use and violence prevention).

We also believe that the simultaneous application of different strategies (for example, classroom nutrition education and altered food choice availability) may leave the investigator unable to determine the relative efficacy of each strategy. Those who wish to go on and implement components of a studied, multifaceted intervention may be unable to assess which components of the intervention were most potent.

Given these considerations, we decided on two interventions (increased availability of low-fat foods and menu labeling), applied them in succession, and determined the relatively greater impact of the former. Both interventions are still in place in this school district 2 years after the end of data collection. Our findings do not deny the potential value of attempting to influence nutrition knowledge, attitudes, and beliefs. However, had either of our interventions also concurrently attempted to change these predisposing factors, we would have been unable to say "what worked."

Robert C. Whitaker, MD, MPH
Jeffrey A. Wright, MD
Department of Pediatrics
University of Washington School of Medicine
Seattle, WA 98195

Thomas D. Koepsell, MD, MPH
Bruce M. Psaty, MD, PhD
Department of Epidemiology
University of Washington School of Public Health and Community Medicine
Seattle, WA 98195

Anita J. Finch, MS, RD
Bellevue Public Schools, District No. 405
Bellevue, WA 98009
9/35/63155

REFERENCES

1. Green LW. Prevention and health education. In: Last JM, Wallace RB, eds. Maxcy-Rosenau-Last public health and preventive medicine. 13th ed. Norwalk, Connecticut: Appleton & Lange, 1992:787-802.
2. Contento IR, Manning AD, Shannon B. Research perspective on school-based nutrition education. J Nutr Educ 1992;24:247-60.

Congenital nephrotic syndrome in neonatal lupus syndrome

To the Editor:

Massengil et al.[1] reported the occurrence of nephrotic syndrome in one 6-week-old and one 3-month-old child with infantile systemic lupus erythematosus (SLE), simulating a congenital nephrotic syndrome. Both children were born to mothers without clinical or serologic evidence of SLE or other connective tissue disease. The authors stressed the importance of distinguishing infantile SLE from the neonatal lupus syndrome (NLS), a condition occurring in children born to mothers with SLE or some other connective tissue disease.[2, 3] Most children with NLS have congenital heart block or cutaneous SLE caused by transplacental transport of antibodies to the fetus. Deposition of immunoglobulins and complement in cardiac tissue has been reported and implicated in the pathogenesis of congenital heart block.[4, 5] However, to the best of our knowledge, nephrotic syndrome or nephritis has not been reported in NLS. An explanation could be that there is no antibody deposition in the fetal kidney, perhaps because the renal antigens involved are not yet present.

We studied renal tissue from an 18-week-old fetus born to a 28-year-old woman with SLE Test results for anti–double-stranded DNA, anticardiolipin, anti-IgG, and anti-ribonucleoprotein antibodies were positive, and the patient had low levels of the third and fourth components of complement. The woman had a good response to prednisone therapy and never had clinical signs of renal disease. A renal biopsy was never performed. Eight months before, her first pregnancy ended in a stillbirth at 15 weeks. In the eighteenth week of her second pregnancy, she had HELLP syndrome (hemolysis, elevated liver enzymes, and low platelets), and labor was induced. At that time she was still receiving a high dose of prednisone and had no clinical signs of active disease. Autopsy of the fetus did not show macroscopic or microscopic abnormalities. Renal histologic findings were in accordance with fetal age, and no pathologic changes were observed. Immunofluorescence microscopy demonstrated focal deposition of IgG, the third component of complement and fibrin along capillary loops and in the mesangium of maturing deep cortical glomeruli, without deposits of IgM, IgA, or the C1q subunit of the first component of complement. No deposits were found in primitive superficial cortical glomeruli. Studies with antibodies against IgA, IgG, IgM, the third component of complement, the c1q subunit of the first component of complement, and fibrin showed no glomerular staining in another 18-week and a 19-week-old fetus.

These data suggest that glomerular immunodeposits are probably present in at least some neonates born to mothers with SLE. Their presence is apparently not sufficient to cause clinical symptoms, because nephritis has never been reported in NLS. Alternatively, lupus nephritis may occur in NLS but be unnoticed.

P. J. Westenend, MD
Department of Pathology
University Hospital Nijmegen
PO Box 9101
6500 HB Nijmegen, The Netherlands
9/35/62986

REFERENCES

1. Massengil SF, Richard GA, Donnelly WH. Infantile systemic lupus erythematosus with onset simulating congenital nephrotic syndrome. J PEDIATR 1994;124:27-31.
2. Kitridou RC, Mintz G. The neonatal lupus syndrome. In: Wallace DJ, Hahn BH, Quismorio JP Jr, Klinenberg JR, eds. Dubois' lupus erythematosus. 4th ed. Philadelphia: Lea & Febiger, 1993:516-22.
3. Buyon JL. Neonatal lupus syndromes. Am J Reprod Immunol 1992;28:259-63.
4. Litsey SE, Noonan JA, O'Connor WN, Cottrill CM, Mitchell B. Maternal connective tissue disease and congenital heart block. Demonstration of immunoglobulin in cardiac tissue. N Engl J Med 1985;312:98-100.
5. Taylor PV, Scott JS, Gerlis LM, Esscher E, Scott O. Maternal antibodies against fetal cardiac antigens in congenital complete heart block. N Engl J Med 1986;315:667-72.

Pancreatitis and organic acidemias

To the Editor:

Kahler et al. (J PEDIATR 1994;124:239-43) report a collaborative investigation on "Pancreatitis in Patients with Organic Acidemia," and conclude that pancreatitis may be a complication of branched-chain organic acidemias. Pancreatitis was also previously reported by Wilson et al.[1] in a patient with 3-methylglutaryl–coenzyme A lyase deficiency, which cleaves 3-hydroxy-3-methylglutaric acid to acetoacetate and acetyl–coenzyme A.

We saw a 10-month-old infant with 3-methylglutaconic (3-MGC) aciduria; he was the third child born to nonconsanguineous Italian parents. The parents had previously had a son with microcephaly, mental retardation, and seizures. Cerebellar vermis hypoplasia was observed with computed tomographic scanning; recurrent episodes of hematemesis and melena were the causes of his death at the age of 2 years.

Our patient was referred for the evaluation of psychomotor delay. Laboratory investigations revealed increased transaminase values. Plasma amino acids, lactate, free and acylcarnitines were all normal. Urine organic acid analysis revealed the consistent elimination of 3-MGC acid and 3-methylglutaric acid. Mithochondrial respiratory chain enzymes (complex IV, II, and III) were normal. Computed tomographic scanning of the brain revealed severe cerebellar vermis hypoplasia. During admission, the child suddenly had diarrhea and vomiting followed by severe hematemesis and melena. Acute pancreatitis was found by laparoscopy. During the following days, renal insufficiency developed; a few days after the operation, the child died with signs of intravascular disseminated coagulation. Evidence is growing that many conditions with brain involvement may be associated with 3-MGC aciduria, and further studies are still in progress to determine whether in our patient this was a primary or a secondary phenomenon (mitochondrial disorder, anomalies of polyisoprenoid metabolism?). At any rate, to our knowledge this case represents the first observation of pancreatitis in a patient with 3-MGC aciduria. The mechanism of damage to the pancreas in patients with organic acidurias is unknown. It is may be supposed that, as in patients with Reye syndrome, metabolic disarrangement may cause damage to the pancreatic tissue, activating pancreatic enzymes in an inappropriate location.

A. Fiumara
R. Barone
F. Nigro
A. Ribes
L. Pavone
Department of Pediatrics, University of Catania
Catania, Italy
Institut of Biochemistry
Barcelona, Spain
9/35/62712

REFERENCE

1. Wilson WG, Cass MB, Sovik O, Gibson KM, Sweetman L. A child with acute pancreatitis and recurrent hypoglycemia due to 3-hydroxy-3-methylglutaryl-CoA lyase deficiency. Eur J Pediatr 1984;142:289-91.

THE JOURNAL OF
PEDIATRICS

JUNE 1995 Volume 126 Number 6

MEDICAL PROGRESS

Recent developments in the pathophysiology and treatment of persistent pulmonary hypertension of the newborn

John P. Kinsella, MD, and Steven H. Abman, MD

From the Department of Pediatrics, Divisions of Neonatology and Pulmonary Medicine, Children's Hospital and the University of Colorado School of Medicine, Denver, Colorado

Persistent pulmonary hypertension of the newborn is a complex disorder associated with a wide array of cardiopulmonary diseases, which are characterized by marked pulmonary hypertension and altered vasoreactivity, leading to right-to-left shunting of blood across the patent ductus arteriosus and foramen ovale.[1-3] Extrapulmonary shunting associated with high pulmonary vascular resistance in severe PPHN can cause critical hypoxemia, which is often poorly responsive to inspired oxygen or pharmacologic vasodilation.[4] However, the syndrome of PPHN is often associated with severe parenchymal lung disease (e.g., lung hypoplasia, meconium aspiration pneumonitis, bacterial pneumonia, and surfactant deficiency), which causes intrapulmonary shunting and further complicates the clinical course and response to treatment. Moreover, disturbances in cardiac performance, hypovolemia, and decreased systemic vascular resistance may compromise the tenuous balance between the systemic and pulmonary circulation in PPHN. Thus effective therapy for neonatal hypoxemic respiratory failure complicated by extrapulmonary venoarterial admixture requires vigilant attention to all aspects of these cardiopulmonary interactions (Fig. 1).

Submitted for publication Aug. 8, 1994; accepted Feb. 10, 1995.

Reprint requests: John P. Kinsella, MD, Division of Neonatology, Box B-070, Children's Hospital, 1056 E. 19th Ave., Denver, CO 80218-1088.

THE JOURNAL OF PEDIATRICS 1995;126:853-64

0022-3476/95/$3.00 + 0 **9/18/64030**

Treatment of PPHN has been limited by the lack of vasodilator agents with selective pulmonary vascular effects and by the ineffectiveness of therapies for severe parenchymal lung disease and systemic hemodynamic collapse (e.g., bacterial sepsis syndromes). The treatment of PPHN has been influenced by recent insights into fetal and transitional pulmonary vasoregulation, newer approaches to management of severe parenchymal lung disease in newborn infants, and the potential role of inhaled nitric oxide as a selective pulmonary vasodilator. We will review (1) recent develop

CDH	Congenital diaphragmatic hernia
ECMO	Extracorporeal membrane oxygenation
ET	Endothelin
HFOV	High-frequency oscillatory ventilation
HMD	Hyaline membrane disease
NO	Nitric oxide
PPHN	Persistent pulmonary hypertension of the newborn

ments in vascular biology concerning the endothelial-derived products NO and endothelin and (2) the potential applications (and limitations) of inhalational NO in the management of PPHN.

FETAL AND TRANSITIONAL PULMONARY VASOREGULATION

The fetal circulation is characterized by high pulmonary vascular resistance; pulmonary blood flow accounts for less than 10% of combined ventricular output in the late-gesta-

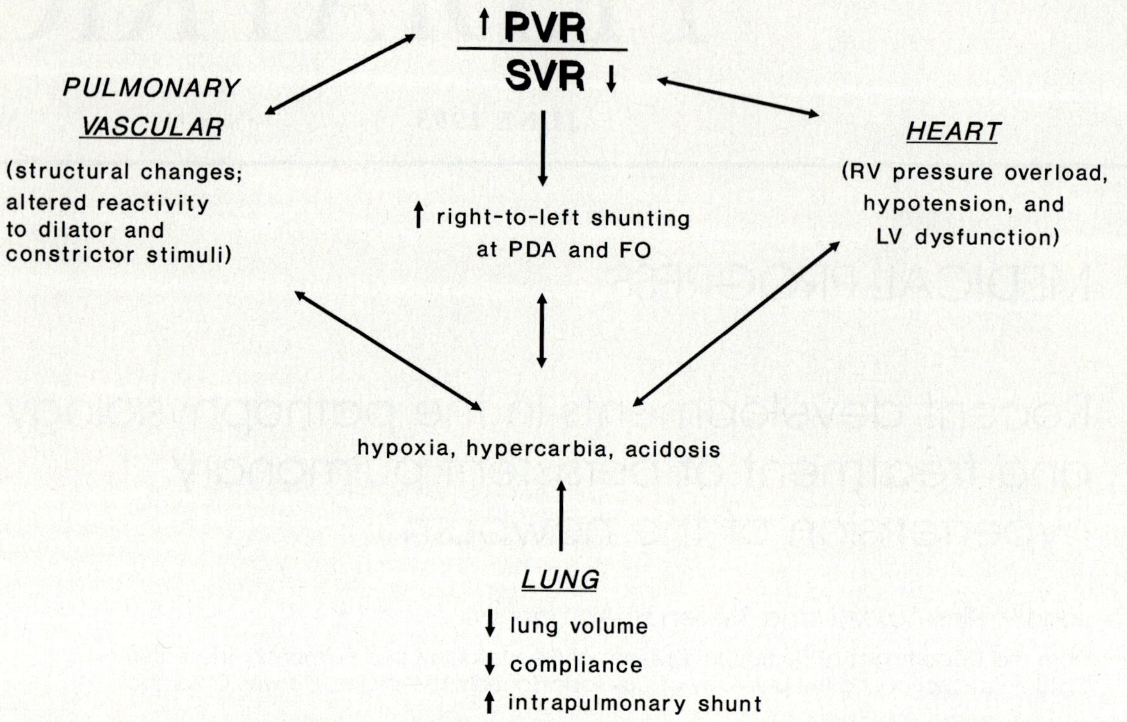

Fig. 1. Cardiopulmonary interactions in PPHN. *PVR*, Pulmonary vascular resistance; *SVR*, systemic vascular resistance; *PDA*, patent ductus arteriosus; *FO*, foramen ovale; *RV*, right ventricular; *LV*, left ventricular.

tion ovine fetus.[5] Mechanisms responsible for maintaining high fetal pulmonary vascular resistance and causing sustained pulmonary vasodilation at birth are incompletely understood; however, studies in fetal and transitional pulmonary vasoregulation have led to increased understanding of the normal physiologic control of pulmonary vascular resistance. Fetal and neonatal pulmonary vascular tone is modulated through a balance between vasoconstrictor and vasodilator stimuli, including mechanical factors (e.g., lung volume) and endogenous mediators (Table). Among multiple vasoactive mediators involved in perinatal pulmonary vasoregulation, recent interest has focused on endothelin. Endothelin type 1 is a vasoactive peptide produced by vascular endothelium that is unique in its ability to cause potent and sustained vasoconstriction.[6] In the late-gestation ovine fetal lung, brief infusions of ET-1 cause transient vasodilation; however, with prolonged infusion, pulmonary vascular resistance increases.[7] Similar to the effects of other vasoactive mediators, the effects of ET-1 on pulmonary vascular resistance are also tone dependent, causing pulmonary vasoconstriction in the ventilated lung.[8] The effects of endothelin on pulmonary vascular resistance in the normal fetus are mediated through distinct receptor subtypes,[9] two of which have been identified. The ET_A receptor has been localized to the vascular smooth muscle cell,[10] and the ET_B receptor is present on the vascular endothelial cell.[11]

In the late-gestation ovine fetus, intrapulmonary infusions of BQ 123 (a selective ET_A receptor antagonist) caused sustained reductions in pulmonary vascular resistance, which suggests that endogenous endothelin formation contributes to basal pulmonary vascular tone in the fetus. In contrast, selective ET_B receptor stimulation (sarafotoxin S6c) causes pulmonary vasodilation through endothelial cell NO release. Similarly, inhibition of endogenous NO formation attenuates the dilator response to exogenous ET-1.[12] It is likely that endogenous production of ET-1 by vascular endothelium primarily causes pulmonary vasoconstriction by its action on the A receptor of the vascular smooth muscle cell.[13]

It is possible that endothelin contributes to the altered vasoreactivity in the pulmonary circulation of patients with PPHN. Severe hypoxia stimulates endothelin secretion and gene expression in vitro,[14] and the pulmonary vasoconstriction associated with compression of the ductus arteriosus in the late-gestation ovine fetus is caused in part by endothelin stimulation of the pulmonary vascular smooth muscle cell.[15] Moreover, circulating ET-1 levels in human neonates with PPHN are markedly elevated, correlate with disease severity, and decline with resolution of the PPHN.[16] Understanding the role of endothelin in the functional and structural changes characterizing PPHN will be a critical component in studies of this complex disorder.

The vasoconstrictor effects of endothelin are offset by dilator substances produced by the pulmonary vascular endothelium, including the recently described endothelium-de-

Table. Factors that modulate pulmonary vascular resistance in the near-term and term transitional and neonatal pulmonary circulation

Lowers PVR	Increases PVR
Endogenous mediators and mechanisms	Endogenous mediators and mechanisms
Oxygen	Hypoxia
Nitric oxide	Acidosis
PGI_2, E_2, D_2	Endothelin-1
Adenosine, ATP, magnesium	Leukotrienes
Bradykinin	Thromboxanes
Atrial natriuretic factor	Platelet activating factor
Alkalosis	Ca^{++} channel activation
K^+ channel activation	α-Adrenergic stimulation
Histamine	$PGF_{2\alpha}$
Vagal nerve stimulation	Mechanical factors
Acetylcholine	Overinflation or underinflation
β-Adrenergic stimulation	Excessive muscularization, vascular remodeling
Mechanical factors	Altered mechanical properties of smooth muscle
Lung inflation	Pulmonary hypoplasia
Vascular cell structural changes	Alveolar capillary dysplasia
Interstitial fluid and pressure changes	Pulmonary thromboemboli
Shear stress	Main pulmonary artery distention
	Ventricular dysfunction, venous hypertension

PVR, Pulmonary vascular resistance; *PGI_2, E_2, D_2*, prostaglandins I_2, E_2, and D_2; *ATP*, adenosine triphosphate; *$PGF_{2\alpha}$*, prostaglandin $F_{2\alpha}$.

rived relaxing factor, NO. The pharmacologic activity of nitrovasodilators derives from the release of NO, and NO was recognized as a potent vascular smooth muscle relaxant as early as 1979.[17] In 1987 investigators from two separate laboratories reported that the endothelium-derived relaxing factor was NO or an NO-containing substance.[18, 19] Recent reports have described the physiologic role of NO in fetal and transitional pulmonary vasoregulation. NO modulates basal pulmonary vascular tone in the late-gestation fetus; pharmacologic NO blockade inhibits endothelium-dependent pulmonary vasodilation and attenuates the rise in pulmonary blood flow at delivery, implicating endogenous NO formation in postnatal adaptation after birth.[20] Increased fetal oxygen tension augments endogenous NO release,[21, 22] and the increase in pulmonary blood flow in response to rhythmic distention of the lung and high inspired oxygen concentrations are mediated in part by endogenous NO release.[23] However, in these studies the pulmonary circulation was structurally normal. Studies using a model of PPHN in which marked structural pulmonary vascular changes are induced by prolonged fetal ductus arteriosus compression demonstrated that the structurally abnormal pulmonary circulation was also functionally abnormal.[24, 25] Despite the progressive loss of endothelium-dependent (acetylcholine) vasodilation with prolonged ductus compression in this model, the response to endothelium-independent (ANP, NO) vasodilation was intact.[24]

Exogenous (inhaled) NO causes potent, sustained, and selective pulmonary vasodilation in the late-gestation ovine fetus.[26] On the basis of the long-term ambient levels considered to be safe for adults by regulatory agencies in the United States,[27] studies were performed in near-term lambs with the use of inhaled NO at doses of 5, 10, and 20 ppm. Inhaled NO caused a dose-dependent increase in pulmonary blood flow in newborn lambs undergoing mechanical ventilation. Inhaled NO at 20 ppm did not decrease coronary arterial or cerebral blood flow in this model.

Roberts et al.[28] studied the effects of inhaled NO on pulmonary hemodynamics in newborn lambs whose lungs were mechanically ventilated; inhaled NO reversed hypoxic pulmonary vasoconstriction, and maximum vasodilation occurred at doses of greater than 80 ppm. They also found that the vasodilation caused by inhaled NO during hypoxia was not attenuated by respiratory acidosis in this model. Berger et al.[29] investigated the effects of inhaled NO on pulmonary vasodilation during the course of group B streptococcal sepsis in piglets; inhaled NO at 150 ppm for 30 minutes caused marked pulmonary vasodilation but was associated with physiologically significant increases in methemoglobin concentrations. Corroborating studies in other animal models support the observations that inhaled NO is a selective pulmonary vasodilator at low doses (≤20 ppm).[30-31]

CLINICAL TRIALS OF INHALED NO IN INFANTS WITH PPHN

Recent studies have demonstrated that inhaled NO causes marked improvement in oxygenation in many newborn infants with PPHN. Roberts et al.[33] reported that brief (30 minutes) inhalation of NO at 80 ppm improved oxygenation in patients with PPHN, but this response was sustained in only one patient after NO was discontinued. In another report, rapid improvement in oxygenation in neonates with severe PPHN was demonstrated with the use of doses of 20 ppm NO for 4 hours, after which the dose was decreased to 6 ppm for the duration of treatment[34]; this strategy resulted in sustained improvement in oxygenation. In a subsequent study, this low-dose NO strategy was used in an additional nine patients with severe PPHN, including two patients with congenital diaphragmatic hernia.[35] The management incorporated the use of high-frequency oscillatory ventilation to achieve optimal lung inflation during the use of NO. Eight patients had resolution of the underlying PPHN, but one patient with overwhelming sepsis, despite an initial improvement in oxygenation, subsequently required treatment with extracorporeal membrane oxygenation for hemodynamic support. In these pilot studies, we found that 13 of 15 infants with severe PPHN recovered without the need for ECMO.[36] Inhaled NO may also be a useful adjunctive therapy in patients who require early decannulation because of severe complications during ECMO (before reactive pulmonary hypertension has resolved). We have succesfully employed NO in such infants for as long as 21 days after ECMO, at doses as low as 0.35 ppm.

The efficacy of low dose NO ($\leq$20 ppm) in causing acute improvement in oxygenation in patients with severe PPHN has been corroborated in a recent study by Finer et al.[37] These investigators measured the improvement in oxygenation associated with doses of NO ranging from 5 to 80 ppm and found that the acute improvement in oxygenation in PPHN was similar at all doses of NO studied. They also found that oxygen levels increased in patients who did not have extrapulmonary shunting as indicated by echocardiography, which suggests that NO could acutely improve oxygenation in some cases of neonatal hypoxemic respiratory failure without severe PPHN.

MANAGEMENT STRATEGIES IN PPHN

Increasing clinical experience with inhaled NO in PPHN has led to improved understanding of the potential role of this potent and selective pulmonary vasodilator. Although consensus on diagnostic criteria is lacking,[38] for the purposes of this discussion PPHN is defined as severe neonatal hyoxemic respiratory failure associated with extrapulmonary right-to-left shunting of blood across the foramen ovale or patent ductus arteriosus or both. Patients with idiopathic PPHN have severe pulmonary hypertension without apparent parenchymal lung disease. In idiopathic PPHN (i.e., without significant lung disease) the pulmonary management should be directed at minimizing overzealous mechanical ventilation and avoiding lung overinflation. Selective pulmonary vasodilation with inhaled NO may cause marked improvement in oxygenation in patients with idiopathic PPHN. However, myriad pathophysiologic disturbances can cause pulmonary hypertension. PPHN frequently complicates the course of more common causes of neonatal respiratory distress, which are marked by severe lung disease (e.g., lung hypoplasia, meconium aspiration, pneumonitis, and surfactant deficiency). Disturbances in cardiac performance can cause further clinical deterioration.[39] Recognizing the relative roles of the pulmonary vascular, pulmonary parenchymal, and cardiac components contributing to hypoxemic respiratory failure is vital in an assessment of the effects of new therapies in PPHN.

Rudolph,[40] Geggel and Reid,[41] and others have described classifications of PPHN based predominantly on structural abnormalities of the lung and the pulmonary vascular smooth muscle. Severe PPHN has been associated with (1) underdevelopment of the pulmonary circulation (e.g., congenital diaphragmatic hernia), (2) maldevelopment with excessive muscularization of pulmonary arteries, and (3) maladaptation or failure of the pulmonary vascular resistance to decline after birth in an otherwise structurally normal pulmonary vascular bed. As pathologic classifications, these descriptions are important, but the clinical manifestations of severe neonatal hypoxemic respiratory failure are infrequently attributable to a single pathophysiologic or structural classification. It is likely that all cases reflect some measure of "maladaptation" related to the multisystem involvement of this disorder. A limitation of such classifications is exemplified in the syndrome of meconium aspiration. The clinical manifestations of this disease may reflect severe reactive pulmonary hypertension, but the pulmonary parenchymal disease may be variable. Progressive deterioration in oxygenation may be the result of disturbances in cardiac, hemodynamic, or pulmonary function. For example, the chest radiograph may be initially marked by patchy parahilar consolidation associated with aspiration of particulate meconium, but subsequent progression of diffuse parenchymal disease may complicate the clinical course (perhaps related to a "secondary" surfactant deficiency or surfactant inactivation).[42, 43] A subset of patients with this syndrome has predominantly large airways disease associated with aspiration of particulate meconium, leading to the "check valve" type of obstruction, focal overinflation, and air leak. Moreover, decreased cardiac performance and reduced left ventricular output can decrease systemic vascular resistance, exacerbating the right-to-left shunting of blood at the ductus arteriosus.

Another disease category in which severe hypoxemia may be caused by multiple factors is congenital diaphragmatic hernia. In infants with CDH, increased pulmonary vascular resistance is related to the small cross-sectional area of pulmonary vessels causing a fixed component of high pulmonary vascular resistance, and altered pulmonary vasoreac-

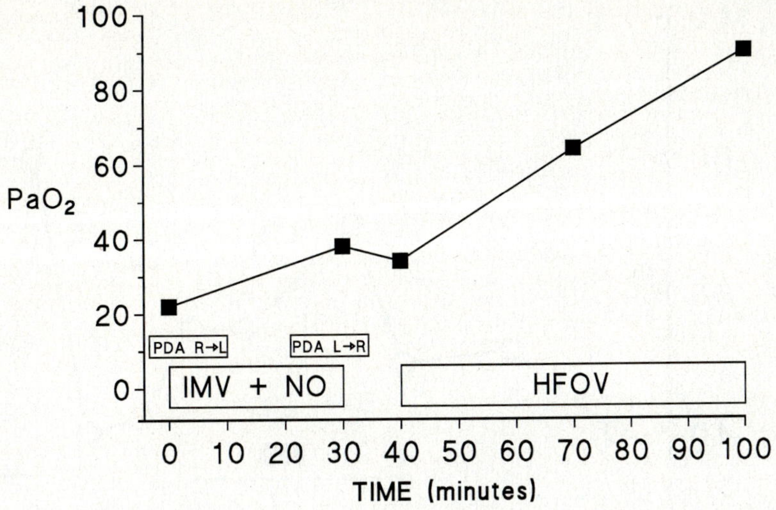

Fig. 2. Role of intrapulmonary shunting in severe PPHN: effects of inhaled NO and HFOV in a patient with PPHN and severe parenchymal lung disease. Before treatment with inhaled NO (20 ppm), echocardiography demonstrated right-to-left shunting at the patent ductus arteriosus (*PDA R → L*). After 30 minutes of NO therapy during conventional mechanical ventilation, the extrapulmonary shunting had reversed (*PDA L → R*); however, improvement in oxygenation was insufficient. This response to inhaled NO demonstrated the contribution of intrapulmonary shunting in this patient, who responded well to lung recruitment using HFOV. *PaO_2*, Partial pressure of oxygen, arterial; *IMV*, intermittent mandatory ventilation.

tivity leads to reactive pulmonary hypertension. In some patients with CDH, left ventricular mass is diminished,[44, 45] which may also contribute to pulmonary hypertension and decreased left ventricular output. Moreover, lung immaturity, underinflation, and susceptibility to lung injury during mechanical ventilation further complicate the management of patients with CDH. In these settings, therapies that target only a single pathophysiologic component of the syndrome will often be ineffective.

Alternative approaches to mechanical ventilation of the newborn infant with PPHN have attracted considerable interest. Alkalosis induced by mechanical hyperventilation has decreased pulmonary arterial pressure and improved oxygenation in some patients with PPHN. However, concerns have been raised regarding the potential complications associated with volu-trauma, and sustained hypocapneic alkalosis may have adverse neurologic effects.[46, 47] Wung et al.[48] described an approach to management of PPHN that is characterized by individualized ventilator strategies based on the underlying disease state, minimal use of paralysis, pulmonary vasodilation using tolazoline, and avoidance of hypocapneic alkalosis. A corroborating study using a similar strategy reported survival in five of six infants with PPHN[49]; however, controlled trials have not been conducted.

Exogenous surfactant therapy is another promising adjunctive treatment for near-term and term neonates with severe hypoxemic respiratory failure. There is evidence that surfactant deficiency contributes to decreased lung compliance and atelectasis in some patients with PPHN.[50-52] Recent studies have suggested that exogenous surfactant therapy can cause sustained clinical improvement in term infants with pneumonia and meconium aspiration syndrome,[53] and can reduce the duration of ECMO.[54] A multicenter trial to study the role of surfactant treatment in term neonates with severe respiratory failure is ongoing.

Considering the important role of parenchymal lung disease in many cases of PPHN, one might not expect pharmacologic pulmonary vasodilation alone to cause sustained clinical improvement. The effects of inhaled NO may be suboptimal when lung volume is decreased in association with pulmonary parenchymal disease.[55] Atelectasis and air space disease (pneumonia, pulmonary edema) will decrease effective delivery of this inhalational agent to its site of action in terminal lung units. In PPHN associated with heterogeneous (patchy) parenchymal lung disease, inhaled NO may be effective in achieving optimal ventilation-perfusion matching by preferentially causing vasodilation in lung units that are well ventilated. The effects of inhaled NO on ventilation-perfusion matching appear to be optimal at low doses (<20 ppm).[56, 57] However, in cases complicated by homogeneous (diffuse) parenchymal lung disease and underinflation, pulmonary hypertension may be exacerbated because of the adverse mechanical effects of underinflation on pulmonary vascular resistance, resulting in functional hypoplasia. In this setting, effective treatment of the underlying lung disease is essential (and sometimes sufficient) to cause resolution of the accompanying pulmonary hypertension.

In cases complicated by severe lung disease, inhaled NO

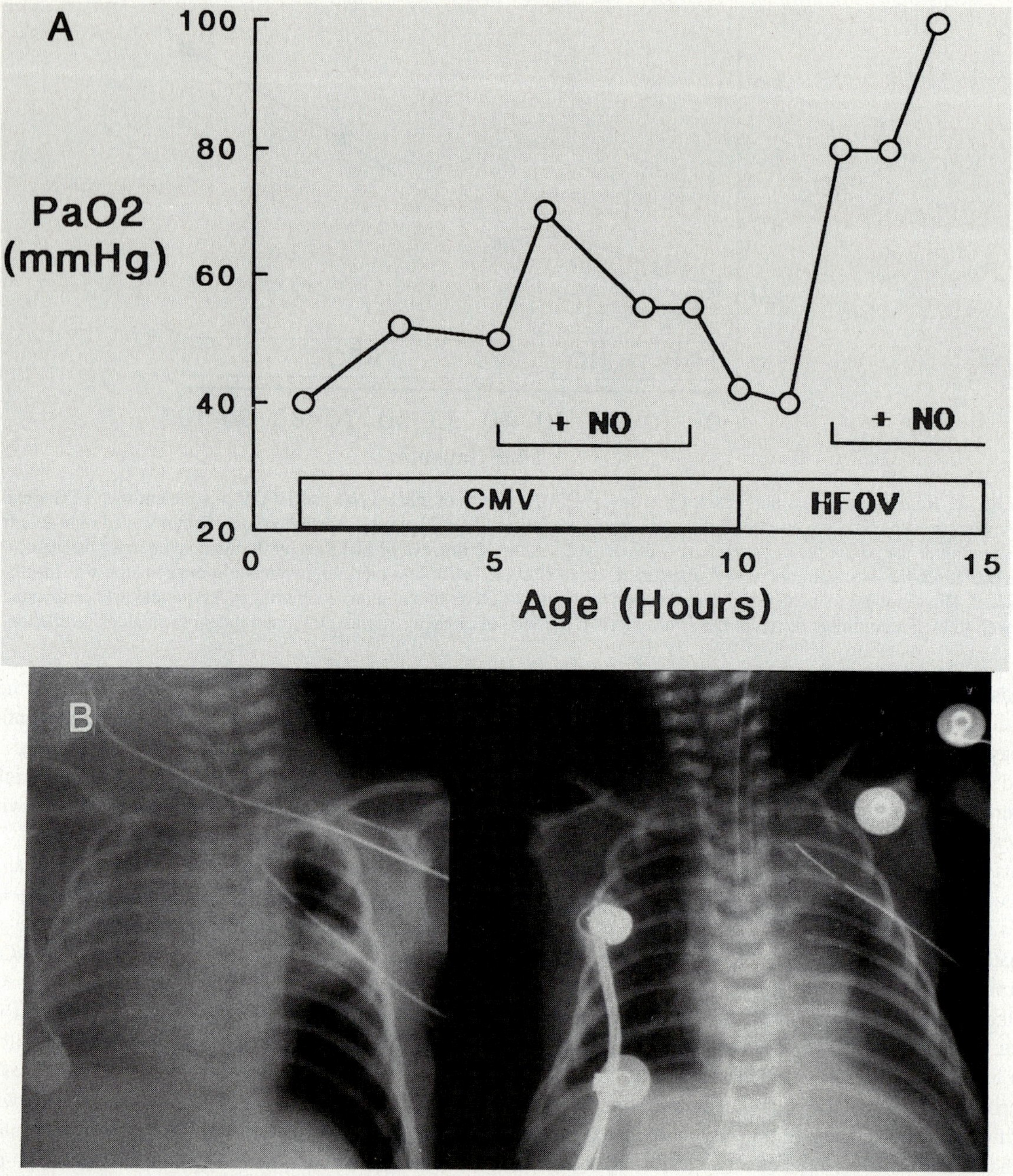

Fig. 3. A, Independent and combined effects of inhaled NO and HFOV on PaO_2 in a patient with congenital diaphragmatic hernia and PPHN. Although this patient had an initial response to inhaled NO during conventional mechanical ventilation (*CMV*), this response was not sustained. Oxygenation did not improve during 1 hour of HFOV, but marked improvements in lung volume were noted on chest radiograph. After adequate lung inflation was achieved, there was a marked and sustained improvement in oxygenation in response to inhaled NO therapy. **B,** Radiographic changes in lung inflation associated with HFOV. Marked improvement in oxygenation with inhaled NO occurred only after adequate lung inflation was achieved with HFOV.

alone will likely be ineffective without optimal pulmonary management and adequate alveolar recruitment. We employed high-frequency oscillatory ventilation to achieve optimal lung inflation and to cause minimal lung injury from tidal volume mechanical breaths (Fig. 2). When HFOV has been used with a strategy designed to recruit atelectatic lung and sustain lung volume, it has been more efficacious than conventional mechanical ventilation in severe neonatal hypoxemic respiratory failure.[58] HFOV allows for effective alveolar ventilation and recruitment while reducing the potential parenchymal and airway injury associated with large phasic pressure and lung volume changes.[59] High end-inspiratory lung volume (such as occurs during conventional ventilation) has been implicated in the development of pulmonary edema and lung injury.[60] However, the strategy employed during HFOV is critically important for optimal lung inflation and minimal risk of adverse cardiopulmonary interactions.[61, 62] If a strategy that does not adequately recruit and sustain lung volume is used, HFOV treatment will often be ineffective.[63] Because of marked attenuation of airway pressure across the endotracheal tube and airways during HFOV, the proximal airway pressure measurements do not accurately reflect the pressure transmitted to the lung.[64] Therefore the conventional indexes of severity of illness (oxygenation index, ventilation index) may not be applicable during HFOV. An effective strategy during HFOV often requires stepwise increases in mean airway pressure (3 to 5 cm H_2O increments) and pressure amplitude until improvement in oxygenation occurs, with rapid reduction in airway pressure in response to improved oxygenation and lung volume. Airway pressure is poorly transmitted to the pleural space in the underinflated and poorly compliant lung. However, as lung inflation and compliance improve, ventilator support must be reduced to avoid injury.

Because of the diverse nature of diseases complicating PPHN, there is no single approach to mechanical ventilation. Ventilator adjustments must be made with attention to radiographic changes of the accompanying lung disease and to hemodynamic status. Although the optimal roles for HFOV and NO are unclear, some patients appear to benefit from combination treatment without adverse effects.[65] In patients with severe PPHN and parenchymal lung disease or pulmonary hypoplasia (CDH), optimal management may include HFOV to recruit and maintain lung volume, thus promoting effective delivery of the inhalational vasodilator NO (Fig. 3).

Serial echocardiographic measurements may prove useful during NO treatment to determine the effects of therapy on extrapulmonary shunting. The cause of suboptimal or transient improvement in oxygenation associated with inhaled NO therapy may be difficult to interpret without adequate assessment of the severity of extrapulmonary shunting. Inhaled NO may eliminate the extrapulmonary right-to-left shunting (as measured with echocardiography) but not result in adequate improvement in oxygenation. In this setting the primary pathophysiologic disturbance is likely caused by severe intrapulmonary shunting, and effective alveolar recruitment is essential.

In some patients the effects of inhaled NO may be time dependent, with gradual improvement in oxygenation for a period of several hours. The rate of response to inhaled NO is likely dependent on several factors, including the nature of the underlying lung disease, the presence of circulating vasoconstrictor agents, cardiac performance, and structural changes in the pulmonary vasculature. Although some patients have rapid improvement in oxygenation with NO therapy, others have a slower, gradual response (Fig. 4).

Potential mechanisms for suboptimal NO responses and loss of NO responsiveness require further study. Serial echocardiographic determinations of cardiac performance may yield predictors for refractory cardiac dysfunction and may indicate the need for the cardiac support provided by ECMO. Circulating vasoconstrictor substances could potentially abate the vasodilatory effects of inhaled NO. Moreover, both structural and functional (e.g., decreased soluble guanylate cyclase activity) changes in the pulmonary vascular smooth muscle cell may alter responsiveness to exogenous NO. It is also possible that the combination of other agents with inhaled NO (e.g., the phospodiesterase inhibitor dipyridamole) could augment pulmonary vascular cyclic guanosine monophosphate concentrations and allow for more effective vasodilation at lower doses of NO.[66-68]

NITRIC OXIDE IN THE PREMATURE INFANT'S PULMONARY CIRCULATION

The fetus is characterized by both structural and functional pulmonary immaturity, including surfactant deficiency. Pulmonary immaturity and hyaline membrane disease lead to respiratory failure after premature delivery, and exogenous surfactant therapy can decrease the severity of the respiratory insufficiency.[69] However, exogenous surfactant therapy results in suboptimal responses in up to 50% of human neonates thought to have HMD,[70] which suggests that other problems of prematurity (e.g., structural lung immaturity or altered vascular responses to dilator stimuli) or complications of mechanical ventilation contribute to respiratory failure.

In some experimental models of HMD, pulmonary vascular resistance falls in response to mechanical ventilation alone, and surfactant therapy does not change the direction or magnitude of sytemic-to-pulmonary shunting across the patent ductus arteriosus.[71, 72] However, progressive deterioration after surfactant therapy occurs in a subset of premature human neonates with HMD, leading to severe pulmonary hypertension with right-to-left shunting across the ductus arteriosus.[73-76] Recent studies have shown that the association of pulmonary hypertension with severe HMD leads to increased mortality rates despite surfactant therapy.[77]

We recently reported that endogenous NO production modulates basal pulmonary vascular tone as early as 115 days of gestational age (term = 147 days) in the ovine fetus

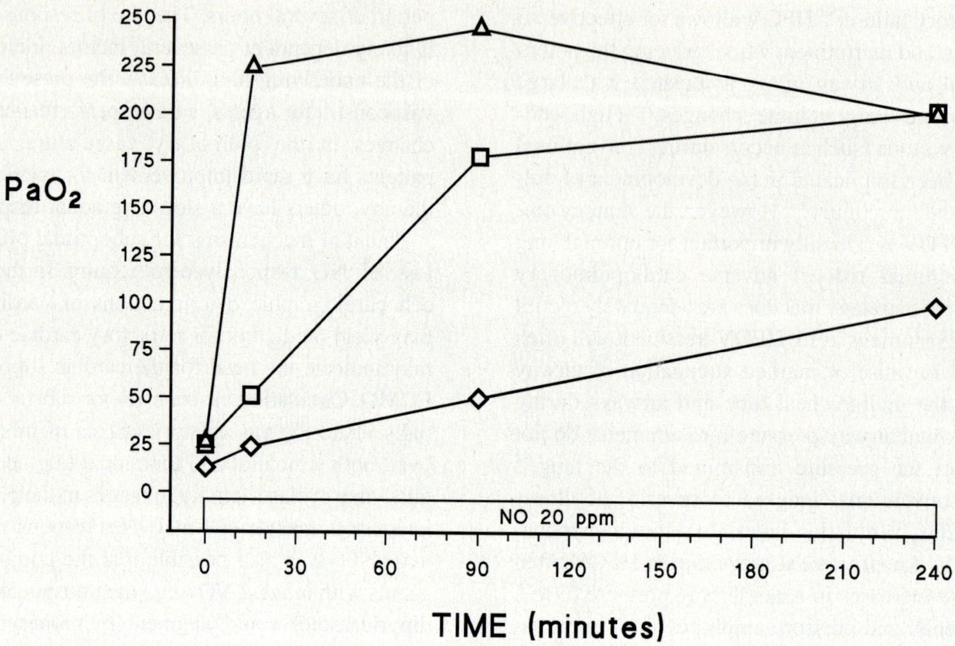

Fig. 4. Variability in time-dependent responses to inhaled NO in PPHN: Change in PaO_2 for three patients with severe PPHN treated with inhaled NO. Note variability in responses and time-dependent improvement in oxygenation. All patients recovered without the need for ECMO. (Mean baseline $PaO_2 = 19 \pm 3$; FiO_2 at 4-hour time point = 0.96.)

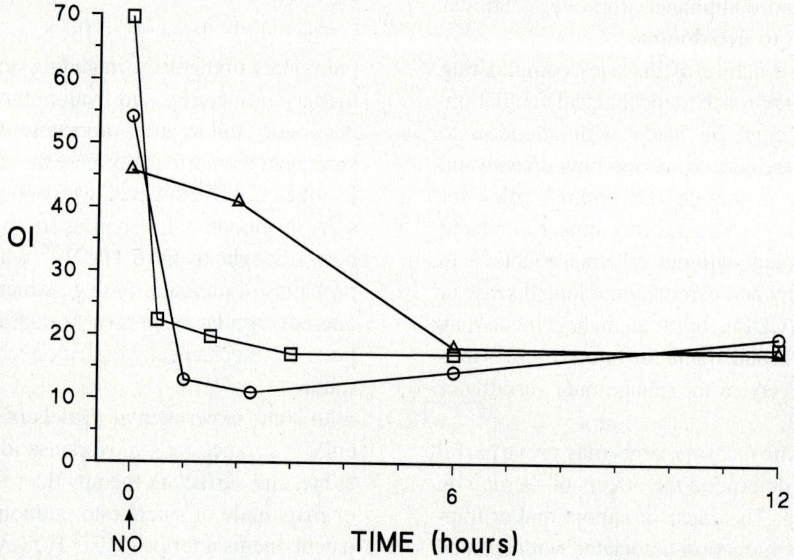

Fig. 5. Response to inhaled NO in premature infants with severe hypoxemic respiratory failure: Oxygenation index (*OI*) is shown for three premature infants (26 to 28 weeks of gestation). All patients had sustained improvement in oxygenation during inhaled NO therapy, but the most rapid improvement in oxygenation occurred in patients with extrapulmonary shunting at the foramen ovale and ductus arteriousus (patients ○ and n).

and contributes to the increase in pulmonary blood flow after extremely premature delivery.[78] In addition, inhaled NO caused marked increases in pulmonary blood flow after NO synthase inhibition, demonstrating marked responsiveness of the vascular smooth muscle cell to NO very early in gestation. We also found that during tidal-volume mechanical ventilation with high inspired oxygen concentrations after delivery of extremely premature lambs, altered pulmonary vasoregulation leads to increased pulmonary vascular resistance, decreased pulmonary blood flow, and worsening gas exchange despite a good initial response to exogenous surfactant. The pulmonary hypertension associated with severe HMD in the extremely premature lamb is responsive to exogenous NO. Continuous treatment with low-dose NO attenuates the decline in gas exchange and pulmonary perfusion during prolonged mechanical ventilation.[79]

These findings have potential implications for the clinical management of severe respiratory failue in premature infants. The immature pulmonary circulation is responsive to inhaled NO, which suggests a potential therapeutic role in the management of the preterm infant with pulmonary hypertension. It is possible that the early use of low-dose inhaled NO could play a role in the management of the premature subject with severe respiratory failure unresponsive to exogenous surfactant therapy,[80] by improving ventilation-perfusion matching and reducing pulmonary vascular resistance (Fig. 5). However, little is known of the potential pulmonary and systemic toxic effects that could occur in the premature subject exposed to inhalational NO, and studies designed to carefully assess such effects are essential before routine clinical application.

TOXICITY

The clinical studies described above were designed to investigate the hemodynamic effects of inhaled NO within ''nontoxic'' concentrations, but concerns remain regarding potential toxic effects, including methemoglobinemia and lung injury caused by NO_2, peroxynitrite, and hydroxyl radical formation.[81, 82] Although little evidence exists for NO toxicity at low concentrations in adult animals,[83-85] further studies in the neonatal lung are needed. Of particular concern are the potential effects of NO on inhibition of DNA synthesis and deamination of DNA.[86, 87] Moreover, long-term exposure to high concentrations of NO may cause down-regulation of endogenous NO synthesis.[88] However, inhaled NO may also have a protective effect by attenuating the increases in capillary permeability associated with oxidant-induced acute lung injury.[89]

The effects of inhaled NO may not be limited to the pulmonary vasculature. Preliminary evidence suggests that NO at high doses may modify the inflammatory response of alveolar macrophages,[90] and the possibility exists that circulating NO-adducts could have adverse extrapulmonary effects including neurotoxic effects in the developing brain.[91]

Another potentially important effect of NO inhalation is the prolongation in bleeding time at doses of 30 to 300 ppm.[92] Endogenous NO inhibits platelet adhesion to the vascular endothelium, and this effect may be related to the formation of stable *S*-nitroso-proteins.[93, 94] However, in a small study of premature infants treated with inhaled NO, no change in bleeding time occurred.[95] Moreover, as with most therapeutic agents, the complications associated with NO are likely dose dependent, and NO should be used in the lowest effective dose. However, the safe and effective application of inhalational nitric oxide therapy to neonates with severe cardiopulmonary failure must also take into account decreased antioxidant host defenses in the immature lung and the potential risk of surfactant inactivation.[96] Controlled clinical trials are ongoing to clarify the potential toxic effects of this new therapy, including NO-induced target cell toxic effects, pulmonary inflammatory cell function, and pathologic consequences of long-term exposure.[97]

SUMMARY

Successful management of severe PPHN depends on the application of appropriate strategies to manage the cardiopulmonary interactions that characterize this syndrome. Manifestations of PPHN often involve dysfunctional pulmonary vasoregulation, with suprasystemic pulmonary vascular resistance causing extrapulmonary shunting, pulmonary parenchymal disease causing intrapulmonary shunting, and systemic hemodynamic deterioration. Inhaled NO can cause marked improvement in oxygenation when optimal lung inflation is achieved and systemic blood volume and vascular resistance are adequate. Although concern has been expressed regarding potential increases in costs associated with this new therapy,[98] we have found that the successful application of inhaled NO in PPHN has reduced costs of hospitalization and duration of hospital stay by approximately 50% and 40%, respectively. However, inhaled NO alone is unlikely to cause sustained improvement in oxygenation in neonatal hypoxemic respiratory failure associated with severe parenchymal lung disease without extrapulmonary shunting. Inhaled NO may be an important tool in the management of severe PPHN when its application is limited to patients with severe extrapulmonary shunting and vigilant attention is given to changes in the clinical course.

REFERENCES

1. Gersony WM, Duc GV, Sinclair JC. ''PFC''syndrome (persistence of the fetal circulation). Circulation 1969;40(suppl 3):87.
2. Gersony WM. Neonatal pulmonary hypertension: pathophysiology, classification and etiology. Clin Perinatol 1984;11:517-24.
3. Drummond WH, Peckam GJ, Fox WW. The clinical profile of the newborn with persistent pulmonary hypertension. Clin Pediatr 1977;16:335-41.
4. Levin DL, Heymann MA, Kitterman JA, Gregory GA, Phibbs RH. Persistent pulmonary hypertension of the newborn infant. J Pediatr 1976;89:626-30.
5. Rudolph AM, Heymann MA. Circulation changes during growth in the fetal lamb. Circ Res 1970;26:289-99.
6. Yanagisawa M, Masaki T. Endothelin, a novel endothelium derived peptide. Pharmacological activities, regulation and possible roles in cardiovascular control. Biochem Pharmacol 1989;38:1877-83.
7. Chatfield BA, McMurtry IF, Hall SL, Abman SH. Hemody-

namic effects of endothelin-1 on ovine fetal pulmonary circulation. Am J Physiol 1991;261:R182-7.

8. Cassin S, Kristova T, Davis T, Kadowitz PP, Gause G. Tone-dependent responses to endothelin in the isolated perfused fetal sheep pulmonary circulation in situ. J Appl Physiol 1991; 70:1228-34.
9. Ivy DD, Kinsella JP, Abman SH. Physiologic characterization of endothelin A and B receptor activity in the ovine fetal pulmonary circulation. J Clin Invest 1994;93:2141-8.
10. Lin HY, Kaji EH, Winkel GK, Ives HE, Lodish HR. Cloning and functional expression of a vascular smooth muscle endothelin-1 receptor. Proc Natl Acad Sci USA 1991:88;3185-9.
11. Sakimoto A, Yanagisawa M, Sakurai T, Takuwa Y, Yanagisawa H, Masaki T. Cloning and functional expression of human cDNA for the ETa endothelin receptor. Biochem Biophys Res Commun 1991:178;656-63.
12. Tod ML, Cassin S. Endothelin-1–induced pulmonary arterial dilation is reduced by AP-nitro-L-arginine in fetal lambs. J Appl Physiol 1992:72;1730-4.
13. Jones OW, Abman SH. Systemic and pulmonary hemodynamic effects of big endothelin-1 and phosphoramidon in the ovine fetus. Am J Physiol 1994:266;R929-35.
14. Kourembanas S, Marsden PA, McQuillan LP, Fuller DV. Hypoxia induces endothelin gene expression and secretion in cultured human endothelium. J Clin Invest 1991;88:1054-7.
15. Ivy DD, Kinsella JP, Abman SH. Role of endothelin in autoregulation of blood flow in the ovine fetal lung [Abstract]. Pediatr Res 1994;35:2013A.
16. Rosenberg AA, Kennaugh J, Koppenhafer SL, Loomis M, Chatfield BA, Abman SH. Elevated immunoreactive endothelin-1 levels in newborn infants with persistent pulmonary hypertension. J PEDIATR 1993;123:109-14.
17. Gruetter CA, Barry BK, McNamara DB, Gruetter DY, Kadowitz P J, Ignarro LJ. Relaxation of bovine coronary artery and activation of coronary arterial guanylate cyclase by nitric oxide, nitroprusside and a carcinogenic nitrosoamine. J Cyclic Nucleotide Res 1979;5:211-24.
18. Palmer RMJ, Ferrige AG, Moncada S. Nitric oxide release accounts for the biological activity of endothelium-derived relaxing factor. Nature 1987;327:524-6.
19. Ignarro LJ, Buga GM, Wood KS, Byrns RE, Chaudhuri G. Endothelium-derived relaxing factor produced and released from artery and vein in nitric oxide. Proc Natl Acad Sci USA 1987;84:9265-9.
20. Abman SH, Chatfield BA, Hall SL, McMurtry IF. Role of endothelium-derived relaxing factor activity during transition of pulmonary circulation at birth. Am J Physiol (Heart Circ Physiol 28) 1990;259:H1921-7.
21. Tiktinsky MH, Morin FC. Increasing oxygen tension dilates fetal pulmonary circulation via endothelium-derived relaxing factor. Am J Physiol 1993;265:H376-80.
22. McQueston JA, Cornfield DN, McMurtry IF, Abman SH. Effects of oxygen and exogenous L-arginine on EDRF activity in fetal pulmonary circulation. Am J Physiol (Heart Circ Physiol) 1993;264:865-71.
23. Cornfield DN, Chatfield BA, McQueston JA, McMurtry IF, Abman SH. Effects of birth related stimuli on L-arginine–dependent vasodilation in the ovine fetus. Am J Physiol (Heart Circ Physiol 31) 1992;262:H1474-81.
24. McQueston JA, Kinsella JP, Ivy DD, Abman SH. Chronic intrauterine pulmonary hypertension impairs endothelium-dependent vasodilation in fetal lambs. Am J Physiol 1995;268: H288-94.
25. Zayek M, Cleveland D, Morin FC. Treatment of persistent pulmonary hypertension in the newborn lamb by inhaled nitric oxide. J PEDIATR 1993;122:743-50.
26. Kinsella JP, McQueston JA, Rosenberg AA, Abman SH. Hemodynamic effects of exogenous nitric oxide in ovine transitional pulmonary circulation. Am J Physiol 1992;262:H875-80.
27. Centers for Disease Control. Recommendations for occupational safety and health standards. MMWR Morb Mortal Wkly Rep 1988;37:S7-21.
28. Roberts JD, Chen TY, Kawai N, et al. Inhaled nitric oxide reverses pulmonary vasoconstriction in the hypoxic and acidotic newborn lamb. Circ Res 1993;72:246-54.
29. Berger JI, Gibson RL, Redding GJ, et al. Effect of inhaled nitric oxide during group B streptococcal sepsis in piglets. Am Rev Respir Dis 1993;147:1080-6.
30. Zayek M, Wild L, Roberts JD, et al. Effect of nitric oxide on the survival rate and incidence of lung injury in newborn lambs with persistent pulmonary hypertension. J PEDIATR 1993; 123:947-52.
31. Etches PC, Finer NN, Barrington KJ, et al. Nitric oxide reverses acute hypoxic pulmonary hypertension in the newborn piglet. Pediatr Res 1994;35:15-9.
32. Nelin LD, Moshin J, Thomas C, et al. The effect of inhaled nitric oxide on the pulmonary circulation of the neonatal pig. Pediatr Res 1994;35:20-4.
33. Roberts JD, Polaner DM, Lang P, et al. Inhaled nitric oxide in persistent pulmonary hypertension of the newborn. Lancet 1992;340:818-9.
34. Kinsella JP, Neish SR, Shaffer E, Abman SH. Low-dose inhalational nitric oxide in persistent pulmonary hypertension of the newborn. Lancet 1992;340:819-20.
35. Kinsella JP, Neish SR, Ivy DD, Shaffer E, Abman SH. Clinical responses to prolonged treatment of persistent pulmonary hypertension of the newborn with low doses of inhaled nitric oxide. J PEDIATR 1993;123:103-8.
36. Kinsella JP, Abman SH. Inhalational nitric oxide therapy for persistent pulmonary hypertension of the newborn. Pediatrics 1993;91:997-8.
37. Finer NN, Etches PC, Kamstra B, et al. Inhaled nitric oxide in infants referred for extracorporeal membrane oxygenation: dose response. J PEDIATR 1994;124:302-8.
38. Walsh-Sukys MC. Persistent pulmonary hypertension of the newborn: the black box revisited. Clin Perinatol 1993;20:127-43.
39. Kinsella JP, McCurnin DC, Clark RH, Lally K, Null DM. Cardiac performance in ECMO candidates: echocardiographic predictors for ECMO. J Pediatr Surg 1992;27:44-7.
40. Rudolph AM. High pulmonary vascular resistance after birth. Clin Pediatr 1980;19:585-90.
41. Geggel RL, Reid LM. The structural basis of PPHN. Clin Perinatol 1984;11:525-49.
42. Clark DA, Nieman GF, Thompson AM, et al. Surfactant displacement by meconium free fatty acids: an alternate explanation for atelectasis in meconium aspiration syndrome. J PEDIATR 1987;110:765-70.
43. Moses D, Holm BA, Spitale P, Liu M, Enhorning G. Inhibition of pulmonary surfactant function by meconium. Am J Ob Gynecol 1991;164:477-81.
44. Siebert H, Haas J, Beckwith J. Left ventricular hypoplasia in

congenital diaphragmatic hernia. J Pediatr Surg 1984:19;567-71.

45. Schwart SM, Vermillion RP, Hirschl RB. Evaluation of left ventricular mass in children with left-sided congenital diaphragmatic hernia. J PEDIATR 1994:125;447-51.
46. Bifano EM, Pfannenstiel A. Duration of hyperventilation and outcome in infants with persistent pulmonary hypertension. Pediatrics 1988;81:657-61.
47. Hendricks-Munoz KD, Walton JP. Hearing loss in infants with persistent fetal circulation. Pediatrics 1988;81:650-6.
48. Wung JT, James LS, Kilchevsky E, et al. Management of infants with severe respiratory failure and persistence of the fetal circulation, without hyperventilation. Pediatrics 1985; 76:488-94.
49. Dworetz AR, Moya FR, Sabo B, Gross I. Survival of infants with PPHN without ECMO. Pediatrics 1989;84:1-6.
50. Hallmann M, Kankaanpaa K. Evidence of surfactant deficiency in persistence of the fetal circulation. Eur J Pediatr 1980; 134:129-34.
51. James DK, Chiswick JL, Havier A, Williams M, Hallworth J. Nonspecificity of surfactant deficiency in neonatal respiratory disorders. BMJ 1985;105:1635-7.
52. Lotze A, Whitsett JA, Kammerman LA, Ritter M, Taylor GA, Short BL. Surfactant protein A concetrations in tracheal aspirate fluid from infants requiring extracorporeal membrane oxygenation. J PEDIATR 1990;116:435-40.
53. Auten RL, Notter RH, Kendig JW, Davis JM, Shapiro DL. Surfactant treatment of full-term newborns with respiratory failure. Pediatrics 1991;87:101-7.
54. Lotze A, Knight FR, Martin GR, et al. Improved pulmonary outcome after exogenous surfactant therapy for respiratory failure in term infants requiring extracorporeal membrane oxygenation. J PEDIATR 1993;122:261-8.
55. Antunes MJ, Greenspan JS, Holt WJ, Vallieu DS, Spitzer AR. Assessment of lung function pre-nitric oxide therapy: a predictor of response? [Abstract]. Pediatr Res 1994;35:212A.
56. Rossaint R, Falke KJ, Lopez F, et al. Inhaled nitric oxide for the adult respiratory distress syndrome. N Engl J Med 1993; 328:399-405.
57. Gerlach H, Rossaint R, Pappert D, Falke KJ. Time-course and dose-response of nitric oxide inhalation for systemic oxygenation and pulmonary hypertension in patients with adult respiratory distress syndrome. Eur J Clin Invest 1993;23:499-502.
58. Clark RH, Yoder BA, Sell MS. Prospective, randomized comparison of high-frequency oscillation and conventional ventilation in candidates for extracorporeal membrane oxygenation. J PEDIATR 1994;124:447-54.
59. Clark RH. High-frequency ventilation. J PEDIATR 1994;124: 661-70.
60. Dreyfuss D, Saumon G. Role of tidal volume, FRC, and end-inspiratory volume in the development of pulmonary edema following mechanical ventilation. Am Rev Respir Dis 1993; 148:1194-203.
61. Meredith KS, deLemos RA, Coalson JJ, et al. Role of lung injury in the pathogenesis of hyaline membrane disease in premature baboons. J Appl Physiol 1989;66:2150-8.
62. Kinsella JP, Gerstmann DR, Clark RH, et al. HFOV vs. IMV: early hemodynamic effects in the premature baboon with HMD. Pediatr Res 1991;29:160-6.
63. Froese AB, McCulloch PR, Sugiura M, Vaclavik S, Possmayer F, Moller F. A comparison of ventilation strategies for the use of high-frequency oscillatory ventilation in the treatment of hyaline membrane disease. Acta Anaesthesiol Scand 1989; 33:102-7.
64. Gerstmann DR, Fouke JM, Winter DC, Taylor AF, deLemos RA. Proximal, tracheal, and alveolar pressures during high frequency oscillatory ventilation in a normal rabbit model. 1990; 28:367-73.
65. Kinsella JP, Abman SH. Methaemoglobin during nitric oxide therapy with high frequency ventilation [Letter]. Lancet 1993; 342:615.
66. Braner DA, Fineman JR, Change R, Soifer SJ. M&B 22948, a cGMP phosphodiesterase inhibitor, is a pulmonary vasodilator in lambs. Am J Physiol 1993;264:H252-8.
67. Ziegler JW, Ivy DD, Kinsella JP, Clarke WR, Abman SH. Dipyridamole, a cGMP phospodiesterase inhibitor augments inhaled nitric oxide–induced pulmonary vasodilation in the ovine transitional circulation [Abstract] Pediatr Res 1994; 35:90A.
68. Steinhorn RH, Thusu KG, Russell JA, Gugino SF, Paradisis M, Morin FC. The cGMP specific phosphodiesterase inhibitor M&B 22948 enhances the effect of nitric oxide in newborn lambs with persistent pulmonary hypertension [Abstract]. Pediatr Res 1994;35:89A.
69. Jobe AH. Pulmonary surfactant therapy. N Engl J Med 1993; 328:861-8.
70. Jobe AH. Surfactant in the perinatal period. Early Hum Dev 1992;26:57-62.
71. Kinsella JP, Gerstmann DR, deLemos RA. Circulatory changes following premature delivery in a baboon model of hyaline membrane disease. Am J Physiol (Heart Circ Physiol) 1991; 261:H1148-54.
72. Kinsella JP, Gerstmann DR, Gong AK, deLemos RA. Ductal shunting and effective systemic blood flow following single dose surfactant treatment in the premature baboon model of hyaline membrane disease. Biol Neonate 1991;60:283-91.
73. Chu J, Clements JA, Cotton EK, Klass MH, Sweet AY, Tooley WH. Neonatal pulmonary ischemia. I. Clinical and physiological studies. Pediatrics 1967;40:109-82.
74. Stahlman M, Blankenship WJ, Shepard FM, Gray J, Young WC, Malan AF. Circulatory studies in clinical hyaline membrane disease. Biol Neonate 1972;20:300-20.
75. Evans NJ, Archer LNJ. Doppler assessment of pulmonary artery pressure and extrapulmonary shunting in the acute phase of hyaline membrane disease. Arch Dis Child 1991;66:6-11.
76. Skinner JR, Boys RJ, Hunter S, Hey EN. Pulmonary and systemic arterial pressure in hyaline membrane disease. Arch Dis Child 1992;67:366-73.
77. Walther FJ, Benders MJ, Leighton JO. Persistent pulmonary hypertension in premature neonates with severe respiratory distress syndrome. Pediatrics 1992;90:899-904.
78. Kinsella JP, Ivy DD, Abman SH. Ontogeny of NO activity and response to inhaled NO in the developing ovine pulmonary circulation. Am J Physiol 1994;267:H1955-61.
79. Kinsella JP, Ivy DD, Abman SFI. Inhaled nitric oxide lowers pulmonary vascular resistance and improves gas exchange in severe experimental hyaline membrane disease. Pediatr Res 1994;36:402-8.
80. Abman SH, Kinsella JP, Schaffer MS, Wilkening RB. Inhaled nitric oxide therapy in a premature newborn with severe respiratory distress and pulmonary hypertension. Pediatrics 1993; 92:606-9.

81. Beckman JS, Beckman TW, Chen J, Marshall PA, Freeman BA. Apparent hydroxyl radical production by peroxynitrite: implications for endothelial injury from nitric oxide and superoxide. Proc Nat Acad Sci USA 1990;87:1620-4.
82. Gaston B, Drazen JM, Loscalzo J, Stamler JS. The biology of nitrogen dioxides in the airways. Am J Respir Crit Care Med 1994;149:538-51.
83. Stavert DM, Lehnert BE. Nitric oxide and nitrogen dioxide as inducers of acute pulmonary injury when inhaled at relatively high concentrations for brief periods. Inhalation Toxicology 1990;2:53-67.
84. Hugod C. Effect of exposure to 43 ppm nitric oxide and 3.6 ppm nitrogen dioxide on rabbit lung. Int Arch Occup Environ Health 1979;42:159-67.
85. Fukase O, Isomura K, Watanabe H. Effects of nitrogen oxides on peroxidative metabolism of mouse lung. Journal of the Japanese Society on Air Pollution 1976;11:65-9.
86. Lepoivre M, Fieschi F, Coves J, Thelander L, Fontecave M. Inactivation of ribonucleotide reductase by nitric oxide. Blochem Biophys Res Commun 1991;179:442-8.
87. Wink DA, Kasprzak KS, Maragos CM, et al. DNA deaminating ability and genotoxicity of nitric oxide and its progenitors. Science 1991;254:1001-3.
88. Bult H, Meyer GRY, Jordaens FH, Herman AG. Chronic exposure to exogenous nitric oxide may suppress its endogenous release and efficacy. J Cardiovasc Pharmacol 1991;17:S79-82.
89. Kavanagh BP, Mouchawar A, Goldsmith J, Pearl RG. Effects of inhaled NO and inhibition of endogenous NO sythesis in oxidant-induced acute lung injury. J Appl Physiol 1994;76:1324-9.
90. Turbow R, Waffarn F, Hallman M, et al. Inflammatory responses and suppressed macrophage function following inhaled nitric oxide [Abstract]. Pediatr Res 1994;35:356A.
91. Stamler JS, Simon DI, Osborne JA, et al. *S*-Nitrosylation of proteins with NO: synthesis and characterization of biologically active compounds. Proc Natl Acad Sci USA 1992; 89:444-8.
92. Hogman M, Frostell C, Arnberg H, Hedenstierna G. Bleeding time prolongation and NO inhalation. Lancet 1993;341:1664-5.
93. Radomski MW, Palmer RMJ, Moncada S. Endogenous nitric oxide inhibits human platelet adhesion to vascular endothelium. Lancet 1987;2:1057-8.
94. Simon DI, Stamler JS, Jaraki O, et al. Antiplatelet properties of protein S–nitrosothiols derived from nitric oxide and endothelium-derived relaxing factor. Arterioscler Thromb 1993; 13:791-9.
95. Ahluwalia J, Kelsall A, Raine J, et al. Nitric oxide improves oxygenation in neonates with respiratory distress syndrome and pulmonary hypertension [Abstract]. Pediatr Res 1994; 36:3A.
96. Haddad IY, Ischiropoulos H, Holm BA, et al. Mechanisms of peroxynitrite-induced injury to pulmonary surfactants. Am J Physiol 1993;265:L555-64.
97. Freeman B. Free radical chemistry of nitric oxide. Chest 1994; 150:79S-84S.
98. Sahni R, Wung JT, James LS. Controversies in management of persistent pulmonary hypertension of the newborn. Pediatrics 1994;94:307-9.

Vertical transmission of human immunodeficiency virus type 1: Autologous neutralizing antibody, virus load, and virus phenotype

Robert N. Husson, MD, Yan Lan, MD, Eiji Kojima, MS, David Venzon, PhD, Hiroaki Mitsuya, MD, PhD, and Kenneth McIntosh, MD

From the Division of Infectious Diseases, Children's Hospital, Department of Pediatrics, Harvard Medical School, Boston, Massachusetts, and the Experimental Retrovirology Section, Medicine Branch, and the Biostatistics and Data Management Section, National Cancer Institute, Bethesda, Maryland

Objective: To evaluate immunologic and virologic correlates of vertical transmission of human immunodeficiency virus type 1 (HIV-1).
Design: Case-control study.
Patients: Women who were prospectively enrolled in a natural history study of HIV-1 infection in women and infants. Sixteen HIV-1–infected women whose infants became infected were matched by CD4+ cell percentage and use of zidovudine during pregnancy with women whose infants did not become infected.
Measurements: Maternal autologous neutralizing antibody, virus load determined by RNA-polymerase chain reaction (RNA-PCR), and virus phenotype.
Results: Most women in both groups had low titers of autologous neutralizing antibody, and no difference in neutralizing titers was observed (range, <4 to 181 in both groups). The HIV-1 copy number in maternal plasma was not significantly different in the two groups but was inversely correlated with maternal CD4+ cell percentage ($p < 0.005$). Five women in the transmitting group and four in the nontransmitting group had syncytium-inducing (SI) phenotype virus. Two infected infants had SI phenotype virus. The SI phenotype virus was associated with a greater HIV-1 copy number in maternal plasma ($p < 0.05$) and an increase in the mortality rate for the infants ($p < 0.01$).
Conclusions: In women matched for CD4+ cell percentage, low titers of autologous neutralizing antibody, high virus load, and SI phenotype virus were not associated with an increased risk of transmission of HIV-1 to their infants. (J PEDIATR 1995;126:865-71)

Supported by grants from the Pediatric AIDS Foundation (50291-14-PG), the Charles H. Hood Foundation, and the Milton Fund of Harvard University, and by Women and Infants Transmission Study contract NO1 AI-82507 from the National Institutes of Health. Dr. Husson was the recipient of a Markey Scholar Award.

Presented in part at the 33rd Interscience Conference on Antimicrobial Agents and Chemotherapy, October 1993, Anaheim, Calif. (Abstract No. 1138).

Reprint requests: Robert N. Husson, MD, Division of Infectious Diseases, Children's Hospital, 300 Longwood Ave., Boston, MA 02115.

9/20/64351

Although reported rates of vertical transmission of immunodeficiency virus type 1 have varied widely, only a small proportion of infants born to infected women become infected. Two large prospective studies of infants born to HIV-1–infected women in Europe found vertical transmission rates of 14.4% and 18.3%, respectively.[1, 2] In the ongoing Women and Infants Transmission Study in the United States, the overall transmission rate is less than 20%.[3] In Africa, reported rates of transmission are higher, although infection occurs in substantially fewer than half of the infants.[4, 5] The recently demonstrated efficacy of zidovudine in

HIV-1	Human immunodeficiency virus type 1
NSI	Non-syncytium-inducing
RNA-PCR	Polymerase chain reaction of reverse transcribed ribonucleic acid
SI	Syncytium-inducing
$TCID_{50}$	Fifty percent tissue culture infectivity dose

reducing the rate of vertical transmission is likely to decrease transmission in populations where this drug is available and the HIV-1 status of women of childbearing age is known.[6]

Despite the importance of the pathogenesis of vertical transmission of HIV-1 and the variables that determine why some infants born to HIV-1–infected women become infected and others do not, relatively little is known about these phenomena. Among the variables that have been consistently associated with an increased likelihood of transmission are advanced maternal clinical disease or markers of advanced disease such as low $CD4^+$ cell counts and high $CD8^+$ cell counts, and markers of high maternal virus burden, such as p24 antigenemia or HIV-1 culture positivity.[1, 5, 7-9] Other variables that may play a role are premature birth, placental inflammation, mode of delivery, and breast-feeding.[1, 2, 5, 7, 10-14] The role of maternal HIV-1–specific immunity in vertical transmission remains unclear, with conflicting results regarding the association of maternal anti-HIV-1 antibody and transmission.[10, 15-20]

A better understanding of the correlates of mother-to-infant transmission of HIV-1 would provide information highly relevant to the prevention of both vertical and horizontal transmission. We therefore conducted a case-control study to assess the role of immunologic and virologic factors in relation to mother-to-infant transmission of HIV-1.

METHODS

Study population. The HIV-1–infected women enrolled in the Boston centers for the Women and Infants Transmission Study between January 1990 and November 1992, who had given birth to infants known to be infected with HIV-1, were identified by study number through a review of the study records. Infants were defined as infected if they had two or more positive HIV-1 culture results, excluding cord blood, from samples obtained at different times in the first year of life.[3] Of the 20 mother-infant pairs identified, 16 were found to have appropriate virus isolates and plasma or serum samples available for study. From the same study population, women whose infants were known not to be infected were identified, and control mother-infant pairs were selected by matching for maternal $CD4^+$ cell percentage, for use of zidovudine during pregnancy, and, if possible, for mode of delivery. Infants were defined as being uninfected if at least three cultures, including at least two when an infant was more than 1 month of age, were negative for HIV-1.[3] Additional data on maternal age, prior pregnancies, infant birth weight, gestational age, and breast-feeding were obtained. The Women and Infants Transmission Study research protocols were approved by the human experimentation review boards of the participating institutions. Written informed consent was obtained from all women enrolled in the study, and from the parent or legal guardian of all infants.

Virus isolates and neutralization assay. Each patient's primary HIV-1 isolate was amplified once in phytohemagglutinin-stimulated normal donor peripheral blood mononuclear cell coculture, the supernatant was harvested, and aliquots were frozen at –70° C. Each virus isolate was titered, and a fresh aliquot of titered frozen virus stock was used in each neutralization experiment. For the mothers, the virus isolate obtained from the delivery blood sample, or from the sample obtained as close as possible to the time of delivery, was used. For the infected infants, the first isolate containing virus, excluding cord blood isolates, was used.

Neutralization by maternal plasma or serum of maternal and infant HIV-1 isolates was determined with modifications of reported methods.[21-24] Maternal plasma or serum samples from the time of delivery were used except in five cases for which samples obtained during the second or third trimester were used. Plasma or serum was separated from whole blood on the day the blood was drawn (usually within 4 hours), and frozen at –70° C until use. Samples were heat inactivated at 56° C for 30 minutes, and fourfold serial dilutions from 1:4 to 1:1024 were prepared in a final volume of 50 ml. These dilutions were then incubated in 96-well plates at 37° C for 60 minutes with 50 ml of virus supernatant containing an inoculum of 100 $TCID_{50}$, followed by the addition of 2×10^5 phytohemagglutinin-stimulated peripheral blood mononuclear cells in 100 ml of medium. The medium was changed on days 1 and 4, and the p24 antigen concentration in the supernatant was determined by enzyme-linked immunosorbent assay (DuPont, Wilmington, Del.) on day 7. Neutralization assays were performed in quadruplicate. The neutralizing titer was defined as the dilution of plasma or serum that resulted in a 50% reduction in p24 concentration compared with the no-serum control, and was calculated by the Karber method.[25] The assay was validated by means of a polyclonal HIV-1 immune globulin of defined titer from the National Institutes of Health AIDS Research and Reference Reagent Program (catalog No. 192). This antibody was used as a positive control, and HIV-1–seronegative plasma served as a negative control in each assay.

Syncytium-inducing phenotype determination. Virus phenotype was determined as described.[26] Briefly, 100 $TCID_{50}$ of each virus stock was used to infect 5×10^4 MT-2 cells and the syncytium-inducing–non-syncytium-inducing phenotype was determined by visual inspection, with syncytium formation defined as more than three syncytia per well. The cultures were continued for 14 days, after which time the virus was scored NSI if syncytia were not observed.

Quantitative RNA polymerase chain reaction, virus culture, and p24 antigen determination. Viral RNA quantification in plasma was performed by reverse transcription of viral RNA followed by amplification by polymerase chain reaction of viral *pol* sequences as previously described.[27] The HIV-1 cultures of maternal and infant cells were grown in phytohemagglutinin-stimulated peripheral blood mononuclear cells as described.[3] Immune complex–dissociated p24 antigen concentration in plasma was determined with a commercial enzyme-linked immunosorbent assay kit (DuPont) according to the manufacturer's directions.

Statistical analysis. Maternal age, $CD4^+$ cell percentages, $CD8^+$ cell percentages, number of prior pregnancies, birth weights, gestational ages, viral copy number determined by ribonucleic acid–PCR, and p24 concentration in plasma were compared between the two groups by means of the Wilcoxon signed rank test. The RNA-PCR data were log-transformed before analysis. Neutralizing titers, mode of delivery, ethnicity, virus phenotype, and the maternal mortality rate were compared by means of the McNemar test. The relation between virus phenotype and neutralizing titers, and between virus phenotype and mortality rate for the infected infants, was analyzed with the Fisher Exact Test. The Mann-Whitney U test was used to compare viral copy number of SI versus NSI phenotype virus. The Spearman rank correlation was computed to determine the intersample correlation in the RNA-PCR assay and to assess the relation between neutralizing antibody titers against maternal and infant virus, between maternal $CD4^+$ cell percentage and viral copy number, and between neutralizing antibody titer and viral copy number.

RESULTS

Study population. The study population, consisting of 16 HIV-1–infected women whose infants also became infected, was matched for $CD4^+$ cell percentage and use of zidovudine during pregnancy with a control population, consisting of 16 HIV-1–infected women whose infants did not become infected. As expected from the matching, there was no significant difference in the two groups in maternal $CD4^+$ cell percentage, use of zidovudine, or mode of delivery of the infant. One case-control pair was discordant for zidovudine use because the case mother was enrolled in a masked trial of zidovudine versus placebo during pregnancy. In addition to the matched variables, there was no significant difference between the groups in maternal $CD8^+$ cell count, maternal age at the time of delivery, ethnicity, number of prior pregnancies, infant birth weight, or infant gestational age. None of the infants in either group was breast fed. Of 16 infected infants, two had positive culture results at birth, another had positive results at day 6 of life, and another at day 14. The one very low birth weight infant (745 gm) was in the infected group.

Virus isolation and neutralization of autologous and infant isolates. Human immunodeficiency virus type 1 was grown and titered from the 32 infected women and from the 16 infected infants. For four isolates, two from women in the transmitting group and two from the infants born to these two women, a titer of at least 100 $TCID_{50}/50\ \mu l$ (2×10^3/ml) was not obtained, so a lower titer was used in the neutralization assay (69 $TCID_{50}$ for the two maternal isolates and 24 and 41 $TCID_{50}$ for the infant isolates).

The neutralizing titer of each woman's serum or plasma against her own (autologous) virus for the transmitting and nontransmitting women is shown in the Table. In both groups most neutralizing titers were low. The median for the transmitting group was 8 (range, <4 to 181), and the median for the nontransmitting group was 6 (range, <4 to 181); six titers in the transmitting group and seven in the nontransmitting group were below the limit of detection of the assay. There was no statistically significant difference in autologous neutralization between the two groups ($p = 1.0$), and no significant difference if the case patient and the control subject who were not matched for use of zidovudine during pregnancy were excluded.

No difference was observed between the neutralizing titers obtained against the maternal isolates versus the titers against the infant isolates (Table). The neutralizing titer of maternal antibody against maternal virus was highly correlated with the titer of the mother's antibody against her infant's virus ($\rho = 0.84$; $p = 0.001$), with one striking exception, mother-infant pair T-12, for whom the titer against the infant isolate was repeatedly higher than the titer against the maternal isolate.

Quantitative RNA-PCR, plasma p24 antigen concentration, and viral culture. The median quantitative RNA-PCR–determined viral copy number per milliliter of plasma was 785 (range, <100 to 24,000) in the transmitting group and 1240 (range, <100 to 122,500) in the nontransmitting group ($p = 0.08$). The results obtained from the duplicate samples for each individual were highly correlated ($\rho = 0.98$; $p < 0.001$), indicating excellent intersample reproducibility of this assay. Significant negative correlations were observed between the RNA-PCR–determined plasma viral load and maternal $CD4^+$ cell percentage ($\rho = -0.53$; $p < 0.005$) and between plasma viral load and maternal autologous neutralizing titer ($\rho = -0.37$; $p < 0.05$).

The p24 antigen concentration in plasma was determined after acid dissociation of immune complexes for 15 of the 16 pairs of women. The concentration was below the limit of detection in the majority of samples from both groups (11 of

Table. Neutralization of maternal and infant virus isolates

Transmitting mother	CD4+ cell percentage	Neutralizing titer: Autologous virus	Neutralizing titer: Infant virus	Nontransmitting mother	CD4+ cell percentage	Neutralizing titer of autologous virus
T-1*	3	<4†	<4‡	NT-1	7	<4
T-2	4	181	512	NT-2	11	<4
T-3	9	4	11	NT-3	12	32
T-4	15	<4	<4	NT-4	19	<4
T-5	16	128	181	NT-5	21	<4
T-6*	19	32	64	NT-6	15	<4
T-7*	22	8	<4	NT-7	17	<4
T-8	26	<4	6	NT-8	22	45
T-9	27	<4†	<4§	NT-9	27	8
T-10	29	11	45	NT-10	24	8
T-11	29	128	128	NT-11	28	<4
T-12	35	8	>1024	NT-12	31	181
T-13	35	23	23	NT-13	36	32
T-14	37	128	128	NT-14	37	45
T-15	41	<4	<4	NT-15	44	16
T-16*	46	<4	<4	NT-16	43	4

*Infant culture positive for HIV-1 at 14 days of age or younger.
†Virus inoculum of 69 $TCID_{50}$.
‡Virus inoculum of 41 $TCID_{50}$.
§Virus inoculum of 24 $TCID_{50}$.

15 in the transmitting group and 9 of 15 in the nontransmitting group; *p* value not significant). No significant difference between the groups was observed. Samples for nonquantitative HIV-1 culture were obtained from women enrolled in the Women and Infants Transmission Study at up to four visits during pregnancy: first, second, and third trimesters and delivery. Most women in both groups had at least two cultures. There was no difference in the rate of culture positivity between the transmitting and the nontransmitting women (29 of 34 vs 26 of 32 cultures grew HIV-1).

Virus phenotype. Five of sixteen isolates from the transmitting group of women and 4 of 16 from the nontransmitting group of women had the SI phenotype. Virus isolates from two of the five infected infants whose mothers had SI phenotype virus were SI and three were NSI. The SI phenotype virus was less likely than the phenotype virus to be neutralizable by maternal antibody; autologous maternal antibody had a neutralizing titer of 4 or less against 7 of 9 SI isolates, in comparison with 8 of 23 NSI isolates ($p < 0.05$). The SI virus was also associated with greater replication in vivo. The median number of HIV-1 particles per milliliter of plasma in the nine women with SI virus was 8650 (range, 980 to 122,500), compared with 410 (range, <100 to 66,000) in the 23 women with NSI virus ($p < 0.05$).

Maternal and infant mortality rates. The median duration of follow-up of the women enrolled in this study from the time of delivery was 1.7 years for the mothers whose infants became infected and 2.4 years for the women whose infants did not become infected. Despite the longer follow-up in the nontransmitting women, all the women who died during the follow-up period were those whose infants became infected (4/16 vs 0/16; $p = 0.13$). There were no deaths in the HIV-1–uninfected infants during the follow-up period. Among the 16 infected infants, two died during the follow-up period. One very low birth weight infant died at 2 weeks of age, and the other child died at 2 years of age. Both infants who died had SI phenotype virus; all 14 infants who survived had NSI virus ($p < 0.01$).

DISCUSSION

In this study of mother-to-infant transmission of HIV-1, in which the transmitting and nontransmitting mothers were matched by maternal CD4+ cell count and use of zidovudine, we did not find an association between HIV-1 transmission and the titer of maternal autologous neutralizing antibody. The lack of association between titers of maternal autologous neutralizing antibody and transmission is consistent with the findings of a small European study in which there was no association between maternal autologous neutralizing antibody and vertical transmission.[28] That study did suggest that mothers whose infants did not become infected were more likely to have neutralizing antibody against one or more heterologous primary isolates. In that study, however, there was a significant difference in CD4+ cell counts and p24 antigen positivity between the transmitting and nontransmitting mothers, which suggests that the observed difference in heterologous neutralizing titers may not have been independent of disease stage and viral load. This interpretation is supported by the inverse correlation between maternal plasma virus load and autologous neutralizing antibody observed in this study, and by previous studies of children and adults that correlate advanced disease with low titers of neutralizing antibody.[29, 30]

Another study found a trend toward lower titers of autologous neutralizing antibody in transmitting versus nontransmitting women.[31] The reason for the difference between the results of that study and our results may be related to differences in the neutralization assays, or to differences in virus phenotype or virus load in the two groups of women in that study. In addition, although we examined a larger number of transmitting and nontransmitting women than were examined in previous studies, the relatively small sample size, the low titers, and the large proportion of titers below the limit of detection of the neutralization assay reduce the power of our study to detect small differences in autologous neutralization.

Other studies of functional maternal anti-HIV-1 antibody in vertical HIV-1 transmission have also failed to identify differences in titer between transmitting and nontransmitting women. A study of neutralizing antibody against the IIIB strain of HIV-1 found no difference in titer between transmitting and nontransmitting women.[10] A study of maternal anti-SI antibody, an antibody function that correlates with neutralization, and a study of maternal antibody–dependent cellular cytotoxicity both failed to observe differences in titers between transmitting and nontransmitting mothers.[32, 33]

Although the low autologous neutralizing titers in both groups limit the power of this study to detect differences between the groups, the finding of low titers in both groups is itself striking. The low titers of autologous anti-HIV-1 neutralizing antibody observed in this and other studies[28, 34] suggest that passive immunization with immunoglobulin preparations containing high titers of neutralizing antibodies against a broad spectrum of HIV-1 isolates has the potential to increase endogenous humoral immunity. This rationale is the basis of an ongoing AIDS Clinical Trials Group study to prevent vertical transmission.

The titer of maternal autologous neutralizing antibody and the titer of maternal neutralizing antibody against the infant's first virus isolate were highly correlated in all but one mother-infant pair. This result indicates that the virus transmitted to the infant is not an unusual variant of the maternal virus population. This interpretation is consistent with the observation of Kliks et al.[31] that the replication kinetics of maternal and infant viruses were highly similar. We also did not observe an association of maternal virus load and vertical transmission as measured by quantitative RNA-PCR, immune-complex–disrupted p24 antigen concentration in plasma, or HIV-1 culture positivity. This result contrasts with recent studies of unmatched transmitting and nontransmitting women that demonstrated a correlation between maternal virus load and vertical HIV-1 transmission.[8, 9] The absence of association between viral load and transmission in our study is likely the result of matching for $CD4^+$ cell percentage between the two groups. This interpretation is supported by the highly significant inverse correlation between $CD4^+$ cell percentage and RNA-PCR–determined viral load observed in this study, a finding that is consistent with known associations between high viral load, low $CD4^+$ cell counts and advanced disease stage.[35-37]

We also did not observe a difference in virus phenotype between the transmitting and nontransmitting women. The SI phenotype has been associated with more advanced disease, but its role in transmission is not known. The phenotype discordance between women with SI virus and infants with NSI virus indicates that the SI phenotype is not transmitted preferentially. This discordance of transmitted phenotype has also been observed in horizontal transmission.[38, 39] This finding suggests that there is selection against expression of this phenotype in newly infected infants, either at the level of transmission or by suppression of SI phenotype virus replication by the infant immune system.

As has been observed in adults, SI phenotype virus in the infant appears to be associated with a poor prognosis. In older children, SI phenotype has been associated with lower $CD4^+$ cell counts, although this association was not independent of age.[40] Consistent with the in vitro phenotype, we found that SI phenotype virus was associated with increased viral load in vivo, and this phenotype occurred predominantly in women with low $CD4^+$ cell counts.

The low titers of autologous neutralizing antibody in this and other studies, and the absence of a difference in titers between the groups in our matched case-control study, suggest that neutralizing antibody against autologous virus is unlikely to play a major role in determining the probability of vertical transmission. The results of several studies, together with the efficacy of zidovudine in decreasing the rate of vertical transmission of HIV-1, suggest that maternal virus load is a major determinant of the probability of transmission. Our study and others, however, demonstrate that infants of women with low viral loads may become infected, and infants of women with high viral burdens may escape infection. Thus the pathogenesis of vertical HIV-1 transmission is likely to be multifactorial, and other viral and immune variables, systemically and at the mucosal surface of the infant and the mother, are likely to play a role in determining whether an infant born to an HIV-infected woman becomes infected.

We thank the Women and Infants Transmission Study investigators, research nurses, and laboratory personnel, including Ruth Tuomola, Arlene Buck, Rosemary Galvin, Patrick Donegan, Steven Pelton, Ellen Cooper, Ethel Hudson, Kathy Khoury, Elizabeth Jones, Martha Muehlmann, and Jenifer Davis.

REFERENCES

1. European Collaborative Study. Risk factors for mother-to-child transmission of HIV-I. Lancet 1992;339:1007-12.
2. Gabiano C, Pier-Angelo T, de Martino M, et al. Mother-to-child transmission of human immunodeficiency virus type I: risk of infection and correlates of transmission. Pediatrics 1992;90: 369-74.
3. McIntosh K, Pitt J, Brambilla D, et al. Blood culture in the first six months of life for the diagnosis of vertically transmitted human immunodeficiency virus infection. J Infect Dis 1994; 170:996-1000.5
4. Ryder R, Nsa W, Hassig S, et al. Perinatal transmission of the human immunodeficiency virus type I to infants of seropositive women in Zaire. N Engl J Med 1989;320:1637-42.
5. St. Louis M, Kamenga M, Brown C, et al. Risk for perinatal HIV-I transmission according to immunologic, virologic, and placental factors. JAMA 1993;269:2853-9.
6. Connor E, Sperling R, Gelber R, et al. Reduction of maternal-infant transmission of human immunodeficiency virus type I with zidovudine treatment. N Engl J Med 1994;331:1173-80.
7. Thomas P, Weedon J, Krasinski K, et al. Maternal predictors of perinatal human immunodeficiency virus transmission. Pediatr Infect Dis J 1994;13:489-95.
8. Borkowsky W, Krasinski K, Cao Y, et al. Correlation of perinatal transmission of human immunodeficiency virus type 1 with maternal viremia and lymphocyte phenotypes. J PEDIATR 1994;125:345-51.
9. Weiser B, Nachman S, Tropper P, et al. Quantitation of human immunodeficiency virus type I during pregnancy: relationship of viral titer to mother-to-child transmission and stability of viral load. Proc Natl Acad Sci USA 1994;91:8037-41.
10. Goedert JJ, Mendez H, Drummond JE, et al. Mother-to-infant transmission of human immunodeficiency virus type I: association with prematurity or low anti-gp120. Lancet 1989;2: 1351-4.
11. Blanche S, Rouzioux C, Moscato MG, et al. A prospective study of infants born to women seropositive for human immunodeficiency virus type I. N Engl J Med 1989;320:1643-8.
12. Van de Perre P, Simonon A, Msellati P, et al. Postnatal transmission of human immunodeficiency virus type I from mother to infant: a prospective cohort study in Kigali, Rwanda. N Engl J Med 1991;325:593-8.
13. Dunn D, Newell M, Ades A, Peckham C. Risk of human immunodeficiency virus type 1 transmission through breastfeeding. Lancet 1992;340:585-8.
14. Palasanthiran P, Ziegler J, Steward G, et al. Breast-feeding during primary maternal human immunodeficiency virus infection and risk of transmission from mother to infant. J Infect Dis 1993;167:441-4.
15. Devash Y, Calvelli T, Wood DG, Reagan KJ, Rubinstein A. Vertical transmission of human immunodeficiency virus is correlated with absence of high affinity/avidity maternal antibodies to the gp120 principal neutralizing domain. Proc Natl Acad Sci USA 1990;87:3445-9.
16. Rossi P, Moschese V, Broliden PA, et al. Presence of maternal antibodies to human immunodeficiency virus I envelope glycoprotein gp120 epitopes correlates with the uninfected status of children born to seropositive mothers. Proc Natl Acad Sci USA 1989;86:8055-8.
17. Parekh B, Shaffer N, Pau C-P, et al. Lack of correlation between maternal antibodies to V3 loop peptides of gp120 and perinatal HIV-I transmission. AIDS 1991;5:1179-84.
18. Robertson C, Mok J, Froebel D, et al. Maternal antibodies to gp120 V3 sequence do not correlate with protection against vertical transmission of human immunodeficiency virus. J Infect Dis 1992;166:704-9.
19. Halsey N, Markham R, Wahren B, Boulos R, Rossi P, Wigzell H. Lack of association between maternal antibodies to V3 loop peptides and maternal-infant HIV-I transmission. J Acquir Immune Defic Syndr 1992;5:153-7.
20. Lallement M, Baillou A, Lallemant-LeCoeur S, et al. Maternal antibody response at delivery and perinatal transmission of human immunodeficiency virus type I in African women. Lancet 1994;343:1001-5.
21. Ho D, Sarngadharan M, Hirsch M, et al. Human immunodeficiency virus neutralizing antibodies recognize several conserved domains on the envelope glycoproteins. J Virol 1987; 61:2024-8.
22. Palker T, Clark M, Langlois A, et al. Type-specific neutralization of the human immunodeficiency virus with antibodies to env-encoded synthetic peptides. Proc Natl Acad Sci USA 1988;85:1932-6.
23. Scott C Jr., Silver S, Profy A, et al. Human monoclonal antibody that recognizes the V3 region of human immunodeficiency virus gp120 and neutralizes the human T-lymphotropic virus type IIIMN strain. Proc Natl Acad Sci USA 1990;87: 8597-601.
24. Mascola J, Louwagie J, McCutchan F, et al. Two antigenically distinct subtypes of human immunodeficiency virus type I: viral genotype predicts neutralization serotype. J Infect Dis 1994;169:48-54.
25. Leland D, French M. Virus isolation and identification. In: Lennette E, Halonen P, Murphy F, eds. Laboratory diagnosis of infectious diseases; vol 2: Viral, rickettsial and chlamydial diseases; vol. 2. New York: Springer-Verlag, 1988.
26. Japour A, Fiscus S, Arduino J-M, Mayers D, Reichelderfer P, Kuritzkes D. Standardized microtiter assay for determination of syncytium-inducing phenotype of clinical human immunodeficiency virus type-I isolates. J Clin Microbiol 1994;32: 2291-4.
27. Kojima E, Shirasaka T, Anderson B, et al. HIV-I viremia changes and development of drug-related mutations in patients with symptomatic human immunodeficiency virus type I infection receiving alternating or simultaneous zidovudine and didanosine therapy. J Infect Dis 1995;171:1152-8.
28. Scarlatti G, Albert J, Rossi P, et al. Mother-to-child transmission of human immunodeficiency virus type 1: correlation with neutralizing antibodies against primary isolates. J Infect Dis 1993;168:207-10.
29. Robert-Guroff M, Goedert J, Naugle C, Jennings A, Blattner W, Gallo R. Spectrum of HIV-I neutralizing antibodies in a cohort of homosexual men: results of a 6-year prospective study. AIDS Res Hum Retroviruses 1988;4:343-50.
30. Robert-Guroff M, Roilides E, Muldoon R, et al. Human immunodeficiency virus (HIV) type I strain MN neutralizing anti-

body in HIV-infected children: correlation with clinic status and prognostic value. J Infect Dis 1993;167:538-46.
31. Kliks S, Wara D, Landers D, Levy J. Features of HIV-I that could influence maternal-child transmission. JAMA 1994;272: 467-74.
32. Bal A, Zhang J, Viscarello R, Miller G, Andiman W. Lack of correlation between maternal HIV-I syncytium inhibiting antibody and vertical transmission [Abstract 954]. Society for Pediatric Research, Baltimore, Maryland, 1993.
33. Jenkins M, Landers D, Williams-Herman D, et al. Association between anti-human immunodeficiency virus type I (HIV-I) antibody–dependent cellular cytotoxicity antibody titers at birth and vertical transmission of HIV-I. J Infect Dis 1994; 170:308-12.
34. Wrin T, Crawford L, Sawyer L, Weber P, Sheppard H, Hanson C. Neutralizing antibody responses to autologous and heterologous isolates of human immunodeficiency virus. J Acquir Immune Defic Syndr 1994;7:211-9.
35. Fahey J, Taylor J, Detels R, et al. The prognostic value of cellular and serologic markers in infection with human immunodeficiency virus type I. N Engl J Med 1990;322:166-72.
36. Ho DD, Moudgil T, Alam M. Quantitation of human immunodeficiency virus type I in the blood of infected persons. N Engl J Med 1989;321:1621-5.
37. Holodniy M, Katzenstein D, Sengupta S, et al. Detection and quantification of human immunodeficiency virus RNA in patient serum by use of the polymerase chain reaction. J Infect Dis 1991;163:862-6.
38. Roos M, Lange J, de Goede R, et al. Viral phenotype and immune response in primary human immunodeficiency virus type I infection. J Infect Dis 1992;165:427-32.
39. Zhu T, Mo H, Wang N, et al. Genotypic and phenotypic characterization of HIV-I in patients with primary infection. Science 1993;261:1179-81.
40. Spencer L, Ogino M, Dankner W, Spector S. Clinical significance of human immunodeficiency virus type I phenotypes in infected children. J Infect Dis 1994;169:491-5.

Cytokine elevations in infants with bacterial and aseptic meningitis

Susan J. Dulkerian, MD, Laurie Kilpatrick, PhD,
Andrew T. Costarino, Jr., MD, Lisa McCawley, BS, Joel Fein, MD,
Linda Corcoran, BSN, Sharon Zirin, BSN, and Mary Catherine Harris, MD

From the Divisions of Neonatology, Allergy, Immunology and Infectious Diseases, the Department of Pediatrics, and the Department of Anesthesia and Critical Care Medicine, Children's Hospital of Philadelphia, University of Pennsylvania School of Medicine

We sought to determine whether the detection of cytokines, produced during the inflammatory response, would aid in the diagnosis of meningitis in young infants. We measured cerebrospinal fluid (CSF) and plasma levels of interleukin-6 (IL-6) and tumor necrosis factor (TNF) in 62 infants less than 6 months of age whose condition was evaluated for meningitis. Twenty infants had culture-proved meningitis, 22 had aseptic meningitis, and 20 control infants had no evidence of meningitis. The CSF IL-6 levels were elevated in all 20 infants with bacterial meningitis and in 9 of 22 infants with aseptic meningitis but were undetectable in all control subjects. Furthermore, CSF IL-6 levels were 10 times greater in infants with bacterial versus aseptic meningitis (*p* <0.001). Levels of TNF in CSF were detected in 12 of 20 infants with bacterial meningitis and were undetectable in infants with aseptic meningitis and in control infants (*p* <0.02). Plasma IL-6 and TNF levels were unreliable for the detection of meningitis in this patient population. We conclude that the presence of IL-6 in the CSF reliably identifies infants with meningitis and that the presence of CSF TNF is a highly specific indicator of bacterial meningeal inflammation. (J PEDIATR 1995;126:872-6)

Recent studies indicate that the host's inflammatory response may be more important in tissue damage than the infecting organism. Tumor necrosis factor and interleukin-6 are two of the endogenous mediators produced by mononuclear phagocytes that play an essential role in the development of tissue injury during infection.[1-11] Recent studies in our laboratory have demonstrated increased plasma levels of TNF and IL-6 during bacterial sepsis in older children and increased IL-6 levels in infected neonates.[12, 13] In children with bacterial meningitis, McCracken et al. and other investigators[14-16] have reported elevated TNF and interleukin-1 levels in the cerebrospinal fluid. Rusconi et al.[17] and other investigators[18] have noted increased CSF IL-6 levels in children with this disease.

Supported by National Institutes of Health grant RR-00240, and the Ethel B. Foederer Fund for Excellence.

Presented in part at the annual meeting of the Society for Pediatric Research, Baltimore, Md., May 1992, and the Fifteenth Annual Conference on Shock, Point Clear, Ala., June 1992.

Submitted for publication June 17, 1994; accepted Jan. 10, 1995.

Reprint requests: Susan J. Dulkerian, MD, University of Maryland School of Medicine, Division of Neonatology, Room N5W68, 22 S. Greene St., Baltimore, MD 21201.

0022-3476/95/$3.00 + 0 **9/20/63319**

CSF	Cerebrospinal fluid
ELISA	Enzyme-linked immunosorbent assay
IL-1	Interleukin-1
IL-6	Interleukin-6
TNF	Tumor necrosis factor

We hypothesized that cytokines are produced locally in the central nervous system during meningitis and that the magnitude of their elevation may distinguish bacterial infection from aseptic causes. The purpose of this study was to determine whether TNF and IL-6 are elevated in the CSF of young infants with meningeal inflammation and to determine whether cytokine production differed in bacterial ver-

Table I. Study population

Infant group	Mean ± SD (range): Gestational age (wk)	Postnatal age (wk)	WBC CSF (cells/mm^3)	Positive blood cultures	Long-term hospitalization*	Foreign body
Bacterial meningitis (n = 20)	37.0 ± 4.4 (24-40)	8.6 ± 6.3 (1-24)	3375 ± 7826† (0-33,300)	12/19‡	7/20	7/20
Aseptic meningitis (n = 22)	39.2 ± 1.8 (33-40)	6.2 ± 4.4 (1-17)	360 ± 351† (50-1495)	0/22	0/22	0/22
Nonmeningitis control (n = 20)	37.2 ± 4.2 (23-42)	5.5 ± 4.5 (1-20)	7 ± 10 (0-49)	0/20	5/20	5/20

*Hospitalization more than 7 days at the time of diagnosis.
†For bacterial meningitis versus aseptic meningitis, and bacterial meningitis versus control subjects, $p < 0.05$.
‡In one infant a blood culture was not drawn before antibiotic administration.

sus aseptic meningitis. In addition, we sought to determine the relationship of CSF to plasma levels of cytokines.

METHODS

Study population. During the study period from November 1990 to December 1993 all infants less than 6 months of age with suspected meningitis were eligible for enrollment. Study infants included those seen in the emergency department and inpatients who were examined for infection. Subjects were enrolled at the time of or immediately after examination for sepsis and meningitis. The decision to perform an examination for sepsis was made by the members of the medical team responsible for the care of each infant. No infant had a spinal tap solely for the purpose of study sample collection.

Infants were subsequently divided into three groups: those with bacterial meningitis, those with aseptic meningitis, and the nonmeningitis control group. Bacterial meningitis was identified by a positive bacterial CSF culture result associated with either abnormal cytologic findings, abnormal glucose and protein values, or both. Aseptic meningitis was identified by a CSF leukocyte count of greater than 50×10^6 cells/L (>50 cells/mm^3), abnormal glucose and protein values, but negative results on bacterial culture of CSF and blood specimens. Because viral cultures of CSF samples were not routine, we cannot comment on the presence or absence of viral disease in this group. Infants whose subsequent examination for infection yielded negative systemic culture results and normal CSF cytologic and chemistry values served as the nonmeningitis control group.

The study was approved by the Children's Hospital of Philadelphia Committee for the Protection of Human Subjects. Informed consent was obtained from parents or guardians of all subjects.

Cytokine determinations. Blood and CSF samples were obtained from infants at the time of examination for sepsis. Blood samples were collected in plastic syringes treated with ethylenediaminetetraacetic acid and aprotinin (0.43 trypsin inhibitory units per milliliter of blood) according to the method of Cannon et al.[19] Plasma was separated by centrifugation at 400*g* for 10 minutes at 4° C. Plasma was then spun at 10,000*g* for 5 minutes to remove platelets and other cellular debris. Samples of CSF were collected in sterile tubes, and the cells and cellular debris were removed by centrifugation at 10,000*g* for 5 minutes. Blood and CSF samples were divided into aliquots and stored at −70° C until assay.

Cytokine determinations were performed with ELISA. Tumor necrosis factor–α and IL-6 analyses were performed with ELISA kits obtained from Genzyme Corp. (Cambridge, Mass.). Duplicate determinations were performed for each CSF and plasma sample. Plasma samples for TNF analysis were extracted twice with double volumes of chloroform, according to the method described by Cannon et al.,[19] to remove interfering lipids and high molecular weight proteins. Samples of CSF did not require chloroform extraction. The limits of detection were 60 pg/ml for TNF-α and 0.160 ng/ml for IL-6.

Statistical analysis. Cytokine levels and other variables in the three groups were compared by factorial analysis of variance and the Student independent *t* test. Analysis of samples for the presence or absence of cytokines was performed with the chi-square test with the Yates correction. Probability of less than 0.05 was considered significant.

RESULTS

Study population. Sixty-two infants with suspected meningitis who met inclusion criteria were enrolled. The study population consisted of 20 infants with bacterial meningitis, 22 infants with aseptic meningitis, and 20 control infants without meningitis (Table I). No differences were found in the mean ages of the three groups in the mean peripheral leukocyte or platelet counts (data not shown). As expected, the infants with bacterial meningitis had significantly higher CSF leukocyte counts than in those with aseptic meningitis or no meningitis ($p < 0.05$). The mean CSF glucose value of 1.33 mmol/L (mean ± SD, 24 ± 18 mg/dl)

Table II. Infants with bacterial meningitis

Patient No.	Postnatal age (wk)	CSF analysis: Leukocyte (cells/mm^3)	CSF analysis: Glucose (mmol/L)	CSF analysis: Protein (gm/L)	Cytokines: IL-6 (ng/ml)	Cytokines: TNF (pg/ml)	Organism	Positive blood culture	Foreign body
1	1	33,300	0.61	11.38	8.5	625	α-Hemolytic streptococcus	+	–
2	2	20	0.06	9.02	9.0	5621	Group B streptococcus	+	–
3	16	6700	3.55	1.74	9.8	0	Group B streptococcus	+	–
4	7	NA	0.56	4.64	20.7	3830	Group B streptococcus	+	–
5	4	12,200	NA	NA	5.1	44	Group D streptococcus*	–	VPS
6	16	2101	0.56	2.78	5.9	0	*Streptococcus pneumoniae*	+	–
7	5	1060	0.56	2.37	17.8	149	*S. pneumoniae*	+	–
8	12	208	0.61	1.75	5.1	130	*S. pneumoniae*	+	–
9	14	1200	2.89	2.83	4.1	0	*S. pneumoniae*	–	–
10	8	0†	1.55	2.48	4.3	1175	*Staphylococcus epidermidis*	–	VPS, ETT
11	2	1913	2.78	9.34	2.8	140	*S. epidermidis*	–	VPS
12	16	605	0.89	2.71	20.4	8034	*S. epidermidis*	–	VPS
13	4	1115	0.89	6.93	4.8	0.2	*Listeria monocytogenes*	+	–
14	24	285	1.39	0.87	2.9	0	*Haemophilus influenzae*	+	–
15	8	604	0.56	1.89	4.8	0	*H. influenzae*	+	–
16	4	900	1.83	0.37	1.7	0	*Escherichia coli*	–	–
17	5	1688	2.50	4.26	12.2	6460	*E. coli*	–	ETT, CVL
18	15	80	1.22	11.15	4.5	2007	*Neisseria meningitidis*	+	–
19	4	30	2.22	0.67	0.5	0	*Klebsiella pneumoniae*	–	CVL
20	4	NA	NA	NA	1.3	0	*Serratia marcescens*	+	ETT, CVL

+, Positive; –, negative; *CVL*, central venous line; *ETT*, endotracheal tube; *NA*, not available; *VPS*, ventriculoperitoneal shunt.
*A blood culture was not drawn before antibiotic administration.
†Subsequent CSF analyses revealed CSF pleocytosis and persistently positive cultures.

was lower in the bacterial meningitis group than the mean value of 2.39 mmol/L (43 ± 5 mg/dl) in the aseptic meningitis group and 2.79 mmol/L (49 ± 13 mg/dl) in the nonmeningitis control group ($p < 0.05$). The difference in mean CSF glucose values between the aseptic meningitis and control groups was not significant. Similarly, the mean CSF protein value of 3.75 gm/L (mean ± SD, 375 ± 325 mg/dl) for the bacterial meningitis group was significantly higher than the mean value of 0.66 gm/L (66 ± 28 mg/dl) for the aseptic meningitis group and 0.66 gm/L (66 ± 38 mg/dl) for the nonmeningitis control group ($p < 0.05$). No significant difference was found in the mean CSF protein values between the aseptic meningitis and control groups.

Within the entire group of study infants the most common signs of infection or meningitis included fever (97%), lethargy or irritability (94%), poor feeding or food intolerance (80%), or respiratory decompensation (30%). None of the infants was receiving corticosteroids at the time of the sepsis evaluation, and none had immunodeficiencies, malignancies, or kidney disease. Six infants had preexisting pulmonary disease, including respiratory distress syndrome or bronchopulmonary dysplasia in three, congenital heart disease in one; two infants had undergone extracorporeal membrane oxygenation.

Table II shows the demographic characteristics and laboratory findings of the infants with bacterial meningitis. Sixty-three percent of the infants with bacterial meningitis had the identical organism isolated from blood and CSF cultures; 35% had foreign bodies present at the time of the studies for meningitis.

Cytokine determinations. All infants with bacterial meningitis had IL-6 in their CSF (Table III). In contrast, only 41% of the infants with aseptic meningitis and none of the control infants had detectable CSF IL-6 levels. The infants with bacterial meningitis had significantly higher levels of CSF IL-6 when compared with both the group of infants with aseptic meningitis and the nonmeningitis control group ($p < 0.001$). In addition, those IL-6 levels were 10 times higher than those from the group of infants with aseptic meningitis. The presence of detectable levels of IL-6 in CSF was 100% sensitive and 79% specific, with a 100% negative predictive value and a 69% positive predictive value, for bacterial meningitis.

Sixty percent of the infants with bacterial meningitis had TNF present in the CSF, whereas none of the patients with aseptic meningitis or control infants had detectable CSF TNF levels (Table III). The mean TNF levels were significantly higher in the group with bacterial meningitis ($p < 0.02$). The presence of detectable levels of TNF in CSF was 60% sensitive and 100% specific, with 100% positive predictive value and 84% negative predictive value, for bacterial meningitis.

All seven infants with IL-6 in their plasma were in the bacterial meningitis group and had bacteremia at the time of sample collection (Table III). Plasma TNF was not consistently detected in the infants with either bacterial or aseptic meningitis. No infant in the control group had IL-6 or TNF in the CSF or plasma. No significant relationship was found between elevations of plasma or CSF TNF and IL-6 levels, and peripheral or CSF leukocyte counts, nor was a difference found in cytokine levels in gram-negative versus gram-positive bacterial meningitis.

DISCUSSION

Our results demonstrate that neonates and young infants respond to pathogen invasion with the release of cytokines at comparable levels to those found in older children and adolescents.[16, 17, 20, 21] Our findings are consistent with previous studies showing elevated cytokine levels in older children with meningitis. In a study of dexamethasone therapy for gram-negative bacterial meningitis, Mustafa et al.[16, 20] demonstrated elevated levels of TNF and IL-1 in the CSF of infants and children. Rusconi et al.[17] found elevated CSF IL-6 levels in children with bacterial meningitis (mean age, 2½ years). In contrast, cytokine elevations have not been consistently reported in aseptic meningitis.[18, 22-25] These conflicting results may be due to differences in cytokine elaboration, which are dependent on the infecting viral pathogen.

We found that CSF cytokine levels may be valuable in distinguishing patients with bacterial from aseptic meningitis. All patients with bacterial meningitis had IL-6 present in the CSF, whereas no infant with aseptic meningitis had detectable CSF TNF levels. Thus, in the prediction of bacterial meningitis, CSF IL-6 was 100% sensitive and had a 100% negative predictive value; CSF TNF was less sensitive (60%) but 100% specific for this diagnosis. These data corroborate previous studies in adults and extend their usefulness to the prediction of bacterial disease in young infants.[18, 26, 27] In a series of eight adults with bacterial meningitis Chavanet et al.[18] found CSF IL-6 to be 100% sensitive in diagnosis. Similarly, Lopez-Cortes et al.[26] found that TNF was a highly specific (100%) indicator of bacterial meningitis in adults and noted its absence in nonbacterial disease.

We found no significant relationship between elevations of TNF or IL-6 and other indicators of inflammation, such as peripheral or CSF leukocyte counts. These findings are similar to those from a recent study by Glimaker et al.[27] but differ from the results of other studies in adults.[18, 26] This lack of correlation of CSF cytokine levels with other indicators of meningeal inflammation suggests a local source of cytokine production that is independent of leukocyte activity in the CSF. This separate and independent source of cytokine production is further corroborated by our findings of a lack of correlation between CSF and plasma cytokine levels in infants with either bacterial or aseptic meningitis. Moreover, our results suggest that in young infants cytokine determinations may be even more useful in the identification of infected infants than traditional indices of inflammation.

Table III. Presence of cytokines in study infants

	No. (%) of patients		
	Bacterial meningitis	Aseptic meningitis	Control
CSF			
IL-6*	20/20 (100)	9/22 (41)	0/20 (0)
TNF†	12/20 (60)	0/22 (0)	0/20 (0)
Plasma			
IL-6‡	7/18 (39)	0/18 (0)	0/20 (0)
TNF§	1/18 (6)	2/15 (13)	0/20 (0)

*For bacterial meningitis versus control group and bacterial versus aseptic meningitis, $p <0.001$; for aseptic meningitis versus control group, $p <0.02$.
†For bacterial meningitis versus control group and bacterial versus aseptic meningitis, $p <0.001$; for aseptic meningitis versus control group, p not significant.
‡For bacterial versus aseptic meningitis, $p <0.02$; for bacterial meningitis versus control group, $p <0.01$; for aseptic meningitis versus control group, p not significant.
§Among all patient groups, p not significant.

We conclude that cytokine measurements may differentiate between bacterial and aseptic meningitis in young infants and that the presence of IL-6 in CSF was uniformly sensitive in the prediction of bacterial meningitis. Moreover, among infants with elevations of TNF the likelihood of bacterial meningitis was extremely high. Detection of cytokines in CSF is more likely to be due to local production rather than to be a reflection of increased plasma levels, because plasma IL-6 and TNF levels did not reliably identify infants with meningitis. Finally, because no infant in the control group had detectable cytokines in the CSF or plasma, the absence of cytokines probably indicates the absence of meningeal inflammation. Future studies with larger samples should explore the clinical applications of these observations.

REFERENCES

1. Klein JO, Feigin RD, McCracken HG Jr, et al. Report of the task force on diagnosis and management of meningitis. Pediatrics 1986;78:959-82.
2. Tunkel AR, Scheld WM. Pathogenesis and pathophysiology of bacterial meningitis. Annu Rev Med 1993;44:103-20.
3. Saukkonen K, Sande S, Cioffe C, et al. The role of cytokines in the generation of inflammation and tissue damage in experimental gram-positive meningitis. J Exp Med 1990;171:439-48.
4. Ohga S, Aoki T, Okada K, et al. Cerebrospinal fluid concentrations of interleukin-1β, tumor necrosis factor-alpha, and in-

terferon gamma in bacterial meningitis. Arch Dis Child 1994; 70:123-5.
5. Teti G, Mancuso G, Tomasello F, Chiofalo MS. Production of tumor necrosis factor-alpha and interleukin-6 in mice infected with group B streptococci. Circ Shock 1992;38:138-44.
6. Aggarwal BB, Kohr WJ, Hass PE, et al. Human tumor necrosis factor: production, [purification and characterization]. J Biol Chem 1985;260:2345-54.
7. Beutler B, Cerami A. Cachectin: more than a tumor necrosis factor. N Engl J Med 1987;316:379-85.
8. Helfgott DC, Tatter SB, Santhanam U, et al. Multiple forms of IFN-β_2/IL-6 in serum and body fluids during acute bacterial infection. J Immunol 1989;142:948-53.
9. Houssiau FA, Bukasa K, Sindic CJM, Van Damme J, Van Snick J. Elevated levels of 26K human hybridoma growth factor (interleukin-6) in cerebrospinal fluid of patients with acute infection of the central nervous system. Clin Exp Immunol 1988;71:320-3.
10. Tracey KJ, Beutler B, Lowry SF, et al. Shock and tissue injury induced by recombinant human cachectin. Science 1986; 234:470-4.
11. Fong Y, Lowry SF. Tumor necrosis factor in the pathophysiology of infection and sepsis. Clin Immunol Immunopathol 1990;55:157-70.
12. Sullivan JS, Kilpatrick L, Costarino AT Jr, Lee SC, Harris MC. Correlation of plasma cytokine elevations with mortality rate in children with sepsis. J PEDIATR 1992;120:510-5.
13. Harris MC, Costarino AT Jr, Sullivan JS, et al. Cytokine elevations in critically ill infants with sepsis and necrotizing enterocolitis. J PEDIATR 1994;124:105-11.
14. Lebel MM, Freij BJ, Syrogiannapoulos GA, et al. Dexamethasone therapy for bacterial meningitis: results of two double-blind, placebo-controlled trials. N Engl J Med 1988;319:964-71.
15. McCracken, GH Jr, Mustafa MM, Ramilo O, Olsen KD, Risser RC. Cerebrospinal fluid interleukin 1-β and tumor necrosis factor concentrations and outcome from neonatal gram-negative enteric bacillary meningitis. Pediatr Infect Dis J 1989;8: 155-9.
16. Mustafa MM, Lebel MH, Ramilo O, et al. Correlation of interleukin-1β and cachectin concentrations in cerebrospinal fluid and outcome from bacterial meningitis. J PEDIATR 1989;115: 208-13.
17. Rusconi F, Parizzi F, Garlaschi L, et al. Interleukin-6 activity in infants and children with bacterial meningitis. Pediatr Infect Dis J 1991;10:117-21.
18. Chavanet P, Bonnotte B, Guiguet M, et al. High concentrations of intrathecal interleukin-6 in human bacterial and nonbacterial meningitis. J Infect Dis 1992;166:428-31.
19. Cannon JG, Van Der Meer JWM, Kwiatowski D, et al. Interleukin 1-β in human plasma: optimization of blood collection, plasma extraction, and radioimmunoassay methods. Lymphokine Res 1988;7:457-67.
20. Mustafa MM, Mertsola J, Ramilo O, Saez-Llorens X, Risser R, McCracken GH Jr. Cerebrospinal fluid prostaglandins, interleukin-1, and tumor necrosis factor in bacterial meningitis: clinical and laboratory correlations in placebo-treated and dexamethasone-treated patients. Am J Dis Child 1990; 144:883-7.
21. Arditi M, Manogue KR, Caplan M, Yogev R. Cerebrospinal fluid cachectin/tumor necrosis factor and platelet activating factor concentrations and severity of bacterial meningitis. J Infect Dis 1990;162:139-47.
22. Ramilo O, Mustafa MM, Porter J, et al. Detection of IL-1β, but not TNF-alpha in cerebrospinal fluid of children with aseptic meningitis. Am J Dis Child 1990;144:349-52.
23. Leist TP, Frei K, Kam-Hansen S, Zinkernagel RM, Fontana A. TNF in CSF during bacterial but not viral meningitis: evaluation in murine model infections and in patients. J Exp Med 1988;167:1743-8.
24. Aderka D, Holtman H, Toker L, Hanh T, Wallach D. Tumor necrosis factor induced by Sendai virus. J Immunol 1987;136: 2938-42.
25. Wainberg MA, Numazaki K, Destaphano L, Wong I, Goldman H. Infection of human epithelial cells by human cytomegalovirus and other viruses: effect on secretion of IL-1 like activity. Clin Exp Immunol 1988;72:415-21.
26. Lopez-Cortes LF, Cruiz-Ruiz M, Gomez-Mateos J, Jimenez-Hernandez D, Palomino J, Jimenez E. Measurement of levels of tumor necrosis factor–alpha and interleukin 1β in the CSF of patients with meningitis of different etiologies: utility in the differential diagnosis. Clin Infect Dis 1993;16:534-9.
27. Glimaker M, Kragsberg P, Forsgren M, Olcen P. Tumor necrosis factor–α in cerebrospinal fluid from patients with meningitis of different etiologies: high levels of TNF-alpha indicate bacterial meningitis. J Infect Dis 1993;167:882-9.

Efficacy of an observation scale in detecting bacteremia in febrile children three to thirty-six months of age, treated as outpatients

Stephen J. Teach, MD, MPH, Gary R. Fleisher, MD, and the Occult Bacteremia Study Group[a]

From the Division of Emergency Medicine and the Department of Pediatrics, Children's Hospital of Buffalo and the School of Medicine and Biomedical Sciences, State University of New York at Buffalo, and the Division of Emergency Medicine and the Department of Pediatrics, Children's Hospital, Boston, and Harvard Medical School, Boston, Massachusetts

Objective: **To assess the efficacy of the Yale Observation Scale (YOS) in detecting occult bacteremia in febrile, ambulatory pediatric patients with no apparent signs or symptoms of severe infection and with no focal infection.**
Design: **YOS scores were assigned as part of a prospective, multicenter, randomized, interventional trial of oral and intramuscular antibiotics in preventing the complications of occult bacteremia in febrile children.**
Setting: **Pediatric emergency departments at eight urban medical centers.**
Participants: **Children, 3 to 36 months of age with a temperature at least 39.0° C, a nonfocal, non-toxic-appearing illness (or uncomplicated otitis media), treated as outpatients.**
Interventions: **None.**
Results: **There were 6611 assessable patients, who had both a blood culture result and a YOS score assigned. The median YOS score for both patients with bacteremia (n = 192) and patients without bacteremia (n = 6419) was 6, but the mean rank among patients with bacteremia was significantly higher (*p* <0.0001). The sensitivity, specificity, and positive and negative predictive values for a YOS score greater than 10 were 5.2%, 96.7%, 4.5%, and 97.1%, respectively.**
Conclusions: **The YOS scores are higher among patients with bacteremia than among patients without bacteremia, but the difference is not clinically useful in detecting occult bacteremia in febrile children, with nonfocal, apparently nontoxic infection, treated as outpatients in this age group. (J PEDIATR 1995; 126:877-81)**

Numerous studies have attempted to define the role of several different laboratory variables in identifying which young, febrile patients have bacteremia.[1-7] Other investigators have examined the efficacy of observation scales on the basis of appearance and behavior.[8-18] In a series of articles beginning in 1980, McCarthy et al.[10, 12, 14, 16, 17] developed and applied a 6-point clinical assessment system for febrile children that has come to be known as the Yale Observation Scale (Table I). They have demonstrated the utility of the Scale in identifying those febrile children who have the most toxic illness and those who have serious illness.[14, 17] The

YOS	Yale Observation Scale

Submitted for publication Aug. 8, 1994; accepted Dec. 29, 1994.

Reprint requests: Stephen J. Teach, MD, MPH, Division of Emergency Medicine, Children's Hospital of Buffalo, 219 Bryant St., Buffalo, NY 14222.

[a]For members of Occult Bacteremia Study Group, see list at end of text.

0022-3476/95/$3.00 + 0 **9/20/62984**

Table I. Yale Observation Scales

Observation	Normal (1 point)	Moderate impairment (3 points)	Severe impairment (5 points)
Quality of cry	Strong with normal tone *or* content and not crying	Whimpering *or* sobbing	Weak *or* moaning *or* high-pitched
Reaction to parent stimulation	Cries briefly then stops *or* content and not crying	Cries off and on	Continual cry *or* hardly responds
State variation	If awake, stays awake, *or* if asleep and stimulated, wakes up quickly	Eyes close briefly, then awakes *or* awakes with prolonged stimulation	Falls to sleep *or* will not arouse
Color	Pink	Pale extremities *or* acrocyanosis	Pale *or* cyanotic *or* mottled *or* ashen
Hydration	Skin and eyes normal *and* mucous membranes moist	Skin and eyes normal *and* mouth slightly dry	Skin doughy *or* tented *and* dry mucous membranes *and/or* sunken eyes
Response (talk, smile) to social overtures	Smiles *or* alerts (≤2 mo)	Smiles briefly *or* alert briefly (≤2 mo)	No smile, face anxious, dull, expressionless, *or* not alerted (≤2 mo)

From McCarthy PL, Lembo RM, Baron MA, Fink HD, Cicchetti DV. Pediatrics 1985;76:167-71. Reproduced by permission of Pediatrics.

purpose of our study was to attempt to extend the findings of McCarthy et al. to a subset of febrile children who appeared less ill at initial examination and to determine the efficacy of the YOS in detecting occult bacteremia in such a group. We therefore studied a large cohort of children 3 to 36 months of age, who had non-toxic-appearing illness and a temperature of at least 39.0° C, all of whom were electively treated as outpatients.

METHODS

The study population was drawn from 6680 patients prospectively enrolled in a prior multicenter trial of the use of parenteral versus oral antibiotics for the prevention of bacterial complications in children with occult bacteremia between November 1987 and May 1991.[19] Criteria for inclusion were age from 90 days to 36 months, a temperature of at least 39.0° C, and a nonfocal febrile illness as determined by a physical examination and a blood sample taken for culture at the time of initial examination. A nonfocal febrile illness was defined as excluding a focal, defined bacterial illness (e.g., pharyngitis, cellulitis, pneumonia). Uncomplicated otitis media was acceptable for inclusion at six of eight centers. Exclusionary criteria included a toxic clinical appearance such that in the opinion of the attending pediatrician the child required admission to the hospital and intravenous antibiotic therapy, a known or suspected allergy to amoxicillin or ceftriaxone, a focal bacterial infection other than otitis media, a specific viral infection (e.g., varicella), a known immunodeficiency or underlying chronic disease that would affect the approach to an uncomplicated febrile illness, antibiotic therapy or immunization during the prior 48 hours, or lack of informed consent. Informed consent was obtained in accordance with the institutional review board at each participating institution.

As part of the initial multicenter study design, an attending pediatrician enrolled and examined each patient in standard fashion with the YOS before patients were randomly assigned to receive an antibiotic regimen. Isolates from blood cultures that were considered pathogens have been described previously.[19]

Data were analyzed with the Mann-Whitney U Test for unpaired nonparametric data. Aggregate mean ranks were compared by the Statistical Package for the Social Sciences/PC statistical software package (SPSS Inc., Chicago, Ill.). Significance was defined at a p value less than 0.05.

RESULTS

Patient population. The eight study centers enrolled 6680 patients who received medication; 6329 (96%) had nonfocal febrile illness and 351 (4%) had otitis media. A detailed description of this population and of its sampling procedures has been previously reported.[19] The mean age was 14.5 ± 8.3 months, and the median age was 12.4 months. The mean temperature was 39.8° ± 0.56° C, with a median of 39.7° C.

Of the 6680 patients who received medication, 43 were excluded from analysis because of lost blood cultures, 23 were excluded because of incomplete YOS scores, and three were excluded because of failure to meet enrollment criteria (two patients) or insufficient follow-up (one). Of the remaining 6611 assessable patients with a blood culture result and a calculated YOS, 6419 patients did not have bacteremia (either a negative blood culture result or nonpathogenic organisms isolated) and 192 had bacteremia (2.9%).

Observation scores. The range of YOS scores was 6 to

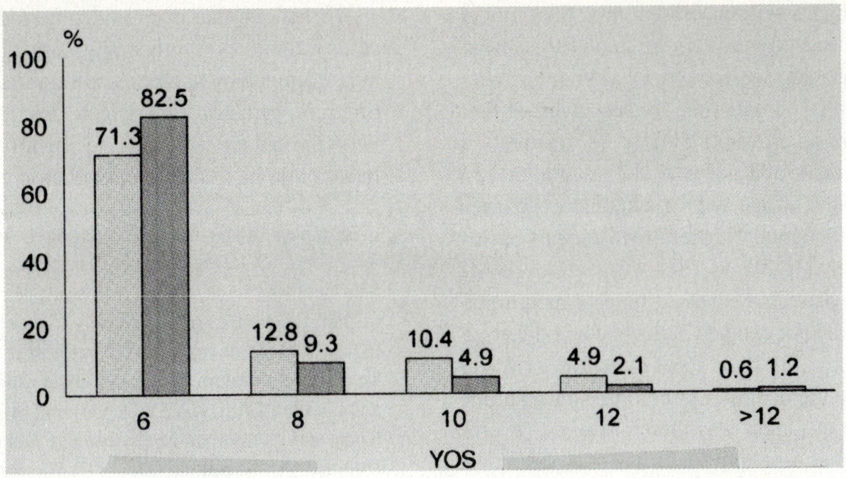

Figure. YOS scores according to blood culture result. *Lightly shaded bars* indicate patients with bacteremia; *darker bars* indicate patients without bacteremia.

Table II. Efficacy of an elevated YOS score in detecting occult bacteremia in a cohort of 6611 febrile patients, 3 to 36 months of age

	Patients with bacteremia		Patients without bacteremia					
YOS score	No.	%	No.	%	Sensitivity (%)	Specificity (%)	PPV (%)	NPV (%)
>6	55	28.6	1122	17.5	28.6	82.5	4.7	97.4
>8	32	16.7	522	8.1	16.7	91.9	5.8	97.3
>10	10	5.2	210	3.3	5.2	96.7	4.5	97.1
>12	1	0.5	75	1.2	0.5	98.8	1.3	97.1

PPV, Positive predictive value; *NPV*, negative predictive value.

14 for patients with bacteremia and 6 to 24 for patients without bacteremia (Figure). The median for both groups was 6, but the mean rank (by Mann-Whitney U test) for patients with bacteremia (3678) was significantly greater than the mean rank for those without bacteremia (3295; $p < 0.0001$). The sensitivity, specificity, and positive and negative predictive values varied at each level of YOS score and are listed in Table II.

DISCUSSION

The YOS[16] is a composite ordinal scoring system with the use of observation variables for the assessment of febrile children. The standard outcome measure used by McCarthy et al.[14, 16] was the detection of serious illness (pneumonia, urinary tract infection, occult bacteremia, a focal complication of occult bacteremia, severe gastroenteritis, aseptic meningitis, and others). It was among the first attempts to recognize and to quantify the physician's overall assessment of toxicity in ill children.

The current study is an attempt to extend the principles of objective assessment of McCarthy et al. to a narrower problem—the detection of occult bacteremia in ambulatory, febrile patients from 3 to 36 months of age who are considered to have neither a toxic nor a serious focal illness. We therefore applied the YOS to a population for whom it was not originally designed. The treatment of such patients is difficult because a finite number have bacteremia and are at risk of focal complications. Such risks are low (very likely <1% for focal complications), but they remain of great concern and controversy,[20] resulting in a recent attempt to establish practice guidelines.[21]

We conclude from our results that the YOS is a poor means of detecting occult bacteremia in this specific, selected patient population. Our very large series enabled us to demonstrate conclusively that the YOS score was significantly higher in patients with bacteremia than in patients without bacteremia ($p < 0.0001$). Nonetheless, because more than half the patients with bacteremia had a YOS score of 6 and because the prevalence of occult bacteremia was low, the sensitivity and positive predictive value of an elevated YOS score were extremely poor. Although patients with bacteremia were judged on the whole to be marginally more ill appearing than patients without bacteremia, the clinical usefulness of this distinction was very limited. The overlap in appearance between the two groups was too great.

The only other published data that we are aware of that address the efficacy of an elevated YOS score in detecting occult bacteremia are those of Baker et al.[18] They studied 154 children 3 to 24 months of age with a temperature greater than 39.4° C and found a much higher prevalence of bacteremia than in our study (12.3% vs 2.9%, respectively). Although they excluded patients with overt signs of meningitis or septic shock, they did not exclude patients who otherwise had an apparently toxic illness or focal infection, or those who were admitted to the hospital. In comparison with our study, their spectrum of illness was therefore more severe, and they found a higher sensitivity and positive predictive value of a YOS score greater than 10 in detecting occult bacteremia (68% vs 5.2% and 30% vs 4.5%, respectively). Given the conclusion of our study that patients with bacteremia have higher YOS scores than patients without bacteremia, it follows that as one includes a greater percentage of children with apparently toxic illness with a higher prevalence of bacteremia, the sensitivity and positive predictive value of an elevated YOS score will increase. In short, the YOS is more useful when the suspected disease is more overt and more common.

In addition to their inclusion of patients who appeared to have more toxic-appearing illness than those in our study, Baker et al.[18] found a higher range of YOS scores for a second reason: they assigned a YOS score before antipyresis. As their study demonstrated, antipyresis lowers the YOS score. Because conventional treatment of febrile children in our participating pediatric emergency departments included administration of antipyretics at the time of triage and before examination by a physician, the range of our scores was probably lower than if antipyretics had routinely been withheld. The effect of antipyretics is the same in patients with and without bacteremia,[22] however, and we believe that the mean ranks of the two groups would be the same whether or not antipyretics were administered.

Other investigators have attempted to detect occult bacteremia with the use of different scales incorporating some of the same observational principles inherent to the YOS. Like Baker et al.,[18] these prior investigators noted higher sensitivities and positive predictive values than those observed among our patients. As described previously, we believe that these differences are due to higher prevalences of bacteremia in these studies (3.6% to 12.0%) and the inclusion of patients with overt focal infection or "toxic" appearance.[8, 13, 15] These prior studies also included fewer patients examined by one person,[15] or by several physicians within a single institution or small group of allied institutions,[8, 13] conditions that might permit a systematic observer bias.

We believe that our multicenter design and much larger sample should minimize any such potential observer bias. When applied by numerous different physicians in numerous different pediatric emergency departments, the YOS was very limited in its ability to identify patients with occult bacteremia in a selected population of febrile children.

Members of the Occult Bacteremia Study Group are Norman Rosenberg, DO, Department of Pediatrics, Wayne State University School of Medicine, Detroit, Mich.; Robert Vinci, MD, Department of Pediatrics, Boston University School of Medicine, Boston, Mass.; Joel Steinberg, MD, Department of Pediatrics, University of Texas Southwestern Medical Center, Dallas; Keith Powell, MD, and Cynthia Christy, MD, Department of Pediatrics, University of Rochester School of Medicine and Dentistry, Rochester, N.Y.; Douglas A. Boenning, MD, Department of Pediatrics, George Washington University School of Medicine, Washington, D.C.; Gary Overturf, MD, Department of Pediatrics, University of New Mexico School of Medicine, Albuquerque; David Jaffe, MD, Department of Pediatrics, Washington University School of Medicine, St. Louis, Mo.; Richard Platt, MD, Department of Medicine, Brigham and Women's Hospital, Harvard Medical School, Boston, Mass.

REFERENCES

1. Jaffe DM, Fleisher GR. Temperature and total white blood cell count as indicators of bacteremia. Pediatrics 1991;87:670-4.
2. Stanley TV, Barrett D, Salmond CE. Viral and bacterial infection in childhood: the value of C reactive protein. N Z Med J 1991;104:138-9.
3. Bennish M, Breem MO, Ormiste V. C-reactive protein and zeta sedimentation ratio as indicators of bacteremia in pediatric patients. J PEDIATR 1984;104:729-32.
4. Morens DM. WBC count and differential: value in predicting bacterial diseases in children. Am J Dis Child 1979;133:25-7.
5. Todd JK. Childhood infections: diagnostic value of peripheral white blood cell and differential cell counts. Am J Dis Child 1974;127:810-6.
6. Saladino R, Erikson M, Levy N, Bachman D, Silber GR, Fleisher GR. Utility of serum interleukin-6 for diagnosis of invasive bacterial disease in children. Ann Emerg Med 1992; 21:1413-6.
7. Rubin LG, Carmody L. Pneumococcal and *Haemophilus influenzae* type b antigen detection in children at risk for occult bacteremia. Pediatrics 1987;80:92-6.
8. Dershewitz RA, Wigder HN, Wigder CM, Nadelman DH. A comparative study of the prevalence, outcome, and prediction of bacteremia in children. J PEDIATR 1983;103:352-7.
9. Bass JW, Steele RW, Wittler RR, et al. Antimicrobial treatment of occult bacteremia: a multicenter cooperative study. Pediatr Infect Dis J 1993;12:446-73.
10. McCarthy PL, Jekel JF, Stashwick CA, Spiesel SZ, Dolan TF. History and observation variables in assessing febrile children. Pediatrics 1980;65:1090-5.
11. Nelson KG. An index of severity for acute pediatric illness. Am J Public Health 1980;70:804-7.
12. McCarthy PL, Jekel JF, Stashwick CA, et al. Further definition of history and observation variables in assessing febrile children. Pediatrics 1981;67:687-93.

13. Waskerwitz S, Berkelhamer JE. Outpatient bacteremia: clinical findings in children under two years with initial temperatures of 39.5° C or higher. J PEDIATR 1981;99:231-3.
14. McCarthy PL, Sharpe MR, Spiesel SZ, et al. Observation scales to identify serious illness in febrile children. Pediatrics 1982; 70:802-9.
15. Schwartz RH, Wientzen RL. Occult bacteremia in toxic-appearing, febrile infants. Clin Pediatr 1982;21:659-63.
16. McCarthy PL, Lembo RM, Baron MA, Fink HD, Cicchetti DV. Predictive value of abnormal physical examination findings in ill-appearing and well-appearing febrile children. Pediatrics 1985;76:167-71.
17. McCarthy PL, Lembo RM, Fink HD, Baron MA, Cicchetti DV. Observation, history, and physical examination in diagnosis of serious illnesses in febrile children ≤24 months. J PEDIATR 1987;110:26-30.
18. Baker RC, Tiller T, Bausher JC, et al. Severity of disease correlated with fever reduction in febrile infants. Pediatrics 1989; 83:1016-9.
19. Fleisher GR, Rosenberg N, Vinci R, et al. Intramuscular versus oral antibiotic therapy for the prevention of meningitis and other bacterial sequelae in young, febrile children at risk for occult bacteremia. J PEDIATR 1994;124:504-12.
20. Liu TA, Schwartz JS, Jaffe DM, Fleisher GR. Strategies for diagnosis and treatment of children at risk for occult bacteremia: clinical effectiveness and cost-effectiveness. J PEDIATR 1991; 118:21-9.
21. Baraff LJ, Bass JW, Fleisher GR, et al. Practice guidelines for the management of infants and children 0 to 36 months of age with fever without source. Pediatrics 1993;92:1-12.
22. Torrey SB, Henretig F, Fleisher GR, et al. Response to antipyretic therapy of temperature in children with and without bacteremia. Am J Emerg Med 1985;3:190-2.

Clinical characteristics and risk factors for *Vibrio cholerae* infection in children

Juan M. Fukuda, MD, Augusto Yi, MD, Luis Chaparro, MD, Miguel Campos, MD, PhD, and Elsa Chea, MD

From the Pediatric Emergency, Pediatric, Microbiology, and Public Health Departments, Universidad Peruana Cayetano Heredia, and Hospital Nacional Cayetano Heredia, Lima, Peru

Surveillance was conducted during February and March 1991 in the pediatric emergency department of Cayetano Heredia Hospital, Lima, Peru, to contrast the characteristics of children with epidemic cholera with those of children with non-cholera-associated diarrhea. Among 626 patients 14 years of age or younger, *Vibrio cholerae* O1 was isolated from stool specimens of 310 patients (49%), more commonly from children older than 24 months of age (66%; *p* <0.0001) than from younger children. Cholera was clinically characterized by a more sudden onset; watery diarrhea; and associated abdominal pain, muscle cramps, and vomiting, which led to more severe dehydration and hospitalization more often than in noncholera cases. Only one patient with cholera died, for a case-fatality rate of 3.2 deaths per 1000 persons. Nonpotable water and uncooked foods were identified as probable vehicles for *V. cholerae*. The frequency of diarrhea among relatives of patients with cholera suggested intrafamily transmission. This study of epidemic cholera describes the clinical features and the risk factors for acquisition of the infection, and points out the low case-fatality rate with prompt and appropriate treatment. (J Pediatr 1995;126:882-6)

The seventh pandemic of cholera started in Indonesia in 1961 and spread in 1991 to the Americas, where the first cases were detected in the Valley of Chancay in Lima, Peru. The epidemic spread rapidly throughout Peru and neighboring countries; more than 500,000 cases and 4000 deaths were reported by the end of 1992.[1]

Cayetano Heredia Hospital, a tertiary-care center located in a poor periurban area north of Lima, has provided care and treatment of patients with cholera since the beginning of the epidemic. This report describes the clinical characteristics and risk factors of the patients examined for diarrhea during the first 2 months of the epidemic.

METHODS

Patients. On Feb. 1, 1991, a week after cholera was first reported in Lima, the Pediatric Emergency Department of the Cayetano Heredia Hospital initiated a microbiologic surveillance program. All patients 14 years of age or younger with the main problem of diarrhea who sought medical care during the daytime hours (8 AM to 2 PM) were enrolled in the study. Diarrhea was defined as any decrease in the consistency or increase in frequency of the stools, as perceived by the child or child's caretaker. Informed consent was obtained from the parents or caretaker of all patients. The study protocol was approved by the ethics committee of Universidad Peruana Cayetano Heredia.

ORS	Oral rehydration solution

Procedures. Stool was obtained by rectal swabbing, placed in a vial containing Cary-Blair transport medium, and transported to the microbiology laboratory the same day. Specimens were then incubated in alkaline peptone water for enrichment and inoculated in thiosulfate-citrate-bile-sucrose according to standard techniques.[2] Standardized questionnaire forms were used to record demographic and clinical data, and probable risk factors associated with acquisition of *V. cholerae* infection.

Submitted for publication May 25, 1994; accepted Dec. 19, 1994.

Reprint requests: Juan M. Fukuda, MD, Universidad Peruana Cayetano Heredia, Av. Honorio Delgado 430, Lima 31, A.P. 4314, Lima 100, Peru.

0022-3476/95/$3.00 + 0 **9/20/62889**

Table I. Characteristics of patients with cholera-associated and non-cholera-associated diarrhea

	No. (%) of patients				
Characteristic	Cholera	Noncholera	OR	95% CI	p
Illness ≤24 hr	212/310 (68)	174/316 (55)	1.77	1.26-2.48	0.001
Age ≤24 mo	40/70 (57)	88/196 (45)	1.64	0.91-2.96	NS
Age >24 mo	172/240 (72)	86/120 (72)	1.00	0.59-1.68	NS
Watery stools	251/308 (81)	202/311 (65)	2.38	1.61-3.51	<0.0001
Age ≤24 mo	44/70 (63)	121/193 (63)	0.99	0.54-1.83	NS
Age >24 mo	207/238 (87)	81/118 (69)	0.33	0.18-0.59	<0.0001
Rice-water	88/195 (45)	27/167 (16)	4.26	2.51-7.29	<0.0001
Age ≤24 mo	5/33 (15)	11/111 (10)	1.61	0.44-5.71	NS
Age >24 mo	83/162 (51)	16/56 (29)	2.63	1.29-5.38	<0.05
Blood and mucus	8/303 (3)	15/309 (5)	0.53	0.20-1.37	NS
Age ≤24 mo	5/70 (7)	13/194 (7)	1.07	0.32-3.43	NS
Age >24 mo	3/233 (1)	2/115 (1)	0.74	0.10-6.49	NS
Vomiting	258/310 (83)	205/313 (65)	2.61	1.75-3.90	<0.0001
Age ≤24 mo	47/70 (67)	127/195 (65)	1.09	0.59-2.05	NS
Age >24 mo	211/240 (88)	78/118 (66)	3.73	2.08-6.71	<0.0001
Abdominal pain	217/285 (76)	190/279 (68)	1.49	1.01-2.21	<0.05
Age ≤24 mo	32/59 (54)	90/160 (56)	0.92	0.48-1.76	NS
Age >24 mo	185/226 (82)	100/119 (84)	0.86	0.45-1.63	NS
Muscle cramp	59/193 (30)	4/157 (3)	16.48	5.58-56.00	<0.0001
Age ≤24 mo	0/36 (0)	0/79 (0)			NS
Age >24 mo	59/157 (38)	4/78 (5)	11.14	3.63-38.22	<0.0001
Subjective fever	58/289 (20)	133/312 (43)	0.34	0.23-0.50	<0.0001
Age ≤24 mo	26/69 (38)	93/195 (48)	0.66	0.36-1.21	NS
Age >24 mo	32/220 (15)	40/117 (34)	0.33	0.18-0.58	0.0001
Fever	14/207 (7)	41/204 (20)	0.29	0.14-0.57	<0.0001
Age ≤24 mo	7/41 (17)	33/125 (26)	0.57	0.21-1.53	NS
Age >24 mo	7/166 (4)	8/79 (10)	0.39	0.12-1.26	NS
Severe dehydration	111/309 (36)	1/316 (0.3)	176	26.15-3493	<0.0001
Age ≤24 mo	11/70 (16)	0/196			<0.0001
Age >24 mo	100/239 (42)	1/120 (1)	85.61	12.51-1706	<0.0001
Hospitalization	122/309 (39)	24/316 (7)	7.94	4.80-13.20	<0.0001
Age ≤24 mo	17/70 (24)	22/196 (11)	2.54	1.18-5.46	<0.05
Age >24 mo	105/239 (44)	2/120 (2)	46.23	10.8-280.39	<0.0001

CI, Confidence interval; *NS*, not significant; *OR*, odds ratio.

Treatment. The degree of dehydration was determined according to World Health Organization guidelines.[3] Rehydration was performed as follows: those patients with mild and moderate dehydration were examined in a holding area for about 4 hours to ensure adequate intake (<20 ml/kg per hour) of oral rehydration soluation–World Health Organization formula (containing sodium, 90 mmol/L; potassium, 20 mmol/L; bases, 30 mmol/L; and glucose, 111 mOsm/L) and then treated as outpatients. Patients with poor oral intake of ORS or severe dehydration were hospitalized. If shock was present, as evidenced by poor peripheral perfusion and low systolic blood pressure (<80 mm Hg + [age in years × 2]), rehydration was initiated with 20 to 60 ml/kg intravenously administered isotonic saline solution (0.9% sodium chloride); followed by the rapid intravenous administration of polyelectrolyte solution (containing the same electrolyte composition as ORS) at 25 ml/kg per hour for the next 4 hours. In all cases 2 hours after the start of intravenous infusion, ORS was offered freely to replace the ongoing losses. After dehydration was resolved, maintenance fluid replacement was continued with ORS. Intravenous administration of fluids was continued only if vomiting was persistent or if the losses were greater than the oral intake. Early feeding was encouraged. Antibiotic treatment was administered with trimethoprim-sulfamethoxazole (trimethoprim component, 8 to 10 mg/kg per day) for 3 days.

Statistical analysis. The EPI-Info program (Centers for Disease Control and Prevention, Atlanta, Ga., and World Health Organization, Geneva, Switzerland) was used for statistical analysis. Continuous variables were compared by the Student *t* test and chi-square test for proportions. Odds ratios and confidence intervals were calculated with the Cornfield approximation.[4] All analyses were interpreted in a two-tailed fashion.

RESULTS

During February and March 1991, of 1571 children with diarrhea, 626 (40%) were enrolled in the present study. *V.*

Table II. Risk factors affecting the rate of isolation of *V. cholerae* from diarrheal stools

	No. (%) of patients				
Risk factor	Cholera	Noncholera	OR	95% CI	*p*
Breast-feeding*	19/30 (63)	67/92 (73)	0.64	0.25-1.70	NS
Lack of potable water	140/218 (64)	61/174 (35)	3.32	2.14-5.18	<0.0001
Age ≤24 mo	23/50 (46)	38/107 (36)	1.55	0.73-3.26	NS
Age >24 mo	117/168 (70)	23/67 (34)	4.39	2.29-8.45	<0.0001
Drinking unboiled water	122/241 (51)	43/241 (18)	4.72	3.04-7.34	<0.0001
Age ≤24 mo	9/48 (19)	13/146 (9)	2.36	0.85-6.53	NS
Age >24 mo	113/193 (59)	30/95 (32)	3.06	1.76-5.35	<0.0001
Eating raw fish	21/238 (9)	7/256 (3)	3.44	1.34-9.17	<0.05
Age ≤24 mo	2/48 (4)	3/154 (2)	2.19	0.24-17.00	NS
Age >24 mo	19/190 (10)	4/102 (4)	2.72	0.83-9.86	NS
Eating raw vegetables	42/225 (19)	26/244 (11)	1.92	1.10-3.39	<0.05
Age ≤24 mo	5/44 (11)	13/148 (9)	1.33	0.38-4.40	NS
Age >24 mo	37/181 (20)	13/96 (14)	1.64	0.78-3.48	NS
Relative with diarrhea	112/239 (47)	51/213 (24)	2.80	1.83-4.30	<0.0001
Age ≤24 mo	17/49 (35)	26/127 (20)	2.06	0.93-4.59	<0.05
Age >24 mo	95/190 (50)	25/86 (29)	2.44	1.36-4.40	<0.05

CI, Confidence interval; *NS*, not significant; *OR*, odds ratio.
*Children less than 12 months of age.

cholerae O1, biotype El Tor, serotype Inaba, was isolated from the stools of 310 of the patients (49%). The age distribution differed between the cholera and noncholera cases (68 ± 48 months vs 34 ± 35 months, respectively; $p < 0.00001$). The rates of cholera isolation were 70 (26%) of 266, 98 (61%) of 160, and 142 (71%) of 200 for children up to 24 months, 25 to 60 months, and older than 60 months of age, respectively (p for trend <0.00001).

Clinical characteristics (Table I). Overall, patients with cholera had a more sudden onset of illness; more profuse watery diarrhea; and associated abdominal pain, muscle cramps, and vomiting, leading to more severe dehydration and requiring hospitalization more often than for those with non-cholera-associated diarrhea. Conversely fever was less common among patients with cholera. Among children 24 months of age or younger, only the presence of severe dehydration and the need for hospitalization were associated with the isolation of *V. cholerae*. Among children older than 24 months, characteristics of the stool and initial symptoms were also important in predicting cholera. The rates of severe dehydration for children with cholera were 11 (16%) of 70, 31 (32%) of 98, and 69 (49%) of 141 at ages up 24 months, 25 to 60 months, and older than 60 months of age, respectively ($p < 0.00001$). Among the patients with non-cholera-associated diarrhea, only one had severe dehydration.

Only one patient with cholera died during the study period, for a case-fatality rate of 3.2 per 1000 cases (Poisson 95% CI = 0.08 to 17.97). This patient was a 7-month-old girl with severe dehydration and shock who died 36 hours after admission with clinical findings compatible with multilobar pneumonia.

Risk factors (Table II). Use of nonpotable water (i.e., no tap water in the house) and uncooked food was associated with cholera among children older than 24 months of age. In addition, significantly more cases of diarrhea occurred among relatives of patients with cholera than among those of patients without cholera, suggesting intrafamily transmission in the former group.

Analysis of the demographic and clinical characteristics as predictors of *V. cholerae* isolation showed that vomiting was the most sensitive (0.83) variable but had a low specificity (0.34). Severe dehydration, on the contrary, was the most specific (0.99) but had low sensitivity (0.36). The combination of acute watery diarrhea and age more than 24 months had a sensitivity of 0.67 and a specificity of 0.74, with negative and positive predictive values of 0.72 and 0.74, respectively. The addition of dehydration improved sensitivity to 0.70, maintaining the other values.

DISCUSSION

Cholera was the most important cause of diarrhea during the study and accounted for half the cases of diarrhea in children 14 years of age or younger. Cholera caused more severe dehydration than did other causes of diarrhea, required hospitalization in a significantly larger number of cases, and hence added a considerable burden to our already overloaded services. The initial clinical features were useful in children older than 24 months to identify the cases likely to be cholera. In younger children, regardless of the cause, the clinical presentation was similar, but cholera was still a cause of more severe dehydration and required hospitalization more frequently.

Despite the large number of cases and their severity, the case-fatality rate was low (3.2 deaths per 1000 cases); in other countries rates of 10% to 20% have been reported.[5, 6] Reasons for the lower rate are unknown but may reflect the organized response at all levels (government, medical personnel, and community) to the epidemic and the widespread and early use of ORS,[7] which has long been known to be an inexpensive and effective way of treating all but the most severe cases of dehydration, regardless of the cause. In Amazon areas of Peru, where medical care was scarce, the mortality rate resulting from cholera increased to 10% to 20%.[8]

Cholera is a noninvasive disease; death occurs as a result of the complications of dehydration. Renal complications are the most common and lethal.[9-11] Neurologic damage also can occur as a result of severe hyponatremic dehydration or hypoglycemia.[12] Thus the management of cholera should focus on overcoming dehydration as quickly as possible. On arrival at our hospital, the pediatric patients were treated with a single uncomplicated scheme applicable to most cases. Efforts were made to reverse shock immediately (within the first 10 to 15 minutes) and then to restore of hydration status within 4 hours, followed by a continuous replacement of losses, volume for volume, preferably orally. We believe that the keys to the low case-fatality rate in our hospital were simplification of the treatment scheme and close clinical monitoring. The treatment of cholera in adults was similar to that in children, except for the rehydration phase isotonic saline solution and ORS were used instead of polyelectrolyte solution and ORS. This treatment regimen also resulted in a low case-fatality rate of 0.65 deaths per 1000 cases.[13] Even though isotonic saline solution is inexpensive and widely available, we do not recommend this solution, at least not alone, for pediatric patients, because it does not replace potassium. If it is used, we suggest that isotonic saline solution be given concomitantly with ORS. Finally, antibiotics were not deemed an essential part of our protocol but rather as an adjunct to decrease the spread of *V. cholerae* and to decrease ongoing losses.[14, 15]

Cholera was a more common cause of diarrhea in children older than 24 months. This could be a result of increased exposure; ambulating increases the potential of reaching contaminated sources. Breast-feeding also might have had a role in protecting against acquisition of cholera in younger children, as demonstrated by other investigators.[16, 17] In our study population, however, we could not demonstrate that breast-feeding was less common among patients of cholera than in those without cholera. We believe that this was due to the small sample and to the fact that cases of cholera were compared with cases of non-cholera-associated diarrhea and not to nondiarrhea cases, as reported by others. Breast-feeding has a protective effect against diarrhea in general,[18, 19] so the effect on cholera might have been diluted.

These data also suggest that lack of potable water, and consumption of unboiled water and raw fish, might be implicated in the acquisition of cholera, in accordance with previous evaluations in different cities of Peru.[20, 21] Among cholera cases, a higher proportion of family members with diarrhea concurrently or within the previous 48 hours was reported than among noncholera cases. We did not investigate the cause involved in these additional cases, but household environment is known to pose an increased risk of cholera infection.[22, 23]

One limitation of our study was the inclusion of only 40% of the patients with diarrhea seen at our pediatric emergency department. This was not a random selection but rather a convenience sample based on the enrollment of cases during morning hours, when most of the working staff was available. The lack of personnel and materials made it impossible to perform surveillance 24 hours a day, as originally planned. For the same reason, only *V. cholerae* was systematically cultured, and we do not know the causes of the noncholera cases.

In summary, our study shows that during epidemic cholera children 14 years of age or younger were affected by *V. cholerae* and that those older than 24 months were most frequently and severely affected. They had watery diarrhea, vomiting, and severe dehydration that required hospitalization more frequently than in children with non-cholera-associated diarrhea. Identified risk factors included lack of potable water, consumption of unboiled water, and a relative with diarrhea. With a simple and rapid rehydration scheme, the treatment of these children with cholera was successful and achieved a low case-fatality rate.

We thank Dr. Rodolfo Begue for critical review of the manuscript.

REFERENCES

1. Centers for Disease Control. Update: cholera—Western Hemisphere, 1992. MMWR 1993;42:89-93.
2. Kelly MT, Hickman-Brenner FW, Farmer JJ. Vibrio. In: Belows A, Hausler WJ, Harrman KL, Isenberg HD, Shadomy HJ, eds. Manual of clinical microbiology. 5th ed. Washington, DC: American Society for Microbiology, 1991:384-95.
3. WHO guidelines for defining degrees of dehydration In: Pan-American Health Office, ed. Manual de tratamiento de la diarrea. Washington, D.C.: Pan American Health Office, 1987.
4. Dean AG, Dean JA, Burton AH, Dicker RC. Epi Info, version 5: a word processing, database, and statistics program for epidemiology on microcomputers. Stone Mountain, Georgia: USD, 1990.
5. Chapman JA, Collocott LP. Cholera in children at Eshowe Hospital. S Afr Med J 1985;68:249-56.
6. Tauxe V, Holmberg SD, Dodin A, Well JV, Blake PA. Epidemic cholera in Mali: high mortality and multiple routes

of transmission in a famine area. Epidemiol Infect 1988;100: 279-89.
7. Carpenter CJ. The treatment of cholera: clinical science at bedside. J Infect Dis 1992;166:2-14.
8. Quick RE, Vargas R, Moreno D, et al. Epidemic cholera in the amazon: the challenge of preventing death. Am J Trop Med Hyg 1993;48:597-602.
9. Cieza J, Gutierrez R, Estremadoiro L, Miyahira J. Insuficiencia renal aguda secundaria a cólera: aspectos epidemiológicos. Rev Med Hered 1992;3:140-7.
10. Gotuzzo E, Cieza J, Estremadoyro L, Seas C. Cholera: lessons from the epidemic in Peru. Infect Dis Clin North Am 1994; 8:183-205.
11. Carpenter CCJ, Mitra PP, Sack RB. Clinical studies in Asiatic cholera. I. Preliminary observations: November 1962-March 1963. Bull Johns Hopkins Hosp 1966;118:165-73.
12. Barua D, Greenough WB III, eds. Current topics in infectious disease—cholera. New York: Plenum, 1992.
13. Cieza J, Gamarra G, Torres C. Letalidad y riesgo de insuficiencia renal por cólera en el Hospital Nacional Cayetano Heredia de Lima, Perú. Rev Med Hered 1991;2:75-8.
14. Burans JP, Podgore J, Mansour MM, et al. Comparative trial of erythromycin and sulphatrimethoprim in the treatment of tetracycline-resistant *Vibrio cholerae* O1. Trans R Soc Trop Med Hyg 1989;83:836-8.
15. Rabbani GH, Butler T, Shahrier M, Mazamdar RR, Islam MR. Efficacy of a single dose of furazolidone for treatment of cholera in children. Antimicrob Agents Chemother 1991;35:1864-7.
16. Glass RI, Svennerholm A-M, Stoll BJ, et al. Protection against cholera in breast-fed children by antibodies in breast milk. N Engl J Med 1983;308:1389-92.
17. Clemens JD, Sack DA, Harris JR, et al. Breast feeding and the risk of severe cholera in rural Bangladeshi children. Am J Epidemiol 1990;131:400-11.
18. Khin-Maung-U, Nyunt-Nyunt-WAI, Myo-Khin, Mu-Mu-Khin, Tin-U, Thane-TOE. Effects on clinical outcome of breast feeding during acute diarrhoea. Br Med J 1985;290:587-9.
19. Brown KH, Black RE, Lopez de Romaña G, Kanashiro HC. Infant-feeding practices and their relationship with diarrheal and other diseases in Huascar (Lima), Peru. Pediatrics 1989; 83:31-40.
20. Ries AA, Vugia DJ, Beingolea L, et al. Cholera in Piura, Peru: a modern urban epidemic. J Infect Dis 1992;166:1429-33.
21. Swerdlow DL, Mintz ED, Rodriguez M, et al. Waterborne transmission of epidemic cholera in Trujillo, Peru: lessons for a continent at risk. Lancet 1992;340:28-33.
22. Oseashon R, Ahmad S, Islam M, Rahman A. Clinical and bacteriological findings among families of cholera patients. Lancet 1966;1:340-2.
23. Gotuzzo E, Seas C, Cabezas C, Carrillo C, Ruiz R. Estudio de transmision intrafamiliar en pacientes con cólera en Lima 1991. Rev Med Hered 1991;1:117-20.

A reexamination of the risk factors for the sudden infant death syndrome

James A. Taylor, MD, and Maureen Sanderson, MPH, RD

From the Departments of Pediatrics and Epidemiology, University of Washington, Seattle

Objective: To determine which risk factors are specific for the sudden infant death syndrome (SIDS) rather than characteristic of postneonatal deaths in general.
Study population: The live births and infant death cohorts of the 1988 National Maternal and Infant Health Survey.
Methods: Information on live births, deaths from SIDS, and postneonatal deaths from other causes was abstracted from the National Maternal and Infant Health Survey. To account for oversampling of certain populations, the data were weighted to reflect national counts. Risk factors were defined as black race, birth weight less than 1500 gm, birth weight less than 2500 gm, gestational age at birth less than 37 weeks, 5-minute Apgar score less than 7, male gender, more than two previous pregnancies, maternal age less than 20 years, maternal education level less than 12 years, multiple births, and maternal smoking during pregnancy. Odds ratios (ORs) and 95% confidence intervals (CIs) were calculated to compare the SIDS with the live births cohort, infants who died of other causes with the live births cohort, and SIDS with non-SIDS deaths. The population-attributable risk percentage was computed for risk factors independently associated with SIDS when compared with other postneonatal deaths.
Results: For all characteristics other than a 5-minute Apgar score less than 7, the ORs comparing infants who died of SIDS with the live births cohort were significantly greater than 1.0. Similarly, ORs comparing infants who died of other causes with the live births cohort were also greater than 1.0, except for male gender. When the two infant death cohorts were compared, only maternal smoking during pregnancy and low maternal education level were significantly more common among the SIDS group. After we controlled for cigarette smoking, the adjusted OR for low maternal education level was not significantly greater than 1.0. However, even after control for low maternal education level, prenatal exposure to tobacco was significantly more common among the SIDS group than in infants dying of other causes (OR = 1.97; 95% CI, 1.59 to 2.45). On the basis of an adjusted OR of 2.92 when the SIDS group was compared with the live births cohort, the population-attributable risk percentage for maternal smoking as a risk factor for SIDS was 30%.
Conclusion: Among characteristics generally thought to be risk factors, only maternal smoking during pregnancy was independently associated with SIDS. Data from this nationally representative sample indicate that if women refrained from smoking while pregnant, up to 30% of SIDS might be prevented. (J PEDIATR 1995;126:887-91)

Presented at the Thirty-fourth Annual Meeting of the Ambulatory Pediatrics Association, Seattle, Wash., May 5, 1994.

Submitted for publication Sept. 14, 1994; accepted Dec. 20, 1994.

Reprint requests: James A. Taylor, MD, Department of Pediatrics (RD-20), University of Washington, Seattle, WA 98195.

0022-3476/95/$3.00 + 0 **9/20/62885**

In one of the first large-scale epidemiologic studies of its kind, Bergman et al.[1] identified risk factors for sudden infant death syndrome. Victims of SIDS were said to be born in disproportionate numbers to young, poor mothers of minority race. Prematurity, low birth weight, and maternal cigarette smoking were also thought to increase the risk of SIDS. During the next 20 years other investigators corroborated these findings and expanded the list of risk factors.[2-6]

Evidence has accumulated, however, to suggest that these risk factors may not be specific for SIDS. Peterson et al.[7] reported that in Washington State the prevalence of risk factors among infants who died of SIDS was not different from that in infants who died of other causes. A New York State study had similar results.[8] In an earlier study, we reviewed the clinical histories and autopsy records of more than 1100 children whose causes of death were classified as SIDS during a 25-year period.[9] Risk factors (other than young maternal age) were more common in infants for whom the diagnosis of SIDS was most questionable; the remaining infants (whose deaths were termed as ''classic'' SIDS) more closely resembled those in the control population.

The 1988 National Maternal and Infant Health Survey (NMIHS) offers an opportunity to evaluate the significance of the risk factors for SIDS. The survey contains information on more than 9000 live births and 5000 infant deaths throughout the United States. From the data it is possible to compare the prevalence of risk factors among infants dying of SIDS with those in a live births cohort and with babies dying of other causes. Additionally, the proportion of SIDS deaths that can be attributed to any of these risk factors can be calculated.

METHODS

The 1988 NMIHS was conducted by the National Center for Health Statistics to study factors related to poor pregnancy outcomes.[10] Data were abstracted from birth and death certificates of selected infants. Additionally, mothers of these children completed a questionnaire of approximately 200 items regarding health practices, prenatal care, perinatal events, and subsequent health of their babies, together with demographic information. After stratification by race and birth weight infants in the survey were randomly selected from 48 states, the District of Columbia, and New York City. Three separate cohorts were included in the sample. The live births cohort consisted of 9953 infants born in 1988. The infant death cohort included 5332 infants less than 1 year of age who died in 1988; some of these infants were born in 1987. Finally, the fetal death cohort contained information on 3309 fetuses of more than 28 weeks of gestational age who died in 1988. Only the live births and infant death components of the survey were analyzed in our study.

Data for the following variables were abstracted from birth certificate information: birth weight; gender; gestational age; 5-minute Apgar score; and maternal age, race, and parity. Maternal education level and history of cigarette smoking during pregnancy were obtained from the mother's questionnaire. Additionally, if the gestational age on the birth certificate was missing or implausible, the gestational age of the infant was derived from responses on the maternal questionnaire. Information on the cause of death was obtained from death certificates. Infants were included in the study if they were at least 28 days of age at the time of death. Deaths were classified as SIDS deaths on the basis of the International Classification of Diseases, Ninth Revision (ICD-9 code 798.0).

Risk factors for SIDS were based on the definitions used in the large-scale National Institute of Child Health and Human Development (NICHD) study.[6] Thus low birth weight was defined as less than 2500 gm, very low birth weight as less than 1500 gm, prematurity as gestational age less than 37 weeks, perinatal asphyxia as a 5-minute Apgar score less han 7, low maternal age as less than 20 years of age at the time of delivery, high parity as more than two previous pregnancies, and low maternal education as completion of fewer than 12 years of school.

CI	Confidence interval
LBW	Low birth weight
OR	Odds ratio
VLBW	Very low birth weight

In the NMIHS black infants were oversampled for the live births and infant death cohorts, and LBW infants were oversampled for the live births cohort, to increase the reliability of estimates for these groups. Additionally, survey response rates varied in different subpopulations.[10] For our study estimates derived from the NMIHS were weighted to generate a nationally representative sample. The weighting adjusted for the unequal chance of certain subpopulations of infants being included in the survey compared with the relative proportions of these groups of infants (defined by race and birth weight) in the entire population of children born in the United States in 1988, and for the differential response rate. A computer program designed to estimate sampling variances in complex surveys was used to perform logistic regression (SUDAAN software, version 6.0, Research Triangle Institute, Research Triangle Park, N.C.). From the regression analyses odds ratios were obtained; ORs were considered significant when 1.0 was not included in the 95% confidence interval. The population-attributable risk percentage was calculated for potentially modifiable risk factors such as maternal smoking on the basis of the adjusted OR and the weighted proportion of infants in the live births cohort with that risk factor.

Table I. Prevalence of risk factors among infants who died of SIDS, infants who died in postneonatal period of other causes, and live births cohort

Risk factor	SIDS (%)	OR* (95% CI)	Live births (%)	OR* (95% CI)	Non-SIDS (%)
Black race	27.7	1.90 (1.62-2.22)	17.1	1.93 (1.75-2.13)	28.2
VLBW	9.2	8.41 (6.27-11.29)	1.2	33.45 (29.16-38.37)	28.6
LBW	21.1	3.67 (3.02-4.46)	6.8	11.36 (10.10-12.78)	45.5
Prematurity	21.5	2.80 (2.26-3.48)	8.8	5.53 (4.73-6.47)	34.9
Perinatal asphyxia	2.5	1.65 (0.92-2.97)	1.6	15.96 (12.13-21.00)	20.2
Male gender	60.0	1.38 (1.15-1.64)	52.1	1.12 (0.97-1.28)	55.1
High parity	44.1	1.45 (1.19-2.38)	35.2	1.36 (1.19-1.56)	42.4
Young maternal age	21.1	1.92 (1.54-2.38)	12.2	1.55 (1.30-1.85)	17.8
Low maternal education level	36.2	2.29 (1.89-2.79)	20.2	1.77 (1.51-2.07)	30.6
Maternal smoking during pregnancy	46.2	3.06 (2.57-3.66)	22.3	1.51 (1.29-1.76)	30.1
Multiple births	5.1	2.69 (1.82-3.98)	2.0	2.75 (2.01-3.76)	5.3

*Based on comparisons of adjacent groups.

RESULTS

Data on 15,285 infants in the NMIHS were reviewed. Eighty-eight infants in the live births cohort were also in the infant death group, the cause of death of five infants was missing, eight children had missing gestational ages, and 12 neonates had birth weights and gestational ages that were implausible (birth weight <1000 gm in an infant with gestational age of 46 weeks, or gestational ages <27 weeks with birth weights >2700 gm). Information on all these children was excluded. Additionally, 3457 neonates died before 1 month of age and were not included in the analysis. The final sample size was thus 11,734 infants. Among these, 649 deaths were due to SIDS, 1221 postneonatal deaths were from other causes, and 9864 infants were in the live births cohort. Autopsies were performed in 92% of the SIDS cases and in 54.2% of non-SIDS cases.

The prevalence of most previously identified risk factors was higher in infants dying of SIDS than in the live births cohort (Table I). The highest OR between these two groups was for the prevalence of VLBW; 9.2% of SIDS infants weighed less than 1500 gm at birth compared to 1.2% of children in the live births cohort. Similarly, 21.1% in the SIDS group had birth weights less than 2500 gm versus 6.8% of those in the live births cohort. Despite the disproportionate number of LBW neonates, the rate of perinatal asphyxia was not significantly higher in infants dying of SIDS; only 2.5% of the SIDS group had a 5-minute Apgar score less than 7 versus 1.6% of children in the live births cohorts. Other than male gender, the risk factor with the highest prevalence among those who died of SIDS was maternal smoking during pregnancy. More than 46% of mothers of infants with SIDS smoked during their pregnancy; 22.3% of infants in the live births cohort had prenatal exposure to tobacco.

Similar data for the non-SIDS group are shown in Table I. For every variable analyzed, other than male gender, the ORs comparing infants in the non-SIDS group with the live births cohort were significantly greater than 1.0. For perinatal risk factors, including prematurity, LBW, VLBW, and perinatal asphyxia, the prevalence among infants with causes of death in the postneonatal period other than SIDS was striking. Among these infants 45.5% weighed less than 2500 gm at birth and 34.9% had birth weights less than 1500 gm. Perinatal asphyxia was common among the non-SIDS group, with 20.2% having received a 5-minute Apgar score less than 7. Compared with the ORs of infants in the live birth cohort, the ORs for these perinatal risk factors were relatively high, ranging from 5.53 to 33.45.

Table II. ORs comparing SIDS deaths with non-SIDS postneonatal deaths

Characteristic	OR	95% CI
Black race	0.98	0.81-1.19
VLBW	0.25	0.18-0.34
LBW	0.32	0.25-0.40
Prematurity	0.52	0.39-0.65
Perinatal asphyxia	0.10	0.06-0.18
Male gender	1.22	0.98-1.52
High parity	1.07	0.86-1.33
Young maternal age	1.23	0.96-1.59
Low maternal education level	1.30	1.05-1.61
Maternal smoking during pregnancy	2.03	1.64-2.52
Multiple births	0.98	0.61-1.57

The ORs for multiple births, young maternal age, high parity, male gender, and black race were not significantly different from 1.0 when infants who died of other causes were compared with the SIDS group (Table II). Those dying of other causes were significantly more likely to have been premature, to have a birth weight less than 2500 gm or less than 1500 gm, and to have a 5-minute Apgar score of less than 7. Infants in the SIDS group were more likely to have been born to mothers with less than a high school education and to mothers who smoked during pregnancy. However, when maternal smoking was controlled for, the prevalence of mothers with low education levels was not significantly higher in the SIDS group (OR = 1.15; 95% CI, 0.93 to 1.43). Conversely, even after control for maternal education level, a history of maternal cigarette smoking was more common in the SIDS group than in those dying of other causes (OR = 1.97; 95% CI, 1.59 to 2.45). Thus maternal smoking was the only variable studied that was significantly more common in the SIDS group than in infants dying of other causes. After adjustment for the other risk factors, the OR for maternal smoking, comparing infants dying of SIDS with the live births cohort, was 2.92 (95% CI, 2.30 to 3.69). The population-attributable risk percentage for maternal smoking as a risk factor for SIDS was 30%.

DISCUSSION

There is a perception that the majority of SIDS deaths are the result of prenatal or perinatal events, or are caused by problems associated with social disadvantage. Programs have been initiated to identify neonates at high risk and, by modifying these risk factors, to attempt to prevent SIDS.[11, 12] However, data from a nationally representative sample demonstrate that, with the exception of maternal smoking during pregnancy, these risk factors are not specific for SIDS but characterize all postneonatal deaths.

The lack of specificity of risk factors such as prematurity, LBW, and VLBW calls into question any causal relationship of these perinatal outcomes with SIDS. It is possible that prematurity, LBW, and VLBW are important in the pathogenesis of both SIDS and non-SIDS deaths, acting through different mechanisms. However, the apparent increased prevalence of these risk factors among infants with SIDS as compared with the live births cohort may largely be the result of misclassification. The diagnosis of SIDS is often difficult to establish firmly. Although 92% of deaths in this study were classified as SIDS after autopsies, Emery et al.[13] found that review of postmortem examinations of cases of SIDS by pediatric pathologists frequently yielded alternative causes of death. Additionally, the diagnosis of SIDS is more questionable in premature infants than in term babies.[9] We found that ORs comparing non-SIDS infants and the live births cohort for prematurity, LBW, and VLBW were extremely high. Thus the classification as SIDS of a relatively small number of deaths from other causes might skew the apparent characteristics of the entire SIDS group.

In this study the rate of perinatal asphyxia, as evidenced by a 5-minute Apgar score less than 7, was not significantly higher in the SIDS group than in the live births cohort. Previous data on the association between perinatal asphyxia and SIDS have been inconsistent. Buck et al.[14] found a significant trend between lower Apgar scores and SIDS but reported an adjusted OR of 1.2 (95% CI, 0.3 to 4.9) for a 5-minute Apgar score less than 7. In the NICHD study a 5-minute Apgar score less than 7 was significantly more common in the SIDS group than in control subjects matched for location and date of birth but not when matching included birth weight and race.[6] Low 5-minute Apgar scores were not associated with SIDS in Washington State.[9] These data, considered together, indicate that low Apgar scores may not significantly increase the risk of SIDS.

The most striking finding of our study is the association between maternal cigarette smoking during pregnancy and SIDS. Bergman and Wiesner[15] identified maternal tobacco use as a risk factor for SIDS in 1976. Several researchers have corroborated this finding.[4-6, 16, 17] Schoendorf and Kiely,[18] who also analyzed the NMIHS data but stratified the analysis by race, and included only normal birth weight babies, demonstrated that maternal smoking is a more significant risk factor for SIDS than for non-SIDS postneonatal deaths. Our results provide further evidence of the possible role of tobacco in causing SIDS. Maternal smoking during pregnancy was the only characteristic evaluated that was significantly more prevalent in the SIDS group than in infants dying of other causes, suggesting that prenatal tobacco exposure has a more direct relationship than other risk factors to SIDS. This result is intriguing because Kinney et al.[19] found that prenatal exposure to nicotine might alter the infant's arousal mechanisms; this might explain some of the increased risk of SIDS associated with the prone sleep position.[20-23] Maternal smoking is a modifiable risk factor; our data indicate that the elimination of smoking during pregnancy could reduce SIDS by as much as 30%.

By comparing the epidemiologic features of SIDS victims with those of infants dying of other causes, it is possible to distinguish risk factors that might have a causal relationship with SIDS from those that are merely part of the milieu in which postneonatal deaths occur with disproportionate frequency. Neither perinatal or sociodemographic risk factors are independently associated with SIDS, and it is unlikely that future studies on infants with these characteristics will be productive. Conversely, our data indicate that maternal smoking during pregnancy has a causal role in a significant proportion of SIDS deaths. Future research efforts should be directed at understanding the pathophysiologic mechanisms by which in utero exposure to tobacco places an infant at risk, in hopes that a greater understanding of all SIDS deaths can be elucidated.

We thank Dr. Noel S. Weiss for assistance in analyzing the study data and Dr. Abraham B. Bergman for his critical review of the manuscript.

REFERENCES

1. Bergman AB, Ray CG, Pomeroy MA, Wahl PW, Beckwith JB. Studies of the sudden infant death syndrome in King County, Washington. III. Epidemiology. Pediatrics 1972; 49:860-70.
2. Protestos CD, Carpenter RG, McWeeny PM, Emery JL. Obstetric and perinatal histories of children who died unexpectedly ("cot death"). Arch Dis Child 1973;48:835-41.
3. Standfast SJ, Jereb S, Janerich DT. The epidemiology of sudden infant death in upstate New York. II. Birth characteristics. Am J Public Health 1980;70:1061-7.
4. Lewak N, van den Berg BJ, Beckwith JB. Sudden infant death syndrome risk factors. Clin Pediatr 1979;18:404-10.
5. Kraus JF, Greenland S, Bultreys M. Risk factors for sudden infant death syndrome in the US Colloborative Perinatal Project. Int J Epidemiol 1989;18:113-20.
6. Hoffman HJ, Hunter JC, Damus K, et al. Diphtheria-tetanus-pertussis immunization and sudden infant death: results of the National Institute of Child Health and Human Development cooperative epidemiological study of risk factors. Pediatrics 1987;79:598-611.
7. Peterson DR, van Belle GE, Chinn NM. Epidemiologic comparisons of the sudden infant death syndrome with other major components of infant mortality. Am J Epidemiol 1979; 110:699-707.
8. Buck GM, Cookfair DZ, Michalek AM, et al. Intrauterine growth retardation and risk of sudden infant death syndrome (SIDS). Am J Epidemiol 1989;129:874-8.
9. Haas JE, Taylor JA, Bergman AB, et al. Relationship between epidemiologic risk factors and clinicopathologic findings in the sudden infant death syndrome. Pediatrics 1993;91:106-12.
10. Sanderson M, Placek PJ, Keppel KG. The 1988 National Maternal and Infant Health Survey: design, content, and data availability. Birth 1991;18:26-32.
11. Carpenter RG, Gardber A, McWeeny PM, Emery JL. Multistage scoring system for identifying infants at risk of unexpected death. Arch Dis Child 1977;52:606-12.
12. Carpenter RG, Emery JL. Final results of study of infants at risk for sudden death. Nature 1977;268:724-5.
13. Emery JL, Chandra S, Gilbert-Barness EF. Findings in child deaths registered as sudden infant death syndrome (SIDS) in Madison, Wisconsin. Pediatr Pathol 1988;8:171-8.
14. Buck GM, Michalek AM, Kramer AA, Balt RE. Labor and delivery events and risk of sudden infant death syndrome (SIDS). Am J Epidemiol 1991;133:900-6.
15. Bergman AB, Wiesner LA. Relationship of passive cigarette-smoking to sudden infant death syndrome. Pediatrics 1976; 58:665-8.
16. Naeye RL, Ladis B, Drage JS. Sudden infant death syndrome: a prospective study. Am J Dis Child 1976;130:1207-10.
17. Haglund B, Cnattigius S. Cigarette smoking as a risk factor for sudden infant death syndrome. Am J Public Health 1990;80:29-32.
18. Schoendorf KC, Kiely JL. Relationship of sudden infant death syndrome to maternal smoking during and after pregnancy. Pediatrics 1992;90:905-8.
19. Kinney HC, O'Donnel TJ, Kriger P, White Ws. Early developmental changes in [^{3}H] nicotine binding in the human brainstem. Neuroscience 1993;55:1127-30.
20. de Jonge GA, Engelberts AC, Komeen-Liefting AJM, Kostense PJ. Cot death and prone sleeping position in The Netherlands. Br Med J 1989;298:722.
21. Dwyer T, Ponsonby AB, Newman NM, Gibbons LE. Prospective cohort study of prone sleeping position and the sudden infant death syndrome. Lancet 1991;337:1244-7.
22. Fleming PJ, Gilbert R, Azaz Y, et al. Interaction between bedding and sleeping position in the sudden infant death syndrome: a population based case-control study. Br Med J 1990;301:85-9.
23. Mitchell EA, Scragg R, Stewart AW, et al. Results from the first year of the New Zealand cot death study. N Z Med J 1991;104:71-6.

Economic comparison of a tissue adhesive and suturing in the repair of pediatric facial lacerations

Martin H. Osmond, MD, CM, Terry P. Klassen, MD, and Jim V. Quinn, MD

From the Department of Pediatrics, University of Ottawa, and the Division of Emergency Medicine, University of Ottawa, Ottawa, Ontario, Canada

Objective: **To determine, from the societal perspective, the most cost efficient of the three methods commonly used to repair pediatric facial lacerations: nondissolving sutures, dissolving sutures, or a tissue adhesive (Histoacryl blue).**
Design: **Cost-minimization analysis and willingness-to-pay survey.**
Setting: **Tertiary-care pediatric emergency department.**
Methods: **All differential costs relevant to equipment utilization, pharmaceutical use, health care worker time, and parental loss of income for follow-up visits were calculated for each method. On the basis of previous research, our model assumes equal cosmetic outcome for the three methods. In addition, a convenience sample of 30 parents were surveyed in the emergency department to rank their preferences and willingness to pay for the three methods of wound closure.**
Results: **The reduction in cost (in Canadian dollars) per patient of switching from the standard nondissolving sutures was $49.60 for switching to tissue adhesive and $37.90 for dissolving sutures. Sensitivity analyses performed on key variables did not significantly alter our conclusions. Of those parents surveyed, 90% (95% confidence interval, 74% to 98%) chose tissue adhesive and 10% (95% confidence interval, 2% to 26%) chose dissolving sutures as their first choice for wound closure. Nondissolving sutures were ranked third by 29 of 30 parents. Parents were willing to pay a median (25th to 75th percentile) of $40 ($25 to $100) for tissue adhesive and $25 ($10 to $56) for dissolving sutures if only nondissolving sutures were provided by the health care system ($p = 0.1$).**
Conclusions: **Tissue adhesive is the preferred method of closure of pediatric facial lacerations because it results in the most efficient use of resources and is preferred by the majority of parents. (J Pediatr 1995;126:892-5)**

Facial lacerations are one of the most common pediatric problems seen in emergency departments.[1] Until recently the standard method of laceration closure has been nondissolving sutures. During the last 6 years a tissue adhesive, *n*-butyl-2-cyanoacrylate (Histoacryl blue), has been shown to be a faster and less painful method of facial laceration repair.[2-5] Its cosmetic results are similar to those of sutures,[2] and there are no differences in the rate of dehiscence or infection between the two methods.[2, 5] The major disadvantage of Histoacryl blue tissue adhesive is that it is a relatively expensive material ($31.61 for a 0.5 ml vial).

CI	Confidence interval
ED	Emergency department

A third proposed method of laceration closure is the use of fast-absorbing, dissolvable sutures. These have the same benefits of nondissolving sutures without the need for physician follow-up for suture removal. Preliminary evidence

Submitted for publication Nov. 1, 1994; accepted Jan. 19, 1995.

Reprint requests: Martin H. Osmond, MD, CM, Division of Emergency Medicine, Children's Hospital of Eastern Ontario, 401 Smyth Rd., Ottawa, Ontario K1H 8L1, Canada.

0022-3476/95/$3.00 + 0 **9/20/63480**

suggests that the cosmetic result and complications of dissolvable suture repair of facial lacerations are equivalent to those for nondissolving sutures.[6]

In choosing which of these techniques to use, the costs and consequences of each method of repair must be compared.[7-9] Because the efficacy, complication rate, and cosmetic outcome are approximately equal among the three methods, the incremental cost becomes an important factor in making this choice.[7] In addition, the value that the parents place on one method of laceration closure over another is an important consideration for the physician deciding which technique to use.

To address these issues, cost-minimization analysis and a parental willingness-to-pay model were applied to the three methods of treating simple pediatric facial lacerations: nondissolving sutures, dissolving sutures, and tissue adhesive.

METHODS

Cost minimization analysis. The techniques used for this economic evaluation were based on existing methodologic standards, namely, comparative analysis of the costs to society of alternative courses of action that have identical outcomes.[7, 9] In this study cost-minimization analysis was used to determine the additional cost generated by one method of laceration closure over another (i.e., the incremental cost). This analysis is based on a previously healthy child, less than 18 years of age, being treated for a simple facial laceration in a tertiary-care pediatric hospital ED with 47,000 visits per year located in Ottawa, Ontario, Canada. A simple facial laceration was defined as meeting the following criteria: a clean laceration, length less than 4 cm, width less than 0.5 cm, and no need for deep-layer closure. Three alternative courses of action were compared.

Nondissolving sutures. A physician treating a laceration with nondissolving sutures performs the procedure with the assistance of a nurse or porter. Analgesia is provided by local injection of 1% lidocaine with epinephrine. After a 5-minute wait, a minor suture tray is opened, the wound is cleansed with an antiseptic solution, and 5-0 or 6-0 nondissolving sutures are inserted to approximate the wound edges. The wound is covered with a bandage. The sutures are removed in 5 to 7 days in a physician's office.

Dissolving sutures. When dissolving sutures are used, the procedure is identical to that used with nondissolving sutures except that 6-0 dissolving sutures (fast-absorbing plain gut) are used. Routine physician follow-up is not needed unless there are complications.

Tissue adhesive. When a physician performs closure with tissue adhesive, the procedure is done with the assistance of a nurse or porter. In a method previously described,[2] the wound is cleansed with an antiseptic solution, and hemostasis is achieved with dry gauze and pressure. The wound edges are approximated, and a few drops of tissue adhesive are applied to the opposed edges. Manual approximation of the wound is maintained for 30 seconds until full polymerization takes place. The wound is covered with a bandage. Routine physician follow-up is not needed unless there are complications.

Table I. Sensitivity analysis

Variable	Estimate*	Range†
Cost of physician ($/hr)	30	24-65
Cost of assistant ($/hr)	10	5-27
Cost of tissue adhesive ($/patient)	3	2.50-6
Parental hr of lost wages	2	0-4

*Estimate used in primary analysis.
†Range of values used for the variables in the sensitivity analysis.

Identification and measurement of costs. Cost identification and measurement were performed by using data from the literature and by using informed clinical opinion when other data were unavailable. Costs were measured in 1993 Canadian dollars (one Canadian dollar = $0.75 in U.S. currency). All costs that differed between treatment alternatives, from the initial presentation in the ED until 1 week after treatment, were included.

Material costs were valued by using the purchase price charged to the pharmacy, stores, and purchasing departments of the Children's Hospital of Eastern Ontario. The cost of using a minor suture tray was calculated by adding the labor, materials, and sterilizing costs for reprocessing the tray. Each 0.5 ml vial of Histoacryl blue adhesive was estimated to treat 10 patients at an approximate cost of $3 per patient.[2] Physician services in the ED were valued by using the respective hourly wage paid to interns, residents, and attending staff, and by estimating the percentage of lacerations treated by each group. Nurse and porter services in the ED were valued by using their respective hourly wage and estimating the percentage of times each group assisted with a laceration repair. The time required to complete each procedure has been previously studied and is estimated to be approximately 7.9 minutes for tissue adhesive and 15.6 minutes for suture repair.[2] Community physician services were valued by using the Ontario Ministry of Health Schedule of Benefits for Physician Services. The costs incurred by society for time off work were tabulated by considering the length of time required for a follow-up physician visit. The average hourly industrial wage for Ontario was used for this calculation.[10] It was assumed that both mothers and fathers would be reimbursed for their time.

The following costs were considered to be equal for the three methods of treatment: (1) the overhead expenses of the ED, (2) the cost of registering to be seen in the ED, and (3)

Table II. Estimated cost per patient in each treatment groups

	Cost per patient ($)		
	Nondissolving sutures	Dissolving sutures	Tissue adhesive
ED physician	7.80	7.80	3.95
ED assistant	2.60	2.60	1.32
Pharmacy	0.14	0.14	3.00
Supplies	5.13	9.76	0.33
Follow-up physician visit	16.25	—	—
Parental costs	26.28	—	—
TOTAL*	58.20	20.30	8.60
Incremental cost†	—	($37.90)	($49.60)
Cost per year‡	36,084	12,586	5,332
Incremental cost per year†	—	(23,498)	(30,752)

*Excluding costs of ED registration and overhead, and parental wage loss during the initial ED visit.
†Values in parentheses indicate that by changing treatments fewer resources would be consumed.
‡Based on 620 simple facial lacerations per year.

parental time off work for the initial ED visit. Because we were interested only in the incremental cost, these equal costs were not included in the analysis. Thus the total cost we report is not the absolute cost to society for each alternative but rather the sum of the costs that differ for each procedure.

Sensitivity analysis. Sensitivity analysis is an important part of any economic evaluation.[8, 9] In a sensitivity analysis specific variables are altered through a range of possibilities to examine the robustness of the results. Table I itemizes the variables and the ranges of the estimates that were used for the sensitivity analysis.

Willingness-to-pay survey. To ascertain and to place a monetary value on parental preferences for method of wound closure, a willingness-to-pay survey was conducted.[11] This technique measures the value that persons are willing to pay to reduce perceived risks to themselves or others. A convenience sample of 30 parents were approached with the survey. All parents were visiting the ED with a child who had a problem other than a laceration. The survey comprised two parts. The first part provided an outline of the three repair techniques, and described, on the basis of previous studies, the cosmetic outcome, complications, and level of pain to be expected with each. The second part was a series of questions. The parents were asked to name the first, second, and third choice of treatment method they would want for their child. They were then asked how much they would be willing to pay for their first and second choice, if only their third choice was provided by the health care system. The final questions asked were (1) the ages of their children, (2) whether their children had previously had stitches or tissue adhesive, and (3) annual family income.

Table III. Parental preference and willingness to pay for each treatment group

	Nondissolving sutures	Dissolving sutures	Tissue adhesive
Parental choice			
First	—	3	27
Second	1	27	2
Third	29	—	1
Willingness to pay for choices ($)			
Median	—	25	40
25th-75th Percentile		10-56	25-100

Statistical analysis. Categoric data were analyzed with the chi-square statistic or the Fisher Exact Test. Nonparametric data were analyzed with the Mann-Whitney U test. The Pearson correlation coefficient was used to measure the association between the parent's willingness to pay and their family income. Ninety-five percent confidence intervals were calculated according to the method of Gardner and Altman.[12] Data were analyzed with Statistical Package for the Social Sciences/PC+ version 4.01 software (SPSS Inc., Chicago, Ill.).

RESULTS

The total cost per alternative for treating one patient is shown in Table II. The nondissolving suture group had the highest total cost, and the tissue adhesive group the lowest. The cost of patient follow-up (physician fee and parental lost wages) was the major reason for the cost difference between nondissolving sutures and the two other alternatives. Dissolving sutures are more costly to use than tissue adhesive, mainly because of the expense of fast-absorbing sutures and the increased demand on physician and assistant time. When compared with nondissolving sutures, cost to society per patient is reduced by $37.90 for dissolving sutures and $49.60 for tissue glue. On the basis of an estimate of 620 simple facial lacerations per year seen at the Children's Hospital of Eastern Ontario, dissolving sutures and tissue glue would save $23,498 and $30,752, respectively, over the conventional nondissolving sutures.

Sensitivity analysis. When individual variables were varied within the ranges listed in Table I, tissue adhesive remained superior to dissolving and nondissolving sutures. The ranges for total cost are $6.65 to $18.44 for tissue adhesive, $17.44 to $33.82 for dissolving sutures, and $29.06 to $98.00 for nondissolving sutures.

Willingness-to-pay survey. Thirty parents were approached with the survey, and all agreed to participate. Table III shows the parental treatment preferences and their willingness to pay for those preferences if only their third choice were provided by the health care system. Ninety percent of parents (95% CI, 74% to 98%) chose tissue adhesive as the preferred method of treatment. Forty-three percent of parents (95% CI, 26% to 63%) had a child who previously had stitches, but only 3% (95% CI, 0% to 18%) had a child previously treated with a tissue adhesive. There was no association between experience with stitches ($p = 0.6$) or tissue adhesive ($p = 0.1$) and choice of treatment. Parents were willing to pay a median (25th to 75th percentile) of $40 ($25 to $100) for tissue adhesive and $25 ($10 to $56) for dissolving sutures if only nondissolving sutures were provided by the health care system ($p = 0.1$). The parents' willingness to pay showed no association with the magnitude of family income (correlation coefficient, 0.01).

DISCUSSION

This economic evaluation has shown that use of tissue adhesive is the most efficient of the three methods of closing simple facial lacerations in children, largely because of lower costs of physician and assistant services in the ED, consumption of less material during the procedure, and absence of routine follow-up costs. The superiority of tissue adhesive was still apparent after key variables were varied in a sensitivity analysis. The cost reduction of $49.60 per child treated demonstrates that tissue adhesive represents considerable savings over the standard nondissolvable sutures. In our hospital this would mean a cost savings of more than $30,000 per year. We estimate, by extrapolating our data to the rest of Canada, that the use of a tissue adhesive for simple pediatric facial lacerations would result in a cost savings to society of approximately $1 million.

In addition, this study has revealed that the majority of parents, given the choice, would prefer a tissue adhesive for the treatment of their child's laceration. This is not surprising, because previous research has shown that parents find the tissue adhesive method to be significantly less painful for their child and significantly faster to perform, thus requiring less restraint of the child.[2]

The willingness-to-pay portion of the survey shows that parents can assign a monetary value to the perceived benefits of the tissue adhesive (in this case, $40). Whether this willingness to pay should be included in the total cost is controversial.[9, 11] Conceivably, parents' willingness to pay may not represent an accurate value, because they may not feel constrained by their ability to pay in the survey's hypothetic scenario.[11] Because of this uncertainty, we chose not to include the value of parents' preferences in our cost analysis. However, even without adding the value of this clear parental preference, tissue adhesive remains the best choice from the societal perspective, because it costs less than the other two alternatives and has an equivalent outcome.

Dissolving sutures are also a more efficient use of resources than nondissolving sutures because of the cost savings of no routine physician follow-up. This method costs $11.70 more per patient than tissue adhesive and was ranked as the second choice by the majority of parents. However, although dissolving sutures cannot be recommended for routine closure of simple facial lacerations, they may be the treatment of choice for lacerations that cannot be closed by a tissue adhesive (i.e., deep lacerations requiring multilayer closure). Future studies are needed to define the role of dissolving sutures.

One possible limitation of a cost-minimization analysis is that it relies on the assumption that all outcomes are equivalent. However, the current evidence, which is of high quality, demonstrates equivalent outcomes between tissue adhesive and sutures.

In summary, this economic analysis has shown that a tissue adhesive is the preferred method of closure of pediatric facial lacerations because it results in the most efficient use of resources and is preferred by the majority of parents.

We thank Conrad Barber-Dueck for his assistance in providing important data.

REFERENCES

1. Sibert JR, Maddocks GB, Brown BM. Childhood accidents. Arch Dis Child 1981;56:225-7.
2. Quinn JV, Drzewiecki A, Li MM, et al. A randomized, controlled trial comparing a tissue adhesive with suturing in the repair of pediatric facial lacerations. Ann Emerg Med 1993; 22:1130-5.
3. Applebaum JS, Zalut T, Applebaum D. The use of tissue adhesion for traumatic laceration repair in the emergency department. Ann Emerg Med 1993;22:1190-2.
4. Watson DP. Use of cyanoacrylate tissue adhesive for closing facial lacerations in children. Br Med J 1989;299:1014.
5. Mizrahi S, Bickel A, Ben-Layish E. Use of tissue adhesives in the repair of lacerations in children. J Pediatr Surg 1988; 23:312-3.
6. Lubitz D, Coyne C, Windle B. Use of fast-absorbable sutures for the repair of pediatric facial lacerations [Abstract]. Arch Pediatr Adolesc Med 1994;148:42.
7. Department of Clinical Epidemiology and Biostatistics. How to read clinical journals. VII. To understand an economic evaluation [Part A]. Can Med Assoc J 1984;130:1428-33.
8. Department of Clinical Epidemiology and Biostatistics. How to read clinical journals. VII. To understand an economic evaluation [Part B]. Can Med Assoc J 1984;130:1542-9.
9. Drummond MF, Stoddart GL, Torrance GW. Methods for the economic evaluation of health care programmes. Toronto: Oxford University Press, 1990.
10. Employment earnings and hours: March 1993. Statistics Canada. Ottawa: 1993:89.
11. Gafni A. Willingness-to-pay as a measure of benefits: relevant questions in the context of public decisionmaking about health care programs. Med Care 1991;29:1246-52.
12. Gardner MJ, Altman DG, eds. Statistics with confidence: confidence intervals and statistical guidelines. London: British Medical Journal, 1989.

Risk of recurrent stroke in patients with sickle cell disease treated with erythrocyte transfusions

Charles H. Pegelow, MD, Robert J. Adams, MD, Virgil McKie, MD, Miguel Abboud, MD, Brian Berman, MD, Scott T. Miller, MD, Nancy Olivieri, MD, Elliott Vichinsky, MD, Winfred Wang, MD, and Donald Brambilla, PhD

From the Department of Pediatrics, University of Miami School of Medicine, Miami, Florida; the Departments of Neurology and Pediatrics, Medical College of Georgia, Augusta; the Department of Pediatrics, Medical University of South Carolina, Charleston; the Department of Pediatrics, Case Western Reserve University, Cleveland, Ohio; the Department of Pediatrics, State University of New York, Brooklyn; the Department of Pediatrics, University of Toronto, Toronto, Ontario, Canada; Children's Hospital Oakland, Oakland, California; the Department of Pediatrics, University of Tennessee, Memphis; and the New England Research Institute, Watertown, Massachusetts

Objective: **To determine the effect of a transfusion program on risk of stroke recurrence in children with sickle cell disease.**
Design: **The clinical course and experience with transfusion therapy at eight centers were reviewed for subjects whose initial stroke occurred after January 1988.**
Results: **Sixty subjects were observed for 191.7 patient-years. Eight had a single recurrent stroke (two intracranial hemorrhages and six infarctions) for a prevalence of 13.3%, or one recurrence for each 24 patient-years of observation. Thirteen subjects had 15 transient neurologic events; two of these had subsequent strokes, but the overall risk was similar for those who did and those did not have transient events. Hemoglobin S levels were greater than the desired maximum of 30% at the time of 7 of 16 transient events and five of six recurrent infarctions. The stroke recurrence rate was similar to those in previous reports of children receiving long-term transfusion therapy but significantly less than that reported for children who did not receive transfusions (p <0.001).**
Conclusions: **We conclude that maintenance of hemoglobin S at a level less than 30% appears to be effective in reducing the rate of recurrent infarction but does not prevent transient neurologic events. Transient neurologic events are common but do not appear to be related to recurrent stroke. (J PEDIATR 1995;126:896-9)**

Stroke occurs in 5% to 10% of children with sickle cell anemia who are less than 15 years of age[1-3] and less often in those with hemoglobin SC disease or sickle cell–thalassemia. Cerebral infarction accounts for the majority of these events; hemorrhage is considerably less frequent. The risk of recurrent stroke in these children has been estimated to be 47% to 93%.[1, 2, 4, 5] Lusher et al.[6] initially reported that recurrent strokes could be prevented by long-term transfusion therapy designed to maintain hemoglobin S levels at less than 40%. Others subsequently reported similar degrees of protection,[2, 7, 8] although current recommendations are that hemoglobin S levels be kept at less than 30%.[9] To define better the risk of recurrent stroke, we undertook a review of the combined experience at eight centers providing medical care for large populations of such children.

Submitted for publication June 3, 1994; accepted Jan. 25, 1995.

Reprint requests: Charles H. Pegelow, MD, Department of Pediatrics (R-131), University of Miami School of Medicine, P.O. Box 016860, Miami, FL 33101.

0022-3476/95/$3.00 + 0 **9/20/63692**

Table. Description of time to recurrent stroke and hematologic status at recurrence

Age at first CVA (yr)	Time to recurrence (mo)	Recurrent event	Hemoglobin at recurrence (gm/L)	Hemoglobin S at recurrence (%)
2.7	22	H	84	28
3.4	37	I	97	70
1.9	43	I	94	41
7.9	37	I	100	30
9.1	2	H	95	15
9.8	27	I	88	22
11.9	13	I	88	44
24.1	13	I	81	42

CVA, Cerebrovascular accident; *H*, intracerebral hemorrhage; *I*, infarction.

METHODS

Subjects included all patients with sickle cell disease who were examined for their first stroke after January 1988 at participating centers. All children known to have stroke were included. All were treated with long-term transfusion therapy designed to maintain hemoglobin S levels at less than 30%. In two patients, hemoglobin S levels were allowed to increase to 60% after an initial period of stability.[10]

A questionnaire was completed for all 60 subjects. Data collected included hematologic diagnosis, age at first stroke, and associated clinical and reported radiographic manifestations. Data regarding any subsequent neurologic event, including reports of imaging studies, associated blood cell counts, and hemoglobin S percentage, were also obtained.

Recurrent strokes were defined as neurologic events associated with radiographic evidence of hemorrhage or new areas of infarction. Transient events were defined as focal neurologic symptoms such as weakness or hypoesthesia of brief duration and without radiographic changes.

The incidence of recurrence was compared with historical data from the two reports[1, 2] in which the periods of observation were presented. Calculating recurrence rates per unit of time is important because longer periods of observation might be expected to uncover more events.

RESULTS

The study population included 36 girls and 24 boys, 20 months to 24 years of age at the time of the initial stroke. Fifty-seven patients had sickle cell anemia, two with hemoglobin S–β+ thalassemia, and one had hemoglobin S–β^0-thalassemia. The cumulative observation time was 191.7 patient-years. Individual subjects were observed for a mean and median duration of 38 and 36 months, respectively; the longest period of observation was 71 months.

Recurrent strokes were documented in eight subjects (Table), for a prevalence of 13.3%, or one event for each 24 patient-years of observation. Two children had fatal intracerebral hemorrhages at 3 weeks and 14 months after the initial cerebral infarct, while they were receiving transfusion therapy. Cerebral infarcts occurred in six subjects (10%), one event per 32 patient-years of observation. All survived, and none had more than one recurrent stroke.

Patients had varied neurologic abnormalities, but radiographic reports of new ischemic damage were present in all children. Two children with intracerebral hemorrhage had hemoglobin S levels of 15% and 28%, respectively. Five of the children with infarcts had hemoglobin S values of at least 30%.

The rate of stroke recurrence was compared with the time of the first recurrent stroke for the patients not receiving transfusion described by Powars et al.[1] and by Moohr et al.,[2] by the use of Kaplan-Meier estimates of the distribution of time without recurrence, and by the log-rank statistical test[11] (Figure). Patients who received transfusion therapy after stroke were less likely to have a recurrence, at least during approximately 6 years of observation ($p < 0.001$). Three additional strokes occurred after more than 71 months in seven subjects who were not given transfusions.

Thirteen of our subjects had 15 transient neurologic events (Table). Radiographic examinations of 12 children were reported to be unchanged from previous studies. No imaging studies were obtained for the remaining child, whose mild symptoms occurred in conjunction with a transfusion. Hemoglobin S levels at the time of these events ranged from 4% to 78%; six were greater than 30%. These subjects were observed for 2 to 27 months (median, 8 months) after the transient event. One child had a second infarction 2 months later, and another died of an intraventricular hemorrhage 14 months after a transient event. This frequency of recurrent strokes (2/13) was not significantly different from that encountered by the subjects who did not have transient events (7/47; *p* not significant, Fisher Exact Test). Three subjects had more than one transient event.

DISCUSSION

Early reports of the natural history of stroke in patients with sickle cell disease indicated a recurrence rate of 67% to more than 90%.[1, 2] More recently, 47% of Jamaican chil-

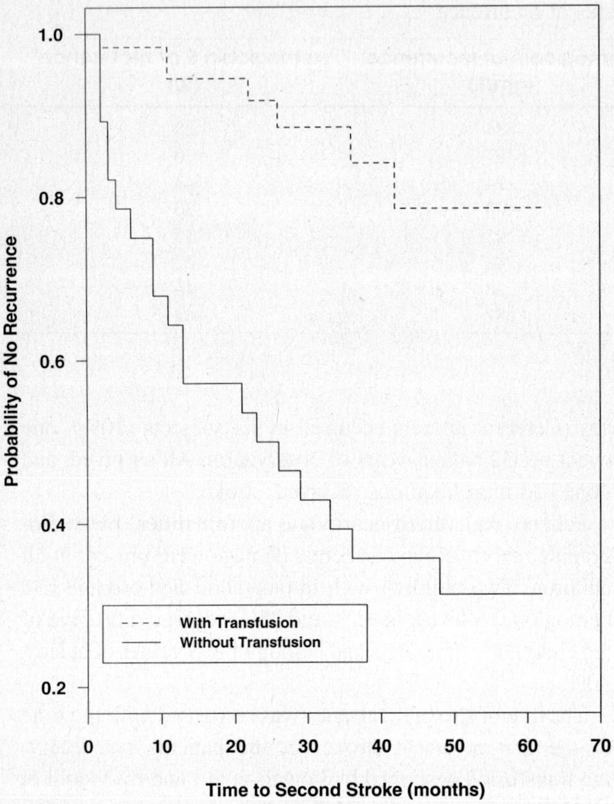

Figure. Comparison of stroke recurrence with time for study population with transfusion and historical control subjects without transfusion.[1,2] Probability of recurrence is significantly different at 71 months (p <0.001). Follow-up was censored at 62 months.

dren who did not receive transfusion therapy had recurrent strokes, although the duration of their observation was not stated.[5] Early reports of decreased recurrence rates in children given long-term transfusion therapy led to general acceptance of transfusion therapy without evaluation by a controlled trial.[4,6,7]

Our experience, although retrospective and compared with historical control subjects without transfusion, corroborates the success of long-term transfusion therapy and provides additional information regarding recurrence risk. The effect of transfusion therapy on intracranial hemorrhage is unclear.[12] We include it in our analysis to allow comparison with data reported by Powars et al.[1] and by Moohr et al.,[2] whom both indicated the interval from first cerebral infarction to subsequent strokes, which included either infarction or hemorrhage. Our subjects had significantly fewer recurrent strokes than those authors reported during a comparable observation period. Their data indicate that longer periods of observation would lower the cumulative risk because the majority of the recurrences were noted within 3 years. Previous reports of long-term transfusion therapy[2,4,7,8] found recurrence rates comparable to those we observed.

Previous publications characterized the stroke recurrence rate as the percentage of subjects who do not receive transfusion who have a stroke during the entire observation period.[1,2,4,5,7] This approach is misleading because it makes no adjustment for the length of observation, and longer periods might be expected to yield more events. Determination of the incidence allows a more meaningful comparison of rates.

Four recurrent infarctions occurred more than 2 years after the initial stroke, indicating that the risk of recurrence does not disappear with prolonged transfusion therapy. This is consistent with the recent report of five recurrent strokes in 10 patients whose long-term transfusion therapy was stopped after a median duration of 8 uneventful years.[13]

Hemoglobin S levels were less than 30% in the two patients with intracranial hemorrhage. Levels were at or greater than 30% in five of the six patients with recurrent infarction. The fact that one had recurrent infarction with hemoglobin S level less than 30% provides further support for the observation that maintenance of a low hemoglobin S level does not provide complete protection.[14] Our analysis includes children with hemoglobin S values greater than 30% (one whose hemoglobin S level was 70% at the time of recurrent infarction) because compliance with prolonged transfusion is often imperfect and levels greater than the desired 30% are often found when the child is brought for transfusion.

Fifteen transient ischemic events occurred in 13 of our subjects. Hemoglobin S level was more than 30% for only six, suggesting that aggressive transfusion therapy does not always prevent such events. However, subsequent strokes were not more frequent in those who had transient events.

Although only two intracranial hemorrhages were encountered, both occurred with hemoglobin S levels less than 30%. Similarly, the majority of transient events (9/15) occurred when hemoglobin S level was less than 30%. In contrast, hemoglobin S level was at least 30% in five of six children with recurrent infarction. This observation is similar to those in previous reports, in which two of the three recurrences occurred in children whose hemoglobin S levels were greater than 30%.[4,7] Unfortunately, neither our report nor those allow determination of a safe hemoglobin S level.

We conclude that transfusion therapy should be provided for all children with sickle cell disease who have had a cerebral infarction. Intracranial hemorrhage and transient neurologic events may not be prevented by transfusion, but maintenance of hemoglobin S level less than 30% provides significant protection against recurrent infarction. Further study is required to determine the optimal intensity and duration of this therapy and the relative efficacy of other treatment approaches.

REFERENCES

1. Powars D, Wilson B, Imbus C, Pegelow C, Allen J. The natural history of stroke in sickle cell disease. Am J Med 1978; 65:461-71.
2. Moohr JW, Wilson H, Pang EJ-M. Strokes and their management in sickle cell disease. In: Fried W, ed. Comparative clinical aspects of sickle cell disease. Amsterdam: Elsevier North Holland, 1982:101-11.
3. Portnoy BA, Herion JC. Neurologic manifestations in sickle cell disease. Ann Intern Med 1972;76:643-52.
4. Sarnaik S, Soorya D, Kim J, Ravindranath Y, Lusher J. Periodic transfusions for sickle cell anemia and CNS infarction. Am J Dis Child 1979;133:1254-7.
5. Balkaran B, Char G, Morris JS, Thomas PW, Serjeant BE, Serjeant GR. Stroke in a cohort of patients with homozygous sickle cell disease. J PEDIATR 1992;120:360-6.
6. Lusher JM, Haghighat H, Khalifa AS. A prophylactic transfusion program for children with sickle cell anemia complicated by CNS infarction. Am J Hematol 1976;1:265-73.
7. Russell MO, Goldberg HI, Hodson A, et al. Effect of transfusion therapy on arteriographic abnormalities and on recurrence of stroke in sickle cell disease. Blood 1984;63:162-9.
8. Willimas J, Goff JR, Anderson HR, Langston JW, Thompson E. Efficacy of transfusion therapy for one to two years in patients with sickle cell disease and cerebrovascular accidents. J PEDIATR 1980;96:205-8.
9. Charache S, Lubin B, Reid CD, eds. Management and therapy of sickle cell disease, U.S. Department of Public Health and Human Services, 1992:22-4, NIH publication No. 92-2117.
10. Miller ST, Jensen D, Rao SP. Less intensive long-term transfusion therapy for sickle cell anemia and cerebrovascular accident. J PEDIATR 1992;120:54-7.
11. Cox DR, Oakes D. Analysis of survival data. New York: Chapman and Hill, 1984.
12. Powars D, Adams RJ, Nichols FT, Milner P, Charache S, Sarnaik S. Delayed intracranial hemorrhage following cerebral infarction in sickle cell anemia. J Acad Minority Phys 1990;1:79-82.
13. Wang WC, Kovnar EH, Tonkin IL, et al. High risk of recurrent stroke after discontinuance of five to twelve years of transfusion therapy in patients with sickle cell disease. J PEDIATR 1991;118:377-82.
14. Buchanan GR, Bowman WP, Smith SJ. Recurrent cerebral ischemia during hypertransfusion therapy in sickle cell anemia. J PEDIATR 1983;103:921-3.

Coagulation factor deficiencies during initiation of extracorporeal membrane oxygenation

Michael L. McManus, MD, Sherwin V. Kevy, MD, Lynne K. Bower, RRT, and Paul R. Hickey, MD

From the Multidisciplinary Intensive Care Unit and the Departments of Laboratory Medicine (Hemotherapy Division) and Anesthesia, Children's Hospital, and the Department of Pediatrics, Harvard Medical School, Boston, Massachusetts

Objective: We examined the hypothesis that critically ill patients receiving extracorporeal membrane oxygenation (ECMO) have reduced clotting factor levels, which may contribute to the risk of hemorrhagic complications.
Methods: Blood samples were collected from 19 patients before and 1 hour after initiation of ECMO. Heparin present in samples was removed by ECTEOLA (epichlorohydrin triethanolamine) cellulose resin adsorption, and coagulation factors were assayed by automated techniques. Factor deficiency was defined as levels at least 2 SD less than published age-adjusted reference values.
Results: Thirteen patients (68%) had deficiencies of two or more factors before ECMO. Despite inclusion of factor-containing blood products in the ECMO priming solution, 10 patients (53%) had deficiencies of two or more factors after initiation of ECMO. Four patients had intracranial hemorrhages and were found to be deficient in five or more factors at the time of cannulation.
Conclusions: Severe coagulation factor deficiencies are often present in patients requiring ECMO, and coagulation factors provided through the circuit prime are insufficient to ensure correction of these deficiencies. Deficiency of multiple coagulation factors may contribute to the risk of intracranial hemorrhage during ECMO; the practice of excluding factor-containing solutions from the circuit prime should be examined prospectively. (J Pediatr 1995;126:900-4)

Hemorrhage is among the most frequent and serious complications encountered in the use of extracorporeal membrane oxygenation.[1-4] The reported incidence of intracranial hemorrhage during ECMO has ranged from as high as 52% in early studies[2] to approximately 15% today.[5] Together with chronic lung disease, neurologic injury associated with intracranial hemorrhage is the primary determinant of long-term morbidity in survivors of ECMO,[6] and concern regarding hemorrhage has hampered widespread application of this therapy in the care of premature infants and patients with a preexisting coagulopathy.[7,8]

Predisposition to hemorrhage in patients receiving ECMO is presumed to be related largely to heparin anticoagulation, but other factors, including preexisting hypoxia, acidosis, carotid ligation, and impaired cerebral autoregulation,[9] may contribute. Additionally, neonates, the most frequent recipients of ECMO, possess coagulation factor levels substantially less than adult levels,[10-12] so that these patients are particularly vulnerable to hemorrhage on further reduction of coagulation factor concentrations.

ECMO	Extracorporeal membrane oxygenation
IVH	Intraventricular hemorrhage
PT	Prothrombin time

Submitted for publication Aug. 31, 1994; accepted Dec. 28, 1994.

Reprint requests: Michael L. McManus, MD, Multidisciplinary Intensive Care Unit Office, Farley 517, Children's Hospital, 300 Longwood Ave., Boston, MA 02115.

0022-3476/95/$3.00 + 0 **9/20/62988**

Table I. Coagulation factor levels* for 19 patients before and after cannulation for ECMO

Factor	Before cannulation (U/ml)		After cannulation (U/ml)	
	Mean ± SD	Range	Mean ± SD	Range
II	0.39 ± 0.27	0.05-0.91	0.53 ± 0.19	0.14-1.00
V	0.50 ± 0.35	0.10-1.47	0.46 ± 0.27	0.10-1.06
VII	0.49 ± 0.26	0.12-0.96	0.50 ± 0.25	0.16-1.18
VIII	0.70 ± 0.50	0.03-2.06	0.48 ± 0.20	0.18-0.87
IX	0.42 ± 0.26	0.04-1.04	0.41 ± 0.15	0.12-0.61
X	0.42 ± 0.24	0.07-0.83	0.52 ± 0.19	0.14-0.94
XI	0.32 ± 0.19	0.01-0.76	0.37 ± 0.16	0.11-0.72
XII	0.24 ± 0.18	0.02-0.64	0.22 ± 0.13	0.02-0.53

*Normal pooled plasma has a factor level of 1.0 U/ml.

Despite the importance of the coagulation system, surprisingly little is known regarding its alterations during ECMO. We hypothesized that, as one basis for predisposition toward hemorrhage, patients receiving ECMO have severe clotting factor deficiencies that precede, and are potentially exacerbated by, initiation of ECMO. We therefore measured the concentrations of clotting factors in plasma taken from patients before and 1 hour after initiation of bypass for ECMO.

METHODS

Subjects. Twenty patients, from neonates (>36 weeks of gestational age) to children 3 years of age, who had been referred to our intensive care unit for ECMO were studied. After initial examination the decision to proceed with ECMO was made by the primary medical-surgical team on the basis of institutional criteria (oxygenation index [(Fraction of inspired oxygen × Mean airway pressure) ÷ Arterial oxygen pressure] >0.4, despite maximal therapy). Study consent and consent for ECMO were then obtained from parents in accordance with protocol established by the Children's Hospital Committee on Clinical Investigation. Patients receiving factor-containing blood products, other than those administered according to ECMO initiation protocol, during the 2 hours preceding or hour after initiation of ECMO, were excluded.

Extracorporeal membrane oxygenation. The ECMO circuit priming solution contained 150 ml fresh-frozen plasma, 400 ml packed erythrocytes, 12 ml calcium gluconate, 75 ml tromethamine and 600 U heparin. During cannulation 0.25 U/kg platelets suspended in plasma (~10 ml/kg) were administered intravenously. Activated clotting time was measured soon after initiation of ECMO, and systemic heparin was administered to maintain activated clotting time between 180 and 200 seconds. No blood products other than packed erythrocytes were given during cannulation or during the first hour of ECMO.

Laboratory tests. Blood was obtained from each patient by way of indwelling arterial catheters before cannulation and 1 hour after the start of ECMO. Samples were collected into citrated tubes on ice and separated by centrifugation at 1700*g*. Plasma was then treated with ECTEOLA (epichlorohydrin triethanolamine) cellulose resin (Sigma Diagnostics, St. Louis, Mo.) for in vitro heparin adsorption before storage at –80° C. In control experiments with plasma from normal volunteers, it has been demonstrated that in vitro heparin adsorption successfully reverses the effects of heparin.[13] This was also verified in our laboratory with plasma from normal volunteers (data not shown).

Each patient sample was assayed for prothrombin time, fibrinogen, and activities of coagulation factors II, V, VII, VIII, IX, X, XI, and XII with the ACL 300 automated coagulation laboratory (Instrumentation Laboratories, Lexington, Mass.). Before all assays, calibration was accomplished by way of internally generated *R* values with commercial control plasma and then further validated through parallel analysis of samples from normal volunteers whose factor levels were verified by other techniques.

Data analysis. Unless otherwise noted, factor activities are expressed as units per milliliter, where pooled plasma contains 1.0 U/ml. For reference, activities were compared with published age-based control values[10-12] and deficiency defined as levels less than or equal to 2 SD below the mean for age. Values for pre-ECMO and post-ECMO PT and fibrinogen are presented as means (n = 19) ± SD. Comparisons of mean pre-ECMO and post-ECMO values were made with the two-tailed Student *t* test.

RESULTS

Blood samples were taken from 20 patients; one patient was excluded from analysis because of incomplete data. Fourteen newborn and five pediatric subjects receiving ECMO were enrolled, encompassing a variety of primary diagnoses including congenital diaphragmatic hernia (five patients), meconium aspiration with persistent pulmonary hypertension (four), pneumonia or sepsis (five), acute respi-

Table II. Deficient coagulation factors before and after initiation of ECMO

Patient No.	Deficient coagulation factors: Before cannulation	After cannulation
1*	II, VIII, IX, X, XI, XII	VIII, IX, XI, XII
2	II, X, XII, F	II, X, XI, XII
3	VIII, XII	V
4	VII, XII	VII, F
5	F	V, VIII, F
6*	II, V, VII, VIII, IX, X, XI, XII	F
7	VIII, XII	XII
8*	II, V, VII, VIII, IX, X, XI, XII	II, V, VII, VIII, IX, XII
9	F	—
10	II	V
11	VIII, IX, XII, F	V, IX, XII, F
12	II, V, VII, X, F	F
13	II, V, VII, F	V, F
14	—	XII
15	II, VIII	XII
16*	II, V, VII, X, F	V, VII, XII, F
17	II, V, F	V, F
18	F	F
19	XII	V, VII, VIII, XI, XII

Measurements were made from samples taken immediately before and 1 hour after initiation of ECMO. Deficiency was defined as levels at least 2 SD less than published means for age.[10]

F, Fibrinogen.

*Patients with hemorrhages. Patient 6 had a grade IIVH before cannulation but had no further extension (see text).

ratory distress syndrome (four), and persistent air leak (one). Overall survival rate was 63%; three patients (16%) died as a direct result of intracranial hemorrhage. Of these, two were newborn infants having signs of hemorrhage by intracranial ultrasound study within 24 hours of cannulation. In the third patient, 3 years of age, a large brain parenchymal hemorrhage developed later in the course of ECMO. One patient with congenital diaphragmatic hernia was cannulated despite the presence of a grade I intraventricular hemorrhage. Although hemorrhage extension was not observed, the patient ultimately died as a result of pulmonary hypoplasia. All newborn infants received vitamin K before ECMO.

Mean factor concentrations for all 19 patients before and after initiation of ECMO are presented in Table I. Wide variability in factor concentrations was observed, as evidenced by large ranges and SD. For the population, differences in factor levels before and after ECMO cannulation did not reach statistical significance, and no consistent global pattern of factor deficiency or destruction was revealed. However, examination of individual patient data revealed frequent and marked abnormalities of coagulation. As detailed in Table II, specific factor deficiencies were identified in nearly all patients before and after initiation of ECMO. Before cannulation 18 patients (95%) were deficient in at least one clotting factor or fibrinogen, and 13 (68%) in more than one factor as defined by levels that were at least 2 SD less than mean for age. Approximately half the patients studied were deficient in factors II and XII; one third were found to be deficient in factors V, VII, and X. All four patients with hemorrhagic complications had concurrent deficiencies in five or more factors (range, five to eight factors), whereas all but one of those without hemorrhage were deficient in four or fewer (range, zero to five factors).

One hour after initiation of ECMO, deficiencies of at least one factor persisted in 17 patients and a new deficiency of factor IX appeared in one patient (Table II). The overall frequency of most specific factor deficiencies decreased after initiation of ECMO; the incidence of deficiency increased only for factor V. However, 10 of 19 patients (53%) continued to lack adequate concentrations of at least two factors, with the mildest deficiencies (e.g., cases 5 and 19) often worsening. Because of large interpatient variability, overall changes in hematologic profile were not reflected in significant ($p < 0.05$) alterations of the mean PT (18.4 ± 5.9 seconds vs 18.6 ± 4.8 seconds) or plasma fibrinogen concentration (1.96 ± 1.20 gm/L vs 1.98 ± 1.20 gm/L). However, as a gross measure of overall clotting, the number of patients with PT prolonged more than 2 SD beyond the mean for age increased from 10 (53%) to 16 (84%).

DISCUSSION

These data demonstrate that critically ill infants and children receiving ECMO often have extensive coagulation factor deficiencies and that the initiation of bypass according to a generally accepted protocol is not consistently a remedy. These heretofore unrecognized factor deficiencies are of sufficient breadth and magnitude as to be clinically worrisome.

A role for coagulopathy in the pathogenesis of neonatal intracranial hemorrhage has been suggested,[14-16] yet these discussions have been largely limited to premature infants. Chessells and Wigglesworth[14] found coagulopathies to be more prevalent in newborn infants with IVH than in those without IVH. Later, McDonald et al.[16] observed hypocoagulability (defined as hypofibrinogenemia, thrombocytopenia, or prolonged clotting time) in 11 of 15 infants in whom IVH occurred and in only 5 of 35 with no IVH. Few data are available concerning the coagulation status of patients receiving prolonged extracorporeal support, but extrapolation from studies such as these have led many institutions to consider the presence of a coagulopathy to be a contraindication to ECMO.[7,8] Nevertheless, numerous other factors are believed to contribute to the risk of intracranial hemorrhage during ECMO, including prolonged hypoxia, ischemia, acidosis, carotid ligation, and fluctuations in cerebral blood flow superimposed on impaired cerebral autoregulation.[9] Although it is likely that all such factors play a role, their individual relative contributions are difficult to ascertain.

Although usually having "normal" surgical hemostasis, healthy neonates, as compared with adults, have markedly diminished concentrations of most procoagulant proteins. For some factors the lower 95% confidence limit of normal values reaches 10% to 15% of adult values. Clinically these differences combine with other factors to produce prolongation of clotting times and, it has been suggested, a sensitiv ity to further minor reductions in factor concentrations.[12] For our study factor deficiency was defined as levels at least 2 SD less than published means for age, to ensure that this term was applied only to very severe factor reductions. It is likely, however, that even less severe reductions, particularly when present across multiple factors, will result in significant impairment of coagulation.[12, 17, 18] For example, to ensure surgical hemostasis in infants and children with hemophilia, it is generally recommended that factor VIII levels be maintained at 50% or more of normal *adult* levels.[19]

In this investigation patients receiving ECMO were found to have coagulation factor levels substantially less than even the normally depleted levels of early infancy. With the use of a factor-containing prime solution, the initiation of ECMO was found to have variable effects on the coagulation profiles of individual patients. Qualitative examination of the data suggests that the priming protocol employed in our institution tended to benefit the patients with the most severe depletion and to lower factor levels in the patients with less depletion. Because our protocol includes administration of platelets in plasma and a circuit prime solution containing small amount of fresh-frozen plasma, it might be expected that the most severe factor deficiencies before ECMO would be ameliorated somewhat by transfusion during ECMO initiation. Conversely, because the priming solution is factor depleted as compared with normal whole blood, patients with relatively normal factor profiles might be expected to have factor reductions through hemodilution alone.

During cardiopulmonary bypass for pediatric open heart surgery, circuit priming solutions devoid of plasma lead to significant hemodilution and as much as 50% reduction in coagulation protein levels.[20] The ECMO priming solution used in our institution has evolved empirically and at the time of this study contained approximately 20% fresh-frozen plasma. Although the factors supplied in this solution were often insufficient to raise overall factor levels into the normal range, it is likely that more precipitous falls in factor concentrations were prevented. A survey of hematologic support practices during ECMO is now in progress; preliminary data obtained from 58 centers in the United States indicate that fewer than one third routinely include *any* factor-containing blood products in the circuit prime. Several centers now using fresh-frozen plasma in their prime have indicated intentions to replace this with simpler and less costly albuminated solutions. Our data call into question the advisability of such practice and represent a starting point for further investigation.

We conclude that pediatric patients undergoing ECMO often have multiple severe, previously unrecognized coagulation factor deficiencies before cannulation and that these deficiencies may persist beyond or even be exacerbated by the initiation of bypass. We speculate that these coagulation factor deficiencies may contribute to the risk of hemorrhage during ECMO, and suggest that the widespread practice of using factor-deficient priming solutions should be reevaluated.

We are indebted to Nicholas J. Morana and John J. Sears for preparation and performance of factor assays.

REFERENCES

1. Watson JW, Brown DM, Lally KP, Null D, Clark R. Complications of extracorporeal membrane oxygenation in neonates. South Med J 1990;83:1262-5.
2. Sell LL, Cullen ML, Whittlesey GC, et al. Hemorrhagic complications during extracorporeal membrane oxygenation: prevention and treatment. J Pediatr Surg 1986;21:1087-91.
3. Bui KC, LaClair P, Vanderkerhove J, Bartlett RH. ECMO in premature infants: review of factors associated with mortality. ASAIO Trans 1991;37:54-9.
4. Cilley RE, Zwischenberger JB, Andrews AF, et al. Intracranial hemorrhage during extracorporeal membrane oxygenation in neonates. Pediatrics 1986;78:699-704.
5. Extracorporeal Life Support Organization. International ECMO registry report. June 1994.
6. Glass P, Miller M, Short B. Morbidity for survivors of extracorporeal membrane oxygenation: neurodevelopmental outcome at 1 year of age. Pediatrics 1989;83:72-8.
7. Kanto WP. A decade of experience with neonatal extracorporeal membrane oxygenation. J PEDIATR 1994;124:335-47.
8. Clark RH, Yoder BA, Sell MS. Prospective, randomized comparison of high-frequency oscillation and conventional ventilation in candidates for extracorporeal membrane oxygenation. J PEDIATR 1994;124:447-54.
9. Short B, Walker L, Traysman R. Impaired cerebral autoregulation in the newborn lamb during recovery from severe, prolonged hypoxia combined with carotid artery and jugular vein ligation. Crit Care Med 1994;22:1262-8.
10. Andrew M, Paes B, Johnston M, et al. Development of the human coagulation system in the full-term infant. Blood 1987; 70:165-72.
11. Andrew M, Paes B, Milner R, et al. Development of the human

coagulation system in the healthy premature infant. Blood 1988;75:1651-7.
12. Andrew M, Paes B, Johnston M. Development of the hemostatic system in the neonate and young infant. Am J Pediatr Hematol Oncol 1990;12:95-104.
13. Thompson AR, Counts RB. Removal of heparin and protamine from plasma. J Lab Clin Med 1976;88:922-9.
14. Chessells J, Wigglesworth J. Coagulation studies in preterm infants with respiratory distress and intracranial hemorrhage. Arch Dis Child 1972;47:564-70.
15. Cole V, Durbin G, Olaffson A, et al. Pathogenesis of intraventricular haemorrhage in newborn infants. Arch Dis Child 1974;49:722-8.
16. McDonald M, Johnson M, Rumack C, et al. Role of coagulopathy in newborn intracranial hemorrhage. Pediatrics 1984; 74:26-31.
17. Seegers WH. Prothrombin complex. Semin Thromb Hemost 1981;7:291.
18. Bick RL. Physiology of hemostasis. In: Johnson KD, ed. Disorders of thrombosis and hemostasis. Chicago: ASCP [American Society of Clinical Pathologists] Press, 1992:1-26.
19. Montgomery R, Scott J. Hemostasis: diseases of the fluid phase. In: Nathan D, Oski F, ed. Hematology of infancy and childhood. 4th ed. Philadelphia: WB Saunders, 1993:1605.
20. Kern FH, Morana NJ, Sears JJ, Hickey PR. Coagulation defects in neonates during cardiopulmonary bypass. Ann Thorac Surg 1992;54:541-6.

FELLOWSHIPS

Fellowships available in pediatric subspecialties and those for general academic pediatric training are listed once a year, in **January,** in THE JOURNAL OF PEDIATRICS. Each **June,** forms for listing fellowships available for the academic year beginning 18 months after publication are sent to the Chairman of the Department of Pediatrics at major hospitals in the United States and Canada. In addition, **a copy of the application form appears in the July, August, and September issues** of THE JOURNAL (please use the current form). Should you desire to list fellowships, a separate application must be made *each* year for *each* position. All applications must be returned to Mosby–Year Book, Inc., by **October 15** preceding the listing year to ensure publication. Additional forms will be supplied on request from the Journal Editing Department, Mosby–Year Book, Inc., 11830 Westline Industrial Drive, St. Louis, MO 63146-3318/800-325-4177, ext. 4317, or 314-453-4317.

Prediction of the outcome of growth hormone therapy in children with idiopathic short stature

A multivariate discriminant analysis

Anna Spagnoli, MD, Gian Luigi Spadoni, MD, Stefano Cianfarani, MD, Anna Maria Pasquino, MD, Simonetta Troiani, MD, and Brunetto Boscherini, MD

From the Departments of Pediatrics, Tor Vergata University and La Sapienza University, Rome, Italy

Objective: To identify, with the use of pretreatment clinical data, the children with idiopathic short stature responsive to treatment with growth hormone (GH).
Design: Open, prospective study in a university hospital.
Subjects: Patients admitted to the study met the following criteria: birth weight at least 2.5 kg, no sign of dysmorphic disease, stature less than the 3rd percentile for chronologic age (CA), linear growth velocity (GV) less than the 25th percentile for bone age (BA), no sign of puberty, maximal GH response to pharmacologic stimulation greater than 10 μg/L, no evidence of organic disease, treatment with daily subcutaneous administration of GH at a dose of 12 to 16 IU/m^2 per week.
Main outcome measures: Eight pretreatment growth variables and the increase of GV after 6 months of therapy were measured. Children with a change in GV that was greater than 2.5 cm/yr after 6 months of GH therapy were considered responders to GH.
Results: We studied 67 patients (44 boys). Forty patients (60%) were responders. With univariate analysis the variables found to have predictive value were GV (*z* score for gender and CA), bone age (*z* score for gender and CA), and percentage of ideal body weight. These variables were employed in a multivariate discriminant analysis. Growth velocity and BA showed the best independent discriminant significance in predicting responsiveness to the initial 6 months of GH therapy. The obtained equation was as follows: Score = $-0.40 + 0.92X_1 - 0.87X_2$, where X_1 is the GV *z* value for CA and X_2 is the BA *z* value for CA). Using this scoring system, we obtained a specificity of 96.3% and a sensitivity of 92.5% in predicting responsiveness to GH (chi-square with Yates correction, 48.2; $p < 0.001$).
Conclusions: Discriminant analysis may permit the pretreatment prediction of responsiveness to the initial 6 months of GH therapy in short children without GH deficiency. (J PEDIATR 1995;126:905-9)

Presented in part at the Fourth Joint Meeting of the Lawson Wilkins Pediatric Endocrine Society and the European Society for Paediatric Endocrinology, San Francisco, Calif., June 1993.

Submitted for publication June 24, 1994; accepted Jan. 27, 1995.

Reprint requests: Anna Spagnoli, MD, Dipartimento di Sanità Pubblica, Clinica Pediatrica, Università Tor Vergata, Via di Tor Vergata 135, 00133 Roma, Italia.

0022-3476/95/$3.00 + 0 **9/20/63722**

Despite several studies[1-8] that have attempted to differentiate otherwise healthy short children who will respond to growth hormone therapy from those who will not, a 6-month therapeutic trial seems to be the only definitive tool for identifying those who should continue the GH therapy, as measured by an increase in linear growth velocity greater than 2 cm/yr.[9, 10]

Multifactor scoring systems are established as a way to predict the presence of disease or expected response to therapy. They permit the simultaneous use of several risk factors, enabling more information to be included in a single evaluation.[11-18]

The aims of our study were (1) to identify with simple univariate analysis, in otherwise healthy children with idiopathic short stature, pretreatment clinical factors with predictive value for the response to the initial 6 months of GH therapy and (2) to develop, with multivariate statistical analysis, a scoring system based on the variables selected by univariate analysis that could be employed in the prediction of the responsiveness of short, healthy children to the initial 6 months of GH therapy.

METHODS

Study population. The subjects were selected consecutively from children referred to the Tor Vergata University Center of Pediatric Endocrinology, Rome, Italy, and to the La Sapienza University Center of Pediatric Endocrinology, Rome, Italy, during a 5-year period (1989 to 1993) for evaluation of short stature. Patients admitted to the study met the following inclusion criteria: birth weight greater than 2.5 kg; no sign of dysmorphic disease; karyotype 46,XX for the girls; no clinical or biochemical evidence of organic disease, including hypothyroidism, psychologic problems, or malnutrition; no long-term medication; no sign of puberty at the beginning and during the initial 6 months of therapy; stature less than the 3rd percentile for chronologic age; GV, as determined during the 6 months before the beginning of GH treatment, less than the 25th percentile for sex and bone age; maximal GH response greater than 10 μg/L to pharmacologic stimulation; treatment with daily subcutaneous administration of GH at a dosage of 12 to 16 IU/m² per week continuously for 6 months.

BA	Bone age
CA	Chronologic age
GH	Growth hormone
GV	Growth velocity [linear]

Study design. Patients' height was measured every 6 months and expressed as a z score for CA and gender, according to the standards of Tanner et al.[19] Height was determined by the average of at least two consecutive measurements that did not differ by more than 0.4 cm, taken by two trained independent observers with the use of the Harpenden stadiometer.

The z scores were calculated with the following formula:

$$z \text{ Score} = \frac{X - \text{Average } X}{\text{SD}}$$

where X is the observed measurement, average X is the mean of this measurement at the relevant age, and SD is the standard deviation from the mean.[20] Growth velocity was evaluated during the 6 months before (GV_0) and the 6 months after (GV_6) the beginning of the treatment. Growth velocity was expressed as centimeters per year and z scores for CA and BA_1 according to the standards of Tanner et al.[19] Changes in GV ($GV_6 - GV_0$), expressed in centimeters per year, and z scores were also evaluated. Patients with a GV change greater than 2.5 cm/yr were defined as responders and the others as nonresponders. Bone age was determined from a radiograph of the left hand and wrist, performed not more than 1 month before the beginning of the treatment, according to the method of Greulich and Pyle[21]; BA was expressed as BA/CA ratio and as z score for CA and gender. Mean parental height was determined, according to the method of Tanner et al.[22] by using the mean of the parents' height and adding 6.5 cm in men or subtracting 6.5 cm in women. Predicted adult height was evaluated according to the method of Bayley and Pinneau.[23] Paternal and maternal height, mean parental height, and predicted adult height were expressed as z score for gender and adult height with the standards of Tanner et al.[19] Weight/height ratio was expressed as percentage of ideal body weight.[19, 24] The pharmacologic stimuli for the evaluation of GH adequacy were insulin (0.1 IU/kg of body weight; administered intravenously), arginine (0.5 gm/kg of body weight; administered intravenously for 30 minutes), or clonidine (100 μg/m² of body surface; administered orally).

Data analysis. Univariate analysis was performed with the chi-square test with Yates correction, and the Student t test (two-tailed) was used to compare the pretreatment data from the responders with data from the nonresponders; simple linear regression analysis was used to test correlations between variables. Variables that were significantly (probability < 0.01) associated with response to GH entered into the multivariate discriminant analysis. The discriminant model developed a scoring system for estimating the probability of responsiveness to therapy. Data are presented as mean ± SD unless otherwise stated. Values of p less than 0.01 were considered significant. The Statgraphics (STSC Inc., Rockville, Md.) statistical software package was used for statistical analysis.

Table I. Pretreatment clinical data (n = 67)

Variable	Mean ± SD
CA (yr)	9.0 ± 1.7
Height (z score for CA)	−2.5 ± 0.3
GV (cm/yr)	4.2 ± 0.7
GV (z score for CA)	−1.7 ± 0.8
GV (z score for BA)	−2.0 ± 0.7
BA (z score for CA)	−2.2 ± 0.9
BA/CA ratio	0.8 ± 0.09
Paternal height (z score for adult height)	−1.6 ± 0.7
Maternal height (z score for adult height)	−1.6 ± 0.9
Mean parental height (z score for adult height)	−1.6 ± 0.6
Ideal body weight (%)	102.7 ± 12.6
Predicted adult height (z score for adult height) (n = 40)	−2.0 ± 0.8

RESULTS

Study population. Sixty-seven patients were eligible, and all were included in the study; 23 were girls (34.3%) (Table I). During the first 6 months of GH therapy, 40 patients (60%) had a GV change greater than 2.5 cm/yr (responders); 27 (40%) had a GV change less than 2.5 cm/yr (nonresponders). The mean dosage of GH was 14.0 ± 1.4 IU/m^2 per week (range, 12.2 to 15.9 IU/m^2 per week). The HV of the whole population expressed as z scores for CA, increased from −1.7 ± 0.8 to 1.8 ± 1.5.

Univariate analysis. Patients who responded to therapy had a lower GV (p <0.001), a less pronounced BA retardation (p <0.001), and a higher percentage of ideal body weight (p <0.01) in comparison with nonresponders (Table II). Age, gender, height, mean parental height, maternal height, paternal height, and predicted adult height were not significantly associated with responsiveness to GH therapy and were excluded from further analysis.

Across the whole population, the change in GV ($GV_6 - GV_0$), expressed as z score for CA, was inversely related to pretreatment GV expressed as centimeters per year, z score for CA, and z score for BA (p <0.001), and directly related to BA as z score for CA (p <0.001). Similar results were obtained when the change in GV ($GV_6 - GV_0$) was expressed as centimeters per year.

Multivariate analysis. The variables with a predictive significance (p <0.01) on univariate analysis were GV (expressed as z score for CA, and as centimeters per year and z score for BA), BA (expressed as z score and BA/CA ratio) and percentage of ideal body weight. These variables were analyzed by discriminant analysis. Growth velocity expressed as z score for CA and BA expressed as z score for

Table II. Results of univariate analysis of pretreatment data in relation to responsiveness to GH therapy

Variable	Responders (n = 40)	Nonresponders (n = 27)	p
CA (yr)	9.0 ± 1.7	8.8 ± 1.8	NS
Gender (n)			
F	10	13	NS
M	30	14	
BA (z score for CA)	−1.7 ± 0.8	−2.9 ± 0.9	<0.001
Height (z score for CA)	−2.5 ± 0.3	−2.6 ± 0.4	NS
GV (z score for CA)	−2.1 ± 0.9	−1.0 ± 0.6	<0.001
GV (z score for BA)	−2.3 ± 0.8	−1.6 ± 0.6	<0.001
Paternal height (z score for adult height)	−1.7 ± 0.7	−1.6 ± 0.8	NS
Maternal height (z score for adult height)	−1.6 ± 1.0	−1.6 ± 0.8	NS
Mean parental height (z score for adult height)	−1.6 ± 0.6	−1.7 ± 0.5	NS
Ideal body weight (%)	106.2 ± 14.0	97.4 ± 9.8	<0.01
Predicted adult height (z score for adult height) (n = 40)	−2.1 ± 0.6 (n = 26)	1.7 ± 1.1 (n = 14)	NS

All values for responders and nonresponders expressed as mean ± SD, except for gender.
NS, Not significant.

CA had a better independent discriminant significance in terms of predicting responsiveness to therapy. The importance of variables in the discriminant analysis was evaluated by the percentage of the relative contribution of each individual variable to the total variance; GV contributed 49.9%, and BA contributed 50.1%.

The equation obtained by discriminant analysis was as follows:

$$\text{Score} = -0.40 + 0.92X_1 - 0.87X_2$$

where X_1 is GV z score for CA and X_2 is BA z score for CA. The Wilks λ for the discriminant function was 0.48 (chi-square, 46.9; p <0.001).

The diagnostic score for an individual patient was calculated by substituting the predictive variables in the discriminant equation. The mean scores were 1.25 and − 0.84 for nonresponders and responders, respectively. The cutoff point that divided responders and nonresponders was 0.20. Patients with a discriminant score greater than the cutoff value

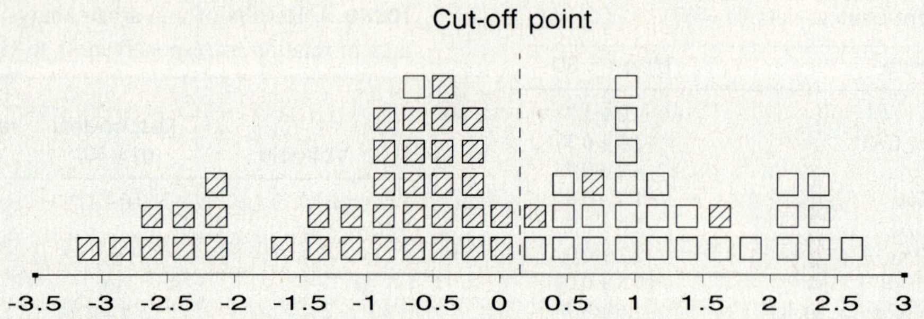

Figure. Distribution of patients by outcome, with score predicted by discriminant equation. *Hatched squares* indicate responders; nonresponders are indicated by *open squares*.

were considered to have a low possibility of responding to the initial 6 months of GH therapy. With this cutoff point the scoring system had a sensitivity of 92.5% and a specificity of 96.3% in predicting the responsiveness to GH therapy in children with idiopathic short stature (chi-square value with Yates correction, 48.2; $p < 0.001$) (Figure).

To test robustness of the model, we employed two procedures:

1. A jackknifed classification was carried out. The jackknife method is based on the "leave one out" principle, where the discriminant function is fitted to repeatedly drawn samples of the original sample.[18, 25] Each patient thus was singled out on the basis of a discriminant function generated from the other subjects. This procedure was repeated for all 67 patients. After jackknifing, only one more patient was misclassified. Thus specificity decreased only marginally to 92.6%, and sensitivity remained unaltered.
2. By randomly selecting two thirds of the cases, a subset was used to generate the discriminant function, which was then used to classify the remaining cases. This test subset contained 14 responders and nine nonresponders. The discriminant function derived from the remaining 44 patients correctly classified 90.9% of its own cases (88.5% of responders; 94.4% of nonresponders), and when tested on the test subset, it correctly predicted 91.3% of the 23 patients (85.7%) of responders; 100% of nonresponders).

DISCUSSION

Many short, otherwise healthy children have been treated with GH, but the growth rate has been enhanced in only some of them.[2-8] Several studies have attempted to define clinical and laboratory criteria for identifying before treatment those children who will respond to GH. The effectiveness of these criteria as prognostic factors was limited by the use of univariate statistical analysis, and a short-term (6-month) trial of GH therapy has been proposed to identify the responders to GH.[9-10] However, the treatment with GH of short but healthy children raises medical, ethical, and economic questions.

In our study we used multivariate discriminant analysis to provide a relatively specific and precise pretreatment prediction of responsiveness to GH therapy for 6 months in children with idiopathic short stature. In individual patients no predictive model can substitute for qualified clinical judgment, but a statistical model may be of some help in better understanding the relative importance of factors that contribute to the identification of patients responsive to any therapy.

The value of our study includes, besides the statistical method used, the narrow range of GH dosage and the large number of children studied. Other investigators, using univariate analysis, have evaluated a smaller number of subjects[3] or a wider GH dosage range.[4]

When we used univariate analysis, an inverse correlation between pretreatment growth velocity and change in growth velocity during treatment was observed. This correlation has been reported by other investigators.[4, 5, 26]

The lower percentage of ideal body weight and the higher degree of delay of BA observed in our nonresponsive patients indicates that suboptimal caloric intake could be the cause of their growth retardation. Rudman *et al.*[2] previously observed[27] a lower height/weight ratio in children with no GH deficiency who did not respond to GH. Probably, as suggested by Crawford,[27] in short, otherwise healthy children initial attention should be given to nutritional status rather than to treatment with GH.

Among the pretreatment variables analyzed, GV and BA were the significant predictors. The combination of these variables in the discriminant analysis provided an acceptable fit for a predictive model. Such precise pretreatment knowledge of statistical probability of a response to the initial 6 months of GH therapy may be particularly valuable in identifying patients who will not respond. In these patients the medical, psychologic, ethical, and economic implications of the decision to begin treatment must be considered, and not recommending therapy could be appropriate.

The main advantage of the discriminant analysis is that it enables the discriminatory value of several features to be considered simultaneously.[17, 18] Our discriminant formula is specific and sensitive in identifying short, healthy children who will respond to 6 months of GH therapy. A limitation of this study, however, is that the model was derived from and tested on the same 67 patients. We could have created the mathematical model from a segment of our study group and tested the model on the remainder, but we chose to use the power of a large patient population to create the model and to use cross-validation to reinforce the results. It would be ideal to test the discriminant function by applying it to another large group of patients and then estimating the error. Short of this possibility, cross-validation with the jackknife procedure is the best compromise.[18, 25] The resulting negligible decreases in diagnostic sensitivity and specificity of the discriminant analysis suggest that the mathematic model is robust for clinical application.[25, 28]

We conclude that the discriminant formula described can provide guidelines for selecting short, otherwise healthy children who will probably respond to short-term GH treatment, although its reliability awaits further testing. We recommend that GH treatment be considered only in those patients who, by discriminant analysis of the appropriate data, are predicted to be responders to therapy.

REFERENCES

1. Cara JF, Johanson AJ. Growth hormone for short stature not due to classic growth hormone deficiency. Pediatr Clin North Am 1990;37:1229-54.
2. Rudman D, Kutner MH, Blackston RD, Cushman RA, Bain RP, Patterson JH. Children with normal-variant short stature: treatment with human growth hormone for six months. N Engl J Med 1981;305:123-31.
3. Van Vliet G, Styne DM, Kaplan S, Grumbach MM. Growth hormone treatment for short stature. N Engl J Med 1983; 301:1016-22.
4. Hindmarsh PC, Brook CGD. Effect of growth hormone on short normal children. Br Med J 1987;295:573-7.
5. Schwartz D, Cheng-Shih S, Shulman DI, Root AW, Bercu BB. Linear growth response to exogenous growth hormone in children with short stature. Am J Dis Child 1990;144:1092-7.
6. Saggese G, Graziano C. Criteria for recognition of the growth inefficient child who may respond to treatment with growth hormone. Am J Dis Child 1989;143:1287-93.
7. Zadik Z, Landau H, Limoni Y, Lieberman E. Predictors of growth response to growth hormone in otherwise normal short children. J Pediatr 1992;121:44-8.
8. Moore KC, Donaldson DL, Ideus PL, Gifford RA, Moore WV. Clinical diagnoses of children with extremely short stature and their response to growth hormone. J Pediatr 1993;122:687-92.
9. Milner RDG. Proper use of growth hormone. Arch Dis Child 1990;65:70-1.
10. Grumbach MM. Growth hormone therapy and the short end of the stick. N Engl J Med 1988;319:238-41.
11. Farinon AM, Grande M, Torquati A, D'Antini P. Multivariate analysis for predicting the presence of bacteria in bile in patients with acute cholecystitis. Eur J Surg 1993;160:184-7.
12. Fung KP, Lau SP. Differentiation between extrahepatic and intrahepatic cholestasis by discriminant analysis. J Paediatr Child Health 1990;26:132-5.
13. Gigot JF, Leese T, Dereme T, Coutinho J, Castaing D, Bismuth H. Acute cholangitis: multivariate analysis of risk factors. Ann Surg 1989;209:435-7.
14. Neoptolemos JP, Shaw DE, Carr-Locke DL. A multivariate analysis of preoperative risk factors in patients with common bile duct stones. Ann Surg 1989;209:157-61.
15. Lee PKD, Wilson DM, Rountree L, Hintz R, Rosenfeld RG. Efficacy of insulin-like growth factor I levels in predicting the response to provocative growth hormone testing. Pediatr Res 1990;27:45-51.
16. Corcoran JD, Patterson CC, Thomas PS, Halliday HL. Reduction in the risk of bronchopulmonary dysplasia from 1980-1990: results of a multivariate logistic regression analysis. Eur J Pediatr 1993;152:677-81.
17. Morrison DF. Multivariate statistical methods. New York: McGraw-Hill, 1967:220-1.
18. Hair JF, Anderson RE, Tatham RL, Black WC. Multivariate data analysis. New York: Macmillan, 1992:1-18.
19. Tanner JM, Whitehouse RH, Takaishi M. Standards from birth to maturity for height, weight, height velocity, weight velocity: British children, 1965—part II. Arch Dis Child 1966; 41:613-35.
20. Armitage P, Berry G. Statistical methods in medical research. 2nd ed. Oxford: Blackwell, 1987.
21. Greulich WW, Pyle SI. Radiographic atlas of skeletal development of the hand and wrist. Palo Alto, Calif: Stanford University Press, 1973.
22. Tanner JM, Goldstein H, Whitehouse RH. Standards for children's height at ages 2-9 years allowing for height of parents. Arch Dis Child 1970;45:755-62.
23. Bayley N, Pinneau SR. Tables for predicting adult height from skeletal age: revised for use with the Greulich-Pyle hand standards. J Pediatr 1952;40:423-41.
24. Passmore R, Eastwood MA. Human nutrition and dietetics. Edinburgh; Churchill Livingstone, 1986.
25. Miller RG. The jackknife: a review. Biometrika 1974;61:1-15.
26. Cianfarani S, Spadoni GL, Scirè G, et al. Pretreatment growth velocity and response to GH (hGH) therapy. Minerva Pediatr 1987;39:757-61.
27. Crawford JD. Meat, potatoes and growth hormone. N Engl J Med 1981;305:164-5.
28. Efron B. Estimating the error rate of a prediction rule: improvement on cross-validation. J Am Stat Assoc 1983;78:316-21.

Clinical and biochemical characterization of short-chain acyl–coenzyme A dehydrogenase deficiency

Ajay Bhala, BS, Steven M. Willi, MD, Piero Rinaldo, MD, Michael J. Bennett, PhD, MRCPath, Eberhard Schmidt-Sommerfeld, MD, and Daniel E. Hale, MD

From the Department of Pediatrics, University of Pennsylvania School of Medicine, Philadelphia; the Department of Pediatrics, Medical University of South Carolina, Charleston; the Department of Genetics, Yale University School of Medicine, New Haven, Connecticut; the Departments of Pathology and Pediatrics, University of Texas Southwestern Medical Center at Dallas; and the Department of Pediatrics, Louisiana State University School of Medicine, New Orleans

***Objective*: We identified two additional patients with short-chain acyl–coenzyme A (CoA), further characterized the clinical and biochemical features of this defect, and compared it with other fatty acid oxidation defects.**

***Design*: We have measured the in vitro short-chain acyl–coenzyme A dehydrogenase (SCAD) activity in six affected persons with the electron-transfer flavoprotein-linked assay in the presence and absence of anti–medium-chain acyl-CoA dehydrogenase antibody. Urine organic acids, acylglycines, acylcarnitines, and radiolabeled substrate catabolism by skin fibroblasts were also examined.**

***Results*: All patients had some neurologic abnormalities, including hypotonia, hypertonia, or seizures. None of the patients had episodes of hypoglycemia; in the only patient tested, fasting ketogenesis was not impaired. Four patients were initially seen in the neonatal period, two with profound metabolic acidosis and two with mild acidemia; the other two cases were recognized in infancy. Enzymatic analysis of cultured skin fibroblasts demonstrated approximately 10% activity of SCAD when compared with control fibroblasts. Gas chromatography and mass spectrometry of urine revealed that ethylmalonic acid was present in all samples but not always at elevated concentrations; methylsuccinic acid and butyrylglycine were sporadically elevated. n-Butyrylcarnitine was often found in urine and plasma. Radiolabeled substrate metabolism was reduced to 40% to 60% of control values.**

***Conclusions*: Because affected persons do not consistently excrete characteristic metabolites, the diagnosis of this enzymatic deficiency is difficult. It is necessary to collect and analyze several urine and plasma specimens when the diagnosis is being considered in patients with neurologic abnormalities suggestive of this disorder. (J PEDIATR 1995;126:910-5)**

Supported by National Institutes of Health grant F32 DK08475 (S. M. W.) and the Joseph Stokes, Jr., Research Institute Fatty Acid Oxidation Research Fund (D. E. H.).

Presented in part at the Thirty-first Annual Symposium of the Society for the Study of Inborn Errors of Metabolism, Manchester, United Kingdom, September 1993.

Submitted for publication July 11, 1994; accepted Jan. 27, 1995.

Reprints requests: Daniel E. Hale, MD, Department of Pediatrics, Division of Endocrinology and Diabetes, University of Texas Health Science Center at San Antonio, 7703 Floyd Curl Dr., San Antonio, TX 78248-7806.

0022-3476/95/$3.00 + 0 **9/20/63721**

Fatty acid metabolism provides an alternative source of fuel during periods of fasting and stress. The first step in the mitochondrial β-oxidation spiral involves three members of the family of flavin-linked acyl–coenzyme A dehydrogenases: long chain, medium chain, and short chain. These three chain length–specific enzymes act on C20-C12, C12-C4, and C6-C4 fatty acyl-CoA, respectively, to form a 2,3-enoyl-CoA product from the saturated precursor.

Since the 1980s the number of reports of defects in ACD has risen because of increased awareness of these disorders. Medium-chain acyl-CoA dehydrogenase deficiency is the most common and well characterized; more than 200 cases are known to us. Approximately 20 cases of defects in long-chain acyl-CoA dehydrogenase[1] or very long chain acyl-CoA dehydrogenase are known.[2] To date, only four cases of short-chain acyl-CoA dehydrogenase deficiency have been confirmed.[3-5] We describe the clinical and biochemical findings in six enzyme-confirmed patients with SCAD deficiency and compare these with the findings in patients with other ACD defects to provide a perspective on the clinical and biochemical manifestations of this disease.

ACD	Acyl-CoA dehydrogenase
CoA	Coenzyme A
EMA	2-Ethylmalonic acid
HPLC	High-performance liquid chromatography
LCAD	Long-chain acyl-CoA dehydrogenase
MCAD	Medium-chain acyl-CoA dehydrogenase
SCAD	Short-chain acyl-CoA dehydrogenase

CASE REPORTS

Clinical details of patients 1,[4] 2 (Amendt et al.,[3] neonate 1), 3 (Amendt et al., neonate 2), and 4[5] have been reported previously. The clinical histories of two new patients (patients 5 and 6; Table I) are described.

Case 5. A 5-year-old girl had increased urinary excretion of 2-ethylmalonic acid in the neonatal period, found by routine neonatal organic acid screening. Repeated urine organic acid analysis at 3 months and at 1 year of age showed increased 2-ethylmalonic acid, whereas that at 6 months was normal. At approximately 2 years of age she had delayed speech development and was modestly hyperactive.

Case 6. A black male infant was the 3545 gm product of a term pregnancy. Born by spontaneous vaginal delivery, he was noted to have a shaking-staring spell on the first day of life. Studies for sepsis yielded negative results. The infant continued to have nystagmus, hypertonia, and sluggishly reactive pupils. Serum lactic acid concentration was 4.7 mmol/L (normal, 0.5 to 1.6 mmol/L); plasma lactic acid values ranged from 1.5 to 7.3 mmol/L. After discharge, plasma lactic acid and urinary EMA measurements were consistently elevated. At 14 days of age the patient was noted to be slightly jittery but in no apparent distress; he had mild hypertonia and hyperreflexia. Results of a laboratory investigation, including a complete blood cell count with differential cell count and determination of levels of serum electrolytes, liver enzymes, blood urea nitrogen, creatinine, venous blood gases, pyruvate, ammonia, and amino acids, all were normal. Blood lactate concentration was normal at 0.1 mmol/L, and an initial urine organic acid profile showed increased excretion of EMA and a slight increase in glutaric acid. Lactic acid values on follow-up were 7.3 and 9.9 mmol/L, respectively. The patient is currently in stable condition and no episodes of metabolic decompensation have been reported.

METHODS

Organic acid and acylglycine analysis. Urinary organic acid and acylglycine levels were measured in samples from asymptomatic and symptomatic periods as previously described, with gas chromatography and mass spectrometry with either electron-impact or chemical ionizations, in the selected ion monitoring modes.[6-9]

Acylcarnitine analysis. Plasma and urine acylcarnitines were detected by a radioisotopic exchange–high-performance liquid chromatography method.[10] Separation of C4-acylcarnitine isomers was achieved by the use of a solvent system designed for this purpose.[11]

Fibroblast cultures. Skin fibroblast cultures from patient and control subjects, at passages less than 15, were grown and prepared for enzymatic analysis as previously described.[12]

Enzyme analysis. Straight-chain ACD activities were measured in fibroblasts as previously described.[4, 12] Samples were assayed with only octanoyl-CoA and butyryl-CoA as substrates. We[4] and others[13] have shown that half the activity toward butyryl-CoA comes from MCAD. To determine the contribution of SCAD in catalysis of this short-chain substrate, we incubated supernatant with polyclonal monospecific rabbit anti-human MCAD antibody (gift of Dr. Arnold W. Strauss, Washington University, St. Louis, Mo.). The activity was measured as described previously. Proteins were measured with the use of the Folin-phenol reagent.

Carbon 14–labeled butyric acid metabolism. Incorporation of carbon 14–labeled butyric acid (Amersham, Arlington Heights, Ill.) into cellular protein was carried out by a modification of the method described by Wendel.[14] Dulbecco minimal essential medium with 10% (vol/vol) fetal calf serum was used as growth medium. Fibroblasts were seeded at a density of 25,000 cells/cm^2; after 24 hours in growth medium, the monolayers were exposed to ^{14}C-labeled substrate in phosphate-buffered saline solution containing 0.1 mmol/L butyrate with a specific activity of 10 mCi/mmol. The cells were then incubated at 37° C for 12, 24, and 36 hours. Incubations were terminated by rapid cooling to 0° C and monolayers were rinsed twice with ice-cold saline solution. After being treated with 6% trichloroacetic acid for 10 minutes and rinsed three times with cold saline solution, protein was solubilized with 2N sodium hydroxide. Carbon 14 incorporation into protein was measured by scintillation counting and total proteins assayed with the Folin-phenol reagent.

Table I. Clinical features

Patient No.	Age at onset	Ethnicity	Consanguinity	Abnormal neurologic findings at presentation	Present status
1	Neonate	Unknown	–	Poor feeding, listlessness	Reportedly normal
2	Neonate	Italian and Portuguese, French-Canadian	–	Lethargy and hypertonia	Dead
3	At 2 mo	Hispanic, French and Irish	–	Progressive skeletal muscle weakness	Dead
4	At 15 mo	Turkish	+ (2nd cousins)	Severe skeletal hypotonia	Dead
5	Neonate	Unknown	Unknown	Possible hyperactivity	Normal
6	Neonate	Black American	Unknown	Probable seizure activity	Reportedly normal

Table II. Biochemical features

		Urinary organic acids (mmol/mol creatinine)			Urinary acylglycine (μg/mg creatinine)		Acylcarnitine (urine, μmol/gm creatinine; serum, nmol/ml)	
Patient No.	Metabolic status	EMA	Methyl-succinate	Glutarate	Butyryl-glycine	Hexanoyl-glycine	Butyryl-carnitine	Isobutyryl-carnitine
1	Acute	732						
	Asymptomatic	48-192 (545 ?)	7-46		1.35-5.0	0.2-1.1		
2*	Acute							
	Asymptomatic						Trace (urine) 0.1 (serum)	Not measurable
3	Acute							
	Asymptomatic	8-14	6-8		0.4-1.0	1.6-4.7		
4	Acute	68.4	26.3	18.2	0.5	2.44		
	Asymptomatic	76.8	10.4	5.3	<0.01	2.63		
5†	Acute							
	Asymptomatic							
6	Acute	3900	630	<10	0.56		79.3 (urine)	Not measureable
	Asymptomatic	16-175	<10-215	<10	<0.01	<0.3		

Normal means (ranges) for organic acids and acylglycines: EMA, 8.1 ± 5.6 mmol/mol (0.5 to 20.2 mmol/mol); methylsuccinate, 5.0 ± 3.0 mmol/mol (0.4 to 13.8 mmol/mol); glutarate, 5.8 ± 3.8 mmol/mol (0.6 to 15.2 mmol/mol); butyrylglycine, 0.8 ± 0.7 mmol/mol (0.03 to 2.1 mmol/mol); hexanoylglycine, 0.9 ± 0.4 mmol/mol (0.2 to 1.9 mmol/mol). Butyrylcarnitine is not detected in normal human urine.
In all samples isobutyrylcarnitine could not be measured.
*Quantitative data not available; see report of Amendt et al.[3] for qualitative data.
†Quantitative data not available; see Case Reports section, above, for qualitative data.

RESULTS

Urine organic acids and acylglycines. The major organic acids found were EMA and 2-methylsuccinic acid (Table II). Glutaric acid excretion was modestly increased in one patient. The prominent acylglycine species was n-butyrylglycine. A small amount of isovalerylglycine was found in one patient. Levels of EMA, 2-methylsuccinic acid, and n-butyrylglycine were intermittently elevated, particularly in patients who were not metabolically stressed (Table II).

Urine and serum acylcarnitines. Two urine samples (from patients 3 and 6) and serum from patient 3 were available for acylcarnitine analysis. In both patients substantial amounts of C4-acylcarnitine were found by radioisotopic exchange–HPLC and confirmed in the serum of patient 6 by fast atom bombardment–tandem mass spectrometry (S. Kahler, Duke University, Durham, N.C.). Separation of C4-acylcarnitine isomers by HPLC revealed n-butyrylcarnitine as the main isomer (Figure). Patient 3 had a total plasma carnitine level of 43 μmol/L with 67% free carnitine in the fed state (normal, 40 to 60 μmol/L total; 80% to 90% free) and patient 4 had a total plasma carnitine of 60 μmol/L with 57% free.

Enzyme activity. Table III lists the enzyme activities of MCAD and SCAD with octanoyl-CoA and butyryl-CoA as the substrates. All patients had normal activity with octanoyl-CoA and half-normal activity with butyryl-CoA when compared with control values. The activity toward butyryl-CoA was reduced by approximately 90% in all but

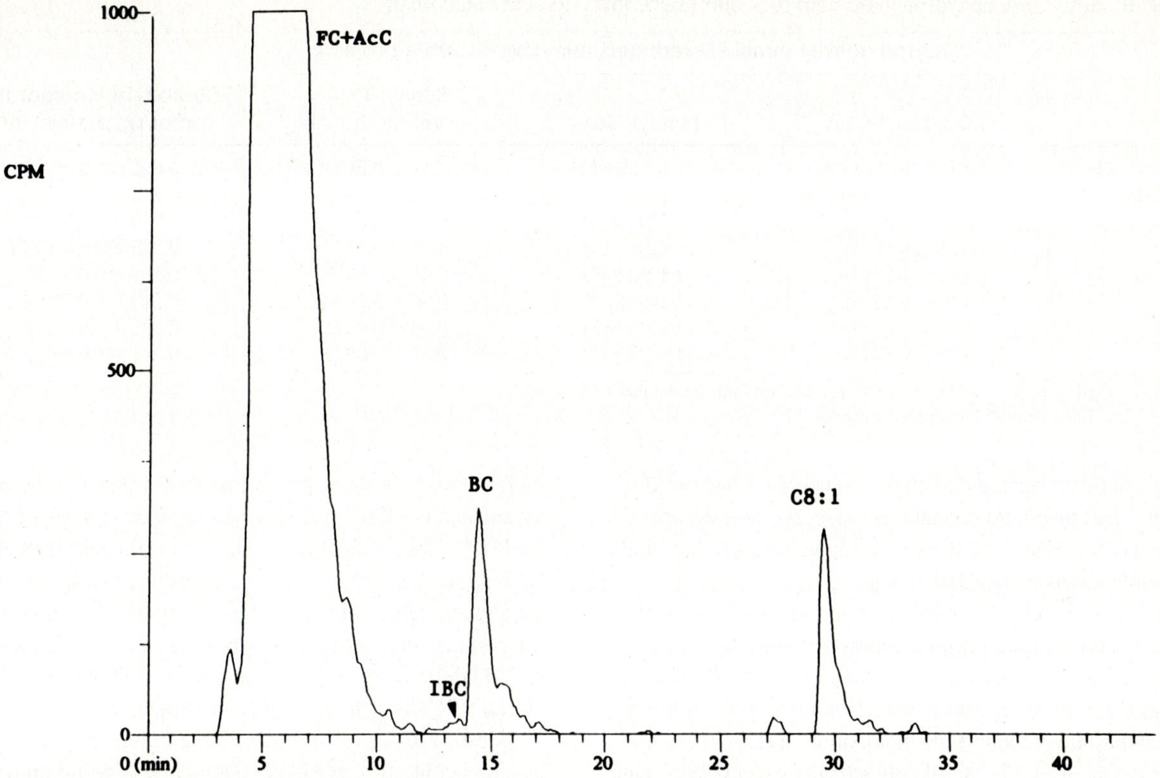

Figure. Patient 6. Urinary acylcarnitine HPLC profile. *AcC*, Acetylcarnitine; *BC*, n-butyrylcarnitine; *C8:1*, octenoylcarnitine; *CPM*, counts per minute; *FC*, free carnitine; *IBC*, isobutyrylcarnitine. Separation of C4-acylcarnitine isomers was achieved with a special solvent system.[11] Carnitine esters were identified by their retention times.

one patient when their tissues were incubated with anti-MCAD antibody.

Carbon 14–labeled butyrate metabolism. The metabolism of [1-^{14}C]butyric acid and radioactive carbon incorporation into cellular protein was measured by quantitation of β-radiation in cell homogenates. Incorporation was reduced to 40% to 60% of control values in all patient fibroblasts (Table III).

DISCUSSION

Short-chain acyl-CoA dehydrogenase deficiency is a rarely described and potentially lethal inborn error of intermediary metabolism. When this defect is compared clinically with other well-known fatty acid oxidation disorders, such as MCAD and LCAD deficiency, several features become apparent. The latter defects typically are manifested as hypoketotic hypoglycemia, but patients with SCAD deficiency may not have hypoglycemia as an important clinical sign. This may reflect stimulation of gluconeogenesis and ketogenesis by the unimpaired oxidation of long-chain and medium-chain fatty acyl-CoA. In a fasting study, patient 4 produced a plasma ketone body concentration of 5 mmol/L,[5] which supports this hypothesis.

In the few persons with SCAD deficiency examined, there has been no secondary hypocarnitinemia, in contrast to MCAD and LCAD deficiency. However, the esterified carnitine/free carnitine ratio has been increased, as in other inborn errors of metabolism.

Most of our patients had neurologic signs such as hypotonia, hypertonia, hyperactivity, or developmental delay, whereas patients with MCAD and LCAD deficiency have no primary neurologic signs. Because an abnormal neurologic pattern appears to be the most common sign in this disorder, we speculate that short-chain organic acid accumulation causes central nervous system deficits rather than muscular problems. Supporting this idea are the neurologic abnormalities in children with congenital lactic acidosis,[15] methylmalonic and propionic acidemia,[16] and glutaric acidemia type II.[17] In terms of age at onset, most of the defects in long-chain and medium-chain fatty acid oxidation become apparent in the first year of life, whereas with SCAD deficiency four of our patients had a neonatal onset (two with profound acidosis and two with mild acidemia); two had disease during onset infancy. Lactic acidosis has also been seen in MCAD deficiency as a secondary phenomenon. The degree of abnormal neurologic findings and acidosis in SCAD defi-

Table III. Acyl-CoA dehydrogenase activities and [1-^{14}C]butyric acid catabolism

	Enzyme activity (nmol ETF reduced/min · mg^{-1} soluble protein)			
	Octanoyl-CoA	Butyryl-CoA	Butyryl-CoA + anti-MCAD Ab	Carbon-14 incorporation (pmol/μg protein · hr^{-1})
Control subjects	4.34 ± 0.05 (142)	2.44 ± 0.27 (126)	1.12 ± 0.08 (30)	0.662 ± 0.059 (29)
Patients				
1	4.16 ± 0.49 (9)	1.06 ± 0.05 (9)	0.12 ± 0.06 (9)	0.270 ± 0.030 (8)
2	4.43 ± 0.10 (3)	1.15 ± 0.18 (4)	0.45 ± 0.12 (3)	0.373 ± 0.098 (≥2)
3	4.14 ± 0.15 (3)	1.09 ± 0.18 (2)	0.08 ± 0.00 (3)	0.369 ± 0.079 (8)
4	3.83 ± 0.25 (4)	0.94 ± 0.02 (3)	0.16 ± 0.09 (4)	0.319 ± 0.043 (9)
5	4.20 ± 0.23 (4)	1.20 ± 0.16 (3)	0.00 ± 0.00 (3)	0.378 ± 0.015 (4)
6	3.75 ± 0.14 (4)	1.00 ± 0.02 (2)	0.07 ± 0.00 (3)	0.281 ± 0.098 (6)

Values expressed as mean ± SEM. Values in parentheses indicate number of analyses.
Ab, Antibody; *ETF*, electron transfer flavoprotein.

ciency did not correspond to clinical outcome. For example, patient 1 had profound neonatal acidosis but was described as normal, whereas patient 3 did not have acidosis but died of complications of her deficiency.

The variable excretion pattern of organic acids when the more common electron-impact ionization–mass spectrometry method is used may make the diagnosis difficult. Use of the more sensitive chemical ionization–mass spectrometry method may aid in identifying metabolites in relatively small amounts that are important diagnostically, especially if stable isotope dilution is used. We have also noted the utility of radioisotopic exchange–HPLC analysis of acylcarnitines in diagnosing this short-chain defect; analysis with this method is superior to fast atom bombardment–tardem mass spectrometry because of isomer resolution. Because isobutyrylcarnitine is excreted by metabolically normal persons[18] and is found in plasma and urine of patients with a defect in branched-chain acyl-CoA oxidation[19] and in those who may have a defect in oxidative phosphorylation,[20] resolution of the isomers is important. It remains to be established whether determination of butyrylcarnitine in plasma or urine is a reliable marker of SCAD deficiency.

We also have demonstrated the usefulness of radiolabeled-substrate metabolism as a general screening tool for short-chain fatty acid oxidation defects. Evidence suggests that the only test that can, in and of itself, be used to make the diagnosis of SCAD deficiency is the electron-transport flavoprotein-linked enzymatic assay, with butyryl-CoA as the substrate in combination with immunoinactivation of MCAD.

Several patients described as having SCAD deficiency appear not to have this disorder. The patient described by Turnbull et al.[21] had decreased activity of SCAD in muscle but not in her fibroblasts.[22] Further investigations have revealed that she may have a riboflavin-responsive multiple ACD variant similar to that reported by DiDonato et al.[23] Amendt et al.[24] suggested that, at least in mice, the SCAD in the muscle is the same as that in fibroblasts. The patient described in 1986[25] not only had reduced activity of SCAD and [1-^{14}C]butyrate oxidation in muscle but had also reduced activity of LCAD and [1-^{14}C]palmitate oxidation, which suggests a defect similar to that in glutaric acidemia type II. In contrast, an additional patient of ours with presumed SCAD deficiency had reduced levels of SCAD activity but normal LCAD activity (data not shown).

Because of the intermittent nature of the organic aciduria, it remains likely that SCAD deficiency is being underdiagnosed. Investigators should consider this diagnosis in the metabolic examination of children with abnormal neurologic findings, particularly when children have central nervous system abnormalities in an acute and intermittent manner. The analysis of organic acids during acute decompensation may be of benefit, but we suggest the inclusion of the more sensitive assays for butyrylglycine and acylcarnitines in the initial evaluation.

We thank Dr. Duna Penn, Louisiana State University Medical Center, for her help with the acylcarnitine analysis; Dr. Charles Stanley, University of Pennsylvania, for his insightful comments; and Drs. Susan Winter, Valley Children's Hospital, Fresno, Calif., Adrian Sewell, Frankfurt Children's Hospital, Frankfurt, Germany, and Harvey Levy, Massachusetts General Hospital, Boston, for providing us with clinical and biochemical data from their patients.

REFERENCES

1. Hale DE, Bennett MJ. Fatty acid oxidation disorders: a new class of metabolic diseases. J PEDIATR 1992;121:1-11.
2. Yamaguchi S, Indo Y, Coates PM, Hashimoto T, Tanaka K. Identification of very-long-chain acyl-CoA dehydrogenase deficiency in three patients previously diagnosed with long-chain acyl-CoA dehydrogenase deficiency. Pediatr Res 1993;34:111-3.
3. Amendt BA, Greene C, Sweetman L, et al. Short-chain acyl-CoA dehydrogenase deficiency. J Clin Invest 1987;79:1303-9.
4. Coates PM, Hale DE, Finocchiaro G, Tanaka K, Winter SC. Genetic deficiency of short-chain acyl-CoA dehydrogenase in cultured fibroblast from a patient with muscle carnitine defi-

ciency and severe skeletal muscle weakness. J Clin Invest 1988; 81:171-5.

5. Sewell AC, Herwig J, Böhles H, Rinaldo P, Bhala A, Hale DE. A new case of short-chain acyl-CoA dehydrogenase deficiency with isolated ethylmalonic aciduria. Eur J Pediatr 1993; 152:922-4.
6. Rinaldo P, Welch RD, Previs SF, et al. Ethylmalonic/adipic aciduria: effects of oral medium chain triglycerides, carnitine, and glycine on urinary excretion of organic acids, acylcarnitines, and acylglycines. Pediatr Res 1991;30:216-21.
7. Tuchman M, McCann MT, Johnson PE, Lemieux B. Screening newborns for multiple organic acidurias in dried filter paper urine samples: method development. Pediatr Res 1991; 30:315-21.
8. Yamaguchi S, Shimizu N, Orii T, et al. Prenatal diagnosis and neonatal monitoring of a fetus with glutaric aciduria type II due to electron transfer flavoprotein (β-subunit) deficiency. Pediatr Res 1991;30:439-43.
9. Rinaldo P, O'Shea JJ, Coates PM, Hale DE, Stanley CA, Tanaka K. Medium-chain acyl-CoA dehydrogenase deficiency: diagnosis by stable isotope dilution measurement of urinary n-hexanoylglycine and 3-phenylpropionylglycine. N Engl J Med 1988;319:1308-13.
10. Schmidt-Sommerfeld E, Penn D, Duran M, Bennett MJ, Santer R, Stanley CA. Detection of inborn errors of fatty acid oxidation from acylcarnitine analysis of plasma and blood spots with the radioisotopic exchange-high performance liquid chromatographic method. J PEDIATR 1993;122:708-14.
11. Bieber LL, Kerner J. Short-chain acyl carnitines: identification and quantitation. In: Chytil D, McCormick FD, eds. Methods in enzymology. Orlando, Fla: Academic Press, 1986: 264-76.
12. Hale DE, Batshaw ML, Coates PM, et al. Long-chain acyl-coenzyme A dehydrogenase deficiency: an inherited cause of non-ketotic hypoglycemia. Pediatr Res 1985;19:666-71.
13. Ikeda Y, Tanaka K. Purification and characterization of five acyl-CoA dehydrogenases from rat liver mitochondria. In: Tanaka K, Coates PM, eds. Fatty acid oxidation: clinical, biochemical and molecular aspects. New York: Alan R Liss, 1990:37-54.
14. Wendel U. Prenatal detection of defects in propionate metabolism. Clin Chim Acta 1980;108:475-7.
15. Robinson BH. Lactic acidemia. In: Scriver CR, Beaudet AL, Sly WS, Valle D, eds. The metabolic basis of inherited disease. New York: McGraw-Hill, 1989:869-88.
16. Heidenreich R, Natowicz M, Hainline BE, et al. Acute extrapyramidal syndrome in methylmalonic acidemia: "metabolic stroke" involving the globus pallidus. J PEDIATR 1988; 113:1022-7.
17. Chow CW, Frerman FE, Goodman SI, Brown GK, Pitt JJ, Danks DM. Striatal degeneration in glutaric acidemia type II. Acta Neuropathol 1989;77:554-6.
18. Schmidt-Sommerfeld E, Penn D, Kerner J, Bieber LL. Analysis of acylcarnitines in normal human urine with the radioisotopic exchange-high performance liquid chromatography (HPLC). Clin Chim Acta 1989;181:231-8.
19. Burlina AB, Zacchello F, Dionisi-Vici C, et al. New clinical phenotype of branched-chain acyl-CoA oxidation defect. Lancet 1991;338:1522-3.
20. Burlina AB, Dionisi-Vici C, Bennett MJ, et al. A new syndrome with ethylmalonic aciduria and normal fatty acid oxidation in fibroblasts. J PEDIATR 1994;124:79-86.
21. Turnbull DM, Bartlett K, Stevens DL, et al. Short-chain acyl-CoA dehydrogenase deficiency associated with a lipid-storage myopathy and secondary carnitine deficiency. N Engl J Med 1984;311:1232-6.
22. Turnbull DM, Sheperd IM, Bartlett K, Sherratt HSA. Short chain acyl-CoA dehydrogenase deficiency. In: Tanaka K, Coates PM, eds. Fatty acid oxidation: clinical, biochemical, and molecular aspects. New York: Alan R Liss, 1990:313-24.
23. DiDonato S, Gellera C, Peluchetti D, et al. Normalization of short-chain acylcoenzyme A dehydrogenase activity after riboflavin treatment in a girl with multiple acylcoenzyme A dehydrogenase deficient myopathy. Ann Neurol 1989;25:479-84.
24. Amendt BA, Freneaux E, Reece C, Wood PA, Rhead WJ. Short-chain acyl-coenzyme A activity, antigen, and biosynthesis are absent in the BALB/cByJ mouse. Pediatr Res 1992; 31:552-6.
25. DiDonato S, Cornelio F, Gellera C, Peluchetti D, Rimoldi M, Taroni F. Short-chain acyl-CoA dehydrogenase deficient myopathy, with secondary carnitine deficiency. Muscle Nerve 1986;9(suppl):178.

Neonatal-onset propionic acidemia: Neurologic and developmental profiles, and implications for management

Kathryn N. North, MD, Mark S. Korson, MD, Yasodha R. Gopal, MD, Frances J. Rohr, MS, RD, T. Berry Brazelton, MD, Susan E. Waisbren, PhD, and Matthew L. Warman, MD

From the Department of Medicine, Children's Hospital, Boston, Massachusetts

Objectives: **To document the clinical and neurodevelopmental profiles of a cohort of patients with neonatal-onset propionic acidemia and to determine the efficacy of current therapy with respect to outcome.**
Method: **The clinical, neurologic, and developmental status of six patients was prospectively evaluated during a 15-month period. Previous clinical and biochemical data were ascertained from hospital records to determine longitudinal nutritional status, number of episodes of hyperammonemia with ketoacidosis, and developmental performance with respect to age.**
Results: **No deaths resulted from propionic acidemia since the identification of the oldest patient in the series in 1980. Therapeutic intervention (e.g., gastrostomy tube feeding) resulted in improved nutritional status and possibly contributed to improved survival. All children had hypotonia, resulting in a significant effect on motor development; however, focal neurologic deficits and evidence of movement or seizure disorder were absent. Mild cortical atrophy was evident on cranial magnetic resonance imaging in four patients. All children, including two patients with no significant episodes of hyperammonemia and normal growth since the neonatal period, had a mild to moderate degree of intellectual impairment.**
Conclusions: **The results of our study suggest that current therapy for neonatal-onset propionic acidemia is associated with improved survival and nutritional status, and an absence of focal neurologic deficits. However, hypotonia and cognitive delay were still present, even in children with "optimal" metabolic control. Additional therapeutic advances are required to improve the developmental and cognitive outcome. (J PEDIATR 1995;126:916-22)**

Propionic acidemia is a disorder of organic acid metabolism caused by a deficiency of propionyl coenzyme A carboxylase. Inherited in an autosomal recessive fashion, the disorder most commonly is manifested in the neonatal period with vomiting, poor feeding, lethargy, hypotonia, metabolic ketoacidosis, and hyperammonemia.[1] Other clinical patterns have been described in older infants, children, and adults.[1-4] The reason for this phenotypic variation is undetermined; it does not correlate with in vitro propionyl CoA carboxylase activity, although it may be related to alternate pathways for in vivo propionate oxidation.[5]

CoA	Coenzyme A
CT	Computed tomography
IQ	Intelligence quotient
MRI	Magnetic resonance imaging

Propionic acidemia is rare (estimated incidence, 1 in 350,000[1]), making assessment of outcome difficult because

Submitted for publication June 3, 1994; accepted Jan. 25, 1995.

Reprint requests: Kathryn North, MD, Department of Neurology, Children's Hospital, Pyrmont Bridge Rd., Camperdown, New South Wales 2050, Australia.

0022-3476/95/$3.00 + 0 **9/20/63690**

even specialized centers follow up few patients. A retrospective survey of 65 patients with the disorder (both early- and late-onset disease) found that most children incurred permanent neurologic damage with markedly delayed development, seizures, and cerebral atrophy on computed tomography.[1] Two further reviews revealed high mortality rates for patients with neonatal onset of symptoms (85%[6] and 41.5%[7]). Only one retrospective study has focused specifically on neurologic outcome[8] (some of these cases were also reviewed earlier[9]); of the 20 patients, 11 were seen during the first week of life. Despite early diagnosis and vigorous treatment, this early-onset group had a median survival time of only 3 years and no patient had an IQ greater than 60. In three patients a movement disorder (chorea or dystonia) developed, and cerebral atrophy was present in three of four patients in whom CT scans were performed.

The treatment of the organic acidemias has evolved during the past decade with the improvement of formula mixtures restricted in isoleucine, valine, methionine, and threonine; the availability of protein-modified foods; the use of gastrostomy tube feeding to guarantee nutritional intake; and the use of carnitine to replete serum and tissue carnitine and to facilitate the excretion of propionylcarnitine.[10] Recent advances in therapy are not reflected in previous studies in which patient ascertainment occurred during several decades, and outcome has not been systematically evaluated.

We report the results from an ongoing prospective study of six children with neonatal-onset propionic acidemia who are being followed up at Children's Hospital, Boston. Prospective evaluation allows for comparisons to be made and conclusions to be drawn from concurrent assessment of all patients within a short period. Through sequential assessment of clinical and neurodevelopmental status, we aimed to determine the efficacy of current therapy and the implications for long-term management.

METHODS

Study population. The study population consisted of three boys and three girls with neonatal-onset propionic acidemia, now 22, 24, 26, 37, 48, and 166 months of age, respectively. Five patients had the diagnosis made and were followed up at Children's Hospital since birth; one patient was initially seen at another center and has been followed up at Children's Hospital since 6 months of age. Another patient (currently 50 months of age) was followed at Children's Hospital for a 6-month period in 1993 before transfer to another center and was excluded from the study because of insufficient longitudinal data. A search of medical records at the Children's Hospital since 1980 revealed no additional patients with a diagnosis of propionic acidemia. The diagnosis was based on the identification of typical metabolites by urine organic acid analysis and confirmed by assay of propionyl CoA carboxylase activity in all patients.

Current management. The Metabolism Service, Children's Hospital, Boston, is a multidisciplinary team consisting of biochemical geneticists, nutritionists, psychologists, a nurse, and a social worker. Current treatment of all patients includes daily carnitine supplements (50 to 200 mg/kg per day) and a protein-modified diet. Approximately half the protein needs of patients is supplied as natural protein (usually in the form of regular infant formula), and half is supplied as medical food restricted in methionine, threonine, isoleucine, and valine. The medical food used depends on the patient's age and product availability (Table I). Additional calories are supplied with Product 80056 (Mead Johnson, Evansville, Ind.) or ProPhree (Ross Products, Columbus, Ohio). All patients received biotin in the neonatal period, which was discontinued when they were determined to be unresponsive. L-Isoleucine supplementation (100 mg/day) is necessary in most patients to correct a relative isoleucine deficiency.

Growth, and plasma amino acids and ammonia levels, are monitored at least monthly on an outpatient basis and more frequently during periods of poor growth or unsatisfactory metabolic control. Total serum protein and albumin levels, and complete blood cell count, are measured at least four times a year. Urinary ketone levels are monitored on a daily basis at home. Dietary changes are made if growth rate is not satisfactory, plasma amino acid values are abnormally high or low, or ammonia level is high.

During mild illnesses without ketonuria, parents are advised to increase the patient's fluid and caloric intakes. When slight to moderate ketonuria is present and persistent, the protein sources in the diet are reduced by half, with an increase in calories and fluid by 20% to 25% greater than normal. Often continuous feedings or overnight feedings are recommended through the gastrostomy tube. Clinical symptoms and urine ketone production are closely monitored, and daily contact is made with clinic staff. If ketone production does not clear or worsens, blood electrolyte and ammonia levels are measured, and if a hospital admission is not indicated, a protein-free diet with added calories and fluid may be recommended for no more than 24 to 48 hours.

Persistent moderate to severe ketonuria accompanied by vomiting, dehydration, lethargy, acidosis, or hyperammonemia demand closer monitoring and are treated in the hospital with intravenously administered dextrose, and bicarbonate if necessary. Maximal calories and fluid are supplied by providing up to one and one-half times the maintenance requirements. Protein intake is recommenced within 36 to 48 hours to help minimize catabolic proteolysis, usually at 25% to 50% of the patient's regular natural protein intake; protein consumption is then increased gradually. Parenteral nutrition

Table I. Clinical and biochemical features

Feature	Patient No. 1	2	3	4	5	6
Current age (mo)	166	49	37	26	24	22
Gender	M	F	F	M	M	F
Ethnic origin	African-American	Portuguese	Hispanic	Czech	Hispanic	Polish
Initial presentation						
Ammonia (μmol/L)	NA	299	56	532	429	265
Glucose (mmol/L)	NA	3.2	6.2	1.2	4.6	6.7
Blood pH	7.10	7.23	7.46	7.35	7.33	7.30
Hospital stay (days)	14	14	16	24	10	21
Enzyme activity (pmol/min/mg protein) (range, 156-348)*	4	5	5	8	6	8
Hospital days†	78	22	31	0	7	0
Current protein intake						
Total protein (gm/kg)	1.1	1.46	1.5	2.48	1.7	1.8
% as natural protein	63	47	54	52	57	46
Current medical foods	OS-1 (MJ)	Maxamaid XMTVI (SHS)	Maxamaid XMTVI (SHS)	OS-1 (MJ)	Analog XMTVI (SHS)	Propimex (Ross)
Current serum albumin (gm/L) (range, 30-45)	34	41	39	36	26	36
Current head circumference (percentile)	25th	5th-10th	25th-50th	75th	5th-10th	75th
Growth percentile before insertion of gastrostomy tube						
Weight	<3rd	25th	5th	50th	<<5th	50th
Height	<3rd	10th	<5th	10th	<5th	50th
Current growth percentile						
Weight	50th	95th	75th	65th	25th	75th
Height	25th	50th	5th	20th	10th	50th
Cortical atrophy on MRI	+	NA	+	NA	+	+

MJ, Mead Johnson (Evansville, Ind.); *NA*, not available; *Ross*, Ross Products (Columbus, Ohio); *SHS*, Scientific Hospital Supplies (Gaithersburg, Md.).
*Propionyl CoA carboxylase activity.
†Days in hospital specifically for ketoacidosis or hyperammonemia or both (excluding initial presentation). Patient 3 required admission on four occasions with hyperchloremic alkalosis associated with vomiting and constipation.

is used to supply protein if enteral feedings are not tolerated. Metronidazole is also given to reduce endogenous propionate production from the gastrointestinal tract. When constipation is present, gut motility agents are employed. Signs of infection are investigated aggressively, and antibiotic or antiviral coverage are initiated when appropriate.

Members of the metabolism service maintain regular contact with the primary pediatrician and community-based support services (including visiting nursing services, developmental intervention, and physical and occupational therapy) to ensure that appropriate therapeutic regimens continue at home. In general, compliance with therapy and follow-up during the period of the study was considered good for all patients.

Study protocol. The study was prospective for 15 months (July 1993 to October 1994). During this period all children were seen on a regular basis in the clinic and detailed neurodevelopmental assessments were performed at least twice. Neurodevelopmental assessment included examination by a neurologist (K. N. N.) and intelligence testing with either the Bayley Scales of Infant Development, the McCarthy Scales of Children's Abilities, or the Wechsler Intelligence Scale for Children–III. Patients 2 to 6 were also observed during play by a developmental pediatrician (T. B. B.). This qualitative assessment was aimed at evaluating the current status of each child's cognitive, linguistic, and affective development in a way that might be underappreciated during standard neurodevelopmental testing. Cranial magnetic resonance imaging examinations were performed in four children (Nos. 1, 3, 5, and 6) during the study period.

In addition, previous clinical and biochemical data were ascertained from hospital records, to determine the nature of clinical onset, longitudinal growth and nutritional status, and the number of episodes of hyperammonemia with ketoacidosis. Previous psychologic assessments, performed at least

Table II. Results of sequential developmental assessments

Assessment by age	Patient No. 1	2	3	4	5	6
At 6 mo						
Mental scale	84	106	<50	123	81	116
Motor scale	86	94	60	72	54	83
At 12 mo						
Mental scale	77	NA	76	89	NA	NA
Motor scale	57	NA	56	69	NA	NA
At 18-24 mo						
Mental scale	55	50	NA	50	50	70
Motor scale	67	50	NA	<50	50	60
At 30-36 mo						
Mental scale	64	NA	<50			
Motor scale	63	NA	<50			
At 42-48 mo						
Cognitive index	74	50				
Verbal scale	79	50				
Perceptual scale	61	50				
At 13 yr						
Full-scale IQ	56					
Verbal IQ	67					
Performance IQ	53					

Results are expressed as standard scores. Test instruments were Bayley Scales of Infant Development (<3 years; mean, 100; SD = 15), McCarthy Scales of Children's Abilities (3 to 6 years; mean, 100; SD = 16), and Wechsler Intelligence Scale for Children–III (<6 years; mean, 100; SD = 15).
NA, Not available.

annually in the clinic, were reviewed to determine developmental performance with respect to age.

RESULTS

There were no deaths from propionic acidemia, nor were any patients lost to follow-up since the identification of the oldest patient in the series in 1980. However, patient 1 had an older sibling who died in the neonatal period with metabolic acidosis and presumed sepsis at another center; this may represent an undiagnosed case of propionic acidemia. Clinical and biochemical characteristics at the time of diagnosis are summarized in Table I. All patients had lethargy, poor feeding, and hyperammonemia during the first week of life; none required hemodialysis. Patient 1 had the most severe neonatal course with hyperammonemic coma and severe prolonged metabolic acidosis. Patient 3 also had bacterial meningitis, which responded to antibiotic therapy. In all patients propionyl CoA carboxylase activity was less than 3% of control values.

Nutrition and growth. The clinical and biochemical features of the study population, including growth percentiles before and after insertion of a gastrostomy tube, are summarized in Table I. Feeding difficulties emerged as the major treatment problem during the latter half of the first year of life in all patients. During this time all children had increasing anorexia with frequent vomiting, and parents had greater difficulty maintaining metabolic stability at home and meeting caloric requirements during intercurrent infection. In three children growth percentiles decreased outside the normal range. Therapy with cyproheptadine was attempted in all children during the period of the study and resulted in transient improvement in oral intake in only one child (patient 6). All patients required placement of a gastrostomy tube to facilitate feeding, usually during the second year of life.

In all cases parents reported that, after the institution of gastrostomy tube feeding, home care was easier and less stressful to the family and that the children were less lethargic and apathetic. Minor episodes of metabolic decompensation (e.g., persistent ketonuria) could be managed at home, and hence the frequency of hospital admissions decreased. Although intermittent episodes of hyperammonemia continued to occur (particularly in patients 2 and 3), a general increase in metabolic stability was observed. For example, during the first 30 months of life, patient 1 was hospitalized on eight occasions with ketoacidosis and sepsis, and linear growth during this period was less than the 5th percentile. After gastrostomy tube placement, linear growth accelerated to the normal range during a 6-month period and his metabolic status stabilized; he was admitted to the hospital only twice during the next 10 years (one admission was during the period of the study). Oral intake improved in mid childhood, and he has not required gastrostomy tube feeding for 6 years (except during periods of metabolic decompensation).

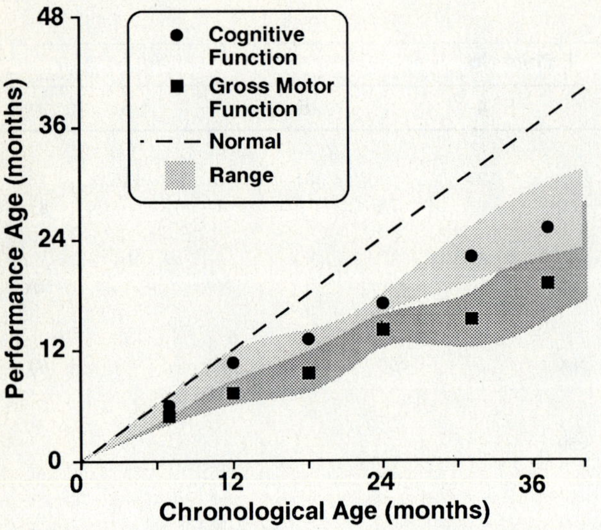

Figure. Results of sequential developmental assessments (Bayley Scales of Infant Development, McCarthy Scales of Children's Abilities). Developmental age for cognitive and motor function is derived from raw-score equivalent tables available with each test instrument. Mean performance age is shown as function of chronologic age. *Shaded area* indicates range of performance for study group. All patients demonstrated delayed acquisition of new skills during second year of life. At all ages motor function was more significantly delayed than cognitive function.

In patient 4 growth was maintained within the normal range during the first 16 months of life despite increased difficulties with oral feeding, frequent vomiting, and recurrent episodes of ketonuria (managed at home). At 16 months of age, he fractured his right radius after minimal trauma and radiologic examination revealed moderately severe osteoporosis. After insertion of a gastrostomy tube at 18 months of age and a regimen of continuous overnight feeding, he has had one subsequent episode of ketonuria (managed successfully at home) and there has been partial resolution of the osteoporosis.

Current growth percentiles are within the normal range in all cases. Serum albumin levels were maintained within the normal range during the period of the study in all patients but patient 5. During the first year of life this patient had anorexia, severe recurrent vomiting, chronic constipation, and poor weight gain, resulting in protein malnutrition with hypoalbuminemia, skin breakdown, and poor hair growth. Initial refusal of gastrostomy tube placement and poor compliance with the feeding regimen complicated his treatment. Serum albumin concentration increased from 20 to 30 gm/L (normal range, 30 to 45 gm/L) after the institution of continuous overnight gastrostomy tube feeding, with normalization of skin and hair texture and linear growth. However, he has continued to have episodic vomiting, and the most recent serum albumin concentration was only 26 gm/L. Oral feeding is encouraged in all children after gastrostomy placement, but patients 2, 3, and 5 continue to refuse all oral intake. Serum glycine concentrations are consistently elevated in all patients and have ranged between 500 to 1800 μmol/L on sequential measurements (normal range, for children 3 months to 6 years of age, 125 to 318 μmol/L). Variations in glycine levels did not correlate with metabolic control. For example, glycine levels were paradoxically lower in some patients during episodes of ketoacidosis and hyperammonemia than during periods of otherwise good metabolic control.

Developmental outcome. On sequential neurologic examinations all patients had generalized hypotonia, with normal power and deep tendon reflexes. No evidence of focal neurologic deficits or movement disorder was present, and no patient had epilepsy. Cranial MRI examinations were performed in four children. The findings were similar in all cases, with slight prominence of the cerebrospinal fluid spaces, suggestive of mild cortical atrophy, and thinning of the corpus callosum; maturation of myelin appeared to be within normal limits. In the oldest patient (No. 1) a CT scan had been performed 4 years previously and findings were reported as normal. The MRI was performed during an episode of hyperammonemia; increased signal intensity of the basal ganglia bilaterally was seen on T2 and proton density images.

The results of sequential developmental and psychologic examinations are summarized in Table II. Motor function was generally more delayed than cognitive development at all ages, presumably because of the effect of hypotonia. Developmental progress slowed in all children as a product of age (Figure), including patients 4 and 6, who have had no significant episodes of hyperammonemia or ketoacidosis, and whose growth has been normal. Cognitive impairment became more pronounced during the second year of life; delays in language acquisition became evident during the third and fourth years.

In the oldest patient (No. 1) performance in all areas of development reached a plateau at 8 years of age. At 13 years of age he has a moderate degree of intellectual impairment (full-scale IQ, 56 according to Wechsler Intelligence Scale for Children–III) with a discrepancy between verbal and performance IQ (verbal IQ, 67; performance IQ, 53). He is friendly and outgoing but has significant behavioral problems. He has symptoms of attention deficit, which are not responsive to methylphenidate, and he receives special educational services in a regular school.

Assessment during play (patients 2 to 6) suggested that the children performed much better on cognitive tasks (adaptive function, social interaction, object permanence) than on tasks that required coordination or motor control. Hypotonia had a marked effect on both fine and gross motor performance, but the children often could compensate partially for their hypotonia, particularly in their ability to manipulate small objects. Several of the children had hypersensitivity to environmental stimuli (both auditory and tactile) and were easily distractable. Despite marked delays in some areas, the children had many positive qualities such as curiosity, self-motivation and a desire to succeed, frustration by failure to conquer a task (a sign of self-awareness and motivation), desire for approval, and interest and "excitement" in their surroundings—qualities that are often absent in children with global developmental delay.

DISCUSSION

The results of our study suggest that current therapy for propionic acidemia is associated with improved survival rates, normalization of growth and nutritional status, and improved neurologic outcome. No deaths caused by propionic acidemia at the Children's Hospital were documented since the identification of the first patient in the series in 1980. All patients currently have linear growth within the normal range and, with one exception, normal serum albumin levels. Movement disorders, epilepsy, or focal neurologic deficits, as have been observed in previous studies,[1, 6-8] were not present in any patient. However, all patients had hypotonia, resulting in a significant effect on motor development, and in all patients the acquisition of cognitive and language skills slowed during the second and third years of life. Consequently, all the children have a mild to moderate degree of intellectual impairment.

No individual clinical or biochemical feature was consistently associated with delays in development. Patients were listless and apathetic during periods of poor nutrition and recurrent metabolic instability, and qualitative improvements were noted after therapeutic intervention. However, this observation was not reflected in the quantitative psychologic assessments. A similar decrease in cognitive performance with age was observed in all patients, including the younger patients, who had normal linear growth and no significant episodes of hyperammonemia or ketoacidosis since the neonatal period.

The occurrence of hypotonia and developmental delay may be attributable to the metabolic instability in the neonatal period and in some cases to recurrent episodes of hyperammonemic ketoacidosis. However, the occurrence of similar developmental profiles in all children suggests that other etiologic factors, such as long-term exposure to abnormal metabolites, may affect developmental outcome. Even "good" metabolic control may be associated with elevations of organic acids in the cerebrospinal fluid, resulting in persistent derangement of brain metabolism.[11] Additionally, normal flux through the pathway from propionyl CoA to succinyl CoA may be necessary to maintain normal brain energy metabolism.

The differences in survival, and neurologic and nutritional status, between this and previous series of children with propionic acidemia may be attributable to improved therapeutic regimens. All patients in our series had the onset of symptoms during the first week of life and hence, by definition, have the classic form of the disorder. However, we cannot exclude genotypic heterogeneity as a possible contributing factor to the observed differences in outcome. In the study of Surtees et al.[8] the majority of patients were of Indo-Pakistani or Arab descent; it is possible that the phenotype in these ethnic groups is associated with a more deleterious enzymatic defect and higher mortality rates than in our patients, whose ethnic origins were more varied.

Implications for management. Anorexia and vomiting are universal problems in children with propionic acidemia, particularly late in the first year and early in the second year of life. The reason for these symptoms is unknown, although we have noted that the children with propionic and other organic acidemias (e.g., methylmalonic acidemia) have a marked increase in unprovoked gagging during episodes of ketoacidosis; it is possible that the abnormal accumulation of organic acids and their metabolites affect central regulation of the gag reflex and appetite. A therapeutic trial of cyproheptadine as a therapy for anorexia was largely unsuccessful (T. Sagie: personal communication, 1994); its antiserotinergic effect is postulated to increase appetite and promote oral motor development.[12] Its use resulted in an improvement in oral intake in only one patient, and the effect was transient, delaying the need for gastrostomy tube placement by 8 months.

The placement of a gastrostomy tube greatly facilitates routine feeding and home management of minor illnesses associated with persistent ketonuria and increased caloric requirements. At present, gastrostomy tube placement is frequently delayed until anorexia affects growth or interferes with the ability to treat early infection or ketosis aggressively. The elective insertion of a gastrostomy tube early during the first year of life may not only prevent some episodes of metabolic decompensation during the crucial early years of development but also the guilt that many parents feel when they "fail" to treat their child without the need for alternative enteral feeding.

Gastrostomy tube feeding may also provide a resource for modifying current therapy regimens. The production of propionic acid and its metabolites occurs in the catabolic degradation of specific amino acids and odd-chain fats.[10] Exposure of the developing central nervous system to abnormal metabolites may contribute to the developmental delays observed in propionic acidemia; thus a long-term prospective trial of frequent daytime and continuous overnight feeding would be worthwhile to determine whether avoidance of recurrent catabolic periods inherent in a regular feeding schedule leads to improved developmental outcome.

Glycine levels were consistently elevated in all patients but did not always increase during hyperammonemic episodes. Propionyl CoA likely inhibits the glycine cleavage system, resulting in hyperglycinemia.[13] However, during episodes of hyperammonemic ketoacidosis, glycine conjugation to intermediary metabolites (e.g., propionylglycine) facilitates their excretion, so that glycine levels may be paradoxically lowered. Hence we have not found glycine levels to be useful as a measure of metabolic stability.

Our experience with the oldest patient supports the observation of Luder et al.[14] that metabolic stability may be easier to maintain as the child becomes older. The reason may be increased metabolic "reserves," the availability of alternative pathways to assist or compensate for defective propionate metabolism, and/or a developing resistance to associated biochemical decompensation (i.e., acid-base status, glucose regulation) with increased age and body weight.

Most of our patients are too young for us to determine whether current management strategies have any effect on ultimate intelligence. However, during the early years of life, when motor performance is the principal means of assessing development, these children appear to have more severely delayed development because of the presence of hypotonia. It may be beneficial to anticipate the occurrence of motor deficits, to communicate this to parents during counseling, and to provide early intervention in the form of physical therapy.

Although current therapy improves growth and minimizes episodes of hyperammonemia and ketoacidosis, which may be life threatening or result in acute neurologic deterioration, it does not appear to alter significantly the cognitive outcome in children with propionic acidemia. Organ transplantation has been used to correct other inborn errors of metabolism and could be considered for propionic acidemia. In the future there is a potential for gene therapy[15]; early and complete correction of the biochemical defect may be the only way to prevent the developmental sequelae of deranged organic acid metabolism.

REFERENCES

1. Wolf B, Hsia YE, Sweetman L, Gravel R, Harris DJ, Nyhan WI. Propionic acidemia: a clinical update. J PEDIATR 1981; 99:835-46.
2. Wolf B, Paulsen EP, Hsia YE. Asymptomatic propionyl CoA carboxylase deficiency in a 13 year old girl. J PEDIATR 1979; 95:563-5.
3. Brandt IK, Hsia E, Clement DH, Provence SA. Propionicacidemia (ketotic hyperglycinemia): dietary treatment resulting in normal growth and development. Pediatrics 1974;53: 391-5.
4. Sethi KD, Ray R, Roesel RA, et al. Adult-onset chorea and dementia with propionic acidemia. Neurology 1989;39:1343-5.
5. Thompson GN, Walter JH, Bresson JL, et al. In vivo propionate oxidation as a prognostic indicator in disorders of propionate metabolism. Eur J Pediatr 1990;149:408-11.
6. Rousson R, Guibaud P. Long term outcome of organic acidurias: survey of 105 French cases (1967-1983). J Inher Metab Dis 1984;7:10-2.
7. Van der Meer SB, Poggi F, Spada M, et al. Clinical outcome and long term management of seventeen patients with propionic acidemia [Abstract]. Sixth International Congress of Inborn Errors of Metabolism, Milan, Italy, 1994.
8. Surtees RAH, Matthews EE, Leonard JV. Neurologic outcome of propionic acidemia. Pediatr Neurol 1992;8:333-7.
9. Leonard JV, Daish P, Naughten ER, Bartlett K. The management and long term outcome of organic acidemias. J Inher Metab Dis 1984;7(suppl 1):13-7.
10. Nyhan WL, Rice-Asaro M, Acosta P. Advances in the treatment of amino acid and organic acid disorders. In: Desnick RJ, ed. Treatment of genetic disease. New York: Churchill Livingstone, 1991:45-67.
11. Hoffman GF, Meier-Augenstein W, Stockler S, et al. Physiology and pathophysiology of organic acids in cerebrospinal fluid. J Inher Metab Dis 1993;16:648-69.
12. Hyman SL, Porter CA, Page TJ, et al. Behavior management of feeding disturbances in urea cycle and organic acid disorders. J PEDIATR 1987;111:558-62.
13. Ugarte M, Lopez-Lahoya J, Garcia ML, et al. Possible explanation for hyperglycinemia in propionic acidemia and methylmalonic acidemia: propionate and methylmalonate inhibit liver and brain mitochondrial transport. J Inher Metab Dis 1979;2: 93-6.
14. Luder AS, Yannicelli S, Green CL. Normal growth and development with unrestricted protein intake after severe infantile propionic acidemia. J Inher Metab Dis 1989;12:307-11.
15. Stankovics J, Ledley FD. Cloning of functional alpha propionyl CoA carboxylase and correction of enzyme deficiency in pccA fibroblasts. Am J Hum Genet 1993;52:144-51.

Prolonged dysphagia caused by congenital pharyngeal dysfunction

Elie Mbonda, MD, Dominique Claus, MD, C. Bonnier, MD, P. Evrard, MD, J. F. Gadisseux, MD, and G. Lyon, MD

From the Service of Pediatric Neurology and the Department of Radiology, St. Luc Hospital, University of Louvain Medical School, Brussels, Belgium

We describe two patients with severe, isolated, congenital dysphagia caused by paralysis of the pharyngeal muscles, who recovered at the ages of 40 months and 20 months, respectively. No other evidence of neurologic or muscular dysfunction was present except for a transient paralysis of the adductors of the vocal cords in one child. Radiocinematographic studies showed paralysis of the pharyngeal stage of swallowing, with minimal involvement of the oral stage. One child refused oral feeding for several months after apparent radiologic recovery. Two other patients with a similar disorder died of tracheal aspiration at the ages of 8 months and 4 months, respectively. Autopsies showed no abnormality of the central nervous system, and the cranial nerves involved in swallowing were normal. Only five other well-studied cases of this syndrome have been reported. These observations demonstrate the existence of a type of severe, idiopathic, congenital dysphagia related to paralysis of the constrictor muscles of the pharynx, with a propensity to recover after several months or years if properly managed. The cause of the disorder is obscure, but it is probably related to a dysfunction of the central nervous system. (J Pediatr 1995;126:923-7)

Congenital incapacity to swallow is a life-threatening condition in neonates and infants. Transitory dysphagia lasting a few days or weeks, possibly related to immaturity of the swallowing reflexes, is common in the premature infant, especially those with birth weights less than 1500 gm,[1, 2] and may occasionally occur in children born at term.[3] A prolonged inability to swallow is much more rare and can be due to various causes (Table).

Another life-threatening congenital swallowing disorder of unknown origin is caused by paralysis of the pharyngeal muscles. The disorder lasts several months or years, but recovery eventually occurs if it is correctly managed. This condition, the subject of our study, has been reported only rarely and, to our knowledge, is not mentioned in review articles or textbooks concerning swallowing disorders in neonates and infants.

Submitted for publication March 21, 1994; accepted Jan. 27, 1995.

Reprint requests: Gilles Lyon, MD, Service of Pediatric Neurology, St. Luc Hospital, University of Louvain Medical School, 10 avenue Hippocrate, 1200 Brussels, Belgium.

0022-3476/95/$3.00 + 0 **9/20/63723**

CASE REPORTS

Case 1. A boy was born at 38 weeks of gestational age by cesarean section because of prenatal asphyxia. The parents were healthy and nonconsanguineous. The infant's brother and sister were healthy. At 8 weeks of gestational age, hydramnios was discovered. At birth the child weighed 3500 gm, was 51 cm in length, and had a head circumference of 36 cm. The Apgar score was 6 at 5 minutes.

From the outset the infant was unable to swallow. Each attempt at oral feeding caused choking, nasal regurgitation, inspiratory dyspnea, and cyanosis. Pharyngeal accumulation of bucconasal secretions and salivation were present.

Clinical examination of the oral cavity at the age of 1 month showed paralysis of the pharyngeal muscles and soft palate. No contraction of these muscles could be elicited by mechanical stimulation. Sucking and tongue movements appeared to be normal. Other cranial nerves were normal. No other neurologic abnormalities were present except for moderate hypotonia. The morphologic characteristics of the face, jaw, and oropharyngeal cavity were unremarkable. Frequent aspiration of the pharynx and tube feeding were necessary. Administration of neostigmine had no effect. When the patient was 8 months of age, a gastrostomy was performed.

Videofluoroscopy of swallowing performed at the ages of 4 days, 6 days, and 6 months gave identical results (Figure). The oral stage of swallowing was normal, although lingual retropulsion move-

Table. Causes of persistent dysphagia in the neonate

Nasal-oropharyngeal malformations
Choanal atresia
Cleft lip or palate
Craniofacial syndromes (e.g., Pierre Robin syndrome, Crouzon syndrome)
Hypopharyngeal stenosis
Nasopharyngeal tumors
Foreign bodies
Esophageal and tracheoesophageal malformations
Tracheoesophageal fistula*
Esophageal stenosis*
Achalasia of cricopharyngeal muscle*
Esophageal achalasia
Esophageal atony
Gastroesophageal reflux
Vascular malformations
Aberrant right subclavian artery
Double aortic arch
Right aortic arch with left ligament
Neurologic causes
Supranuclear bulbar palsy: Pseudobulbar syndrome*
Dystonic syndromes
Chiari malformation with myelomeningocele
Werdnig-Hoffmann spinal muscular atrophy
Möbius syndrome
Duosyndrome of laryngeal nerve
Bilateral laryngeal paralysis
Riley-Day syndrome
Willi-Prader syndrome*
Muscular causes*
Familial infantile myasthenia
Myotonic dystrophy*
Congenital muscular dystrophy
Facioscapulohumeral dystrophy
Nemaline myopathy*
Myotubular myopathy
Disproprotion, congenital fiber type
Syndrome of congenital persistent idiopathic paralysis of the pharynx

Adapted from Weiss MH (Otolaryngol Clin North Am 1988;21:727-35) and Volpe JJ (Neurology of the newborn. Philadelphia: WB Saunders, 1987:88-9).
*Most frequent causes.

ments were somewhat slow. When the bolus was pushed into the pharynx, pharyngeal contractions were not induced, and there was reflux into the nasal cavity with tracheal aspiration. The movements of the esophagus were normal. Laryngoscopy showed paresis of the adductors of the vocal cords. The electromyogram of pharyngeal and facial muscles was normal. Chest x-ray studies showed evidence of aspiration pneumonia. The cerebral computed tomographic scan was unremarkable.

Dysphagia and inability to feed orally persisted unchanged until the patient was 18 months of age. However, no serious pulmonary infections occurred and the child gained weight normally. Independent walking was achieved at 20 months. Intellectual development seemed satisfactory, but language skills were retarded.

When the patient was 20 months of age, a radiologic study showed considerable improvement: pharyngeal peristalsis had reappeared, and tracheal aspiration was no longer present. However, the child refused oral feeding.

During the next 18 months, the patient progressively learned first to feed himself and then to be fed by mouth with solid food and later with liquids. When the patient was 3 years of age, the gastrostomy was closed, and at 3½ years of age, he no longer had any clinical evidence of swallowing difficulties. His voice was normal, and radiologic signs of vocal cord paresis were no longer detected. He retained for some time peculiar obsessive feeding habits concerning the nature, form, and consistency of food. Although he continued to make steady progress, language skills remained poor. At the age of 3½ years, with the Borel-Maisonny test, comprehension of language was at the 2- to 3-year age level and expression was at 2 years. When the patient was 6 years of age, his language performance had somewhat improved. His intellectual development was within normal limits. A brother also had delayed development of language.

Case 2. A girl, born normally at term, weighed 2870 gm and measured 50 cm in length, with a head circumference of 34 cm. Her parents and a prematurely born sister were in good health. Absence of swallowing, salivation, and oral cyanosis was noted during the first hours of life. The pharynx was filled with liquid, and complete paralysis of the pharyngeal muscles and velum was observed. Findings of a neurologic examination were otherwise normal. The patient had no facial, mandibular, or oropharyngeal abnormalities.

Endoscopy showed no abnormality of the larynx, trachea, or esophagus. Videofluoroscopy revealed the absence of pharyngeal contractions, and passive passage of the contrast medium in the esophagus and trachea was observed. When the patient was 4 months of age, an electromyogram of the pharyngeal muscles, facial muscles, tongue, and skeletal muscle was normal. The electroencephalogram and brain CT scan were unremarkable.

The infant had several serious episodes of tracheal aspiration and was fed by gavage. When she was 9 months of age, her dysphagia was unchanged. A videofluoroscopic study showed poorly coordinated movements of the tongue, delay in the induction of the pharyngeal stage of swallowing, absence of contraction of the caudal portion of the pharyngeal muscles, and no laryngeal ascension; tracheal aspiration was present. At the age of 16 months, the patient was able to take thick food orally, and by 20 months she ate and swallowed normally. Her motor and mental development were normal.

Case 3. A girl weighing 3600 gm was born at term after a normal pregnancy and an uneventful delivery. She was the only child of healthy parents. At the first feeding attempts, complete paralysis of swallowing was detected. She had total immobility of the pharyngeal muscles and soft palate. No other neurologic or muscular abnormalities, and no malformations of the face, mandible, or oropharynx, were present. Laryngoscopic and esophagoscopic findings were normal. She was fed by tube. Aspiration and pulmonary infection were frequent and severe. The infant died at the age of 8 months of bronchopneumonia. Dysphagia was unchanged at the time of death.

At autopsy the esophagus, heart, and large vessels of the neck were normal. Both vagus nerves were present and of normal size. No abnormality was found in the central nervous system. In the brain stem, nuclei of nerves involved in swallowing and mastication (the ambiguous nucleus, the dorsal nucleus of the vagus nerve

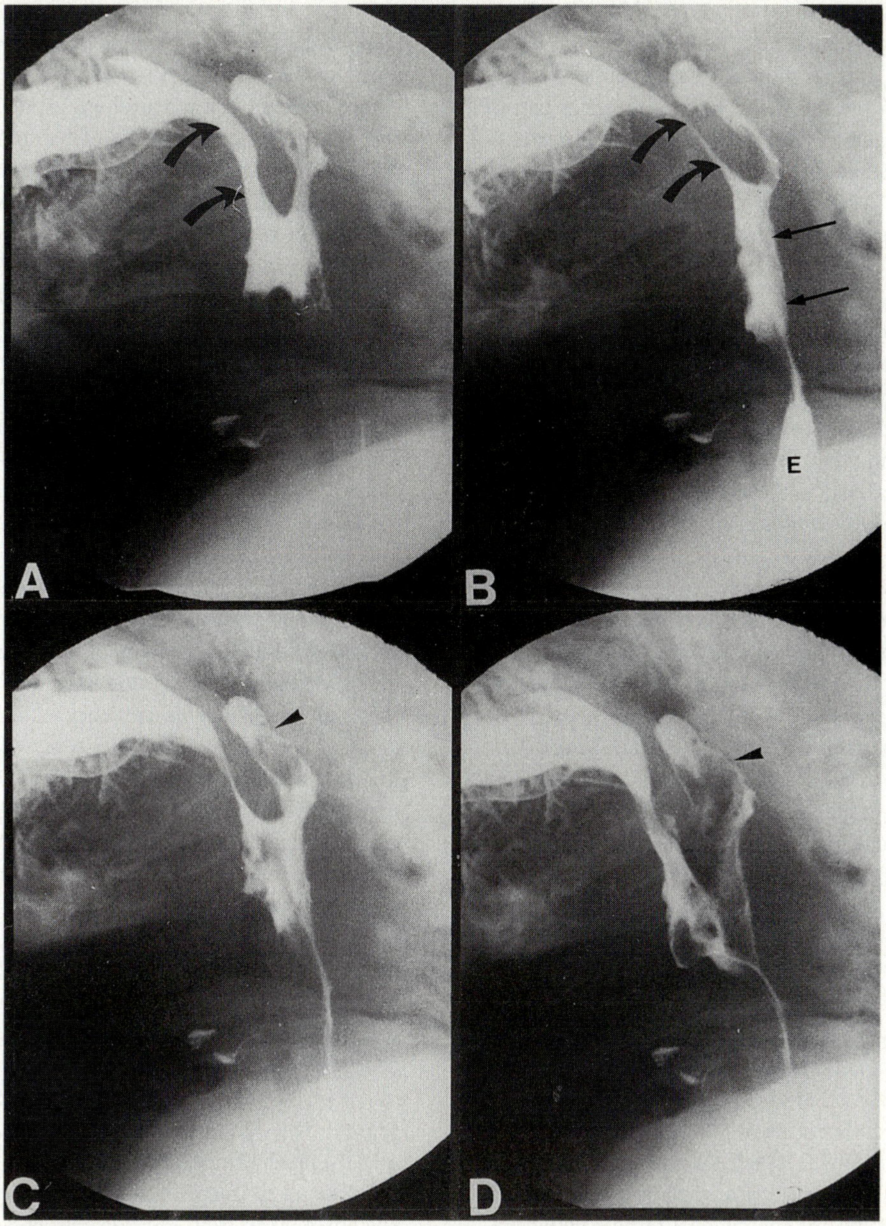

Figure. Case 1. Videoscopy of swallowing. Sequential lateral views were taken when patient was 6 months old. **A,** Propulsion of barium bolus into pharynx by normal lingual movements. Posterosuperior surface of tongue is indicated by *curved arrows*. **B,** Barium bolus fills pharynx and reaches esophagus *(E)*, but no pharyngeal contractions are present. Posterior wall of pharynx *(straight arrows)* is motionless. **C** and **D,** Persistence of pharyngeal stasis and nasal reflux *(arrowhead)*.

(cranial nerve X), the nuclei of cranial nerves V, VII, and XII), and all other cranial nerve nuclei were normal.

Case 4. A girl, born normally at term, had complete and isolated paralysis of swallowing from the time of birth. She died at the age of 4 months of tracheal aspiration. At autopsy the esophagus and neck vessels were normal. No lesions were found in the central nervous system. Serial sections of the brainstem showed no abnormality of the ambiguous nucleus or of the nuclei of the other cranial nerves involved in swallowing and mastication (nerves X, IX, VII, and V).

DISCUSSION

These four patients had a severe, isolated, and persistent congenital dysphagia related to a paralysis of the constrictor muscles of the pharynx. Very few similar cases have been reported. Benson[2] described a girl who could not swallow. The condition was present at birth and lasted for 6 months. When the patient was 3 months old, videofluoroscopy showed paralysis of the soft palate and the superior part of the pharynx. Lingual retropulsion was poor. An electromyelogram EMG of the palate was normal. Her developmental quotient was 92 at 13 months of age. During the discussion of this presentation at the Royal Society of Medicine, Macaulay said that he had observed a similar case in which tube feeding was required for 19 months.

Ardran et al.[4] described five patients with congenital dysphagia resulting from a dysfunction of the pharyngeal musculature. In three patients no other neuromuscular abnormality was present. Swallowing became possible at 6½ months, 4 years, and 5 months, respectively. Videofluoroscopy revealed paralysis of the constrictor muscle of the pharynx. Tongue movements were weak in two patients.

Bellmaine et al.[3] reported a case in a girl born at term with "pharyngeal incoordination" at birth. Dysphagia appeared to be intermittent. Motor and speech development were slow. Radiologic examination showed ineffective tongue retropulsion, and a flaccid pharynx and soft palate. The patient recovered the ability to swallow at the age of 4 years.

Illingsworth[5] described two infants with congenital "incoordination of the swallowing mechanism," one of whom died of pneumonia at the age of 9 months; the other patient achieved normal deglutition at the age of 27 weeks. A cineradiologic examination showed "incoordination of swallowing and tongue movements."

Our patients, together with the five other well-studied patients described,[2-4] demonstrate the existence of a special type of congenital dysphagia characterized by persistent paralysis of the pharyngeal muscles with minimal and inconstant involvement of the first stage of swallowing. Complete clinical recovery or considerable improvement of swallowing occur after several months or years if the life-threatening accidents inherent in this condition are prevented by rigorous symptomatic treatment and feeding by nasal or gastric tubes. Myotomy of the cricopharyngeal muscle could possibly be considered in selected cases that do not resolve spontaneously, because this surgical procedure has been successful in various disorders involving the second stage of swallowing in adults.[6]

Some discrepancy existed between the clinical and radiologic signs of pharyngeal dysfunction; the latter remained long after apparent clinical recovery in patients described by Benson[2] and Ardran et al.[4] Because of insufficient follow-up, we were not able to confirm this finding in our patients. Benson and Ardran et al. believe that one element of clinical recovery in their patients was a good recuperation of tongue movements. In our first patient, however, the oral stage of swallowing has always been practically normal.

Of the nine patients, eight were girls. All were born normally at term. Mild neonatal respiratory difficulties were noted in three infants. Dysphagia was not associated with any clinical evidence of a neurologic or muscular disorder, except for a transient paralysis of the adductors of the vocal cords in one of our patients and a mild unilateral facial palsy in another.[4] Motor retardation, clumsiness, and speech delay were noted in three patients.

These cases do not fit into any of the etiologic categories of persistent congenital dysphagia listed in the Table, and their cause remains unknown. All cases were sporadic. In our first patient the presence of hydramnios points to a prenatal origin of the disorder. No abnormality of the esophagus was detected on radiologic examination or at autopsy, and idiopathic cricopharyngeal achalasia[7, 8] could be excluded.

Congenital muscle disorders also may give rise to swallowing difficulties at birth (Table), together with other signs of a myopathy such as hypotonia, weakness, contractures, involvement of the facial and extraocular muscles, or breathing difficulties. In some patients with nemaline myopathy, dysphagia is the predominant abnormality in early infancy and indisputable evidence of a widespread muscle disorder becomes evident only somewhat later (V. Dubowitz: personal communication, 1994). Therefore a congenital myopathy cannot totally be ruled out in our two patients who died in infancy, in the absence of morphologic studies of skeletal and pharyngeal muscles. Of the seven patients who survived, three had some delay in their motor development and remained clumsy but none had muscle weakness or atrophy, arthrogryposis, or bilateral involvement of facial or external ocular muscles, and it seems highly improbable that they had a generalized muscle disorder. Nemaline rods and aberrant mitochondria have been described in biopsy specimens of the cricopharyngeal muscle obtained during myotomy in five adult patients with long-standing cricopharyngeal dysphagia and gastroesophageal reflux.[9] These findings are difficult to interpret: none of the patients had a biopsy specimen taken from skeletal muscle, and the normal ultrastructure of the pharyngeal muscles is not known. The microscopic examination of the pharyngeal muscles could also be an occasion to explore the state of the myenteric plexus, which lies at the external surface of the constrictor muscle of the pharynx,[6, 10] and which could possibly be affected in cases of congenital dysphagia.

In case 1, paresis of the vocal cords was discovered by laryngoscopy but did not cause dyspnea. In perinatal lesions of the laryngeal nerve and especially in the so-called duosyndrome of the laryngeal nerve,[11] paralysis of the adductors of the vocal cords results in severe breathing difficulties associated with more minor difficulties in swallowing.

No sign of cerebral palsy, a pseudobulbar syndrome (by involvement of the corticobulbospinal tracts), or a dystonic syndrome was present in these patients. In these conditions, only the oral phase of swallowing is affected; dysphagia is usually milder than in our cases and is not fully expressed at birth.

No evidence could be found to suggest that the oropharyngeal muscles were deprived of their motor innervation. No signs of denervation atrophy were present on the electromyogram, and the ambiguous nucleus that supplies the motor innervation of the pharynx was normal in the two patients who died in infancy. However, the caudal portion of the ambiguous nucleus is composed of irregularly arranged small cell groups that are difficult to delineate accurately.[12] Therefore a moderate numeric reduction of the neurons of this nucleus cannot be ruled out. Moreover, the simultaneous involvement of the pharynx and vocal cords in patient 1 could favor a diagnosis of dysfunction of the ambiguous nucleus, because this nucleus provides the motor innervation of both muscle groups, by way of the vagal and glossopharyngeal nerves.

In most patients with prolonged congenital dysphagia the dysfunction was not strictly limited to the pharynx and soft palate, but extended more or less to the motility of the tongue. This raises the possibility of a derangement of the supranuclear mechanisms controlling swallowing, although their anatomic structures remain largely unknown in human beings. The tendency for the disorder to improve with time is more in keeping with the progressive adaptation of a central command than with lesions of peripheral nerves or of muscles.

REFERENCES

1. Morgan J. Neuromuscular incoordination of swallowing in the newborn. J Laryngol 1956;70:295-300.
2. Benson PF. Transient dysphagia due to muscular incoordination. Proc R Soc Med 1962;55:237-8.
3. Bellmaine SP, McCredie J, Storey B. Pharyngeal incoordination from birth to three years with recurrent bronchopneumonia and ultimate recovery. Aust Paediat J 1972;8:137-9.
4. Ardran GM, Benson PF, Butler NR, Ellis HL, McKendrick T. Congenital dysphagia resulting from dysfunction of the pharyngeal musculature. Dev Med Child Neurol 1965;7:157-66.
5. Illingsworth RS. Sucking and swallowing difficulties in infancy: diagnostic problems of dysphagia. Arch Dis Child 1969;44:655-65.
6. Blakely WR, Garety EJ, Smith DE. Section of the cricopharyngeus muscle for dysphagia. Arch Surg 1968;96:745-60.
7. Farriaux JP, Walbaum R, Fovet-Poingt O. Trouble de la déglutition à début néonatal. Presse Med 1964;72:759-62.
8. Shapiro J, Haely GB. Dysphagia in infants. Otolaryngol Clin North Am 1988;21:737-41.
9. Hanna W, Henderson RD. Nemaline rods in cricopharyngeal dysphagia. Am J Clin Pathol 1980;74:186-91.
10. Mitchell GAG. The autonomic nerve supply to the throat, nose and ear. J Laryngol 1954;68:495-516.
11. Chapple CC. A duosyndrome of the laryngeal nerve. Am J Dis Child 1956;91:14-8.
12. Olszewski J, Baxter D. Cytoarchitecture of the human brain stem. Philadelphia: JB Lippincott, 1954:65.
13. Weiss MH. Dysphagia in infants and children. Otolaryngol Clin North Am 1988;21:727-35.
14. Volpe JJ. Neurology of the newborn. Philadelphia: WB Saunders, 1987:88-9.

Book review

Educational care

Levine M. Cambridge: Educators Publishing Service, 1994. 325 pages.

"This book is dedicated to innocent children whose stifled struggles to succeed have been misinterpreted." This poignant dedication introduces a unique addition to the growing body of literature designed to facilitate understanding and treatment of children with learning problems. Much of what is presented will be valuable for parents, clinicians, teachers, and certainly for children who struggle daily with atypical learning styles.

The guiding principles of this book are clearly enumerated in the first chapter. Informed observation and description are always superior to labeling and evaluating in the management of children's learning problems. Identifying and encouraging innate strengths of children with learning problems are essential not only in helping to overcome the problems but also in ameliorating pervasively low self-esteem. Although it is commonly accepted in the adult world that many different kinds of minds can function successfully, only during childhood in the educational setting is a mind expected to be reasonably adept at everything. Such an expectation discriminates against children with uneven abilities and, in the classroom, commonly causes variations to be misinterpreted as deviations.

The next six chapters of this book describe 26 commonly observable phenomena, grouped according to particular educational themes such as weak attention controls, reduced remembering, chronic misunderstanding, deficient output in language production, motor performance, and organization, delayed skill acquisition, and poor adaptation.

Chapters follow a specific format. Each begins with a description of the specific function or process involved in learning (including descriptive tables or figures), followed by a definition of and elaboration on specific variations or problems associated with function or process. I found these chapter portions to be the most difficult to understand, perhaps because much of what clinicians have been taught in the past about learning problems used constructs dissimilar from those presented in this text. Each chapter subsequently outlines collaborative suggestions for parents and for schools to help children cope with learning variations. Along with management suggestions, each chapter includes a section on demystification, which the author describes as "the process through which adults talk to children about the nature of their learning disorders and strengths." The value and power of this text emanate from these management and demystification portions.

The text includes diagrams (to help children organize information when they are reading or writing), self-assessment forms, and questionnaires (addressing ability in mathematics and writing). The concluding portions of the book offer a series of appendixes with examples of interview formats to be used with children. Included are a problem-solving format, a mathematics interview, a writing interview, a report developer, a story developer, a form to help adults understand children's reading problems, and a collaboration worksheet to help teachers, parents, and clinicians work together in planning a child's educational program. A directory of resources for parents and schools (with addresses and explanations) and an annotated list of suggested readings follow.

The last two chapters of the book discuss assessment and management of educational problems, and policy issues for schools and communities in addressing learning problems. The author argues that a good assessment is a form of treatment and that after such an assessment "children and their parents should feel uplifted, energized, and more optimistic about the future." When as a clinician did you last feel these emotions after reviewing standard educational testing of a patient? Helpful suggestions are offered for use in discussing with the child the assessment results (once again providing demystification for the child). Resistance and denial of parents, children, and school officials in addressing educational concerns are described. The use of medication is outlined in a helpful table.

The final chapter addresses the need to change public attitudes regarding children's educational issues. According to the author, multiple pathways need to be created to encourage successful learning in childhood, schools need to be attuned to neurodevelopmental diversity, and parents, clinicians, and children need to achieve a new understanding of dissimilar learning styles. The author includes a footnote on a national project called "Schools Attuned." This project provides curriculum materials and educational videotapes to help teachers become more responsive to learning diversity.

This book works best as a resource manual. Attempting to master all the concepts offered will be overwhelming. However, assimilating information in the introductory and closing chapters will be essential to understand the author's philosophy and to effectively use information in other parts of the book. In a subsequent edition, it would be helpful for the author to offer a specific case example and to demonstrate how this book can be used to address the issues presented in the example. This book will be especially valuable if readers can pinpoint a symptom or learning dysfunction and locate it in the index or table of contents. Parents with limited education will need assistance in using this book.

Educational Care presents at least three challenges: to clinicians to rethink attitudes regarding assessing and treating children with learning variations; to schools to develop multidisciplinary teams to adapt educational curricula without unnecessary labeling of children; and to clinicians, schools, and communities to establish adequate funding. Despite these challenges, this book represents a fascinating and essential resource for all who are dedicated to ensuring that children with school-related issues can strive to become successful, responsible, and self-assured adults.

Greg E. Prazar, MD
Exeter Pediatric Associates
Exeter, NH 03833

EDITOR'S COLUMN

Prevention of recurrent febrile seizures

Disorders of high prevalence but low morbidity rates, such as febrile seizures, are rich sources of controversy. Four percent of children will have a first febrile seizure, and 30% to 40% will have at least one recurrence.[1, 2] There is nearly universal agreement that the vast majority of febrile seizures cause no physical harm to the child. The most impressive evidence has come from the National Collaborative Perinatal Project.[3] This prospective cohort study identified 431 sibling pairs who were discordant for febrile seizures. When they were assessed at age 7 years, there was no difference in intelligence or academic achievement. On the other hand, most parents are extremely upset by what they perceive as a near-death event for their child.[4] To date, studies of the risks and benefits of medical treatment designed to prevent recurrent febrile seizures have failed to address the effect of these treatments on parental anxiety.

We suspect that the most common medical treatment aimed at reducing febrile seizure recurrences is the use of antipyretic agents. The essential precursor of a febrile seizure is fever, usually a high fever. Therefore physicians have intuitively concluded that antipyretic measures should prevent recurrences, but there is abundant evidence to the contrary. Because sponging febrile children with cool water is ineffective for fever reduction, the use of acetylsalicylic acid or acetaminophen is the only logical potential intervention.[5] The recurrence rate in the first year after a first ''simple'' febrile seizure was 25% in a group of children receiving intensive antipyretic instruction and placebo.[6] In a British study of 89 children with a febrile seizure, half had received an appropriate dose of antipyretics within an hour of a febrile seizure.[7] In this issue of THE JOURNAL, Uhari et al.[8] report a randomized trial of alternating acetaminophen versus placebo during subsequent illnesses, for Finnish children who had had a first febrile seizure. The authors observed no reduction in recurrences with acetaminophen. Acetaminophen was prescribed as 10 mg/kg per dose, a reasonable though not enormous dose.[9] From this study we also learn that after a first febrile seizure the risk of a recurrence appears to be 5.6% to 11.1% per febrile illness. Intuition is therefore misguided, and there is no evidence that the usual methods of fever control have any effect on recurrences of febrile seizures. For physicians to continue to recommend meticulous documentation of fever and abundant use of antipyretic agents seems destined to increase parental anxiety and ''fever phobia.'' [10]

Prescription of anticonvulsant medications is the alternative approach to the prevention of recurrences. Daily administration of phenobarbital may or may not be efficacious but does appear to alter cognitive abilities and behavior frequently—a large price for the prevention of a benign disorder.[11-13] Anticonvulsant medication administered only at the time of illness might be more acceptable. Intermittent use of phenobarbital at the time of illness appears ineffective, probably because of the delay in achieving appropriate serum levels. The only placebo-controlled trials of intermittent administration of medication have been with orally administered diazepam.[8, 14, 15] Again, the meticulous Uhari study[8] showed no benefit in recurrence when orally administered diazepam, 0.2 mg/kg per dose, was given every 8 hours while the child was ''feverish.'' Furthermore, the investigators examined the combined effect of this dose of diazepam plus acetaminophen and found the combination no better than placebo. A French randomized study of 185 patients treated with orally administered diazepam at the time of illness also found the drug to be ineffective[14]; the dose was 0.5 mg/kg as an initial dose, and then 0.2 mg/kg every 12 hours if the temperature was greater than 38° C. The authors concluded that the failure was related to the difficulties of early recognition of fever and the logistics of administering medication intermittently to children with multiple caretakers, asopposed to the ineffectiveness of orally administered diazepam. Some investigators have noted that febrile seizures may be the initial manifestation of fever, an observation that predicts some failures for all intermittent regimens.[16]

See related article, p. 991.

A randomized, placebo-controlled American study of 406 children with febrile seizures found intermittent oral administration of diazepam at a dosage of 0.33 mg/kg per dose to reduce the incidence of recurrent febrile seizures ''significantly.''[15] On the basis of an intention-to-treat survival curve analysis, the percentage of children with at least one recurrence who received diazepam was 23% compared

Reprint requests: Peter Camfield, MD, FRCP(C), IWK Children's Hospital, Box 3070, Halifax, Nova Scotia B3J 3G9, Canada.
THE JOURNAL OF PEDIATRICS 1995;126:929-30

0022-3476/95/$3.00 + 0 **9/21/64615**

with 31% of those given placebo ($p = 0.064$). This represents a rather modest reduction in the risk of recurrence of 26%.

The way that results are presented may influence the perception of utility of a treatment.[17-19] An alternative and perhaps more practical technique is to calculate the number of patients requiring treatment for one successful outcome.[17-19] Using the data from the U.S. study, one can calculate that 12 children would have to be treated with intermittent oral administration of diazepam to prevent a single recurrent febrile seizure. In addition, the use of intermittent diazepam could be viewed as self-defeating because 40% of the children treated with a 0.33 mg/kg dose had "moderately severe" side effects, including somnolence and ataxia. Although these side effects were apparently eliminated by dose reduction, we now know that a lower dose, 0.2 mg/kg, is ineffective.[8]

We conclude that physicians must counsel parents that currently available oral intermittent medication regimens (diazepam or acetaminophen or both) will not prevent recurrent febrile seizures in most children. Antipyretic agents may be useful in making a febrile child more comfortable, but this is the only benefit in relation to febrile seizures. Our efforts should focus on strategies to reduce parental anxiety about this benign disorder, rather than offering children ineffective medication.

Peter R. Camfield, MD, FRCP(C)
Carol S. Camfield, MD, FRCP(C)
Kevin Gordon, MD, FRCP(C)
Joseph M. Dooley, MB, FRCP(C)
Department of Pediatrics, Division of Neurology
Isaak Walton Killam Children's Hospital
and Dalhousie University
Halifax, Nova Scotia B3J 3G9, Canada

REFERENCES

1. Nelson K, Ellenberg J. Prognosis in children with febrile seizures. Pediatrics 1978;61:720-7.
2. Annegers JF, Hauser WA, Shirto S, et al. Factors prognostic of unprovoked seizures after febrile convulsions. N Engl J Med 1987;316:493-8.
3. Ellenberg JH, Nelson KB. Febrile seizures and later intellectual performance. Arch Neurol 1978;35:17-21.
4. Baumer JH, David TJ, Valentine SJ, Roberts JE, Hughes BR. Many parents think their child is dying when having a first febrile convulsion. Dev Med Child Neurol 1981;23:462-4.
5. Newman J. Evaluation of sponging to reduce body temperature in febrile children. Can Med Assoc J 1985;132:641-2.
6. Camfield PR, Camfield CS, Shapiro S, Cummings C. The first febrile seizure: antipyretic instruction plus either phenobarbital or placebo to prevent a recurrence. J PEDIATR 1980; 97:16-21.
7. Rutter N, Metcalfe DH. Febrile convulsions: what do parents do? BMJ 1978;2:1345-6.
8. Uhari M, Rantala H, Vainionpää, Kurttila R. Effect of acetaminophen and of low intermittent doses of diazepam on prevention of recurrences of febrile seizures. J PEDIATR 1995; 126:991-5.
9. Compendium of pharmaceuticals and specialities; Toronto: CK Productions, 1994;12:15-6.
10. Schmitt BD. Fever phobia. Am J Dis Child 1980;134:176-81.
11. Newton RW. Randomized controlled trials of phenobarbitone and valproate in febrile convulsions. Arch Dis Child 1988; 63:1189-92.
12. Camfield CS, Chaplin S, Doyle AB, et al. Side effects of phenobarbital in toddlers: behavioral and cognitive aspects. J PEDIATR 1979;95:361-5.
13. Farwell J, Lee YJ, Hirtz DG, Sulzbacher SI, Ellenberg JH, Nelson KB. Phenobarbital for febrile seizures: effects on intelligence and on seizure recurrence. N Engl J Med 1990; 322:364-9.
14. Autret E, Billard C, Bertrand P, Motte J, Pouplard F, Jonville AP. Double-blind randomized trial of diazepam versus placebo for prevention of recurrence of febrile seizures. J PEDIATR 1990;117:490-5.
15. Rosman NP, Colton T, Labazzo J, et al. A controlled trial of diazepam administered during febrile illnesses to prevent recurrence of febrile seizures. N Engl J Med 1993;329:79-85.
16. Wolf SM, Carr A, David DC, et al. The value of phenobarbital in the child who has had a single febrile seizure: a controlled prospective study. Pediatrics 1977;59:378-85.
17. Naylor CD, Chen E, Strauss B. Measured enthusiasm: does the method of reporting trial results alter perceptions of therapeutic effectiveness? Ann Intern Med 1992;117:916-21.
18. Forrow L, Taylor WC. Absolutely relative: how research results are summarized can affect treatment decisions. Am J Med 1992;92:121-4.
19. Sackett DL, Cook RJ. Understanding clinical trials. BMJ 1994;309:755-6.

Comparison of an optical immunoassay technique with two culture methods for the detection of group A streptococci in a pediatric office

Oliver F. Roddey, Jr., MD, Herbert W. Clegg, MD, Edward S. Martin, MD, Raymond L. Swetenburg, MD, and Elizabeth W. Koonce, MD

In private practice, Charlotte, North Carolina

For detecting group A β-hemolytic streptococci in an office setting, an optical immunoassay method was compared with two culture methods. The sensitivity and specificity of OIA as compared with 5% sheep blood agar cultures were 91.4% and 95.6%, and as compared with a Todd-Hewitt broth method were 90.4% and 94.1%, respectively. (J PEDIATR 1995;126:931-3)

A new method for the rapid detection of group A β-hemolytic streptococci from throat swabs has been developed and is being marketed as Strep A OIA test (Biostar Inc., Boulder, Colo.). The principle of this optical immunoassay is that the reflection of light changes when an antigen binds to antibody on a reflecting surface, and this can be directly visualized. The OIA test has been found to be sensitive in hospital laboratories,[1-4] but studies have not been reported from pediatric offices. The present study, from our five-physician pediatric office, compares both the OIA test and a standard throat culture method with each other and with an enhanced THB method.

METHODS

In a private pediatric practice, 301 patients with acute pharyngitis who had not used antibiotics during the preceding week were enrolled between November 1993 and March 1994. Throat cultures were taken by simultaneously rubbing two dry, sterile, rayon-tipped swabs (Culturette II Collection and Transport System, Becton Dickinson Microbiology Systems, Cockeysville, Md.) over both tonsillar areas. The first swab was inserted into a dry, sterile paper packet and left at room temperature for 2 to 6 hours. A medical office assistant then inoculated it onto a sheep blood agar plate (TSA II, 5% sheep blood; BBL Microbiology Systems, Cockeysville, Md.) with standard technique. Six to eight stabs were made into the agar, and a bacitracin disk was applied at the junction of the primary and secondary streaks. The swab was then used by the same person to perform and interpret the OIA test according to the manufacturer's recommendations. Test results were recorded as negative or positive (1+ to 4+, depending on the degree of gray to blue hue that developed).

See related article, p. 933.

CFU	Colony-forming units
GAS	Group A β-hemolytic streptococci
OIA	Optical immunoassay [test]
SBA	5% Sheep blood agar
THB	Todd-Hewitt broth

The culture plates were incubated overnight aerobically at 35° C and read the next day by one of the physicians (O. F. R. or H. W. C.). All plates were also reread in a masked fashion by a registered, hospital-based microbiologist. Cultures that were negative for β-hemolysis the first day were reincubated and reinterpreted the next day. If isolated colonies suggestive of β-hemolytic streptococci were present either on the original plate or after subculturing, these were serologically grouped by the microbiologist (BBL Strep Grouping Kit).

Supported by a grant from the Research in Pediatrics Practice Fund of the American Academy of Pediatrics. Biostar Inc. furnished the Strep A OIA devices and the training of our personnel through Patty L. Childers of their staff. BBL Microbiological Systems supplied the blood agar plates and Strep Grouping Kits.

Submitted for publication Sept. 20, 1994; accepted Nov. 28, 1994.

Reprint requests: Oliver F. Roddey, Jr., MD, Eastover Pediatrics, 2711 Randolph Rd., Suite 501, Charlotte, NC 28207.

0022-3476/95/$3.00 + 0 **9/22/62354**

Table. Comparison of OIA with two culture methods for recovery of GAS

OIA	SBA result	THB result
OIA result		
Positive	107 positive, 8 negative	104 positive, 11 negative
Negative	10 positive, 176 negative	11 positive, 175 negative
Sensitivity (%; 95% CI)	91.4 (86.4-96.5)	90.4 (85.1-95.8)
Specificity (%; 95% CI)	95.6 (92.7-98.6)	94.1 (90.7-97.5)
Positive predictive value (%; 95% CI)	93.0 (88.4-97.7)	90.4 (85.1-95.8)
Negative predictive value (%; 95% CI)	94.6 (91.4-97.9)	94.1 (90.7-97.5)

CI, Confidence interval.

Immediately after the swabs were obtained, the second swab was inserted into the Culturette collection tube and the system activated by crushing the ampule of transport medium. Between 2 and 6 hours later the pledget at the interface of the swab and the transport medium was extracted and placed in THB as described.[1] The THB was incubated for 16 to 20 hours and then refrigerated for 2 to 6 hours (to arrest overgrowth of normal flora) before being inoculated onto an SBA plate. It was then incubated aerobically overnight at 35° C and examined for β-hemolytic colonies the next day.

Measurement of β-hemolytic colonies was as follows: 1+, 1 to 10 colony-forming units per plate; 2+, 11 to 50 CFU/plate; 3+, more than 50 CFU/plate but not the predominant organism; 4+, more than 50 CFU/plate and the predominant growth or pure culture.

RESULTS

Of the 301 sets of swabs processed, 122 (41%) were positive for GAS by at least one of the two culture methods. Of the 122 positive by either culture method, 116 were positive on the SBA plates, 115 in the THB, and 107 by the OIA method. Another eight were positive by OIA but negative with both culture methods. Of the eight SBA plates that were 1+, the corresponding OIA result was positive only once. For those 108 cultures which were scored as 2+ or more, OIA's sensitivity was 97% and specificity was 96%. A period of 8 to 10 minutes was required for the performance of the OIA when a single test was run.

In the Table the OIA method is compared with the SBA and THB methods, with the latter two as the standards. Of the 10 OIA false-negative results, the corresponding SBA cultures had the following scores: seven were 1+, two were 2+, and one was 3+. Of the eight OIA results read as positive when the SBA cultures were negative, seven of the OIA devices were read as 1+ and one as 2+.

When the SBA and THB methods were compared with the latter as the standard, the sensitivity was 94.8% and the specificity was 96.2%. These cultures were from different swabs and were both negative or both positive for GAS in 96.0% of the pairs.

Of the 10 patients whose cultures were positive for non–group A streptococci, those of two adolescents who were strongly suspected clinically of having streptococcal illness were scored 4+. All 10 patients with non–group A streptococci had negative OIA results.

DISCUSSION

Although only one of the eight SBA cultures with a 1+ score was detected by the OIA method, more results might have been positive had the swabs been used for the OIA before rather than after having been rolled over the SBA plates in the inoculation process. For those 108 SBA cultures with more than 10 CFU/plate, the OIA was extremely sensitive and specific. Moreover, its specificity might be higher, because any culture that was positive for GAS was considered a true positive, whereas an OIA-positive but culture-negative specimen was considered to be a false-positive OIA result.

Among rapid antigen detection methods, the advantages of the OIA test are that (1) the color change is permanent, thus allowing the results to be checked by different examiners, and (2) should there be an error or an equivocal test, there is sufficient test solution for a repeated test to be done without obtaining an additional swab. Disadvantages are that (1) the test takes longer than others to perform and (2) because more steps are involved, the initial training period can be more complicated than for some others.

General drawbacks to the use of antigen detection for GAS as opposed to culture methods include the following: (1) they are more expensive; (2) more personnel time is required; (3) the waiting time for results increases crowding of the office with patients, usually at the busiest times of the day; and (4) methods specific for group A streptococcal antigen fail to detect the occasional patient with non–group A streptococcal illness who might benefit from antibiotic treatment.[5,6]

Our standard method of aerobic incubation of SBA plates after the swabs are allowed to dry before inoculation was found to be sensitive as compared with both the OIA and THB methods. A possible explanation for our better results with aerobic incubation than those which others have reported in recent years[1, 7, 8] is our allowing the swabs to dry for 2 to 6 hours rather than holding them in transport medium before inoculation of the plates. Drying of the swabs promotes better growth of GAS on the plates because the more fragile normal flora, which may be inhibitory to GAS, survive less well on dried swabs.[9, 10] In our office, where sample antibiotics can be given until the next day when indicated, and where follow-up by telephone is usually easily accomplished, the SBA method is preferable for the majority of our patients. When a more prompt result is needed, such as with a severely ill or vomiting child who may need parenteral therapy, the OIA test is adequately sensitive and specific. However, in our study approximately 9% of cultures positive for GAS and a few strongly positive ones for non–group A streptococci would have been missed by the OIA; we believe that a throat culture should be processed in the case of a negative OIA result.

The microbiologists involved in the study were Virginia Monigold, BS, MT(ASCP), and Fran Reichard, BS, RM(ASM). Statistical assistance was provided by James Norton, PhD, and Cheryl Pulliam, BA.

REFERENCES

1. Harbeck RJ, Teague J, Crossen GR, Maul DM, Childers PL. Novel, rapid optical immunoassay technique for detection of group A streptococci from pharyngeal specimens: comparison with standard culture methods. J Clin Microbiol 1993;31:839-44.
2. Daly JA, Korgensk EK, Munson AC, Llausas-Magana E. Optical immunoassay for streptococcal pharyngitis: evaluation of accuracy with routine and mucoid strains associated with acute rheumatic fever outbreak in the intermountain area of the United States. J Clin Microbiol 1994;32:531-2.
3. Della-Latta P, Whittier S, Hosmer M, Agre F. Rapid detection of group A streptococcal pharyngitis in a pediatric population with optical immunoassay. Pediatr Infect Dis J 1994; 13:742-3.
4. Dale JC, Vetter EA, Contezac JM, Iverson LK, Wollan PC, Cockerill FR. Evaluation of two rapid antigen assays, Biostar strep A OIA and Pacific Biotech CARDS O.S., and culture for detection of group A streptococci in throat swabs. J Clin Microbiol 1994;32:2698-701.
5. Gerber MA, Markowitz M. Streptococcal pharyngitis: clearing up the controversies. Contemp Pediatr 1992;118-31.
6. Miller JM, Phillips HL, Graves RK, Facklam RR. Evaluation of the Directigen group A strep test kit. J Clin Microbiol 1984; 20:846-8.
7. Wegner DL, Witte DL, Schrantz RD. Insensitivity of rapid antigen detection methods and single blood agar plate culture for diagnosing streptococcal pharyngitis. JAMA 1992;267: 695-7.
8. Kellogg JA. Suitability of throat culture procedures for detection of group A streptococci as reference standards for evaluation of streptococcal antigen detection kits. J Clin Microbiol 1990;28:165-9.
9. Breese BB. The use of cotton-tipped swabs as a simple method of transporting cultures of beta hemolytic streptococci. Pediatrics 1965;36:599-603.
10. Roddey OF, Mauney CU, Clegg HW, Martin ES, Swetenburg RL. Comparison of immediate and delayed culture methods for isolation of group A streptococci. Pediatr Infect Dis J 1989; 8:710-2.

Diagnosis of group A streptococcal pharyngitis in a private clinic: Comparative evaluation of an optical immunoassay method and culture

Stephen M. Fries, MD

From Boulder Medical Center, Boulder, Colorado

We compared the sensitivity and specificity of the Strep A Optical ImmunoAssay (OIA) method with our routine trypticase soy agar with 5% sheep blood (TSA) culture technique and with a broth-enhanced culture in the diagnosis of group A β-hemolytic streptococcal infection. Compared with broth-enhanced culture, the Strep A OIA had a sensitivity and specificity of 94.8% and 98.8%, respectively; TSA culture had a sensitivity and specificity of 92.5% and 99.4%, respectively. The Strep A OIA, which takes 10 minutes to perform, offered sensitivity and specificity equivalent to that of TSA culture in the diagnosis of group A β-hemolytic streptococcal pharyngitis. (J Pediatr 1995;126:933-6)

Supported by BioStar Inc., Boulder, Colo.
Submitted for publication Sept. 8, 1994; accepted Feb. 7, 1995.
Reprint requests: Stephen M. Fries, MD, Boulder Medical Center, 2750 Broadway, Boulder, CO 80304.

0022-3476/95/$3.00 + 0 **9/22/63975**

Rapid antigen detection tests for group A β-hemolytic streptococcus have become popular because of the short time required to obtain a result. However, rapid tests have lacked sensitivity in comparison with throat culture and thus have not been an acceptable alternative to culture when used alone.[1,2] A committee of the American Academy of Pediatrics has recommended culture confirmation, although physician practice in this area varies widely.[3] The requirement for culture backup compromises the usefulness and cost effectiveness of some rapid antigen detection tests. Thus the availability of an immediate test for GABHS that has sensitivity and specificity comparable to those of culture should be a valuable diagnostic tool. Such a test would enhance the physician's ability to avoid unnecessary antibiotic treatment and provide appropriate antibiotic treatment sooner than is possible with culture, effectively shortening the patient's period of communicability and the duration of his or her illness.

This study evaluated a new type of antigen detection test, Strep A Optical ImmunoAssay (BioStar Inc., Boulder, Colo.), in comparison with our standard trypticase soy agar with 5% sheep blood (BBL Becton Dickinson Microbiology Systems, Cockeysville, Md.) throat culture method and to a broth-enhanced culture method.

See related article, p. 931.

GABHS	Group A β-hemolytic streptococcus
OIA	Optical ImmunoAssay
THB	Todd-Hewitt broth
TSA	Trypticase soy agar with 5% sheep blood

METHODS

Study design. This study was conducted in the pediatric department at Boulder Medical Center, a multispecialty group practice in Boulder, Colo. Four physicians obtained throat swabs from pediatric patients with symptoms of pharyngitis during two periods (low-prevalence period from Aug. 21 through Sept. 30, 1992, and high-prevalence period from Nov. 12, 1992, through Jan. 20, 1993). A combined total of 505 samples were obtained, 91 during the low-prevalence period and 414 during the high-prevalence period.

Throat swab samples were collected with a single synthetic fiber swab (S/P Culturette System, Baxter Diagnostics, Deerfield, Ill.) with modified Stuart transport medium in the collection tube. Immediately after sampling, the swab was placed in the collection-transport tube. The physician who collected the samples inoculated and subsequently interpreted the TSA culture plates. After inoculation of the plates, swabs were reinserted in the transport tubes and held for Strep A OIA testing. To simplify study logistics, these samples were batched and tested with the Strep A OIA method once a day by one medical technologist (American Society of Clinical Pathologists) in the pediatric office. After the OIA this medical technologist aseptically removed the pledget from the transport tube and placed it into THB (BBL Microbiology Systems) for the broth-enhanced culture. Broths were incubated and processed by a second medical technologist. Thus results for each test method were read in blinded fashion by a different person. Each technique is briefly described.

Trypticase soy agar culture. Each swab was inoculated onto a TSA culture plate. A 0.04 U bacitracin disk (BBL, Taxo A) was applied to the initial inoculation area of the primary plate. All plates were incubated in ambient air at 35° to 37° C for 18 to 24 hours and then inspected for the presence of β-hemolytic colonies. Negative plates were held and inspected again 24 hours later. Positive plates were interpreted on the basis of inhibition of β-hemolytic growth surrounding the bacitracin disk. Colony counts were categorized as rare, few, moderate, or many, on the basis of growth in the inoculum, second, third, and fourth quadrants, respectively. For colony counts categorized as rare, the presence of fewer than 10 colonies was noted. Plates that were difficult to interpret were subcultured and evaluated after 24 hours. The medical technologist who read the broth-enhanced cultures also performed serogrouping to confirm organisms on positive plates (PathoDx Strep Grouping Kit, Diagnostic Products Corp., Los Angeles, Calif.).

Strep A OIA. After the plating step, a medical technologist used the same swab to perform the Strep A OIA, which provides visual detection of group A streptococcal antigen. The OIA kit comprises a gold silicon wafer to which a thin film optical coating and an anti-GABHS polyclonal rabbit antibody are attached. When a liquid sample containing GABHS antigen is placed directly on the wafer, an antigen-antibody complex is formed, resulting in increased thickness or mass, which is visually seen as a change in the color of light refracted through the optical coating from gold to purple-blue. If GABHS antigen is not present in the sample, the surface remains gold. A procedural control has been incorporated onto each test surface to validate each assay. The Strep A OIA procedure can be completed in 10 minutes and has been described in detail elsewhere.[4]

Broth-enhanced culture. To optimize recovery of GABHS organisms in the pharyngeal swabs, a broth-enhanced culture was performed with the pledget from the collection-transport tube. The pledget is a cotton plug that abuts the swab and separates the swab from the transport medium in the tube. The pledget was aseptically removed and placed in THB. The THB was incubated in ambient air at 35° to 37° C for 18 to 24 hours and then subcultured to

Table. Comparison of Strep A OIA method, TSA culture, and broth-enhanced culture results from assay of 505 pediatric throat swab samples*

A. Comparison between Strep A OIA, and broth-enhanced and TSA cultures

	Strep A OIA			
	Positive	**Negative**	**Sensitivity (%)**	**Specificity (%)**
Broth-enhanced culture			94.8	98.8
Positive	164	9		
Negative	4	328		
TSA culture			93.2	95.0
Positive	151	11		
Negative	17†	326		

B. Comparison between TSA culture and broth-enhanced culture

	TSA			
	Positive	**Negative**	**Sensitivity (%)**	**Specificity (%)**
Broth-enhanced culture			92.5	99.4
Positive	160	13		
Negative	2	330		

*Percent agreement between Strep A OIA and TSA culture was 94.5%.
†Thirteen of these samples were confirmed as positive by broth-enhanced culture for a corrected sensitivity and specificity of 93.7% and 98.8%, respectively.

a TSA agar plate. The TSA subcultures were performed exactly as the primary TSA cultures were performed on the swab. This technique has been shown to be more sensitive than conventional culturing methods[4] and has been used as an optimized control in other studies.[5, 6]

Analysis. In this analysis the broth-enhanced culture results were considered to be the standard. The sensitivity of routine TSA culture and of the Strep A OIA were calculated in comparison with broth-enhanced culture by dividing the number of broth-enhanced culture and OIA-positive (or TSA-positive) results by the total number of broth-enhanced–positive results. The specificity of each method was calculated by dividing the number of broth-enhanced culture and OIA-negative (or TSA-negative) results by the total number of broth-enhanced culture–negative results. The percentage of agreement between the Strep A OIA and TSA culture was calculated as the sum of the results that were positive and negative by both tests, divided by the total number of samples. All cultures, regardless of colony counts, were included in this analysis. Differences between the sensitivities of the test methods were evaluated with the McNemar Test.

RESULTS

Of the 505 samples processed in this study, 173 (34.3%) were positive by the broth-enhanced culture method. The Strep A OIA detected 164, and TSA culture detected 160 of these positive samples (Table). Strep A OIA sensitivity, compared with the broth-enhanced culture, was 94.8% and its specificity was 98.8%. The OIA method's sensitivity was not significantly different from that of broth-enhanced culture (McNemar factor = 3.2). The sensitivity and specificity of TSA culture compared with broth-enhanced culture were 92.5% and 99.4%, respectively. The TSA culture sensitivity was significantly lower than that of broth-enhanced culture (McNemar factor = 8.8). Compared with TSA culture, the Strep A OIA had a sensitivity and a specificity of 93.2% and 95.0%, respectively. The sensitivities of the Strep A OIA method and TSA culture were not significantly different (McNemar factor = 1.3) after correction of the TSA results. However, 13 of the 17 apparent OIA false-positive results were confirmed by broth-enhanced culture as true positives, resulting in a corrected OIA sensitivity and specificity compared with TSA culture of 93.7% and 98.8%, respectively. The percentage of agreement between TSA culture and the Strep A OIA was 94.5%.

Of 10 samples with results initially read as TSA culture–positive, and OIA- and broth-enhanced culture–negative, eight were found to be non-GABHS organisms by serogrouping. Various organisms were identified in these samples: *Staphylococcus aureus*, group G and C streptococcus, and non-GABHS. These samples were not included as TSA culture–positive in the data analysis. Of 11 samples with results read as positive by TSA culture but as negative by OIA, colony counts were categorized as rare for six samples (five with <10 colonies and one with <10 colonies on the original culture plate), few for four samples, and many for one sample (organisms in this sample were not serogrouped and thus not confirmed as GABHS).

DISCUSSION

The sensitivities of the Strep A OIA and TSA culture compared with broth-enhanced culture were equivalent (94.8% and 92.5%, respectively; McNemar factor = 1.3). The Strep A OIA sensitivity observed was similar to that obtained by Harbeck et al.[4] However, Harbeck et al. found the sensitivity of TSA compared with broth-enhanced culture to be 76.3%—much lower than in the current study. They evaluated the environment (temperature) and duration of sample transport to the laboratory and observed that these factors significantly affected the viability of organisms and thus the sensitivity of the culture; variation in these factors may have been responsible for the relatively low sensitivity for TSA culture in that study.

In this study a single swab was used for both the TSA culture and the Strep A OIA. Five samples were encountered with low colony counts that were TSA and broth-enhanced culture positive but OIA negative. As a result of the single-swab technique, the presence of antigen at a level less than the assay's limit of detection may have been due to the deposition of available organisms on the culture plate and the pledget before the OIA. The observed Strep A OIA false-positive results may be attributed to the presence of GABHS antigen in the absence of viable organisms. Up to 12% of children with pharyngitis are seen by their physicians after having received some antibiotic therapy, which may reduce the viability of collected organisms[7]; we did not include an assessment of antibiotic use before testing.

The results of this study suggest that the Strep A OIA method has a sensitivity and specificity equivalent to those of routine culture as practiced at this study site. In addition, we found that this test was easy to use and to read. By providing an immediate and accurate diagnosis while the patient is still in the physician's office, the Strep A OIA may simplify the physician's approach to the treatment of patients with pharyngitis. Potential therapeutic and cost-related benefits include avoidance of inappropriate antibiotic therapy and provision of appropriate antibiotic treatment sooner than possible with culture, effectively shortening the patient's period of communicability and duration of illness.

I thank Mary Ann Becker, Ginger Fedak, Gretchen Crossen, and the staff of the Boulder Medical Center pediatrics and research departments for their assistance with this study.

REFERENCES

1. Facklam RR. Specificity studies of kits for detection of group A streptococci directly from throat swabs. J Clin Microbiol 1987;25:504-8.
2. Wegner DL, Witte DL, Schrantz RD. Insensitivity of rapid antigen detection methods and single blood agar plate culture for diagnosing streptococcal pharyngitis. JAMA 1992;267: 695-7.
3. Redd SC, Facklam RR, Collin S, Cohen ML. Rapid group A streptococcal antigen detection kit: effect on antimicrobial therapy for acute pharyngitis. Pediatrics 1988;82:576-81.
4. Harbeck RJ, Teague J, Crossen GR, Maul DM, Childers PL. Novel, rapid optical immunoassay technique for detection of group A streptococci from pharyngeal specimens: comparison with standard culture methods. J Clin Microbiol 1993;31:839-44.
5. Della-Latta P, Whittier S, Hosmer M, Agre F. Rapid detection of group A streptococcal pharyngitis in a pediatric population with optical immunoassay. Pediatr Infect Dis J 1994; 13:742-3.
6. Daly JA, Korgenski EK, Munson AC, Llausas-Magana E. Optical immunoassay for streptococcal pharyngitis: evaluation of accuracy with routine and mucoid strains associated with acute rheumatic fever outbreak in the intermountain area of the United States. J Clin Microbiol 1994;32:531-2.
7. Cunningham DG, Malliswari C, O'Keefe P, et al. Unprescribed use of antibiotics in common childhood infections. J PEDIATR 1983;103:747-9.

Relationship between parental occupation and children's oropharyngeal colonization with *Neisseria meningitidis*

W. James King, MD, FRCP(C), Noni E. MacDonald, MD, FRCP(C), George Wells, PhD, Doug Manion, MD, FRCP(C), Frank Chan, MSc, and Upton D. Allen, MD, FRCP(C)

From the Department of Pediatrics, Children's Hospital of Eastern Ontario, University of Ottawa, and the Clinical Epidemiology Unit, Ottawa Civic Hospital, Ottawa, Ontario, Canada

We explored, during an outbreak of meningococcal disease, whether children of parents with workplace exposure to children were at increased risk of oropharyngeal colonization with *Neisseria meningitidis*. In comparison with children of parents without workplace exposure to children, the risk of colonization was not increased (odds ratio = 1.62; 95% confidence interval, 0.56 to 4.72). Therefore a parent's occupation does not appear to increase the risk of their children's colonization with *N. meningitidis*. (J PEDIATR 1995;126:937-9)

An outbreak of invasive group C meningococcal disease among adolescents in our community was associated with considerable anxiety regarding the risk of disease acquisition.[1, 2] A frequently asked question was whether parents with occupational exposure to children were at increased risk of bringing this organism home to their own children. This was of particular concern to health care workers and schoolteachers in the community. Although previous carriage studies have shown that age, crowded sleeping arrangements, and upper respiratory tract infections influence colonization rates,[3-5] the effect of parental occupation on colonization rates has not been explored. Therefore we examined whether children whose parents had workplace exposure to children were at increased risk of oropharyngeal colonization with *Neisseria meningitidis* versus children whose parents had no WEC.

METHODS

Subjects. This cross-sectional study, nested within a meningococcal vaccine trial, was conducted in January 1992 during a public health mass vaccination campaign in eastern Ontario and western Quebec, Canada; 1922 healthy children, 6 months to 19 years of age, were recruited through newspaper advertisement or through referral by their primary care physician, and were examined at the Children's Hospital of Eastern Ontario. A questionnaire regarding demographic information (numbers of adults and children in the household, adult WEC, sleeping arrangements, smoking history, and attendance at day care, school, or college) was completed. Parents were grouped by occupation involving WEC or no WEC. The WEC parent group was then further partitioned into health care workers, schoolteachers, day-care workers, and other occupations with exposure to children (e.g., school bus drivers, school janitors, clerical staff in pediatric hospitals or schools).

CI	Confidence interval
OR	Odds ratio
WEC	Workplace exposure to children

Protocol. Subjects had throat swabs (deep sweep of tonsillar and posterior pharyngeal region) taken with Starswab rayon-tipped swabs and transported in modified Stuart medium (Starplex Scientific, Etobicoke, Ontario, Canada). Specimens were kept at room temperature to optimize recovery of *N. meningitidis*. A modified Thayer-Martin agar plate (PML Microbiologicals, Mississauga, Ontario, Canada) was incubated in 5% carbon dioxide and examined after 2 and 3 days for the presence of *N. meningitidis*. With standard microbiologic procedures,[6] *N. meningitidis* was identified by oxidase carbohydrate utilization and *o*-nitrophenyl β-D-galactopyranoside tests. All *N. meningitidis* isolates were also identified by the Vitek system (BioMérieux, St. Laurent, Quebec, Canada) and forwarded to the Bureau

Presented at a meeting of the Society for Pediatric Research, Washington, D.C., May 1993.

Submitted for publication Sept. 6, 1994; accepted Dec. 20, 1994.

Reprint requests: W. James King, MD, FRCPC, Ambulatory Care, Department of Pediatrics, Children's Hospital of Eastern Ontario, 401 Smyth Rd., Ottawa, Ontario, Canada K1H 8L1.

0022-3476/95/$3.00 + 0 **9/22/62887**

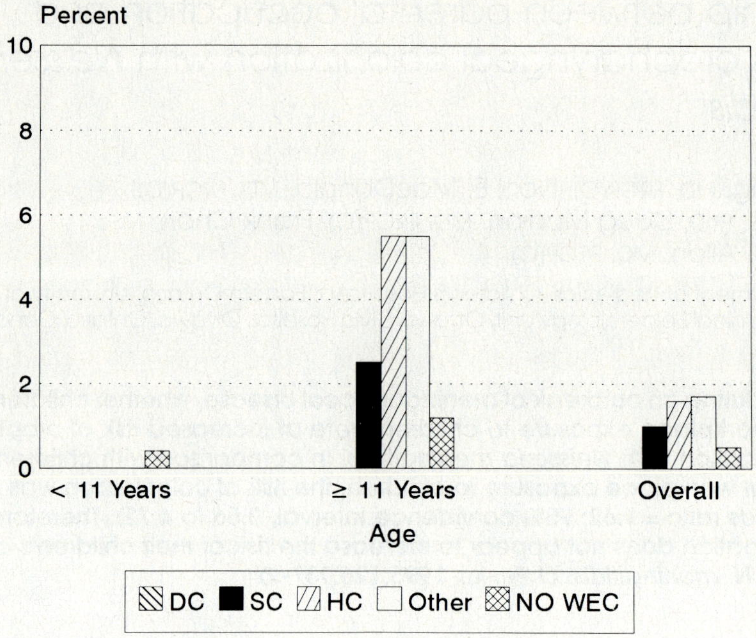

Figure. Child oropharyngeal colonization rates (expressed as percentage) for *N. meningitidis* by age and specific parental WEC: day-care *(DC)*, school *(SC)*, health care *(HC)*, and other. In WEC group no isolates of *N. meningitidis* were found in children less than 11 years old.

Table. Demographic characteristics of study groups

	WEC (n = 371)	No WEC (n = 1551)	p
Mean age (yr)	7.4	7.2	NS
Gender (% female)	51.0	52.3	NS
Family size (total No.)	4.2	4.1	NS
Children with own room (%)	75.1	69.5	<0.01*
Smoking in home (%)	30.3	37.6	<0.01*

NS, Not significant.
*Chi-square analysis.

of Microbiology, Laboratory Center for Disease Control, Ottawa, Canada, for confirmation.

Analysis. Statistical analyses were performed with Statistical Package for the Social Sciences/PC+, version 3.0 (SPSS Inc., Chicago, Ill.). Categoric variables (day-care attendance, gender, children with own room, percentage of smokers) were compared by chi-square analysis; numeric variables (age, family size) were compared by the independent *t* test. To account for different parental WEC, analysis was performed by looking at colonization rates in three groups: rates in children of parents without WEC were first compared with those in all children of parents with WEC, then with those in children who had one parent with WEC, and finally with those in children who had two parents with WEC. Oropharyngeal colonization rates for the two groups were compared by logistic regression analyses and reported as odds ratios with 95% confidence interval. Covariant adjustment was performed to control for factors found to influence oropharyngeal carriage.

RESULTS

Demographic information for the two groups is given in the Table; 1551 children (78%) had parents with no WEC and 371 (22%) had one or both parents with WEC. Among these 371 children, 59 had both parents with WEC; 34% of the parents with WEC worked in health care, 27% in schools, 8% in day-care centers, and 31% in other occupations. The Figure shows the oropharyngeal colonization rate of *N. meningitidis* by age and parental occupation. No significant difference was found with respect to *N. meningitidis* carriage within each parental WEC category.

Two factors were found independently to influence colonization rate: age and number of children sleeping in the same room (p <0.05). For the parental WEC group, logistic regression with covariant adjustment to control for these factors did not demonstrate a significant risk of *N. meningitidis* colonization, regardless of exposure risk (OR = 1.62; 95% Cl; 0.56 to 4.72).

DISCUSSION

This study of almost 2000 healthy children without respiratory symptoms explored whether parental occupation influenced the children's risk of being colonized with *N. meningitidis* during an outbreak of meningococcal disease. Previous reports had suggested that parents may be the initial source for colonization for their children,[7, 8] and the concern expressed by health care workers and schoolteachers about bringing this organism home was understandable. However, even when age and crowded sleeping conditions were taken into account, we did not demonstrate an increased risk of *N. meningitidis* colonization for children of parents with WEC, even if both parents had WEC.

Several factors may have influenced the ability of this study to demonstrate a significant difference in colonization rates between the groups. The first is the low carriage rate that we observed for *N. meningitidis* (1.1%; 95% Cl; 0.9% to 1.3%). During previous community-based disease outbreaks the population carriage rate for *N. meningitidis* has varied from 1% to 10%.[9, 12] The large number of study participants is supportive that our study cohort is representative of the *N. meningitidis* oropharyngeal carriage in our community at the time of the study. On the basis of an observed carriage rate of 1% in the no-WEC group, the power of this study to detect an increase in the *N. meningitidis* carriage rate to 5% in the WEC group was 95% ($\alpha = 0.05$). Thus it is unlikely that a true difference exists between the two groups that we were unable to demonstrate in this study, even when a conservative estimate of increased risk (5%) is used. Finally, because this was a cross-sectional survey, trends in organism acquisition in time cannot be taken into account. However, this study occurred during a regional outbreak of meningococcal disease, when one would assume that the risk for *N. meningitidis* acquisition, was increased.

We conclude that during an outbreak of meningococcal disease among children, parents who have WEC can be reassured that their occupation does not appear to increase the risk of their own children being colonized with *N. meningitidis*.

REFERENCES

1. Gemmill I. An outbreak of meningococcal disease in Ottawa-Carleton December 1991-February 1992. Can J Public Health 1992;83:134-7.
2. Manion I, Davidson S, Harrison M, King J, MacDonald N. Knowledge, psychosocial impact and health behaviours during an outbreak of meningococcal disease [Abstract]. Clin Invest Med 1993;16:A36.
3. Gold R, Goldschneider I, Lepow ML, Draper TF, Randolph M. Carriage of *Neisseria meningitidis* and *Neisseria lactamica* in infants and children. J Infect Dis 1978;137:112-21.
4. Olcen P, Kjellander J, Danielsson D, Lindquist BL. Culture diagnosis of meningococcal carriers. J Clin Pathol 1979;32:1222-5.
5. Moore P, Hierholzer J, DeWitt W, et al. Respiratory viruses and mycoplasma as cofactors for epidemic group A meningococcal meningitis. JAMA 1990;26:1271-5.
6. Balows A, Hausler WJ Jr, Hermann KJ, Isenberg HD, Shadomy HJ, eds. Manual of clinical microbiology. 5th ed. Washington, DC: American Society for Microbiology, 1991.
7. Greenfield S, Feldman HA. Familial carriers and meningococcal meningitis. N Engl J Med 1967;277:497-502.
8. Olsen S, Djurhuus B, Rasmussen K, et al. Pharyngeal carriage of *Neisseria meningitidis* and *Neisseria lactamica* in households with infants within areas with high and low incidences of meningococcal disease. Epidemiol Infect 1991;106:445-57.
9. LeSaux N, Ashton F, Rahman M, et al. Carriage of *Neisseria* species in communities with different rates of meningococcal disease. Can J Infect Dis 1992;3:60-4.
10. Greenfield S, Sheehe PR, Feldman HA. Meningococcal carriage in a population of "normal" families. J Infect Dis 1971;123:67-73.
11. Marks MI, Frasch CE, Shapera RM. Meningococcal colonization and infection in children and their household contacts. Am J Epidemiol 1979;109:563-71.
12. Broome CV. The carrier state: *Neisseria meningitidis*. J Antimicrob Chemother 1986;18(suppl A):25-34.

Consumption of soft drinks with phosphoric acid as a risk factor for the development of hypocalcemia in children: A case-control study

Efraín Mazariegos-Ramos, MD, Fernando Guerrero-Romero, MD, Martha Rodríguez-Morán, MD, Gloria Lazcano-Burciaga, MD, Ramón Paniagua, MD, and Dante Amato, MD, DSc

From Hospital General de Zona No. 1 Durango, Mexico, and Unidad de Investigación Médica en Enfermedades Nefrológicas, Hospital de Especialidades Centro Médico Nacional Siglo XXI, Instituto Mexicano del Seguro Social, Mexico City, Mexico

A comparison of 57 cases (in children with serum calcium concentration <2.2 mmol/L) and 171 controls (in children with serum calcium level ≥2.2 mmol/L) was carried out to assess whether the intake of at least 1.5 L/wk of soft drinks containing phosphoric acid is a risk factor for the development of hypocalcemia. A significant association was found: odds ratio = 5.27; 95% confidence interval, 3.17 to 8.75; *p* <0.001. The hypothesis of a causal relationship between intake of phosphoric acid–containing soft drinks and hypocalcemia warrants further investigation. (J PEDIATR 1995;126:940-2)

Recently we described five children who consumed large amounts of soft drinks and who had hypocalcemic tetany, whose clinical and biochemical abnormalities disappeared after discontinuing consumption of soft drinks, and a case series of 43 children who drank at least 1.5 L/wk of soft drinks, 18 (42%) of whom had hypocalcemia (serum calcium, <2.1 mmol/L [≤8.7 mg/dl]).[1] From these data the hypothesis of a causal relationship between soft drink consumption and hypocalcemia was established. The potential of exogenous phosphorus loads to cause hypocalcemia has been widely recognized,[2] but soft drinks with phosphoric acid are not considered among the sources of exogenous P that may cause hypocalcemia in the standard texts of mineral metabolism.[3, 4] On the other hand, several articles address the health risks or damage that soft drink consumption may cause, including dental caries,[5] urinary lithiasis,[6] and peptic disease.[7] This study was carried out to assess the hypothesis that intake of at least 1.5 L of soft drinks with phosphoric acid per week is a risk factor for the development of hypocalcemia in children.

Submitted for publication Nov. 9, 1994; accepted Jan. 17, 1995.

Reprint requests: Dante Amato, MD, Jefatura de Servicios de Investigación Médica, Instituto Mexicano del Seguro Social, Bloque B, Unidad de Congresos, Centro Médico Nacional Siglo XXI, Av. Cuauhtémoc 330, Col. Doctores, C.P. 06720, México D.F., México.

0022-3476/95/$3.00 + 0 **9/22/63489**

METHODS

Study design. A case-control study of children was designed with a case/control ratio of 1:3. Cases were defined as a serum Ca level less than 2.2 mmol/L (8.8 mg/dl), and controls as serum Ca levels of at least 2.2 mmol/L. The study was planned to include 51 cases and 153 controls, a number 10% higher than that required to meet the following criteria: $\alpha = 0.05$; power, 80%; frequency of exposure in the cases, 43%. The protocol was approved by the research and ethics committee of the hospital. Children of either sex, 18 months to 14 years of age, were recruited from primary care facilities of the Mexican Institute of Social Security and from elementary schools belonging to the government educational system in the urban area of Durango. Children with malnutrition, chronic diseases, or a history of having received drugs or other medical treatments within the past 3 months were excluded from the study. Nutritional status was assessed only by somatometry. No paraclinical studies were done to rule out chronic diseases. Children recruited from primary-care facilities were eligible only if they had been seen for healthy-child examinations, vaccination, minor trauma, or mild upper respiratory tract infections. After we obtained informed consent of the children, their parents, and, in the case of children recruited from schools, the school authorities, a 3 ml blood sample was obtained without venous stasis from each child, to measure serum Ca, P, and albumin. For age matching, children aged 3 months more or less than the corresponding case were considered. When 51 cases were obtained, we had identified 209 potential control sub-

Table. Sex, age, number of bottles of soft drink consumed each week, and serum Ca, P, and albumin concentrations in case and control groups

	Mean ± SD (range)	
	Case	Control
Sex ratio (M/F)*	29/28	87/84
Age (mo)	67.5 ± 29.3 (18-142)	67.5 ± 29.0 (18-142)
Soft drink use (bottles/wk)†	6 ± 8 (0-21)	2 ± 3 (0-9)
Ca (mmol/L; mg/dl)	2.1 ± 0.1 (1.7-2.1); 8.3 ± 0.3 (7.0-8.7)	2.4 ± 0.1 (2.2-2.9); 9.2 ± 0.6 (8.8-11.8)
P (mmol/L; mg/dl)	1.7 ± 0.4 (1.2-3.0); 5.3 ± 1.3 (3.6-9.4)	1.6 ± 0.3 (0.7-2.6); 5.0 ± 1.0 (2.3-7.9)
Albumin (μmol/L; gm/dl)	517 ± 57 (356-620); 4.5 ± 0.5 (3.1-5.4)	528 ± 35 (414-666); 4.6 ± 0.3 (3.6-5.8)

*Values expressed as ratio, not as mean ± SD and range.
†The values shown are median (instead of mean) and inner quartile range (instead of S.D.); case is significantly different from control group (p ⟨0.001, Mann-Whitney U test).

jects. Only 119 of them fulfilled the matching criteria, so he rest of the control subjects were sought among children matched for age and sex to cases lacking controls. During this search, six more cases with hypocalcemia were identified, and appropriate controls were obtained for them. Children with a serum Ca concentration of at least 3.0 mmol/L (12.0 mg/dl) were excluded. When the matching procedure was completed, an office visit was scheduled. If a participant did not come for the scheduled visit, he or she was contacted and invited to attend, so we did not lose any participant. The objective and the hypothesis of the study were not told to the participating children or to their parents. In a masked and independent manner one of the researchers (E. M. R.) interviewed all the children and their mothers to determine the number of bottles (1 bottle = 375 ml) of soft drink with phosphoric acid (Coca-Cola or Pepsi-Cola) that they drank per week and to perform a directed short history and physical examination including measurement of height and weight. The presence of seizures or cramps was also determined. We did not have to exclude any participant in this phase of the study because of inclusion or exclusion criteria. All the interviews were done within 3 weeks of the blood sampling. Finally, 57 cases and 171 controls were included; 123 subjects were recruited from primary medical care facilities and the remaining 105 from schools.

It was also possible to follow up 17 children (from both case and control groups) who drank four or more bottles of soft drink each week, who agreed to discontinue soft drink consumption and to have repeated measurements of serum Ca, Ps, and albumin 30 days later.

Laboratory measurements. Levels of Ca, P, and albumin were measured with a clinical chemistry automatic analyzer (Ciba Corning Diagnostic Corp., Overling, Ohio) with colorimetric techniques. Serum Ca was corrected for albumin concentration with the following formula: Corrected Ca (in milligrams per deciliter) = (Total Ca [milligrams per deciliter] – Albumin [grams per deciliter]) + 5.[8]

Statistics. For calculation of odds ratio and 95% confidence interval, the consumption of four or more bottles of soft drink per week was considered as a risk factor for hypocalcemia. To assess statistical significance, a method of analysis for matched data with a 1:3 case/control ratio and a dichotomous exposure was used.[9]

The proportions of children with seizures in case and control groups were compared by the Fisher Exact Test, and proportions of children with cramps were compared by the chi-square test.

For all 228 children (including case and control groups) serum Ca levels were plotted against the number of bottles of soft drink that they consumed each week. A logarithmic transformation of the serum Ca values was done to calculate the Pearson r correlation coefficient.

Basal Ca and P levels of the 17 children who were followed up were compared with the values obtained 30 days after withdrawal of soft drink consumption with a one-tailed Student t test for paired data. Data are shown as mean ± SD. Differences were considered statistically significant if p values were 0.05 or less.

RESULTS

Comparative data for sex; age; number of bottles of soft drink consumed each week; and serum Ca, P, and albumin are shown in the Table. Of the 57 children with serum Ca levels less than 2.2 mmol/L (8.8 mg/dl), 38 (66.7%) drank more than four bottles of soft drink per week, but only 48 (28%) of the 171 children with serum Calcium levels of at least 2.2 mmol/L did so (odds ratio = 5.27; 95% confidence interval, 3.17 to 8.75; p <0.001).

Four (7%) of the 57 subjects in the case group and 1 (0.6%) of the 171 subjects in the control group had one or more episodes of seizures within the 3 months before the interview (p <0.02). Cramps were present in 13 children (23%) in the case group and in eight (5%) of the control subjects (p <0.001).

For all 228 children, including case and control subjects

in a single group, a significant negative correlation ($r = -0.41$; $p < 0.001$) between the serum Ca level and the number of bottles of soft drink consumed each week was found.

In the 17 children that were followed up, basal serum Ca levels rose from 2.17 ± 0.25 mmol/L (8.7 ± 1.0 mg/dl) to 2.35 ± 0.15 mmol/L (9.4 ± 0.6 mg/dl; $p < 0.003$) and serum P levels dropped from 1.84 ± 0.42 mmol/L (5.7 ± 1.3 mg/dl) to 1.52 ± 1.9 mmol/L (4.7 ± 0.6 mg/dl; $p < 0.002$) 30 days after soft drink intake was discontinued.

DISCUSSION

Exogenous administration of phosphate can cause hyperphosphatemia and hypocalcemia. This situation commonly develops during parenteral alimentation, oral or intravenous administration of phosphate salts, feeding of newborn infants with formula with a high P content and a low Ca/P ratio, and the use of phosphate enemas.[3, 4] Hyperphosphatemia can cause hypocalcemia by inhibiting 1α-hydroxylase, which results in diminished 1α,25-dihydroxyvitamin D_3 formation.[10] Inhibition of bone resorption[11] and precipitation of Ca-P complexes in soft tissues[12] also occur. On the other hand, hydrogen ion loads can produce metabolic acidosis, a condition that also may be a cause of hypocalcemia.[4]

Ingestion of formula with high P content is known to cause hypocalcemic seizures in infants less than 1 year of age.[2] Cow milk contains more Ca and P than does human milk; the Ca/P ratio in cow milk is 1.3:1 and that in human milk is 2.3:1. The P content of human milk is 14 mg per 100 gm.[13] The P content of Coca-Cola is 19.7 mg/dl, and that of Pepsi-Cola is 16.1 mg/dl,[14] with virtually no Ca, which facilitates P absorption.

The United States is ranked first among the countries with higher soft drink consumption. In Mexico, ranked second, the consumption of soft drinks has reached 142 L/yr per capita.[1] The soft drink consumption patterns in Mexico have not been studied, but the sales of these products in the country show a rising trend. In the United States, soft drink consumption patterns show that exposure is frequent in all age groups of the American population, including children up to 4 years of age.[15] In Mexico some mothers have substituted soft drinks for milk to feed their infants.[1] This phenomenon may be related to low educational and income levels and to the fact that in Mexico soft drink prices are three to five times lower than in the United States. As our data show, not only infants but older children of school age who consume soft drinks are at risk of hypocalcemia.

Serum Ca levels such as those described in the case in this study group may be clinically significant. In addition to tetany and seizures, hypocalcemia may cause subnormal intelligence, papilledema, cardiovascular electrophysiologic disorders eventually leading to cardiac arrest or congestive heart failure, and intestinal malabsorption.[3, 4]

The appropriate examination and treatment of a child with hypocalcemia should include monitoring of soft drinks with phosphoric acid and other dietary sources of P.

In this study the criteria supporting the hypothesis of a causal relationship between ingestion of soft drinks containing phosphoric acid and hypocalcemia—a strong relationship, a biologic gradient, a temporal relationship, and a coherent explanation—seem to be present. However, this hypothesis requires further investigation and awaits confirmation from studies with different designs and other populations.

REFERENCES

1. Mazariegos-Ramos E, Rodríguez-Morán M, Guerrero-Romero JF, Paniagua R, Amato D. Alteraciones en el metabolismo del calcio y fosfatos secundarias a la ingestión de refrescos fosforados. Bol Med Hosp Infant Mex 1995;52:5-9.
2. Mizraki A, London RD, Gribetz D. Neonatal hypocalcemia: its causes and treatment. N Engl J Med 1968;278:1163-5.
3. Carpenter TO, Key LL Jr. Disorders of the metabolism of calcium, phosphorus and other divalent ions. In: Ichikawa I, ed. Pediatric textbook of fluids and electrolytes. Baltimore: Williams & Wilkins, 1990:237-68.
4. Benabe JE, Martínez-Maldonado M. Disorders of calcium metabolism. In: Narins RG, ed. Maxwell & Kleeman's clinical disorders of fluid and electrolyte metabolism. 5th ed. New York: McGraw-Hill, 1994:1009-44.
5. Meurman JH, Frank RM. Progression and surface ultrastructure of in vitro caused erosive lesions in human and bovine enamel. Caries Res 1991;25:81-7.
6. Shuster J, Jenkins A, Logan C, et al. Soft drink consumption and urinary stone recurrence: a randomized prevention trial. J Clin Epidemiol 1992;45:911-6.
7. Holcombe C, Kaluba J, Lucas SB. Non-ulcer dyspepsia in Nigeria: a case control study. Trans R Soc Trop Med Hyg 1991; 85:553-5.
8. Garabedian M, Balsan S. Troubles du metabolisme calcique en dehors du rachitisme. In: Encyclopedie médico chirurgicale. Paris: Editions Techniques, 1979:4057A.
9. Breslow NE, Day NE. Statistical methods in cancer research; vol 1. The analysis of case-control studies. Lyon: International Agency for Research on Cancer, Scientific publication No. 32, 1980:169-74.
10. Haussler MR, McCain TA. Basic and clinical concepts related to vitamin D metabolism and action. N Engl J Med 1977; 297:974-83.
11. Raisz LG. Physiologic and pharmacologic regulation of bone resorption. N Engl J Med 1970;282:909-16.
12. Carey RW. Massive extraskeletal calcification during phosphate treatment of hypercalcemia. Arch Intern Med 1968; 122:150-5.
13. National Research Council. Recommended dietary allowances. 10th ed. Washington, D.C.: National Academy Press, 1989:184-7.
14. Massey LK, Strang MM. Soft drink consumption, phosphorus intake, and osteoporosis. J Am Diet Assoc 1982;80:581-3.
15. Morgan KJ, Stults VJ, Stampley GL. Soft drink consumption patterns of the U.S. population. J Am Diet Assoc 1985; 85:352-4.

Cerebral artery stenoses in Williams syndrome cause strokes in childhood

Paige Kaplan, MBBCh, Martin Levinson, MD, and Bernard S. Kaplan, MBBCh

From the Divisions of Genetics and Nephrology, Children's Hospital of Philadelphia and University of Pennsylvania and Sinai Hospital, Detroit, Michigan

Extensive narrowing of lumens of many cerebral arteries caused strokes with brain damage and chronic hemipareses in two children with Williams syndrome. Increased irritability, loss of consciousness, and seizures were initial signs. Arterial stenoses are not limited to the supravalvular aorta and pulmonary arteries in patients with Williams syndrome. (J Pediatr 1995;126:943-5)

The cardiovascular system is affected in 60% of patients with Williams syndrome; the most common problem is narrowing (stenosis, hypoplasia, coarctation) of the lumens of the supravalvular aorta and peripheral pulmonary arteries. Stenoses of cerebral arteries have not been considered part of the spectrum of vascular disease in Williams syndrome. We describe two patients with extensive narrowing of cerebral arteries and neurologic sequelae.

Submitted for publication Nov. 4, 1994; accepted Jan. 27, 1995.

Reprint requests: Paige Kaplan, MBBCh, Children's Hospital of Philadelphia, 34th Street and Civic Center Boulevard, Philadelphia, PA 19104-4399.

0022-3476/95/$3.00 + 0 **9/22/63716**

CASE REPORTS

Case 1. A 22-year-old woman was recognized as having Williams syndrome at age 19 years. She had had marked hypertension and congestive heart failure at 10 weeks of age. Cardiac catheterization showed peripheral pulmonic stenosis, a thickened pulmonic

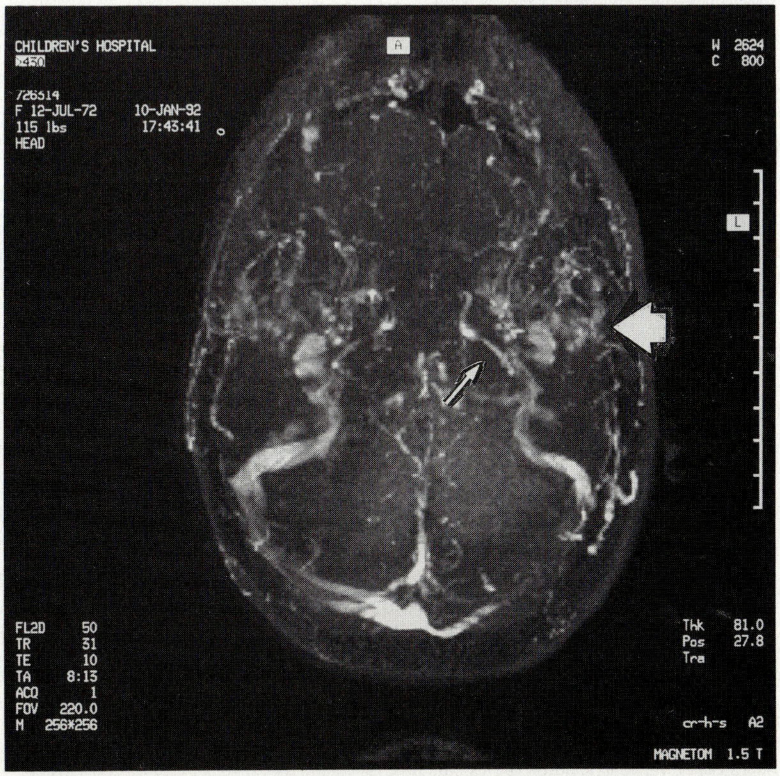

Fig. 1. Case 1. Magnetic resonance angiography of brain at 19½ years showing narrow lumens of internal carotid arteries at bifurcation into anterior and middle cerebral arteries *(small arrow)* and collateral vessels *(wide arrow)*.

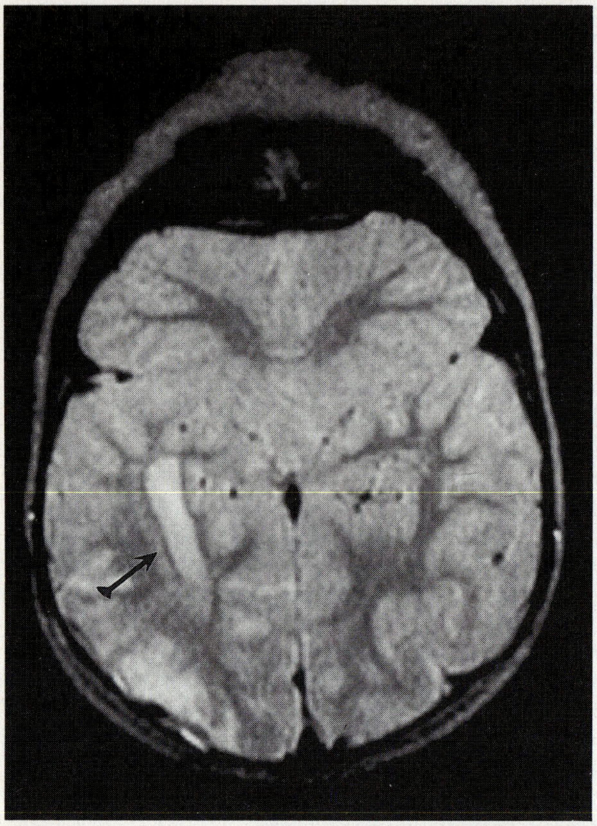

Fig. 2. Case 2. Magnetic resonance imaging of brain at 3 years showing infarction in area of left middle cerebral area *(arrow)*.

See related article, p. 945.

MRI	Magnetic resonance imaging

valve, and right-sided ventricular hypertrophy; aortic narrowing was absent. She had three episodes of cerebrovascular insufficiency: at 3 years of age she suddenly became more irritable and lost consciousness, and an acute left hemiparesis developed, with greater involvement of the upper limb than the lower. Blood pressure was 120 to 140/90 mm Hg. Cranial bruits were heard over the parietal and left carotid arteries. Arteriography showed occlusion of the right anterior and middle cerebral arteries with "abnormal blushing" in the diencephalon. Moyamoya was diagnosed. The electroencephalogram showed abnormal asymmetric intermittent interhemispheric activity. The patient was treated with acetylsalicylic acid, 7.5 mg/day. The hemiparesis resolved but recurred a few weeks later on the right side. Focal and generalized seizures developed subsequently. She lost the ability to recite the alphabet and numbers, and to recognize colors. At 6½ years of age she had another episode of hemiparesis and had residual, permanent bilateral spastic hemiparesis. At 12 years of age she had intermittent pain and discoloration in the left arm. Severe narrowing of the left subclavian artery and moderate narrowing of the origin of the left renal artery were seen with arteriography. Magnetic resonance imaging was done when she was 19½ years old because she had severe headaches and chronic hypertension (198/100 mm Hg). Magnetic resonance imaging of the brain showed old watershed infarcts in the areas supplied by the left and right anterior and middle cerebral arteries. Magnetic resonance angiography (Fig. 1) demonstrated that the internal carotid arteries had fairly normal calibers in the cavernous parts but very narrow lumens in the supraclinoid parts at the bifurcation into anterior and middle cerebral arteries. The basilar artery was narrow. Multiple small collateral vessels coursed from the external to internal circulations over the scalp, midface, skull base, and area adjacent to the incisure of the tentorium. The left vertebral artery originated from the aortic arch instead of from the subclavian artery. Magnetic resonance imaging showed normal caliber of the ascending and descending aorta. Mild dilatation of the left coronary and main pulmonary arteries was present. The peripheral pulmonary arteries had normal caliber. She has severe mental handicaps, functions at the level of an 8-year-old child, and has episodes of intense verbal and physical aggression.

Case 2. A 5-year-old boy was found in the neonatal period to have extensive, severe narrowing of the ascending and descending aorta; aortic arch; coronary, subclavian, common carotid, and pulmonary arteries; and to have a ventricular septal defect. At 25 months of age, 5 weeks after graft reconstruction of the aortic arch, he became more irritable and had a prolonged right-sided seizure. He then had right hemiparesis and loss of speech, which eventually improved after several months. Magnetic resonance imaging of the head demonstrated an acute left middle cerebral artery infarct (Fig. 2). At 34 months of age he had recurrent episodes of projectile vomiting together with headaches, irritability, and loss of consciousness, thought to be due to transient ischemia. Angiography when the patient was 40 months of age showed an abnormal, narrow common origin of the left common carotid and innominate arteries. The left middle cerebral artery was narrow, with diminished blood flow to the parietal and temporal areas. The left vertebral artery was very narrow. The entire posterior cerebral circulation was served by the right vertebral artery. Collateral vessels had developed.

DISCUSSION

Only three cases of Williams syndrome with cerebral artery narrowing, cerebrovascular insufficiency, acute decompensation, and strokes have been reported.[1-3] A 2-year-old boy, who had a viral infection, became unresponsive within 3 hours[1]; magnetic resonance angiography showed stenoses of the left common carotid artery, midcervical areas of the internal carotid arteries bilaterally, and right internal carotid and posterior cerebral arteries. Collateral vessels connected the ophthalmic artery with cerebral arteries. Another 2-year-old boy had prolonged seizures and hemiplegia and was found to have narrow cerebral arteries.[2] An 18-year-old woman, who had the same diagnoses of Williams syndrome and Moyamoya as in case 1, died suddenly of an intraventricular hemorrhage.[3] At autopsy the circle of Willis, internal carotid arteries, anterior and middle cerebral arteries, and ascending aorta were narrow. In our opinion, the vascular narrowing in this woman and in patient 1 was misclassified as Moyamoya.

The onset of clinical signs of cerebrovascular insufficiency in early childhood is ominous. The presence of collateral arteries in all the patients with cerebrovascular insufficiency suggests that the main cerebral vessels were narrow for long periods before the strokes occurred. No obvious precipitating causes of the acute decompensation were found. It is unlikely that chronic hypertension, acute infection, or thrombi or emboli precipitated the strokes. Cerebral arterial stenoses may be more prevalent in Williams syndrome than previously realized but may not be manifesting with acute cerebral infarction. For example, in the brain of a 31-year-old man who was severely retarded but without strokes or hemiplegia, intracortical patches of cell loss and gliosis were consistent with small vessel ischemia.[4] Abnormal origin of arteries is another unusual aspect of the vascular anomalies in Williams syndrome.[5]

Narrowing of the carotid, cerebral, or vertebral arteries may cause serious, chronic morbidity in early childhood and premature death. It may be the first problem demanding medical attention and must be considered in a child with Williams syndrome who suddenly becomes more irritable or has seizures with hemiparesis or severe hypertension. Conversely, the diagnosis of Williams syndrome should be considered in a child having a stroke or the manifestations described in our patients.

REFERENCES

1. Ardinger RH Jr, Goertz KK, Mattioli LF. Cerebrovascular stenoses with cerebral infarction in a child with Williams syndrome [Abstract]. Am J Med Genet 1994;51:200-2.
2. Greally JM, Soper R, Chaloupka JC, et al. Multivessel cerebral arteriopathy causing stroke in Williams syndrome [Abstract]. Am J Hum Genet 1994;55:81A.
3. Kawai M, Nishikawa T, Tanaka M, et al. An autopsied case of Williams syndrome complicated by moyamoya disease. Acta Paediatr Jpn 1993;35:63-7.
4. Galaburda AM, Wang PP, Bellugi U, Rossen ML. Cytoarchitectonic anomalies in a genetically based disorder: Williams syndrome. Neuroreport 1994;5:753-7.
5. Ottesen OE, Antia AU, Rowe RD. Peripheral vascular anomalies associated with the supravalvular aortic stenosis syndrome. Radiology 1966;86:430-5.

Ischemic stroke and intracranial multifocal cerebral arteriopathy in Williams syndrome

Robert Soper, MD, John C. Chaloupka, MD, Pierre B. Fayad, MD, John M. Greally, MB,BCh, BAO, Bennett A. Shaywitz, MD, Issam A. Awad, MD, and Barbara R. Pober, MD

From the Departments of Genetics, Diagnostic Radiology and Neurosurgery, Neurology, Pediatric Neurology, and Neurovascular Surgery, Yale University, New Haven, Connecticut

We describe an otherwise healthy 2-year-old patient with Williams syndrome who had a stroke as a result of intracranial multivessel focal and segmental stenotic disease. The diagnosis of Williams syndrome was confirmed by elastin gene deletion testing. Combined magnetic resonance imaging and magnetic resonance angiography, and transcranial Doppler flow studies, were used in diagnosing and monitoring the course of the disease. (J PEDIATR 1995;126:945-8)

Submitted for publication Nov. 7, 1994; accepted Feb. 8, 1995.

Reprint requests: Robert Soper, MD, Department of Genetics, Yale University School of Medicine, P.O. Box 208005, New Haven, CT 06520-8005.

0022-3476/95/$3.00 + 0 **9/22/64038**

Williams syndrome is a genetic disorder with manifestations including vasculopathy, originally described as supravalvular aortic stenosis[1] but now recognized to involve many areas of the arterial circulation.[2] We describe a 2-year-old boy with WS and ischemic stroke resulting from multifocal intracranial arterial stenoses without discernable premor-

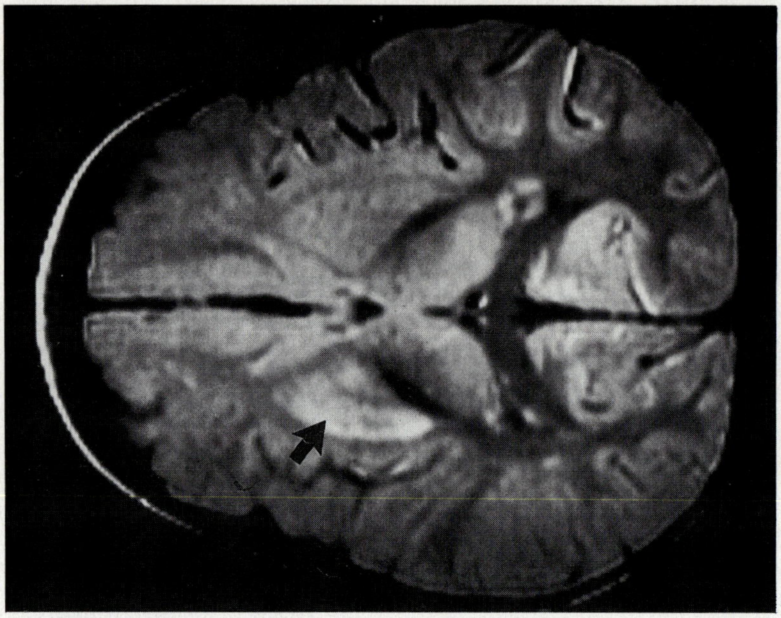

Fig. 1. Axial MRI with long repetition time and (TR) short echo time (TE) of brain shows increased signal within right putamen and globus pallidus, consistent with striatocapsular infarction *(arrow)*.

See related article, p. 943.

MRA	Magnetic resonance angiography
MRI	Magnetic resonance imaging
TCD	Transcranial Doppler
WS	Williams syndrome

bid cardiovascular abnormalities or other predisposing factors.

CASE REPORT

The patient was recognized at 1 month of age to have dysmorphic facies, mild supravalvular pulmonary stenosis, peripheral pulmonary stenosis, mild hypercalcemia, and irritability, characteristic of WS. During follow-up the pulmonary stenosis resolved, height and weight remained at less than the 3rd percentile, and developmental delays appeared. Elastin deletion testing with a fluorescently labeled cDNA elastin probe, was performed in the laboratory of Dr. Lap-Chee Tsui, Hospital for Sick Children, Toronto, Ontario, Canada, and demonstrated hemizygosity for the elastin locus at chromosome 7q11.2.

At 2½ years of age, the patient was hospitalized because of decreased speech and activity, the onset of a hemifacial droop, and drooling. Physical examination revealed a slightly irritable child; blood pressure was 110/80 mm Hg and pulse was 130 beats/min. Neurologic examination revealed a left facial droop, flattening of the left nasolabial fold, drooling, independent gait but with left-sided weakness, decreased left appendicular movements, a left visual field defect, and a left extensor plantar reflex.

Computed tomography indicated an acute infarction, prompting magnetic resonance imaging and magnetic resonance angiography of the brain. These showed abnormally high signal intensity on long repetition time and echo time sequences within the right putamen, internal capsule, head of the caudate nucleus, centrum semiovale, and the optic radiation, compatible with infarction (Fig. 1). Loss of normal flow void was seen in the right supraclinoid internal carotid artery, proximal segments of the right anterior cerebral artery, and middle cerebral artery. Cerebral angiography showed long segmental stenoses of these vessels (Fig. 2) and two focal basilar artery stenoses, consistent with partially recanalized thrombus or severely obstructive vasculopathy. Extensive pial-pial collateralization to the middle cerebral territory from the ipsilateral anterior and posterior cerebral arteries was present. The extracranial carotid and vertebral arteries, and supravalvular portion of the aortic arch, were not stenotic. A transcranial Doppler study (Medasonics, Fremont, Calif.) of the circle of Willis demonstrated abnormalities in cerebral blood velocities consistent with these findings.

Results of all routine laboratory studies were normal. Rheumatoid factor, and antinuclear and anticardiolipin antibodies were absent. Coagulation studies, including prothrombin time, partial thromboplastin time, and antithrombin III and plasminogen levels, were normal. A transthoracic echocardiogram was normal.

The patient was treated with low doses of aspirin (80 mg/day) and has slowly improved during the subsequent year. Speech and facial asymmetry have improved, he drools only when excited, and he is able to run. The patient receives physiotherapy for residual palmar

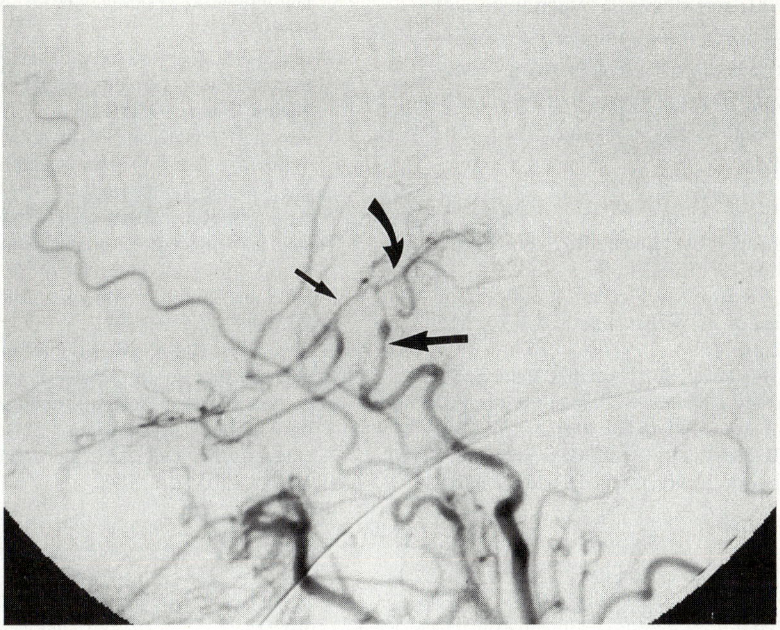

Fig. 2. Cerebral angiography from right common carotid injection, lateral projection shows long segmental stenoses of right supraclinoid internal carotid artery *(large arrow)*, right M-1 segment of middle cerebral artery *(curved arrow)*, and right A-1 *(small arrow)* segment of anterior cerebral artery.

wrist flexion and mild hip flexion contractures. Follow-up MRI at 6 and 12 months of age has shown no progression of parenchymal ischemic damage; MRA and TCD studies revealed no progression of the vasculopathy, within the limits of resolution of these techniques.

DISCUSSION

Vascular disease in WS, originally recognized as supravalvular aortic stenosis,[1] is now known to include diffuse and localized stenoses of the thoracic and abdominal aorta, and coronary and visceral arteries.[2] Vessel wall thickening has been confirmed in vivo with intravascular ultrasonography[3] and is seen at surgery or pathologic examination. The microscopic appearance, described as medial fibroelastic dysplasia,[4] shows marked medial wall thickening, hypertrophied smooth muscle cells, and variable disorganization of elastin fibers in an excessive, loose collagenous stroma. These pathologic changes are most likely caused by elastin insufficiency resulting from the deletion of one copy of the elastin gene in patients with WS.[5]

Kawai et al.[6] described an 18-year-old girl with WS who died suddenly after hemorrhagic stroke. She had cerebral moyamoya disease with severe hypoplasia of the vessels of the circle of Willis and long-segment stenosis of the ascending aorta. The authors suggested that moyamoya vessels were a secondary phenomenon, a compensatory collateral circulation in response to the restricted vascular supply in the circle of Willis. A 2-year-old child with WS had a nonhemorrhagic infarction of both middle cerebral arteries and the left posterior cerebral artery, that affected the left occipital lobe and both parietal and temporal lobes.[7] A persistently elevated erythrocyte sedimentation rate prompted corticosteroid therapy for a tentative diagnosis of vasculitis. This patient also had hypertension, supravalvular aortic stenosis, narrowing of both the ascending and descending aorta, and narrowing of the left common carotid artery in the neck, that extended to the base of the skull. We also know of ischemic stroke occurring in one other patient with WS.[8]

Our patient has had an otherwise benign medical course. Physicians caring for patients with WS should be aware that stroke may be an isolated vascular complication of this condition. The presence of new or worsening neurologic symptoms should prompt MRI to reveal the extent and sites of any intracerebral parenchymal injury, followed by angiography to demonstrate associated vasculopathy. In follow-up, disease progression can be monitored by TCD studies, which do not demand either an immobile subject or the technology necessary for satisfactory MRA.[9] MRA does, however, permit the study of arterial segments that cannot be evaluated by TCD. We consider TCD and MRA complementary techniques; further study is needed on their relative sensitivities for long-term monitoring.

Our patient differs from the two previously described patients in a number of important ways. He represents the first patient with WS and stroke who has a proved elastin gene deletion. Furthermore, he has no signs of independent risk factors such as systemic vascular stenoses, hypertension, or laboratory evidence of vasculitis or of an underlying angiogenic process (i.e., moyamoya disease). The growing recognition of WS and its complications suggests that this condition should now be included in any consideration of the causes of childhood stroke.[10]

REFERENCES

1. Williams JCP, Barratt-Boyes BG, Lowe JB. Supravalvular aortic stenosis. Circulation 1961;24:1311-8.
2. Zalzstein E, Moes CAF, Musewe NN, Freedom RM. Spectrum of cardiovascular anomalies in Williams-Beuren syndrome. Pediatr Cardiol 1991;12:219-23.
3. Rein AJJT, Preminger TJ, Perry SB, Lock JE, Sanders SP. Generalized arteriopathy in Williams syndrome: an intravascular ultrasound study. J Am Coll Cardiol 1993;21:1727-30.
4. O'Connor WN, Davis JB, Geissler R, Cottrill CM, Noonan JA, Todd EP. Supravalvular aortic stenosis: clinical and pathological observations in six patients. Arch Pathol Lab Med 1985; 109:179-85.
5. Ewart AK, Morris CA, Atkinson D, et al. Hemizygosity at the elastin locus in a developmental disorder, Williams syndrome. Nature Genet 1993;5:11-6.
6. Kawai M, Nishikawa T, Tanaka M, et al. An autopsied case of Williams syndrome complicated by moyamoya disease. Acta Paediatr Jpn 1993;35:63-7.
7. Ardinger RH, Goertz KK, Matteoli LF. Cerebrovascular stenosis with cerebral infarction in a child with Williams syndrome. Am J Med Genet 1994;51:200-2.
8. Williams Syndrome Association. Case report of strokes (Adam Berman). August 1992.
9. Fayad PB, Brass LM. Doppler ultrasonography in occlusive vascular disease. In: Awad IA, ed. Cerebrovascular occlusive disease and brain ischemia: neurosurgical topics. Parkridge, Illinois: American Association of Neurological Surgeons, 1992.
10. Natowicz M, Kelley RI. Mendelian etiologies of stroke. Ann Neurol 1987;22:175-92.

Pancreatic glucagon levels in infants and children with hyperinsulinemia

Ewa Pronicka, MD, PhD, Beata Gruszczyńska, MD, Bogdan Woźniewicz, Andrzej Cedro, MD, Wojciech Kamiński, MD, and Anna Leśniewska

From the Departments of Metabolic Diseases, Pathology, Surgery, and Nuclear Medicine, Child Health Center, Warsaw, Poland

Serum concentrations of pancreatic glucagon were measured in 40 patients with hyperinsulinemic hypoglycemia. In infants with severe disease the glucagon levels were markedly elevated; lower levels were observed in children with episodic hypoglycemia. During diazoxide treatment and after pancreatectomy, the glucagon levels decreased proportionally to suppression of the insulin secretion. Thus the secretion of glucagon seems to be retained in hyperinsulinism in proportion to the insulin hypersecretion, and an increased glucagon level indicates long duration and severity of hyperinsulinemic hypoglycemia. (J PEDIATR 1995;126:948-51)

Hypoglycemia caused by hyperinsulinism is particularly dangerous because of the possibility of brain damage resulting from the energy deficit. An elevated insulin concentration makes impossible the reduction of glucose utilization by insulin-dependent tissues and suppresses glucose release from hepatic glycogen, whereas the levels of alternative substrates such as free fatty acids and ketone bodies are low. The elevated insulin level is believed to suppress glucagon activity, resulting in a further decrease of glycogenolysis and gluconeogenesis.[1-3]

Our aim was to determine to what extent the levels of pancreatic glucagon in children with hyperinsulinemia reflect the characteristics of the condition, and the mode and efficacy of treatment.

Submitted for publication Dec. 2, 1994; accepted Jan. 27, 1995.

Reprint requests: Ewa Pronicka, MD, PhD, Department of Metabolic Diseases, Child Health Center, Al. Dzieci Polskich 20, 04-736 Warsaw, Poland.

0022-3476/95/$3.00 + 0 **9/22/63771**

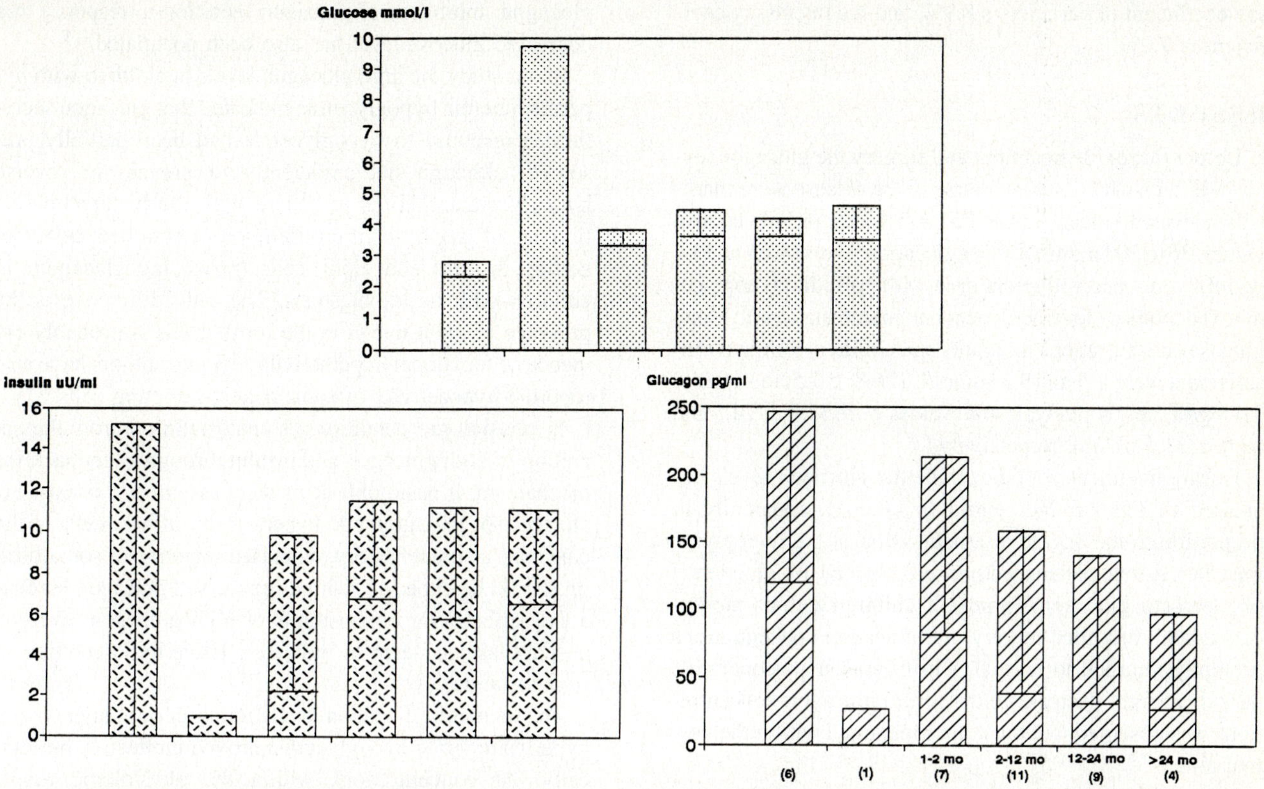

Figure. Glucose, insulin, and glucagon concentrations of patients with hyperinsulinemic hypoglycemia after pancreatectomy. Values are mean ± SD; number of measurements is shown in *parentheses*. In the *lower right panel*, the glucagon concentrations are shown after partially successful pancreatectomy *(first bar)*, in a patient with postsurgical diabetes *(second bar)*, and after fully successful pancreatectomy *(remaining four bars)*.

METHODS

Patients. Forty children with hyperinsulinemic hypoglycemia (24 boys and 16 girls, 3 weeks to 19 years of age) have been studied (details of the clinical, biochemical, and histopathologic findings are available from us on request). Spontaneous or fasting hypoketotic hypoglycemia was observed in 38 patients. In the remaining two patients, hypoglycemic manifestations were evoked by leucine.

The diagnostic tests were performed in the following order: glucose and insulin concentrations during spontaneous hypoglycemia (ratio of glucose [in milligrams per decileter] to insulin [in micro units per milliliter] ⟨3), a 24-hour glycemia profile, a test with glucagon (0.03 mg/kg) during hypoglycemia, a fasting test, an orally administered leucine load (0.15 gm/kg), and a tolbutamide test.

The treatment of hypoglycemia was in each case tailored to the needs of the particular patient. Treatment began with a special diet and additional orally administered glucose and, when necessary, 10% glucose infusions at a rate greater than 8 mg/kg per minute. Once hyperinsulinism had been diagnosed, patients with a more severe course of the disease were immediately referred for surgery; in milder cases, diet and diazoxide therapy were tried first. Of the 40 patients, 29 underwent nearly total pancreatectomy, and two had enucleation of adenomas. Eight patients needed reoperation because of persistent hypoglycemia.

A single adenoma of the pancreas was found in three patients. In the remaining patients the lesions were diffuse or dispersed except in one infant, who had lesions confined to the head. Demonstration of beta cells with giant nuclei was found to be of particular diagnostic value.

Laboratory procedures. Glucagon concentrations were measured in serum, usually at the beginning of hospitalization during spontaneous hypoglycemia or at the end of the fasting test. At the same time, glucose and insulin levels were determined. In selected patients the measurements of glucagon, insulin, and glucose after an overnight fast were carried out several times at intervals before and after the pancreatectomy. Kits manufactured by Biodata (Montecelio, Italy) were used throughout the study. The kits employ a very specific antiserum for assay of pancreatic glucagon without crossreaction with gastrointestinal compounds. The intraassay coefficient of variation is 8.9%, and the interassay coefficient is 9.0%.

RESULTS

Before diazoxide treatment and surgery the glucagon levels in infants with a severe course of the disease were markedly elevated (mean value, 351.4 ± 179.9 pg/ml; control values, 36 to 200 pg/ml). Lower glucagon levels (80.3 ± 23.1 pg/ml) were observed in children with episodic hypoglycemia (adenomas, leucine-dependent manifestations). Mean glucose concentrations in infants and children with hyperinsulinemia were 1.5 and 1.1 mmol/L (26.8 ± 7.5 and 19.0 ± 9.4 mg/dl), respectively; insulin values were 34.8 ± 24.5 and 88.0 ± 31.5 μU/ml, respectively.

During treatment with diazoxide the glucagon levels decreased to 111.1 ± 26.2 pg/ml ($p < 0.001$), apparently in proportion to the degree of amelioration of the hypoglycemia. Nearly total pancreatectomy did not lead to a deficiency of pancreatic glucagon (Figure). In children with normoglycemia achieved after surgery, the glucagon concentrations promptly returned to normal. During longer postoperative periods a slight decrease in the serum glucagon concentrations was observed, but the values remained within the normal range.

In the patients whose pancreatectomy was not fully successful, who required diazoxide postoperatively for persistent hypoglycemia, the serum glucagon levels were higher than those found in normoglycemic patients.

Postpancreatectomy hypoglucagonemia was observed in only one patient with postoperative diabetes.

DISCUSSION

There are few data on serum pancreatic glucagon concentrations in children with hyperinsulinemic hypoglycemia. Single reports have mentioned normal or slightly increased glucagon values.[3-6] On the other hand, the test with exogenous glucagon has been generally recognized as a valuable diagnostic tool.[7,8]

During acute hypoglycemia, glucagon is the most important counterregulatory hormone. The threshold for glucagon secretion has been estimated as a decrease of glucose concentration to about 3.6 mmol/L (65 mg/dl).[2] Initially glucagon mainly stimulates glycogenolysis; gluconeogenesis becomes more important subsequently. Glucagon also increases lipolysis and ketogenesis and has a feedback stimulation effect on insulin secretion.[1,9]

During prolonged hypoglycemia the biologic effectiveness of glucagon is reduced. Glucose production may be decreased substantially even though the glucagon concentration remains raised. There is evidence that an elevated insulin concentration may suppress the biologic effects of glucagon. Inhibition of glucagon secretion in response to a decreased glucose level has also been postulated.[1,9]

In our study the high glucagon levels in children with hyperinsulinemic hypoglycemia indicated that glucagon secretion in response to hypoglycemia had been partially preserved, although not sufficiently to prevent or reverse hypoglycemia. This is in accord with the histopathologic findings of proportional proliferation of both beta cells (secreting insulin) and alpha cells (producing glucagon) in children with nesidioblastosis. The only difference is the presence of giant nuclei in the former; this is probably evidence of functional hyperactivity.[10] Some authors have also reported hypoactivity of somatostatin-secreting cells.[5,6]

In physiologic conditions, somatostatin controls the secretion of both glucagon and insulin through a feedbacklike mechanism. If nesidioblastosis were assumed to consist exclusively of the automatic hyperactivity of beta cells of the pancreas, a compensatory, increased secretion of somatostatin should be expected, with a suppressed glucagon level as a side effect. Our observations of high glucagon levels in nesidioblastosis seem to indicate relative hyposecretion of somatostatin.

The increased glucagon levels found in our patients with hyperinsulinemic hypoglycemia proved ineffective biologically. At concentrations within the physiologic range, glucagon exerts hyperglycemic effects only when insulin is absent.

On the basis of these findings we conclude that the activity of alpha cells of the pancreas (i.e., production and secretion of glucagon as reflected by serum pancreatic glucagon concentrations) seems to be retained in proportion to the activity of beta cells, both in the preoperative insulin hypersecretion phase and after subtotal pancreatectomy. However, the response of the target tissue (liver) to endogenous glucagon is entirely overcome by the coexistent increased level of insulin. We also conclude that, in clinical practice, raised serum glucagon concentrations in children with hyperinsulinemic hypoglycemia seem to be evidence of the severity and long duration of the low blood glucose concentration, whereas postoperatively they may indicate that pancreatectomy has not been fully effective.

REFERENCES

1. Bondy PK, Rosenberg LE. Metabolic control and disease. Philadelphia: WB Saunders, 1980:297-9.
2. Butler PC, Rizza RA. Regulation of carbohydrate metabolism and response to hypoglycemia. Endocrinol Metab Clin North Am 1989;18:1-25.
3. Vidnes J, Oyasaeter S. Reduced gluconeogenesis due to hyperinsulinism: hormonal and metabolic studies in an infant with hypoglycemia. Pediatr Res 1978;12:619-24.
4. D'Arcangues C, Awoke S, Lawrence G. Metastatic insulinoma with long survival and glucagonoma syndrome. Ann Intern Med 1984;100:233-5.

5. Hirsch HJ, Loo S, Evans N, Crigler JF, Filler RM, Gabbay KM. Hypoglycemia of infancy and nesidioblastosis: studies with somatostatin. N Engl J Med 1977;296:1323-6.
6. Roe TF, Kogut MD. Idiopathic leucine-sensitive hypoglycemia syndrome: insulin and glucagon responses and effect of diasoxide. Pediatr Res 1982;16:1-4.
7. Amendt P, Kohnert KD, Kunz J. The hyperinsulinaemic hypoglycaemias in infancy: a study of six cases. Eur J Pediatr 1988;148:107-12.
8. Finegold DN, Stanley CA, Baker L. Glycemic response to glucagon during fasting hypoglycemia: an aid in the diagnosis of hyperinsulinism. J PEDIATR 1980;96:257-9.
9. Sperling MA, Grajwer L, Leake RD, Fisher DA. Effects of somatostatin (SRIF) infusion on glucose homeostasis in newborn lambs: evidence for a significant role of glucagon. Pediatr Res 1977;11:962-7.
10. Rahier J. Relevance of endocrine pancreas nesidioblastosis to hyperinsulinemic hypoglycemia. Diabetes 1989;12:1964-6.

Chronic pancreatitis in a patient with cystic fibrosis and clinical pancreatic insufficiency

J. Fernando del Rosario, MD, Philip E. Putnam, MD, and David M. Orenstein, MD

From the Divisions of Pediatric Gastroenterology and Pediatric Pulmonology, Department of Pediatrics, University of Pittsburgh School of Medicine, Children's Hospital of Pittsburgh, Pittsburgh, Pennsylvania

Pancreatitis occurs in up to 15% of patients with cystic fibrosis and pancreatic sufficiency, but the possibility of its occurrence in patients with pancreatic insufficiency has not been recognized. We describe a patient with homozygous ΔF508 cystic fibrosis and typical symptoms of pancreatic insufficiency (greasy, fatty stools) in whom pancreatitis developed. (J PEDIATR 1995;126:951-2)

Pancreatitis occurs in 2% to 15% of patients with cystic fibrosis who retain pancreatic function, but the possibility of its occurrence in patients with pancreatic insufficiency has not been generally recognized.[1-3] We describe a patient who had pancreatitis with CF and clinical evidence of pancreatic insufficiency.

CASE REPORT

A 4-year-old white boy with genotypically homozygous ΔF508 CF was examined at our hospital for a 1½-week history of periumbilical pain and vomiting. He had no fever, respiratory symptoms, diarrhea, or other illness. He had been exposed to well water and had swum in a lake. His medications included trimethoprim (80 mg)-sulfamethoxazole (400 mg) twice daily, inhaled albuterol (2.5 mg) and cromolyn (20 mg) twice daily, α-tocopheryl (53 IU/day), and pancrelipase (two to three capsules per meal) for chronic cough and steatorrhea. Before the present episode he had had up to three stools per day, described as "greasy" and malodorous, particularly after greasy meals or when he failed to take the enzymes. He had no family history of pancreatitis. Physical examination revealed a well-developed and well-nourished boy in the 25th to 50th percentile for weight and height. He was afebrile and had stable vital signs and clear lungs on auscultation. His abdomen was nontender with no organomegaly. Findings of the rest of his examination were normal. Laboratory evaluation revealed elevated serum lipase (353 IU/L; normal, <200 IU/L) and normal amylase (45 IU/L; normal, <100 IU/L) values.

CF	Cystic fibrosis

Five days later he was admitted to the hospital because of increased abdominal pain. He was given nothing by mouth. Complete blood cell count and serum electrolyte, blood urea nitrogen, creatinine, cholesterol, triglyceride, and amylase levels were normal. Serum lipase level was elevated to 348 IU/L. Liver enzyme values were normal except for aspartate aminotransferase (68 IU/L; normal, <40 IU/L). Results of stool studies were negative for ova and parasites. Chest and abdominal radiographs were normal. Ab-

Submitted for publication Nov. 21, 1994; accepted Dec. 30, 1994.
Request reprints: J. Fernando del Rosario, MD, Division of Pediatric Gastroenterology, Children's Hospital of Pittsburgh, 3705 Fifth Avenue at DeSoto Street, Pittsburgh, PA 15213-2583.

0022-3476/95/$3.00 + 0 **9/22/62985**

dominal ultrasonography revealed the biliary system and pancreatic head and body to be normal, but the pancreatic tail was not adequately visualized because of overlying intestinal gas. Administration of intravenous fluids and ranitidine was started; his other medications were withheld. After 5 days his lipase level decreased to 241 IU/L. However, initiation of enteral feeding resulted inrecurrence of abdominal pain and an increase in the lipase level to 404 IU/L. A catheter was placed to provide total parenteral nutrition. Repeated abdominal ultrasonography revealed no pseudocyst formation. After 1 week of total parenteral nutrition the lipase level declined, and reintroduction of a low-fat, low-protein diet did not lead to a recurrence of pain. Twenty days after admission he was discharged to receive pancrelipase and a diet with 30 gm fat. His lipase level was still elevated at 362 IU/L.

Although he initially had no abdominal pain and his serum lipase activity decreased while he was receiving a diet of a 40 gm protein and 30 gm fat, his lipase level increased to 404 IU/L 2 months after discharge. An endoscopic retrograde cholangiopancreatographic study, performed to rule out obstructive causes of recurrent pancreatitis, showed only pancreatic ductular irregularities consistent with chronic pancreatitis; no evidence of a long common channel was found. A cholangiogram was normal. No peptic ulcer disease was noted on endoscopy. The same diet was continued, and pancreatic enzymes were measured periodically. He has remained free of symptoms 6 months later with a liberal diet and has a serum amylase level of 54 IU/L and a lipase level of 36 IU/L.

DISCUSSION

Pancreatitis occurs in as many as 15% of patients with CF and pancreatic sufficiency.[1-3] It is thought to develop because of hyperconcentration of pancreatic secretions, resulting in obstruction of the pancreatic duct and autodigestion of the pancreas by activated pancreatic proteolytic enzymes.[1] It is thought not to occur in patients with CF who have pancreatic insufficiency,[4] because these persons lack the proteolytic enzymes necessary to promote autodigestion and perhaps because they lack sufficient viable pancreatic tissue to become inflamed.

We describe a young patient with CF who had pancreatitis despite having typical symptoms of pancreatic insufficiency (greasy, fatty stools). Although no formal studies were carried out to determine his exocrine pancreatic function, his history was typical for pancreatic insufficiency. Furthermore, his genotype (homozygous ΔF508) is nearly always (97%) associated with pancreatic insufficiency.[5] We are aware of only two other patients homozygous for ΔF508 who have been reported to have pancreatitis, but no details of their clinical course were provided.

Although trimethoprim-sulfamethoxazole can cause pancreatitis, it is not likely the cause of this child's disease, because he had recurrent pancreatitis even when not taking the medication. It is also unlikely that the elevated lipase level was due to impaired renal clearance or biliary disease, because he had normal renal function and cholangiogram, and his serum bilirubin and γ-glutamyl transpeptidase levels were normal.

This case illustrates the importance of considering pancreatitis in the differential diagnosis of a child with CF and abdominal pain, even if the child has typical pancreatic insufficiency.

REFERENCES

1. Atlas AB, Orenstein SR, Orenstein DM. Pancreatitis in young children with cystic fibrosis. J PEDIATR 1992;120:756-9.
2. Durie, PR. The pathophysiology of pancreatic defect in cystic fibrosis. Acta Paediatr Scand [Suppl] 1989;363:41-4.
3. Shwachman H, Lebenthal E, Khaw K. Recurrent acute pancreatitis in patients with cystic fibrosis with normal pancreatic enzymes. Pediatrics 1975;55:86-94.
4. Kopelman HR. Cystic fibrosis. In: Wyllie R, Hyams JS, eds. Pediatric gastrointestinal disease: pathophysiology, diagnosis and management. Philadelphia: WB Saunders, 1993:854-65.
5. Hamosh A, Corey M. Correlation between genotype and phenotype in patients with cystic fibrosis. N Engl J Med 1993; 329:1308-13.

Beneficial effect of growth hormone on atherogenic risk in children with growth hormone deficiency

Hitoshi Kohno, MD, Nami Ueyama, MD, Shinji Yanai, MD, Koutaro Ukaji, MD, and Sunao Honda, MD

From the Department of Endocrinology and Metabolism, Fukuoka Children's Hospital, Fukuoka, Japan

We studied changes in the atherogenic index (total cholesterol ÷ high-density lipoprotein cholesterol) in 12 prepubertal boys with growth hormone (GH) deficiency during 9 months of GH treatment. High-density lipoprotein cholesterol level increased until 5 months without significant changes in total cholesterol level; thus GH therapy may be beneficial in reducing the atherogenic index in boys with GH deficiency. (J Pediatr 1995;126:953-5)

Growth hormone is important in the regulation of fat, carbohydrate, and protein metabolism. These metabolic effects subsequently affect body composition and atherogenic risk factors. Growth hormone deficiency is associated with obesity which reportedly responds to GH treatment.[1-3] In addition, children[4] and adults[5] with GH deficiency often have hypercholesterolemia and thus might be at increased risk of having atherosclerotic diseases in later life. In fact, patients with GH deficiency have been reported to have increased morbidity and mortality rates as a result of cardiovascular disease.[6] We evaluated the atherogenic index in children with GH deficiency before and during GH treatment to determine the effect of GH on atherogenic risk factors.

METHODS

We studied 12 boys, 7 to 14 years of age, with GH deficiency. Their heights were 2.01 to 3.55 SD less than normal on the basis of growth charts produced by the Japanese Ministry of Health and Welfare, and the Ministry of Education. All children were prepubertal, and none had any sign of puberty during the study period. No evidence of kidney disease was present, and all patients were euthyroid before and during GH treatment. One hundred twenty-eight lean boys, 12 to 13 years of age, served as control subjects.

Peak GH levels after overnight fasting were determined by insulin hypoglycemia (0.1 U/kg), arginine infusion (0.5 gm/kg), and/or L-dopa (10 mg/kg) to be less than 10 ng/ml in all patients. Growth hormone was measured in duplicate by a conventional radioimmunoassay kit (Dinabot, Tokyo, Japan). Growth hormone was given daily by subcutaneous injection of methionine-free recombinant GH in a weekly dosage of 0.5 IU/kg (approximately 0.19 mg/kg).

Body mass index was calculated from the anthropometric measurements. Body fat was measured by bioelectrical impedance analysis (BIA 101, RJL Systems, Detroit, Mich.) because this method was validated for use in children.[7]

The AI, an important atherogenic risk factor,[8] is calculated as follows: AI = Total cholesterol ÷ High-density lipoprotein cholesterol. The TC concentrations were determined with fully enzymatic methods (TCHO-RXR1; Kokusai Siyaku, Kobe, Japan) with an automatic analyzer (model JCA-RX 20; JEOL, Tokyo, Japan). Both the intraassay and interassay coefficients of variation were less than 1.0%. The HDLC concentrations were determined enzymatically after precipitation of low-density lipoprotein cholesterol and very low density lipoprotein cholesterol with dextran sulfate and magnesium chloride (HDL-O_2; Daiichi Pure Chemicals, Tokyo, Japan). Both the intraassay and interassay coefficients of variation were less than 2.0%.

AI	Atherogenic index
GH	Growth hormone
HDLC	High-density lipoprotein cholesterol
TC	Total cholesterol

Differences in cholesterol between the control group and the GH-deficient group were assessed by unpaired *t* test. Responses to treatment were analyzed by analysis of

Supported in part by a grant from the Clinical Research Foundation, Fukuoka Children's Hospital.

Submitted for publication Aug. 8, 1994; accepted Jan. 11, 1995.

Reprint requests: Hitoshi Kohno, MD, Department of Endocrinology and Metabolism, Fukuoka Children's Hospital, 2-5-1 Tojinmachi, Chuo-ku, Fukuoka 810, Japan.

0022-3476/95/$3.00 + 0 **9/22/63321**

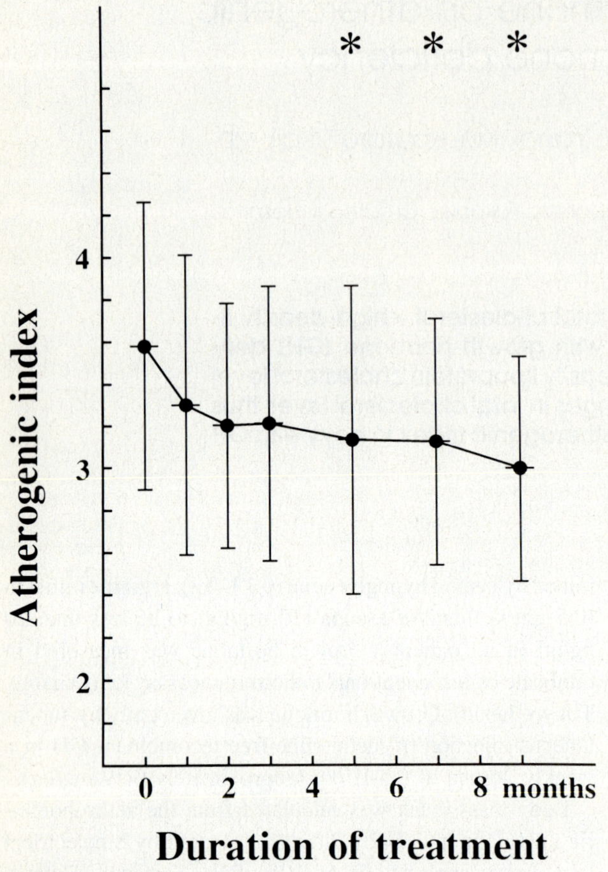

Figure. Decrease in AI during GH replacement therapy in 12 boys with GH deficiency. *Bars* represent SD. *Asterisks* denote significant differences ($p < 0.05$) versus pretreatment values.

variance for repeated measures. When the F value was significant ($p < 0.05$), pairs of time periods of treatment were compared by the Dunnett t test. The results were given as the mean ± SD. A p value less than 0.05 was considered to be significant.

This protocol was approved by the clinical research committee of Fukuoka Children's Hospital, and informed consent was obtained from all parents of the patients and control subjects.

RESULTS

During the GH treatment, both height and weight increased linearly, resulting in no significant changes in body mass index. However, percentage of body fat decreased after 1 month from 16.1% to 14.5%, and reached 13.4% by the end of the study. Fat mass decreased after 2 months of treatment from 4.2 to 3.5 kg. The lean body mass increased steadily from 21.8 to 25.1 kg during 9 months of treatment. The ratio of lean body mass versus fat mass also increased from 5.56 to 7.07 at 1 month of GH treatment and remained high thereafter.

Values for TC and HDLC in the control group were 4.22 ± 0.64 mmol/L (163 ± 25 mg/dl) and 1.46 ± 0.33 mmol/L (56 ± 13 mg/dl), respectively. In the GH-deficient group TC and HDLC before GH treatment were 4.71 ± 0.90 mmol/L (182 ± 35 mg/dl) and 1.36 ± 0.34 mmol/L (53 ± 13 mg/dl), respectively. The differences between the two groups were not significant.

In the GH-deficient group HDLC gradually increased and the increase reached statistical significance (18% increase, from 1.36 to 1.61 mmol/L [53 to 62 mg/dl]) after 5 months of GH therapy and remained constant thereafter; TC did not change significantly during the entire course of treatment. Consequently, the AI decreased significantly at 5 months of treatment, from 3.58 to 3.13 (Figure).

DISCUSSION

We have demonstrated an improvement in body composition and a reduction in AI after the initiation of GH therapy in children with GH deficiency. A rapid decrease of upper arm and calf fat was previously shown during the first 3 months after GH therapy with radiologic measurements in 63 patients with GH deficiency.[1] The skin-fold thickness also decreased during the first 6 to 10 weeks after the initiation of GH treatment and remained constant thereafter.[2] Exogenous GH administration in children with GH deficiency was associated with the redistribution of adipose tissue from an abdominal to a more peripheral area, which may lead to decreases in obesity-related diseases such as hypertension, diabetes, stroke, and myocardial infarction.[9] In addition, an increase in the amount of body fat was also observed after discontinuing GH therapy both before and after the completion of height growth.[3] These results indicate that GH replacement therapy may have a physiologic role in reducing obesity in children with GH deficiency.

The effects of GH treatment on serum lipids in children with GH deficiency have been conflicting. In some studies the TC level decreased after GH administration.[10] In other reports, however, no significant changes were observed.[11] Furthermore, there has been disagreement as to the HDLC level after GH treatment. In one study HDLC decreased after 3 days of GH administration[10]; in another, no changes were reported after 7 days of GH treatment[12]; and in a third, an increase was reported after 26 weeks of GH treatment.[13] In our study the values of HDLC in patients with GH deficiency were not different from those in the control subjects. However, HDLC progressively increased during GH therapy without significant changes in TC. Consequently, the AI decreased gradually.

We conclude that GH replacement therapy may have a

beneficial effect on atherogenic risk factors in children with GH deficiency. Long-term studies on lipid metabolism during GH replacement therapy in boys and girls with GH deficiency, and further investigations on the changes in health risk factors after discontinuation of GH therapy, are needed.

REFERENCES

1. Tanner JM, Hughes PCR, Whitehouse RH. Comparative rapidity of response of height, limb muscle and limb fat to treatment with human growth hormone in patients with and without growth hormone deficiency. Acta Endocrinol (Copenh) 1977;84:681-96.
2. Collipp PJ, Curti V, Thomas J, Sharma RK, Maddaiah VT, Cohn SH. Body composition changes in children receiving human growth hormone. Metabolism 1973;22:589-95.
3. Van der Werff ten Bosch JJ, Bot A. Effects of human pituitary growth hormone on body composition. Neth J Med 1987; 30:220-7.
4. LaFranchi S, Hanna CE, Illingworth DR. Effect of growth hormone replacement on development of hypothyroidism and hyperlipidemia. J PEDIATR 1985;106:588-93.
5. Libber SM, Plotnick LP, Johanson AJ, Blizzard RM, Kwiterovich PO, Migeon CJ. Long-term follow-up of hypopituitary patients treated with human growth hormone. Medicine 1990; 69:46-55.
6. Rosén T, Bengtsson B-Å. Premature mortality due to cardiovascular disease in hypopituitarism. Lancet 1990;336:285-8.
7. Houtkooper LB, Lohman TG, Going SB, Hall MC. Validity of bioelectric impedance for body composition assessment in children. J Appl Physiol 1989;66:814-21.
8. Castelli WP, Abbott RD, McNamara PM. Summary estimates of cholesterol used to predict coronary heart disease. Circulation 1983;67:730-4.
9. Rosenbaum M, Gertner JM, Leibel RL. Effects of systemic growth hormone (GH) administration on regional adipose tissue distribution and metabolism in GH-deficient children. J Clin Endocrinol Metab 1989;69:1274-81.
10. Asayama K, Amemiya S, Kusano S, Kato K. Growth-hormone-induced changes in postheparin plasma lipoprotein lipase and hepatic triglyceride lipase activities. Metabolism 1984;33:129-31.
11. Winter RJ, Green OC. Effect of thyroxine and growth hormone on the hypercholesterolemia of growth hormone deficiency. Metabolism 1984;33:54-7.
12. Møller A, Rasmussen LM, Thuesen L, Christiansen JS. Impact of human growth hormone on plasma lipoprotein concentrations. Horm Metab Res 1989;21:207-9.
13. Edén S, Wiklund O, Oscarsson J, Rosén T, Bengtsson B-Å. Growth hormone treatment of growth hormone-deficient adults results in a marked increase in Lp(a) and HDL cholesterol concentrations. Arterioscler Thromb 1993;13:296-301.

Bayley-Pinneau method of height prediction in girls with central precocious puberty: Correlation with adult height

A. Bar, MD, B. Linder, MD, E. H. Sobel, MD, P. Saenger, MD, and J. DiMartino-Nardi, MD

From the Albert Einstein College of Medicine/Montefiore Medical Center, Department of Pediatrics, Bronx, New York

One of the sequelae of idiopathic central precocious puberty (ICPP) can be short adult stature. In this retrospective study adult height was normal in 90% of girls with untreated ICPP (mean, 161.4 ± 7.7 cm). The height prediction made at the time of initial examination and the height age correlated with adult height. Therefore the initial height prediction can be useful in identifying those girls with ICPP at risk for short stature. (J PEDIATR 1995;126:955-8)

Presented at the seventy-sixth Annual Meeting of the Society for Pediatric Research, Seattle, Wash., May 1994.

Submitted for publication Oct. 25, 1994; accepted Jan. 23, 1995.

Reprint requests: Joan DiMartino-Nardi, MD, Department of Pediatrics, Division of Pediatric Endocrinology, Montefiore Medical Center, 111 E. 210th St., Bronx, NY 10467.

0022-3476/95/$3.00 + 0 **9/22/63688**

In 95% of girls the onset of puberty occurs between the ages of 8 and 13 years.[1] Most girls who have precocious puberty with pubertal onset before the age of 8 years do not have an identifiable lesion and are designated as having idiopathic central precocious puberty. Children with sexual precocity may be short as adults because of early maturation of the bones. Therapy with long-acting analogs of luteinizing hormone–releasing hormone is available to halt pubertal pro-

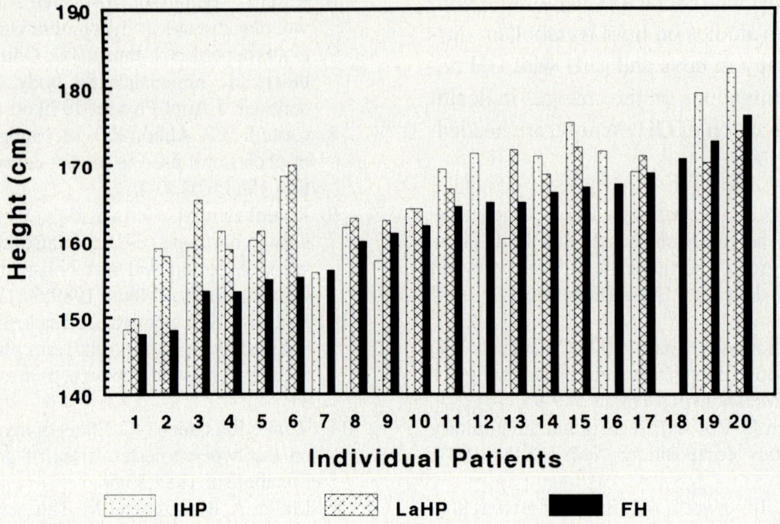

Fig. 1. Individual initial HP *(iHP)*, last available HP *(LaHP)*, and FH are shown. Values for FH are scattered around mean. Initial HP overestimated FH by 4.2 ± 4.4 cm.

FH	Final height
HP	Height prediction
ICPP	Idiopathic central precocious puberty

gression, but information regarding the effect on increasing final height is still evolving.[2]

The reported heights of untreated girls with ICPP are variable.[3-6] Girls with mild variants of ICPP have a normal initial predicted height that does not decrease after 2 years of observation.[7, 8] However, the adult height of these girls has not been not reported.

Therapy to halt pubertal progression and improve FH might not be warranted in all girls with ICPP. The purpose of this study is to report the FH in untreated girls with ICPP and to identify those factors which can predict FH.

METHODS

Records of 72 girls with untreated ICPP who were followed in Bronx Municipal Hospital Center from 1955 to 1994 were reviewed. Idiopathic central precocious puberty was defined as the appearance and progression of breast development before the age of 8 years. Excluded were girls with peripheral precocious puberty, premature thelarche, or lesions of the central nervous system. The patients included were of Hispanic, black, or white ethnic origin.

Height measurements were obtained with the recumbent Harpenden stadiometer (Seritex Inc., Carlstadt, N.J.). Bone age was assessed by the method of Greulich and Pyle.[9] Height predictions were made with the Bayley-Pinneau method,[10] which is based on the child's bone age and concurrent height. The initial HP was made at the time of initial evaluation. The FH was achieved if height did not change during at least a 3-month interval or if the bone age or chronologic age or both were more than 16 years. The near-FH was defined by a change in height of less than 1 cm/yr or by a bone age or chronologic age, or both, of at least 14 years. The last available HP was based on the last available height and bone age. The height age is the age at which the child's height can be plotted at the 50th percentile. Height age advancement represents the difference between the height age and the chronologic age.

Exploratory data analysis and regression analysis were done to evaluate FH and the factors that may predict FH. The differences between the initial HP and FH or near-FH were tested with the paired t test. A p value less than 0.05 was considered to indicate statistical significance. All data are expressed as mean ± SD.

RESULTS

Final height data were available for 20 patients, and near-FH data were available for seven. We were able to compare the initial height with a follow-up HP up to 5 years after the initial examination for 62 patients, including 42 patients in whom FH and near-FH data were not available.

For those girls in whom FH data were available, the appearance of breast tissue occurred at 5.6 ± 1.6 years; the first evaluation was performed at 7 ± 2.4 years. Six children were less than 6 years of age at the time of the initial evaluation. Although the mean bone age was 8.4 ± 3 years, one third of the girls had a bone age at least 2 years (range, 2 to 3.7 years) greater than their chronologic age. For those girls with near-FH data, the mean chronologic age and bone ages were

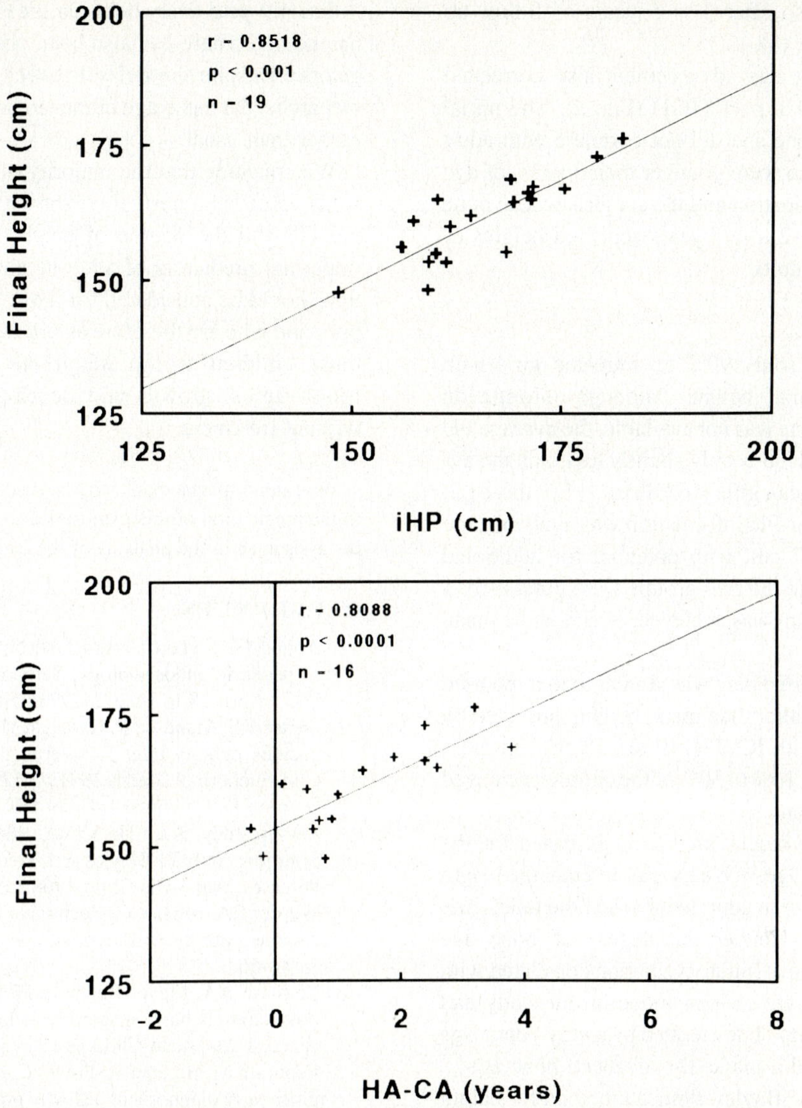

Fig. 2. Final height significantly correlated with initial HP *(iHP)* ($r = 0.85$; $p < 0.001$) and with degree of height age advancement *(HA – CA)* ($r = 0.8$; $p < 0.001$).

similar to those of patients with FH data. Menarche occurred 4.9 ± 2.4 years (range, 3 to 13 years) after thelarche, at a mean age of 10.5 ± 1.2 years. Seventy-five percent of these girls were not obese when first seen. However, during follow-up, 40% of the children were overweight.

The mean FH and near-FH were 161.4 ± 7.7 cm (32nd percentile) and 165 cm (59th percentile), respectively. The FH values were distributed in a manner similar to a normal distribution curve with most of the heights scattered around the mean (Fig. 1). Ninety percent of the girls achieved a height of more than 153 cm (3rd percentile, or –1.8 SD). Only 10% were shorter than 150 cm (1st percentile, or –2.3 SD).

The initial HP, last available HP, and FH for each patient are shown in Fig. 1. (Patient 14 did not have an initial HP available for comparison.) The range of differences between the initial HP and the FH was +4.6 to –13.2 cm (mean, –4.2 ± 4.4 cm). In five girls, although the initial HP overestimated the FH by more than 6.3 cm (2.5 SD of the Bayley-Pinneau method), the girls achieved a normal adult stature. In one patient the initial HP was normal (159 cm) but the ultimate height was short at 148.3 cm.

There was a significant correlation between the initial HP and the FH ($r = 0.85$; $p < 0.001$) (Fig. 2). The correlation between the initial HP and the last available HP was preserved during short-term follow-up (0.9 to 3 years) ($r = 0.69$; *p*

<0.001; n = 44) and also after 3 to 5 years of follow-up ($r = 0.72$; $p < 0.001$; n = 18).

The degree of height age advancement also correlated with adult height ($r = 0.8$; $p < 0.0001$) (Fig. 2). The initial chronologic age and bone age did not correlate with adult height. The six girls who were younger than 6 years of age at the time of initial evaluation and the six girls whose bone ages were advanced by 2 to 3.7 years achieved heights of more than 153 cm as adults.

DISCUSSION

In this retrospective study 90% of untreated girls with ICPP achieved a normal height. Although information regarding parental heights was not available, the average FH was 161.4 ± 7.7 cm, which is only slightly less than the average for healthy American girls (163.8 cm).[11] For those patients in whom only near-FH information was available, the near-FH was 165 ± 8.7 cm, with potential for additional growth. When data from the two groups were combined, a FH or near-FH of 163 cm was achieved, which is the mean for normal girls.

The adult height reported here was similar to that reported by Ehrhardt et al.[6] but taller than mean heights provided by other studies of girls with ICCP (149 to 155 cm). In these latter reports as many as 20% to 30% of the children achieved a FH of less than 150 cm.[3-5]

The Bayley-Pinneau height prediction is based on the child's height and bone age.[10] We have found that the height age has an important role in adult height (i.e., the taller girls become taller adults). Neither the degree of bone age advancement nor the age at initial evaluation correlated with FH. However, none of the girls included in our study had severe precocious puberty characterized by a very young age at the time of onset and a markedly advanced bone age.

In normal children the Bayley-Pinneau method for height prediction is accurate with an SD of 2.54 cm (at the age we measured).[10] Therefore 99% of normal children achieve an adult height within ± 6.3 cm (2.5 SD) of their initial HP.[11] Seventy-five percent of the girls achieved a height within 6.3 cm of the initial HP (99% within 10.5 cm). One girl who did not reach her initial HP within 6.3 cm achieved a height of 148.3 cm, which was 10.7 cm less than her initial HP. Therefore careful follow-up and reassessment of growth and development should be made because other factors can influence growth.

The 4.9-year delay between breast development and menarche noted here has also been observed by other investigators.[5] Despite the delay between onset of thelarche and menarche, the mean age of menarche was 10.5 years, 2 years earlier than usual.

We conclude that the majority of girls with ICPP in this study achieved a normal height without treatment. The initial HP and the degree of height age advancement were important predictors of adult height. Therapeutic intervention should be considered for those girls whose initial HP is poor and who are therefore at risk for short adult stature. For those children whose initial HP is acceptable, careful follow-up of growth and development should continue without treatment.

We extend special thanks to Ms. Zaida Fajardo for her assistance in the preparation of this manuscript and to Mr. Robert Varner for his assistance in the analysis of the data.

REFERENCES

1. August GP. Puberty: normal mechanisms. In: A current review of pediatric endocrinology. Serono symposium, Washington, D.C., April 28 to May 2, 1993:45-50.
2. Oerter KE, Manasco P, Barnes KM, et al. Adult height in precocious puberty after long-term treatment with deslorelin. J Clin Endocrinol Metab 1991;73:1235-40.
3. Murram D, Dewhurst J, Grant DB. Precocious puberty: a follow-up study. Arch Dis Child 1984;59:77-8.
4. Sigurjonsdottir TJ, Hayles AB. Precocious puberty: a report of 96 cases. Am J Dis Child 1968;115:309-21.
5. Werder EA, Mueset G, Zachmann M, et al. Treatment of precocious puberty with cyproterone acetate. Pediatr Res 1974; 8:248-56.
6. Ehrhardt AA, Meyer-Bahlburg HFL, Bell JJ, et al. Idiopathic precocious puberty in girls: psychiatric follow-up in adolescence. J Am Acad Child Psychiatry 1984;23:23-33.
7. Fontoura M, Brauner R, Prevot C, et al. Precocious puberty in girls: early diagnosis of a slowly progressing variant. Arch Dis Child 1989;64:1170-6.
8. Kreiter M, Burstein S, Rosenfield RL, et al. Preserving adult height potential in girls with idiopathic true precocious puberty. J J PEDIATR 1990;117:364-70.
9. Greulich WW, Pyle SI. Radiographic atlas of skeletal development of the hand and wrist. 2nd ed. Stanford, California: Stanford University Press, 1959.
10. Bayley N, Pinneau S. Tables for predicting adult height from skeletal age. J PEDIATR 1952;14:432-41.
11. Hamill PVV, Drizd TA, Johnson CL, Reed RB, Roch AF, Moore WM. Physical growth: National Center for Health Statistics percentiles. Am J Clin Nutr 1979;32:607-29.

Acquired platelet dysfunction with eosinophilia in white children

Man-Chiu Poon, MD, FRCP(C), Soo Chin Ng, MBBS, FRCPA(A), and Max J. Coppes, MD, PhD

From the Departments of Medicine, Pediatrics, Oncology and Laboratory Medicine, University of Calgary, Foothills Hospital, Alberta Children's Hospital, Tom Baker Cancer Centre, and the Canadian Red Cross Blood Services, Calgary, Alberta, Canada, and Subang Jaya Medical Centre, Petaling Jaya, Selangor, Malaysia

Acquired platelet dysfunction associated with eosinophilia has been described mainly in indigenous Southeast Asian and East Indian children. We describe two white boys in whom this disorder developed after they had lived in Malaysia for 12 to 18 months. Acquired platelet dysfunction associated with eosinophilia should therefore be considered in children who, after a visit to this region, have easy bruising and eosinophilia. (J PEDIATR 1995;126:959-61)

Acquired platelet dysfunction associated with eosinophilia is a syndrome characterized by transient mild bleeding symptoms of ecchymoses, epistaxis, or gingival bleeding, normal platelet count with variable platelet aggregation defects, and eosinophilia.[1-8] Since the 1970s it has commonly been recognized in indigenous children in tropical Southeast Asia[1-3, 6-8] and India,[4] but has been described only once in a white child visiting Malaysia.[5] It has not been reported in other geographic areas. We describe two white boys who had been living in Malaysia for 12 to 18 months and who had APDE. In one patient APDE developed after he returned to Canada.

CASE REPORTS

Case 1. A 5-year-old white Australian boy who had lived in Malaysia for 18 months was seen at the Subang Jaya Clinic in Petaling Jaya, Malaysia, with a 3-week history of recurrent bruises. He was otherwise well and taking no medication. He had no history of easy bruising or bleeding. There was no family history of bleeding disorders. Physical examination revealed an otherwise healthy boy with several recent ecchymoses on the arms, legs, and anterior aspect of the chest. No hepatosplenomegaly or lymphadenopathy was noted. A hemogram showed the following values: hemoglobin, 110 gm/L; platelet count, 284×10^9 cells/L; leukocyte count 7.4×10^9 cells/L, with 37% neutrophils, 42% lymphocytes, 1% basophils, 20% eosinophils (absolute count, 1.5×10^9 cells/L; normal, $<0.4 \times 10^9$ cells/L). Coagulation studies showed a prolonged Duke bleeding time of 10 minutes (normal, <5 minutes) and normal prothrombin time, activated partial thromboplastin time, thrombin time, and fibrinogen level. Platelet function was not studied. Stool examinations did not show ova and parasites; nonetheless, the patient was treated empirically with one 400 mg dose of albendazole (Zental, SmithKline & French, Rizal, the Philippines). His bruises disappeared spontaneously after 1 month. He has remained well since.

Case 2. A 6-year-old white boy was seen at the Alberta Children's Hospital in Calgary with a 4-week history of easy bruising. He was otherwise healthy and receiving no medication; he had not taken aspirin recently. He had no previous bleeding problems and had no family history of a bleeding disorder. He had been living in Malaysia for 1 year with his parents and two sisters and had come back to Calgary for vacation 5 weeks previously. Unusually large bruises were observed after the patient had fallen during skating. He had had an abscessed tooth extracted the day before and had continuing oozing for 18 hours. Physical examination revealed a healthy boy with ecchymoses on the chest, back, and thighs. He had no petechiae, mucous membrane bleeding, subconjunctival or retinal hemorrhage, deep hematomas, icterus, rash, hepatosplenomegaly, or lymphadenopathy. The tooth socket was dry. A hemogram showed the following values: hemoglobin, 126 gm/L; platelet count, 274×10^9 cells/L; leukocyte count, 9.5×10^9 cells/L, with 27% neutrophils, 33% lymphocytes, 5% monocytes, 29% eosinophils (absolute count, 2.8×10^9 cells/L), and 1% basophils. Three stool examinations failed to detect ova and parasites. Coagulation studies showed a Template bleeding time of 17.5 minutes (normal, <9 minutes), and normal prothrombin time, activated partial thrombo-

APDE	Acquired platelet dysfunction associated with eosinophilia

Submitted for publication Nov. 23, 1994; accepted Jan. 19, 1995.
Reprint requests: Man-Chiu Poon, MD, University of Calgary Foothills Hospital, 1403 29th St. NW, Calgary, Alberta T2N 2T9, Canada.

0022-3476/95/$3.00 + 0 **9/22/63481**

plastin time, thrombin time, fibrinogen, factor XIII, factor VIII (1.06 U/ml), and von Willebrand factor (antigen, 0.87 U/ml; ristocetin cofactor activity, 0.87 U/ml). The bleeding time did not shorten ½ hour after the intravenous infusion of 0.3 μg/kg 1-desamino-8-D-arginine vasopressin (DDAVP, desmopressin). Platelet aggregation studies showed a lack of secondary wave response to 4 μmol/L adenosine diphosphate and 10 μmol/L epinephrine, no response to 0.0016 gm/L collagen, and a disaggregation response to 0.5 gm/L arachidonic acid. Platelet aggregation to 1.5 gm/L ristocetin was normal. Results of platelet aggregation studies of both parents were normal. Flow cytometry analyses for platelet surface IgG, IgA, and IgM showed increased IgG (mean channel fluorescence, 369, compared with 173, 192, and 166 for control, mother, and father platelets, respectively). Normal platelets incubated with the patient's serum but not with another normal serum, acquired an increased level of platelet surface IgG. Serum immune complex composed of IgG and IgM at a concentration of 2.71 gm/L was present in the serum.

The patient returned to Malaysia several weeks later without specific treatment. Two months later his hemogram showed a leukocyte count of 8.6×10^9 cells/L with 0.9×10^9 cells/L eosinophils. The easy bruising disappeared spontaneously during the next several months. Ten months later he had a leukocyte count of 7.3×10^9 cells/L with an eosinophil count of 0.3×10^9 cells/L.

DISCUSSION

Both our patients had a mild, transient hemorrhagic disorder typical of the syndrome of APDE, which thus far has been mainly described in indigenous children and young adults in Thailand,[1-3, 7, 8] Singapore,[6] and India.[4] Suvatte et al.[2] reported heterogeneous functional platelet defects in 62 children (56 Thai, five Chinese, one Japanese) living in Thailand with eosinophilia and spontaneous painless ecchymoses, and suggested the term *APDE*. Since then, additional patients have been described.[5-8] Acquired platelet dysfunction with eosinophilia occurs mainly in children or adolescents,[1-8] and less frequently in young adults.[6] The most common initial problem is painless ecchymoses. Approximately half the children also have epistaxis; less common are gingival bleeding and petechiae. Patients with APDE have not been described to have severe bleeding except after trauma, including extraction of teeth.[2] No central nervous system hemorrhages have been reported.

The pathogenesis of APDE is unknown. It has been suggested that this syndrome might reflect an unusual immunologic response to an inflammatory or infectious process peculiar to Asian countries; a parasitic infection has been reported in more than half the patients with APDE.[2, 6, 8] The parasites most commonly identified are *Ascaris lumbricoides, Enterobius vermicularis* (pinworm), and *Ancylostoma duodenale* (Old World hookworm). Patients with intestinal parasitic infection or eosinophilia, without easy bruising, do not have platelet dysfunction.[2, 6] In our patients repeated stool collections failed to detect ova or parasites. However, the platelet surface IgG level of patient 2 was increased. Subsequent analysis revealed that control platelets incubated with this patient's serum also acquired increased platelet surface IgG. This suggests that the patient's serum contained an IgG fraction capable of reacting with normal platelets. We hypothesize that the platelet-reactive IgG may have developed as a reaction to an underlying condition that also resulted in the observed eosinophilia and that the platelet-reactive IgG may play a pathogenic role in causing the acquired platelet-release defect. Acquired impairment of platelet-release reaction, with or without a deficiency of the platelet pool constituents, has been observed in immunologic disorders associated with the presence of platelet-reactive IgG and immune complexes.[9, 10]

The hemorrhagic diathesis in APDE typically disappears within 6 to 12 months.[2, 8] No therapeutic agent has been proven of value. Trauma or elective surgery should be avoided while the bleeding time is prolonged. If excessive bleeding occurs, a platelet transfusion can be considered,[2, 3] but the in vitro results obtained with the serum of patient 2 indicate that it may not be useful in all patients. For patients with a proved parasitic infection, appropriate antihelminthic therapy is indicated. Whether antihelminthic therapy shortens the duration of hemorrhagic diathesis, as suggested in one report,[2] remains to be determined. Once the syndrome is resolved, recurrence is apparently rare.[2, 8]

We conclude that APDE should be considered in children with easy bruising, eosinophilia, and a history of a recent visit to tropical Southeast Asian countries.

REFERENCES

1. Mitrakul C. Transient spontaneous bruising with long bleeding time and normal platelet count. Am J Clin Pathol 1975; 63:81-6.
2. Suvatte V, Mahasandana C, Tanphaichitr V, Tuchinda S. Acquired platelet dysfunction with eosinophilia: study of platelet function in 62 cases. Southeast Asian J Trop Med Public Health 1979;10:368-72.
3. Hathirat P, Bintadish P, Sasanakul W, Isarangkura P. Blood components therapy in acquired platelet dysfunction with eosinophilia: a preliminary report. Southeast Asian J Trop Med Public Health 1979;10:358-67.
4. Krishna Das KV. Haematology in India, present status and future prospect. Indian J Paediatr 1981;48:481-4.
5. Muthiah MM, Mitchell TR, Thorn CT. Acquired platelet dysfunction with eosinophilia. BMJ 1984;289:1044.
6. Kueh YK, Teo CG. Eosinophilic purpura: the syndrome of acquired platelet dysfunction with eosinophilia—a tropical phenomenon. Ann Acad Med 1986;15:262-7.
7. Ramanathan M, Duraisamy G. Acquired platelet dysfunction with eosinophilia (APDE): an underdiagnosed condition. Med J Malaysia 1987;42:53-5.

8. Ng SC, Koong PL. A study of 31 patients with easy bruising from University Hospital, Kuala Lumpur. Med J Malaysia 1990;45:325-8.
9. Karpatkin S, Lackner HL. Association of antiplatelet antibody with functional platelet disorders: autoimmune thrombocytopenic purpura, systemic lupus erythematosus and thrombopathia. Am J Med 1975;59:599-604.
10. Weiss HJ, Rosove MH, Lages BA, Kaplan KL. Acquired storage pool deficiency with increased platelet-associated IgG: report of five cases. Am J Med 1980;69:711-7.

Effect of airway pressure on inferior vena cava pressure as a measure of central venous pressure in children

Zacharia Reda, MD, Sion Houri, MD, Alan L. Davis, MD, and Victor C. Baum, MD

From the Departments of Pediatrics and Anesthesiology, University of California, Los Angeles, and Miller Children's Hospital, Long Beach, California

We evaluated the effect of elevated airway pressure on the validity of intravascular pressure obtained in the distal inferior vena cava (IVC) as a measure of central venous pressure (CVP) in a group of children receiving mechanical ventilation. The IVC pressure correlated well with CVP in the patients without abdominal distention, but the disparity was wider in those with abdominal distention. Elevated mean airway pressure or positive end-expiratory pressure had no effect on the relationship of IVC to CVP. (J PEDIATR 1995;126:961-5)

Catheterization of the femoral vein in children has been shown to be safe,[1, 2] but the comparability of pressure measured in the abdominal inferior vena cava as compared with the right atrium in patients receiving mechanical ventilation with increased intrathoracic pressure remains undetermined. In addition, the relationship of IVC and central venous pressure measured from within the thorax in the face of abdominal distention has not been evaluated. Three reports have evaluated the correlation of IVC and superior vena cava pressures.[3-5] However, these studies were done in dogs[3] or in children in the cardiac catheterization laboratory[4] or the intensive care unit[5] who did not have pulmonary disease or high airway pressures. This study was designed to address the appropriateness of using IVC catheters as a reflection of CVP in pediatric patients receiving mechanical ventilation at high airway pressures.

Critically ill pediatric patients occasionally require multiple central venous catheters. We took advantage of this clinical practice to compare pressures obtained via femoral and thoracic venous catheters in patients whose lungs were mechanically ventilated with the use of routine clinical equipment in a clinical setting. We hypothesized that these pressures would be similar. In addition, we analyzed separately data from a group of pediatric patients receiving mechanical ventilation who were judged clinically to have increased intraabdominal pressure. It was expected that the disparity between IVC and SVC pressures in this group would be increased, making IVC pressure measurements unreliable as an indicator of CVP.

CVP	Central venous pressure
IVC	Inferior vena cava
MAP	Mean airway pressure
PEEP	Positive end-expiratory pressure
SVC	Superior vena cava

Presented in part at the annual meeting of the Society for Pediatric Research, Seattle, Wash., May 1994.

Submitted for publication Sept. 30, 1994; accepted Jan. 20, 1995.

Reprint requests: Victor C. Baum, MD, Department of Anesthesiology, Box 238, University of Virginia Medical Center, Charlottesville, VA 22908.

0022-3476/95/$3.00 + 0 **9/22/63483**

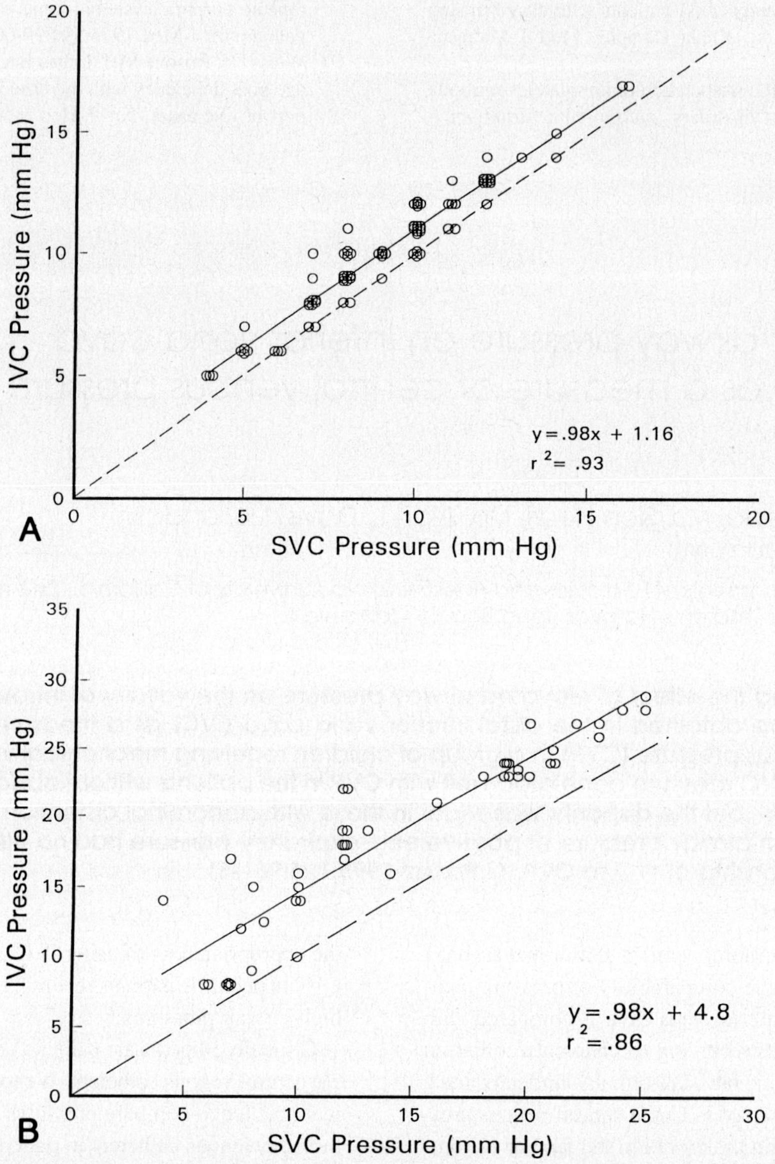

Fig. 1. Correlation of IVC and SVC pressures in group 1 with no abdominal distention (**A**), and in group 2 with adominal distention (**B**). *Dashed line* is line of identity, and *solid line* is regression line.

METHODS

This study was approved by the appropriate human subject protection committees. The need for informed consent was waived by these institutional review boards. No interventions were done solely for the purpose of the study. All patients had had percutaneous placement of 4F 8 cm double-lumen catheters (Cook Critical Care, Bloomington, Ind.) into a femoral vein and into the SVC through either the internal jugular or subclavian veins. Multiple data points were collected at different levels of positive end-expiratory pressure and mean airway pressure for each patient. Each data point represented a mean of three readings done at least 30 minutes after any interventions. Catheter positions were verified radiographically. Femoral catheter tips were in the iliac vein and the SVC catheters were at the SVC–right atrium junction.

All data were collected while patients with mechanically ventilated lungs were in the supine position. We previously documented that CVP as measured by our bedside monitors reliably reproduces measurements of CVP made manually at end-exhalation.[5] Auto-PEEP was measured by introducing an expiratory hold during mechanical ventilation. Patients

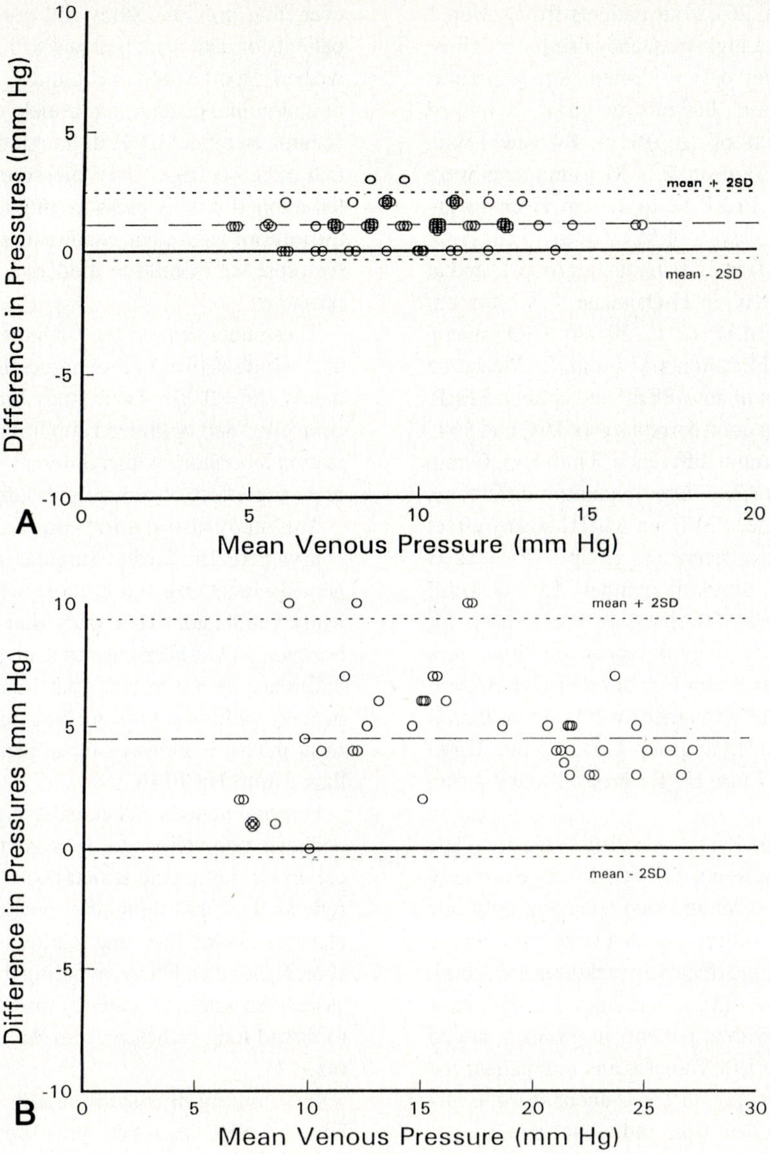

Fig. 2. Difference in pressures (IVC – SVC) versus MAP in patients with no abdominal distention (**A**) (bias, 1.0 mm Hg) and in patients with abdominal distention (**B**) (bias, 4.5 mm).

were divided into two groups: group 1 had no apparent abdominal distention, and group 2 had apparent abdominal distention. The diagnosis of abdominal distention was made clinically, and no attempt was made to measure intraabdominal pressure. Diagnoses in group 2 included recuperation from liver transplantation, abdominal mass, tension pneumoperitoneum, and massive ascites. No attempt was made to measure venous pressure at different subjective levels of abdominal pressure.

Bias (mean of differences) and precision (SD of differences) of venous pressures were determined for both groups of patients.[6] Data were compared by the two-tailed paired *t* test. Statistical significance was considered at a *p* level less than 0.05. On the basis of preliminary data showing a variance of 1.63 in the difference between measurements obtained in the two catheter positions, there was a 91% chance of detecting a difference as small as 1 mm Hg with a sample size of 20 patients, and a 98% chance with a sample size of 30. Data are expressed as mean ± SEM.

RESULTS

Patients in group 1 ranged from 14 days to 16 years of age (mean, 4.3 years) with PRISM (pediatric risk of mortality) scores of 12 to 48 (mean, 26). Four patients from group 1 received ventilation from a high-frequency oscillator. Three of these patients also had data collected during periods of conventional ventilation. Patients in group 2 ranged from 7 months to 16 years of age (mean, 4.4 years) with PRISM scores of 12 to 42 (mean, 22). Measurements were obtained at 47 levels of PEEP (2 to 12 cm H_2O; mean, 7.1 ± 0.4 cm H_2O) and 76 levels of MAP (4 to 35 cm H_2O; mean, 18.3 ± 0.9 cm H_2O) in 17 patients in group 1, and at 41 levels of PEEP (0 to 16 cm H_2O; mean, 7.7 ± 0.5 cm H_2O) and 47 levels of MAP (2 to 29 cm H_2O; mean, 16.3 ± 1.0 cm H_2O) in 11 patients in group 2. Measured PEEP represented the sum of auto-PEEP and applied PEEP.

Patients in group 1 had a good correlation of IVC and SVC pressure ($R^2 = 0.93$; maximum difference, 3 mm Hg). Group 2 showed wider variation ($R^2 = 0.86$; maximum difference, 10 mm Hg) (Fig. 1). Neither PEEP nor MAP had any effect on the IVC-SVC pressure difference in group 1 ($R^2 = 0.003$ and <0.001, respectively). Similarly, neither PEEP or MAP had any effect on the IVC-SVC pressure relationship for group 2 ($R^2 = 0.1$ and 0.05). Only two pressure differences in group 1 were as large as 3 mm Hg. In group 2, however, 50% of IVC-SVC pressure differences were greater than 3 mm Hg. Bias was 1.0 mm Hg in group 1 and 4.5 mm Hg in group 2. Precision was 0.7 mm Hg for group 1 and 2.4 mm Hg for group 2 (Fig. 2).

Data from individual patients were also evaluated. The IVC and SVC data from patients in group 1 were extremely close. For all data points from any single patient, only one patient had any IVC-SVC differences that were more than 1 mm Hg apart across the range of airway pressures measured. One patient had differences of 0, 1, and 2 mm Hg. The variances of the data for individual patients in group 1 ranged from 0.0 to 0.47 (mean, 0.19). Thus for any one patient the relationship of IVC to SVC pressure was unchanging as airway pressure varied. The data from individual group 2 patients were more widely dispersed. Variances for this group were from 0.06 to 7.36 (mean, 1.65).

DISCUSSION

This study compared the effects of PEEP and MAP on the reliability of CVP as measured in the iliac vein in patients with and without abdominal distention. We have shown that high airway pressure (both PEEP and MAP) does not affect this pressure as a valid measure of CVP; the difference was always 3 mm Hg or less in group 1. The two measurements with a difference of 3 mm Hg occurred in one patient early in the study, and we cannot exclude the possibility that this patient was not completely supine at the time data were collected. Unlike the situation in group 1, we found that the SVC-IVC pressure correlation in patients with abdominal distention was poor, in contrast to a previous report.[4] However, that previous study did not specifically describe the patients or data from patients with abdominal distention. As we had hypothesized, we found that IVC pressure in the face of abdominal distention routinely overestimated and did not accurately reflect CVP, although the possibility had existed that increased right atrial pressure and CVP from transmitted applied airway pressure might in some way keep open the inferior vena cava, equalizing IVC and SVC pressures in the presence of mild to moderate increased intraabdominal pressure.

These data support the findings of the study by Lloyd et al.,[4] which showed close agreement between the measurements ($R^2 = 0.99$). Their study was done under the highly controlled and optimized conditions of the cardiac catheterization laboratory with a different technique, and did not address the effect of airway pressure on IVC.

This study also confirms our previous findings in postoperative pediatric cardiac surgical patients who were spontaneously breathing and in those whose lungs were mechanically ventilated.[5] That study documented good correlation between IVC and right atrial pressures, with a maximum difference of 3 mm Hg. That study, however, was done in patients without significant lung disease or elevated intrathoracic pressure. None of those patients was receiving more than 3 mm Hg PEEP.

Femoral venous catheters have been used successfully in pediatric populations to decrease the risk of injuring cervical and intrathoracic structures.[1,2] If IVC pressure reliably reflects SVC and right atrial pressure and is not affected by elevated airway pressure, it allows monitoring of CVP from short femoral catheters, avoiding the potential complications associated with SVC catheter insertion and avoiding the need to thread long catheters from the femoral vein into the thorax.

In summary, this study reports the excellent correlation between SVC and IVC pressures in patients undergoing mechanical ventilation with high PEEP, and MAP. This excellent correlation is valid only for supine patients with no abdominal distention.

We acknowledge the gracious help of the nurses and fellows of UCLA's and Miller Children's Hospital's pediatric intensive care units.

REFERENCES

1. Stenzel JP, Green TP, Furhrman BP. Percutaneous femoral venous catheterizations: a prospective study of complications. J PEDIATR 1989;114:411-5.
2. Stenzel JP, Green TP, Furhrman BP. Percutaneous femoral venous catheterization in a pediatric intensive care unit: a survival analysis of complications. Crit Care Med 1989;17:984-8.
3. Berg RA, Lloyd TR, Donnerstein RL. Accuracy of central

venous pressure monitoring in the intraabdominal vena cava: a canine study. J PEDIATR 1992;120:67-71.
4. Lloyd TR, Donnerstein RL, Berg RA. Accuracy of central venous pressure monitoring in the intraabdominal inferior vena cava. Pediatrics 1992;89:506-8.
5. Chait HI, Kuhn MA, Baum VC. Inferior vena caval pressure reliably predicts right atrial pressure in pediatric cardiac surgical patients. Crit Care Med 1994;22:219-24.
6. Bland JM, Altman DG. Statistical methods for assessing agreement between two methods of clinical measurement. Lancet 1986;1:307-10.

Peutz-Jeghers syndrome in a neonate

M. J. Fernandez Seara, MD, M. I. Martinez Soto, MD, J. R. Fernandez Lorenzo, MD, S. Trabazo, MD, E. Gamborino, MD, and J. Forteza Vila, MD

From the Departments of Pediatrics and Pathology, Hospital General de Galicia, Santiago de Compostela, Spain

A 15-day-old girl was found to have generalized gastrointestinal polyposis resulting from Peutz-Jeghers syndrome. Her manifestations included abdominal distention, hematemesis, bloody diarrhea, and edema. She died at 1 year of age of multiple complications of her disease. (J PEDIATR 1995;126:965-7)

Submitted for publication July 11, 1994; accepted Dec. 20, 1994.

Reprint requests: M. Jose Fernandez Seara, MD, Republica del Salvador No. 29-5° C, Santiago de Compostela 15701, La Coruña, Spain.

0022-3476/95/$3.00 + 0 **9/22/62888**

Peutz-Jeghers syndrome is characterized by mucocutaneous pigmentations and gastrointestinal polyps of the hamartomatous type; most polyps (50% to 90%) are located in the small intestine.[1] A family history of autosomal dominant transmission with incomplete penetrance is noted in 50% of the cases.[2] The clinical manifestations are recurrent abdom-

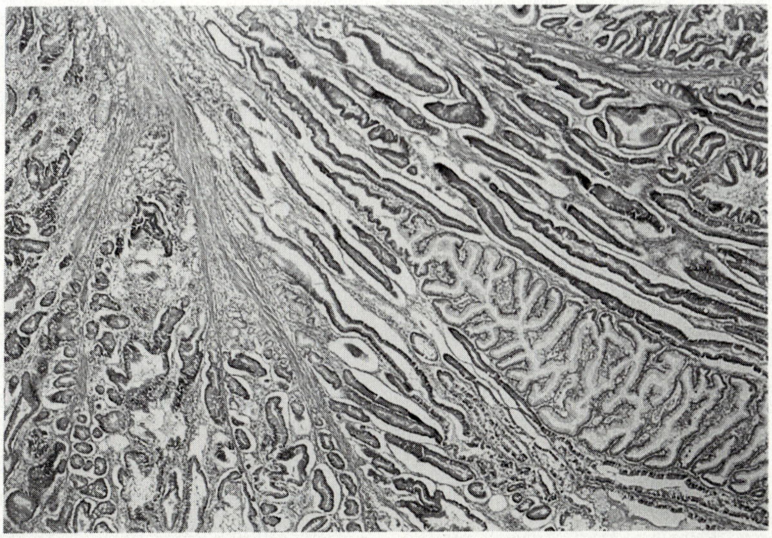

Fig. 1. Jejunal polyp composed of intestinal crypts and villi with abnormal architectural arrangement. Note band of smooth muscle running between segments of this lesion. Gastric and colonic polyps had similar appearance. (Hematoxylin-eosin stain; original magnification, ×40.)

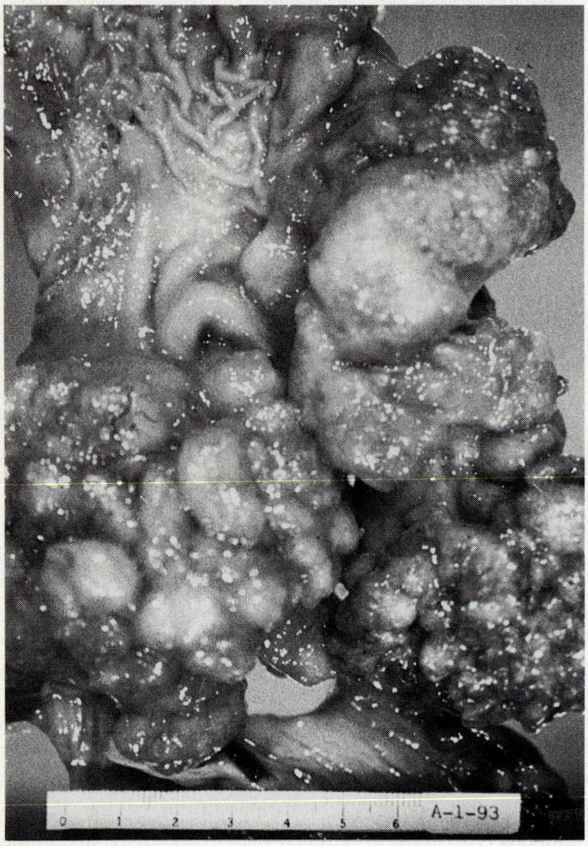

Fig. 2. Jejunum at autopsy shows typical multiple hamartomatous polyps.

inal pain, intestinal intussusception, rectal bleeding, and, more rarely, prolapse of a polyp. Symptoms usually commence in adolescence.[3]

We report an unusual case in a 1-month-old girl of generalized Peutz-Jeghers polyposis of the gastrointestinal tract.

CASE REPORT

A 2-day-old girl was admitted to our hospital because of heart failure resulting from congenital heart disease (ostium secundum atrial septal defect and persistent ductus arteriosus). The patient was the product of a normal pregnancy and delivery. Birth weight was 2490 gm. Diuretic and indomethacin therapy improved her clinical situation. When the patient was 15 days of age, intestinal obstruction was detected and diagnosed radiologically as ileocecal intussusception; it did not reduce after hydrostatic enema and required ileocecal surgical resection. At that time no polyps were found in the compromised intestine.

When the patient was 1 month of age, profuse hematemesis and rectal prolapse developed with a large polyp in its mucosa. Resection of this polyp was performed. Pathologic study showed typical features of a hamartomatous polyp. Esophagogastroscopy revealed the presence of polyps in the stomach; one in the antrum partially obstructed the lumen. At colonoscopy small polyps were observed in the rectosigmoid colon. At that time the patient weighed 2400 gm. The heart murmur had disappeared. No hyperpigmentation of the lips or oral mucosa was observed.

No polypectomies were performed because too many polyps were present to allow their complete removal. Medical treatment included parenteral nutrition, administration of H_2-blockers, and repeated blood transfusions. Enteral feeding was then gradually introduced. After slight clinical improvement, she was discharged from the hospital at 4 months of age.

Colonoscopy of the patient's parents revealed no polyps.

At 6 months of age, the patient was readmitted to the hospital because of abdominal distention, hepatomegaly, a left lower abdominal quadrant mass, and profuse bloody diarrhea. The clinical course included intestinal malabsorption, protein-losing enteropathy, and chronic diarrhea with secondary hypoalbuminemia, hypokalemia, and severe anemia. She required frequent supplementary blood transfusions, daily administration of human serum albumin, and parenteral feeding.

A barium gastrointestinal study performed when the patient was 9 months of age revealed multiple intraluminal masses of irregular surface located in the body of the stomach, duodenal bulb, and distal aspect of the duodenum. A double-contrast barium enema radiogram showed a large intraluminal polyp in the sigmoid colon. The rectal mucosa appeared nodular, characteristic of small polyps. Pathologic examination of a rectal polyp biopsy confirmed the diagnosis of Peutz-Jeghers syndrome–associated polyps. A liver biopsy was interpreted as showing reactive hepatitis and hemosiderosis.

Anasarca and hepatic encephalopathy subsequently developed, and the patient died at 12 months of age.

Histologic study of a jejunal polyp showed connective tissue containing smooth muscle fibers, which spread to the edges of the polyp. The lesion consisted of glandular lumens lined by the indigenous cells to the intestinal mucosa (Fig. 1). All the polyps examined showed similar findings. At autopsy macroscopic findings included multiple polyps, mainly in the distal part of the stomach and rectosigmoid colon. Polyps were less frequent in the small intestine (Fig. 2). The histologic findings were consistent with these observations. In the liver areas of massive centrolobular necrosis of vascular origin were observed; only the periportal areas were preserved.

DISCUSSION

Multiple polyps in the gastrointestinal tract have been classified differently according to their respective histologic characteristics, location, clinical manifestations, and any associated abnormalities. Mucocutaneous pigmentation, characteristic of Peutz-Jeghers polyposis, was absent in our patient and her relatives. These maculae may be present at birth or later in life. A search for them in the autopsy produced a negative result. Even so, not all the clinical manifestations of the syndrome are always present in the affected patients; some patients have been described who had only mucocutaneous pigmentation, and others had only intestinal polyposis.[4, 5] This case was sporadic because no family members were identified to have Peutz-Jeghers syndrome.

Among the frequent clinical manifestations of the illness are attacks of recurrent intestinal intussusception, abdominal pain, and, more rarely, diarrhea with hematemesis and melena, or a malabsorption syndrome with weight loss.[6,7] Our patient had all these symptoms and recurrent rectal prolapse in the first year of life. In a few patients these symptoms occur in infancy,[5] but more frequently the manifestations appear from puberty onward. Our experience with this patient shows that Peutz-Jeghers syndrome may become clinically apparent during the neonatal period.

REFERENCES

1. Stringer DA, ed. Pediatric gastrointestinal imaging. Philadelphia: BC Decker, 1989:434-69.
2. Dodds WJ, Schulte WJ, Hensley GT, et al. Peutz-Jeghers syndrome and gastrointestinal malignancy. AJR Am J Roentgenol 1972;115: 374-7.
3. Howell J, Pringle K, Kirschner B, et al. Peutz-Jeghers polyps causing colocolic intussusception in infancy. J Pediatr Surg 1981;16:82-4.
4. Erbe RW. Current concepts in genetics: inherited gastrointestinal polyposis syndromes. N Engl J Med 1976;294:1101-4.
5. Keating MA, Young RH, Lillehei CW, Retik AB. Hamartoma of the bladder in a 4 year old girl with hamartomatous polyps of the gastrointestinal tract. J Urol 1987;138:366-9.
6. Peri L, Falaschi F, Sbragia P, Colombo S. Sindrome di Peutz-Jeghers: descrizione de un caso. Radiol Med 1989;77:137-8.
7. Franchi M, Lopez M, Sturlese P. La malatia di Peutz-Jeghers: considerazioni a distanza sopra un caso seguito per 19 anni. Pathologica 1976;68:445-7.

FELLOWSHIPS

Fellowships available in pediatric subspecialties and those for general academic pediatric training are listed once a year, in **January,** in THE JOURNAL OF PEDIATRICS. Each **June,** forms for listing fellowships available for the academic year beginning 18 months after publication are sent to the Chairman of the Department of Pediatrics at major hospitals in the United States and Canada. In addition, **a copy of the application form appears in the July, August, and September issues** of THE JOURNAL (please use the current form). Should you desire to list fellowships, a separate application must be made *each* year for *each* position. All applications must be returned to Mosby–Year Book, Inc., by **October 15** preceding the listing year to ensure publication. Additional forms will be supplied on request from the Journal Editing Department, Mosby–Year Book, Inc., 11830 Westline Industrial Drive, St. Louis, MO 63146-3318/800-325-4177, ext. 4317, or 314-453-4317.

New books received

Essentials of critical care pharmacology. 2nd ed.
Chernow B, ed. York, Pennsylvania: Waverly, 1994. 613 pages. $59.

Pediatric orofacial medicine and pathology
Hall RK. London: Chapman & Hall Medical, 1994. 413 pages. $199.

Pediatric diagnosis
Beasley SW, Hutson JM, Myers NA. London: Chapman & Hall Medical, 1993. 392 pages. $275.

Biomaterials, medical devices, and tissue engineering: an integrated approach
Silver FH. London: Chapman & Hall Medical, 1994. 303 pages. $89.95.

Anthropometry of the head and face. 2nd ed.
Farkas LG. New York: Raven Press, 1994. 405 pages. $145.

Mother and child health. 3rd ed.
Williams CD, Baumslag N, Jelliffe DB. New York: Oxford University Press, 1994. 392 pages. $59.95/$35.

Fundamentals of pediatrics. 1st ed.
Rudolph AM, Kamei RK, eds. Norwalk, Connecticut: Appleton & Lange, 1994. 701 pages. No price listed.

Prenatal exposure to toxicants
Needleman HL, Bellinger D. Baltimore: Johns Hopkins University Press, 1994. 321 pages. $90.

Protein and energy: a study of changing ideas in nutrition
Carpenter KJ. New York: Cambridge University Press, 1994. 280 pages. $39.95.

Handbook of child behavior therapy in the psychiatric setting
Ammerman RT, Hersen M. New York: Wiley, 1994. 512 pages. $75.

Double-blind, randomized trial of one versus three prophylactic doses of synthetic surfactant in 826 neonates weighing 700 to 1100 grams: Effects on mortality rate

Anthony Corbet, MB, FRACP, Jeffrey Gerdes, MD, Walker Long, MD, Emilio Avila, MD, Asha Puri, MD, Adam Rosenberg, MD, Kathleen Edwards, MSc, Larry Cook, MD, and American Exosurf Neonatal Study Groups I and II[a]

From the Departments of Pediatrics, Emory University, Atlanta, Georgia; Pennsylvania Hospital and University of Pennsylvania, Philadelphia; University of North Carolina at Chapel Hill; Cedar Sinai Medical Center, Los Angeles, California; Children's Hospital and University of Colorado Health Sciences Center, Denver; Alaska Neonatology Associates, Anchorage; the Department of Clinical Statistics, Burroughs Wellcome Co., Research Triangle Park, North Carolina; Kosair Children's Hospital and University of Louisville, Louisville, Kentucky; and participating centers

At 33 hospitals in the United States, a double-blind, randomized clinical trial was performed to compare one versus three prophylactic doses of synthetic surfactant in 700 to 1100 gm inborn infants. All 826 infants received an initial prophylactic dose of surfactant within 30 minutes of birth. Subsequently 410 infants received two doses of placebo (air) 12 and 24 hours later, and 416 infants received two additional doses of surfactant. By the age of 28 days, 70 infants who received one dose of surfactant and 40 infants who received three doses were dead, a 43% relative reduction in the mortality rate (30 fewer deaths; *p* = 0.002). By the age of 1 year after term, 87 infants who received one dose and 62 infants who received three doses were dead: a 29% relative reduction in the mortality rate (25 fewer deaths; *p* = 0.027). Infants who received three doses of surfactant required significantly less oxygen and less mean airway pressure for the first week of life. Necrotizing enterocolitis (9 vs 25 infants; *p* = 0.005), and use of high-frequency ventilation (13 vs 26 infants; *p* = 0.037); pancuronium (43 vs 62 infants; *p* = 0.045); and leukocyte transfusions (0 vs 4 infants; *p* = 0.042) were less frequent in the three-dose group, but air leak, bronchopulmonary dysplasia, intraventricular hemorrhage, patent ductus arteriosus, pulmonary hemorrhage, and infections were not different. These results indicate that physiologic findings, mortality rates, and probably morbidity rates are improved by two additional prophylactic doses of synthetic surfactant. (J PEDIATR 1995;126:969-78)

Supported by Burroughs Wellcome Co., Research Triangle Park, N.C.

Submitted for publication Nov. 10, 1993; accepted Jan. 6, 1995.

Reprint requests: Walker Long, MD, CB 7220, Department of Pediatrics, University of North Carolina at Chapel Hill, Chapel Hill, NC 27599-7220.

[a]Members of the study groups are listed after the text.

0022-3476/95/$3.00 + 0 **9/23/63159**

Surfactant replacement is now well established in the management of respiratory distress syndrome, but several important issues remain unresolved.[1] Recently the controversial issue of prophylaxis versus rescue was decided by two large randomized trials in favor of prophylaxis.[2,3] The trial described here, reported elsewhere in preliminary form,[4] was designed to address the question of whether administration of two additional doses 12 and 24 hours after the first prophylactic dose of synthetic surfactant in infants at high risk of RDS would improve outcome.

METHODS

The trial was conducted with a common protocol at 33 hospitals in the United States. The first patient was enrolled on March 4, 1989, and the last patient was enrolled on May 28, 1990. This double-blind prophylactic trial, which used a fixed dosing schedule (the first dose was administered shortly after birth, and the second and third doses were administered 12 and 24 hours later to all infants who continued to receive mechanical ventilation at those times) originally had three treatment arms: (1) three doses of air placebo; (2) one dose of surfactant, followed by two doses of air placebo; and (3) three doses of surfactant. However, as soon as evidence became available that a single prophylactic dose of this synthetic surfactant reduced mortality in this weight class,[5] the treatment arm with three doses of air was abandoned. The 59 babies who were enrolled in the treatment arm receiving three doses of air are not considered further in this report.

BPD	Bronchopulmonary dysplasia
CI	Confidence interval
IVH	Intraventricular hemorrhage
NEC	Necrotizing enterocolitis
PDA	Patent ductus arteriosus
Po_2	Oxygen pressure
RDS	Respiratory distress syndrome

Hypothesis. The hypothesis for this trial was that two additional prophylactic doses of surfactant at 12-hour intervals after the first dose in 700 to 1100 gm infants would improve neonatal survival rates. Stated more formally, the trial was designed to reject the null hypothesis that the overall neonatal mortality rate was not different for 700 to 1100 gm infants receiving one and three prophylactic doses of synthetic surfactant.

Surfactant preparation. The surfactant used in the trial—dipalmitoyl phosphatidylcholine, cetyl alcohol, and tyloxapol (Exosurf Neonatal, Burroughs Wellcome Co., Research Triangle Park, N.C.)—is a totally synthetic surfactant, invented by Clements at the University of California, that has been formulated with sodium chloride as a lyophilized powder.[6-8] The material is vacuum packaged in 10 ml glass vials and stored at room temperature; immediately before use, 8 ml sterile, preservative-free water is added to the vial.[8] The resulting suspension contains dipalmitoyl phosphatidylcholine, 13.5 mg/ml, hexadecanol, 1.5 mg/ml, and tyloxapol, 1.0 mg/ml, in 0.1N sodium chloride.

Trial mechanics. Methods of patient recruitment, masking, dosing, and data collection, and inclusion and exclusion criteria and definitions of all outcomes, were identical to those reported previously in a double-blind trial of a single prophylactic dose of synthetic surfactant versus air placebo conducted in 446 infants.[5] One difference was that the first dose of surfactant was administered openly in this trial, whereas the first (and only) dose of synthetic surfactant or air placebo was administered in a double-masked fashion in the previous trial. Masking was maintained for the second and third doses of synthetic surfactant or air placebo throughout this trial.

Outcome measures. The principal efficacy outcome measure of the trial was prospectively designated as the overall mortality rate at 28 days of age. Secondary measures of efficacy were incidence of bronchopulmonary dysplasia, survival through 28 days without BPD, incidence of RDS, severity of RDS, and incidence of death resulting from RDS. All other outcome variables were considered safety measures.

Definitions of key outcomes. Intraventricular hemorrhage, patent ductus arteriosus, RDS, BPD, transient tachypnea of the newborn, and congenital pneumonia were defined and evaluated as described for the previous trial.[5] The criteria for the diagnosis of RDS and BPD are reiterated here for the convenience of the reader: RDS was diagnosed at 7 days of age by review of the hospital course. Infants who died at less than 12 hours were considered to have RDS if autopsy confirmed the diagnosis or, in the absence of autopsy, if death was attributed to RDS by the masked attending neonatologist. For those alive at 12 hours, all the following criteria had to be met for diagnosis of RDS: (1) 30% oxygen or more required to maintain an arterial oxygen pressure of 50 mm Hg after the age of 12 hours, (2) mean airway pressure of 6 cm H_2O or more required after the age of 12 hours, (3) chest radiograph at age 24 hours considered by the attending physician to be consistent with RDS, and (4) after complete evaluation of the neonatal course the lung disease not attributable to another cause.

In surviving infants the diagnosis of BPD was made at 28 days of age by the following criteria: (1) presence of tachypnea and retractions, (2) need for supplemental oxygen to maintain the skin surface oxygen pressure at less than 60 mm Hg or the pulse oximeter reading at more than 80% saturation, and (3) chest radiographic abnormalities rating a score of 4 or more by the Edwards classification.[9]

Among infants who died and had autopsies, BPD was diagnosed by the histologic criteria of Bonikos et al.[10] If infants died between 10 and 28 days and did not have an autopsy, BPD was diagnosed if, at the time of death, they required more than 60% oxygen and 7 cm H_2O mean airway pressure, they had persistently abnormal chest radiographs, and there was no other explanation for respiratory failure.

Follow-up phase. All infants were followed throughout their hospital course. After the patients' discharge from the hospital, contact was maintained by correspondence, by telephone, and by appointment to the outpatient clinics until the age of 1 year after term. At this time, pertinent information with regard to hospital admissions, surgical operations, oxygen and ventilator use, and retinal examinations was obtained, and a complete physical examination and neurodevelopmental assessment were performed. Hospital charges through the first year of life were also collected. These results of follow-up will be reported separately, except for the survival data, which are included in the present report.

Causes of death. If a death occurred, the primary cause was determined by a masked investigator who took into account the clinical history. For patients who died and had autopsies, the cause of death, as determined by postmortem examination, was substituted for the clinically determined cause of death in the tabulations.

Sample size. When the trial was originally designed, it was calculated that 768 infants, one third in each group, would be required to provide a 90% chance of detecting a 20% change in the incidence of survival without BPD between the one-dose group and air placebo group, and between the three-dose group and the one-dose group.[11] However, when the initial multicenter prophylactic trial of synthetic surfactant in this weight class demonstrated a 39% relative reduction in the neonatal mortality rate after a single dose (from an absolute rate of 19.8% in the placebo group to an absolute rate of 12.0% in the single prophylactic dose group[5]), the present trial was formally amended to abandon the arm with three doses of air, and to change the hypothesis to a further reduction in the neonatal mortality rate with two additional prophylactic doses of synthetic surfactant. The sample size was not changed; the target of 768 patients was estimated to provide 90% power to detect an additional relative reduction in the neonatal mortality rate of 33% (from an expected absolute neonatal mortality rate of 12% with one dose to a projected 8% absolute neonatal mortality rate with three doses).

Stopping rules. An independent advisory panel monitored conduct of the trial and was empowered to stop the trial for safety but not for efficacy. The panel reviewed masked data from the trial at 6-month intervals and was empowered to unmask the trial if a statistically significant difference in severe IVH (grade III or periventricular echodensities or both) occurred in the two groups, and to stop the trial if the excess in severe IVH occurred in the three-dose group. Early stopping for reduction in the neonatal mortality rate was not part of the trial's design because of convictions that (1) some outcomes of premature infants are worse than death, (2) apparent reductions in the mortality rate during the neonatal period may not be maintained subsequently, and (3) completion of the targeted sample size of 768 patients was critically important for evaluation of safety and efficacy.

Statistical methods

Efficacy end points. The protocol specified two analyses of the principal efficacy end point—the overall mortality rate through 28 days: (1) an intention-to-treat analysis, with all patients grouped as originally randomly selected regardless of treatment and (2) a supplemental analysis in which all patients were grouped as actually treated (one dose vs more than one dose) but from which patients who had unrecognized congenital pneumonia or unrecognized major anomalies at the time of randomization were excluded. The other major efficacy end points of BPD and survival without BPD were analyzed similarly. All secondary efficacy end points (including incidence of RDS, death resulting from RDS, and severity of RDS [as assessed by gas exchange and ventilatory requirements]) were analyzed as actually treated without any exclusions.

Safety end points. All safety end points were analyzed as actually treated without any exclusions.

Statistical tests. Incidence comparisons were made with the Cochran-Mantel-Haenszel test and controlled for the four randomization strata[12]; in addition, relative risks and 95% confidence intervals based on the Cochran-Mantel-Haenszel test were calculated.[13] Gas exchange and ventilatory support data were compared by *t* tests on the area under the curve for the entire first week of life. "Time to first event" comparisons were made and survival was displayed graphically with Kaplan-Meier techniques. All tests were two tailed and differences were considered significant at a p value less than 0.05.

RESULTS

The independent advisory panel reviewed interim data from the trial three times, and on each occasion recommended that the trial continue. During the period of enrollment 1687 infants who were eligible by weight were born at the 33 participating hospitals. Of these, 801 were not enrolled for the reasons given in Table I. Of the 886 enrolled patients, 59 patients were randomly assigned to receive three doses of air (before that arm was abandoned), 412 were randomly assigned to receive one dose of surfactant, and 415 were randomly assigned to receive three doses of surfactant.

Ten infants did not receive the treatment allocated by the randomization procedure. One patient randomly assigned to the one-dose group received nothing, and another four received more than one dose. Five patients randomly assigned to the three-dose group did not receive more than one dose despite continuing artificial ventilation for at least 13 hours after the first dose. The other 876 patients received the treatment assigned.

The randomization procedure was successful in that the infants who received one and three doses of surfactant were comparable in terms of their demographic, physical, and clinical features (Table II).

Table I. Derivation of population enrolled in trial

	No.	%
Infants eligible by birth weight	1687	100
Not enrolled: Legitimate reasons		
Consent refused	39	2
Failure to meet prenatal inclusion/exclusion	188	11
Failure to meet postnatal inclusion/exclusion	58	3
Outborn	228	14
Total not enrolled for legitimate reasons	513	30
Not enrolled: Other reasons		
Missed/precipitous delivery	273	16
Too unstable to randomly assign at birth	15	1
Total not enrolled for other reasons	288	17
Enrolled and randomly assigned	886	53
TOTAL	1687	100

Infants treated with three doses of surfactant required significantly less oxygen and mean airway pressure, and had significantly lower arterial/alveolar Po_2 ratios for the first week of life than infants treated with only one dose (Fig. 1). In both groups, among survivors, the median time to permanent removal from all forms of ventilatory support, including constant positive airway pressure and supplemental oxygen, was 24 days.

Effects on mortality rates. In the intention-to-treat analysis, 70 infants in the one-dose group and 40 infants in the three-dose group died during the neonatal period; the relative reduction in the neonatal mortality rate was 43% (absolute mortality rate, 17% vs 12%; $p = 0.002$). Similarly, in the intention-to-treat analysis at 1 year after term, 87 infants died in the one-dose group and 62 infants died in the three-dose group; the relative reduction in the mortality rate was 29% (absolute mortality rate, 21% vs 15%; $p = 0.027$). Differences in neonatal survival were maintained through 1 year after term, as displayed graphically in Fig. 2. The supplemental analysis confirmed these results (data not shown).

Effects on BPD, other complications of prematurity, and RDS. The incidence of BPD (relative risk, 1.21; 95% CI, 0.84 to 1.76); the incidence of the combined outcome, death or BPD (relative risk, 0.87; 95% CI, 0.68 to 1.10); and the incidence of survival without BPD were not changed by treatment with two additional prophylactic doses of synthetic surfactant in either the intention-to-treat analysis (Table III) or in the supplemental analysis (data not shown).

Other complications of prematurity and RDS were also largely unchanged by treatment with two additional doses of synthetic surfactant. However, a significant reduction in the incidence of necrotizing enterocolitis was observed in the three-dose group (9 vs 25 infants, $p = 0.005$) (Table IV). In addition, infants treated with three doses of surfactant required use of high-frequency ventilation (13 vs 26 infants, $p = 0.037$), pancuronium (43 vs 62 infants, $p = 0.045$) and leukocyte transfusions (zero vs four infants, $p = 0.042$) significantly less frequently than infants treated with only one dose of surfactant (Table V). Other measures of morbidity were not different.

Table II. Characteristics of enrolled infants

	One dose (n = 410)	Three doses (n = 416)
Birth weight (gm)*	898 ± 121	906 ± 128
Gestational age (wk)*	27.0 ± 1.7	27.1 ± 1.8
No. (%) of infants		
Race		
White	207 (50)	232 (56)
Black	159 (39)	139 (33)
Hispanic	20 (5)	26 (7)
Other	24 (6)	19 (5)
Gender		
M	228 (56)	235 (56)
F	182 (44)	181 (44)
Delivery		
Abdominal	233 (57)	246 (59)
Vaginal	177 (43)	170 (41)
Multiple gestation	76 (19)	83 (20)
Labor present	303 (74)	301 (72)
Tocolytic therapy	186 (45)	183 (44)
Prenatal steroids given >24 hr before delivery	86 (21)	92 (22)
Apgar score at 1 min (median)	4	4
Apgar score at 5 min (median)	7	7

*Expressed as mean ± SD.

Causes of death. Deaths during the neonatal period are listed in Table VI. The differences in the one-dose and three-dose groups in death resulting from NEC (zero vs seven infants, $p < 0.001$) and in death resulting from pulmonary hemorrhage (five vs one infant, $p < 0.05$) were statistically significant. Although neonatal deaths resulting from BPD were equivalent in the two groups (zero vs two infants) (Table VI), fewer babies in the three-dose group who died in the first 28 days of life died with BPD (two vs seven infants) (Table III).

The numbers of deaths after the neonatal period (29 days to 1 year after term), accounting for 26% of the total mortality rate in the study, were not different in the two groups; the only significant difference in postneonatal deaths was that more infants died of BPD after 28 days of age in the three-dose group (one vs eight infants, $p < 0.01$) (Table VI).

DISCUSSION

The trial we conducted is the second-largest double-masked randomized clinical trial of synthetic surfactant replacement reported to date; the largest such trial was a placebo-controlled rescue trial in which 1237 infants were enrolled.[14] The question addressed in our current trial was whether two additional doses at 12-hour intervals could further improve the neonatal mortality rate in 700 to 1100 gm infants who receive a single prophylactic dose of synthetic surfactant at birth. The 43% relative reduction in the neonatal mortality rate and 29% relative reduction in the mortality rate at 1 year after term observed in the three-dose group provide strong evidence that the survival of babies treated prophylacticaly with synthetic surfactant can be improved by repeated "prophylactic" dosing 12 and again 24 hours after the first dose in infants who continue to receive artificial ventilation.

Except in trials with large samples,[5] very large single doses of surfactant,[15] high mortality rates in the control group,[15, 16] or very large reductions in the mortality rate in the treated group,[17] single doses of a variety of surfactants have failed to improve survival rates in most trials.[18-23] In contrast, randomized placebo-controlled trials of more than one dose of surfactant have consistently shown reductions in overall mortality rate, regardless of the type of surfactant used.[14, 24-28] However, the optimal schedule for redosing may vary for the different surfactants, because both the chemical composition and the amount of phospholipid contained per dose vary substantially.

Redosing in our trial was based on continued access to the airway (i.e., infants who continue intubation and artificial ventilation were given additional doses). This approach has the appeal of redosing at a time when the benefits of the first dose have not yet begun to wear off and most infants are doing well. In our trial the second and third doses not only reduced the mortality rate but also accelerated physiologic recovery, at least as judged from the improved gas exchange and ventilator settings during the first week of life in the three-dose group. One other trial also compared one and three doses of surfactant given at 12-hour intervals on the basis of continued access to the airway.[29] The surfactant used in that trial was porcine, the trial was not masked, and redosing was studied in infants who had established RDS (i.e., it was a rescue study, not a prophylaxis study). Despite these differences, that trial also showed improved physiologic measurements and reduced the mortality rate in the three-dose group. One difference in the two trials was that three doses of porcine surfactant, unlike three doses of synthetic surfactant, reduced the incidence of pneumothorax further. However, given the 12.6% incidence of pneumothorax in the one-dose group in our trial, it would have taken a sample size many times larger to have documented that the 9% lower rate of pneumothorax observed in the three-dose group was significant.

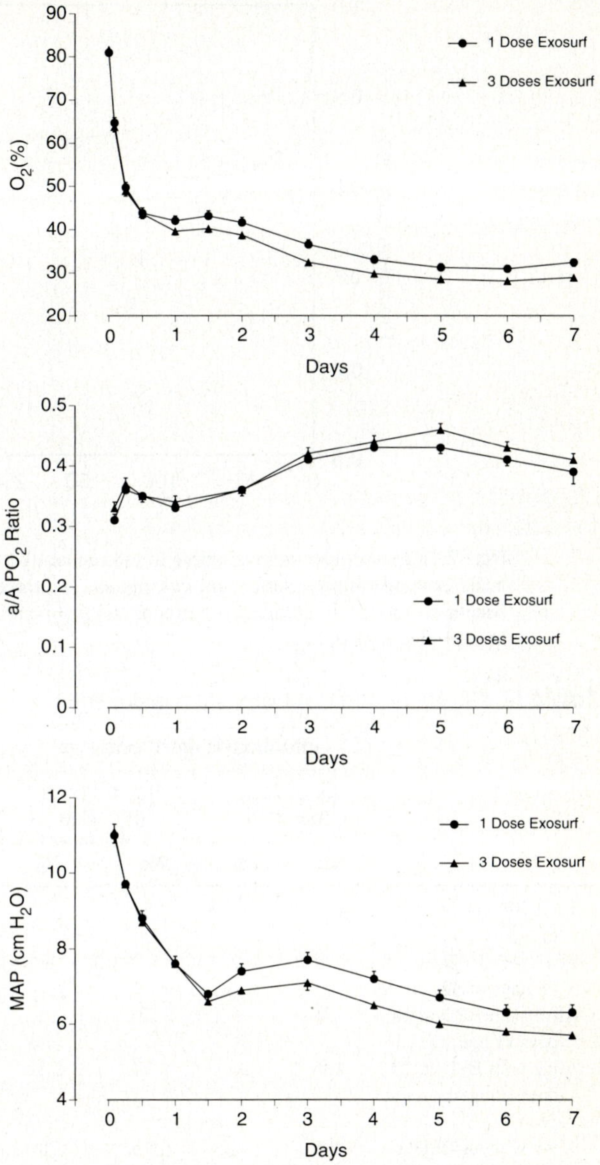

Fig. 1. Inspired oxygen concentration *(O_2)*, alveolar-arterial oxygen tension gradient *(A-a Po_2)*, and mean airway pressure *(MAP)* for enrolled infants through day 7 of life. For infants who died during this time, values are included until event. *Circles*, one dose of synthetic surfactant followed by two doses of air placebo (n = 410); *triangles*, three doses of synthetic surfactant (n = 416). Values represent means ± SEM and were compared by *t* tests on areas under curve during entire first 7 days of life for three groups. Differences during first 7 days of life are significant for both groups for all three measurements ($p < 0.005$).

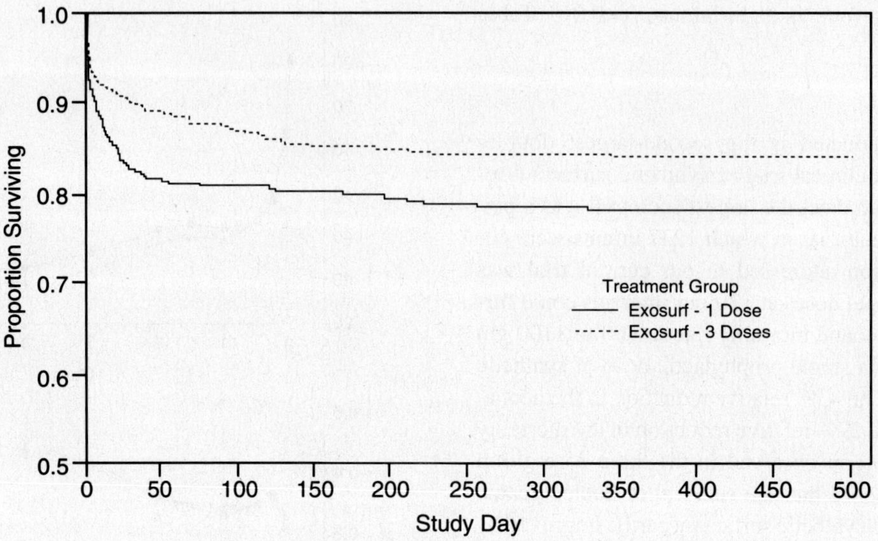

Fig. 2. Kaplan-Meier survival curve for all randomly assigned infants through 1 year after term. *Solid line*, One prophylactic dose of synthetic surfactant; *interrupted line*, three prophylactic doses of synthetic surfactant. Most of the survival benefit accrued early in three dose group, and that benefit was maintained through 1 year after term ($p = 0.027$, Cochran-Mantel-Haenszel test).

Table III. Effects on BPD and survival without BPD

	Intention-to-treat analysis			
	One dose (n = 412)		Three doses (n = 415)	
	No.	%	No.	%
Total BPD at 28 days of age	43	10	52	13
Dead with BPD by 28 days of age	7	2	2	1
Alive with BPD at 28 days of age	36	9	50	12
Alive with BPD at 28 days of age or dead	106	26	90	22
Alive without BPD at 28 days of age	306	74	325	78

Other investigators have also studied the optimal number of doses for prophylactic treatment of RDS with synthetic surfactant. In the OSIRIS trial, a large randomized comparison of two versus up to four doses of synthetic surfactant for both prophylactic and rescue use, no benefits were documented with the additional doses for either prophylaxis or rescue, but neither were deleterious effects seen.[2] However, that trial included babies in the prophylaxis arm who were far larger than those in our trial. In any case, it seems doubtful that additional benefit accrues with more than three doses, on the basis of the OSIRIS results[2] and the preliminary results from a trial of three versus up to six doses we conducted in 500 to 750 gm infants.[30]

The gains in the neonatal survival rate in the group receiving three prophylactic doses of synthetic surfactant not only were maintained through at least 1 year after term but also were not exacted at the price of excess morbidity. Most major safety outcomes such as air leak, BPD, IVH, PDA, sepsis, and pulmonary hemorrhage were not significantly different in the two groups. Indeed, morbidity was somewhat less in the three-dose group: reductions in NEC and in use of high-frequency ventilation, pancuronium, and leukocyte transfusions were observed in the three-dose group.

Bronchopulmonary dysplasia was not reduced by two additional prophylactic doses of synthetic surfactant in our trial, as was also true for two additional rescue doses of porcine surfactant.[29] Both these observations are consistent with recently published metaanalyses that demonstrate no changes in the incidence of BPD after prophylactic use of synthetic surfactant,[31-33] and no changes in the incidence of BPD after both prophylactic and rescue use of mammalian surfactants. One possible explanation for the failure of prophylactic use of both types of surfactant to reduce BPD is that prophylaxis saves the lives of infants who cannot be saved with rescue therapy,[1, 2, 34] and these extra survivors are at increased risk of BPD. The fact that rescue use of synthetic surfactant reduces both the incidence[31-33] and severity[33, 35] of BPD, whereas rescue use of mammalian surfactants does not, remains unexplained, but the definition of BPD in the trials of synthetic surfactant required moderate to severe radiographic abnormalities.

In previous placebo-controlled prophylactic and rescue trials of this same synthetic surfactant, we have consistently observed significant reductions in death resulting from

Table IV. Complications of prematurity

	No. (%) of patients		
	One dose (n = 410)	Three doses (n = 416)	Relative risk (95% CI)
RDS	263 (64)	278 (67)	1.03 (0.94-1.13)
Congenital pneumonia	5 (1)	6 (1)	1.19 (0.66-3.85)
Nosocomial pneumonia	54 (13)	64 (15)	1.17 (0.84-1.63)
Nonpulmonary infections	138 (34)	138 (33)	0.98 (0.81-1.19)
Sepsis	120 (29)	110 (26)	0.91 (0.73-1.13)
Meningitis	4 (1)	7 (2)	1.70 (0.53-5.50)
Pulmonary air leak	123 (30)	108 (27)	0.88 (0.71-1.09)
Pneumothorax	58 (14)	48 (12)	0.84 (0.59-1.19)
Pneumomediastinum	12 (3)	10 (2)	0.85 (0.37-1.93)
Pulmonary interstitial emphysema	99 (24)	91 (22)	0.92 (0.72-1.18)
IVH	126 (31)	128 (31)	0.99 (0.82-1.21)
Grade III IVH	32 (8)	24 (6)	0.74 (0.45-1.22)
PVED	36 (9)	28 (7)	0.76 (0.47-1.21)
Grade III IVH or PVED	42 (10)	35 (8)	0.81 (0.53-1.24)
Seizures	30 (7)	22 (5)	0.74 (0.44-1.26)
Hypotension	218 (53)	208 (50)	0.95 (0.83-1.08)
PDA	234 (57)	241 (58)	1.01 (0.90-1.14)
NEC	25 (6)	9 (2)	0.36 (0.18-0.74)*
Pulmonary hemorrhage	19 (5)	24 (6)	1.28 (0.72-2.28)
Apnea of prematurity	254 (67)	281 (68)	1.08 (0.98-1.19)

Relative risk <1 indicates decreased risk with three doses.
PVED, Periventricular echodensities.
*For a reduction in NEC in three-dose group, $p = 0.005$.

Table V. Other outcomes

	No. (%) of patients		
	One dose (n = 410)	Three doses (n = 416)	Relative risk (95% CI)
HFV	26 (6)	13 (3)	0.51 (0.27-0.96)*
Drug use			
Pancuronium	62 (15)	43 (10)	0.69 (0.48-0.99)†
Methylxanthines	313 (76)	339 (81)	1.06 (0.99-1.14)
Tolazoline	8 (2)	3 (1)	0.39 (0.11-1.37)
Exchange transfusions	11 (3)	4 (1)	0.37 (0.12-1.09)
Erythrocyte transfusion‡	59 (14)	54 (13)	0.91 (0.65-1.28)
Leukocyte transfusion	4 (1)	0 (0)	0 (not calculated)§
Reduction in [glucose]‖	165 (40)	142 (35)	0.85 (0.71-1.01)
K administration¶	21 (5)	14 (3)	0.67 (0.35-1.28)
K restriction#	26 (6)	40 (10)	1.55 (0.97-2.48)

Relative risk <1 indicates decreased risk with three doses.
HFV, High-frequency ventilation.
*For less frequent use of high-frequency ventilation in the three-dose group, $p = 0.037$.
†For less frequent use of pancuronium in the three-dose group, $p = 0.045$.
‡Erythrocyte transfusions for documented anemia or hypotension, not for blood loss.
§For less frequent use of leukocyte transfusions in the three dose group, $p = 0.042$.
‖Reduction intravenous fluid glucose concentration because of hyperglycemia.
¶Increase in intravenous fluid potassium concentration because of hypokalemia.
#Decrease in intravenous fluid potassium concentration because of hyperkalemia.

RDS[5, 14, 17, 22, 23, 26] and from air leak[5, 14, 26] during the neonatal period. After the neonatal period we have also observed significant reductions in deaths resulting from BPD.[5, 14, 26] In the current trial death resulting from NEC during the neonatal period was significantly reduced in the three-dose group, and death from pulmonary hemorrhage was significantly increased (although the incidence of pulmonary hemorrhage was not significantly different in the two groups). Differ-

Table VI. Primary causes of death

Cause of death	No. (%) of patients	
	One dose (n = 410)	Three doses (n = 416)
Deaths during first 28 days of life		
RDS	14 (3)	8 (2)
IVH/PVED	11 (3)	4 (1)
Pulmonary air leaks	7 (2)	3 (1)
BPD	0 (0)	2 (1)
Sepsis	11 (3)	7 (2)
NEC	7 (2)	0* (0)
Pulmonary hypoplasia	6 (1)	2 (1)
Pulmonary hemorrhage	1 ((1)	5† (1)
Other	13 (3)	9 (2)
TOTAL	70 (17)	40 (10)
Deaths 29 days to 1 yr after term		
IVH	2 (1)	0 (0)
BPD	1 ((1)	8‡ (2)
Sepsis	2 (1)	4 (1)
NEC	5 (1)	3 (1)
Sudden infant death syndrome	2 (1)	3 (1)
Other	5 (1)	5 (1)
TOTAL	17 (4)	23 (6)

PVED, Periventricular echodensities.
*Compared with one dose; $p < 0.001$.
†Compared with one dose; $p < 0.05$.
‡Compared with one dose; $p < 0.01$.

ences in the causes of death were also observed after the neonatal period. Significantly more infants in the three-dose group died of BPD between 29 days and 1 year after term, although the overall mortality rate during follow-up was not different in the one-dose and three-dose groups.

We believe that the explanation for the excess neonatal deaths resulting from pulmonary hemorrhage and late deaths from BPD in the three-dose group may lie in the fact that the two additional prophylactic doses of synthetic surfactant save lives. If the extra survivors in the three-dose group are a high-risk group and if they are no longer dying of RDS, IVH, or air leak during the neonatal period, it would not be unexpected that more of them might die of the complications that arise from either recovering too quickly after receiving surfactant (pulmonary hemorrhage) or not recovering fully (BPD). In the case of excess late deaths resulting from BPD, the reverse was observed: during the neonatal period two babies in the three-dose group and seven babies in the one-dose group died of BPD.

The incidence of RDS was not reduced with three doses of synthetic surfactant in our present trial but was reduced after multiple doses of a modified bovine surfactant.[27] A reduction in the incidence of RDS has been observed with prophylactic use of synthetic surfactant in only two trials, one in which the definition of RDS was the same as in this trial,[22] and another (a double-masked, randomized European trial comparing prophylactic and rescue treatment) in which RDS was defined by an alveolar-arterial Po_2 ratio less than 0.22 after 2 hours of age in infants receiving mechanically ventilation.[36] Thus, prevention of RDS may be a benefit more consistently demonstrable with mammalian surfactants. The failure of prophylactic administration of this synthetic surfactant to reduce the incidence of RDS,[33] despite reductions in both the severity of RDS and death from RDS,[5, 17, 22, 23, 37] remains unexplained; the explanation could have something to do with both less severe criteria for diagnosis of RDS and a more rapid onset of action of protein-containing surfactants. The ultimate importance of preventing RDS also remains unclear, because the reductions in overall mortality with prophylactic use of the two types of surfactant are the same.[31, 33] In any case, the severity of RDS was improved in the three-dose group in our current trial.

This trial had insufficient power to study the effects of three doses on pulmonary hemorrhage. The explanation we favor for the higher rates of clinical pulmonary hemorrhage observed after use of surfactant is hemorrhagic pulmonary edema. Surfactant improves ventilation and reduces pulmonary vascular resistance in infants with RDS; the ductus is patent in the first days of life in virtually all infants with RDS,[38] and the net result is increased systemic-to-pulmonary shunt through the PDA.[39, 40] Many investigators believe that early closure of the ductus may prevent the increase in clinical pulmonary hemorrhage associated with surfactant replacement, but this hypothesis remains unproved.

We conclude that three prophylactic doses of synthetic surfactant, given at 12-hour intervals starting soon after birth, produced significant reductions in the severity of RDS and in the morbidity and mortality rates in small premature infants, compared with similar treatment with only one dose at birth.

We thank the parents of the participating infants for permitting their children to enroll and thereby help answer the question the trial was designed to address. We also thank the clinical and research staffs of each participating institution and the clinical research, clinical data processing, and clinical statistics staffs at Burroughs Wellcome Co., Research Triangle Park, N.C.

Members of *American Exosurf Neonatal Study Group I* are David Stevenson, MD, Stanford University Medical Center, Palo Alto, Calif.; Steven Goldman, MD, Children's Hospital of San Francisco, San Francisco, Calif.; Frans Walther, MD, Women's Hospital, University of Southern California, Los Angeles; Stephen Boros, MD, and Mark Mammel, MD, Children's Hospital of St. Paul, St. Paul, Minn.; Theodore Thompson, MD, University of Minnesota, Minneapolis; Richard Bucciarelli, MD, and David Burchfield, MD, University of Florida, Gainesville; Anthony Corbet, MB, FRACP, Baylor College of Medicine, Houston, Tex; Martha Mullett, MD, West Virginia University Medical Center, Morgantown; Robert Cotton, MD, and Hakan Sundell, MD, Vanderbilt University Medical Center, Nashville, Tenn.; Ross Vaughn, MD, Wake Area Health Education Center, Raleigh, N.C.; Michael LeBlanc, MD, University of Mississippi Medical Center, Jackson; Carl Bose, MD, University of North Carolina at Chapel Hill; Donnal Walter, MD, Arkansas Children's Hospital, Little Rock; Thomas Pauley, MD, Albert Chandler Medical Center, University of Kentucky, Lexington; Robert Schumacher, MD, C. S. Mott Children's Hospital, University of Michigan, Ann Arbor; Alice Gong, MD, Santa Rosa Hospital, University of Texas Health Sciences Center, San Antonio; Matthew Sell, MD, St. Luke's Regional Medical Center, Boise, Idaho; Sherry Courtney, MD, The Children's Medical Center, Wright State University, Dayton, Ohio; Jeffrey Gerdes, MD, Pennsylvania Hospital, University of Pennsylvania, Philadelphia; Douglas Derleth, MD, Mayo Medical Center, Rochester, Minn.; Endla Anday, MD, Hospital of the University of Pennsylvania, Philadelphia; and Frank Volberg, MD, Bowman Gray School of Medicine, Wake Forest University, Winston Salem, N.C.

Members of *American Exosurf Neonatal Study Group II* are David Easa, MD, Kapiolani Women and Children's Medical Center, University of Hawaii, Honolulu; Arun Pramanik, MD, Louisiana State University Medical Center, Shreveport; R. Dhanireddy, MD, Georgetown University Medical Center, Washington, D.C.; Emilio Avila, MD, Alaska Neonatal Association, Anchorage; Arthur Kopelman, MD, and John Wimmer, MD, Pitt Memorial Hospital, East Carolina University School of Medicine, Greenville, N.C.; David Berry, MD, Forsyth Memorial Hospital, Bowman Gray School of Medicine, Wake Forest University, Winston Salem, N.C.; Keith Kanarek, MD, Tampa General Hospital, University of South Florida, Tampa; Larry Cook, MD, Kosair Children's Hospital and Humana Hospital, University of Louisville, Louisville, Ky.; Asha Puri, MD, Cedar Sinai Medical Center, Los Angeles, Calif.; Dona S. Buchter, MD, Grady Memorial Hospital, Emory University School of Medicine, Atlanta, Ga.; Robert Jarrett, DO, Tripler Army Medical Center, Honolulu, Hawaii; Frank Volberg, MD, Bowman Gray School of Medicine, Wake Forest University, Winston Salem, N.C.

REFERENCES

1. Merritt TA, Soll RF, Hallman M. Overview of exogenous surfactant replacement therapy. J Intensive Care Med 1993;8:205-28.
2. The OSIRIS Collaborative Group. Early versus delayed neonatal administration of synthetic surfactant: the judgment of OSIRIS. Lancet 1992;340:1363-9.
3. Kattwinkel J, Bloom BT, Delmue P, et al. Prophylactic administration of calf lung surfactant extract is more effective than early treatment of respiratory distress syndrome in newborns of 29 through 32 weeks gestation. Pediatrics 1993; 92:90-8.
4. Gerdes J, Cook L, Beaumont E, Corbet A, Long W, and the U.S. Exosurf Neonatal Study Groups I and II. Effects of three vs one prophylactic doses of Exosurf Neonatal in 700-1100 gram infants [Abstract]. Pediatr Res 1991;29:214A.
5. Corbet A, Bucciarelli R, Goldman S. Decreased mortality in small premature infants treated at birth with a single dose of synthetic surfactant: a multi-center controlled trial. J PEDIATR 1991;118:277-84.
6. Durand DJ, Clyman RI, Heymann MA, et al. Effects of a protein-free synthetic surfactant on the survival and pulmonary function of preterm lambs. J PEDIATR 1985;107:775-80.
7. Tooley WH, Clements JA, Muramatsu K, Brown CL, Schlueter MA. Lung function in prematurely delivered rabbits treated with a synthetic surfactant. Am Rev Resp Dis 1987;136:651-6.
8. Long WA, Sanders RL. New treatment methods in idiopathic respiratory distress syndrome: replacement of surface active material. Clin Crit Care Med 1988;13:21-56.
9. Edwards DK. Radiology of hyaline membrane disease, transient tachypnea of the newborn, and bronchopulmonary dysplasia. In: Farrell PM, ed. Lung development: biological and clinical perspectives; vol 2. New York: Academic Press, 1982: 47-89.
10. Bonikos DS, Bensch KG, Northway WH, et al. Bronchopulmonary dysplasia: the pulmonary pathologic sequel of necrotizing bronchiolitis and pulmonary fibrosis. Hum Pathol 1976; 7:643-66.
11. Friedman LM, Furberg CD, DeMets DL. Fundamentals of clinical trials. Littleton, Mass: PSF, 1985:83-107.
12. Fleiss JL. Statistical methods for rates and proportions. New York: John Wiley & Sons, 1981:160-87.
13. Dixon WJ, Massey F. Introduction to statistical analysis. New York: McGraw-Hill, 1969:222-236.
14. Long WA, Corbet AJ, Cotton R, et al. A controlled trial of synthetic surfactant in infants weighing 1250g or more with respiratory distress syndrome. N Engl J Med 1991;325:1696-703.
15. Collaborative European Multicenter Study Group. Surfactant replacement therapy for severe neonatal respiratory distress syndrome: an international randomized clinical trial. Pediatrics 1988;82:683-91.
16. Fujiwara T, Onishi M, Nanby H, et al. Surfactant supplemen-

tation treatment of neonatal respiratory distress syndrome (RDS): results of a multifacility cooperative comparative control trial. Shonika Rinsho 1987;40:549-68.

17. Corbet AJ, Long WA, Murphy DJ, Garcia-Prats JA, Lombardy LR, Wold DE. Reduced mortality in small premature infants treated at birth with a single dose of synthetic surfactant. J Paediatr Child Health 1991;27:245-9
18. Hallman M, Merritt TA, Jarvenpaa A-L, et al. Exogenous human surfactant for treatment of severe respiratory distress syndrome: a randomized clinical trial. J PEDIATR 1985;106: 963-9.
19. Horbar JD, Soll RF, Schachinger H, et al. A European multicenter randomized controlled trial of single dose surfactant therapy for idiopathic respiratory distress syndrome. Eur J Pediatr 1990;149:416-23.
20. Soll RF, Hoekstra RE, Fangman JJ et al. Multicenter trial of single dose modified bovine surfactant extract (Survanta) for prevention of respiratory distress syndrome. Pediatrics 1990;85: 1092-102.
21. Horbar JD, Soll RF, Sutherland JM, et al. A multicenter placebo-controlled randomized trial of surfactant therapy for respiratory distress syndrome. N Engl J Med 1989;320:959-65.
22. Bose C, Corbet A, Bose G, et al. Improved outcome at 28 days of very low birth weight infants treated with a single dose of synthetic surfactant. J PEDIATR 1990;117:947-53.
23. Stevenson D, Walther F, Long W, et al. Controlled trial of a single dose of synthetic surfactant at birth in premature infants weighing 500 to 699 grams. J PEDIATR 1992;120(suppl):3-12.
24. Merritt TA, Hallman M, Bloom BT, et al. Prophylactic treatment of very premature infants with human surfactant. N Engl J Med 1986;315:785-90.
25. Ten Centre Study Group. Ten centre trial of artificial surfactant (artificial lung expanding compound) in very premature babies. Br Med J 1987;294:991-6.
26. Long WA, Thompson T, Sundell H, Schumacher R, Volberg F, Guthrie R. Effects of two rescue doses of a synthetic surfactant on mortality in 700-1500 gram infants with RDS. J PEDIATR 1991;118:595-605.
27. Hoekstra RE, Jackson JC, Myers TF, et al. Improved neonatal survival following multiple doses of bovine surfactant in very premature infants at risk for respiratory distress syndrome. Pediatrics 1991;88:10-8.
28. Liechty EA, Donovan E, Purohit D, et al. Reduction of neonatal mortality after multiple doses of bovine surfactant in low birth weight neonates with respiratory distress syndrome. Pediatrics 1991;88:19-28.
29. Speer CP, Robertson B, Curostedt T, et al. Randomized European multicenter trial of surfactant replacement for severe neonatal respiratory distress syndrome: single versus multiple doses of Curosurf. Pediatrics 1992;89:13-20.
30. Long WA, Merritt A, Kanto W, et al. Randomized comparison of three vs six doses of synthetic surfactant in 348 infants weighing ⟨750 grams [Abstract]. Pediatr Res 1992;31:314A.
31. Jobe AH. Pulmonary surfactant therapy. N Engl J Med 1993; 328:861-8.
32. Mercier CE, Soll RF. Clinical trials of natural surfactant extract in respiratory distress syndrome. Clin Perinatol 1993; 20:711-36.
33. Long WA. Synthetic surfactant. Semin Perinatol 1993;17:275-84.
34. Kendig J, Notter RH, Cox C, et al. A comparison of surfactant as immediate prophylaxis and as rescue therapy in newborns of less than 30 weeks gestation. N Engl J Med 1991; 324:865-71.
35. Corbet A. Clinical trials of synthetic surfactant in the respiratory distress syndrome of premature infants. Clin Perinatol 1993;20:737-60.
36. European Exosurf Study Group. Early or selective surfactant (colfosceril palmitate, Exosurf) for intubated babies at 26 to 29 weeks gestation. On Line J Clin Trials 1992;document 28.
37. Phibbs RH, Ballard RA, Clements JA, et al. Initial clinical trial of Exosurf, a protein-free synthetic surfactant, for prophylaxis and early treatment of hyaline membrane disease. Pediatrics 1991;88:1-9.
38. Murphy DJ, Corbet AJ, Long WA. The ''natural'' history of patent ductus arteriosus (PDA) [Abstract]. Pediatr Res 1991; 29:245A.
39. Heldt GP, Pesonen E, Merritt TA, Elias W, Sahn DJ. Closure of the ductus arteriosus and mechanics of breathing in preterm infants after surfactant replacement therapy. Pediatr Res 1989; 25:305-10.
40. Balsan MJ, Jones JG, Guthrie RD. Effects of a clinically detectable PDA on pulmonary mechanics measures in VLBW infants with RDS. Pediatr Pulmonol 1991;111:161-5.

Clinical and laboratory observations

Effects of central apnea on cerebral blood flow velocity in healthy term infants

Virender K. Rehan, MD, MRCP, MRCPI, Ruben E. Alvaro, MD, Jaques Belik, MD, FRCPC, Doug W. Allen, RRT, Kim Kwiatkowski, RN, and Carlos A. Fajardo, MD

From the Department of Pediatrics, University of Manitoba, Winnipeg, Manitoba, Canada

We evaluated a new method of monitoring cerebral blood flow velocity (CBFV) and described changes in CBFV in relation to central apnea in 17 healthy term infants. The area under the velocity curve during apnea did not change, whereas area under the velocity curve per the waveform showed a significant difference, suggesting that stability is maintained through an increase in CBFV with each heartbeat. The maintenance of cerebral hemodynamics during isolated central apnea supports the assumption that these episodes are benign. (J PEDIATR 1995;126:979-82)

Apnea occurs commonly in term infants during early postnatal life.[1, 2] The implications of these episodes are incompletely understood. It has been suggested that they are normal developmental events resulting from oscillations in the respiratory control system because of immature neuronal and chemoreceptor development.[1]

Cerebral blood flow velocity, as measured by the Doppler technique, has been frequently used as a marker of cerebral blood flow both in preterm and term infants,[3] but previous studies have obtained measurements on a semicontinuous basis.[4] Because inherent drawbacks of intermittent monitoring exist, we carried out a prospective, descriptive study in healthy term infants to determine the feasibility of continuous CBFV monitoring and studied the effects of isolated central apnea on CBFV. In relation to the latter, we hypothesized that the CBFV would be altered during these episodes of isolated apnea.

Supported in part by Manitoba Medical Services Foundation.

Presented at the 103rd Annual Meeting of the Society for Pediatric Research, Washington, D.C., May 1993.

Submitted for publication June 30, 1994; accepted Dec. 21, 1994.

Reprint requests: Carlos Alfonso Fajardo, MD, Women's Hospital, WR004, 735 Notre Dame Ave., Winnipeg, Manitoba R3E 0L8, Canada.

0022-3476/95/$3.00 + 0 **9/24/62892**

METHODS

After parental consent, healthy term infants with no clinical evidence of cardiorespiratory compromise or any other illness were studied in the nursery within 24 hours of delivery. A transcranial-range gated Doppler technique (TC2-64, TECA Corp., Pleasantville, N.Y.) was used for CBFV measurement. The Doppler probe was positioned to obtain the best visual signals from the middle cerebral artery, placed within a plastic ring, and held at the desired site with hook-and-loop (Velcro) bands. Visual quality control was maintained during signal acquisition.

AUVC	Area under the velocity curve
CBF	Cerebral blood flow
CBFV	Cerebral blood flow velocity
PI	Pulsatility index

An acquisition program, written with proprietary software (Pix Software, Winnipeg, Manitoba, Canada), allowed simultaneous and continuous acquisition of CBFV and cardiorespiratory signals, which were directly fed into the computer and stored for later analysis (Figure). After acquisition, each file was reviewed and edited by an investigator (K.K.) in a systematic manner. Later, data were independently analyzed by two investigators (C.A.F. and V.K.R.). An isolated central apnea was defined as cessation of airflow

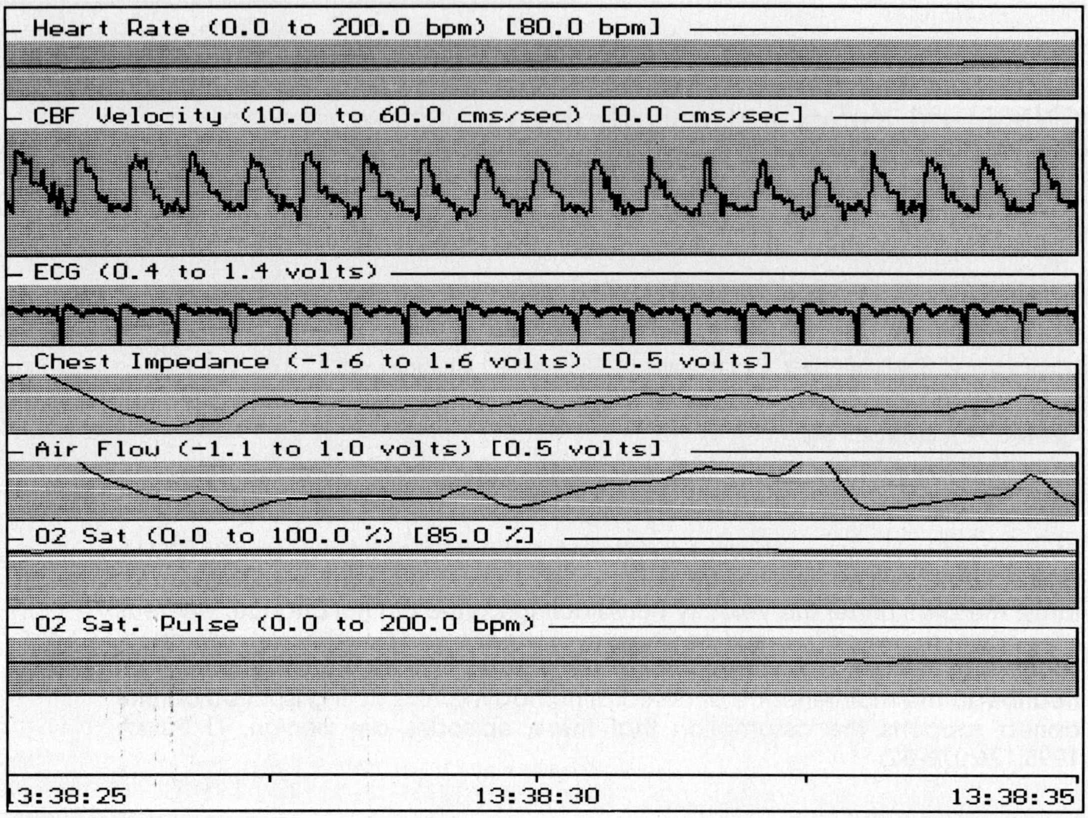

Figure. Representative tracing of CBFV and cardiorespiratory measurements (heart rate, electrocardiogram [*ECG*] chest impedance, air flow, oxygen saturation [*O_2 Sat.*] and oxygen saturation pulse [*O_2 Sat. Pulse*]). Customized seven-channel computer program with Hewlett-Packard (model 78304A) cardiorespiratory monitor (Hewlett-Packard Co., Palo Alto, Calif.), Nellcor pulse oximeter (model 100C; Nellcor Inc., Hayward, Calif.), and thermistor probe with three wings, which was positioned to sense airflow from both nostrils and from mouth was used. Pulse oximeter was used in mode 2 to acquire pulse rate and oxygen saturation signals.

Table. Changes in CBFV and heart rate in relation to isolated central apnea

	Isolated central apnea (n = 96)		
	Before	During	After
AUVC (cm/sec)	29.7 ± 3.2	29.1 ± 3.1	29.8 ± 3.2
AUVC per waveform	14.2 ± 2.4	15.1 ± 3.1*	14.6 ± 2.5
Heart rate (beats/min)	127 ± 14	119 ± 16†	124 ± 13
PI per epoch	0.92 ± 0.02	0.94 ± 0.02	0.92 ± 0.02

Values expressed as mean ± SEM.
*In relation to before apnea, p ⟨0.05.
†In relation to both before and after apnea, $p \leq 0.05$.

for 5 or more seconds without respiratory effort as assessed by chest impedance and no other apnea, bradycardia, hypoxemia, or miscellaneous event occurred within 1 minute before or after this cessation. Only epochs of apnea with acceptable Doppler waveforms were analyzed. Criteria for acceptable Doppler waveform were (1) the presence of uninterrupted recording in all seven channels for the whole apneic episode, (2) concordance of electrocardiogram wave to CBFV waveforms, and (3) smooth waveform configuration for at least seven waveforms immediately before, during, and after the apnea. The mean CBFV during apnea was compared with the mean CBFV for the 10 waveforms immediately before and the 10 waveforms immediately after the cessation of apnea.

Mean CBFV was calculated according to a previously described method[4] and given in centimeters per second, and pulsatility index was calculated for each epoch of the waveforms analyzed according to the formula (Maximum frequency shift – minimum frequency shift)/Mean frequency shift. The area under the velocity curve was also expressed as centimeters per waveform to control for changes in heart rate.

Statistical comparisons were made by analysis of variance

and the Fisher Least Significant Difference Test (when indicated). In all comparisons a p value of less than 0.05 was considered significant and all results are expressed as mean ± SD.

RESULTS

We studied 17 infants (birth weight, 3.61 ± 0.49 kg [mean ± SD]; median gestational age, 39 weeks [range, 37 to 41 weeks]), nine boys and eight girls with ages ranging between 2½ and 18 hours. Infants were monitored for a mean duration of 194 ± 8.2 minutes (range, 156 to 240 minutes). During this time (almost 55 hours), 267 episodes of central apnea of at least 5 seconds in duration were recorded. Of the 267 episodes of central apnea, 96 (36%) were classified as "isolated" according to the criteria outlined earlier. Of these, 90 (94%) lasted 5 to 10 seconds and six (6%) lasted more than 10 seconds. No apnea recorded was more than 15 seconds in duration.

We were able to obtain CBFV signals of acceptable quality during 90% to 97% of the time of monitoring, even when the infant was handled for routine care. The interobserver agreement between independent analyses of CBFV by the two investigators was high ($r = 0.96$).

Results are summarized in the Table. The CBFV, measured as AUVC (in centimeters per second) during apnea, was not significantly different from values before and after apnea. When these AUVC changes were controlled for heart rate (AUVC in centimeters per waveform), a significant difference was observed during apnea as compared with before apnea ($p < 0.05$). Heart rate decreased significantly during apnea compared with before and after apnea ($p < 0.05$). The PI did not change significantly before, during, or after the apnea.

DISCUSSION

Many investigators have studied CBFV with the intermittent Doppler technique in newborn infants.[3] Even with the on-line Doppler technique the data have been acquired semicontinuously at best.[5] Inherent drawbacks to intermittent monitoring exist with the Doppler technique because of the inevitable changes in insonation angle on repeated recordings. We attempted to overcome these drawbacks by acquiring data continuously, to maintain a stable insonation angle for the duration of monitoring.[6] Assembly of the system was simple, and an acceptable quality of CBFV and other signals could be obtained for most of the monitoring period, even while the infant was gently handled for routine needs. No side effects or complications were apparent, and infants were not unduly fussy once the probe had been applied.

We restricted our analysis to isolated central apnea, because this is the most frequent type of apnea in term infants[1] and because we could exclude the confounding of CBFV changes caused by associated events. The dynamic relationship between CBFV and apnea in healthy term infants has not been reported before. We observed no significant differences in the mean CBFV during apnea. When the CBFV was corrected for heart rate, we noted a significant but transient increase in the mean CBFV per waveform during apnea, whereas PI did not change.

The rapid changes in CBFV observed in relation to heart rate suggest that a neural reflex mechanism may be involved. Other possible mechanisms for the increase in CBFV per heartbeat are the vasodilating effects of an increase in arterial carbon dioxide pressure and a fall in arterial oxygen pressure during the apneic episode.[7, 8] However, this is unlikely because the changes observed appear to have abated almost instantaneously at the end of the apnea, whereas abnormalities in carbon dioxide and oxygen must take some time to return to normal.

The measurement of CBFV with Doppler technique is dependent not only on the blood flow but also on the cross-sectional area of the vessel; thus the observed increase in CBFV per heartbeat could have been due to vasoconstriction of the cerebral circulation. However, this possibility is unlikely because the AUVC has been shown to correlate directly with CBF in piglets.[9]

Concern may be raised over the safety of continuous ultrasound monitoring of neonates. Published evidence with traditional monitoring does not point toward any harmful effect in human beings.[10-12] Because the range-gated device emits pulses only intermittently, the exposure to ultrasound waves is only a fraction of what it would be with continuous devices; for example, the calculated exposure to incoming energy is only 24 seconds during 6 hours of continuous monitoring with a range-gated device.

This study specifically focuses on alterations in cerebral circulation during isolated apneic episodes less than 15 seconds long in healthy term neonates. The results provide new information about the CBFV changes that occur in relation to the most common type of apnea observed in these infants. We cannot extrapolate these results to the episodes of apnea observed in some abnormal conditions or to those apneic events associated with bradycardia or desaturation.

We conclude that the system described is practical, because we obtained adequate CBFV signals for 90% to 97% of the time, for periods up to 6 hours or more. We found that the mean CBFV did not change significantly during apnea. This stability was maintained through an increase in CBFV with each heartbeat to compensate for the relative bradycardia observed during these episodes of apnea. The mean CBFV measured by AUVC per waveform returned to baseline values after the apnea. We speculate that healthy term infants during the first day of life are able to maintain cerebral hemodynamics by increasing CBF per heartbeat during apnea. This regulation may be affected by superimposed bradycardia and/or hypoxemia. The later implications of these CBFV alterations remain to be studied.

REFERENCES

1. Lee D, Caces R, Kwiatkowski K, Cates D, Rigatto H. A developmental study on types and frequency distribution of short apneas (3 to 15 seconds) in term and preterm infants. Pediatr Res 1987;22:344-9.
2. Albani M, Bentele KHP, Budde C, Schulte FJ. Infant sleep apnea profile: preterm vs term infants. Eur J Pediatr 1985; 143:261-8.
3. Perlman JM. Neonatal cerebral blood flow velocity measurement. Clin Perinatol 1985;12:179-93.
4. Fenton A, Evans DH, Levene MI. On line cerebral blood flow velocity and blood pressure measurement in neonates: a new method. Arch Dis Child 1990;65:11-4.
5. Rosenkrantz TS, Oh W. Cerebral blood flow velocity in infants with polycethymia and hyperviscocity: effects of partial exchange transfusion with Plasmanate. J Pediatr 1982;101: 94-8.
6. Padayachee TS, Kirkham FJ, Lewis RR, et al. Transcranial measurement of blood velocities in the basal cerebral arteries using pulsed Doppler ultrasound: a method of assessing the circle of Willis. Ultrasound Med Biol 1986;12:5-14.
7. Archer LNJ, Evans DH, Paton JY, Levene MI. Controlled hypercapnia and neonatal cerebral artery Doppler ultrasound waveforms. Pediatr Res 1986;20:218-21.
8. Koehler RC, Jones MD Jr, Traystman RJ. Cerebral circulatory response to carbon monoxide and hypoxic hypoxia in the lamb. Am J Physiol 1982;243:H27-H32.
9. Hansen NB, Stonestreet BS, Rosenkrantz TS, Oh W. Validity of Doppler measurements of anterior cerebral artery blood flow velocity: correlation with flow in piglets. Pediatrics 1983;72: 526-31.
10. American Institute of Ultrasound in Medicine Bioeffects Committee Report. J Ultrasound Med 1988;7:S1-S38.
11. American Institute of Ultrasound in Medicine Bioeffects Committee. Safety standard for diagnostic ultrasound equipment. J Ultrasound Med 1983;2(suppl):S1-S50.
12. Brown BSJ. How safe is diagnostic ultrasonography? Can Med Assoc J 1984;131:307-11.

Soluble interleukin-2 receptor as a predictor of neonatal sepsis

Michael L. Spear, MD, John L. Stefano, MD, Paul Fawcett, PhD, and Roy Proujansky, MD

From the Division of Neonatology, Department of Pediatrics, Medical Center of Delaware, Newark; the Divisions of Gastroenterology and Immunology, A. I. duPont Institute, Wilmington, Delaware; and the Department of Pediatrics, Jefferson Medical College, Philadelphia, Pennsylvania

We prospectively measured soluble interleukin-2 receptor levels in 56 premature infants with suspected sepsis and demonstrated significant differences between those with positive results on blood, urine, or cerebrospinal fluid cultures, and those with negative results. Soluble interleukin-2 receptor levels can be used to facilitate the diagnosis of sepsis in premature infants with negative blood culture results. (J Pediatr 1995;126:982-5)

Soluble interleukin-2 receptor has been demonstrated in vitro to be important in lymphocyte activation and mobilization. In vivo the cell-associated receptor for this factor is transiently expressed after in vivo lymphocyte activation. This cell-associated receptor consists of distinct glycoproteins that link noncovalently to form a receptor complex that mediates interleukin-2 signal transduction. A soluble form of the IL-2 receptor is shed from the cell surface, increases in time, and persists in serum.[1,2] The soluble receptor is a 45 kd molecule that is thought to be the product of a proteolytic cleavage of the cell-associated receptor complex.[3] In human

IL-2	Interleukin-2
IL-6	Interleukin-6
sIL2R	Soluble interleukin-2 receptor

Submitted for publication Oct. 27, 1994; accepted Jan. 15, 1995.

Reprint requests: Michael L. Spear, MD, Division of Neonatology, Christiana Hospital, PO Box 6001, Newark, DE 19718.

0022-3476/95/$3.00 + 0 **9/24/63486**

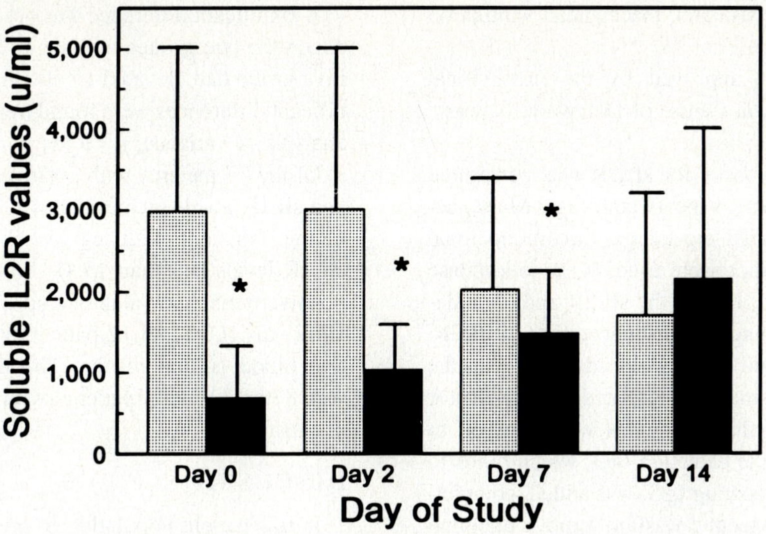

Figure. Soluble IL-2 receptor values in patients with positive culture results (*shaded blocks*) versus those with negative results (*dark blocks*), from time of initial sepsis evaluation through day 14. Values are expressed as means ± SD. *$p < 0.05$.

Table. Patient characteristics

	Total population	Group 1 (n = 17)	Group 2 (n = 39)	p
Birth weight (gm)	1085 ± 448	943 ± 388	1146 ± 462	0.12
Gestational age (wk)	28 ± 3	27 ± 3	29 ± 3	0.14
Postconceptional age (wk)	29 ± 1	27 ± 1	30 ± 1	0.06
Leukocyte count ($\times 10^6$ cells/L)		17.1 ± 11.1	14.8 ± 8.4	0.09
Hemoglobin (gm/L)		117 ± 22	137 ± 28	0.001
Platelets ($\times 10^6$ cells/L)		230 ± 155	299 ± 144	0.02
Maternal antibiotics (No. of patients)	21	8	13	0.12

infants cord blood mononuclear cells are capable of producing sIL2R at adult levels.[4] Soluble interleukin receptor levels are elevated in infants with or at risk of bronchopulmonary dysplasia.[5] In a preliminary retrospective investigation in premature infants, sIL2R levels were elevated in patients with active or recent bacterial infection.[6]

Because of the increasing use of intrapartum antibiotics to treat the woman who is delivered of a child prematurely, it is difficult to rely solely on the presence of bacteremia to confirm sepsis in the premature infant. The purpose of this investigation was to determine whether sIL2R levels can identify bacterial infection in premature infants as part of the initial laboratory evaluation for sepsis.

METHODS

Study population. Eligible patients included hospitalized premature infants (<36 weeks of gestational age) at Christiana Hospital, Medical Center of Delaware, who were being examined for suspected bacterial infection by the clinicians caring for the patients. The patients had one or more risk factors for infection: maternal disease (fever, leukocytosis, uterine tenderness, or other infectious illnesses such as pneumonia, bacterial endocarditis, or bacteremia), rupture of membranes for more than 24 hours before delivery, unexplained prematurity, respiratory distress, cardiovascular instability, abnormal level of activity, abnormal leukocyte count (absolute neutrophil count, $<1.5 \times 10^9$ cells/L), or immature/total polymorphonuclear cell ratio greater than 0.20, hypoglycemia (<2.2 mmol/L [40 mg/dl]) or hyperglycemia (>6.6 mmol/L [120 mg/dl]) of new onset.

Samples for sIL2R were drawn at the time of the initial investigation and on 2, 7 and 14 days later. Group 1 was retrospectively defined as patients who were infected (i.e., positive blood, urine, or cerebrospinal fluid cultures). Group 2, the control group, was defined as patients who were not infected. Additional data collected included birth weight, gestational age, postnatal age, complete blood cell counts, nutritional intake, diagnosis, and mechanical ventilation data.

This investigation was approved by the institutional review board at the Medical Center of Delaware, Newark, Del.

Assay for sIL2R. The assay for sIL2R was performed with a kit from T Cell Sciences Inc. (Cambridge, Mass.) according to the recommended procedure. Two monoclonal anti–IL-2 receptor antibodies were used: (1) a solid-phase IgG coating antibody that binds to the sIL2R and (2) a detection IgG antibody that binds at a distinct epitope of sIL2R. Patient samples were added to the wells adsorbed with the coating IgG antibody. Plasma was incubated in the wells for 2 hours at 37° C. After the leukocytes were washed to remove unbound sIL2R, the detection IgG, which binds to the IL2R captured by the coating IgG, was added, completing the sandwich. After a second wash to remove unbound detection antibody, a substrate (*o*-phenylenediamine) was added to form a colored product that was proportional to the amount of sIL2R present (determined by reading at 490 nm with a Titertek Multiscan spectrophotometer, Flow Laboratories, McLean, Va.). The units (per milliliter) of sIL2R present were calculated from a standard curve from known standards.

Statistical analysis. Within each group the levels of sIL2R were compared by repeated-measures analysis of variance to determine the effect of day of sampling on this measurement. To determine the effect of sepsis on sIL2R, we compared each sampling time (baseline and days 2, 7, and 14) by the Student *t* test between groups 1 and 2. In addition, the birth weight, gestational age, and postnatal age of the infants in each group were compared by the Student *t* test.

RESULTS

Study population. Fifty-six premature infants were enrolled. All patients had hyaline membrane disease and initially received mechanical ventilation, and all were examined for sepsis during the first 2 weeks of life. None of the patients received corticosteroids. Seventeen patients had blood cultures positive for the following organisms: coagulase-negative staphylococcus, eight patients; group B streptococcus, two; *Klebsiella pneumoniae*, two; *Staphylococcus aureus*, two; *Escherichia coli*, one; *Enterobacter cloacae*, one; and *Serratia marcescens*, one. No significant differences were found between the two groups in birth weight, gestational age, or postnatal age. No difference was found in the number of infants whose mothers were treated intrapartum with antibiotics. No significant differences were observed between the two groups in leukocyte counts; the hemoglobin and platelet counts in the culture-negative group were significantly higher (Table) ($p <0.05$, Student *t* test).

A significant difference was observed in sIL2R values between the two groups on days 0, 2, and 7; the culture-positive group had elevated levels (Figure). By day 14, no significant differences were found (repeated-measures one-way analysis of variance; $p <0.05$).

Of the 17 patients with positive blood culture results, 12 had sIL2R levels greater than 1500 U/ml (71% sensitivity). Of the 39 patients with negative blood culture results, all had sIL2R levels less than 1500 U/ml (100% specificity). The positive predictive value of a sIL2R level greater than 1500 U/ml was 100%; all 12 patients with high levels had positive blood culture results. The negative predictive value was 87%; 39 of 44 patients with low levels had negative results.

DISCUSSION

In this patient population of premature infants examined for sepsis, we demonstrated a significant elevation in sIL2R values in patients with positive blood culture results, in comparison with values in patients with negative results. An elevation of sIL2R values in the sepsis group persisted 7 daysafter the initial blood culture specimen was drawn. By day 14 after the initial evaluation, the values were no longer significantly different. At the time of the initial evaluation for sepsis, all the patients with negative blood culture results had a sIL2R value less than 1500 U/ml (100% specificity) and all the patients with a sIL2R value of greater than 1500 U/ml had positive results (100% positive predictive value). The differences in sIL2R values persisted for at least 7 days. A rise in sIL2R values in the culture-negative patients occurred by 14 days of age. This suggests that the normal course of sIL2R is to rise postnatally and that infection causes an acute elevation in this soluble receptor, although no data are presented for normal premature infants. Patients with bronchopulmonary dysplasia have an elevation in sIL2R levels, which may account for the rate of rise in premature infants.

Harris et al.[7] investigated premature infants with sepsis or necrotizing enterocolitis or both and measured tumor necrosis factor and interleukin-6 during the first 48 hours after the initial evaluation for sepsis. They demonstrated a difference between patients with positive culture results and those with negative results. Groll et al.[8] investigated the role of IL-6 in neonates with early-onset sepsis. As in our investigation, infants with documented sepsis had acute elevations in IL-6 values, which returned to normal by the end of the antibiotic therapy. We measured changes for 14 days, which is longer than the investigations of Harris et al. and of Groll et al.

Although a sIL2R level greater than 1500 U/ml correctly identified all infants with bacteremia, the sensitivity of 71% does not allow the sIL2R value to be used as an initial screening test. However, the 100% specificity, if confirmed in larger studies, could allow the clinician to decrease the number of infants treated for an entire course of antibiotics in the face of a negative blood culture result, when infants are treated for suspected sepsis. The other laboratory markers of infection have not been demonstrated to be useful to monitor the effectiveness of therapy. This use of the sIL2R could lessen the number of infants treated for a full course, although not the number of infants initially examined.

We recommend the use of the sIL2R level to aid in determining whether premature infants examined for sepsis have bacteremia. We speculate that the sIL2R level may be helpful in determining whether therapy is effective during the first 14 days after the initial evaluation for sepsis.

REFERENCES

1. Rubin LA, Jurman CC, Biddison WE, et al. A monoclonal antibody 7G7/B6, binds to an epitope on the human interleukin-2 (IL-2) receptor that is distinct from that recognized by IL-2 or anti-Tac. Hybridoma 1985;4:91-101.
2. Uchiyama T, Nelson DL, Fleisher TA, et al. A monoclonal antibody (anti-Tac) reactive with activated and functionally mature human T cells. II. Expression of Tac antigen on activated cytotoxic killer T cells, suppressor cells, and on one of two types of helper T cells. J Immunol 1981;4:1398-403.
3. Smith KA. The bimolecular structure of the interleukin 2 receptor. Immunol Today 1988;9:36-7.
4. Nelson DL, Kurman CC, Fritz ME, et al. The production of soluble and cellular interleukin-2 receptors by cord blood mononuclear cells following in vitro activation. Pediatr Res 1986;20:136-9.
5. Stefano JL, Spear ML, Pearlman SA, Fawcett P, Proujansky R. Soluble interleukin-2 receptors in infants with BPD [Abstract]. Pediatr Res 1991;29:331A.
6. Spear ML, Stefano JL, Fawcett P, Proujansky R. Interleukin-2 receptor levels in premature neonates [Abstract]. Pediatr Res 1991;29:235A.
7. Harris MC, Costarino AT, Sullivan JS. Cytokine elevations in critically ill infants with sepsis and necrotizing enterocolitis. J Pediatr 1994;124:105-11.
8. Groll AH, Meiser A, Weise M, et al. Interleukin 6 as early mediator in neonatal sepsis. Pediatr Infect Dis J 1992;11:495-6.

Reference ranges for serum cortisol and 17-hydroxyprogesterone levels in preterm infants

Saad Al Saedi, MD, FRCPC, Heather Dean, MD, FRCPC, William Dent, MSc, and Catherine Cronin, MD, MRCPI, FRCPC

From the Department of Paediatrics, Sections of Neonatology and Paediatric Endocrinology, and Division of Laboratory Medicine and Pathology, Health Sciences Centre, University of Manitoba, Winnipeg, Manitoba, Canada

Reference ranges for cortisol and 17-hydroxyprogesterone were developed with sera from 39 healthy preterm infants less than 31 weeks of gestational age, collected weekly until 37 weeks of corrected age. (J Pediatr 1995;126:985-7)

The adrenal cortex facilitates postnatal adaptation of the newborn infant.[1] In C21-hydroxylase deficiency, 17-hydroxyprogesterone is increased in serum.[2] Although normative data on cortisol and 17-OHP are available for term infants,[3] no such data exist for "healthy" very low birth weight infants. Delineation of neonatal glucocorticoid levels is essential to understand neonatal adrenal physiology and to assess adrenocortical malfunction. We attempted to define reference ranges for cortisol and 17-OHP in well preterm infants, by sequential sampling from the first week of life to 37 weeks of postconceptional age.

Supported by the Manitoba Medical Services Foundation and the Children's Hospital Research Foundation of Winnipeg.

Submitted for publication Nov. 3, 1994; accepted Jan. 31, 1995.

Reprint requests: Catherine Cronin, MD, MRCPI, FRCPC, E3003 Section of Neonatology, St. Boniface General Hospital, 409 Taché Ave., Winnipeg, Manitoba R2H 2A6, Canada.

0022-3476/95/$3.00 + 0 **9/24/63861**

METHODS

Patients. Between July 1992 and December 1993, we studied 39 preterm infants in the neonatal intensive care units at Health Sciences Centre and St. Boniface Hospital, Winnipeg, Manitoba, Canada. Subjects were less than 31 weeks of gestational age and had no congenital anomalies, or family history of adrenal disorders or current major acute illnesses, and had not received inotropes or hormone therapy within 48 hours. Infants whose mothers had prenatally received corticosteroids and those with mild hyaline membrane disease or apnea of prematurity were included.

17-OHP	17-Hydroxyprogesterone
PCA	Postconceptional age

Table I. Median, 10th, and 90th percentiles for cortisol, 17-OHP and, cortisol/17-OHP ratio in healthy preterm infants less than 31 weeks of gestational age, versus PCA

	Postconceptional age							
Percentile	<30 wk	30 wk	31 wk	32 wk	33 wk	34 wk	35 wk	≥36 wk
90th								
Cortisol (nmol/L)	375	346	320	302	234	204	212	316
17-OHP (nmol/L)	36	25.3	44.3	26	15.7	14.2	10	8.85
Cortisol/17-OHP ratio	33	36.6	45.5	40.8	47.6	42.4	35.1	76.2
50th								
Cortisol (nmol/L)	137	140	104	84	67	72	36	76
17-OHP (nmol/L)	14.4	12.3	12.9	8.6	7.2	7.55	5.9	5.15
Cortisol/17-OHP ratio	11.6	13.9	7.8	10.9	9.5	8.4	8.4	11.5
10th								
Cortisol (nmol/L)	51	56	37	30	30	33	29	30
17-OHP (nmol/L)	5	3.6	4	3.8	3.1	2.2	2.2	2.95
Cortisol/17-OHP ratio	2.6	3.3	2.4	1.7	2.5	3.8	3.7	4.5

Table II. Distribution of cortisol and 17-OHP in healthy infants less than 31 weeks of gestational age

	Concentration in nmol/L (μ/dl)	No. (%) of samples
Cortisol	≤30 (≤1.1)	28* (12.3)
	≤100 (≤3.6)	124 (54.6)
	≤350 (≤12.7)	218 (96)
	≤450 (≤16.3)	225 (99.1)
17-OHP	≤10 (≤0.4)	133 (58.6)
	≤25 (≤0.9)	210 (98.7)
	≤50 (≤1.8)	224 (98.7)
	>50 (>1.8)	3† (1.3)

*From 15 infants (38.5% of patients
†Levels were 69 to 82.5 nmol/L (2.5 to 3.0 μg/dl) from three different infants, 7–23 days old.

Each infant had a 1.0 ml heel-stick blood sample taken between 8 and 10 AM, 1 hour after feeding. Sampling was repeated weekly until 37 weeks of PCA or discharge from hospital. No sample was taken before day 5 of life. Any acute illness led to exclusion from the study until the illness was fully resolved. Samples taken within 48 hours before onset of sepsis were excluded from analysis.

The study was approved by the University of Manitoba Committee on the Use of Human Subjects in Research. Written informed parental consent was obtained.

Laboratory procedures. Serum was frozen at –20° C until analyzed in lots of 50 or more. Serum cortisol and 17-OHP were measured by standard radioimmunoassays (Coat-A-Count; Diagnostic Products Corp., Los Angeles, Calif.[4]). To remove steroid sulfates and glucuronides that crossreact with the 17-OHP antibody, measurement of 17-OHP was preceded by specimen extraction with toluene as follows.

Seven calibration standards, each containing 1 to 50 nmol of 17-OHP per liter, were prepared. Then, 0.1 ml of standard, control, and patient serum were transferred to 12 × 75 mm polypropylene tubes. Toluene, 1.0 ml, was added to each tube. Extraction was performed by 2 minutes of shaking, followed by 10 minutes of standing, to allow organic and aqueous phase separation. Two hundred fifty microliters of the toluene phase of each standard, control, and patient specimen was transferred in duplicate to the kit manufacturer's 17-OHP antibody-coated tubes. The solvent was evaporated under flowing nitrogen at 37° C. Iodine 125–labeled 17-OHP reagent, 1.0 ml, was added to all tubes and incubated for 2 hours at room temperature. Contents were decanted before determination of radioactivity with an LKB Multigamma counter (Pharmacia Inc., Piscataway, N.J.). Determinations of 17-OHP were generated directly by Multigamma data reduction software.

Interassay coefficients of variation were 14.4% for 17-OHP and 10.7% for cortisol. Sensitivities were 0.3 nmol/L (0.01 μg/dl) for 17-OHP and 8.5 nmol/L (0.3 μg/dl) for cortisol.

Statistics. Thirty samples within each subgroup of age enabled definition of confidence limits. Initial samples were used to calculate reference ranges with respect to PCA according to the method of Royston.[5]

RESULTS

Thirty-nine patients (23 boys) provided 227 samples (mean ± SD, 4 ± 2.3 samples/patient). Gestational age was 29 ± 1.5 weeks; birth weight was 1250 ± 280 gm. All but two patients had apnea of prematurity. Gender, history of hyaline membrane disease, bronchopulmonary dysplasia, patent ductus arteriosus, or intraventricular hemorrhage did not influence results, which were pooled for analysis. Tables I and II summarize the results.

Cortisol. Cortisol levels ranged from 20 to 680 nmol/L (0.7 to 24.6 μg/dl), with a mean ± SD of 125.4 ± 107 nmol/L (4.5 ± 3.9 μg/dl). With the use of the Royston method,[5] predicted initial cortisol levels were 134 to 201 nmol/L (4.9 to 7.3 μg/dl). Lowest morning cortisol levels occurred at 35 to 56 days of age (predicted levels, 25 to 144 nmol/L [0.9 to 5.2 μg/dl]).

17-Hydroxyprogesterone. Levels of 17-OHP ranged from 1.4 to 82.5 nmol/L (0.05 to 3.0 μg/dl), with a mean ± SD of 11.4 ± 11.1 nmol/L (0.4 ± 0.4 μg/dl). Predicted levels were 9.4 to 13 nmol/L (0.3 to 0.47 μg/dl) for initial 17-OHP and 5.2 to 5.3 nmol/L (0.188 to 0.19 μg/dl) at 35 to 56 days of age.

DISCUSSION

Cortisol. Glucocorticoid hormone levels decrease rapidly during the first days of life.[6] Lee et al.[7] documented random cortisol levels of 190 ± 29 nmol/L (6.9 ± 1.1 μg/dl) in well preterm infants on days 2 to 5. Similar results were reported in sick preterm infants with elevated levels of steroid precursors; many infants responded poorly to adrenocorticotrophic hormone.[8] Rokicki et al.[9] found that free cortisol levels decreased from 32% to 21% in the second month in term infants and from 37% to 24% in preterm infants. We were unable to measure free cortisol levels, but on the basis of the data of Rokicki et al., free cortisol in our patients can be estimated at less than 70 nmol/L (2.5 μg/dl) in the first sample and less than 50 nmol/L (1.8 μg/dl) at 35 to 56 days of age.

17-Hydroxyprogesterone. Concentrations of 17-OHP in cord serum exceed those of older children. Values in term infants decrease to adult levels by 2 to 7 days of age. Values observed in preterm infants depend on the use and type of extraction procedure.[4] We found high 17-OHP levels compared with those reported in term infants.[3] The absence of symptoms and the normalization of 17-OHP in time suggest that these infants did not have adrenal disease.

Definition of upper limits for 17-OHP is important in view of its measurement for screening purposes. Patients with classic congenital adrenal hyperplasia have much higher values than do healthy preterm infants, but values from patients with nonclassic congenital adrenal hyperplasia and from premature infants overlap.[10] Because only three of our samples had values greater than 50 nmol/L (1.8 μg/dl) when measured by radioimmunoassay with toluene extraction, an upper limit of 50 nmol/L (1.8 μg/dl) is suggested for this population.

We used strict exclusion criteria for infants with any evidence of current illness; thus our data reflect the best estimate so far of the statistical normal values for healthy very low birth weight infants after the first 5 days of postnatal life.

The existence of diurnal rhythm in the neonate is disputed. Establishment of a 24-hour sleep-wake cycle takes many weeks from discharge from the hospital. The rhythms of hospitalized preterm infants, if any, may not be diurnal. In older patients cortisol levels peak between 8 and 10 AM. Persistently low cortisol levels in the absence of primary adrenal dysfunction suggest that the hypothalamic-pituitary-adrenal axis may operate at a low setting up to several weeks after birth.

Conclusions. Cortisol levels in healthy preterm infants may be low or undetectable without signifying adrenal disease. Levels of 17-OHP less than 50 nmol/L (1.8 μg/dl), measured by extracted quantitative radioimmunoassay, are normal and do not suggest C21-hydroxylase deficiency. Future studies should document the response of the adrenal cortex to physiologic stimuli, maturation of the glucocorticoid biosynthetic pathway, and development of day-night cycling.

The assistance of Valerie Cook with specimen and data collection and of Mary Cheang with statistical advice is gratefully acknowledged.

REFERENCES

1. Helbock HJ, Insoft RM, Conte FA. Glucocorticoid-responsive hypotension in extremely low birth weight newborns. Pediatrics 1993;92:715-7.
2. Hughes IA, Read GF. Control in congenital adrenal hyperplasia monitored by frequent saliva 17 OH-progesterone determinations. Horm Res 1984;19:79-85.
3. Wiener D, Smith J, Dahlem S, Berg G, Moshang T. Serum adrenal steroid levels in healthy full term 3-day-old infants. Pediatrics 1987;110:122-4.
4. Coat-A-Count 17-hydroxyprogesterone and cortisol product information. Los Angeles: Diagnostic Products Corp., 1992.
5. Royston P. Constructing time-specific reference ranges. Stat Med 1991;10:675-90.
6. Kojima S, Yanaihara T, Nakayama T. Serum steroid levels in children at birth and in early neonatal period. Am J Obstet Gynecol 1981;140:961-5.
7. Lee MM, Rajagopalan L, Berg GJ, Moshang T. Serum adrenal steroid concentrations in premature infants. J Clin Endocrin Metab 1989;69:1133-6.
8. Hingre RV, Gross SJ, Hingre KS, Mayes DM, Richman RA. Adrenal steroidogenesis in very low birth weight preterm infants. J Clin Endocrinol Metab 1994;78:266-70.
9. Rokicki W, Forest MG, Loras B, Bonnet H, Bertrand J. Free cortisol of human plasma in the first three months of life. Biol Neonate 1990;57:21-9.
10. Lee A, Ellis G. Serum 17α-hydroxyprogesterone in infants and children as measured by a direct radioimmunoassay kit. Clin Biochem 1991;24:505-11.

Conjugated hyperbilirubinemia in a newborn infant after maternal (transplacental) treatment with flecainide acetate for fetal tachycardia and fetal hydrops

Andre L. Vanderhal, MD, Jose Cocjin, MD, Thomas V. Santulli, Jr., MD, Dru E. Carlson, MD, and Philip Rosenthal, MD

From the Divisions of Neonatology, Pediatric Gastroenterology, and Pediatric Cardiology, Ahmanson Pediatric Center, the Department of Obstetrics and Gynecology, Cedars-Sinai Medical Center, Los Angeles, California, and the Department of Pediatrics, University of California–Los Angeles School of Medicine

An infant with intrauterine supraventricular tachycardia and fetal hydrops, successfully treated with administration of flecainide acetate to the mother had conjugated hyperbilirubinemia shortly after birth. An extensive evaluation failed to disclose a known cause. We believe that in utero exposure to flecainide acetate resulted in conjugated hyperbilirubinemia in this infant. (J PEDIATR 1995; 126:988-90)

Conjugated hyperbilirubinemia in the newborn infant is always abnormal, sometimes is the result of drug therapy, and always requires evaluation.[1] We describe a newborn infant in whom conjugated hyperbilirubinemia developed after maternal transplacental therapy with flecainide acetate for fetal tachycardia, an association not previously described in childhood.

CASE REPORT

A male infant (birth weight, 2843 gm; length, 51.5 cm; head circumference, 35.5 cm) was born by normal spontaneous vaginal delivery at 36 weeks of gestational age. His mother was referred to Cedars-Sinai Medical Center at 28 weeks of gestation for fetal supraventricular tachycardia. Ultrasound examination revealed polyhydramnios, fetal ascites, pericardial effusion, cardiomegaly, and tricuspid and mitral valve regurgitation. Intravenous administration of digoxin to the mother was ineffective, and transcutaneous intraumbilical adenosine only transiently resulted in conversion to sinus rhythm. Treatment of the mother with orally administered flecainide acetate, 150 mg twice daily, was begun. After 24 hours fetal sinus rhythm was predominant. After 1 week the mother discontinued flecainide acetate therapy. At 30 weeks of gestation a recurrence of fetal tachycardia and ascites were noted and maternal flecainide acetate therapy was resumed, with resolution of fetal ascites but persistence of fetal cardiomegaly. The mother's serum flecainide level 11 days before delivery was 0.54 mg/L (therapeutic range, 0.2 to 1.0 mg/L), and her liver enzyme levels were normal (total bilirubin, 8.6 μmol/L [0.5 mg/dL]); alkaline phosphatase, 176 U/L; aspartate aminotransferase, 15 U/L; and alanine aminotransferase, 12 U/L.

The infant required oxygen in the delivery room. Physical examination revealed a systolic murmur and hepatomegaly, with a heart rate of 140 beats/min, respiratory rate of 56 breaths/min, temperature of 36.7° C, and blood pressure of 79/41 mm Hg. Electrocardiography showed normal sinus rhythm without preexcitation, right atrial and ventricular enlargement, first-degree atrioventricular

Table I. Liver function tests

	Bilirubin (mg/dl*)		AST	ALT
	Total	Direct	(U/L)	(U/L)
Age-specific normal value	<11.7	<1.2	<140	<60
Days of age				
1	4.9	1.3	110	<10
2	13.2	1.8		
3	17.1			
4	15.4	2.9		
5	13.7	6.2	51	15
7	9.1	3.9		
9	8.9	4.5		
11	6.9	4.0	144	59
60	0.9		48	36

ALT, Alanine aminotransferase; *AST*, aspartate aminotransferase.
*Bilirubin conversion: milligrams per deciliter × 17.1 = micromoles per liter.

Submitted for publication Aug. 2, 1994; accepted Jan. 27, 1995.

Reprint requests: Andre L. Vanderhal, MD, Division of Neonatology, Cedars-Sinai Medical Center, Room 4310, 8700 Beverly Blvd., Los Angeles, CA 90048.

0022-3476/95/$3.00 + 0 **9/26/63717**

Table II. Laboratory findings

Test	Result	Normal value
Hepatitis A antibody (IgM)	Negative	
Hepatitis B surface antigen	Negative	
Hepatitis C antibody	Negative	
Hemoglobin (gm/L)	218	
Hematocrit	0.65	
Platelet count (cells/dl)	134×10^{12}	
Leukocyte count (cells/dl)	9.6×10^{9}	
Differential (%)		
Polymorphonuclear	70	
Lymphocytes	26	
Monocytes	3	
Eosinophils	1	
Nucleated erythrocyte count	1/100 WBC	
Reticulocytes (%)	1.2	
Prothrombin time (sec)	12.4	
Partial thromboplastin time (sec)	42	
Fibrinogen (gm/L)	1.01	2.00-4.00
D-Dimer (ng/ml)	<500	
Blood type	Type A; Rh^+; direct $Coombs^-$	
Cord blood IgM (mg/dl)	4	5-19
Cytomegalovirus urine culture	Negative	
Total protein (gm/L)	54	60-85
Albumin (gm/L)	26	35-55

block (PR interval, 0.18 milliseconds) and precordial ST depression. Echocardiography demonstrated bilaterally enlarged atria, tricuspid and mitral regurgitation, patent ductus arteriosus, and increased papillary muscle mass. The infant's serum flecainide level on day 1 was 0.14 mg/L. When the infant was 9 hours of age, episodes of paroxysmal atrial and ventricular contractions (confirmed with a Holter recording) developed and treatment with digoxin was started. On the first day after birth the direct-reacting fraction was 27% of the total bilirubin value and diminished during the following days (Table I). Clinically apparent jaundice prompted phototherapy at 2 days of age. By day 5 the direct-reacting bilirubin fraction increased to 45% and phototherapy was discontinued. An evaluation for causes of conjugated hyperbilirubinemia failed to demonstrate a known cause (Table II).

The infant responded well to digoxin therapy and was discharged home at 10 days of age. On follow-up at 2 months of age, hepatomegaly, conjugated hyperbilirubinemia, and elevated transaminase values had resolved (Table I). The digoxin therapy was discontinued at 2 years of age, and at 28 months of age he continues to do well, with no recurrence of tachycardia or hyperbilirubinemia.

DISCUSSION

Conjugated hyperbilirubinemia is defined by a direct-reacting bilirubin fraction greater than 30% of the total serum bilirubin level.[1] In the first week of life conjugated hyperbilirubinemia has been associated with fetal hydrops caused by severe hemolysis from blood group incompatibility but not with nonimmune hydrops.[2] Neither hydrops from congestive heart failure caused by induced tachycardia in fetal sheep experiments nor hydrops with fetal tachycardia in human beings has resulted in conjugated hyperbilirubinemia.[1, 3, 4] Although medications have been associated with conjugated hyperbilirubinemia in newborn infants, the agents used in transplacental or transumbilical treatment of fetal tachycardias are not known to cause neonatal conjugated hyperbilirubinemia.[1]

In adults the hepatic effects of flecainide acetate include asymptomatic isolated elevations of alkaline phosphatase and serum transaminases, cholestasis, and hepatic failure.[5, 6] The mechanisms leading to these effects are unresolved. In such instances flecainide acetate should be discontinued.[5]

Although flecainide acetate therapy has been associated with conjugated hyperbilirubinemia in adults, its use for maternal, fetal, or childhood arrhythmias has not resulted in conjugated hyperbilirubinemia, even after toxic effects of flecainide acetate have become evident.[7-10] Other causes or nonrecognized pathophysiologic processes for the conjugated hyperbilirubinemia, including additive effects such as congestive liver damage (rather than heart failure) and flecainide acetate therapy, are, in the light of the evaluation and follow-up, speculative at best.

This is to our knowledge the first reported case of transient conjugated hyperbilirubinemia associated with transplacental flecainide acetate treatment in a newborn infant. We suggest that flecainide acetate be added to the list of agents that can cause conjugated hyperbilirubinemia in infants. No long-term deleterious effects on hepatic function were observed in our patient after flecainide acetate therapy was discontinued.

We thank Dr. J. J. Pomerance for his helpful comments and review, and Dr. Don N. Smith for the follow-up data on the patient.

REFERENCES

1. Rosenthal P, Sinatra F. Jaundice in infancy. Pediatr Rev 1989; 11:79-86.
2. Cashore WJ. Hyperbilirubinemia. In: Pomerance JJ, Richardson CJ, eds. Neonatology for the clinician. Norwalk, Conn: Appleton & Lange, 1993:231-41.
3. Gest AL, Martin CG, Moise AA, Hansen TN. Reversal of venous blood flow with atrial tachycardia and hydrops in fetal sheep. Pediatr Res 1990;28:223-6.
4. Gest AL, Hansen TN, Moise AA, Hartley CJ. Atrial tachycardia causes hydrops in fetal lambs. Am J Physiol 1990;258: H1159-63.
5. Flecainide acetate (TAMBOCOR) [Package insert]. St Paul MN: 3M Pharmaceuticals, 1994.
6. Kühlkamp V, Haasis R, Seipel L. Flecainidinduzierte Hepatitis. Z Kardiol 1988;77:678-80.
7. Perry JC, McQuinn RL, Smith RT, Gothing CG, Fredell P, Garson A. Flecainide acetate for resistant arrhythmias in the young: efficacy and pharmacokinetics. J Am Coll Cardiol 1989;14:185-91.
8. Russell GAB, Martin RP. Flecainide toxicity. Arch Dis Child 1989;64:860-2.
9. Zeigler VL, Peterson J. Flecainide toxicity in a neonate with supraventricular tachycardia. Heart Lung 1991;20:689-91.
10. Palmer CM, Norris MC. Placental transfer of flecainide. Am J Dis Child 1990;144:144.

Effect of acetaminophen and of low intermittent doses of diazepam on prevention of recurrences of febrile seizures

M. Uhari, MD, H. Rantala, MD, L. Vainionpää, MD, and R. Kurttila, BM

From the Department of Pediatrics, University of Oulu, Oulu, Finland

Acetaminophen and low doses of diazepam were evaluated for the prevention of recurrences of febrile seizures in a placebo-controlled, double-blind trial. Children after their first febrile seizure were assigned to receive either one dose of rectally administered diazepam, and then, after 6 hours, oral doses of 0.2 mg/kg three times a day for the first 2 days if the fever stayed greater than 38.5° C, or a placebo similarly during forthcoming febrile episodes. In addition, each febrile episode was randomly assigned to be treated with acetaminophen or the placebo. Thus four groups were examined for 2 years: patients receiving two kinds of placebo, patients receiving diazepam and a placebo, patients receiving acetaminophen and a placebo, and patients receiving both diazepam and acetaminophen. Of a total of 180 patients (102 boys), 161 were followed for the 2-year period and 157 were seen at the last outpatient examination: 80 in the diazepam group and 77 in the placebo group. The final analysis of the efficacy of the drugs was made on the basis of the data from 153 patients who had had at least one febrile episode during follow-up. There were 641 fever events during this period, and 38 children (21.1%) had 55 recurrences of febrile seizures. Acetaminophen had no effect on the recurrence rate. Seizures recurred at least once in 21 patients (28.4%) receiving diazepam and 17 (21.5%) receiving a placebo ($p = 0.4138$, log-rank test). The combination of antipyretic agents with anticonvulsant medication did not reduce the recurrence of febrile seizures. Our results show that low doses of acetaminophen or diazepam or both are ineffective for preventing febrile seizures. (J Pediatr 1995;126:991-5)

Febrile convulsions recur in about one fifth to one third of children affected.[1-4] Although benign, they are frightening for parents, and long-term medication has been used to prevent their recurrence.[5] The effectiveness of phenobarbital is controversial, and continuous treatment cannot be recommended, because phenobarbital depresses cognitive performance in children treated for febrile seizures.[6, 7]

Supported by the Alma and K.A. Snellman Foundation, Finland.

Submitted for publication Nov. 15, 1994; accepted Jan. 31, 1995.

Reprint requests: M. Uhari, MD, PhD, MSc, Associate Professor of Pediatrics, Department of Pediatrics, University of Oulu, FIN-90220 Oulu, Finland.

0022-3476/95/$3.00 + 0 **9/25/63860**

It has also been generally assumed that antipyretic agents can prevent recurrences of febrile seizures, but Schnaiderman et al.[8] could not show any effect of antipyretics in preventing the immediate recurrence of seizures when given regularly as compared with sporadic use, even though the children with a regular regimen received significantly more acetaminophen than the others. Their sample was small, however, and seizures rarely recur during the same febrile illness.[9] To our knowledge no controlled clinical trials have evaluated the efficacy of antipyretics in preventing febrile seizures.

See commentary, p. 929.

In 1978 diazepam given rectally every 8 hours was found to be as effective as continuous administration of phenobarbital,[10] and this was recently confirmed in a selected series of patients given diazepam orally.[11] Knudsen,[12] however, showed that the prophylactic use of diazepam was ineffective in children with no risk factors, and other investigators have reported similar findings.[13]

We wanted to see whether diazepam is effective among unselected patients and whether acetaminophen, an antipyretic, has any effect alone or in combination with diazepam in preventing recurrences of febrile seizures. We thus performed a randomized, double-blind trial involving both drugs.

METHODS

The parents of all children seeking medical help from the University of Oulu Department of Pediatrics for their first febrile seizures between November 1986 and September 1990 were offered the possibility of participating in a 2-year follow-up study. The parents of all but three patients expressed willingness to participate; in addition to these unwilling parents, only those patients known to be unable to attend the follow-up visit at the end of the 2-year period were excluded. All children from the primary catchment area of our hospital are sent to the department of pediatrics after their first febrile seizure.

The criteria for eligibility were no history of afebrile seizures, no anticonvulsant medication, and absence of any chronic disease requiring continuous medication. Baseline physical, developmental, and neurologic assessments were conducted by a pediatrician and repeated by a pediatric neurologist at the end of the 2 years.

The patients participating in the trial were randomly assigned to receive either a placebo or diazepam during all their febrile infections, by blocks of varying sizes of four, six, or eight patients within each stratum. Only the biostatistician knew the details of the randomization schedule. The medication was started with a solution for rectal use (rectiol) containing 2.5 mg of diazepam or placebo for children weighing less than 7 kg, 5 mg diazepam for children weighing 7 to 15 kg, and 10 mg diazepam for children weighing more than 15 kg, and then continued after 6 hours with oral doses of 0.2 mg/kg three times a day for the first 2 days if the patient's temperature stayed at greater than 38.5° C. This dose of diazepam is the lowest reported to be effective in preventing febrile seizures.[12]

Each child received antipyretic agents, and the febrile episodes were assigned so that every other episode was treated with acetaminophen and every other one with a placebo; the first febrile episode was assigned randomly to management with acetaminophen or placebo. Acetaminophen was given at a dose of 10 mg/kg four times per day, a dose shown to reduce temperature by about 1.5° C.[14] Parents were advised to give their child acetaminophen at a dose of 10 mg/kg if the temperature rose to greater than 40° C. If the child had a seizure, the parents were advised to give the active preparation of diazepam rectiol at the dose given previously. The families were sent new supplies of medication as needed, with adjustments in the dose according to changes in the child's body weight. At the end of the 2-year follow-up period, we had records of febrile events in four groups of patients: those receiving two kinds of placebo, patients receiving diazepam and a placebo, patients receiving acetaminophen and a placebo, and patients receiving both diazepam and acetaminophen.

The parents were asked to fill in a predesigned symptom sheet for each infectious and febrile event during the 2 years of follow-up. If no event was recorded in the course of 1 month, parents were contacted by the study nurse. The medication for each episode was recorded, and the parents measured the child's temperature twice a day as long as the fever continued. The parents were told about the possibility of the child's receiving only a placebo; whenever they believed that they should administer acetaminophen, they were allowed to do so and to report it to us.

The main end point for analysis was a febrile seizure reported by the parents; only one seizure per episode of fever was counted in the analysis. We had found in our earlier surveys that the recurrence rate among our patients was about 20%, and we regarded a reduction to 5% as clinically important. For a power of 80% and a type I error of 0.05, the calculated sample size for each group was 66 children. To ensure samples of this size even after some subjects dropped out, we included 90 patients in each anticonvulsive treatment group.

The data were stored in a microcomputer and analyzed with SPSSWin, version 6 (Statistical Package for the Social Sciences, Chicago, Ill.). The differences in frequencies between the patients and episodes in each stratum were assessed with the chi-square test; the time to the first recurrence of a febrile seizure was analyzed with the Kaplan-Meier method for plotting the cumulative incidence curves and the log-rank test to compare the groups. The Cox proportional-hazards regression model was used to adjust the survival rates for age, gender, and background risk factors (Table I).

The study protocol was approved by the ethical committee of the University of Oulu Medical Faculty, and informed consent was obtained from the parents.

Of the total of 180 patients (102 boys), 161 were followed for the 2-year period and 157 came to the last outpatient examination, 80 in the diazepam group and 77 in the placebo group (Table I). The final analysis of the efficacy of the drugs was based on the data for 65 girls and 88 boys who had had

Table I. Withdrawals, background information, and number of febrile episodes during follow-up of 161 children for 2 years after their first febrile seizure

	Treatment	
	Diazepam	Placebo
Reasons for withdrawal (n)		
Moved abroad or contact lost	1	2
Did not want to continue	8	8
Did not come to last follow-up	1	3
No. of children followed 2 yr	81	80
No. (%) of girls	32 (39.5)	39 (48.8)
Age (yr)		
Mean	1.8	1.6
Range	0.5-4.5	0.3-4.6
Risk factors (n)		
Type of first febrile seizure		
Simple	57	59
Complex	24	21
Family history of febrile seizures	41	31
Family history of nonfebrile seizures	11	11
Delayed psychomotor development	0	0
No. of febrile seizures during follow-up		
1	15	12
2	3	4
3	2	1
5	1	—

One hundred fifty-seven patients were present for the last follow-up visit; of these, 153 had had at least one febrile episode.

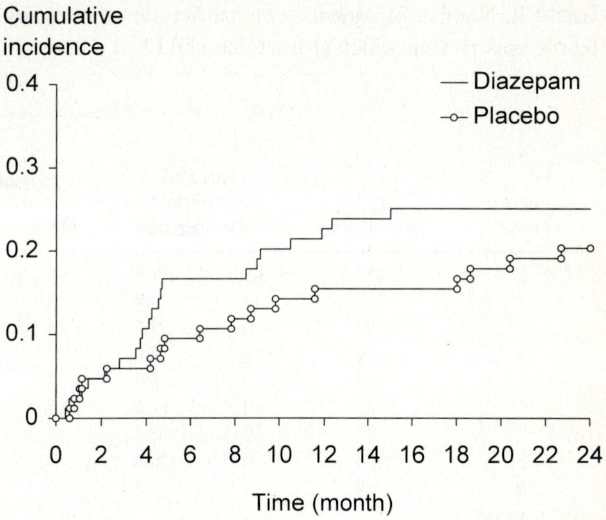

Figure. Cumulative incidence of recurrent febrile seizures, by treatment group. Difference between curves was not significant ($p = 0.4138$).

at least one febrile episode and had thus used the medicines supplied. The age range of the patients was 0.8 to 4.6 years. Nineteen patients dropped out after up to 18 months; nine dropped out so before their first febrile event, and 10 others dropped out after 1 to 18 months of follow-up. Their data, when available, are included in the Kaplan-Meier analysis.

RESULTS

Altogether 153 children of the total of 180 (85.0%) had at least one febrile event during the follow-up, and the total number of such events during that period was 641. Of the 180 children, 38 (21.1%) had a total of 55 recurrences of febrile seizures; 27 had one such recurrence, and one child had as many as five (Table I). Thirty-two of the children (17.8%) had seizures during the first year of the follow-up, and 15 (9.8%) of the 153 children had a seizure during their first febrile event. The frequency of seizures relative to febrile events varied from 5.6% to 11.1% (Table II).

During their first febrile episode, 79 of the 153 children received acetaminophen (Table II). Acetaminophen had no effect on the recurrence of febrile seizures (Tables II and III). Parents gave similar amounts of extra antipyretic agents to children receiving either acetaminophen or the placebo. The mean temperature during each febrile episode was 0.5° higher among those children who had seizures than among those who did not; the mean difference in highest temperatures between the acetaminophen and placebo groups for all febrile episodes was not significant (difference, 0.03° C; $p > 0.05$). Even though acetaminophen reduced mean temperatures, it had no effect on the highest temperatures or on the temperatures in those patients who had febrile seizures.

Febrile seizures recurred at least once in 21 patients receiving diazepam (28.4%) and in 17 receiving the placebo (21.5%); analysis of the timing of the first recurrence by the Kaplan-Meier method showed no difference between the anticonvulsant treatment groups ($p = 0.4138$ by the log-rank test; Figure). Similarly, no differences were observed between the diazepam and placebo groups during any given febrile episode taken in rank order (Table II).

When the occurrences for each febrile episode are considered according to the treatment regimen, none of the differences was significant. The combination of antipyretic and anticonvulsant medication did not reduce the recurrence of febrile seizures (Table III). Temperature and the number of febrile episodes were the only explanatory factors associated with recurrences of febrile seizures in the Cox regression model.

Findings of the neurologic assessment were normal in all the patients. Parents of five children, three in the placebo

Table II. Number of patients who had febrile seizures, by febrile episodes and medication received during the first nine febrile episodes, in which at least one child had a convulsion

				Patients receiving medication							
				Antipyretic agents				Anticonvulsant agents			
		No. (%) of children with seizures		Placebo		Acetaminophen		Placebo		Diazepam	
Order of episode	Total No. of children			No.	%	No.	%	No.	%	No.	%
1	153	15	9.8	7	9.5	8	10.1	5	6.3	10	13.5
2	117	11	9.4	6	9.7	5	9.1	6	10.0	5	8.8
3	94	9	9.6	5	10.4	4	8.7	4	8.2	5	11.1
4	68	4	5.9	2	5.1	2	6.9	3	8.3	1	3.1
5	54	3	5.6	2	8.7	1	3.2	3	9.4	0	
6	45	5	11.1	5	20.0	0		1	3.7	4	22.2
7	32	2	6.3	1	5.6	1	7.1	0		2	14.3
8	24	5	20.8	3	30.0	2	14.3	1	7.7	4	36.4
9	19	1	5.3	1	9.1	0		0		1	14.3
All episodes*				32	9.8	23	7.3	23	6.7	32	10.7

A total of 641 febrile episodes were recorded, and one child had as many as 20. One patient may have had more than one febrile convulsion and thus may appear in more than one febrile episode.
*The same child may have had several episodes. The differences between the groups are statistically not significant.

Table III. Number of patients who had febrile seizures, by febrile episodes and medication received, during the first nine febrile episodes in which at least one child had a seizure

	Patients receiving treatment regimen							
	Placebo + placebo		Placebo + acetaminophen		Diazepam + acetaminophen		Diazepam + placebo	
Order of episode	No.	%	No.	%	No.	%	No.	%
1	3	7.7	2	5.0	6	15.4	4	11.4
2	4	12.5	2	7.1	3	11.1	2	6.7
3	2	8.7	2	7.7	2	10.0	3	12.0
4	1	5.3	2	11.8	0		1	5.0
5	2	13.3	1	5.9	0		0	
6	1	7.7	0		0		4	33.3
7	0		0		1	16.7	1	12.5
8	1	20.0	0		2	33.3	2	40.0
9	0		0		0		1	25.0
All episodes*	14	8.2	9	5.2	14	9.9	18	11.5

Each child received both the placebo and acetaminophen as antipyretic drugs, and thus one individual child may contribute an event to both the placebo and the acetaminophen column.
*The same child may have had several episodes. The differences between the groups are not significant.

group and two in the diazepam group, reported side effects associated with high fever.

DISCUSSION

Both acetaminophen as an antipyretic agent and the prophylactic use of diazepam appeared to be ineffective in preventing recurrences of febrile seizures. Even though such seizures are associated with the degree of fever, surprisingly few surveys have analyzed the importance of the temperature for their occurrence. Even high doses of antipyretics have been shown to be ineffective for preventing a new rise in temperature among children hospitalized for febrile convulsions[8]; during the first day the mean dose of acetaminophen employed by Schnaiderman et al.[8] varied from 73.9 to 105.9 mg per kilogram of body weight in the high-dose group, in comparison with 44.1 to 59.4 mg/kg in the comparison group. Our results support this finding. Camfield et al.[15] compared the efficacy of antipyretics with or without phenobarbital and found that the group receiving both antipyretics and phenobarbital had fewer recurrences than those receiving placebo and antipyretics. The effect of antipyretics thus could not be evaluated, although the authors concluded that antipyretic therapy was not likely to reduce recurrences of febrile convulsions.

Antipyretic agents differ in the mechanism by which they lower body temperature.[16] Acetaminophen acts on the central nervous system by lowering the thermoregulation set point, whereas most of the modern antipyretic and analgesic agents are more clearly prostaglandin inhibitors. The effect of more effective prostaglandin inhibitors on reduction of febrile seizures deserves further study.

The best results regarding the preventive efficacy of diazepam have been reported among patients with a high frequency of recurrence,[11, 12] and no effect has been reported in an unselected series of patients.[13] Our patients were unselected and had a low frequency of recurrence during the first year of follow-up; this may be one explanation for our results.

Our results contradict the most recent report, in which diazepam given orally was found to be effective in preventing recurrences of febrile seizures.[11] At least two important differences exist between our trial and the study reported by Rosman et al.[11]: the dose of the diazepam used and the selection of the patients. Our dose of diazepam, 0.2 mg per kilogram of body weight every 8 hours, was significantly lower than that given by Rosman et al. (0.33 mg/kg). Rosman et al. had chosen this dose because it produces blood drug levels of 150 to 300 μg/ml within an hour, levels that have been found to prevent seizures in children.[17] Plasma levels of diazepam correlate positively with the frequency of seizures in the quaking mouse.[18] We chose our dose on the basis of earlier reports showing the dose of 0.2 mg/kg to be effective when given rectally; orally administered diazepam seems to be as effective as the rectally administered preparation.[12, 19]

About half the patients studied by Rosman et al.[11] were recruited after recurrences and not after their first febrile seizure, and the unexpected finding that the children who received diazepam had more fevers than those in the placebo group was explained by the possibility that parents could identify differences between the treatment regimens and reported the results more carefully after administration of diazepam. In our group receiving diazepam, the number of seizure recurrences was equal to that in the group receiving placebo, and there were no differences in the incidence of fevers between the treatment groups. We did not use any marker to check the medication used. When Rosman et al. restricted their analysis to those patients who had actually received diazepam, most recurrences were seen to have been prevented. Thus, if diazepam is recommended, the dose should be 0.33 mg per kilogram of body weight every 8 hours. We saw few side effects, but it is probable that when the higher dose is used, the frequency of side effects will increase.

Our results demonstrate that the routine use of acetaminophen to prevent febrile seizures was not effective and that perhaps prostaglandin inhibitors or a larger dose of acetaminophen should be used. We currently restrict the use of diazepam to those patients who have risk factors for recurrence and then prescribe a dose of at least 0.33 mg/kg every 8 hours.

REFERENCES

1. Bethune P, Gordon K, Dooley J, Camfield C, Camfield P. Which child will have a febrile seizure? Am J Dis Child 1993; 147:35-9.
2. Annegers JF, Blakley SA, Hauser WA, Kurland LT. Recurrence of febrile convulsions in a population-based cohort. Epilepsy Res 1990;5:209-16.
3. Nelson KB, Ellenberg JH. Prognosis in children with febrile seizures. Pediatrics 1978;61:720-7.
4. Forsgren L, Sidenvall R, Blomquist HK, Heijbel J, Nystrom L. An incident case-referent study of febrile convulsions in children: genetical and social aspects. Neuropediatrics 1990; 21:153-9.
5. Millichap JG, Colliver JA. Management of febrile seizures: survey of current practice and phenobarbital usage. Pediatr Neurol 1991;7:243-8.
6. Newton RW. Randomised controlled trials of phenobarbitone and valproate in febrile convulsions. Arch Dis Child 1988; 63:1189-91.
7. Farwell JR, Lee YJ, Hirtz D, Sulzbacher SI, Ellenberg JH, Nelson KB. Phenobarbital for febrile seizures: effects on intelligence and on seizure recurrence. N Engl J Med 1990;322: 364-9.
8. Schnaiderman D, Lahat E, Sheefer T, Aladjem M. Antipyretic effectiveness of acetaminophen in febrile seizures: ongoing prophylaxis versus sporadic usage. Eur J Pediatr 1993;152: 747-9.
9. Green AL, Macfaul R. Duration of admission for febrile convulsions? Arch Dis Child 1985;60:1182-4.
10. Knudsen FU, Vestermark S. Prophylactic diazepam or phenobarbitone in febrile convulsions: a prospective, controlled study. Arch Dis Child 1978;53:660-3.
11. Rosman NP, Colton T, Labazzo J, et al. A controlled trial of diazepam administered during febrile illnesses to prevent recurrence of febrile seizures. N Engl J Med 1993;329:79-84.
12. Knudsen FU. Recurrence risk after first febrile seizure and effect of short term diazepam prophylaxis. Arch Dis Child 1985;60:1045-9.
13. Autret E, Billard C, Bertrand P, Motte J, Pouplard F, Jonville AP. Double-blind, randomized trial of diazepam versus placebo for prevention of recurrence of febrile seizures. J Pediatr 1990;117:490-4.
14. Keinänen S, Hietula M, Similä S, Kouvalainen K. Antipyretic therapy: comparison of rectal and oral paracetamol. Eur J Clin Pharmacol 1977;12:77-80.
15. Camfield PR, Camfield CS, Shapiro SH, Cummings C. The first febrile seizure: antipyretic instruction plus either phenobarbital or placebo to prevent recurrence. J Pediatr 1980; 97:16-21.
16. Wilkinson MF, Kasting NW. Central vasopressin V1-blockade prevents salicylate but not acetaminophen antipyresis. J Appl Physiol 1990;68:1793-8.
17. Agurell S, Berlin A, Ferngren H, Hellström B. Plasma levels of diazepam after parenteral and rectal administration in children. Epilepsia 1975;16:277-83.
18. Taylor SM, Bennet GD, Abbott LC, Finnel RH. Seizure control following administration of anticonvulsant drugs in the quaking mouse. Eur J Pharmacol 1985;118:163-70.
19. Ravnborg M, Hasselström L, Ostergård D. Premedication with oral and rectal diazepam. Acta Anaesthesiol Scand 1986; 30:132-8.

Benign intracranial hypertension in children with growth hormone deficiency treated with growth hormone

Saul Malozowski, MD, PhD, L. Ann Tanner, RPh, MPH,* Diane K. Wysowski, PhD, G. Alexander Fleming, MD, and Bruce V. Stadel, MD, MPH

From the Division of Metabolism and Endocrine Drug Products and the Division of Epidemiology and Surveillance, Center for Drug Evaluation and Research, U.S. Food and Drug Administration, Rockville, Maryland

We report 13 cases of benign intracranial hypertension (IH) in children with growth hormone (GH) deficiency treated with GH in the United States. The group consisted of eight boys and five girls, 3 to 16 years of age (median, 9 years). The interval from starting GH therapy to diagnosis of IH was 2 weeks or less in six patients, between 2 and 12 weeks in four, 8 months in one, 5 years in one, and unknown in one. Seven patients were not known to have previously described IH risk factors; the other six had at least one factor each. All patients but one had headache, nausea, vomiting, and visual changes. All had papilledema, and cerebrospinal fluid pressures were elevated (>250 mm H_2O) in all nine patients tested. The GH dosage range was 0.17 to 0.35 mg per kilogram body weight per week (median, 0.30 mg/kg per week) for the 11 patients with dosage data. After discontinuation of GH and treatment with lumbar punctures and/or medications, signs and symptoms resolved in eight children; in two of these children signs and symptoms reappeared when GH therapy was restarted. In four patients signs and symptoms resolved while GH therapy was continued; one child was treated with a ventriculoperitoneal shunt because of an arachnoid cyst, after which GH was restarted without subsequent IH. In the 12 patients with idiopathic GH deficiency the course of IH was benign, with complete resolution of all signs and symptoms. Because doses and scheduling of GH administration have changed since the introduction of recombinant GH, higher doses and increased frequency of administration may be contributing to the development of IH in some patients. We suggest beginning therapy at the lowest recommended dose, with gradual titration to higher doses, and the performance of routine funduscopic examinations during initiation of GH therapy and whenever signs or symptoms of IH develop. (J Pediatr 1995;126:996-9)

"Benign" intracranial hypertension, or pseudotumor cerebri, is defined as IH in the absence of a space-occupying lesion.[1] It is characterized by increased cerebrospinal fluid pressure with normal CSF composition, papilledema, visual changes, headaches, nausea, and vomiting. Dysfunction of extraocular muscles with strabismus, dizziness, ataxia, back or neck pain, mood changes, irritability, and somnolence may also be present.[2-4] Benign IH occurs more often in female than in male patients and in adults is associated with

CSF	Cerebrospinal fluid
GH	Growth hormone
IGF-I	Insulin-like growth factor-I
IH	Intracranial hypertension

This article represents the views of the authors and does not constitute an official position of the U.S. Food and Drug Administration.

Submitted for publication Sept. 30, 1994; accepted Dec. 2, 1994.

Reprint requests: Saul Malozowski, MD, 5600 Fishers Lane, HFD-510, Rockville, MD 20857.

*Now at Marion Merrell Dow Inc., Kansas City, Mo.

9/25/62526

Table. Clinical characteristics of patients with IH

Patient No.	Sex/age (yr)	Height (cm)	Weight (kg)	GH dosage (mg/kg/wk)	Onset time	Risk factors	Dechallenge	Rechallenge
1	M/16	155	58	0.30	2 wk	Obesity, thyroid hormone (T_4) therapy	NA*	NA
2	M/15	158	61	0.29	6 wk	Obesity, sinusitis	+	+
3	M/12	Unk	Unk	Unk	2 wk	T_4 therapy	+	Unk
4	M/9	108	39	0.35	2 wk	Obesity, mastoiditis	+	Unk
5	M/8	103	16	0.25	1 wk	None	+	Unk
6	M/7	Unk	Unk	0.17	6 wk	Unk	+	–
7	M/6	Unk	22	0.30	1 wk	Unk	+	Unk
8†	M/3	Unk	Unk	0.30	34 wk	Unk	–	–
9	F/14	Unk	85	0.17	12 wk	Obesity, prednisone	NA*	NA
10	F/12	Unk	Unk	Unk	Unk	Unk	NA*	NA
11	F/10	123	25	0.28	1 wk	None	+	+
12	F/9	125	Unk	0.30	3 wk	Unk	+	Unk
13	F/7	Unk	30	0.25	5 yr	Obesity, T_4 therapy, hydrocortisone	NA*	NA

+, Positive; –, negative; *NA*, not applicable; *T_4*; thyroxine; *Unk*, unknown.
*Drug continued and symptoms resolved.
†Patient with arachnoid cyst.

obesity, achieving a peak incidence in 20- to 44-year-old obese women.[5, 6] Intracranial hypertension has been related to the use of numerous medications such as thyroid hormone,[7] corticosteroids,[8, 9] retinol (vitamin A),[10] and tetracycline.[11] (Lessell[4] provides a detailed list.) In a recent report of IH in children, the sex ratio was reported as equal and obesity was a feature in about one third of the patients.[12] Previously reported causes include ear infections, dural sinus thrombosis, head injury, and tetracycline and retinol overdose.[2, 10]

We recently reported briefly an international series of 23 cases of benign IH associated with growth hormone treatment in children who either had GH deficiency or were short because of chronic kidney failure, Prader-Willi syndrome, Turner syndrome, or delayed puberty.[13] One adult patient also had IH during GH therapy for control of hypoglycemic symptoms. Since our initial report, in which we identified five cases of IH in patients with GH deficiency in the United States, we have identified eight more and now report in greater detail these 13 cases in children with GH deficiency.

METHODS

The initial two patients were identified through the Food and Drug Administration MedWatch Spontaneous Reporting System and the remaining 11 through direct communication between one of us and the pharmaceutic companies that market GH in the United States. About 4 months were required to obtain the data presented in this report, which are as complete as the companies were able to supply after inquiries to physicians and providers of care.

RESULTS

The Table summarizes data for the 13 patients by sex, age, height, weight, GH dose, time to onset of IH, the presence or absence of known risk factors for benign IH, response to withdrawal of therapy, and rechallenge. There were eight boys and five girls, 3 to 16 years of age (median, 9 years). The height range was 103 to 158 cm (median, 123 cm) for the six patients with height data, and the weight range was 16 to 85 kg (median, 34.5 kg) for the eight with weight data. All patients except one had idiopathic GH deficiency; patient 8 had an arachnoid cyst.

The GH dosage range was 0.17 to 0.35 mg/kg body weight per week (median, 0.30 mg/kg per week) for the 11 children with dosage data; weekly doses ranged from about 4 to 23 mg (12 to 68 IU). The time from starting GH to diagnosis of IH was 2 weeks or less in six patients, between 2 and 12 weeks in four, 8 months in one, and 5 years in one; the time was unknown in one patient.

Seven patients had no mention of the previously described risk factors for benign IH; six had at least one factor each: two were taking thyroid hormone, one was taking thyroid hormone and hydrocortisone, one was taking prednisone, one had sinusitis, and one had minimal bilateral mastoiditis. Five of the eight patients with weight information were obese. All patients except one (patient 13) had some or all of the following symptoms of IH: visual disturbances, headache, nausea, vomiting, and mood changes. In addition, in two patients (Nos. 5 and 7) lateral rectus muscle paralysis developed as a result of compression of the sixth cranial nerve. In one patient (No. 1) ankle edema and other signs of fluid retention were reported to have developed. In the one patient without symptoms (No. 13) papilledema was found during a routine physical examination.

The CSF pressures ranged between 260 and 600 mm H_2O in the nine patients tested; CSF chemistry values were normal. Findings of computed axial tomography and magnetic resonance imaging studies were normal in the 10 patients who underwent studies.

In eight patients the signs and symptoms of IH disappeared when administration of GH was stopped; in two of them (Nos. 2 and 11) the signs and symptoms reappeared when GH was restarted (positive rechallenge), but in one (No. 6) they did not (negative rechallenge). Effects of GH reintroduction were unknown in the other five patients whose condition improved once GH was first discontinued. Four patients had resolution of symptoms with continued GH treatment. The patient with an arachnoid cyst was treated by placement of a ventriculoperitoneal shunt, after which the IH resolved; GH therapy was then restarted without subsequent IH.

Most of the patients were treated with spinal fluid removal through lumbar punctures and with medications. The course of IH was benign in the 12 patients with idiopathic GH deficiency, who had complete resolution of all signs and symptoms. Clinical improvement occurred within 8 weeks in six patients; one report indicated improvement in a "few months," one in 7 months, and one in 10 months. Information regarding the remaining four patients was not available.

DISCUSSION

To our knowledge GH treatment has been associated with IH in only two patients reported by Otten et al.[14] and in our prior brief communication.[13] However, we have now identified a total of 13 U.S. cases of IH that, according to the reporting physicians, developed during GH treatment of children with GH deficiency. Several observations support a causal relationship with GH therapy. First, in two patients the signs and symptoms of IH disappeared when GH therapy was stopped and reappeared when it was restarted. The absence of recurrent signs and symptoms of IH when GH was restarted in one patient, and the resolution of IH while GH was continued in four, do not preclude GH therapy as the initiating event in the development of IH, because resolution of IH might have been related to homeostatic adjustments. Second, 10 of the 13 cases developed within the first 12 weeks of GH treatment; this temporal clustering is consistent with a causal relationship between GH therapy and IH. Third, seven of the 13 patients had no known predisposing condition for IH. Five of the eight patients with weight information were obese, but presumably obesity was a preexisting condition. Furthermore, treatment with corticosteroids or thyroid hormone was also preexistent. These drugs have been used for decades in the treatment of GH deficiency[15] and to our knowledge have not been reported as possible causes of IH in children with GH deficiency, although they have been implicated in the development of IH in patients with other disorders.[7-9] Finally, although IH is most commonly seen in obese, sexually mature women,[4-6] eight of our 13 patients were boys and the median age for the entire series was 9 years.

Although the pathogenesis of IH is uncertain, it is thought to involve increased production of CSF, decreased drainage, or both.[1, 2] Growth hormone induces rapid changes in fluid balance,[16] and in adults treated with GH, clinically apparent edema tends to develop even when the starting dosage is 0.09 mg/kg body weight per week,[17, 18] or approximately half the lowest dosage reported in our 13 patients. Although clinical edema was reported in only one of our patients, the possibility should be considered that GH may exert more subtle, clinically inapparent effects on body fluid distribution that lead to development of IH.

Johansson et al.[19] reported that GH passes the blood-brain barrier and induces increased levels of insulin-like growth factor–I in the CSF of adults with GH deficiency. Relatively large amounts of both IGF-I and IGF-I receptors have been found in rat choroid plexus.[20] The choroid plexus is thought to be the main site of CSF production. Thus direct action of GH at this level, augmenting IGF-I and in turn CSF production, could be advanced as an additional hypothesis for the pathogenesis of IH. Supportive of this hypothesis, we have reported three cases of IH treated with IGF-I for GH insensitivity (a very rare disorder) within the first 4 months of therapy.[13]

It may be significant that IH was not recognized as a complication of GH treatment in children with GH deficiency until abundant supplies of the hormone became available in 1985, with the introduction of GH produced by DNA recombinant techniques. Between 1960 and 1985, when supplies were limited to the amounts obtainable from human pituitary glands, the typical dosage schedule was 2 IU three times per week, for a total weekly dose of 6 IU, or about 2 mg. However, GH is now being given as frequently as six to seven times per week, at total weekly doses of 0.18 to 0.3 mg/kg.[21, 22] In our series the total weekly dose ranged from 4 to 23 mg, or approximately 12 to 68 IU. The fact that most of the cases occurred within 3 months of beginning GH therapy suggests a temporal association. Aggressive GH dosing appears to be a common risk factor in these cases, but the manner in which GH therapy is initiated may be more important than the ultimate dose. It is possible that a gradual dose escalation during GH therapy might eliminate or at least decrease the risk of IH in children with GH deficiency, even if the final dose is relatively high. It would also be prudent to perform funduscopic examinations routinely during initiation of GH therapy and whenever signs or symptoms of IH develop. Finally, the association between GH therapy and IH is not confined to patients with GH deficiency[13, 14]; all patients receiving GH may be at risk of this complication.

We thank the staffs of Genentech, Lilly, Novo-Nordisk, Pharmacia, and Serono, and the members of the National Cooperative Growth Study, for their assistance in collecting and sharing the data for this manuscript.

REFERENCES

1. Miller NR. Papilledema. In: Miller NR, ed. Walsh and Hoyt's neuro-ophthalmology; vol 1. Baltimore: Williams & Wilkins, 1982:175-211.
2. Radhakrishnan K, Ahlskog JE, Garrity JA, Kurland LT. Idiopathic intracranial hypertension. Mayo Clin Proc 1994;69: 169-80.
3. Dhiravibulya K, Ouvrier R, Johnston I, Procopis P, Antony J. Benign intracranial hypertension in childhood: a review of 23 patients. J Paediatr Child Health 1991;27:304-7.
4. Lessell S. Pediatric pseudotumor cerebri (idiopathic intracranial hypertension). Surv Ophthalmol 1992;37:155-66.
5. Durcan FJ, Corbett JJ, Wall M. The incidence of pseudotumor cerebri: population studies in Iowa and Louisiana. Arch Neurol 1988;45:875-7.
6. Wall M, George D. Idiopathic intracranial hypertension: a prospective study of 50 patients. Brain 1991;114:155-80.
7. Huseman CA, Torkelson RD. Pseudotumor cerebri following treatment of hypothalamic and primary hypothyroidism. Am J Dis Child 1984;138:927-31.
8. Cohn GA. Pseudotumor cerebri in children secondary to administration of adrenal steroids. J Neurosurg 1963;20:784-6.
9. Greer M. Benign intracranial hypertension (pseudotumor cerebri). Pedriatr Clin North Am 1967;14:819-30.
10. Weisberg LA, Chutorian AM. Pseudotumor cerebri in childhood. Am J Dis Child 1977;131:1243-8.
11. Fields JP. Bulging fontanel: a complication of tetracycline therapy in infants. J Pediatr 1961;58:74-6.
12. Babikian P, Corbett J, Bell W. Idiopathic intracranial hypertension in children: the Iowa experience. J Child Neurol 1994; 9:144-9.
13. Malozowski S, Tanner LA, Wysowski D, Fleming GA. Growth hormone, insulin-like growth factor I, and benign intracranial hypertension. N Engl J Med 1993;329:665-6.
14. Otten BJ, Rottevel JJ, Cruysberg JRM. Pseudotumor cerebri following treatment with growth hormone [Abstract]. Horm Res 1992; 37:16.
15. Goodman HG, Grumbach MM, Kaplan SL. Growth and growth hormone. II. A comparison of isolated growth hormone deficiency and multiple pituitary-hormone deficiencies in 35 patients with idiopathic pituitary dwarfism. N Engl J Med 1968;278:57-68.
16. Aloia JF, Zanzi I, Ellis K, et al. Effects of growth hormone in osteoporosis. J Clin Endocrinol Metab 1976;43:992-9.
17. Rudman D, Feller AG, Nagraj HS, et al. Effects of human growth hormone in men over 60 years old. N Engl J Med 1990;323:1-6.
18. Marcus R, Butterfield G, Holloway L, et al. Effects of short term administration of recombinant growth hormone to elderly people. J Clin Endocrinol Metab 1990;70:519-27.
19. Johansson JO, Larson G, Andersson M, et al. Growth hormone treatment results in an increase in GH, IGF-I, IGFBP-3 and β-endorphin concentrations in the cerebrospinal fluid. Endocrinol Metab 1994;1(suppl B):32.
20. Bondy C, Werner H, Roberts CT Jr, LeRoith D. Cellular pattern of type I insulin-like growth factor receptor gene expression during maturation in the rat brain: comparisons with insulin-like growth factors I and II. Neuroscience 1992;46:909-23.
21. Kastrup KW, Christiansen SJ, Andersen KJ, Orskov H. Increased growth rate following transfer to daily sc administration from three weekly im injections of hGH in growth hormone deficient children. Acta Endocrinol Copenh 1983; 104:148-52.
22. Jorgensen JOL. Human growth hormone replacement therapy: pharmacological and clinical aspects. Endoc Rev 1991; 12:189-207.

Comparative safety and efficacy of two immune globulin products in Kawasaki disease

Elaine A. Rosenfeld, MD, Stanford T. Shulman, MD, Kathleen E. Corydon, RN, William Mason, MD, Masato Takahashi, MD, and Chieko Kuroda, BS

From the Department of Pediatrics, Northwestern University Medical School, Children's Memorial Hospital, Chicago, Illinois, and the Department of Pediatrics, University of Southern California, Childrens Hospital of Los Angeles, Los Angeles, California

Objective: To compare the safety and efficacy of various intravenously administered immune globulin (IVGG) products in patients with Kawasaki disease.
Methods: We performed a retrospective matched-pair study of 45 pairs of patients, matched by age, gender, hospital, and illness day when IVGG therapy was initiated. All patients received aspirin, 80 to 100 mg/kg per day; one of each pair received Venoglobulin, 2 gm/kg (product A), and the other received Iveegam, 2 gm/kg (product B). Safety was assessed during and after IVGG infusion by recording rigors, pruritus, hypotension, urticaria, and nausea. Treatment efficacy was evaluated by posttreatment height and duration of fever, and subsequent echocardiographic changes.
Results: Untoward reactions during infusions occurred more often with product A (25%) than with product B (2%) ($p < 0.025$); most reactions were rigors (18% vs 2%) ($p < 0.05$). Therapy was completed in all patients. Height of fever and proportion of patients febrile each day after product A or B did not differ significantly. No differences were found in the frequency of coronary artery abnormalities 1 year after illness.
Conclusions: No significant differences in efficacy appeared between the two IVGG products, but they differed significantly in non-life-threatening adverse reactions, especially infusion-related rigors. Other IVGG products should be evaluated in a similar fashion. (J PEDIATR 1995;126:1003-3)

Published reports of trials of intravenously administered immune globulin for treatment of Kawasaki disease have included few of the preparations commercially available in the United States.[1, 2] It is unclear whether the IVGG products of various manufacturers are equally efficacious in KD and whether they differ with respect to adverse reaction rate. To assess both therapeutic efficacy and the safety profile of two IVGG products available in the United States, we studied patients with acute KD who were treated with a single 2 gm/kg dose of either Venoglobulin-I (Alpha Therapeutics, Los Angeles, Calif.; product A) or Iveegam (Immuno AG, Vienna, Austria; product B), and each with high-dose aspirin therapy.

CAA	Coronary artery abnormality
IVGG	Intravenously administered immune globulin
KD	Kawasaki disease

Submitted for publication Sept. 16, 1994; accepted Jan. 27, 1995.

Reprint requests: Elaine A. Rosenfeld, MD, Children's Memorial Hospital, Department of Infectious Diseases, 2300 Children's Plaza Box 20, Chicago, IL 60614.

0022-3476/95/$3.00 + 0 **9/25/63720**

METHODS

We performed a retrospective matched-pair study of 45 pairs of patients hospitalized with KD at Children's Memorial Hospital, Chicago, or Children's Hospital of Los Angeles between January 1986 and December 1993. Kawasaki disease was defined as an acute febrile illness with fever for at least 5 days and at least four of the following manifestations: bilateral conjunctival injection, edema and erythema of hands and feet, acute nonpurulent cervical adenopathy, polymorphous exanthem, and erythema of lips and oral mucosa.[3] We diagnosed KD before the fifth day of fever in five of these patients who had classic manifestations of KD.

All patients had been treated by the day 10 of illness with aspirin (80 to 100 mg/kg per day) and a single dose of IVGG (2 gm/kg) administered for 10 to 12 hours. One of each patient pair had received product A and the other received product B.

Product A is a sterile, highly purified lyophilized preparation of intact, unmodified immune globulin. The manufacturing process includes cold alcohol fractionation plus purification by polyethylene glycol fractionation and diethylaminoethyl-Sephadex ion exchange adsorption. In the preparation of product B, pooled plasma is also fractionated by a modified cold ethanol process. Cohn fraction II is treated with immobilized trypsin and purified by sequential precipitation steps with polyethylene glycol, which may be present in the final product at levels less than 0.5 gm/dl. The products differ somewhat in IgG-subclass distribution, in the range of IgG antibodies represented in the pool, in the proportions of IgG aggregates and fragments of IgG, and in the degree of contamination by non-IgG molecules, such as IgA and others[4-7] (Table I).

Patients were matched by age, gender, hospital, and illness day when IVGG treatment was initiated. Patients less than 24 months of age were matched by age within 3 months, those 24 to 84 months within 6 months, and patients older than 84 months within 24 months. We infused IVGG at 1.2 ml/kg per hour for 15 minutes, then at 2.4 ml/kg per hour for 15 minutes, and then 4.8 ml/kg per hour for the remainder of the infusion. Vital signs were measured every 15 minutes for the first hour, then every 30 minutes for the next hour, and then hourly for the remainder of the infusion.

Treatment efficacy was evaluated by assessing posttreatment height and duration of fever, and the development of coronary artery abnormalities detected by echocardiography. A coronary artery was defined as aneurysmal if the internal lumen diameter was at least 3 mm in a child less than 5 years of age or at least 4 mm in a child 5 years of age or older, or if the internal diameter of a segment was at least one and one-half times that of an adjacent segment.[2] Echocardiograms were obtained at the time of diagnosis and at 2 weeks, 4 to 6 weeks, 6 weeks to 12 months, and approximately 1 year after the diagnosis of KD. Echocardiograms were interpreted by an echocardiographer masked to the patient's treatment group. Fever was defined as rectal temperature at least 38.0° C. Safety was assessed during and after IVGG infusion by recording the occurrence of rigors with fever, pruritus, hypotension, urticaria, and nausea.

Table I. Manufacturing and content information of IVGG products A and B[4-7]

	Product A	Product B
Manufacturer (trade name)	Alpha Therapeutics (Venoglobulin-I)	Immuno AG (Iveegam)
Preparation	Cold ethanol-PEG fractionation, DEAE-Sephadex treatment, plasmin digestion	Cold ethanol-sequential PEG preparation, ion exchange, immobilized trypsin
Formulation	5% IgG with 2% mannitol, 10% albumin; lyophilized	5% IgG with 5% glucose; lyophilized
pH	6.8	6.8
IgG1 (%)	62.3	64.1
IgG2 (%)	32.8	30.3
IgG3 (%)	2.9	4.0
IgG4 (%)	2.0	1.5
IgA content (μg/ml)	24.3	10
MWT (%)		
Polymers, >300 kd	0.1	0
Dimers, 300 kd	8.9	5.7
Monomers, 150 kd	91	81
Fragments	0	9.3

DEAE, Diethylaminoethyl; *MWD*, molecular weight density; *PEG*, polyethylene glycol.

Categoric data were analyzed statistically by chi-square analysis with the Yates correction for small numbers. Continuous data were analyzed by the Student *t* test. Odds ratio and confidence intervals were calculated on the basis of the Cochran test, and extension of the Fisher Exact Test that is employed when minimum expected frequencies do not exceed 5 for the 2 × 2 table. Significance was defined at a *p* level less than 0.05.

RESULTS

No statistically significant differences were found between the patients in the product A and product B groups in distribution by race, gender, age, or illness day when first seen (Table II).

Safety. A significant difference was found in the incidence of rigors in the two treatment groups (Table III) ($p < 0.05$). These were not severe, and no IVGG infusions were terminated because of adverse reactions. Two infusions of prod-

Table II. Demographic data of patients treated with one of two IVGG products for KD

	Product A	Product B
Total No. of patients	45	45
Chicago	27	27
Los Angeles	18	18
Age (mo)		
Median	37	38
Mean	41.6	42.1
Range	4-112	4-110
Gender, No. (%)		
M	29 (64)	29 (64)
F	16 (36)	16 (36)
Race, No. (%)		
White	21 (44)	36 (58)
Asian	11 (24)	9 (20)
Black	9 (20)	3 (7)
Hispanic	5 (11)	7 (16)
Illness day when seen		
Median	6.0	6.2
Mean	6.3	6.2
Range	3-10	2-10

No differences between groups were statistically significant.

uct A were halted temporarily because of rigors with fever and pruritus and were then resumed at a slower rate of infusion, without further difficulty.

More patients treated with product A than product B had at least one adverse reaction during IVGG infusion ($p < 0.025$) (Table III). Patients who did or did not have untoward effects did not differ significantly with regard to age, gender, race, illness day of IVGG treatment, or subsequent development of echocardiographic changes.

Efficacy. As shown in Table IV, the percentage of patients who were febrile at the time of initiation of IVGG, the percentage of febrile patients on each day after treatment, and the maximum temperature attained each day after treatment did not differ significantly between the two treatment groups. The mean febrile days of illness before initiation of IVGG was 6.3 days with product A and 6.2 days with product B.

A total of 5 of 45 patients (11%) treated with product A and 3 of 45 patients (7%) given product B had CAA at some time in the course of their illness. The odds that a CAA will develop after treatment with product A was 1.75 compared with product B (95% confidence interval, 0.39 to 7.80) on the basis of the Fisher Exact Test. Seven of the eight patients with CAA, including five treated with product A and two with product B, had echocardiographic evidence of CAA before IVGG treatment. No significant difference was found in the timing of treatment in those with and without pretreatment CAA. The only patient with a normal pretreatment echocardiogram in whom a CAA developed after IVGG therapy received product B. No giant (internal diameter, <8 mm) or persistent (≥1 year) CAA developed in either treatment group; all observed abnormalities resolved.

Table III. Adverse reactions with IVGG in treatment of KD

Side effect	No. (%) of patients: Product A (n = 45)	Product B (n = 45)	
Rigors	8 (18)	1 (2)	<0.05
Pruritus	2 (4)	0 (0)	
Urticaria	0 (0)	0 (0)	
Nausea	0 (0)	0 (0)	
Hypotension	0 (0)	0 (0)	
Total with ≥1 side effect	9/45 (20)*	1/45 (2)	<0.025

*One patient had both rigors and pruritus.

Of 90 study patients, three (3%) were retreated with IVGG because of persistent fever and unresolved clinical signs and symptoms after the first dose. Two patients received a second 2 gm/kg dose of product A, and a third patient received a repeated 2 gm/kg dose of product A, followed by a 2 gm/kg dose of product B. That all three retreated patients had been treated initially with product A was not statistically significant.

DISCUSSION

The IVGG produced by Immuno AG, licensed in the United States as Iveegam (product B in this study), was very well tolerated in the U.S. multicenter clinical trials of KD and was associated with very few adverse reactions.[1,2] Newburger et al.[1] reported congestive heart failure in 4%, and 1% each with rigors, sepsis, and neutropenia associated with treatment with product B. Newburger et al.[2] reported adverse effects in 2.7% of those treated with product B, including new or worsening congestive heart failure or pruritus (each in 0.4% of patients); edema (0.2%); and nasal congestion, cough, and nausea (each in 0.1%). Rigors were not reported in this population.

We found a significantly greater incidence of adverse reactions during IVGG infusions (rigors and/or pruritus) with product A (20%) compared with product B (2%). None of these reactions were serious or life threatening, but patients were uncomfortable and two required temporary discontinuation of the infusion until their symptoms resolved. All infusions were completed satisfactorily, some at a reduced rate.

Potential biases may affect any two-center, retrospective study. Most patients were enrolled in earlier noncomparative trials of clinical efficacy of IVGG treatment in KD. Studies

Table IV. Percentage of febrile patients and mean maximum temperatures on day of treatment and on days after treatment with product A or product B

		Day after treatment		
	Day of treatment	Day 1	Day 2	Day 3
Product A				
Febrile patients (%)	93	87	49	33
Patients febrile at initiation of IVGG (%)	100	88	48	36
Mean maximum temperature (° C)	39.5	39.4	38.2	37.7
Product B				
Febrile patients (%)	82	71	31	27
Patients febrile at initiation of IVGG (%)	100	78	38	30
Mean maximum temperature (° C)	39.2	38.8	37.8	37.6

of product B were initiated 6 years before initiation of those of product A. Although we carefully assessed the medical record and study records, use of historical data may be affected by nonstandardized collection.

Several studies have documented the striking efficacy of IVGG to prevent development of CAA and to induce rapid resolution of fever and other clinical signs and laboratory indexes of inflammation in patients with KD.[1, 2, 8] In the present study the proportion of patients treated with a single dose of each brand of IVGG in whom CAA developed was consistent with these reports. In only one of 90 patients (2%) did CAA develop after IVGG therapy. In our small sample we detected no difference in efficacy of CAA prevention in the two treatment groups; however, a sample size of 910 patients would be required to detect, with a power of 80%, a true difference between the observed 7% and 11% CAA incidence rates.

Multicenter studies of IVGG treatment of KD in the United States demonstrated considerably greater antiinflammatory activity, as measured by amount and degree of fever, with IVGG and aspirin compared with aspirin alone.[1, 2] We did not demonstrate a significant difference in maximum temperatures after treatment with product B when compared with product A.

The basis for the difference in adverse reaction rates to the two IVGG products is not clear. Commercial IVGG products are prepared from large plasma pools by somewhat different methods. Differences in adverse reaction rates may be related to these factors, particularly to the degree of IgG aggregates, and possibly to the degree of IgA contamination when IVGG is inadvertently administered to the rare persons with severe IgA deficiency.

To minimize risk of adverse effects of IVGG, we recommend infusion of IVGG at a slow rate and frequent monitoring. In the event of an adverse reaction, particularly manifested by fever and rigors, one should slow or even stop the infusion. A cooling blanket may benefit the patient with rigors, and diphenhydramine may relieve pruritus during an infusion. In our experience resumption of the infusion at a slower rate is almost always feasible without additional reaction.

Since documentation of the efficacy of IVGG for KD, there has been speculation that various commercial IVGG products might differ in efficacy and frequency of adverse reactions. We have demonstrated that products A and B appear to be comparably effective in prevention of CAA but that they differ in frequency of adverse effects, none of which was life threatening. This study demonstrates the need for further studies to address the issues of comparable efficacy and safety for other commercial IVGG products in the treatment of KD.

We thank Dr. Anne H. Rowley for her critical reading of this manuscript and Mark Donovan for his assistance with statistical analysis.

REFERENCES

1. Newburger JW, Takahashi M, Burns JC, et al. The treatment of Kawasaki syndrome with intravenous gamma globulin. N Engl J Med 1986;315:341-7.
2. Newburger JW, Takahashi M, Beiser AS, et al. A single intravenous infusion of gamma globulin as compared with four infusions in the treatment of acute Kawasaki syndrome. N Engl J Med 1991;324:1633-9.
3. Centers for Disease Control: Kawasaki disease—New York. MMWR 1980;29:61-3.
4. Siegel J. Comparison of commercially available intravenous immune globulins. Pharm Immunol 1990;4:1-4.
5. Fischer GW. Uses of intravenous globulin to prevent or treat infections. Adv Pediatr Infect Dis 1992;7:85-108.
6. Hooper JA, Alpern M, Mankarious S. Immunoglobulin manufacturing procedures. In: Krijnen HW, Strengers PFW, Van Aken WG, eds. Immunoglobulins, Leiden. Central Laboratory of The Netherlands Red Cross Blood Transfusion Service, 1988.
7. Nielsen H. Immunoglobulin preparations for intravenous administration. Allergy 1994;49:69-73.
8. Rowley AH, Duffy E, Shulman ST. Prevention of giant coronary artery aneurysms in Kawasaki disease by intravenous gamma globulin. J Pediatr 1988;113:290-4.

A randomized trial comparing the efficacy of epinephrine with salbutamol in the treatment of acute bronchiolitis

Kusum Menon, MD, Teresa Sutcliffe, RN, and Terry P. Klassen, MD

From the Department of Pediatrics, University of Ottawa, and Children's Hospital of Eastern Ontario, Ottawa, Ontario, Canada

This randomized, double-blind trial compared the efficacy of nebulized epinephrine with salbutamol in the treatment of infants with acute bronchiolitis. The mean percent oxygen saturation at 60 minutes was significantly higher in the epinephrine group. Thirty-three percent of the patients in epinephrine group were admitted to the hospital compared with 81% of the salbutamol group ($p = 0.003$). We conclude that nebulized epinephrine is more efficacious than salbutamol for infants with acute bronchiolitis seen in an emergency department. (J PEDIATR 1995;126:1004-7)

The optimal treatment for bronchiolitis has been controversial; much of the uncertainty centers on the role of bronchodilators for treatment of this disease. Recent clinical trials with β_2-agonists have measured some improvement with clinical scoring systems,[1-3] but the clinical importance of this change has been questioned.[4] Concern has also been expressed about the oxygen desaturation observed in some infants with bronchiolitis after the administration of salbutamol.[5-7]

Wohl and Chernick[8] proposed that epinephrine may be the ideal bronchodilator because of its α- and β-receptor agonist properties. Recent clinical trials have shown epinephrine to be superior to placebo in acute bronchiolitis.[9-11] Sanchez et al.[12] compared salbutamol with racemic epinephrine, and showed that hospitalized patients who received epinephrine had a greater decrease in respiratory rate and pulmonary resistance. The purpose of our study was to examine the efficacy of epinephrine compared with salbutamol in outpatients with acute bronchiolitis.

Supported by grant No. R93-47 from the Physicians Services Incorporated Foundation.

Submitted for publication Aug. 10, 1994; accepted Nov. 17, 1994.

Reprint requests: Terry P. Klassen, MD, Division of Emergency Medicine, Children's Hospital of Eastern Ontario, 401 Smyth Rd., Ottawa, Ontario, K1H 8L1, Canada.

0022-3476/95/$3.00 + 0 **9/26/61904**

METHODS

Study setting. The Children's Hospital of Eastern Ontario is a regional tertiary care pediatric hospital. Each year approximately 50,000 patients visit the emergency department, which is staffed 24 hours a day by 10 full-time emergency pediatricians. These pediatricians also care for patients in a holding unit, where children's care is managed awaiting hospitalization or improvement to the point of being discharged home.

RDAI	Respiratory Distress Assessment Instrument

Selection of patients. Patients who came to the emergency department between Jan. 1, 1994, and March 30, 1994, were eligible for the study if they met the following criteria: age 6 weeks to 1 year, oxygen saturation $\geq$85% and $\leq$96%, Respiratory Distress Assessment Instrument[11] score $\geq$4, first episode of wheezing, and clinical symptoms of viral respiratory infection (temperature $\geq$38.0° C or coryza). Patients were excluded from the study if they had any chronic cardiac or pulmonary disease, a diagnosis of asthma by a physician or any previous use of bronchodilators, severe disease requiring resuscitation room care or heart rate <200 beats/min, or had received glucocorticoids within the previous 24 hours. The study was approved by the research ethics committee at the Children's Hospital of Eastern Ontario. Informed, written consent was obtained from all parents before enrollment of patients.

Outcome measures. All patients had measurements at baseline and at 30, 60, and 90 minutes by one of three research assistants trained by the investigators; these measurements consisted of the RDAI, respiratory rate, heart rate, and oxygen saturation. Oxygen saturation, which was the primary outcome measure, was measured noninvasively by pulse oximeter (model N20, Nellcor, Inc., Hayward, Calif.) after the infant had been in room air for 10 minutes.

Our secondary outcome measures included the RDAI, which, using an ordinal scale from 0 to 17, measures expiratory wheezing (0 to 4 points), inspiratory wheezing (0 to 2 points), location of wheeze (0 to 2 points), supraclavicular indrawing (0 to 3 points), intercostal indrawing (0 to 3 points), and subcostal indrawing (0 to 3 points).[11] The interobserver reliability, as measured by the weighted kappa value, was previously established by this study team to be 0.94.[2] Other secondary outcome measures included admission rates and side effects.

Study design. Eligible patients were randomly assigned to receive a dose (at 0 and 30 minutes) of either 0.3 ml of a 5 mg/ml solution of salbutamol (Ventolin) (1.5 mg) combined with 2.7 ml of 0.9% saline solution to make a total of 3 ml, or 3 ml of 1:1000 epinephrine (Adrenalin) solution (3 mg) by nebulizer with continuous flow of oxygen at 5 to 6 L/min. Doses were based on the maximum dose used in previous clinical trials of patients with either bronchiolitis or croup.[3, 9, 10, 13] Observers were unable to distinguish between the two nebulized solutions by odor, color, or any other characteristic. Randomization was performed in blocks of four by the pharmacy department according to a random numbers table. The list was concealed until after the calculated sample size was reached. Both drugs were packaged in syringes that were identical and identified with only a study number.

Emergency pediatricians followed the patients throughout the study period and were free to withdraw the patients from the study and to use other interventions, such as a higher concentration of oxygen or extra doses of salbutamol, if they deemed it clinically necessary. Any pallor, vomiting, or tremors were recorded. An admission was defined as any patient admitted directly to the inpatient wards or kept in the holding unit for longer than 6 hours. During the respiratory virus season, it is unusual for patients to be admitted directly to the hospital wards because of limited inpatient bed space. At the end of the 90-minute study period, all management decisions were made by the emergency pediatrician, who was unaware of the treatment allocation.

Table. Comparison of outcome variables at 30, 60, and 90 minutes

Variable time	Salbutamol	Epinephrine	*p*
Heart rate (beats/min)			
30 min	160 ± 17	159 ± 17	0.88
60 min	163 ± 15	159 ± 16	0.12
90 min	165 ± 13	151 ± 16	0.003
Respiratory rate (breaths/min)			
30 min	57 ± 15	51 ± 16	—
60 min	55 ± 16	50 ± 13	—
90 min	54 ± 12	49 ± 11	—
RDAI			
30 min	7.8 ± 2.2	7.6 ± 1.8	—
60 min	6.7 ± 2.1	6.4 ± 2.6	—
90 min	7.5 ± 1.7	6.6 ± 2.5	—
Oxygen saturation (%)			
30 min	96 ± 3	96 ± 2	0.88
60 min	94 ± 4	96 ± 3	0.02
90 min	95 ± 3	95 ± 4	0.80

All values are expressed as mean ± SD.

Sample size estimate. A 3% difference in oxygen saturation was considered to be a clinically important improvement. On the basis of our pilot study of 11 patients during the 1993 respiratory syncytial virus season, we calculated the standard deviation to be 3%. With an α level of 0.05 (two-tailed test), 90% power, a sample size of 21 patients per group would be required.

Statistical analysis. Data were analyzed with SPSS/PC + V4.01 software (Statistical Package for the Social Sciences, SPSS Inc., Chicago, Ill.). The analyst was unaware of the actual drug preparation because the two groups were labeled Drug 1 or Drug 2. Repeated measures analysis of variance was used to analyze the mean oxygen saturation, RDAI, respiratory rate, and heart rate for the effect of time (baseline, 30, 60 and 90 minutes), the effect of the group (salbutamol or epinephrine), and the interaction between the two (group × time). When significant differences were detected, independent, two-tailed *t* tests were used to assess the differences related to the group effect. Categoric data were analyzed with the chi-square statistic, or the Fisher Exact Test if numbers were small. Kaplan-Meier survival analysis was used to determine the difference in discharge rates between the two groups using the Breslow test on SPSS for MS Windows, Release 6.0.

RESULTS

Patient characteristics. During the study period, 81 patients were seen in our emergency department and met the eligibility criteria of our study. Of these, four were seen when the study team was not on call; for 33 patients the emergency physicians failed to contact the study team. Of the 44 par-

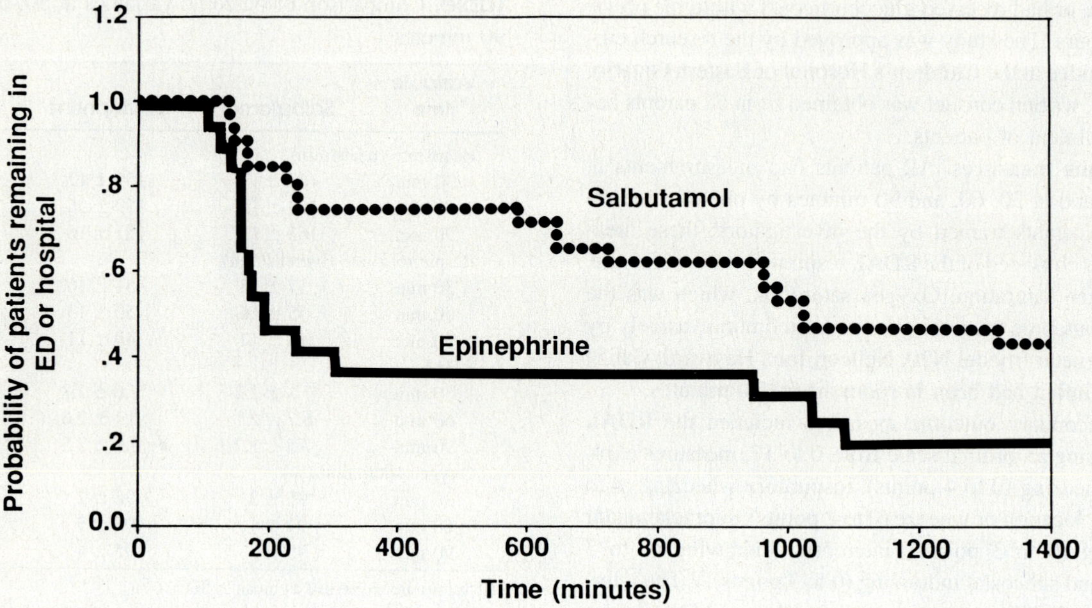

Figure. Survival curve illustrating significantly shorter time of epinephrine-treated patients in emergency department of hospital compared with those given salbutamol ($p = 0.02$).

ents of patients approached for study participation, 42 agreed to participate.

Twenty-one patients were randomly assigned to the epinephrine group and 21 to the salbutamol group. However, it was discovered after randomization that one of the patients in the epinephrine group had previously received a bronchodilator and therefore was excluded. All baseline demographic and clinical variables were evenly distributed between the two groups except for an age difference (salbutamol 0.4 ± 0.2 years vs epinephrine 0.5 ± 0.2 years) that was not considered clinically significant. (Data available from authors on request.)

Outcome variables. Repeated measures analysis of variance showed that there was a significant interaction between time and group ($p = 0.04$) for the mean oxygen saturation because patients treated with nebulized epinephrine had a significantly higher oxygen saturation at 60 minutes (96% vs 94%; $p = 0.02$; Table). There was a significant effect of time for heart rate ($p = 0.03$) and RDAI ($p < 0.0001$), but there was no significant interaction between time and group because the conditions of infants in both groups were improving over time from baseline. The effect of group did not reach traditional levels of statistical significance ($p = 0.07$), but a significantly lower mean heart rate was found in the epinephrine group when compared with the salbutamol group at 90 minutes ($p = 0.003$; Table). For the mean respiratory rate, there was no significant effect of time, group, or interaction between group and time.

Patient follow-up. Seventeen (81%) of the patients in the salbutamol group were admitted compared with 7 (33%) in the epinephrine group ($p = 0.003$). The mean duration of admission in the salbutamol group was 30.4 ± 27.8 hours compared with a mean of 41.5 ± 30.4 hours in the epinephrine group ($p = 0.40$). The Figure demonstrates a significantly faster rate of discharge for epinephrine-treated patients than for the salbutamol group ($p = 0.02$) within the first 4 hours.

In the 6 hours before admission, not including the 90-minute study period, the salbutamol group received 1.4 ± 1.6 salbutamol administrations compared with 0.4 ± 0.9 salbutamol administrations in the epinephrine group ($p = 0.03$). No one in either group received glucocorticoids during this time. There were four return visits within 24 hours of discharge from the hospital in each group ($p = 0.94$).

Adverse effects. A higher incidence of pallor was found in the epinephrine group than in the salbutamol group at 30 minutes (10 patients vs 3; $p = 0.01$) and at 60 minutes (8 patients vs 3; $p = 0.06$). However, this difference had diminished by 90 minutes (4 patients vs 1; $p = 0.13$). No vomiting was noted in either group, and no significant differences in tremor were present. No patient required withdrawal from the study or interventions that were not part of the protocol.

DISCUSSION

This randomized, controlled trial has shown that nebulized epinephrine causes increased clinical benefit compared with salbutamol in the treatment of acute bronchiolitis in infancy. This benefit is reflected primarily in the markedly reduced admission rates but is also supported by the improved oxygen saturation at 60 minutes, a lower heart rate at 90 minutes, and a faster rate of discharge from the emergency department. These findings are consistent with the findings of Sanchez et al.,[12] who documented an improvement in the epinephrine group compared with the salbutamol group when a decrease in pulmonary resistance is used as the primary outcome measure. Other studies have shown epinephrine to be superior to placebo,[9-11] but have not compared epinephrine with salbutamol, although salbutamol has become the agent of choice in acute bronchiolitis if physicians have decided to use pharmacologic treatment.

The most significant changes in this study were those based on decisions by physicians (such as hospitalization rates, discharge rates from the emergency department, and number of supplemental salbutamol treatments) compared with the more modest changes in heart rate and oxygen saturation. This may be because vital signs, oxygen saturation, and clinical scoring systems are less sensitive to changes in the patient's clinical status. Experienced emergency physicians, who were unaware of the treatment allocation, apparently noticed something in the patient's clinical status that prompted them to send patients home sooner and to administer fewer supplemental salbutamol treatments. Ultimately, if an intervention decreases health care utilization, it has a greater probability of reducing health care costs.

There has been some concern about the potential for more frequent side effects from epinephrine compared with salbutamol, especially the side effect of tachycardia. This was not seen in our study, and at 90 minutes the heart rate was significantly lower in the epinephrine group. Pallor was noted more frequently in the epinephrine group but is of no known clinical significance.

The nebulized form of epinephrine most commonly used is racemic epinephrine, which contains equal parts of the L- and D-isomers. It was originally thought that the D-form of the preparation blocked the cardiovascular β_1-adrenergic receptors, resulting in fewer cardiac side effects. The L-epinephrine formulation costs less than racemic epinephrine ($0.76 vs $1.74 per dose).

Concern has been expressed about the possible irritant or allergenic property of metabisulfites, present as a preservative in 1:1000 L-epinephrine preparations. However, in a previous clinical trial in patients with croup (n = 31),[13] in our pilot study (n = 11), and in this randomized controlled trial (n = 41), no patient experienced deterioration in his or her condition. In addition, racemic epinephrine also contains metabisulfites and has been used widely for the treatment of croup.

On the basis of the decrease in the number of admissions and a faster rate of discharge from the emergency department, we conclude that nebulized epinephrine is a more effective and equally safe medication when compared with salbutamol for infants with acute bronchiolitis. Future studies are needed to confirm these results and to develop measurement tools that are more sensitive to changes in the patient's clinical status.

We thank Pat Harman and Joanne Momy for their work as research assistants, Tara Tucker and Solange Wolfe for their invaluable assistance in the pilot study, Colline Blanchard for randomization and drug preparation, Dr. Marilyn Li, and all the emergency department pediatricians and nurses for their help with patient recruitment. We also thank Dr. Peter C. Rowe and Grace Dueck for reviewing this manuscript.

REFERENCES

1. Alario AJ, Lewander WJ, Dennehy P, Seifer R, Mansell AL. The efficacy of nebulized metaproterenol in wheezing infants and young children. Am J Dis Child 1992;146:412-8.
2. Klassen TP, Rowe PC, Sutcliffe T, Ropp LJ, McDowell IW, Li MM. Randomized trial of salbutamol in acute bronchiolitis [published erratum appears in J PEDIATR 1991;119:1010]. J PEDIATR 1991;118:807-11.
3. Schuh S, Canny G, Reisman JJ, et al. Nebulized albuterol in acute bronchiolitis. J PEDIATR 1990;117:633-7.
4. Goodman BT, Chambers TL. Bronchodilators for bronchiolitis? Lancet 1993;341:1380.
5. Ho L, Collis G, Landau LI, Le Souef PN. Effect of salbutamol on oxygen saturation in bronchiolitis. Arch Dis Child 1991; 66:1061-4.
6. Seidenberg J, Mir Y, von der Hardt H. Hypoxaemia after nebulised salbutamol in wheezy infants: the importance of aerosol acidity. Arch Dis Child 1991;66:672-5.
7. Prendiville A, Rose A, Maxwell DL, Silverman M. Hypoxaemia in wheezy infants after bronchodilator treatment. Arch Dis Child 1987;62:997-1000.
8. Wohl ME, Chernick V. State of the art: bronchiolitis. Am Rev Respir Dis 1978;118:759-81.
9. Wennergren G, Kristjánsson S, Sten G, Bjure J, Engström I. Nebulized racemic adrenaline for wheezy bronchitis. Acta Paediatr Scand 1991;80:375-7.
10. Kristjánsson S, Lodrup Carlsen KC, Wennergren G, Strannegard I-L, Carlsen K-H. Nebulized racemic adrenaline in the treatment of acute bronchiolitis in infants and toddlers. Arch Dis Child 1993;69:650-4.
11. Lowell DI, Lister G, Von Koss H, McCarthy P. Wheezing in infants: the response to epinephrine. Pediatrics 1987;79:939-45.
12. Sanchez I, De Koster J, Powell RE, Wolstein R, Chernick V. Effect of racemic epinephrine and salbutamol on clinical score and pulmonary mechanics in infants with bronchiolitis. J PEDIATR 1993;122:145-51.
13. Waisman Y, Klein BL, Boenning DL, et al. Prospective randomized double-blind study comparing L-epinephrine and racemic epinephrine aerosols in the treatment of laryngotracheitis (croup). Pediatrics 1992;89:302-6.

Antibiotic-associated hemorrhagic colitis without *Clostridium difficile* toxin in children

Seiichi Kato, MD, Kyoko Ebina, MD, Akira Ozawa, MD, Hiroshi Naganuma, MD, and Hiroshi Nakagawa, MD
From the Departments of Pediatrics and Pathology, Sendai City Hospital, Sendai, Japan

We describe nine children with antibiotic-associated hemorrhagic colitis without *Clostridium difficile* toxin. The onset was usually sudden, with severe hematochezia and abdominal cramps. The illness quickly resolved and required no specific treatment except discontinuation of the implicated antibiotic. Early proctosigmoidoscopy was a useful diagnostic adjunct. It appears that antibiotic-associated hemorrhagic colitis is a distinct entity rather than a variant of antibiotic-associated colitis in children. (J PEDIATR 1995;126:1008-10)

Antibiotic therapy can cause several diarrheal diseases. Since toxin-producing *Clostridium difficile* was established as the cause of pseudomembranous colitis, it has been the major factor identified in cases of antibiotic-associated diarrhea or colitis. Infections with *C. difficile* have a broad clinical spectrum, ranging from the asymptomatic carrier state to fulminant colitis.[1] In recent years, antibiotic-associated hemorrhagic colitis without pseudomembranes has been reported in adults.[2-6] In Japan, AHC rather than PMC has become a major clinical problem. Although pediatric cases of AHC have been mentioned in studies of Japanese adults,[7] few details concerning the clinical features are available. The purpose of this study was to review retrospectively nine children in whom AHC developed without *C. difficile* toxin.

METHODS

Between December 1988 and March 1994, nine patients aged 1 to 15 years (mean, 10.7 years) with AHC were referred to Sendai City Hospital (Table I). A diagnosis of AHC was made on the basis of each history and negative fecal cultures.[3] With a PCF 20 fiberscope or a PCF 200 videoscope (Olympus, Tokyo, Japan) colonoscopy was performed 1 to 5 days (mean, 2.7 days) after the onset of illness in all patients. Seven patients had endoscopic biopsies for pathologic study of the affected mucosa. A double-contrast enema was performed an average of 6.6 days (range, 4 to 11 days) after onset in all patients. Enteric pathogens, including *Shigella*, *Salmonella*, *Campylobacter*, and diarrheogenic *Escherichia coli*, were sought by conventional methods in the stool cultures. Fecal samples from all but one patient were also analyzed for the presence of *C. difficile* enterotoxin D_1 with the rapid latex agglutination method (C. D. Check D_1; Shionogi Pharmaceutical Co., Ltd., Osaka, Japan). With this method a value of 500 ng/ml or more of enterotoxin D_1 is considered positive. In addition, lymphocyte stimulation tests were done with the implicated antibiotics to study allergic hypersensitivity in six patients; a stimulation index of less than 200% was considered negative for enhanced blastogenesis.

AHC	Antibiotic-associated hemorrhagic colitis
PMC	Pseudomembranous colitis

RESULTS

Clinical manifestations. None of the patients had any underlying diseases. All antibiotics were administered orally, and the majority of implicated antibiotics (88.9%) were penicillin derivatives, most commonly amoxicillin (Table I). The initial and chief symptoms were hematochezia and abdominal cramps, which began either during therapy or within 1 to 2 days after therapy was stopped. Hematochezia was severe (≥20 stools per day in six patients), but it did not result in anemia. In five patients diarrhea was initially watery but progressed to bloody within a few hours. Abdominal cramps were localized in the left or lower part of the abdomen in six patients and in the periumbilical area in three. Vomiting, which occurred in four patients, was mild. Fever occurred in three patients, with temperatures of 37.5° to 38.0° C, but this subsided within 1 to 2 days.

Laboratory and bacteriologic examinations. Leukocyte count was elevated to greater than 10×10^9 cells/L (≥10,000

Submitted for publication Sept. 6, 1994; accepted Jan. 24, 1995.
Reprint requests: Seiichi Kato, MD, Department of Pediatrics, Sendai City Hospital, 3-1 Shimizukoji Wakabayashi-ku, Sendai 980, Japan.

0022-3476/95/$3.00 + 0 **9/26/63689**

Table I. Clinical data for patients with AHC

Patient No.	Sex/age (yr)	Implicated drug	Dosage (mg)	Duration (days)	Indication for antibiotic	Time to onset (days)*	Duration of symptoms (days)
1	F/5	Amoxicillin	400	3	URI	4	4
2	M/8	Amoxicillin	300	3	Dog bite	4	4
3	F/6	Amoxicillin	700	4	URI	4	2
4	F/13	Amoxicillin	600	3	URI	4	4
5	M/10	Amoxicillin	750	3	URI	5	5
6	M/13	Ampicillin	1200	5	Epididymitis	5	3
7	M/12	Sultamicillin†	1125	4	Furuncle	6	5
8	M/15	Lenampicillin	750	3	Dental caries	2	4
9	M/14	Cefdinir	300	1	Enteritis	1	3
Mean	10.7			3.2		3.9	3.8

URI, Upper respiratory tract infection.
*Interval between start of oral antibiotic administration and the onset of colitis.
†Combination drug comprising ampicillin and sulbactam.

Table II. Laboratory data and distribution of colonoscopic findings

Patient No.	Leukocyte count ($\times 10^9$/L)	ESR (mm/hr)	Stool culture*	Colonoscopic findings: Rectum	Sigmoid colon	Descending colon
1	12.9	22	*Klebsiella pneumoniae*	+	+	ND
2	19.4	7	*Streptococcus faecalis*	−	+	+
3	12.2	30	*Klebsiella oxytoca*	−	ND	ND
4	6.0	4	*K. pneumoniae*	−	+	ND
5	9.1	5	*K. oxytoca*	+	+	+
6	18.3	ND	*K. oxytoca*	−	+	+
7	11.5	20	*Escherichia coli*	−	+	ND
8	9.7	2	*S. faecalis*	−	+	+
9	4.7	7	*E. coli*	−	+	−

+, Positive; −, negative; *ESR*, erythrocyte sedimentation rate; *ND*, not done.
*Main bacteria cultured are listed.

cells/mm^3) in five patients (Table II). About half the patients had neutrophilia, but none had eosinophilia. Erythrocyte sedimentation rate was normal in five of eight patients. No imbalance in serum electrolyte values or hypoalbuminemia occurred in any patient. Urinalysis revealed no abnormality during the course of the illness in any patient. Results of lymphocyte stimulation tests were negative in all six patients studied. Although *Klebsiella oxytoca* was cultured from stools of three patients, no enteric pathogens were found in the others.

Colonoscopic examination and double-contrast enema. Because of severe gastrointestinal symptoms, colonoscopic observation was extended to the sigmoid colon as a rule, whereas it was extended to the descending colon in five patients (Table II). Colonoscopic findings included, to varying degrees, redness, petechiae, bleeding, swelling, or erosions. However, neither pseudomembranes nor frank ulcerations were visible. The sigmoid colon was frequently stenotic because of mucosal swelling or spasms or both. Findings involving the rectum, if affected, tended to be milder than those involving the more proximal aspect of the colon. Rates of lesions with positive findings for the rectum, sigmoid colon, and descending colon were 22%, 100%, and 80%, respectively. Proctosigmoidoscopy was repeated 7 to 9 days after onset of symptoms in three patients and confirmed marked improvement in findings.

Barium contrast studies showed segmental spasm of the descending colon in patient 6 and a saw-toothed appearance of the sigmoid colon in patient 9 but failed to demonstrate any gross abnormalities in the other patients.

The biopsy specimens of the colon showed a decrease in goblet cells, hemorrhage with congestion beneath the superficial epithelium, and mild inflammatory changes in the lamina propria. In patient 8 detachment of the superficial epithelium was found.

Treatment and clinical course. Oral antibiotic therapy was stopped if the patient was still receiving it. Some patients needed pentazocin for severe abdominal cramps. Other than this drug the only treatments given were parenteral hydration and fasting for 1 to 2 days. Symptoms completely disappeared within a mean of 3.8 days (range, 2 to 5 days). No serious complications occurred during the course of the illness. All patients made an uneventful recovery without sequelae.

DISCUSSION

Since the reports published by Toffler et al.[2] and Sakurai et al.,[3] AHC has been recognized as being an unique entity distinct from PMC. This study defines several characteristic features of AHC: (1) the onset is sudden, with hematochezia and abdominal cramps, which are commonly severe; (2) systemic manifestations are rare or nonexistent; (3) colonoscopic examination demonstrates no pseudomembranes; (4) no specific treatment other than discontinuing the antibiotic is needed; and (5) the illness quickly resolves without any complications. These points are fairly consistent with the evidence in previous reports.[2-6, 8]

Proctosigmoidoscopy is sufficient for visualizing colonic changes in the majority of cases of antibiotic-associated colitis.[9] However, the necessity for early total colonoscopy has been emphasized, because in AHC the proximal aspect of the colon is generally affected and the proctosigmoid colon is frequently spared.[5, 6] Although this study was limited in its ability to determine the distribution of lesions, the results suggested that the distal aspect of the colon may be more commonly affected. We believe that early proctosigmoidoscopy is safe and useful for confirming the diagnosis of childhood AHC.

Ampicillin and amoxicillin are the most common offenders, but nearly all antibiotics can result in the development of AHC, irrespective of route of administration.[8] However, the pathogenesis remains unclear. One report indicated that *C. difficile* toxin was present in 10 of 27 patients with AHC.[7] During our study we found two patients in whom AHC developed, with *C. difficile* toxin present but without pseudomembranes, who were treated with orally administered vancomycin. *C. difficile*, which is thought to overpopulate because of the change in intestinal flora induced by antibiotic use, is responsible for virtually all cases of PMC and for up to 20% of cases of antibiotic-associated diarrhea without colitis.[1] Further study is required to determine the relationship between AHC and *C. difficile* infection. Although one author has suggested *K. oxytoca* as an etiologic factor,[10] its detection may imply only opportunistic overgrowth caused by antibiotic administration. Virologic investigation, including rotavirus testing, was not done in this study; we cannot rule out viral agents as an etiologic factor.

Sakurai et al.[3] found no mucosal changes after local application of ampicillin solution in patients with ampicillin-associated hemorrhagic colitis. Although patient 5 in our study was treated with amoxicillin at least twice before the onset of colitis, he had no prior symptoms. These observations support the contention that an allergic mechanism does not play a role in AHC.

Differential diagnosis should include infectious colitis, necrotizing enterocolitis, ischemic colitis, inflammatory bowel disease, Henoch-Schönlein purpura, hemolytic-uremic syndrome, and cow milk allergy. No specific diagnostic tools are available for AHC. In patients with sudden onset of hematochezia and abdominal cramps, a history of recent antibiotic use is the essential diagnostic clue.

REFERENCES

1. Triadafilopoulos G, LaMont JT. Pseudomembranous colitis. In: Walker WA, Durie PR, Hamilton JR, Walker-Smith JA, Watkins JB, eds. Pediatric gastrointestinal disease. Philadelphia: BC Decker, 1991:619-29.
2. Toffler RB, Pingoud EG, Burrell MI. Acute colitis related to penicillin and penicillin derivatives. Lancet 1978;2:707-9.
3. Sakurai Y, Tsuchiya H, Ikegami F, Funatomi T, Takasu S, Uchikoshi T. Acute right-sided hemorrhagic colitis associated with oral administration of ampicillin. Dig Dis Sci 1979; 24:910-5.
4. Iida M, Matsui T, Fuchigami T, Iwashita A, Omae T. Radiographic and endoscopic findings in penicillin-related nonpseudomembranous colitis. Endoscopy 1985;17:64-8.
5. Rimmer MJ, Freeman AH, Low FM. The barium enema diagnosis of penicillin associated colitis. Clin Radiol 1982;33:529-33.
6. Gould PC, Khawaja FI, Rosenthal WS. Antibiotic-associated hemorrhagic colitis. Am J Gastroenterol 1982;77:491-3.
7. Arai T, Matsumoto J, Odajima H, Shimojo H, Kosugi H, Kondo T. A clinical study of antibiotic-associated acute hemorrhagic colitis, with special reference of *Clostridium difficile*. Jpn J Gastroenterol 1985;82:78-85 (in Japanese).
8. Tada M, Tanaka Y, Watanabe Y, Kawamoto Y, Kawai K. Clinical studies on antibiotic associated colitis. Stomach and Intestine 1983;18:133-43 (in Japanese).
9. Chang TW. Antibiotic-associated injury to the gut. In: Haubrich WS, Kalser MH, Roth JLA, Schaffner F, eds. Gastroenterology. Philadelphia: WB Saunders, 1985;2538-92.
10. Totani T. Acute hemorrhagic enteritis by *Klebsiella oxytoca*. Nihon Rinsho 1978;36:1308-9 (in Japanese).

Abnormalities in control of ventilation in newborn infants with myelomeningocele

Mario C. Petersen, MD, Mark Wolraich, MD, Andrea Sherbondy, MD, and Jeff Wagener, MD

From the Division of Developmental Disabilities, Department of Pediatrics, University of Iowa, Iowa City, the Division of Child Development, Department of Pediatrics, Vanderbilt University, Nashville, Tennessee, and the Department of Pediatrics, University of Colorado Medical School, Denver

Objective: **The objective of this study was to assess respiratory responses of newborn infants with myelomeningocele through pneumograms and carbon dioxide challenge, and to evaluate the possibility of predicting which patients with myelomeningocele acquired respiratory symptoms related to the Arnold-Chiari deformity and brain-stem dysfunction.**
Methods: **All surviving infants with spina bifida who were born at the University of Iowa Hospitals and Clinics (UIHC) or were transferred there on the first day of life between January 1987 and January 1991 were assessed with a pneumogram and CO_2 challenge once they were medically stable, and were followed for a mean of 30 months (10 to 53 months).**
Results: **Thirty patients met the inclusion criteria for this study; four died before being studied. Of the 26 remaining patients, 12 were born at the UIHC and 14 were transferred to the UIHC on the first day of life. Of the 26 infants studied, 12 (46%) had abnormalities on the pneumogram, including 2 with significant periodic breathing and 10 with episodes of desaturation below 87%. Of the 26 infants studied, 4 had no detectable response to an increasing fraction of CO_2 in inspired air on the CO_2 challenge and 12 had an increase in exhaled minute ventilation per increase in the alveolar fraction of CO_2 in exhaled air more than 2 SD below the mean. Only 10 patients (38.5%) had normal ventilatory responses to the increasing fraction of CO_2 in inspired air. On follow-up, only one study patient had symptoms related to Arnold-Chiari deformity and brain-stem dysfunction (bilateral vocal cord paralysis). His neonatal CO_2 challenge results and his pneumogram were normal.**
Conclusion: **We conclude that these two tests are not useful in predicting which patients will have symptoms related to Arnold-Chiari deformity. Specificity for the pneumogram and the CO_2 challenge was 0.52 and 0.36, respectively. Sensitivity was zero for both tests, although this result is limited by the low incidence of symptomatic Arnold-Chiari deformity in this sample. As previous investigators have found, a significant number of patients with meningomyelocele had abnormal ventilatory patterns. These ventilatory abnormalities indicate that even in the absence of severe symptoms, the control of the ventilatory response is somewhat impaired in many patients with meningomyelocele. This alteration in ventilatory control is probably related to abnormalities in the development of the brain stem. (J PEDIATR 1995;126:1011-5)**

Submitted for publication Feb. 19, 1994; accepted Dec. 20, 1994.

Reprint requests: Mark Wolraich, MD, Child Development Director, Vanderbilt University, Nashville, TN 37232.

0022-3476/95/$3.00 + 0 **9/73/62886**

The Arnold-Chiari malformation is present in 95% of patients with myelomeningocele.[1] The Arnold-Chiari II deformity is characterized by an abnormal position of the cerebellum and the brain stem. The cerebellum is caudally displaced, extending into the foramen magnum. In some cases

ACD	Arnold-Chiari deformity
$FICO_2$	Fraction CO_2 in inspired air
FIO_2	Fraction of O_2 in inspired air
MMC	Myelomeningocele
$PACO_2$	Alveolar fraction CO_2 in expired air
$TcPO_2$	Transcutaneous pressure of O_2
$\dot{V}E$	Minute ventilation

the cerebellum can reach the lower cervical vertebrae. The brain stem is also elongated and extends through the foramen magnum into the cervical spine. ACD produces an obstruction of cerebrospinal fluid flow, which results in hydrocephalus in 85% of patients with MMC.[2]

Symptoms caused by bulbar involvement, such as central apnea, vocal cord paralysis, or dysphagia, are present in 5% to 20% of infants with ACD.[3, 4] Three major symptom complexes have been described in infants.[3, 5] The most frequent symptom complex is isolated vocal cord paralysis, which is usually secondary to increased intracranial pressure, and generally resolves after a ventriculoperitoneal shunt is placed.[6, 7] The second symptom complex is vocal cord paralysis with other cranial nerve deficits, such as swallowing problems. Swallowing problems can result in a significant mortality rate (20%).[7] The third symptom complex includes stridor or dysphagia associated with apnea and/or cyanosis.[5] Central ventilatory dysfunction, which may include stridor, respiratory distress, aspiration, increased periodic breathing during sleep, and central apnea, was present in approximately 6% of patients with ACD and MMC in a study by Hays et al.,[8] all seen before 12 months of age and the majority before 6 months of age; central ventilatory dysfunction was the leading cause of death in that series of patients. The rate of death as a consequence of respiratory symptoms can be very high (60%).[3] Some uncontrolled clinical studies suggest that posterior fossa decompression, when done early, might improve the outcome.[4, 9] Historically, the diagnosis of ACD complications has depended on the presence of symptoms. These symptoms do not always disappear after surgical intervention; however, early detection may improve outcome and decrease the mortality rate in this population.

The objective of this study was to assess the respiratory responses of newborn infants with MMC by using a pneumogram and a CO_2 challenge, and to evaluate the possibility of predicting which patients with MMC would acquire symptoms related to ACD.

METHODS

All newborn infants with spina bifida born at University of Iowa Hospitals and Clinics (UIHC) or transferred there on the first day of life between January 1987 and January 1991 were included in the study. There were 106 infants with spina bifida born in the state of Iowa during this 4-year period; 66 of them (62%) had hydrocephalus (Iowa Birth Defects Registry, University of Iowa). The UIHC is the only tertiary level hospital in eastern Iowa; most, if not all, newborn infants with MMC who were born in eastern Iowa and some from western Iowa or bordering states are referred to UIHC. Thirty patients met the inclusion criteria for this study. Patients were assessed once they were medically stable and ready for discharge (mean age, 27.1 days). The following data were recorded: birth weight, gestational age, Apgar scores at 1 and 5 minutes, and anatomic and functional levels of the spinal defect. Segmental motor level determination was used as described by Kendall et al.[10] and corresponded to the lowest level of purposeful movement with strength enough to move a segment at least against gravity. The sensory level corresponded to the lowest dermatome with sensation to touch or pain or both. Anatomic level was defined by the level of the upper limit of the defect seen on the x-ray study of the spine. Anatomic and functional levels were grouped into cervical, thoracic, high lumbar, low lumbar, and sacral levels. The degree of hydrocephalus was based on the most severe radiologic study result (brain computed tomography, magnetic resonance imaging, or ultrasonography) obtained before shunting. Hydrocephalus was estimated as mild, moderate, or severe on the basis of the report by the radiologist. These studies were requested on the basis of clinical needs. The time between shunt placement and respiratory study was also recorded. The children were followed for a mean of 30 months (10 to 53 months) to detect any clinical symptoms.

Pneumograms entailed continuous recordings of heart rate, nasal airflow (Yellow Springs Thermistor, Yellow Springs Instrument Co., Inc., Yellow Springs, Ohio), chest movements (thoracic impedance), and O_2 saturation (Nellcor oximeter, Nellcor Inc., Hayward, Calif.) during sleep. The infant was studied in a quiet, darkened room with an ambient temperature of 21° to 23° C. All tests were done during quiet sleep, 3 to 4 hours after a feeding, to create a standardized, nonstimulating environment. Studies were hand scored according to the following definitions: *apnea* was defined as cessation of nasal airflow for 15 seconds or more,[11] and *periodic breathing* was defined as three or more episodes of no nasal airflow for 3 seconds or more, separated by periods of 20 seconds or less.[12] Pneumograms were classified as showing abnormalities (1) if there was any apnea; (2) if periodic breathing occurred for <5% of total sleep time,[12] or (3) if oxygen saturation as measured by pulse oximetry was <0.87.[13]

The CO_2 challenge evaluated the ventilatory response to increasing levels of inspired CO_2 during sleep.[14] Sleep was obtained by sleep deprivation for a couple of hours or by chloral hydrate, or both (nine patients; 50 to 75 mg/kg). No differences were found between the two methods of obtain-

Table I. Description of the cohort (N = 26)

	Mean	SD	Range	
Gestational age (wk)	38.73	1.12	36	40
Birth weight (kg)	3.14	0.44	2.37	4.05
Apgar score				
At 1 min	6	2.48	1	9
At 5 min	8	0.71	7	10
Shunt age (days)	9	5	11	22
Study age (days)	27	10	11	98
Follow up (mo)	30	12	10	53

ing sleep. Studies were done in the morning in a quiet, darkened room with an ambient temperature of 21° to 23° C. An MGC System 4000 (Medical Graphics Corp., St. Paul, Minn.) was used to measure ventilatory response. This system consists of (1) a pneumotachygraph with a pressure transducer and a carrier demodulator to measure instantaneous flow, (2) an infrared CO_2 analyzer, and (3) a waveform analyzer that samples at a speed of 100 samples per second and calculates tidal volume, fraction CO_2 in inspired air, alveolar fraction of CO_2 in exhaled air, breathing frequency, exhaled minute ventilation, and the increase in $\dot{V}E$ increase in $PACO_2$ ($D\dot{V}E/CO_2$). With the child asleep, a baseline ventilatory measurement, including $PACO_2$ and transcutaneous pressure of O_2, was obtained in room air. The $FICO_2$ was gradually increased by 0.01 every 2 minutes. The $D\dot{V}E/CO_2$ was measured by regression analysis of the change in expired ventilation volume in milliliters per kilogram per minute for each 1 mm Hg increase in $PACO_2$. The normal value of this slope is 64 ml/kg per minute per millimeter of mercury of CO_2, with a standard deviation of 19[15]; values less than 25 were considered abnormal.

To validate this procedure and confirm these normal values, we compared the results against the CO_2 challenge results in seven infants referred during the same period for study as symptom-free siblings of victims of sudden infant death syndrome. Their mean age was 48 days (SD = 23). The difference in age was not statistically significant, although the power to detect a significant difference was only 0.64 (for a p value of ≤ 0.05). The comparison group had a mean $D\dot{V}E/CO_2$ of 32.4 ml/kg per minute per millimeter of mercury of CO_2 pressure (SD = 19.04), with a range of 16.6 to 69.1 ml/kg per minute per millimeter of mercury of CO_2 pressure.

We employed the t test and the chi-square test for continuous and categorical data, respectively. Regression analysis was used to evaluate the association of continuous data ($D\dot{V}E/CO_2$) with continuous data (birth weight, gestational age, $PACO_2$, $TcPO_2$), and rank Spearman correlation was used for comparison with ordinal data (level of lesion, degree of hydrocephalus).

Table II. Hydrocephalus and level of the lesion

	No.	%
Hydrocephalus		
None	1	3.8
Mild	6	23.0
Moderate	12	46.2
Severe	7	26.9
Level of lesion		
Cervical	1	3.8
Thoracic	6	23.0
High lumbar (L1-L3)	8	30.8
Low lumbar (L4-L5)	9	43.6
Sacral	2	7.7

RESULTS

Of the 30 newborn candidates for the study, four died during the first 48 hours of life (one with hydranencephaly and myeloschisis from the first thoracic vertebra to the third sacral vertebra; a premature infant with severe hydrocephalus, grade IV intraventricular hemorrhage, and sepsis; an 1850 gm twin with a single multicystic kidney, bladder agenesis, and ambiguous genitalia; and a term infant with holoprosencephaly, omphalocele, and ambiguous genitalia). Of the 26 infants included in this study, 12 were born at UIHC and 14 were transferred there on the first day of life. All but one of the infants had surgical repair of the myelomeningocele within the first 24 hours of life. All but one had hydrocephalus requiring ventriculoperitoneal shunting. The mean age at shunt placement was 9.2 days (range, 1 to 22 days). In all cases the shunt was placed before the respiratory study. Tables I and II describe the characteristics of the infants.

Pneumogram. Of the 26 infants studied, 12 (46%) had abnormal results. Two had significant periodic breathing, and 10 had episodes of desaturation of less than 87%. Most of these episodes of desaturation occurred during or soon after respiratory pauses 6 to 10 seconds in duration. None of the patients had apnea (either central or obstructive).

CO_2 challenge. Of the 26 patients studied, 16 (61.5%) had abnormal ventilatory responses to the increase of $FICO_2$. Of these, 4 had no detectable response to increasing $FICO_2$ and 12 had a $D\dot{V}E/CO_2$ that was more than 2 SD below the mean. Only 10 (38.5%) of the 26 patients had ventilatory responses within the normal range, although no responses reached the normal mean. These 10 patients had a mean ventilatory response of 19.0 ml/kg per millimeter of mercury of CO_2 pressure (SD = 12.54), which was significantly lower than that in the comparison group (t test = 2.24; $p < 0.05$). Arousal responses were tested in 18 patients. Of the 18 patients, 7 (39%) did not arouse with an $FICO_2$ of 0.07 and documented alveolar hypoventilation.

On follow-up, symptoms related to ACM developed in

Table III. Relation between pneumogram and CO_2 challenge response

	Pneumogram results	
CO_2 challenge response	**Normal**	**Abnormal**
Normal	4	6
⟨2 SD	8	4
⟨3 SD	2	2

only one patient. He had bilateral vocal cord paralysis diagnosed by direct laryngoscopy. His CO_2 challenge response in the newborn period was normal ($\dot{D}V_E/CO_2 = 38.4$ ml/kg per millimeter of mercury of CO_2 pressure). His pneumogram also showed no abnormalities.

Patients with or without abnormalities on pneumograms had similar responses to the CO_2 challenge (mean $\dot{D}V_E/CO_2$, 17.6 [SD = 12.5] and 20.6 ml/kg per millimeter of mercury of CO_2 pressure [SD = 12.4], respectively) ($p = 0.62$) (Table III). The only significant correlation between breathing tests and clinical variables was a positive correlation between CO_2 challenge response and Apgar score at 1 minute ($r = 0.41$; $p < 0.05$). There was no association between CO_2 challenge response or pneumogram results and the following: birth weight; gestational age; Apgar score at 5 minutes; degree of hydrocephalus; anatomic, motor, or sensory level; use of chloral hydrate; baseline $PaCO_2$ or $TcPO_2$; or time between shunting and respiratory study.

DISCUSSION

The results reported here were obtained in 26 consecutively treated infants with MMC. One patient eventually had bilateral vocal cord paralysis—an incidence of 3.9% with symptomatic ACD. This incidence is lower than in previous reports[3, 4] and may reflect a difference in case identification when previous studies were not prospective. More likely, this low incidence occurred by chance. Two patients with severe symptoms of ACD and brain-stem dysfunction, born a few months before the initiation of this study, provided the motivation for this study. Soon after the study ended, another patient was born who later had symptoms related to ACD. If these patients had been included in the study, the incidence of symptomatic ACD would have been 14%.

Given the high number of abnormal results in our study, we conclude that these two tests are not useful in predicting which patients will eventually have symptoms related to ACD. Specificity of the pneumogram and the CO_2 challenge was 0.52 and 0.36, respectively. Sensitivity was zero for both tests, although this result is limited by the low incidence of symptomatic ACD in our study sample.

As previous investigators have found,[16-20] a significant number of patients with MMC had abnormal ventilatory patterns. More than 60% of our patients had a poor response to CO_2 challenge; four patients had no response to the increase of $FiCO_2$. An arousal response was absent in 39% of the patients tested. There was a lack of association between $\dot{D}V_E/CO_2$ and baseline $PaCO_2$ and $TcPO_2$, which suggests that the abnormal response to CO_2 challenge was not related to pulmonary problems such as hypoxemia, atelectasis, or limited pulmonary volumes caused by scoliosis. The CO_2 challenge result, despite having been abnormal in these patients, did not correlate with the clinical outcome or with the pneumogram.

Our results differ from those of Krieger et al.,[18] who found normal ventilatory patterns and normal ventilatory responses to CO_2 challenge in seven of eight patients with MMC. The one patient in their study who had periodic breathing and apnea had symptoms, stridor, and a normal response to CO_2 challenge. This difference between studies may be due to different methods of assessing ventilatory response; Kreiger et al. used a baseline FiO_2 of 1.0 and an FiO_2 of 0.9 with an $FiCO_2$ of 0.05 for the CO_2 challenge, compared with our protocol, with a baseline FiO_2 of 0.21 and a gradually increasing $FiCO_2$.

Worley and Oakes[19] evaluated the ventilatory response to CO_2 challenge in 31 patients with MMC; 19 had abnormal responses. Six of the patients with abnormal responses had signs of brain-stem dysfunction at the time of the study, and three other patients later had signs of brain-stem dysfunction. Only 1 of the 12 patients with normal responses had symptomatic ACD with mild dysphagia. In our patients the CO_2 challenge response did not correlate with symptomatic outcome. None of our patients with abnormal response to CO_2 challenge had symptoms of ACD, and the only patient with symptoms had a normal response. One would have to conclude that the CO_2 challenge response, despite having been abnormal in a significant number of newborn infants with MMC, is not a useful predictor of symptomatic ACD in infants.

Additional abnormalities of ventilation control in patients with MMC have been described before, even in symptom-free patients. The hypoxic arousal response is abnormal in infants with MMC,[16] and the hypercapnic ventilation response is lower in adolescents.[20] Davidson Ward et al.[17] compared the pneumograms of 18 symptom-free infants with MMC (1.4 to 24 months of age) with the pneumograms of 64 healthy control subjects. Patients with MMC had a greater duration of respiratory pauses lasting more than 6 seconds as a percentage of sleep time. Seventy-two percent of the patients had abnormalities on pneumograms, compared with 6% in the healthy control group.

Twelve of our patients (46%) had abnormalities on pneumograms. Many of these patients had relatively minor abnormalities that probably are not clinically significant for individual patients. However, when the entire cohort is taken into consideration, the number of patients with periodic breathing or frequent episodes of brief desaturation is remarkable. The clinical significance of these findings is not clear. Two patients had excessive periodic breathing, a finding that is more frequent in patients with near-miss sudden infant death syndrome[12] and in siblings of infants who died as a result of the syndrome.[21] Additionally, 10 of our patients had an abnormal amount of desaturation during sleep.

The ventilatory abnormalities found in this and previous studies show that even in the absence of severe symptoms the control of the ventilatory response is somewhat impaired in many patients with MMC. This alteration in ventilatory control is probably related to abnormalities in the development of the brain stem.[5] Learning problems have been reported in patients with congenital central hypoventilation syndrome[22] in whom desaturation and/or failure to respond to CO_2 challenge occurred; the effect of these ventilatory abnormalities on intellectual development and long-term morbidity in patients with MMC also needs to be considered. However, the abnormal results need to be interpreted cautiously because the reproducibility of the findings have yet to be established and more long-term follow-up is required.

We are grateful to Deb Thies, RRT, for performing the studies, and to all the families who participated in this project.

REFERENCES

1. Emery JL, MacKenzie N. Medullo-cervical dislocation deformity (Chiari II deformity) related to neurospinal dysraphism (myelomeningocele). Brain 1973;96:155-62.
2. Patet JD, Lapras C, Guilburd JN, Lapras C. Spina bifida aperta–myelomeningocele: hydrocephalus. Neurochirurgie 1988; 34(suppl 1):47-52.
3. Hesz N, Wolraich M. Vocal-cord paralysis and brainstem dysfunction in children with spina bifida. Dev Med Child Neurol 1985;27:528-31.
4. Park TS, Hoffman HJ, Hendrick EB, Humphreys RP. Experience with surgical decompression of the Arnold-Chiari malformation in young infants with myelomeningocele. Neurosurgery 1983;13:147-52.
5. Charney EB, Rorke LB, Sutton LN, Schut L. Management of Chiari II complications in infants with myelomeningocele. J Pediatr 1987;111:364-71.
6. Bluestone CD, Delerme AN, Samuelson GH. Airway obstruction due to vocal cord paralysis in infants with hydrocephalus and meningomyelocele. Ann Otol 1972;81:778-83.
7. Holschneider AM, Bliesener JA, Abel M. The brain stem dysfunction in Arnold-Chiari II syndrome. Zeitschrift für Kinderchirurgie 1990;45:67-71.
8. Hays RM, Jordan RA, McLaughlin JF, Nickel RE, Fisher LD. Central ventilatory dysfunction in myelodysplasia: an independent determinant of survival. Dev Med Child Neurol 1989; 31:366-70.
9. Dyste GN, Menezes AH, Van Gilder JC. Symptomatic Chiari malformations: an analysis of presentation, management and long-term outcome. J Neurosurg 1989;71:159-68.
10. Kendall HO, Kendall PK, Wadsworth GE. Muscle testing and function. Baltimore: Williams & Wilkins, 1971.
11. Hunt CE, Brouillette RT, Hanson D, David RJ, Stein IM, Weissbluth M. Home pneumograms in normal infants. J Pediatr 1985;106:551-5.
12. Kelly DH, Shannon DC. Periodic breathing in infants with near-miss sudden infant death syndrome. Pediatrics 1979; 63:355-60.
13. Mok JY, McLaughlin FJ, Pintar M, Hak H, Amaro-Galvez R, Levison H. Transcutaneous monitoring of oxygenation: what is normal? J Pediatr 1986;108:365-71.
14. Avery ME, Chernik V, Dutton RE, et al. Ventilatory response to inspired carbon dioxide in infants and adults. J Appl Physiol 1963;18:895-903.
15. Shannon DC, Kelly D. Abnormal ventilatory response to CO_2 during quiet sleep in aborted SIDS. Chest 1978;73(suppl):301.
16. Ortega M, Davidson Ward SL, Swaminathan S, Jacobs RA, Keens TG. Abnormal hypoxic arousal response in myelomeningocele infants without apneas [Abstract]. Pediatr Res 1988; 23:324A.
17. Davidson-Ward SL, Jacobs RA, Gates EP, Hart LD, Keens TG. Abnormal ventilatory patterns during sleep in infants with myelomeningocele. J Pediatr 1986;109:631-4.
18. Krieger AJ, Detwiler JS, Trooskin SZ. Respiratory function in infants with Arnold-Chiari malformation. Laryngoscope 1976; 86:718-23.
19. Worley G, Oakes WJ. The CO_2 response test in children with spina bifida. Dev Med Child Neurol 1986;28:88.
20. Swaminathan S, Paton JY, Davidson Ward SL, Jacobs RA, Sargent CW, Keens TG. Abnormal control of ventilation in adolescents with myelodysplasia. J Pediatr 1989;115:898-903.
21. Kelly DH, Walker AM, Cahen L, Shannon DC. Periodic breathing in siblings of sudden infant death syndrome victims. Pediatrics 1980;66:515-20.
22. Marcus CL, Jansen MT, Poulsen MK, et al. Medical and psychosocial outcome of children with congenital central hypoventilation syndrome. J Pediatr 1991;119:888-95.

THE BOOK SHELF

André D. Lascari, *Editor*

New books received

Blindness and children: an individual differences approach
Warren DH. New York: Cambridge University Press, 1994. 380 pages. $59.95.

Current: pediatric diagnosis and treatment. 12th ed.
Hay WW, Groothuis JR, Hayward AR, Levin MJ, eds. Norwalk, Connecticut: Appleton & Lange, 1994. 1295 pages. $41.95.

Cognitive effects of early brain injury
Dorman C, Katzir B. Baltimore: Johns Hopkins University Press, 1994. 325 pages. $55.

Development and clinical uses of *Haemophilus* b conjugate vaccines
Ellis RW, Granoff DM. New York: Marcel Dekker, 1994. 520 pages. $175.

Meeting early intervention challenges. 2nd ed.
Johnson LJ, Gallagher RJ, LaMontagne MJ, Jordan JB, Gallagher JJ, eds. Baltimore: Paul H. Brookes, 1994. 307 pages. $30.

The projective use of mother-and-child drawings: a manual for clinicians
Gillespie J. New York: Brunner/Mazel, 1994. 156 pages. $28.95.

Creative scripts for hypnotherapy
Hunter ME. New York: Brunner/Mazel, 1994. 234 pages. $25.95.

Textbook of pharmacotherapy for child and adolescent psychiatric disorders
Rosenberg DR, Holttum J, Gershon S. New York: Brunner/Mazel, 1994. 570 pages. $65.

Annals of child development; vol 9.
Vasta R, ed. London: Jessica Kingsley, 1993. 204 pages. $75.

Children, teenagers and health: the key data
Woodroffe C, Glickman M, Barker M, Power C. Bristol, Pennsylvania: Open University Press, 1993. 193 pages. $36.

EDITORIAL CORRESPONDENCE

Discordance for hyperinsulinemic hypoglycemia in monozygotic twins

To the Editor:

Data from two recent studies provide no clinical and histologic evidence of distinct familial and sporadic types of persistent hyperinsulinemic hypoglycemia of infancy (PHHI). Segregation analyses suggest that most if not all cases of diffuse islet cell disease (nesidioblastosis) are genetically determined and transmitted by an autosomal recessive trait.[1, 2] However, we have identified PHHI in one identical twin. Monozygosity was demonstrated by conventional and molecular biologic methods with single-locus and multilocus DNA probes.

The affected twin had increased weight gain compared with his nonaffected brother at 7 months of age. At 9 months, he was admitted to a hospital with hypoketotic hypoglycemia with clinical symptoms often observed after feedings. Inadequate elevation of plasma insulin (with a maximum insulin [in microunits per milliliter]/glucose [in milligrams per deciliter] ratio of 5.5 [normal <0.4]) was documented repeatedly in both the fed and fasted states. Oral administration of L-leucine resulted in severe hyperinsulinemic hypoglycemia in the affected twin but had no effect in the healthy brother. Hyperinsulinemia and leucine sensitivity have persisted for more than 2 years. Dietary treatment with frequent feedings and leucine restriction has been sufficient to prevent severe hypoglycemia in the patient. Nesidioblastosis has not been proved by histologic methods. No tumor has been found by repeated thin-section computed tomographic scans of the pancreas.

In recent years this clinical pattern, formerly termed "leucine-sensitive hypoglycemia," is believed to represent a mild late-onset variant of the broad spectrum of PHHI.[3] The observation of PHHI in only one identical twin weakens the hypothesis that genetic factors are solely responsible for this disorder. The possibility that a postzygotic event can cause PHHI means that, at least for a subgroup of cases, the recurrence risk for PHHI in subsequent children may be lower than the one-in-four risk for autosomal recessive inheritance.

René Santer, MD
Heike Hoffmann, MD
Meinolf Suttorp, MD
Eva Simeoni, MD
Jürgen Schaub, MD
Departments of Pediatrics and Forensic Medicine
University of Kiel
Kiel, Germany
9/35/63322

REFERENCES

1. Thornton PS, Sumner AE, Ruchell ED, et al. Familial and sporadic hyperinsulinism: histopathologic findings and segregation analysis support a single autosomal recessive disorder. J PEDIATR 1991;119:721-4.
2. Woolf DA, Leonhard JV, Trembath RC, et al. Nesidioblastosis: evidence for autosomal recessive inheritance. Arch Dis Child 1991;66:529-30.
3. Sperling MA. Hypoglycemia. In: Behrman RE, ed. Nelson textbook of pediatrics. Philadelphia: Saunders, 1992:409-19.

Reply

To the Editor:

Santer et al. suggest that their observation of hyperinsulinism in one identical twin weakens the hypothesis that congenital hyperinsulinism (HI) is a genetic disorder.[1] The clinical diagnosis and laboratory features as given raise serious concerns about the diagnosis of HI. The patient was not large for gestational age, did not have symptoms until late in the first year of life, and did not have fasting hypoglycemia, but rather had increased weight gain and postprandial hypoglycemia. The course was also unusual for HI in that diet alone controlled the hypoglycemia. Moreover, an insulin/glucose ratio of 5.5 implies insulin levels of 220 to 440 μU/ml for glucose values between 40 to 80 mg/dl. These markedly elevated insulin concentrations are not typical in patients with HI. Such extraordinary insulin levels would be expected to make control of hypoglycemia very difficult. In more than 75 children treated for HI, we have never had a single child whose problem could be controlled with diet alone. These findings make the diagnosis of HI unlikely, and raise concern about surreptitious insulin administration or the presence of insulin antibodies that interfere with the insulin assay. Acquired insulinoma remains a possibility in view of the late onset of symptoms.

Since our earlier report of possible autosomal recessive inheritance of HI based on recurrence in families, we have demonstrated by linkage analysis that a locus for HI exists on chromosome 11p15.1.[2] This further supports the concept that HI is a genetic disorder and underlines the suggestion that suitable genetic counseling should be given to families with an affected child.

Paul S. Thornton, MBBCh, MRCPI
Lester Baker, MD
Charles A. Stanley, MD
Department of Pediatrics
Children's Hospital of Philadelphia
Philadelphia, PA 19104-9786
9/35/63323

REFERENCES

1. Thornton PS, Alter CA, Levit Katz LE, Baker L, Stanley CA. Acute and long-term treatment of congenital hyperinsulinism with octreotide. J PEDIATR 1993;123:637-43.
2. Glaser B, Chiu KC, Anker R, et al. Familial hyperinsulinism maps to human chromosome 11p14-15.1, 30 cM centromeric to the insulin gene. Nature Genetics 1994;7:2:185-8.

Comparison of fiberoptic and conventional phototherapy for neonatal hyperbilirubinemia

To the Editor:

We were interested in the comparison of fiberoptic and conventional phototherapy for neonatal hyperbilirubinemia reported by Tan.[1] He reported that fluid intake was increased during phototherapy to offset the increased fluid loss during exposure but did not indicate whether the extent of this problem varied according to the mode of phototherapy. Increased fluid loss during phototherapy is a significant clinical problem in the term infant when the mother is trying to establish breast-feeding and in very low birth weight infants, in whom dehydration may lead to hypernatrenia. Transdermal water loss, respiratory water loss, and gastrointestinal water loss can all be involved.[2, 3]

Because it is possible to give fiberoptic phototherapy (using the Biliblanket; Ohmeda Critical Care, Columbia, Md.) with the infant clothed, we hypothesized that transdermal water loss would be less because the presence of clothing would create a microclimate with increased local humidity. We also had surmised that there might be less heating of the skin because the fiberoptic light plate is not hot. We have compared fluid loss during fiberoptic phototherapy and conventional phototherapy. Twenty-four infants (birth weight 831 to 4520 gm) with a clinical indication for phototherapy were randomly assigned in a crossover trial design; each infant received 12 hours of treatment with the Biliblanket and 12 hours of conventional phototherapy (blue/white lamps; Air-Shields Vickers, Hatboro, Pa.) 40 cm distance from the infant's abdomen. Total fluid loss (transdermal, respiratory, urinary, and gastrointestinal) and insensible fluid loss (transdermal plus respiratory) were measured by repeated weighing before and after each treatment, careful recording of fluid input during each treatment, and weighing of diapers (to measure gastrointestinal and urinary losses).

Total fluid loss was 138.7 gm/12 hours (SD $\pm$ 59.0) during Biliblanket treatment and 140.9 gm/12 hours (SD $\pm$ 78.1) during conventional phototherapy (p =0.78). Insensible fluid loss during Biliblanket treatment was 55.1 gm/12 hours (SD $\pm$ 39.3) compared with 43.8 gm/12 hours (SD $\pm$ 35.2) during conventional phototherapy (p =0.129). Total fluid loss in 10 infants with birth weights ⟨1500 gm during Biliblanket treatment was 111.5 gm/12 hours compared with 105.4 gm/12 hours during conventional phototherapy (p =0.61). Insensible loss during Biliblanket treatment was 47 gm/12 hours (SD $\pm$ 45.2) compared with 29.7 gm/12 hours (SD $\pm$ 35.6) during conventional phototherapy (confidence interval for difference between means 4.5 to 29.9, p 0.026).

These results show that term infants had no overall difference in fluid loss with the two modes of phototherapy, but there was evidence of increased insensible water loss during Biliblanket treatment in the infants <1500 gm. They appear to have compensated by decreasing urine volume. Although some nurses believed that the fiberoptic plate caused local warming, axillary temperature measurements did not show a significant difference between the two treatments. The opinions of our nurses in the neonatal intensive care unit were substantially different from those reported in Tan's article. They commented that the noise of the fan was troublesome and the light plate was uncomfortable for preterm infants to lie on. In contrast, the nurses and mothers on the postnatal wards were enthusiastic about the Biliblanket because it is much easier for the mother to breast-feed during phototherapy; the lack of eyepads was also viewed as very positive.

We conclude that the Biliblanket is a useful alternative (or adjunct) to conventional phototherapy, but attention to adequate hydration is just as important during Biliblanket treatment as with conventional phototherapy.

Jakob Larsen, MD
Andrew Whitelaw, MD, FRCP
Department of Pediatrics
University of Oslo
Oslo, Norway
9/35/63487

REFERENCES

1. Tan KL. Comparison of the efficacy of fiberoptic and conventional phototherapy for neonatal hyperbilirubinemia. J PEDIATR 1994;125:607-12.
2. Oh W, Karechi H. Phototherapy and sensible water loss in the newborn infant. Am J Dis Child 1972;124:230-2.
3. Wu PYK, Moosa A. Effect of phototherapy on nitrogen and electrolyte levels and water balance in jaundiced preterm infants. Pediatrics 1978;61:193-8.

Reply

To the Editor:

Increased fluid intake was necessary to offset increased fluid loss during phototherapy. No attempt was made to evaluate the amount of fluid loss during this particular study. However, to maintain adequate hydration (as assessed clinically and by regular weight observations and the use of biochemical measurements), we had to increase fluid intake almost equally in preterm babies exposed to fibreoptic or conventional phototherapy. Intake was further increased in those who had combination phototherapy. Similarly, we found that increased fluid intake was also needed in term infants exposed to conventional or fiberoptic phototherapy, again with a further increase required for those who received combination phototherapy but less than in preterm infants.

Our nurses in both the neonatal intensive care unit and those in the normal nurseries gave favorable responses to the use of fiberoptic phototherapy from the point of ease of usage and freedom from obstruction. Parents were also enthusiastic about this device. Our neonatal intensive care nurses did not find the fan noise from the fiberoptic device significantly disturbing; they became accustomed to it shortly after fiberoptic phototherapy was started.

K. L. Tan, MBBS, FRCPE, FRACP, DCH
Department of Neonatology
National University Hospital
Singapore, Republic of Singapore
9/35/63488

Single-day therapy for rickets

To the Editor:

Shah and Finberg reported their 10-year experience of treating vitamin D–deficiency rickets with a single, large dose (600,000 IU) ("stosstherapy") of ergocalciferol (J PEDIATR 1994;125:487-90). They claim this form of treatment is safe (no hypercalcemia or hypocalcemia), eliminates problems of noncompliance, and is diagnostically useful because rapid correction of hypophosphatemia confirms the diagnosis of vitamin D deficiency, whereas its persistence should raise the possibility of another form of rickets. They conclude that stosstherapy is the "preferred method of treatment for vitamin D–deficiency rickets".

Although I do not argue with the compliance issue, all other claims of this article are debatable:

1. "Stosstherapy does not cause hypercalcemia." In the absence of any data, this statement is difficult to verify; when, and how often, was serum calcium (and preferably ionized calcium, because many of these patients may have also had hypoproteinemia) measured? Did the patients become hypercalciuric? (Was urine calcium tested, and how often?)

2. "Stosstherapy, in contrast to small doses of vitamin D, does not expose the child to the risk of hypocalcemia (hungry bone syndrome)." Here again, the data are not shown. Maybe the authors missed the window during which hypocalcemia may develop. The authors refer to Harrison,[1] a book chapter that may reflect more the authors' opinion rather than irrefutable research data. Furthermore, Venkataraman et al.[2] treated vitamin D–deficiency rickets with daily physiologic doses (400 IU), and never observed hypercalcemia or hypocalcemia.

3. "Rapid correction of hypophosphatemia allows for quick differential diagnosis." This statement would not be unique to stosstherapy. Venkataraman et al.[2] demonstrated that daily administration of 400 IU of vitamin D in vitamin D-deficient children with rickets raised the mean serum phosphate concentration from 3.5 to 5.2 mg/dl in 7 days, and normalized bone mineral content in 8 weeks and serum levels of parathyroid hormone in 8 weeks.

In view of this, I regret that there is no randomized, clinical trial (gold standard of modern medical research) comparing the risks versus benefits of stosstherapy versus low-dose daily vitamin D therapy. In the meantime, I remain unconvinced that stosstherapy is the preferred approach. I will continue to use it with caution, and only when parental compliance appears questionable. I also am concerned that practitioners who use stosstherapy, unlike Shah et al., might use a propylene glycol preparation, exposing the patient to the risk of toxicity.

F. Mimouni, MD
Department of Pediatrics
Maimonides Medical Center
Brooklyn, NY 11219
9/35/63485

REFERENCES

1. Harrison HE, Harrison HC. Rickets and osteomalacia. In: Schaffer AJ, Marcowitz M, eds. Disorders of calcium and phosphate metabolism in childhood and adolescence. Philadelphia: WB Saunders, 1979:141-256.
2. Venkataraman PS, Tsang RC, Buckley DD, Ho M, Steichen JJ. Elevation of serum 1,25-dihydroxyvitamin D in response to physiologic doses of vitamin D in vitamin D–deficient infants. J PEDIATR 1983;103:416-9.

Reply

To the Editor:

The letter from Dr. Mimouni gives us the opportunity to expand our concepts and to clarify further any doubts about the safety of a single large dose of ergocalciferol (vitamin D_2) for nutritional vitamin D–deficiency rickets. Although the randomized, controlled clinical trial is an excellent and powerful tool for most therapeutic comparisons, it is not always either necessary or appropriate. Our study constituted such an instance because both therapies under consideration, the small daily dose with good compliance and the large single dose, are known to be fully effective.

The combined experience with the single large dose by H. E. Harrison and ourselves spans more than 50 years and hundreds of patients. We wrote our article because of concerns about safety and because we had data for all patients described for levels of calcidiol, calcitriol, and parathormone (at least before and after treatment) and serial values for calcium, phosphate, and sometimes ionized calcium. We could not publish all of our laboratory data because of space considerations for data that were "negative."

Nutritional rickets may occur at an early stage, before secondary hyperparathyroidism compensates with a low calcium level, or at a later stage with a normal calcium level. When our patients had hypocalcemia, they were monitored daily after stosstherapy until the serum calcium level became normal. We did not obtain a 24-hour urine calcium measurement (we thought it is unnecessary and technically difficult because most of our patients were younger than 24 months). In all our patients with hypocalcemia (54.8%), the serum calcium level became normal within 48 to 72 hours; none had tetany (either latent or manifest). Ionized calcium levels, which followed the same pattern, were also available for some of these patients. In patients with normocalcemia (45.2%), a second determination was done in 4 days. No patient (a total of 45 "stoss" treatments) had hypocalcemia or hypercalcemia. No patients in this study had hypoalbuminemia.

In the study of only five patients by Venkataraman et al.[1] (quoted by Dr. Mimouni), serum calcium values were reported at 1, 2, and 8 weeks after a daily small dose of vitamin D (400 IU). Four of the five patients who had serum calcium measurements at 1 week had a mean value of 8.3 ± 0.7 mg/dL (still in the hypocalcemic range). Thus we cannot draw any conclusion whether a further decrease in serum calcium (which may be seen in the initial phases of healing with a very small dose of vitamin D) occurred. Also, with a small dose of vitamin D therapy, hypocalcemia persisted longer in these patients.

With stosstherapy (barring malabsorption) the phosphate concentration usually rises in 72 to 96 hours and always by 7 days. If the expected phosphate level increase does not occur, then metabolic bone disease becomes likely and we continue to find new variants thereby. Our experience from referred patients has shown that for most patients with nutritional rickets who receive a small daily dose of vitamin D (1000 IU), the phosphate concentration may not increase for several weeks and radiologic improvement may not occur for several weeks.

We thank Dr. Mimouni for emphasizing, as we had already noted, that one should not use a dilute preparation of ergocalciferol in propylene glycol for large-dose treatments because the vehicle solvent will be toxic to children.

Because safety is ensured and compliance is a major issue with this disorder (in the article by Venkataraman et al.,[1] two of the five patients were lost to follow-up after 8 weeks), and because of the usefulness in differential diagnosis of the occasional puzzling patient, we believe that single-dose therapy is the preferred treatment for these patients.

Binita R. Shah, MD
Laurence Finberg, MD
Children's Medical Center of Brooklyn
SUNY, Health Science Center at Brooklyn
Brooklyn, NY
9/35/63484

REFERENCE

1. Venkataraman PS, Tsang RC, Buckley DD, Ho M, Steichen JJ. Elevation of serum 1,25-dihydroxyvitamin D in response to physiologic doses of vitamin D in vitamin D–deficient infants. J PEDIATR 1983;103:416-9.

Hemoglobin A_{1c} levels in young patients with diabetes beyond the "honeymoon" period

To the Editor:

The Diabetes Control and Complications Trial Research Group (DCCT) reported the effects of "intensive" and "conventional" diabetes treatments on hemoglobin A_{1c} (HbA_{1c}) values and on the development of long-term complications in young diabetic subjects.[1] A significant difference in mean HbA_{1c} levels was observed between the "intensive" and the "conventional" treatment groups, but mean HbA_{1c} levels were substantially higher in intensively treated adolescents than in adults, even if patients of both age groups received care from the same multidisciplinary team at each center.[2] In the Editor's Column, Geffner[3] wrote: "An obvious question that arises from this study is, How universally applicable are the results to all children and adolescents with diabetes?" This letter presents our results in terms of HbA_{1c} levels that can be achieved in an unselected population of young diabetic patients without any residual insulin secretion.[4]

A total of 129 patients aged 17.7 ± 6.4 years (mean ± SD) were followed for 1 year by the same pediatric diabetologist (6.6 ± 1.9 visits/year per patient). The patients had a duration of diabetes from 2 to 27 years (mean, 9.7 years; median, 8.0 years). Mean age at onset was 8.1 ± 3.7 years. C-peptide was undetectable in all patients. Mean (SD) annual HbA_{1c} levels were 6.9% ± 1.5% (median, 6.6%), which is similar to that obtained in the adult cohort of the DCCT receiving "intensive" therapy, but better than in the adolescent subgroup. The frequency of home blood glucose monitoring was between 0 and 250 measurements (77 ± 49) per month. The HbA_{1c} value was not related to gender, ethnic origin, age, or duration of diabetes. No difference was observed in metabolic control between the 84 patients receiving only two or (rarely) three daily insulin injections, and the 45 patients receiving four injections with the basal-bolus regimen (rapid-acting insulin before the three main meals; long-acting insulin at bedtime). The regression analysis showed a weak but significant inverse correlation between HbA_{1c} and the frequency of home blood glucose monitoring, (HBGM) as well as the frequency of outpatient clinic attendance. The yearly incidence rates of severe hypoglycemia were 0.10 in the two-injection group, and 0.31 in the four-injection group (lower than in the DCCT) without relationship to HbA_{1c} levels. The explanation for this difference could be the older age (mean, 22.5 vs 15.1 years), associated with a longer diabetes duration (mean, 13.7 vs 7.5 years) and awareness of hypoglycemia, and the lack of snacks in the four-injection group. Frequency of subclinical complications was 15% for nephropathy (24-hour microalbuminuria), 31% for neuropathy (sensitive and motor nerve conduction velocities), and 39% for retinopathy (fluorescein angiography). The minimum age at which incipient complications appeared was 13 years for one complication, 17 years for two complications, and 23 years for three complications, after a diabetes duration of 3, 7, and 15 years, respectively. Only the presence of subclinical neuropathy was related to mean annual levels of HbA_{1c}. Our results[4] with two, three, or four injections are close to those of Ludvigsson,[5] whose patients received four or five injections or used insulin pumps. In other studies, HbA_{1c} levels are higher regardless of the type of treatment.[1, 2, 6-8]

We conclude that frequent home blood glucose monitoring and outpatient clinic attendance does help to obtain better metabolic control, but the multiple-injection insulin regimen does not necessarily improve HbA_{1c} levels. It is inadequate to equate the multiple-injection regimen to "intensified insulin therapy" and the "conventional" two-injection regimen to nonintensive insulin therapy. A multiple-injection regimen not associated with intensified patient education, as well as with the application of the acquired knowledge, may have deleterious effects on HbA_{1c} levels. On the other hand, the proper use of blood and urine glucose monitoring, insulin dose alteration, and allocation of diet may lead to "intensive conventional therapy" and good metabolic control. Successful glycemic control in young patients depends mainly on the quality and intensity of diabetes education by an experienced multidisciplinary team in the outpatient clinic and by specialized nurses visiting the children's homes and schools.[9, 10]

Harry Dorchy, MD, PhD
Clinique de Pédiatrie Ambulatoire et de Diabétologie
Hôpital Universitaire des Enfants Reine Fabiola
Brussels, Belgium
9/35/63775

REFERENCES

1. Diabetes Control and Complications Trial Research Group. Effect of intensive diabetes treatment on the development and

progression of long-term complications in adolescents with insulin-dependent diabetes mellitus: the Diabetes Control and Complications Trial. J PEDIATR 1994;125:177-88.
2. Diabetes Control and Complications Trial Research Group. The effect of intensive treatment of diabetes on the development and progression of long-term complications in insulin-dependent diabetes mellitus. N Engl J Med 1993;329:977-86.
3. Geffner ME. Reviewing the Diabetes Control and Complications Trial: one member of the "control panel" speaks. J PEDIATR 1994;125:228-9.
4. Dorchy H. Quel contrôle glycémique peut-il être obtenu chez des jeunes diabétiques sans sécrétion résiduelle d'insuline endogène? Quelle est la fréquence des hypoglycémies sévères et des complications subcliniques? Arch Pediatr 1994;1:970-81.
5. Ludvigsson J. Successful glycemic control in diabetic adolescents. In: Rifkin H, Colwell JA, Taylor SI, eds. Diabetes 1991. Amsterdam: Elsevier Science, 1991:822-7.
6. Bougnères PF, Landais P, Mairesse AM, et al. Improvement of diabetic control and acceptability of a three-injection insulin regimen in diabetic adolescents. Diabetes Care 1993;16:94-102.
7. Delamater AM, Albrecht DR, Postellon DC, Gutai JP. Racial differences in metabolic control of children and adolescents with type I diabetes mellitus. Diabetes Care 1991;14:20-5.
8. Virtanen SM. Metabolic control and diet in Finnish diabetic adolescents. Acta Paediatr 1992;81:239-43.
9. Czernichow P, Dorchy H. Traitement et insulinothérapie. In: Czernichow P, Dorchy H, eds. Diabétologie pédiatrique. Paris: Doin, 1989:445-96.
10. Dorchy H. Dorchy's recipes explaining the "intriguing efficacy of Belgian conventional therapy." Diabetes Care 1994; 17:458-60.

Reply

To the Editor:

One of the advantages of a randomized, controlled clinical trial, such as the Diabetes Control and Complications Trial (DCCT), is the ability to test specific hypotheses in a scientifically and statistically valid fashion. The major study question posed, and answered, by the DCCT was whether an intensive treatment regimen aimed at achieving glycemic control as close to the nondiabetic range as possible would prevent the onset and/or slow the progression of long-term complications in insulin-dependent diabetes mellitus, compared with a conventional treatment regimen. The primary analysis compared the effects of the randomly assigned treatments.

In the DCCT, intensive therapy had a consistent, beneficial effect in delaying the onset and slowing the progression of diabetic complications. Intensive therapy was composed of many components, including treatment with multiple daily insulin injections or insulin pumps, frequent visits, self-glucose monitoring, and dietary interventions. Although we cannot identify which component(s) of the treatment package reduced the risk of complications, secondary analyses suggest that lowering hemoglobin A_{1c} levels was particularly important. If a similar reduction of hemoglobin A_{1c} can be safely achieved and maintained in young patients with "intensified conventional therapy" as suggested by Dr. Dorchy, it is reasonable to assume that such patients will have a corresponding improvement in prognosis regarding diabetic complications. However, it is incumbent on the proponents of such treatment regimens to compare, in a rigorous and scientifically valid fashion, their efficacy in lowering hemoglobin A_{1c} levels and the accompanying frequency and severity of treatment-related adverse events with the results of intensive therapy as conducted in the DCCT. In the absence of a satisfactory controlled clinical study of such regimens, intensive therapy as practiced in the DCCT continues to be the treatment of choice for most patients with insulin-dependent diabetes mellitus.

William V. Tamborlane, MD
David M. Nathan, MD
for the DCCT Research Group
Box NDIC/DCCT
Bethesda, MD 20892
9/35/63774

Lactic acidosis in a patient with acute lymphoblastic leukemia

To the Editor,

Ali et al.[1] report an interesting clinical observation in a patient with acute lymphoblastic leukemia who had lactic acidosis. Several aspects of the acid-base abnormalities observed in this patient require clarification. The authors state that the "lactate values again returned to normal (4.0 mmol/L)." A normal serum lactate concentration is less than 2.0 mmol/L. There was therefore continuing evidence of lactic acidosis in their patients. Is it possible that the continuing lactic acidosis was a sign of persistent acute lymphoblastic leukemia?

The authors state that the urine pH was inappropriately low at 5.0. This urine pH is appropriately low for a patient with systemic acidemia. With chronic acidemia, the kidney responds by increasing the excretion of hydrogen ions including free hydrogen ions, ammonium, and titratable acid. The authors mention that a contributing factor to the metabolic acidosis "may have been high doses of alkaline therapy," which does not cause metabolic acidosis. The authors may be referring to the modest increase in serum lactate observed in patients with alkalemia. The anion gap was elevated at 32 mmol/L. The elevation in serum lactate concentration explained only 12 mmol/L of the elevated anion gap; there was 8 mmol/L of further unexplained anions.

William Lane M. Robson, MD, FRCP(C), FRSH, MRCP(Glasg)
Children's Hospital Greenville Hospital System
Department of Pediatrics
University of South Carolina School of Medicine
Greenville, SC 29605-4253

Alexander K. C. Leung, MBBS, FRCP(C), FRCP(Edin)
Department of Pediatrics
University of Calgary and the Alberta Children's Hospital
Calgary, Alberta, Canada
9/35/64044

REFERENCE

1. Ali AA, Flombaum CD, Brochstein JA, Gillio AP, Bussel JB, Boulad F. Lactic acidosis and renal enlargement at diagnosis and relapse of acute lymphoblastic leukemia. J PEDIATR 1994; 125:584-6.

True hermaphroditism with 46,XY karyotype and a point mutation in the *SRY* gene

To the Editor:

We read with interest the article by Hadjiathanasiou et al.[1] regarding the genetic variants and clinical management of true hermaphrodites. The authors discuss 22 patients with respect to their karyotypes and the presence of the *SRY* gene. We studied a patient with similar clinical features, but a 46,XY karyotype. The individual was born at term, small for gestational age. A urogenital sinus with a large phallus of 3.8 cm and bilateral hernias were present. The patient had a normal-appearing vagina, but no evidence of a cervix on laparotomy. The left gonad was in the labioscrotal fold, and the right gonad was just distal to the superficial inguinal ring. At surgical correction for female sex of rearing, the gonads were removed; one of them was an ovotestis on histologic examination.

We studied the presence of the *SRY* gene in blood leukocyte DNA of this patient. The sequence encoding for the DNA-binding motif was amplified by polymerase chain reaction and screened for point mutations with a nonisotopic single-strand conformation polymorphism analysis.[2] In contrast to 200 control DNAs from phenotypically normal male subjects, this patient carried a variation in the amplified *SRY* fragment. Sequencing revealed a thymidine to cytidine base exchange in the third codon of the DNA-binding motif, leading to a substitution of the normally present valine by alanine. Braun et al.[3] reported a similar case of true hermaphroditism with 46,XY karyotype and two mutations in the *SRY* gene. One silent mutation was present; the second mutation led to an amino acid substitution of leucine to histidine in position 44 of the DNA-binding motif.

We believe it to be noteworthy that a subset of patients with true hermaphroditism has a 46,XY karyotype. In these individuals one should not only look for the presence of *SRY*, but characterize this gene carefully for point mutations in the highly conserved coding sequences.

Olaf Hiort, MD
Britta Gramss
Department of Pediatrics
Medical University of Lübeck
Lübeck, Germany

George T. Klauber, MD
Division of Pediatric Urology
Tufts University School of Medicine
Boston, Mass.
9/35/64045

REFERENCES

1. Hadjiathanasiou CG, Brauner R, Lortat-Jacob S, et al. True hermaphroditism: genetic variants and clinical management. J PEDIATR 1994;125:738-44.
2. Hiort O, Wodtke A, Struve D, Zöllner A, Sinnecker GHG. Detection of androgen receptor gene mutations using non-isotopic single strand conformation polymorphism analysis. Hum Mol Genet 1994;3:1163-6.
3. Braun A, Kammerer S, Cleve H, Löhrs U, Schwarz HP, Kuhnle U. True hermaphroditism in a 46,XY individual, caused by a postzygotic somatic point mutation in the male gonadal sex-determining locus (SRY): molecular genetics and histological findings in a sporadic case. Am J Hum Genet 1993; 52:578-85.

INDEX TO VOLUME 126

Author index*

A

Abboud M (*see* Basco et al). 1995;126:847-8 (Letter)
—— (*see* Pegelow et al). 1995;126:896-9
Abelson HT (*see* Colina and Abelson). 1995;126:395-7 (CLO)
Abman SH (*see* Kinsella and Abman). 1995;126:853-64
Abraham SK (*see* Rosh et al). 1995;126:143-5 (CLO)
Abrahamov A (*see* Zimran et al). 1995;126:596-7 (CLO)
Abrams SA (*see* Schanler and Abrams). 1995;126:441-7
Abramson JS, O'Shea TM, Ratledge DL, Lawless MR, Givner LB. Development of a vaccine tracking system to improve the rate of age-appropriate primary immunization in children of lower socioeconomic status. 1995;126:583-6 (CLO)
Abzug MJ, Loeffelholz M, Rotbart HA. Diagnosis of neonatal enterovirus infection by polymerase chain reaction. 1995; 126:447-50 (CLO)
Accurso FJ (*see* Bronstein et al). 1995;126:28-33
Adams LM, Emery JR, Clark SJ, Carlton EI, Nelson JC. Reference ranges for newer thyroid function tests in premature infants. 1995;126:122-7
Adams M (*see* Andrew et al). 1995;126:358-63
Adams RJ (*see* Pegelow et al). 1995;126:896-9
Akimoto K (*see* Ino et al). 1995;126:304-8
Akinbi H, Bhutani V, Abbasi S. Blood flow velocities and neonatal asphyxia. 1995;126:676 (Letter reply)
Al Saedi S, Dean H, Dent W, Cronin C. Reference ranges for serum cortisol and 17-hydroxyprogesterone levels in preterm infants. 1995;126:985-7 (CLO)
Albanese A, Stanhope R. Predictive factors in the determination of final height in boys with constitutional delay of growth and puberty. 1995;126:545-50
Allen A (*see* Smyth et al). 1995;126:S81-9 (Symposium)
Allen DW (*see* Rehan et al). 1995;126:979-82 (CLO)
Allen UD (*see* King et al). 1995;126:937-9 (CLO)
Alpan O (*see* La Gamma et al). 1995;126:457-9 (CLO)
Alvaro RE (*see* Rehan et al). 1995;126:979-82 (CLO)
Amato D (*see* Mazariegos-Ramos et al). 1995;126:940-2 (CLO)
Ament ME (*see* Baron et al). 1995;126:397-400 (CLO)
American and Canadian Exosurf Neonatal Study Groups (*see* Courtney et al). 1995;126:S43-52 (Symposium)
—— (*see* Sauve et al). 1995;126:S75-80 (Symposium)
American Exosurf Neonatal Study Group I (*see* Corbet et al). 1995;126:S5-12 (Symposium)
—— (*see* Gong et al). 1995;126:S68-74 (Symposium)
—— (*see* Sell et al). 1995;126:S20-5 (Symposium)
—— (*see* Walther et al). 1995;126:S13-9 (Symposium)
American Exosurf Neonatal Study Groups I and II (*see* Corbet et al). 1995;126:969-78
—— (*see* Gerdes et al). 1995;126:S26-32 (Symposium)
Ames BN (*see* Helbock and Ames). 1995;126:747-8 (Editor's column)
Amini S (*see* Furman et al). 1995;126:434-40
Amir N (*see* Elpeleg et al). 1995;126:72-4 (CLO)
Amos CI (*see* Duliège et al). 1995;126:625-32
Amyot K (*see* Lascari and Amyot). 1995;126:816-7 (CLO)
Anday E (*see* Gong et al). 1995;126:S68-74 (Symposium)

*January, pp. 1-162; February, pp. 163-332; March, pp. 333-506; April, pp. 507-682; May, pp. 683-852 and S1-S102; June, pp. 853-1064 and S103-S134.

Anderson CE (*see* Rabinowitz et al). 1995;126:266-9 (CLO)
Andrew M, Marzinotto V, Pencharz P, Zlotkin S, Burrows P, Ingram J, Adams M, Filler R. A cross-sectional study of catheter-related thrombosis in children receiving total parenteral nutrition at home. 1995;126:358-63
—— (*see* Uziel et al). 1995;126:722-7
Andria G (*see* Parenti et al). 1995;126:246-51
Antoniazzi F (*see* Zamboni et al). 1995;126:756-8 (CLO)
Antonioli DA (*see* Odze et al). 1995;126:163-70
Arav-Boger R, Reif S, Bujanover Y. Portal vein thrombosis caused by protein C and protein S deficiency associated with cytomegalovirus infection. 1995;126:586-8 (CLO)
Arslanian S (*see* Gschwend et al). 1995;126:178-84
Asbill D (*see* Kraybill et al). 1995;126:S33-42 (Symposium)
Atchison J (*see* Gschwend et al). 1995;126:178-84
Atherton HD (*see* Kotagal et al). 1995;126:88-93
Atkinson SA (*see* Halton et al). 1995;126:557-64
Aughton DJ (*see* Polack et al). 1995;126:261-3 (CLO)
Austin NC (*see* Inder et al). 1995;126:128-31 (CLO)
Avila E (*see* Corbet et al). 1995;126:969-78
Awad IA (*see* Soper et al). 1995;126:945-8 (CLO)

B

Bachrach S (*see* Proujansky et al). 1995;126:850 (Letter reply)
Backhouse ME (*see* Mauskopf et al). 1995;126:94-101
Baker L (*see* Thornton et al). 1995;126:1017 (Letter reply)
Baley J (*see* Furman et al). 1995;126:434-40
Baley JE (*see* Heggie et al). 1995;126:503-4 (Letter reply)
Balfour HH Jr (*see* Schwebke et al). 1995;126:293-5 (CLO)
Balsamo A, Tassoni P, Cassio A, Colli C, Tassinari D, Cicognani A, Cacciari E. Response to growth hormone therapy in patients with growth hormone deficiency who were small or appropriate in size for gestational age at birth. 1995;126:474-7
Balsan MJ (*see* Brozanski et al). 1995;126:769-76
Bancalari E (*see* Rojas et al). 1995;126:605-10
Bandini LG, Puelzl-Quinn H, Morelli JA, Fukagawa NK. Estimation of energy requirements in persons with severe central nervous system impairment. 1995;126:828-32
Bar A, Linder B, Sobel EH, Saenger P, DiMartino-Nardi J. Bayley-Pinneau method of height prediction in girls with central precocious puberty: correlation with adult height. 1995;126:955-8 (CLO)
Barash V (*see* Elpeleg et al). 1995;126:72-4 (CLO)
Barbé T, Losay J, Grimon G, Devictor D, Sardet A, Gauthier F, Houssin D, Bernard O. Pulmonary arteriovenous shunting in children with liver disease. 1995;126:571-9
Bard H (*see* Courtney et al). 1995;126:S43-52 (Symposium)
—— (*see* McMillan et al). 1995;126:S90-8 (Symposium)
—— (*see* Sauve et al). 1995;126:S75-80 (Symposium)
Bardeguez A (*see* Palumbo et al). 1995;126:592-5 (CLO)
Bar-Haim Y (*see* Tully et al). 1995;126:S105-11
Barker G (*see* Beca et al). 1995;126:44-9
Bar-Maor JA (*see* Zimran et al). 1995;126:596-7 (CLO)
Barnett JL (*see* Klein et al). 1995;126:252-6
Baron HI, Beck DC, Vargas JH, Ament ME. Overinterpretation of gastroduodenal motility studies: two cases involving Munchausen syndrome by proxy. 1995;126:397-400 (CLO)
Barone R (*see* Fiumara et al). 1995;126:852 (Letter)
Barr RD (*see* Halton et al). 1995;126:557-64
Barsanti S (*see* Saggese et al). 1995;126:468-73
Barton LL. Infectious hazards of immune globulin. 1995;126:321-2 (Letter)

Barton NW (*see* Zimran et al). 1995;126:596-7 (CLO)
Basco WT Jr, Abboud M, Holden KR. Opsoclonus-myoclonus and recurrent neuroblastoma. 1995;126:847-8 (Letter)
Bass N, Wyllie E, Comair Y, Kotagal P, Ruggieri P, Holthausen H. Supplementary sensorimotor area seizures in children and adolescents. 1995;126:537-44
Battezzati PM (*see* Colombo et al). 1995;126:155-6 (Letter reply)
Baum VC (*see* Reda et al). 1995;126:961-5 (CLO)
Beaudry M, Dufour R, Marcoux S. Relation between infant feeding and infections during the first six months of life. 1995; 126:191-7
Beaumont E (*see* Gerdes et al). 1995;126:S26-32 (Symposium)
Beca J, Cox PN, Taylor MJ, Bohn D, Butt W, Logan WJ, Rutka JT, Barker G. Somatosensory evoked potentials for prediction of outcome in acute severe brain injury. 1995;126:44-9
Beck DC (*see* Baron et al). 1995;126:397-400 (CLO)
Becker D (*see* Gschwend et al). 1995;126:178-84
Bejar R (*see* Greenberg et al). 1995;126:633-5 (CLO)
Bélanger S (*see* Chessex et al). 1995;126:619-24
Belik J (*sec* Rehan et al). 1995;126:979 82 (CLO)
Belknap WM (*see* Polack et al). 1995;126:261-3 (CLO)
Bell LM (*see* Wiley et al). 1995;126:392-5 (CLO)
Bennett MJ (*see* Bhala et al). 1995;126:910-5
—— (*see* Dawson et al). 1995;126:69-71 (CLO)
Benoist MR (*see* Rufin et al). 1995;126:161-2 (Letter)
Berde CB (*see* Collins et al). 1995;126:653-7
Berman B (*see* Pegelow et al). 1995;126:896-9
Bernard O (*see* Barbé et al). 1995;126:571-9
Bernheim J (*see* Pomeranz et al). 1995;126:140-2 (CLO)
Bernheim J (*see* Pomeranz et al). 1995;126:140-2 (CLO)
Bernini JC, Mustafa MM, Sutor LJ, Buchanan GR. Fatal hemolysis induced by ceftriaxone in a child with sickle cell anemia. 1995;126:813-5 (CLO)
Bernstein G (*see* Cleary et al). 1995;126:407-11
Berry P (*see* Ellis et al). 1995;126:40-3
Beydon N (*see* Delacourt et al). 1995;126:703-9
Bhala A, Willi SM, Rinaldo P, Bennett MJ, Schmidt-Sommerfeld E, Hale DE. Clinical and biochemical characterization of short-chain acyl–coenzyme A dehydrogenase deficiency. 1995; 126: 910-5
Bhatia V (*see* Gupta et al). 1995;126:389-92 (CLO)
Bhutani V (*see* Akinbi and Bhutani). 1995;126:676 (Letter reply)
Bierman CW. Venom immunotherapy: Who should receive it? 1995;126:257-8 (Editor's column)
Biggar RJ (*see* Duliège et al). 1995;126:625-32
Bingham W (*see* Casiro et al). 1995;126:S53-60 (Symposium)
—— (*see* Saigal et al). 1995;126:S61-7 (Symposium)
Blaiss MS (*see* Herrod et al). 1995;126:530-6
Blanche S (*see* Tardieu et al). 1995;126:375-9
Blanchette VS. Short-term, high-dose corticosteroid therapy in childhood acute immune thrombocytopenic purpura. 1995; 126:156-7 (Letter reply)
Blanco CE (*see* Foreman–van Drongelen et al). 1995;126:611-8
Blaser S (*see* Uziel et al). 1995;126:722-7
Blau N, Ichinose H, Nagatsu T, Heizmann CW, Zacchello F, Burlina AB. A missense mutation in a patient with guanosine triphosphate cyclohydrolase I deficiency missed in the newborn screening program. 1995;126:401-5 (CLO)
Bodensteiner JB (*see* Sheth et al). 1995;126:259-61 (CLO)
Bohn D (*see* Beca et al). 1995;126:44-9
Bonner CM, DeBrie KL, Hug G, Landrigan E, Taylor BJ. Effects of parenteral L-carnitine supplementation on fat metabolism and nutrition in premature neonates. 1995;126:287-92
Bonnier C (*see* Mbonda et al). 1995;126:923-7
Borawski-Clark E (*see* Furman et al). 1995;126:434-40
Borg WP (*see* Jones et al). 1995;126:171-7
Boros S (*see* Gong et al). 1995;126:S68-74 (Symposium)
Boscherini B (*see* Spagnoli et al). 1995;126:905-9
Bose CL (*see* Kraybill et al). 1995;126:S33-42 (Symposium)
—— (*see* Makhlouf et al). 1995;126:454-56 (CLO)
Boulware SD (*see* Jones et al). 1995;126:171-7
Bower LK (*see* McManus et al). 1995;126:900-4
Boxerbaum B (*see* Heggie et al). 1995;126:503-4 (Letter reply)
Bradley RL (*see* Tully et al). 1995;126:S105-11
Brady RO (*see* Zimran et al). 1995;126:596-7 (CLO)
Brambilla D (*see* Pegelow et al). 1995;126:896-9
Braselton WE (*see* Rajaram et al). 1995;126:791-6
Brazelton TB (*see* North et al). 1995;126:916-22
Broecker EB (*see* Hentschel et al). 1995;126:61-4 (CLO)
Broemeling LD (*see* Klein et al). 1995;126:252-6
Bronstein MN, Davies PSW, Hambidge KM, Accurso FJ. Normal energy expenditure in the infant with presymptomatic cystic fibrosis. 1995;126:28-33
Brook CGD (*see* Crowley et al). 1995;126:297-303
Brown AK (*see* Slusher et al). 1995;126:102-8
Brozanski BS, Jones JG, Gilmour CH, Balsan MJ, Vazquez RL, Israel BA, Newman B, Mimouni FB, Guthrie RD. Effect of pulse dexamethasone therapy on the incidence and severity of chronic lung disease in the very low birth weight infant. 1995;126:769-76
Brunstrom JE (*see* Schlesinger et al). 1995;126:234-41
Bryant D (*see* Roberts et al). 1995;126:481-9
Bucciarelli R (*see* Gong et al). 1995;126:S68-74 (Symposium)
Buchanan GR (*see* Bernini et al). 1995;126:813-5 (CLO)
Buchino JJ (*see* Jones and Buchino). 1995;126:663-8
Buck GM (*see* Rogers et al). 1995;126:496-8 (CLO)
Buck R (*see* Garland et al). 1995;126:272-9
Buckley D (*see* Li et al). 1995;126:353-7
Bucolo S (*see* Thomson et al). 1995;126:21-7
Bujanover Y (*see* Arav-Boger et al). 1995;126:586-8 (CLO)
Buller RS (*see* Schlesinger et al). 1995;126:234-41
Burchfield D (*see* Gong et al). 1995;126:S68-74 (Symposium)
Burchinal MR (*see* Roberts et al). 1995;126:481-9
Burlina AB (*see* Blau et al). 1995;126:401-5 (CLO)
Burrows P (*see* Andrew et al). 1995;126:358-63
Burt R (*see* Mueller et al). 1995;126:749-52 (CLO)
Butler RB (*see* Maris et al). 1995;126:269-71 (CLO)
Butler VT (*see* Heggie et al). 1995;126:503-4 (Letter reply)
Butt W (*see* Beca et al). 1995;126:44-9

C

Cabral H (*see* Mirochnick et al). 1995;126:636-8 (CLO)
Cacciari E (*see* Balsamo et al). 1995;126:474-7
Caldwell MB (*see* Lobato et al). 1995;126:710-5
Callahan S (*see* Schuh et al). 1995;126:639-45
Camfield CS (*see* Camfield et al). 1995;126:929-30 (Editor's column)
Camfield PR, Camfield CS, Gordon K, Dooley JM. Prevention of recurrent febrile seizures. 1995;126:929-30 (Editor's column)
Campana S (*see* Taccetti et al). 1995;126:848-9 (Letter)
Campos M (*see* Fukuda et al). 1995;126:882-6
Canadian Exosurf Neonatal Follow-Up Group (*see* Casiro et al). 1995;126:S53-60 (Symposium)
Canadian Exosurf Neonatal Study Group (*see* Casiro et al). 1995; 126:S53-60 (Symposium)
—— (*see* McMillan et al). 1995;126:S90-8 (Symposium)
—— (*see* Saigal et al). 1995;126:S61-7 (Symposium)
—— (*see* Smyth et al). 1995;126:S81-9 (Symposium)
Canny G (*see* Schuh et al). 1995;126:639-45
Cantarero MD (*see* Iacono et al). 1995;126:34-9
Carlson DE (*see* Vanderhal et al). 1995;126:988-90 (CLO)
Carlson SE (*see* Rajaram et al). 1995;126:791-6
Carlton EI (*see* Adams et al). 1995;126:122-7
Carr AC (*see* Inder et al). 1995;126:128-31 (CLO)
Carroccio A (*see* Iacono et al). 1995;126:34-9
Casado-Flores J (*see* Martinez-Azagra et al). 1995;126:678 (Letter)
Casella SJ, Finberg L. A new defect in vitamin D metabolism. 1995;126:677 (Letter reply)

Casiro O, Bingham W, MacMurray B, Whitfield M, Saigal S, Vincer M, Long W, Canadian Exosurf Neonatal Study Group, Canadian Exosurf Neonatal Follow-Up Group. One-year follow-up of 89 infants with birth weights of 500 to 749 grams and respiratory distress syndrome randomized to two rescue doses of synthetic surfactant or air placebo. 1995;126:S53-60 (Symposium)
—— (*see* Saigal et al). 1995;126:S61-7 (Symposium)
Cassell GH (*see* Waites et al). 1995;126:502 (Letter)
Cassidy SB (*see* Hákonarson et al). 1995;126:565-70
Cassio A (*see* Balsamo et al). 1995;126:474-7
Castro-Gago M (*see* Fuster-Siebert and Castro-Gago). 1995;126:506 (Letter)
Cavataio F (*see* Iacono et al). 1995;126:34-9
Cedar E (*see* Hählen et al). 1995;126:309-13
Cedro A (*see* Pronicka et al). 1995;126:948-51 (CLO)
Cesaretti G (*see* Saggese et al). 1995;126:468-73
Chaloupka JC (*see* Soper et al). 1995;126:945-8 (CLO)
Chamberlain MC. Opsoclonus-myoclonus, ataxia, and coincident neuroblastoma. 1995;126:675 (Letter)
Chan F (*see* King et al). 1995;126:937-9 (CLO)
Chan GM, Hoffman K, Wiebke G, McMurry M. Effects of dairy products on bone and body composition in pubertal girls. 1995;126:551-6
Chang M-H (*see* Lee et al). 1995;126:716-21
—— (*see* Lin et al). 1995;126:589-91 (CLO)
Chang S-J (*see* Greenberg et al). 1995;126:206-11
—— (*see* Lieberman et al). 1995;126:198-205
Chaparro L (*see* Fukuda et al). 1995;126:882-6
Charney EB (*see* Stallings et al). 1995;126:833-9
Charrow J (*see* Habiby et al). 1995;126:364-7
Chea E (*see* Fukuda et al). 1995;126:882-6
Chen D-S (*see* Lin et al). 1995;126:589-91 (CLO)
Chen P-J (*see* Lin et al). 1995;126:589-91 (CLO)
Chernick V (*see* McMillan et al). 1995;126:S90-8 (Symposium)
Chessex P, Bélanger S, Piedboeuf B, Pineault M. Influence of energy substrates on respiratory gas exchange during conventional mechanical ventilation of preterm infants. 1995;126:619-24
Chew FJ (*see* Kjolhede et al). 1995;126:807-12
Chipman M (*see* Perlman et al). 1995;126:75-87
Chiu C-Y (*see* Greenberg et al). 1995;126:206-11
—— (*see* Lieberman et al). 1995;126:198-205
Chonmaitree T (*see* Patel et al). 1995;126:799-806
Chretien D (*see* Rötig et al). 1995;126:597-601 (CLO)
Christensen RD (*see* Ohls et al). 1995;126:421-6
Christodoulou J, Hoare J, Hammond J, Ip WC, Wilcken B. Neonatal onset of medium-chain acyl–coenzyme A dehydrogenase deficiency with confusing biochemical features. 1995;126:65-8 (CLO)
Chureau C (*see* Delacourt et al). 1995;126:703-9
Cianfarani S (*see* Spagnoli et al). 1995;126:905-9
Cicognani A (*see* Balsamo et al). 1995;126:474-7
Claris O (*see* Perlman et al). 1995;126:75-87
Clark SJ (*see* Adams et al). 1995;126:122-7
Claure N (*see* Rojas et al). 1995;126:605-10
Claus D (*see* Mbonda et al). 1995;126:923-7
Cleary JP, Bernstein G, Mannino FL, Heldt GP. Improved oxygenation during synchronized intermittent mandatory ventilation in neonates with respiratory distress syndrome: a randomized, crossover study. 1995;126:407-11
Clegg HW, Riopel DA. Furosemide-associated fever. 1995;126:817-8 (CLO)
—— (*see* Roddey et al). 1995;126:931-3 (CLO)
Clerici M (*see* Viganó et al). 1995;126:368-74
Cleveland DC (*see* Rogers et al). 1995;126:496-8 (CLO)
Cloutier MM (*see* Hákonarson et al). 1995;126:565-70
Clyne M (*see* Gormally et al). 1995;126:753-6 (CLO)
Cocjin J (*see* Vanderhal et al). 1995;126:988-90 (CLO)
Cockshott WP (*see* Halton et al). 1995;126:557-64
Cohen AR (*see* Maris et al). 1995;126:269-71 (CLO)
Cohen RB (*see* Lanchoney et al). 1995;126:762-4 (CLO)
Colina KF, Abelson HT. Resolution of breath-holding spells with treatment of concomitant anemia. 1995;126:395-7 (CLO)
Colli C (*see* Balsamo et al). 1995;126:474-7
Collins JJ, Grier HE, Kinney HC, Berde CB. Control of severe pain in children with terminal malignancy. 1995;126:653-7
Colombo C, Giunta A, Battezzati PM. Incidence of liver disease in patients with cystic fibrosis and meconium ileus. 1995;126:155-6 (Letter reply)
Comair Y (*see* Bass et al). 1995;126:537-44
Connor EM (*see* Palumbo et al). 1995;126:592-5 (CLO)
Conway B (*see* Courtney et al). 1995;126:S43-52 (Symposium)
Cook L (*see* Corbet et al). 1995;126:969-78
—— (*see* Gerdes et al). 1995;126:S26-32 (Symposium)
Coppes MJ (*see* Poon et al). 1995;126:959-61 (CLO)
Corbet A, Gerdes J, Long W, Avila E, Puri A, Rosenberg A, Edwards K, Cook L, American Exosurf Neonatal Study Groups I and II. Double-blind, randomized trial of one versus three prophylactic doses of synthetic surfactant in 826 neonates weighing 700 to 1100 grams: effects on mortality rate. 1995;126:969-78
——, Long W, Schumacher R, Gerdes J, Cotton R, American Exosurf Neonatal Study Group I. Double-blind developmental evaluation at 1-year corrected age of 597 premature infants with birth weights from 500 to 1350 grams enrolled in three placebo-controlled trials of prophylactic synthetic surfactant. 1995;126:S5-12 (Symposium)
—— (*see* Kraybill et al). 1995;126:S33-42 (Symposium)
Corcoran L (*see* Dulkerian et al). 1995;126:872-6
Corydon KE (*see* Rosenfeld et al). 1995;126:524-9
—— (*see* Rosenfeld et al). 1995;126:1000-3
Costarino AT Jr (*see* Dulkerian et al). 1995;126:872-6
Cotton R (*see* Corbet et al). 1995;126:S5-12 (Symposium)
—— (*see* Sell et al). 1995;126:S20-5 (Symposium)
Courtney SE, Long W, McMillan D, Walter D, Thompson T, Sauve R, Conway B, Bard H, American and Canadian Exosurf Neonatal Study Groups. Double-blind 1-year follow-up of 1540 infants with respiratory distress syndrome randomized to rescue treatment with two doses of synthetic surfactant or air in four clinical trials. 1995;126:S43-52 (Symposium)
Cox PN (*see* Beca et al). 1995;126:44-9
Crane RT (*see* Schwebke et al). 1995;126:293-5 (CLO)
Cronin C (*see* Al Saedi et al). 1995;126:985-7 (CLO)
Cronk CE (*see* Stallings et al). 1995;126:833-9
Crouse DT, Reese JM. Isolation of *Ureaplasma urealyticum* from low birth weight infants. 1995;126:502-3 (Letter)
Crowley S, Hindmarsh PC, Matthews DR, Brook CGD. Growth and the growth hormone axis in prepubertal children with asthma. 1995;126:297-303
Crump SR. Promotion of healthy eating habits in children. 1995;126:850 (Letter)
Crupi L (*see* Viganó et al). 1995;126:368-74
Cutfield WS, Webster D. Newborn screening for congenital adrenal hyperplasia in New Zealand. 1995;126:118-21
Cutler GB Jr (*see* Ross et al). 1995;126:242-5
Cystic Fibrosis Foundation Prednisone Trial Group (*see* Eigen et al). 1995;126:515-23

D

Daigle KL (*see* Hákonarson et al). 1995;126:565-70
Daly LE (*see* Gormally et al). 1995;126:753-6 (CLO)
Dampier CD, Setty BNY, Logan J, Ioli JG, Dean R. Intravenous morphine pharmacokinetics in pediatric patients with sickle cell disease. 1995;126:461-7
Darlow BA (*see* Inder et al). 1995;126:128-31 (CLO)
—— (*see* Neužil et al). 1995;126:785-90
David M (*see* Rivard et al). 1995;126:646-52

David R (*see* Rapaport et al). 1995;126:759-61 (CLO)
Davies PSW (*see* Bronstein et al). 1995;126:28-33
Davis AL (*see* Reda et al). 1995;126:961-5 (CLO)
Davis SL. Adult respiratory distress syndrome in children associated with miliary tuberculosis. 1995;126:678-9 (Letter reply)
Dawson DB, Waber L, Hale DE, Bennett MJ. Transient organic aciduria and persistent lacticacidemia in a patient with short-chain acyl–coenzyme A dehydrogenase deficiency. 1995;126: 69-71 (CLO)
Dean H (*see* Al Saedi et al). 1995;126:985-7 (CLO)
Dean R (*see* Dampier et al). 1995;126:461-7
de Blic J (*see* Delacourt et al). 1995;126:703-9
—— (*see* Rufin et al). 1995;126:161-2 (Letter)
DeBrie KL (*see* Bonner et al). 1995;126:287-92
de Graeff-Meeder ER (*see* Wulffraat et al). 1995;126:849 (Letter reply)
Delacourt C, Poveda J-D, Chureau C, Beydon N, Mahut B, de Blic J, Scheinmann P, Garrigue G. Use of polymerase chain reaction for improved diagnosis of tuberculosis in children. 1995;126: 703-9
del Rosario JF, Putnam PE, Orenstein DM. Chronic pancreatitis in a patient with cystic fibrosis and clinical pancreatic insufficiency. 1995;126:951-2 (CLO)
Demarini S, Specker BL, Sierra RI, Miodovnik M, Tsang RC. Evidence of increased intrauterine bone resorption in term infants of mothers with insulin-dependent diabetes. 1995;126:796-8 (CLO)
Dent W (*see* Al Saedi et al). 1995;126:985-7 (CLO)
Derleth D (*see* Sauve et al). 1995;126:S75-80 (Symposium)
Desgres J (*see* Semama et al). 1995;126:742-6
Devictor D (*see* Barbé et al). 1995;126:571-9
De Vivo DC (*see* Elpeleg et al). 1995;126:72-4 (CLO)
Dewey KG, Heinig MJ, Nommsen-Rivers LA. Differences in morbidity between breast-fed and formula-fed infants. 1995;126:696-702
Dhanireddy R (*see* Gerdes et al). 1995;126:S26-32 (Symposium)
Dilks S (*see* Schlager et al). 1995;126:490-6
Diller PM, Huster GA, Leach AD, Laskarzewski PM, Sprecher DL. Definition and application of the discretionary screening indicators according to the National Cholesterol Education Program for Children and Adolescents. 1995;126:345-52
DiMartino-Nardi J (*see* Bar et al). 1995;126:955-8 (CLO)
Doi A (*see* Yuki et al). 1995;126:55-7 (CLO)
Donovan EF (*see* Kotagal et al). 1995;126:88-93
Dooley JM (*see* Camfield et al). 1995;126:929-30 (Editor's column)
Dorchy H. Hemoglobin A_{1c} levels in young patients with diabetes beyond the "honeymoon" period. 1995;126:1020-1 (Letter)
Doron MW (*see* Makhlouf et al). 1995;126:454-56 (CLO)
Drumm B (*see* Gormally et al). 1995;126:753-6 (CLO)
Dudley R (*see* Osterhoudt et al). 1995;126:819-21 (CLO)
Duffy LB (*see* Waites et al). 1995;126:502 (Letter)
Dufour R (*see* Beaudry et al). 1995;126:191-7
Duliège A-M, Amos CI, Felton S, Biggar RJ, International Registry of HIV-Exposed Twins, Goedert JJ. Birth order, delivery route, and concordance in the transmission of human immunodeficiency virus type 1 from mothers to twins. 1995;126:625-32
Dulkerian SJ, Kilpatrick L, Costarino AT Jr, McCawley L, Fein J, Corcoran L, Zirin S, Harris MC. Cytokine elevations in infants with bacterial and aseptic meningitis. 1995;126:872-6
Dungy CI (*see* Losch et al). 1995;126:507-14
Durnin MT (*see* Gormally et al). 1995;126:753-6 (CLO)
Dusdieker LB (*see* Losch et al). 1995;126:507-14
Dyke JW (*see* Karna et al). 1995;126:322 (Letter reply)

E

Easa D (*see* Walther et al). 1995;126:S13-9 (Symposium)
Ebina K (*see* Kato et al). 1995;126:1008-10 (CLO)
Edwards K (*see* Corbet et al). 1995;126:969-78
—— (*see* Kraybill et al). 1995;126:S33-42 (Symposium)
Ehrlich RM (*see* Rovet and Ehrlich). 1995;126:380-6
Eigen H, Rosenstein BJ, FitzSimmons S, Schidlow DV, Cystic Fibrosis Foundation Prednisone Trial Group. A multicenter study of alternate-day prednisone therapy in patients with cystic fibrosis. 1995;126:515-23
Elliott SJ. Blood flow velocities and neonatal asphyxia. 1995;126: 675-6 (Letter)
Ellis EN, Wood EG, Berry P. Spectrum of disease associated with anti-neutrophil cytoplasmic autoantibodies in pediatric patients. 1995;126:40-3
Elpeleg ON, Ruitenbeek W, Jakobs C, Barash V, De Vivo DC, Amir N. Congenital lacticacidemia caused by lipoamide dehydrogenase deficiency with favorable outcome. 1995;126:72-4 (CLO)
Elstein D (*see* Zimran et al). 1995;126:596-7 (CLO)
Emans SJ. Adolescent medicine 1995. 1995;126:387-8 (Editor's column)
Emery JR (*see* Adams et al). 1995;126:122-7
Englund JA, Piedra PA, Gilbert BE. Cost of ribavirin therapy for respiratory syncytial virus infection. 1995;126:847 (Letter reply)
Erenberg A. Perspectives on infant feeding: Introduction. 1995; 126:S104
—— (*see* Nowak et al). 1995;126:S130-4
Erkul I (*see* Yavûz et al). 1995;126:156 (Letter)
Etches PC (*see* Peliowski et al). 1995;126:450-53 (CLO)
Evans CS (*see* Lee et al). 1995;126:280-6
Evrard P (*see* Mbonda et al). 1995;126:923-7

F

Faix RG. Hypotension in preterm infants. 1995;126:160-1 (Letter reply)
Fajardo CA (*see* Rehan et al). 1995;126:979-82 (CLO)
Farber SD, Van Fossen RL, Koontz SW. Quantitative and qualitative video analysis of infants feeding: angled- and straight-bottle feeding systems. 1995;126:S118-24
Farrar HC (*see* Marshall et al). 1995;126:657-9 (CLO)
Farrell C (*see* Rivard et al). 1995;126:646-52
Fawcett P (*see* Spear et al). 1995;126:982-5 (CLO)
Fayad PB (*see* Soper et al). 1995;126:945-8 (CLO)
Feig SA (*see* Sager et al). 1995;126:59-61 (CLO)
Fein J (*see* Dulkerian et al). 1995;126:872-6
Feldmann E (*see* Kruse and Feldmann). 1995;126:145-8 (CLO)
Felton S (*see* Duliège et al). 1995;126:625-32
Feuillan P (*see* Ross et al). 1995;126:242-5
Filler R (*see* Andrew et al). 1995;126:358-63
Finberg L (*see* Casella and Finberg). 1995;126:677 (Letter reply)
—— (*see* Shah and Finberg). 1995;126:1019-20 (Letter reply)
Finch AJ (*see* Whitaker et al). 1995;126:850-1 (Letter reply)
Finer N (*see* McMillan et al). 1995;126:S90-8 (Symposium)
—— (*see* Peliowski et al). 1995;126:450-53 (CLO)
—— (*see* Ryan and Finer). 1995;126:317-9
FitzSimmons S (*see* Eigen et al). 1995;126:515-23
Fiumara A, Barone R, Nigro F, Ribes A, Pavone L. Pancreatitis and organic acidemias. 1995;126:852 (Letter)
Fleisher GR (*see* Teach et al). 1995;126:877-81
Fleming GA (*see* Malozowski et al). 1995;126:996-9
Foreman–van Drongelen MMHP, van Houwelingen AC, Kester ADM, Hasaart THM, Blanco CE, Hornstra G. Long-chain polyunsaturated fatty acids in preterm infants: status at birth and its influence on postnatal levels. 1995;126:611-8
Forleo V (*see* Tonini et al). 1995;126:159 (Letter)
Forster J (*see* Hauk et al). 1995;126:185-90
Fraher L (*see* Halton et al). 1995;126:557-64
Frank DA (*see* Mirochnick et al). 1995;126:636-8 (CLO)
Freij BJ (*see* Polack et al). 1995;126:261-3 (CLO)

Friedl K (*see* Hauk et al). 1995;126:185-90
Friedrich W (*see* Hentschel et al). 1995;126:61-4 (CLO)
Fries SM. Diagnosis of group A streptococcal pharyngitis in a private clinic: comparative evaluation of an optical immunoassay method and culture. 1995;126:933-6 (CLO)
Frosch M (*see* Hentschel et al). 1995;126:61-4 (CLO)
Fuhrman BP (*see* Leach et al). 1995;126:412-20
Fukagawa NK (*see* Bandini et al). 1995;126:828-32
Fukuda JM, Yi A, Chaparro L, Campos M, Chea E. Clinical characteristics and risk factors for *Vibrio cholerae* infection in children. 1995;126:882-6
Fulginiti VA. C. Henry Kempe. 1995;126:152-4 (Profiles)
Funck-Brentano I (*see* Tardieu et al). 1995;126:375-9
Furman L, Hack M, Watts C, Borawski-Clark E, Baley J, Amini S, Hook B. Twenty-month outcome in ventilator-dependent, very low birth weight infants born during the early years of dexamethasone therapy. 1995;126:434-40
Fuster-Siebert M, Castro-Gago M. Electrocardiographic findings in Rett syndrome. 1995;126:506 (Letter)

G

Gadisseux JF (*see* Mbonda et al). 1995;126:923-7
Gadomski AM (*see* Kjolhede et al). 1995;126:807-12
Galant SP. Placebo-controlled versus comparative studies of drug effects. 1995;126:681 (Letter reply)
Gamborino E (*see* Seara et al). 1995;126:965-7 (CLO)
Garcia-Prats J (*see* Kraybill et al). 1995;126:S33-42 (Symposium)
Gardner MH (*see* Goldberg et al). 1995;126:682 (Letter reply)
Garfunkel JM. Placebo-controlled versus comparative studies of drug effects. 1995;126:681 (Letter reply)
Garland JS, Buck R, Leviton A. Effect of maternal glucocorticoid exposure on risk of severe intraventricular hemorrhage in surfactant-treated preterm infants. 1995;126:272-9
Garrigue G (*see* Delacourt et al). 1995;126:703-9
Gauthier F (*see* Barbé et al). 1995;126:571-9
Gerdes J, Gerdes M, Beaumont E, Cook L, Dhanireddy R, Kopleman A, Jarrett R, Long W, American Exosurf Neonatal Study Groups I and II. Health and neurodevelopmental outcome at 1-year adjusted age in 508 infants weighing 700 to 1100 grams who received prophylaxis with one versus three doses of synthetic surfactant. 1995;126:S26-32 (Symposium)
—— (*see* Corbet et al). 1995;126:969-78
—— (*see* Corbet et al). 1995;126:S5-12 (Symposium)
Gerdes M (*see* Gerdes et al). 1995;126:S26-32 (Symposium)
Gibson LE (*see* Goldberg et al). 1995;126:682 (Letter reply)
Gilbert BE (*see* Englund et al). 1995;126:847 (Letter reply)
Gilbert-Barness E. Edith Potter. 1995;126:845-6 (Profiles)
Gilmour CH (*see* Brozanski et al). 1995;126:769-76
Gingell RL (*see* Rogers et al). 1995;126:496-8 (CLO)
Giunta A (*see* Colombo et al). 1995;126:155-6 (Letter reply)
Givner LB (*see* Abramson et al). 1995;126:583-6 (CLO)
Goedert JJ (*see* Dulìège et al). 1995;126:625-32
Goldberg AI, Gardner MH, Gibson LE. Standards for home care of sick children. 1995;126:682 (Letter reply)
Goldberg M (*see* Zimran et al). 1995;126:596-7 (CLO)
Gong A, Anday E, Boros S, Bucciarelli R, Burchfield D, Zucker J, Long W, American Exosurf Neonatal Study Group I. One-year follow-up evaluation of 260 premature infants with respiratory distress syndrome and birth weights of 700 to 1350 grams randomized to two rescue doses of synthetic surfactant or air placebo. 1995;126:S68-74 (Symposium)
Gonzalez A (*see* Rojas et al). 1995;126:605-10
Gopal YR (*see* North et al). 1995;126:916-22
Goran MI, Johnson R. Techniques for measurement of resting energy expenditure in children. 1995;126:679-80 (Letter reply)
Gordon K (*see* Camfield et al). 1995;126:929-30 (Editor's column)
Gormally SM, Prakash N, Durnin MT, Daly LE, Clyne M, Kierce BM, Drumm B. Association of symptoms with *Helicobacter pylori* infection in children. 1995;126:753-6 (CLO)
Goutieres F (*see* Rötig et al). 1995;126:597-601 (CLO)
Gouyon J-B (*see* Semama et al). 1995;126:742-6
Gramss B (*see* Hiort et al). 1995;126:1022 (Letter)
Grayson GH (*see* Sager et al). 1995;126:59-61 (CLO)
Greally JM (*see* Soper et al). 1995;126:945-8 (CLO)
Greenberg DP, Lieberman JM, Marcy SM, Wong VK, Partridge S, Chang S-J, Chiu C-Y, Ward JI. Enhanced antibody responses in infants given different sequences of heterogeneous *Haemophilus influenzae* type b conjugate vaccines. 1995;126:206-11
—— (*see* Lieberman et al). 1995;126:198-205
Greenberg F (*see* Scheuerle et al). 1995;126:764-7 (CLO)
Greenberg M, Movahed H, Peterson B, Bejar R. Placement of umbilical venous catheters with use of bedside real-time ultrasonography. 1995;126:633-5 (CLO)
Grier HE (*see* Collins et al). 1995;126:653-7
Grimon G (*see* Barbé et al). 1995;126:571-9
Groisman G (*see* Rosh et al). 1995;126:143-5 (CLO)
Gross S (*see* Herrod et al). 1995;126:530-6
Gruszcyńska B (*see* Pronicka et al). 1995;126:948-51 (CLO)
Gschwend S, Ryan C, Atchison J, Arslanian S, Becker D. Effects of acute hyperglycemia on mental efficiency and counterregulatory hormones in adolescents with insulin-dependent diabetes mellitus. 1995;126:178-84
Gubler M-C (*see* Rötig et al). 1995;126:597-601 (CLO)
Guerrero-Romero F (*see* Mazariegos-Ramos et al). 1995;126:940-2 (CLO)
Guest G (*see* Rötig et al). 1995;126:597-601 (CLO)
Gujral RB (*see* Gupta et al). 1995;126:389-92 (CLO)
Gulick L (*see* Mueller et al). 1995;126:749-52 (CLO)
Gupta RK, Bhatia V, Poptani H, Gujral RB. Brain metabolite changes on in vivo proton magnetic resonance spectroscopy in children with congenital hypothyroidism. 1995;126:389-92 (CLO)
Guthrie R (*see* Brozanski et al). 1995;126:769-76
—— (*see* Mauskopf et al). 1995;126:94-101
—— (*see* Sell et al). 1995;126:S20-5 (Symposium)
Guzzetta PC (*see* Zimran et al). 1995;126:596-7 (CLO)

H

Habiby R, Silverman B, Listernick R, Charrow J. Precocious puberty in children with neurofibromatosis type 1. 1995;126:364-7
Hack M (*see* Furman et al). 1995;126:434-40
Hählen K, Quintana E, Pinkerton CR, Cedar E. A randomized comparison of intravenously administered granisetron versus chlorpromazine plus dexamethasone in the prevention of ifosfamide-induced emesis in children. 1995;126:309-13
Hákonarson H, Moskovitz J, Daigle KL, Cassidy SB, Cloutier MM. Pulmonary function abnormalities in Prader-Willi syndrome. 1995;126:565-70
Hale DE (*see* Bhala et al). 1995;126:910-5
—— (*see* Dawson et al). 1995;126:69-71 (CLO)
Hall RB (*see* Schelonka et al). 1995;126:505-6 (Letter reply)
Halton JM, Atkinson SA, Fraher L, Webber CE, Cockshott WP, Tam C, Barr RD. Mineral homeostasis and bone mass at diagnosis in children with acute lymphoblastic leukemia. 1995;126: 557-64
Hambidge KM (*see* Bronstein et al). 1995;126:28-33
Hammond J (*see* Christodoulou et al). 1995;126:65-8 (CLO)
Hao Y (*see* Perlman et al). 1995;126:75-87
Harms E (*see* Hentschel et al). 1995;126:61-4 (CLO)
Harris MC (*see* Dulkerian et al). 1995;126:872-6
Hasaart THM (*see* Foreman–van Drongelen et al). 1995;126:611-8

Hauk P, Friedl K, Kaufmehl K, Urbanek R, Forster J. Subsequent insect stings in children with hypersensitivity to Hymenoptera. 1995;126:185-90
Heggie AD, Jacobs MR, Butler VT, Baley JE, Boxerbaum B. Isolation of *Ureaplasma urealyticum* from low birth weight infants. 1995;126:503-4 (Letter reply)
Heikkinen T, Ruuskanen O, Ziegler T, Waris M, Puhakka H. Short-term use of amoxicillin clavulanate during upper respiratory tract infection for prevention of acute otitis media. 1995; 126:313-6 (CLO)
Heinig MJ (*see* Dewey et al). 1995;126:696-702
Heizmann CW (*see* Blau et al). 1995;126:401-5 (CLO)
Helbock HJ, Ames BN. Use of intravenous lipids in neonates. 1995;126:747-8 (Editor's column)
Heldt GP (*see* Cleary et al). 1995;126:407-11
Henderson FW (*see* Roberts et al). 1995;126:481-9
Hendley JO (*see* Schlager et al). 1995;126:490-6
Henretig FM (*see* Osterhoudt et al). 1995;126:819-21 (CLO)
—— (*see* Wiley et al). 1995;126:392-5 (CLO)
Henry K (*see* Schwebke et al). 1995;126:293-5 (CLO)
Hentschel R, Broecker EB, Kolde G, Frosch M, Friedrich W, Holzgreve W, Westphal E, Harms E. Intact survival with transfusion-associated graft-versus-host disease proved by human leukocyte antigen typing of lymphocytes in skin biopsy specimens. 1995;126:61-4 (CLO)
Hergenroeder AC. Bone mineralization, hypothalamic amenorrhea, and sex steroid therapy in adolescents and young adults. 1995; 126:683-9
Hernan LJ (*see* Leach et al). 1995;126:412-20
Herndon DN (*see* Klein et al). 1995;126:252-6
Herrod HG, Blaiss MS, Valenski WR, Gross S. Cell-mediated immune status of children with recurrent infection. 1995;126:530-6
Hickey PR (*see* McManus et al). 1995;126:900-4
Hindmarsh PC (*see* Crowley et al). 1995;126:297-303
Hiort O, Gramss B, Klauber GT. True hermaphroditism with 46,XY karyotype and a point mutation in the *SRY* gene. 1995;126:1022 (Letter)
Hirata T (*see* Sell et al). 1995;126:S20-5 (Symposium)
Hjelte L (*see* Lindblad et al). 1995;126:155 (Letter)
Hoare J (*see* Christodoulou et al). 1995;126:65-8 (CLO)
Hoberman A, Wald ER. Diagnostic accuracy of urinary tract infection and subsequent development of renal scars. 1995;126:158-9 (Letter reply)
Hoffman K (*see* Chan et al). 1995;126:551-6
Hoffmann H (*see* Santer et al). 1995;126:1017 (Letter)
Holden KR (*see* Basco et al). 1995;126:847-8 (Letter)
Holm B (*see* Leach et al). 1995;126:412-20
Holmes LB. Possible fetal effects of cervical dilation and uterine curettage during the first trimester of pregnancy. 1995;126:131-4 (CLO)
Holthausen H (*see* Bass et al). 1995;126:537-44
Holzgreve W (*see* Hentschel et al). 1995;126:61-4 (CLO)
Holzman BH (*see* McLaughlin et al). 1995;126:821-4 (CLO)
Honda S (*see* Kohno et al). 1995;126:953-5 (CLO)
—— (*see* Sato et al). 1995;126:109-13
Hook B (*see* Furman et al). 1995;126:434-40
Hooper S (*see* Roberts et al). 1995;126:481-9
Horne M (*see* Mueller et al). 1995;126:749-52 (CLO)
Hornstra G (*see* Foreman–van Drongelen et al). 1995;126:611-8
Houri S (*see* Reda et al). 1995;126:961-5 (CLO)
Houssin D (*see* Barbé et al). 1995;126:571-9
Howie V (*see* Patel et al). 1995;126:799-806
Hsu H-Y (*see* Lin et al). 1995;126:589-91 (CLO)
Huang L-M (*see* Lee et al). 1995;126:716-21
Huang S-C (*see* Lin et al). 1995;126:589-91 (CLO)
Huet BA (*see* Zwiener et al). 1995;126:728-35
Huet F (*see* Semama et al). 1995;126:742-6
Hug G (*see* Bonner et al). 1995;126:287-92
Husson RN, Lan Y, Kojima E, Venzon D, Mitsuya H, McIntosh K. Vertical transmission of human immunodeficiency virus type I: autologous neutralizing antibody, virus load, and virus phenotype. 1995;126:865-71
Huster GA (*see* Diller et al). 1995;126:345-52
Hwang L-H (*see* Lin et al). 1995;126:589-91 (CLO)

I

Iacono G, Carroccio A, Cavataio F, Montalto G, Cantarero MD, Notarbartolo A. Chronic constipation as a symptom of cow milk allergy. 1995;126:34-9
Ichikawa H (*see* Yuki et al). 1995;126:55-7 (CLO)
Ichinose H (*see* Blau et al). 1995;126:401-5 (CLO)
Incerti B (*see* Parenti et al). 1995;126:246-51
Inder TE, Carr AC, Winterbourn CC, Austin NC, Darlow BA. Vitamin A and E status in very low birth weight infants: development of an improved parenteral delivery system. 1995;126:128-31 (CLO)
—— (*see* Neužil et al). 1995;126:785-90
Ingram J (*see* Andrew et al). 1995;126:358-63
Ino T, Okubo M, Akimoto K, Nishimoto K, Yabuta K, Kawai S, Okada R. Corticosteroid therapy for ventricular tachycardia in children with silent lymphocytic myocarditis. 1995;126:304-8
International Registry of HIV-Exposed Twins (*see* Duliège et al). 1995;126:625-32
Ioli JG (*see* Dampier et al). 1995;126:461-7
Ip WC (*see* Christodoulou et al). 1995;126:65-8 (CLO)
Israel BA (*see* Brozanski et al). 1995;126:769-76
Iwao H (*see* Sato et al). 1995;126:109-13

J

Jackson TM (*see* Lee et al). 1995;126:280-6
Jacobs MR (*see* Heggie et al). 1995;126:503-4 (Letter reply)
Jacobsen F (*see* Mueller et al). 1995;126:749-52 (CLO)
Jakobs C (*see* Elpeleg et al). 1995;126:72-4 (CLO)
James-Herry A (*see* Weinblatt et al). 1995;126:263-5 (CLO)
Jarrett R (*see* Gerdes et al). 1995;126:S26-32 (Symposium)
Johnson DW (*see* Schuh et al). 1995;126:639-45
Johnson R (*see* Goran and Johnson). 1995;126:679-80 (Letter reply)
Jones D (*see* Mauskopf et al). 1995;126:94-101
Jones JG (*see* Brozanski et al). 1995;126:769-76
Jones TW, Borg WP, Boulware SD, McCarthy G, Sherwin RS, Tamborlane WV. Enhanced adrenomedullary response and increased susceptibility to neuroglycopenia: mechanisms underlying the adverse effects of sugar ingestion in healthy children. 1995;126:171-7
Jones VF, Buchino JJ. A three-month-old girl with fever and hepatomegaly. 1995;126:663-8
Jordan MC (*see* Schwebke et al). 1995;126:293-5 (CLO)

K

Kamiński W (*see* Pronicka et al). 1995;126:948-51 (CLO)
Kao J-H (*see* Lin et al). 1995;126:589-91 (CLO)
Kaplan BS (*see* Kaplan et al). 1995;126:943-5 (CLO)
Kaplan FS (*see* Lanchoney et al). 1995;126:762-4 (CLO)
Kaplan P, Levinson M, Kaplan BS. Cerebral artery stenoses in Williams syndrome cause strokes in childhood. 1995;126:943-5 (CLO)
—— (*see* Rabinowitz et al). 1995;126:266-9 (CLO)

Kaplowitz PB. Effect of growth hormone therapy on final versus predicted height in short twelve- to sixteen-year-old boys without growth hormone deficiency. 1995;126:478-80 (CLO)
Karna P, Murray DL, Dyke JW. Infectious hazards of immune globulin. 1995;126:322 (Letter reply)
Karpen SJ (*see* Shrier et al). 1995;126:57-9 (CLO)
Katch V (*see* Steinberger et al). 1995;126:690-5
Kato S, Ebina K, Ozawa A, Naganuma H, Nakagawa H. Antibiotic-associated hemorrhagic colitis without *Clostridium difficile* toxin in children. 1995;126:1008-10 (CLO)
Kaufmehl K (*see* Hauk et al). 1995;126:185-90
Kaul S, Sockalosky JJ. Human synthetic calcitonin therapy for hypercalcemia of immobilization. 1995;126:825-7 (CLO)
Kawai S (*see* Ino et al). 1995;126:304-8
Kearns GL (*see* Marshall et al). 1995;126:657-9 (CLO)
Kester ADM (*see* Foreman–van Drongelen et al). 1995;126:611-8
Kevy SV (*see* McManus et al). 1995;126:900-4
Kierce BM (*see* Gormally et al). 1995;126:753-6 (CLO)
Kilpatrick L (*see* Dulkerian et al). 1995;126:872-6
King WJ, MacDonald NE, Wells G, Manion D, Chan F, Allen UD. Relationship between parental occupation and children's oropharyngeal colonization with *Neisseria meningitidis*. 1995;126:937-9 (CLO)
Kinney HC (*see* Collins et al). 1995;126:653-7
Kinsella JP, Abman SH. Recent developments in the pathophysiology and treatment of persistent pulmonary hypertension of the newborn. 1995;126:853-64
Kiser WR (*see* Warren and Kiser). 1995;126:321 (Letter)
Kjolhede CL, Chew FJ, Gadomski AM, Marroquin DP. Clinical trial of vitamin A as adjuvant treatment for lower respiratory tract infections. 1995;126:807-12
Klassen TP (*see* Menon et al). 1995;126:1004-7 (CLO)
—— (*see* Osmond et al). 1995;126:892-5
Klauber GT (*see* Hiort et al). 1995;126:1022 (Letter)
Klaus G (*see* Nützenadel et al). 1995;126:676-7 (Letter)
Klein GL, Herndon DN, Langman CB, Rutan TC, Young WE, Pembleton G, Nusynowitz M, Barnett JL, Broemeling LD, Sailer DE, McCauley RL. Long-term reduction in bone mass after severe burn injury in children. 1995;126:252-6
Klein RZ (*see* Mitchell and Klein). 1995;126:673 (Letter)
Kochen J (*see* Weinblatt et al). 1995;126:263-5 (CLO)
Kocherlakota P (*see* La Gamma et al). 1995;126:457-9 (CLO)
Koepsell TD (*see* Whitaker et al). 1995;126:850-1 (Letter reply)
Kohno H, Ueyama N, Yanai S, Ukaji K, Honda S. Beneficial effect of growth hormone on atherogenic risk in children with growth hormone deficiency. 1995;126:953-5 (CLO)
Kojima E (*see* Husson et al). 1995;126:865-71
Kolde G (*see* Hentschel et al). 1995;126:61-4 (CLO)
Komoroski EM (*see* Valentine and Komoroski). 1995;126:135-40
Kondo T (*see* Sato et al). 1995;126:109-13
Koo WWK (*see* Rajaram et al). 1995;126:791-6
Kooistra L (*see* Vulsma and Kooistra). 1995;126:673-4 (Letter reply)
Koonce EW (*see* Roddey et al). 1995;126:931-3 (CLO)
Koontz SW (*see* Farber et al). 1995;126:S118-24
Kopleman A (*see* Gerdes et al). 1995;126:S26-32 (Symposium)
Korson MS (*see* North et al). 1995;126:916-22
Korzets Z (*see* Pomeranz et al). 1995;126:140-2 (CLO)
Koskimies O. Diagnostic accuracy of urinary tract infection and subsequent development of renal scars. 1995;126:157-8 (Letter)
Kotagal P (*see* Bass et al). 1995;126:537-44
Kotagal UR, Perlstein PH, Atherton HD, Donovan EF. Acuity scores as predictors of cost-related outcomes of neonatal intensive care. 1995;126:88-93
Kowal K (*see* Ross et al). 1995;126:242-5
Krafte-Jacobs B, Sivit CJ, Mejia R, Pollack MM. Catheter-related thrombosis in critically ill children: comparison of catheters with and without heparin bonding. 1995;126:50-4
——, Williams J, Soldin SJ. Plasma erythropoietin reference ranges in children. 1995;126:601-3 (CLO)
Kraybill E, Bose CL, Corbet A, Garcia-Prats J, Asbill D, Edwards K, Long W. Double-blind evaluation of developmental and health status to age 2 years of infants weighing 700 to 1350 grams treated prophylactically at birth with a single dose of synthetic surfactant or air placebo. 1995;126:S33-42 (Symposium)
—— (*see* Long et al). 1995;126:S1-4 (Symposium)
Kruse K. Pathophysiology of calcium metabolism in children with vitamin D–deficiency rickets. 1995;126:736-41
——, Feldmann E. Healing of rickets during vitamin D therapy despite defective vitamin D receptors in two siblings with vitamin D–dependent rickets type II. 1995;126:145-8 (CLO)
Krzeski R (*see* McMillan et al). 1995;126:S90-8 (Symposium)
Kuis W (*see* Wulffraat et al). 1995;126:849 (Letter reply)
Kuroda C (*see* Rosenfeld et al). 1995;126:1000-3
Kurttila R (*see* Uhari et al). 1995;126:991-5
Kushner H (*see* Ross et al). 1995;126:242-5
Kwiatkowski K (*see* Rehan et al). 1995;126:979-82 (CLO)
Kwok S (*see* Palumbo et al). 1995;126:592-5 (CLO)

L

La Gamma EF, Alpan O, Kocherlakota P. Effect of granulocyte colony-stimulating factor on preeclampsia-associated neonatal neutropenia. 1995;126:457-9 (CLO)
Lallemant C (*see* Semama et al). 1995;126:742-6
Lan Y (*see* Husson et al). 1995;126:865-71
Lanchoney TF, Cohen RB, Rocke DM, Zasloff MA, Kaplan FS. Permanent heterotopic ossification at the injection site after diphtheria-tetanus-pertussis immunizations in children who have fibrodysplasia ossificans progressiva. 1995;126:762-4 (CLO)
Landrigan E (*see* Bonner et al). 1995;126:287-92
Langman CB (*see* Klein et al). 1995;126:252-6
Larsen J, Whitelaw A. Comparison of fiberoptic and conventional phototherapy for neonatal hyperbilirubinemia. 1995;126:1018 (Letter)
Lascari AD, Amyot K. Fatal hemolysis caused by ceftriaxone. 1995;126:816-7 (CLO)
Laskarzewski PM (*see* Diller et al). 1995;126:345-52
Law BJ (*see* Wang et al). 1995;126:212-9
Lawless MR (*see* Abramson et al). 1995;126:583-6 (CLO)
Lawrence R. The clinician's role in teaching proper infant feeding techniques. 1995;126:S112-7
—— (*see* Neifert et al). 1995;126:S125-9
Laxer RM (*see* Uziel et al). 1995;126:722-7
Lazcano-Burciaga G (*see* Mazariegos-Ramos et al). 1995;126:940-2 (CLO)
Leach AD (*see* Diller et al). 1995;126:345-52
Leach CL, Holm B, Morin FC III, Fuhrman BP, Papo MC, Steinhorn D, Hernan LJ. Partial liquid ventilation in premature lambs with respiratory distress syndrome: efficacy and compatibility with exogenous surfactant. 1995;126:412-20
LeBlanc M (*see* Sell et al). 1995;126:S20-5 (Symposium)
Lee C-Y (*see* Lee et al). 1995;126:716-21
Lee DA, Slagle TA, Jackson TM, Evans CS. Reducing blood donor exposures in low birth weight infants by the use of older, unwashed packed red blood cells. 1995;126:280-6
Lee P-I, Lee C-Y, Huang L-M, Chang M-H. Long-term efficacy of recombinant hepatitis B vaccine and risk of natural infection in infants born to mothers with hepatitis B e antigen. 1995;126: 716-21
Leichtner AM (*see* Odze et al). 1995;126:163-70
Leśniewska A (*see* Pronicka et al). 1995;126:948-51 (CLO)
Leung AKC (*see* Robson and Leung). 1995;126:1021 (Letter)
Levinson M (*see* Kaplan et al). 1995;126:943-5 (CLO)
Levison H (*see* Schuh et al). 1995;126:639-45

Leviton A (*see* Garland et al). 1995;126:272-9
Lewis D (*see* Palumbo et al). 1995;126:592-5 (CLO)
Lewison LJ (*see* Slusher et al). 1995;126:102-8
Lewno MJ (*see* Maxson et al). 1995;126:321 (Letter reply)
Li R, O'Connor L, Buckley D, Specker B. Relation of activity levels to body fat in infants 6 to 12 months of age. 1995;126:353-7
Lieberman JM, Greenberg DP, Wong VK, Partridge S, Chang S-J, Chiu C-Y, Ward JI. Effect of neonatal immunization with diphtheria and tetanus toxoids on antibody responses to *Haemophilus influenzae* type b conjugate vaccines. 1995;126:198-205
—— (*see* Greenberg et al). 1995;126:206-11
Lin H-H, Kao J-H, Hsu H-Y, Ni Y-H, Chang M-H, Huang S-C, Hwang L-H, Chen P-J, Chen D-S. Absence of infection in breast-fed infants born to hepatitis C virus–infected mothers. 1995;126:589-91 (CLO)
Lin J-S (*see* Lin et al). 1995;126:114-7
Lin J-Y, Lin J-S, Tsai C-H. Use of the urine-to-blood carbon dioxide tension gradient as a measurement of impaired distal tubular hydrogen ion secretion among neonates. 1995;126:114-7
Lindblad A, Strandvik B, Hjelte L. Incidence of liver disease in patients with cystic fibrosis and meconium ileus. 1995;126:155 (Letter)
Linder B (*see* Bar et al). 1995;126:955-8 (CLO)
Liptak GS (*see* McConnochie et al). 1995;126:220-9
Listernick R (*see* Habiby et al). 1995;126:364-7
Liu P (*see* Perlman et al). 1995;126:75-87
Lobato MN, Caldwell MB, Ng P, Oxtoby MJ, Pediatric Spectrum of Disease Clinical Consortium. Encephalopathy in children with perinatally acquired human immunodeficiency virus infection. 1995;126:710-5
Loeffelholz M (*see* Abzug et al). 1995;126:447-50 (CLO)
Logan J (*see* Dampier et al). 1995;126:461-7
Logan WJ (*see* Beca et al). 1995;126:44-9
Long LM (*see* Ross et al). 1995;126:242-5
Long W, Zucker J, Kraybill E. Symposium on Synthetic Surfactant II: perspective and commentary. 1995;126:S1-4 (Symposium)
—— (*see* Casiro et al). 1995;126:S53-60 (Symposium)
—— (*see* Corbet et al). 1995;126:969-78
—— (*see* Corbet et al). 1995;126:S5-12 (Symposium)
—— (*see* Courtney et al). 1995;126:S43-52 (Symposium)
—— (*see* Gerdes et al). 1995;126:S26-32 (Symposium)
—— (*see* Gong et al). 1995;126:S68-74 (Symposium)
—— (*see* Kraybill et al). 1995;126:S33-42 (Symposium)
—— (*see* Mauskopf et al). 1995;126:94-101
—— (*see* McMillan et al). 1995;126:S90-8 (Symposium)
—— (*see* Saigal et al). 1995;126:S61-7 (Symposium)
—— (*see* Sauve et al). 1995;126:S75-80 (Symposium)
—— (*see* Sell et al). 1995;126:S20-5 (Symposium)
—— (*see* Smyth et al). 1995;126:S81-9 (Symposium)
—— (*see* Walther et al). 1995;126:S13-9 (Symposium)
Lorenzo JRF (*see* Seara et al). 1995;126:965-7 (CLO)
Losay J (*see* Barbé et al). 1995;126:571-9
Losch M, Dungy CI, Russell D, Dusdieker LB. Impact of attitudes on maternal decisions regarding infant feeding. 1995;126:507-14
Luke A (*see* Schoeller and Luke). 1995;126:679 (Letter)
Lynch A, Tobias JD. Life-threatening infection in two children with hemoglobin S–beta-thalassemia. 1995;126:581-2 (CLO)
Lyon G (*see* Mbonda et al). 1995;126:923-7
Lyon NR (*see* Rogers et al). 1995;126:496-8 (CLO)

M

MacDonald NE (*see* King et al). 1995;126:937-9 (CLO)
MacGregor GL (*see* Rosenfeld and MacGregor). 1995;126:504-5 (Letter)
MacMurray B (*see* Casiro et al). 1995;126:S53-60 (Symposium)
—— (*see* Saigal et al). 1995;126:S61-7 (Symposium)
—— (*see* Smyth et al). 1995;126:S81-9 (Symposium)
Maffeis C, Pinelli L, Schutz Y. Increased fat oxidation in prepubertal obese children: A metabolic defense against further weight gain? 1995;126:15-20
Mahut B (*see* Delacourt et al). 1995;126:703-9
Makhlouf RA, Doron MW, Bose CL, Price WA, Stiles AD. Administration of granulocyte colony-stimulating factor to neutropenic low birth weight infants of mothers with preeclampsia. 1995;126:454-56 (CLO)
Malozowski S, Stadel BV. Prepubertal gynecomastia during growth hormone therapy. 1995;126:659-61 (CLO)
——, Tanner LA, Wysowski DK, Fleming GA, Stadel BV. Benign intracranial hypertension in children with growth hormone deficiency treated with growth hormone. 1995;126:996-9
Mammel M (*see* Mauskopf et al). 1995;126:94-101
—— (*see* Sell et al). 1995;126:S20-5 (Symposium)
Mancini MA (*see* Pasquino et al). 1995;126:11-4
Manion D (*see* King et al). 1995;126:937-9 (CLO)
Mannino FL (*see* Cleary et al). 1995;126:407-11
Marcoux S (*see* Beaudry et al). 1995;126:191-7
Marcy SM (*see* Greenberg et al). 1995;126:206-11
Marianelli L (*see* Taccetti et al). 1995;126:848-9 (Letter)
Marinoni S (*see* Tonini et al). 1995;126:159 (Letter)
Maris JM, Butler RB, Cohen AR. Loss of detectable antibody to hepatitis B surface antigen in immunized patients with hemophilia but without human immunodeficiency virus infection. 1995;126:269-71 (CLO)
Marquardt ED. Cost of ribavirin therapy for respiratory syncytial virus infection. 1995;126:847 (Letter)
Marroquin DP (*see* Kjolhede et al). 1995;126:807-12
Marshall JD, Farrar HC, Kearns GL. Diarrhea associated with enteral benzodiazepine solutions. 1995;126:657-9 (CLO)
Martin ES (*see* Roddey et al). 1995;126:931-3 (CLO)
Martinez-Azagra A, Serrano A, Casado-Flores J. Adult respiratory distress syndrome in children associated with miliary tuberculosis. 1995;126:678 (Letter)
Marzinotto V (*see* Andrew et al). 1995;126:358-63
Mason W (*see* Rosenfeld et al). 1995;126:1000-3
Matthews DR (*see* Crowley et al). 1995;126:297-303
Mauk JE. *Helicobacter pylori* infection in neurologically impaired children. 1995;126:849 (Letter)
Mauskopf JA, Backhouse ME, Jones D, Wold DE, Mammel MC, Mullett M, Guthrie R, Long WA. Synthetic surfactant for rescue treatment of respiratory distress syndrome in premature infants weighing from 700 to 1350 grams: impact on hospital resource use and charges. 1995;126:94-101
Maxson MS, Lewno MJ, Schutze GE. Usefulness of cerebrospinal fluid bacterial antigen tests. 1995;126:321 (Letter reply)
Mayaux M-J (*see* Tardieu et al). 1995;126:375-9
Mayer L (*see* Rosh et al). 1995;126:143-5 (CLO)
Mazariegos-Ramos E, Guerrero-Romero F, Rodriguez-Morán M, Lazcano-Burciaga G, Paniagua R, Amato D. Consumption of soft drinks with phosphoric acid as a risk factor for the development of hypocalcemia in children: a case-control study. 1995;126:940-2 (CLO)
Mazur A (*see* Rabinowitz et al). 1995;126:266-9 (CLO)
Mbonda E, Claus D, Bonnier C, Evrard P, Gadisseux JF, Lyon G. Prolonged dysphagia caused by congenital pharyngeal dysfunction. 1995;126:923-7
McCabe ERB (*see* Scheuerle et al). 1995;126:764-7 (CLO)
McCarthy G (*see* Jones et al). 1995;126:171-7
McCauley RL (*see* Klein et al). 1995;126:252-6
McCawley L (*see* Dulkerian et al). 1995;126:872-6
McConnell MS, Perkin RM. Standards for home care of sick children. 1995;126:681-2 (Letter)
McConnochie KM, Roghmann KJ, Liptak GS. Hospitalization for lower respiratory tract illness in infants: variation in rates among counties in New York State and areas within Monroe County. 1995;126:220-9
McEvoy C (*see* Shrier et al). 1995;126:57-9 (CLO)

McIntosh K (*see* Husson et al). 1995;126:865-71
McKenzie NE. Accuracy of aural infrared temperature device. 1995;126:324 (Letter)
McKie V (*see* Pegelow et al). 1995;126:896-9
McKinney N (*see* Palumbo et al). 1995;126:592-5 (CLO)
McLaren DW (*see* Slusher et al). 1995;126:102-8
McLaughlin GE, Virdee SS, Schleien CL, Holzman BH, Scott GB. Effect of corticosteroids on survival of children with acquired immunodeficiency syndrome and *Pneumocystis carinii*–related respiratory failure. 1995;126:821-4 (CLO)
McManus ML, Kevy SV, Bower LK, Hickey PR. Coagulation factor deficiencies during initiation of extracorporeal membrane oxygenation. 1995;126:900-4
McMillan D, Chernick V, Finer N, Schiff D, Bard H, Watts J, Krzeski R, Long W, Canadian Exosurf Neonatal Study Group. Effects of two rescue doses of synthetic surfactant in 344 infants with respiratory distress syndrome weighing 750 to 1249 grams: a double-blind, placebo-controlled multicenter Canadian trial. 1995;126:S90-8 (Symposium)
—— (*see* Courtney et al). 1995;126:S43-52 (Symposium)
McMurry M (*see* Chan et al). 1995;126:551-6
Medley LP (*see* Roberts et al). 1995;126:481-9
Mehls O (*see* Nützenadel et al). 1995;126:676-7 (Letter)
Mejia R (*see* Krafte-Jacobs et al). 1995;126:50-4
Menon K, Sutcliffe T, Klassen TP. A randomized trial comparing the efficacy of epinephrine with salbutamol in the treatment of acute bronchiolitis. 1995;126:1004-7 (CLO)
Mikol J (*see* Rötig et al). 1995;126:597-601 (CLO)
Miller RW. Josef Warkany. 1995;126:669-72 (Profiles)
Miller ST (*see* Pegelow et al). 1995;126:896-9
Milstein JM. Hypotension in preterm infants. 1995;126:160 (Letter)
Mimouni F. Single-day therapy for rickets. 1995;126:1019 (Letter)
Mimouni FB (*see* Brozanski et al). 1995;126:769-76
—— (*see* Ozolek et al). 1995;126:322-3 (Letter reply)
Miodovnik M (*see* Demarini et al). 1995;126:796-8 (CLO)
Mirochnick M, Frank DA, Cabral H, Turner A, Zuckerman B. Relation between meconium concentration of the cocaine metabolite benzoylecgonine and fetal growth. 1995;126:636-8 (CLO)
Mitchell ML, Klein RZ. Motor and cognitive development in children with congenital hypothyroidism. 1995;126:673 (Letter)
Mitsuya H (*see* Husson et al). 1995;126:865-71
Montalto G (*see* Iacono et al). 1995;126:34-9
Moorehead C (*see* Steinberger et al). 1995;126:690-5
Moran CJ (*see* Schlesinger et al). 1995;126:234-41
Morelli JA (*see* Bandini et al). 1995;126:828-32
Morin FC III (*see* Leach et al). 1995;126:412-20
Moskovitz J (*see* Hákonarson et al). 1995;126:565-70
Movahed H (*see* Greenberg et al). 1995;126:633-5 (CLO)
Msall ME (*see* Rogers et al). 1995;126:496-8 (CLO)
Mueller BU, Burt R, Gulick L, Jacobsen F, Pizzo PA, Horne M. Disseminated intravascular coagulation associated with granulocyte colony-stimulating factor therapy in a child with human immunodeficiency virus infection. 1995;126:749-52 (CLO)
——, Pizzo PA. Cancer in children with primary or secondary immunodeficiencies. 1995;126:1-10
Mullett M (*see* Mauskopf et al). 1995;126:94-101
—— (*see* Walther et al). 1995;126:S13-9 (Symposium)
Mundy M (*see* Roberts et al). 1995;126:481-9
Municchi G (*see* Pasquino et al). 1995;126:11-4
Munnich A (*see* Rötig et al). 1995;126:597-601 (CLO)
Murray DL (*see* Karna et al). 1995;126:322 (Letter reply)
Mustafa MM (*see* Bernini et al). 1995;126:813-5 (CLO)

N

Naganuma H (*see* Kato et al). 1995;126:1008-10 (CLO)
Nagatsu T (*see* Blau et al). 1995;126:401-5 (CLO)
Nakagawa H (*see* Kato et al). 1995;126:1008-10 (CLO)
Nathan DM (*see* Tamborlane and Nathan). 1995;126:1021 (Letter reply)
Neely EK, Wilson DM. Local reactions to luteinizing hormone releasing hormone analog therapy. 1995;126:159-60 (Letter reply)
Neifert M, Lawrence R, Seacat J. Nipple confusion: toward a formal definition. 1995;126:S125-9
Nelson JC (*see* Adams et al). 1995;126:122-7
Neuspiel DR. Screening neonates for intrauterine cocaine exposure. 1995;126:323 (Letter)
Neužil J, Darlow BA, Inder TE, Sluis KB, Winterbourn CC, Stocker R. Oxidation of parenteral lipid emulsion by ambient and phototherapy lights: potential toxicity of routine parenteral feeding. 1995;126:785-90
Newman B (*see* Brozanski et al). 1995;126:769-76
Ng P (*see* Lobato et al). 1995;126:710-5
Ng SC (*see* Poon et al). 1995;126:959-61 (CLO)
Ni Y-H (*see* Lin et al). 1995;126:589-91 (CLO)
Niaudet P (*see* Rötig et al). 1995;126:597-601 (CLO)
Nigro F (*see* Fiumara et al). 1995;126:852 (Letter)
Nishimoto K (*see* Ino et al). 1995;126:304-8
Nommsen-Rivers LA (*see* Dewey et al). 1995;126:696-702
Norris MK (*see* Rogers et al). 1995;126:496-8 (CLO)
North KN, Korson MS, Gopal YR, Rohr FJ, Brazelton TB, Waisbren SE, Warman ML. Neonatal-onset propionicacidemia: neurologic and developmental profiles, and implications for management. 1995;126:916-22
Notarbartolo A (*see* Iacono et al). 1995;126:34-9
Nowak AJ, Smith WL, Erenberg A. Imaging evaluation of breastfeeding and bottle feeding systems. 1995;126:S130-4
Nussbaum J (*see* Wiley et al). 1995;126:392-5 (CLO)
Nusynowitz M (*see* Klein et al). 1995;126:252-6
Nützenadel W, Mehls O, Klaus G. A new defect in vitamin D metabolism. 1995;126:676-7 (Letter)

O

Oberfield SE (*see* Rapaport et al). 1995;126:759-61 (CLO)
Occult Bacteremia Study Group (*see* Teach et al). 1995;126:877-81
O'Connor L (*see* Li et al). 1995;126:353-7
Odze RD, Wershil BK, Leichtner AM, Antonioli DA. Allergic colitis in infants. 1995;126:163-70
Ohls RK, Osborne KA, Christensen RD. Efficacy and cost analysis of treating very low birth weight infants with erythropoietin during their first two weeks of life: a randomized, placebo-controlled trial. 1995;126:421-6
Okada R (*see* Ino et al). 1995;126:304-8
Okubo M (*see* Ino et al). 1995;126:304-8
Oleske JM (*see* Palumbo et al). 1995;126:592-5 (CLO)
Olivieri N (*see* Pegelow et al). 1995;126:896-9
Olson D (*see* Schwebke et al). 1995;126:293-5 (CLO)
Orenstein DM (*see* del Rosario et al). 1995;126:951-2 (CLO)
Osborne KA (*see* Ohls et al). 1995;126:421-6
O'Shea TM (*see* Abramson et al). 1995;126:583-6 (CLO)
Osmond MH, Klassen TP, Quinn JV. Economic comparison of a tissue adhesive and suturing in the repair of pediatric facial lacerations. 1995;126:892-5
Osterhoudt KC, Wiley CC, Dudley R, Sheen S, Henretig FM. Rebound severe methemoglobinemia from ingestion of a nitroethane artificial fingernail remover. 1995;126:819-21 (CLO)
Owen M (*see* Patel et al). 1995;126:799-806
Oxtoby MJ (*see* Lobato et al). 1995;126:710-5
Ozawa A (*see* Kato et al). 1995;126:1008-10 (CLO)
Ozel A (*see* Yavûz et al). 1995;126:156 (Letter)
Ozolek JA, Watchko JF, Mimouni FB. Differences in clinical significance of maternal-infant blood group incompatibility in mothers with blood type O, A, or B. 1995;126:322-3 (Letter reply)

P

Palumbo PE, Kwok S, Waters S, Wesley Y, Lewis D, McKinney N, Bardeguez A, Connor EM, Oleske JM. Viral measurement by polymerase chain reaction–based assays in human immunodeficiency virus–infected infants. 1995;126:592-5 (CLO)
Pandit P (*see* Perlman et al). 1995;126:75-87
Paniagua R (*see* Mazariegos-Ramos et al). 1995;126:940-2 (CLO)
Papo MC (*see* Leach et al). 1995;126:412-20
Parenti G, Sebastio G, Strisciuglio P, Incerti B, Pecoraro C, Terracciano L, Andria G. Lysinuric protein intolerance characterized by bone marrow abnormalities and severe clinical course. 1995;126:246-51
Partridge S (*see* Greenberg et al). 1995;126:206-11
—— (*see* Lieberman et al). 1995;126:198-205
Pasquino AM, Pucarelli I, Passeri F, Segni M, Mancini MA, Municchi G. Progression of premature thelarche to central precocious puberty. 1995;126:11-4
—— (*see* Spagnoli et al). 1995;126:905-9
Passeri F (*see* Pasquino et al). 1995;126:11-4
Patel JA, Reisner B, Vizirinia N, Owen M, Chonmaitree T, Howie V. Bacteriologic failure of amoxicillin-clavulanate in treatment of acute otitis media caused by nontypeable *Haemophilus influenzae*. 1995;126:799-806
Pauly T (*see* Sauve et al). 1995;126:S75-80 (Symposium)
Pavone L (*see* Fiumara et al). 1995;126:852 (Letter)
Pecoraro C (*see* Parenti et al). 1995;126:246-51
Pediatric Investigators Collaborative Network on Infections in Canada (*see* Wang et al). 1995;126:212-9
Pediatric Spectrum of Disease Clinical Consortium (*see* Lobato et al). 1995;126:710-5
Pegelow CH, Adams RJ, McKie V, Abboud M, Berman B, Miller ST, Olivieri N, Vichinsky E, Wang W, Brambilla D. Risk of recurrent stroke in patients with sickle cell disease treated with erythrocyte transfusions. 1995;126:896-9
Peliowski A, Finer NN, Etches PC, Tierney AJ, Ryan CA. Inhaled nitric oxide for premature infants after prolonged rupture of the membranes. 1995;126:450-53 (CLO)
—— (*see* Smyth et al). 1995;126:S81-9 (Symposium)
Pembleton G (*see* Klein et al). 1995;126:252-6
Pencharz P (*see* Andrew et al). 1995;126:358-63
Perkin RM (*see* McConnell and Perkin). 1995;126:681-2 (Letter)
Perl H. Differences in clinical significance of maternal-infant blood group incompatibility in mothers with blood type O, A, or B. 1995;126:322 (Letter)
Perlman M, Claris O, Hao Y, Pandit P, Whyte H, Chipman M, Liu P. Secular changes in the outcomes to eighteen to twenty-four months of age of extremely low birth weight infants, with adjustment for changes in risk factors and severity of illness. 1995; 126:75-87
Perlstein PH (*see* Kotagal et al). 1995;126:88-93
Petersen MC, Wolraich M, Sherbondy A, Wagener J. Abnormalities in control of ventilation in newborn infants with myelomeningocele. 1995;126:1011-5
Peterson B (*see* Greenberg et al). 1995;126:633-5 (CLO)
Petruska ML (*see* Zwiener et al). 1995;126:728-35
Phelps DL (*see* Ryan and Phelps). 1995;126:324 (Letter reply)
Philip AGS. Neonatal mortality rate: Is further improvement possible? 1995;126:427-33
Piedboeuf B (*see* Chessex et al). 1995;126:619-24
Piedra PA (*see* Englund et al). 1995;126:847 (Letter reply)
Pieroni DR (*see* Rogers et al). 1995;126:496-8 (CLO)
Pineault M (*see* Chessex et al). 1995;126:619-24
Pinelli L (*see* Maffeis et al). 1995;126:15-20
Pinkerton CR (*see* Hählen et al). 1995;126:309-13
Pizzo PA (*see* Mueller and Pizzo). 1995;126:1-10
—— (*see* Mueller et al). 1995;126:749-52 (CLO)
Pober BR (*see* Soper et al). 1995;126:945-8 (CLO)
Polack FP, Transue DJ, Belknap WM, Freij BJ, Aughton DJ. Transient elevation of sweat chloride concentration in a malnourished girl with the Mauriac syndrome. 1995;126:261-3 (CLO)
Pollack MM (*see* Krafte-Jacobs et al). 1995;126:50-4
Pomeranz A, Wolach B, Bernheim J, Korzets Z, Bernheim J. Successful treatment of Finnish congenital nephrotic syndrome with captopril and indomethacin. 1995;126:140-2 (CLO)
Poole C (*see* Rojas et al). 1995;126:605-10
Poon M-C, Ng SC, Coppes MJ. Acquired platelet dysfunction with eosinophilia in white children. 1995;126:959-61 (CLO)
Poptani H (*see* Gupta et al). 1995;126:389-92 (CLO)
Poveda J-D (*see* Delacourt et al). 1995;126:703-9
Prakash N (*see* Gormally et al). 1995;126:753-6 (CLO)
Price WA (*see* Makhlouf et al). 1995;126:454-56 (CLO)
Prince A (*see* Rosh et al). 1995;126:143-5 (CLO)
—— (*see* Zar et al). 1995;126:230-3
Principi N (*see* Viganó et al). 1995;126:368-74
Pronicka E, Gruszczyńska B, Woźniewicz B, Cedro A, Kamiński W, Leśniewska A. Pancreatic glucagon levels in infants and children with hyperinsulinemia. 1995;126:948-51 (CLO)
Proujansky R, Shaffer S, Vinton N, Bachrach S. *Helicobacter pylori* infection in neurologically impaired children. 1995;126:850 (Letter reply)
—— (*see* Spear et al). 1995;126:982-5 (CLO)
Pryse-Phillips WEM (*see* Sheth et al). 1995;126:259-61 (CLO)
Psaty BM (*see* Whitaker et al). 1995;126:850-1 (Letter reply)
Pucarelli I (*see* Pasquino et al). 1995;126:11-4
Puelzl-Quinn H (*see* Bandini et al). 1995;126:828-32
Puhakka H (*see* Heikkinen et al). 1995;126:313-6 (CLO)
Puri A (*see* Corbet et al). 1995;126:969-78
Putnam PE (*see* del Rosario et al). 1995;126:951-2 (CLO)

Q

Quinn JV (*see* Osmond et al). 1995;126:892-5
Quintana E (*see* Hählen et al). 1995;126:309-13
Quirk P (*see* Thomson et al). 1995;126:21-7
Quittell L (*see* Zar et al). 1995;126:230-3

R

Rabinowitz LG, Williams LR, Anderson CE, Mazur A, Kaplan P. Painful keratoderma and photophobia: hallmarks of tyrosinemia type II. 1995;126:266-9 (CLO)
Rajaram S, Carlson SE, Koo WWK, Braselton WE. Plasma mineral concentrations in preterm infants fed a nutrient-enriched formula after hospital discharge. 1995;126:791-6
Rantala H (*see* Uhari et al). 1995;126:991-5
Rao J (*see* Rapaport et al). 1995;126:759-61 (CLO)
Rapaport R, Oberfield SE, Robison L, Salisbury S, David R, Rao J, Redmond GP. Relation of growth hormone deficiency and leukemia. 1995;126:759-61 (CLO)
Ratledge DL (*see* Abramson et al). 1995;126:583-6 (CLO)
Reda Z, Houri S, Davis AL, Baum VC. Effect of airway pressure on inferior vena cava pressure as a measure of central venous pressure in children. 1995;126:961-5 (CLO)
Redmond GP (*see* Rapaport et al). 1995;126:759-61 (CLO)
Reese JM (*see* Crouse and Reese). 1995;126:502-3 (Letter)
Rehan VK, Alvaro RE, Belik J, Allen DW, Kwiatkowski K, Fajardo CA. Effects of central apnea on cerebral blood flow velocity in healthy term infants. 1995;126:979-82 (CLO)
Reif S (*see* Arav-Boger et al). 1995;126:586-8 (CLO)
Reisner B (*see* Patel et al). 1995;126:799-806
Ribes A (*see* Fiumara et al). 1995;126:852 (Letter)
Riggs JE (*see* Sheth et al). 1995;126:259-61 (CLO)
Rijkers GT (*see* Wulffraat et al). 1995;126:849 (Letter reply)
Rinaldo P (*see* Bhala et al). 1995;126:910-5
Riopel DA (*see* Clegg and Riopel). 1995;126:817-8 (CLO)

Riva C (*see* Viganó et al). 1995;126:368-74
Rivard GE, David M, Farrell C, Schwarz HP. Treatment of purpura fulminans in meningococcemia with protein C concentrate. 1995;126:646-52
Roberts JE, Burchinal MR, Medley LP, Zeisel SA, Mundy M, Roush J, Hooper S, Bryant D, Henderson FW. Otitis media, hearing sensitivity, and maternal responsiveness in relation to language during infancy. 1995;126:481-9
Robertson C (*see* Saigal et al). 1995;126:S61-7 (Symposium)
—— (*see* Sauve et al). 1995;126:S75-80 (Symposium)
Robison L (*see* Rapaport et al). 1995;126:759-61 (CLO)
Robson WLM, Leung AKC. Lactic acidosis in a patient with acute lymphoblastic leukemia. 1995;126:1021 (Letter)
Rocchini AP (*see* Steinberger et al). 1995;126:690-5
Rocke DM (*see* Lanchoney et al). 1995;126:762-4 (CLO)
Roddey OF Jr, Clegg HW, Martin ES, Swetenburg RL, Koonce EW. Comparison of an optical immunoassay technique with two culture methods for the detection of group A streptococci in a pediatric office. 1995;126:931-3 (CLO)
Rodriguez WJ (*see* Schwartz and Rodriguez). 1995;126:677-8 (Letter)
Rodriguez-Morán M (*see* Mazariegos-Ramos et al). 1995;126:940-2 (CLO)
Rogers BT, Msall ME, Buck GM, Lyon NR, Norris MK, Roland J-MA, Gingell RL, Cleveland DC, Pieroni DR. Neurodevelopmental outcome of infants with hypoplastic left heart syndrome. 1995;126:496-8 (CLO)
Roghmann KJ (*see* McConnochie et al). 1995;126:220-9
Rohr FJ (*see* North et al). 1995;126:916-22
Rojas MA, Gonzalez A, Bancalari E, Claure N, Poole C, Silva-Neto G. Changing trends in the epidemiology and pathogenesis of neonatal chronic lung disease. 1995;126:605-10
Roland J-MA (*see* Rogers et al). 1995;126:496-8 (CLO)
Rosenberg A (*see* Corbet et al). 1995;126:969-78
Rosenblum LS (*see* Wiley et al). 1995;126:392-5 (CLO)
Rosenfeld CR, MacGregor GL. Band neutrophil counts in neonates. 1995;126:504-5 (Letter)
Rosenfeld EA, Corydon KE, Shulman ST. Kawasaki disease in infants less than one year of age. 1995;126:524-9
——, Shulman ST, Corydon KE, Mason W, Takahashi M, Kuroda C. Comparative safety and efficacy of two immune globulin products in Kawasaki disease. 1995;126:1000-3
Rosenstein BJ (*see* Eigen et al). 1995;126:515-23
Rosenthal P (*see* Vanderhal et al). 1995;126:988-90 (CLO)
Rosh JR, Tang HB, Mayer L, Groisman G, Abraham SK, Prince A. Treatment of intractable gastrointestinal manifestations of chronic granulomatous disease with cyclosporine. 1995;126:143-5 (CLO)
Ross JL, Feuillan P, Long LM, Kowal K, Kushner H, Cutler GB Jr. Lipid abnormalities in Turner syndrome. 1995;126:242-5
Rossi A (*see* Saggese et al). 1995;126:468-73
Rotbart HA (*see* Abzug et al). 1995;126:447-50 (CLO)
Rötig A, Goutieres F, Niaudet P, Rustin P, Chretien D, Guest G, Mikol J, Gubler M-C, Munnich A. Deletion of mitochondrial DNA in patient with chronic tubulointerstitial nephritis. 1995;126:597-601 (CLO)
Roush J (*see* Roberts et al). 1995;126:481-9
Rovet JF, Ehrlich RM. Long-term effects of L-thyroxine therapy for congenital hypothyroidism. 1995;126:380-6
Rufin P, Benoist MR, de Blic J, Scheinmann P. Terbutaline powder for acute asthma. 1995;126:161-2 (Letter)
Ruggieri P (*see* Bass et al). 1995;126:537-44
Ruitenbeek W (*see* Elpeleg et al). 1995;126:72-4 (CLO)
Russell D (*see* Losch et al). 1995;126:507-14
Rustico M (*see* Tonini et al). 1995;126:159 (Letter)
Rustin P (*see* Rötig et al). 1995;126:597-601 (CLO)
Rutan TC (*see* Klein et al). 1995;126:252-6
Rutka JT (*see* Beca et al). 1995;126:44-9
Ruuskanen O (*see* Heikkinen et al). 1995;126:313-6 (CLO)
Ryan C (*see* Gschwend et al). 1995;126:178-84
Ryan CA, Finer NN. Antenatal corticosteroid therapy to prevent respiratory distress syndrome. 1995;126:317-9
—— (*see* Peliowski et al). 1995;126:450-53 (CLO)
Ryan RM, Phelps DL. Screening neonates for intrauterine cocaine exposure. 1995;126:324 (Letter reply)

S

Saenger P (*see* Bar et al). 1995;126:955-8 (CLO)
Sager S, Grayson GH, Feig SA. Methemoglobinemia associated with acidosis of probable renal origin. 1995;126:59-61 (CLO)
Saggese G, Cesaretti G, Barsanti S, Rossi A. Combined treatment with growth hormone and gonadotropin-releasing hormone analogs in short normal girls. 1995;126:468-73
Sahdev I (*see* Weinblatt et al). 1995;126:263-5 (CLO)
Saigal S, Robertson C, Sankaran K, Bingham W, Casiro O, MacMurray B, Whitfield M, Long W, Canadian Exosurf Neonatal Study Group. One-year outcome in 232 premature infants with birth weights of 750 to 1249 grams and respiratory distress syndrome randomized to rescue treatment with two doses of synthetic surfactant or air placebo. 1995;126:S61-7 (Symposium)
—— (*see* Casiro et al). 1995;126:S53-60 (Symposium)
Sailer DE (*see* Klein et al). 1995;126:252-6
Saiman L (*see* Zar et al). 1995;126:230-3
Salisbury S (*see* Rapaport et al). 1995;126:759-61 (CLO)
Sanderson M (*see* Taylor and Sanderson). 1995;126:887-91
Sankaran K (*see* Saigal et al). 1995;126:S61-7 (Symposium)
—— (*see* Smyth et al). 1995;126:S81-9 (Symposium)
Santer R, Hoffmann H, Suttorp M, Simeoni E, Schaub J. Discordance for hyperinsulinemic hypoglycemia in monozygotic twins. 1995;126:1017 (Letter)
Santulli TV Jr (*see* Vanderhal et al). 1995;126:988-90 (CLO)
Sardet A (*see* Barbé et al). 1995;126:571-9
Sato K, Kondo T, Iwao H, Honda S, Ueda K. Internal potassium shift in premature infants: cause of nonoliguric hyperkalemia. 1995;126:109-13
Sauve R, Long W, Vincer M, Bard H, Derleth D, Stevenson D, Pauly T, Robertson C, American and Canadian Exosurf Neonatal Study Groups. Outcome at 1-year adjusted age of 957 infants weighing more than 1250 grams with respiratory distress syndrome randomized to receive synthetic surfactant or air placebo. 1995;126:S75-80 (Symposium)
—— (*see* Courtney et al). 1995;126:S43-52 (Symposium)
Schanler RJ, Abrams SA. Postnatal attainment of intrauterine macromineral accretion rates in low birth weight infants fed fortified human milk. 1995;126:441-7
Schaub J (*see* Santer et al). 1995;126:1017 (Letter)
Scheinmann P (*see* Delacourt et al). 1995;126:703-9
—— (*see* Rufin et al). 1995;126:161-2 (Letter)
Schelonka RL, Yoder BA, Hall RB. Band neutrophil counts in neonates. 1995;126:505-6 (Letter reply)
Scheuerle A, Greenberg F, McCabe ERB. Dysmorphic features in patients with complex glycerol kinase deficiency. 1995;126:764-7 (CLO)
Schidlow DV (*see* Eigen et al). 1995;126:515-23
Schiff D (*see* McMillan et al). 1995;126:S90-8 (Symposium)
Schiffmann R (*see* Zimran et al). 1995;126:596-7 (CLO)
Schlager TA, Dilks S, Trudell J, Whittam TS, Hendley JO. Bacteriuria in children with neurogenic bladder treated with intermittent catheterization: natural history. 1995;126:490-6
Schleien CL (*see* McLaughlin et al). 1995;126:821-4 (CLO)
Schlesinger Y, Buller RS, Brunstrom JE, Moran CJ, Storch GA. Expanded spectrum of herpes simplex encephalitis in childhood. 1995;126:234-41
Schmidt-Sommerfeld E (*see* Bhala et al). 1995;126:910-5
Schneider R (*see* Uziel et al). 1995;126:722-7

Schoeller DA, Luke A. Techniques for measurement of resting energy expenditure in children. 1995;126:679 (Letter)
Schuh S, Johnson DW, Callahan S, Canny G, Levison H. Efficacy of frequent nebulized ipratropium bromide added to frequent high-dose albuterol therapy in severe childhood asthma. 1995;126:639-45
Schulze A, Whyte RK, Way RC, Sinclair JC. Effect of the arterial oxygenation level on cardiac output, oxygen extraction, and oxygen consumption in low birth weight infants receiving mechanical ventilation. 1995;126:777-84
Schumacher R (*see* Corbet et al). 1995;126:S5-12 (Symposium)
—— (*see* Walther et al). 1995;126:S13-9 (Symposium)
Schutz Y (*see* Maffeis et al). 1995;126:15-20
Schutze GE (*see* Maxson et al). 1995;126:321 (Letter reply)
Schwartz RH, Rodriguez WJ. Criteria for studies of antibiotic therapy for acute otitis media. 1995;126:677-8 (Letter)
Schwarz HP (*see* Rivard et al). 1995;126:646-52
Schwebke K, Henry K, Balfour HH Jr, Olson D, Crane RT, Jordan MC. Congenital cytomegalovirus infection as a result of nonprimary cytomegalovirus disease in a mother with acquired immunodeficiency syndrome. 1995;126:293-5 (CLO)
Scimeca P (*see* Weinblatt et al). 1995;126:263-5 (CLO)
Scott GB (*see* McLaughlin et al). 1995;126:821-4 (CLO)
Seacat J (*see* Neifert et al). 1995;126:S125-9
Seara MJF, Soto MIM, Lorenzo JRF, Trabazo S, Gamborino E, Vila JF. Peutz-Jeghers syndrome in a neonate. 1995;126:965-7 (CLO)
Searcey KB (*see* Waites et al). 1995;126:502 (Letter)
Sebastio G (*see* Parenti et al). 1995;126:246-51
Segni M (*see* Pasquino et al). 1995;126:11-4
Seibel N (*see* Tardieu et al). 1995;126:375-9
Sell MS, Cotton R, Hirata T, Guthrie R, LeBlanc M, Mammel M, Long W, American Exosurf Neonatal Study Group I. One-year follow-up of 273 infants with birth weights of 700 to 1100 grams after prophylactic treatment of respiratory distress syndrome with synthetic surfactant or air placebo. 1995;126:S20-5 (Symposium)
Semama DS, Huet F, Gouyon J-B, Lallemant C, Desgres J. Use of peritoneal dialysis, continuous arteriovenous hemofiltration, and continuous arteriovenous hemodiafiltration for removal of ammonium chloride and glutamine in rabbits. 1995;126:742-6
Seri I. Cardiovascular, renal, and endocrine actions of dopamine in neonates and children. 1995;126:333-44
Serrano A (*see* Martinez-Azagra et al). 1995;126:678 (Letter)
Setty BNY (*see* Dampier et al). 1995;126:461-7
Shaffer S (*see* Proujansky et al). 1995;126:850 (Letter reply)
Shah BR, Finberg L. Single-day therapy for rickets. 1995;126:1019-20 (Letter reply)
Shaywitz BA (*see* Soper et al). 1995;126:945-8 (CLO)
Shearer GM (*see* Viganó et al). 1995;126:368-74
Sheen S (*see* Osterhoudt et al). 1995;126:819-21 (CLO)
Shelov S. Perspectives on infant feeding: Guest Editor's note. 1995;126:S103
Shepherd RW (*see* Thomson et al). 1995;126:21-7
Sherbondy A (*see* Petersen et al). 1995;126:1011-5
Sherwin RS (*see* Jones et al). 1995;126:171-7
Sheth RD, Pryse-Phillips WEM, Riggs JE, Bodensteiner JB. Critical illness neuromuscular disease in children manifested as ventilatory dependence. 1995;126:259-61 (CLO)
Shrier LA, Karpen SJ, McEvoy C. Acute pancreatitis associated with acute hepatitis A in a young child. 1995;126:57-9 (CLO)
Shukla A (*see* Smyth et al). 1995;126:S81-9 (Symposium)
Shulman ST (*see* Rosenfeld et al). 1995;126:524-9
—— (*see* Rosenfeld et al). 1995;126:1000-3
Sierra RI (*see* Demarini et al). 1995;126:796-8 (CLO)
Silva-Neto G (*see* Rojas et al). 1995;126:605-10
Silverman B (*see* Habiby et al). 1995;126:364-7
Silverman ED (*see* Uziel et al). 1995;126:722-7
Simeoni E (*see* Santer et al). 1995;126:1017 (Letter)
Sinclair JC (*see* Schulze et al). 1995;126:777-84
Sivit CJ (*see* Krafte-Jacobs et al). 1995;126:50-4
Slagle TA (*see* Lee et al). 1995;126:280-6
Sluis KB (*see* Neužil et al). 1995;126:785-90
Slusher TM, Vreman HJ, McLaren DW, Lewison LJ, Brown AK, Stevenson DK. Glucose-6-phosphate dehydrogenase deficiency and carboxyhemoglobin concentrations associated with bilirubin-related morbidity and death in Nigerian infants. 1995;126:102-8
Smith WL (*see* Nowak et al). 1995;126:S130-4
Smyth J, Allen A, MacMurray B, Peliowski A, Sankaran K, Volberg F, Shukla A, Long W, Canadian Exosurf Neonatal Study Group. Double-blind, randomized, placebo-controlled Canadian multicenter trial of two doses of synthetic surfactant or air placebo in 224 infants weighing 500 to 749 grams with respiratory distress syndrome. 1995;126:S81-9 (Symposium)
Sobel EH (*see* Bar et al). 1995;126:955-8 (CLO)
Sockalosky JJ (*see* Kaul and Sockalosky). 1995;126:825-7 (CLO)
Soldin SJ (*see* Krafte-Jacobs et al). 1995;126:601-3 (CLO)
Soper R, Chaloupka JC, Fayad PB, Greally JM, Shaywitz BA, Awad IA, Pober BR. Ischemic stroke and intracranial multifocal cerebral arteriopathy in Williams syndrome. 1995;126:945-8 (CLO)
Soto MIM (*see* Seara et al). 1995;126:965-7 (CLO)
Spadoni GL (*see* Spagnoli et al). 1995;126:905-9
Spagnoli A, Spadoni GL, Cianfarani S, Pasquino AM, Troiani S, Boscherini B. Prediction of the outcome of growth hormone therapy in children with idiopathic short stature: a multivariate discriminant analysis. 1995;126:905-9
Spear ML, Stefano JL, Fawcett P, Proujansky R. Soluble interleukin-2 receptor as a predictor of neonatal sepsis. 1995;126:982-5 (CLO)
Specker B (*see* Demarini et al). 1995;126:796-8 (CLO)
—— (*see* Li et al). 1995;126:353-7
Sprecher DL (*see* Diller et al). 1995;126:345-52
Stadel BV (*see* Malozowski and Stadel). 1995;126:659-61 (CLO)
—— (*see* Malozowski et al). 1995;126:996-9
Stallings VA, Cronk CE, Zemel BS, Charney EB. Body composition in children with spastic quadriplegic cerebral palsy. 1995;126:833-9
Stanhope R (*see* Albanese and Stanhope). 1995;126:545-50
Stanley CA (*see* Thornton et al). 1995;126:1017 (Letter reply)
Stefano JL (*see* Spear et al). 1995;126:982-5 (CLO)
Steinberger J, Moorehead C, Katch V, Rocchini AP. Relationship between insulin resistance and abnormal lipid profile in obese adolescents. 1995;126:690-5
Steinhorn D (*see* Leach et al). 1995;126:412-20
Stephens D (*see* Wang et al). 1995;126:212-9
Stevenson D (*see* Sauve et al). 1995;126:S75-80 (Symposium)
Stevenson DK (*see* Slusher et al). 1995;126:102-8
Stiles AD (*see* Makhlouf et al). 1995;126:454-56 (CLO)
Stocker R (*see* Neužil et al). 1995;126:785-90
Storch GA (*see* Schlesinger et al). 1995;126:234-41
Strandvik B (*see* Lindblad et al). 1995;126:155 (Letter)
Straub E (*see* Tardieu et al). 1995;126:375-9
Strisciuglio P (*see* Parenti et al). 1995;126:246-51
Sundell H (*see* Walther et al). 1995;126:S13-9 (Symposium)
Sutcliffe T (*see* Menon et al). 1995;126:1004-7 (CLO)
Sutor LJ (*see* Bernini et al). 1995;126:813-5 (CLO)
Suttorp M (*see* Santer et al). 1995;126:1017 (Letter)
Swetenburg RL (*see* Roddey et al). 1995;126:931-3 (CLO)

T

Taccetti G, Campana S, Marianelli L, Turchini S. Cystic fibrosis and episodic arthritis. 1995;126:848-9 (Letter)
Takahashi M (*see* Rosenfeld et al). 1995;126:1000-3
Tam C (*see* Halton et al). 1995;126:557-64
Tamborlane WV, Nathan DM. Hemoglobin A_{1c} levels in young patients with diabetes beyond the "honeymoon" period. 1995;126:1021 (Letter reply)

—— (*see* Jones et al). 1995;126:171-7
Tan KL. Comparison of fiberoptic and conventional phototherapy for neonatal hyperbilirubinemia. 1995;126:1018 (Letter reply)
Tang HB (*see* Rosh et al). 1995;126:143-5 (CLO)
Tanner LA (*see* Malozowski et al). 1995;126:996-9
Tardieu M, Mayaux M-J, Seibel N, Funck-Brentano I, Straub E, Teglas J-P, Blanche S. Cognitive assessment of school-age children infected with maternally transmitted human immunodeficiency virus type 1. 1995;126:375-9
Tassinari D (*see* Balsamo et al). 1995;126:474-7
Tassoni P (*see* Balsamo et al). 1995;126:474-7
Tató L (*see* Zamboni et al). 1995;126:756-8 (CLO)
Taylor BJ (*see* Bonner et al). 1995;126:287-92
Taylor JA, Sanderson M. A reexamination of the risk factors for the sudden infant death syndrome. 1995;126:887-91
Taylor MJ (*see* Beca et al). 1995;126:44-9
Teach SJ, Fleisher GR, Occult Bacteremia Study Group. Efficacy of an observation scale in detecting bacteremia in febrile children three to thirty-six months of age, treated as outpatients. 1995; 126:877-81
Teglas J-P (*see* Tardieu et al). 1995;126:375-9
Terracciano L (*see* Parenti et al). 1995;126:246-51
Thompson T (*see* Courtney et al). 1995;126:S43-52 (Symposium)
Thomson MA, Bucolo S, Quirk P, Shepherd RW. Measured versus predicted resting energy expenditure in infants: a need for reappraisal. 1995;126:21-7
Thornton PS, Baker L, Stanley CA. Discordance for hyperinsulinemic hypoglycemia in monozygotic twins. 1995;126:1017 (Letter reply)
Tierney AJ (*see* Peliowski et al). 1995;126:450-53 (CLO)
Tobias JD (*see* Lynch and Tobias). 1995;126:581-2 (CLO)
Tobin R (*see* Wiley et al). 1995;126:392-5 (CLO)
Tonini G, Marinoni S, Forleo V, Rustico M. Local reactions to luteinizing hormone releasing hormone analog therapy. 1995;126: 159 (Letter)
Trabattoni D (*see* Viganó et al). 1995;126:368-74
Trabazo S (*see* Seara et al). 1995;126:965-7 (CLO)
Transue DJ (*see* Polack et al). 1995;126:261-3 (CLO)
Troiani S (*see* Spagnoli et al). 1995;126:905-9
Trudell J (*see* Schlager et al). 1995;126:490-6
Tsai C-H (*see* Lin et al). 1995;126:114-7
Tsang RC (*see* Demarini et al). 1995;126:796-8 (CLO)
Tsujino Y (*see* Yuki and Tsujino). 1995;126:162 (Letter)
Tully SB, Bar-Haim Y, Bradley RL. Abnormal tympanography after supine bottle feeding. 1995;126:S105-11
Turchini S (*see* Taccetti et al). 1995;126:848-9 (Letter)
Turner A (*see* Mirochnick et al). 1995;126:636-8 (CLO)

U

Uauy R (*see* Zwiener et al). 1995;126:728-35
Ueda K (*see* Sato et al). 1995;126:109-13
Ueyama N (*see* Kohno et al). 1995;126:953-5 (CLO)
Uhari M, Rantala H, Vainionpää L, Kurttila R. Effect of acetaminophen and of low intermittent doses of diazepam on prevention of recurrences of febrile seizures. 1995;126:991-5
Ukaji K (*see* Kohno et al). 1995;126:953-5 (CLO)
Urbanek R (*see* Hauk et al). 1995;126:185-90
Uziel Y, Laxer RM, Blaser S, Andrew M, Schneider R, Silverman ED. Cerebral vein thrombosis in childhood systemic lupus erythematosus. 1995;126:722-7

V

Vainionpää L (*see* Uhari et al). 1995;126:991-5
Valenski WR (*see* Herrod et al). 1995;126:530-6
Valentine JL, Komoroski EM. Use of a visual panel detection method for drugs of abuse: clinical and laboratory experience with children and adolescents. 1995;126:135-40
Vanderhal AL, Cocjin J, Santulli TV Jr, Carlson DE, Rosenthal P. Conjugated hyperbilirubinemia in a newborn infant after maternal (transplacental) treatment with flecainide acetate for fetal tachycardia and fetal hydrops. 1995;126:988-90 (CLO)
van der Laag H (*see* Wulffraat et al). 1995;126:849 (Letter reply)
Van Fossen RL (*see* Farber et al). 1995;126:S118-24
van Houwelingen AC (*see* Foreman–van Drongelen et al). 1995; 126:611-8
Vargas JH (*see* Baron et al). 1995;126:397-400 (CLO)
Vazquez RL (*see* Brozanski et al). 1995;126:769-76
Venzon D (*see* Husson et al). 1995;126:865-71
Vichinsky E (*see* Pegelow et al). 1995;126:896-9
Viganó A, Principi N, Villa ML, Riva C, Crupi L, Trabattoni D, Shearer GM, Clerici M. Immunologic characterization of children vertically infected with human immunodeficiency virus, with slow or rapid disease progression. 1995;126:368-74
Vila JF (*see* Seara et al). 1995;126:965-7 (CLO)
Villa ML (*see* Viganó et al). 1995;126:368-74
Vincer M (*see* Casiro et al). 1995;126:S53-60 (Symposium)
—— (*see* Sauve et al). 1995;126:S75-80 (Symposium)
Vinton N (*see* Proujansky et al). 1995;126:850 (Letter reply)
Virdee SS (*see* McLaughlin et al). 1995;126:821-4 (CLO)
Vizirinia N (*see* Patel et al). 1995;126:799-806
Volberg F (*see* Smyth et al). 1995;126:S81-9 (Symposium)
Vreman HJ (*see* Slusher et al). 1995;126:102-8
Vulsma T, Kooistra L. Motor and cognitive development in children with congenital hypothyroidism. 1995;126:673-4 (Letter reply)

W

Waber L (*see* Dawson et al). 1995;126:69-71 (CLO)
Wagener J (*see* Petersen et al). 1995;126:1011-5
Waisbren SE (*see* North et al). 1995;126:916-22
Waites KB, Cassell GH, Duffy LB, Searcey KB. Isolation of *Ureaplasma urealyticum* from low birth weight infants. 1995;126:502 (Letter)
Wald ER (*see* Hoberman and Wald). 1995;126:158-9 (Letter reply)
Walter D (*see* Courtney et al). 1995;126:S43-52 (Symposium)
Walther FJ, Mullett M, Schumacher R, Sundell H, Easa D, Long W, American Exosurf Neonatal Study Group I. One-year follow-up of 66 premature infants weighing 500 to 699 grams treated with a single dose of synthetic surfactant or air placebo at birth: results of a double-blind trial. 1995;126:S13-9 (Symposium)
Wang EEL, Law BJ, Stephens D, Pediatric Investigators Collaborative Network on Infections in Canada. Pediatric Investigators Collaborative Network on Infections in Canada (PICNIC) prospective study of risk factors and outcomes in patients hospitalized with respiratory syncytial viral lower respiratory tract infection. 1995;126:212-9
Wang W (*see* Pegelow et al). 1995;126:896-9
Ward JI (*see* Greenberg et al). 1995;126:206-11
—— (*see* Lieberman et al). 1995;126:198-205
Waris M (*see* Heikkinen et al). 1995;126:313-6 (CLO)
Warman ML (*see* North et al). 1995;126:916-22
Warren CR, Kiser WR. Usefulness of cerebrospinal fluid bacterial antigen tests. 1995;126:321 (Letter)
Watchko JF (*see* Ozolek et al). 1995;126:322-3 (Letter reply)
Waters S (*see* Palumbo et al). 1995;126:592-5 (CLO)
Watts C (*see* Furman et al). 1995;126:434-40
Watts J (*see* McMillan et al). 1995;126:S90-8 (Symposium)
Way RC (*see* Schulze et al). 1995;126:777-84
Webber CE (*see* Halton et al). 1995;126:557-64
Webster D (*see* Cutfield and Webster). 1995;126:118-21
Weinberger MW. Placebo-controlled versus comparative studies of drug effects. 1995;126:680-1 (Letter)

Weinblatt ME, Scimeca P, James-Herry A, Sahdev I, Kochen J. Transformation of congenital neutropenia into monosomy 7 and acute nonlymphoblastic leukemia in a child treated with granulocyte colony-stimulating factor. 1995;126:263-5 (CLO)
Wells G (*see* King et al). 1995;126:937-9 (CLO)
Wershil BK (*see* Odze et al). 1995;126:163-70
Wesley Y (*see* Palumbo et al). 1995;126:592-5 (CLO)
Westenend PJ. Congenital nephrotic syndrome in neonatal lupus syndrome. 1995;126:851 (Letter)
Westphal E (*see* Hentschel et al). 1995;126:61-4 (CLO)
Whitaker RC, Wright JA, Koepsell TD, Psaty BM, Finch AJ. Promotion of healthy eating habits in children. 1995;126:850-1 (Letter reply)
Whitelaw A (*see* Larsen and Whitelaw). 1995;126:1018 (Letter)
Whitfield M (*see* Casiro et al). 1995;126:S53-60 (Symposium)
—— (*see* Saigal et al). 1995;126:S61-7 (Symposium)
Whittam TS (*see* Schlager et al). 1995;126:490-6
Whyte H (*see* Perlman et al). 1995;126:75-87
Whyte RK (*see* Schulze et al). 1995;126:777-84
Wiebke G (*see* Chan et al). 1995;126:551-6
Wilcken B (*see* Christodoulou et al). 1995;126:65-8 (CLO)
Wiley CC (*see* Osterhoudt et al). 1995;126:819-21 (CLO)
Wiley JF II, Bell LM, Rosenblum LS, Nussbaum J, Tobin R, Henretig FM. Lead poisoning: low rates of screening and high prevalence among children seen in inner-city emergency departments. 1995;126:392-5 (CLO)
Willi SM (*see* Bhala et al). 1995;126:910-5
Williams J (*see* Krafte-Jacobs et al). 1995;126:601-3 (CLO)
Williams LR (*see* Rabinowitz et al). 1995;126:266-9 (CLO)
Wilson DM (*see* Neely and Wilson). 1995;126:159-60 (Letter reply)
Winterbourn CC (*see* Inder et al). 1995;126:128-31 (CLO)
—— (*see* Neužil et al). 1995;126:785-90
Wolach B (*see* Pomeranz et al). 1995;126:140-2 (CLO)
Wold DE (*see* Mauskopf et al). 1995;126:94-101
Wolraich M (*see* Petersen et al). 1995;126:1011-5
Wong VK (*see* Greenberg et al). 1995;126:206-11
—— (*see* Lieberman et al). 1995;126:198-205
Wood EG (*see* Ellis et al). 1995;126:40-3
Woźniewicz B (*see* Pronicka et al). 1995;126:948-51 (CLO)
Wright JA (*see* Whitaker et al). 1995;126:850-1 (Letter reply)
Wulffraat NM, de Graeff-Meeder ER, Rijkers GT, van der Laag H, Kuis W. Cystic fibrosis and episodic arthritis. 1995;126:849 (Letter reply)
Wyllie E (*see* Bass et al). 1995;126:537-44
Wysowski DK (*see* Malozowski et al). 1995;126:996-9

Y

Yabuta K (*see* Ino et al). 1995;126:304-8
Yanai S (*see* Kohno et al). 1995;126:953-5 (CLO)
Yavûz H, Ozel A, Erkul I. Short-term, high-dose corticosteroid therapy in childhood acute immune thrombocytopenic purpura. 1995;126:156 (Letter)
Yetman R. Accuracy of aural infrared temperature device. 1995;126:324-5 (Letter reply)
Yi A (*see* Fukuda et al). 1995;126:882-6
Yoder BA (*see* Schelonka et al). 1995;126:505-6 (Letter reply)
Young WE (*see* Klein et al). 1995;126:252-6
Yuki N, Ichikawa H, Doi A. Fisher syndrome after *Campylobacter jejuni* enteritis: human leukocyte antigen and the bacterial serotype. 1995;126:55-7 (CLO)
——, Tsujino Y. Familial Guillain-Barré syndrome subsequent to *Campylobacter jejuni* enteritis. 1995;126:162 (Letter)

Z

Zacchello F (*see* Blau et al). 1995;126:401-5 (CLO)
Zamboni G, Antoniazzi F, Tató L. Use of the gonadotropin-releasing hormone agonist triptorelin in the diagnosis of delayed puberty in boys. 1995;126:756-8 (CLO)
Zar H, Saiman L, Quittell L, Prince A. Binding of *Pseudomonas aeruginosa* to respiratory epithelial cells from patients with various mutations in the cystic fibrosis transmembrane regulator. 1995;126:230-3
Zasloff MA (*see* Lanchoney et al). 1995;126:762-4 (CLO)
Zeisel SA (*see* Roberts et al). 1995;126:481-9
Zemel BS (*see* Stallings et al). 1995;126:833-9
Ziegler T (*see* Heikkinen et al). 1995;126:313-6 (CLO)
Zimran A, Elstein D, Schiffmann R, Abrahamov A, Goldberg M, Bar-Maor JA, Brady RO, Guzzetta PC, Barton NW. Outcome of partial splenectomy for type I Gaucher disease. 1995;126:596-7 (CLO)
Zirin S (*see* Dulkerian et al). 1995;126:872-6
Zlotkin S (*see* Andrew et al). 1995;126:358-63
Zucker J (*see* Gong et al). 1995;126:S68-74 (Symposium)
—— (*see* Long et al). 1995;126:S1-4 (Symposium)
Zuckerman B (*see* Mirochnick et al). 1995;126:636-8 (CLO)
Zwiener RJ, Uauy R, Petruska ML, Huet BA. Low-density lipoprotein apheresis as long-term treatment for children with homozygous familial hypercholesterolemia. 1995;126:728-35

Subject index*

A

Abnormalities
Possible fetal effects of cervical dilation and uterine curettage during the first trimester of pregnancy (Holmes). 1995;126:131-4 (CLO)
Prolonged dysphagia caused by congenital pharyngeal dysfunction (Mbonda et al). 1995;126:923-7
Acetaminophen
Effect of acetaminophen and of low intermittent doses of diazepam on prevention of recurrences of febrile seizures (Uhari et al). 1995;126:991-5
Prevention of recurrent febrile seizures (Camfield et al). 1995; 126:929-30 (Editor's column)
Acid-base imbalance
Pancreatitis and organic acidemias (Fiumara et al). 1995;126:852 (Letter)
Acidosis
Methemoglobinemia associated with acidosis of probable renal origin (Sager et al). 1995;126:59-61 (CLO)
Acidosis, lactic
Lactic acidosis in a patient with acute lymphoblastic leukemia (Robson and Leung). 1995;126:1021 (Letter)
Acidosis, renal tubular
Use of the urine-to-blood carbon dioxide tension gradient as a measurement of impaired distal tubular hydrogen ion secretion among neonates (Lin et al). 1995;126:114-7
Aciduria
Transient organic aciduria and persistent lactic acidemia in a patient with short-chain acyl–coenzyme A dehydrogenase deficiency (Dawson et al). 1995;126:69-71 (CLO)
Acknowledgment of reviewers
Reviewers. 1995;126:327-32
Acoustic impedance tests
"Abnormal" tympanography after supine bottle feeding (Tully et al). 1995;126:S105-11
Acquired immunodeficiency syndrome
Congenital cytomegalovirus infection as a result of nonprimary cytomegalovirus disease in a mother with acquired immunodeficiency syndrome (Schwebke et al). 1995;126:293-5 (CLO)
Effect of corticosteroids on survival of children with acquired immunodeficiency syndrome and *Pneumocystis carinii*–related respiratory failure (McLaughlin et al). 1995;126:821-4 (CLO)
Encephalopathy in children with perinatally acquired human immunodeficiency virus infection (Lobato et al). 1995;126:710-5
Activity levels; *see* Exercise
Acuity index method
Acuity scores as predictors of cost-related outcomes of neonatal intensive care (Kotagal et al). 1995;126:88-93
Acute lymphoblastic leukemia; *see* Leukemia, lymphocytic, acute
Acyl–coenzyme A dehydrogenases; *see* Fatty acid desaturases
Administration, inhalation
Inhaled nitric oxide for premature infants after prolonged rupture of the membranes (Peliowski et al). 1995;126:450-53 (CLO)
Adolescence
Adolescent medicine 1995 (Emans). 1995;126:387-8 (Editor's column)

*January, pp. 1-162; February, pp. 163-332; March, pp. 333-506; April, pp. 507-682; May, pp. 683-852 and S1-S102; June, pp. 853-1064 and S103-S134.

Adolescence—cont'd
Bone mineralization, hypothalamic amenorrhea, and sex steroid therapy in adolescents and young adults (Hergenroeder). 1995; 126:683-9
Definition and application of the discretionary screening indicators according to the National Cholesterol Education Program for Children and Adolescents (Diller et al). 1995;126:345-52
Effect of growth hormone therapy on final versus predicted height in short twelve- to sixteen-year-old boys without growth hormone deficiency (Kaplowitz). 1995;126:478-80 (CLO)
Effects of acute hyperglycemia on mental efficiency and counterregulatory hormones in adolescents with insulin-dependent diabetes mellitus (Gschwend et al). 1995;126:178-84
Hemoglobin A_{1c} levels in young patients with diabetes beyond the "honeymoon" period (Dorchy) (Letter); (Tamborlane and Nathan) (Reply). 1995;126:1020-1
Relationship between insulin resistance and abnormal lipid profile in obese adolescents (Steinberger et al). 1995;126:690-5
Supplementary sensorimotor area seizures in children and adolescents (Bass et al). 1995;126:537-44
Use of a visual panel detection method for drugs of abuse: clinical and laboratory experience with children and adolescents (Valentine and Komoroski). 1995;126:135-40
Adrenal cortex hormones
Antenatal corticosteroid therapy to prevent respiratory distress syndrome (Ryan and Finer). 1995;126:317-9
Corticosteroid therapy for ventricular tachycardia in children with silent lymphocytic myocarditis (Ino et al). 1995;126:304-8
Effect of corticosteroids on survival of children with acquired immunodeficiency syndrome and *Pneumocystis carinii*–related respiratory failure (McLaughlin et al). 1995;126:821-4 (CLO)
Growth and the growth hormone axis in prepubertal children with asthma (Crowley et al). 1995;126:297-303
Short-term, high-dose corticosteroid therapy in childhood acute immune thrombocytopenic purpura (Yavûz et al) (Letter); (Blanchette) (Reply). 1995;126:156-7
Adrenal hyperplasia, congenital
Newborn screening for congenital adrenal hyperplasia in New Zealand (Cutfield and Webster). 1995;126:118-21
Adult respiratory distress syndrome; *see* Respiratory distress syndrome, adult
Air placebos; *see* Placebos
Airway resistance
Effect of airway pressure on inferior vena cava pressure as a measure of central venous pressure in children (Reda et al). 1995;126:961-5 (CLO)
Albuterol
Efficacy of frequent nebulized ipratropium bromide added to frequent high-dose albuterol therapy in severe childhood asthma (Schuh et al). 1995;126:639-45
A randomized trial comparing the efficacy of epinephrine with salbutamol in the treatment of acute bronchiolitis (Menon et al). 1995;126:1004-7 (CLO)
Allergens
Allergic colitis in infants (Odze et al). 1995;126:163-70
Allergic colitis; *see* Colitis
Amenorrhea
Bone mineralization, hypothalamic amenorrhea, and sex steroid therapy in adolescents and young adults (Hergenroeder). 1995;126:683-9
Ammonium chloride
Use of peritoneal dialysis, continuous arteriovenous hemofiltration, and continuous arteriovenous hemodiafiltration for removal of ammonium chloride and glutamine in rabbits (Semama et al). 1995;126:742-6
Amoxicillin
Bacteriologic failure of amoxicillin-clavulanate in treatment of acute otitis media caused by nontypeable *Haemophilus influenzae* (Patel et al). 1995;126:799-806

Amoxicillin—cont'd
Criteria for studies of antibiotic therapy for acute otitis media (Schwartz and Rodriguez). 1995;126:677-8 (Letter)
Short-term use of amoxicillin clavulanate during upper respiratory tract infection for prevention of acute otitis media (Heikkinen et al). 1995;126:313-6 (CLO)
Anemia
Resolution of breath-holding spells with treatment of concomitant anemia (Colina and Abelson). 1995;126:395-7 (CLO)
Anemia, sickle cell
Fatal hemolysis induced by ceftriaxone in a child with sickle cell anemia (Bernini et al). 1995;126:813-5 (CLO)
Intravenous morphine pharmacokinetics in pediatric patients with sickle cell disease (Dampier et al). 1995;126:461-7
Risk of recurrent stroke in patients with sickle cell disease treated with erythrocyte transfusions (Pegelow et al). 1995;126:896-9
Antibiotics
Antibiotic-associated hemorrhagic colitis without *Clostridium difficile* toxin in children (Kato et al). 1995;126:1008-10 (CLO)
Criteria for studies of antibiotic therapy for acute otitis media (Schwartz and Rodriguez). 1995;126:677-8 (Letter)
Short-term use of amoxicillin clavulanate during upper respiratory tract infection for prevention of acute otitis media (Heikkinen et al). 1995;126:313-6 (CLO)
Antibodies
Effect of neonatal immunization with diphtheria and tetanus toxoids on antibody responses to *Haemophilus influenzae* type b conjugate vaccines (Lieberman et al). 1995;126:198-205
Enhanced antibody responses in infants given different sequences of heterogeneous *Haemophilus influenzae* type b conjugate vaccines (Greenberg et al). 1995;126:206-11
Vertical transmission of human immunodeficiency virus type I: autologous neutralizing antibody, virus load, and virus phenotype (Husson et al). 1995;126:865-71
Antibodies to hepatitis B; *see* Hepatitis B antibodies
Anticonvulsants
Prevention of recurrent febrile seizures (Camfield et al). 1995; 126:929-30 (Editor's column)
Antigens, bacterial
Usefulness of cerebrospinal fluid bacterial antigen tests (Warren and Kiser) (Letter); (Maxson et al) (Reply). 1995;126:321
Antigens, surface
Loss of detectable antibody to hepatitis B surface antigen in immunized patients with hemophilia but without human immunodeficiency virus infection (Maris et al). 1995;126:269-71 (CLO)
Anti-neutrophils; *see* Neutrophils
Apheresis; *see* Blood component removal
Apnea
Effects of central apnea on cerebral blood flow velocity in healthy term infants (Rehan et al). 1995;126:979-82 (CLO)
Arnold-Chiari deformity
Abnormalities in control of ventilation in newborn infants with myelomeningocele (Petersen et al). 1995;126:1011-5
Arteriovenous hemofiltration; *see* Hemofiltration
Arthritis
Cystic fibrosis and episodic arthritis (Taccetti et al) (Letter); (Wulffraat et al) (Reply). 1995;126:848-9
Aseptic meningitis; *see* Meningitis, aseptic
Asphyxia neonatorum
Blood flow velocities and neonatal asphyxia (Elliott) (Letter); (Akinbi and Bhutani) (Reply). 1995;126:675-6
Asthma
Efficacy of frequent nebulized ipratropium bromide added to frequent high-dose albuterol therapy in severe childhood asthma (Schuh et al). 1995;126:639-45
Growth and the growth hormone axis in prepubertal children with asthma (Crowley et al). 1995;126:297-303
Asthma—cont'd
Terbutaline powder for acute asthma (Rufin et al). 1995;126:161-2 (Letter)
Ataxia
Opsoclonus-myoclonus, ataxia, and coincident neuroblastoma (Chamberlain). 1995;126:675 (Letter)
Atherogenic diet; *see* Diet, atherogenic
Attitude
Impact of attitudes on maternal decisions regarding infant feeding (Losch et al). 1995;126:507-14
Aural infrared temperature; *see* Body temperature
Autoantibodies
Spectrum of disease associated with anti-neutrophil cytoplasmic autoantibodies in pediatric patients (Ellis et al). 1995;126:40-3
Autologous neutralizing antibody; *see* Antibodies

B

Bacteremia
Efficacy of an observation scale in detecting bacteremia in febrile children three to thirty-six months of age, treated as outpatients (Teach et al). 1995;126:877-81
Bacteria
Association of symptoms with *Helicobacter pylori* infection in children (Gormally et al). 1995;126:753-6 (CLO)
Bacteriologic failure of amoxicillin-clavulanate in treatment of acute otitis media caused by nontypeable *Haemophilus influenzae* (Patel et al). 1995;126:799-806
Fisher syndrome after *Campylobacter jejuni* enteritis: human leukocyte antigen and the bacterial serotype (Yuki et al). 1995;126:55-7 (CLO)
Bacterial infections
Cytokine elevations in infants with bacterial and aseptic meningitis (Dulkerian et al). 1995;126:872-6
Bacterial vaccines
Effect of neonatal immunization with diphtheria and tetanus toxoids on antibody responses to *Haemophilus influenzae* type b conjugate vaccines (Lieberman et al). 1995;126:198-205
Enhanced antibody responses in infants given different sequences of heterogeneous *Haemophilus influenzae* type b conjugate vaccines (Greenberg et al). 1995;126:206-11
Bacteriuria
Bacteriuria in children with neurogenic bladder treated with intermittent catheterization: natural history (Schlager et al). 1995;126:490-6
Bayley-Pinneau method
Bayley-Pinneau method of height prediction in girls with central precocious puberty: correlation with adult height (Bar et al). 1995;126:955-8 (CLO)
Behavior
Enhanced adrenomedullary response and increased susceptibility to neuroglycopenia: mechanisms underlying the adverse effects of sugar ingestion in healthy children (Jones et al). 1995;126:171-7
Long-term effects of L-thyroxine therapy for congenital hypothyroidism (Rovet and Ehrlich). 1995;126:380-6
Benign intracranial hypertension; *see* Pseudotumor cerebri
Benzodiazepines
Diarrhea associated with enteral benzodiazepine solutions (Marshall et al). 1995;126:657-9 (CLO)
Benzoylecgonine
Relation between meconium concentration of the cocaine metaboiite benzoylecgonine and fetal growth (Mirochnick et al). 1995;126:636-8 (CLO)
Beta-thalassemia
Life-threatening infection in two children with hemoglobin S–beta-thalassemia (Lynch and Tobias). 1995;126:581-2 (CLO)

Beverages
Consumption of soft drinks with phosphoric acid as a risk factor for the development of hypocalcemia in children: a case-control study (Mazariegos-Ramos et al). 1995;126:940-2 (CLO)
Bilirubin
Glucose-6-phosphate dehydrogenase deficiency and carboxyhemoglobin concentrations associated with bilirubin-related morbidity and death in Nigerian infants (Slusher et al). 1995;126:102-8
Biochemical phenomena
Neonatal onset of medium-chain acyl–coenzyme A dehydrogenase deficiency with confusing biochemical features (Christodoulou et al). 1995;126:65-8 (CLO)
Biopsy
Intact survival with transfusion-associated graft-versus-host disease proved by human leukocyte antigen typing of lymphocytes in skin biopsy specimens (Hentschel et al). 1995;126:61-4 (CLO)
Birth; *see* Labor
Birth order
Birth order, delivery route, and concordance in the transmission of human immunodeficiency virus type 1 from mothers to twins (Duliège et al). 1995;126:625-32
Birth weight
Response to growth hormone therapy in patients with growth hormone deficiency who were small or appropriate in size for gestational age at birth (Balsamo et al). 1995;126:474-7
Bladder, neurogenic
Bacteriuria in children with neurogenic bladder treated with intermittent catheterization: natural history (Schlager et al). 1995;126:490-6
Blood
Use of the urine-to-blood carbon dioxide tension gradient as a measurement of impaired distal tubular hydrogen ion secretion among neonates (Lin et al). 1995;126:114-7
Blood coagulation
Treatment of purpura fulminans in meningococcemia with protein C concentrate (Rivard et al). 1995;126:646-52
Blood coagulation factors
Coagulation factor deficiencies during initiation of extracorporeal membrane oxygenation (McManus et al). 1995;126:900-4
Blood component removal
Low-density lipoprotein apheresis as long-term treatment for children with homozygous familial hypercholesterolemia (Zwiener et al). 1995;126:728-35
Blood component transfusion
Risk of recurrent stroke in patients with sickle cell disease treated with erythrocyte transfusions (Pegelow et al). 1995;126:896-9
Blood donors
Reducing blood donor exposures in low birth weight infants by the use of older, unwashed packed red blood cells (Lee et al). 1995;126:280-6
Blood flow velocity
Blood flow velocities and neonatal asphyxia (Elliott) (Letter); (Akinbi and Bhutani) (Reply). 1995;126:675-6
Effects of central apnea on cerebral blood flow velocity in healthy term infants (Rehan et al). 1995;126:979-82 (CLO)
Blood group incompatibility
Differences in clinical significance of maternal-infant blood group incompatibility in mothers with blood type O, A, or B (Perl) (Letter); (Ozolek et al) (Reply). 1995;126:322-3
Blood grouping and crossmatching
Differences in clinical significance of maternal-infant blood group incompatibility in mothers with blood type O, A, or B (Perl) (Letter); (Ozolek et al) (Reply). 1995;126:322-3
Blood platelets
Acquired platelet dysfunction with eosinophilia in white children (Poon et al). 1995;126:959-61 (CLO)
Blood transfusion
Efficacy and cost analysis of treating very low birth weight infants with erythropoietin during their first two weeks of life: a randomized, placebo-controlled trial (Ohls et al). 1995;126:421-6
Intact survival with transfusion-associated graft-versus-host disease proved by human leukocyte antigen typing of lymphocytes in skin biopsy specimens (Hentschel et al). 1995;126:61-4 (CLO)
Body composition
Body composition in children with spastic quadriplegic cerebral palsy (Stallings et al). 1995;126:833-9
Effects of dairy products on bone and body composition in pubertal girls (Chan et al). 1995;126:551-6
Increased fat oxidation in prepubertal obese children: A metabolic defense against further weight gain? (Maffeis et al). 1995;126:15-20
Normal energy expenditure in the infant with presymptomatic cystic fibrosis (Bronstein et al). 1995;126:28-33
Body fat
Relation of activity levels to body fat in infants 6 to 12 months of age (Li et al). 1995;126:353-7
Body height
Bayley-Pinneau method of height prediction in girls with central precocious puberty: correlation with adult height (Bar et al). 1995;126:955-8 (CLO)
Combined treatment with growth hormone and gonadotropin-releasing hormone analogs in short normal girls (Saggese et al). 1995;126:468-73
Effect of growth hormone therapy on final versus predicted height in short twelve- to sixteen-year-old boys without growth hormone deficiency (Kaplowitz). 1995;126:478-80 (CLO)
Prediction of the outcome of growth hormone therapy in children with idiopathic short stature: a multivariate discriminant analysis (Spagnoli et al). 1995;126:905-9
Predictive factors in the determination of final height in boys with constitutional delay of growth and puberty (Albanese and Stanhope). 1995;126:545-50
Body temperature
Accuracy of aural infrared temperature device (McKenzie) (Letter); (Yetman) (Reply). 1995;126:324-5
Bone density
Effects of dairy products on bone and body composition in pubertal girls (Chan et al). 1995;126:551-6
Long-term reduction in bone mass after severe burn injury in children (Klein et al). 1995;126:252-6
Mineral homeostasis and bone mass at diagnosis in children with acute lymphoblastic leukemia (Halton et al). 1995;126:557-64
Postnatal attainment of intrauterine macromineral accretion rates in low birth weight infants fed fortified human milk (Schanler and Abrams). 1995;126:441-7
Bone marrow
Lysinuric protein intolerance characterized by bone marrow abnormalities and severe clinical course (Parenti et al). 1995;126:246-51
Bone mineralization; *see* Calcification, physiologic
Bone resorption
Evidence of increased intrauterine bone resorption in term infants of mothers with insulin-dependent diabetes (Demarini et al). 1995;126:796-8 (CLO)
Book reviews
The book shelf. 1995;126:296, 320, 460, 580, 604, 768, 840, 928
Bottle feeding
Abnormal tympanography after supine bottle feeding (Tully et al). 1995;126:S105-11
The clinician's role in teaching proper infant feeding techniques (Lawrence). 1995;126:S112-7
Imaging evaluation of breast-feeding and bottle-feeding systems (Nowak et al). 1995;126:S130-4

Bottle feeding—cont'd
Nipple confusion: toward a formal definition (Neifert et al). 1995;126:S125-9
Perspectives on infant feeding: Guest Editor's note (Shelov). 1995;126:S103
Perspectives on infant feeding: Introduction (Erenberg). 1995; 126:S104
Quantitative and qualitative video analysis of infants feeding: angled- and straight-bottle feeding systems (Farber et al). 1995;126:S118-24

Brain
Brain metabolite changes on in vivo proton magnetic resonance spectroscopy in children with congenital hypothyroidism (Gupta et al). 1995;126:389-92 (CLO)

Brain diseases
Encephalopathy in children with perinatally acquired human immunodeficiency virus infection (Lobato et al). 1995;126:710-5

Brain injuries
Somatosensory evoked potentials for prediction of outcome in acute severe brain injury (Beca et al). 1995;126:44-9

Breast
Progression of premature thelarche to central precocious puberty (Pasquino et al). 1995;126:11-4

Breast-feeding
Absence of infection in breast-fed infants born to hepatitis C virus–infected mothers (Lin et al). 1995;126:589-91 (CLO)
The clinician's role in teaching proper infant feeding techniques (Lawrence). 1995;126:S112-7
Differences in morbidity between breast-fed and formula-fed infants (Dewey et al). 1995;126:696-702
Imaging evaluation of breast-feeding and bottle feeding systems (Nowak et al). 1995;126:S130-4
Impact of attitudes on maternal decisions regarding infant feeding (Losch et al). 1995;126:507-14
Nipple confusion: toward a formal definition (Neifert et al). 1995;126:S125-9
Perspectives on infant feeding: Guest Editor's note (Shelov). 1995;126:S103
Perspectives on infant feeding: Introduction (Erenberg). 1995; 126:S104
Relation between infant feeding and infections during the first six months of life (Beaudry et al). 1995;126:191-7

Breath-holding spells; *see* Respiration disorders

Bronchiolitis
A randomized trial comparing the efficacy of epinephrine with salbutamol in the treatment of acute bronchiolitis (Menon et al). 1995;126:1004-7 (CLO)

Bronchopulmonary dysplasia
Influence of energy substrates on respiratory gas exchange during conventional mechanical ventilation of preterm infants (Chessex et al). 1995;126:619-24

Burns
Long-term reduction in bone mass after severe burn injury in children (Klein et al). 1995;126:252-6

C

Calcification, physiologic
Bone mineralization, hypothalamic amenorrhea, and sex steroid therapy in adolescents and young adults (Hergenroeder). 1995;126:683-9

Calcitonin
Human synthetic calcitonin therapy for hypercalcemia of immobilization (Kaul and Sockalosky). 1995;126:825-7 (CLO)

Calcium
Effects of dairy products on bone and body composition in pubertal girls (Chan et al). 1995;126:551-6

Calcium—cont'd
Postnatal attainment of intrauterine macromineral accretion rates in low birth weight infants fed fortified human milk (Schanler and Abrams). 1995;126:441-7

Calcium metabolism disorders
Pathophysiology of calcium metabolism in children with vitamin D–deficiency rickets (Kruse). 1995;126:736-41

Caloric intake
Normal energy expenditure in the infant with presymptomatic cystic fibrosis (Bronstein et al). 1995;126:28-33

Campylobacter jejuni
Familial Guillain-Barré syndrome subsequent to *Campylobacter jejuni* enteritis (Yuki and Tsujino). 1995;126:162 (Letter)
Fisher syndrome after *Campylobacter jejuni* enteritis: human leukocyte antigen and the bacterial serotype (Yuki et al). 1995;126:55-7 (CLO)

Cancer; *see* Neoplasms

Captopril
Successful treatment of Finnish congenital nephrotic syndrome with captopril and indomethacin (Pomeranz et al). 1995; 126:140-2 (CLO)

Carbohydrates, adverse effects
Enhanced adrenomedullary response and increased susceptibility to neuroglycopenia: mechanisms underlying the adverse effects of sugar ingestion in healthy children (Jones et al). 1995;126:171-7

Carbon dioxide
Use of the urine-to-blood carbon dioxide tension gradient as a measurement of impaired distal tubular hydrogen ion secretion among neonates (Lin et al). 1995;126:114-7

Carboxyhemoglobin
Glucose-6-phosphate dehydrogenase deficiency and carboxyhemoglobin concentrations associated with bilirubin-related morbidity and death in Nigerian infants (Slusher et al). 1995; 126:102-8

Cardiac output
Effect of the arterial oxygenation level on cardiac output, oxygen extraction, and oxygen consumption in low birth weight infants receiving mechanical ventilation (Schulze et al). 1995;126: 777-84

Cardiovascular diseases
Definition and application of the discretionary screening indicators according to the National Cholesterol Education Program for Children and Adolescents (Diller et al). 1995;126: 345-52

Cardiovascular system
Cardiovascular, renal, and endocrine actions of dopamine in neonates and children (Seri). 1995;126:333-44

Carnitine
Effects of parenteral L-carnitine supplementation on fat metabolism and nutrition in premature neonates (Bonner et al). 1995;126:287-92

Catheterization
Bacteriuria in children with neurogenic bladder treated with intermittent catheterization: natural history (Schlager et al). 1995;126:490-6

Catheters, indwelling
Catheter-related thrombosis in critically ill children: comparison of catheters with and without heparin bonding (Krafte-Jacobs et al). 1995;126:50-4
A cross-sectional study of catheter-related thrombosis in children receiving total parenteral nutrition at home (Andrew et al). 1995;126:358-63
Placement of umbilical venous catheters with use of bedside real-time ultrasonography (Greenberg et al). 1995;126:633-5 (CLO)

Ceftriaxone
Fatal hemolysis caused by ceftriaxone (Lascari and Amyot). 1995;126:816-7 (CLO)

Ceftriaxone—cont'd
Fatal hemolysis induced by ceftriaxone in a child with sickle cell anemia (Bernini et al). 1995;126:813-5 (CLO)
Cell-mediated immunity; *see* Immunity, cellular
Cells, cultured
Comparison of an optical immunoassay technique with two culture methods for the detection of group A streptococci in a pediatric office (Roddey et al). 1995;126:931-3 (CLO)
Diagnosis of group A streptococcal pharyngitis in a private clinic: comparative evaluation of Optical ImmunoAssay method and culture (Fries). 1995;126:933-6 (CLO)
Central nervous system diseases
Estimation of energy requirements in persons with severe central nervous system impairment (Bandini et al). 1995;126:828-32
Central venous pressure
Effect of airway pressure on inferior vena cava pressure as a measure of central venous pressure in children (Reda et al). 1995;126:961-5 (CLO)
Cerebral artery diseases
Cerebral artery stenoses in Williams syndrome cause strokes in childhood (Kaplan et al). 1995;126:943-5 (CLO)
Ischemic stroke and intracranial multifocal cerebral arteriopathy in Williams syndrome (Soper et al). 1995;126:945-8 (CLO)
Cerebral palsy
Body composition in children with spastic quadriplegic cerebral palsy (Stallings et al). 1995;126:833-9
Cerebral veins
Cerebral vein thrombosis in childhood systemic lupus erythematosus (Uziel et al). 1995;126:722-7
Cerebrospinal fluid
Usefulness of cerebrospinal fluid bacterial antigen tests (Warren and Kiser) (Letter); (Maxson et al) (Reply). 1995;126:321
Cerebrovascular disorders
Cerebral artery stenoses in Williams syndrome cause strokes in childhood (Kaplan et al). 1995;126:943-5 (CLO)
Ischemic stroke and intracranial multifocal cerebral arteriopathy in Williams syndrome (Soper et al). 1995;126:945-8 (CLO)
Risk of recurrent stroke in patients with sickle cell disease treated with erythrocyte transfusions (Pegelow et al). 1995;126:896-9
Cervical dilation and uterine curettage; *see* Dilation and curettage
Charges; *see* Fees and charges
Child development
Double-blind evaluation of developmental and health status to age 2 years of infants weighing 700 to 1350 grams treated prophylactically at birth with a single dose of synthetic surfactant or air placebo (Kraybill et al). 1995;126:S33-42 (Symposium)
Health and neurodevelopmental outcome at 1-year adjusted age in 508 infants weighing 700 to 1100 grams who received prophylaxis with one versus three doses of synthetic surfactant (Gerdes et al). 1995;126:S26-32 (Symposium)
Neonatal-onset propionicacidemia: neurologic and developmental profiles, and implications for management (North et al). 1995;126:916-22
Neurodevelopmental outcome of infants with hypoplastic left heart syndrome (Rogers et al). 1995;126:496-8 (CLO)
Chlorides
Transient elevation of sweat chloride concentration in a malnourished girl with the Mauriac syndrome (Polack et al). 1995;126:261-3 (CLO)
Chlorpromazine
A randomized comparison of intravenously administered granisetron versus chlorpromazine plus dexamethasone in the prevention of ifosfamide-induced emesis in children (Hählen et al). 1995;126:309-13
Cholesterol
Beneficial effect of growth hormone on atherogenic risk in children with growth hormone deficiency (Kohno et al). 1995;126:953-5 (CLO)
Cholesterol—cont'd
Definition and application of the discretionary screening indicators according to the National Cholesterol Education Program for Children and Adolescents (Diller et al). 1995;126:345-52
Lipid abnormalities in Turner syndrome (Ross et al). 1995;126:242-5
Chronic granulomatous disease; *see* Granulomatous disease, chronic
Cicatrix
Diagnostic accuracy of urinary tract infection and subsequent development of renal scars (Koskimies) (Letter); (Hoberman and Wald) (Reply). 1995;126:157-9
Clarithromycin
Criteria for studies of antibiotic therapy for acute otitis media (Schwartz and Rodriguez). 1995;126:677-8 (Letter)
Clinical trial
Clinical trial of vitamin A as adjuvant treatment for lower respiratory tract infections (Kjolhede et al). 1995;126:807-12
Clostridium difficile
Antibiotic-associated hemorrhagic colitis without *Clostridium difficile* toxin in children (Kato et al). 1995;126:1008-10 (CLO)
Coagulation factors; *see* Blood coagulation factors
Cocaine
Relation between meconium concentration of the cocaine metabolite benzoylecgonine and fetal growth (Mirochnick et al). 1995;126:636-8 (CLO)
Screening neonates for intrauterine cocaine exposure (Neuspiel) (Letter); (Ryan and Phelps) (Reply). 1995;126:323-4
Cognition
Cognitive assessment of school-age children infected with maternally transmitted human immunodeficiency virus type 1 (Tardieu et al). 1995;126:375-9
Congenital lacticacidemia caused by lipoamide dehydrogenase deficiency with favorable outcome (Elpeleg et al). 1995;126:72-4 (CLO)
Effects of acute hyperglycemia on mental efficiency and counterregulatory hormones in adolescents with insulin-dependent diabetes mellitus (Gschwend et al). 1995;126:178-84
Enhanced adrenomedullary response and increased susceptibility to neuroglycopenia: mechanisms underlying the adverse effects of sugar ingestion in healthy children (Jones et al). 1995;126:171-7
Motor and cognitive development in children with congenital hypothyroidism (Mitchell and Klein) (Letter); (Vulsma and Kooistra) (Reply). 1995;126:673-4
Colitis
Allergic colitis in infants (Odze et al). 1995;126:163-70
Antibiotic-associated hemorrhagic colitis without *Clostridium difficile* toxin in children (Kato et al). 1995;126:1008-10 (CLO)
Congenital adrenal hyperplasia; *see* Adrenal hyperplasia, congenital
Congenital defects; *see* Abnormalities
Constipation
Chronic constipation as a symptom of cow milk allergy (Iacono et al). 1995;126:34-9
Convulsions, febrile
Effect of acetaminophen and of low intermittent doses of diazepam on prevention of recurrences of febrile seizures (Uhari et al). 1995;126:991-5
Prevention of recurrent febrile seizures (Camfield et al). 1995;126:929-30 (Editor's column)
Correspondence
Letters. 1995;126:155-62, 321-5, 502-6, 673-82, 847-52, 1017-22
Corticosteroids; *see* Adrenal cortex hormones
Cortisol; *see* Hydrocortisone
Cost-benefit analysis
Acuity scores as predictors of cost-related outcomes of neonatal intensive care (Kotagal et al). 1995;126:88-93

Cost-benefit analysis—cont'd
Efficacy and cost analysis of treating very low birth weight infants with erythropoietin during their first two weeks of life: a randomized, placebo-controlled trial (Ohls et al). 1995;126: 421-6
Symposium on Synthetic Surfactant II: perspective and commentary (Long et al). 1995;126:S1-4 (Symposium)
Synthetic surfactant for rescue treatment of respiratory distress syndrome in premature infants weighing from 700 to 1350 grams: impact on hospital resource use and charges (Mauskopf et al). 1995;126:94-101
Usefulness of cerebrospinal fluid bacterial antigen tests (Warren and Kiser) (Letter); (Maxson et al) (Reply). 1995;126:321
Costs and cost analysis
Economic comparison of a tissue adhesive and suturing in the repair of pediatric facial lacerations (Osmond et al). 1995; 126:892-5
Hospitalization for lower respiratory tract illness in infants: variation in rates among counties in New York State and areas within Monroe County (McConnochie ct al). 1995;126: 220-9
Counterregulatory hormones; *see* Hormones
Cow milk allergy; *see* Milk hypersensitivity
Critical illness
Catheter-related thrombosis in critically ill children: comparison of catheters with and without heparin bonding (Krafte-Jacobs et al). 1995;126:50-4
Coagulation factor deficiencies during initiation of extracorporeal membrane oxygenation (McManus et al). 1995;126:900-4
Critical illness neuromuscular disease in children manifested as ventilatory dependence (Sheth et al). 1995;126:259-61 (CLO)
Cultured cells; *see* Cells, cultured
Cyclosporine
Treatment of intractable gastrointestinal manifestations of chronic granulomatous disease with cyclosporine (Rosh et al). 1995; 126:143-5 (CLO)
Cystic fibrosis
Binding of *Pseudomonas aeruginosa* to respiratory epithelial cells from patients with various mutations in the cystic fibrosis transmembrane regulator (Zar et al). 1995;126:230-3
Chronic pancreatitis in a patient with cystic fibrosis and clinical pancreatic insufficiency (del Rosario et al). 1995;126:951-2 (CLO)
Cystic fibrosis and episodic arthritis (Taccetti et al) (Letter); (Wulffraat et al) (Reply). 1995;126:848-9
Incidence of liver disease in patients with cystic fibrosis and meconium ileus (Lindblad et al) (Letter); (Colombo et al) (Reply). 1995;126:155-6
Measured versus predicted resting energy expenditure in infants: a need for reappraisal (Thomson et al). 1995;126:21-7
A multicenter study of alternate-day prednisone therapy in patients with cystic fibrosis (Eigen et al). 1995;126:515-23
Normal energy expenditure in the infant with presymptomatic cystic fibrosis (Bronstein et al). 1995;126:28-33
Cytokines
Cytokine elevations in infants with bacterial and aseptic meningitis (Dulkerian et al). 1995;126:872-6
Immunologic characterization of children vertically infected with human immunodeficiency virus, with slow or rapid disease progression (Viganó et al). 1995;126:368-74
Cytomegalic inclusion disease
Congenital cytomegalovirus infection as a result of nonprimary cytomegalovirus disease in a mother with acquired immunodeficiency syndrome (Schwebke et al). 1995;126:293-5 (CLO)
Portal vein thrombosis caused by protein C and protein S deficiency associated with cytomegalovirus infection (Arav-Boger et al). 1995;126:586-8 (CLO)
Cytoplasm
Spectrum of disease associated with anti-neutrophil cytoplasmic autoantibodies in pediatric patients (Ellis et al). 1995;126:40-3

D

Dairy products
Effects of dairy products on bone and body composition in pubertal girls (Chan et al). 1995;126:551-6
Death, infant; *see* Infant death
Deglutition disorders
Prolonged dysphagia caused by congenital pharyngeal dysfunction (Mbonda et al). 1995;126:923-7
Delayed puberty; *see* Puberty, delayed
Deletion of gene; *see* Gene deletion
Delivery
Birth order, delivery route, and concordance in the transmission of human immunodeficiency virus type 1 from mothers to twins (Duliège et al). 1995;126:625-32
Developmental profiles; *see* Child development
Dexamethasone
Effect of pulse dexamethasone therapy on the incidence and severity of chronic lung disease in the very low birth weight infant (Brozanski et al). 1995;126:769-76
A randomized comparison of intravenously administered granisetron versus chlorpromazine plus dexamethasone in the prevention of ifosfamide-induced emesis in children (Hählen et al). 1995;126:309-13
Twenty-month outcome in ventilator-dependent, very low birth weight infants born during the early years of dexamethasone therapy (Furman et al). 1995;126:434-40
Dextran sulfate
Low-density lipoprotein apheresis as long-term treatment for children with homozygous familial hypercholesterolemia (Zwiener et al). 1995;126:728-35
Diabetes mellitus
Transient elevation of sweat chloride concentration in a malnourished girl with the Mauriac syndrome (Polack et al). 1995;126:261-3 (CLO)
Diabetes mellitus, insulin-dependent
Effects of acute hyperglycemia on mental efficiency and counterregulatory hormones in adolescents with insulin-dependent diabetes mellitus (Gschwend et al). 1995;126:178-84
Evidence of increased intrauterine bone resorption in term infants of mothers with insulin-dependent diabetes (Demarini et al). 1995;126:796-8 (CLO)
Diabetes mellitus, juvenile-onset
Hemoglobin A_{1c} levels in young patients with diabetes beyond the "honeymoon" period (Dorchy) (Letter); (Tamborlane and Nathan) (Reply). 1995;126:1020-1
Diagnosis
Diagnosis of group A streptococcal pharyngitis in a private clinic: comparative evaluation of an optical immunoassay method and culture (Fries). 1995;126:933-6 (CLO)
Diagnostic accuracy of urinary tract infection and subsequent development of renal scars (Koskimies) (Letter); (Hoberman and Wald) (Reply). 1995;126:157-9
Use of polymerase chain reaction for improved diagnosis of tuberculosis in children (Delacourt et al). 1995;126:703-9
Diarrhea
Diarrhea associated with enteral benzodiazepine solutions (Marshall et al). 1995;126:657-9 (CLO)
Diazepam
Effect of acetaminophen and of low intermittent doses of diazepam on prevention of recurrences of febrile seizures (Uhari et al). 1995;126:991-5

Diazoxide
Pancreatic glucagon levels in infants and children with hyperinsulinemia (Pronicka et al). 1995;126:948-51 (CLO)
Diet
Chronic constipation as a symptom of cow milk allergy (Iacono et al). 1995;126:34-9
Promotion of healthy eating habits in children (Crump) (Letter); (Whitaker et al) (Reply). 1995;126:850-1
Transient elevation of sweat chloride concentration in a malnourished girl with the Mauriac syndrome (Polack et al). 1995;126:261-3 (CLO)
Diet, atherogenic
Beneficial effect of growth hormone on atherogenic risk in children with growth hormone deficiency (Kohno et al). 1995; 126:953-5 (CLO)
Dietary fats
Promotion of healthy eating habits in children (Crump) (Letter); (Whitaker et al) (Reply). 1995;126:850-1
Dilation and curettage
Possible fetal effects of cervical dilation and uterine curettage during the first trimester of pregnancy (Holmes). 1995;126: 131-4 (CLO)
Diphtheria-tetanus-pertussis vaccines
Permanent heterotopic ossification at the injection site after diphtheria-tetanus-pertussis immunizations in children who have fibrodysplasia ossificans progressiva (Lanchoney et al). 1995;126:762-4 (CLO)
Diphtheria toxoid
Effect of neonatal immunization with diphtheria and tetanus toxoids on antibody responses to *Haemophilus influenzae* type b conjugate vaccines (Lieberman et al). 1995;126:198-205
Discriminant analysis
Prediction of the outcome of growth hormone therapy in children with idiopathic short stature: a multivariate discriminant analysis (Spagnoli et al). 1995;126:905-9
Disease
Immunologic characterization of children vertically infected with human immunodeficiency virus, with slow or rapid disease progression (Viganó et al). 1995;126:368-74
Disease susceptibility
Enhanced adrenomedullary response and increased susceptibility to neuroglycopenia: mechanisms underlying the adverse effects of sugar ingestion in healthy children (Jones et al). 1995;126:171-7
Disseminated intravascular coagulation
Disseminated intravascular coagulation associated with granulocyte colony-stimulating factor therapy in a child with human immunodeficiency virus infection (Mueller et al). 1995;126: 749-52 (CLO)
Distal tubules; *see* Kidney tubules, distal
DNA, mitochondrial
Deletion of mitochondrial DNA in patient with chronic tubulointerstitial nephritis (Rötig et al). 1995;126:597-601 (CLO)
Dopamine
Cardiovascular, renal, and endocrine actions of dopamine in neonates and children (Seri). 1995;126:333-44
Dose-response relationship, drug
Double-blind, randomized trial of one versus three prophylactic doses of synthetic surfactant in 826 neonates weighing 700 to 1100 grams: effects on mortality rate (Corbet et al). 1995; 126:969-78
Health and neurodevelopmental outcome at 1-year adjusted age in 508 infants weighing 700 to 1100 grams who received prophylaxis with one versus three doses of synthetic surfactant (Gerdes et al). 1995;126:S26-32 (Symposium)
Long-term effects of L-thyroxine therapy for congenital hypothyroidism (Rovet and Ehrlich). 1995;126:380-6
Dose-response relationship, drug—cont'd
A multicenter study of alternate-day prednisone therapy in patients with cystic fibrosis (Eigen et al). 1995;126:515-23
Single-day therapy for rickets (Mimouni) (Letter); (Shah and Finberg) (Reply). 1995;126:1019-20
Drug hypersensitivity
Local reactions to luteinizing hormone releasing hormone analog therapy (Tonini et al) (Letter); (Neely and Wilson) (Reply). 1995;126:159-60
Drugs
Placebo-controlled versus comparative studies of drug effects (Weinberger) (Letter); (Galant) (Reply); (Garfunkel) (Reply). 1995;126:680-1
Drugs of abuse; *see* Street drugs
Duodenal ulcer
Association of symptoms with *Helicobacter pylori* infection in children (Gormally et al). 1995;126:753-6 (CLO)
Dysphagia; *see* Deglutition disorders

E

Eating habits; *see* Food habits
Economic comparison; *see* Costs and cost analysis
Edema
Conjugated hyperbilirubinemia in a newborn infant after maternal (transplacental) treatment with flecainide acetate for fetal tachycardia and fetal hydrops (Vanderhal et al). 1995;126: 988-90 (CLO)
Electrocardiography
Electrocardiographic findings in Rett syndrome (Fuster-Siebert and Castro-Gago). 1995;126:506 (Letter)
Emergency medical services
Lead poisoning: low rates of screening and high prevalence among children seen in inner-city emergency departments (Wiley et al). 1995;126:392-5 (CLO)
Emesis; *see* Vomiting
Encephalitis
Expanded spectrum of herpes simplex encephalitis in childhood (Schlesinger et al). 1995;126:234-41
Encephalopathy; *see* Brain diseases
Endocrine glands
Cardiovascular, renal, and endocrine actions of dopamine in neonates and children (Seri). 1995;126:333-44
Endothelins
Recent developments in the pathophysiology and treatment of persistent pulmonary hypertension of the newborn (Kinsella and Abman). 1995;126:853-64
Energy metabolism
Estimation of energy requirements in persons with severe central nervous system impairment (Bandini et al). 1995;126:828-32
Influence of energy substrates on respiratory gas exchange during conventional mechanical ventilation of preterm infants (Chessex et al). 1995;126:619-24
Measured versus predicted resting energy expenditure in infants: a need for reappraisal (Thomson et al). 1995;126:21-7
Normal energy expenditure in the infant with presymptomatic cystic fibrosis (Bronstein et al). 1995;126:28-33
Relation of activity levels to body fat in infants 6 to 12 months of age (Li et al). 1995;126:353-7
Techniques for measurement of resting energy expenditure in children (Schoeller and Luke) (Letter); (Goran and Johnson) (Reply). 1995;126:679-80
Enteral nutrition
Diarrhea associated with enteral benzodiazepine solutions (Marshall et al). 1995;126:657-9 (CLO)
Enteritis
Familial Guillain-Barré syndrome subsequent to *Campylobacter jejuni* enteritis (Yuki and Tsujino). 1995;126:162 (Letter)

Enteritis—cont'd
Fisher syndrome after *Campylobacter jejuni* enteritis: human leukocyte antigen and the bacterial serotype (Yuki et al). 1995;126:55-7 (CLO)
Enterovirus infections
Diagnosis of neonatal enterovirus infection by polymerase chain reaction (Abzug et al). 1995;126:447-50 (CLO)
Eosinophilia
Acquired platelet dysfunction with eosinophilia in white children (Poon et al). 1995;126:959-61 (CLO)
Epidemiology
Changing trends in the epidemiology and pathogenesis of neonatal chronic lung disease (Rojas et al). 1995;126:605-10
Epinephrine
A randomized trial comparing the efficacy of epinephrine with salbutamol in the treatment of acute bronchiolitis (Menon et al). 1995;126:1004-7 (CLO)
Episodic arthritis; *see* Arthritis
Epithelial cells
Binding of *Pseudomonas aeruginosa* to respiratory epithelial cells from patients with various mutations in the cystic fibrosis transmembrane regulator (Zar et al). 1995;126:230-3
Ergocalciferols
Single-day therapy for rickets (Mimouni) (Letter); (Shah and Finberg) (Reply). 1995;126:1019-20
Erythrocyte transfusion; *see* Blood component transfusion
Erythropoietin
Efficacy and cost analysis of treating very low birth weight infants with erythropoietin during their first two weeks of life: a randomized, placebo-controlled trial (Ohls et al). 1995;126:421-6
Plasma erythropoietin reference ranges in children (Krafte-Jacobs et al). 1995;126:601-3 (CLO)
Evoked potentials, somatosensory
Somatosensory evoked potentials for prediction of outcome in acute severe brain injury (Beca et al). 1995;126:44-9
Exercise
Relation of activity levels to body fat in infants 6 to 12 months of age (Li et al). 1995;126:353-7
Extracorporeal membrane oxygenation
Coagulation factor deficiencies during initiation of extracorporeal membrane oxygenation (McManus et al). 1995;126:900-4
Extremely low birth weight infant; *see* Infant, low birth weight
Eye
Painful keratoderma and photophobia: hallmarks of tyrosinemia type II (Rabinowitz et al). 1995;126:266-9 (CLO)

F

Facial lacerations; *see* Wounds and injuries
Familial hypercholesterolemia; *see* Hypercholesterolemia, familial
Fat emulsions, intravenous
Oxidation of parenteral lipid emulsion by ambient and phototherapy lights: potential toxicity of routine parenteral feeding (Neužil et al). 1995;126:785-90
Fats
Effects of parenteral L-carnitine supplementation on fat metabolism and nutrition in premature neonates (Bonner et al). 1995;126:287-92
Increased fat oxidation in prepubertal obese children: A metabolic defense against further weight gain? (Maffeis et al). 1995;126:15-20
Techniques for measurement of resting energy expenditure in children (Schoeller and Luke) (Letter); (Goran and Johnson) (Reply). 1995;126:679-80
Fatty acid desaturases
Clinical and biochemical characterization of short-chain acyl–coenzyme A dehydrogenase deficiency (Bhala et al). 1995; 126:910-5
Fatty acid desaturases—cont'd
Neonatal onset of medium-chain acyl–coenzyme A dehydrogenase deficiency with confusing biochemical features (Christodoulou et al). 1995;126:65-8 (CLO)
Transient organic aciduria and persistent lacticacidemia in a patient with short-chain acyl–coenzyme A dehydrogenase deficiency (Dawson et al). 1995;126:69-71 (CLO)
Fatty acids, unsaturated
Long-chain polyunsaturated fatty acids in preterm infants: status at birth and its influence on postnatal levels (Foreman–van Drongelen et al). 1995;126:611-8
Febrile children; *see* Fever
Febrile seizures; *see* Convulsions, febrile
Feeding behavior
Abnormal tympanography after supine bottle feeding (Tully et al). 1995;126:S105-11
The clinician's role in teaching proper infant feeding techniques (Lawrence). 1995;126:S112-7
Imaging evaluation of breast-feeding and bottle feeding systems (Nowak et al). 1995;126:S130-4
Impact of attitudes on maternal decisions regarding infant feeding (Losch et al). 1995;126:507-14
Nipple confusion: toward a formal definition (Neifert et al). 1995;126:S125-9
Perspectives on infant feeding: Guest Editor's note (Shelov). 1995;126:S103
Perspectives on infant feeding: Introduction (Erenberg). 1995; 126:S104
Quantitative and qualitative video analysis of infants feeding: angled- and straight-bottle feeding systems (Farber et al). 1995;126:S118-24
Relation between infant feeding and infections during the first six months of life (Beaudry et al). 1995;126:191-7
Fees and charges
Synthetic surfactant for rescue treatment of respiratory distress syndrome in premature infants weighing from 700 to 1350 grams: impact on hospital resource use and charges (Mauskopf et al). 1995;126:94-101
Fetal development
Possible fetal effects of cervical dilation and uterine curettage during the first trimester of pregnancy (Holmes). 1995;126: 131-4 (CLO)
Relation between meconium concentration of the cocaine metabolite benzoylecgonine and fetal growth (Mirochnick et al). 1995;126:636-8 (CLO)
Fetal hydrops; *see* Edema
Fetus, drug effects
Effect of maternal glucocorticoid exposure on risk of severe intraventricular hemorrhage in surfactant-treated preterm infants (Garland et al). 1995;126:272-9
Fever
Efficacy of an observation scale in detecting bacteremia in febrile children three to thirty-six months of age, treated as outpatients (Teach et al). 1995;126:877-81
Furosemide-associated fever (Clegg and Riopel). 1995;126:817-8 (CLO)
A three-month-old girl with fever and hepatomegaly (Jones and Buchino). 1995;126:663-8
Fibrodysplasia ossificans progressiva; *see* Myositis ossificans
Fingernail remover; *see* Poisons
Finland
Successful treatment of Finnish congenital nephrotic syndrome with captopril and indomethacin (Pomeranz et al). 1995; 126:140-2 (CLO)
First trimester of pregnancy; *see* Pregnancy trimester, first
Fisher syndrome
Fisher syndrome after *Campylobacter jejuni* enteritis: human leukocyte antigen and the bacterial serotype (Yuki et al). 1995;126:55-7 (CLO)

Flecainide
Conjugated hyperbilirubinemia in a newborn infant after maternal (transplacental) treatment with flecainide acetate for fetal tachycardia and fetal hydrops (Vanderhal et al). 1995; 126: 988-90 (CLO)
Fluticasone
Placebo-controlled versus comparative studies of drug effects (Weinberger) (Letter); (Galant) (Reply); (Garfunkel) (Reply). 1995;126:680-1
Follow-up studies
Double-blind developmental evaluation at 1-year corrected age of 597 premature infants with birth weights from 500 to 1350 grams enrolled in three placebo-controlled trials of prophylactic synthetic surfactant (Corbet et al). 1995;126:S5-12 (Symposium)
Double-blind evaluation of developmental and health status to age 2 years of infants weighing 700 to 1350 grams treated prophylactically at birth with a single dose of synthetic surfactant or air placebo (Kraybill et al). 1995;126:S33-42 (Symposium)
Double-blind, randomized, placebo-controlled Canadian multicenter trial of two doses of synthetic surfactant or air placebo in 224 infants weighing 500 to 749 grams with respiratory distress syndrome (Smyth et al). 1995;126:S81-9 (Symposium)
Double-blind 1-year follow-up of 1540 infants with respiratory distress syndrome randomized to rescue treatment with two doses of synthetic surfactant or air in four clinical trials (Courtney et al). 1995;126:S43-52 (Symposium)
Effects of two rescue doses of synthetic surfactant in 344 infants with respiratory distress syndrome weighing 750 to 1249 grams: a double-blind, placebo-controlled multicenter Canadian trial (McMillan et al). 1995;126:S90-8 (Symposium)
Health and neurodevelopmental outcome at 1-year adjusted age in 508 infants weighing 700 to 1100 grams who received prophylaxis with one versus three doses of synthetic surfactant (Gerdes et al). 1995;126:S26-32 (Symposium)
One-year follow-up evaluation of 260 premature infants with respiratory distress syndrome and birth weights of 700 to 1350 grams randomized to two rescue doses of synthetic surfactant or air placebo (Gong et al). 1995;126:S68-74 (Symposium)
One-year follow-up of 66 premature infants weighing 500 to 699 grams treated with a single dose of synthetic surfactant or air placebo at birth: results of a double-blind trial (Walther et al). 1995;126:S13-9 (Symposium)
One-year follow-up of 89 infants with birth weights of 500 to 749 grams and respiratory distress syndrome randomized to two rescue doses of synthetic surfactant or air placebo (Casiro et al). 1995;126:S53-60 (Symposium)
One-year follow-up of 273 infants with birth weights of 700 to 1100 grams after prophylactic treatment of respiratory distress syndrome with synthetic surfactant or air placebo (Sell et al). 1995;126:S20-5 (Symposium)
One-year outcome in 232 premature infants with birth weights of 750 to 1249 grams and respiratory distress syndrome randomized to rescue treatment with two doses of synthetic surfactant or air placebo (Saigal et al). 1995;126:S61-7 (Symposium)
Outcome at 1-year adjusted age of 957 infants weighing more than 1250 grams with respiratory distress syndrome randomized to receive synthetic surfactant or air placebo (Sauve et al). 1995;126:S75-80 (Symposium)
Symposium on Synthetic Surfactant II: perspective and commentary (Long et al). 1995;126:S1-4 (Symposium)
Food
Techniques for measurement of resting energy expenditure in children (Schoeller and Luke) (Letter); (Goran and Johnson) (Reply). 1995;126:679-80
Food habits
Promotion of healthy eating habits in children (Crump) (Letter); (Whitaker et al) (Reply). 1995;126:850-1
Formula, infant; *see* Infant food
Fractures
Long-term reduction in bone mass after severe burn injury in children (Klein et al). 1995;126:252-6
Furosemide
Furosemide-associated fever (Clegg and Riopel). 1995;126:817-8 (CLO)

G

Gastritis
Association of symptoms with *Helicobacter pylori* infection in children (Gormally et al). 1995;126:753-6 (CLO)
Gastrointestinal diseases
Peutz-Jeghers syndrome in a neonate (Seara et al). 1995;126:965-7 (CLO)
Relation between infant feeding and infections during the first six months of life (Beaudry et al). 1995;126:191-7
Treatment of intractable gastrointestinal manifestations of chronic granulomatous disease with cyclosporine (Rosh et al). 1995; 126:143-5 (CLO)
Gastrointestinal motility
Overinterpretation of gastroduodenal motility studies: two cases involving Munchausen syndrome by proxy (Baron et al). 1995;126:397-400 (CLO)
Gaucher's disease
Outcome of partial splenectomy for type I Gaucher disease (Zimran et al). 1995;126:596-7 (CLO)
Gene deletion
Deletion of mitochondrial DNA in patient with chronic tubulointerstitial nephritis (Rötig et al). 1995;126:597-601 (CLO)
Genes
Dysmorphic features in patients with complex glycerol kinase deficiency (Scheuerle et al). 1995;126:764-7 (CLO)
True hermaphroditism with 46,XY karyotype and a point mutation in the *SRY* gene (Hiort et al). 1995;126:1022 (Letter)
Genes, regulator
Binding of *Pseudomonas aeruginosa* to respiratory epithelial cells from patients with various mutations in the cystic fibrosis transmembrane regulator (Zar et al). 1995;126:230-3
Gestational age
Response to growth hormone therapy in patients with growth hormone deficiency who were small or appropriate in size for gestational age at birth (Balsamo et al). 1995;126:474-7
Glomerulonephritis
Spectrum of disease associated with anti-neutrophil cytoplasmic autoantibodies in pediatric patients (Ellis et al). 1995;126: 40-3
Glucagon
Pancreatic glucagon levels in infants and children with hyperinsulinemia (Pronicka et al). 1995;126:948-51 (CLO)
Glucocorticoids
Effect of maternal glucocorticoid exposure on risk of severe intraventricular hemorrhage in surfactant-treated preterm infants (Garland et al). 1995;126:272-9
Glucose
Enhanced adrenomedullary response and increased susceptibility to neuroglycopenia: mechanisms underlying the adverse effects of sugar ingestion in healthy children (Jones et al). 1995;126:171-7
Influence of energy substrates on respiratory gas exchange during conventional mechanical ventilation of preterm infants (Chessex et al). 1995;126:619-24
Glucose phosphate dehydrogenase deficiency
Glucose-6-phosphate dehydrogenase deficiency and carboxyhemoglobin concentrations associated with bilirubin-related morbidity and death in Nigerian infants (Slusher et al). 1995; 126:102-8

Glutamine
Use of peritoneal dialysis, continuous arteriovenous hemofiltration, and continuous arteriovenous hemodiafiltration for removal of ammonium chloride and glutamine in rabbits (Semama et al). 1995;126:742-6
Glycerol kinase
Dysmorphic features in patients with complex glycerol kinase deficiency (Scheuerle et al). 1995;126:764-7 (CLO)
Gonadorelin
Combined treatment with growth hormone and gonadotropin-releasing hormone analogs in short normal girls (Saggese et al). 1995;126:468-73
Use of the gonadotropin-releasing hormone agonist triptorelin in the diagnosis of delayed puberty in boys (Zamboni et al). 1995;126:756-8 (CLO)
Gonadotropin-releasing hormone; *see* Gonadorelin
Graft vs host disease
Intact survival with transfusion-associated graft-versus-host disease proved by human leukocyte antigen typing of lymphocytes in skin biopsy specimens (Hentschel et al). 1995;126:61-4 (CLO)
Granisetron
A randomized comparison of intravenously administered granisetron versus chlorpromazine plus dexamethasone in the prevention of ifosfamide-induced emesis in children (Hählen et al). 1995;126:309-13
Granulocyte colony-stimulating factor
Administration of granulocyte colony-stimulating factor to neutropenic low birth weight infants of mothers with preeclampsia (Makhlouf et al). 1995;126:454-56 (CLO)
Disseminated intravascular coagulation associated with granulocyte colony-stimulating factor therapy in a child with human immunodeficiency virus infection (Mueller et al). 1995;126:749-52 (CLO)
Effect of granulocyte colony-stimulating factor on preeclampsia-associated neonatal neutropenia (La Gamma et al). 1995;126:457-9 (CLO)
Transformation of congenital neutropenia into monosomy 7 and acute nonlymphoblastic leukemia in a child treated with granulocyte colony-stimulating factor (Weinblatt et al). 1995;126:263-5 (CLO)
Granulomatous disease, chronic
Treatment of intractable gastrointestinal manifestations of chronic granulomatous disease with cyclosporine (Rosh et al). 1995;126:143-5 (CLO)
Group A streptococci; *see Streptococcus pyogenes*
Growth
Growth and the growth hormone axis in prepubertal children with asthma (Crowley et al). 1995;126:297-303
Growth disorders
Predictive factors in the determination of final height in boys with constitutional delay of growth and puberty (Albanese and Stanhope). 1995;126:545-50
Growth hormone, pituitary; *see* Somatotropin
GTP cyclohydrolase
A missense mutation in a patient with guanosine triphosphate cyclohydrolase I deficiency missed in the newborn screening program (Blau et al). 1995;126:401-5 (CLO)
Guanosine triphosphate cyclohydrolase; *see* GTP cyclohydrolase
Guillain-Barré syndrome; *see* Polyradiculoneuritis
Gynecomastia
Prepubertal gynecomastia during growth hormone therapy (Malozowski and Stadel). 1995;126:659-61 (CLO)

H

Haemophilus influenzae
Bacteriologic failure of amoxicillin-clavulanate in treatment of acute otitis media caused by nontypeable *Haemophilus influenzae* (Patel et al). 1995;126:799-806
***Haemophilus influenzae* vaccine; *see* Bacterial vaccines**
Health
Double-blind evaluation of developmental and health status to age 2 years of infants weighing 700 to 1350 grams treated prophylactically at birth with a single dose of synthetic surfactant or air placebo (Kraybill et al). 1995;126:S33-42 (Symposium)
Health and neurodevelopmental outcome at 1-year adjusted age in 508 infants weighing 700 to 1100 grams who received prophylaxis with one versus three doses of synthetic surfactant (Gerdes et al). 1995;126:S26-32 (Symposium)
Health resources
Synthetic surfactant for rescue treatment of respiratory distress syndrome in premature infants weighing from 700 to 1350 grams: impact on hospital resource use and charges (Mauskopf et al). 1995;126:94-101
Hearing
Otitis media, hearing sensitivity, and maternal responsiveness in relation to language during infancy (Roberts et al). 1995;126:481-9
Hearing tests
Abnormal tympanography after supine bottle feeding (Tully et al). 1995;126:S105-11
Heart defects, congenital
Neurodevelopmental outcome of infants with hypoplastic left heart syndrome (Rogers et al). 1995;126:496-8 (CLO)
Height; *see* Body height
Helicobacter pylori
Association of symptoms with *Helicobacter pylori* infection in children (Gormally et al). 1995;126:753-6 (CLO)
Helicobacter pylori infection in neurologically impaired children (Mauk) (Letter); (Proujansky et al) (Reply). 1995;126:849-50
Hematocrit
Reducing blood donor exposures in low birth weight infants by the use of older, unwashed packed red blood cells (Lee et al). 1995;126:280-6
Hemofiltration
Use of peritoneal dialysis, continuous arteriovenous hemofiltration, and continuous arteriovenous hemodiafiltration for removal of ammonium chloride and glutamine in rabbits (Semama et al). 1995;126:742-6
Hemoglobin, sickle
Life-threatening infection in two children with hemoglobin S–beta-thalassemia (Lynch and Tobias). 1995;126:581-2 (CLO)
Hemoglobin A, glycosylated
Hemoglobin A_{1c} levels in young patients with diabetes beyond the "honeymoon" period (Dorchy) (Letter); (Tamborlane and Nathan) (Reply). 1995;126:1020-1
Hemolysis
Fatal hemolysis caused by ceftriaxone (Lascari and Amyot). 1995;126:816-7 (CLO)
Fatal hemolysis induced by ceftriaxone in a child with sickle cell anemia (Bernini et al). 1995;126:813-5 (CLO)
Hemophilia
Loss of detectable antibody to hepatitis B surface antigen in immunized patients with hemophilia but without human immunodeficiency virus infection (Maris et al). 1995;126:269-71 (CLO)
Hemorrhage
Coagulation factor deficiencies during initiation of extracorporeal membrane oxygenation (McManus et al). 1995;126:900-4
Effect of maternal glucocorticoid exposure on risk of severe intraventricular hemorrhage in surfactant-treated preterm infants (Garland et al). 1995;126:272-9
Hemorrhagic colitis; *see* Colitis
Heparin
Catheter-related thrombosis in critically ill children: comparison of catheters with and without heparin bonding (Krafte-Jacobs et al). 1995;126:50-4
Hepatitis A
Acute pancreatitis associated with acute hepatitis A in a young child (Shrier et al). 1995;126:57-9 (CLO)

Hepatitis antibodies
Infectious hazards of immune globulin (Barton) (Letter); (Karna et al) (Reply). 1995;126:321-2
Hepatitis B antibodies
Loss of detectable antibody to hepatitis B surface antigen in immunized patients with hemophilia but without human immunodeficiency virus infection (Maris et al). 1995;126:269-71 (CLO)
Hepatitis B e antigens
Long-term efficacy of recombinant hepatitis B vaccine and risk of natural infection in infants born to mothers with hepatitis B e antigen (Lee et al). 1995;126:716-21
Hepatitis B vaccines
Long-term efficacy of recombinant hepatitis B vaccine and risk of natural infection in infants born to mothers with hepatitis B e antigen (Lee et al). 1995;126:716-21
Hepatitis C virus
Absence of infection in breast-fed infants born to hepatitis C virus–infected mothers (Lin et al). 1995;126:589-91 (CLO)
Hepatomegaly
A three-month-old girl with fever and hepatomegaly (Jones and Buchino). 1995;126:663-8
Hermaphroditism
True hermaphroditism with 46,XY karyotype and a point mutation in the *SRY* gene (Hiort et al). 1995;126:1022 (Letter)
Herpes simplex
Expanded spectrum of herpes simplex encephalitis in childhood (Schlesinger et al). 1995;126:234-41
Heterotopic ossification; *see* Ossification, heterotopic
HIV
Disseminated intravascular coagulation associated with granulocyte colony-stimulating factor therapy in a child with human immunodeficiency virus infection (Mueller et al). 1995;126: 749-52 (CLO)
Encephalopathy in children with perinatally acquired human immunodeficiency virus infection (Lobato et al). 1995;126: 710-5
Immunologic characterization of children vertically infected with human immunodeficiency virus, with slow or rapid disease progression (Viganó et al). 1995;126:368-74
Loss of detectable antibody to hepatitis B surface antigen in immunized patients with hemophilia but without human immunodeficiency virus infection (Maris et al). 1995;126:269-71 (CLO)
Viral measurement by polymerase chain reaction–based assays in human immunodeficiency virus–infected infants (Palumbo et al). 1995;126:592-5 (CLO)
HIV-1
Birth order, delivery route, and concordance in the transmission of human immunodeficiency virus type 1 from mothers to twins (Duliège et al). 1995;126:625-32
Cognitive assessment of school-age children infected with maternally transmitted human immunodeficiency virus type 1 (Tardieu et al). 1995;126:375-9
Vertical transmission of human immunodeficiency virus type I: autologous neutralizing antibody, virus load, and virus phenotype (Husson et al). 1995;126:865-71
HLA antigens
Fisher syndrome after *Campylobacter jejuni* enteritis: human leukocyte antigen and the bacterial serotype (Yuki et al). 1995;126:55-7 (CLO)
Intact survival with transfusion-associated graft-versus-host disease proved by human leukocyte antigen typing of lymphocytes in skin biopsy specimens (Hentschel et al). 1995;126:61-4 (CLO)
Home nursing
Standards for home care of sick children (McConnell and Perkin) (Letter); (Goldberg et al) (Reply). 1995;126:681-2
Homeostasis
Mineral homeostasis and bone mass at diagnosis in children with acute lymphoblastic leukemia (Halton et al). 1995;126:557-64
Hormone analogs; *see* Hormones, synthetic
Hormones
Effects of acute hyperglycemia on mental efficiency and counterregulatory hormones in adolescents with insulin-dependent diabetes mellitus (Gschwend et al). 1995;126:178-84
Hormones, synthetic
Local reactions to luteinizing hormone releasing hormone analog therapy (Tonini et al) (Letter); (Neely and Wilson) (Reply). 1995;126:159-60
Hospital discharge; *see* Patient discharge
Hospitalization
Hospitalization for lower respiratory tract illness in infants: variation in rates among counties in New York State and areas within Monroe County (McConnochie et al). 1995;126:220-9
Hospitals
Synthetic surfactant for rescue treatment of respiratory distress syndrome in premature infants weighing from 700 to 1350 grams: impact on hospital resource use and charges (Mauskopf et al). 1995;126:94-101
Human immunodeficiency virus; *see* HIV
Human leukocyte antigens; *see* HLA antigens
Human milk; *see* Milk, human
Hydrocortisone
Reference ranges for serum cortisol and 17-hydroxyprogesterone levels in preterm infants (Al Saedi et al). 1995;126:985-7 (CLO)
Hydrogen ions; *see* Protons
Hydroxyprogesterones
Reference ranges for serum cortisol and 17-hydroxyprogesterone levels in preterm infants (Al Saedi et al). 1995;126:985-7 (CLO)
Hymenoptera
Subsequent insect stings in children with hypersensitivity to Hymenoptera (Hauk et al). 1995;126:185-90
Venom immunotherapy: Who should receive it? (Bierman). 1995;126:257-8 (Editor's column)
Hyperbilirubinemia
Comparison of fiberoptic and conventional phototherapy for neonatal hyperbilirubinemia (Larsen and Whitelaw) (Letter); (Tan) (Reply). 1995;126:1018
Conjugated hyperbilirubinemia in a newborn infant after maternal (transplacental) treatment with flecainide acetate for fetal tachycardia and fetal hydrops (Vanderhal et al). 1995;126: 988-90 (CLO)
Hypercalcemia
Human synthetic calcitonin therapy for hypercalcemia of immobilization (Kaul and Sockalosky). 1995;126:825-7 (CLO)
Hypercholesterolemia, familial
Low-density lipoprotein apheresis as long-term treatment for children with homozygous familial hypercholesterolemia (Zwiener et al). 1995;126:728-35
Hyperglycemia
Effects of acute hyperglycemia on mental efficiency and counterregulatory hormones in adolescents with insulin-dependent diabetes mellitus (Gschwend et al). 1995;126:178-84
Hyperinsulinism
Discordance for hyperinsulinemic hypoglycemia in monozygotic twins (Santer et al) (Letter); (Thornton et al) (Reply). 1995; 126:1017
Pancreatic glucagon levels in infants and children with hyperinsulinemia (Pronicka et al). 1995;126:948-51 (CLO)
Hyperkalemia
Internal potassium shift in premature infants: cause of nonoliguric hyperkalemia (Sato et al). 1995;126:109-13
Hypersensitivity
Subsequent insect stings in children with hypersensitivity to Hymenoptera (Hauk et al). 1995;126:185-90
Venom immunotherapy: Who should receive it? (Bierman). 1995;126:257-8 (Editor's column)
Hypocalcemia
Consumption of soft drinks with phosphoric acid as a risk factor for the development of hypocalcemia in children: a case-control study (Mazariegos-Ramos et al). 1995;126:940-2 (CLO)

Hypocalcemia—cont'd
Healing of rickets during vitamin D therapy despite defective vitamin D receptors in two siblings with vitamin D–dependent rickets type II (Kruse and Feldmann). 1995;126:145-8 (CLO)
Hypoglycemia
Discordance for hyperinsulinemic hypoglycemia in monozygotic twins (Santer et al) (Letter); (Thornton et al) (Reply). 1995; 126:1017
Effects of acute hyperglycemia on mental efficiency and counterregulatory hormones in adolescents with insulin-dependent diabetes mellitus (Gschwend et al). 1995;126:178-84
Enhanced adrenomedullary response and increased susceptibility to neuroglycopenia: mechanisms underlying the adverse effects of sugar ingestion in healthy children (Jones et al). 1995;126:171-7
Pancreatic glucagon levels in infants and children with hyperinsulinemia (Pronicka et al). 1995;126:948-51 (CLO)
Hypoplastic left heart syndrome; *see* Heart defects, congenital
Hypotension
Hypotension in preterm infants (Milstein) (Letter); (Faix) (Reply). 1995;126:160-1
Hypothalamus
Bone mineralization, hypothalamic amenorrhea, and sex steroid therapy in adolescents and young adults (Hergenroeder). 1995;126:683-9
Hypothyroidism
Brain metabolite changes on in vivo proton magnetic resonance spectroscopy in children with congenital hypothyroidism (Gupta et al). 1995;126:389-92 (CLO)
Long-term effects of L-thyroxine therapy for congenital hypothyroidism (Rovet and Ehrlich). 1995;126:380-6
Motor and cognitive development in children with congenital hypothyroidism (Mitchell and Klein) (Letter); (Vulsma and Kooistra) (Reply). 1995;126:673-4

I

Ifosfamide
A randomized comparison of intravenously administered granisetron versus chlorpromazine plus dexamethasone in the prevention of ifosfamide-induced emesis in children (Hählen et al). 1995;126:309-13
IgE
Immunologic characterization of children vertically infected with human immunodeficiency virus, with slow or rapid disease progression (Viganó et al). 1995;126:368-74
IgG
Differences in clinical significance of maternal-infant blood group incompatibility in mothers with blood type O, A, or B (Perl) (Letter); (Ozolek et al) (Reply). 1995;126:322-3
Ileus; *see* Intestinal obstruction
Immobilization
Human synthetic calcitonin therapy for hypercalcemia of immobilization (Kaul and Sockalosky). 1995;126:825-7 (CLO)
Immune globulin; *see* Immunoglobulins, intravenous
Immune thrombocytopenic purpura; *see* Purpura, thrombocytopenic
Immunity, cellular
Cell-mediated immune status of children with recurrent infection (Herrod et al). 1995;126:530-6
Immunization
Development of a vaccine tracking system to improve the rate of age-appropriate primary immunization in children of lower socioeconomic status (Abramson et al). 1995;126:583-6 (CLO)
Effect of neonatal immunization with diphtheria and tetanus toxoids on antibody responses to *Haemophilus influenzae* type b conjugate vaccines (Lieberman et al). 1995;126:198-205
Loss of detectable antibody to hepatitis B surface antigen in immunized patients with hemophilia but without human immunodeficiency virus infection (Maris et al). 1995;126:269-71 (CLO)
Immunoassay
Comparison of an optical immunoassay technique with two culture methods for the detection of group A streptococci in a pediatric office (Roddey et al). 1995;126:931-3 (CLO)
Diagnosis of group A streptococcal pharyngitis in a private clinic: comparative evaluation of an optical immunoassay method and culture (Fries). 1995;126:933-6 (CLO)
Immunodeficiency; *see* Immunosuppression
Immunogenetics
Enhanced antibody responses in infants given different sequences of heterogeneous *Haemophilus influenzae* type b conjugate vaccines (Greenberg et al). 1995;126:206-11
Immunoglobulins, intravenous
Comparative safety and efficacy of two immune globulin products in Kawasaki disease (Rosenfeld et al). 1995;126:1000-3
Infectious hazards of immune globulin (Barton) (Letter); (Karna et al) (Reply). 1995;126:321-2
Kawasaki disease in infants less than one year of age (Rosenfeld et al). 1995;126:524-9
Immunosuppression
Cancer in children with primary or secondary immunodeficiencies (Mueller and Pizzo). 1995;126:1-10
Immunotherapy
Venom immunotherapy: Who should receive it? (Bierman). 1995;126:257-8 (Editor's column)
Indomethacin
Successful treatment of Finnish congenital nephrotic syndrome with captopril and indomethacin (Pomeranz et al). 1995;126: 140-2 (CLO)
Infant
Long-term efficacy of recombinant hepatitis B vaccine and risk of natural infection in infants born to mothers with hepatitis B e antigen (Lee et al). 1995;126:716-21
Measured versus predicted resting energy expenditure in infants: a need for reappraisal (Thomson et al). 1995;126:21-7
Normal energy expenditure in the infant with presymptomatic cystic fibrosis (Bronstein et al). 1995;126:28-33
Otitis media, hearing sensitivity, and maternal responsiveness in relation to language during infancy (Roberts et al). 1995; 126:481-9
Oxidation of parenteral lipid emulsion by ambient and phototherapy lights: potential toxicity of routine parenteral feeding (Neužil et al). 1995;126:785-90
Relation between infant feeding and infections during the first six months of life (Beaudry et al). 1995;126:191-7
Relation of activity levels to body fat in infants 6 to 12 months of age (Li et al). 1995;126:353-7
Infant, diseases
Cytokine elevations in infants with bacterial and aseptic meningitis (Dulkerian et al). 1995;126:872-6
Efficacy of an observation scale in detecting bacteremia in febrile children three to thirty-six months of age, treated as outpatients (Teach et al). 1995;126:877-81
Furosemide-associated fever (Clegg and Riopel). 1995;126:817-8 (CLO)
Hospitalization for lower respiratory tract illness in infants: variation in rates among counties in New York State and areas within Monroe County (McConnochie et al). 1995;126: 220-9
Kawasaki disease in infants less than one year of age (Rosenfeld et al). 1995;126:524-9
A three-month-old girl with fever and hepatomegaly (Jones and Buchino). 1995;126:663-8
Infant, low birth weight
Administration of granulocyte colony-stimulating factor to neutropenic low birth weight infants of mothers with preeclampsia (Makhlouf et al). 1995;126:454-56 (CLO)
Effect of the arterial oxygenation level on cardiac output, oxygen extraction, and oxygen consumption in low birth weight infants receiving mechanical ventilation (Schulze et al). 1995;126: 777-84

Infant, low birth weight—cont'd
Effect of pulse dexamethasone therapy on the incidence and severity of chronic lung disease in the very low birth weight infant (Brozanski et al). 1995;126:769-76
Efficacy and cost analysis of treating very low birth weight infants with erythropoietin during their first two weeks of life: a randomized, placebo-controlled trial (Ohls et al). 1995;126:421-6
Isolation of *Ureaplasma urealyticum* from low birth weight infants (Waites et al) (Letter); (Crouse and Reese) (Letter); (Heggie et al) (Reply). 1995;126:502-4
Postnatal attainment of intrauterine macromineral accretion rates in low birth weight infants fed fortified human milk (Schanler and Abrams). 1995;126:441-7
Reducing blood donor exposures in low birth weight infants by the use of older, unwashed packed red blood cells (Lee et al). 1995;126:280-6
Secular changes in the outcomes to eighteen to twenty-four months of age of extremely low birth weight infants, with adjustment for changes in risk factors and severity of illness (Perlman et al). 1995;126:75-87
Twenty-month outcome in ventilator-dependent, very low birth weight infants born during the early years of dexamethasone therapy (Furman et al). 1995;126:434-40
Vitamin A and E status in very low birth weight infants: development of an improved parenteral delivery system (Inder et al). 1995;126:128-31 (CLO)

Infant, newborn
Band neutrophil counts in neonates (Rosenfeld and MacGregor) (Letter); (Schelonka et al) (Reply). 1995;126:504-6
Cardiovascular, renal, and endocrine actions of dopamine in neonates and children (Seri). 1995;126:333-44
Effect of neonatal immunization with diphtheria and tetanus toxoids on antibody responses to *Haemophilus influenzae* type b conjugate vaccines (Lieberman et al). 1995;126:198-205
Neonatal mortality rate: Is further improvement possible? (Philip). 1995;126:427-33
Newborn screening for congenital adrenal hyperplasia in New Zealand (Cutfield and Webster). 1995;126:118-21
Screening neonates for intrauterine cocaine exposure (Neuspiel) (Letter); (Ryan and Phelps) (Reply). 1995;126:323-4
Soluble interleukin-2 receptor as a predictor of neonatal sepsis (Spear et al). 1995;126:982-5 (CLO)
Use of the urine-to-blood carbon dioxide tension gradient as a measurement of impaired distal tubular hydrogen ion secretion among neonates (Lin et al). 1995;126:114-7

Infant, newborn, diseases
Abnormalities in control of ventilation in newborn infants with myelomeningocele (Petersen et al). 1995;126:1011-5
Acuity scores as predictors of cost-related outcomes of neonatal intensive care (Kotagal et al). 1995;126:88-93
Blood flow velocities and neonatal asphyxia (Elliott) (Letter); (Akinbi and Bhutani) (Reply). 1995;126:675-6
Changing trends in the epidemiology and pathogenesis of neonatal chronic lung disease (Rojas et al). 1995;126:605-10
Comparison of fiberoptic and conventional phototherapy for neonatal hyperbilirubinemia (Larsen and Whitelaw) (Letter); (Tan) (Reply). 1995;126:1018
Congenital nephrotic syndrome in neonatal lupus syndrome (Westenend). 1995;126:851 (Letter)
Conjugated hyperbilirubinemia in a newborn infant after maternal (transplacental) treatment with flecainide acetate for fetal tachycardia and fetal hydrops (Vanderhal et al). 1995;126:988-90 (CLO)
Diagnosis of neonatal enterovirus infection by polymerase chain reaction (Abzug et al). 1995;126:447-50 (CLO)
Double-blind, randomized trial of one versus three prophylactic doses of synthetic surfactant in 826 neonates weighing 700 to 1100 grams: effects on mortality rate (Corbet et al). 1995;126:969-78

Infant, newborn, diseases—cont'd
Effect of granulocyte colony-stimulating factor on preeclampsia-associated neonatal neutropenia (La Gamma et al). 1995;126:457-9 (CLO)
Improved oxygenation during synchronized intermittent mandatory ventilation in neonates with respiratory distress syndrome: a randomized, crossover study (Cleary et al). 1995;126:407-11
A missense mutation in a patient with guanosine triphosphate cyclohydrolase I deficiency missed in the newborn screening program (Blau et al). 1995;126:401-5 (CLO)
Neonatal onset of medium-chain acyl–coenzyme A dehydrogenase deficiency with confusing biochemical features (Christodoulou et al). 1995;126:65-8 (CLO)
Neonatal-onset propionicacidemia: neurologic and developmental profiles, and implications for management (North et al). 1995;126:916-22
Peutz-Jeghers syndrome in a neonate (Seara et al). 1995;126:965-7 (CLO)
Placement of umbilical venous catheters with use of bedside real-time ultrasonography (Greenberg et al). 1995;126:633-5 (CLO)
Recent developments in the pathophysiology and treatment of persistent pulmonary hypertension of the newborn (Kinsella and Abman). 1995;126:853-64
Use of intravenous lipids in neonates (Helbock and Ames). 1995;126:747-8 (Editor's column)

Infant, premature
Double-blind developmental evaluation at 1-year corrected age of 597 premature infants with birth weights from 500 to 1350 grams enrolled in three placebo-controlled trials of prophylactic synthetic surfactant (Corbet et al). 1995;126:S5-12 (Symposium)
Double-blind evaluation of developmental and health status to age 2 years of infants weighing 700 to 1350 grams treated prophylactically at birth with a single dose of synthetic surfactant or air placebo (Kraybill et al). 1995;126:S33-42 (Symposium)
Double-blind, randomized, placebo-controlled Canadian multicenter trial of two doses of synthetic surfactant or air placebo in 224 infants weighing 500 to 749 grams with respiratory distress syndrome (Smyth et al). 1995;126:S81-9 (Symposium)
Double-blind, randomized trial of one versus three prophylactic doses of synthetic surfactant in 826 neonates weighing 700 to 1100 grams: effects on mortality rate (Corbet et al). 1995;126:969-78
Double-blind 1-year follow-up of 1540 infants with respiratory distress syndrome randomized to rescue treatment with two doses of synthetic surfactant or air in four clinical trials (Courtney et al). 1995;126:S43-52 (Symposium)
Effect of maternal glucocorticoid exposure on risk of severe intraventricular hemorrhage in surfactant-treated preterm infants (Garland et al). 1995;126:272-9
Effects of parenteral L-carnitine supplementation on fat metabolism and nutrition in premature neonates (Bonner et al). 1995;126:287-92
Effects of two rescue doses of synthetic surfactant in 344 infants with respiratory distress syndrome weighing 750 to 1249 grams: a double-blind, placebo-controlled multicenter Canadian trial (McMillan et al). 1995;126:S90-8 (Symposium)
Health and neurodevelopmental outcome at 1-year adjusted age in 508 infants weighing 700 to 1100 grams who received prophylaxis with one versus three doses of synthetic surfactant (Gerdes et al). 1995;126:S26-32 (Symposium)
Hypotension in preterm infants (Milstein) (Letter); (Faix) (Reply). 1995;126:160-1
Influence of energy substrates on respiratory gas exchange during conventional mechanical ventilation of preterm infants (Chessex et al). 1995;126:619-24
Inhaled nitric oxide for premature infants after prolonged rupture of the membranes (Peliowski et al). 1995;126:450-53 (CLO)
Internal potassium shift in premature infants: cause of nonoliguric hyperkalemia (Sato et al). 1995;126:109-13

Infant, premature—cont'd
Long-chain polyunsaturated fatty acids in preterm infants: status at birth and its influence on postnatal levels (Foreman–van Drongelen et al). 1995;126:611-8
One-year follow-up evaluation of 260 premature infants with respiratory distress syndrome and birth weights of 700 to 1350 grams randomized to two rescue doses of synthetic surfactant or air placebo (Gong et al). 1995;126:S68-74 (Symposium)
One-year follow-up of 66 premature infants weighing 500 to 699 grams treated with a single dose of synthetic surfactant or air placebo at birth: results of a double-blind trial (Walther et al). 1995;126:S13-9 (Symposium)
One-year follow-up of 89 infants with birth weights of 500 to 749 grams and respiratory distress syndrome randomized to two rescue doses of synthetic surfactant or air placebo (Casiro et al). 1995;126:S53-60 (Symposium)
One-year follow-up of 273 infants with birth weights of 700 to 1100 grams after prophylactic treatment of respiratory distress syndrome with synthetic surfactant or air placebo (Sell et al). 1995;126:S20-5 (Symposium)
One-year outcome in 232 premature infants with birth weights of 750 to 1249 grams and respiratory distress syndrome randomized to rescue treatment with two doses of synthetic surfactant or air placebo (Saigal et al). 1995;126:S61-7 (Symposium)
Outcome at 1-year adjusted age of 957 infants weighing more than 1250 grams with respiratory distress syndrome randomized to receive synthetic surfactant or air placebo (Sauve et al). 1995;126:S75-80 (Symposium)
Partial liquid ventilation in premature lambs with respiratory distress syndrome: efficacy and compatibility with exogenous surfactant (Leach et al). 1995;126:412-20
Plasma mineral concentrations in preterm infants fed a nutrient-enriched formula after hospital discharge (Rajaram et al). 1995;126:791-6
Reference ranges for newer thyroid function tests in premature infants (Adams et al). 1995;126:122-7
Reference ranges for serum cortisol and 17-hydroxyprogesterone levels in preterm infants (Al Saedi et al). 1995;126:985-7 (CLO)
Symposium on Synthetic Surfactant II: perspective and commentary (Long et al). 1995;126:S1-4 (Symposium)
Synthetic surfactant for rescue treatment of respiratory distress syndrome in premature infants weighing from 700 to 1350 grams: impact on hospital resource use and charges (Mauskopf et al). 1995;126:94-101

Infant death
Congenital cytomegalovirus infection as a result of nonprimary cytomegalovirus disease in a mother with acquired immunodeficiency syndrome (Schwebke et al). 1995;126:293-5 (CLO)
Double-blind developmental evaluation at 1-year corrected age of 597 premature infants with birth weights from 500 to 1350 grams enrolled in three placebo-controlled trials of prophylactic synthetic surfactant (Corbet et al). 1995;126:S5-12 (Symposium)
Double-blind, randomized trial of one versus three prophylactic doses of synthetic surfactant in 826 neonates weighing 700 to 1100 grams: effects on mortality rate (Corbet et al). 1995; 126:969-78
Glucose-6-phosphate dehydrogenase deficiency and carboxyhemoglobin concentrations associated with bilirubin-related morbidity and death in Nigerian infants (Slusher et al). 1995; 126:102-8
Neonatal mortality rate: Is further improvement possible? (Philip). 1995;126:427-33
A reexamination of the risk factors for the sudden infant death syndrome (Taylor and Sanderson). 1995;126:887-91
Secular changes in the outcomes to eighteen to twenty-four months of age of extremely low birth weight infants, with adjustment for changes in risk factors and severity of illness (Perlman et al). 1995;126:75-87

Infant death—cont'd
Symposium on Synthetic Surfactant II: perspective and commentary (Long et al). 1995;126:S1-4 (Symposium)

Infant feeding; *see* Feeding behavior

Infant food
Differences in morbidity between breast-fed and formula-fed infants (Dewey et al). 1995;126:696-702
Plasma mineral concentrations in preterm infants fed a nutrient-enriched formula after hospital discharge (Rajaram et al). 1995;126:791-6

Infection
Absence of infection in breast-fed infants born to hepatitis C virus–infected mothers (Lin et al). 1995;126:589-91 (CLO)
Bacteriuria in children with neurogenic bladder treated with intermittent catheterization: natural history (Schlager et al). 1995;126:490-6
Band neutrophil counts in neonates (Rosenfeld and MacGregor) (Letter); (Schelonka et al) (Reply). 1995;126:504-6
Cell-mediated immune status of children with recurrent infection (Herrod et al). 1995;126:530-6
Efficacy of an observation scale in detecting bacteremia in febrile children three to thirty-six months of age, treated as outpatients (Teach et al). 1995;126:877-81
Infectious hazards of immune globulin (Barton) (Letter); (Karna et al) (Reply). 1995;126:321-2
Life-threatening infection in two children with hemoglobin S–beta-thalassemia (Lynch and Tobias). 1995;126:581-2 (CLO)
Long-term efficacy of recombinant hepatitis B vaccine and risk of natural infection in infants born to mothers with hepatitis B e antigen (Lee et al). 1995;126:716-21
Relation between infant feeding and infections during the first six months of life (Beaudry et al). 1995;126:191-7

Inferior vena cava; *see* Vena cava, inferior

Infusions, intravenous
Intravenous morphine pharmacokinetics in pediatric patients with sickle cell disease (Dampier et al). 1995;126:461-7
A randomized comparison of intravenously administered granisetron versus chlorpromazine plus dexamethasone in the prevention of ifosfamide-induced emesis in children (Hählen et al). 1995;126:309-13
Use of intravenous lipids in neonates (Helbock and Ames). 1995;126:747-8 (Editor's column)

Inhaled administration; *see* Administration, inhalation

Injections
Permanent heterotopic ossification at the injection site after diphtheria-tetanus-pertussis immunizations in children who have fibrodysplasia ossificans progressiva (Lanchoney et al). 1995;126:762-4 (CLO)

Inner city health; *see* Urban health

Insect bites and stings
Subsequent insect stings in children with hypersensitivity to Hymenoptera (Hauk et al). 1995;126:185-90
Venom immunotherapy: Who should receive it? (Bierman). 1995;126:257-8 (Editor's column)

Insulin-dependent diabetes; *see* Diabetes mellitus, insulin-dependent

Insulin-like growth factor
Growth and the growth hormone axis in prepubertal children with asthma (Crowley et al). 1995;126:297-303

Insulin resistance
Relationship between insulin resistance and abnormal lipid profile in obese adolescents (Steinberger et al). 1995;126: 690-5

Intelligence
Long-term effects of L-thyroxine therapy for congenital hypothyroidism (Rovet and Ehrlich). 1995;126:380-6

Intensive care units, neonatal
Acuity scores as predictors of cost-related outcomes of neonatal intensive care (Kotagal et al). 1995;126:88-93

Interleukin-2 receptors; *see* Receptors, interleukin-2

Interleukin-6
Cytokine elevations in infants with bacterial and aseptic meningitis (Dulkerian et al). 1995;126:872-6
Intestinal obstruction
Incidence of liver disease in patients with cystic fibrosis and meconium ileus (Lindblad et al) (Letter); (Colombo et al) (Reply). 1995;126:155-6
Intravenous infusions; *see* Infusions, intravenous
Intubation, intratracheal
Improved oxygenation during synchronized intermittent mandatory ventilation in neonates with respiratory distress syndrome: a randomized, crossover study (Cleary et al). 1995;126:407-11
Ipratropium
Efficacy of frequent nebulized ipratropium bromide added to frequent high-dose albuterol therapy in severe childhood asthma (Schuh et al). 1995;126:639-45
Ischemic stroke; *see* Cerebrovascular disorders
Italy
Lysinuric protein intolerance characterized by bone marrow abnormalities and severe clinical course (Parenti et al). 1995;126:246-51

J

Jaundice
Glucose-6-phosphate dehydrogenase deficiency and carboxyhemoglobin concentrations associated with bilirubin-related morbidity and death in Nigerian infants (Slusher et al). 1995;126:102-8
Jaundice, neonatal
Comparison of fiberoptic and conventional phototherapy for neonatal hyperbilirubinemia (Larsen and Whitelaw) (Letter); (Tan) (Reply). 1995;126:1018

K

Karyotyping
True hermaphroditism with 46,XY karyotype and a point mutation in the *SRY* gene (Hiort et al). 1995;126:1022 (Letter)
Kawasaki disease; *see* Mucocutaneous lymph node syndrome
Kempe, C Henry
C. Henry Kempe (Fulginiti). 1995;126:152-4 (Profiles)
Keratoderma, palmoplantar
Painful keratoderma and photophobia: hallmarks of tyrosinemia type II (Rabinowitz et al). 1995;126:266-9 (CLO)
Kidney
Cardiovascular, renal, and endocrine actions of dopamine in neonates and children (Seri). 1995;126:333-44
Diagnostic accuracy of urinary tract infection and subsequent development of renal scars (Koskimies) (Letter); (Hoberman and Wald) (Reply). 1995;126:157-9
Methemoglobinemia associated with acidosis of probable renal origin (Sager et al). 1995;126:59-61 (CLO)
Kidney tubules, distal
Use of the urine-to-blood carbon dioxide tension gradient as a measurement of impaired distal tubular hydrogen ion secretion among neonates (Lin et al). 1995;126:114-7

L

Labor
Long-chain polyunsaturated fatty acids in preterm infants: status at birth and its influence on postnatal levels (Foreman–van Drongelen et al). 1995;126:611-8
Possible fetal effects of cervical dilation and uterine curettage during the first trimester of pregnancy (Holmes). 1995;126:131-4 (CLO)
Laboratory experience; *see* Research
Lactates
Congenital lacticacidemia caused by lipoamide dehydrogenase deficiency with favorable outcome (Elpeleg et al). 1995;126:72-4 (CLO)
Lactic acid; *see* Lactates
Transient organic aciduria and persistent lacticacidemia in a patient with short-chain acyl–coenzyme A dehydrogenase deficiency (Dawson et al). 1995;126:69-71 (CLO)
Lactic acidosis; *see* Acidosis, lactic
Language
Otitis media, hearing sensitivity, and maternal responsiveness in relation to language during infancy (Roberts et al). 1995;126:481-9
Lead poisoning
Lead poisoning: low rates of screening and high prevalence among children seen in inner-city emergency departments (Wiley et al). 1995;126:392-5 (CLO)
Letters
Letters. 1995;126:155-62, 321-5, 502-6, 673-82, 847-52, 1017-22
Leukemia
Fatal hemolysis caused by ceftriaxone (Lascari and Amyot). 1995;126:816-7 (CLO)
Relation of growth hormone deficiency and leukemia (Rapaport et al). 1995;126:759-61 (CLO)
Leukemia, lymphocytic, acute
Lactic acidosis in a patient with acute lymphoblastic leukemia (Robson and Leung). 1995;126:1021 (Letter)
Mineral homeostasis and bone mass at diagnosis in children with acute lymphoblastic leukemia (Halton et al). 1995;126:557-64
Leukemia, nonlymphocytic, acute
Transformation of congenital neutropenia into monosomy 7 and acute nonlymphoblastic leukemia in a child treated with granulocyte colony-stimulating factor (Weinblatt et al). 1995;126:263-5 (CLO)
Leukocyte count
Band neutrophil counts in neonates (Rosenfeld and MacGregor) (Letter); (Schelonka et al) (Reply). 1995;126:504-6
Leuprolide
Local reactions to luteinizing hormone releasing hormone analog therapy (Tonini et al) (Letter); (Neely and Wilson) (Reply). 1995;126:159-60
LH
Local reactions to luteinizing hormone releasing hormone analog therapy (Tonini et al) (Letter); (Neely and Wilson) (Reply). 1995;126:159-60
Lipids
Lipid abnormalities in Turner syndrome (Ross et al). 1995;126:242-5
Oxidation of parenteral lipid emulsion by ambient and phototherapy lights: potential toxicity of routine parenteral feeding (Neužil et al). 1995;126:785-90
Relationship between insulin resistance and abnormal lipid profile in obese adolescents (Steinberger et al). 1995;126:690-5
Use of intravenous lipids in neonates (Helbock and Ames). 1995;126:747-8 (Editor's column)
Lipoamide dehydrogenase
Congenital lacticacidemia caused by lipoamide dehydrogenase deficiency with favorable outcome (Elpeleg et al). 1995;126:72-4 (CLO)
Lipoproteins, LDL
Low-density lipoprotein apheresis as long-term treatment for children with homozygous familial hypercholesterolemia (Zwiener et al). 1995;126:728-35
Liver cirrhosis
Pulmonary arteriovenous shunting in children with liver disease (Barbé et al). 1995;126:571-9
Liver diseases
Incidence of liver disease in patients with cystic fibrosis and meconium ileus (Lindblad et al) (Letter); (Colombo et al) (Reply). 1995;126:155-6

Liver diseases—cont'd
Pulmonary arteriovenous shunting in children with liver disease (Barbé et al). 1995;126:571-9
Local reaction to drugs; *see* Drug hypersensitivity
Low birth weight infant; *see* Infant, low birth weight
Low-density lipoproteins; *see* Lipoproteins, LDL
Lower respiratory tract infections; *see* Respiratory tract infections
Lung diseases
Changing trends in the epidemiology and pathogenesis of neonatal chronic lung disease (Rojas et al). 1995;126:605-10
Effect of pulse dexamethasone therapy on the incidence and severity of chronic lung disease in the very low birth weight infant (Brozanski et al). 1995;126:769-76
Twenty-month outcome in ventilator-dependent, very low birth weight infants born during the early years of dexamethasone therapy (Furman et al). 1995;126:434-40
Lupus erythematosus, systemic
Cerebral vein thrombosis in childhood systemic lupus erythematosus (Uziel et al). 1995;126:722-7
Congenital nephrotic syndrome in neonatal lupus syndrome (Westenend). 1995;126:851 (Letter)
Luteinizing hormone; *see* LH
Lymphocytes
Cognitive assessment of school-age children infected with maternally transmitted human immunodeficiency virus type 1 (Tardieu et al). 1995;126:375-9
Intact survival with transfusion-associated graft-versus-host disease proved by human leukocyte antigen typing of lymphocytes in skin biopsy specimens (Hentschel et al). 1995;126:61-4 (CLO)
Lymphocytic myocarditis; *see* Myocarditis
Lysinuric protein intolerance
Lysinuric protein intolerance characterized by bone marrow abnormalities and severe clinical course (Parenti et al). 1995; 126:246-51

M

Macromineral accretion; *see* Calcium; Phosphorus
Malaysia
Acquired platelet dysfunction with eosinophilia in white children (Poon et al). 1995;126:959-61 (CLO)
Malignancy; *see* Neoplasms
Malnutrition; *see* Nutrition disorders
Mass screening
Definition and application of the discretionary screening indicators according to the National Cholesterol Education Program for Children and Adolescents (Diller et al). 1995;126:345-52
Lead poisoning: low rates of screening and high prevalence among children seen in inner-city emergency departments (Wiley et al). 1995;126:392-5 (CLO)
A missense mutation in a patient with guanosine triphosphate cyclohydrolase I deficiency missed in the newborn screening program (Blau et al). 1995;126:401-5 (CLO)
Screening neonates for intrauterine cocaine exposure (Neuspiel) (Letter); (Ryan and Phelps) (Reply). 1995;126:323-4
Maternal behavior
Impact of attitudes on maternal decisions regarding infant feeding (Losch et al). 1995;126:507-14
Otitis media, hearing sensitivity, and maternal responsiveness in relation to language during infancy (Roberts et al). 1995; 126:481-9
Maternal death
Congenital cytomegalovirus infection as a result of nonprimary cytomegalovirus disease in a mother with acquired immunodeficiency syndrome (Schwebke et al). 1995;126:293-5 (CLO)
Maternal-fetal exchange
Birth order, delivery route, and concordance in the transmission of human immunodeficiency virus type 1 from mothers to twins (Duliège et al). 1995;126:625-32
Cognitive assessment of school-age children infected with maternally transmitted human immunodeficiency virus type 1 (Tardieu et al). 1995;126:375-9
Conjugated hyperbilirubinemia in a newborn infant after maternal (transplacental) treatment with flecainide acetate for fetal tachycardia and fetal hydrops (Vanderhal et al). 1995; 126:988-90 (CLO)
Effect of maternal glucocorticoid exposure on risk of severe intraventricular hemorrhage in surfactant-treated preterm infants (Garland et al). 1995;126:272-9
Maternal-infant blood group incompatibility; *see* Blood group incompatibility
Mauriac syndrome
Transient elevation of sweat chloride concentration in a malnourished girl with the Mauriac syndrome (Polack et al). 1995;126:261-3 (CLO)
Mechanical ventilation; *see* Respiration, artificial
Meconium
Incidence of liver disease in patients with cystic fibrosis and meconium ileus (Lindblad et al) (Letter); (Colombo et al) (Reply). 1995;126:155-6
Relation between meconium concentration of the cocaine metabolite benzoylecgonine and fetal growth (Mirochnick et al). 1995;126:636-8 (CLO)
Membranes
Inhaled nitric oxide for premature infants after prolonged rupture of the membranes (Peliowski et al). 1995;126:450-53 (CLO)
Meningitis, aseptic
Cytokine elevations in infants with bacterial and aseptic meningitis (Dulkerian et al). 1995;126:872-6
Meningococcal infections
Treatment of purpura fulminans in meningococcemia with protein C concentrate (Rivard et al). 1995;126:646-52
Meningomyelocele
Abnormalities in control of ventilation in newborn infants with myelomeningocele (Petersen et al). 1995;126:1011-5
Mental health
Effects of acute hyperglycemia on mental efficiency and counterregulatory hormones in adolescents with insulin-dependent diabetes mellitus (Gschwend et al). 1995;126:178-84
Metabolism
Effects of parenteral L-carnitine supplementation on fat metabolism and nutrition in premature neonates (Bonner et al). 1995;126:287-92
Enhanced adrenomedullary response and increased susceptibility to neuroglycopenia: mechanisms underlying the adverse effects of sugar ingestion in healthy children (Jones et al). 1995;126:171-7
Increased fat oxidation in prepubertal obese children: A metabolic defense against further weight gain? (Maffeis et al). 1995; 126:15-20
Methemoglobinemia
Methemoglobinemia associated with acidosis of probable renal origin (Sager et al). 1995;126:59-61 (CLO)
Rebound severe methemoglobinemia from ingestion of a nitroethane artificial fingernail remover (Osterhoudt et al). 1995; 126:819-21 (CLO)
Miliary tuberculosis; *see* Tuberculosis, miliary
Milk, human
Postnatal attainment of intrauterine macromineral accretion rates in low birth weight infants fed fortified human milk (Schanler and Abrams). 1995;126:441-7
Milk hypersensitivity
Allergic colitis in infants (Odze et al). 1995;126:163-70
Chronic constipation as a symptom of cow milk allergy (Iacono et al). 1995;126:34-9

Minerals
Mineral homeostasis and bone mass at diagnosis in children with acute lymphoblastic leukemia (Halton et al). 1995;126:557-64
Plasma mineral concentrations in preterm infants fed a nutrient-enriched formula after hospital discharge (Rajaram et al). 1995;126:791-6
Postnatal attainment of intrauterine macromineral accretion rates in low birth weight infants fed fortified human milk (Schanler and Abrams). 1995;126:441-7
Mitochondrial DNA; *see* DNA, mitochondrial
Monosomy
Transformation of congenital neutropenia into monosomy 7 and acute nonlymphoblastic leukemia in a child treated with granulocyte colony-stimulating factor (Weinblatt et al). 1995;126:263-5 (CLO)
Morbidity
Differences in morbidity between breast-fed and formula-fed infants (Dewey et al). 1995;126:696-702
Glucose-6-phosphate dehydrogenase deficiency and carboxyhemoglobin concentrations associated with bilirubin-related morbidity and death in Nigerian infants (Slusher et al). 1995;126:102-8
Pediatric Investigators Collaborative Network on Infections in Canada (PICNIC) prospective study of risk factors and outcomes in patients hospitalized with respiratory syncytial viral lower respiratory tract infection (Wang et al). 1995;126:212-9
Morphine
Intravenous morphine pharmacokinetics in pediatric patients with sickle cell disease (Dampier et al). 1995;126:461-7
Mortality, infant; *see* Infant death
Motor activity
Motor and cognitive development in children with congenital hypothyroidism (Mitchell and Klein) (Letter); (Vulsma and Kooistra) (Reply). 1995;126:673-4
Mucocutaneous lymph node syndrome
Comparative safety and efficacy of two immune globulin products in Kawasaki disease (Rosenfeld et al). 1995;126:1000-3
Kawasaki disease in infants less than one year of age (Rosenfeld et al). 1995;126:524-9
Munchausen syndrome by proxy
Overinterpretation of gastroduodenal motility studies: two cases involving Munchausen syndrome by proxy (Baron et al). 1995;126:397-400 (CLO)
Muscular dystrophy
Dysmorphic features in patients with complex glycerol kinase deficiency (Scheuerle et al). 1995;126:764-7 (CLO)
Mutation
Binding of *Pseudomonas aeruginosa* to respiratory epithelial cells from patients with various mutations in the cystic fibrosis transmembrane regulator (Zar et al). 1995;126:230-3
A missense mutation in a patient with guanosine triphosphate cyclohydrolase I deficiency missed in the newborn screening program (Blau et al). 1995;126:401-5 (CLO)
True hermaphroditism with 46,XY karyotype and a point mutation in the *SRY* gene (Hiort et al). 1995;126:1022 (Letter)
Myelomeningocele; *see* Meningomyelocele
Myocarditis
Corticosteroid therapy for ventricular tachycardia in children with silent lymphocytic myocarditis (Ino et al). 1995;126:304-8
Myoclonus
Opsoclonus-myoclonus, ataxia, and coincident neuroblastoma (Chamberlain). 1995;126:675 (Letter)
Opsoclonus-myoclonus and recurrent neuroblastoma (Basco et al). 1995;126:847-8 (Letter)
Myositis ossificans
Permanent heterotopic ossification at the injection site after diphtheria-tetanus-pertussis immunizations in children who have fibrodysplasia ossificans progressiva (Lanchoney et al). 1995;126:762-4 (CLO)

N

Narcotics
Control of severe pain in children with terminal malignancy (Collins et al). 1995;126:653-7
Intravenous morphine pharmacokinetics in pediatric patients with sickle cell disease (Dampier et al). 1995;126:461-7
National Cholesterol Education Program for Children and Adolescents
Definition and application of the discretionary screening indicators according to the National Cholesterol Education Program for Children and Adolescents (Diller et al). 1995;126:345-52
Nebulizers and vaporizers
Efficacy of frequent nebulized ipratropium bromide added to frequent high-dose albuterol therapy in severe childhood asthma (Schuh et al). 1995;126:639-45
Terbutaline powder for acute asthma (Rufin et al). 1995;126:161-2 (Letter)
Neisseria meningitidis
Relationship between parental occupation and children's oropharyngeal colonization with *Neisseria meningitidis* (King et al). 1995;126:937-9 (CLO)
Neonatal asphyxia; *see* Asphyxia neonatorum
Neonatal hyperbilirubinemia; *see* Jaundice, neonatal
Neonatal intensive care units; *see* Intensive care units, neonatal
Neonatal screening
Newborn screening for congenital adrenal hyperplasia in New Zealand (Cutfield and Webster). 1995;126:118-21
Neonate; *see* Infant, newborn
Neoplasms
Cancer in children with primary or secondary immunodeficiencies (Mueller and Pizzo). 1995;126:1-10
Control of severe pain in children with terminal malignancy (Collins et al). 1995;126:653-7
Nephritis, interstitial
Deletion of mitochondrial DNA in patient with chronic tubulointerstitial nephritis (Rötig et al). 1995;126:597-601 (CLO)
Nephrotic syndrome
Congenital nephrotic syndrome in neonatal lupus syndrome (Westenend). 1995;126:851 (Letter)
Successful treatment of Finnish congenital nephrotic syndrome with captopril and indomethacin (Pomeranz et al). 1995;126:140-2 (CLO)
Nervous system neoplasms
Opsoclonus-myoclonus, ataxia, and coincident neuroblastoma (Chamberlain). 1995;126:675 (Letter)
Opsoclonus-myoclonus and recurrent neuroblastoma (Basco et al). 1995;126:847-8 (Letter)
Neuroblastoma
Opsoclonus-myoclonus, ataxia, and coincident neuroblastoma (Chamberlain). 1995;126:675 (Letter)
Opsoclonus-myoclonus and recurrent neuroblastoma (Basco et al). 1995;126:847-8 (Letter)
Neurodevelopmental outcome; *see* Child development
Neurofibromatosis 1
Precocious puberty in children with neurofibromatosis type 1 (Habiby et al). 1995;126:364-7
Neurogenic bladder; *see* Bladder, neurogenic
Neuroglycopenia; *see* Hypoglycemia
Neurologic manifestations
Clinical and biochemical characterization of short-chain acyl–coenzyme A dehydrogenase deficiency (Bhala et al). 1995; 126:910-5
Helicobacter pylori infection in neurologically impaired children (Mauk) (Letter); (Proujansky et al) (Reply). 1995;126:849-50
Neonatal-onset propionicacidemia: neurologic and developmental profiles, and implications for management (North et al). 1995;126:916-22
Neuromuscular diseases
Critical illness neuromuscular disease in children manifested as ventilatory dependence (Sheth et al). 1995;126:259-61 (CLO)

Neutropenia
Administration of granulocyte colony-stimulating factor to neutropenic low birth weight infants of mothers with preeclampsia (Makhlouf et al). 1995;126:454-56 (CLO)
Effect of granulocyte colony-stimulating factor on preeclampsia-associated neonatal neutropenia (La Gamma et al). 1995; 126:457-9 (CLO)
Transformation of congenital neutropenia into monosomy 7 and acute nonlymphoblastic leukemia in a child treated with granulocyte colony-stimulating factor (Weinblatt et al). 1995;126: 263-5 (CLO)
Neutrophils
Band neutrophil counts in neonates (Rosenfeld and MacGregor) (Letter); (Schelonka et al) (Reply). 1995;126:504-6
Spectrum of disease associated with anti-neutrophil cytoplasmic autoantibodies in pediatric patients (Ellis et al). 1995;126:40-3
New books received
The book shelf. 1995;126:326, 406, 662, 968, 1016
New Zealand
Newborn screening for congenital adrenal hyperplasia in New Zealand (Cutfield and Webster). 1995;126:118-21
Newborn infant; *see* Infant, newborn
Nigeria
Glucose-6-phosphate dehydrogenase deficiency and carboxyhemoglobin concentrations associated with bilirubin-related morbidity and death in Nigerian infants (Slusher et al). 1995; 126:102-8
Nipples
Imaging evaluation of breast-feeding and bottle feeding systems (Nowak et al). 1995;126:S130-4
Nipple confusion: toward a formal definition (Neifert et al). 1995;126:S125-9
Nitric oxide
Inhaled nitric oxide for premature infants after prolonged rupture of the membranes (Peliowski et al). 1995;126:450-53 (CLO)
Recent developments in the pathophysiology and treatment of persistent pulmonary hypertension of the newborn (Kinsella and Abman). 1995;126:853-64
Nitroethane
Rebound severe methemoglobinemia from ingestion of a nitroethane artificial fingernail remover (Osterhoudt et al). 1995; 126:819-21 (CLO)
Nonoliguric hyperkalemia; *see* Hyperkalemia
Nuclear magnetic resonance
Brain metabolite changes on in vivo proton magnetic resonance spectroscopy in children with congenital hypothyroidism (Gupta et al). 1995;126:389-92 (CLO)
Nutrient-enriched formula; *see* Infant food
Nutrition
Body composition in children with spastic quadriplegic cerebral palsy (Stallings et al). 1995;126:833-9
Effects of parenteral L-carnitine supplementation on fat metabolism and nutrition in premature neonates (Bonner et al). 1995;126:287-92
Nutrition disorders
Transient elevation of sweat chloride concentration in a malnourished girl with the Mauriac syndrome (Polack et al). 1995;126:261-3 (CLO)

O

Obesity
Increased fat oxidation in prepubertal obese children: A metabolic defense against further weight gain? (Maffeis et al). 1995;126:15-20
Relationship between insulin resistance and abnormal lipid profile in obese adolescents (Steinberger et al). 1995;126:690-5
Observer variation
Accuracy of aural infrared temperature device (McKenzie) (Letter); (Yetman) (Reply). 1995;126:324-5
Occupational exposure
Relationship between parental occupation and children's oropharyngeal colonization with *Neisseria meningitidis* (King et al). 1995;126:937-9 (CLO)
Oligohydramnios
Inhaled nitric oxide for premature infants after prolonged rupture of the membranes (Peliowski et al). 1995;126:450-53 (CLO)
Opsoclonus
Opsoclonus-myoclonus, ataxia, and coincident neuroblastoma (Chamberlain). 1995;126:675 (Letter)
Opsoclonus-myoclonus and recurrent neuroblastoma (Basco et al). 1995;126:847-8 (Letter)
Optic pathway tumors
Precocious puberty in children with neurofibromatosis type 1 (Habiby et al). 1995;126:364-7
Optical immunoassay; *see* Immunoassay
Organic acidemia; *see* Acid-base imbalance
Ossification, heterotopic
Permanent heterotopic ossification at the injection site after diphtheria-tetanus-pertussis immunizations in children who have fibrodysplasia ossificans progressiva (Lanchoney et al). 1995;126:762-4 (CLO)
Otitis media
Abnormal tympanography after supine bottle feeding (Tully et al). 1995;126:S105-11
Bacteriologic failure of amoxicillin-clavulanate in treatment of acute otitis media caused by nontypeable *Haemophilus influenzae* (Patel et al). 1995;126:799-806
Criteria for studies of antibiotic therapy for acute otitis media (Schwartz and Rodriguez). 1995;126:677-8 (Letter)
Otitis media, hearing sensitivity, and maternal responsiveness in relation to language during infancy (Roberts et al). 1995; 126:481-9
Short-term use of amoxicillin clavulanate during upper respiratory tract infection for prevention of acute otitis media (Heikkinen et al). 1995;126:313-6 (CLO)
Outpatients
Efficacy of an observation scale in detecting bacteremia in febrile children three to thirty-six months of age, treated as outpatients (Teach et al). 1995;126:877-81
Oxidation
Increased fat oxidation in prepubertal obese children: A metabolic defense against further weight gain? (Maffeis et al). 1995;126:15-20
Oxygen
Effect of the arterial oxygenation level on cardiac output, oxygen extraction, and oxygen consumption in low birth weight infants receiving mechanical ventilation (Schulze et al). 1995;126: 777-84
Improved oxygenation during synchronized intermittent mandatory ventilation in neonates with respiratory distress syndrome: a randomized, crossover study (Cleary et al). 1995;126:407-11

P

Packed red blood cells; *see* Hematocrit
Pain
Control of severe pain in children with terminal malignancy (Collins et al). 1995;126:653-7
Painful keratoderma and photophobia: hallmarks of tyrosinemia type II (Rabinowitz et al). 1995;126:266-9 (CLO)
Pancreas
Pancreatic glucagon levels in infants and children with hyperinsulinemia (Pronicka et al). 1995;126:948-51 (CLO)

Pancreatic insufficiency
Chronic pancreatitis in a patient with cystic fibrosis and clinical pancreatic insufficiency (del Rosario et al). 1995;126:951-2 (CLO)
Pancreatitis
Acute pancreatitis associated with acute hepatitis A in a young child (Shrier et al). 1995;126:57-9 (CLO)
Chronic pancreatitis in a patient with cystic fibrosis and clinical pancreatic insufficiency (del Rosario et al). 1995;126:951-2 (CLO)
Pancreatitis and organic acidemias (Fiumara et al). 1995;126:852 (Letter)
Parenteral lipid emulsion; *see* Fat emulsions, intravenous
Parenteral nutrition
Effects of parenteral L-carnitine supplementation on fat metabolism and nutrition in premature neonates (Bonner et al). 1995;126:287-92
Oxidation of parenteral lipid emulsion by ambient and phototherapy lights: potential toxicity of routine parenteral feeding (Neužil et al). 1995;126:785-90
Vitamin A and E status in very low birth weight infants: development of an improved parenteral delivery system (Inder et al). 1995;126:128-31 (CLO)
Parenteral nutrition, home total
A cross-sectional study of catheter-related thrombosis in children receiving total parenteral nutrition at home (Andrew et al). 1995;126:358-63
Partial liquid ventilation; *see* Ventilation
Patient discharge
Plasma mineral concentrations in preterm infants fed a nutrient-enriched formula after hospital discharge (Rajaram et al). 1995;126:791-6
Pediatric Investigators Collaborative Network on Infections in Canada
Pediatric Investigators Collaborative Network on Infections in Canada (PICNIC) prospective study of risk factors and outcomes in patients hospitalized with respiratory syncytial viral lower respiratory tract infection (Wang et al). 1995; 126:212-9
Peritoneal dialysis
Use of peritoneal dialysis, continuous arteriovenous hemofiltration, and continuous arteriovenous hemodiafiltration for removal of ammonium chloride and glutamine in rabbits (Semama et al). 1995;126:742-6
Persistent fetal circulation syndrome
Recent developments in the pathophysiology and treatment of persistent pulmonary hypertension of the newborn (Kinsella and Abman). 1995;126:853-64
Peutz-Jeghers syndrome
Peutz-Jeghers syndrome in a neonate (Seara et al). 1995;126:965-7 (CLO)
Pharmacokinetics
Intravenous morphine pharmacokinetics in pediatric patients with sickle cell disease (Dampier et al). 1995;126:461-7
Pharnygeal diseases
Prolonged dysphagia caused by congenital pharyngeal dysfunction (Mbonda et al). 1995;126:923-7
Pharyngitis
Diagnosis of group A streptococcal pharyngitis in a private clinic: comparative evaluation of an optical immunoassay method and culture (Fries). 1995;126:933-6 (CLO)
Phenotype
Lysinuric protein intolerance characterized by bone marrow abnormalities and severe clinical course (Parenti et al). 1995; 126:246-51
Vertical transmission of human immunodeficiency virus type I: autologous neutralizing antibody, virus load, and virus phenotype (Husson et al). 1995;126:865-71
Phenylalanine
A missense mutation in a patient with guanosine triphosphate cyclohydrolase I deficiency missed in the newborn screening program (Blau et al). 1995;126:401-5 (CLO)
Phenylketonuria
A missense mutation in a patient with guanosine triphosphate cyclohydrolase I deficiency missed in the newborn screening program (Blau et al). 1995;126:401-5 (CLO)
Phosphoric acids
Consumption of soft drinks with phosphoric acid as a risk factor for the development of hypocalcemia in children: a case-control study (Mazariegos-Ramos et al). 1995;126:940-2 (CLO)
Phosphorus
Postnatal attainment of intrauterine macromineral accretion rates in low birth weight infants fed fortified human milk (Schanler and Abrams). 1995;126:441-7
Photophobia
Painful keratoderma and photophobia: hallmarks of tyrosinemia type II (Rabinowitz et al). 1995;126:266-9 (CLO)
Phototherapy
Comparison of fiberoptic and conventional phototherapy for neonatal hyperbilirubinemia (Larsen and Whitelaw) (Letter); (Tan) (Reply). 1995;126:1018
Oxidation of parenteral lipid emulsion by ambient and phototherapy lights: potential toxicity of routine parenteral feeding (Neužil et al). 1995;126:785-90
PICNIC; *see* Pediatric Investigators Collaborative Network on Infections in Canada
Placebos
Double-blind developmental evaluation at 1-year corrected age of 597 premature infants with birth weights from 500 to 1350 grams enrolled in three placebo-controlled trials of prophylactic synthetic surfactant (Corbet et al). 1995;126:S5-12 (Symposium)
Double-blind evaluation of developmental and health status to age 2 years of infants weighing 700 to 1350 grams treated prophylactically at birth with a single dose of synthetic surfactant or air placebo (Kraybill et al). 1995;126:S33-42 (Symposium)
Double-blind, randomized, placebo-controlled Canadian multicenter trial of two doses of synthetic surfactant or air placebo in 224 infants weighing 500 to 749 grams with respiratory distress syndrome (Smyth et al). 1995;126:S81-9 (Symposium)
Double-blind 1-year follow-up of 1540 infants with respiratory distress syndrome randomized to rescue treatment with two doses of synthetic surfactant or air in four clinical trials (Courtney et al). 1995;126:S43-52 (Symposium)
Effects of two rescue doses of synthetic surfactant in 344 infants with respiratory distress syndrome weighing 750 to 1249 grams: a double-blind, placebo-controlled multicenter Canadian trial (McMillan et al). 1995;126:S90-8 (Symposium)
One-year follow-up evaluation of 260 premature infants with respiratory distress syndrome and birth weights of 700 to 1350 grams randomized to two rescue doses of synthetic surfactant or air placebo (Gong et al). 1995;126:S68-74 (Symposium)
One-year follow-up of 66 premature infants weighing 500 to 699 grams treated with a single dose of synthetic surfactant or air placebo at birth: results of a double-blind trial (Walther et al). 1995;126:S13-9 (Symposium)
One-year follow-up of 89 infants with birth weights of 500 to 749 grams and respiratory distress syndrome randomized to two rescue doses of synthetic surfactant or air placebo (Casiro et al). 1995;126:S53-60 (Symposium)
One-year follow-up of 273 infants with birth weights of 700 to 1100 grams after prophylactic treatment of respiratory distress syndrome with synthetic surfactant or air placebo (Sell et al). 1995;126:S20-5 (Symposium)

Placebos—cont'd
One-year outcome in 232 premature infants with birth weights of 750 to 1249 grams and respiratory distress syndrome randomized to rescue treatment with two doses of synthetic surfactant or air placebo (Saigal et al). 1995;126:S61-7 (Symposium)
Outcome at 1-year adjusted age of 957 infants weighing more than 1250 grams with respiratory distress syndrome randomized to receive synthetic surfactant or air placebo (Sauve et al). 1995;126:S75-80 (Symposium)
Placebo-controlled versus comparative studies of drug effects (Weinberger) (Letter); (Galant) (Reply); (Garfunkel) (Reply). 1995;126:680-1
Plasma
Plasma erythropoietin reference ranges in children (Krafte-Jacobs et al). 1995;126:601-3 (CLO)
Plasma mineral concentrations in preterm infants fed a nutrient-enriched formula after hospital discharge (Rajaram et al). 1995;126:791-6
Platelets; *see* Blood platelets
Pneumocystis carinii
Congenital cytomegalovirus infection as a result of nonprimary cytomegalovirus disease in a mother with acquired immunodeficiency syndrome (Schwebke et al). 1995;126:293-5 (CLO)
Effect of corticosteroids on survival of children with acquired immunodeficiency syndrome and *Pneumocystis carinii*–related respiratory failure (McLaughlin et al). 1995;126:821-4 (CLO)
Poisons
Rebound severe methemoglobinemia from ingestion of a nitroethane artificial fingernail remover (Osterhoudt et al). 1995; 126:819-21 (CLO)
Polymerase chain reaction
Diagnosis of neonatal enterovirus infection by polymerase chain reaction (Abzug et al). 1995;126:447-50 (CLO)
Expanded spectrum of herpes simplex encephalitis in childhood (Schlesinger et al). 1995;126:234-41
Use of polymerase chain reaction for improved diagnosis of tuberculosis in children (Delacourt et al). 1995;126:703-9
Viral measurement by polymerase chain reaction–based assays in human immunodeficiency virus–infected infants (Palumbo et al). 1995;126:592-5 (CLO)
Polyradiculoneuritis
Familial Guillain-Barré syndrome subsequent to *Campylobacter jejuni* enteritis (Yuki and Tsujino). 1995;126:162 (Letter)
Polyunsaturated fatty acids; *see* Fatty acids, unsaturated
Portal vein
Portal vein thrombosis caused by protein C and protein S deficiency associated with cytomegalovirus infection (Arav-Boger et al). 1995;126:586-8 (CLO)
Postnatal care
Long-chain polyunsaturated fatty acids in preterm infants: status at birth and its influence on postnatal levels (Foreman–van Drongelen et al). 1995;126:611-8
Potassium
Internal potassium shift in premature infants: cause of nonoliguric hyperkalemia (Sato et al). 1995;126:109-13
Potter, Edith
Edith Potter (Gilbert-Barness). 1995;126:845-6 (Profiles)
Prader-Willi syndrome
Pulmonary function abnormalities in Prader-Willi syndrome (Hákonarson et al). 1995;126:565-70
Precocious puberty; *see* Puberty, precocious
Predictive value of tests
Measured versus predicted resting energy expenditure in infants: a need for reappraisal (Thomson et al). 1995;126:21-7
Prediction of the outcome of growth hormone therapy in children with idiopathic short stature: a multivariate discriminant analysis (Spagnoli et al). 1995;126:905-9
Predictive value of tests—cont'd
Predictive factors in the determination of final height in boys with constitutional delay of growth and puberty (Albanese and Stanhope). 1995;126:545-50
Soluble interleukin-2 receptor as a predictor of neonatal sepsis (Spear et al). 1995;126:982-5 (CLO)
Somatosensory evoked potentials for prediction of outcome in acute severe brain injury (Beca et al). 1995;126:44-9
Viral measurement by polymerase chain reaction–based assays in human immunodeficiency virus–infected infants (Palumbo et al). 1995;126:592-5 (CLO)
Prednisone
A multicenter study of alternate-day prednisone therapy in patients with cystic fibrosis (Eigen et al). 1995;126:515-23
Preeclampsia
Administration of granulocyte colony-stimulating factor to neutropenic low birth weight infants of mothers with preeclampsia (Makhlouf et al). 1995;126:454-56 (CLO)
Effect of granulocyte colony-stimulating factor on preeclampsia-associated neonatal neutropenia (La Gamma et al). 1995; 126:457-9 (CLO)
Pregnancy, multiple
Birth order, delivery route, and concordance in the transmission of human immunodeficiency virus type 1 from mothers to twins (Duliège et al). 1995;126:625-32
Discordance for hyperinsulinemic hypoglycemia in monozygotic twins (Santer et al) (Letter); (Thornton et al) (Reply). 1995; 126:1017
Pregnancy complications, cardiovascular
Administration of granulocyte colony-stimulating factor to neutropenic low birth weight infants of mothers with preeclampsia (Makhlouf et al). 1995;126:454-56 (CLO)
Effect of granulocyte colony-stimulating factor on preeclampsia-associated neonatal neutropenia (La Gamma et al). 1995;126: 457-9 (CLO)
Pregnancy trimester, first
Possible fetal effects of cervical dilation and uterine curettage during the first trimester of pregnancy (Holmes). 1995;126: 131-4 (CLO)
Premature infant; *see* Infant, premature
Premature thelarche; *see* Thelarche
Prepuberty; *see* Puberty
Preterm infant; *see* Infant, premature
Profiles
C. Henry Kempe (Fulginiti). 1995;126:152-4 (Profiles)
Edith Potter (Gilbert-Barness). 1995;126:845-6 (Profiles)
Josef Warkany (Miller). 1995;126:669-72 (Profiles)
Propanediols
Diarrhea associated with enteral benzodiazepine solutions (Marshall et al). 1995;126:657-9 (CLO)
Prophylaxis
Double-blind developmental evaluation at 1-year corrected age of 597 premature infants with birth weights from 500 to 1350 grams enrolled in three placebo-controlled trials of prophylactic synthetic surfactant (Corbet et al). 1995;126:S5-12 (Symposium)
Double-blind evaluation of developmental and health status to age 2 years of infants weighing 700 to 1350 grams treated prophylactically at birth with a single dose of synthetic surfactant or air placebo (Kraybill et al). 1995;126:S33-42 (Symposium)
Double-blind, randomized trial of one versus three prophylactic doses of synthetic surfactant in 826 neonates weighing 700 to 1100 grams: effects on mortality rate (Corbet et al). 1995; 126:969-78
Health and neurodevelopmental outcome at 1-year adjusted age in 508 infants weighing 700 to 1100 grams who received prophylaxis with one versus three doses of synthetic surfactant (Gerdes et al). 1995;126:S26-32 (Symposium)

Prophylaxis—cont'd
One-year follow-up of 273 infants with birth weights of 700 to 1100 grams after prophylactic treatment of respiratory distress syndrome with synthetic surfactant or air placebo (Sell et al). 1995;126:S20-5 (Symposium)
Propionic acids
Neonatal-onset propionic acidemia: neurologic and developmental profiles, and implications for management (North et al). 1995;126:916-22
Protein C
Portal vein thrombosis caused by protein C and protein S deficiency associated with cytomegalovirus infection (Arav-Boger et al). 1995;126:586-8 (CLO)
Treatment of purpura fulminans in meningococcemia with protein C concentrate (Rivard et al). 1995;126:646-52
Protein S
Portal vein thrombosis caused by protein C and protein S deficiency associated with cytomegalovirus infection (Arav-Boger et al). 1995;126:586-8 (CLO)
Proton magnetic resonance spectroscopy; *see* Nuclear magnetic resonance
Protons
Use of the urine-to-blood carbon dioxide tension gradient as a measurement of impaired distal tubular hydrogen ion secretion among neonates (Lin et al). 1995;126:114-7
Pseudomonas aeruginosa
Binding of *Pseudomonas aeruginosa* to respiratory epithelial cells from patients with various mutations in the cystic fibrosis transmembrane regulator (Zar et al). 1995;126:230-3
A multicenter study of alternate-day prednisone therapy in patients with cystic fibrosis (Eigen et al). 1995;126:515-23
Pseudotumor cerebri
Benign intracranial hypertension in children with growth hormone deficiency treated with growth hormone (Malozowski et al). 1995;126:996-9
Puberty
Effects of dairy products on bone and body composition in pubertal girls (Chan et al). 1995;126:551-6
Growth and the growth hormone axis in prepubertal children with asthma (Crowley et al). 1995;126:297-303
Increased fat oxidation in prepubertal obese children: A metabolic defense against further weight gain? (Maffeis et al). 1995;126:15-20
Prepubertal gynecomastia during growth hormone therapy (Malozowski and Stadel). 1995;126:659-61 (CLO)
Puberty, delayed
Predictive factors in the determination of final height in boys with constitutional delay of growth and puberty (Albanese and Stanhope). 1995;126:545-50
Use of the gonadotropin-releasing hormone agonist triptorelin in the diagnosis of delayed puberty in boys (Zamboni et al). 1995;126:756-8 (CLO)
Puberty, precocious
Bayley-Pinneau method of height prediction in girls with central precocious puberty: correlation with adult height (Bar et al). 1995;126:955-8 (CLO)
Precocious puberty in children with neurofibromatosis type 1 (Habiby et al). 1995;126:364-7
Progression of premature thelarche to central precocious puberty (Pasquino et al). 1995;126:11-4
Pulmonary arteriovenous shunts; *see* Shunts
Pulmonary function; *see* Respiratory function tests
Pulmonary gas exchange
Influence of energy substrates on respiratory gas exchange during conventional mechanical ventilation of preterm infants (Chessex et al). 1995;126:619-24
Purpura
Treatment of purpura fulminans in meningococcemia with protein C concentrate (Rivard et al). 1995;126:646-52
Purpura, thrombocytopenic
Short-term, high-dose corticosteroid therapy in childhood acute immune thrombocytopenic purpura (Yavûz et al) (Letter); (Blanchette) (Reply). 1995;126:156-7

Q

Quadriplegia
Body composition in children with spastic quadriplegic cerebral palsy (Stallings et al). 1995;126:833-9
Human synthetic calcitonin therapy for hypercalcemia of immobilization (Kaul and Sockalosky). 1995;126:825-7 (CLO)
Quality of health care
Acuity scores as predictors of cost-related outcomes of neonatal intensive care (Kotagal et al). 1995;126:88-93
Adolescent medicine 1995 (Emans). 1995;126:387-8 (Editor's column)
Hospitalization for lower respiratory tract illness in infants: variation in rates among counties in New York State and areas within Monroe County (McConnochie et al). 1995;126:220-9
Standards for home care of sick children (McConnell and Perkin) (Letter); (Goldberg et al) (Reply). 1995;126:681-2
Usefulness of cerebrospinal fluid bacterial antigen tests (Warren and Kiser) (Letter); (Maxson et al) (Reply). 1995;126:321
Quality of life
Neurodevelopmental outcome of infants with hypoplastic left heart syndrome (Rogers et al). 1995;126:496-8 (CLO)

R

Receptors, interleukin-2
Soluble interleukin-2 receptor as a predictor of neonatal sepsis (Spear et al). 1995;126:982-5 (CLO)
Recombinant vaccines; *see* Vaccines, synthetic
Rectum
Allergic colitis in infants (Odze et al). 1995;126:163-70
Recurrent stroke; *see* Cerebrovascular disorders
Reference values
Plasma erythropoietin reference ranges in children (Krafte-Jacobs et al). 1995;126:601-3 (CLO)
Reference ranges for newer thyroid function tests in premature infants (Adams et al). 1995;126:122-7
Reference ranges for serum cortisol and 17-hydroxyprogesterone levels in preterm infants (Al Saedi et al). 1995;126:985-7 (CLO)
Renal abnormalities; *see* Kidney
Renal scars; *see* Cicatrix
Research
Adolescent medicine 1995 (Emans). 1995;126:387-8 (Editor's column)
Use of a visual panel detection method for drugs of abuse: clinical and laboratory experience with children and adolescents (Valentine and Komoroski). 1995;126:135-40
Resources, health; *see* Health resources
Respiration, artificial
Effect of airway pressure on inferior vena cava pressure as a measure of central venous pressure in children (Reda et al). 1995;126:961-5 (CLO)
Effect of the arterial oxygenation level on cardiac output, oxygen extraction, and oxygen consumption in low birth weight infants receiving mechanical ventilation (Schulze et al). 1995;126:777-84
Influence of energy substrates on respiratory gas exchange during conventional mechanical ventilation of preterm infants (Chessex et al). 1995;126:619-24
Respiration disorders
Abnormalities in control of ventilation in newborn infants with myelomeningocele (Petersen et al). 1995;126:1011-5

Respiration disorders—cont'd
Resolution of breath-holding spells with treatment of concomitant anemia (Colina and Abelson). 1995;126:395-7 (CLO)
Respiratory distress syndrome
Antenatal corticosteroid therapy to prevent respiratory distress syndrome (Ryan and Finer). 1995;126:317-9
Double-blind, randomized, placebo-controlled Canadian multicenter trial of two doses of synthetic surfactant or air placebo in 224 infants weighing 500 to 749 grams with respiratory distress syndrome (Smyth et al). 1995;126:S81-9 (Symposium)
Double-blind 1-year follow-up of 1540 infants with respiratory distress syndrome randomized to rescue treatment with two doses of synthetic surfactant or air in four clinical trials (Courtney et al). 1995;126:S43-52 (Symposium)
Effects of two rescue doses of synthetic surfactant in 344 infants with respiratory distress syndrome weighing 750 to 1249 grams: a double-blind, placebo-controlled multicenter Canadian trial (McMillan et al). 1995;126:S90-8 (Symposium)
Hypotension in preterm infants (Milstein) (Letter); (Faix) (Reply). 1995;126:160-1
Improved oxygenation during synchronized intermittent mandatory ventilation in neonates with respiratory distress syndrome: a randomized, crossover study (Cleary et al). 1995;126:407-11
One-year follow-up evaluation of 260 premature infants with respiratory distress syndrome and birth weights of 700 to 1350 grams randomized to two rescue doses of synthetic surfactant or air placebo (Gong et al). 1995;126:S68-74 (Symposium)
One-year follow-up of 89 infants with birth weights of 500 to 749 grams and respiratory distress syndrome randomized to two rescue doses of synthetic surfactant or air placebo (Casiro et al). 1995;126:S53-60 (Symposium)
One-year follow-up of 273 infants with birth weights of 700 to 1100 grams after prophylactic treatment of respiratory distress syndrome with synthetic surfactant or air placebo (Sell et al). 1995;126:S20-5 (Symposium)
One-year outcome in 232 premature infants with birth weights of 750 to 1249 grams and respiratory distress syndrome randomized to rescue treatment with two doses of synthetic surfactant or air placebo (Saigal et al). 1995;126:S61-7 (Symposium)
Outcome at 1-year adjusted age of 957 infants weighing more than 1250 grams with respiratory distress syndrome randomized to receive synthetic surfactant or air placebo (Sauve et al). 1995;126:S75-80 (Symposium)
Partial liquid ventilation in premature lambs with respiratory distress syndrome: efficacy and compatibility with exogenous surfactant (Leach et al). 1995;126:412-20
Symposium on Synthetic Surfactant II: perspective and commentary (Long et al). 1995;126:S1-4 (Symposium)
Synthetic surfactant for rescue treatment of respiratory distress syndrome in premature infants weighing from 700 to 1350 grams: impact on hospital resource use and charges (Mauskopf et al). 1995;126:94-101
Respiratory distress syndrome, adult
Adult respiratory distress syndrome in children associated with miliary tuberculosis (Martinez-Azagra et al) (Letter); (Davis) (Reply). 1995;126:678-9
Respiratory function tests
A multicenter study of alternate-day prednisone therapy in patients with cystic fibrosis (Eigen et al). 1995;126:515-23
Pulmonary function abnormalities in Prader-Willi syndrome (Hákonarson et al). 1995;126:565-70
Respiratory gas exchange; *see* Pulmonary gas exchange
Respiratory insufficiency
Effect of corticosteroids on survival of children with acquired immunodeficiency syndrome and *Pneumocystis carinii*–related respiratory failure (McLaughlin et al). 1995;126:821-4 (CLO)
Respiratory syncytial viruses
Cost of ribavirin therapy for respiratory syncytial virus infection (Marquardt) (Letter); (Englund et al) (Reply). 1995;126:847
Pediatric Investigators Collaborative Network on Infections in Canada (PICNIC) prospective study of risk factors and outcomes in patients hospitalized with respiratory syncytial viral lower respiratory tract infection (Wang et al). 1995; 126:212-9
Respiratory tract infections
Cell-mediated immune status of children with recurrent infection (Herrod et al). 1995;126:530-6
Clinical trial of vitamin A as adjuvant treatment for lower respiratory tract infections (Kjolhede et al). 1995;126:807-12
Hospitalization for lower respiratory tract illness in infants: variation in rates among counties in New York State and areas within Monroe County (McConnochie et al). 1995;126:220-9
Pediatric Investigators Collaborative Network on Infections in Canada (PICNIC) prospective study of risk factors and outcomes in patients hospitalized with respiratory syncytial viral lower respiratory tract infection (Wang et al). 1995; 126:212-9
Relation between infant feeding and infections during the first six months of life (Beaudry et al). 1995;126:191-7
Short-term use of amoxicillin clavulanate during upper respiratory tract infection for prevention of acute otitis media (Heikkinen et al). 1995;126:313-6 (CLO)
Resting energy expenditure; *see* Energy metabolism
Rett syndrome
Electrocardiographic findings in Rett syndrome (Fuster-Siebert and Castro-Gago). 1995;126:506 (Letter)
Rhinitis
Placebo-controlled versus comparative studies of drug effects (Weinberger) (Letter); (Galant) (Reply); (Garfunkel) (Reply). 1995;126:680-1
Ribavirin
Cost of ribavirin therapy for respiratory syncytial virus infection (Marquardt) (Letter); (Englund et al) (Reply). 1995;126:847
Rickets
Healing of rickets during vitamin D therapy despite defective vitamin D receptors in two siblings with vitamin D–dependent rickets type II (Kruse and Feldmann). 1995;126:145-8 (CLO)
A new defect in vitamin D metabolism (Nützenadel et al) (Letter); (Casella and Finberg) (Reply). 1995;126:676-7
Pathophysiology of calcium metabolism in children with vitamin D–deficiency rickets (Kruse). 1995;126:736-41
Single-day therapy for rickets (Mimouni) (Letter); (Shah and Finberg) (Reply). 1995;126:1019-20
Risk factors
Beneficial effect of growth hormone on atherogenic risk in children with growth hormone deficiency (Kohno et al). 1995; 126:953-5 (CLO)
Cancer in children with primary or secondary immunodeficiencies (Mueller and Pizzo). 1995;126:1-10
Clinical characteristics and risk factors for *Vibrio cholerae* infection in children (Fukuda et al). 1995;126:882-6
Consumption of soft drinks with phosphoric acid as a risk factor for the development of hypocalcemia in children: a case-control study (Mazariegos-Ramos et al). 1995;126:940-2 (CLO)
Effect of maternal glucocorticoid exposure on risk of severe intraventricular hemorrhage in surfactant-treated preterm infants (Garland et al). 1995;126:272-9
Pediatric Investigators Collaborative Network on Infections in Canada (PICNIC) prospective study of risk factors and outcomes in patients hospitalized with respiratory syncytial viral lower respiratory tract infection (Wang et al). 1995; 126:212-9
A reexamination of the risk factors for the sudden infant death syndrome (Taylor and Sanderson). 1995;126:887-91

Risk factors—cont'd
Risk of recurrent stroke in patients with sickle cell disease treated with erythrocyte transfusions (Pegelow et al). 1995;126:896-9
Secular changes in the outcomes to eighteen to twenty-four months of age of extremely low birth weight infants, with adjustment for changes in risk factors and severity of illness (Perlman et al). 1995;126:75-87
Rupture
Inhaled nitric oxide for premature infants after prolonged rupture of the membranes (Peliowski et al). 1995;126:450-53 (CLO)

S

Salbutamol; *see* Albuterol
Screening; *see* Mass screening
Seizures
Supplementary sensorimotor area seizures in children and adolescents (Bass et al). 1995;126:537-44
Sepsis; *see* Septicemia
Septicemia
Band neutrophil counts in neonates (Rosenfeld and MacGregor) (Letter); (Schelonka et al) (Reply). 1995;126:504-6
Soluble interleukin-2 receptor as a predictor of neonatal sepsis (Spear et al). 1995;126:982-5 (CLO)
Severity of illness index
Secular changes in the outcomes to eighteen to twenty-four months of age of extremely low birth weight infants, with adjustment for changes in risk factors and severity of illness (Perlman et al). 1995;126:75-87
Sex steroids; *see* Steroids
Short stature; *see* Body height
Shunts
Pulmonary arteriovenous shunting in children with liver disease (Barbé et al). 1995;126:571-9
Sickle cell anemia; *see* Anemia, sickle cell
Skin biopsy; *see* Biopsy
Social class
Development of a vaccine tracking system to improve the rate of age-appropriate primary immunization in children of lower socioeconomic status (Abramson et al). 1995;126:583-6 (CLO)
Socioeconomic status; *see* Social class
Soft drinks; *see* Beverages
Somatosensory evoked potentials; *see* Evoked potentials, somatosensory
Somatotropin
Beneficial effect of growth hormone on atherogenic risk in children with growth hormone deficiency (Kohno et al). 1995; 126:953-5 (CLO)
Benign intracranial hypertension in children with growth hormone deficiency treated with growth hormone (Malozowski et al). 1995;126:996-9
Combined treatment with growth hormone and gonadotropin-releasing hormone analogs in short normal girls (Saggese et al). 1995;126:468-73
Effect of growth hormone therapy on final versus predicted height in short twelve- to sixteen-year-old boys without growth hormone deficiency (Kaplowitz). 1995;126:478-80 (CLO)
Growth and the growth hormone axis in prepubertal children with asthma (Crowley et al). 1995;126:297-303
Prediction of the outcome of growth hormone therapy in children with idiopathic short stature: a multivariate discriminant analysis (Spagnoli et al). 1995;126:905-9
Prepubertal gynecomastia during growth hormone therapy (Malozowski and Stadel). 1995;126:659-61 (CLO)
Relation of growth hormone deficiency and leukemia (Rapaport et al). 1995;126:759-61 (CLO)

Somatotropin—cont'd
Response to growth hormone therapy in patients with growth hormone deficiency who were small or appropriate in size for gestational age at birth (Balsamo et al). 1995;126:474-7
Spastic quadriplegia; *see* Quadriplegia
Spleen
Outcome of partial splenectomy for type I Gaucher disease (Zimran et al). 1995;126:596-7 (CLO)
Steroids
Bone mineralization, hypothalamic amenorrhea, and sex steroid therapy in adolescents and young adults (Hergenroeder). 1995;126:683-9
Effect of maternal glucocorticoid exposure on risk of severe intraventricular hemorrhage in surfactant-treated preterm infants (Garland et al). 1995;126:272-9
Street drugs
Use of a visual panel detection method for drugs of abuse: clinical and laboratory experience with children and adolescents (Valentine and Komoroski). 1995;126:135-40
Streptococcus pneumoniae
Life-threatening infection in two children with hemoglobin S–beta-thalassemia (Lynch and Tobias). 1995;126:581-2 (CLO)
Streptococcus pyogenes
Comparison of an optical immunoassay technique with two culture methods for the detection of group A streptococci in a pediatric office (Roddey et al). 1995;126:931-3 (CLO)
Diagnosis of group A streptococcal pharyngitis in a private clinic: comparative evaluation of an optical immunoassay method and culture (Fries). 1995;126:933-6 (CLO)
Substance abuse
Relation between meconium concentration of the cocaine metabolite benzoylecgonine and fetal growth (Mirochnick et al). 1995;126:636-8 (CLO)
Screening neonates for intrauterine cocaine exposure (Neuspiel) (Letter); (Ryan and Phelps) (Reply). 1995;126:323-4
Substance abuse detection
Use of a visual panel detection method for drugs of abuse: clinical and laboratory experience with children and adolescents (Valentine and Komoroski). 1995;126:135-40
Sucking behavior
Imaging evaluation of breast-feeding and bottle feeding systems (Nowak et al). 1995;126:S130-4
Nipple confusion: toward a formal definition (Neifert et al). 1995;126:S125-9
Sudden infant death
A reexamination of the risk factors for the sudden infant death syndrome (Taylor and Sanderson). 1995;126:887-91
Sugar, adverse effects; *see* Carbohydrates, adverse effects
Supine position
Abnormal tympanography after supine bottle feeding (Tully et al). 1995;126:S105-11
Surface-active agents
Double-blind developmental evaluation at 1-year corrected age of 597 premature infants with birth weights from 500 to 1350 grams enrolled in three placebo-controlled trials of prophylactic synthetic surfactant (Corbet et al). 1995;126:S5-12 (Symposium)
Double-blind evaluation of developmental and health status to age 2 years of infants weighing 700 to 1350 grams treated prophylactically at birth with a single dose of synthetic surfactant or air placebo (Kraybill et al). 1995;126:S33-42 (Symposium)
Double-blind, randomized, placebo-controlled Canadian multicenter trial of two doses of synthetic surfactant or air placebo in 224 infants weighing 500 to 749 grams with respiratory distress syndrome (Smyth et al). 1995;126:S81-9 (Symposium)

Surface-active agents—cont'd
Double-blind, randomized trial of one versus three prophylactic doses of synthetic surfactant in 826 neonates weighing 700 to 1100 grams: effects on mortality rate (Corbet et al). 1995; 126:969-78
Double-blind 1-year follow-up of 1540 infants with respiratory distress syndrome randomized to rescue treatment with two doses of synthetic surfactant or air in four clinical trials (Courtney et al). 1995;126:S43-52 (Symposium)
Effect of maternal glucocorticoid exposure on risk of severe intraventricular hemorrhage in surfactant-treated preterm infants (Garland et al). 1995;126:272-9
Effects of two rescue doses of synthetic surfactant in 344 infants with respiratory distress syndrome weighing 750 to 1249 grams: a double-blind, placebo-controlled multicenter Canadian trial (McMillan et al). 1995;126:S90-8 (Symposium)
Health and neurodevelopmental outcome at 1-year adjusted age in 508 infants weighing 700 to 1100 grams who received prophylaxis with one versus three doses of synthetic surfactant (Gerdes et al). 1995;126:S26-32 (Symposium)
One-year follow-up evaluation of 260 premature infants with respiratory distress syndrome and birth weights of 700 to 1350 grams randomized to two rescue doses of synthetic surfactant or air placebo (Gong et al). 1995;126:S68-74 (Symposium)
One-year follow-up of 66 premature infants weighing 500 to 699 grams treated with a single dose of synthetic surfactant or air placebo at birth: results of a double-blind trial (Walther et al). 1995;126:S13-9 (Symposium)
One-year follow-up of 89 infants with birth weights of 500 to 749 grams and respiratory distress syndrome randomized to two rescue doses of synthetic surfactant or air placebo (Casiro et al). 1995;126:S53-60 (Symposium)
One-year follow-up of 273 infants with birth weights of 700 to 1100 grams after prophylactic treatment of respiratory distress syndrome with synthetic surfactant or air placebo (Sell et al). 1995;126:S20-5 (Symposium)
One-year outcome in 232 premature infants with birth weights of 750 to 1249 grams and respiratory distress syndrome randomized to rescue treatment with two doses of synthetic surfactant or air placebo (Saigal et al). 1995;126:S61-7 (Symposium)
Outcome at 1-year adjusted age of 957 infants weighing more than 1250 grams with respiratory distress syndrome randomized to receive synthetic surfactant or air placebo (Sauve et al). 1995;126:S75-80 (Symposium)
Partial liquid ventilation in premature lambs with respiratory distress syndrome: efficacy and compatibility with exogenous surfactant (Leach et al). 1995;126:412-20
Symposium on Synthetic Surfactant II: perspective and commentary (Long et al). 1995;126:S1-4 (Symposium)
Synthetic surfactant for rescue treatment of respiratory distress syndrome in premature infants weighing from 700 to 1350 grams: impact on hospital resource use and charges (Mauskopf et al). 1995;126:94-101
Surface antigens; *see* Antigens, surface
Surfactants; *see* Surface-active agents
Survival
Effect of corticosteroids on survival of children with acquired immunodeficiency syndrome and *Pneumocystis carinii*–related respiratory failure (McLaughlin et al). 1995;126:821-4 (CLO)
Encephalopathy in children with perinatally acquired human immunodeficiency virus infection (Lobato et al). 1995;126:710-5
Intact survival with transfusion-associated graft-versus-host disease proved by human leukocyte antigen typing of lymphocytes in skin biopsy specimens (Hentschel et al). 1995;126:61-4 (CLO)
Neonatal mortality rate: Is further improvement possible? (Philip). 1995;126:427-33
Susceptibility; *see* Disease susceptibility
Suture techniques
Economic comparison of a tissue adhesive and suturing in the repair of pediatric facial lacerations (Osmond et al). 1995; 126:892-5
Sweat
Transient elevation of sweat chloride concentration in a malnourished girl with the Mauriac syndrome (Polack et al). 1995;126:261-3 (CLO)
Symposium
Symposium on synthetic surfactant II: health and developmental outcomes at one year. 1995;126:S1-102
Synthetic surfactant; *see* Surface-active agents
Systemic lupus erythematosus; *see* Lupus erythematosus, systemic

T

Tachycardia
Conjugated hyperbilirubinemia in a newborn infant after maternal (transplacental) treatment with flecainide acetate for fetal tachycardia and fetal hydrops (Vanderhal et al). 1995;126: 988-90 (CLO)
Tachycardia, ventricular
Corticosteroid therapy for ventricular tachycardia in children with silent lymphocytic myocarditis (Ino et al). 1995;126:304-8
Terbutaline
Terbutaline powder for acute asthma (Rufin et al). 1995;126:161-2 (Letter)
Terminal care
Control of severe pain in children with terminal malignancy (Collins et al). 1995;126:653-7
Tetanus toxoid
Effect of neonatal immunization with diphtheria and tetanus toxoids on antibody responses to *Haemophilus influenzae* type b conjugate vaccines (Lieberman et al). 1995;126:198-205
Thelarche
Progression of premature thelarche to central precocious puberty (Pasquino et al). 1995;126:11-4
Thrombosis
Catheter-related thrombosis in critically ill children: comparison of catheters with and without heparin bonding (Krafte-Jacobs et al). 1995;126:50-4
Cerebral vein thrombosis in childhood systemic lupus erythematosus (Uziel et al). 1995;126:722-7
A cross-sectional study of catheter-related thrombosis in children receiving total parenteral nutrition at home (Andrew et al). 1995;126:358-63
Portal vein thrombosis caused by protein C and protein S deficiency associated with cytomegalovirus infection (Arav-Boger et al). 1995;126:586-8 (CLO)
Thyroid function tests
Reference ranges for newer thyroid function tests in premature infants (Adams et al). 1995;126:122-7
Thyroxine
Long-term effects of L-thyroxine therapy for congenital hypothyroidism (Rovet and Ehrlich). 1995;126:380-6
Tissue adhesives
Economic comparison of a tissue adhesive and suturing in the repair of pediatric facial lacerations (Osmond et al). 1995; 126:892-5
Total parenteral nutrition, home; *see* Parenteral nutrition, home total
Toxins
Antibiotic-associated hemorrhagic colitis without *Clostridium difficile* toxin in children (Kato et al). 1995;126:1008-10 (CLO)

Transfusion; *see* Blood transfusion
Transient organic aciduria; *see* Aciduria
Transmembrane regulator gene; *see* Genes, regulator
Transmission, transplacental; *see* Maternal-fetal exchange
Transplacental treatment; *see* Maternal-fetal exchange
Triptorelin
Use of the gonadotropin-releasing hormone agonist triptorelin in the diagnosis of delayed puberty in boys (Zamboni et al). 1995;126:756-8 (CLO)
Tuberculosis
Use of polymerase chain reaction for improved diagnosis of tuberculosis in children (Delacourt et al). 1995;126:703-9
Tuberculosis, miliary
Adult respiratory distress syndrome in children associated with miliary tuberculosis (Martinez-Azagra et al) (Letter); (Davis) (Reply). 1995;126:678-9
Tubulointerstitial nephritis; *see* Nephritis, interstitial
Tumor necrosis factor
Cytokine elevations in infants with bacterial and aseptic meningitis (Dulkerian et al). 1995;126:872-6
Turner's syndrome
Lipid abnormalities in Turner syndrome (Ross et al). 1995;126: 242-5
Twins
Birth order, delivery route, and concordance in the transmission of human immunodeficiency virus type 1 from mothers to twins (Duliège et al). 1995;126:625-32
Discordance for hyperinsulinemic hypoglycemia in monozygotic twins (Santer et al) (Letter); (Thornton et al) (Reply). 1995; 126:1017
Twins, monozygotic
Discordance for hyperinsulinemic hypoglycemia in monozygotic twins (Santer et al) (Letter); (Thornton et al) (Reply). 1995; 126:1017
Tympanography; *see* Acoustic impedance tests
Tyrosine
Painful keratoderma and photophobia: hallmarks of tyrosinemia type II (Rabinowitz et al). 1995;126:266-9 (CLO)

U

Ultrasonography
Placement of umbilical venous catheters with use of bedside real-time ultrasonography (Greenberg et al). 1995;126:633-5 (CLO)
Umbilical arteries
Placement of umbilical venous catheters with use of bedside real-time ultrasonography (Greenberg et al). 1995;126:633-5 (CLO)
Urban health
Lead poisoning: low rates of screening and high prevalence among children seen in inner-city emergency departments (Wiley et al). 1995;126:392-5 (CLO)
Ureaplasma urealyticum
Isolation of *Ureaplasma urealyticum* from low birth weight infants (Crouse and Reese) (Letter); (Heggie et al) (Reply). 1995;126:502-4
Urinary tract infections
Diagnostic accuracy of urinary tract infection and subsequent development of renal scars (Koskimies) (Letter); (Hoberman and Wald) (Reply). 1995;126:157-9
Urine
Use of the urine-to-blood carbon dioxide tension gradient as a measurement of impaired distal tubular hydrogen ion secretion among neonates (Lin et al). 1995;126:114-7

V

Vaccines; *see also* Bacterial vaccines
Development of a vaccine tracking system to improve the rate of age-appropriate primary immunization in children of lower socioeconomic status (Abramson et al). 1995;126:583-6 (CLO)
Vaccines, synthetic
Long-term efficacy of recombinant hepatitis B vaccine and risk of natural infection in infants born to mothers with hepatitis B e antigen (Lee et al). 1995;126:716-21
Vasculitis
Spectrum of disease associated with anti-neutrophil cytoplasmic autoantibodies in pediatric patients (Ellis et al). 1995;126:40-3
Vena cava, inferior
Effect of airway pressure on inferior vena cava pressure as a measure of central venous pressure in children (Reda et al). 1995;126:961-5 (CLO)
Venoms
Venom immunotherapy: Who should receive it? (Bierman). 1995;126:257-8 (Editor's column)
Ventilation
Abnormalities in control of ventilation in newborn infants with myelomeningocele (Petersen et al). 1995;126:1011-5
Improved oxygenation during synchronized intermittent mandatory ventilation in neonates with respiratory distress syndrome: a randomized, crossover study (Cleary et al). 1995;126:407-11
Partial liquid ventilation in premature lambs with respiratory distress syndrome: efficacy and compatibility with exogenous surfactant (Leach et al). 1995;126:412-20
Ventilators, mechanical
Critical illness neuromuscular disease in children manifested as ventilatory dependence (Sheth et al). 1995;126:259-61 (CLO)
Twenty-month outcome in ventilator-dependent, very low birth weight infants born during the early years of dexamethasone therapy (Furman et al). 1995;126:434-40
Ventricular tachycardia; *see* Tachycardia, ventricular
Very low birth weight infant; *see* Infant, low birth weight
Vibrio cholerae
Clinical characteristics and risk factors for *Vibrio cholerae* infection in children (Fukuda et al). 1995;126:882-6
Virus phenotype; *see* Phenotype
Viruses
Vertical transmission of human immunodeficiency virus type I: autologous neutralizing antibody, virus load, and virus phenotype (Husson et al). 1995;126:865-71
Visual panel detection of drug abuse; *see* Substance abuse detection
Vitamin A
Clinical trial of vitamin A as adjuvant treatment for lower respiratory tract infections (Kjolhede et al). 1995;126:807-12
Vitamin A and E status in very low birth weight infants: development of an improved parenteral delivery system (Inder et al). 1995;126:128-31 (CLO)
Vitamin D deficiency
Healing of rickets during vitamin D therapy despite defective vitamin D receptors in two siblings with vitamin D–dependent rickets type II (Kruse and Feldmann). 1995;126:145-8 (CLO)
A new defect in vitamin D metabolism (Nützenadel et al) (Letter); (Casella and Finberg) (Reply). 1995;126:676-7
Pathophysiology of calcium metabolism in children with vitamin D–deficiency rickets (Kruse). 1995;126:736-41
Single-day therapy for rickets (Mimouni) (Letter); (Shah and Finberg) (Reply). 1995;126:1019-20
Vitamin E
Vitamin A and E status in very low birth weight infants: development of an improved parenteral delivery system (Inder et al). 1995;126:128-31 (CLO)

Vomiting
A randomized comparison of intravenously administered granisetron versus chlorpromazine plus dexamethasone in the prevention of ifosfamide-induced emesis in children (Hählen et al). 1995;126:309-13

W

Warfarin
Cerebral vein thrombosis in childhood systemic lupus erythematosus (Uziel et al). 1995;126:722-7
A cross-sectional study of catheter-related thrombosis in children receiving total parenteral nutrition at home (Andrew et al). 1995;126:358-63

Warkany, Joseph
Josef Warkany (Miller). 1995;126:669-72 (Profiles)

Weight gain
Increased fat oxidation in prepubertal obese children: A metabolic defense against further weight gain? (Maffeis et al). 1995;126:15-20

Whites
Acquired platelet dysfunction with eosinophilia in white children (Poon et al). 1995;126:959-61 (CLO)

Williams syndrome
Cerebral artery stenoses in Williams syndrome cause strokes in childhood (Kaplan et al). 1995;126:943-5 (CLO)
Ischemic stroke and intracranial multifocal cerebral arteriopathy in Williams syndrome (Soper et al). 1995;126:945-8 (CLO)

Wounds and injuries
Economic comparison of a tissue adhesive and suturing in the repair of pediatric facial lacerations (Osmond et al). 1995; 126:892-5

Y

Yale Observation Scale
Efficacy of an observation scale in detecting bacteremia in febrile children three to thirty-six months of age, treated as outpatients (Teach et al). 1995;126:877-81

Supplement to
THE JOURNAL OF
PEDIATRICS

May 1995 *Volume 126* *Number 5, Part 2*

SYMPOSIUM ON SYNTHETIC SURFACTANT II: HEALTH AND DEVELOPMENTAL OUTCOMES AT ONE YEAR

Guest Editors:
Walker A. Long, MD
Janet A. Zucker, PhD
Ernest N. Kraybill, MD

Supplement to

THE JOURNAL OF PEDIATRICS

Mosby

Contents

MAY 1995 PART 2

SYMPOSIUM ON SYNTHETIC SURFACTANT II: HEALTH AND DEVELOPMENTAL OUTCOMES AT ONE YEAR

Symposium on Synthetic Surfactant II: Perspective and commentary S1
Walker Long, MD, Janet Zucker, PhD, and Ernest Kraybill, MD, Chapel Hill and Research Triangle Park, North Carolina

Double-blind developmental evaluation at 1-year corrected age of 597 premature infants with birth weights from 500 to 1350 grams enrolled in three placebo-controlled trials of prophylactic synthetic surfactant S5
Anthony Corbet, MB, FRACP, Walker Long, MD, Robert Schumacher, MD, Jeffrey Gerdes, MD, Robert Cotton, MD, and the American Exosurf Neonatal Study Group I (see Appendix I), Houston, Texas; Chapel Hill, North Carolina; Ann Arbor, Michigan; Philadelphia, Pennsylvania; and Nashville, Tennessee

One-year follow-up of 66 premature infants weighing 500 to 699 grams treated with a single dose of synthetic surfactant or air placebo at birth: Results of a double-blind trial S13
Frans J. Walther, MD, PhD, Martha Mullett, MD, Robert Schumacher, MD, Hakan Sundell, MD, David Easa, MD, Walker Long, MD, and the American Exosurf Neonatal Study Group I (see Appendix I), Los Angeles, California; Morgantown, West Virginia; Ann Arbor, Michigan; Nashville, Tennessee; Honolulu, Hawaii; and Chapel Hill, North Carolina

One-year follow-up of 273 infants with birth weights of 700 to 1100 grams after prophylactic treatment of respiratory distress syndrome with synthetic surfactant or air placebo S20
Matthew Sell, MD, Robert Cotton, MD, Toshiko Hirata, MD, Robert Guthrie, MD, Michael LeBlanc, MD, Mark Mammel, MD, Walker Long, MD, and the American Exosurf Neonatal Study Group I (see Appendix I), Boise, Idaho; Nashville, Tennessee; San Francisco, California; Pittsburgh, Pennsylvania; Jackson, Mississippi; St. Paul, Minnesota; and Chapel Hill, North Carolina

Continued on page 4A

Vol. 126, No. 5, Part 2, May 1995. The Journal of Pediatrics (ISSN 0022-3476) is published monthly (six issues per volume, two volumes per year) by Mosby–Year Book, Inc., 11830 Westline Industrial Dr., St. Louis, MO 63146-3318. Second-class postage paid at St. Louis, Mo., and additional mailing offices. POSTMASTER: Send changes of address to The Journal of Pediatrics, Mosby–Year Book, Inc., 11830 Westline Industrial Dr., St. Louis, MO 63146-3318, (800)453-4351. Annual subscription rates: domestic, $102.00 for individuals and $211.00 for institutions. Printed in U.S.A.

CONTENTS *continued*

Health and neurodevelopmental outcome at 1-year adjusted age in 508 infants weighing 700 to 1100 grams who received prophylaxis with one versus three doses of synthetic surfactant S26
Jeffrey Gerdes, MD, Marsha Gerdes, PhD, Ed Beaumont, MD, Larry Cook, MD, R. Dhanireddy, MD, Arthur Kopleman, MD, Robert Jarrett, DO, Walker Long, MD, and the American Exosurf Neonatal Study Groups I and II (see Appendixes I and II), Philadelphia, Pennsylvania; Grand Rapids, Michigan; Louisville, Kentucky; Washington, D.C.; Honolulu, Hawaii; and Greenville and Chapel Hill, North Carolina

Double-blind evaluation of developmental and health status to age 2 years of infants weighing 700 to 1350 grams treated prophylactically at birth with a single dose of synthetic surfactant or air placebo S33
Ernest N. Kraybill, MD, Carl L. Bose, MD, Anthony J. Corbet, MB, FRACP, Jose Garcia-Prats, MD, Diane Asbill, RN, Kathleen Edwards, MPH, and Walker Long, MD, Chapel Hill, North Carolina; Houston, Texas; and Research Triangle Park, North Carolina

Double-blind 1-year follow-up of 1540 infants with respiratory distress syndrome randomized to rescue treatment with two doses of synthetic surfactant or air in four clinical trials S43
Sherry E. Courtney, MD, Walker Long, MD, Douglas McMillan, MD, Donnal Walter, MD, Theodore Thompson, MD, Reginald Sauve, MD, Brent Conway, Harry Bard, MD, and the American and Canadian Exosurf Neonatal Study Groups (see Appendixes I-IV), Dayton, Ohio; Chapel Hill, North Carolina; Little Rock, Arkansas; Minneapolis, Minnesota; Calgary, Alberta, Canada; Research Triangle Park, North Carolina; and Montreal, Quebec, Canada

One-year follow-up of 89 infants with birth weights of 500 to 749 grams and respiratory distress syndrome randomized to two rescue doses of synthetic surfactant or air placebo S53
Oscar Casiro, MD, William Bingham, MD, Brock MacMurray, MD, Michael Whitfield, MD, Saroj Saigal, MD, Michael Vincer, MD, Walker Long, MD, the Canadian Exosurf Neonatal Study Group, and the Canadian Exosurf Neonatal Follow-Up Group (see Appendixes III and IV), Winnipeg, Manitoba, Canada; Saskatoon, Saskatchewan, Canada; Ottawa, Ontario, Canada; Vancouver, British Columbia, Canada; Hamilton, Ontario, Canada; Halifax, Nova Scotia, Canada; and Chapel Hill, North Carolina

CONTENTS *continued*

One-year outcome in 232 premature infants with birth weights of 750 to 1249 grams and respiratory distress syndrome randomized to rescue treatment with two doses of synthetic surfactant or air placebo S61
Saroj Saigal, MD, Charlene Robertson, MD, Koravangattu Sankaran, MD, William Bingham, MD, Oscar Casiro, MD, Brock MacMurray, MD, Michael Whitfield, MD, Walker Long, MD, and the Canadian Exosurf Neonatal Study Group (see Appendix III), Hamilton, Ontario, Canada; Edmonton, Alberta, Canada; Saskatoon, Saskatchewan, Canada; Winnipeg, Manitoba, Canada; Ottawa, Ontario, Canada; Vancouver, British Columbia, Canada; and Chapel Hill, North Carolina

One-year follow-up evaluation of 260 premature infants with respiratory distress syndrome and birth weights of 700 to 1350 grams randomized to two rescue doses of synthetic surfactant or air placebo S68
Alice Gong, MD, Endla Anday, MD, Stephen Boros, MD, Richard Bucciarelli, MD, David Burchfield, MD, Janet Zucker, PhD, Walker Long, MD, and the American Exosurf Neonatal Study Group I (see Appendix I), San Antonio, Texas; Philadelphia, Pennsylvania; St. Paul, Minnesota; Gainesville, Florida; and Research Triangle Park and Chapel Hill, North Carolina

Outcome at 1-year adjusted age of 957 infants weighing more than 1250 grams with respiratory distress syndrome randomized to receive synthetic surfactant or air placebo S75
Reginald Sauve, MD, Walker Long, MD, Michael Vincer, MD, Harry Bard, MD, Doug Derleth, MD, David Stevenson, MD, Thomas Pauly, MD, Charlene Robertson, MD, and the American and Canadian Exosurf Neonatal Study Groups (see Appendixes I and III), Calgary, Alberta, Canada; Chapel Hill, North Carolina; Halifax, Nova Scotia, Canada; Montreal, Quebec, Canada; Rochester, Minnesota; Palo Alto, California; Lexington, Kentucky; and Edmonton, Alberta, Canada

Double-blind, randomized, placebo-controlled Canadian multicenter trial of two doses of synthetic surfactant or air placebo in 224 infants weighing 500 to 749 grams with respiratory distress syndrome S81
John Smyth, MD, Alexander Allen, MD, Brock MacMurray, MD, Abraham Peliowski, MD, Koravangatu Sankaran, MD, Frank Volberg, MD, Arvind Shukla, MD, Walker Long, MD, and the Canadian Exosurf Neonatal Study Group (see Appendix III), Vancouver, British Columbia, Canada; Halifax, Nova Scotia, Canada; Ottawa, Ontario, Canada; Edmonton, Alberta, Canada; Saskatoon, Saskatchewan, Canada; Winston-Salem, North Carolina; Calgary, Alberta, Canada; and Chapel Hill, North Carolina

Continued on page 6A

CONTENTS *continued*

Effects of two rescue doses of synthetic surfactant in 344 infants with respiratory distress syndrome weighing 750 to 1249 grams: A double-blind, placebo-controlled multicenter Canadian trial S90
Douglas McMillan, MD, Victor Chernick, MD, Neil Finer, MD, David Schiff, MD, Harry Bard, MD, John Watts, MD, Robert Krzeski, MD, Walker Long, MD, and the Canadian Exosurf Neonatal Study Group (see Appendix III), Calgary, Alberta, Canada; Winnipeg, Manitoba, Canada; Edmonton, Alberta, Canada; Montreal, Quebec, Canada; Hamilton, Ontario, Canada; and Chapel Hill, North Carolina

APPENDIX I S99

APPENDIX II S100

APPENDIX III S101

APPENDIX IV S102

Annual subscription prices (effective through September 30, 1995)	U.S.A.	International surface mail		International airmail		
		All regions*	Canada†	Canada†	Mexico	All other*
Institutions	$211.00	$238.00	$254.66	$289.97	$271.00	$276.00
Individuals‡	$102.00	$129.00	$138.03	$173.34	$162.00	$167.00
Students, residents‡	$ 51.00	$ 78.00	$ 83.46	$118.77	$111.00	$116.00
Bound volumes§	$ 77.00	$ 93.00	$ 99.51	—	—	—
Single issues	$ 10.00	$ 10.00	$10.00	—	—	—

Subscription rates include supplements. Remittances should be made by check, draft, post office or express money order, in U.S. funds, drawn through a U.S. bank, payable to this JOURNAL. Claims for missing issues will be serviced only within 3 months (6 months international) of mail date. Single-copy prices will be charged on missing issues older than 3 months (6 months international) from mail date. Back issues generally are available for the previous 5 years. Subscriptions may begin at any time. Contact Mosby–Year Book, Inc., Subscription Services, 11830 Westline Industrial Dr., St. Louis, MO 63146-3318, U.S.A.; telephone (800)453-4351 or (314)453-4351; fax (314)432-1158.

*Contact exclusive agents in Japan and India for subscription information. Igaku-Shoin MYW Ltd., 3-23-14 Hongo, Bunkyo-ku, Tokyo 113, Japan. Universal Subscription Agency Pvt. Ltd., 18-19 Community Ctr/P.O. Box 8, Malviya Nagar Extn/Saket, New Delhi 110017, India.

†Canadian 7% Goods and Services Tax calculated on U.S. base rate has been added and will be paid by Mosby to Revenue Canada under GST No. R127341295.

‡Individual subscriptions and all student-rate subscriptions must be in the names of, billed to, and paid by individuals. All student-rate requests must indicate training status and name of institution.

§Available only to subscribers.

Supplement to

THE JOURNAL OF PEDIATRICS

May 1995 *Volume 126* *Number 5, Part 2*

Symposium on Synthetic Surfactant II: Perspective and commentary

Walker Long, MD, Janet Zucker, PhD, and Ernest Kraybill, MD

From the Department of Pediatrics, School of Medicine, University of North Carolina at Chapel Hill, Kenan Institute Of Private Enterprise, Kenan Flagler Business School, University of North Carolina at Chapel Hill, and the Clinical Research Division, Wellcome Research Laboratories, Research Triangle Park, North Carolina

The introduction of surfactant replacement 5 years ago has proved to be an important milestone in pediatrics in a number of ways. First, the clinical trials of surfactant have set a new standard for the clinical testing of potential innovations in the health care of children. No longer will champions of new "breakthroughs" for sick children delude themselves and others with the results from small, brief clinical trials conducted at a center or two. It is now clear that large multicenter trials with sufficient statistical power to answer the questions posed must be conducted. In addition, follow-up studies over periods long enough to know what really happened to the children who participated in the trials must be completed if we are to know whether the posited "breakthrough" is both safe and effective. After surfactant we pediatricians will be far less likely to do unwitting harm to the children we would like to help by adopting new therapies and techniques on insufficient evidence. To do no harm must remain our fundamental commitment. Large randomized trials are the only safeguard against getting lost in (1) enthusiasm for what is new and (2) desperation to do something. Therapeutic misadventure will continue to tarnish the checkered history of pediatrics unless we all moor to the safe bulwark of randomized clinical trials. This fundamental insight is perhaps the greatest legacy of the advent of surfactant replacement.

Reprint requests: Walker Long, MD, Division of Pediatric Cardiology, Department of Pediatrics, CB #7220, 311 Burnett Womack, Bldg, University of North Carolina at Chapel Hill, Chapel Hill, NC 27599-7220.

J PEDIATR 1995;126:S1-4.

0022-3476/95/$3.00 + 0 **9/0/64446**

Second, without doubt, surfactants are saving the lives of premature infants around the world. The largest drop in infant mortality observed in 20 years in the United States occurred in 1990,[1] the year in which surfactant was first released for commercial distribution. Both the Surgeon General and the Centers For Disease Control attributed that sudden drop in infant mortality to surfactant's reduction of mortality among premature infants. Significant improvements in the survival rates of premature infants have been observed in virtually every country in which surfactant has been introduced.[2, 3]

Third, the acute morbidity of premature infants has also been reduced substantially by surfactant.[4-6] The severity of respiratory distress syndrome and the frequency of air leak are universally recognized to be lessened by surfactant. Reductions in both the incidence and severity of bronchopulmonary dysplasia are also increasingly acknowledged as benefits of surfactant therapy.[5, 7, 8] Reductions in intraventricular hemorrhage are more controversial, but are without doubt documented at least for rescue use of synthetic-surfactant.[5, 7-9] We believe that reductions in intraventricular hemorrhage by surfactant will be accepted as fact once the effects of surfactant on IVH are analyzed by meta-analysis of all placebo-controlled, randomized trials of surfactant. The power and utility of meta-analysis were recently demonstrated to neonatology by Sinclair and Bracken[10] in their ground-breaking book.

IVH	Intraventricular hemorrhage
RDS	Respiratory distress syndrome

Fourth, the health economic consequences of using surfactant are becoming clear. Gains in survival that cost less than $100,000 per life-year gained are considered to be cost-effective. Gains in survival that cost less than $20,000 per life-year gained are considered to be highly cost-effective. Several retrospective studies have suggested that surfactant is highly cost-effective in larger infants but not in smaller infants.[11-16] This misimpression has been corrected by recently published, prospective, randomized, placebo-controlled health economic studies of synthetic surfactant.[17-19]

Synthetic surfactant proved to be highly cost-effective in infants weighing 700 to 1350 gm who had RDS.[18] Total first-year hospital charges were $206 more per surfactant-treated infant when compared with placebo-treated infants among 419 infants weighing 700 to 1350 gm with RDS who were randomized to two rescue doses of synthetic surfactant or air placebo.[18] The extra cost per surfactant-treated infant was small but the gains in survival were large in the surfactant group; the cost per life-year gained was $28[18]—three orders of magnitude less than the $20,000 price per life-year gained considered to be the threshold for high cost-effectiveness.

In infants who weighed more than 1250 gm, a cost-effectiveness analysis was not possible because there was no cost to using synthetic surfactant.[19] Instead, synthetic surfactant actually saved money.[19] Infants who received surfactant required 9 days less in the hospital during the first year of life, 5 days less in the ICU, 14 days less on oxygen, and 4 days less on mechanical ventilation.[19] Total first-year hospital charges were $12,761 *less* per surfactant-treated infant than per placebo-treated infant among 1237 infants with RDS weighing more than 1249 gm randomized to two rescue doses of synthetic surfactant or air placebo.[19] The 50% relative reduction in mortality observed in that trial, clearly statistically significant,[9] was 2% in absolute terms.[19] Thus only a relatively small number of new life-years were added by synthetic surfactant, but a great deal less money was spent on each surfactant-treated infant. The net result, although not presented in the article,[19] was that all life-years gained were gained at a net *savings* of $8286 per added life-year. Very few interventions have been documented to save money as well as lives; only vaccines have been shown to have comparable health economic effects.

These studies[17-19] have set a new standard for health economic studies in children. In the future, the health economic effects of new therapies for children, like the clinical effects, will have to be evaluated prospectively as part of large randomized clinical trials.[20, 21] The substantial savings caused by use of surfactant in the larger infants with RDS, combined with the minimal cost (high cost-effectiveness) of using surfactant in middle-sized infants, more than pays for the higher costs incurred in using surfactant in tiny infants. Thus, for the population as whole, surfactant saves lives, reduces morbidity, and also saves money. It is therefore a costly mistake, not only in morbidity and mortality but also in money, to withhold surfactant in larger infants with RDS; those are the infants in whom the greatest cost savings occur. Similarly, it is a mistake for governments or health authorities to limit funding for use of surfactant, which should be a high priority in allocation of scarce health-care resources, as surfactant saves those resources for use in other diseases.

The articles collected in this issue of the *Journal* reflect a fifth and equally important aspect of the introduction of surfactant—how do surfactant-treated infants fare at late follow-up? Despite saving lives, reducing acute morbidity, and saving money, does surfactant add to the burden of infants with impairments destined to be cared for by society? Numerous studies have examined outcomes of surfactant-treated infants at late follow-up, but the answers provided to that question have conflicted. On the other hand, most such studies were either not double-blind or were too small for definitive conclusions. The best follow-up data published to date were from Morely and Morely.[22]

The ten articles on follow-up published in this supplement[23-32] represent double-blind follow-up at 1-year adjusted age on more than 2000 infants randomized in one of seven placebo-controlled trials[24-26, 29-32] and more than 500 infants randomized in a trial of one versus three prophylactic doses in infants weighing 700 to 1100 gm.[27] In addition, double-blind follow-up at 2 years of age is described for more than 100 infants enrolled in a placebo-controlled trial of a single prophylactic dose of synthetic surfactant or air in infants weighing 700 to 1350 gm.[26]

When we first analyzed these data, we not only analyzed each study individually but also combined all patients into a single overview to maximize the chances of detecting real but small differences in outcomes. That analysis, published elsewhere,[33] documented significant gains in Bayley Scales of Infant Development scores and rates of mild impairment in infants weighing less than 750 gm, significant reductions in retinopathy of prematurity in infants weighing more than 1250 gm, and significant reductions in numbers of infants on respiratory support at 1 year in both the entire cohort and in infants weighing more than 1250 gm. However, because of concerns over significantly higher impairment rates in the group treated prophylactically in a randomized comparison of prophylaxis and rescue using a different surfactant,[34] we decided to break the overview down into two summaries, one for infants enrolled in placebo-controlled trials of prophylactic administration of synthetic surfactant[23] and one for infants enrolled in placebo-controlled trials of rescue administration of synthetic surfactant.[28] This approach caused a loss of power, and several of the beneficial effects observed in the entire cohort were lost when the population was split in this way.

In any case, the data contained in this supplement demonstrate that developmental and health outcomes of surfactant-treated infants are at least as good as those of placebo-treated infants, and that infants treated prophylactically fare at least as well as those who received rescue treatment. Indeed, late respiratory morbidity as measured by the number of infants receiving oxygen at 1-year adjusted age was still significantly less in infants weighing more than 1249 gm,[28, 32] and there were probably modest reductions in mild impairments among infants weighing less than 750 gm.[24, 29] Furthermore, both the proportions and absolute numbers of infants with impairments were lower in the surfactant group in 9 of the 10 articles on follow-up in this supplement, despite more survivors with surfactant. These findings indicate that surfactant does not result in more survivors with impairments, at least through 1 year of age. Data from double-blind follow-up at 2 and 3 years of age from the placebo-controlled Canadian rescue studies should shed additional light on the developmental and health outcomes of surfactant-treated infants.

The supplement is completed by two previously unpublished placebo-controlled rescue studies, both of which were conducted in Canada.[35, 36] The first is the only prospective rescue study of any surfactant targeted at very tiny infants with RDS (500 to 749 gm)[35]; synthetic surfactant improved physiology but not morbidity or mortality. Prophylaxis is by far the superior way to manage infants of this size.[37-41] The second[36] was a rescue study conducted in infants weighing 750 to 1249 gm that was halted short of targeted sample size because of positive results from other rescue trials.[9, 42] Despite premature termination, physiology, several forms of air leak, and survival without bronchopulmonary dysplasia were improved significantly,[36] as was true in both other placebo-controlled rescue trials of synthetic surfactant in infants with RDS weighing more than 700 gm.[9, 42]

REFERENCES

1. Wegman EM. Annual summary of vital statistics-1990. Pediatrics 1991;88:1081-92.
2. Ho NK. Surfactant replacement therapy: the Singapore experience. J Singapore Paediatr Soc 1993;35:58-67.
3. Tapia JL, Oto MA, Ramírez R, Henriquez MT, Fernández P, Alvarez J. Terapia con surfactante exógeno en recién nacidos con enfermedad de membrana hialina. Rev Chil Pediatr 1994; 65:137-42.
4. Soll RF, McQueen MM. Respiratory distress syndrome. In: Sinclair J, Bracken M, eds. Effective care of the newborn infant. Oxford: Oxford University Press, 1992:325-58.
5. Jobe AH. Pulmonary surfactant therapy. N Engl J Med 1993; 328:861-8.
6. Merritt TA, Soll RF, Hallman M. Overview of exogenous surfactant replacement therapy. J Inten Care Med 1993;8: 205-28.
7. Long WA. Synthetic surfactant. Semin Perinatol 1993;17:275-84.
8. Corbet A. Clinical trials of synthetic surfactant in the respiratory distress syndrome of premature infants. Clin Perinatol 1993;20:737-60.
9. Long W, Cotton R, Corbet A, et al. A controlled trial of synthetic surfactant in infants weighing 1250 G or more with respiratory distress syndrome. N Engl J Med 1991;325:1696-703.
10. Sinclair JC, Bracken MB, eds. Effective care of the newborn infant. Oxford: Oxford University Press, 1992.
11. Tubman TRJ, Halliday HL, Norman C. Cost of surfactant replacement treatment for severe neonatal respiratory distress syndrome: a randomized controlled trial. BMJ 1990;301:842-5.
12. Mugford M, Piercy J, Chalmers I. Cost implications of different approaches to the prevention of respiratory distress syndrome. Arch Dis Child 1991;68:757-64.
13. Merritt TA, Hallman M, Vaucher Y, et al. Impact of surfactant treatment on cost of neonatal intensive care: a cost-benefit analysis. J Perinatol 1991;10:416-9.
14. Mugford M, Howard S. Cost effectiveness of surfactant replacement in preterm babies. Pharmacoeconomics 1993;3: 362-73.
15. Soll RF, Jacobs J, Pashko S, et al. Cost effectiveness of beractant in the prevention of respiratory distress syndrome. Pharmacoeconomics 1993;4:278-86.
16. Schwartz RM, Luby AM, Scanlon JW, et al. Effect of surfactant on morbidity mortality and resource use in newborn infants weighing 500 to 1500 g. N Engl J Med 1994;330:1476-80.
17. Phibbs CS, Phibbs RH, Wakeley A, et al. Cost effects of surfactant therapy for neonatal respiratory distress syndrome. J PEDIATR 1993;123:953-62.
18. Mauskopf JA, Backhouse ME, Jones D, et al. Synthetic surfactant for rescue treatment of respiratory distress syndrome in premature infants weighing from 700 to 1350 grams: impact on hospital resource use and charges. J PEDIATR 1995;125:94-101.
19. Backhouse ME, Mauskopf JA, Jones D, et al. Economic outcomes of synthetic surfactant rescue therapy in infants weighing 1250 grams or more with respiratory distress syndrome: results from a randomized trial. Pharmacoeconomics 1994; 6:358-69.
20. Bryson HM, Whittington R. Colfosceril palmitate: a pharmacoeconomic evaluation of a synthetic surfactant preparation (Exosurf Neonatal) in infants with respiratory distress syndrome. Pharmacoeconomics 1994;6:563-77.
21. Long WA, Zeng G, Henry GW. New drugs for perinatal practice: the role of industry-sponsored clinical trials. In: Sinclair JC, ed. *Evidence-based perinatal practice*, Seminars in Perinatology 1995;19:132-43.
22. Morely CJ, Morely R. Follow up of premature babies treated with artificial surfactant (ALEC). Arch Dis Child 1990; 65:667-9.
23. Corbet A, Long W, Schumacher R, et al. Double-blind developmental evaluation at 1-year corrected age of 597 premature infants with birth weights from 500 to 1350 grams enrolled in three placebo-controlled trials of prophylactic synthetic surfactant. J PEDIATR 1995;126:S5-12.
24. Walther FJ, Mullett M, Schumacher R, Sundell H, Easa D, Long W. One-year follow-up of 66 premature infants weighing 500 to 699 grams treated with a single dose of synthetic surfactant or air placebo at birth: results of a double-blind trial. J PEDIATR 1995;126:S13-9.

25. Sell M, Cotton R, Hirata T, Guthrie R, LeBlanc M, Mammel M, Long W. One-year follow-up of 273 infants with birth weights of 700 to 1100 grams after prophylactic treatment of respiratory distress syndrome with synthetic surfactant or air placebo. J PEDIATR 1995;126:S20-5.
26. Kraybill EN, Bose C, Corbet A, Garcia Prats J, Asbill D, Edwards K, Long W. Double-blind evaluation of developmental and health status to age 2 years of infants weighing 700 to 1350 grams treated prophylactically at birth with a single dose of synthetic surfactant or air placebo. J PEDIATR 1995;126:S33-42.
27. Gerdes J, Gerdes M, Beaumont E, Cook L, Dhanireddy R, Kopleman A, Jarrett R, Long W. Health and neurodevelopmental outcome at 1-year adjusted age in 508 infants weighing 700 to 1100 grams who received prophylaxis with one versus three doses of synthetic surfactant. J PEDIATR 1995;126:S26-32.
28. Courtney SE, Long W, McMillan D, et al. Double-blind 1-year follow-up of 1540 infants with respiratory distress syndrome randomized to rescue treatment with two doses of synthetic surfactant or air in four clinical trials. J PEDIATR 1995;126:S43-52.
29. Casiro O, Bingham W, MacMurray B, et al.. One-year follow-up of 89 infants with birth weights of 500 to 749 grams and respiratory distress syndrome randomized to two rescue doses of synthetic surfactant or air placebo. J PEDIATR 1995;126:S53-60.
30. Saigal S, Robertson C, Sankaran K, Bingham W, Casiro O, MacMurray B, Whitfield M, Long W. One-year outcome in 232 premature infants with birth weights of 750 to 1249 grams and respiratory distress syndrome randomized to rescue treatment with two doses of synthetic surfactant or air placebo. J PEDIATR 1995;126:S61-7.
31. Gong A, Anday E, Boros S, Bucciarelli R, Burchfield D, Zucker J, Long W. One-year follow-up evaluation of 260 premature infants with respiratory distress syndrome and birth weights of 700 to 1350 grams randomized to two rescue doses of synthetic surfactant or air placebo. J PEDIATR 1995;126:S68-74.
32. Sauve R, Long W, Vincer M, et al. Outcome at 1-year adjusted age of 957 infants weighing more than 1250 grams with respiratory distress syndrome randomized to receive synthetic surfactant or air placebo. J PEDIATR 1995;126:S75-80.
33. Sauve RS. Developmental outcome at one year of infants treated with Exosurf Neonatal. In: Long WA, Tilson HH, eds. Proceedings of the Exosurf Neonatal Treatment IND Investigators' Meeting. Langhorne, Pa.: Adis International Inc., 1992:57-64.
34. Vaucher YE, Harker L, Merritt TA. Outcome at twelve months adjusted age in very low birth weight infants with lung immaturity: a randomized placebo controlled trial of human surfactant. J PEDIATR 1993;122:126-32.
35. Smyth J, Allen A, MacMurray B, Peliowski A, Sankaran K, Volberg F, Shukla A, Long W. Double-blind, randomized, placebo-controlled Canadian multicenter trial of two doses of synthetic surfactant or air placebo in 224 infants weighing 500 to 749 gm with respiratory distress syndrome. J PEDIATR 1995;126:S81-9.
36. McMillan D, Chernick V, Finer N, Schiff D, Bard H, Watts J, Krzeski R, Long W. Effects of two rescue doses of synthetic surfactant in 344 infants with respiratory distress syndrome weighing 750 to 1249 grams: a double-blind, placebo-controlled multicenter Canadian trial. J PEDIATR 1995;126:S90-8.
37. Kendig J, Notter RH, Cox C, et al. A comparison of surfactant as immediate prophylaxis and as rescue therapy in newborns of less than 30 weeks gestation. N Engl J Med 1991; 324:865-71.
38. Kattwinkel J, Bloom BT, Delmue P, et al. Prophylactic administration of calf lung surfactant extract is more effective than early treatment of respiratory distress syndrome in newborns of 29 through 32 weeks gestation. Pediatr 1993;92: 90-8.
39. Soll RF, Sinclair JC, Bracken MB. Meta analysis of surfactant trials: the effect of prophylactic surfactant vs surfactant treatment of established RDS [Abstract]. Pediatr Res 1992;33: 276A.
40. European Exosurf Study Group. Early or selective surfactant (colfosceril palmitate Exosurf) for intubated babies at 26 to 29 weeks gestation. On Line J Clin Trials 1992;Document no. 28.
41. The OSIRIS Collaborative Group. Early versus delayed neonatal administration of synthetic surfactant: the judgment of OSIRIS. Lancet 1992;340:1363-9.
42. Long WA, Thompson T, Sundell H, Schumacher R, Volberg F, Guthrie R. Effects of two rescue doses of a synthetic surfactant on mortality in 700-1350 gm infants with RDS. J PEDIATR 1991;118:595-605.

Double-blind developmental evaluation at 1-year corrected age of 597 premature infants with birth weights from 500 to 1350 grams enrolled in three placebo-controlled trials of prophylactic synthetic surfactant

Anthony Corbet, MB, FRACP, Walker Long, MD, Robert Schumacher, MD, Jeffrey Gerdes, MD, Robert Cotton, MD, and the American Exosurf Neonatal Study Group I (see Appendix I)

From the Departments of Pediatrics, Baylor College of Medicine, Houston, Texas; University of North Carolina at Chapel Hill; C.S. Mott Children's Hospital, University of Michigan, Ann Arbor; Pennsylvania Hospital, University of Pennsylvania, Philadelphia; Vanderbilt University, Nashville, Tennessee; and participating centers

Infants enrolled in three clinical trials of prophylactic treatment for respiratory distress syndrome with a single dose of synthetic surfactant (Exosurf Neonatal) or air placebo were monitored through 1-year adjusted age. A total of 1046 infants with birth weights from 500 to 1350 gm were enrolled in the three trials; of the 735 infants who survived to 1 year of age, follow-up evaluations were completed for 597 (80%, air placebo group; 82%, synthetic surfactant group). Infants in the air placebo and synthetic surfactant treatment groups had no differences in general health, growth, or neurodevelopmental outcomes or impairments. These follow-up results at 1-year adjusted age for infants who received a single dose of synthetic surfactant indicate that a single dose of synthetic surfactant reduces mortality without increasing the absolute number or proportion of infants with impairments at 1 year of age. (J Pediatr 1995;126:S5-12)

Respiratory distress syndrome is caused by deficiency of pulmonary surfactant in terminal air spaces of the lung.[1] Many clinicians now treat small premature infants with an instillation of exogenous surfactant into the lungs at birth, usually within half an hour after delivery. This preventive approach contrasts with a more selective rescue strategy of waiting until infants develop definite signs of RDS before providing treatment with exogenous surfactant. Several controlled clinical trials have suggested that a single prophylactic dose of surfactant at birth can reduce the mortality of small premature infants.[2-4] However, improved survival rates may be associated with either increased or decreased rates of subsequent impairment. In this report we describe the outcome at 1-year adjusted age of infants enrolled in three clinical trials[3-6] that examined the effects of a single prophylactic dose of synthetic surfactant at birth.

CI	Confidence interval
CP	Cerebral palsy
MDI	Mental development index
RDS	Respiratory distress syndrome
ROP	Retinopathy of prematurity

Supported by funds from Burroughs Wellcome Co., Research Triangle Park, North Carolina.

Reprint requests: Anthony Corbet, MD, Santa Rosa Childrens Hospital, 519 W. Houston St., San Antonio, TX 78207.

0022-3476/95/$3.00 + 0 **9/0/61823**

Table I. Clinical trials included in the 1-year analysis of prophylactic synthetic surfactant

Study No.	Birth weight (gm)	Patient entry	Study site	Reference	
				Days 1-28	1 Yr*
01/02	700-1350	385	USA	5	7
03	500-699	215	USA	6	8
04	700-1100	446	USA	4	9

*Articles for each individual trial also appear in this supplement.

METHODS

Study design and patient enrollment. Three multicenter, prospective, double-blind, randomized, parallel comparisons of a synthetic surfactant (colfosceril palmitate, cetyl alcohol, and tyloxapol; Exosurf Neonatal, Burroughs Wellcome Co., Research Triangle Park, N.C.) with air placebo in the prophylactic treatment of RDS were conducted in the United States (Table I; participants are listed in Appendix I). In these trials, infants born alive with qualifying birth weights were intubated and assigned randomly to receive a 5 ml/kg endotracheal dose of synthetic surfactant or air placebo as soon as possible after birth.

The trials were conducted with a common protocol and consisted of two evaluation periods: days 1 to 28 and 1-year follow-up. The effects of a single prophylactic dose of this synthetic surfactant on acute morbidity and mortality of infants with RDS have been published previously.[3-6] The follow-up studies, which are presented individually in this supplement[7-9] and have been combined for this article, consisted of double-blind evaluations conducted at 1-year adjusted age. The protocols were approved by the Institutional Review Board at each hospital, and informed consent was obtained from the parents of each patient who was enrolled in the studies. Patients were entered into the studies between April 1986 and December 1989.

Ophthalmologic examination. Ophthalmologic examinations were performed during the first year of life. Many infants had several ophthalmologic examinations, and data were collected for both the worst and last examination before the 1-year follow-up date. If only one examination was performed, it was recorded as both the worst and last examination. For each eye, retinopathy of prematurity was evaluated and the requirements for surgery, cryotherapy, and laser therapy were recorded. Data for the worst eye are reported. ROP was classified according to the Committee for Classification of Retinopathy.[10] Mild/moderate ROP was diagnosed if the disease did not exceed stage 3; ROP that was classified as stage 3+ and greater was considered severe.

ONE-YEAR FOLLOW-UP EVALUATION

Infants were scheduled for evaluation within 6 weeks of 1-year adjusted age, defined as the chronologic age minus the number of weeks the infant was premature. Evaluators and parents were both masked as to which infants had received synthetic surfactant or air placebo.

Health status. A complete physical examination was performed. Height, weight, and head circumference measurements were obtained and plotted in relation to adjusted age on National Center for Health Statistics charts.[11] Pertinent information with regard to intervening medical complications, hospital admissions, surgical operations, use of medications for chronic lung and neurologic diseases, the highest required level of respiratory support, and the presence or absence of various allergies was documented on the day of the 1-year follow-up examination.

Neurodevelopmental outcome. A child developmental specialist at each institution assessed mental and motor development using the Bayley Scales of Infant Development.[12] Both the mental and psychomotor developmental indices have a mean of 100 and an SD of 16 in normal populations. A period of 6 weeks on either side of the 1-year adjusted-age target date was allowed for performance of the examinations. Bayley Scales of Infant Development examinations were not performed for infants considered by the examiner to be too delayed to be tested.

Impairments. The degree of impairment was graded for all children as none, mild to moderate, or severe, similar to the method of Kitchen et al.[13] Mild to moderate impairment was diagnosed if one of the following criteria was present: mild cerebral palsy, Bayley Scales of Infant Development MDI score of 69 to 84 (between one and two SD below the mean), sensorineural deafness not requiring amplification, or significant visual defect without blindness. Serious impairment was diagnosed if more than one of the aforementioned criteria or any of the following criteria were present: moderate or severe CP, Bayley Scales of Infant Development MDI score less than 69 (>2 SD below the mean), bilateral sensorineural deafness requiring amplification, or bilateral blindness.

For each child CP was recorded as being absent, mild, or moderate/severe according to the definitions suggested by Nelson and Ellenberg.[14] Mild CP was considered present if the infant had a definite abnormality of neuromuscular physical findings (increased tone, increased deep tendon re-

Table II. Patient accountability*

	Air placebo (*n* = 524)	Synthetic surfactant (*n* = 522)
Alive at 1 yr	352 (67)	383 (73)
Completed follow-up	283 (54) [80]	314 (60) [82]
Lost to follow-up	69 (13) [20]†	69 (13) [18]†

Numbers in parentheses represent the percentage of enrolled infants; numbers in brackets represent the percentage of survivors at 1-year adjusted age.
*Includes all patients as treated without exclusion.
†Includes approximately 13% of patients whose survival status was assessed by telephone contact.

flexes, positive Babinski's sign) but no or minimal functional defect. Moderate/severe CP was considered to be present if significant interference with independent function existed in addition to a definite abnormality of neuromuscular findings.

Developmental delay was determined by the Bayley Scales for Infant Development MDI score for adjusted age. An infant with an MDI score less than 69 was considered to have a severe developmental delay; an infant with an MDI score of 69 to 84 was considered to have a moderate developmental delay.

Hearing evaluations were performed during the first year, although the methods of assessing hearing loss and timing of the evaluations varied among institutions. Hearing loss was considered present if any degree of loss was recorded; deafness was considered present if the hearing threshold was more than 90 decibels.

Infants were considered to have a significant visual defect if they required surgical intervention or their vision could not be corrected to normal. Blindness was considered present if vision could not be corrected to better than legal blindness (≤20/200).

Data analyses and statistical methods. Categorical data were summarized by treatment group using frequency counts and percentages. Numeric data were summarized by treatment group using mean, SD, median, minimum, and maximum; mean differences were calculated. Incidence comparisons were expressed using relative risks and 95% confidence intervals. Relative risks and CI for the ophthalmologic and Bayley Scales of Infant Development examinations, impairment, and medical history assessments were based on the Cochran-Mantel-Haenszel test. In the analyses for the individual studies, the Cochran-Mantel-Haenszel test controlled for the randomization strata, that is, sex and birth weight classes. In the across-study analyses, the Cochran-Mantel-Haenszel test controlled for the original protocol. The CIs for these assessments are statistically significant when they exclude the ratio of "1." The number of patients is not consistent across all tables because all patients were not assessed for every measurement.

Table III. Entry characteristics and major neonatal complications of infants who completed the 1-year follow-up evaluations

	Air placebo (*n* = 283)	Synthetic surfactant (*n* = 314)
Birth weight (gm)*	931 ± 191	934 ± 179
Birth weight distribution (%)		
500-750 gm	52 (18)	54 (17)
750-1249 gm	217 (77)	244 (78)
1250 gm or more	14 (5)	16 (5)
Gestational age (wk)*	27 ± 2	27 ± 2
Multiple birth (%)	23	24
Inborn (%)	65	69
Race distribution (%)		
White	46	41
Black	36	37
Hispanic	14	16
Other	4	6
Maternal age (yr)*	25 ± 6	26 ± 6
Maternal education (yr)*	12 ± 3	12 ± 3
Gender (%)		
Male	50	50
Female	50	50
Apgar score (median)		
1 min	5	5
5 min	7	7
IVH during days 1-28 (%)		
Grade I/II	68 (24)	77 (25)
Grade III/IV	27 (10)	27 (9)
No IVH	185 (66)	209 (67)
BPD at day 28 (%)	55 (19)	66 (21)

IVH, Intraventricular hemorrhage; *BPD*, bronchopulmonary dysplasia.
*Values are mean ± SD. Differences are not significant.

RESULTS

Of 1046 infants enrolled at birth in the three clinical trials, 311 infants died before 1-year adjusted age (Table II). Of 735 survivors, 597 had neurodevelopmental assessments at 1-year adjusted age (81%), and 138 were lost to follow-up (19%). Of the 597 infants examined at the age of 1 year, 283 (47%) had received air placebo and 314 (53%) had received synthetic surfactant at birth; these two groups of infants were very similar with regard to their maternal demographics and clinical characteristics in the neonatal period (Table III).

Mean measurements of height (74 cm), weight (9.1 kg), and head circumference (46 cm) were equivalent in the two treatment groups; in addition, the distributions by percentile for weight, height, and head circumference were also equivalent (Table III; Fig. 1).

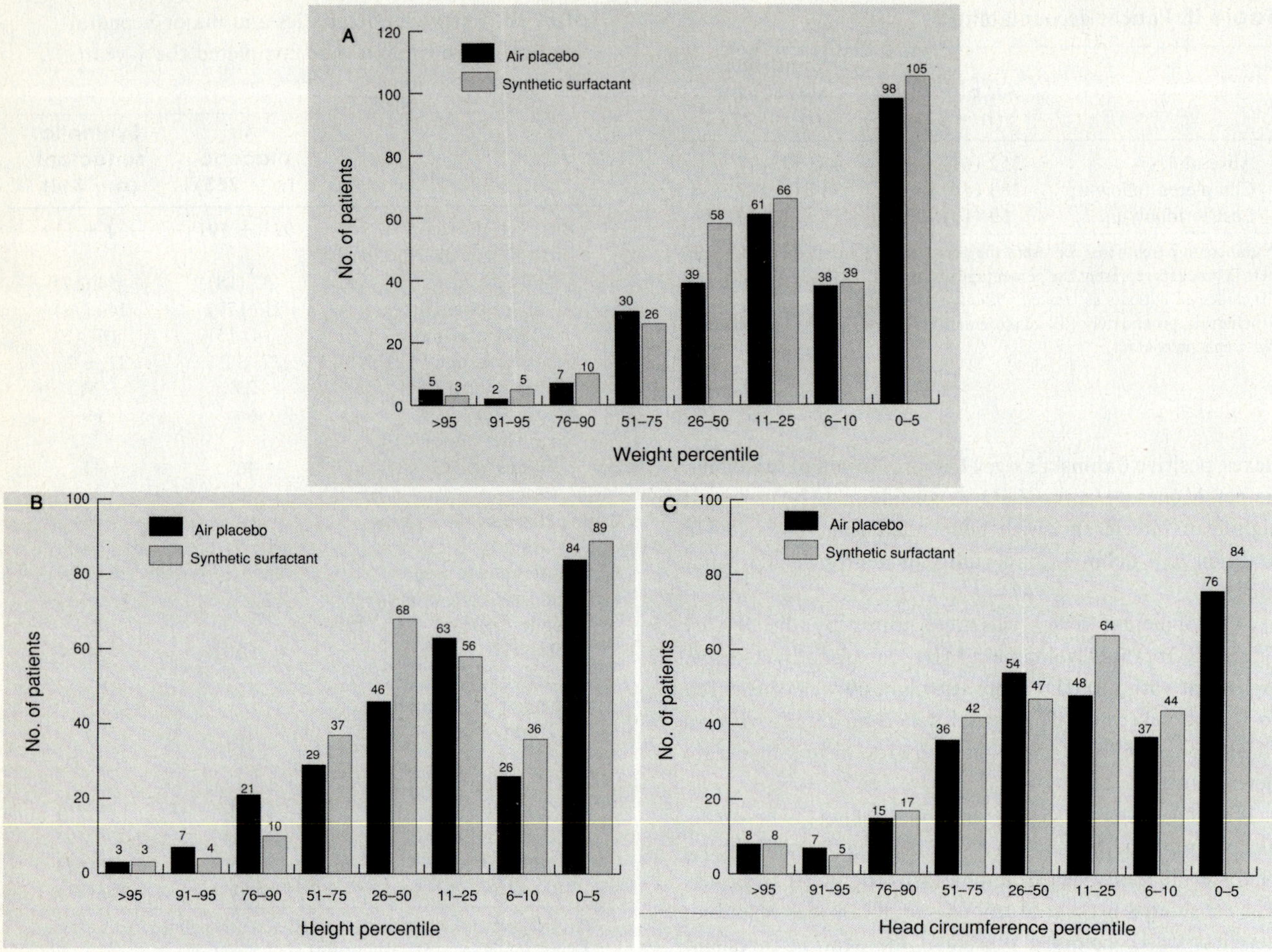

Fig. 1. Combined controlled trials of synthetic surfactant used prophylactically at birth in premature infants: the percentile distribution of growth parameters in control and treated infants at the age of 1 year.

The number of hospital readmissions, the number of surgical operations, the incidence of allergic complications, and the incidence of chronic lung disease requiring oxygen, ventilator support, or medications were equivalent in the two groups (Table IV). Asthma was reported significantly less frequently in the infants who were treated with synthetic surfactant.

Of 1046 infants enrolled at birth in the three clinical trials, 396 infants had retinal examinations reported during the follow-up period. Infants were often transferred to other hospitals before their eye examinations; data from these later examinations (performed outside the study protocol) were not collected. Based on both the worst and the last examination, the overall incidence of ROP and the incidence of severe ROP in the two treatment groups were the same (Table V).

Bayley Scales of Infant Development scores were also equivalent in the two groups (Table VI). Rates of impairment were similar in infants treated with air placebo (43%) and synthetic surfactant (37%) (Table VII). Furthermore, there were no differences between the two treatment groups in the incidence or severity of visual defects, auditory defects, CP, or neurodevelopmental delay (Table VII).

The proportion of infants with functional impairments, expressed in terms of all infants originally entered into the clinical trials at birth, was not different in the two treatment groups (Fig. 2).

Subdividing infants by birth weight into the categories of tiny (500 to 749 gm), middle-sized (750 to 1249 gm), and large (1250 gm or more) revealed a significant reduction in the proportion of infants with mild to moderate impair-

Table IV. Health status between day 29 and 1-year corrected age

	Air placebo (%) (*n* = 283)	Synthetic surfactant (%) (*n* = 314)	Relative risk*	95% Confidence interval
Surgery	94 (33)	106 (34)	1.05	0.84-1.31
Readmission to hospital	126 (45)	123 (39)	0.90	0.75-1.09
Physical evidence of CLD	31 (11)	30 (10)	0.90	0.56-1.45
Medications for CLD	23 (14)	24 (14)	0.99	0.58-1.76
Respiratory support on examination day	11 (4)	5 (2)	0.46	0.17-1.26
Medications: Chronic neurologic disease	2 (1)	4 (2)	2.11	0.37-12.2
Allergies	24 (15)	15 (9)	0.56	0.30-1.02
Asthma	15 (9)	6 (3)	0.35	0.14-0.83*
Eczema	3 (2)	1 (1)	0.28	0.03-2.32

CLD, Chronic lung disease.
*A relative risk of <1.00 indicates a decreased risk for the event with synthetic surfactant; if the CI does not include 1.00, then the change is significant, as in the case of asthma.

Table V. Retinopathy of prematurity*

	Air placebo (%) (*n* = 189)	Synthetic surfactant (%) (*n* = 207)	Relative risk†	95% Confidence interval
Worst examination				
No ROP	56 (30)	68 (33)	1.10	0.83-1.47
Mild/moderate ROP	100 (53)	108 (52)		
Severe ROP	33 (17)	31 (15)	0.86	0.56-1.34
Treatment‡	24 (11)	30 (13)		
Surgery	18 (10)	25 (12)		
Cryotherapy	10 (5)	12 (6)		
Last examination				
No ROP	131 (69)	148 (72)	1.03	0.91-1.17
Mild/moderate ROP	49 (26)	46 (22)		
Severe ROP	9 (5)	13 (6)	1.33	0.58-3.01
Treatment‡	7 (5)	11 (7)		
Surgery	5 (4)	8 (4)		
Cryotherapy	3 (2)	7 (3)		

*Based on worst and last examination for all infants who received ophthalmologic examinations under study protocol. Mild/moderate ROP = grades 1-3; severe ROP = grades 3+ and greater.
†A relative risk of <1.00 indicates a reduced risk for the event with synthetic surfactant treatment; if the CI includes 1.00, then the increase is not significant.
‡Some patients received more than one treatment.

ments among the tiny infants who received synthetic surfactant, and a corresponding increase in the proportion of infants surviving without significant impairment in that weight class (Fig. 3).

DISCUSSION

The results of this analysis indicate that infants who survive after treatment at birth with a single prophylactic dose of synthetic surfactant fare at least as well in terms of growth, development, and late morbidities as infants who survive without such treatment. There were no differences in the medical history during the first year of life, there were no differences in growth, and there were no differences in the incidence of visual defects, auditory defects, CP, or neurodevelopmental delay at 1-year adjusted age between control subjects and infants treated with synthetic surfactant. The only exception was a significant reduction in the incidence of asthma among infants treated with synthetic surfactant. Although this finding may have resulted from chance, it may also be real. Synthetic surfactant helps protect the airways of small premature infants from injury during mechanical ventilation,[15] and a reduction in asthma could be a late benefit.

The proportion of surviving infants with severe impairments was 23% in both treatment groups. The absolute number of impaired survivors was five less in the surfactant group (120 vs 115), despite the evaluation of 31 more survivors at follow-up in the surfactant group (278 vs 309). In

Table VI. Mental and psychomotor development indices, as determined by Bayley Scales of Infant Development

	Air placebo (*n* = 272)	Synthetic surfactant (*n* = 301)	Relative risk*	95% Confidence interval
Mental development index				
Analysis I†	90 ± 23	93 ± 22		
Analysis II†	94 ± 20	95 ± 21		
Index >2 SD below the mean (%)	27 (10)	36 (12)	1.20	0.75-1.94
Psychomotor development index				
Analysis I†	85 ± 20	88 ± 21		
Analysis II†	89 ± 18	91 ± 19		
Index >2 SD below the mean (%)‡	26 (10)	33 (11)	1.17	0.72-1.91

*A relative risk of <1.00 indicates a reduced risk for the event with synthetic surfactant; if the CI includes 1.00, then the increase is not significant.
†Values are means ± SD. In analyses I and II, index values <50 were set at 49. In analysis II, infants with severe impairments were excluded.
‡Bayley Scales of Infant Development scores <69.

Table VII. Impairments

	Air placebo (*n* = 278)	Synthetic surfactant (*n* = 309)	Relative risk*	95% Confidence interval
Impairment present	120 (43)	115 (37)	0.87	0.71-1.06
No impairment	158 (57)	194 (63)		
Severity of impairment				
Mild/moderate	56 (20)	43 (14)		
Serious	64 (23)	72 (23)	1.02	0.76-1.37
Type of impairment†‡				
MDI <69	47 (17)	48 (16)	0.94	0.66-1.36
MDI 69-84	51 (18)	42 (14)	0.74	0.51-1.08
CP				
Moderate/severe	20 (7)	23 (7)	1.05	0.59-1.86
Mild	24 (8)	21 (7)	0.79	0.45-1.40
Bilateral sensorineural deafness	0 (0)	2 (1)	0	—,—
Deafness not needing amplification	1 (0)	3 (1)	2.71	0.35-21.3
Bilateral blindness	9 (3)	7 (2)	0.73	0.29-1.84
Visual defect	22 (8)	24 (8)	1.01	0.58-1.77

*A relative risk of <1.00 indicates a reduced risk for the event with synthetic surfactant treatment; if the CI includes 1.00, then the increase is not significant.
†Infants may have more than one impairment.
‡Bayley Scales of Infant Development MDI scores <50 set to 49.

the group that received synthetic surfactant, there were eight more severely impaired survivors than in the control group, but there were 13 fewer mild-to-moderately impaired survivors.

In the infants treated with synthetic surfactant, the severe impairments were distributed in the same way as in the control infants: 15% of the infants treated with synthetic surfactant who returned for evaluation had severe mental retardation, 7% had moderate to severe CP, 2% had bilateral blindness, and 1% had severe deafness. For the purpose of reference, these findings represent a contemporary population of small premature infants treated with synthetic surfactant; the mean birth weight was 934 gm, 95% weighed less than 1250 gm at birth, the mean gestational age was 27 weeks, and the incidence of severe intraventricular hemorrhage was 9%.

The aforementioned estimates represent percentages of infants who returned for evaluation. In Figs. 2 and 3, the data are expressed as percentages of all those originally enrolled at birth; overall, it can be seen that with synthetic surfactant treatment fewer infants died, approximately the same number of infants survived with significant impairments, and more infants survived without impairments. The latter was especially the case in infants who weighed 500 to 750 gm at birth; for this reason, there appears to be an advantage in late outcome after use of synthetic surfactant in tiny infants, perhaps in part because surfactant replacement does not greatly improve overall mortality significantly in this weight group, as discussed elsewhere in this supplement.[8]

The neurodevelopmental evaluation of infants at the age of 1 year may not be absolutely reliable for the estimation

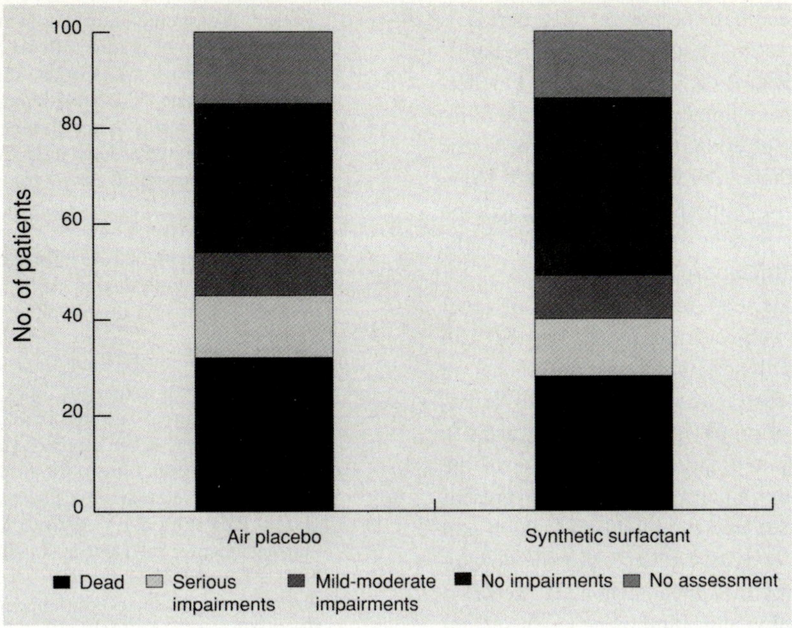

Fig. 2. Combined controlled trials of synthetic surfactant used prophylactically at birth in premature infants: outcomes in control and treated infants at the age of 1 year, expressed as percentages of the number of infants enrolled at birth.

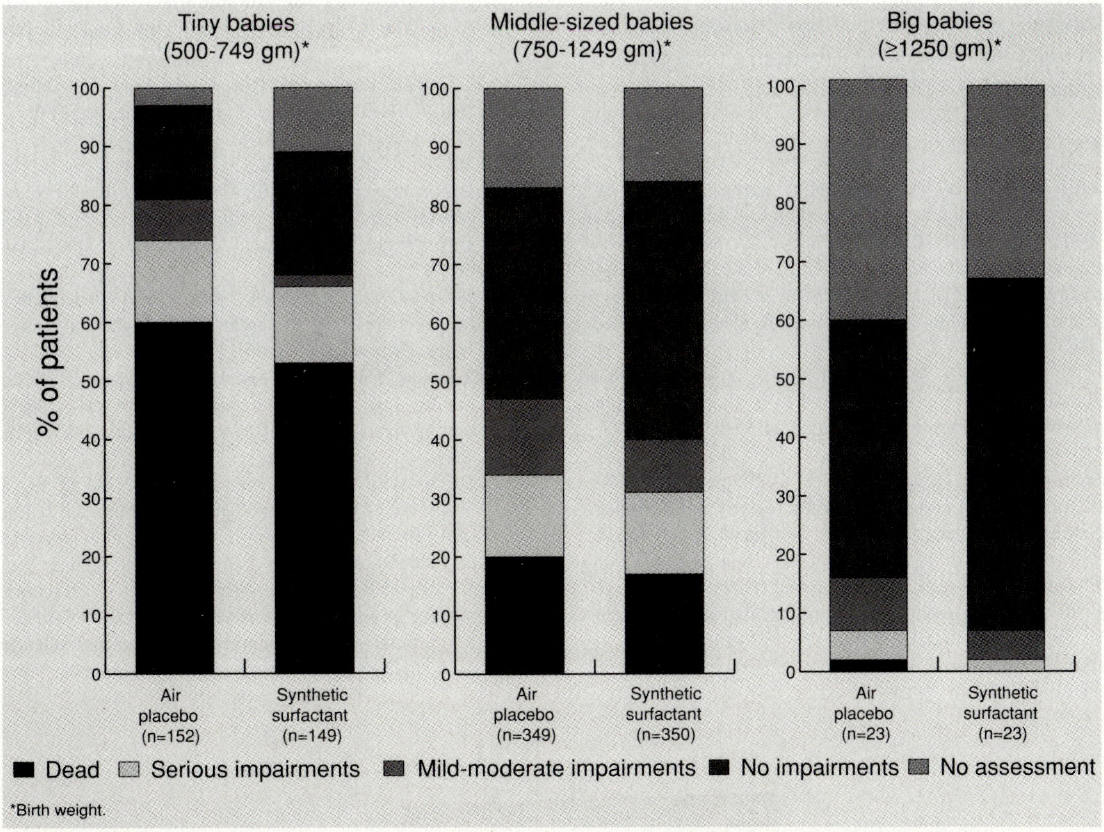

Fig. 3. Combined controlled trials of synthetic surfactant used prophylactically at birth in premature infants: outcomes in control and treated infants at the age of 1 year, separated into birth weight categories and expressed as percentages of the number of infants enrolled at birth.

of later outcome. The estimate of mental retardation is likely to be low[16] and the estimate of CP is likely to be high[14] compared with estimates at 2 or 3 years of age. Furthermore, the incidence of severe impairments in the 19% of infants who did not return for evaluation at the age of 1 year may be higher than in those who were evaluated.[17] However, there is no reason to suppose that these phenomena would have biased the present results in favor of the synthetic surfactant treatment group.

These findings are consistent with the results of other studies in which control subjects and infants treated with surfactant were examined and important differences in neurodevelopmental outcomes were not found.[18-20] It has been suggested that use of prophylactic surfactant at birth may be accompanied by a proportionate increase in the number of children with impairments.[21, 22] The present data, which were collected in a double-blind fashion and represent a much larger body of evidence, provide no support for the occurrence of this phenomenon. However, it does not appear that prophylactic administration of surfactant is associated with a decreased proportion of infants with severe impairments, as was hoped when surfactant therapy was first introduced. On the other hand, prophylactic administration of synthetic surfactant provides enhanced survival rates without additional numbers of impaired survivors, and it does so while reducing the incidence of mild to moderate impairment, particularly in tiny infants.

REFERENCES

1. Jackson JC, Palmer S, Truog WE, et al. Surfactant quantity and composition during recovery from hyaline membrane disease. Pediatr Res 1986;20:1243-7.
2. Enhorning G, Shennan A, Possmayer F, et al. Prevention of neonatal respiratory distress syndrome by tracheal instillation of surfactant: a randomized clinical trial. Pediatrics 1985; 76:145-53.
3. Corbet AJ, Long WA, Murphy DJ, et al. Reduced mortality in small premature infants treated at birth with a single dose of synthetic surfactant. J Paediatr Child Health 1991;27: 245-9.
4. Corbet A, Bucciarelli R, Goldman S, et al. Decreased mortality rate among small premature infants treated at birth with a single dose of synthetic surfactant: a multicenter controlled trial. J PEDIATR 1991;118:277-84.
5. Bose C, Corbet A, Bose G, et al. Improved outcome at 28 days of age for very low birthweight infants treated with a single dose of synthetic surfactant. J PEDIATR 1990;117:947-53.
6. Stevenson D, Walther F, Long WA, et al. Controlled trial of single dose of synthetic surfactant at birth in premature infants weighing 500-699 grams. J PEDIATR 1992;120:S3-12.
7. Kraybill EN, Bose CL, Corbet AJ, Garcia-Prats J, Asbill D, Edwards K, Long W. Double-blind evaluation of developmental and health status to age 2 years of infants weighing 700 to 1350 grams treated prophylactically at birth with a single dose of synthetic surfactant or air placebo. J PEDIATR 1995;126: S33-42.
8. Walther FJ, Mullett M, Schumacher R, et al. One-year follow-up of 66 premature infants weighing 500 to 699 grams treated with a single dose of synthetic surfactant or air placebo at birth: results of a double-blind trial. J PEDIATR 1995;126: S13-9.
9. Sell M, Cotton R, Hirata T, et al. One-year follow-up of 273 infants with birth weights of 700 to 1100 grams after prophylactic treatment of respiratory distress syndrome with synthetic surfactant or air placebo. J PEDIATR 1995;126:S20-5.
10. International Committee. An international classification of retinopathy of prematurity. Pediatrics 1984;74:127-33.
11. Hamill PVV, Drizd TA, Johnson CL, et al. Physical growth: National Center for Health Statistics percentiles. Am J Clin Nutr 1979;32:607-29.
12. Bayley N. Bayley scales of infant development. New York: The Psychological Corp, 1969.
13. Kitchen W, Ford G, Orgill A, et al. Outcome in infants with birth weight 500 to 999 gm: a regional study of 1979 and 1980 births. J PEDIATR 1984;104:921-7.
14. Nelson KB, Ellenberg JH. Children who "outgrew" cerebral palsy. Pediatrics 1982;69:529-36.
15. Long WA. Synthetic surfactant. Clin Perinatol 1993;17:275-84.
16. Tyson JE, Laskey RE, Rosenfeld CR, et al. An analysis of potential biases in the loss of indigent infants to follow-up. Early Hum Dev 1988;111:651-9.
17. Wariyar UK, Richmond S. Morbidity and preterm delivery: importance of 100% follow-up. Lancet 1989;1:387-8.
18. Morley CJ, Morley R. Follow up of premature babies treated with artificial surfactant (ALEC). Arch Dis Child 1990;65: 667-9.
19. Ware J, Taeusch HW, Soll RF, et al. Health and developmental outcomes of a surfactant controlled trial: follow-up at 2 years. Pediatrics 1990;85:1103-7.
20. Vaucher YE, Merritt TA, Hallman M, et al. Neurodevelopmental and respiratory outcome in early childhood after human surfactant treatment. Am J Dis Child 1988;142:927-30.
21. Dunn MS, Shennan AT, Hoskins EM, et al. Two year follow-up of infants enrolled in a randomized trial of surfactant replacement therapy for prevention of neonatal respiratory distress syndrome. Pediatrics 1988;82:543-7.
22. Vaucher YE, Harker L, Merritt TA, et al. Outcome at twelve months of adjusted age in very low birth weight infants with lung immaturity: a randomized placebo controlled trial of human surfactant. J PEDIATR 1993;122:126-32.

One-year follow-up of 66 premature infants weighing 500 to 699 grams treated with a single dose of synthetic surfactant or air placebo at birth: Results of a double-blind trial

Frans J. Walther, MD, PhD, Martha Mullett, MD, Robert Schumacher, MD, Hakan Sundell, MD, David Easa, MD, Walker Long, MD, and the American Exosurf Neonatal Study Group I (see Appendix I)

From the Departments of Pediatrics, King/Drew Medical Center and UCLA School of Medicine, Los Angeles, California; West Virginia University School of Medicine, Morgantown; University of Michigan Hospitals, Ann Arbor; Vanderbilt University Medical Center, Nashville, Tennessee; Kapiolani Medical Center for Women and Children, Honolulu, Hawaii; University of North Carolina at Chapel Hill; and participating centers

In a multicenter, double-blind, placebo-controlled trial that enrolled 215 premature infants with birth weights of 500 to 699 gm, 106 infants were treated prophylactically with a single 5 ml/kg dose of synthetic surfactant and 109 infants were given an equivalent dose of air placebo shortly after birth. In each group, 40 children survived infancy: 36 children in the air placebo group and 30 children in the synthetic surfactant group were available for follow-up. Weight, height, and head circumference measurements were similar for both groups at 1-year adjusted age. Infants who received synthetic surfactant at birth had statistically similar Bayley Scales of Infant Development scores (mental developmental index, 92 vs 83; psychomotor developmental index, 87 vs 82) compared with controls. Mild to moderate impairments in the synthetic surfactant group were 7% versus 29% in the control group; these differences were not statistically significant. The incidence of retinopathy of prematurity, the number of hospital readmissions, the need for surgery after day 28, evidence of chronic lung disease, the need for respiratory support at 1-year adjusted age, and the incidence of allergies were also not different between the two groups. However, the proportion of infants surviving without impairment was modestly higher in the synthetic surfactant group (8%, air placebo group; 23%, synthetic surfactant group). The findings from this small study indicate that infants weighing 500 to 699 gm who receive a single prophylactic dose of synthetic surfactant at birth have neurodevelopmental outcomes at least equivalent to those of infants given air placebo at 1-year follow-up. (J Pediatr 1995;126:S13-9)

Randomized clinical trials have shown that both prophylactic and rescue surfactant replacement therapy reduce morbidity and overall mortality in premature infants.[1, 2] We recently reported the neonatal morbidity and infant mortality of 215 infants with birth weights of 500 to 699 gm who received a single prophylactic dose of synthetic surfactant or air placebo at birth as part of a randomized, double-blind

CLD	Chronic lung disease
RDS	Respiratory distress syndrome
ROP	Retinopathy of prematurity

Reprint requests: Frans J. Walther, MD, Department of Pediatrics, King/Drew Medical Center, 12021 S. Wilmington Ave, Los Angeles, CA 90059.

0022-3476/95/$3.00 + 0 9/0/61826

Table I. Patient accountability*

	Air placebo (n = 109)	Synthetic surfactant (n = 106)
Alive at 1-year adjusted age	40 (37)	40 (38)
Lost to follow-up	4 (4) [10]†	10 (9) [25]†
Completed follow-up	36 (33) [90]	30 (28) [75]

Numbers in parentheses represent the percentage of enrolled infants; numbers in brackets represent the percentage of patients who survived.
*Includes all patients as treated without exclusions.
†Includes approximately 10% of patients whose survival status was assessed by telephone contact.

trial.[3] One dose of prophylactic synthetic surfactant was associated with improved lung function and a reduced incidence of air leaks and death from respiratory distress syndrome but did not appear to affect overall mortality. This report presents data on growth, mental and motor development, functional impairment, and medical problems of the survivors at 1-year adjusted age.

METHODS

This single-dose prophylactic trial in infants weighing 500 to 699 gm was conducted with a common protocol at 23 hospitals in the United States. Between October 1987 and December 1989, 215 infants were enrolled in the study; 109 infants were treated with air placebo, and 106 were treated with synthetic surfactant (Exosurf Neonatal, Burroughs Wellcome Co., Research Triangle Park, N.C.). Assessment methods used at 1-year adjusted age included physical and neurologic examinations, measurement of height, weight, and head circumference, and the Bayley Scales of Infant Development. Determinations were made of retinopathy of prematurity, impairments, hospital readmissions and surgery after day 28, lung disease, respiratory support, and presence of allergies. The details regarding data collection and analyses are described elsewhere in this supplement. The protocol was approved by the Institutional Review Board at each hospital. Participants in this study are listed in Appendix I.

Patient recruitment and enrollment. Liveborn infants with birth weights of greater than or equal to 500 gm and less than 700 gm were eligible for entry in the study. The prenatal and postnatal exclusion criteria for this study have been previously published.[3]

Infants whose mothers had given consent before delivery were stratified according to birth weight (500 to 599 gm or 600 to 699 gm) and gender into four strata and were randomly assigned to receive a dose of either synthetic surfactant or air placebo as soon after birth as possible.

RESULTS

Of the 215 infants enrolled in the trial, 80 (37%) survived infancy: 40 of 109 (37%) in the control group and 40 of 106 (38%) in the synthetic surfactant group (Table I). Fourteen infants were lost to follow-up or their families failed to return for follow-up; thus 36 (90%) of the infants who survived in the control group and 30 (75%) of the infants who survived in the surfactant group were examined at 1-year adjusted age. The birth weights and gestational ages were similar for both groups (Table II). The differences for intraventricular hemorrhage and bronchopulmonary dysplasia were not statistically significant.

Mean adjusted ages at the 1-year examination were comparable (375 vs 371 days for the air placebo and synthetic surfactant groups, respectively). At 1-year adjusted age, mean weight (7.86 kg vs 8.06 kg), height (69.9 cm vs 70.9 cm), and head circumference (44.1 cm vs 44.3 cm) for the air placebo and synthetic surfactant groups, respectively, were not significantly different. Weights below the 10th percentile for adjusted age were found in 67% of the subjects in the control group and 67% of subjects in the surfactant group; for height, these percentages were 55% and 67%; and for head circumference, these percentages were 64% and 67% (Fig. 1).

The incidence of hospital readmissions and surgery after day 28 and the incidence of chronic lung disease did not differ between the two groups (Table III). Similarly, the need for respiratory support at 1-year adjusted age, the need for medication for CLD, and the incidence of allergies were not different in the two groups (Table III).

The two groups had similar rates of absence of ROP, mild to moderate ROP, and severe ROP at the worst and last ophthalmologic examinations (Table IV). Similarly, the incidence of treatment (surgery or cryotherapy) for ROP was not different in the two groups.

Infants who received surfactant at birth had statistically similar Bayley Scales of Infant Development scores for both mental and psychomotor development when compared with the control group (Table V). These findings were not affected by exclusion of low index values or by exclusion of infants who were severely impaired because of bilateral blindness or deafness or who had moderate to severe cerebral palsy (n = 3, control group; n = 5, surfactant group).

Overall, 60% of subjects in the control group and 43% in the surfactant group had impairments (Table VI); the difference was not statistically significant. The types and degree of impairment are shown in Table VI. The incidence of hearing and visual impairments was not different in the two groups. Fig. 2 demonstrates the overall status of the group given air placebo and the group treated with synthetic surfactant at 1-year adjusted age; the proportion of infants who survived without impairment was modestly higher in the synthetic surfactant group.

DISCUSSION

Prophylactic treatment with a single dose of synthetic surfactant in infants with birth weights of 500 to 699 gm reduces neonatal mortality caused by RDS, the incidence of

Table II. Baseline characteristics and major neonatal complications of infants who completed 1-year follow-up evaluation*

Characteristic	Air placebo (n = 36)	Synthetic surfactant (n = 30)
Birth weight (gm)†	628 ± 51	637 ± 51
Gestational age (wk)†	25.3 ± 1.8	25.4 ± 1.7
Multiple birth (%)	8 (22)	4 (13)
Race (%)		
White	16 (44)	13 (43)
Black	14 (39)	10 (33)
Hispanic	5 (14)	4 (13)
Other	1 (3)	3 (10)
Maternal age (yr)†	28 ± 7	29 ± 5
Maternal education (yr)† ‡	13 ± 2	14 ± 3
Sex		
Male	14 (39)	16 (53)
Female	22 (61)	14 (47)
Apgar score (median)		
1 min	3	3
5 min	6	6
IVH during days 1-28 (%)		
Grade I/II	9 (25)	12 (40)
Grade III/PVED	7 (19)	2 (7)
No IVH	20 (56)	16 (53)
BPD at day 28 (%)	9 (27)	14 (47)

IVH, Intraventricular hemorrhage; *PVED*, periventricular echodensities; *BPD*, bronchopulmonary dysplasia.
*Infants are classified in groups according to the treatment they received.
†Mean values ± SD.
‡For maternal education: n = 30, air placebo group; n = 21, synthetic surfactant group.

Table III. Health status*

Condition	Air placebo (%) (n = 35)	Synthetic surfactant (%) (n = 30)	Relative risk†	95% Confidence interval
Surgery	17 (49)	18 (60)	1.194	0.759, 1.879
Readmitted to hospital	20 (57)	18 (60)	1.030	0.667, 1.591
Physical evidence of CLD	7 (20)	7 (23)	1.104	0.473, 2.794
Medication for CLD	8 (23)	7 (23)	0.950	0.377, 2.395
Respiratory support on day of examination	4 (11)	2 (7)	0.491	0.095, 2.522
Medication for chronic neurologic disease	2 (6)	1 (3)	0.462	0.049, 4.344
Allergies‡	6 (17)	1 (3)	0.182	0.027, 1.216
Asthma	2 (6)	0 (0)	—§	—, —§
Milk allergy	2 (6)	1 (3)	0.567	0.043, 7.425

*Includes data on health status between day 29 and 1-year adjusted age.
†Relative risk <1.000 indicates decreased risk of event with synthetic surfactant treatment.
‡No patient was reported to have dermatitis, rhinitis, eczema, or hay fever.
§Counts were too low for a valid estimate.

pulmonary air leaks, and the need for ventilatory assistance and oxygen requirements through 3 days of age,[3] indicating a positive effect on lung function in extremely premature infants. Infants in this weight category are near the threshold of viability, and the long-term prognosis of survivors is guarded. Infant mortality is high despite treatment with a single dose of synthetic surfactant at birth[3]; furthermore, the prevalence of impairments among survivors is also high. Long-term follow-up data on survivors of surfactant replacement therapy are limited,[4-12] especially for infants with birth weights between 500 and 699 gm, who were the subjects of this study.

Dunn et al.[5] monitored 55 of 60 survivors from a randomized trial of bovine surfactant therapy used prophylactically in infants of less than 30 weeks gestation with a mean birth weight of ~950 grams. The treated group had a lower neonatal mortality than the control group, but a disturbing trend toward more neurodevelopmental impair-

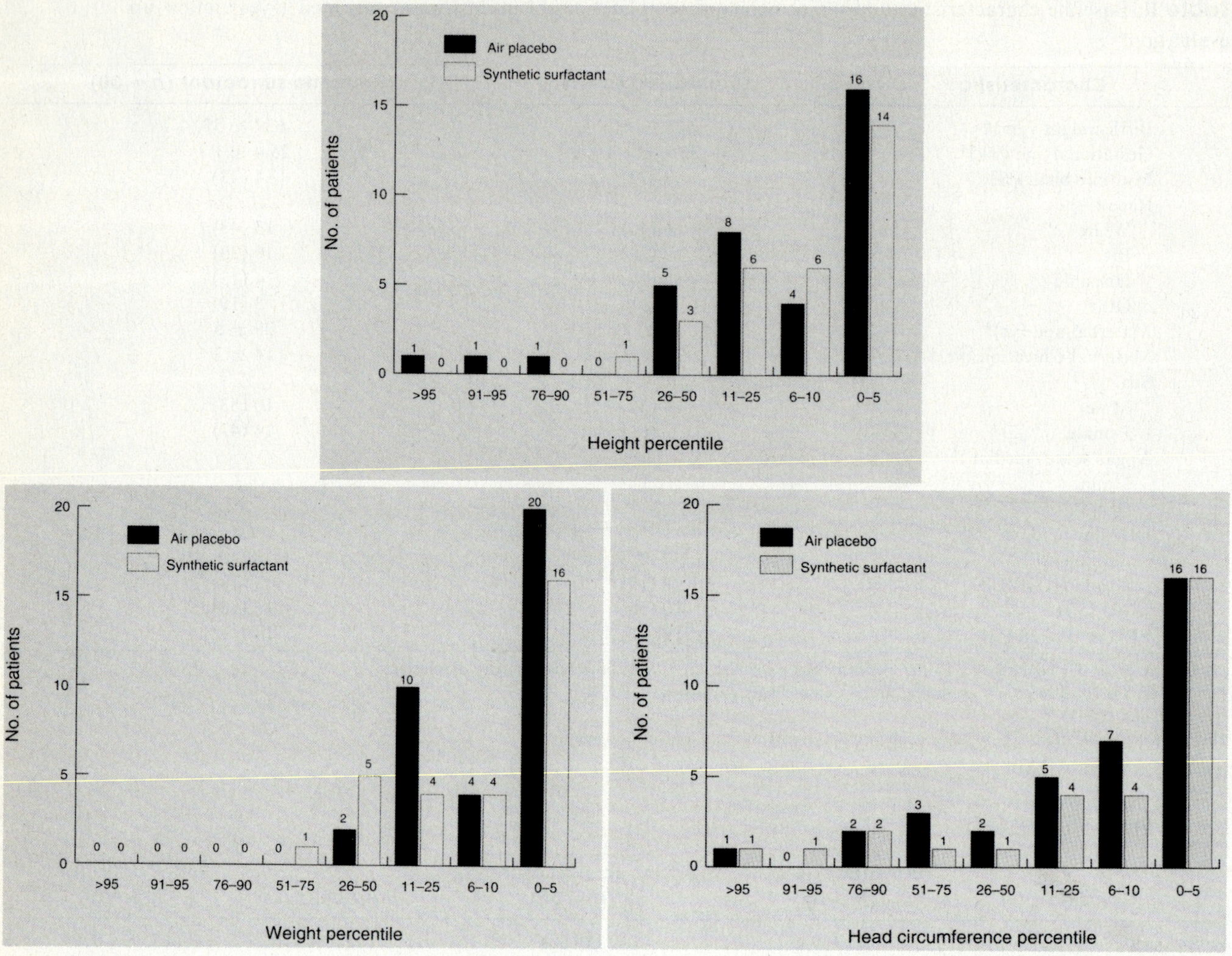

Fig. 1. Height, weight, and head circumference measurements for infants treated with synthetic surfactant and air placebo at 1-year adjusted age. (Percentile rankings based on growth charts for the National Center for Health Statistics.)

ments appeared at 2 years of age. The incidence of late respiratory or allergic disease was comparable in both groups. Vaucher et al.[6] studied 46 surviving infants with similar birth weights who were enrolled in separate placebo-controlled, randomized trials of prophylactic and rescue treatment with human surfactant. No adverse effects of surfactant therapy on growth or neurologic or developmental outcomes were detected at 12 to 24 months of age. More recently, Vaucher et al.[7] reported the neurodevelopmental outcome at 1 year of age of 145 premature infants with mean birth weights of ~1000 to 1100 gm who were treated with either prophylactic human surfactant, rescue human surfactant, or air placebo. Prophylactic surfactant administration was associated with lower mean Bayley Scales of Infant Development mental developmental index and psychomotor developmental index scores and more CLD than rescue surfactant treatment. Ware et al.[8] examined 32 survivors (mean birth weight: 1249 gm) of a randomized, controlled trial of rescue treatment with modified bovine surfactant at 12 and 24 months of age and also found no differences in growth, abnormal physical findings, and mental and psychomotor scores of the Bayley Scales of Infant Development. The Collaborative European Multicentre Study Group[9] monitored, until 2 years of age, 73 infants who weighed 700 to 2000 gm at birth and were randomized to rescue treatment with porcine surfactant or a short period of manual ventilation, and they also found no differences between subjects treated with surfactant and control subjects.

Morley and Morley[10] monitored 231 infants from a prophylactic trial of the synthetic surfactant ALEC (artificial lung expanding compound, Pumactant, Britania Pharmaceuticals, Cambridge, United Kingdom), composed of dipalmitoyl phosphatidylcholine and phosphatidylglycerol in a ratio of 7:3, at 9 and/or 18 months of age and did not detect differences in the incidence of neurologic impair-

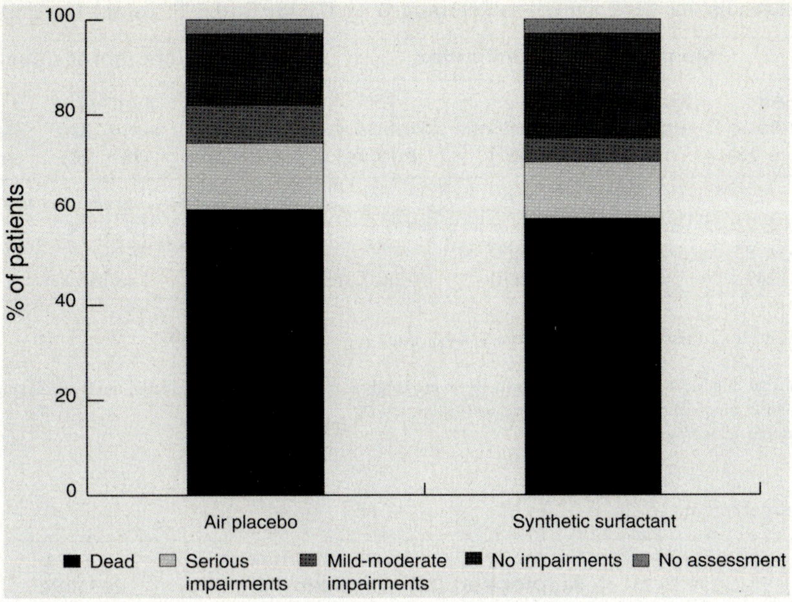

Fig. 2. Infant mortality and severity of impairments for infants treated with synthetic surfactant and air placebo at 1-year adjusted age follow-up (all patients).

Table IV. Retinopathy of prematurity*

	Worst examination				Last examination			
	Air placebo (%) (n = 38)	Synthetic surfactant (%) (n = 40)	Relative risk†	95% Confidence interval	Air placebo (%) (n = 38)	Synthetic surfactant (%) (n = 40)	Relative risk†	95% Confidence interval
No ROP	3 (8)	3 (8)	0.968	0.201, 4.653	20 (53)	27 (68)	1.282	0.881, 1.866
Mild/moderate ROP	21 (55)	22 (55)			16 (42)	7 (18)		
Severe ROP	14 (37)	15 (38)	0.963	0.562, 1.651	2 (5)	6 (15)	2.692	0.624, 11.61
Treatment‡	7 (18)	9 (23)			1 (3)	3 (8)		
Surgery	1 (3)	5 (13)			0 (0)	1 (3)		
Cryotherapy	7 (18)	8 (20)			1 (3)	2 (5)		

*Based on worst and last examination for all infants who received ophthalmologic examinations under study protocol. Mild/moderate ROP = grades 1-3; severe ROP = grades ≥3+.
†Relative risk <1.000 indicates decreased risk of event with synthetic surfactant treatment.
‡Some patients received more than one treatment.

ment, mental impairment, respiratory infections, allergies, or hospital admissions. Halliday et al.[11] monitored 80 premature infants who participated in a controlled trial of prophylactic instillation of relatively low doses of a synthetic surfactant, consisting of dipalmitoyl phosphatidylcholine and high-density lipoprotein, and found that surfactant treatment was not associated with adverse long-term effects.

Our 1-year follow-up study of extremely low birth weight infants is best compared with that of Ferrara et al.,[12] who reported on 54 infants from selected study centers with birth weights of 600 to 750 gm who survived multiple-dose prophylactic bovine surfactant or air placebo treatment. Ferrara's report, a post hoc subanalysis from 4 to 10 participating centers, showed that infant mortality was lower in the infants treated with surfactant and that the percentage of healthy survivors was higher at 12 months of age. However, when the entire cohort of infants weighing 600 to 750 gm who were enrolled at all 10 participating centers was analyzed, overall mortality was not different in the two groups.[13]

In any case, in our study no significant differences in neurodevelopmental outcome were observed at 1-year adjusted age. Somatic growth in both of our groups was equivalent; the incidence of mild to moderate impairments was not different in the infants treated with synthetic sur-

Table V. Mental and psychomotor development as determined by Bayley Scales of Infant Development

	Mental development index				Psychomotor development index			
	Air placebo (n = 35)	Synthetic surfactant (n = 27)	Relative risk*†	95% Confidence interval	Air placebo (n = 35)	Synthetic surfactant (n = 26)	Relative risk*†	95% Confidence interval
Developmental index*								
Analysis I‡	80 ± 22	86 ± 23			80 ± 20	81 ± 24		
Analysis II‡ §	83 ± 20	92 ± 20			82 ± 19	87 ± 21		
Index <2 SD‖ (%)	8 (24%)	4 (15%)	0.880	0.328, 2.358	6 (18%)	4 (15%)	1.103	0.364, 3.343

*Mean ± SD.
†Relative risk <1.000 indicates decreased risk of event with synthetic surfactant.
‡Index values <50 set to 49.
§Severe impairments (e.g., bilateral blindness or deafness, moderate or severe cerebral palsy) were excluded from analyses. Mental development index and psychomotor development index scores: air placebo, n = 32; synthetic surfactant, n = 22.
‖Bayley Scales of Infant Development scores <69.

Table VI. Functional impairments

	Air placebo (%) (n = 35)	Synthetic surfactant (%) (n = 30)	Relative risk*	95% Confidence interval
Impairment present	21 (60)	13 (43)	0.733	0.450, 1.193
No impairment	14 (40)	17 (57)		
Severity of impairments				
Mild to moderate	10 (29)	2 (7)		
Serious	11 (31)	11 (37)	0.935	0.493, 1.773
Type of impairment†				
Mental development index <69‡	11 (31)	8 (27)	0.832	0.380, 1.818
Mental development index 69-84‡	6 (17)	2 (7)	0.441	0.106, 1.844
Moderate to severe cerebral palsy	2 (6)	4 (13)	1.882	0.394, 8.998
Mild cerebral palsy	6 (17)	2 (7)	0.425	0.104, 1.742
Bilateral sensorineural deafness	0	2 (7)	—§	—, —§
Deafness not requiring amplification	0	1 (3)	—§	—, —§
Bilateral blindness	1 (3)	3 (10)	3.648	0.394, 33.75
Visual defect	5 (14)	4 (13)	0.884	0.263, 2.971

*Relative risk <1.000 indicates decreased risk of event with synthetic surfactant treatment.
†Infants may have more than one impairment.
‡Bayley Scales of Infant Development mental development index scores <50 set to 49.
§Counts were too low for a valid estimate.

factant at birth. Similarly, the somewhat higher Bayley Scales of Infant Development scores observed in the synthetic surfactant group were not significantly different. The overall results indicate that infants weighing 500 to 700 gm who receive a single prophylactic dose of synthetic surfactant at birth are possibly more likely to survive without impairments than infants treated with air placebo (8%, air placebo group; 23%, synthetic surfactant group). In other studies, infants treated with prophylactic human surfactant,[7] other synthetic surfactants,[10, 11] and animal-derived surfactant preparations either did more poorly or no better than control subjects.[5, 8, 9]

Although overall infant mortality in our study of infants weighing 500 to 699 gm was not affected by treatment with a single prophylactic dose of synthetic surfactant at birth, neonatal morbidity and death from RDS were less, and at 1-year follow-up neurodevelopmental outcomes were at least equivalent and possibly slightly better. These observations may warrant aggressive use of surfactant in this birth weight category, despite the lack of evidence of a clear benefit on overall mortality. Considering that three prophylactic doses of synthetic surfactant in infants with birth weights of 700 to 1100 gm[14] further reduce overall mortality in comparison with a single dose, a more extensive administration scheme might prove more beneficial in infants who weigh 500 to 699 gm as well. Preliminary data from a randomized trial that used three versus six doses of synthetic surfactant in infants weighing less than 750 gm at birth indicate no benefit in this weight class from more than three doses.[15]

REFERENCES

1. Jobe AH. Pulmonary surfactant therapy. N Engl J Med 1993;328:861-8.
2. Mercier CE, Boll RF. Clinical trials of natural surfactant extract in respiratory distress syndrome. Clin Perinatol 1992; 20:711-36.
3. Stevenson D, Walther F, Long W, et al. Controlled trial of a single dose of synthetic surfactant at birth in premature infants weighing 500 to 699 grams. J PEDIATR 1992;120:S3-12.
4. Corbet A, Bose C, Long W, Schumacher R, Gerdes J, Cotton R, and the American Exosurf Neonatal Study Group I. Double-blind developmental evaluation at 1-year corrected age of 597 premature infants with birth weights of 500 to 1350 grams enrolled in three placebo-controlled trials of prophylactic synthetic surfactant. J PEDIATR 1995;126:S5-12.
5. Dunn MS, Shennan AT, Hoskins EM, Lennox K, Enhorning G. Two-year follow-up of infants enrolled in a randomized trial of surfactant replacement therapy for prevention of neonatal respiratory distress syndrome. Pediatrics 1988;82:543-47.
6. Vaucher YE, Merritt TA, Hallman M, Jarvenpaa A-L, Telsey AM, Jones BL. Neurodevelopmental and respiratory outcome in early childhood after human surfactant treatment. Am J Dis Child 1988;142:927-30.
7. Vaucher YE, Harker L, Merritt TA, et al. Outcome at twelve months of adjusted age in very low birth weight infants with lung immaturity: a randomized, placebo-controlled trial of human surfactant. J PEDIATR 1993;122:126-32.
8. Ware J, Taeusch HW, Soll RF, McCormick MC. Health and developmental outcomes of a surfactant controlled trial: follow-up at 2 years. Pediatrics 1990;85:1103-7.
9. Collaborative European Multicentre Study Group. A 2-year follow up of babies enrolled in a European multicentre trial of porcine surfactant replacement for severe neonatal respiratory distress syndrome. Eur J Pediatr 1992;151:372-6.
10. Morley CJ, Morley R. Follow up of premature babies treated with artificial surfactant (ALEC). Arch Dis Child 1990;65: 667-9.
11. Halliday HL, McClure G, Reid MM. Growth and development two years after artificial surfactant replacement at birth. Early Hum Dev 1986;13:323-7.
12. Ferrara TB, Hoekstra RE, Couser RJ, et al. Effects of surfactant therapy on outcome of infants with birth weights of 600 to 750 grams. J PEDIATR 1991;119:455-7.
13. Berry D. Should tiny babies be treated with surfactant? In: Long WA, Tilson HH, eds. Proceedings of the Exosurf Neonatal Treatment IND Investigators' Meeting, November 13-14, 1991. Langhorne, PA.: Adis International, 1992:37-44.
14. Gerdes J, Gerdes M, Beaumont E, et al. Health and neurodevelopmental outcome at 1-year adjusted age in 508 infants weighing 700 to 1100 grams who received prophylaxis with one versus three doses of synthetic surfactant. J PEDIATR 1995; 126:S26-32.
15. Long WA, Merritt A, Kanto W, et al. Randomized comparison of three vs six doses of synthetic surfactant in 348 infants weighing < 750 grams [Abstract]. Pediatr Res 1992;31:314A.

One-year follow-up of 273 infants with birth weights of 700 to 1100 grams after prophylactic treatment of respiratory distress syndrome with synthetic surfactant or air placebo

Matthew Sell, MD, Robert Cotton, MD, Toshiko Hirata, MD, Robert Guthrie, MD, Michael LeBlanc, MD, Mark Mammel, MD, Walker Long, MD, and the American Exosurf Neonatal Study Group I (see Appendix I)

From the Departments of Pediatrics, St. Luke's Regional Medical Center, Boise, Idaho; Vanderbilt University, Nashville, Tennessee; California Medical Center, San Francisco; Magee-Women's Hospital, Pittsburgh, Pennsylvania; University of Mississippi Medical Center, Jackson; St. Paul's Children's Hospital, St. Paul, Minnesota; University of North Carolina at Chapel Hill; and participating centers

A single dose of synthetic surfactant was administered prophylactically to premature neonates with birth weights between 700 and 1100 gm. The effects of this treatment on neurodevelopmental, neurologic, and ophthalmologic outcomes, impairments, and general health status were examined during a follow-up evaluation at 1-year adjusted age. The study was a multicenter, parallel, randomized, double-blind comparison of 446 infants who received either air placebo ($n = 222$) or synthetic surfactant ($n = 224$). Follow-up evaluations were completed for 82% of surviving infants in both treatment groups. Neurodevelopmental outcome and growth were equivalent in the infants treated with synthetic surfactant and in the infants given air placebo. Impairments occurred in 38% of the infants treated with air placebo compared with 31% of those given synthetic surfactant; the difference was not statistically significant (relative risk 0.809, 95% confidence interval 0.585, 1.119). The incidence of asthma was significantly higher in the group of infants given air placebo (4% vs 10% for surfactant and air placebo, respectively, relative risk 0.391, 95% confidence intervals 0.157, 0.972). Other outcomes, including retinopathy of prematurity, hospital readmissions, surgery, and evidence of chronic lung disease, were not different. Administration of a single prophylactic dose of synthetic surfactant increases survival in infants with birth weights between 700 and 1100 gm without increasing the number or proportion of impaired survivors. (J Pediatr 1995;126:S20-5)

Both prophylactic and rescue use of synthetic surfactant have been shown to reduce mortality and morbidity in premature infants.[1,2] There is little information, however, concerning the long-term developmental outcomes of the infants who received synthetic surfactant. The potential for long-term disability in the increasing numbers of high-risk premature infants who are surviving is an essential safety issue in surfactant-replacement therapy. Either the proportion or absolute number of infants with chronic disabilities

MDI	Mental development index
PDI	Psychomotor development index
ROP	Retinopathy of prematurity

Reprint requests: Matthew S. Sell, MD, Department of Pediatrics, St. Luke's Hospital, 190 East Bannock St., Boise, ID 83712.

0022-3476/95/$3.00 + 0 **9/0/61820**

such as cerebral palsy, mental retardation, and sensory impairment could be increased in premature infants who are surviving.

The purpose of this study was to determine whether the improved survival rates of premature infants who receive prophylactic surfactant treatment for respiratory distress syndrome alter the number of impaired infants or infants with other adverse outcomes at 1-year adjusted age. The results of the first 28 days have been reported elsewhere.[3]

METHODS

The study was a multicenter, randomized, double-blind, parallel comparison of the effects of a single dose of either air placebo or synthetic surfactant (colfosceril palmitate, cetyl alcohol, and tyloxapol; Exosurf Neonatal, Burroughs Wellcome Co., Research Triangle Park, N.C.) administered prophylactically to premature infants with birth weights of 700 to 1100 gm.[3] This report presents the results of the double-blind, follow-up evaluation conducted at 1-year adjusted age. The protocol was approved by the Institutional Review Board at each of the 23 participating centers (participants are listed in Appendix I). Patient entry occurred from October 1987 through December 1988.

Patient recruitment and enrollment. Patient screening, treatment, and posttreatment phases for days 1 to 28 have been previously reported.[3] Briefly, all premature infants born at participating institutions with birth weights between 700 and 1100 gm were eligible for the trial. Consent for enrollment was sought from all mothers who were likely to deliver a live infant in the weight range. The details of data collection, ophthalmologic examination, 1-year follow-up evaluation, and data analyses are described elsewhere.[3, 4]

RESULTS

Patient accountability. As shown in Table I, similar proportions of surviving infants given air placebo (125 of 153 [82%]) and synthetic surfactant (148 of 179 [83%]) returned for follow-up at 1-year adjusted age. Baseline characteristics of the children who completed the 1-year follow-up evaluation were not different in the air placebo and synthetic surfactant treatment groups at the time of enrollment (Table II).

Health status. There were no significant differences between the air placebo and synthetic surfactant treatment groups with respect to surgery, hospital readmissions, chronic lung or neurologic disease, or respiratory support on the day of the follow-up examination (Table III). The incidence of asthma was significantly lower in the group treated with synthetic surfactant compared with the group that was given air placebo (6 of 148 [4%] vs 13 of 125 [10%]; relative risk 0.391, 95% confidence interval 0.157, 0.972).

Table I. Patient accountability for 1-year follow-up evaluation*

	Air placebo (n = 222)	Synthetic surfactant (n = 224)
Survivors at follow-up	153 (69)	179 (80)
Lost to follow-up	28 (13) [18]†	31 (14) [17]†
Assessed at follow-up	125 (56) [82]	148 (66) [83]

Numbers in parentheses represent the percentage of enrolled infants; numbers in brackets represent the percentage of survivors at 1-year adjusted age.
*Includes all patients as treated, no exclusions.
†Includes approximately 12% of patients whose survival status was assessed by telephone contact.

Table II. Characteristics and major neonatal complications of infants who completed 1-year follow-up*

Characteristic	Air placebo (n = 125)	Synthetic surfactant (n = 148)
Birth weight (gm)†	924 ± 116	915 ± 116
Gestational age (wk)†	27.4 ± 1.7	27.4 ± 1.7
Multiple birth	15 (12)	33 (22)
Race (%)		
White	72 (58)	88 (60)
Black	38 (30)	35 (24)
Hispanic	8 (6)	15 (10)
Other	7 (6)	10 (7)
Maternal age (yr)†	25 ± 6	27 ± 6
Maternal education (yr)‡	12 ± 3	13 ± 3
Sex (%)		
Male	63 (50)	73 (49)
Female	62 (50)	75 (51)
Apgar score (median)		
1 min	4	5
5 min	7	7
IVH during days 1-28 (%)		
Grade I/II	32 (26)	35 (24)
Grade III/PVED	11 (9)	18 (12)
No IVH	81 (65)	95 (64)
BPD at day 28 (%)	15 (12)	28 (19)
1-year survival without BPD (%)	104 (83)	127 (86)

IVH, Intraventricular hemorrhage; *PVED*, periventricular echodensities; *BPD*, bronchopulmonary dysplasia.
*Infants are classified according to the treatment they received.
†Mean ± SD.
‡For maternal education: n = 116, air placebo; n = 136, synthetic surfactant.

Weight, height, and head circumference percentiles were similar in both treatment groups (Fig. 1).

Ophthalmologic examination. No differences were observed in the incidence of retinopathy of prematurity

Table III. Health status

Condition	Air placebo (%) (*n* = 125)	Synthetic surfactant (%) (*n* = 148)	Relative risk*	95% Confidence interval
Surgery	38 (30)	43 (29)	0.962	0.674, 1.373
Readmitted to hospital	60 (48)	61 (41)	0.858	0.659, 1.116
Physical evidence of CLD	16 (13)	13 (9)	0.696	0.349, 1.386
Medication for CLD	15 (12)	17 (11)	0.965	0.501, 1.861
Respiratory support on day of examination	3 (2)	1 (<1)	0.283	0.035, 2.306
Medication for chronic neurologic disease	0 (0)	3 (2)	—†	—, —†
Allergies	18 (14)	14 (9)	0.663	0.343, 1.281
Asthma	13 (10)	6 (4)	0.391	0.157, 0.972‡
Dermatitis	1 (<1)	6 (4)	5.141	0.775, 3.411
Eczema	3 (2)	1 (<1)	0.288	0.035, 2.343
Milk	3 (2)	1 (<1)	0.275	0.031, 2.399

CLD, Chronic lung disease.
*Relative risk <1.000 indicates decreased risk of event with synthetic surfactant.
†Counts too low for valid estimate.
‡Less than one patient in each treatment had rhinitis or hay fever.

Table IV. Retinopathy of prematurity: Ophthalmologic data based on worst and last examinations for infants who completed follow-up

	Worst examination				Last examination			
	Air placebo (%) (*n* = 137)	Synthetic surfactant (%) (*n* = 155)	Relative risk*	95% Confidence interval	Air placebo (%) (*n* = 137)	Synthetic surfactant (%) (*n* = 155)	Relative risk*	95% Confidence interval
No ROP	48 (35)	61 (39)	1.130	0.845, 1.513	103 (75)	114 (74)	0.976	0.853, 1.117
Mild/moderate ROP	72 (53)	78 (50)			29 (21)	36 (23)		
Severe ROP	17 (12)	16 (10)	0.835	0.441, 1.581	5 (4)	5 (3)	0.917	0.275, 3.060
Treatment†	9 (7)	8 (5)			2 (1)	1 (<1)		
Surgery	5	2			0	1		
Cryotherapy	6	7			2	2		

*Relative risk <1.000 indicates decreased risk of event with synthetic surfactant.
†Patients may have received more than one treatment.

Table V. Mental and psychomotor development as determined by Bayley Scales of Infant Development at 1-year adjusted age

	Mental development index				Psychomotor development index			
	Air placebo (*n* = 119)	Synthetic surfactant (*n* = 141)	Relative risk*	95% Confidence interval	Air placebo (*n* = 119)	Synthetic surfactant (*n* = 141)	Relative risk*	95% Confidence interval
Development index†,‡								
Analysis I	94 ± 21	97 ± 19			88 ± 19	89 ± 18		
Analysis II§	97 ± 19	99 ± 17			90 ± 17	92 ± 16		
Index >−2 SD (%)‖	8 (7)	8 (6)	0.834	0.320, 2.176	9 (8)	11 (8)	0.987	0.424, 2.299

*Relative risk <1.000 indicates decreased risk of event with synthetic surfactant.
†Mean ± SD.
‡Index values <50 set to 49.
§Patients with severe impairments (e.g., bilateral blindness or deafness or moderate or severe cerebral palsy) were excluded from analysis; placebo, *n* = 112; synthetic surfactant, *n* = 132.
‖Bayley Scales of Infant Development scores <69.

between the infants given air placebo and those treated with synthetic surfactant at either the worst or last ophthalmologic examination (Table IV). At the worst examination, severe ROP was reported in similar proportions of patients in the air placebo group (17 of 137 [12%]) and synthetic surfactant treatment group (16 of 155 [10%]). At the last examination, fewer patients were reported to have ROP, but the proportions with ROP were similar in both treatment groups (5 of 137 [4%] in the air placebo group vs 5 of 155 [3%] in the synthetic surfactant group).

Neurodevelopmental evaluation. The mean values for the Bayley Scales of Infant Development mental and psychomotor development indices were similar for both treatment groups whether or not patients with severe impairments were included (Group I: MDI 94, air placebo group, vs 97, synthetic surfactant group; PDI 88, air placebo group, vs 89, synthetic surfactant group) or excluded (Group II: MDI 97, air placebo group, vs 99, synthetic surfactant group; PDI 90, air placebo group, vs 92, synthetic surfactant group) (Table V). Approximately equal proportions of infants given air placebo and infants treated with synthetic surfactant had prematurity-adjusted scores that were less than 69 (2 SD below the mean score of 100 in normal populations).

Impairments. Impairment occurred in 46 of 148 (31%) of the infants treated with synthetic surfactant and in 48 of 125 (38%) of the infants treated with air placebo; the difference was not statistically significant (relative risk 0.809; 95% confidence interval 0.585, 1.119) (Table VI). Similar proportions of infants had impairments that were classified as serious. None of the patients had bilateral sensorineural deafness that either required or did not require amplification. Fig. 2 illustrates the overall outcome for all infants enrolled in the study; the proportion of infants without impairments was greater in the synthetic surfactant group than in the air placebo group. In addition, a greater proportion of the infants treated with air placebo were either dead or had a serious impairment at 1-year adjusted age.

DISCUSSION

Corbet et al.[3] reported a significant improvement in both neonatal and 1-year survival rates for infants weighing 700 to 1100 gm who received a single dose of synthetic surfactant. The present study was a part of the original protocol reported by Corbet et al.,[4] and designed to investigate the impact of a single prophylactic dose of synthetic surfactant on growth, developmental outcome, and morbidity at 1 year adjusted age.

Smaller premature infants are at high risk for neurologic and developmental impairments. Gains in survival in this patient population could lead to an increase in either the proportion or absolute number of impaired survivors. Two reports suggest that there may be a trend toward a larger number of severely impaired survivors after surfactant

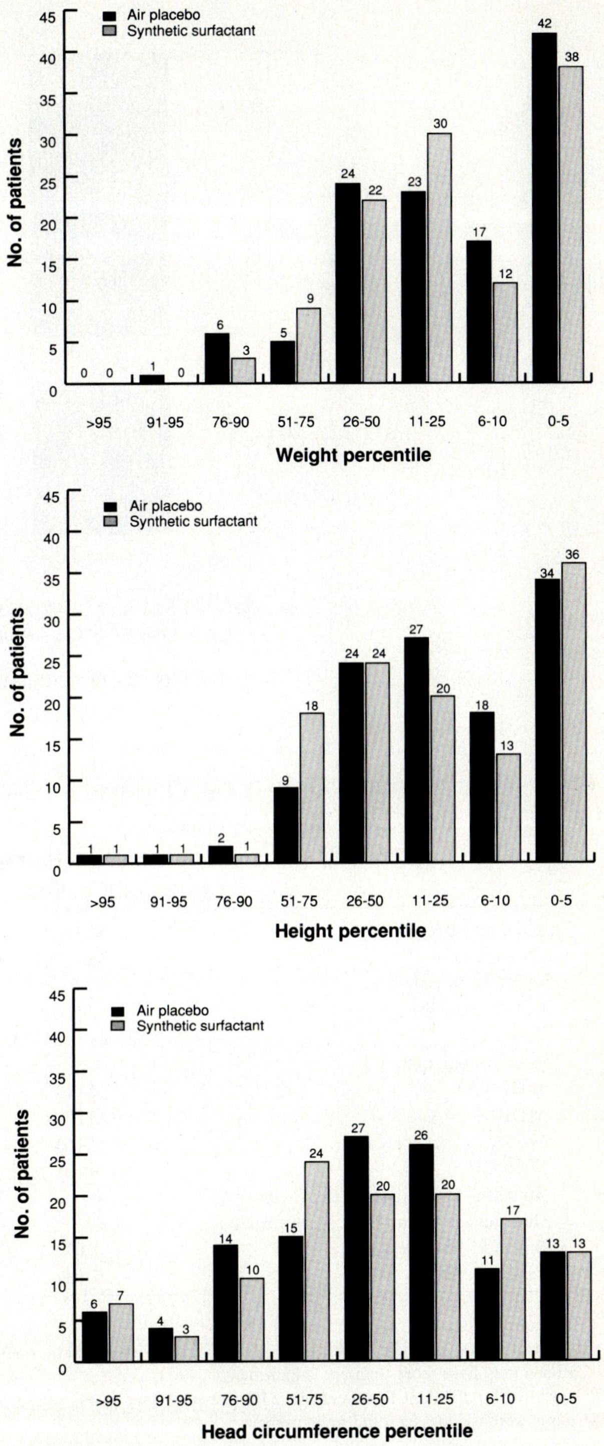

Fig. 1. Height, weight, and head circumference measurements for infants given synthetic surfactant and air placebo at 1-year adjusted age. (Percentile rankings based on growth charts from the National Center for Health Statistics.)

treatment.[5,6] The European Collaborative Group[5] reported a somewhat higher incidence of major disability (severe cerebral palsy, blindness, and deafness requiring hearing aids)

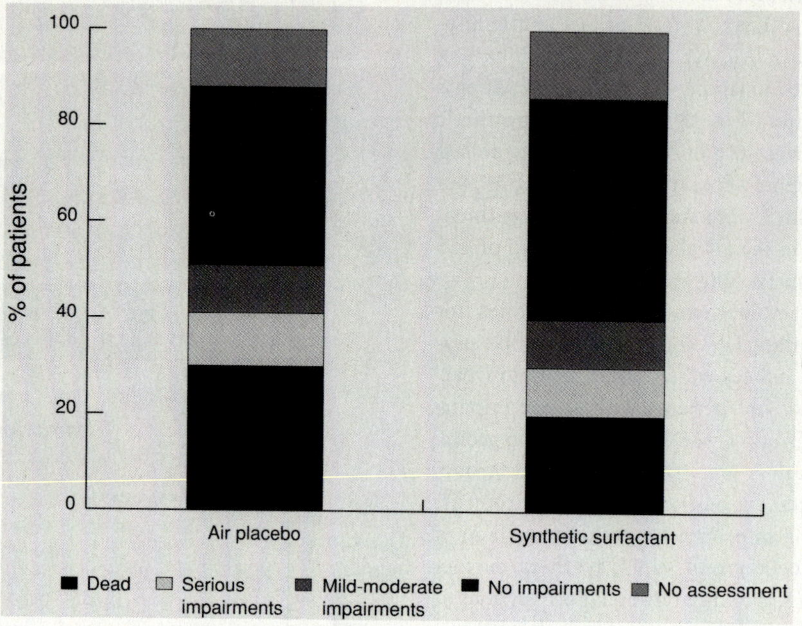

Fig. 2. Overall outcome for all infants enrolled.

Table VI. Impairments of infants who completed a 1-year follow-up evaluation

	Air placebo (%) (*n* = 125)	Synthetic surfactant (%) (*n* = 148)	Relative risk*	95% Confidence interval
Impairment present	48 (38)	46 (31)	0.809	0.585, 1.119)
No impairment	75 (60)	99 (67)		
Severity of impairment				
Mild/moderate	25 (20)	21 (14)		
Serious	23 (18)	24 (16)	0.829	0.499, 1.377
Type of impairment† ‡				
MDI <69	14 (11)	13 (9)	0.782	0.381, 1.608
MDI 69-84	25 (20)	20 (14)	0.676	0.398, 1.150
Moderate/severe CP	8 (6)	10 (7)	1.065	0.431, 2.631
Mild CP	8 (6)	7 (5)	0.730	0.274, 1.947
Bilateral sensorineural deafness	0	0	—§	—, —§
Deafness not requiring amplification	0	0	—§	—, —§
Bilateral blindness	4 (3)	2 (1)	0.400	0.078, 2.050
Visual defect	7 (6)	11 (8)	1.332	0.537, 3.304

CP, Cerebral palsy.
*Relative risk <1.000 indicates decreased risk of event with synthetic surfactant.
†Patients may have more than one impairment.
‡Bayley Scales of Infant Development MDI scores <50 set to 49.
§Counts were too low for valid measurement.

in infants treated with porcine surfactant at 2-year follow-up. Dunn et al.[6] observed a somewhat higher rate of severe handicap in infants treated with bovine surfactant compared with those who received a placebo. In both studies, the differences observed were not statistically significant, possibly because of the small number of patients reported. Other studies with similar small sample sizes have found no long-term increase in neurologic impairment.[7-11]

Most recently, Vaucher et al.[12] suggested that infants treated prophylactically with human surfactant fared worse on developmental follow-up than infants who received rescue treatment. Infants who received surfactant prophylactically had lower MDI and PDI scores than infants who received rescue surfactant treatment. On the basis of these results, Vaucher et al.[12] suggested that the timing of surfactant treatment may be an important variable in developmental outcome.

In our study, prophylactic treatment with a single dose of synthetic surfactant did not increase the risk for retinal abnormalities, developmental delay of mental or motor skills, impairments, medical problems, or abnormal growth. The only statistically significant difference in the treated and control groups was a lower incidence of asthma in infants who received synthetic surfactant. Not only was the proportion of impaired survivors the same in the two groups, but the total number of impaired survivors was less despite a significant increase in survival rate. These results indicate that, at least for synthetic surfactant, improvements in survival rates of infants weighing 700 to 1100 gm are not accompanied by an increased number of impaired infants.

REFERENCES

1. Jobe AH. Pulmonary surfactant therapy. N Engl J Med 1993;328:861-8.
2. Merritt TA, Boll RF, Hallman M. Overview of exogenous surfactant replacement therapy. J Intensive Care Med 1993; 8:205-28.
3. Corbet A, Bucciarelli R, Goldman S, et al. Decreased mortality rate among small premature infants treated at birth with a single dose of synthetic surfactant: a multicenter controlled trial. J PEDIATR 1991;118:277-84.
4. Corbet A, Long W, Schumacher R, Gerdes J, Cotton R, the American Exosurf Neonatal Study Group I. Double-blind developmental evaluation at 1-year corrected age of 597 premature infants with birth weights from 500 to 1350 grams enrolled in three placebo-controlled trials of prophylactic synthetic surfactant. J PEDIATR 1995;126:S5-12.
5. Robertson B, Curstedt T, Tubman R, et al. A 2-year follow-up of babies enrolled in a European multicenter trial of porcine surfactant replacement for severe neonatal respiratory distress syndrome. Eur J Pediatr 1992;151:372-6.
6. Dunn MS, Shennan AT, Hoskins EM, et al. Two year follow-up of infants enrolled in a randomized trial of surfactant therapy for prevention of neonatal respiratory distress syndrome. Pediatrics 1988;82:543-7.
7. Ferrara TB, Hoekstra RE, Couser RJ, et al. Effects of surfactant therapy on outcome of infants with birth weights of 600 to 750 grams. J PEDIATR 1991;119:455-7.
8. Halliday HL, McClure BG, Reid MM. Growth and development two years after artificial surfactant replacement at birth. Early Hum Dev 1986;13:323-7.
9. Morley CJ, Morley R. Follow-up of premature babies treated with artificial surfactant (ALEC). Arch Dis Child 1990; 65:667-9.
10. Vaucher YE, Merritt TA, Hallman M, et al. Neurodevelopmental and respiratory outcome in early childhood after human surfactant treatment. Am J Dis Child 1988;142:927-30.
11. Wave J, Taeusch HW, Soll RF, et al. Health and developmental outcomes of a surfactant controlled trial: follow-up at 2 years. Pediatrics 1990;85:1103-7.
12. Vaucher YE, Harker L, Merritt TA, et al. Outcome at twelve months of adjusted age in very low birth weight infants with lung immaturity: a randomized, placebo-controlled trial of human surfactant. J PEDIATR 1993;122:126-32.

Health and neurodevelopmental outcome at 1-year adjusted age in 508 infants weighing 700 to 1100 grams who received prophylaxis with one versus three doses of synthetic surfactant

Jeffrey Gerdes, MD, Marsha Gerdes, PhD, Ed Beaumont, MD, Larry Cook, MD, R. Dhanireddy, MD, Arthur Kopleman, MD, Robert Jarrett, DO, Walker Long, MD, and the American Exosurf Neonatal Study Groups I and II (see Appendixes I and II)

From the Departments of Pediatrics, Pennsylvania Hospital, University of Pennsylvania, Philadelphia; Butterworth Hospital, Grand Rapids, Michigan; Kosair Children's Hospital, University of Louisville, Kentucky; Georgetown University Hospital, Washington, D.C.; Pitt County Memorial Hospital, East Carolina University, Greenville, North Carolina; Tripler Army Medical Center, Honolulu, Hawaii; University of North Carolina at Chapel Hill; and participating centers

A three-dose prophylactic regimen of synthetic surfactant replacement has been shown to improve neonatal and 1-year survival rates in infants of 700 to 1100 gm birth weight when compared with a single prophylactic dose. The purpose of this study was to evaluate the growth, development, and late morbidity at 1 year adjusted age among the survivors of the 826 patients enrolled in the protocol. Complete follow-up data were obtained for 75% of the survivors in both groups. Chronic lung disease, need for respiratory support, neurologic disease requiring medication, visual or auditory impairments, and the incidence and severity of retinopathy of prematurity were equivalent in the two groups. The frequency of neurodevelopmental impairment was also comparable in the groups that received one dose versus three doses: moderate to severe cerebral palsy was found in 9% versus 6%, mental retardation assessed by Bayley Scales of Infant Development scores less than 69 was found in 16% vs 14%, and moderate to severe impairments of any kind were found in 33% vs 24%, respectively. Furthermore, the absolute number of impaired survivors was 92 in the three-dose group versus 106 in the one-dose group, despite a higher survival rate in the three-dose group. This study demonstrates that developmental outcomes of infants weighing 700 to 1100 gm who received three prophylactic doses of synthetic surfactant are at least as good as those of infants receiving a single dose, and that improving survival rates of very premature infants with synthetic surfactant does not result in increased numbers of infants with impairments. (J Pediatr 1995;126:S26-32)

Reprint requests: Jeffrey J. Gerdes, MD, Section on Newborn Pediatrics, Pennsylvania Hospital, 800 Spruce St., Philadelphia, PA 19107.

0022-3476/95/$3.00 + 0 **9/0/61825**

New therapies introduced into clinical use in the intensive care nursery must satisfy three major criteria before they are accepted into the clinician's armamentarium. The treatment should produce short-term improvements in morbidity or mortality, have an acceptable risk/benefit ra-

BPD	Bronchopulmonary dysplasia
CI	Confidence interval
CLD	Chronic lung disease
CP	Cerebral palsy
MDI	Mental development index
PDI	Psychomotor development index
ROP	Retinopathy of prematurity
RR	Relative risk

tio, and improve or at least leave unchanged the long-term health and neurodevelopmental outcome in survivors of the disease and its treatment. Surfactant replacement therapy has been shown to reduce mortality and short-term morbidity associated with preterm birth and respiratory distress syndrome. However, we are still in the process of ascertaining the long-term consequences of surfactant therapy. One important question is whether reductions in mortality result in more survivors with impairments.

Single-dose prophylactic treatment with synthetic surfactant has been shown to reduce mortality in infants weighing 700 to 1100 gm[1] without increasing adverse long-term outcome in survivors.[2] Several surfactant preparations have been shown to reduce morbidity and mortality when multidose treatment was compared with placebo, but the optimal dosage regimen remains unknown.[3-6] A recent comparison of one versus three prophylactic doses of synthetic surfactant showed a reduction in the severity of respiratory distress syndrome and in mortality at 28 days and 1 year of age in neonates weighing 700 to 1100 gm who received prophylactic surfactant treatment with the three-dose regimen.[7] In that study of 886 preterm neonates who weighed 700 to 1100 gm at birth, mortality at age 1 year was reduced from 21.0% in the group that received one dose to 15.1% in the group that received three doses, a reduction of 29%.[7] The purpose of this study was to compare the outcome at 1-year adjusted age of infants receiving the one- and three-dose regimens.

METHODS

Study design. The trial was designed as a multicenter, prospective, double-blind, randomized, parallel comparison of the effects of one versus three doses of 5 ml/kg of synthetic surfactant (colfosceril palmitate, cetyl alcohol, and tyloxapol; Exosurf Neonatal, Burroughs Wellcome Co., Research Triangle Park, N.C.). The trial involved a common protocol at 33 hospitals in the United States; participants are listed in Appendixes I and II. The follow-up study consisted of a double-blind evaluation conducted at 1-year adjusted age. The protocol was approved by the Institutional Review Board at each hospital. Patients were entered in the trial from March 1989 to April 1990.

Patient recruitment and enrollment. Informed consent was obtained prenatally from mothers who were expected to deliver premature infants with birth weights between 700 and 1100 gm. Prenatal and postnatal exclusion criteria were identical to those used in an earlier prophylactic trial of this synthetic surfactant.[1] At birth, neonates who met all criteria underwent intubation and ventilation in the delivery room with standardized ventilator support and were given a dose of 5 ml/kg synthetic surfactant through an endotracheal tube adaptor within 30 minutes of birth. The three-dose group received two additional 5 ml/kg synthetic sur-

Table I. Patient accountability*

	Synthetic surfactant	
	One dose (n = 410)	Three doses (n = 416)
Alive at 1-year adjusted age	324 (79)	353 (85)
Lost to follow-up	80 (20) [25]	89 (21) [25]
Completed follow-up	244 (60) [75]	264 (63) [75]

Numbers in parentheses represent the percentage of enrolled infants; numbers in brackets represent the percentage of survivors at 1-year adjusted age.
*Includes all patients as treated without exclusions.

Table II. Baseline characteristics and major neonatal complications of infants who completed 1-year follow-up*

	Synthetic surfactant	
Characteristic	One dose (n = 244)	Three doses (n = 264)
Birth weight (gm)†	907 ± 121	911 ± 125
Gestational age (wk)†	27.2 ± 1.7	27.2 ± 1.8
Multiple birth (%)	46 (19)	55 (21)
Race (%)		
White	134 (55)	160 (60)
Black	90 (37)	80 (30)
Hispanic	9 (4)	12 (5)
Other	11 (5)	13 (5)
Maternal age (yr)*	26 ± 6	26 ± 7
Maternal education (yr)†	13 ± 3	12 ± 3
Sex (%)		
Male	135 (55)	149 (56)
Female	109 (45)	116 (44)
Apgar score (median)		
1 min	4	4
5 min	7	7
IVH during days 1-28 (%)		
Grade I/II	53 (22)	67 (26)
Grade III/PVED	24 (10)	18 (7)
BPD day 28 (%)	20 (8)	26 (10)

IVH, Intraventricular hemorrhage; *PVED*, periventricular echodensities.
*Infants are classified according to the treatment they received.
†For maternal education: n = 179, air placebo; n = 179, synthetic surfactant.

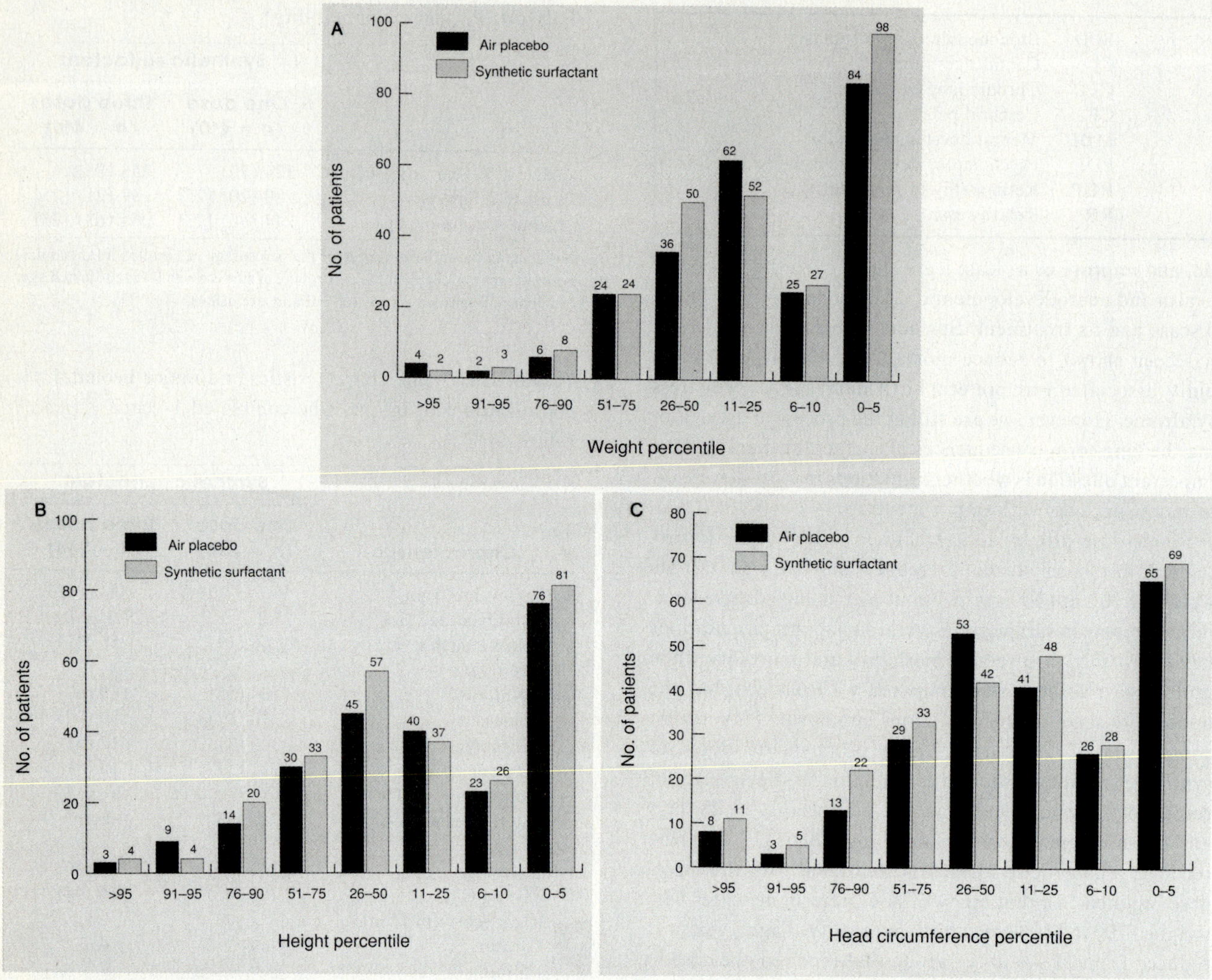

Fig. 1. Weight, height, and head circumference measurements at 1-year adjusted age for infants treated with one or three prophylactic doses of synthetic surfactant. (Percentile rankings based on growth charts from the National Center for Health Statistics.)

factant doses at 12-hour intervals; the one-dose group received two additional doses of air placebo at the same intervals.

The details of data collection, ophthalmologic examination, 1-year follow-up examination, and data analyses are described elsewhere in this supplement.[8]

RESULTS

The three-dose regimen proved to be substantially more effective than the one-dose regimen and, at least acutely, equally safe. The group that received three doses had lower oxygen and ventilator requirements and better neonatal and 1-year survival rates; a detailed report has been published.[7]

Complete follow-up data were obtained for 244 of 324 surviving patients who received one dose (75.3%) and for 264 of 353 surviving patients who received three doses (74.8%) (Table I). The two groups were balanced in terms of maternal and demographic characteristics and diagnosis of intraventricular hemorrhage and BPD (Table II). The patients for whom a follow-up examination was refused had been comparable at the day 28 assessments with respect to the diagnosis of BPD and respiratory support (data not shown).

Physical examination. The mean adjusted age at the time of the double-blind, follow-up evaluation was 379 days for both the one-dose and three-dose synthetic surfactant groups. Mean height (73 cm), weight (8.7 kg), and head circumference (45.3 cm) were the same for both treatment groups. The distribution percentiles for these measurements also were equivalent in the two groups at the 1-year

Table III. Health status*

Condition	Synthetic surfactant: One dose (%) (n = 243)	Three doses (%) (n = 264)	Relative risk†	95% Confidence interval
Surgery	96 (40)	86 (33)	0.822	(0.659, 1.027)
Readmitted to hospital	108 (44)	110 (42)	0.931	(0.763, 1.137)
Physical evidence of CLD	43 (18)	40 (15)	0.859	(0.580, 1.272)
Medication for CLD	35 (14)	30 (11)	0.805	(0.512, 1.267)
Respiratory support on day of examination	8 (3)	5 (2)	0.586	(0.190, 1.811)
Medication for chronic neurologic disease	12 (5)	3 (1)	0.216	(0.067, 0.697)
Allergies	21 (9)	26 (10)	1.147	(0.659, 1.995)
Asthma	13 (5)	16 (6)	1.127	(0.548, 2.316)
Rhinitis	3 (1)	6 (2)	1.903	(0.487, 7.435)

*RR <1.000 indicates decreased risk of event with three doses of synthetic surfactant treatment.
†Includes data on health status between day 29 and 1-year adjusted age.

Table IV. Retinopathy of prematurity*

	Worst examination				Last examination			
	Synthetic surfactant				Synthetic surfactant			
	One dose (%) (n = 300)	Three doses (%) (n = 317)	Relative risk†	95% Confidence interval	One dose (%) (n = 300)	Three doses (%) (n = 317)	Relative risk†	95% Confidence interval
No ROP	114 (38)	115 (36)	0.941	(0.771, 1.149)	213 (71)	221 (70)	0.980	(0.885, 1.085)
Mild/moderate ROP	139 (46)	167 (53)			73 (24)	85 (27)		
Severe ROP	47 (16)	35 (11)	0.733	(0.495, 1.085)	14 (5)	11 (3)	0.773	(0.361, 1.654)
Treatment‡	26 (9)	20 (6)			7 (2)	6 (2)		
Surgery	12	10			4	6		
Cryotherapy	23	19			6	7		
Laser	1	0			0	0		

*Based on worst and last examination for all infants who received ophthalmologic examinations under study protocol. Mild/moderate ROP = grades 1-3; severe ROP = grades >3.
†RR <1.000 indicates decreased risk of event with three doses of synthetic surfactant.
‡Some patients received more than one treatment.

follow-up examination (Fig. 1). However, in the total study group, 36% of infants were below the 5th percentile in weight, 31% were below the 5th percentile in height, and 27% were below the 5th percentile in head circumference.

Health status. The needs for surgery and hospital readmission after day 28 were not different in the two groups (Table III). Only a small number of infants in either group had evidence of chronic lung disease. In the one-dose versus the three-dose groups, 18% versus 15% had physical evidence of CLD, 14% versus 11% received medications for CLD, and 3% versus 2% were receiving respiratory support. Of the infants with CLD, two babies in the one-dose group required continuous positive airway pressure or mechanical ventilation at 1-year adjusted age. None of the babies in the three-dose group required mechanical support. The only significant difference in health outcome between the two study groups was a significantly lower use of medication for seizures in the three-dose group (12 of 243 vs 3 of 264: relative risk 0.216; 95% confidence interval 0.067-0.697).

Ophthalmologic examination. There were no differences in the incidence of any grade of retinopathy of prematurity between the study groups. At the time of the worst examination results, 47 of 300 (16%) of the babies in the one-dose group had severe ROP, versus 35 of 317 (11%) of the babies in the three-dose group (RR 0.733; 95% CI 0.495-1.085). By the time of the last examination, resolution of ROP had occurred for most infants, at which time 14 of 300 (5%) of the babies who received one dose and 11 of 317 (3%) of the babies who received three doses had severe ROP (Table IV).

Table V. Mental and psychomotor development as determined by Bayley Scales of Infant Development

	Mental development index				Psychomotor development index			
	Synthetic surfactant				Synthetic surfactant			
	One dose (*n* = 205)	Three doses (*n* = 235)	Relative risk*	95% Confidence interval	One dose (*n* = 198)	Three doses (*n* = 229)	Relative risk*	95% Confidence interval
Developmental index† ‡								
Analysis I	92 ± 23	92 ± 22			88 ± 19	89 ± 20		
Analysis II§	94 ± 22	94 ± 21			91 ± 17	90 ± 19		
Index <2 SD (%)‖	29 (15)	30 (13)	0.898	(0.558, 1.444)	18 (10)	26 (12)	1.248	(0.704, 2.214)

*Relative risk <1.000 indicates decreased risk of event with synthetic surfactant.
†Mean ± SD.
‡Index values <50 were set to 49.
§Severe impairments (e.g., bilateral blindness or deafness or moderate or severe CP) were excluded from analyses (MDI and PDI: 193, one dose; 223, three doses).
‖Bayley Scales of Infant Development score <69.

Table VI. Impairments

	Synthetic surfactant			
	One dose (%) (*n* = 243)	Three doses (%) (*n* = 264)	Relative risk*	95% Confidence interval
Impairment present†	106 (44)	92 (35)	0.81	(0.652, 1.000)
No impairment	123 (51)	155 (59)		
Severity of impairment				
Mild/moderate	40 (17)	39 (15)		
Serious	66 (27)	53 (20)	0.76	(0.555, 1.032)
Type of impairment† ‡				
MDI <69	40 (16)	38 (14)	0.89	(0.595, 1.344)
MDI 69-84	29 (12)	33 (13)	1.03	(0.645, 1.643)
Moderate/severe CP	22 (9)	16 (6)	0.71	(0.386, 1.299)
Mild CP	16 (7)	15 (6)	0.90	(0.454, 1.781)
Bilateral sensorineural deafness	5 (2)	1 (0)	0.18	(0.026, 1.287)
Deafness not requiring amplification	5 (2)	2 (1)	0.37	(0.078, 1.709)
Bilateral blindness	10 (4)	4 (2)	0.39	(0.131, 1.136)
Visual defect	24 (10)	22 (8)	0.88	(0.509, 1.512)

*RR <1.000 indicates decreased risk of event with three doses of synthetic surfactant.
†Infants may have more than one impairment.
‡Bayley Scales of Infant Development MDI scores <50 set to 49.

Neurodevelopmental status. The percentage of children with neurodevelopmental impairments did not differ between the two study groups (Table V). The incidence of cerebral palsy was not different between the one- versus three-dose groups (Table VI). Moderate or severe CP was documented in 9% (one-dose group) versus 6% (three-dose group), and mild CP was documented in 7% (one-dose group) versus 6% (three-dose group). The incidence of sensorineural hearing impairment was low, and no significant differences were found between the two study groups.

No significant differences were observed between the two groups on Bayley Scales of Infant Development mental and psychomotor development indices at 1-year adjusted age. The mean MDI was 92 ± 23 and 92 ± 22, and the mean PDI was 88 ± 19 and 89 ± 20 in the one-dose and three-dose groups, respectively. A similar percentage of children in both groups had serious delays in mental and motor skills as indicated by MDI or PDI scores less than 69 (Table VI).

Impairments. Infants who received three doses had a 35% rate of any impairments, versus infants in the one-dose group, who had a 44% rate (RR 0.807; 95% CI 0.652, 1.000) and those who received three doses had a 20% rate of severe impairments versus those given one dose, who had a 27% rate (RR 0.757; 95% CI 0.555-1.032). The percentage of children who experienced mild to moderate impairment was similar in the two groups (17% vs 15% with one and three doses, respectively). At 1-year adjusted age, the majority of patients in both groups had no impairments and were functionally normal (51% vs 59% with one and three doses, respectively). Fig. 2 and Table VI summarize the proportions of patients with different degrees of functional impairments.

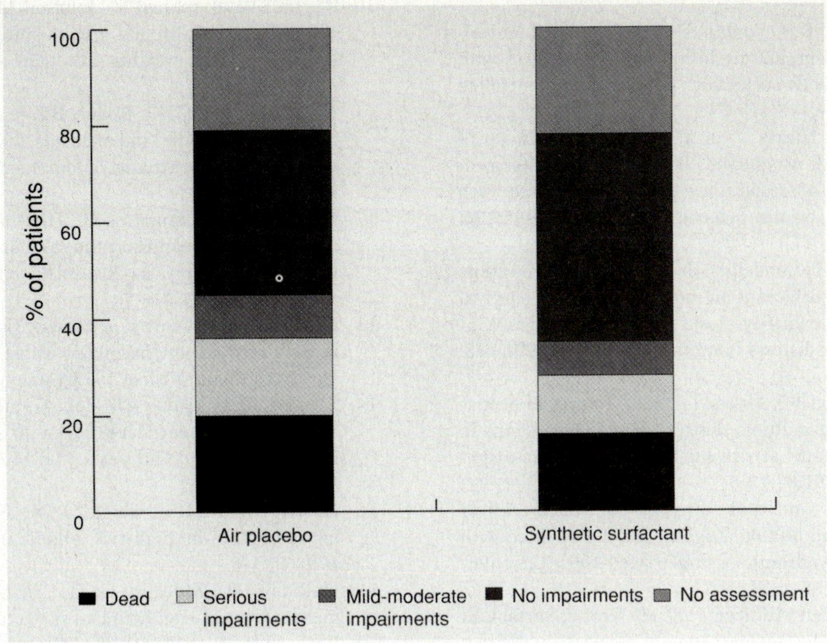

Fig. 2. Incidence of death and serious or mild to moderate functional handicaps at 1-year adjusted age in patients who received one or three prophylactic doses of synthetic surfactant.

DISCUSSION

The most important finding of this large, double-blind, follow-up study is that developmental and late morbidity outcomes of infants randomized to one or three prophylactic doses of synthetic surfactant were equivalent. It may be of some clinical importance (although the differences were not statistically significant) that in the three-dose group the proportion and absolue number of impaired infants were somewhat lower than in the one-dose group, despite significantly more survivors in the three-dose group. Thus the improvement in survival rates with the three-dose regimen was not associated with extra survivors with impairments.

In both study groups, more than half of the infants were developmentally normal at 1-year adjusted age. This finding represents an acceptable outcome, considering that the definition of impairments was strict; for instance, an infant with no developmental impairment but hypertonicity in one extremity was considered to be mildly impaired. The incidence of moderate to severe CP was low and was comparable with the expected rates of CP in this birth weight group.[9] The incidence of mental retardation (MDI scores <69) in the total study group was 15%, again comparable with previous reports from the presurfactant era.[10, 11] Auditory or visual impairments occurred in a small fraction of the study population.

These data obtained at 1-year adjusted age should be interpreted with caution because developmental status at 1 year does not predict long-term outcome for all infants. For example, at 1 year of age, some findings, such as abnormalities of muscle tone, may resolve as the child matures.[12, 13] Similarly, assessment at 1 year of age does not address or predict developmental morbidity such as learning disabilities at school age.[14, 15]

Previous studies that used synthetic surfactants,[16, 17] human surfactant,[18] and bovine-derived surfactant[19, 20] have shown similar health and neurodevelopmental outcomes at 1- or 2-years adjusted age for treated and control populations. However, these earlier studies were far smaller. Comparisons among the various follow-up trials are difficult because of differences in study populations, surfactant preparations and techniques of administration, and follow-up assessments.

In any case, we can conclude that both late morbidity and developmental outcomes of infants weighing 700 to 1100 gm birth who were treated with three prophylactic doses of synthetic surfactant are at least as good as those treated with a single prophylactic dose. Furthermore, the gains in survival observed in the three-dose group were not achieved at the cost of more survivors with impairments. These conclusions can be drawn with some confidence because of the randomized, double-blind design of the trial and its large size.

REFERENCES

1. Corbet A, Bucciarelli R, Goldman S, et al. Decreased mortality rate among small premature infants treated at birth with a single dose of synthetic surfactant: a multicenter controlled trial. J PEDIATR 1991;118:277-84.
2. Sell MS, Cotton R, Hirata T, et al. One-year follow-up of 273 infants with birth weights of 700 to 1100 gm after prophylactic treatment of respiratory distress syndrome with synthetic surfactant or air placebo. J PEDIATR 1995;126: S20-5.
3. Long W, Thompson T, Sundell H, et al. Effects of two rescue doses of a synthetic surfactant on mortality rate and survival without bronchopulmonary dysplasia in 700- to 1350-gram infants with respiratory distress syndrome. J PEDIATR 1991;118: 595-605.
4. Hoekstra RE, Jackson JC, Myers TF, et al. Improved neonatal survival following multiple doses of bovine surfactant in very premature neonates at risk for respiratory distress syndrome. Pediatrics 1991;88:10-8.
5. Long W. Corbet A, Cotton R, et al. A controlled trial of synthetic surfactant in infants weighing 1250 g or more with respiratory distress syndrome. N Engl J Med 1991;325:1696-703.
6. Collaborative European Multicenter Study Group. Surfactant replacement therapy for severe neonatal respiratory distress syndrome: an international randomized clinical trial. Pediatrics 1988;82:693-91.
7. Corbet A, Gerdes J, Long W, et al. Double-blind randomized trial of one versus three prophylactic doses of synthetic surfactant in 826 neonates weighing 700 to 1100 grams: effects on mortality rate. J PEDIATR (in press).
8. Corbet A, Long W, Schumacher R, et al. Double-blind developmental evaluation at 1-year corrected age of 597 premature infants with birth weights from 500 to 1350 grams enrolled in three placebo-controlled trials of prophylactic synthetic surfactant. J PEDIATR 1995;126:S5-12.
9. Bernbaum JC, Hoffmann-Williamson M. Primary care of the preterm infant. In: Neuromuscular assessment and cerebral palsy. St. Louis: Mosby–Year Book, 1991:211-48.
10. Teplin SW, Burchinal M, Johnson-Martin N, et al. Neurodevelopmental, health and growth status at age 6 years of children with birth weights less than 1001 grams. J PEDIATR 1991;118:768-77.
11. Msall ME, Buck GM, Rogers BT, et al. Risk factors for major neurodevelopmental impairments and need for special education resources in extremely premature infants. J PEDIATR 1991; 119:606-14.
12. Georgieff MK, Bernbaum JC, Hoffmann-Williamson M, et al. Abnormal truncal muscle tone as a useful early marker for developmental delay in low-birth-weight infants. Pediatrics 1986;77:659.
13. Drillien CM. Abnormal neurologic signs in the first year of life in low-birth-weight infants: possible prognostic significance. Dev Med Child Neurol 1972;14(suppl):575.
14. Stewart AL, Costello AM deL, Hamilton PA, et al. Relationship between neurodevelopmental status of very preterm infants at one and four years. Dev Med Child Neurol 1989;31: 756-65.
15. Li AKF, Sauve RS, Creighton DE. Early indicators of learning problems in high-risk children. J Dev Behav Pediatr 1990;11:1-6.
16. Halliday HL, McClure G, Reid MM. Growth and development two years after artificial surfactant replacement at birth. Early Hum Dev 1986;13:323-7.
17. Morley CJ, Morley R. Follow-up of premature babies treated with artificial surfactant (ALEC). Arch Dis Child 1990;65: 667-9.
18. Vaucher YE, Merritt TA, Hallman M, et al. Neurodevelopmental and respiratory outcome in early childhood after human surfactant treatment. Am J Dis Child 1988;142:927-30.
19. Dunn MS, Shennan AT, Hoskins EM, et al. Two-year follow-up of infants enrolled in a randomized trial of surfactant replacement therapy for prevention of neonatal respiratory distress syndrome. Pediatrics 1988;82:543-7.
20. Ware J, Taeusch HW, Soll RF, et al. Health and developmental outcomes of a surfactant controlled trial: follow-up at 2 years. Pediatrics 1990;85:1103-7.

Double-blind evaluation of developmental and health status to age 2 years of infants weighing 700 to 1350 grams treated prophylactically at birth with a single dose of synthetic surfactant or air placebo

Ernest N. Kraybill, MD, Carl L. Bose, MD, Anthony J. Corbet, MB, FRACP, Jose Garcia-Prats, MD, Diane Asbill, RN, Kathleen Edwards, MPH, and Walker Long, MD

From the Departments of Pediatrics, University of North Carolina at Chapel Hill and Baylor College of Medicine, Houston, Texas, and the Department of Statistics, Burroughs Wellcome Co., Research Triangle Park, North Carolina

In a previously published article, we reported results of a two-center study of outcome to 28 days of 385 infants with birth weights from 700 to 1350 gm who were assigned randomly to receive a single 5 ml/kg intratracheal dose of either synthetic surfactant or air placebo. Infants treated with surfactant had a higher rate of survival to 28 days without bronchopulmonary dysplasia than did control subjects given an air placebo. The present study assessed survivors in early childhood to determine neurodevelopmental outcome and late morbidity. Two hundred fifty-eight surviving infants from both centers were evaluated at 1-year adjusted age; medical histories were obtained, standard physical and neurologic examinations were performed, and Bayley Scales of Infant Development were administered. Ophthalmologic examinations were performed at various times between 28 days and 1-year adjusted age. At 2-years adjusted age, 118 infants from one center were reevaluated with the same procedures and also had hearing and speech evaluations. Neither the 1-year assessment of the entire population nor the 2-year assessment of the one center's cohort revealed physical or neurodevelopmental differences between treatment groups. We conclude that administration of a single prophylactic dose of synthetic surfactant to premature infants with birth weights from 700 to 1350 grams results in improved survival rates to 28 days without bronchopulmonary dysplasia and is not associated with adverse health or neurodevelopmental effects at 1-year or 2-years adjusted age. (J Pediatr 1995;126:S33-42)

Supported by funds from Burroughs Wellcome Co., Research Triangle Park, North Carolina.

Reprint requests: Ernest N. Kraybill, MD, Department of Pediatrics, The University of North Carolina at Chapel Hill, Chapel Hill, NC 27599-7220.

0022-3476/95/$3.00 + 0 **9/0/61826**

Several mammalian and synthetic surfactants have been shown to reduce the adverse effects of respiratory distress syndrome when given prophylactically or as rescue treatment to premature infants.[1-13] In a previously published article we reported a two-center study of outcome at 28 days of age of infants with birth weights from 700 to 1350 gm who were assigned randomly to receive a single 5 ml/kg

HCHD	Harris County Hospital District
MDI	Mental development index
NCMH	North Carolina Memorial Hospital
PDI	Psychomotor development index
ROP	Retinopathy of prematurity

intratracheal dose of either synthetic surfactant or air placebo as soon as possible after birth.[12] Infants treated with surfactant had a higher rate of survival to 28 days without bronchopulmonary dysplasia than did infants who received air placebo.

We now report the physical and neurodevelopmental status at 1-year adjusted age of surviving infants treated at both study sites, and at 2-years adjusted age of survivors treated at one of the two sites.

METHODS

Study design and patient enrollment. The trials were prospective, double-blind, randomized, parallel comparisons of the effect of a single 5 ml/kg intratracheal dose of either synthetic surfactant (colfosceril palmitate, cetyl alcohol, and tyloxapol; Exosurf Neonatal, Burroughs Wellcome Co., Research Triangle Park, N.C.) or air placebo and were conducted with identical protocols at two study centers, North Carolina Memorial Hospital, Chapel Hill, North Carolina, and the Harris County Hospital District, Houston, Texas. The research was approved by the Institutional Review Board of each hospital, and parents gave informed consent. Subject recruitment and enrollment are described in a previously published article.[12] Subjects were entered in the trial from April 1986 through July 1989.

Assessments at 1-year adjusted age. The 323 surviving infants from both centers were the intended subjects of the 1-year follow-up part of the study. Monitoring of subjects between age 28 days and 1-year adjusted age (including procedures for ophthalmologic assessment) and the 1-year evaluation procedures are described in another article in this supplement.[14]

Assessments at 2-years adjusted age. The 145 subjects who had been treated in the NCMH study center and were not known to have died before 1 year of age were intended subjects of the 2-year follow-up evaluation. The assessments were scheduled to be performed within 6 weeks of subjects becoming 2-years adjusted age. The procedures that comprised the 1-year evaluations were repeated. Audiometry by sound field testing and language evaluation by the Receptive-Expressive Emergent Language Scale[15] were also performed. Specific impairments and overall functional impairments were defined as for the 1-year follow-up evaluation. If subjects were unable to return for 2-year follow-up evaluation, an attempt was made to interview parents by telephone to determine whether the subject was alive.

Methods of data analysis are described in another article in this supplement.[14]

RESULTS

Two hundred fifty-eight (80%) of the 323 eligible survivors were evaluated at 1-year adjusted age; 122 (76%) were from the air placebo group and 136 (83%) were from the surfactant group (Table I). The two groups were similar in demographic and birth characteristics (Table II). Six subjects (four [3%] from the group that received air placebo and two [1%] from the group treated with surfactant) were receiving oxygen in alveolar concentrations of 26% to 40% (estimated from cannula flow rate and oxygen concentration) at the time of the 1-year examination. One of the two oxygen-dependent, surfactant-treated infants was also receiving continuous positive airway pressure. Eight (7%) of the infants given air placebo and 10 (7%) of the infants treated with surfactant were considered to have physical evidence of chronic lung disease. Similar proportions of infants (air placebo group, 31%; surfactant group, 32%) required surgery between day 28 and 1-year adjusted age.

The air placebo and surfactant groups did not differ in distribution among height-for-age, weight-for-age, or head circumference-for-age percentile groupings at 1-year adjusted age (Fig. 1).

During the first year, retinopathy of prematurity was found in 82 of 132 (62%) of the infants given air placebo and in 86 of 143 (60%) of the infants treated with surfactant who survived and received ophthalmologic examinations (Table III). Seven (5%) of the infants given air placebo and 10 (7%) of the infants treated with surfactant received treatment for ROP (surgery or cryotherapy). At the latest examination reported, ROP was present in 29 (22%) of the infants given air placebo and 39 (27%) of the infants treated with surfactant. Two (2%) of the infants given air placebo and two (2%) of the infants treated with surfactant had severe ROP at the last reported examination.

The mean Bayley Scales of Infant Development mental development index scores of the infants given air placebo (85 ± 20) were not different from the mean MDI scores of those who had received surfactant (88 ± 22) (Table IV). The air placebo group also did not differ in the proportion of infants with MDI scores less than 2 SD below the normative mean (air-placebo group, 11 [9%]; surfactant group, 23 [14%]).

Bayley Scales of Infant Development psychomotor development index mean scores (air-placebo group, 89 ± 22; surfactant group, 91 ± 23) and the proportion of scores less than 2 SD below the mean also were similar between treatment groups (Table IV). The MDI and PDI mean scores for each group were similar when scores less than 49 were set to 50 or when patients with severe impairments were excluded.

Table I. Patient accountability*

	1-year NCMH and HCHD		2-year (NCMH only)	
	Air placebo (*n* = 193)	Synthetic surfactant (*n* = 192)	Air placebo (*n* = 84)	Synthetic surfactant (*n* = 83)
Alive at 1-year adjusted age	160 (83)	163 (85)	73 (87)	72 (87)
Lost to follow-up	38 (20) [24]†	27 (14) [17]†	3 (4) [4]	4 (5) [6]
Completed 1-year follow-up	122 (63) [76]	136 (71) [83]	70 (83) [96]	68 (82) [94]
Survivors at 2-year follow-up			69 (82)	67 (81)
Lost to follow-up			8 (10) [12]	10 (12) [15]
Completed 2-year follow-up			61 (73) [88]	57 (69) [85]

Numbers in parentheses represent the percentage of enrolled patients; numbers in brackets represent the percentage of surviving patients.
*Includes all patients as treated without exclusion.
†Includes approximately 10% of patients whose survival status was assessed by telephone contact.

Table II. Baseline characteristics and major neonatal complications of infants who completed 1- and 2-year follow-up*

	1-year (NCMH and HCHD)		2-year (NCMH only)	
Characteristic	Air placebo (*n* = 122)	Synthetic surfactant (*n* = 136)	Air placebo (*n* = 61)	Synthetic surfactant (*n* = 57)
Birth weight (gm)†	1028 ± 184	1022 ± 177	1005 ± 184	1043 ± 165
Gestational age (wk)†	28.1 ± 2.0	28.2 ± 1.9	28.1 ± 1.8	28.3 ± 1.8
Multiple birth (%)	32 (26)	30 (22)	21 (34)	12 (21)
Race (%)				
White	42 (34)	28 (21)	26 (43)	20 (35)
Black	51 (42)	72 (53)	33 (54)	34 (60)
Hispanic	27 (22)	31 (23)		
Other	2 (2)	5 (4)	2 (3)	3 (5)
Maternal age (yr)†	25 ± 6	24 ± 6	25 ± 5	24 ± 5
Maternal education (yr)†,‡	11 ± 4	11 ± 3	12 ± 3	12 ± 2
Sex (%)				
Male	64 (52)	69 (51)	26 (43)	28 (49)
Female	58 (48)	67 (49)	35 (57)	29 (51)
Apgar score (median)				
1 min	5.0	6.0	6.0	6.0
5 min	8.0	8.0	8.0	8.0
IVH during days 1-28 (%)				
Grade I/II	27 (23)	30 (22)	12 (20)	10 (18)
Grade III/PVED	9 (8)	7 (5)	5 (9)	3 (5)
No IVH	84 (70)	98 (73)	42 (71)	43 (77)
BPD at day 28 (%)	31 (25)	24 (18)	17 (28)	13 (23)

IVH, Intraventricular hemorrhage; *PVED*, periventricular echodensities; *BPD*, bronchopulmonary dysplasia.
*Infants classified according to treatment they received.
†Mean ± SD.
‡For maternal education at 1 year: air placebo, *n* = 104; synthetic surfactant, *n* = 117. For maternal education at 2 years: air placebo, *n* = 47; synthetic surfactant, *n* = 41.

Prevalence of impairment at 1-year adjusted age was similar between the treatment groups (Table V). Among the infants given air placebo, 58% had no impairment, 18% had mild to moderate impairment, and 24% had serious impairment; among the infants treated with surfactant, 58% were free of impairment, 14% had mild to moderate impairment, and 28% had serious impairment. Fifteen more survivors were evaluated at 1 year in the surfactant group. There were eight more infants with no impairments, eight more infants with serious impairments, and two fewer infants with mild/moderate impairments in the surfactant group. Specific functional handicaps are shown in Table V. Prevalence of impairment at 1-year adjusted age among the NCMH subset was not different from that of the combined

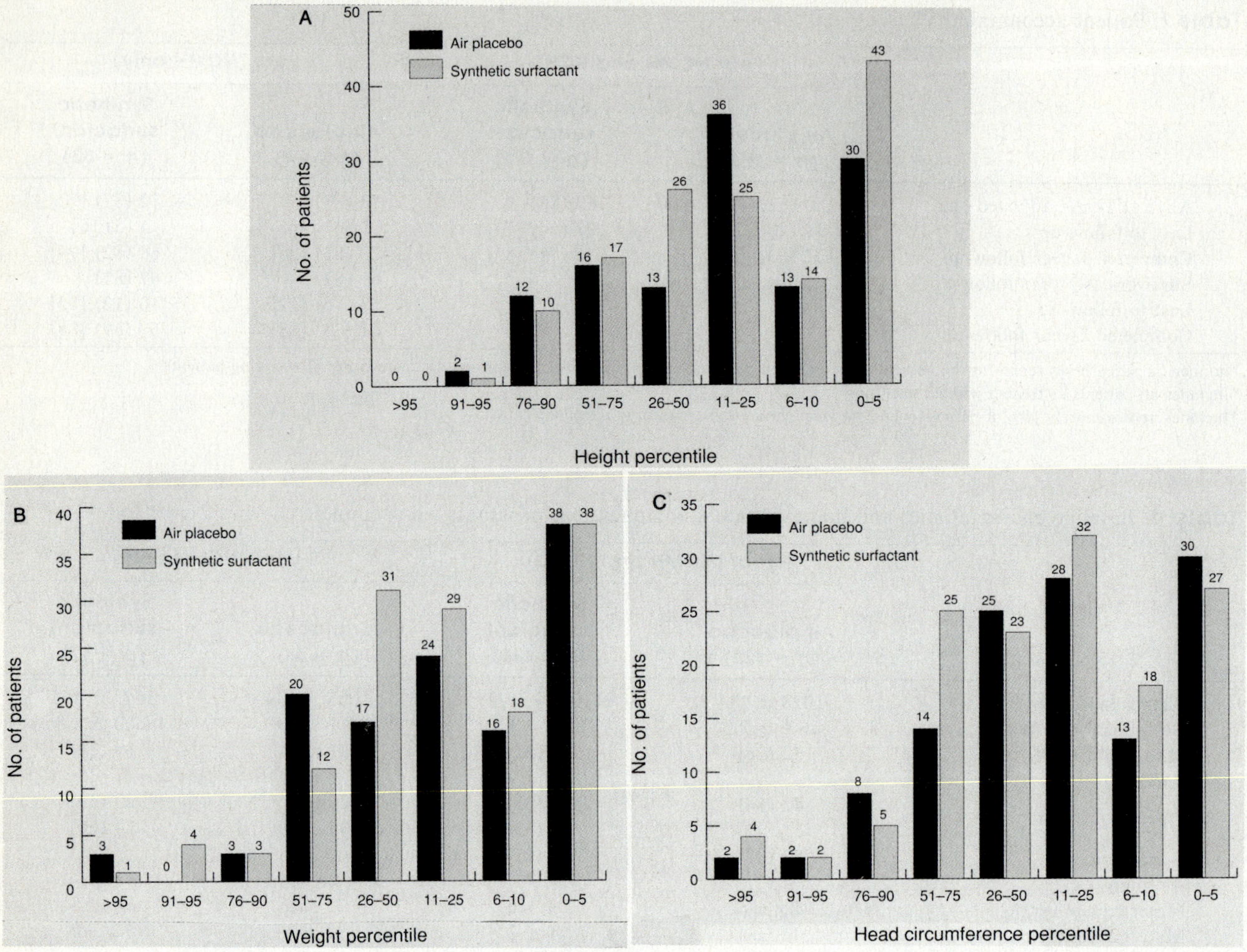

Fig. 1. Height-for-age, weight-for-age, and head circumference-for-age percentiles at 1-year adjusted age of infants treated at birth with air placebo or synthetic surfactant. (Percentile rankings are based on growth charts from the National Center for Health Statistics. Individual percentiles were derived by plotting measurement against chronologic age.)

group (Table VI). Outcome to 1-year adjusted age of all infants, by treatment, is shown in Fig. 2.

Status at 2-years adjusted age (NCMH Cohort). The two treatment groups evaluated at 2-years adjusted age (air-placebo group, 61 [88%]; surfactant group, 57 [85%]) were similar demographically and in birth characteristics. The entire NCMH cohort was similar at birth to the combined NCMH and HCHD group except in racial composition and in the proportion of mothers who had received corticosteroids. The NCMH population contained no Hispanic infants and relatively more infants of both black and white races; more NCMH mothers had received steroids (45% vs 25%).

During the second year of observation, eight infants given air placebo and nine infants treated with surfactant were hospitalized for respiratory illnesses. Ten (16%) of the infants given air placebo and 6 (11%) of the infants treated with surfactant were receiving bronchodilator medications regularly at 2-years adjusted age. Two infants treated with surfactant and none of the infants given air placebo had tracheostomies at the 2-year evaluation. Similar proportions of infants given air placebo (10%) and infants treated with surfactant (9%) required surgery between 1 and 2 years of age.

The infants given air placebo were similar to the infants treated with surfactant in distribution among weight-for-age, height-for-age, and head circumference-for-age percentile groupings (Fig. 3).

At 2-years adjusted age there were no significant differences between the treatment groups in mean Bayley Scales of Infant Development MDI or PDI scores or in the proportion of infants with MDI or PDI scores less than 2 SD below the normative mean (Table VII). The mean Receptive-Expressive Emergent Language Scale receptive quotient (air placebo group, 1.0 ± 0.2; surfactant group, 1.0 ± 0.2), expressive quotient (air placebo group, 1.0 ± 0.2; surfactant group, 0.9 ± 0.3), and language quo-

Table III. Retinopathy of prematurity*

	Worst examination		Last examination	
	Air placebo (%) (*n* = 132)	Synthetic surfactant (%) (*n* = 143)	Air placebo (%) (*n* = 132)	Synthetic surfactant (%) (*n* = 143)
No ROP	50 (38)	57 (40)	103 (78)	104 (73)
Mild/moderate ROP	79 (60)	84 (59)	27 (20)	37 (26)
Severe ROP	3 (2)	2 (2)	2 (2)	2 (2)
Treatment†	7 (5)	10 (7)	4 (3)	6 (4)
Surgery	4 (3)	3 (2)	3 (2)	4 (3)
Cryotherapy	4 (3)	8 (6)	2 (1)	3 (2)

*Based on worst and last examination for all infants who received ophthalmologic examinations under study protocol. Mild/moderate ROP = grades 1-2; severe ROP = grades 3-4. Plus disease was not recorded in this study.
†Some patients received more than one treatment.

Table IV. Mental and psychomotor development according to Bayley Scales of Infant Development at 1-year adjusted age

	Mental development index				Psychomotor development index			
			Estimated difference				Estimated difference	
	Air placebo (*n* = 118)	Synthetic surfactant (*n* = 133)	Relative risk*	95% Confidence interval	Air placebo (*n* = 118)	Synthetic surfactant (*n* = 133)	Relative risk*	95% Confidence interval
Developmental index†,‡								
Analysis I	85 ± 20	88 ± 22			89 ± 22	91 ± 23		
Analysis II§	89 ± 18	90 ± 21			93 ± 20	92 ± 24		
Index <2 SD (%)‖	11 (9)	23 (14)	1.726	0.892, 3.340	11 (9)	18 (14)	1.337	0.665, 2.689

*Relative risk <1.000 indicates decreased risk of event with synthetic surfactant.
†Mean ± SD.
‡Index values <50 were set to 49.
§Severe impairments (e.g., bilateral blindness or deafness or moderate or severe cerebral palsy) were excluded from analyses. Air placebo, *n* = 104; synthetic surfactant, *n* = 124.
‖Bayley Scales of Infant Development scores <69; <2 SD below the normative mean of 100.

Table V. Impairments at 1-year adjusted age for subjects from both centers

	Air placebo (%) (*n* = 119)	Synthetic surfactant (%) (*n* = 134)	Relative risk*	95% Confidence interval
No impairment	69 (58)	78 (58)		
Impairment present	50 (42)	56 (42)	1.002	0.751, 1.338
Severity of impairment				
Mild/moderate	21 (18)	19 (14)		
Serious	29 (24)	37 (28)	1.141	0.755, 1.724
Type of impairment†‡				
MDI <69	22 (18)	27 (20)	1.088	0.655, 1.807
MDI 69-84	19 (16)	20 (15)	0.956	0.537, 1.700
Moderate/severe CP	10 (8)	9 (7)	0.809	0.340, 1.927
Mild CP	10 (8)	12 (9)	1.098	0.492, 2.449
Bilateral sensorineural deafness	0 (0)	0 (0)	—§	—, —§
Deafness not requiring amplification	1 (1)	2 (1)	1.850	0.178, 1.921
Bilateral blindness	4 (3)	2 (1)	0.431	0.085, 2.196
Visual defect	9 (8)	9 (7)	0.892	0.368, 2.163

CP, Cerebral palsy.
*Relative risk <1.000 indicates decreased risk of event with synthetic surfactant treatment.
†Infants may have more than one impairment.
‡Bayley Scales of Infant Development MDI scores <50 set to 49.
§Counts were too low for valid estimate.

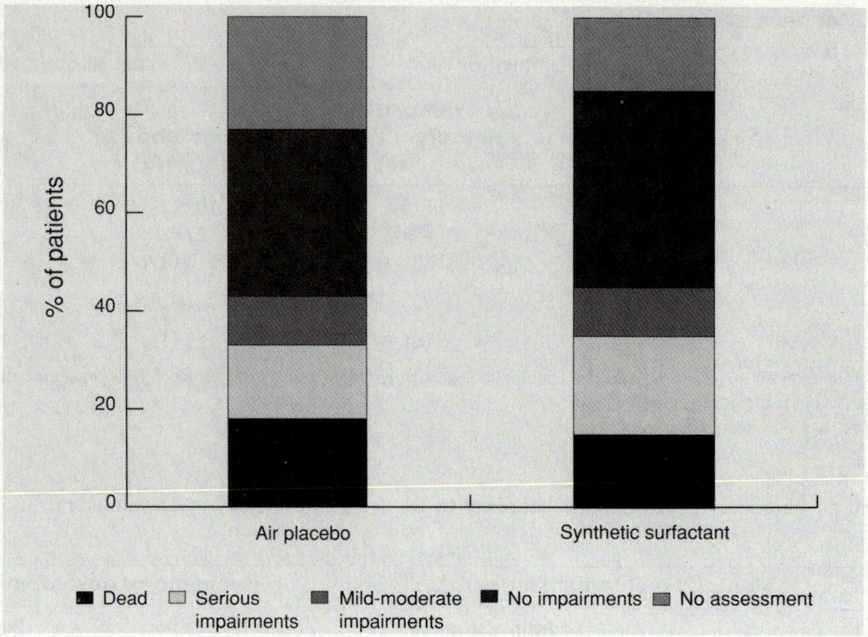

Fig. 2. Summary of outcomes to 1-year adjusted age by treatment group (all patients).

Table VI. Impairments at 1-year adjusted age for subjects from NCMH only

Test	Air placebo (%) (*n* = 61)	Synthetic surfactant (%) (*n* = 61)	Relative risk: Estimate*	Relative risk: 95% Confidence interval
No impairment	37 (61)	36 (59)	—†	
Impairment present	22 (36)	23 (38)	1.057	0.661, 1.690
Severity of impairment				
Mild/moderate	12 (20)	11 (18)		
Serious	10 (16)	12 (20)	1.167	0.559, 2.436
Type of impairment‡§				
Bayley Index <69	9 (15)	9 (15)	0.994	0.423, 2.335
Bayley Index 69-86	9 (15)	11 (18)	1.237	0.553, 2.770
Moderate or severe cerebral palsy	5 (8)	4 (7)	0.802	0.220, 2.925
Mild cerebral palsy	3 (5)	3 (5)	1.031	0.199, 5.330
Bilateral sensorineural deafness	0 (0)	0 (0)	—†	—, —†
Deafness not requiring amplification	0 (0)	1 (2)	—†	—, —†
Bilateral blindness	0 (0)	1 (2)	—†	—, —†
Visual defect	4 (7)	3 (5)	0.736	(0.176, 3.086)

*Estimate <1.000 indicates decreased risk of event with synthetic surfactant.
†Counts too low for valid estimate.
‡Infants may have more than one impairment.
§Bayley Scales of Infant Development MDI scores <50 set to 49.

tient (air placebo group, 1.0 ± 0.2; surfactant group, 0.9 ± 0.3) did not differ between the two treatment groups.

Among the infants given air placebo, 53% had no impairment, 28% had mild to moderate impairment, and 18% had severe impairment at 2-years adjusted age. Among infants treated with surfactant, 46% had no impairment, 40% had mild to moderate impairment, and 13% had severe impairment at 2-years adjusted age (Table VIII). The absolute number of impaired infants was equal (n = 28) in the two groups, but there were four fewer severely impaired infants and four more mildly/moderately impaired infants in the surfactant group. None of the observed differences was statistically significant. Outcome of all infants by treatment group is shown in Fig. 4.

DISCUSSION

At 1-year adjusted age the overall proportion of survivors for whom follow-up was completed was 80%; 10% did not

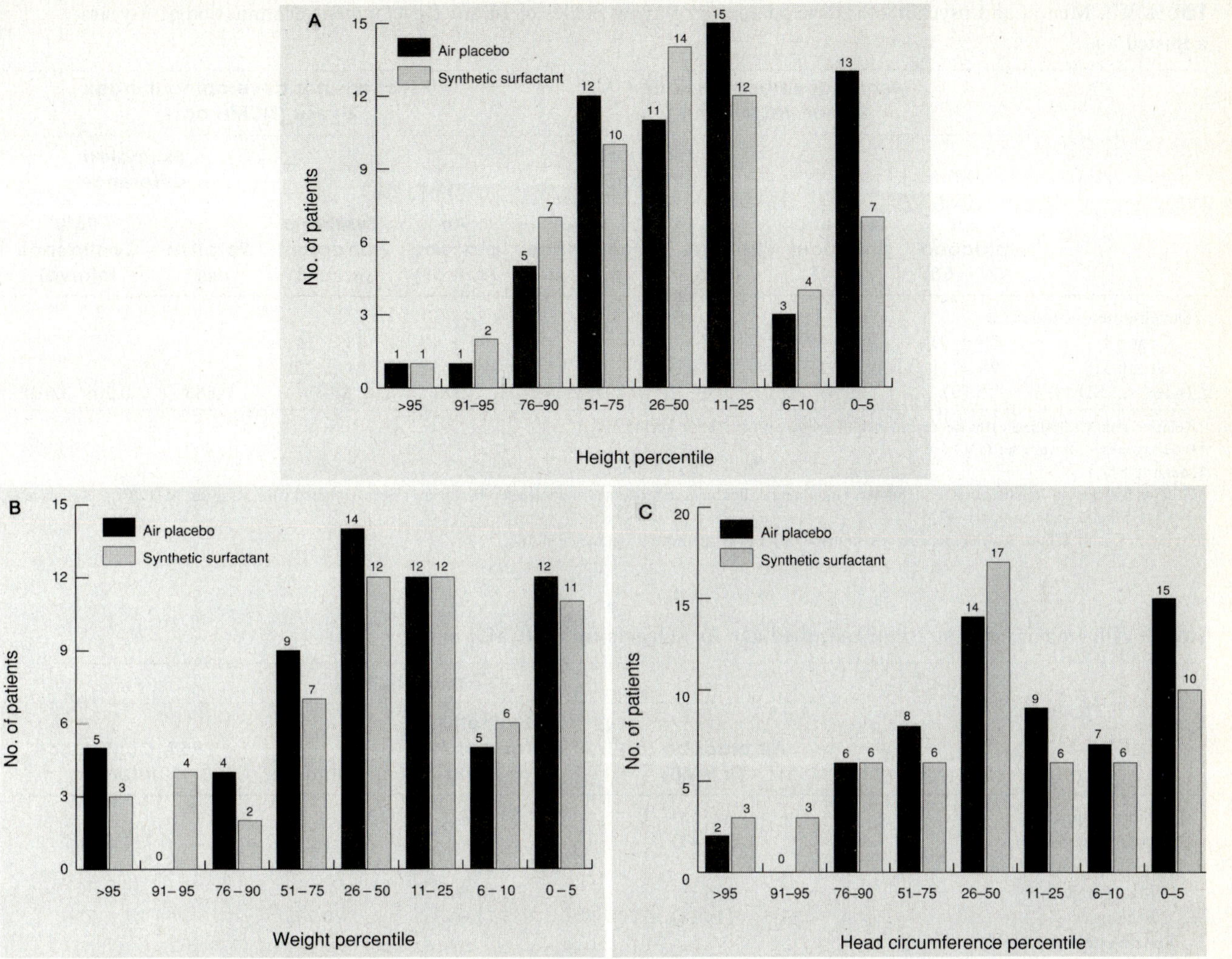

Fig. 3. Height-for-age, weight-for-age, and head circumference-for-age percentiles at 2-years adjusted age of infants treated at birth with air placebo or synthetic surfactant (NCMH only). (Percentile rankings are based on growth charts from the National Center for Health Statistics. Individual percentiles were derived by plotting measurement against chronologic age.)

return for the follow-up examination, but their parents were contacted by telephone. The proportion returning for follow-up at 1-year adjusted age was slightly higher in the surfactant group (83% vs 77%), but this difference does not appear to have influenced the results of the study. At 2-years adjusted age, the overall proportion of surviving infants who completed follow-up was 87%.

Our finding that there are no differences between infants treated with surfactant and control infants in prevalence of developmental impairment at 1-year and 2-years adjusted age is similar to findings reported by others.[16-26] However, only one of these studies evaluated more than 100 children in each group. The other studies reported outcomes for surfactant treatment groups that contained 13 to 45 infants and control groups of 10 to 41 infants, and thus they had limited power to detect moderate differences that may have been present.

In the present two-center study (NCMH and HCHD), we found no differences in neurodevelopmental outcomes at 1-year adjusted age. Evaluation of 118 subjects from one of the two centers at 2-years adjusted age also did not reveal differences. This subset was similar to the original two-center population in perinatal characteristics, except for racial composition and the proportion of mothers who received corticosteroids, and was similar to the entire population in prevalence and severity of impairment at 1 year. In neither the entire population at 1 year nor in the NCMH population at 2 years did we find developmental differences between treatment groups.

The importance of large, well-designed follow-up studies

Table VII. Mental and psychomotor development by Bayley Scales of Infant Development examination at 2-years adjusted age

	Mental development index 2-year (NCMH only)				Psychomotor development index 2-year (NCMH only)			
			Estimated difference				Estimated difference	
	Air placebo (*n* = 58)	Synthetic surfactant (*n* = 48)	Relative risk*	95% Confidence interval	Air placebo (*n* = 58)	Synthetic surfactant (*n* = 48)	Relative risk*	95% Confidence interval
Developmental index†,‡								
Group I	89 ± 21	90 ± 19			89 ± 18	88 ± 16		
Group II§	95 ± 18	92 ± 17			94 ± 13	91 ± 13		
Index <2 SD (%)‖	5 (9)	2 (4)	0.483	0.104, 2.248	4 (8)	3 (7)	0.866	0.208, 3.610

*Relative risk <1.000 indicates decreased risk of event with synthetic surfactant.
†Index values <50 were set to 49.
‡Mean ± SD.
§Patients with severe impairments (e.g., bilateral blindness or deafness or moderate or severe cerebral palsy) were excluded from analysis; MDI, PDI: Air placebo, *n* = 55; synthetic surfactant, *n* = 47.
‖Bayley Scales of Infant Development scores <69; <2 SD below the normative mean of 100.

Table VIII. Impairments at 2-years adjusted age for subjects from NCMH only

	2-year (NCMH)			
	Air placebo (%) (*n* = 60)	Synthetic surfactant (%) (*n* = 52)	Estimate*	95% Confidence interval
No impairment	32 (53)	24 (46)		
Impairment present	28 (47)	28 (54)	1.078	0.734, 1.585
Severity of impairment				
Mild/moderate	17 (28)	21 (40)		
Serious	11 (18)	7 (13)	0.785	0.332, 1.856
Type of impairment†‡				
MDI <69	8 (13)	2 (4)	0.284	0.073, 1.106
MDI 69-84	14 (23)	18 (35)	1.376	0.759, 2.494
Moderate/severe cerebral palsy	6 (10)	5 (10)	0.912	0.275, 3.024
Mild cerebral palsy	2 (3)	3 (6)	1.605	0.264, 9.760
Bilateral sensorineural deafness	0 (0)	0 (0)	—§	—, —§
Deafness not requiring amplification	0 (0)	0 (0)	—§	—, —§
Bilateral blindness	0 (0)	3 (6)	—§	—, —§
Visual defect	8 (13)	2 (4)	0.294	0.075, 1.157

*Estimate <1.000 indicates decreased risk of event with synthetic surfactant treatment.
†Patients may have more than one impairment.
‡Bayley Scales of Infant Development MDI scores <50 set to 49.
§Counts were too low for valid estimate.

to determine whether surfactant therapy may have untoward effects on neurodevelopment is heightened by a report by Hellstrom-Westas et al.[27] They demonstrated a transient decrease in cerebral activity, as shown by continuous electroencephalography, and a transient decrease in mean arterial blood pressure in 21 of 23 neonates with respiratory distress syndrome after endotracheal instillation of a porcine lung extract with surface-active properties.

We found that the children treated with synthetic surfactant were not different from controls given air placebo at 1-year and 2-years adjusted age, which is consistent with findings of other investigators.[16, 17, 22]

We conclude that a single dose of synthetic surfactant given within the first few minutes of life to premature infants with birth weights from 700 to 1350 gm (previously shown to be associated with a higher rate of survival with-

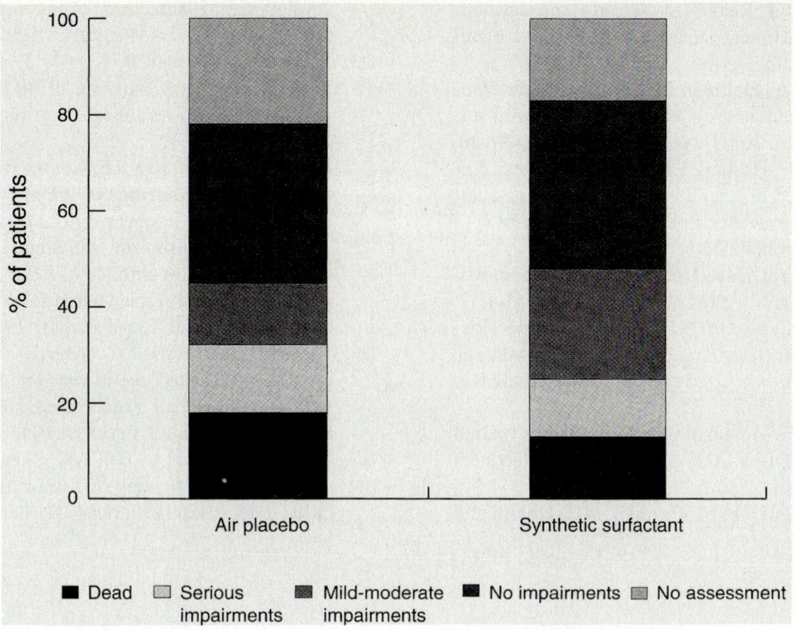

Fig. 4. Summary of outcomes at 2-years adjusted age by treatment group (NCMH only).

out bronchopulmonary dysplasia) is not associated with adverse health or neurodevelopmental effects at 1-year or 2-years adjusted age. Longer follow-up periods of large surfactant-treated and control groups are needed to confirm these findings and to detect other differences that may not appear until later in childhood.

REFERENCES

1. Merritt TA, Hallman M, Berry C, et al. Randomized placebo-controlled trial of human surfactant given at birth versus rescue administration in very low birth weight infants with lung immaturity. J PEDIATR 1991;118:581-94.
2. Kwong MS, Egan EA, Notter RH, et al. Double-blind clinical trial of calf lung surfactant extract administered at birth to very premature infants for prevention of respiratory distress syndrome. Pediatrics 1985;76:585-92.
3. Shapiro DL, Notter RH, Morin FC, et al. Double-blind randomized trial of a calf lung surfactant extract administered at birth to very premature infants for prevention of respiratory distress syndrome. Pediatrics 1985;76:593-9.
4. Collaborative European Multicenter Study Group. Surfactant replacement therapy for severe neonatal respiratory distress syndrome; an international randomized clinical trial. Pediatrics 1988;82:683-91.
5. Horbar JD, Roger MD, Soll F, et al. A multicenter randomized placebo-controlled trial of surfactant therapy for respiratory distress syndrome. N Engl J Med 1989;320:959-65.
6. Hoekstra RE, Jackson JC, Myers TF, et al. Improved neonatal survival following multiple doses of bovine surfactant in very premature neonates at risk for respiratory distress syndrome. Pediatrics 1991;88:10-8.
7. Leichty EA, Donovan E, Purohit D, et al. Reduction of neonatal mortality after multiple doses of bovine surfactant in low birth weight neonates with respiratory distress syndrome. Pediatrics 1991;88:19-28.
8. Morley CJ, Greenough A, Miller NG, et al. Randomized trial of neonatal surfactant (ALEC) given at birth to babies from 23 to 34 weeks gestation. Early Hum Dev 1988;82:683-91.
9. Phibbs RH, Ballard RA, Clements JA, et al. Initial clinical trial of Exosurf, a protein-free synthetic surfactant, for the prophylaxis and early treatment of hyaline membrane disease. Pediatrics 1991;88:1-8.
10. Corbet A, Bucciarelli R, Goldman S, et al. Decreased mortality rate among small premature infants treated at birth with a single dose of synthetic surfactant: a multicenter controlled trial. J PEDIATR 1991;118:277-84.
11. Long W, Thompson T, Sundell H, et al. Effects of two rescue doses of a synthetic surfactant on mortality rate and survival without bronchopulmonary dysplasia in 700-1350 gram infants with respiratory distress syndrome. J PEDIATR 1991; 118:595-605.
12. Bose C, Corbet A, Bose G, et al. Improved outcome at 28 days of age for very low birth weight infants treated with a single dose of a synthetic surfactant. J PEDIATR 1990;117:947-53.
13. Long W, Corbet A, Cotton R, et al. A controlled trial of synthetic surfactant in infants weighing 1250 g or more with respiratory distress syndrome. N Engl J Med 1991;325:1696-703.
14. Corbet A, Long W, Schumacher R, et al. Double-blind developmental evaluation at 1-year corrected age of 597 premature infants with birth weights from 500 to 1350 grams enrolled in three placebo-controlled trials of prophylactic synthetic surfactant. J PEDIATR 1995;126:S5-12.
15. Bzoch KR, League R, eds. Assessing language skills in infancy: a handbook for the multidimensional analysis of emergent language. Baltimore: University Park Press, 1978.

16. Halliday HL, McClure G, Reid MM. Growth and development two years after artificial surfactant therapy at birth. Early Hum Dev 1986;13:323-7.
17. Vaucher YE, Merritt TA, Hallman M, et al. Neurodevelopmental and respiratory outcomes in early childhood after human surfactant treatment. Am J Dis Child 1988;142:927-30.
18. Dunn MS, Shennan ST, Hoskins EM, et al. Two-year follow-up of infants enrolled in a randomized trial of surfactant replacement therapy for prevention of respiratory distress syndrome. Pediatrics 1988;82:543-7.
19. Jain L, Vidyasagar D, Raju TNK. Developmental outcomes of infants from surfactant trials. Pediatr Res 1989;25:255A.
20. Msall ME, Rogers BT, Catanzaro N, et al. Five year developmental outcome of infants less than 28 weeks gestational age enrolled in a surfactant randomized clinical trial. Pediatr Res 1989;25:258A.
21. Morley CJ, Morley R. Follow-up of premature babies treated with artificial surfactant (ALEC). Arch Dis Child 1990;65:667-9.
22. Ware J, Taeusch HW, Soll RF, McCormick MC. Health and developmental outcomes of a surfactant controlled trial: follow-up at 2 years. Pediatrics 1990;85:1103-7.
23. Wagner C, Kramer B, Kendig J, et al. Neurodevelopmental and pulmonary outcome of 40 premature infants at 5-7 years: surfactant versus saline at birth. Pediatr Res 1992;31:263A.
24. Ferrara TB, Hoekstra RE, Couser RJ, et al. Effects of surfactant therapy on outcome of infants with birth weights of 600 to 750 grams. J PEDIATR 1991;119:455-7.
25. Collaborative European Multicentre Study Group. A 2-year follow up of babies enrolled in a European multicentre trial of porcine surfactant replacement for severe neonatal respiratory distress syndrome. Eur J Pediatr 1992;151:372-6.
26. Vaucher YE, Harker L, Merritt TA. Outcome at twelve months of adjusted age in very low birth weight infants with lung immaturity: a randomized, placebo-controlled trial of human surfactant. J PEDIATR 1993;122:126-32.
27. Hellstrom-Westas L, Bell AH, Skov L, et al. Cerebroelectrical depression following surfactant treatment in preterm neonates. Pediatrics 1992;89:643-7.

Double-blind 1-year follow-up of 1540 infants with respiratory distress syndrome randomized to rescue treatment with two doses of synthetic surfactant or air in four clinical trials

Sherry E. Courtney, MD, Walker Long, MD, Douglas McMillan, MD, Donnal Walter, MD, Theodore Thompson, MD, Reginald Sauve, MD, Brent Conway, Harry Bard, MD, and the American and Canadian Exosurf Neonatal Study Groups (see Appendixes I-IV)

From the Departments of Pediatrics, Children's Medical Center and Wright State University, Dayton, Ohio; University of North Carolina at Chapel Hill; Arkansas Children's Hospital, Little Rock; University of Minnesota, Minneapolis; Foothills Hospital and the University of Calgary, Alberta, Canada; the Clinical Research Division, Burroughs Wellcome Co., Research Triangle Park, North Carolina; and the Department of Pediatrics, St. Justine Hospital, University of Montreal, Quebec, Canada

Synthetic surfactant has been shown to reduce neonatal and 1-year mortality and neonatal morbidity in infants with respiratory distress syndrome. However, less is known about the effects of synthetic surfactant on developmental outcome and long-term morbidity. Four multicenter, randomized, placebo-controlled trials of synthetic surfactant administered as rescue therapy were conducted in the United States and Canada, with a total enrollment of 2224 patients. Double-blind developmental evaluations of survivors were conducted at 1 year of age (adjusted for prematurity) in all four trials. Of the 1802 patients enrolled in the placebo-controlled rescue trials who survived to 1 year, 1540 (85%) completed the 1-year follow-up evaluation. Height, weight, and head circumference measurements were not different in the treatment and control groups. Mean and median Bayley Scores of Infant Development for both the Mental Development Index and the Psychomotor Development Index were also equivalent. The incidence of impairments was not different in the two groups (mild to moderate impairment, 12% (92 of 745) for the air placebo group vs 11% (86 of 771) for the synthetic surfactant group; severe impairment, 15% (114 of 745) for the air placebo group vs 13% (102 of 771) for the synthetic surfactant group). No differences in rates of retinopathy of prematurity or hearing impairment were found in the treatment groups. The need for surgery after day 28 of life (relative risk, 0.779; 95% confidence interval, 0.665, 0.927) and the need for respiratory support at 1 year (relative risk, 0.525; 95% confidence intervals, 0.303, 0.911) were both reduced in the synthetic surfactant group. These results indicate that developmental outcome at 1 year of age is at least as good among infants with respiratory distress syndrome who received rescue therapy with synthetic surfactant as it is in infants who received air placebo; the results also indicate that the incidence of long-term morbidity is reduced. (J Pediatr 1995;126:S43-52)

Reprint requests: Walker Long, MD, Department of Pediatrics, CB No. 7220, University of North Carolina at Chapel Hill, Chapel Hill, NC 27599-7220.

0022-3476/95/$3.00 + 0 **9/0/61819**

Reductions in neonatal and 1-year mortality and neonatal morbidity have been documented when synthetic surfactant is administered as rescue therapy.[1, 2] However, less is known about the effects of synthetic surfactant preparations on developmental outcome and long-term morbidity. De-

BPD	Bronchopulmonary dysplasia
CLD	Chronic lung disease
CP	Cerebral palsy
MDI	Mental development index
PDI	Psychomotor development index
RDS	Respiratory distress syndrome
ROP	Retinopathy of prematurity

velopmental follow-up is particularly important to our understanding of how new therapeutic interventions affect long-term infant outcome. The purpose of this study was to assess whether administration of synthetic surfactant as a rescue therapy alters growth, development, or morbidity through 1-year adjusted age.

METHODS

Study design and patient enrollment. Four multicenter, prospective, double-blind, randomized, parallel, placebo-controlled studies of a synthetic surfactant (colfosceril palmitate, cetyl alcohol, and tyloxapol; Exosurf Neonatal, Burroughs Wellcome Co., Research Triangle Park, N.C.) administered as rescue therapy for established respiratory distress syndrome were conducted in the United States and Canada (Table I).[1-4] Participants are listed in Appendixes I-IV. In these trials, infants who required mechanical ventilation for RDS and had an arterial/alveolar oxygen tension ratio below 0.22 in the first 24 hours of life were assigned randomly to receive two 5 ml/kg endotracheal doses (given 12 hours apart) of synthetic surfactant or air placebo.

The trials were conducted with a common protocol and consisted of two evaluation periods: days 1 to 28 and day 29 through 1 year. The effect of this synthetic surfactant on acute morbidity and mortality of infants with RDS has been published previously.[1-4] The follow-up studies, which are presented individually in this supplement and are combined for this article, consisted of a double-blind safety evaluation conducted at 1 year adjusted age.[5-8] The protocols were approved by the Institutional Review Boards at each hospital, and informed consent was obtained from the parents of patients who entered the studies. Patient entry into the studies occurred between October 1987 and September 1990.

One-year follow-up evaluation. Infants were scheduled for evaluation within 6 weeks of 1 year of age, corrected for prematurity by subtracting the number of weeks the infant was premature from the chronologic age. Evaluators and parents were masked as to which infants had received synthetic surfactant or air placebo.

Health status. A complete physical examination was performed. Height, weight, and head circumference measurements were obtained and plotted in relation to adjusted age on physical growth charts compiled by the National Center for Health Statistics.[9] Pertinent information with regard to intervening medical complications, hospital admissions, surgical operations, use of medications for chronic lung and neurologic diseases, the highest required level of respiratory support, and allergies was documented on the day of the 1-year follow-up examination.

Neurodevelopmental outcome. A child developmental specialist at each institution used the Bayley Scales of Infant Development[10] to assess mental and motor development. Both the mental and psychomotor development indices have a mean of 100 and an SD of 16 in normal populations. A period of 6 weeks on either side of the 1-year date was targeted for performance of the examinations. Bayley Scales of Infant Development were not used to examine infants considered too delayed by the examiner to be tested. Because of the difficulty in accurately assigning scores below 50, all scores less than 50 were set at 49.[10]

Impairments. The degree of impairment was graded for all children as none, mild to moderate, or serious, similar to the method used by Kitchen et al.[11] Mild to moderate impairment was diagnosed if one of the following criteria was present: mild cerebral palsy, a Bayley Scales of Infant Development MDI score of 69 to 84 (between 1 and 2 SD below the mean), sensorineural hearing loss that did not require amplification, or significant visual defect but not blindness. Serious impairment was diagnosed if more than one of the aforementioned criteria were present, or if any of the following criteria were present: moderate or severe CP, a Bayley Scales of Infant Development MDI score of less than 69 (>2 SD below the mean), bilateral sensorineural hearing loss requiring amplification, bilateral deafness, or bilateral blindness.

For each child cerebral palsy was recorded as being absent, mild, or moderate to severe according to the definitions suggested by Nelson and Ellenberg.[12] Mild CP was considered to be present if the infant had a definite abnormality of neuromuscular physical findings (increased tone, increased deep tendon reflexes, and/or positive Babinski's sign) but had either no or minimal functional defect. Moderate to severe CP was considered to be present if significant interference with independent function existed in addition to a definite abnormality of neuromuscular findings.

Hearing evaluations were performed during the first year, although the methods of assessing hearing loss and the timing of evaluations varied among institutions. Hearing loss was considered to be present if any degree of loss was recorded; deafness was considered to be present if the hearing threshold was greater than or equal to 90 db. Infants were considered to have a significant visual defect if they required surgical intervention or their vision could not be corrected to normal. Infants were considered to be blind if

Table I. Patient accountability

Study No.	Birth weight (gm)	Sample size	Site	Reference No. Days 1-28	Reference No. 1 yr
05	700-1350	419	USA	1	5
06/09	≥1250	1237	USA (06) Canada (09)	2	6
07	500-749	224	Canada	3	7
08	750-1249	344	Canada	4	8

vision could not be corrected to better than legal blindness (≤20/200).

Ophthalmologic examinations. Ophthalmologic examinations were required in the three studies that enrolled infants with birth weights of 1250 gm or less.[1, 3, 4] Many infants had several ophthalmologic examinations during the first year, and data were collected for both the worst and last examination before the 1-year follow-up date. If only one examination was performed, it was recorded as both the worst and last examination.

For each eye, retinopathy of prematurity was evaluated and the requirements for surgery, cryotherapy, and laser therapy were recorded. Retinopathy of prematurity was classified according to the international classification of ROP.[13] Mild to moderate ROP was diagnosed if the disease did not exceed stage 3; stages 3+ and worse were considered to indicate severe ROP.

Data analyses and statistical methods. Frequency counts and percentages were used to summarize categorical data by treatment group. The mean, SD, median, minimum, and maximum were used to summarize numerical data by treatment group; mean differences were calculated. Relative risks and 95% confidence intervals were used to express incidence comparisons. Relative risks and confidence intervals for the ophthalmologic examinations, impairments, and medical history assessments were based on the Cochran-Mantel-Haenszel test. In the across-study analysis the Cochran-Mantel-Haenszel test controlled for the original protocol. In the analyses for the individual studies the Cochran-Mantel-Haenszel test controlled for the randomization strata (sex and birth weight classes). Confidence intervals for assessments are statistically significant when they exclude "1." The number of patients is not consistent across all tables because all patients were not assessed for every measurement.

RESULTS

Baseline characteristics and major neonatal complications of infants who completed 1-year follow-up were equivalent with one important exception: fewer infants treated with surfactant had bronchopulmonary dysplasia at day 28 ($p = 0.0385$) (Table II). Of the patients who were alive at 1 year, 86% of the air placebo group and 85% of the synthetic surfactant group completed follow-up (Table III). The number of surviving patients lost to follow-up or refusing follow-up was similar for each group

Table II. Baseline characteristics and major neonatal complications of infants who completed follow-up at 1-year adjusted age*

Characteristic	Air placebo (%) ($n = 758$)	Synthetic surfactant (%) ($n = 782$)
Birth weight (gm)†	1586 ± 614	1577 ± 616
Birth weight groups (gm)		
<750	49 (6)	50 (6)
750-1249	188 (25)	210 (27)
≥1250	521 (69)	522 (67)
Gestational age (wk)†	30.6 ± 3.2	30.6 ± 3.0
Multiple birth	170 (23)	185 (24)
Inborn	495 (65)	536 (69)
Race		
White	611 (81)	645 (83)
Black	56 (7)	44 (6)
Hispanic	32 (4)	39 (5)
Native American	16 (2)	17 (2)
Asian	20 (3)	17 (2)
Other	23 (3)	20 (3)
Maternal age (yr)†	26 ± 6	27 ± 6
Maternal education (yr)†	13 ± 3	13 ± 3
Sex		
Male	446 (59)	482 (62)
Female	311 (41)	300 (38)
Apgar score (median)		
1 min	5	5
5 min	7	7
IVH during days 1-28		
Grade I/II	184 (26)	171 (24)
Grade III/PVED	55 (8)	40 (6)
BPD at day 28	95 (13)	71 (9)‡

IVH, Intraventricular hemorrhage; *PVED*, periventricular echodensities.
*Infants are classified into groups according to the treatment received.
†Values are means ± SD.
‡$p = 0.0385$.

Table III. Survival and follow-up status*

	Air placebo ($n = 1108$)	Synthetic surfactant ($n = 1116$)
Alive at 1 year	882 (79)	920 (83)
Lost to follow-up	124 (11) [14]†	138 (12) [15]†
Completed follow-up	758 (68) [86]	782 (71) [85]

Numbers in parentheses represent the percentage of enrolled infants; numbers in brackets represent the percentage of survivors at 1 year adjusted age.
*Includes all patients as treated without exclusions, through 1-year adjusted age.
†Includes approximately 9% of patients whose survival status was determined by telephone.

Table IV. Growth at 1-year adjusted age

	Mean (SD)		Median	
	Air placebo	Synthetic surfactant	Air placebo	Synthetic surfactant
Height (cm)	74.2 (3.9)	74.2 (4.3)	74.3	74.2
(n)	(748)	(767)	(748)	(767)
Weight (kg)	9.2 (1.4)	9.3 (1.4)	9.2	9.3
(n)	(753)	(769)	(753)	(769)
Head circumference (cm)	46.1 (1.9)	46.2 (1.9)	46.0	46.0
(n)	(746)	(764)	(746)	(764)

(14% vs 15%), which included telephone contact to confirm survival status.

Growth status (Table IV; Figs. 1 to 3). Mean and median values for height, weight, and head circumference were nearly identical between the air placebo and synthetic surfactant groups. Numbers of infants at each major percentile grouping were also very similar.

Health evaluations (Table V). The numbers of patients readmitted to the hospital after 28 days of life in the air placebo and synthetic surfactant groups were not different. Physical evidence of lung disease, as defined by the presence of wheezing, tachypnea, or both, was likewise not different between groups at the 1-year examination. However, fewer infants treated with synthetic surfactant were receiving medication for chronic lung disease or continued respiratory support (O_2, continuous positive airway pressure, or ventilator) at 1 year.

Infants in the synthetic surfactant group were also less likely to have had surgery after day 28 and were less likely to be receiving medication for chronic neurologic disease at 1-year adjusted age. No differences in numbers of infants with allergies, asthma, or eczema were found between treatment groups.

Retinopathy of prematurity (Table VI). No differences were evident between treatment groups for ROP at both the worst examination and the last examination during the first year.

Bayley Scales of Infant Development scores (Table VII). Mean and median Bayley Scales of Infant Development scores both with and without exclusion of infants who had severe impairments were equivalent in the treatment groups. The proportions of infants with indices more than 2 SD below the mean were also not different between treatment groups.

Functional impairments (Table VIII). Equivalent numbers of infants in the treatment groups had functional impairments. The absolute numbers of survivors with mild to moderate functional impairments at 1-year follow-up were 92 of 745 (12%) in the air placebo group and 86 of 771 (11%) in the synthetic surfactant group. The numbers of survivors with serious functional impairments included 114 of 745 (15%) in the air placebo group and 102 of 771 (13%) in the synthetic surfactant group, using the definitions described in the Methods section. Seventy-two percent of control subjects and 76% of infants treated with synthetic surfactant had no impairment. Mental delays as diagnosed by the Bayley Scales of Infant Development MDI, the incidence of both mild and moderate to severe CP, and the incidence of hearing loss of any degree were not different between treatment groups. Likewise no differences existed between treatment groups for impairments resulting from visual defects or blindness. Data for eye examinations were not required for the larger infants in trial 06/09.[2] It is therefore possible that some cases of ROP or subtle visual defects may have been missed; it is unlikely that any cases of infants with blindness were missed.

Overall outcome (Figs. 4 and 5). Overall outcome at 1 year for patients enrolled in the rescue studies was certainly no worse in the synthetic surfactant group than in the air placebo group. Use of synthetic surfactant did not increase the number of impaired survivors.

DISCUSSION

Therapies that reduce mortality rates have the potential to increase the number of impaired survivors. The results from this study are encouraging for both parents and society because developmental outcome of infants treated with synthetic surfactant through 1 year of age is at least as good as that of untreated infants, and some measures of long-term morbidity are improved in the synthetic surfactant group.

Similar findings have been reported by others who performed studies with different surfactant preparations. Ware et al.[14] reported 1- and 2-year follow-up findings of 32 infants who had been enrolled in a randomized trial of bovine surfactant.[14] They found comparable frequencies of abnormal findings in both control and treatment groups, but the study had low statistical power because of the small sample size. The Collaborative European Multicentre Study Group[15] recently reported 1- and 2-year follow-up findings

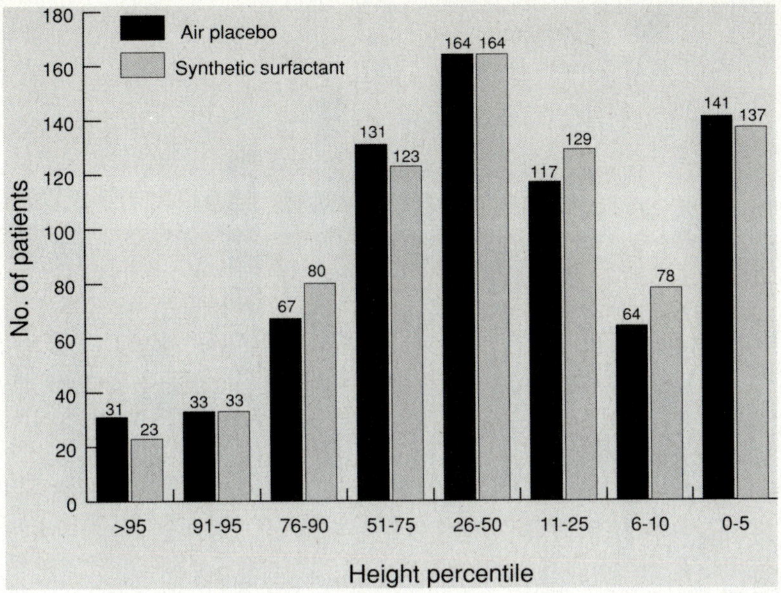

Fig. 1. Distribution of height percentiles by treatment group at 1-year adjusted age.

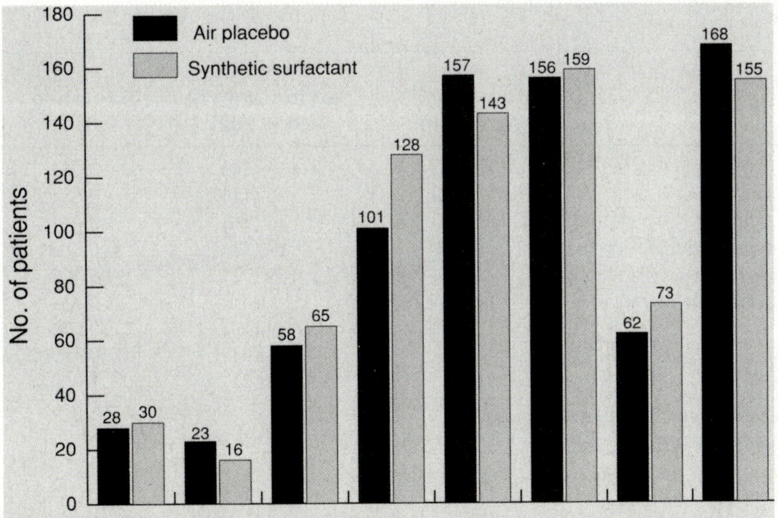

Fig. 2. Distribution of weight percentiles by treatment group at 1-year adjusted age.

of 146 infants with birth weights of 700 to 2000 gm who were randomized to receive porcine surfactant or no treatment. These infants had clinical and radiologic evidence of RDS, and all of the infants were receiving mechanical ventilation with a fractional concentration of oxygen in inspired gas of greater than or equal to 0.60 at study entry. Thus they were largely comparable with the infants described in this report, but were perhaps in slightly more distress (infants in this report had established RDS and an arterial/alveolar oxygen tension ratio of <0.22). The Collaborative Study Group found no differences between control and surfactant treatment groups in growth rates, incidence of CP, incidence of visual or hearing impairment, or overall disability rates at both the 1- and 2-year follow-up evaluations. Other follow-up studies that have compared control subjects and infants treated with surfactant have either combined prophylaxis and rescue groups[16, 17] or only reported results of prophylactic groups versus control groups.[18-22]

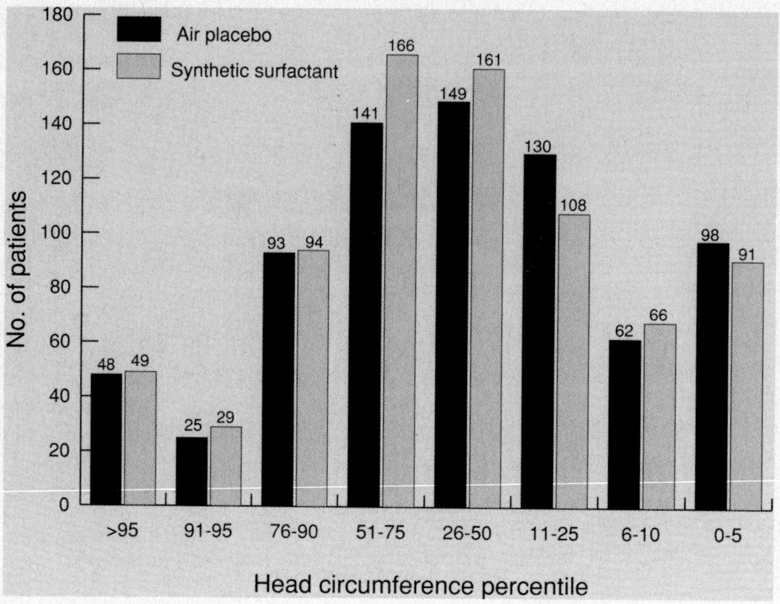

Fig. 3. Distribution of head circumference percentiles by treatment group at 1-year adjusted age.

Table V. Health status*

	Air placebo (%) (n = 758)	Synthetic surfactant (%) (n = 782)	Relative risk†	95% Confidence interval
Readmitted to hospital	140 (35)	139 (34)	0.956	0.791, 1.155
Physical evidence of CLD	90 (12)	82 (11)	0.881	0.666, 1.165
Medication for CLD	109 (14)	76 (10)	0.673	0.514, 0.882‡
Respiratory support on day of examination	33 (4)	18 (2)	0.525	0.303, 0.911‡
Surgery	208 (27)	168 (22)	0.779	0.655, 0.927‡
Medication for chronic neurologic disease	14 (2)	5 (1)	0.334	0.127, 0.883‡
Allergies	77 (10)	79 (10)	0.996	0.739, 1.341
Asthma	47 (6)	44 (6)	0.909	0.610, 1.355
Eczema	11 (1)	12 (2)	1.050	0.468, 2.357

*Includes data on health status between day 29 and 1-year adjusted age.
†Relative risk <1.000 indicates decreased risk of event with surfactant treatment.
‡Statistically significant.

One recent report of 145 infants treated with human surfactant compares those treated prophylactically with those given rescue therapy and suggests that infants treated prophylactically perform less well at the 1-year follow-up evaluation.[23] Thus it may be important to study separately the developmental outcomes of infants treated with surfactant prophylactically and those given rescue treatment. However, follow-up in large randomized trials of prophylaxis versus rescue use of surfactant, such as the OSIRIS trial,[24] will be needed to address this concern appropriately.

The type of surfactant as well as the treatment strategy used (prophylaxis versus rescue) might be important in developmental outcome. A variety of surfactants were used in follow-up studies reported to date, including bovine,[14, 17-20] porcine,[15] human,[16, 23] and synthetic preparations.[22] However, none of these studies demonstrated a statistically significant increase in the frequency of neurodevelopmental impairment in the infants who received surfactant. Nevertheless, it remains unclear whether different surfactants have different effects on developmental outcome, because in most previously published studies the numbers of infants enrolled have been relatively small.

Bayley Scales of Infant Development scores are indicative of current levels of functioning and have some predictive value for future function.[25] The lack of differences in mean and median scores for both the MDI and PDI between air placebo and synthetic surfactant groups in this trial is encouraging but not definitive. Follow-up beyond 1 year is

Table VI. Retinopathy of prematurity*

	Air placebo (%) n = 294	Synthetic surfactant (%) n = 345	Relative risk†	95% Confidence interval
Worst examination				
No ROP	143 (49)	180 (52)	1.076	0.924, 1.254
Mild/moderate ROP	116 (40)	135 (39)		
Severe ROP	35 (12)	30 (8)	0.726	0.460, 1.144
Treatment‡	19 (6)	10 (3)		
Surgery	11 (4)	3 (1)		
Cryotherapy	16 (5)	8 (2)		
Last examination				
No ROP	234 (80)	278 (81)	1.013	0.938, 1.095
Mild/moderate ROP	43 (15)	53 (15)		
Severe ROP	17 (6)	14 (4)	0.698	0.352, 1.382
Treatment‡	5 (2)	3 (1)		
Surgery	6 (2)	2 (1)		
Cryotherapy	4 (1)	1 (1)		

*Based on worst and last examination for all infants who received ophthalmologic examinations under study protocol. Mild/moderate ROP = grades 1-3; severe ROP = ≥ grade 3+.
†Relative risk <1.000 indicates decreased risk of event with surfactant treatment.
‡Patients may have received more than one treatment.

Table VII. Mental and psychomotor development as determined by Bayley Scales of Infant Development at 1-year adjusted age

	Air placebo			Synthetic surfactant			Relative risk* (95% Confidence interval)
	n (%)	Mean†	Median	n (%)	Mean†	Median	
Mental development index							
Analysis I‡	726	98 ± 22	102	761	99 ± 21	102	
Analysis II‡,§	683	100 ± 20	103	731	100 ± 19	103	
Index >2 SD‖	53 (7)			54 (7)			0.933 (0.649,1.341)
Psychomotor development index							
Analysis I‡	725	90 ± 20	92	757	92 ± 20	92	
Analysis II‡,§	683	92 ± 19	92	726	93 ± 18	93	
Index >2 SD‖	74 (10)			71 (9)			0.898 (0.662,1.219)

*Relative risk <1.000 indicates decreased risk of event with synthetic surfactant.
†±SD.
‡Index values <50 were set to 49.
§Patients with bilateral blindness or deafness or moderate to severe cerebral palsy were excluded.
‖Bayley Scales of Infant Development scores <69.

necessary. For the three Canadian trials, evaluation at 2 years corrected age is complete and results are being analyzed, and evaluation at 3 years is ongoing. A full picture of the impact of synthetic surfactant on morbidity and mortality will not be complete until these data are available. Nonetheless, it is encouraging that no extra numbers of survivors with CP, vision loss, hearing loss, and overall incidence of functional impairment at 1-year corrected age were found in the synthetic surfactant group.

Although the number of infants who required surgery in the first year was significantly decreased in the synthetic surfactant group, the type of surgery performed was not recorded. Determining the impact of surfactant therapy on the subsequent need for surgery is an area that future follow-up studies may wish to address.

The number of infants in the synthetic surfactant group who were receiving respiratory support at 1 year was also significantly reduced, as were the numbers of infants receiving medications for CLD and for chronic neurologic disease. These markers of long-term morbidity were not significantly different in the individual studies,[6-9] but combining the 1-year follow-up results for the four rescue trials provides more power to detect real differences. The observed reductions in long-term respiratory morbidity in this trial

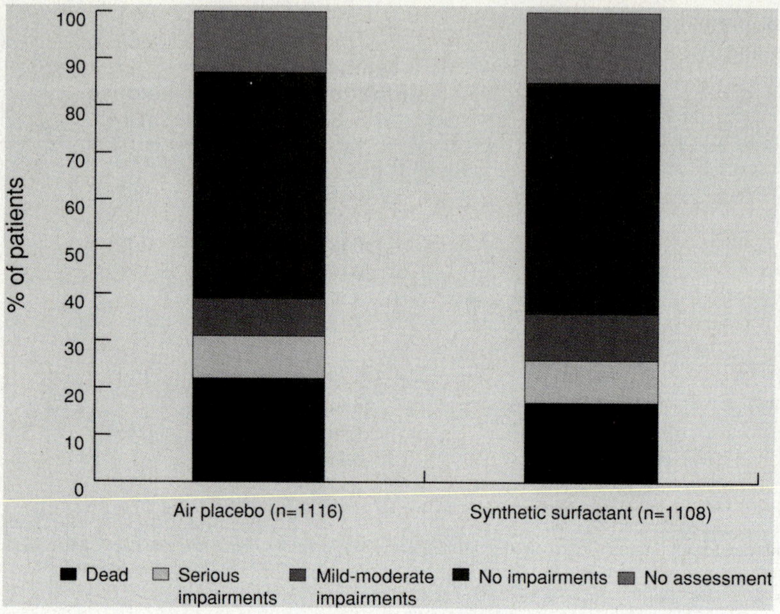

Fig. 4. Overall outcome at 1-year adjusted age.

Table VIII. Impairments for infants who completed follow-up evaluation at 1-year adjusted age

	Air placebo (%) *n* = 745	Synthetic surfactant (%) *n* = 771	Relative risk*	95% Confidence interval
No impairment	539 (72)	583 (76)		
Impairment present	206 (27)	188 (24)	0.879	0.744, 1.034
Mild/moderate	92 (12)	86 (11)		
Serious	114 (15)	102 (13)	0.854	0.670, 1.088
Type of impairment†,‡				
MDI 69-84	86 (11)	76 (10)	0.847	0.633, 1.132
MDI <69	82 (11)	78 (10)	0.914	0.685, 1.221
Mild CP	30 (4)	24 (3)	0.761	0.450, 1.286
Moderate/severe CP	42 (6)	30 (4)	0.690	0.439, 1.085
Hearing loss	3 (<1)	3 (<1)	0.960	0.200, 4.609
Deafness	5 (1)	2 (<1)	0.397	0.082, 1.925
Visual defect	40 (5)	32 (4)	0.761	0.488, 1.187
Blindness	8 (1)	11 (1)	1.281	0.532, 3.087

*Relative risk <1.000 indicates decreased risk of event with surfactant treatment.
†Infants may have more than one impairment.
‡Bayley Scales of Infant Development MDI scores <50 set to 49.

are consistent with both the reduction in the incidence of BPD at day 28 observed in this study in the infants completing follow-up who received synthetic surfactant and with findings of two recent meta-analyses demonstrating that rescue use of synthetic surfactant reduces the incidence of BPD.[26, 27] Furthermore, the reduction in the use of medications for chronic neurologic disease (i.e., seizure medication) in the synthetic surfactant group is consistent with the results of the meta-analyses by Jobe,[26] which showed a reduction in the incidence of brain hemorrhage with rescue use of synthetic surfactant.

The graphic portrayals of overall outcome at 1 year for all infants enrolled in the rescue studies (Fig. 4) and among all three birth weight groups separately (Fig. 5) must be interpreted cautiously. Nevertheless, these figures demonstrate that overall outcome was certainly no worse and, if anything, slightly better in the synthetic surfactant group. For the specific results of each trial, please refer to the individual studies reported in this supplement.

In conclusion, synthetic surfactant administered as rescue therapy does not result in an increased number of impaired survivors at 1-year adjusted age. Growth, scores on

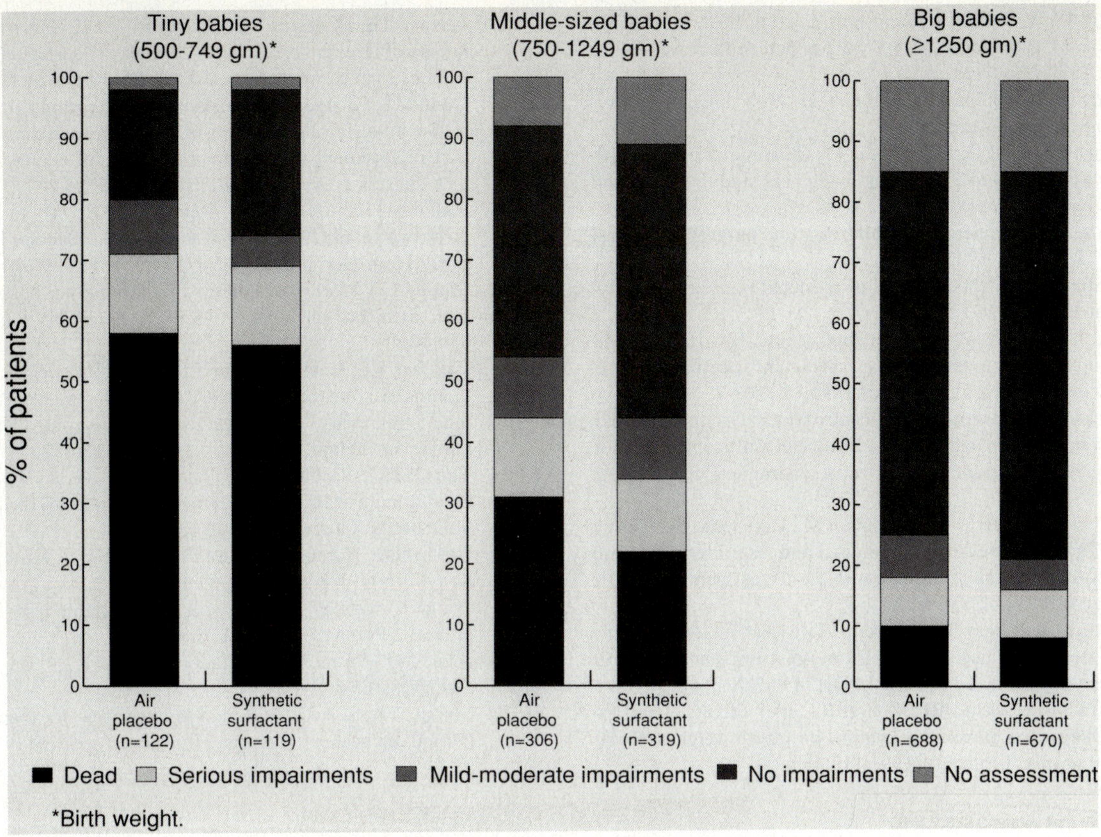

Fig. 5. Outcome at 1-year adjusted age by birth weight.

the Bayley Scales of Infant Development, vision, hearing, and degree of functional impairment were also no worse among the infants who received synthetic surfactant. Infants who received synthetic surfactant were significantly less likely to require oxygen therapy, continuous positive airway pressure, or ventilator support at 1 year of age and were significantly less likely to require medication for CLD or neurologic disease. Morbidity from RDS thus was decreased through at least 1-year adjusted age in the infants who received rescue therapy with synthetic surfactant, with no adverse effects on developmental outcome.

REFERENCES

1. Long W, Thompson T, Sundell H, et al. Effects of two rescue doses of a synthetic surfactant on mortality rate and survival without bronchopulmonary dysplasia in 700-1350 gram infants with respiratory distress syndrome. J PEDIATR 1991; 118:595-605.
2. Long W, Corbet A, Cotton R, et al. A controlled trial of synthetic surfactant in infants weighing 1250 g or more with respiratory distress syndrome. N Engl J Med 1991;325:1696-703.
3. Smyth J, Allen A, MacMurray B, et al. Double-blind, randomized, placebo-controlled Canadian multicenter trial of two doses of synthetic surfactant or air placebo in 224 infants weighing 500 to 749 grams with respiratory distress syndrome. J PEDIATR 1995;126:S81-9.
4. McMillan D, Chernick V, Finer N, et al. Effects of two rescue doses of synthetic surfactant in 344 infants with respiratory distress syndrome weighing 750 to 1249 grams: a double-blind, placebo-controlled multicenter Canadian trial. J PEDIATR 1995;126:S90-8.
5. Gong A, Anday E, Boros S, et al. One-year follow-up evaluation of 260 premature infants with respiratory distress syndrome and birth weights of 700 to 1350 grams randomized to two rescue doses of synthetic surfactant or air placebo. J PEDIATR 1995;126:S68-74.
6. Sauve R, Long W, Vincer M, et al. Outcome at 1-year adjusted age of 957 infants weighing more than 1250 grams with respiratory distress syndrome randomized to receive synthetic surfactant or air placebo. J PEDIATR 1995;126:S75-80.
7. Casiro O, Bingham W, MacMurray B, et al. One-year follow-up of 89 infants with birth weights of 500 to 749 grams and respiratory distress syndrome randomized to two rescue doses of synthetic surfactant or air placebo. J PEDIATR 1995;126:S53-60.
8. Saigal S, Robertson C, Sankaran K, et al. One-year outcome in 232 premature infants with birth weights of 750 to 1249 grams and respiratory distress syndrome randomized to rescue treatment with two doses of synthetic surfactant or air placebo. J PEDIATR 1995;126:S61-7.

9. Hamill PVV, Drizd TA, Johnson CL, et al. Physical growth: National Center for Health Statistics percentiles. Am J Clin Nutr 1979;30:607-29.
10. Bayley Scales of Infant Development. New York: The Psychological Corporation, 1969.
11. Kitchen W, Ford G, Orgill A, et al. Outcome in infants with birth weight 500 to 999 grams: a regional study of 1979 and 1980 births. J PEDIATR 1984;104:921-7.
12. Nelson KB, Ellenberg JH. Children who "outgrew" cerebral palsy. Pediatrics 1982;69:529-36.
13. An international classification of retinopathy of prematurity. Pediatrics 1984;74:127-33.
14. Ware J, Taeusch W, Soll RF, McCormick MC. Health and developmental outcomes of a surfactant controlled trial: follow-up at 2 years. Pediatrics 1990;85:1103-7.
15. Collaborative European Multicentre Study Group. A 2-year follow up of babies enrolled in a European multicentre trial for severe neonatal respiratory distress syndrome. Eur J Pediatr 1992;151:372-6.
16. Vaucher YE, Merritt TA, Hallman M, Jarvenpaa AL, Telsey AM, Jones BL. Neurodevelopmental and respiratory outcome in early childhood after human surfactant treatment. Am J Dis Child 1988;142:927-30.
17. Survanta Multidose Study Group. Two-year follow-up of infants treated for neonatal respiratory distress syndrome with bovine surfactant. J PEDIATR 1994;124:962-7.
18. Ferrara TB, Hoekstra RE, Couser RJ, et al. Effects of surfactant therapy on outcome of infants with birth weights of 600 to 750 grams. J PEDIATR 1991;119:455-7.
19. Ferrara TB, Hoekstra RE, Couser RJ, et al. Survival and follow-up of infants born at 23 to 26 weeks of gestational age: effects of surfactant therapy. J PEDIATR 1994;124:119-24.
20. Dunn MS, Shennan AT, Hoskins EM, Enhorning G. Two-year follow-up of infants enrolled in a randomized trial of surfactant replacement therapy for prevention of neonatal respiratory distress syndrome. Pediatrics 1988;82:543-7.
21. Halliday HL, McClure G, Reid MM. Growth and development two years after artificial surfactant replacement at birth. Early Hum Dev 1986;13:323-7.
22. Morley CJ, Morley R. Follow-up of premature babies treated with artificial surfactant (ALEC). Arch Dis Child 1990; 65:667-9.
23. Vaucher YE, Harker L, Merritt TA, et al. Outcome at twelve months of adjusted age in very low birth weight infants with lung immaturity: a randomized, placebo-controlled trial of human surfactant. J PEDIATR 1993;122:126-32.
24. The OSIRIS Collaborative Group. Early versus delayed neonatal administration of a synthetic surfactant—the judgment of OSIRIS. Lancet 1992;340:1363-9.
25. Teplin SW, Burchinal M, Johnson-Martin N, Humphry RA, Kraybill EN. Neurodevelopmental, health, and growth status at age 6 years of children with birth weights less than 1001 grams. J PEDIATR 1991;118:768-77.
26. Jobe AH. Pulmonary surfactant therapy. N Engl J Med 1993;328:861-8.
27. Merritt TA, Soll RF, Hallman M. Overview of exogenous surfactant replacement therapy. J Intensive Care Med 1993;8:205-28.

One-year follow-up of 89 infants with birth weights of 500 to 749 grams and respiratory distress syndrome randomized to two rescue doses of synthetic surfactant or air placebo

Oscar Casiro, MD, William Bingham, MD, Brock MacMurray, MD, Michael Whitfield, MD, Saroj Saigal, MD, Michael Vincer, MD, Walker Long, MD, the Canadian Exosurf Neonatal Study Group, and the Canadian Exosurf Neonatal Follow-Up Group (see Appendixes III and IV)

From the Departments of Pediatrics, Children's Hospital, University of Manitoba, Winnipeg, Canada; University of Saskatchewan, Saskatoon, Canada; University of Ottawa, Ontario, Canada; British Columbia Children's Hospital, Vancouver, Canada; McMaster University, Hamilton, Ontario, Canada; University of Dalhousie, Halifax, Nova Scotia, Canada; the University of North Carolina at Chapel Hill; and participating centers

Double-blind neurodevelopmental and physical evaluations were conducted at 1-year adjusted age in 89 infants with birth weights of 500 to 749 gm who had respiratory distress syndrome in the neonatal period and were randomized to receive two rescue doses of a synthetic surfactant (Exosurf Neonatal, Burroughs Wellcome Co., Research Triangle Park, N.C.) or air placebo. The trial used a common protocol and was conducted at 13 hospitals; patients were entered in the trial between February 1988 and September 1990. Ninety-five percent of surviving infants were assessed. Growth and development in the two groups were equivalent. Mean Bayley Scales of Infant Development scores were comparable (mental development index, 79 ± 22 vs 87 ± 20; psychomotor development index, 73 ± 18 vs 81 ± 19 for air placebo and synthetic surfactant, respectively). The incidence of severe retinopathy of prematurity was significantly decreased in the surfactant group compared with the air placebo group (15% vs 34%; relative risk 0.428; 95% confidence interval 0.2 to 0.9). Overall, administration of surfactant appeared to increase the probability of a favorable outcome. Confirmation of the trends observed in this study would provide a strong rationale for the rescue use of synthetic surfactant in extremely low birth weight infants with respiratory distress syndrome even if overall mortality is not reduced. (J Pediatr 1995;126:S53-60)

Results from large, randomized, clinical trials indicate that both prophylactic and therapeutic (rescue) administration of pulmonary surfactant improves survival rates and reduces perinatal morbidity in low birth weight infants.[1-6]

Reprint requests: Oscar Casiro, MD, Children's Hospital, 840 Sherbrook St., CK261, Winnipeg, Manitoba, Canada R3A 1S1.

0022-3476/95/$3.00 + 0 **9/0/61827**

Follow-up studies suggest that the improved survival rate of patients treated with surfactant is not associated with impaired neurologic function or an increase in disability rates.[7-13] In extremely low birth weight infants who received exogenous surfactant, a significant reduction in overall mortality was reported in a retrospective study[14] and, more convincingly, a reduction in mortality from respiratory distress[15] was reported in a prospective study. In treating these tiny infants, there is a potential risk of achieving a reduc-

Table I. Patient accountability*

	Air placebo (n = 111)	Synthetic surfactant (n = 113)
Alive at 1-year adjusted age	44 (40) [100]	49 (43) [100]
Lost to follow-up†	2 (2) [5]	2 (1) [2]
Completed follow-up	42 (38) [95]	47 (42) [96]

Numbers in parentheses represent the percentage of enrolled infants; numbers in brackets represent the percentage of survivors at 1-year adjusted age.
*Includes all patients as treated without exclusion.
†No patients were contacted by telephone to assess survival.

a/APo$_2$	Arterial/alveolar oxygen tension ratio
CI	Confidence interval
CP	Cerebral palsy
FiO$_2$	Fractional concentration of oxygen in inspired gas
RDS	Respiratory distress syndrome
ROP	Retinopathy of prematurity
RR	Relative risk

tion in mortality at the expense of an increased rate of disability.

The long-term safety of surfactant replacement in extremely low birth weight infants cannot be inferred from follow-up studies of larger premature infants. As part of the Canadian Exosurf Multicentre Trials, we conducted a follow-up evaluation of a large group of infants with respiratory distress syndrome and with a birth weight of 500 to 749 gm who received two rescue doses of either synthetic surfactant or air placebo. The major conclusion from the neonatal period was that administration of two rescue doses of synthetic surfactant was associated with decreased FiO$_2$ requirements, increased a/APo$_2$ ratio, and decreased a/APo$_2$ gradient from time of administration through day 7 compared with the control group. Mortality, incidence of pulmonary air leaks, bronchopulmonary dysplasia, necrotizing enterocolitis, incidence or severity of intraventricular hemorrhage, or other clinically important adverse consequences associated with prematurity and its treatment were unaltered.[16] The present follow-up study was designed to determine whether two rescue doses of synthetic surfactant in this birth weight group alters late morbidity or developmental outcome at 12-months corrected age.

METHODS

Study design. The trial was designed as a multicenter, prospective, double-blind, randomized, parallel comparison of the effects of two 5 ml/kg endotracheal doses (each 5 ml/kg dose given 12 hours apart) of either synthetic surfactant (colfosceril palmitate, cetyl alcohol, and tyloxapol, Exosurf Neonatal, Burroughs Wellcome Co., Research Triangle Park, N.C.) or air placebo. The trial involved a common protocol and was conducted at 13 hospitals in Canada; participating principal investigators are listed in Appendix III. The protocol was approved by the Institutional Review Board at each hospital, and parents gave informed consent. Patients were enrolled in the trial from February 1988 through September 1990. The follow-up component of the study consisted of a double-blind ophthalmologic examination and a double-blind follow-up evaluation conducted at 1-year adjusted age; participating developmentalists are listed in Appendix IV.

Table II. Baseline characteristics and major neonatal complications of infants who completed follow-up at 1-year adjusted age*

Characteristic	Air placebo (%) (n = 42)	Synthetic surfactant (%) (n = 47)
Birth weight (gm)	661 ± 52	652 ± 64
Gestational age (wk)†	24.8 ± 1.1	25.8 ± 1.6
Inborn	35 (83)	45 (96)
Outborn	7 (17)	2 (4)
Multiple birth	6 (14)	10 (21)
Race		
White	34 (81)	41 (87)
Black	3 (7)	0 (0)
Hispanic	1 (2)	0 (0)
Canadian Native Indian or Aboriginal	1 (2)	0 (0)
Asian	2 (5)	4 (9)
Other	1 (2)	2 (4)
Maternal age (yr)†	29 ± 6	29 ± 6
Maternal education (yr)‡	12 ± 2	13 ± 3
Sex		
Male	17 (40)	19 (40)
Female	25 (60)	28 (60)
Apgar score (median)		
1 min	3	3
5 min	7	7
IVH during days 1-28§		
Grade I/II	11 (26)	13 (28)
Grade III/PVED	6 (14)	3 (6)
No IVH	24 (57)	30 (64)
BPD at day 28	25 (60)	19 (40)

IVH, Intraventricular hemorrhage; *PVED*, periventricular echodensities; *BPD*, bronchopulmonary dysplasia.
*Infants are classified according to the treatment received.
†Mean ± SD.
‡For maternal education: n = 28, air-placebo group; n = 30, synthetic surfactant group.
§For IVH: n = 41, air-placebo group; n = 46, synthetic surfactant group.

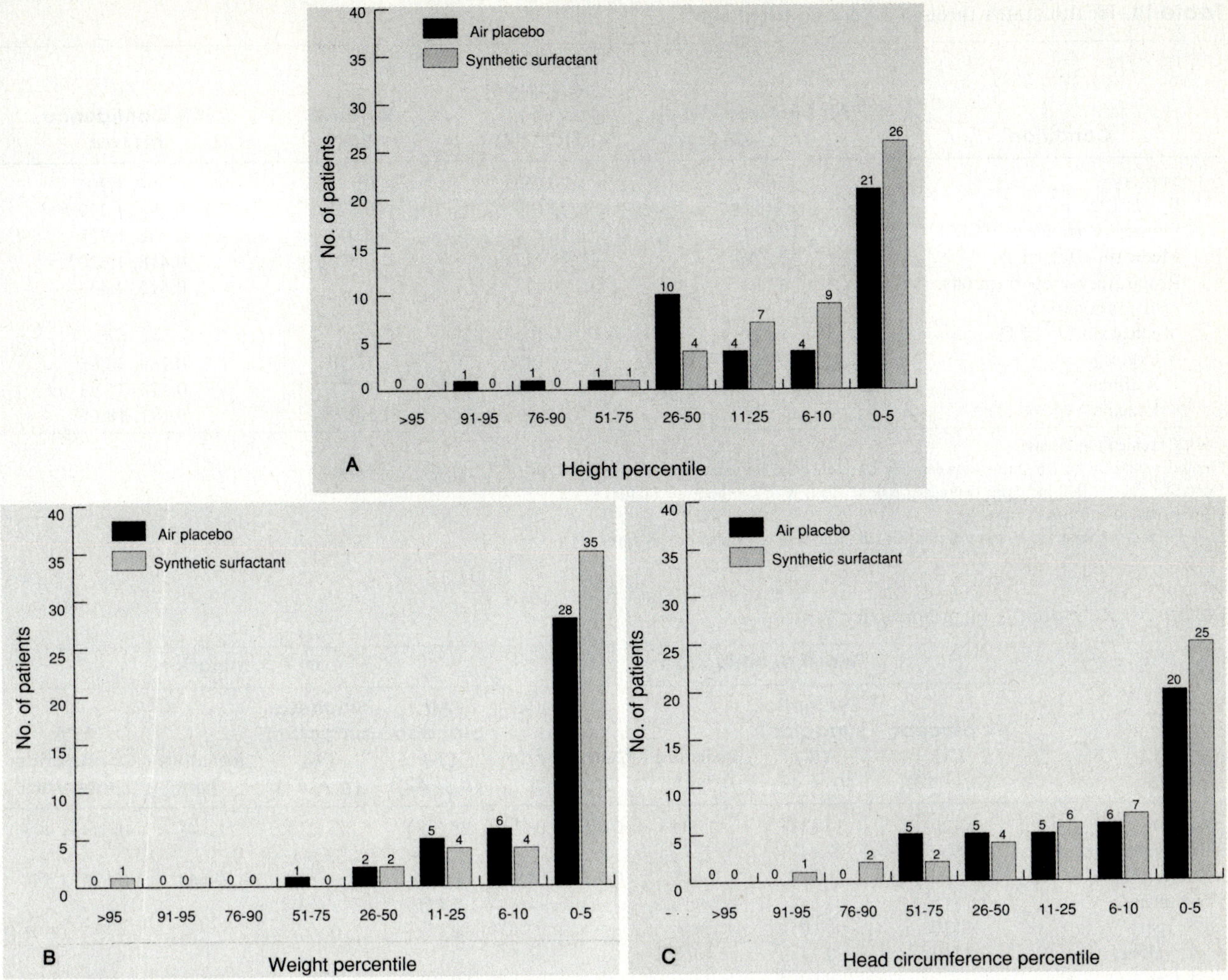

Fig. 1. Distribution of percentiles of physical growth measurements at 1-year adjusted age in infants who received air placebo or synthetic surfactant at birth. **A,** Height percentiles; **B,** weight percentiles; **C,** head circumference percentiles. (Percentile rankings are based on growth charts from the National Center for Health Statistics.)

Patient recruitment and enrollment. Premature infants who weighed 500 to 749 gm at birth and in whom RDS developed within the first 24 hours, who were receiving mechanical ventilation, and who had an a/APo_2 ratio below 0.22 were eligible to enter the study. Exclusion criteria for this study were the same as those used in an earlier trial of synthetic surfactant.[3] Infants whose parents gave consent were stratified by gender and birth weight (500 to 625 gm; 626 to 749 gm) into four strata and randomized to either two doses of synthetic surfactant or air placebo administered 12 hours apart. The details of data collection, ophthalmologic examination, 1-year follow-up, health status evaluation, and data analyses are described elsewhere in this supplement.[17]

RESULTS

This report describes results from data collected from day 29 through 1-year adjusted age. During the enrollment period, 224 patients entered the trial. A total of 111 patients in the air placebo group and 113 patients in the surfactant group were treated (Table I). At 1-year adjusted age, a total of 89 survivors, 42 (95%) in the placebo group and 47 (96%) in the surfactant group, were assessed. Two patients who received the air placebo and two patients treated with surfactant were lost to follow-up.

Baseline comparability (Table II). The baseline characteristics of infants in both treatment groups who completed the 1-year follow-up were similar.

Growth (Fig. 1). Summary statistics for mean height (air

Table III. Health status through 1-year adjusted age*

Condition	Air placebo (%) (*n* = 42)	Synthetic surfactant (%) (*n* = 47)	Relative risk†	95% Confidence interval
Surgery	23 (55)	20 (43)	0.748	0.464, 1.206
Readmitted to hospital	24 (57)	23 (49)	0.871	0.593, 1.279
Physical evidence of CLD	10 (24)	10 (21)	0.912	0.432, 1.929
Medication for CLD	12 (29)	11 (23)	0.823	0.418, 1.620
Respiratory support on day of examination	4 (10)	6 (13)	1.356	0.415, 4.433
Medication for CLD	1 (2)	0 (0)	—‡	—, —‡
Allergies§	2 (5)	4 (9)	1.830	0.369, 9.085
Asthma	1 (2)	2 (4)	1.773	0.175, 17.93
Eczema	1 (2)	2 (4)	1.889	0.191, 18.65

CLD, Chronic lung disease.
*Includes data on health status between day 29 and 1-year adjusted age.
†Relative risk <1.000 indicates decreased risk of event with synthetic surfactant.
‡Counts too low for valid estimate.
§No patient was reported to have dermatitis, rhinitis, milk allergies, or hay fever.

Table IV. Retinopathy of prematurity*

	Worst examination				Last examination			
	Air placebo (%) (*n* = 42)	Synthetic surfactant (%) (*n* = 47)	Relative risk†	95% Confidence interval	Air placebo (%) (*n* = 42)	Synthetic surfactant (%) (*n* = 47)	Relative risk†	95% Confidence interval
No ROP	8 (20)	18 (38)	2.006	0.994, 4.052	28 (68)	37 (79)	1.148	0.893, 1.476
Mild/moderate ROP	20 (48)	22 (47)			8 (19)	7 (15)		
Severe ROP	14 (33)	7 (15)	0.428	0.200, 0.918	6 (14)	3 (6)	0.448	0.128, 1.564
Treatment‡	6 (15)	2 (4)			2 (5)	1 (2)		
Surgery	4 (10)	0 (0)			2 (5)	0 (0)		
Cryotherapy	5 (12)	2 (4)			2 (5)	1 (2)		
Laser	1 (2)	0 (0)			0 (0)	0 (0)		

*Based on worst and last examinations for all infants who received ophthalmologic examinations under study protocol. Mild/moderate ROP = grade 1-3; severe ROP = grades >3+.
†Relative risk <1.000 indicates decreased risk of event with synthetic surfactant.
‡Patients may have received more than one treatment.

placebo group, 70.9 cm; surfactant group, 69.6 cm), weight (air placebo group, 7.69 kg; surfactant group, 7.50 kg), and head circumference (air placebo group, 43.9 cm; surfactant group, 43.7 cm) at the 1-year adjusted age follow-up examination were similar for patients in the air placebo and surfactant groups. When plotted on the National Center for Health Statistics growth charts, the means of these three growth measures were below the 10th percentile for adjusted age. A large proportion of these extremely premature infants remained smaller than the norm, and very few had attained average size by 1-year adjusted age. Height, weight, and head circumference measurements were below the 5th percentile for adjusted age for 47%, 63%, and 45% of the infants, respectively. Conversely, height, weight, and head circumference measurements were above the 25th percentile for adjusted age for only 18%, 6%, and 19% of the infants, respectively.

Health status (Table III). The differences in proportions of patients in the air placebo and surfactant groups who had required surgery (air placebo group, 23 of 42 [55%]; surfactant group, 20 of 47 [43%]) or were readmitted to the hospital after day 28 (air placebo group, 24 of 42 [57%]; surfactant group, 23 of 47 [49%]) were not statistically significant. On the day of the follow-up examination, the proportions of patients who had physical evidence of chronic lung disease, were receiving medication for lung disease or neurologic disease, or required respiratory support also were not significantly different in the two treatment groups. Four patients in the air placebo group and six patients in the surfactant group required supplemental oxygen. Oxygen was

Table V. Mental and psychomotor development as determined by Bayley Scales of Infant Development at 1-year adjusted age

	Mental development index				Psychomotor development index			
	Air placebo (%) (*n* = 39)	Synthetic surfactant (%) (*n* = 45)	Relative risk*	95% Confidence interval	Air placebo (%) (*n* = 38)	Synthetic surfactant (%) (*n* = 45)	Relative risk*	95% Confidence interval
Development index†,‡								
Group I‡	79 ± 22	87 ± 20			73 ± 18	81 ± 19		
Group II§	84 ± 21	89 ± 19			78 ± 16	83 ± 17		
Index <2 SD‖	7 (22)	9 (21)	0.978	0.403, 1.577	9 (29)	8 (19)	0.679	0.293, 2.372

*Relative risk <1.000 indicates decreased risk of event with synthetic surfactant.
†Mean ± SD.
‡Index values <50 set to 49.
§Patients with bilateral blindness or deafness, moderate or severe CP were excluded from analysis. Air placebo, *n* = 32; synthetic surfactant, *n* = 42.
‖Bayley Scales of Infant Development scores <69.

delivered by nasal cannula in all but two patients: one patient in the air placebo group had a tracheostomy tube in place and the other patient, who was in the synthetic surfactant group, was receiving oxygen by hood. None of the infants remained on a ventilator. The incidence of allergies (with asthma and eczema being the only allergies reported) among patients in the surfactant group (4 of 47 [9%]) and air placebo group (2 of 42 [5%]) was not significantly different.

Ophthalmologic examination (Table IV). The incidence of retinopathy of prematurity at worst examination for infants who received an ophthalmologic examination during the first year was 33 of 42 (79%) in the placebo group and 29 of 47 (62%) in the synthetic surfactant group. A significant reduction in the incidence of severe ROP according to the worst ophthalmologic examination was observed in the synthetic surfactant group (7 of 47 [15%]) compared with the air placebo group (14 of 42 [33%]; relative risk 0.428; 95% confidence interval 0.200, 0.918). Six patients in the air placebo group and two patients in the synthetic surfactant group had received treatment (surgery, laser, or cryotherapy) by the time of the worst examination.

At the time of the last ophthalmologic evaluation, the incidence of severe ROP was 6 of 42 (14%) in the air placebo group and 3 of 47 (6%) in the synthetic surfactant group (RR 0.448; 95% CI 0.128, 1.564). Retinopathy of prematurity was not detected at the last ophthalmologic examination in 28 of 42 (67%) of patients who received air placebo and 37 of 47 (79%) of patients treated with synthetic surfactant. At the last ophthalmologic examination, two patients in the air placebo group and one patient in the synthetic surfactant group were reported to have been treated with surgery or cryotherapy.

Developmental outcome (Table V). Mental development index and psychomotor index scores on the Bayley Scales of Infant Development were not significantly different in the two groups. Equivalent numbers of infants had PDI scores (9 [29%] of infants given air placebo and 8 [19%] of infants treated with synthetic surfactant) and MDI scores (7 [22%] of infants given air placebo and 9 [21%] of infants treated with synthetic surfactant) that were greater than 2 SD below the mean.

Types and severity of impairments (Table VI). Forty-five percent of infants treated with synthetic surfactant had impairments versus 62% of those receiving air placebo (RR 0.71; 95% CI 0.48, 1.04). There were no differences in the incidence of serious impairments (17 of 42 [40%] in the air placebo group vs 15 of 47 [32%] in the synthetic surfactant group) or mild impairments (9 of 42 [21%] in the air placebo group vs 6 of 47 [13%] in the synthetic surfactant group). The overall outcome at 1-year adjusted age is depicted in Fig. 2.

No significant differences in the various types of impairments were observed. Seven infants were diagnosed as having mild cerebral palsy, three (7%) in the air placebo group and four (9%) in the synthetic surfactant group. Ten infants had moderate to severe CP, six (4%) treated with air placebo and four (9%) treated with surfactant. None of the air placebo or synthetic surfactant recipients had bilateral sensorineural deafness that either required or did not require amplification. Of the four patients with bilateral blindness, three (7%) were in the air placebo group and one (2%) was in the synthetic surfactant group. Of 18 patients with less severe visual defects, 11 (26%) were in the air placebo group and seven (15%) were in the synthetic surfactant group. These differences were not statistically significant.

DISCUSSION

The present multicenter study was designed to evaluate outcome at 1-year adjusted age after two rescue doses of

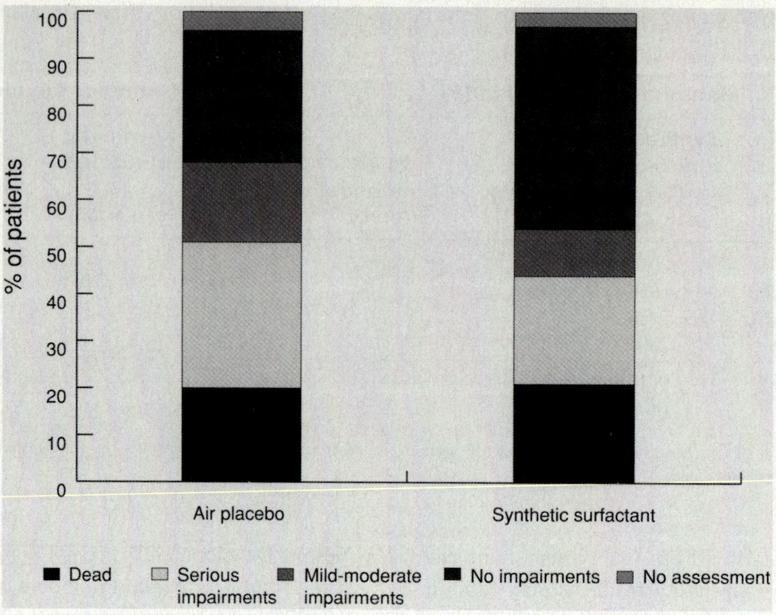

Fig. 2. Overall outcome at 1-year adjusted age for infants who were treated with air placebo or synthetic surfactant at birth.

Table VI. Impairments for infants who completed follow-up evaluation at 1-year adjusted age

	Air placebo (%) (*n* = 42)	Synthetic surfactant (%) (*n* = 47)	Relative risk*	95% Confidence interval
Impairment present	26 (62)	21 (45)	0.710	0.484, 1.041
No impairment	16 (38)	26 (55)		
Severity of impairment				
Mild/moderate	9 (21)	6 (13)		
Serious	17 (41)	15 (32)	0.777	0.442, 1.364
Type of impairment†,‡				
MDI <69	13 (31)	11 (23)	0.750	0.370, 1.517
MDI 69-84	8 (19)	6 (13)	0.647	0.249, 1.681
Moderate/severe CP	6 (14)	4 (9)	0.584	0.170, 2.008
Mild CP	3 (7)	4 (9)	1.206	0.286, 5.086
Bilateral sensorineural deafness	0 (0)	0 (0)	—	—, —§
Deafness not requiring amplification	0 (0)	0 (0)	—	—, —§
Bilateral blindness	3 (7)	1 (2)	0.285	0.037, 2.210
Visual defect	11 (26)	7 (15)	0.571	0.245, 1.331

MDI, Mental development index.
*Relative risk <1.000 indicates decreased risk of event with synthetic surfactant.
†Patients may have more than one impairment.
‡Bayley Scales of Infant Development MDI scores <50 set to 49.
§Counts too low for valid estimate.

synthetic surfactant or air placebo in neonates with RDS whose birth weights were greater than or equal to 500 gm and less than 750 gm. Ninety-five percent of surviving infants in the air placebo group and 96% in the synthetic surfactant group completed the 1-year evaluation. The risk of disability or other adverse outcomes between 29 days postnatal and 12-months adjusted age was not altered by the administration of synthetic surfactant.

Infants with birth weights greater than or equal to 500 gm and less than 750 gm face many risks that inherently accompany prematurity and lung disease. In addition, iatrogenic risks can result from the treatment these infants receive in the neonatal intensive care unit. Therapeutic measures such as surfactant, which reduce mortality, have the potential to increase the number of infants surviving with long-term disabilities. Of concern is a recent report of a transient fall in mean arterial blood pressure followed by acute cerebral dysfunction in neonates receiving exogenous surfactant for the treatment of RDS.[18] A short but significant decrease in cerebral activity was seen in 21 of 23 infants immediately after the instillation of porcine surfactant, in spite of improved pulmonary function. The long-term neurologic effects of this event, if any, are unknown. In contrast, Amato et al.[19] used cerebral ultrasound examinations, measurements of creatine kinase isoenzyme levels, and detection of antibodies to brain antigens as markers for cerebral injury. They found no evidence of any negative influence of surfactant therapy on cerebral function in treated preterm infants.

Data from long-term follow-up studies indicate that improved survival of patients treated with surfactant is not associated with a significant increase in disability rates.[7-13] In a recent retrospective analysis of data from 4 of 10 centers that participated in a randomized multicenter trial, the use of a modified bovine surfactant appeared to improve the likelihood of intact survival of extremely low birth weight infants (600 to 750 gm) at 1 year of age.[14] Late developmental outcomes of this retrospectively selected subset of infants enrolled in the original trial have not been reported. Another single-center retrospective study reported that treatment with a modified bovine surfactant increased survival at time of hospital discharge for infants born at gestational ages between 23 and 26 weeks; no difference in neurologic outcome was found at long-term follow-up examination.[15]

In a recent report that combines all trials, an increase in brain hemorrhage was noted among infants with birth weights less than 750 gm who received this same modified bovine surfactant, which raises questions about subsequent developmental outcome in this weight class.[20] The results of our study demonstrate that extremely low birth weight infants (500 to 749 gm) who received two rescue doses of synthetic surfactant had developmental outcomes at least as good as those of infants who received air placebo; the RR estimates suggested a possible decreased risk of overall impairments, developmental delay, moderate or severe CP, bilateral blindness, and visual defects in patients who received surfactant. Thus at the 1-year follow-up examination, more patients in the surfactant group were free of handicaps (55% vs 38%). In contrast, the Collaborative European Multicentre Study Group[7] and Dunn et al.[10] reported a higher but not statistically significant incidence of handicaps in the groups treated with porcine and bovine surfactant, respectively. However, differences not only in surfactant preparations but also in populations studied and methods of follow-up assessment may explain the apparent difference on the incidence of handicaps.

The significant reduction in the severity of ROP at the worst examination in infants who received synthetic surfactant merits attention, although at the time of the last examination, the difference in prevalence of severe ROP was no longer statistically significant. Regression of neurovascular tissue occurs in some infants who have ROP with engorgement and tortuosity of the posterior vessels. The mechanism that determines which infants will have scar formation and which will experience regression or healing is not well understood.[21] Refraction anomalies, strabismus, amblyopia, and other sequelae are more common than expected in infants with regressed ROP.[21, 22] An increased risk for diminished vision seems to be one of the sequelae of ROP even when the retinopathy appears to have healed completely.[23]

It is not clear why treatment with synthetic surfactant reduced the severity of ROP in our study. Although FiO_2 and $a{:}AP_{O2}$ ratio differences were significantly lower in infants treated with surfactant during the first 7 days of life, length and degree of respiratory support and the incidence of bronchopulmonary dysplasia were similar in both groups. Follow-up at 2 and 3 years of age, which recently has been completed, should provide valuable information regarding further group differences in visual function.

In summary, the developmental outcomes of extremely premature infants with RDS who receive two rescue doses of synthetic surfactant are at least as good at 1-year adjusted age as in those who receive air placebo. Confirmation of the favorable trends in other measurements observed in this study would provide a strong rationale for the rescue use of synthetic surfactant in extremely premature infants with RDS, even if overall mortality is not reduced.

REFERENCES

1. Bose C, Corbet A, Bose G, et al. Improved outcome at 28 days of age for very low birthweight infants treated with a single dose of synthetic surfactant. J PEDIATR 1990;117:947-53.
2. Corbet A, Bucciarelli R, Goldman S, Mammel M, Wold D, Long WA. Decreased mortality rate among small premature infants treated at birth with a single dose of synthetic surfactant: a multicentre controlled trial. J PEDIATR 1991;118:277-84.
3. Long W, Thompson T, Sundell H, Schumacher R, Volberg F, Guthrie R. Effects of two rescue doses of a synthetic surfactant on mortality in 700- to 1350-gram infants with respiratory distress syndrome. J PEDIATR 1991;118:595-605.
4. Long W, Corbet A, Cotton R, et al. A controlled trial of synthetic surfactant in infants weighing 1250 g or more with respiratory distress syndrome. N Engl J Med 1991;325:1696-703.
5. Collaborative European Multicentre Study Group. Surfactant replacement therapy for severe neonatal respiratory distress

syndrome: an international randomized clinical trial. Pediatrics 1988;82:683-91.

6. Hoekstra RE, Jackson JC, Myers TF, et al. Improved neonatal survival following multiple doses of bovine surfactant in very premature neonates at risk for respiratory distress syndrome. Pediatrics 1991;88:10-8.
7. Collaborative European Multicentre Study Group. A 2-year follow up of babies enrolled in a European multicentre trial of porcine surfactant replacement for severe neonatal respiratory distress syndrome. Eur J Pediatr 1992;151:372-6.
8. Ware J, Taeusch HW, Soll RF, McCormick MC. Health and developmental outcomes of a surfactant controlled trial: follow-up at 2-years. Pediatrics 1990;85:1103-7.
9. Halliday HL, McClure G, Reid MM. Growth and development two years after artificial surfactant replacement at birth. Early Hum Dev 1986;13:323-7.
10. Dunn MS, Shennan AT, Hoskins EM, Enhorning G. Two-year follow-up of infants enrolled in a randomized trial of surfactant replacement therapy for the prevention of neonatal respiratory distress syndrome. Pediatrics 1988;82:543-7.
11. Morley CJ, Morley R. Follow up of premature babies treated with artificial surfactant (ALEC). Arch Dis Child 1990;65:667-9.
12. Vaucher YE, Merrit TA, Hallmann M, et al. Neurodevelopmental and respiratory outcome in early childhood after human surfactant treatment. Am J Dis Child 1988;142:927-30.
13. Vaucher YE, Harker L, Merrit TA, et al. Outcome at twelve months of adjusted age in very low birth weight infants with lung immaturity: a randomized, placebo-controlled trial of human surfactant. J PEDIATR 1993;122:126-32.
14. Ferrara TB, Hoekstra RE, Couser RJ, et al. Effects of surfactant therapy on outcome of infants with birth weight of 600 to 750 grams. J PEDIATR 1991;119:455-7.
15. Ferrara TB, Hoekstra RE, Couser RJ, et al. Survival and follow-up of infants born at 23 to 26 weeks of gestational age: effects of surfactant therapy. J PEDIATR 1994;124:119-23.
16. Smyth J, Allen A, MacMurray B, et al. Double-blind, randomized, placebo-controlled Canadian multicenter trial of two doses of synthetic surfactant or air placebo in 224 infants weighing 500 to 749 grams with respiratory distress syndrome. J PEDIATR 1995;126:S81-9.
17. Courtney SE, Long W, McMillan D, et al. Double-blind 1-year follow-up in 1540 infants with respiratory distress syndrome randomized to rescue treatment with two doses of synthetic surfactant or air in four clinical trials. J PEDIATR 1995;126:S43-52.
18. Hellstrom-Westas L, Bell AH, Liselotte S, Greisen G, Svenningsen NW. Cerebroelectrical depression following surfactant treatment in preterm neonates. Pediatrics 1992;89:643-7.
19. Amato M, Huppi P, Markus D, Herschkowitz N. Neurological function of immature babies after surfactant replacement therapy. Neuropediatrics 1991;22:43-4.
20. Gunkel JH, Phillips PLC. Surfactant therapy and intracranial hemorrhage: review of the literature and results of new analyses. Pediatrics 1993;92:775-86.
21. Phelps DL. Retinopathy of prematurity. In: Fanaroff A, Martin R, eds. Neonatal-perinatal medicine: diseases of the fetus and infant. St. Louis: Mosby–Year Book, 1992:1391-5.
22. Gallo J, Holmstrom G, Kugelburg U, Hedquist B, Lennerstrand G. Regressed retinopathy of prematurity and its sequelae in children aged 5-10 years. Br J Ophthalmol 1991;75:527-31.
23. Cats B, Tan K. Prematures with and without regressed retinopathy of prematurity: comparison of long-term (6-10 years) ophthalmological morbidity. J Pediatr Ophthalmol Strabismus 1989;26:271-5.

One-year outcome in 232 premature infants with birth weights of 750 to 1249 grams and respiratory distress syndrome randomized to rescue treatment with two doses of synthetic surfactant or air placebo

Saroj Saigal, MD, Charlene Robertson, MD, Koravangattu Sankaran, MD, William Bingham, MD, Oscar Casiro, MD, Brock MacMurray, MD, Michael Whitfield, MD, Walker Long, MD, and the Canadian Exosurf Neonatal Study Group (see Appendix III)

From Children's Hospital, McMaster University, Hamilton, Ontario, Canada; Royal Alexandra Hospital, University of Alberta, Edmonton, Canada; University of Saskatchewan, Saskatoon, Canada; Children's Hospital, University of Manitoba, Winnipeg, Canada; University of Ottawa, Ontario, Canada; British Columbia Children's Hospital, Vancouver, Canada; the University of North Carolina at Chapel Hill; and participating centers

A randomized, double-blind, placebo-controlled trial was performed in 13 hospitals in Canada to assess whether two rescue doses of a synthetic surfactant (Exosurf Neonatal) would reduce mortality and morbidity rates in neonates with respiratory distress syndrome who weighed from 750 to 1249 gm. As part of the original trial design, double-blind follow-up evaluations were performed at 1-year adjusted age. A total of 118 patients who received air placebo and 114 patients who received synthetic surfactant were evaluated at 1 year. Growth and development in the two groups were equivalent. Scores on the Bayley Scales of Infant Development were within the normal range for both groups (mental development index, 90 ± 22 vs 92 ± 22; psychomotor development index, 81 ± 19 vs 87 ± 22 for the air placebo and synthetic surfactant groups, respectively). However, in both groups the proportion of infants with any impairment (air placebo group, 43 of 118 (36%); synthetic surfactant group, 41 of 114 (36%)) and severe impairment (air placebo group, 29 of 118 (25%); synthetic surfactant group, 21 of 114 (18%)) was substantial. We conclude that two rescue doses of synthetic surfactant in infants with RDS who weighed 750 to 1249 gm had no detrimental effect on developmental outcome or late morbidity. No long-term benefits to 12-months corrected age were observed with the use of surfactant in this weight class. Larger studies or meta-analyses of existing trials will be required to determine if there are any late outcome advantages associated with rescue use of synthetic surfactant in infants weighing 700 to 1249 gm. (J Pediatr 1995;126:S61-7)

Reprint requests: Saroj Saigal, MD, Department of Pediatrics, McMaster University, 1200 Main St. West, Hamilton, Ontario, Canada, L8N 3Z5.

0022-3476/95/$3.00 + 0 **9/0/61828**

Several recent randomized clinical trials of surfactant therapy given prophylactically to infants at risk of respiratory distress syndrome or as rescue treatment to infants with established RDS have shown improvements in pulmonary function, reductions in pulmonary air leak, and reductions

Table I. Patient accountability*

	Air placebo (*n* = 170)	Synthetic surfactant (*n* = 174)
Alive at 1-year adjusted age	123 [72]	127 [72]
Lost to follow-up	5 (3) [4]†	13 (7) [10]†
Completed follow-up	118 (69) [96]	114 (66) [90]

Numbers in parentheses represent the percentage of enrolled infants; numbers in brackets represent the percentage of survivors at 1-year adjusted age.
*Includes all patients as treated.
†Includes patients (2%, air placebo group; 8%, synthetic surfactant group) whose survival status was assessed by telephone contact.

BPD	Bronchopulmonary dysplasia
MDI	Mental development index
PDI	Psychomotor development index
RDS	Respiratory distress syndrome
ROP	Retinopathy of prematurity

in neonatal mortality.[1-6] The beneficial effects on lung function, air leak, and survival demonstrated during the neonatal period with the use of synthetic, bovine, porcine, and human extract surfactants have been similar.[7] However, the results and consequences of surfactant replacement after the newborn period are not as well characterized. Follow-up studies reported to date[8-16] have shown no adverse side effects with the use of surfactant, but sample sizes from most of these studies were relatively small and some of the studies were not double-blind. Definitive data on the late outcomes of infants treated with surfactant are not yet available.

We report 1-year follow-up results of infants enrolled in a double-blind, randomized, placebo-controlled rescue trial of two doses of synthetic surfactant or air placebo in infants with RDS who weighed 750 to 1249 gm. Two questions were posed: First, does the use of synthetic surfactant in infants with RDS who weigh 750 to 1249 gm have any long-term adverse side effects? Second, are there any concomitant benefits with rescue use of synthetic surfactant in this birth-weight group as determined by a decrease in neurodevelopmental and respiratory morbidity at 12 months adjusted age?

METHODS

Study design. The trial was a double-blind, placebo-controlled study conducted in 13 tertiary-level hospitals in Canada, all of which also had follow-up programs. The protocol was approved by the Institutional Review Board at each of the 13 participating centers (participants are listed

Table II. Baseline characteristics and major neonatal complications of infants who completed follow-up at 1-year adjusted age*

Characteristic	Air placebo (%) (*n* = 118)	Synthetic surfactant (%) (*n* = 114)
Birth weight (gm)†	1000 ± 133	1012 ± 145
Gestational age (wk)†	27.7 ± 1.8	27.8 ± 1.9
Multiple birth	40 (34)	39 (34)
Inborn	102 (86)	101 (87)
Race		
White	103 (87)	98 (86)
Black	0 (0)	1 (1)
Asian	6 (5)	9 (8)
Native American	6 (5)	3 (3)
Other	3 (3)	3 (3)
Maternal age (yr)†	27 ± 5	27 ± 5
Maternal education (yr)†,‡	13 ± 3	13 ± 3
Sex		
Male	63 (53)	64 (56)
Female	55 (47)	50 (44)
Apgar score (median)		
1 min	4.0	4.0
5 min	7.0	7.0
IVH during days 1-28		
Grade I/II	43 (36)	34 (30)
PVED and/or Grade III	11 (9)	11 (10)
BPD at day 28	35 (30)	23 (20)

IVH, Intraventricular hemorrhage; *PVED*, periventricular echodensities.
*Infants are classified according to the treatment they received.
†Values are mean ± SD.
‡For maternal education: *n* = 100, air placebo; *n* = 98, synthetic surfactant.

in Appendixes III and IV). Patients were enrolled in the trial from January 1988 through July 1989. The targeted number for entry was 400 patients (200 patients each in the synthetic surfactant and air placebo groups). The study was stopped short of targeted enrollment on June 28, 1989, when another trial in this same birth-weight class showed that rescue use of synthetic surfactant improved survival rates.[3] Details of the assessment measures used and classification of impairments are described elsewhere.[17]

RESULTS

Patient accountability (Table I). During the enrollment period, 344 infants were treated with air placebo (*n* = 170) or synthetic surfactant (*n* = 174). At 1-year adjusted age, 118 air placebo recipients and 114 synthetic surfactant recipients had complete follow-up assessments. Follow-up was completed in 96% of the air placebo recipients and 90% of the synthetic surfactant recipients who survived to 1-year

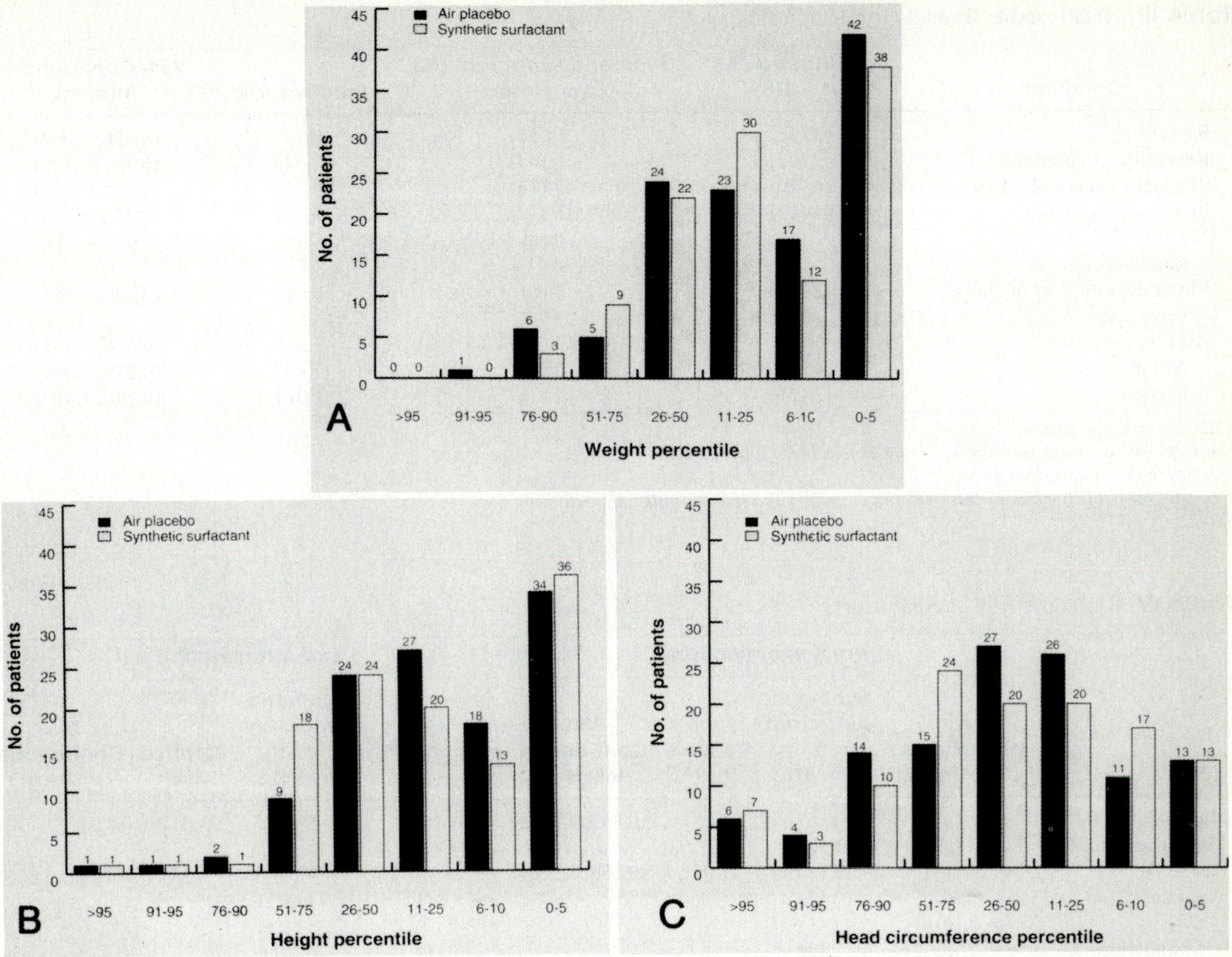

Fig. 1. Distribution of percentiles of physical growth measurements at 1-year adjusted age in infants who received air placebo or synthetic surfactant at birth. **A,** Weight percentiles; **B,** height percentiles; **C,** head circumference percentiles. (Percentile rankings are based on growth charts from the National Center for Health Statistics. Individual percentiles were derived by plotting measurements against chronologic age.)

adjusted age. Five air placebo recipients and 13 synthetic surfactant recipients were lost to follow-up or their families were noncompliant.

Baseline characteristics and major neonatal complications of infants who completed follow-up at 1-year adjusted age (Table II). The two groups were comparable in their sociodemographic characteristics and severity of illness. The incidence of bronchopulmonary dysplasia among the infants evaluated at 1 year was similar between the two groups (placebo group, 35 of 118 [30%]; synthetic surfactant group, 23 of 114 [20%]).

Physical measurements (Fig. 1). Mean anthropometric measurements for weight (placebo group, 8.61 kg; synthetic surfactant group, 8.64 kg), height (placebo group, 72.5 cm; synthetic surfactant group, 72.8 cm) and head circumference (placebo group, 45.9 cm; synthetic surfactant group, 45.9 cm) were almost identical for recipients in both groups. Approximately equal numbers of placebo and surfactant recipients were below the 5th percentile at the 1-year follow-up examination (Fig. 1). No statistically significant differences in anthropometric measurements by gender were found between the treatment groups.

Health status through 1-year adjusted age (Table III). No statistically significant differences in general health status were observed between the synthetic surfactant and placebo groups (Table III). A high percentage of children in both groups were rehospitalized after the neonatal period (placebo group, 42%; surfactant group, 44%). Surgery after 28 days was performed frequently in both groups (placebo group, 36%; synthetic surfactant group, 26%). Physical ev-

Table III. Health status through 1-year adjusted age*

Condition	Air placebo (%) (*n* = 118)	Synthetic surfactant (%) (*n* = 114)	Relative risk*	95% Confidence interval
Surgery	43 (36)	30 (26)	0.735	(0.506, 1.069)
Readmitted to hospital	49 (42)	50 (44)	1.049	(0.777, 1.416)
Physical evidence of CLD	24 (20)	17 (15)	0.726	(0.413, 1.276)
Medication for CLD	22 (19)	16 (14)	0.758	(0.422, 1.360)
Medication for chronic neurologic disease	1 (1)	0 (0)	—†	(—, —)†
Respiratory support on day of examination	12 (10)	7 (6)	0.596	(0.244, 1.457)
Allergies‡	9 (8)	13 (11)	1.522	(0.674, 3.437)
Asthma	4 (3)	7 (6)	1.857	(0.572, 6.028)
Eczema	2 (2)	2 (2)	1.018	(0.140, 7.409)

CLD, Chronic lung disease.
*Includes data on health status between day 29 and 1-year adjusted age.
†Counts too low for valid estimate.
‡Relative risk <1.000 indicates decreased risk of event with synthetic surfactant treatment.

Table IV. Retinopathy of prematurity*

	Worst examination				Last examination			
	Air placebo (%) (*n* = 115)	Synthetic surfactant (%) (*n* = 126)	Relative risk†	95% Confidence interval	Air placebo (%) (*n* = 115)	Synthetic surfactant (%) (*n* = 126)	Relative risk†	95% Confidence interval
No ROP	61 (53)	72 (57)	1.057	(0.842, 1.325)	96 (83)	108 (86)	1.017	(0.913, 1.132)
Mild/moderate ROP	43 (37)	41 (33)			14 (12)	14 (11)		
Severe ROP	11 (10)	13 (10)	1.061	(0.506, 2.226)	5 (4)	4 (3)	0.734	(0.201, 2.685)
Treatment‡	7 (6)	3 (2)			1 (<1)	1 (<1)		
Surgery	5 (5)	1 (1)			2 (2)	1 (<1)		
Cryotherapy	5 (5)	2 (2)			0 (0)	0 (0)		

*Based on worst and last examination for all infants who received ophthalmologic examinations under study protocol. Mild/moderate ROP = grades 1-3; severe ROP = grades >3+.
†Relative risk <1.000 indicates decreased risk of event with synthetic surfactant treatment.
‡Patients may have received more than one treatment.

Table V. Mental and psychomotor development as determined by Bayley Scales of Infant Development at 1-year adjusted age

	Mental development index				Psychomotor development index			
	Air placebo (*n* = 117)	Synthetic surfactant (*n* = 112)	Relative risk*	95% Confidence interval	Air placebo (*n* = 110)	Synthetic surfactant (*n* = 111)	Relative risk*	95% Confidence interval
Development index†,‡								
Analysis I	90 ± 22	92 ± 22			81 ± 19	87 ± 22		
Analysis II§	92 ± 21	96 ± 20			83 ± 18	91 ± 19		
Index <2 SD (%)‖	18 (16)	8 (8)	0.514	(0.235, 1.125)	23 (21)	11 (11)	0.557	(0.289, 1.076)

*Relative risk <1.000 indicates decreased risk of event with synthetic surfactant.
†Mean ± SD.
‡Index values <50 were set to 49.
§Infants with bilateral blindness or deafness or moderate or severe cerebral palsy were excluded from analyses (PDI and MDI: air placebo, *n* = 110; synthetic surfactant, *n* = 101).
‖Bayley Scales of Infant Development scores <69.

Table VI. Impairments for infant who completed follow-up evaluation at 1-year adjusted age

	Air placebo (%) (*n* = 118)	Synthetic surfactant (%) (*n* = 114)	Relative risk*	95% Confidence interval
Impairment present	43 (36)	41 (36)	1.011	(0.719, 1.420)
No impairment	75 (64)	73 (64)		
Severity of impairment				
Mild/moderate	14 (12)	20 (18)		
Severe	29 (25)	21 (18)	0.836	(0.516, 1.355)
Type of impairment†,‡				
MDI <69	24 (20)	18 (16)	0.799	(0.460, 1.391)
MDI 69-84	15 (13)	15 (13)	1.064	(0.549, 2.062)
Moderate/severe CP	6 (5)	8 (7)	1.372	(0.513, 3.671)
Mild CP	7 (6)	4 (4)	0.606	(0.185, 1.981)
Bilateral sensorineural deafness	1 (1)	1 (1)	0.982	(0.077, 12.46)
Deafness not requiring amplification	0	0	—§	(—, —)§
Bilateral blindness	0	5 (4)	—§	(—, —)§
Visual defect	6 (5)	7 (6)	1.207	(0.427, 3.410)

CP, Cerebral palsy.
*Relative risk <1.000 indicates decreased risk of event with synthetic surfactant treatment.
†Patients may have more than one impairment.
‡Bayley Scales of Infant Development MDI scores <50 set to 49.
§Counts were too low for valid estimate.

idence of chronic lung disease at the 1-year evaluation was frequent in both groups (placebo group, 20%; synthetic surfactant group, 15%); 6% of infants in the surfactant group required respiratory support at 1 year versus 10% in the placebo group (relative risk 0.596; 95% confidence interval 0.244 to 1.457). Two infants in the placebo group were intubated at the 1-year assessment (one infant was on mechanical ventilation and the other was on continuous positive airway pressure breathing); all other infants who required respiratory support were receiving oxygen only. There were no significant differences in the proportion of children in each group with allergies.

Retinopathy of prematurity (Table IV). For patients given air placebo, the mean ages at which patients received the worst and last ophthalmologic examination were day 91 and day 220, respectively; for patients treated with synthetic surfactant, the mean ages were similar—day 89 and 201, respectively. Surgery or cryotherapy were reported in seven placebo recipients and in three surfactant recipients at the worst examination; surgery was reported in one patient in each group at the last examination.

At the last ophthalmologic examination, a similar number of patients in the placebo and surfactant groups had mild to moderate ROP. There were no differences between groups in the last or worst ROP examinations (Table IV).

Mental and psychomotor development as determined by Bayley Scales of Infant Development at 1-year adjusted age (Table V). Mean Bayley Scales of Infant Development mental and psychomotor development index scores in the two groups were not different when index values less than 50 were set at 49 or when patients with sensorineural impairments were excluded. The mean PDI scores for the placebo group, however, were below than 1 SD of the mean of the normative sample. Twenty-one percent of the placebo recipients and 11% of the surfactant recipients had a PDI of 2 SD below the average score of 100. The corresponding proportions less than 2 SD below the mean for MDI were 16% and 8%, respectively. None of these differences was statistically significant.

Impairments for infants who completed follow-up evaluation at 1-year adjusted age (Table VI). The proportion of children identified with any impairments was similar for both groups (Fig. 2).

DISCUSSION

Before any innovative treatment is adopted for general use, it is imperative that its safety be evaluated and that both short-term and long-term effects be demonstrated. Because most large surfactant trials to date have shown improvements in survival rates, as well as reductions in air leak and improvements in lung function, surfactant has become standard treatment in neonatal intensive care units. However, the late effects of surfactant replacement are not as well established.

We have shown that premature infants with RDS and birth weights of 750 to 1249 gm who were randomized to receive synthetic surfactant had no increase in long-term adverse side effects compared with patients in the placebo group, as determined by the occurrence of health-related

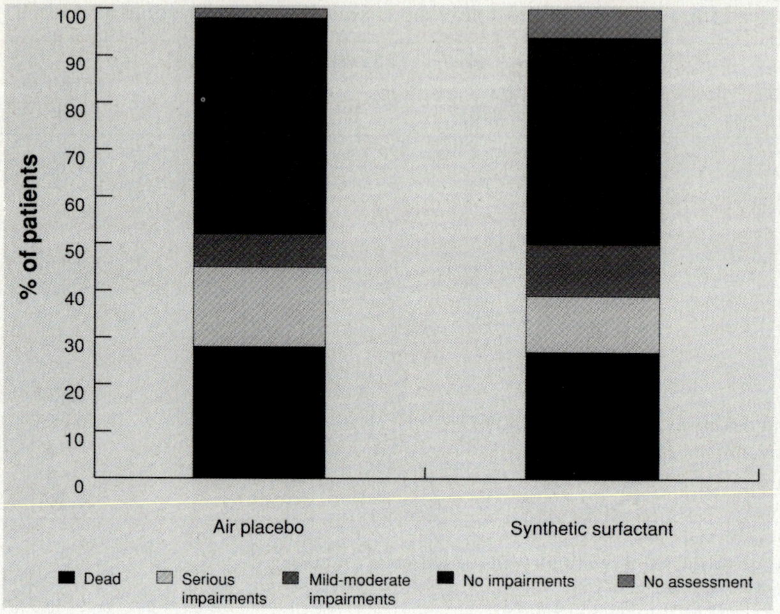

Fig. 2. Overall outcome at 1-year adjusted age for infants who were treated with air placebo or synthetic surfactant at birth.

problems, rehospitalizations, use of medication for chronic chest problems, and allergic symptoms. On the other hand, no significant advantages were observed in long-term morbidity, prevalence and severity of impairments, or in the MDI and PDI scores in the synthetic surfactant group in these infants weighing 750-1249 gm. Thus although the safety of synthetic surfactant is established, improvement in neurodevelopmental outcomes and health status was not observed among survivors at 1-year adjusted age.

The targeted sample size of 400 infants in our study was precalculated specifically to detect differences in intact cardiopulmonary survival, defined as survival at day 28 without BPD. As discussed earlier, the trial was terminated for ethical reasons before that enrollment goal was reached. The study was not designed to detect clinically significant predefined differences in long-term outcome. However, it is one of the larger studies in terms of sample size at follow-up in this birth-weight stratum. Although no benefits were noted at the 12-month assessments, further follow-up performed at 3-year adjusted age may provide more objective measurements of the participants' neurologic and cognitive status, and these findings will be reported in a separate publication.

Several reports have recently been published on the outcome of infants who received surfactant therapy. In a randomized trial of artificial surfactant, Morley and Morley[12] showed a significant improvement in neonatal mortality, with no increase in the rates of neurodevelopmental impairments, respiratory illness, allergies, or rehospitalization among 231 survivors monitored to 18 months of age. Ferrara et al.[13] performed a retrospective analysis of 154 infants treated with surfactant and 156 controls born between 23 and 26 weeks of gestational age. Improved survival rates were observed without an increase in the proportion of impaired survivors. Similar improvements in survival rates without an increase in disability rates were observed in the Collaborative European Multicentre Study Group[14] and in the across-study analysis of all rescue trials of synthetic surfactant.[15] Other investigators[9-11] have reported no neurodevelopmental advantage with the use of surfactant. In one study, prophylactic use of human surfactant replacement was associated with poorer outcome than rescue use, but the sample size was small.[10] Studies by Halliday et al.[8] that used prophylactic artificial surfactant and by Ware et al.[16] that used a bovine surfactant also had inadequate power, thus limiting any definitive conclusions.

Other investigators have evaluated pulmonary function at follow-up of infants treated with surfactant. Most pulmonary function studies at follow-up have shown neither improvements nor adverse effects on the developing respiratory system.[18-20] The studies that have shown an improvement in lung function[21, 22] had an inadequate sample size,[21] and the benefits were observed mainly in larger preterm infants.[22]

The failure to demonstrate any long-term outcome benefits with the use of synthetic surfactant is somewhat surprising, given the fact that synthetic surfactant (unlike animal-derived surfactant) has been shown to reduce the incidence of intraventricular hemorrhage[6, 7] and the incidence[6, 7] and severity[15, 23, 24] of BPD. Nevertheless, an important finding in most studies is that improved survival was not obtained at the expense of an increase in functionally impaired children.[8-14] Larger studies or a meta-analysis of current studies will be required to determine if the use of synthetic surfactant results in any additional long-term benefits in infants weighing 750 to 1249 gm.

We thank Mrs. Barbara Stoskopf, Research Coordinator of the Exosurf Follow-Up Study, for her assistance.

REFERENCES

1. Collaborative European Multicentre Study Group. Surfactant replacement therapy for severe neonatal respiratory distress syndrome: an international randomized clinical trial. Pediatrics 1988;82:683-91.
2. Bose C, Corbet A, Bose G, et al. Improved outcome at 28 days of age for very low birth weight infants treated with a single dose of synthetic surfactant. J Pediatr 1990;117:947-53.
3. Long W, Thompson T, Sundell H, Schumacher R, Volberg F, Guthrie R, and The American Exosurf Neonatal Study Group. Effects of two rescue doses of a synthetic surfactant on mortality rate and survival without bronchopulmonary dysplasia in 700 to 1350-gram infants with respiratory distress syndrome. J Pediatr 1991;118:595-605.
4. Hoekstra RE, Jackson JC, Myers TF, et al. Improved neonatal survival following multiple doses of bovine surfactant in very premature neonates at risk for respiratory distress syndrome. Pediatrics 1991;88:10-8.
5. Liechty EA, Donovan E, Purohit D, et al. Reduction of neonatal mortality after multiple doses of bovine surfactant in low birth weight neonates with respiratory distress syndrome. Pediatrics 1991;88:19-28.
6. Long W, Corbet A, Cotton R, The American Exosurf Neonatal Study Group I, and The Canadian Exosurf Neonatal Study Group. A controlled trial of synthetic surfactant in infants weighing 1250 g or more with respiratory distress syndrome. N Engl J Med 1991;325:1696-703.
7. Jobe A. Pulmonary surfactant therapy. N Engl J Med 1993; 328:861-8.
8. Halliday HL, McClure G, Reid MM. Growth and development two years after artificial surfactant replacement at birth. Early Hum Dev 1986;13:323-7.
9. Vaucher YE, Merritt TA, Hallman M, Jarvenpaa AL, Telsey AM, Jones BL. Neurodevelopmental and respiratory outcome in early childhood after human surfactant treatment. Am J Dis Child 1988;142:927-30.
10. Vaucher YE, Harker L, Merritt TA, et al. Outcome at twelve months of adjusted age in very low birth weight infants with lung immaturity: a randomized, placebo-controlled trial of human surfactant. J Pediatr 1993;122:126-32.
11. Dunn MS, Shennan AT, Hoskins EM, Lennox K, Enhorning G. Two-year follow-up of infants enrolled in a randomized trial of surfactant replacement therapy for prevention of neonatal respiratory distress syndrome. Pediatrics 1988;82:543-7.
12. Morley CJ, Morley R. Follow up of premature babies treated with artificial surfactant (ALEC). Arch Dis Child 1990;65: 667-9.
13. Ferrara TB, Hoekstra RE, Couser RJ, et al. Survival and follow-up of infants born at 23 to 26 weeks of gestational age: effects of surfactant therapy. J Pediatr 1994;124:119-24.
14. Collaborative European Multicentre Study Group. A 2-year follow up of babies enrolled in a European multicentre trial of porcine surfactant replacement for severe neonatal respiratory distress syndrome. Eur J Pediatr 1992;151:372-6.
15. Corbet A. Clinical trials of synthetic surfactant in the respiratory distress syndrome of premature infants. Clin Perinatol 1993;20:737-60.
16. Ware J, Taeusch HW, Soll RF, McCormick MC. Health and developmental outcomes of a surfactant controlled trial: follow-up at 2 years. Pediatrics 1990;85:1103-7.
17. McMillan D, Chernick V, Finer N, et al. Effects of two rescue doses of synthetic surfactant in 344 infants with respiratory distress syndrome weighing 750 to 1249 grams: a double-blind, placebo-controlled multicenter Canadian trial. J Pediatr 1995;126:S90-8.
18. Walti H, Boule M, Moriette G, Relier JP. Pulmonary functional outcome at one year of age in infants treated with natural porcine surfactant at birth. Biol Neonate 1992;61(suppl 1):48-53.
19. Armsby DH, Bellon G, Carlisle K, et al. Delayed compliance increase in infants with respiratory distress syndrome following synthetic surfactant. Pediatr Pulmonol 1992;14:206-13.
20. Couser RJ, Ferrara TB, Wheeler W, et al. Pulmonary follow-up 2.5 years after a randomized, controlled, multiple dose bovine surfactant study of preterm newborn infants. Pediatr Pulmonol 1993;15:163-7.
21. Yuksel B, Greenough A, Gamsu HR. Respiratory function at follow-up after neonatal surfactant replacement therapy. Respir Med 1993;87:217-21.
22. Abbasi S, Bhutani VK, Gerdes JS. Long-term pulmonary consequences of respiratory distress syndrome in preterm infants treated with exogenous surfactant. J Pediatr 1993; 122:446-52.
23. Courtney SE, Long W, McMillan D, et al. Double-blind 1-year follow-up of 1540 infants with respiratory distress syndrome randomized to rescue treatment with two doses of synthetic surfactant or air in four clinical trials. J Pediatr 1995;126: S43-52.
24. Long WA. Synthetic surfactant. Semin Perinatol 1993;17: 275-84.

One-year follow-up evaluation of 260 premature infants with respiratory distress syndrome and birth weights of 700 to 1350 grams randomized to two rescue doses of synthetic surfactant or air placebo

Alice Gong, MD, Endla Anday, MD, Stephen Boros, MD, Richard Bucciarelli, MD, David Burchfield, MD, Janet Zucker, PhD, Walker Long, MD, and the American Exosurf Neonatal Study Group I (see Appendix I)

From the Departments of Pediatrics, Santa Rosa Hospital, University of Texas Health Sciences Center at San Antonio; Hospital of the University of Pennsylvania, Philadelphia; Children's Hospital of St. Paul, University of Minnesota, St. Paul; University of Florida College of Medicine, Gainesville; Burroughs Wellcome Co., Research Triangle Park, North Carolina; the University of North Carolina at Chapel Hill; and participating centers

A multicenter, randomized, double-blind, placebo-controlled trial of synthetic surfactant therapy for premature infants with respiratory distress syndrome (RDS) and birth weights of 700 to 1350 gm demonstrated a reduction in severity of RDS, morbidity, and neonatal and 1-year mortality. Of the 419 infants who were entered in the study, 80% of the surviving infants in both the air placebo group (122) and the synthetic surfactant group (138) returned for the follow-up evaluation at 1-year adjusted age. The only significant difference observed at follow-up was a reduction in the incidence of mild cerebral palsy in the synthetic surfactant group (air placebo group, 8 of 122 (7%); synthetic surfactant group, 3 of 138 (2%); relative risk 0.306; 95% confidence interval 0.094, 0.999). No differences were observed between the air placebo and synthetic surfactant treatment groups with respect to health status of the infants, including the incidence of retinopathy of prematurity and neurodevelopmental delays. The difference in the overall incidence of impairment among the 1-year survivors in the air placebo group (43 of 122 (35%)) and in the synthetic surfactant group (40 of 138 (29%)) was not statistically significant. The results of this 1-year follow-up study show that rescue treatment with synthetic surfactant in infants weighing 700 to 1300 gm is not associated with adverse developmental consequences despite the improvement in survival. (J Pediatr 1995;126:S68-74.)

Reprint requests: Alice Gong, MD, Division of Neonatology, Department of Pediatrics, University of Texas Health Sciences Center at San Antonio, 7705 Floyd Curl Dr., San Antonio, TX 78284-7812.

0022-3476/95/$3.00 + 0 **9/0/61821**

Recent studies have demonstrated that rescue treatment of premature infants with respiratory distress syndrome is effective in improving survival rates and reducing early morbidity.[1-9] However, an increase in the survival rate may result in a potential increase in the number of infants surviving with impairments.

A-aPo2	Alveolar-arterial oxygen tension gradient
CLD	Chronic lung disease
IVH	Intraventricular hemorrhage
RDS	Respiratory distress syndrome
ROP	Retinopathy of prematurity

This study was designed to evaluate late morbidity and developmental outcomes at 1 year of age in infants who were originally enrolled in a previously reported multicenter, randomized, double-blind, placebo-controlled trial.[3] In that trial, two rescue doses of synthetic surfactant or air placebo were given to infants receiving ventilation who had RDS, birth weights of 700 to 1350 gm, and an A-aPo2 ratio of less than 0.22.[3] The group that was randomized to two rescue doses of synthetic surfactant had improvements in oxygenation and ventilator requirements for 1 week, significant reductions in death from RDS, neonatal mortality, and overall 1-year mortality, and an improved survival rate without bronchopulmonary dysplasia. Follow-up through 1 year of age was part of the original protocol and is reported herein.

METHODS

Study design. The trial was designed as a multicenter, prospective, double-blind, randomized, parallel comparison of the effects of two 5 ml/kg doses of synthetic surfactant (colfosceril palmitate, cetyl alcohol, and tyloxapol; Exosurf Neonatal, Burroughs Wellcome Co., Research Triangle Park, N.C.) or air placebo. The trial used a common protocol and was conducted at 21 hospitals (participants are listed in Appendix I). The follow-up study consisted of a double-blind evaluation conducted at 1-year adjusted age. The protocol was approved by the Institutional Review Board at each hospital; parents or guardians gave informed consent before infants entered the study. Patients were entered in the trial between October 1987 and June 1989.

Patient recruitment and enrollment. Premature infants who weighed 700 to 1350 gm at birth and developed RDS within their first 24 hours of life, were receiving mechanical ventilation, and had an A-aPo2 ratio less than 0.22 were eligible to enter the study. Exclusion criteria for this study were the same as those used in other rescue trials of the same surfactant.[5] Infants who met inclusion and exclusion criteria were randomized to receive two doses of either air placebo or synthetic surfactant administered 12 hours apart.

A detailed description of the methods for data collection, ophthalmologic examination, the 1-year follow-up evaluation, and data analyses is provided elsewhere in this supplement.[10]

RESULTS

Patient accountability (Table I). Similar proportions of infants treated with air placebo (122 of 151 [81%]) and synthetic surfactant (138 of 172 [80%]) who were alive at the time of the 1-year follow-up examination were evaluated in this study.

Baseline characteristics (Table II). Follow-up evaluations were completed for 260 infants at 1 year. The two treatment groups had no major differences in birth weight, gestational age, multiple births, inborn or outborn infants, race, maternal age, maternal education, Apgar scores, or incidence of bronchopulmonary dysplasia. However, a greater proportion of male infants were found in the synthetic surfactant group compared with the air placebo group (65% vs 56%). Fewer infants treated with synthetic surfactant than those given air placebo were reported to have severe intraventricular hemorrhage, but the incidence of severe IVH was low in both groups (6% vs 13%).

Health status (Table III). The prevalence of chronic lung disease at 1-year adjusted age, as based on physical evidence or medications for CLD, was 14% in both the air placebo and synthetic surfactant groups. Similarly, there was no statistically significant difference between the air placebo group (19%) and the synthetic surfactant group (12%) in use of medications for CLD. Of the 122 children in the air placebo treatment group, seven (6%) were receiving respiratory support (six, nasal cannula; one, mechanical ventilation) at 1-year adjusted age. Nasal cannula was used as a means of respiratory support at 1-year adjusted age for four (3%) of the 138 children who received synthetic surfactant. The concentrations of supplemental oxygen being received by the children given air placebo ranged from 28% to 50%; the concentrations received by the infants treated with synthetic surfactant ranged from 28% to 35%. Similar proportions of infants had surgery after day 28 (34% vs 28%) or were readmitted to the hospital after discharge (42% vs 41%). No differences in allergic manifestations were found between the two treatment groups.

No differences were detected between the two treatment groups in the mean weight (8.73 kg, air placebo group, vs 8.89 kg, synthetic surfactant group), mean height (73.2 cm, air placebo group, vs 73.9 cm, synthetic surfactant group), and mean head circumference (45.4 cm, air placebo group, vs 45.7 cm, synthetic surfactant group) of the children seen at 1-year adjusted age. Approximately one third of the children had physical measurements below the 5th percentile for age (Fig. 1).

Retinopathy of prematurity (Table IV). The two treatment groups did not differ in the proportions of infants with no ROP, mild ROP, or severe ROP when either the worst or the last ophthalmologic examination was considered. At the last ophthalmologic examination, 19% of the infants given air placebo and 21% of the infants treated with synthetic surfactant had evidence of ROP.

Neurodevelopmental outcome (Table V). No differences

Table I. Patient accountability*

	Air placebo (*n* = 213)	Synthetic surfactant (*n* = 206)
Survivors at 1 yr	151 (71)	172 (83)
Lost to follow-up	29 (13) [19]	34 (17) [20]†
Completed follow-up	122 (57) [81]	138 (67) [80]

Numbers in parentheses represent the percentage of enrolled patients; numbers in brackets represent the percentage of surviving infants.
*Includes all patients as treated.
†Includes approximately 14% of patients whose survival status was assessed by telephone contact.

Table II. Baseline characteristics and major neonatal complications of infants who completed follow-up at 1-year adjusted age*

Characteristic	Air placebo (%) (*n* = 122)	Synthetic surfactant (%) (*n* = 138)
Birth weight (gm)†	1163 ± 163	1167 ± 136
Gestational age (wk)†	29.1 ± 2.1	29.0 ± 1.7
Multiple birth	33 (27)	43 (31)
Inborn	66 (54)	82 (59)
Race		
White	86 (71)	95 (69)
Black	20 (16)	26 (19)
Hispanic	13 (11)	15 (11)
Other	3 (3)	2 (1)
Maternal age (yr)†	25 ± 6	25 ± 6
Maternal education (yr)†,‡	12 ± 2	12 ± 3
Sex		
Male	68 (56)	90 (65)
Female	54 (44)	48 (35)
Apgar score (median)		
1 min	5	5
5 min	7	7
IVH during days 1-28		
Grade I/II	42 (35)	47 (35)
Grade III/PVED	15 (13)	8 (6)
No IVH	62 (52)	81 (60)
BPD at day 28	17 (14)	17 (12)

PVED, Periventricular echodensities; *BPD*, bronchopulmonary dysplasia.
*Infants are classified according to the treatment they received.
†Mean ± SD.
‡For maternal education: *n* = 106, air placebo; *n* = 117, synthetic surfactant.

Table III. Health status through 1-year adjusted age*

Condition	Air placebo (%) (*n* = 122)	Synthetic surfactant (%) (*n* = 138)	Relative risk†	95% Confidence interval
Surgery	41 (34)	38 (28)	0.747	0.523, 1.067
Readmitted to hospital	51 (42)	57 (41)	0.960	0.716, 1.288
Physical evidence of CLD	17 (14)	19 (14)	0.962	0.516, 1.791
Medication for CLD	23 (19)	17 (12)	0.620	0.345, 1.112
Respiratory support on day of examination	7 (6)	4 (3)	0.531	0.163, 1.734
Medication for chronic neurologic disease	5 (4)	3 (2)	0.431	0.105, 1.766
Allergies‡	13 (11)	16 (12)	1.050	0.525, 2.099
Asthma	8 (7)	9 (7)	0.979	0.384, 2.494
Milk allergy	3 (2)	4 (3)	1.016	0.216, 4.747

*Includes data on health status between day 29 and 1-year adjusted age.
†Relative risk <1.000 indicates decreased risk of event with synthetic surfactant.
‡Fewer than two patients in each treatment group were reported to have dermatitis, rhinitis, eczema, or hay fever.

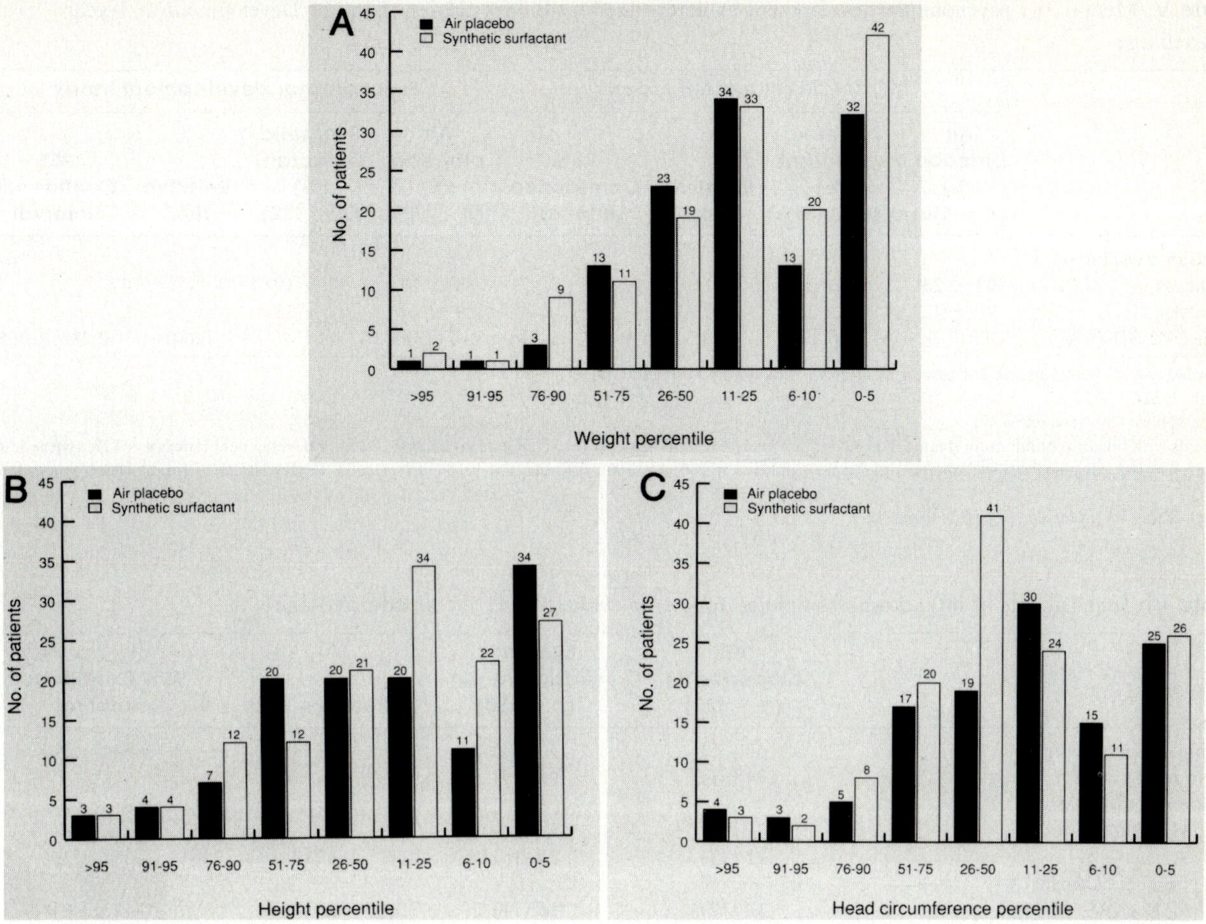

Fig. 1. Distribution of percentiles of physical growth measurements at 1-year adjusted age in infants who received air placebo or synthetic surfactant at birth. **A,** Weight percentiles; **B,** height percentiles; **C,** head circumference percentiles. (Percentile rankings are based on growth charts from the National Center for Health Statistics. Individual percentiles were derived by plotting measurements against chronologic age.)

Table IV. Retinopathy of prematurity*

	Worst examination				Last examination			
	Air placebo (%) ($n = 127$)	Synthetic surfactant (%) ($n = 148$)	Relative risk†	95% Confidence interval	Air placebo (%) ($n = 127$)	Synthetic surfactant (%) ($n = 148$)	Relative risk†	95% Confidence interval
No ROP	69 (54)	77 (52)	0.978	0.798, 1.214	103 (81)	117 (79)	0.983	0.874, 1.105
Mild/moderate ROP	49 (39)	63 (43)			21 (17)	26 (18)		
Severe ROP	9 (7)	8 (5)	0.758	0.314, 1.832	3 (2)	5 (3)	1.480	0.381, 1.832
Treatment‡	6 (5)	2 (1)			2 (2)	0 (0)		
Surgery	2 (2)	0 (0)			2 (2)	0 (0)		
Cryotherapy	6 (5)	2 (1)			2 (2)	0 (0)		

*Based on worst and last examination for all infants who received ophthalmologic examinations under study protocol. Mild/moderate ROP = grades 1-3; severe ROP = grades >3+.
†Relative risk <1.000 indicates decreased risk of event with synthetic surfactant.
‡Patients may have received more than one treatment.

Table V. Mental and psychomotor development as determined by Bayley Scales of Infant Development at 1-year adjusted age

	Mental development index				Psychomotor development index			
	Air placebo (%) (*n* = 110)	Synthetic surfactant (%) (*n* = 131)	Relative risk*	95% Confidence interval	Air placebo (%) (*n* = 111)	Synthetic surfactant (%) (*n* = 132)	Relative risk*	95% Confidence interval
Development index†,‡								
Analysis I	94 ± 23	96 ± 20			88 ± 20	92 ± 19		
Analysis II§	95 ± 22	96 ± 20			89 ± 19	92 ± 18		
Index <2 SD (%)‖	11 (10)	14 (11)	0.92	0.451, 1.875	14 (13)	11 (8)	0.601	0.285, 1.265

*Relative risk <1.000 indicates decreased risk of event with synthetic surfactant.
†Mean ± SD.
‡Index values <50 were set to 49.
§Patients with bilateral blindness or deafness or moderate/severe cerebral palsy were excluded from analysis. Mental development index: *n* = 129, synthetic surfactant; *n* = 103, air placebo. Psychomotor development index: *n* = 130, synthetic surfactant; *n* = 106, air placebo. Bayley Scales of Infant Development scores <69.
‖Bayley Scales of Infant Development scores <69.

Table VI. Impairments of infants who completed follow-up evaluation at 1-year adjusted age

	Air placebo (%) (*n* = 122)	Synthetic surfactant (%) (*n* = 138)	Relative risk*	95% Confidence interval
Impairment present	43 (35)	40 (29)	0.773	0.544, 1.099
No impairment	74 (61)	95 (69)		
Severity of impairment				
Mild/moderate	22 (17)	18 (13)		
Serious	21 (17)	22 (16)	0.769	0.457, 1.294
Type of impairment†,‡				
MDI <69	14 (12)	15 (11)	0.833	0.423, 1.638
MDI 69-84	20 (16)	19 (14)	0.825	0.461, 1.477
Moderate/severe cerebral palsy	6 (5)	3 (2)	0.359	0.094, 1.375
Mild cerebral palsy	8 (7)	3 (2)	0.306	0.094, 0.999*
Bilateral sensorineural deafness	1 (1)	0 (0)	—§	—, —§
Deafness not requiring amplification	2 (2)	0 (0)	—§	—, —§
Bilateral blindness	4 (3)	2 (1)	0.407	0.073, 2.273
Visual defect	4 (3)	6 (4)	1.279	0.365, 4.512

*Relative risk <1.000 indicates decreased risk of event with synthetic surfactant.
†Patients may have more than one impairment.
‡Bayley Scales of Infant Development mental development index scores <50 set to 49.
§Counts too low for valid estimate.

were found between the two treatment groups with respect to the mean mental development index or the mean psychomotor development index of the Bayley Scales of Infant Development.

Impairments (Table VI). Prevalence of impairment among 1-year survivors in the air placebo group was 43 of 122 (35%) compared with 40 of 138 (29%) in the synthetic surfactant group. Fewer children in the synthetic surfactant group had cerebral palsy (mild, moderate, or severe: 6 of 138 [4%] in the synthetic surfactant group vs 14 of 122 [11%] in the air placebo group). The difference in the number of infants with mild cerebral palsy in the two treatment groups was statistically significant (air placebo group, 8 of 122 [7%]; synthetic surfactant group, 3 of 138 [2%]; relative risk 0.306; 95% confidence interval 0.094, 0.999).

The proportion of children surviving without impairments at 1-year adjusted age was 69% in the synthetic surfactant group and 61% in the air placebo group (Fig. 2). Not only was the proportion of children surviving with impairments equivalent in the two treatment groups (35% vs 29%; Table VI), but the absolute numbers of infants with impairments were 40 in the synthetic surfactant group and 43 in the air placebo group, despite significantly better survival in the synthetic surfactant group.

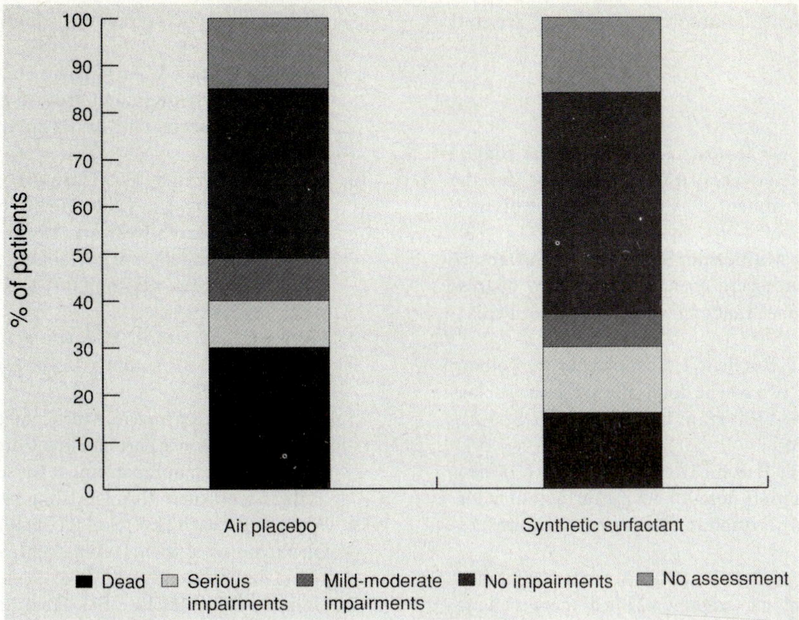

Fig. 2. Overall outcome at 1-year adjusted age for infants treated with air placebo or synthetic surfactant at birth.

DISCUSSION

Multicenter, randomized, placebo-controlled trials have shown that rescue administration of surfactant to infants with RDS reduces morbidity and mortality.[1-9] Fewer studies have addressed the question of whether gains in neonatal survival are maintained through the first year of life. Studies that have examined this question have convincingly shown that 1-year survival rates are also improved by surfactant.[3, 5, 9, 11-13] Whether this reduction in 1-year mortality is associated with an increase in the number of survivors who are impaired is the question addressed by our study. The answer from this double-blind, placebo-controlled study is "no": more infants are not surviving with impairments, either in terms of absolute numbers or proportions. Similar results at follow-up have been reported,[14-19] but in one study an "increase" (not significant) in impairments was noted among infants treated with surfactant.[20]

Although there was a greater percentage of male infants in the synthetic surfactant group in the present study, the proportions of infants with impairments were equivalent in the two treatment groups. Furthermore, the rates of serious impairments were also equivalent for the two groups and were not different from the rates in other reports of babies with similar birth weights.[16, 19]

The lack of reduction of the number of infants with impairments in previous trials has been attributed to small sample sizes that lacked the power to detect significant differences. Differences in developmental outcomes, if such differences exist, may be influenced by several factors, including the different rates of IVH. However, Dunn et al.[20] showed an increase in the number of impairments in infants treated with surfactant despite a lower rate of IVH. Other investigators have proposed that the effects of surfactant and improved ventilation on cerebral circulation may have an adverse effect on the central nervous system, resulting in an increase in neurodevelopmental impairments.[20, 21] The tendency of the synthetic surfactant group in this trial to have lower rates of overall and severe IVH, although not statistically significant, could have contributed to the fact that more infants in the synthetic surfactant group survived at 1 year without neurodevelopmental impairments.

At 1-year adjusted age, neurodevelopmental data represent relatively short-term outcomes. In the short term, perinatal factors have a greater influence on developmental outcomes; in the long term, social, educational, economic, and environmental factors have a greater influence on outcomes. Learning disabilities may become evident as the child grows older; therefore, additional long-term studies are needed to assess fully the impact of surfactant replacement therapy on developmental outcomes.

In summary, the improvement in survival rates of premature infants with RDS and birth weights of 700 to 1350 gm who were treated with two rescue doses of synthetic surfactant did not result in an excess of survivors with impairments. However, additional follow-up assessments at later stages of development will be essential for accurate assessment of developmental outcome of infants treated with surfactant.

REFERENCES

1. Phibbs RH, Ballard RA, Clements JA, et al. Initial clinical trial of Exosurf, a protein-free synthetic surfactant, for the prophylaxis and early treatment of hyaline membrane disease. Pediatrics 1991;88:1-9.
2. Collaborative European Multicenter Study Group. Surfactant replacement therapy for severe neonatal respiratory distress syndrome: an international randomized clinical trial. Pediatrics 1988;82:683-91.
3. Long WA, Thompson T, Sundell H, Schumacher R, Volberg F, Guthrie R. Effects of two rescue doses of a synthetic surfactant on mortality in 700-1300 gram infants with RDS. J PEDIATR 1991;118:595-605.
4. Liechty EA, Donovan E, Purohit D, et al. Reduction of neonatal mortality after multiple doses of bovine surfactant in low birth weight neonates with respiratory distress syndrome. Pediatrics 1991;88:19-26.
5. Long WA, Corbet AJ, Cotton R, et al. A controlled trial of synthetic surfactant in infants weighing 1250g or more with respiratory distress syndrome. N Engl J Med 1991;325:1696-703.
6. Jobe AH. Pulmonary surfactant therapy. N Engl J Med 1993;328:801-58.
7. Merritt TA, Soll RF, Hallman M. Overview of exogenous surfactant replacement therapy. J Intensive Care Med 1993;8:205-28.
8. Mercier CE, Soll RF. Clinical trials of natural surfactant extract in respiratory distress syndrome. Clin Perinatol 1993; 20:711-36.
9. Long WA. Synthetic surfactant. Semin Perinatol 1993;17:275-84.
10. Courtney SE, Long W, McMillan D, et al. Double-blind 1-year follow-up of 1540 infants with respiratory distress syndrome randomized to rescue treatment with two doses of synthetic surfactant or air in four clinical trials. J PEDIATR 1995;126: S43-52.
11. Corbet AJ, Bucciarelli R, Goldman SA, et al. Decreased mortality in small premature infants treated at birth with a single dose of synthetic surfactant: a multicenter trial. J PEDIATR 1991;118:277-84.
12. Corbet AJ, Long WA, Murphy DJ, et al. Reduced mortality in small premature infants treated at birth with a single dose of synthetic surfactant. J Paediatr Child Health 1991;27: 245-9.
13. Horbar JD, Wright EC, Onstad L, and the Members of the National Institute of Child Health and Human Development Neonatal Research Network. Decreasing mortality associated with the introduction of surfactant therapy: an observational study of neonates weighing 601 to 1300 grams at birth. Pediatrics 1993;92:191-6.
14. Morley CJ, Morley R. Follow-up of premature babies treated with artificial surfactant (ALEC). Arch Dis Child 1990;65: 667-9.
15. Collaborative European Multicentre Study Group. A 2-year follow up of babies enrolled in a European multicentre trial of porcine surfactant replacement for severe neonatal respiratory distress syndrome. Eur J Pediatr 1992;151:372-6.
16. Ware J, Taeusch HW, Soll RF, et al. Health and developmental outcomes of a surfactant controlled trial: follow-up at 2 years. Pediatrics 1990;85:1103-7.
17. Halliday HL, McClure BG, Reid MM. Growth and development two years after artificial surfactant replacement at birth. Early Hum Dev 1986;3:323-7.
18. Vaucher YE, Merritt TA, Hallman M, et al. Neurodevelopmental and respiratory outcome in early childhood after human surfactant treatment. Am J Dis Child 1988;142:927-30.
19. Robertson B, Curstedt T, Tubman R, et al. A 2-year follow-up of babies enrolled in a European multicenter trial of porcine surfactant replacement for severe neonatal respiratory distress syndrome. Eur J Pediatr 1992;151:372-6.
20. Dunn MS, Shennan AT, Hoskins EM, et al. Two year follow-up of infants enrolled in a randomized trial of surfactant therapy for prevention of neonatal respiratory distress syndrome. Pediatrics 1988;82:543-7.
21. Vaucher YE, Harker L, Merritt TA, et al. Outcome at twelve months of adjusted age in very low birth weight infants with lung immaturity: a randomized placebo controlled trial of human surfactant. J PEDIATR 1993;122:126-32.

Outcome at 1-year adjusted age of 957 infants weighing more than 1250 grams with respiratory distress syndrome randomized to receive synthetic surfactant or air placebo

Reginald Sauve, MD, Walker Long, MD, Michael Vincer, MD, Harry Bard, MD, Doug Derleth, MD, David Stevenson, MD, Thomas Pauly, MD, Charlene Robertson, MD, and the American and Canadian Exosurf Neonatal Study Groups (see Appendixes I and III)

From the Departments of Pediatrics, Foothills Hospital and the University of Calgary, Alberta, Canada; University of North Carolina at Chapel Hill; Dalhousie University, Halifax, Nova Scotia, Canada; St. Justine Hospital, Montreal, Quebec, Canada; Mayo Clinic, Rochester, Minnesota; Stanford University Medical Center, Palo Alto, California; Albert Chandler Medical Center, University of Kentucky, Lexington; Glenrose Rehabilitation Hospital and the University of Alberta, Edmonton, Canada; and participating centers

This study determined outcomes at 12-months adjusted age of 957 infants weighing more than 1250 gm at birth who were subjects in a randomized, double-blind, controlled trial of synthetic surfactant or air placebo administered in a rescue trial at 23 hospitals in the United States and 13 hospitals in Canada. Follow-up results were available for 475 of 563 surviving infants who received air placebo (84%) and 482 of 571 infants who received synthetic surfactant (84%). Developmental outcome was equivalent in the two groups. Morbidity was less in the synthetic surfactant group as assessed by the need for medication for chronic lung disease (52 of 475 (11%) for the air placebo group vs 32 of 482 (7%) for the synthetic surfactant group) or respiratory support (10 of 475 (2%) for the air placebo group vs 1 of 482 (<1%) for the synthetic surfactant group) at 1-year adjusted age. Bayley Scales of Infant Development (mental development index: 102 for both the air placebo and synthetic surfactant groups; psychomotor development index: 95 for the air placebo group vs 94 for the synthetic surfactant group) and impairment rates (94 of 475 (20%) for the air placebo group vs 86 of 482 (18%) for the synthetic surfactant group) were similar in the two groups. Infants weighing more than 1250 gm who have respiratory distress syndrome have previously been shown to have improved survival rates and lower neonatal morbidity after treatment with synthetic surfactant. These follow-up data confirm that developmental outcome as determined at 12-months adjusted age is at least as good in those receiving synthetic surfactant. (J Pediatr 1995;126:S75-80)

Several reports have documented improved survival rates and decreased perinatal morbidity among ventilated preterm infants with respiratory distress syndrome who were treated with intratracheally administered surfactant.[1-4] In recently reported multicenter trials with preterm infants weighing more than 1250 gm who had RDS,[1] treatment

Reprint requests: Reginald Sauve, MD, Departments of Community Health Sciences and Pediatrics, Faculty of Medicine, University of Calgary, 3330 Hospital Dr. NW, Calgary, Alberta, Canada, T2N 4N1.

0022-3476/95/$3.00 + 0 **9/0/61822**

Table I. Patient accountability*

	Air placebo (*n* = 622)	Synthetic surfactant (*n* = 615)
Alive at 1-year adjusted age	563 (91)	571 (93)
Lost to follow-up	88 (14) [16]†	89 (14) [16]†
Completed follow-up	475 (76) [84]	482 (78) [84]

Numbers in parentheses represent the percentage of enrolled infants; numbers in brackets represent the percentage of survivors at 1-year adjusted age.
*Includes all patients as treated without exclusion.
†Includes approximately 7% of patients whose survival status was assessed by telephone contact.

CLD	Chronic lung disease
MDI	Mental development index
PDI	Psychomotor development index
RDS	Respiratory distress syndrome

with two doses of synthetic surfactant was found to improve 1-year survival rates from 92% to 95%, decrease the frequency of bronchopulmonary dysplasia[5] at 28 days of age from 5% to 2%, and decrease the frequency of intraventricular hemorrhage[6, 7] from 23% to 18%. However, questions remain about whether the improved survival rate brings increased risk of poor long-term outcome and whether the improved perinatal morbidity is associated with decreased long-term morbidity.[1, 8-10]

Our multicenter, prospective, double-blind, randomized, controlled trial of synthetic surfactant provided the opportunity to study long-term health and neurodevelopmental morbidity of a large population of infants with RDS randomized to treatment with air placebo or synthetic surfactant. Our study differed from other studies of the long-term outcome of infants treated with surfactant in that our sample size was larger, the population in our study had a higher birth weight, our follow-up rates were high, and the follow-up investigators in our study remained masked to study group allocation. The primary question we examined was whether treatment with two rescue doses of synthetic surfactant in larger preterm infants with RDS alters neurodevelopmental outcome at 1-year corrected age. An additional question we had was whether the observed decrease in neonatal morbidity is sustained to 1 year of corrected age.

METHODS

The basic study design we used has been detailed elsewhere.[1, 11] The infants described in this study received their neonatal treatment at 1 of 23 United States hospitals (where infants >1350 gm were enrolled) and 13 Canadian hospitals (where infants >1250 gm were enrolled) between October 1987 and June 1989 (participants are listed in Appendixes I and II).[1] The follow-up studies were double-blind, and they were performed at 12-months adjusted age between September 1988 and August 1990 (participants listed in Appendix IV).[1]

The follow-up examinations were conducted in a manner similar to all follow-up studies described in this supplement,[11] but unlike the other studies, the larger infants in this study were not required to have an ophthalmologic examination.

Table II. Baseline characteristics and major neonatal complications of infants who completed follow-up at 1-year adjusted age*

Characteristic	Air placebo (%) (*n* = 475)	Synthetic surfactant (%) (*n* = 482)
Birth weight (gm)†	1922 ± 519	1920 ± 528
Gestational age (wk)†	32.2 ± 2.4	32.2 ± 2.3
Multiple birth	91 (19)	93 (19)
Inborn	292 (62)	307 (64)
Race		
White	388 (82)	410 (85)
Black	33 (7)	17 (4)
Hispanic	18 (4)	24 (5)
Other	36 (8)	21 (6)
Maternal age (yr)†	26 ± 6	27 ± 6
Maternal education (yr)†,‡	13 ± 3	13 ± 3
Sex		
Female	177 (37)	173 (36)
Male	298 (63)	309 (64)
Apgar score (median)		
1 min	6.0	6.0
5 min	8.0	8.0
IVH during days 1-28	111 (23)	95 (20)
Grade I/II	88 (21)	77 (19)
PVED and/or Grade III	23 (5)	18 (4)
BPD at day 28	18 (4)	12 (3)

IVH, Intraventricular hemorrhage; *PVED*, periventricular echodensities; *BPD*, bronchopulmonary dysplasia.
*Infants are classified according to the treatment they received.
†Values are mean ± SD.
‡For maternal education: *n* = 390, air placebo; *n* = 400, synthetic surfactant.

RESULTS

Patient accountability (Table I). A large proportion of infants survived to the time of the 1-year follow-up (air placebo group, 91%; synthetic surfactant group, 93%). Of the surviving infants, equal percentages of the two groups were assessed at follow-up (air placebo group, 84%; synthetic surfactant group, 84%). Infants lost to follow-up did not differ from those who were examined in terms of birth

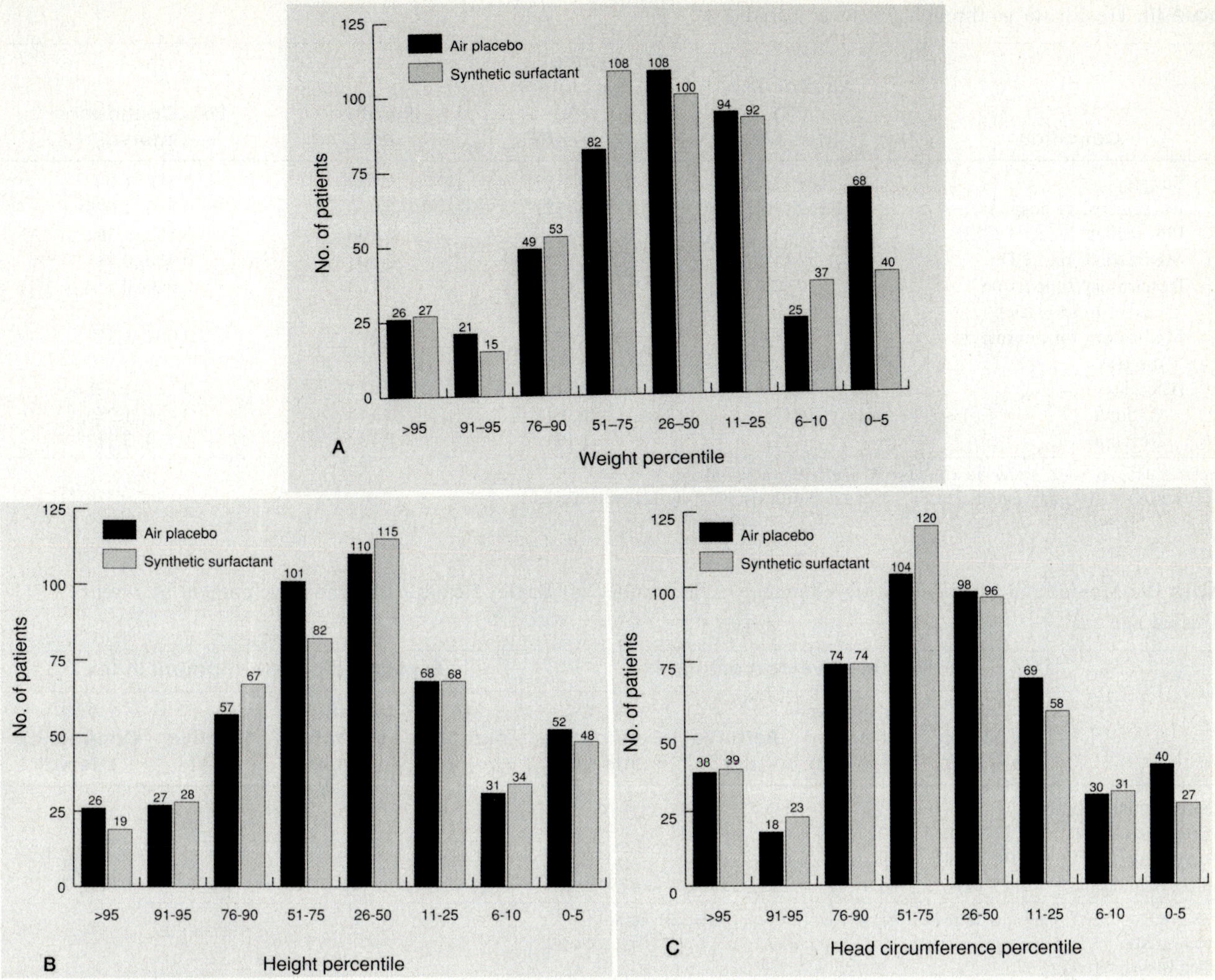

Fig. 1. Distribution of percentiles of physical growth measurements at 1-year adjusted age in infants who received air placebo or synthetic surfactant at birth. **A,** Weight percentiles; **B,** height percentiles; **C,** head circumference percentiles. (Percentile rankings are based on growth charts from the National Center for Health Statistics. Individual percentiles were derived by plotting measurements against chronologic age.)

weight, gestational age, neonatal hospital stay, or frequencies of bronchopulmonary dysplasia or intraventricular hemorrhage (data not shown).

Baseline characteristics and major neonatal complications of infants who completed follow-up at 1-year adjusted age (Table II). The air placebo and synthetic surfactant groups did not differ in terms of demographic characteristics, but a male predominance was evident in both groups. The synthetic surfactant group had fewer infants with bronchopulmonary dysplasia or intraventricular hemorrhage.

Growth (Fig. 1). Growth outcomes of infants in the two groups were similar. Mean weight (air placebo group, 9.66 ± 1.34 kg; synthetic surfactant group, 9.78 ± 1.29 kg), mean height (air placebo group, 75.2 cm; synthetic surfactant group, 75.2 cm), and mean head circumference (air placebo group, 46.5 ± 1.8 cm; synthetic surfactant group, 46.7 ± 1.7 cm) were equivalent.

Health status through 1-year adjusted age (Table III). The application of surgical procedures beyond the neonatal period was noted in 101 of 475 infants treated with air placebo (21%) and 80 of 482 of those who received synthetic surfactant (17%). Rehospitalizations were required for 32% of infants in the group treated with synthetic surfactant versus 36% of infants in the group given air placebo.

Evidence of chronic lung disease was relatively infrequent in both groups of infants and was not significantly different between groups. Overall, 39 of 475 infants given air placebo

Table III. Health status through 1-year adjusted age*

Condition	Air placebo (%) (*n* = 475)	Synthetic surfactant (%) (*n* = 482)	Relative risk†	95% Confidence interval
Surgery	101 (21)	80 (17)	0.774	0.598, 1.002
Readmitted to hospital	169 (36)	156 (32)	0.906	0.760, 1.079
Physical evidence of CLD	39 (8)	36 (7)	0.904	0.588, 1.391
Medication for CLD	52 (11)	32 (7)	0.603	0.400, 0.911
Respiratory support on day of examination	10 (2)	1 (<1)	0.100	0.020, 0.514
Medication for neurologic disease	7 (1)	2 (<1)	0.273	0.064, 1.171
Allergies	53 (11)	46 (10)	0.853	0.587, 1.238
Asthma	34 (7)	26 (5)	0.746	0.456, 1.218
Eczema	7 (1)	8 (2)	1.133	0.413, 3.113

*Includes data on health status between day 29 and 1-year adjusted age.
†Relative risk <1.000 indicates decreased risk of event with synthetic surfactant treatment.

Table IV. Mental and psychomotor development as determined by Bayley Scales of Infant Development at 1-year adjusted age

	Mental development index				Psychomotor development index			
	Air placebo (*n* = 460)	Synthetic surfactant (*n* = 473)	Relative risk*	95% Confidence interval	Air placebo (*n* = 460)	Synthetic surfactant (*n* = 469)	Relative risk*	95% Confidence interval
Developmental index†,‡								
Analysis I	102 ± 20	102 ± 19			95 ± 19	94 ± 19		
Analysis II§	104 ± 18	104 ± 18			96 ± 17	95 ± 18		
Index <2 SD (%)‖	17 (4)	23 (5)	1.253	0.679, 2.313	28 (6)	41 (9)	1.403	0.888, 2.217

*Relative risk <1.000 indicates decreased risk of event with synthetic surfactant.
†Mean ± SD.
‡Index values <50 set to 49.
§Patients with bilateral blindness, deafness, or moderate or severe cerebral palsy were excluded from analyses. (Mental development index: air placebo, *n* = 436; synthetic surfactant, *n* = 459. Psychomotor development index: air placebo, *n* = 436; synthetic surfactant, *n* = 455.)
‖Bayley Scales of Infant Development scores less than 69.

(8%) and 36 of 482 infants treated with synthetic surfactant (7%) had physical evidence of CLD. On the other hand, medication for CLD was used significantly less frequently in patients treated with synthetic surfactant (32 of 482; 7%) than in patients who were given air placebo (52 of 475; 11%). Ten of the infants who received air placebo (2%) but only one of the infants treated with synthetic surfactant (<1%) were receiving respiratory support on the day of the follow-up examination; this difference also was significant. Two patients given air placebo required assisted ventilation, and the others were receiving only oxygen.

Few infants in either group were reported to be receiving medications for seizure control at the time of the examination. Symptoms considered to be allergic in origin also occurred in similar numbers of infants in the two groups (Table III).

Mental and psychomotor development as determined by Bayley Scales of Infant Development at 1-year adjusted age (Table IV). Bayley Scales of Infant Development were largely equivalent in the two groups. Overall, psychomotor development indices were slightly lower than mental development indices. Total group mean indices were equivalent both when all values less than 50 were set at 49 and when Bayley scores of infants with severe impairments (such as bilateral blindness, deafness, and moderate or severe cerebral palsy) were excluded. The percentage of infants with MDI and PDI scores less than 2 SD was similar between the two groups.

Impairments for infants who completed follow-up evaluation at 1-year adjusted age (Table V and Fig. 2). Impairments[12] detected in 180 infants were relatively infrequent in both groups (air placebo group, 20%; synthetic surfactant

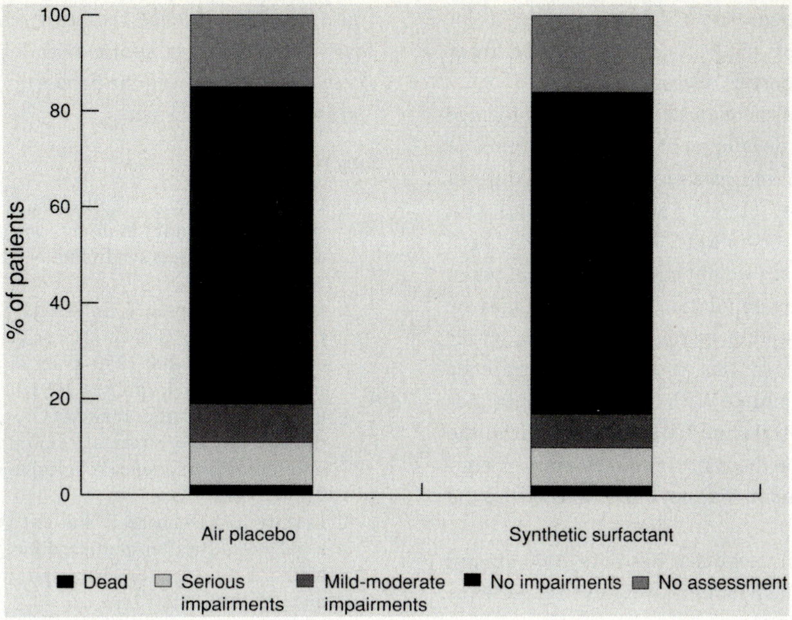

Fig. 2. Overall outcome at 1-year adjusted age for infants who were treated with air placebo or synthetic surfactant at birth.

Table V. Impairments for infants who completed follow-up evaluation at 1-year adjusted age

	Air placebo (%) (n = 475)	Synthetic surfactant (%) (n = 482)	Relative risk*	95% Confidence interval
Impairment present	94 (20)	86 (18)	0.901	0.694, 1.170
No impairment	375 (79)	389 (81)		
Severity of impairment				
Mild/moderate	47 (10)	42 (9)		
Serious	47 (10)	44 (9)	0.917	0.624, 1.347
Type of impairment†,‡				
MDI <69	31 (7)	34 (7)	1.076	0.675, 1.715
MDI 69-84	43 (9)	36 (7)	0.821	0.538, 1.254
Moderate/severe cerebral palsy	24 (5)	15 (3)	0.616	0.331, 1.143
Mild cerebral palsy	12 (3)	13 (3)	1.065	0.492, 2.307
Bilateral sensorineural deafness	3 (1)	1 (<1)	0.334	0.039, 2.852
Deafness not requiring amplification	1 (<1)	3 (1)	2.908	0.343, 24.65
Bilateral blindness	1 (<1)	3 (1)	2.989	0.333, 26.80
Visual defect	19 (4)	12 (2)	0.625	0.311, 1.255

*Relative risk <1.000 indicates decreased risk of event with synthetic surfactant treatment.
†Infants may have more than one impairment.
‡Bayley Scales of Infant Development mental development index scores <50 set to 49.

group, 18%). Serious impairments were even less frequent (air placebo group, 10%; synthetic surfactant group, 9%). The most frequent types of impairment were Bayley MDI scores greater than or equal to 2 SD below population means and the occurrence of cerebral palsy. In all instances, 95% confidence interval of relative risk comparing air placebo and synthetic surfactant groups did not indicate statistical significance.

DISCUSSION

In this population of preterm infants who weighed more than 1250 gm at birth, had severe RDS, and were randomized to treatment with two rescue doses of synthetic surfactant or air placebo, neurodevelopmental morbidity at 12-months adjusted age in those given synthetic surfactant was the same as in those who had received air placebo, despite a greater number of survivors in the surfactant group. The severity of CLD was lower, as indicated by the need for less medication for CLD and lower need for respiratory support at 1 year.

Infants who had RDS as neonates are more likely to have deficits in psychomotor development than are infants of comparable birth weight and gestational age who did not have RDS. However, most follow-up studies of infants with RDS have concentrated on infants with the lowest birth weights and have used birth weight cutoff points that make comparison with our study population difficult.[12] It may be advisable for follow-up studies to routinely include larger infants with RDS because this group may experience increased long-term morbidity. With or without confounders, however, scores on MDIs and PDIs were similar in the two groups of infants. Furthermore, the incidence of neurodevelopmental impairments was not different between the two groups.

Children who had birth weights of less than 2000 gm are more likely than those of heavier birth weights to experience recurrent respiratory symptoms as they grow older, particularly if they had severe neonatal lung disease. As expected, the presence of CLD was less common in the infants treated with synthetic surfactant at 12-months adjusted age than in infants given air placebo.

Several possible confounding factors have been described in studies of recurrent respiratory symptoms in infants. One of these factors is passive smoking; parental smoking was not studied here, and the presence of a differential distribution of parental smoking in the two groups cannot be ruled out. On the other hand, such an imbalance seems unlikely to account for a tenfold difference in the need for respiratory support at 1 year. Another possible confounder is the presence of allergic disorders. In this study, the prevalence of possible clinical signs of allergy symptoms was similar in the two groups, but the study did not include more definitive explorations of allergy such as serum immunoglobulin levels, bronchial responsivity measures, or skin tests.

Because it is not possible to determine final developmental outcomes at 12-months adjusted age, additional evaluations of these infants are taking place at 24 and 36 months adjusted age. However, the follow-up results available to date provide evidence that two rescue doses of synthetic surfactant in larger infants with RDS reduce late morbidity without increasing the proportion or absolute number of infants with impairments.

REFERENCES

1. Long W, Corbet A, Cotton R, et al. A controlled trial of synthetic surfactant in infants weighing 1250 g or more with respiratory distress syndrome. N Engl J Med 1991;325:1696-703.
2. Long W, Thompson T, Sundell H, Schumacher R, Volberg F, Guthrie R. Effects of two rescue doses of synthetic surfactant on mortality in 700-1350–gram infants with respiratory distress syndrome. J PEDIATR 1991;118:595-605.
3. Collaborative European Study Group. Surfactant replacement therapy for severe mental respiratory distress syndrome: an international randomized clinical trial. Pediatrics 1988;82:638-91.
4. Liechty EA, Donovan E, Purohit D, et al. Reduction of neonatal mortality after multiple doses of bovine surfactant in low birth weight neonates with respiratory distress syndrome. Pediatrics 1991;88:19-28.
5. O'Brodovich HM, Mellins RB. Bronchopulmonary dysplasia: unresolved neonatal acute lung injury. Am Rev Respir Dis 1985;132:694-709.
6. Papile L-A, Munsick-Bruno G, Schaefer A. Relationship of cerebral intraventricular hemorrhage and early childhood neurologic handicaps. J PEDIATR 1983;103:273-7.
7. McMenamin JB, Shackelford GD, Volpe JJ. Outcome of neonatal intraventricular hemorrhage with periventricular echodense lesions. Ann Neurol 1984;15:285-90.
8. Vaucher YE, Merritt TA, Hallman M, Jarvenpaa A-L, Telsey AM, Jones BL. Neurodevelopmental and respiratory outcome in early childhood after human surfactant treatment. Am J Dis Child 1988;142:927-30.
9. Ware J, Taeusch W, Soll RF, McCormick MD. Health and developmental outcomes of a surfactant controlled trial: follow-up at 2 years. Pediatrics 1990;85:1103-7.
10. Jobe A, Ikegami M. Surfactant for the treatment of respiratory distress syndrome. Am Rev Respir Dis 1987;136:1256-75.
11. Courtney SE, Long W, McMillan D, et al. Double-blind 1-year follow-up of 1540 infants with respiratory distress syndrome randomized to rescue treatment with two doses of synthetic surfactant or air in four clinical trials. J PEDIATR 1995; 126:S43-52.
12. Kitchen W, Ford G, Orvill A, et al. Outcome in infants with birth weight 500 to 999 gm: a regional study of 1979 and 1980 births. J PEDIATR 1984;104:921-7.

Double-blind, randomized, placebo-controlled Canadian multicenter trial of two doses of synthetic surfactant or air placebo in 224 infants weighing 500 to 749 grams with respiratory distress syndrome

John Smyth, MD, Alexander Allen, MD, Brock MacMurray, MD, Abraham Peliowski, MD, Koravangatu Sankaran, MD, Frank Volberg, MD, Arvind Shukla, MD, Walker Long, MD, and the Canadian Exosurf Neonatal Study Group (see Appendix III)

From British Columbia's Children's Hospital, Vancouver, Canada; Grace Maternity Hospital, Halifax, Nova Scotia, Canada; Children's Hospital of Eastern Ontario, Ottawa General Hospital and Ottawa Civic Hospital, Ontario, Canada; Royal Alexandra Hospital, Edmonton, Alberta, Canada; University of Saskatchewan, Saskatoon, Canada; the Department of Radiology, Bowman Gray School of Medicine, Winston-Salem, North Carolina; Foothills Hospital, Calgary, Alberta, Canada; and the Department of Pediatrics, University of North Carolina at Chapel Hill

In a multicenter, double-masked, placebo-controlled rescue trial conducted at 12 Canadian hospitals, two 5 ml/kg doses of a synthetic surfactant or air placebo were administered to 224 infants with birth weights of 500 to 749 gm who had established respiratory distress syndrome and an arterial/alveolar oxygen tension ratio of less than 0.22. The first dose was given between 2 and 24 hours of age; the second dose was given 12 hours later to the infants continuing to receive mechanical ventilation. Infants were stratified at study entry by birth weight and gender. Infants receiving synthetic surfactant showed significant improvements in alveolar-arterial oxygen tension gradient, arterial/alveolar oxygen tension ratio, and oxygen and ventilator requirements through day 7. In the group randomized to synthetic surfactant, significant improvements were seen in oxygen requirements at the first time point measured (2 hours; $p = 0.02$), in the alveolar-arterial oxygen tension gradient by the second time point measured (6 hours; $p = 0.03$), and in mean airway pressure after 6 hours. Overall mortality at 28 days was not significantly different in the two groups (50% vs 46%, air placebo group vs synthetic surfactant group; $p = 0.586$). Similarly, neither the incidence of bronchopulmonary dysplasia (37% vs 30%, air placebo group vs synthetic surfactant group; $p = 0.089$) nor the incidence of survival without BPD through 28 days (17% vs 26%, respectively; $p = 0.070$) was significantly different in the two groups. No significant differences in the incidence of safety-related outcomes or in adverse effects such as apnea or pulmonary hemorrhage were noted. These findings indicate that rescue therapy with synthetic surfactant results in physiologic improvements in very tiny premature infants, but improvements in overall mortality or other complications of respiratory distress syndrome were not documented in the sample evaluated. (J Pediatr 1995;126:S81-9)

Reprint requests: John Smyth, MD, Newborn Services, Room 1N1, British Columbia's Children's Hospital, 4480 Oak St., Vancouver, British Columbia, Canada V6H 3V4.

0022-3476/$3.00 + 0 9/0/63711

The use of surfactant replacement therapy for both preventive and rescue treatment of respiratory distress syndrome has gained widespread acceptance.[1-6] Data from both individual large randomized trials[1-6] and meta-analyses[7-9] document that both for prevention and rescue use, surfactant therapy results in benefits (physiologic improvements, reduction in overall mortality, and reductions in air leak) that outweigh its possible risks (sepsis, pulmonary hemorrhage, and intraventricular hemorrhage). However, little information is available from randomized trials on the effects of surfactant replacement in infants at the edge of viability, who are at the greatest risk of poor outcome. One report suggested that prophylactic use of a modified bovine surfactant reduced mortality in infants weighing 600 to 750 gm,[10] but the study used a retrospective subgroup analysis from four centers participating in a 10-center trial. Examination of data from the entire cohort[11, 12] showed no reduction in overall mortality. Another report of a double-blind, randomized, placebo-controlled trial of prophylactic treatment with synthetic surfactant in infants weighing 500 to 699 gm demonstrated reductions in air leak and death from RDS but not in overall mortality.[13]

The purpose of this trial was to evaluate the safety and efficacy of two rescue doses of synthetic surfactant in infants at greatest risk for mortality and morbidity—the tiniest infants (500 to 749 gm) with RDS.

A-aPo$_2$	Alveolar-arterial oxygen tension gradient
a/APo$_2$	Arterial/alveolar oxygen tension ratio
AUC	Area under curve
BPD	Bronchopulmonary dysplasia
IVH	Intraventricular hemorrhage
PVED	Periventricular echodensities
RDS	Respiratory distress syndrome

METHODS

This prospective, multicenter, randomized, double-masked trial was conducted at 13 neonatal centers in Canada. Members of the Canadian Exosurf Neonatal Study Group are listed in Appendix III. The protocol was approved by the Ethics Review Board at each individual center in accordance with the guidelines of the Health Protection Branch, Health and Welfare, Canada. Except for birth weights, sample size, and the hypothesis to be tested, the design of this trial was identical to that of previously reported rescue trials with this synthetic surfactant.[5, 6]

Patient recruitment and enrollment. Infants with established RDS and birth weights of 500 to 749 gm who were born either in study hospitals or outside of study hospitals were eligible for study enrollment if they required mechanical ventilation, were at least 2 hours of age and less than 24 hours of age, and had an arterial to alveolar oxygen tension ratio (a/APo$_2$) of less than 0.22. The formula used to calculate alveolar oxygen tension and the inclusion and exclusion criteria for this study were identical to those previously described.[5, 6] On the basis of a predicted mortality of 57% in the control group, it was calculated that an enrollment of 198 patients would be required to provide a 90% chance of detecting a 40% relative reduction in mortality (from 57% to 30%) at the 0.05 level of significance. Eligible infants whose parents had granted informed consent were stratified into four groups according to gender and birth weight (500 to 625 gm and 626 to 749 gm). Within each stratum, infants were randomly assigned to receive up to two doses of either synthetic surfactant or air placebo (5 ml/kg of birth weight). The second dose was administered 12 hours after the initial dose to infants continuing to receive mechanical ventilation. Randomization was performed at each center by the selection of sequentially numbered opaque envelopes.

Preparation and administration of surfactant. The synthetic surfactant used in this trial was a mixture of colfosceril palmitate, cetyl alcohol, and tyloxapol formulated with sodium chloride as a lyophilized powder (Exosurf Neonatal, Burroughs Wellcome Co., Research Triangle Park, N.C.). Details of its formulation, in vitro surface-tension properties, toxicology, and reconstitution have been reported elsewhere.[14-16] The rationale for the choice of dose of synthetic surfactant and the methods of randomization and surfactant administration have been described previously.[5, 6] Synthetic surfactant or air placebo was administered by members of drug-administration teams who did not reveal the treatment administered or participate in the patients' subsequent clinical care.

Data collection. Data for each patient enrolled in the study were collected by a nurse coordinator and a neonatologist. At each participating center, data were collected on maternal demographics, medical and obstetric history, and details of the pregnancy, labor, and delivery. Patient data were collected for 28 days, commencing with the day that the initial dose of synthetic surfactant or air placebo was administered. Requirements for assisted ventilation and data on arterial blood gas values were recorded at 2, 6, and 12 hours after each dose of synthetic surfactant or air placebo and at the end of each 24-hour period after the first dose through 28 days of life. The a/APo$_2$ was calculated daily for the first 7 days. Cranial ultrasound examinations were performed within the first week, between days 12 and 16, and between days 26 and 30 and were repeated as necessary. All copies of cranial sonograms obtained during the first 28 days were sent for evaluation to the same pediatric radiologist (F. Volberg, MD, Bowman Gray School of Medicine, Winston-Salem, N.C.), who was blinded to treatment assignment. The severity of hemorrhage was classified according to the criteria of Papile et al.[17] Other complications of prematurity and the use of a number of medications also were recorded. Criteria for the diagnosis of other outcomes were identical to those reported previously.[5, 6]

Chest radiographs were obtained on days 1 and 28. The radiographs from day 1 were evaluated by attending clinicians, and those from day 28 were evaluated by one pediatric radiologist (F. Volberg, MD), who was blinded to treatment assignment. Each radiograph from day 28 was assigned a score based on the Edwards system of classification for the severity of bronchopulmonary dysplasia.[18] The diagnosis of BPD was based on a combination of clinical[19] and radiographic[20] criteria. Three criteria had to be satisfied: the presence of tachypnea and retractions; the need for supplemental oxygen to maintain the skin-surface oxygen tension at greater than 60 mm Hg or the pulse oximeter reading at greater than 85% saturation; and abnormalities on the chest radiograph with a score of higher than 4 on the Edwards scale. In infants who died before day 28 of life and for whom an autopsy was performed, a diagnosis of BPD was made according to the histologic criteria of Bonikos et al.[20] For the infants who died between days 10 and 28 of life for whom an autopsy was not performed, a diagnosis of BPD was made if, at the time of death, the infant required more than 60% oxygen and a mean airway pressure of 7 cm of water, had persistent abnormalities on chest radiographs, and had no other reason for respiratory failure.

Efficacy outcome measures. The principal efficacy outcome variable was death within 28 days of the initial study treatment. Two other major measures of efficacy included BPD and survival at 28 days without BPD. Secondary measures of efficacy included respiratory status assessments and duration assessments (number of days required to regain birth weight, number of days mechanical ventilation and supplemental oxygen was required, and number of days of hospitalization).

Safety outcome measures. The primary measure of safety was severe IVH, defined as grade III IVH and/or periventricular echodensities. As previously reported, rules for stopping the study were delineated in the protocol, and an independent advisory panel reviewed blinded data from the trial at 6-month intervals. The abnormal hematologic and blood chemistry values that first prompted treatment, the incidence and clinical significance of expected complications of prematurity, including patent ductus arteriosus, pulmonary air leak, necrotizing enterocolitis, IVH, and PVED, and the incidence of expected and unexpected adverse experiences, including pulmonary hemorrhage, were considered secondary measures of safety.

Cause of death. The primary cause of death in each infant was determined clinically by a physician blinded to treatment assignment. When an autopsy was performed, the cause of death reported by the pathologist, if different from the clinically determined cause, was used in the tabulations that follow.

Table I. Reasons for nonenrollment of patients with birth weights of 500 to 749 gm

Enrollment status	No. infants
Eligible by birth weight	491
Enrolled and randomized	224
Infants not entered	
Precipitous delivery/missed	4
Born outside of study hospital	9
Failure to meet inclusion/ exclusion criteria	177
Refused consent	18
Unstable	42
Reason not indicated	14
Entered other study	3
Total patients not enrolled	267

Follow-up. All infants were monitored until they were discharged from the hospital. Afterwards, patient contact was maintained through correspondence, telephone calls, and outpatient clinic visits. Comprehensive follow-up assessments were performed at 1, 2, and 3 years of age (adjusted for prematurity). The 1-year follow-up data are reported elsewhere in this supplement.[21] Only the 28-day outcome is reported here.

Statistical analyses. Incidence comparisons were made with Cochran-Mantel-Haenszel tests that used the original stratum of enrollment in the analysis.[22] Ventilator and oxygen requirements and alveolar-arterial oxygen tension gradients (A-aP_{O_2}) at 2 and 6 hours after entry were compared with use of nonpaired t tests. Ventilator and oxygen requirements and A-aP_{O_2} were compared by calculating the area under the curve, obtaining an average to achieve normal distribution, and then analyzing covariance with the baseline value as the covariate.[23] Results with p values less than 0.05 were accepted as statistically significant.

Efficacy comparisons (comparisons of the incidences of death, BPD, and survival without BPD) were made with all patients grouped according to original random assignments (intention-to-treat analysis). Safety comparisons and secondary efficacy comparisons were made with all patients grouped as actually treated, regardless of randomization, with no exclusions. The p values were calculated with use of Cochran-Mantel-Haenszel tests. Differences were considered significant when p values were less than 0.05.

RESULTS

Study accountability. Patient enrollment began in February 1988 and was completed in September 1990. During

Table II. Baseline characteristics of enrolled infants according to treatment group*

Characteristic	Air placebo (n = 111)	Synthetic surfactant (n = 113)
Birth weight (gm)	647 ± 62	644 ± 69
Gestational age (wk)	24.7 ± 1.5	25.1 ± 1.7
Sex		
Male	52	53
Female	59	60
Race		
White	93	94
Asian	4	9
Black	4	1
Hispanic	1	0
Native American	4	5
Other	5	4
Weight strata by sex (M/F)		
500 to 625 gm	15/25	16/27
626 to 749 gm	37/34	37/33
Delivery		
Abdominal	29	47
Vaginal	82	66
Multiple gestation	26	31
Prenatal cortico-steroids	19	26
Apgar score (median)		
1 min	2	3
5 min	6	6
Age at first dose (hr)	7.4 ± 5.1	7.3 ± 5.1
Peak inspiratory pressure (cm water)	22 ± 6	22 ± 5
Positive-end expiratory pressure (cm water)	4.4 ± 0.9	4.3 ± 0.8
Ventilator rate (breaths/min)	59 ± 20	58 ± 21
Fractional inspired oxygen	0.78 ± 0.21	0.79 ± 0.21
a/APo_2	0.11 ± 0.04	0.12 ± 0.05

*Plus-minus values are means ± SD. Infants are classified according to treatment they actually received.

those 32 months, 491 infants admitted to the 13 participating centers weighed less than 750 gm and had RDS. Of these infants, 267 were not enrolled for the reasons given in Table I. Of the 224 infants who entered the trial, 109 were randomly assigned to receive air placebo and 115 were randomly assigned to receive synthetic surfactant. Two infants randomly assigned to receive synthetic surfactant received the air placebo instead. Thus for the analyses based on actual treatment received (including baseline characteristics, the secondary measures of efficacy, and all safety-related outcomes), 111 infants received air placebo and 113 received synthetic surfactant.

Baseline comparability. The air placebo and synthetic surfactant groups were comparable in terms of the infants' demographic, physical, and clinical characteristics, except for the greater prevalence of abdominal delivery in the group treated with synthetic surfactant (42% vs 26%) (Table II). Age at first dose, ventilator settings, inspired oxygen tension, and a/APo_2 were also comparable (Table II).

Mortality, bronchopulmonary dysplasia, and survival with BPD. There was no significant difference in mortality rates at 28 days. The Kaplan-Meier survival curve appeared to show a slightly better survival rate from day 3 through 1 year of age for infants treated with synthetic surfactant (Fig. 1). Most of the 107 deaths occurred early: 56 deaths occurred within 1 day after treatment, and 89 occurred within 1 week after treatment. The difference in the incidence of BPD was not statistically significant (37% in the air placebo group vs 30% in the synthetic surfactant group, p = 0.089). Survival to 28 days without BPD was also not different in the two groups (17% in the air placebo group vs 26% in the synthetic surfactant group, p = 0.070) (Table III).

Causes of death. For days 1 through 28, the predominant cause of death for both treatment groups, as determined by physicians blinded to treatment assignment, was RDS (28% in the air placebo group vs 26% in the synthetic surfactant group). Death from pulmonary air leak occurred less frequently in the infants treated with surfactant (6% in the air placebo group vs 3% in the synthetic surfactant group), but deaths resulting from other causes occurred with similar frequencies in the two groups (Table IV). Of 29 deaths

Table III. Measures of efficacy in intention-to-treat population

Endpoint	No. patients (%) Air placebo (n = 109)	Synthetic surfactant (n = 115)	p value*
Death by day 10	49 (45)	46 (40)	0.430
Death by day 28	54 (50)	53 (46)	0.586
Death by 1 yr	65 (61)	66 (58)	0.615
BPD by day 28†	40 (37)	35 (30)	0.089
Survival at day 28 without BPD	18 (17)	30 (26)	0.070

*For comparison between treatment groups.
†BPD whether alive or dead at day 28.

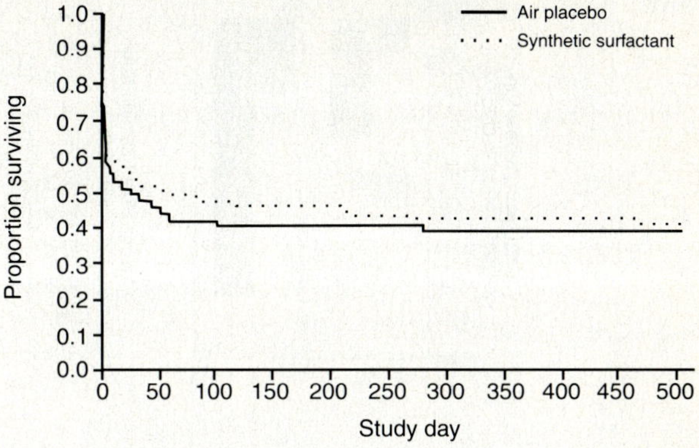

Fig. 1. Kaplan-Meier survival curve for infants with birth weights of 500 to 749 gm in trial of synthetic surfactant or air placebo for established RDS.

Table IV. Causes of death (intention to treat)

Cause of death	Air placebo (n = 109)	Synthetic surfactant (n = 115)
Days 1 to 28		
Sepsis	2	3
IVH	5	4
Pulmonary air leak	7	4
BPD	0	2
Necrotizing enterocolitis	0	1
RDS	30	29
Other	10	10
Total early deaths	54	53
Day 29 to 1-year adjusted age		
Sepsis	0	1
BPD	8	5
RDS	0	1
Other	3	6
Total late deaths	11	13

classified as resulting from other causes, 16 were attributed to "prematurity." BPD was an equally common cause of late death in both treatment groups (day 29 to 1-year adjusted age: 17% in the air placebo group vs 6% in the synthetic surfactant group).

Severity of RDS: Physiologic changes. A significant reduction in inspired oxygen concentration was demonstrated in the synthetic surfactant group at 2 hours after the initial dose, which was the first time point assessed (Fig. 2). A significant difference in A-aPo_2 in the synthetic surfactant group was demonstrated 6 hours after treatment, which was the second time point assessed. Significant differences in mean airway pressure were observed after 6 hours. AUC calculations for oxygen requirements were significantly improved through 7 days (p = 0.008) in the synthetic surfactant group (Fig. 3). The AUCs for a/APo_2 (p = 0.006) and A-aPo_2 (p = 0.008) were also significantly improved through day 7. Peak inspiratory pressure was significantly improved through 48 hours (p = 0.05), and mean airway pressure was significantly improved through 48 hours (p = 0.037) but not through day 7 (p = 0.073). The difference in ventilatory rate through 7 days also was not significant (p = 0.064). The median and mean ages at which infants in the air placebo group and the synthetic surfactant group were removed from various forms of respiratory support were not different.

Safety. There were no differences between the air placebo and synthetic surfactant groups with respect to other complications of prematurity and RDS, including various forms of pulmonary air leak, IVH, PVED, patent ductus arteriosus, sepsis, and necrotizing enterocolitis. The use of various medications in the two groups also did not differ (data not shown). All other safety-related outcomes, including apnea and pulmonary hemorrhage, did not differ significantly (Table V).

DISCUSSION

Two rescue doses of synthetic surfactant given 12 hours apart did not significantly reduce neonatal mortality (50% in the air placebo group vs 46% in the synthetic surfactant group) in premature infants with RDS and birth weights of 500 to 749 gm. Similarly, reductions in the major complications of RDS, including air leak, BPD, and IVH, were not observed. However, two rescue doses of synthetic surfactant resulted in physiologic benefits in these extremely premature infants with RDS.

As in other rescue clinical trials with synthetic surfactant, infants randomly assigned to receive two rescue doses of synthetic surfactant had reduced oxygen requirements and improved a/APo_2, A-aPo_2, mean airway pressures, and mechanical ventilation rates shortly after administration; these beneficial effects persisted for the first days of life.

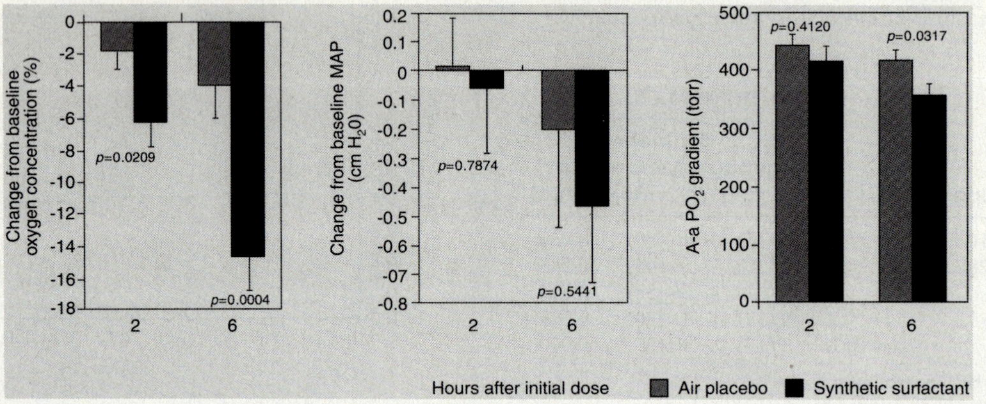

Fig. 2. Changes from baseline values in oxygen concentration, mean airway pressure (MAP), and the A-aPO_2 at 2 and 6 hours after initial dose of synthetic surfactant or air placebo.

Table V. Complications of prematurity and RDS according to treatment received

Outcome	Air placebo (n = 111)	Synthetic surfactant (n = 113)	Relative risk*	95% Confidence interval
Pneumothorax	31	30	1.04	0.68-1.59
Pneumomediastinum	2	4	0.52	0.10-2.67
Pulmonary interstitial emphysema	44	44	1.00	0.73-1.39
Pneumopericardium	2	1	1.94	0.19-20.25
Any form of air leak	58	58	1.04	0.81-1.34
IVH	35	37	0.94	0.67-1.33
Grade III IVH	8	12	0.68	0.29-1.56
PVED	10	7	1.40	0.55-3.56
Grade III IVH or PVED	14	13	1.07	0.53-2.17
Seizures	6	12	0.51	0.20-1.28
Patent ductus arteriosus	65	63	1.05	0.85-1.30
Necrotizing enterocolitis	4	2	1.98	0.38-10.30
Sepsis	20	22	0.91	0.53-1.57
Nosocomial pneumonia	4	4	1.03	0.26-4.07
Meningitis	0	2	0.00	
Arterial hypotension	76	84	0.92	0.78-1.08
Apnea of prematurity	31	26	1.19	0.76-1.86
Pulmonary hemorrhage	3	3	1.02	0.21-4.91

*A relative risk of >1.00 indicates lower risk with synthetic surfactant.

Beneficial effects relating to gas exchange and oxygen requirements persisted for the first 7 days of life, as seen in larger infants.[5, 6] However, in these extremely tiny infants, unlike in larger infants,[5, 6] the beneficial effects of two rescue doses of synthetic surfactant on peak inspiratory pressure, mean airway pressure, and ventilatory rate disappeared after 2 to 3 days. The onset of improvements in mean airway pressures 6 hours after administration in infants in this weight class is consistent with the findings of Stevenson et al.[13] after the administration of a single prophylactic dose of synthetic surfactant in infants weighing 500 to 699 gm. Unlike other randomized trials with this synthetic surfactant, in this trial the physiologic improvements observed were not accompanied by reductions in the common complications of prematurity and RDS such as pneumothorax, pulmonary interstitial emphysema, BPD, IVH, or death.

The major efficacy outcomes that came closest to a significant improvement were BPD and survival at day 28 without BPD. These outcomes are of major clinical significance in extremely low birth weight infants. The criteria for diagnosis of BPD, which were based on a combination of clinical and radiographic findings, were more stringent in this trial than in other surfactant trials (usually the need for supplemental oxygen alone at day 28 or the same plus an

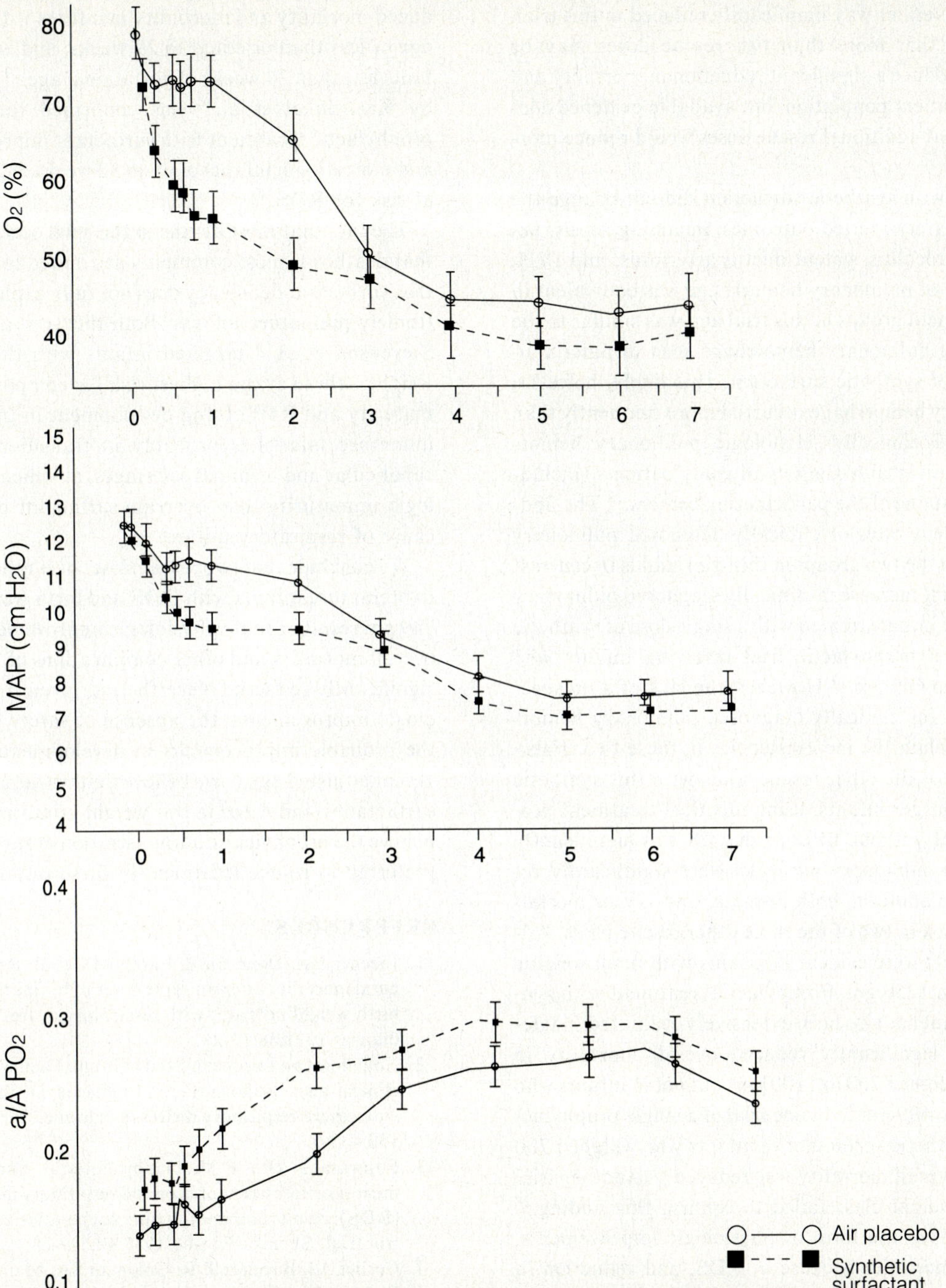

Fig. 3. Fraction of inspired oxygen (FiO_2), mean airway pressure (MAP), and a/APo_2 during a 7-day period in infants given synthetic surfactant or air placebo.

"abnormal" chest radiograph). The ability to detect significant differences in intact cardiopulmonary survival and in other neonatal outcomes was hampered by the relatively small sample size; the chance of a type II error may be high. A prophylactic study with a single dose of this same synthetic surfactant and a similar sample size showed a significant reduction in the incidence of pneumothorax and death from RDS in tiny infants with birth weights of 500 to 699 gm.[13] Neither was significantly reduced in this trial. It is possible that more than two rescue doses may be required to produce a significant reduction in mortality and BPD in this patient population, but available evidence does not suggest that additional rescue doses would reduce mortality.[24, 25]

Treatment with synthetic surfactant did not change the incidence of safety-related outcomes, including sepsis, necrotizing enterocolitis, patent ductus arteriosus, and IVH. The incidence of pulmonary hemorrhage was equivalent in the two treatment groups in this trial and was similar to the overall rate of pulmonary hemorrhage seen in other controlled trials of synthetic surfactant. It is likely, however, that pulmonary hemorrhage occurred more frequently than was diagnosed clinically. Histologic pulmonary hemorrhage was a universal finding in all study patients (including controls) at one of the participating centers.[23] The finding of equivalent rates of clinically diagnosed pulmonary hemorrhage in the two groups in this trial stands in contrast to the significant increase in clinically diagnosed pulmonary hemorrhage in infants treated with a single dose of synthetic surfactant in a prophylactic trial involving infants who weighed 500 to 699 gm.[13] However, the lack of a prospective definition for clinically diagnosed pulmonary hemorrhage may explain the inconsistencies in these two trials.

In all three of the other rescue trials with this synthetic surfactant in larger infants, using identical treatment protocols, survival without BPD at day 28 was significantly improved and pulmonary air leaks were significantly reduced.[5, 6, 26] In addition, both neonatal and 1-year mortality were reduced in two of the three other rescue trials. Additional benefits were evident in infants with birth weights of greater than 1250 gm. Prophylactic treatment with synthetic surfactant has also been extensively evaluated: single-dose therapy significantly reduced overall mortality in infants who weighed 700 to 1100 gm[4] but not in infants who weighed 500 to 699 gm.[13] In one trial of a single prophylactic dose of synthetic surfactant in infants who weighed 700 to 1350 gm, overall mortality was reduced.[27] Another trial in the same weight class failed to confirm this finding.[28] Other benefits, in the form of physiologic improvements, reduction in mortality because of RDS, and reduction in pulmonary air leaks, were demonstrated in all the prophylactic trials.

In a large international open trial, the OSIRIS collaborative group showed that early intervention with synthetic surfactant therapy was more effective than delayed selective administration in more than 6700 infants with an average gestational age of 28 weeks.[25] Advantages of prophylactic therapy versus rescue therapy in very premature infants were also demonstrated by Kendig et al.[29] in a trial of modified bovine surfactant in which prophylactic therapy reduced mortality and morbidity in infants with a gestational age of less than or equal to 29 weeks, and especially in infants less than 26 weeks of gestational age.[29] A larger study by Kattwinkel et al.[30] has confirmed the finding that prophylactic treatment with surfactant improves morbidity and mortality in infants of up to 32 weeks of gestational age at risk for RDS.[30]

The fact that most deaths in this trial occurred early and that death was most commonly attributed to RDS suggests that surfactant deficiency does not fully explain RDS in extremely premature infants. Both this trial and the trial of Stevenson et al.[13] targeted infants with the lowest birth weight—those at the highest risk for complications of prematurity and RDS. Lung development in these extremely immature infants is probably in transition between the canalicular and terminal sac stages, at which time morphologic immaturity may override surfactant deficiency as a cause of respiratory failure.

We conclude that two rescue doses of synthetic surfactant in premature infants with RDS and birth weights of 500 to 749 gm result in acute physiologic improvements. However, overall mortality and other complications of RDS were not significantly reduced. Nevertheless, given the acute physiologic improvements, the absence of safety problems, and the probable improvements in developmental outcome at 1-year adjusted age,[21] we believe that rescue use of synthetic surfactant is indicated in this weight group as well. We also believe the prophylactic administration of surfactant is to be preferred to rescue treatment in these tiny infants.[29, 30]

REFERENCES

1. Liechty EA, Donovan E, Purohit D, et al. Reduction of neonatal mortality after multiple doses of bovine surfactant in low birth weight neonates with respiratory distress syndrome. Pediatrics 1991;88:19-28.
2. Collaborative European Study Group. Factors influencing the clinical response to surfactant replacement therapy in babies with severe respiratory distress syndrome. Eur J Pediatr 1991; 150:433-9.
3. Fujiwara T, Onishi M, Nanby H, et al. Surfactant supplementation treatment of neonatal respiratory distress syndrome (RDS): results of a multifacility cooperative comparative control trial. Shonika Rinsho 1987;40:549-68.
4. Corbet AJ, Bucciarelli R, Goldman SA, Mammel MA, Wold D, Long WA. Decreased mortality in small premature infants treated at birth with a single dose of synthetic surfactant: a multicenter trial. J Pediatr 1991;118:277-84.
5. Long WA, Thompson T, Sundell H, Schumacher R, Volberg F, Guthrie R. Effects of two rescue doses of a synthetic surfactant on mortality in 700-1300 gram infants with RDS. J Pediatr 1991;118:595-605.
6. Long W, Cotton R, Corbet A, et al. A controlled trial of synthetic surfactant in infants weighing 1250 g or more with respiratory distress syndrome. N Engl J Med 1991;325:1696-703.
7. Jobe AH. Pulmonary surfactant therapy. N Engl J Med 1993; 328:861-8.

8. Merritt TA, Soll RF, Hallman M. Overview of exogenous surfactant replacement therapy. J Intens Care Med 1993;8:205-28.
9. Soll RF, McQueen MM. Respiratory distress syndrome. In: Sinclair J, Bracken M, eds. Effective care of the newborn infant. New York: Oxford University Press, 1992;325-58.
10. Ferrara TB, Hoekstra RE, Couser RJ, et al. Effects of surfactant therapy on outcome of infants with birth weights of 600-750 grams. J PEDIATR 1991;119:455-8.
11. Hoekstra RE, Jackson JC, Myers TF, et al. Improved neonatal survival following multiple doses of bovine surfactant in very premature neonates at risk for respiratory distress syndrome. Pediatrics 1991;88:910-8.
12. Berry D. Should tiny babies be treated with surfactant? In: Long WA, Tilson HH, eds. Proceedings of the Exosurf Neonatal Treatment IND Investigators' Meeting, November 13-14, 1991. Langhorne, Pa.: Adis International, 1992:37-44.
13. Stevenson D, Walther F, Long W, et al. Controlled trial of a single dose of synthetic surfactant at birth in premature infants weighing 500 to 699 grams. J PEDIATR 1992;120(suppl):S3-12.
14. Long WA, Sanders RL. New treatment methods in idiopathic respiratory distress syndrome: replacement of surface active material. Clin Crit Care Med 1988;13:21-56.
15. Durand DJ, Clyman RI, Heymann MA, et al. Effects of a protein-free synthetic surfactant on the survival and pulmonary function of preterm lambs. J PEDIATR 1985;107:775-80.
16. Tooley WH, Clements JA, Muramatsu K, Brown CL, Schlueter MA. Lung function in prematurely delivered rabbits treated with a synthetic surfactant. Am Rev Respir Dis 1987; 136:651-6.
17. Papile L, Burstein J, Burstein R, Koffler H. Incidence and evolution of subependymal and intraventricular hemorrhage: a study of infants with birth weights less than 1500 grams. J PEDIATR 1978;92:529-34.
18. Edwards DK. Radiology of hyaline membrane disease transient tachypnea of the newborn and bronchopulmonary dysplasia. In: Farrell PM, ed. Lung development: biological and clinical perspectives, vol 2. New York: Academic Press, 1982:47-89.
19. O'Brodovich HM, Mellins RB. Bronchopulmonary dysplasia. Am Rev Respir Dis 1985;132:694-709.
20. Bonikos DS, Bensch KG, Northway WH, et al. Bronchopulmonary dysplasia: the pulmonary pathologic sequel of necrotizing bronchiolitis and pulmonary fibrosis. Hum Pathol 1976;7:643-66.
21. Casiro O, Bingham W, MacMurray B, et al. One-year follow-up of 89 infants with birth weights of 500 to 749 grams and respiratory distress syndrome randomized to two rescue doses of synthetic surfactant or air placebo. J PEDIATR 1995;126:S53-60.
22. Fleiss JL. Statistical methods for rates and proportions. New York: John Wiley and Sons, 1981:160-87.
23. Smyth J, McFadden D, Fitzgerald C, MacKinnon M. Histological pulmonary hemorrhage in respiratory distress syndrome: effect of Exosurf treatment [Abstract]. Pediatr Res 1991;29:330A.
24. Long WA, Merritt A, Kanto W, et al. Randomized comparison of three vs six doses of synthetic surfactant in 348 infants weighing <750 grams [Abstract]. Pediatr Res 1992;31:314A.
25. The OSIRIS Collaborative Group. Early versus delayed neonatal administration of synthetic surfactant: the judgment of OSIRIS. Lancet 1992;340:1363-9.
26. McMillan D, Chernick V, Finer N, et al. Effects of two rescue doses of synthetic surfactant in 344 infants with respiratory distress syndrome weighing 750 to 1249 grams: a double-blind, placebo-controlled multicenter Canadian trial. J PEDIATR 1995;126:S90-8.
27. Corbet AJ, Long WA, Murphy DJ, Garcia-Prats JA, Lombardy DL, Wold DE. Reduced mortality in small premature infants treated at birth with a single dose of synthetic surfactant. J Paediatr Child Health 1991;27:245-9.
28. Bose C, Corbet A, Bose G, et al. Improved outcome at 28 days of very low birth weight infants treated with a single dose of synthetic surfactant. J PEDIATR 1990;117:947-53.
29. Kendig J, Notter RH, Cox C, et al. A comparison of surfactant as immediate prophylaxis and as rescue therapy in newborns of less than 30 weeks gestation. N Engl J Med 1991; 324:865-71.
30. Kattwinkel J, Bloom T, Delmore P, et al. Prophylactic administration of calf lung surfactant extract is more effective than early treatment of respiratory distress syndrome in neonates of 29 through 32 weeks gestation. Pediatrics 1993;92:90-8.

Effects of two rescue doses of synthetic surfactant in 344 infants with respiratory distress syndrome weighing 750 to 1249 grams: A double-blind, placebo-controlled multicenter Canadian trial

Douglas McMillan, MD, Victor Chernick, MD, Neil Finer, MD, David Schiff, MD, Harry Bard, MD, John Watts, MD, Robert Krzeski, MD, Walker Long, MD, and the Canadian Exosurf Neonatal Study Group (see Appendix III)

From Foothills Hospital, Calgary, Alberta, Canada; Health Sciences Centre and St. Boniface Hospital, Winnipeg, Manitoba, Canada; Royal Alexandra Hospital, Edmonton, Alberta, Canada; Walter MacKenzie Health Sciences Centre, Edmonton, Alberta, Canada; St. Justine Hospital, Montreal, Quebec, Canada; Chedoke-McMaster Hospitals, Hamilton, Ontario, Canada; and the Department of Pediatrics, University of North Carolina at Chapel Hill

In a multicenter, double-blind, placebo-controlled rescue trial conducted at 13 Canadian hospitals, two 5 ml/kg doses of a synthetic surfactant or air placebo were administered to 344 infants with birth weights of 750 to 1249 gm who had established respiratory distress syndrome and an arterial/alveolar oxygen tension ratio less than 0.22. The first dose was given between 2 and 24 hours of age, and the second dose was given 12 hours later to the infants remaining on mechanical ventilation. Infants were stratified at study entry by birth weight and gender. The trial was terminated short of the targeted sample size because significant reductions in mortality were observed in another rescue trial completed in the United States in the same weight class of infants. Despite premature termination of the trial, the rate of survival without bronchopulmonary dysplasia was increased (61% vs 52%; $p = 0.046$) in infants treated with surfactant. In addition, there was a significant reduction in the incidence of overall pulmonary air leak (46% vs 32%; $p = 0.009$), pneumothorax (27% vs 17%; $p = 0.023$), and pulmonary interstitial emphysema (40% vs 28%; $p = 0.018$) in infants treated with synthetic surfactant. There was no difference in the incidence of bronchopulmonary dysplasia, apnea, or pulmonary hemorrhage. Significant improvements in alveolar-arterial oxygen tension gradient, arterial/alveolar oxygen tension ratio, and oxygen and ventilator requirements through day 7 were present. These findings indicate that rescue therapy with synthetic surfactant can improve outcome for premature infants weighing 750 to 1249 gm with respiratory distress syndrome. (J Pediatr 1995;126:S90-8)

The efficacy of exogenous synthetic surfactant treatment in small, middle-sized, and large infants has been demonstrated in large, multicenter, randomized trials.[1-8] Data from these trials show that synthetic surfactant, administered as both prophylactic and rescue therapy, saves lives and decreases the severity and complications of respiratory distress syndrome. Data from one previous open, randomized trial with a bovine surfactant extract indicated that multiple-dose prophylactic treatment was more efficacious than multiple-dose rescue treatment in infants less than 30

Reprint requests: Douglas McMillan, MD, Foothills Hospital, Room C211, 1403 29 Street NW, Calgary, Alberta, Canada T2N 2T9.

0022-3476/95/$3.00 + 0 **9/0/63712**

A-aPo$_2$	Alveolar-arterial oxygen tension gradient
a/APo$_2$	Arterial/alveolar oxygen tension ratio
AUC	Area under curve
BPD	Bronchopulmonary dysplasia
IVH	Intraventricular hemorrhage
PVED	Periventricular echodensities
RDS	Respiratory distress syndrome

weeks of gestational age.[9] Subsequent studies have confirmed that the prophylactic approach in small, premature infants results in a better outcome.[10-12] Nevertheless, some premature infants will be born in centers that are not prepared for prophylactic administration of surfactant, and these infants will have to be treated with the rescue approach.

The objective of this study was to determine if rescue treatment with two doses of synthetic surfactant administered 12 hours apart (with the first dose between 2 and 24 hours of age) to infants weighing 750 to 1249 gm at birth who have RDS and are on mechanical ventilation with an arterial/alveolar oxygen tension ratio (a/APo$_2$) of less than 0.22 would improve the rate of survival without bronchopulmonary dysplasia at 28 days of life, an outcome termed "intact cardiopulmonary survival."

METHODS

The trial, designed as a prospective, multicenter, randomized, double-masked study, was conducted at 13 hospitals in Canada (members of the Canadian Exosurf Neonatal Study Group are listed in Appendix III). The protocol was approved by the Ethics Review Board at each hospital in accordance with the guidelines of the Health Protection Branch, Health and Welfare, Canada. The targeted enrollment was 400 babies, a sample size calculated to provide 90% power in detection of a 40% relative improvement in infant cardiopulmonary survival. Patients were enrolled in the study from January 1988 through July 1989. The study was stopped in July 1989 before completion of its target enrollment because, in another trial in the United States,[1] two rescue doses of synthetic surfactant were shown to improve survival rates of infants with RDS who weighed 700 to 1350 gm.

Patient enrollment. Infants with established RDS who were admitted to a study hospital were eligible for study enrollment at that hospital if they weighed at least 750 gm but less than 1250 gm, were at least 2 hours and less than 24 hours of age, were receiving mechanical ventilation, and had an a/APo$_2$ of less than 0.22. The formulas used to calculate alveolar oxygen tension and the exclusion criteria for this study were identical to those described in earlier rescue trials of synthetic surfactant.[1, 2] Infants whose parents had granted informed consent were stratified into four groups according to birth weight (750 to 999 gm and 1000 to 1249 gm) and gender. Separate boxes of sequential opaque, sealed envelopes for each of the four strata were used to ensure masking. Within each stratum, infants were randomly assigned to receive two doses of either synthetic surfactant or air placebo (5 ml/kg of birth weight). The second dose was administered 12 hours after the initial dose to all infants who remained on the ventilator.

The exogenous surfactant used in this trial was a totally synthetic surfactant (colfosceril palmitate, cetyl alcohol, and tyloxapol; Exosurf Neonatal, Burroughs Wellcome Co., Research Triangle Park, N.C.). Details of its formulation, in vitro surface-tension properties, toxicology, and reconstitution have been reported elsewhere.[13-15] The rationale for the choice of dose of surfactant and the methods of randomization and surfactant administration have been described previously.[1, 2] Treatment with synthetic surfactant or air placebo was administered by study personnel who did not participate in subsequent care of the patient. Masking was maintained through completion of a 3-year follow-up study.

Data collection. Maternal demographics, medical and obstetric history, and details of the pregnancy, labor, and delivery were recorded by the nurse coordinator or neonatologist. Assessments of ventilation settings and arterial blood gas values were recorded at 2, 6, and 12 hours after each administration period and at the end of each 24-hour period after the first dose, through 28 days of life. The a/APo$_2$ ratio was calculated from each arterial blood gas analysis through day 7. Daily fluid intake was recorded through day 7.

Chest radiographs were obtained on days 1 and 28; the radiographs from day 1 were evaluated by attending clinicians, and all the radiographs obtained on day 28 were interpreted by the same pediatric radiologist, who was blinded to treatment. For each radiograph obtained on day 28, a score was assigned on the basis of the Edwards system of classification for the severity of BPD.[16] All infants underwent cranial ultrasound examinations between days 5 and 7, days 12 and 16, and days 26 and 30; ultrasonography was repeated as necessary. Copies of all cranial sonograms obtained during the first 28 days were forwarded to the same pediatric radiologist for double-blind evaluation. The severity of hemorrhage was classified as subependymal hemorrhage (grade I), intraventricular hemorrhage without ventricular dilation (grade II), IVH with dilation (grade III), or periventricular echodensities. Other complications of prematurity and the use of various medications were also recorded. Patent ductus arteriosus was assessed clinically daily through 28 days of life; criteria used for the diagnosis of patent ductus arteriosus, as well as other outcomes, have been described elsewhere.[1, 2]

Intact cardiopulmonary survival. Intact cardiopulmonary

Table I. Enrollment of patients with birth weights of 750 to 1249 gm

Enrollment status	No. patients
Eligible on the basis of weight and diagnosis	924
Enrolled and randomly assigned	344
Not enrolled	
Failure to meet inclusion exclusion criteria	513
Parents declined consent	28
Unstable	24
Missed*	15
Total not enrolled	580

*Missed indicates patients who were eligible but not enrolled.

survival was defined prospectively as survival without BPD at 28 days of life. The diagnosis of BPD was based on a combination of clinical[17] and radiographic[16] criteria. Three criteria had to be satisfied: the presence of tachypnea and retractions; the need for supplemental oxygen to maintain the skin-surface oxygen tension above 60 mm Hg or the pulse oximeter reading above 85% saturation; and abnormalities on a chest radiograph with a score of 4 or higher on the Edwards scale.[16] In infants who died before 28 days of life and for whom autopsies were performed, BPD was diagnosed by the histologic criteria of Bonikos et al.[18] For the infants who died between 10 and 28 days of life and did not undergo a postmortem examination, BPD was diagnosed if, at the time of death, they required more than 60% oxygen and a mean airway pressure of 7 cm of water, they had persistent abnormalities on chest radiographs, and there was no other reason for respiratory failure.

Other complications of prematurity. Other common safety-related outcomes and their respective protocol definitions were described previously.[1, 2] Pulmonary hemorrhage was not defined prospectively, but data on its incidence were collected prospectively.

Efficacy measurements. The principal efficacy outcome was intact cardiopulmonary survival (survival without BPD at day 28). Other major efficacy endpoints included death and BPD. Secondary measures of efficacy included respiratory status assessments and duration assessments (number of days to regain birth weight, number of days mechanical ventilation and supplemental oxygen were required, and number of days of hospitalization).

For all patient deaths, the primary cause of death was determined clinically by a physician who was unaware of the patient's treatment. When a postmortem examination was performed, the cause of death determined at autopsy was substituted for the clinical cause of death in the tabulations that follow.

Safety measurements. The principal measure of safety was severe IVH, defined as grade III IVH and/or PVED. Other secondary measures of safety included the first abnormal hematologic and blood chemistry values that required specific treatment, incidence and severity of expected complications of prematurity, including patent ductus arteriosus, pulmonary air leak, necrotizing enterocolitis, IVH, PVED, BPD, and incidence of expected and unexpected adverse experiences, including pulmonary hemorrhage.

An independent advisory panel monitored the conduct of the trial and could stop the study for safety reasons. The panel, which reviewed double-blind data at 6-month intervals during the study, was empowered to break the code if an excess of cases of severe IVH (grade III and/or PVED) occurred in either group and to stop the study if the excess of cases of severe IVH proved to have occurred in the group treated with surfactant.

Follow-up. All infants were monitored throughout their hospital course. After discharge from the hospital, patient contact was maintained through correspondence, telephone calls, and outpatient clinic visits until the age of 3 years (adjusted for prematurity). At that time pertinent information with regard to hospital readmissions, surgery, oxygen and ventilator requirements, retinal examinations, and a complete physical and neurodevelopmental assessment were performed. Follow-up data through 1-year adjusted age for infants enrolled in this trial are reported elsewhere in this supplement.[19]

Statistical analyses. Incidence comparisons were made with Cochran-Mantel-Haenszel tests that used the original stratum of enrollment in the analysis.[20] Ventilator and oxygen requirements and alveolar-arterial oxygen tension gradients (A-aP_{O_2}) at 2 and 6 hours after entry were compared with use of the nonpaired *t*-test. Ventilator and oxygen requirements and A-aP_{O_2} were compared by calculating areas under the curve, obtaining an average to achieve normal distribution, and then analyzing covariance with the baseline value as the covariant.[21] Results with *p* values less than 0.05 were accepted as statistically significant.

Major efficacy comparisons (comparisons of the incidences of death, BPD, and survival without BPD) were made with all randomized patients grouped as actually treated. Randomized patients who were not treated were grouped with the patients who received air placebo. A supplemental analysis of efficacy was made according to original random assignments (intention-to-treat analysis). Safety comparisons and secondary efficacy comparisons were also made with all patients grouped as actually treated. Safety comparisons were expressed as relative risks with 95% confidence intervals. For 95% confidence intervals that did not overlap 1 (that is, those that were statistically significant), *p* values were calculated with the use of Cochran-Mantel-Haenszel tests.

Table II. Measures of efficacy

	As treated			Intention to treat		
	No. patients (%)			No. patients (%)		
Endpoint	Air placebo (*n* = 170)	Synthetic surfactant (*n* = 174)	*p* value	Air placebo (*n* = 168)	Synthetic surfactant (*n* = 176)	*p* value
Intact cardiopulmonary survival	87 (51)	108 (62)	0.046	87	107*	0.068
Death by day 28	42 (25)	34 (21)	0.266	40	36	0.455
BPD†	46 (34)	38 (26)	0.099	46	38	0.304

*BPD was not assessed in 1 surviving patient.
†Includes infants who died and had BPD as well as infants who survived with BPD.

Table III. Baseline characteristics of enrolled infants according to treatment group*

Characteristic	Air placebo (*n* = 170)	Synthetic surfactant (*n* = 174)
Birth weight (gm)	983 ± 137	992 ± 146
Gestational age (wk)	27.4 ± 1.8	27.5 ± 1.9
Maternal age (yr)	27 ± 6	27 ± 5
Sex		
Male	100	103
Female	70	71
Race		
Non-Hispanic white	146	148
Black	0	1
Asian	9	11
Native American	10	9
Other	5	5
Delivery		
Abdominal	81	87
Vaginal	89	87
Multiple gestation	55	54
Place of birth		
In study hospital	144	150
Outside study hospital	26	24
Membranes ruptured before delivery	66	60
Prenatal corticosteroids >24 hr	33	28
Apgar score (median)		
1 min	3	4
5 min	7	6
Age at first dose (min)	484 ± 291	456 ± 290
Peak inspiratory pressure (cm water)	23 ± 6	23 ± 7
Positive end-expiratory pressure (cm water)	4.7 ± 2.0	4.5 ± 0.8
Ventilator rate (breaths/min)	53 ± 21	52 ± 22
Percent inspired oxygen	75 ± 21	79 ± 19
a/AP_{O_2}†	0.13 ± 0.05	0.12 ± 0.04

*Plus-minus values are mean ± SD. Infants are classified according to the treatment they actually received.
†Up to 4 hr before study entry.

Table IV. Cause of death according to treatment received: day 1 through day 28

Cause of death	Air placebo (*n* = 170)	Synthetic surfactant (*n* = 174)
Days 1 to 28		
RDS	21	13
Pulmonary air leaks	5	7
IVH	4	1
BPD	2	4
Necrotizing enterocolitis	0	2
Sepsis	3	2
Other	7	5
Total early deaths	42	34
Day 29 to 1-year adjusted age		
Sepsis	1	1
IVH	0	1
BPD	3	5
Necrotizing enterocolitis	0	1
Other	1	5
Total late deaths	5	13

RESULTS

In accordance with the original design of the trial, the independent advisory panel reviewed data from the trial on three occasions and determined that the trial should proceed. The trial was stopped jointly by the sponsor (Burroughs Wellcome Inc., Montreal, Canada) and the Health Protection Branch after 344 patients (86%) were enrolled because of reductions in mortality observed in another rescue trial completed in the United States in the same weight class,[1] as well as similar reductions in morbidity and mortality observed in a second rescue trial conducted in larger infants.[2]

During the enrollment period, 924 infants were eligible for the study by virtue of their weight and diagnosis of RDS. Of these infants, 580 were not enrolled for the reasons shown in Table I; the remaining 344 infants entered the trial. A total of 168 infants were randomly assigned to re-

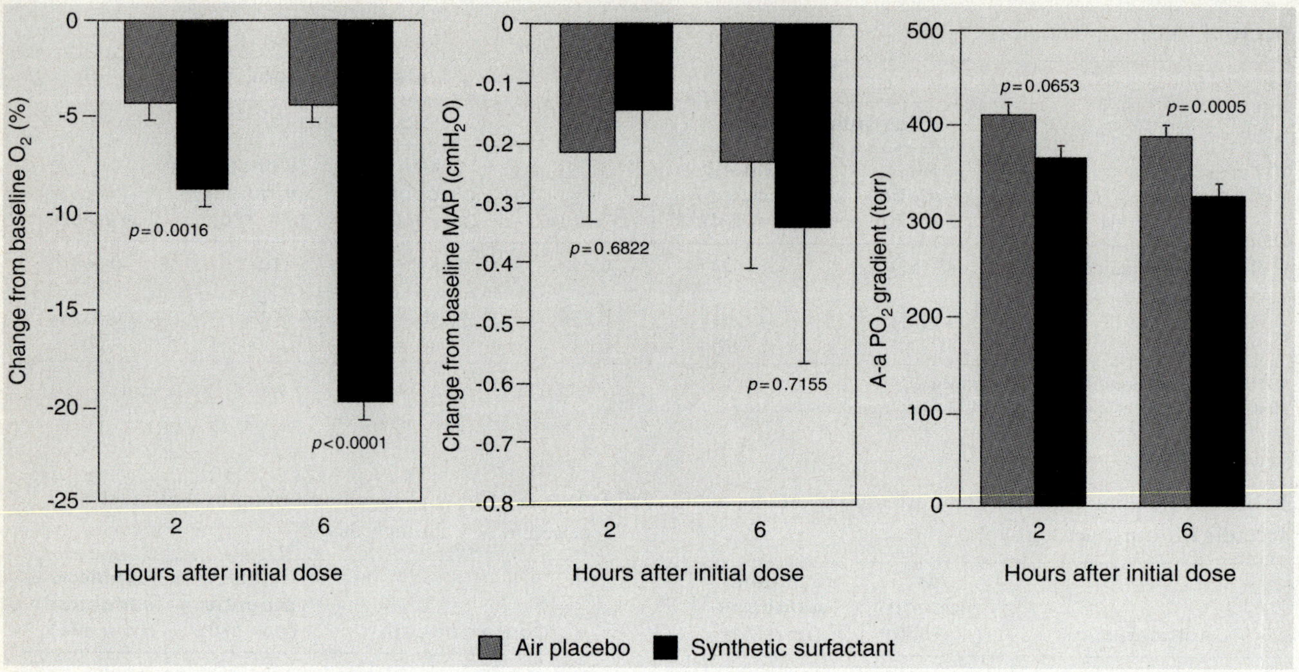

Fig. 1. Changes from baseline values in inspired oxygen concentration (O_2), mean airway pressure (MAP), and A-aPo_2 at 2 and 6 hours after initial dose of air placebo or synthetic surfactant.

ceive air placebo, and 176 were randomly assigned to receive synthetic surfactant; because of errors, two infants received air instead of synthetic surfactant. Thus for the intention-to-treat (as randomized) analysis of the principal efficacy outcome (survival without BPD at 28 days of age and the two other major efficacy endpoints [death and BPD]), there were 168 patients in the placebo group and 176 in the surfactant group (Table II). All other analyses, including the safety analyses and baseline characteristics, were "as treated" with 170 patients in the air placebo group and 174 in the synthetic surfactant group (Tables III, IV, and V).

The randomization procedure was successful in that the air placebo and synthetic surfactant groups were comparable in terms of the infants' demographic, physical, and clinical characteristics, as well as age at baseline, ventilator settings, and inspired oxygen tension (Table III).

Intact cardiopulmonary survival, overall mortality, and neonatal death or survival with BPD. Intact cardiopulmonary survival (survival at day 28 without BPD) was improved in the synthetic surfactant group (as treated analysis, $p = 0.046$); the difference was not statistically significant in the supplemental (intention to treat) analysis ($p = 0.068$). Mortality at days 10 and 28 did not differ between the air placebo and synthetic surfactant groups in either analysis. In addition, there was no difference in the incidence of BPD in either analysis (Table II).

Causes of death. The primary causes of death, as determined by physicians blinded to treatment assignments, are listed in Table IV. There were no significant differences in cause of death between the placebo and surfactant groups through 28 days or from day 29 to 1 year adjusted age. The most common cause of death during the neonatal period was RDS. The most common cause of death during the period from day 29 through 1-year adjusted age was BPD.

Onset and duration of action. Treatment with synthetic surfactant was associated with a significant reduction in inspired oxygen concentration at the first time point recorded, 2 hours (Fig. 1). The A-aPo_2 was improved significantly at 6 hours after treatment, the second time point recorded. Significant improvements in mean airway pressure occurred after 6 hours. These beneficial effects of synthetic surfactant persisted over the first week of life. AUC calculations for oxygen requirements ($p = 0.0001$), peak inspiratory pressure ($p = 0.0078$), mean airway pressure ($p = 0.0017$), and rate of mechanical ventilation ($p = 0.0002$) were significantly improved throughout the first 7 days in the surfactant group (Fig. 2). In addition, the AUC for a/APo_2 ($p = 0.0001$) and A-aPo_2 ($p = 0.0001$) were significantly improved through 7 days. The median and mean ages at which infants were removed from various forms of respiratory support were not different in the placebo and surfactant groups (data not shown).

Safety. Pneumothorax, pulmonary interstitial emphysema, and overall pulmonary air leak were significantly less frequent in the surfactant group (Table V). In addition, the

Table V. Safety-related outcomes according to treatment received

Outcome or medication	No. with outcome (%) Air placebo (n = 170)	Synthetic surfactant (n = 174)	Relative risk*	95% Confidence interval
Pneumothorax	46 (27)	29 (17)†	1.60	1.07-2.39
Pneumomediastinum	12 (7)	6 (3)	2.00	0.80-5.05
Pulmonary interstitial emphysema	68 (40)	48 (28)‡	1.43	1.06-1.91
Pneumopericardium	3 (2)	3 (2)	1.02	0.21-4.87
Any form of air leak	77 (46)	56 (32)§	1.42	1.09-1.85
IVH	70 (47)	67 (42)	1.12	0.87-1.43
Grade III IVH	16 (11)	12 (8)	1.41	0.70-2.86
PVED	16 (11)	18 (11)	0.95	0.50-1.78
Grade III IVH or PVED	21 (14)	20 (13)	1.11	0.63-1.96
Seizures	7 (4)	13 (8)	0.54	0.22-1.29
Patent ductus arteriosus	111 (69)	120 (71)	0.97	0.84-1.12
Necrotizing enterocolitis	3 (2)	9 (5)	0.34	0.10-1.17
Sepsis	28 (17)	30 (17)	0.96	0.60-1.53
Nosocomial pneumonia	5 (3)	2 (1)	2.58	0.53-12.66
Meningitis	1 (1)	1 (1)	1.07	0.07-16.14
Arterial hypotension	101 (59)	96 (55)	1.06	0.89-1.27
Apnea of prematurity	85 (50)	103 (59)	0.85	0.71-1.03
Pulmonary hemorrhage	1 (1)	3 (2)	0.35	0.04-2.90
Antibiotics	170 (100)	172 (99)	1.02	0.99-1.05
Diuretic agents	103 (61)	96 (55)	1.10	0.92-1.32
Anticonvulsant agents	14 (8)	17 (10)	0.84	0.43-1.65
Inotropic agents	49 (29)	43 (25)	1.16	0.82-1.65
Sedatives	113 (66)	106 (61)	1.09	0.93-1.28
Pancuronium bromide	60 (35)	43 (25)‖	1.43	1.03-1.97
Methylxanthines	108 (64)	124 (71)	0.90	0.78-1.04

*Relative risk >1.00 indicates reduced risk with synthetic surfactant.
†$p = 0.023$.
‡$p = 0.018$.
§$p = 0.009$.
‖$p = 0.034$.

use of pancuronium bromide was significantly reduced in the group treated with synthetic surfactant. There were no differences between the air placebo and synthetic surfactant groups with respect to unusual or unexpected adverse events. All other safety-related outcomes, including apnea and pulmonary hemorrhage, did not differ significantly between groups (Table V).

DISCUSSION

The major finding of this prospective, multicenter, double-masked, parallel, placebo-controlled clinical trial was a significant improvement in intact cardiopulmonary survival for infants treated with synthetic surfactant. This result was achieved with two doses of synthetic surfactant given 12 hours apart to middle-sized infants with RDS, despite premature termination of the trial for ethical reasons. Another important finding was the reduction in morbidity associated with RDS. The incidence of overall pulmonary air leak, as well as pneumothorax and pulmonary interstitial emphysema, was reduced. These findings are consistent with similar reductions in pulmonary air leak shown in other trials with synthetic surfactant.[1-8]

The lack of significant improvement in mortality in this trial may be related to the smaller-than-planned sample size, because significant reductions in overall mortality at 28 days and at 1 year were observed in the two other rescue trials involving infants with RDS who weighed more than 700 gm that did reach targeted sample size.[1, 2] Premature termination of this study did not allow for sufficient patient enrollment to detect effects of synthetic surfactant that were evident in other trials in babies of this size.

Bronchopulmonary dysplasia, defined by a combination of clinical and radiographic criteria, was not significantly reduced with two doses of synthetic surfactant in this trial. One possible explanation for this finding is the relatively small sample size, which poses a commensurately greater risk of type II error. One study that used the same synthetic surfactant but had a sample size that was three times larger showed a significant reduction in the incidence of BPD in larger infants with established RDS and birth weights of

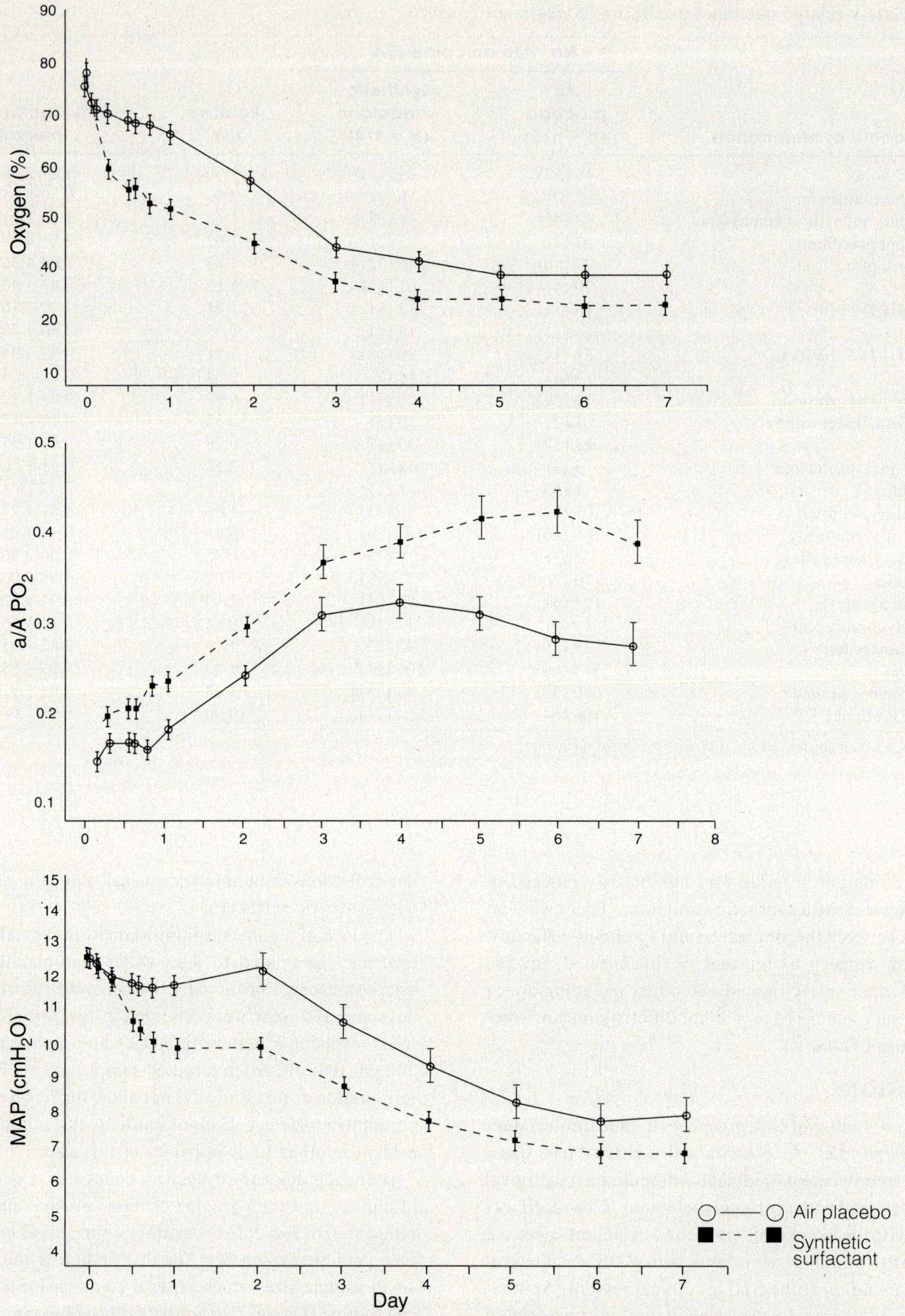

Fig. 2. Oxygen requirements, a/APo$_2$, and mean airway pressure (MAP) during the first days of life in infants given air placebo or synthetic surfactant.

1250 gm or more.[2] However, a similar rescue study in infants with established RDS and birth weights between 700 and 1350 gm did not show a significant reduction in BPD; this latter study included approximately 400 infants.[1] One possible explanation for the failure to see reductions in BPD after rescue use of synthetic surfactant in smaller babies with RDS may be that the extra survivors in this weight class are at higher risk of BPD and thus obscure the reduction in BPD documented in larger infants.

With a reduction in the severity of RDS, as judged by improvements in physiology and reductions in the incidence of pneumothorax, PIE, and overall air leak, as well as use of pancuronium, one would expect to observe a decrease in the incidence of IVH. However, the reduction in mortality seen with surfactant replacement therapy results in survival of more infants at high risk for developing IVH. Previously, these infants would have died without IVH being diagnosed. In this trial in infants weighing 750 to 1249 gm, neither the incidence of any grade of IVH nor the incidence of severe IVH (grade III IVH and/or PVED) was altered by synthetic surfactant. This observation is consistent with other trials of synthetic surfactant in middle-sized babies.[1,4] In the only trial with the same synthetic surfactant conducted in larger infants (birth weights >1250 gm), the incidence of IVH was reduced by 50%.[2] The prophylactic use of animal-derived surfactant preparations has been shown to reduce IVH in a few trials in smaller infants less than 30 weeks of gestational age.[22,23] In contrast, the incidence of IVH was increased in one single-dose trial of rescue administration of a modified bovine surfactant in infants with RDS who weighed 750 to 1750 gm.[24] Across all trials of modified bovine surfactant, the incidence of IVH has been shown to be increased in infants who weigh less than 750 gm.[25] The complex relationships between changes in pulmonary function, cardiac output, ductal shunt, central venous pressure, and cerebral blood flow could account for some of these findings.

In this trial, administration of two doses of synthetic surfactant improved respiratory measurements even though the onset of action was slightly delayed in comparison with that in other rescue studies with synthetic surfactant.[1,2] The lack of significant improvement in mean airway pressure at 2 and 6 hours after the first dose could be related to the small sample size. In similar studies, improvement in the mean airway pressure was significant at 6 hours after the first dose.[1,2] The observed improvements in respiratory measurements such as fractional inspired oxygen, mean airway pressure, and A/aPo_2 during days 1 through 7 were significant. These improvements probably contributed to the significant decreases in pneumothorax and pulmonary interstitial emphysema. The improvement in respiratory status also was supported by the decreased utilization of pancuronium bromide in the group treated with surfactant.

Other clinical or laboratory problems commonly seen in middle-sized infants with RDS occurred at the same rate in both treatment groups. Furthermore, the need for drug therapy was equal in both groups. In contrast to other studies,[1,2] there was no increase in the incidence of apnea in this study. Apnea might be expected to occur more often with less frequent use of pancuronium bromide and reductions in ventilation requirements. The incidence of pulmonary hemorrhage also did not differ between groups in this trial; however, the lack of a prospective definition for pulmonary hemorrhage limits the usefulness of this observation.

Unlike other studies of surfactant replacement therapy, which have shown either increases[26] or decreases[2] in the incidence of patent ductus arteriosus, this study showed no difference in the incidence of this disorder between the placebo and surfactant groups, although clinical findings occur earlier in infants treated with surfactant.[27] The adverse effects of patent ductus arteriosus on long compliance[28-31] prompted protocol-required early diagnosis and treatment of this disorder during this study. There was no significant difference in the incidence of necrotizing enterocolitis or infections between groups. Consideration of infections is important, because pneumonia may be difficult to distinguish from RDS soon after birth. The synthetic surfactant used in this study has been shown to be bacteriostatic and bactericidal in the presence of common perinatal pathogens[32,33]; other rescue studies with this synthetic surfactant also have not shown increases in the incidence of sepsis or nosocomial pneumonia.[1,2] In contrast, a significant increase in sepsis was observed in a cross-study analysis of a modified bovine surfactant.[34]

We conclude that two rescue doses of synthetic surfactant cause physiologic improvements in premature infants weighing 750 to 1249 gm with RDS, reduce pulmonary air leaks, and improve survival rates without BPD at 28 days of life.

REFERENCES

1. Long WA, Thompson T, Sundell H, Schumacher R, Volberg F, Guthrie R. Effects of two rescue doses of a synthetic surfactant on mortality in 700-1350 gram infants with RDS. J PEDIATR 1991;118:595-605.
2. Long W, Cotton R, Corbet A, et al. A controlled trial of synthetic surfactant in infants weighing 1250 g or more with respiratory distress syndrome. N Engl J Med 1991;325:1696-703.
3. Smyth J, Allen A, MacMurray B, et al. A double-blind, randomized, placebo-controlled Canadian multicenter trial of two doses of synthetic surfactant or air placebo in 224 infants weighing 500 to 699 grams with respiratory distress syndrome. J PEDIATR 1995;126:S81-9.
4. Corbet AJ, Bucciarelli R, Goldman SA, Mammel MA, Wold D, Long WA. Decreased mortality in small premature infants

treated at birth with a single dose of synthetic surfactant: a multicenter trial. J PEDIATR 1991;118:277-84.

5. Bose C, Corbet A, Bose G, et al. Improved outcome at 28 days of very low birth weight infants treated with a single dose of synthetic surfactant. J PEDIATR 1990;117:947-53.
6. Phibbs RH, Ballard RA, Clements JA, et al. Initial clinical trial of Exosurf a protein-free synthetic surfactant for prophylaxis and early treatment of hyaline membrane disease. Pediatrics 1991;88:1-9.
7. Corbet AJ, Long WA, Murphy DJ, Garcia-Prats JA, Lombardy DL, Wold DE. Reduced mortality in small premature infants treated at birth with a single dose of synthetic surfactant. J Paediatr Child Health 1991;27:245-9.
8. Corbet A, Gerdes J, Long W, et al. Double-blind randomized trial of one versus three prophylactic doses of synthetic surfactant in 826 neonates weighing 700 to 1100 grams: effects on mortality rate. J PEDIATR (in press).
9. Kendig J, Notter RH, Cox C, et al. A comparison of surfactant as immediate prophylaxis and as rescue therapy in newborns of less than 30 weeks gestation. N Engl J Med 1991; 324:865-71.
10. Kattwinkel J, Bloom T, Delmore P, et al. Prophylactic administration of calf lung surfactant extract is more effective than early treatment of respiratory distress syndrome in neonates of 29 through 32 weeks gestation. Pediatrics 1993;92:90-8.
11. The OSIRIS Collaborative Group. Early versus delayed neonatal administration of synthetic surfactant: the judgment of OSIRIS. Lancet 1992;340:1363-9.
12. Soll RF, Sinclair JC, Bracken MB. Meta-analysis of surfactant trials: the effect of prophylactic surfactant vs. surfactant treatment of established RDS [Abstract]. Pediatr Res 1993; 33:276A.
13. Long WA, Sanders RL. New treatment methods in idiopathic respiratory distress syndrome: replacement of surface active material. Clin Crit Care Med 1988;13:21-56.
14. Durand DJ, Clyman RI, Heymann MA, et al. Effects of a protein-free synthetic surfactant on the survival and pulmonary function of preterm lambs. J PEDIATR 1985;107:775-80.
15. Tooley WH, Clements JA, Muramatsu K, Brown CL, Schlueter MA. Lung function in prematurely delivered rabbits treated with a synthetic surfactant. Am Rev Respir Dis 1987; 136:651-6.
16. Edwards DK. Radiology of hyaline membrane disease transient tachypnea of the newborn and bronchopulmonary dysplasia. In: Farrell PM, ed. Lung development: biological and clinical perspectives, vol 2. New York: Academic Press, 1982: 47-89.
17. O'Brodovich HM, Mellins RB. Bronchopulmonary dysplasia. Am Rev Respir Dis 1985;132:694-709.
18. Bonikos DS, Bensch KG, Northway WH, et al. Bronchopulmonary dysplasia: the pulmonary pathologic sequel of necrotizing bronchiolitis and pulmonary fibrosis. Hum Pathol 1976;7:643-66.
19. Saigal S, Robertson C, Sankaran K, et al. One-year outcome in 232 premature infants with birth weights of 750 to 1249 grams and respiratory distress syndrome randomized to rescue treatment with two doses of synthetic surfactant or air placebo. J PEDIATR 1995;126:S61-7.
20. Fleiss JL. Statistical methods for rates and proportions. New York: John Wiley and Sons, 1981:160-87.
21. Dixon WJ, Massey F. Introduction to statistical analysis. New York: McGraw Hill, 1969:222-36.
22. Fujiwara T, Onishi M, Nanby H, et al. Surfactant supplementation treatment of neonatal respiratory distress syndrome (RDS): results of a multifacility cooperative comparative control trial. Shonika Rinsho 1987;40:549-68.
23. Enhorning G, Grossman G, Robertson B. Tracheal deposition of surfactant in premature rabbit fetuses. Am Rev Respir Dis 1973;107:921-7.
24. Horbar JD, Soll RF, Schachinger H, et al. A European multicenter randomized controlled trial of single dose surfactant therapy for idiopathic respiratory distress syndrome. Eur J Pediatr 1990;149:416-23.
25. Gunkel JH, Banks PLC. Surfactant therapy and intracranial hemorrhage: review of the literature and results of new analyses. Pediatrics 1992;92:775-86.
26. Fujiwara T, Chida S, Watabe Y, Maeta H, Morita T, Abe T. Artificial surfactant therapy in hyaline membrane disease. Lancet 1980;1:55-9.
27. Murphy DJ, Corbet AJ, Long WA. The "natural" history of patent ductus arteriosus (PDA) [Abstract]. Pediatr Res 1991;29:245A.
28. Yeh TF, Thalji A, Luken L, Lilien L, Carr I, Pildes RS. Improved lung compliance following indomethacin therapy in premature infants with patent ductus arteriosus. Chest 1981; 80:698-700.
29. Heldt GP, Pesonen E, Merritt TA, Elias W, Sahn DJ. Closure of the ductus arteriosus and mechanics of breathing in preterm infants after surfactant replacement therapy. Pediatr Res 1989;25:305-10.
30. Stefano JL, Abbasi S, Perlman SA, Spear ML, Esterly KL, Bhutani VK. Closure of the ductus arteriosus with indomethacin in ventilated neonates with respiratory distress syndrome. Am Rev Respir Dis 1991;143:236-9.
31. Balsan MJ, Jones JG, Guthrie RD. Effects of a clinically detectable PDA on pulmonary mechanics measures in VLBW infants with RDS. Pediatr Pulmonol 1991;111:161-5.
32. Sherman MP, Campbell LA, Merritt TA, Shapiro DL, Long WA, Gunkel JH. The infected preterm rabbit lung: a model to test the effect of surfactant replacement on lung host defenses. In: Wichert P, von Muller B, eds. Basic research on lung surfactant: progressive respiratory research, vol 25. Basel: Karger, 1990:204-8.
33. Sherman MP, Campbell LA, Merritt TA, et al. Effect of surfactant on Group B streptococcal infection in premature rabbits. J PEDIATR 1994;125:939-47.
34. Liechty EA, Donovan E, Purohit D, et al. Reduction of neonatal mortality after multiple doses of bovine surfactant in low birth birth weight neonates with respiratory distress syndrome. Pediatrics 1991;88:19-28.

APPENDIX I

Participants in the American Exosurf Neonatal Study Group I were as follows:

Endla Anday, MD, University of Pennsylvania, Philadelphia, Penn.

Stephen Boros, MD, Children's Hospital of St. Paul, St. Paul, Minn.

Carl Bose, MD, University of North Carolina at Chapel Hill, Chapel Hill, N.C.

Richard Bucciarelli, MD, University of Florida, Gainesville, Fla.

David Burchfield, MD, University of Florida, Gainesville, Fla.

Larry N. Cook, MD, Kosair Children's Hospital, University of Louisville, Louisville, Ky.

Anthony Corbet, MB, FRACP, Baylor College of Medicine, Houston, Texas

Robert Cotton, MD, Vanderbilt University, Nashville, Tenn.

Sherry Courtney, MD, MS, Wright State University, Dayton, Ohio

Douglas Derleth, MD, Mayo Clinic, Rochester, Minn.

R. Dhanireddy, MD, Georgetown University Hospital, Washington, D.C.

David Easa, MD, Kapiolani Women and Children's Medical Center, Honolulu, Hawaii

Jeffrey Gerdes, MD, Pennsylvania Hospital, Philadelphia, Penn.

Steven Goldman, MD, Children's Hospital of San Francisco, San Francisco, Calif.

Alice Gong, MD, Santa Rosa Hospital and University of Texas Health Science Center, San Antonio, Texas

Robert Guthrie, MD, Magee-Women's Hospital, Pittsburgh, Penn.

Michael LeBlanc, MD, University of Mississippi, Jackson, Miss.

Mark Mammel, MD, Children's Hospital of St. Paul, St. Paul, Minn.

Gail McGuiness, MD, University of Iowa, Iowa City, Iowa

Martha Mullett, MD, West Virginia University, Morgantown, W.V.

Thomas Pauly, MD, University of Kentucky, Lexington, Ky.

Arun K. Pramanik, MD, Louisiana State University Medical Center, Shreveport, La.

Robert Schumacher, MD, C. S. Mott Children's Hospital, University of Michigan, Ann Arbor, Mich.

Matthew Sell, MD, St. Luke's Regional Medical Center, Boise, Idaho

David Stevenson, MD, Stanford University, Palo Alto, Calif.

Hakan Sundell, MD, Vanderbilt University, Nashville, Tenn.

Theodore Thompson, MD, University of Minnesota, Minneapolis, Minn.

Ross Vaughan, MD, Wake Area Health Education Center, Raleigh, N.C.

Frank Volberg, MD, Bowman Gray School of Medicine, Winston-Salem, N.C.

Donnal Walter, MD, PhD, Children's Hospital, Little Rock, Ark.

Frans Walther, MD, PhD, University of Southern California, Los Angeles, Calif.

APPENDIX II

Participants in the American Exosurf Neonatal Study Group II were as follows:

Emilio Avila, MD, Alaska Neonatal Association, Anchorage, Alaska

Ed Beaumont, MD, Butterworth Hospital, Grand Rapids, Mich.

David Berry, MD, Bowman Gray School of Medicine, Winston-Salem, N.C.

Susie Buchter, MD, Emory University School of Medicine, Atlanta, Ga.

Keith Kanarek, MD, University of South Florida, Tampa, Fla.

Arthur E. Kopelman, MD, East Carolina University School of Medicine, Greenville, N.C.

Joseph Philips, MD, University of Alabama at Birmingham, Birmingham, Ala.

Asha Puri, MD, Cedar Sinai Medical Center, Los Angeles, Calif.

Adam Rosenberg, MD, University of Colorado Health Sciences Center, Denver, Colo.

APPENDIX III

Participants in the Canadian Exosurf Neonatal Study Group were as follows:

Alexander Allen, MD, Grace Maternity Hospital, Halifax, Nova Scotia

Harry Bard, MD, St. Justine's Hospital, Montreal, Quebec

Victor Chernick, MD, Health Sciences Centre and St. Boniface Hospital, Winnipeg, Manitoba

Neil Finer, MD, Royal Alexandra Hospital, Edmonton, Alberta

Brock MacMurray, MD, Children's Hospital of Eastern Ontario, Ottawa General Hospital and Ottawa Civic Hospital, Ottawa, Ontario

Douglas McMillan, MD, Foothills Hospital, Calgary, Alberta

Abraham Peliowski, MD, Royal Alexandra Hospital, Edmonton, Alberta

Koravangattu Sankaran, MD, University Hospital, Saskatoon, Saskatchewan

David Schiff, MD, PhD, Walter MacKenzie Health Sciences Center, Edmonton, Alberta

Arvind Shukla, MD, Foothills Hospital, Calgary, Alberta

John Smyth, MD, British Columbia's Children's Hospital, Vancouver, British Columbia

John Watts, MD, Chedoke-McMaster Hospitals, Hamilton, Ontario

APPENDIX IV

Participants in the Canadian Exosurf Neonatal Follow-Up Study Group were as follows:

Harry Bard, MD, St. Justine's Hospital, Montreal, Quebec

William Bingham, MD, University Hospital, Saskatoon, Saskatchewan

Oscar G. Casiro, MD, University of Manitoba, Winnipeg, Manitoba

Brock MacMurray, MD, Children's Hospital of Eastern Ontario, Ottawa General Hospital, and Ottawa Civic Hospital, Ottawa, Ontario

Diane Moddemann, MD, University of Manitoba, Winnipeg, Manitoba

Charlene Robertson, MD, Northern and Central Alberta Perinatal Program, Edmonton, Alberta

Saroj Saigal, MD, McMaster University, Hamilton, Ontario

Koravangattu Sankaran, MD, University Hospital, Saskatoon, Saskatchewan

Reginald Sauve, MD, University of Calgary, Calgary, Alberta

Michael J. Vincer, MD, University of Dalhousie, Halifax, Nova Scotia

SUPPLEMENT

Perspectives on infant feeding: Controversies, research, and recommendations

Proceedings of a Johnson & Johnson Symposium, ''Controversies in the 1990s: Infant Feeding—Where Do We Go From Here?'' held in Denver, Colorado, April 22, 1994

Editor: Steven P. Shelov, MD

Supported by an educational grant from Johnson & Johnson Consumer Products, Inc.

Guest Editor's Note

The most important advice we can give expectant mothers is to encourage them to breast-feed. Unfortunately, today's realities are such that many mothers find it difficult to breast-feed exclusively for any extended period. Economic and social pressures force women to resume careers, schooling, or other commitments soon after the birth of a child. Consequently, many infants who could benefit from breast-feeding are deprived of this opportunity.

Bottle feeding expressed mother's milk cannot provide the same degree of intimate physical contact and security as breast-feeding, and yet it does supply the same nutritional and health benefits and is thus an acceptable alternative. In fact, mothers who have responsibilities outside the home should be encouraged to have their infants fed in this manner during their absence. In this way, they can continue to provide the benefits of human milk to their children for at least 1 year or longer.

The subject of artificial feeding systems as a method of prolonging the duration of breast-feeding or for mothers who choose to bottle-feed, then, is very timely. However, this is not a topic that has been given much coverage in the medical literature. Yet providing mothers with a basic understanding of artificial feeding systems and instruction in appropriate artificial feeding techniques is essential if we are to encourage breast-feeding in any meaningful way.

This supplement offers an intriguing look at current and future research in these areas. Some of the topics and techniques have not been previously addressed in the medical literature on infant feeding. This supplement provides an unusual opportunity for clinicians to review new findings on artificial feeding systems—a topic that is often overlooked and makes for thought-provoking reading.

Steven Shelov, MD
Professor and Vice Chairman of Pediatrics
Albert Einstein College of Medicine and
Montefiore Medical Center
Bronx, New York

Johnson & Johnson Consumer Products, Inc., is not responsible for any statements or views expressed at the symposium ''Controversies in the 1990s: Infant Feeding—Where Do We Go From Here?'' or in this supplement.

THE JOURNAL OF PEDIATRICS 1995;126:S103.

0022-3476/95/$3.00 + 0 **9/0/64227**

Introduction

Ideally, every infant born in the United States should be breast fed exclusively for the first year of life, in terms of nutrition, immunologic protection, emotional bonding, and psychologic needs. Human milk offers species-specific advantages for the neonate; it contains an appropriate combination of protein, carbohydrate, and fat. Both colostrum and mature milk provide host resistance factors against bacterial and viral infection. Breast-feeding assures intimate physical contact between mother and infant, an important factor in the process of attachment and later psychosocial development.

It is important that we, as pediatricians and health-care professionals, support breast-feeding in our practices and in the institutions we serve. Hospital policies must not undermine the decision to breast-feed by encouraging formula or water supplementation of breast-fed infants. Breast-feeding mothers must have ongoing support and advice when they encounter difficulties at home. They must be able to address breast-feeding problems during office visits or be put in touch with support services in the community, such as visiting nurses, lactation consultants, breast-feeding support groups, and hospital call-in lines.

There are times, however, when feeding with an artificial system is a medical or physiologic necessity or is electively chosen by the mother. In situations in which the breast-feeding mother must be separated from her infant because of work, school, or other commitments, an artificial feeding system is required to provide infant nutrition. New developments in the area of bottle feeding are the subject of this supplement.

Proper positioning of the infant during bottle feeding may prevent certain problems. In the first article, Susan Tully, Yehuda Bar-Haim, and Richard Bradley report on tympanometric studies that demonstrate that supine bottle feeding may predispose an infant to otitis media.

The second article, written by Ruth Lawrence, identifies other problems associated with improper bottle feeding techniques—choking, swallowing air, and gastric discomfort—in addition to reflux of fluid into the middle ear. On the basis of observations of breast-feeding mothers and infants, Dr. Lawrence proposes that transferring many of the natural mechanics of breast-feeding to bottle feeding can help prevent or decrease the incidence of such feeding-related problems.

Can bottle design contribute to a more positive feeding experience? In an ergonomic study, Shereen Farber examined mother-infant teams during feeding, using two different bottles to determine the impact of bottle design on the positioning of the infant, the ease of feeding, and the overall comfort of mother and infant during the feeding session. Her study used qualitative and quantitative video analysis as bases for measurement.

Although proper instruction in bottle feeding and improvements in bottle design can enhance the quality of the feeding experience for the infant, an infant may have difficulty switching between a human nipple and an artificial nipple. Marianne Neifert addresses the problems of nipple confusion and nipple preference from a medical perspective. Although these phenomena have been frequently discussed in the lay press, they have been largely ignored in medical literature. Niefert proposes formal definitions of nipple confusion and nipple preference, examines the possible cause of, and potential risk factors for, these problems, and suggests directions for future research in these areas.

The last article in this supplement discusses practical and design characteristics of artificial feeding systems. Wilbur Smith, Arthur Nowak, and this investigator report on the use of intraoral imaging by ultrasonography during feeding to compare such factors as nipple length and compression of an artificial nipple with those of the human breast.

As the articles in this supplement highlight, it is increasingly important for us to play an active role in encouraging breast-feeding and ensuring proper feeding techniques when artificial feeding systems are required or chosen. We should familiarize ourselves with the different artificial feeding systems available so we can properly guide new mothers and accurately respond to their inquiries.

Allen Erenberg, MD
Professor of Pediatrics
Department of Pediatrics
The University of Kansas Medical Center
Kansas City, Kansas

THE JOURNAL OF PEDIATRICS 1995;126:S104.

0022-3476/95/$3.00 + 0 **9/0/64225**

Abnormal tympanography after supine bottle feeding

Susan B. Tully, MD, Yehuda Bar-Haim, MD, and Richard L. Bradley, PA-C

From the Department of Pediatrics, University of California, Los Angeles, School of Medicine and Olive View–UCLA Medical Center, the Department of Pediatrics B, Kaplan Hospital, Rehovot, Israel, and the Departments of Pediatrics and Family Medicine, Los Angeles County–University of Southern California Medical Center.

***Objective*: To determine whether bottle feeding with the infant in the supine position is related to entry of milk into the middle ear, thereby predisposing the infant to otitis media.**

***Study design*: Ninety children, aged 7 to 24 months, who were free of respiratory infection and had normal tympanograms initially, were bottle fed in either the supine or the semiupright position, and tympanography was repeated immediately afterward.**

***Results*: Thirty-four (59.6%) of the 57 infants fed in the supine position had abnormal postfeeding tympanographic results compared with only five (15%) of the 33 infants fed in the semiupright position ($p<0.005$). In addition, when the infants with abnormal tympanograms were placed in semiupright or prone positions for 15 minutes after feeding, the majority of tympanograms returned to normal.**

***Conclusion*: These data suggest that supine bottle feeding has a significant effect on middle-ear pressure dynamics, probably caused by the aspiration of milk into the ear. The results also suggest that repositioning infants after feeding may mitigate the effects of supine feeding, at least in healthy children. Although this study did not demonstrate that tympanographic abnormality definitely predisposes to otitis media, it provides more evidence to encourage the practice of feeding infants in a semiupright position. (J PEDIATR 1995;126:S105-11)**

For more than 30 years, published studies have reported that otitis media is more common in bottle-fed than in breast-fed infants.[1-6] As early as 1960, Duncan and Wellington[5] suggested that the supine position during bottle feeding might be one of the mechanisms involved in inflammation of the middle-ear cavity and coined the term ''positional otitis media.'' They postulated that the supine position permitted reflux of milk into the postnasal space and that inflammation occurred around the eustachian orifice. They added that nasal obstruction, such as that which occurs with upper respiratory tract infection, played a role in the pathogenesis of the infection.

A few years later, Wittenborg and Neuhauser[7] demonstrated that reflux of fluid into the eustachian tube was possible. They developed a radiographic technique for visualizing the eustachian tube using a radiopaque fluid with a consistency similar to that of milk. The investigators found that when adults in a supine position swallowed this fluid, the fluid spurted into the cartilaginous portion of the eustachian tube. With increased intranasal pressure, the contrast material sometimes entered the middle-ear cavity and remained there for as long as 10 minutes before clearing. The investigators also reported that the eustachian tube was visualized more easily in infants and young children than in older children and adults. They further reported that although the or-

Supported in part by grants from the American Physician Fellowship Inc. for Medicine in Israel and from Johnson & Johnson Consumer Products, Inc., Skillman, N.J.

Based on a study completed at Los Angeles County–University of Southern California Medical Center and reported first in Hebrew by Dr. Bar-Haim in *Harefuah* 1985;109(1-2):8-10 and later in English as an abstract in Am J Dis Child 1986;140:303.

Reprint requests: Susan B. Tully, MD, Olive View–UCLA Medical Center, Department of Pediatrics Room 3A108, 14445 Olive View Dr., Sylmar, CA 91342-1495.

0022-3476/95/$3.00 + 0 **9/0/64228**

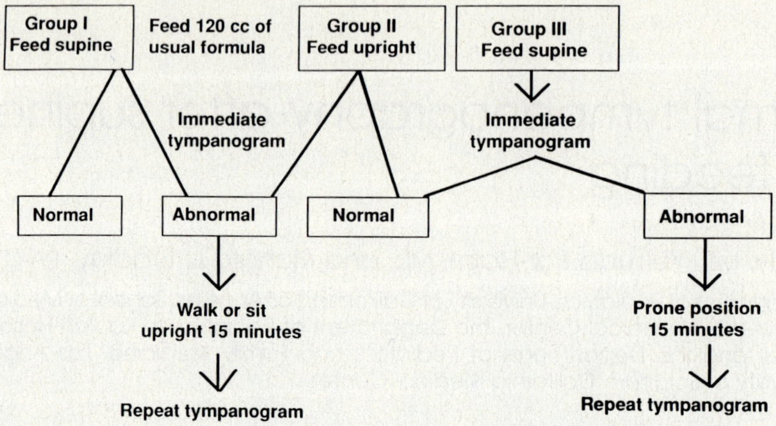

Fig. 1. All children in the three study groups had normal tympanograms initially. After receiving 120 ml of their usual formula, they received another tympanogram. In children with abnormal results after feeding, tympanograms were repeated after repositioning for 15 minutes.

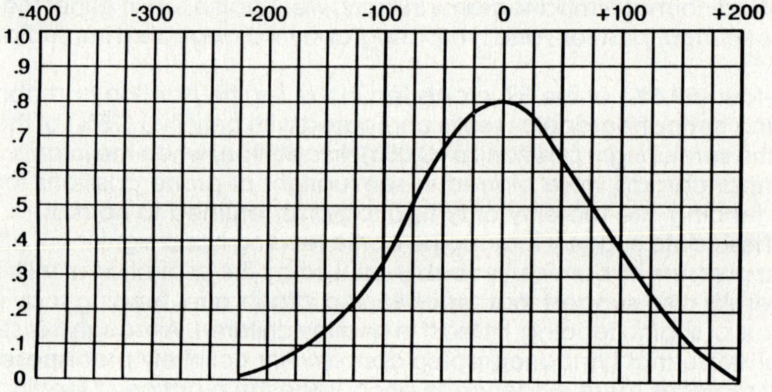

Fig. 2. Tympanograms were interpreted as normal if they showed a clear peak greater than 0.3 at normal pressure (type A). Pressure is expressed as millimeters of water (–400 to +200 mm H_2O). (Vertical axis shows compliance.)

ifice of the eustachian tube normally remained closed, it opened on tensing of the soft palate, an action that occurs during swallowing.

The findings of Wittenborg and Neuhauser[7] were confirmed by other investigators, such as Bluestone et al.,[8] who determined that nasal obstruction contributed to the generation of high-pressure gradients that increased the chance of reflux in patients with recent otitis. Bluestone et al.[9] also suggested that the supine position might increase the chance of eustachian tube obstruction (and consequent negative pressure) by hydrostatic venous pressure and that gravity could also (1) make nasopharyngeal secretions accessible at the tube, (2) allow freer drainage into the middle ear, and (3) allow effusion in the dependent portion of the middle-ear–mastoid system to persist.

Additional evidence that a postural mechanism might be at work in otitis media can be found in several other studies over the years. In 1971, Beauregard[10] noted that bottle propping was more frequently reported by mothers of infants with otitis media than by mothers of infants without otitis media. In 1980, an epidemiologic study of 2565 children concluded that the practice of putting an infant to bed with a bottle was the sole feature associated significantly with the persistence of middle-ear effusion after otitis media; this study did not consider feeding position as a variable.[11] In 1989, Narayanan et al.,[12] while studying the relationship between ear infections and infant feeding patterns in India, reported a high incidence of otitis media even among breast-fed infants but added that the majority of these infants were frequently breast fed while mother and infant were lying down, with the infant's head in a flat position.

In the present study, we sought to investigate the effects of supine feeding on middle-ear pressure dynamics. It was our impression that inordinate numbers of very young infants at our institution had otitis media and that the practice of supine bottle feeding was very common among the Hispanic

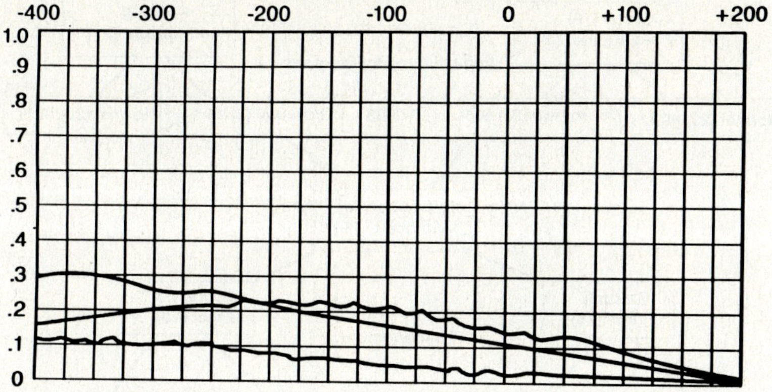

Fig. 3. Tympanograms were interpreted as abnormal if they showed no peak or peaks less than 0.2 at normal pressure (type B). Pressure is expressed as millimeters of water (–400 to +200 mm H_2O).

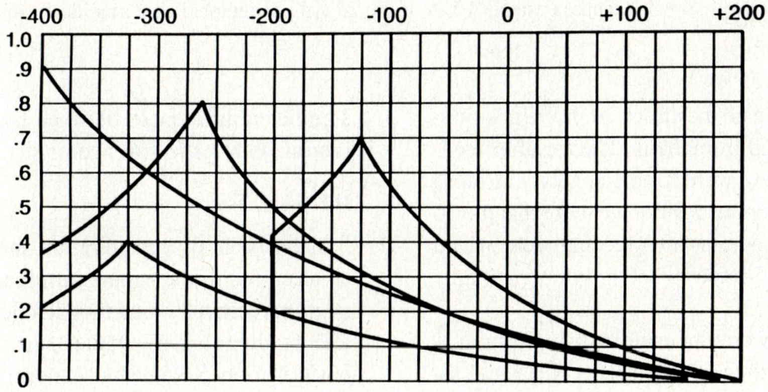

Fig. 4. Tympanograms were excluded if they showed a clear peak at negative pressure (type C). Pressure is expressed as millimeters of water (–400 to +200 mm H_2O).

patients we saw. We used tympanometry as a sensitive and noninvasive technique to determine whether regurgitation of fluid into the middle ear occurs and whether this regurgitation is related to the feeding position.

METHODS

The study population consisted of 90 children between the ages of 7 and 24 months who were ward or clinic patients at the Los Angeles County–University of Southern California Medical Center and who were undergoing treatment for a variety of medical and surgical conditions or were receiving well-child care. All were regularly bottle fed in the supine position at least some of the time. Children with acute current upper respiratory tract infection or a history of otitis media during the past 3 months were specifically excluded. We elected not to observe infants younger than 7 months, because their auditory canals are reportedly distensible and tympanometry is less reliable in diagnosing effusion in this age group.[13] Informed consent was obtained from all parents, and the study protocol was in accord with the guidelines of the Human Research Committee.

More than 90% of the children were Hispanic, a reflection of the hospital's patient population. All subjects were examined initially by pneumatic otoscopy and tympanometry, and only those with normal results were included in the study. There were two study populations; all children were bottle fed with at least 120 ml of their usual formula.

The first study consisted of 66 children. These children were assigned to two groups by using a table of random numbers: group I infants were fed in the supine position, and group II infants in the semiupright position. Tympanograms were recorded for each child immediately after the feeding to detect the presence of fluid in the middle ear. All children had to be restrained in a supine position for the time required to obtain the tympanogram. If the tympanogram was abnormal, the child was allowed to sit up or walk for 15 minutes, after which tympanography was repeated.

An additional 24 subjects were recruited for a second

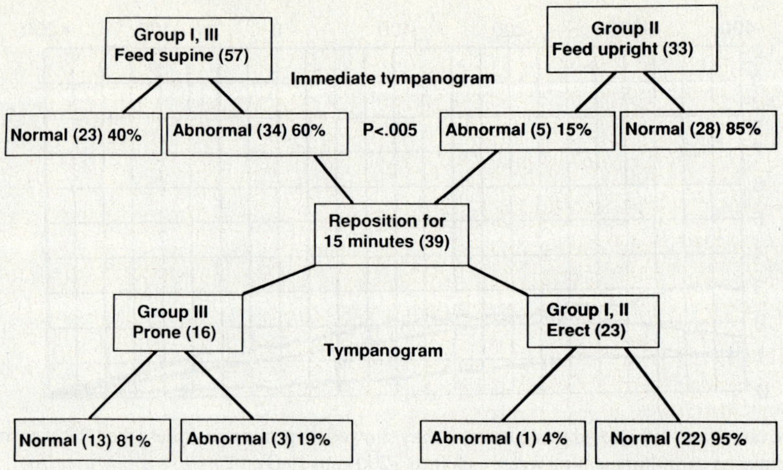

Fig. 5. Summary of results. Significantly more tympanographic abnormalities were observed in infants bottle fed in the supine position than in the semiupright position. When the infants were repositioned in a prone or semiupright posture for 15 minutes after feeding, all but 4 (approximately 10%) of the 39 tympanographic abnormalities resolved.

study population to investigate the effects of prone positioning on the clearance of fluid from the middle ear after feeding. These group III children were handled exactly as those in group I (i.e., fed in the supine position), except that the 20 who had abnormal tympanograms after feeding were placed in the prone position for 15 minutes before tympanography was repeated (Fig. 1).

All the tympanograms were obtained by using a tympanometer (American Electromedics, Amherst, N.H.) and interpreted according to standard tympanographic classifications.[14, 15] The authors were masked to feeding position when interpreting the tympanograms. To be included in the study, the necessary two or three tympanograms from each patient had to be sufficiently free of artifacts that all three authors could agree on their interpretation. Tracings were read as normal when they showed a clear peak greater than 0.3 at normal pressure (±100 mm H_2O), as seen in Fig. 2. Tympanograms that showed no peak, or low peaks less than 0.2, were read as abnormal (Fig. 3). Patients with type C tympanograms (i.e., a clear peak at negative pressure) were excluded from the study because of the lack of agreement among various authorities about the significance of type C tracings (Fig. 4).[15] Because the type C tympanograms and those with artifact were excluded, many more patients were studied than the 90 we report here. However, we have no information on the excluded subjects.

Completed, interpretable studies were obtained in 90 children. Results from the 33 children in group I and the 24 children in group III were combined for statistical analysis because these groups were handled identically except for repositioning after feeding. The results were then compared with results from the 33 children in group II. There were no significant differences between the supine and semiupright groups with respect to age or sex.

RESULTS

The results of the study are shown in Fig. 5. Of the 57 children fed in the supine position, 34 (59.6%) had tympanograms demonstrating fluid in one or both ears immediately after feeding (Fig. 6). Of the 33 infants fed in the semiupright position, only 5 (15%) had abnormal tympanographic results after feeding (Fig. 7). The difference between these two groups was significant, $p < 0.005$.

When the 39 children who had abnormal tympanograms were repositioned for 15 minutes after feeding, 22 (95%) of the 23 infants who were allowed to sit or walk and 13 (81%) of the 16 infants who were kept in the prone position had normal tracings on repeat tympanograms, indicating clearance of fluid from the middle ear. The difference between the results in the erect and prone positions was not significant.

DISCUSSION

To the best of our knowledge, this is the first study to measure and record pressure changes in the middle ear in response to postural changes of the infant during feeding. Tympanometry has been demonstrated to be a reliable method for detecting fluid in the middle ear. We believe that the abnormal tympanographic results seen in this study are related to regurgitation of milk into the middle ear. That a small number of the upright-fed children had abnormal tympanograms after feeding may be related to the necessity of restraining all of them in the supine position for the tympanograms.

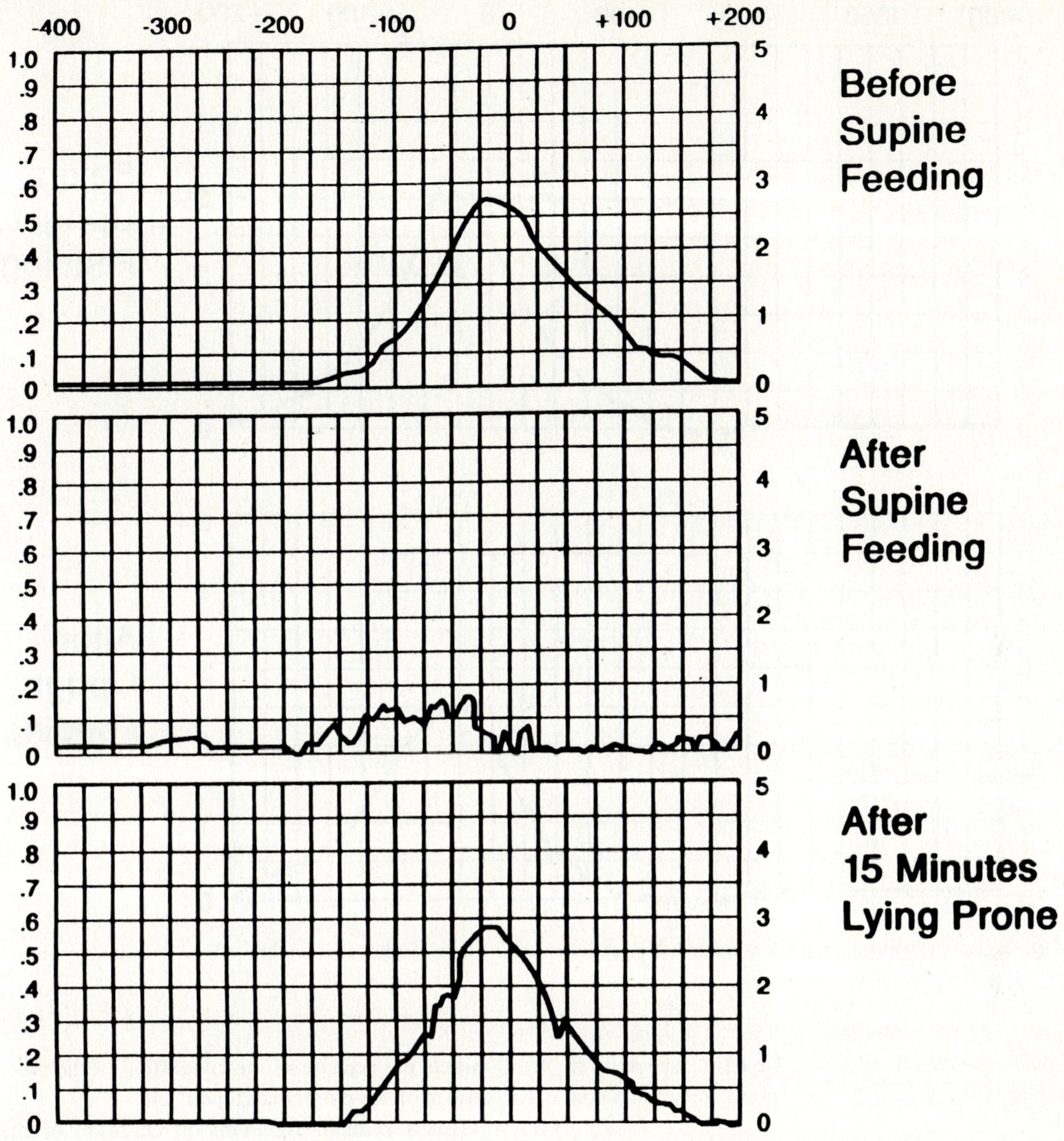

Fig. 6. Sample tympanograms of an infant before and after bottle feeding in the supine position and after spending 15 minutes in the prone position after feeding. Pressure is expressed as millimeters of water.

The finding that supine feeding encourages reflux of milk into the ear is in agreement with the hypotheses of previous studies and provides support for the epidemiologic association between bottle feeding and otitis media. The basis for this association has often been postulated to be allergy or lack of the immunologic protection conferred by breast milk.[1] However, our results suggest that the lower rate of otitis media in breast-fed babies is also at least partially related to feeding position. Although it is possible to breast-feed an infant while he or she is lying flat, this is not the most common breast-feeding position in the United States. When supine breast-feeding is common, otitis media is frequent in breast-fed infants.[12]

The finding that tympanographic abnormality resolved after infants spent 15 minutes in either the upright or prone position is consistent with the results of a report by Compere[16] that demonstrated that fluids introduced into the middle ears of normal adults disappear in about 10 minutes. Spontaneous clearing of fluid from the ear also helps explain why otitis media, although common, does not occur universally with supine feeding. Although most infants probably have reflux of milk into the ear during supine feeding,

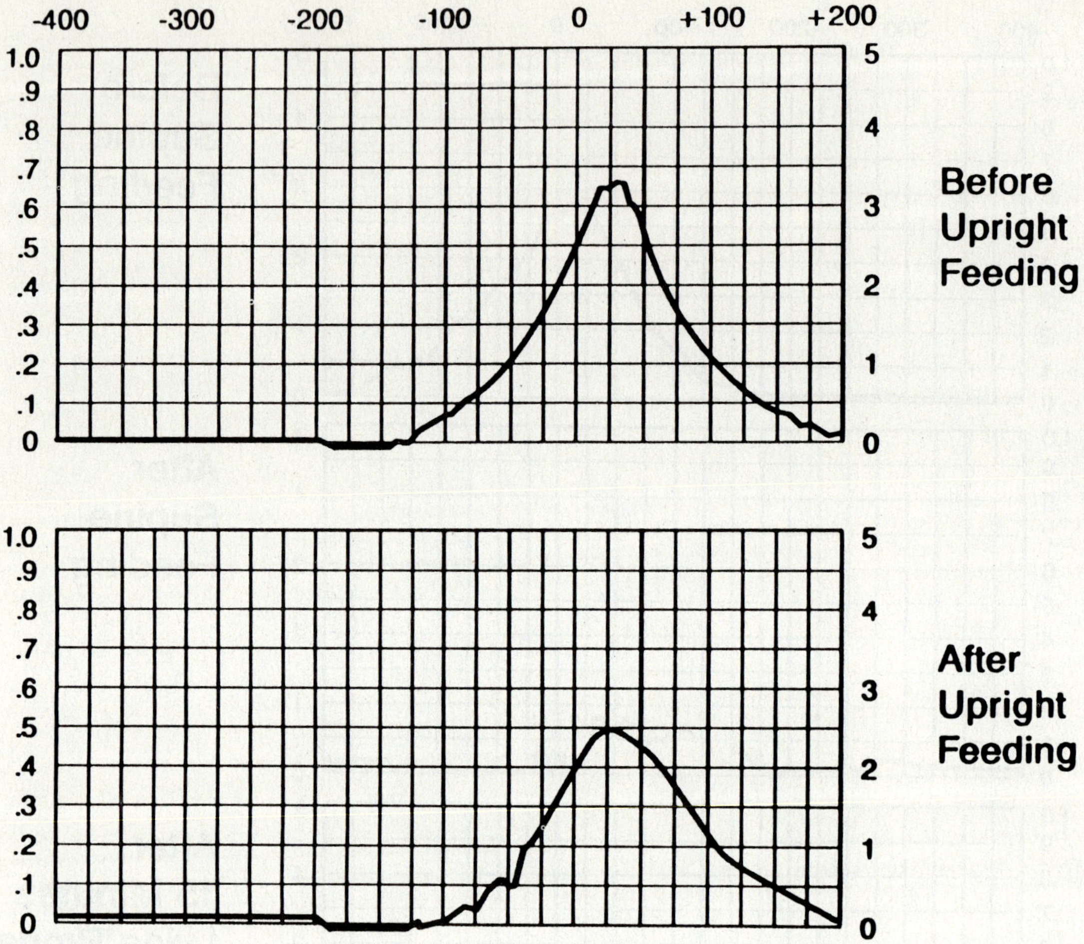

Fig. 7. Sample tympanograms of an infant before and after bottle feeding in the semiupright position. Pressure is expressed as millimeters of water.

healthy infants can usually evacuate the fluid, especially if they are placed in an upright or prone position soon afterward.

Our results also help explain why Teele et al.[11] observed such a strong correlation between the persistence of middle-ear effusion and the practice of putting an infant to bed with a bottle. If a child falls asleep immediately, as many infants do, the supine position is maintained and gravity does not promote drainage of fluid from the ear.

This study did not include infants with upper respiratory tract infection or other causes of nasal obstruction. However, in these situations, it can be presumed that the risk of aspiration of fluids would be higher, because pressure in the postnasal space is increased. Thus liquid occupying the nasopharyngeal region might be even more likely to be forced into the eustachian tube during swallowing. In addition, infants with nasal congestion from colds or allergic rhinitis would have difficulty clearing regurgitated liquid from the middle ear because of the congestion of the mucous membranes of the eustachian tube itself.

Bluestone et al.[8] found middle-ear reflux of fluid instilled in the nasopharynx almost exclusively in children with recent otitis and defined reflux, especially during open-nose swallowing, as ''abnormal.'' They did not specifically evaluate the effect of position, nor did they specify the position in which their patients were studied. We found apparent reflux in normal children fed in the supine position. We did not have sufficiently reliable histories to evaluate ''otitis proneness'' in our study children; however, the exclusion of children with any history of otitis in the last 3 months probably excluded many, if not all, otitis-prone children. The possibility exists that our patients, who were nearly all Hispanic, may have had a genetic, anatomic, or functional predisposition to reflux (i.e., abnormally patent eustachian tubes) not found in the subjects of Bluestone et al. It is also possible that the different results are related to position or to the fact that

Bluestone et al. used a tube to instill radiopaque fluid into the nasopharynx, whereas our subjects were actively sucking (presumably generating higher positive and negative pressures and wider pressure variations).[5, 9]

This study did not address the question of how aspirated fluids increase the risk of otitis media. However, it has been suggested that inflammation may occur through chemical irritation caused by the fluids,[5] a "foreign body granuloma,"[3] or impaired mucociliary function[17] or through transport of nasopharyngeal flora into the middle ear in the presence of a "culture medium" (regurgitated liquids, such as milk) that is highly conducive to bacterial growth and infection.

Finally, this study did not attempt to follow the children in the days after their inclusion in the study because of the difficulty of controlling feeding practices by parents or hospital staff. However, it would have been interesting to learn whether otitis media eventually developed in the approximately 10% of children who had abnormal tympanograms at the end of the study, even after repositioning.

Other questions arose during the course of this study. For example, what is the actual risk of otitis media developing after supine feeding? Are there host factors (such as anatomy) that cause some children to be at more risk to aspirate fluid during sucking? Is the aspirated fluid or the position alone responsible for the tympanographic abnormalities? Does feeding in a semiupright position or repositioning the child after supine feeding help mitigateotitis media even when a child has a cold? These questions can be answered only through further research. However, on the basis of our results and those of others, we believe that bottle feeding mothers should be encouraged to feed their infants in a semiupright position and to keep them semiupright for some time before putting them to bed to avoid increased risk of reflux of fluid into the middle ear and a possible increased risk of otitis media. This practice may be especially important for children with colds, allergic rhinitis, and recurrent or chronic otitis media.

REFERENCES

1. Duncan B, Ey J, Holberg CJ, et al. Exclusive breast-feeding for at least 4 months protects against otitis media. Pediatrics 1993;91:867-72.
2. Schaeffer O. Otitis media and bottle-feeding: an epidemiological study of infant feeding habits and incidence of recurrent and chronic middle ear disease in Canadian Eskimos. Can J Public Health 1971;62:478-89.
3. Timmermans FJW, Gerson S. Chronic granulomatous otitis media in bottle-fed Inuit children. Can Med Assoc J 1980; 122:545-7.
4. Saarinen UM. Prolonged breast feeding as prophylaxis for recurrent otitis media. Acta Paediatr Scand 1982;567-71.
5. Duncan RB, Wellington NZ. Positional otitis media. Arch Otolaryngol 1960;72:454-63.
6. Kero P, Piekkala P. Factors affecting the occurrence of acute otitis media during the first year of life. Acta Paediatr Scand 1987;76:618-23.
7. Wittenborg MH, Neuhauser EBD. Simple roentgenographic demonstration of eustachian tubes and abnormalities. AJR Am J Roentgenol 1963;89:1194-200.
8. Bluestone CD, Paradise JL, Beery QC. Symposium on prophylaxis and treatment of middle ear effusions: IV. Physiology of the eustachian tube in the pathogenesis and management of middle ear effusions. Laryngoscope 1972;82:1654-70.
9. Bluestone CD, Beery QC, Andrus WS. Mechanics of the eustachian tube as it influences susceptibility to and persistence of middle ear effusions in children. Ann Otol Rhinol Laryngol 1974;83(Suppl 11):27-34.
10. Beauregard WG. Positional otitis media. J PEDIATR 1971; 79:294-6.
11. Teele DW, Klein JO, Rosner BA. Epidemiology of otitis media in children. Ann Otol Rhinol Laryngol 1980;89(Suppl 68):5-6.
12. Narayanan I, Singh S, Mathur R, Jain BK. Ear infection and infant feeding practices. Indian J Pediatr 1989;56:399-402.
13. Paradise JL, Smith CD, Bluestone CD. Tympanometric detection of middle ear effusion in infants and young children. Pediatrics 1976;58:198-210.
14. Jerger J. Clinical experience with impedance audiometry. Arch Otolaryngol 1970;92:311-24.
15. Northern JL. Advanced techniques for measuring middle ear function. Pediatrics 1978;61:761-7.
16. Compere WE. The radiologic evaluation of eustachian tube function. Arch Otolaryngol 1960;71:386-9.
17. Paradise JL. Otitis media in infants and children. Pediatrics 1980;65:917-43.

The clinician's role in teaching proper infant feeding techniques

Ruth Lawrence, MD

From the Division of Neonatology, the Department of Pediatrics, University of Rochester, Rochester, New York

The species-specific advantages and significant nutritional and health benefits of breast-feeding are widely acknowledged. Less recognized are the advantages of the process of breast-feeding itself. Adherence to the natural mechanics of breast-feeding will preclude many of the problems associated with improper bottle feeding. For example, the semiupright position of the infant during breast-feeding helps eliminate the entry of milk into the middle ear and reduces choking and regurgitation. The action of suckling during breast-feeding minimizes the intake of air. In addition, the direct eye contact that is natural to breast-feeding fosters bonding, and the close body contact promotes a sense of security in the child. These advantages, so natural to breast-feeding, are likely to be absent from bottle feeding unless some of the natural techniques associated with breast-feeding are adopted. This article describes various aspects of the breast-feeding process with the goal of urging practitioners to instruct patients to transfer these techniques to bottle feeding. In so doing, clinicians may help their patients avoid the hazards of improper bottle feeding. (J Pediatr 1995;126:S112-7)

The reasons to encourage breast-feeding are numerous and reach far beyond its nutritional superiority. Species specificity,[1] host-resistance factors,[2] immunologic protection,[3] and allergy protection[1, 2] are just a few of the advantages that have been cited frequently. Species specificity is the most compelling reason, because human milk is designed uniquely for meeting the growth and development needs of the human infant. The milks of the 4000 mammalian species are all designed specifically for the offspring of each species.[4] The composition of the milk, the timing and method of feeding, and the weaning period are all species specific.

Host-resistance factors include active enzymes, living cells, immunologlubins, hormones, carrier proteins, and nonspecific factors that protect the infant's respiratory and gastrointestinal tract from invasion by bacteria, viruses, and other pathogens. The immunologic protection provided by human milk is attributed to the presence of immunoglobulins, antiinflammatory agents, and immunomodulating agents. Epidemiologic and, more recently, prospective studies have demonstrated the relationship between exclusive breast-feeding for 4 months or longer and the decrease in childhood onset diabetes mellitus, Crohn disease, and childhood cancers (especially acute leukemia). Prospective studies of infants at high risk for allergies such as infantile eczema, infant-onset asthma, and rhinitis have shown a lower-than-predicted onset of symptoms in the first 2 years of life when the infant is breast-fed exclusively for at least 6 months and protected from other known family allergens.[4]

Another important factor that has been, until recently, frequently underestimated is the close interaction between mother and infant at the breast.[1, 3] Considering that the infant develops within the mother's body and complete nourishment is available at the breast after birth, the maternal bond is the strongest human bond. In contrast to some other species, the human infant is totally dependent on mother (or a surrogate) for survival at birth. The mother-infant bond was well detailed by Klaus and Kennell[5] in their studies of early contact after birth. Most of the mothers in their original study were breast-feeding. This work has had a major impact on the way families are treated during the birthing process, re-

Supported by a grant from Johnson & Johnson Consumer Products, Inc., Skillman, N.J.

Reprint requests: Ruth A. Lawrence, MD, University of Rochester, School of Medicine, Department of Pediatrics, 601 Elmwood Ave., Box 777, Rochester, NY 14642.

0022-3476/95/$3.00 + 0 **9/0/64222**

sulting in the elimination of the take-charge rules of the past and the creation of an environment supportive of parent-infant interaction and, as a natural correlate, breast-feeding.[6] Early contact and early breast-feeding enhance the rate and duration of breast-feeding.[6-8]

The natural mechanics of breast-feeding effect a healthful feeding relationship with few, if any, associated problems. Body contact and communication between mother and child foster a sense of security in the child. The close contact inspires the beginnings of confidence and self-esteem. This interaction also affects the mother physiologically. As the infant suckles at the breast, the release of oxytocin and prolactin initiates milk production and let-down. Mothers who breast-feed are not different from those who bottle feed, but breast-feeding makes them different, as reported by Newton[9] in her studies of such women in the first 3 years postpartum. Women who breast-feed are more self-assured, have higher self-esteem, and interact more warmly with their infants, speaking to them in sentences rather than monosyllabic orders.[10]

The focus of this discussion will be on the mechanics of breast-feeding.

THE POSITION OF THE INFANT DURING BREAST-FEEDING

One of the most important advantages of breast-feeding is the natural semiupright positioning of the infant, the most commonly used position. Throughout recorded history, mothers have used this breast-feeding position—the infant facing the breast, the breast held in a scissor grasp (mother's thumb and index finger above the areola, with the other fingers supporting the breast from below).[4]

Although there were references to the risk of ear infections associated with bottle feeding, the first definitive study was reported in 1959 by Duncan.[11] Infants who were exclusively breast-fed did not develop otitis media. The author connected the ear infections to bottle feeding in the supine position when held by the caregiver, or to bottle propping. The article illustrates the proper position to hold the bottle and the importance of always keeping the infant upright. As a result of Duncan's paper, the term "positional otitis media" was coined.[11] A few years later (1964), an angled-neck nursing bottle was developed by Thornton[12] to prevent positional otitis media, crying, colic, and chronic spitting in bottle-fed infants. The author pointed out that the nipple on the human breast points outward from the lower part of the breast and not downward from the most dependent part of the breast, regardless of the shape or size of the breast. Thornton further stated that supine feeding results in forced feeding, "with strangling, gulping, and air swallowing."[12]

Although bottle propping received considerable criticism in the lay press, the medical literature was almost silent on the subject until Taubenhaus[13] published his study in 1968. A questionnaire was distributed to 50 teaching services in the United States; 39 were returned. Responses indicated that both hospital personnel and families practiced bottle propping. However, the risks of bottle propping were believed to be minimal for choking and dying. No mention of otitis media was made in the report, but Beauregard[14] followed with a study showing that 85% of infants who had otitis media had had their bottles propped, whereas only 8% of infants without otitis media were subjected to bottle propping. This clinically confirmed what radiologists Wittenborg and Neuhauser[15] had reported radiographically, which is that the eustachian tube can easily be filled with radiopaque material if the subject swallows it while lying supine; the liquid spurted into the eustachian tubes with an occasional spread into the middle ear.[15] Editorial comment in response to Beauregard's study suggested that the angled-neck bottle was a more anatomically correct means of artificial feeding.[16]

An epidemiologic study of infant feeding habits and incidence of otitis media was reported in Canadian eskimos.[17] The rate of breast-feeding had dropped in recent years, and infants bottle fed from the first month on experienced a 10 times greater incidence of severe otitis than those breast-fed 8 months or longer. Chronic granulomatous otitis media in Inuit children was therefore associated with bottle feeding. More specifically, the study showed that chronic foreign body granuloma of the middle ear developed from the milk introduced into the relatively short and straight eustachian tubes of Inuit infants by the high negative intraoral pressure necessary for bottle-feeding.[18]

Current research is beginning to focus on the connection between the rising incidence of "positional otitis media" among infants and the growing dependence on infant day care. In one study of early day care, Owen et al.[19] found that the commonly used supine feeding position is directly related to the onset and duration of otitis media with effusion in infants 2 years of age or less. However, the much lower incidence of otitis media among breast-fed infants has been largely attributed thus far to the protective qualities of human milk as opposed to the allergic, irritative properties of cow milk.[20-24] More studies must be done to determine the role position alone plays during feeding. For example, the effects of human milk when given in the upright position using an angled-neck bottle need further evaluation.

In breast-feeding, the mother normally holds the baby in the crook of her arm so that the infant's head is in exactly the right relationship to the breast. The infant's ventral surface facing the breast is in contact with the mother's ventral surface (Fig. 1). The infant has no trouble breathing in this position. The nose at birth is designed to fit perfectly with a lactating breast, as is evident in a close-up view of a breast-feeding infant (Fig. 2). Even when the nose appears

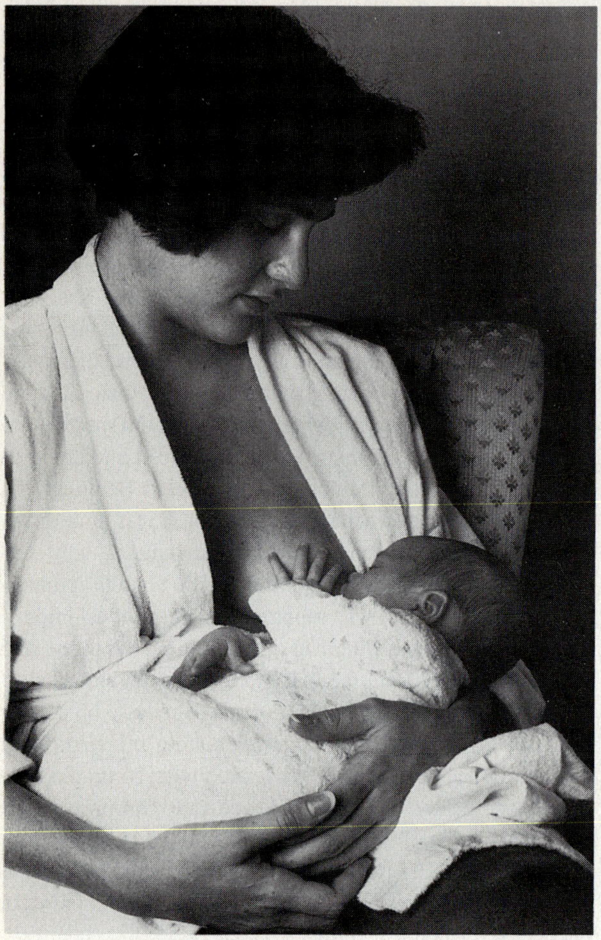

Fig. 1. Proper breast-feeding position: the infant is semiupright with the head supported by the mother's arm. The infant's ventral surface is in contact with the mother's ventral surface.

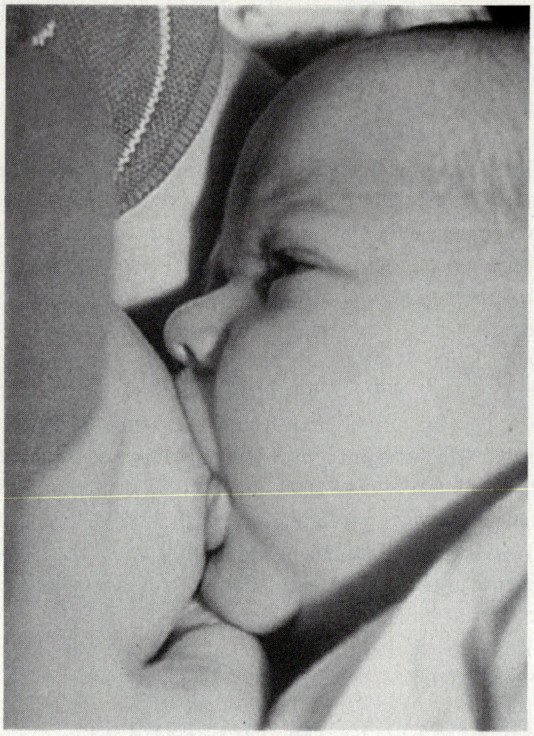

Fig. 2. When positioned properly, the infant has no trouble breathing. The nose at birth is designed to fit perfectly with a lactating breast.

to be pressed against the breast, the curve of the nares allows a full airway.

Semiupright positioning offers several benefits. First, because the infant's head is elevated, suckling and swallowing propel the milk with a peristaltic motion to the stomach in a process that protects the eustachian tube from the entry of milk. This synchronous motion also minimizes choking and regurgitation.[12] Second, semiupright feeding enhances the proper latch-on.

CORRECT LATCH-ON

Correct latch-on is essential to initiate adequate mammary stimulus and to avoid nipple soreness. Latch-on occurs with the help of the rooting reflex. When the lips or cheek are stimulated, the infant moves the mouth and face toward the stimulus. However, when the lower lip in particular is stimulated in the midline by the nipple, the infant's mouth opens wide to draw in the entire nipple and areola.[2] To achieve good latch-on at the breast, the infant should be stimulated centrally on the lower lip rather than on either cheek or either side of the mouth.[2]

The entire nipple and most of the areola should be drawn to the infant's mouth. The nipple and areola elongate into a teat that is compressed by the infant's tongue against the hard palate. The lips provide a seal around the base of the teat to prevent the entrance of air. If the infant does not open his or her mouth wide enough when latching on, and rather than drawing the nipple and areola into the mouth clamps down only on the nipple, the result can be painful for the mother and can interfere with the let-down process (Figs. 3 and 4).

PROPER SUCKLING

By definition, suckling refers to the giving or taking of milk directly from the mammary gland. Sucking, on the other hand, is a more general term that means the drawing of any fluid into the mouth by inhalation, partial vacuum, or licking. Therefore, the specific term suckling is used exclusively in discussions of breast-feeding.

As the process of suckling proceeds, the infant compresses the nipple and areola against the hard palate, and the peri-

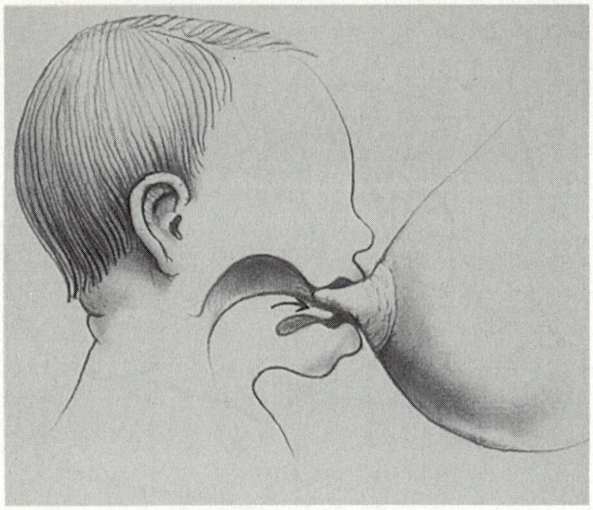

Fig. 3. Proper latch-on: The entire nipple and most of the areola are within the infant's mouth.

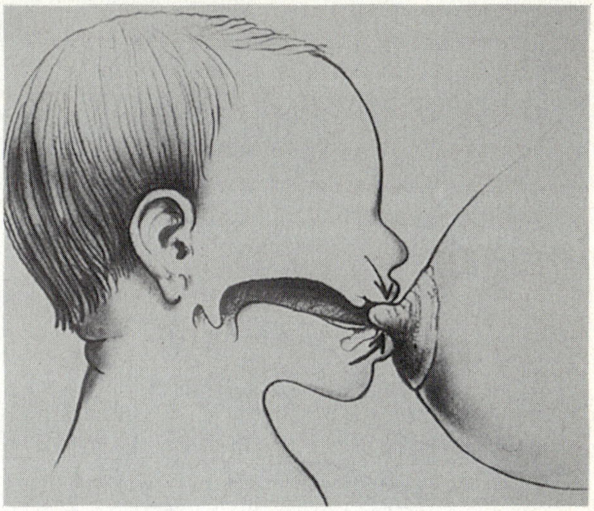

Fig. 4. Poor latch-on: The infant chews on the tip of the nipple alone. The pain to the mother can be so severe that it interferes with the let-down process.

staltic action of the tongue milks the ducts of the breast and helps eject the milk. The peristaltic action continues to the posterior pharynx and esophagus, thus triggering the swallowing reflex. The swallowing reflex then triggers the glottis to close, protecting the airway. The peristaltic action, which extends along the intestinal tract, protects the infant from aspirating fluid and automatically coordinates suck and swallow.

THE LET-DOWN REFLEX

Although the infant's tongue facilitates milk ejection, the mammary gland response is critical to this process. The ejection or let-down reflex is the most important physiologic reaction to suckling (Fig. 5). Suckling sends a message through the spinal column to the mother's hypothalamus and pituitary gland, initiating the release of oxytocin and prolactin—all part of a perfectly balanced plan to satisfy the infant's needs.

Whereas prolactin stimulates the lacteal cells in the breast to produce milk, oxytocin causes the myoepithelial cells in the breast, which surround the alveoli and the lactiferous ducts, to contract. When the myoepithelial cells contract, the milk is propelled from the alveoli through the ducts and out through the nipple.

If the infant is put to the breast immediately after birth, in addition to causing the myoepithelial cells of the breast to contract, oxytocin will cause the myoepithelial cells of the uterus to contract and expel the placenta. For the first few weeks postpartum, the oxytocin stimulates the uterus so that the involution of the uterus occurs much sooner in a woman who is breast-feeding. Normally, the uterus of a lactating woman is back to its prepregnancy size by 6 weeks postpartum.

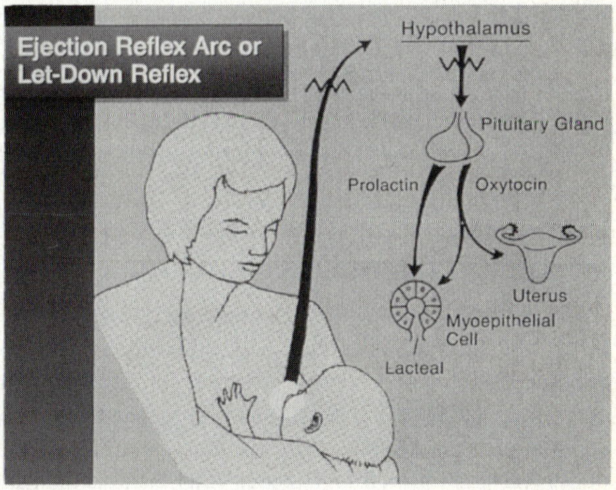

Fig. 5. In the let-down reflex, suckling triggers the release of prolactin and oxytocin from the pituitary gland. Prolactin stimulates the lacteal cells to produce more milk. Oxytocin causes contraction of the myoepithelial cells in the breast, which forces milk from the alveoli into the ducts and out through the mother's nipple.

Various types of sensory input can affect the let-down reflex. For instance, if a mother hears her baby cry, sees a picture of her baby, or happens to look at the clock and notice that it is feeding time, oxytocin may be released, and she may experience a little dripping of the breast. No additional milk will be produced, however, unless prolactin has been released. Prolactin is released only by suckling or pumping the breast.

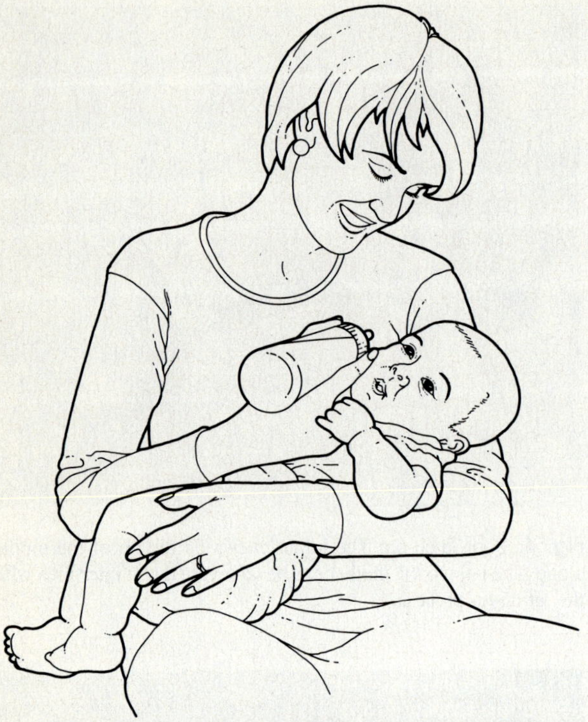

Fig. 6. Improper stimulation of the rooting reflex. The artificial nipple should not stroke the infant's cheek or the side of the mouth; rather, it should stimulate the infant's lips centrally.

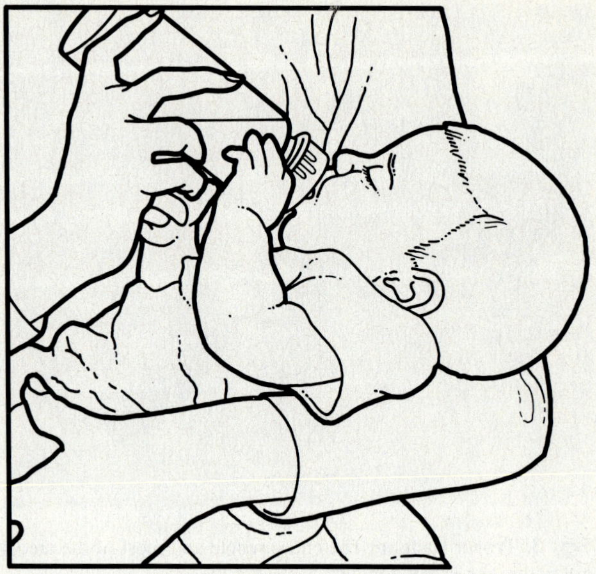

Fig. 7. The nipple and neck of the bottle should remain filled with liquid throughout the feeding.

RECOMMENDATIONS FOR BOTTLE FEEDING THE BREAST-FED INFANT

Ideally, an infant should breast-feed exclusively for the first 6 months[24]; then solids and other foods can be introduced. Infants continue, however, to benefit from breast-feeding for several years. Naturally, depending on the duration of breast-feeding, there are times when the infant must receive nutrition from a source other than the mother. This usually occurs at 8, 12, or more weeks, when the mother returns to school or work. Practitioners should encourage mothers who are breast-feeding to express milk, which can be provided in the mother's absence.

The instructions a family member or caregiver receives on how to bottle feed are extremely important. The adjustment for the breast-fed infant may be easier if some of the techniques that are natural to the phenomenon of breast-feeding are transferred to bottle feeding. For instance, parents and other caregivers should be informed that the infant should be held in a semiupright position during bottle feeding, just as in breast-feeding. The infant's head should be held in the security of the crook of the elbow of the caregiver, and the baby's body should be aligned ventral surface to ventral surface with the caregiver. The bottle then is held along the caregiver's chest. The infant's head should never be flat, and the bottle should never be propped.

As with breast-feeding, it is important that the rooting reflex be elicited by central stimulation. Too often, illustrations of bottle-feeding techniques indicate that the artificial nipple should be stroked against the cheek to stimulate the rooting reflex (Fig. 6). Unfortunately, this will only cause the infant to turn its head toward the stimulus; however, if the central portion of the lower lip is stimulated instead, the infant will move forward and latch on directly. Just as in breast-feeding, in bottle feeding it is important that the infant open his or her mouth wide enough and draw in enough of the artificial nipple to create a tight seal around it and prevent the entry of air.

Holding the bottle properly can also minimize the amount of air the infant swallows. It is essential that the family and caregiver understand that the bottle should be positioned so the nipple and neck remain filled with milk until the end of the feeding. This can help prevent gastric discomfort during and after the feeding (Fig. 7).

Finally, it must be emphasized that bottle feeding, like breast-feeding, should be a social as well as a nutritional event. Too many texts depict bottle feeding without eye contact between the infant and the caregiver. Feeding is a primary method of communication for children during the first year of life, and the social aspects of bottle feeding should not be overlooked by parents or caregivers.

SUMMARY

The pediatrician or other health-care provider who is counseling a family about bottle feeding must carefully instruct family members to simulate the techniques of breast-feeding as much as possible to minimize such feeding-related problems as choking, gastric discomfort, and the flow of fluid to the middle ear. It is essential to address the issues of body position, sucking, and swallowing, as well as the importance of close body contact and communication with the caregiver.

Breast-fed infants often initially refuse a bottle. Families and caregivers should be encouraged to feed their infants expressed milk in a semiupright position when bottle feeding. This position not only reduces the stress of adjusting to a bottle but also avoids many of the problems associated with improper bottle feeding. Semiupright feeding also ensures body contact between infant and caregiver, eye-to-eye communication, and the warmth and cuddling that are the automatic benefits of breast-feeding.

REFERENCES

1. Jelliffe DB, Jelliffe EFP. The uniqueness of human milk. Am J Clin Nutr 1971;24:968-9, 1013-23.
2. Kovar MG, Serdula MK, Marks JS, Fraser DW. Review of the epidemiologic evidence for an association between infant feeding and infant health. Pediatrics 1984;76(suppl):615-38.
3. Howard CR, Weitzman M. Breast or bottle: practical aspects of infant nutrition in the first 6 months. Pediatr Ann 1992; 21:619-21.
4. Lawrence RA. Breastfeeding: a guide for the medical profession. 4th ed. St. Louis: Mosby–Year Book, 1994:438, 462.
5. Klaus M, Kennell J. Parent-infant bonding. St. Louis: Mosby–Year Book, 1982:59-62.
6. Sosa R, Kennell JH, Klaus M. The effect of early mother-infant contact on breast feeding infection and growth. In: Breast feeding and the mother, Ciba Foundation Symposium, no. 45. Amsterdam: Elsevier Scientific, 1976:179-88.
7. Lozoff B, Brittenham GM, Trause MA, et al. The mother-newborn relationship: limits of adaptability. J PEDIATR 1977; 91:1-12.
8. Siegel E. Early and extended maternal-infant contact. Am J Dis Child 1982;136:251-7.
9. Newton N. Psychologic differences between breast and bottle feeding. In: Jelliffe DB, Jelliffe EFR, eds. Symposium, the uniqueness of human milk. Am J Clin Nutr 1971;24:993-1004.
10. Gussler J, Bryant C. Helping mothers breast-feed: program for strategies for minority communities. In: Health Action Papers, vol I. Lexington, Ky.: Lexington Fayette County Health Department, University of Kentucky Medical Behavioral Sciences Department, 1984:1-10.
11. Duncan RB, Wellington NZ. Positional otitis media. Arch Otolaryngol 1960;72:454-63.
12. Thornton HA. New infant nursing bottle with angled neck. Postgrad Med 1964;40(Jul/Aug):174-7.
13. Taubenhaus LJ. Bottle propping for infant feeding. J PEDIATR 1968;72:669-72.
14. Beauregard WG. Positional otitis media. J PEDIATR 1971; 79:294-6.
15. Wittenborg MH, Neuhauer EBD. Simple roentgenographic demonstration of Eustachian tubes and abnormalities. Am J Roentgen 1963;89:1194-200.
16. Nelson JD. Prop the baby, not the bottle. J PEDIATR 1971; 79:348-50.
17. Schaefer O. Otitis media and bottle-feeding: an epidemiological study of infant feeding habits and incidence of recurrent and chronic middle ear disease in Canadian Eskimos. Otitis Media 1971;62:478-89.
18. Timmermans FJW, Stanton G. Chronic granulomatous otitis media in bottle-fed Inuit children. Can Med Assoc J 1980; 122:545-7.
19. Owen MJ, Baldwin CD, Swank PR, et al. Relation of infant feeding practices, cigarette smoke exposure, and group child care to the onset and duration of otitis media with effusion in the first two years of life. J PEDIATR 1993;123:702-11.
20. Backon J. Prolonged breast feeding as a prophylaxis for recurrent otitis media: relevance of prostaglandins. Med Hypotheses 1984;13:161.
21. Duncan RB, Ey J, Holberg CJ, et al. Exclusive breast-feeding for at least 4 months protects against otitis media. Pediatrics 1993;91:867-72.
22. Kero P, Piekkala P. Factors affecting the occurrence of acute otitis media during the first year of life. Acta Paediatr Scand 1987;76:618-23.
23. Saarinen UM. Prolonged breast feeding as prophylaxis for recurrent otitis media. Acta Paediatr Scand 1982;71:567-71.
24. American Academy of Pediatrics Committee on Nutrition: The use of whole cow's milk in infancy. Pediatrics 1992;89: 1105-9.

Quantitative and qualitative video analysis of infants feeding: Angled- and straight-bottle feeding systems

Shereen D. Farber, PhD, OTR, FAOTA, Rory L. Van Fossen, MS, and Stephen W. Koontz, PhD

From Neurorehabilitation Services and Johnson & Johnson Consumer Products, Inc.

Objective: **To determine whether an angled-bottle feeding system is more effective than a straight-bottle feeding system in facilitating the medically recommended semiupright infant posture and to determine whether an angled bottle promotes improved ergonomic alignment and comfort for the feeder.**
Study design: **On two consecutive days, 23 pairs of parent-infant teams, seated in an ergonomic chair, were videotaped at the same time of day, during which infants were fed by their parents with either an angled or a straight bottle (presented in balanced order) fitted with the infants' regular nipple. Infants were given their regular type and amount of formula.**
Results: **The angled bottle provided a higher level of satisfaction compared with the straight bottle. Less gastric discomfort occurred with the angled bottle versus the straight bottle when each was compared with the bottle used at home. In addition, feeders assumed ergonomically sound positions.**
Conclusion: **This study indicates that an angled bottle is preferable to a straight bottle because it encourages more physiologic positioning of the infant, improves the comfort level of the feeder, improves ergonomic feeding performance, and decreases the need for burping. (J PEDIATR 1995;126:S118-24)**

The position in which an infant is held during feeding is physiologically important and can determine the degree of safety in feeding and comfort for mother and infant. Semiupright positioning during bottle feeding is recommended by the American Academy of Pediatricians to decrease the amount of liquid that may enter the middle ear and potentially to reduce the risk of choking. Contrary to semiupright feeding, supine feeding may be associated with colic, chronic regurgitation of milk, and otitis media,[1] as noted by one series of observers.

For many years, straight, reusable bottles (hereafter known as straight bottles) have been the standard in artificial feeding systems. However, during a typical feeding session with a straight bottle, the infant may be progressively reclined as the liquid level is reduced to avoid introduction of air during feeding. Increased recumbent posture serves to keep the nipple filled with fluid.[2] Alternatively, if the infant is not reclined to enhance the liquid flow to the nipple, the feeder may increase the vertical slope of the bottle. This practice changes the slope of the nipple in the infant's mouth from a natural, more horizontal position to an unnatural, more vertical position. During efficient sucking, the nipple is generally parallel to the hard palate and tongue so that the tongue may elevate to the nipple and extract the liquid.[3] When a bottle is propped or an infant is put to bed with a bottle, the infant is often completely recumbent and the problems associated with supine feeding are magnified.

As early as 1964, Thornton[1] suggested that an angled bottle would allow proper upright positioning of an infant, comparable with that seen in breast-feeding. He argued that an angled design would permit a child to swallow at leisure (because of the slower rate that fluid is presented to the mouth) and therefore swallow less air. He urged correction

Supported by a grant from Johnson & Johnson Consumer Products, Inc., Skillman, N.J.

Reprint requests: Rory L. Van Fossen, MS, Johnson & Johnson Consumer Products, Inc., Grandview Road, Skillman, NJ 08558.

0022-3476/95/$3.00 + 0 **9/0/64265**

of the mechanics of infant feeding with an angled design, but his ideas never gained wide acceptance.

Recently, an angled-bottle feeding system has been introduced. This study was designed to examine the angled bottle from an ergonomic vantage point and to determine quantitatively and qualitatively whether it offers advantages over the traditional straight bottle. Five hypotheses were proposed:

Hypothesis 1: Some aspect of the angled bottle will encourage a more physiologic position of the infant during feeding and result in greater infant comfort.

Hypothesis 2: Feeders using the angled bottle will feel greater satisfaction.

Hypothesis 3: Feeders will perceive less need to burp the infant when using an angled bottle as compared with a straight bottle.

Hypothesis 4: Feeders will report increased personal comfort using the angled bottle when posture is controlled by use of an ergonomic chair.

Hypothesis 5: Feeders will demonstrate an improved ergonomic feeding performance with an angled bottle as compared with a straight bottle.

METHODS

The study population consisted of 23 parent-infant subject teams selected on the basis of telephone interviews (22 mother-infant teams, 1 father-infant team). All infants were between 2 and 4 months of age and were regularly bottle fed formula with a nonorthodontic nipple. In this study, infants were fed with their usual nipple.

Each feeder-infant team was videotaped during feeding sessions that were scheduled on two consecutive days, at the same time of day in a noise-, temperature-, and light-controlled room. The video equipment, a recorder video camera (S-VHS; Panasonic Co., Secaucus, N.J.) and monitor (AG450; Panasonic), was situated in a permanent position in a second viewing room, and taping was conducted through a one-way mirror. A standard ergonomic chair, one that has adjustability for height from the floor, seat pan angle, seat depth, seat back height, seat width, and armrest height, was used along with an angled footrest. Position of all furniture in the feeding room was standardized to assure consistency of image size. A posture grid was placed 2 ft behind the chair and mounted on a partition. Feeders were taught to adjust the ergonomic chair and told that, if necessary, they could modify chair settings during the taping. Subjects were issued a hospital gown to standardize clothing worn during taping. White sticky dots were used to locate anatomic landmarks that would be measured from the video analysis. The following anatomic landmarks were identified on all feeders: midline of the forehead, midzygoma bilaterally, midline mentum, sternal notch, and anterior tip of the left and right acromion and on the feeding arm, lateral epicondyle of the humerus, ulnar head, and metacarpal heads. Infants were clothed in a diaper and bib so that clear postural views could be recorded. The following anatomic landmarks were placed on all infants: earlobe that would face the camera, midline tip of the acromion, lateral epicondyle of the infants' humerus, greater trochanter, and lateral patella (Fig. 1).

The research design was a controlled, balanced, paired comparison study. The order of product use was balanced. Feeders using the angled bottle and collar first, and straight bottle and collar second, were identified as cell 1 feeders (N = 12). Feeders using the straight bottle and collar first, and angled bottle and collar second, were identified as cell 2 feeders (N = 11). Chronologically, feeders were placed in one of the two cells in an alternating fashion, beginning with the first feeder being placed in cell 1. The test bottles were packaged and labeled before the initiation of the study.

Subjects signed an informed consent before initiation of the study. Once feeders were positioned comfortably in a hospital gown and with anatomic markers, they were given a standard set of instructions. They were also given an option to drop out during the study should they or their infant have unwanted signs or symptoms that related to the products tested and that compromised health. All subjects completed the study. Once the feeding session began, the camera ran continuously until the session was completed. Feeders answered questions on a consumer perception questionnaire. In addition, after each session feeders answered a series of monadic (rating) questions about the bottle tested on that day. After the second (final) feeding session, feeders answered a series of comparison questions concerning the two bottles tested.

Data analysis

Consumer response. Consumer response data were collected by using a survey tabulation software package (Creative Research Systems, Petaluma, Calif.). Consumer ratings were analyzed by using analysis of variance (ANOVA) two-way without replication. Preference data were analyzed by using the binomial test.

Morphometry. Subjects were videotaped during the feeding. One frame was captured every 3 minutes for each bottle. At least four frames were captured per feeder per bottle. Morphometric image analysis (bottle and torso angles) was performed by use of Jandel software (Jandel Scientific, San Rafael, Calif.). Median angles were used to summarize the multiple frames from each feeding.

Behavioral observations. Behavioral data were collected by viewing the videotape and pausing the tape. Behavioral data sheets were given a code based on the subject team number and initials for angled bottle versus straight bottle. Data were unitized (sorted by specific behaviors), and then

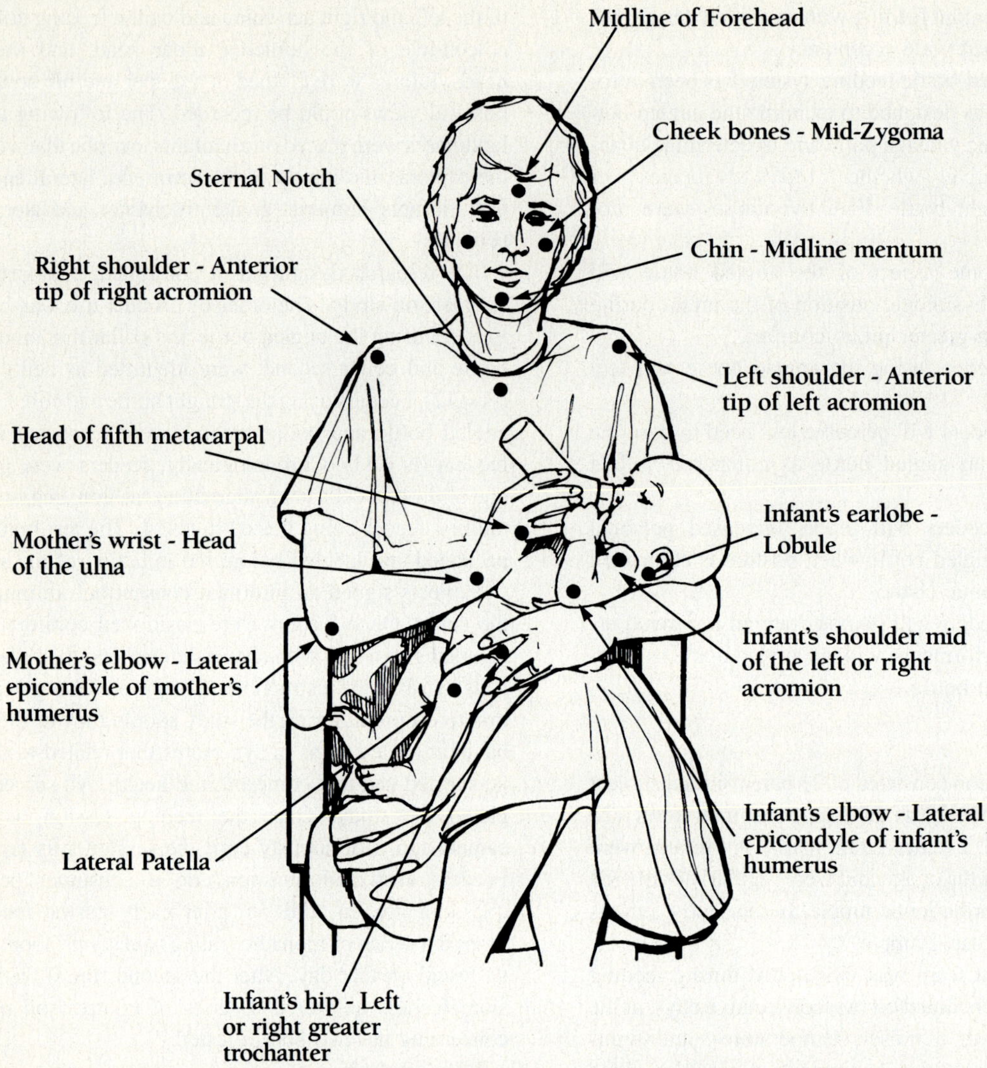

Fig. 1. Locations of anatomic markers worn by feeders and infants during videotaped feeding sessions (angled bottle).

comparisons were made between bottles for recorded behaviors. Typical behaviors recorded included parental postural responses to the chair and the bottle, bottle-holding patterns for feeder and infant, infant movement, infant posture, sucking, and burping activity.

RESULTS

Nipple slope, a quantitatively derived function, was significantly different when the two test bottles were compared (p <0.001, paired t-test). (Figs. 2 and 3). The nipple of the angled bottle sloped in a more horizontal position in infants' mouths. The nipple of the straight bottle had a higher (more vertical) nipple slope, which may make it more difficult for liquid to be extracted from the nipple by the tongue.

The consumer perception rating questions that were asked feeders after each feeding session resulted in a number of statistically significant differences in consumer bottle impression and related behaviors. Regarding the angled bottle, a significant difference (p <0.05, ANOVA) was found for overall satisfaction, comfort in holding the bottle, and increased postural comfort as compared with the straight bottle or the current bottle feeders used at home.

The qualitative behavioral assessment correlated with data obtained through consumer perceptions or morphometry. In total, 108 burping behaviors were noted, 56% of which were recorded during straight-bottle feedings. Feeders using angled bottles were unsuccessful at burping their infants or made no attempt to burp their infants 76% of the time. This behavior occurred 23% of the time with straight-bottle feedings. Quiet sucking was specifically noted during angled-bottle feedings 60.5% of the time as compared with 39% during straight-bottle feedings.

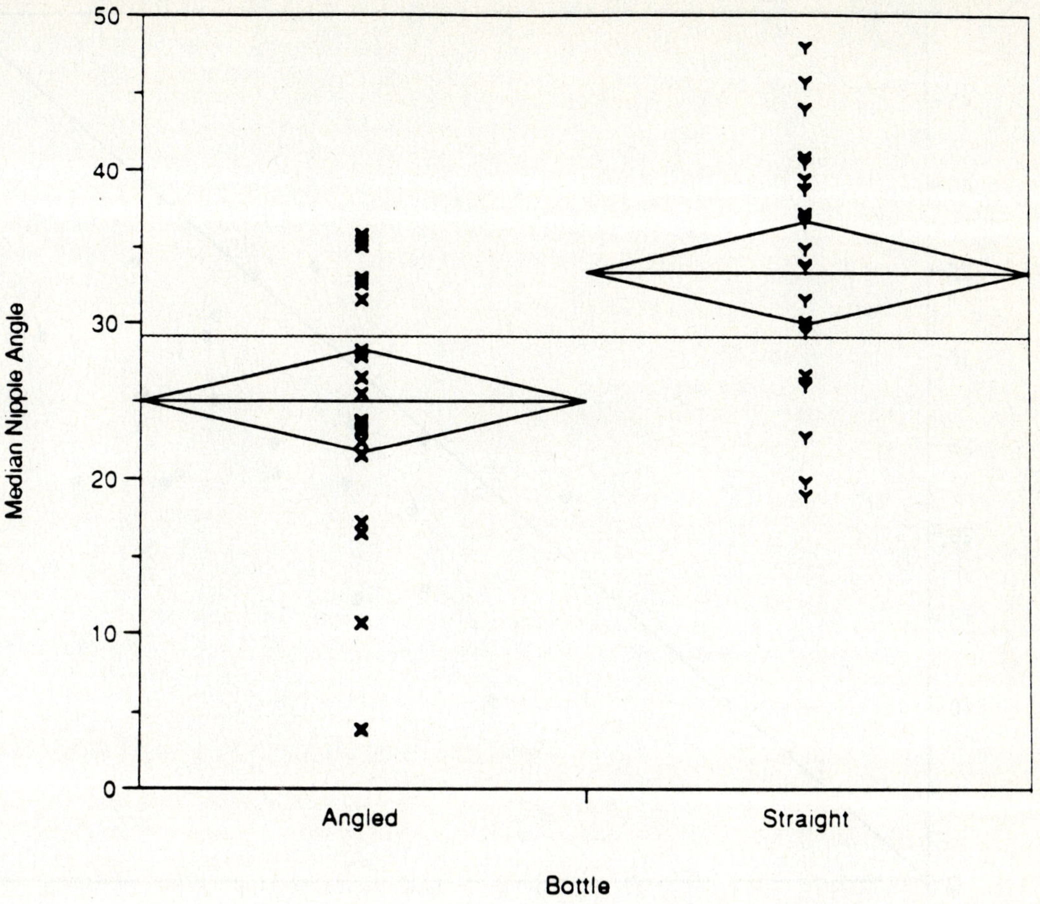

Fig. 2. Comparison of median nipple angles for both bottles indicated that straight bottle had a higher nipple slope than angled bottle. Thus, nipple of straight bottle is in a more vertical position, making it difficult for infant to extract liquid from nipple. Values are expressed as means, with 95% confidence intervals.

After the monadic ratings for the second (final) feeding session were obtained, feeders were asked to compare the two test bottles. When asked their overall preference of the two bottles, 22 of the 23 feeders (96%) selected the angled bottle. Reasons for selecting the angled bottle included ease of holding and feeding the infant, lack of necessity to tip the bottle, and nipples that remained filled with liquid longer during the feeding. Forty-one percent of the feeders specifically mentioned that with the angled bottle, they did not have to worry about the bottle angle, could get closer to the infant, and felt more comfortable during the feeding.

Feeders also were asked to compare each of the test bottles with the bottle they used at home. Twenty-two of the 23 feeders (96%) indicated that they did not prefer their current bottle over the angled bottle. When asked to explain why, 45% mentioned the angle of the test bottle and 41% stated improved comfort for the feeder while holding the angled bottle. For the straight-bottle feeding, 11 feeders (48%) indicated preference for their current bottle and 12 (52%) indicated they did not prefer their current bottle over the straight bottle. Preferences for the angled bottle were significant ($p = 0.001$) for the specific attributes listed in the Table. There was an even distribution regarding the perception of which bottle would be easier for an infant to hold (11 feeders selected the angled bottle, 11 feeders selected the straight bottle, and one feeder expressed no preference).

Regarding parental posture, head position over the midline of the body was graded. Head flexion is increased when the subject moves the chin closer to the sternum. Head rotation is defined as lateral movement of the chin in a horizontal plane, away from the midline about a vertical axis. "Sidebending" is a head position in which the subject moves his or her head so that the ipsilateral earlobe is closer to the shoulder; this represents frontal plane movement about a sagittal axis. Mild flexion and rotation of the head were more commonly seen in those using the angled bottle. The mild sidebent head position was equally split between angled- and straight-bottle feedings. Moderate head flexion and rotation

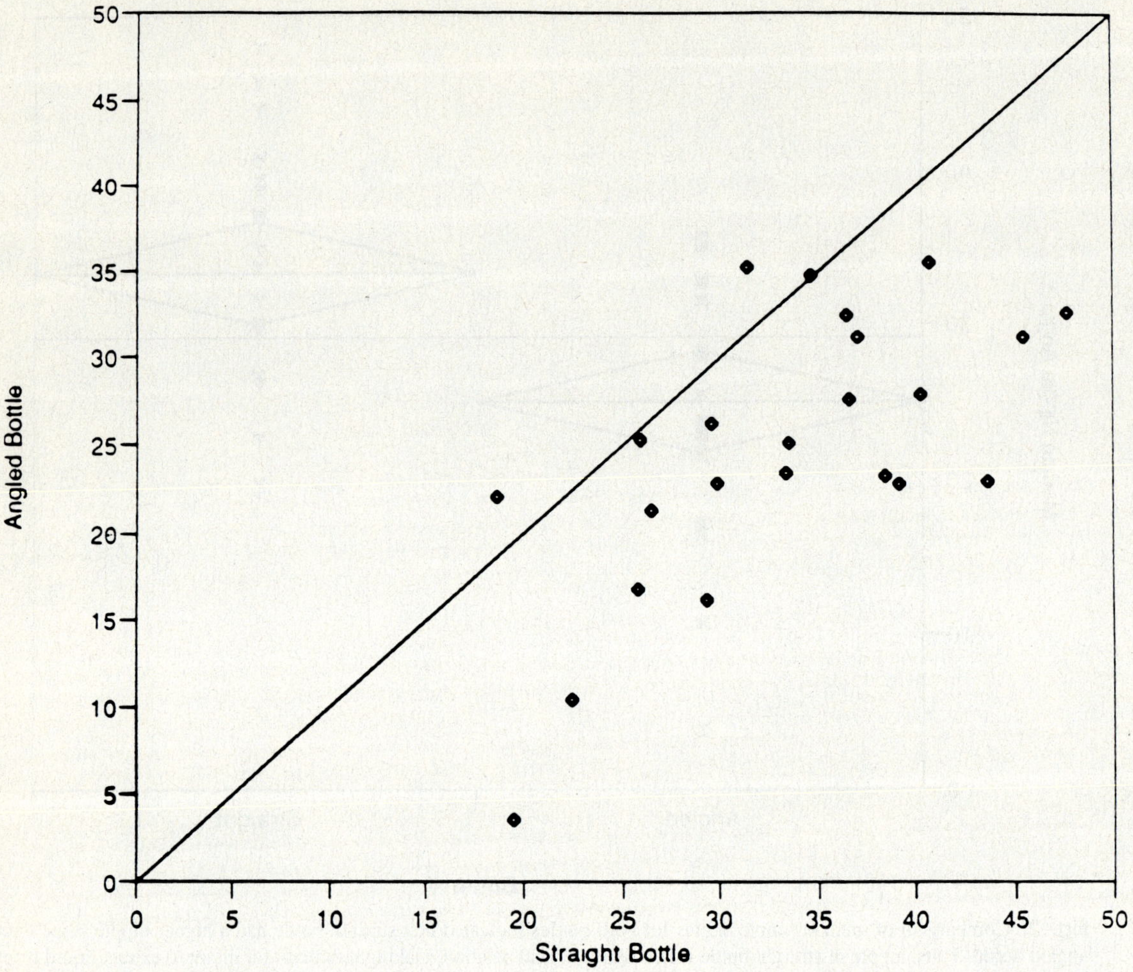

Fig. 3. Median nipple angle of angled bottle, with line of no differences. Nipple of straight bottle was consistently in a more vertical position than nipple of angled bottle.

were equally split between both bottles, but moderate sidebending was more commonly seen in the straight-bottle feeding sessions (60% compared with 40%). Extreme head flexion, rotation, or sidebending occurred only in those using the straight bottle (75% for head flexion, 82% for rotation, and 62.5% for extreme sidebending). Combinations of rotation, flexion, and sidebending were twice as likely to occur during straight-bottle feeding. The neutral positioning of the feeder's head was prevalent in the angled-bottle feeding sessions, while combinations of rotation, flexion, and sidebending were often observed in the straight-bottle feeding sessions. Shoulder position was symmetrical in 68% of feeders using angled bottles, whereas asymmetry of the shoulders occurred in 67% of those using straight bottles. The number of feedings during which the feeder moved from mild to extreme wrist extension was greater with the straight-bottle feedings than with the angled-bottle feedings. Thus those using the angled bottle had improved posture as compared with those using the straight bottle (Fig. 4).

Regarding bottle holding, feeders using the angled bottle tended to maintain their grip on the bottle primarily at the angle of the bottle. In those using a straight bottle, the loci of grip changed frequently throughout the feeding. In terms of holding the infants, the feeders who used the angled bottle placed their infants in a more upright posture 61% of the time. Fifty-seven percent of the feeders who used the straight bottle frequently repositioned their infants.

Regarding infant movement during feeding, total body movement for infants fed with the straight bottle was 60%, whereas in some cases those who fed their babies with angled bottles appeared motionless or the infants had isolated body part movement. Infants held the straight bottle with little assistance more frequently and for a longer period; however, both bottles were touched with equal frequency.

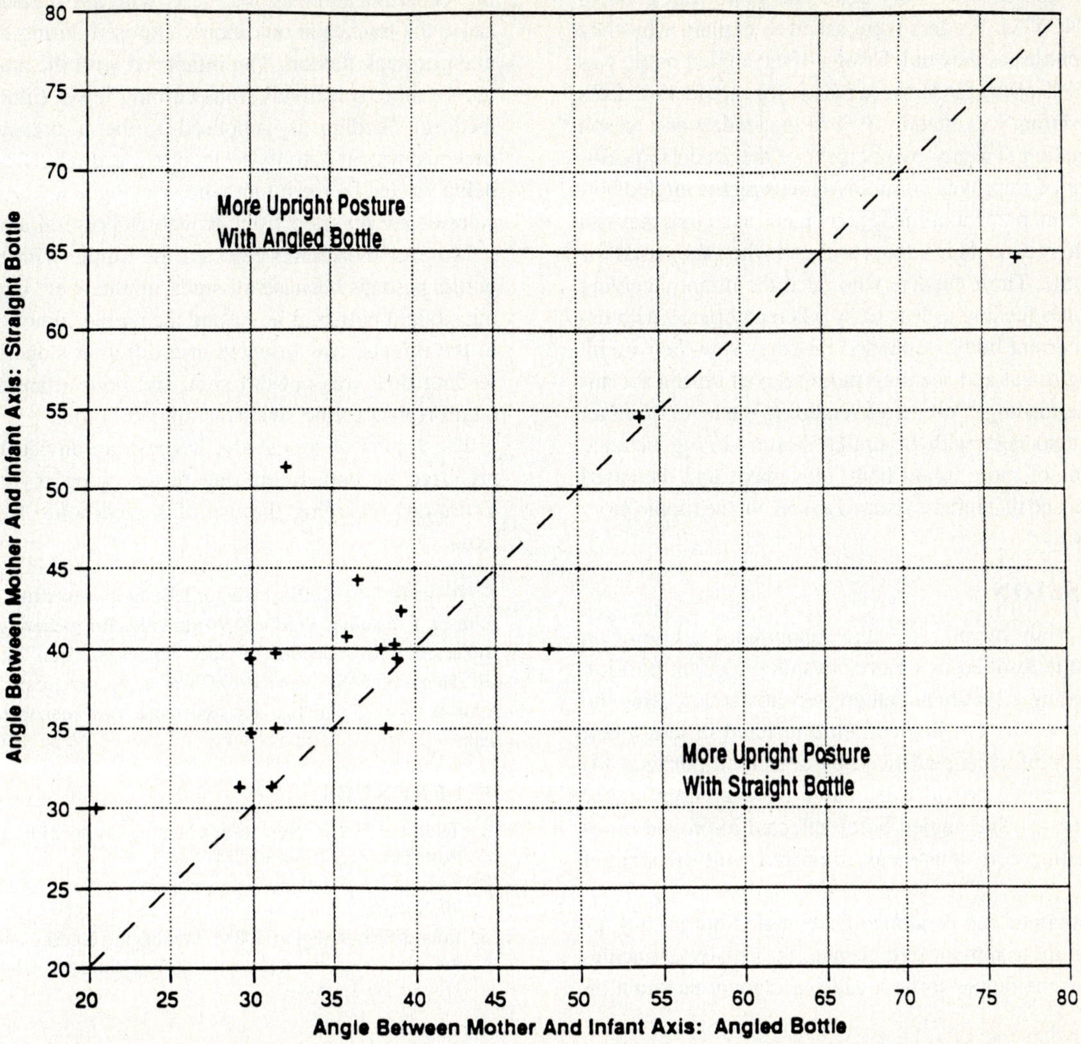

Fig. 4. Measurement of angle, in degrees, formed between feeder's midline axis and infant's axis from hip to ear lobe during feeding sessions with an angled bottle and a straight bottle. Posture was significantly more upright, $p = 0.028$ by signed-rank test, with angled bottle.

More infants had head alignment or slight neck flexion, which would protect the infant from choking, during feeding with the angled bottle as compared with the straight bottle. Equal numbers of infants had slight neck extension, which would expose the trachea to fluid intake.

Feeders reported that the infants' gastric discomfort when using the angled bottle was considered normal to somewhat lower than normal as compared with the bottle used at home ($p < 0.05$, ANOVA). The straight bottle was rated at normal to somewhat higher levels of gastric discomfort when compared with the bottle used at home. The angled-bottle feeding sessions resulted in an overall rating between extremely good and very good, whereas the straight-bottle feeding ses-

Table. Attributes for which feeders preferred angled bottle

Being comfortable to hold when feeding
Being easy to use and hold when feeding
Helps you maintain good posture while using to feed infant
Allows infant to feed easily
Reduces the amount of air swallowed during feeding
Allows you to hold infant comfortably and with less strain when feeding
Being a bottle that has a better shape
Reduces flow of liquid to the middle ear
Allows you to hold infant in a semiupright position during feeding
Being a bottle that can help digestion
Being a bottle that would be recommended by a pediatrician or nurse

sion was rated between very good and somewhat good ($p < 0.05$, ANOVA). Feeders were asked to explain why they rated the bottles as they did. Design of the angled bottle was cited by 52% of the feeders as a reason for satisfaction. Less air for the infant was cited by 39% of the feeders as a reason for satisfaction. Twenty-two percent of the feeders specifically reported improved comfort when using the angled bottle. Seventeen percent of the feeders mentioned that they did not have to recline their infants as much when they used the angled bottle. Those feeders who rated the infant receiving angled-bottle feeding as less fussy when compared with using their current bottle explained that they saw their infant continuing to eat and seeming more relaxed during the angled-bottle feeding. Comments regarding the level of infant fussiness associated with the straight-bottle feeding included perceptions of more infant body movement and increased crankiness and that infants seemed to spit out the nipple more frequently.

DISCUSSION

All the study hypotheses were supported: (1) Use of an angled bottle resulted in a more physiologic infant position during feeding. (2) Parents felt greater satisfaction using the angled bottle. (3) The angled bottle resulted in less infant gastric discomfort as evidenced by decreased burping. (4) The angled bottle provided increased personal comfort for the parents. (5) The angled bottle effected improved ergonomic feeding performance as compared with the straight bottle.

The horizontal nipple slope of the angled bottle may allow the infant to remain semiupright, thus easily extracting liquid from the nipple without causing ergonomic strain on the feeder. Head position is safer with the angled bottle because the trachea is not unduly exposed during head alignment or neck flexion. The infant fed with the angled bottle moves more selectively, thus burning fewer calories during feeding. Feeding is supposed to be a parasympathetic nervous system activity to facilitate growth. If calories are being wasted by the infant who is trying to achieve comfort, calories are diverted from growth to postural adaptation.

More of the infants rejected the nipple with the angled bottle, perhaps because all study infants were currently using straight bottles at home and the nipple, although familiar to the infants, was oriented at a different slope. However, feeding time was not different, and both infant and feeder comfort was greater with the angled bottle.

The results of this study, wherein an angled bottle was preferred by both infant and feeder, support the ideas of Thornton[1] regarding the use of angled-bottle feeding systems.

We thank Julie Kelliher, senior laboratory associate, Johnson & Johnson Consumer Products Worldwide, for gathering pilot data and assisting in collection of video behavioral data. We also thank Gil Henyon, MS, manager of statistical services, Johnson & Johnson, for his patience and assistance with management of the data.

REFERENCES

1. Thornton HA Jr. New infant nursing bottle with angled neck. Postgrad Med 1964;36:174-7.
2. Nelson JD. Prop the baby, not the bottle. J PEDIATR 1971; 79:348-50.
3. Imhoff SM, Wigginton VM. Identifying feeding and swallowing problems in infants and young children. Clin Commun Disord 1991;1:59-67.

Nipple confusion: Toward a formal definition

Marianne Neifert, MD, Ruth Lawrence, MD, and Joy Seacat, RN, CHA, MS

From the Lactation Program, Presbyterian/St. Luke's Medical Center, Denver, Colorado, and the Department of Pediatrics, University of Rochester, Rochester, New York

The purposes of this article are to introduce a formal definition of nipple confusion and to propose various hypotheses concerning its cause. The term nipple confusion refers to an infant's difficulty in achieving the correct oral configuration, latching technique, and suckling pattern necessary for successful breast-feeding after bottle feeding or other exposure to an artificial nipple. Many early breast-feeding failures are attributed to nipple confusion, although scientific data are lacking to document its prevalence, the mechanisms involved, or various factors that predispose an infant to this phenomenon. Two classifications of nipple confusion are recommended to distinguish the impact of artificial nipples during the newborn period from their influence after breast-feeding is well established. Maternal and infant risk factors making an infant more susceptible to nipple confusion are discussed. Future studies are planned to help elucidate the nature of nipple confusion and identify the circumstances under which infants are most vulnerable to this phenomenon. Meanwhile, it would seem prudent for clinicians to identify newborns at risk for nipple confusion and to minimize the use of bottle feedings in such babies. Medically indicated supplements in the early days of life could be provided by alternative methods, such as cup, spoon, or dropper feeding, until breast-feeding can be established. (J Pediatr 1995;126:S125-9)

The Committee on Nutrition of the American Academy of Pediatrics strongly endorses breast-feeding as the optimal source of nutrition for infants during the first 6 months of life.[1] Currently, more than half of mothers in the United States elect to begin breast-feeding their infants, but many women discontinue nursing prematurely.[2] The rapid attrition in breast-feeding during the postnatal period reflects the prevalence of early problems in the establishment of lactation and the frequency with which women encounter difficulties in guiding their infants to nurse effectively. As a result of today's abbreviated postpartum hospital confinements, contemporary mothers receive only minimal support and instruction in proper breast-feeding techniques.

Lactation counselors and lay supporters of breast-feeding attribute many early failures to ''nipple confusion''—the interference of artificial nipples with the successful initiation of breast-feeding. A newborn infant who alternates between the maternal nipple and an artificial nipple may have difficulty nursing correctly and may soon show a preference for artificial feeding. This observation has been validated by clinicians who work with breast-feeding mothers. A common scenario includes the infant who nurses well right after delivery, receives bottles in the nursery during the night, then fusses and frets at the breast in the morning and will not latch on to nurse.

The concept of nipple confusion enjoys tremendous popularity and has been widely disseminated in literature aimed at parents. Many of these texts imply that nipple confusion is the inevitable and ominous consequence of offering even a single bottle to a breast-fed infant before breast-feeding is well established, as these excerpts indicate:

> Using a pacifier, nipple shields, or supplemental bottles of water, formula, or juice can cause nipple confusion and interfere with a baby's ability to suck effectively at the breast. Just one bottle is enough to confuse some babies, especially in the early weeks.[3]

Supported by a grant from Johnson & Johnson Consumer Products, Inc., Skillman. N.J.

Reprint requests: Marianne Neifert, MD, Lactation Program, Presbyterian/St. Luke's Medical Center, 1719 E. 19th Ave., Denver, CO 80218.

0022-3476/95/$3.00 + 0 **9/0/64223**

For some babies, it may take a week of bottles before they become nipple-confused; for other babies, only one or two bottles—or other artificial nipples—will cause it.[4]

In our practices, we periodically encounter parents who are convinced that even a single bottle feeding during the early postpartum weeks will seriously jeopardize their breast-feeding attempts. Such parents may be hesitant to provide supplemental milk to their infants even when a valid medical indication exists because they fear that nipple confusion inevitably will result. (Although other alternatives exist for providing supplemental milk to infants, bottle feeding is still the most widely practiced.) In extreme cases, misguided attempts to avoid nipple confusion have resulted in severe dehydration and malnutrition among breast-fed infants.[5]

However, the notion that offering a single bottle is likely to result in breast-feeding failure runs contrary to experience. Many breast-fed infants receive one or more supplemental feedings by bottle during the first week of life, and yet go on to breast-feed exclusively. Other infants, including some whose mothers are employed outside the home, accept a bottle readily and resume breast-feeding without apparent difficulty. Cronenwett et al.,[6] in a prospective study of 121 breast-feeding couples highly motivated to nurse, found that single daily bottle use in the early weeks after birth had no significant impact on the duration of breast-feeding. On the basis of the study results, the investigators rejected the nipple confusion hypothesis. Both physicians and lactation consultants wrote letters to the editor arguing the existence of nipple confusion and citing early bottles and pacifiers for such diverse breast-feeding maladies as infant latch-on troubles, fussiness, and slow weight gain, as well as maternal sore nipples, engorgement, and decreased milk production.[7-12]

Although nipple confusion usually describes newborn infants who have not learned to nurse well, some practitioners apply the term to older infants who are breast-feeding successfully but who subsequently display difficulties nursing after bottle feeding is introduced. Nipple confusion also has been used to describe the proficiently breast-feeding infant who refuses to drink from a bottle, exhibiting a strong preference for the breast. This type of problem in older infants differs sufficiently from that in newborn infants experiencing difficulty learning to nurse that it warrants a separate classification.

Despite its acceptance in lay circles, nipple confusion has never been formally defined or widely acknowledged within the medical profession. No data exist to document the incidence of nipple confusion, the possible mechanisms involved in its cause, or specific maternal and infant factors that may predispose an infant to difficulty in breast-feeding after exposure to an artificial nipple.

This article will introduce a formal definition of nipple confusion and working hypotheses to explain the phenomenon. It also will attempt to identify the factors that may cause some infants to be more vulnerable than others to nipple confusion. Recommendations for supplementing breast-fed newborns in clinical practice will be discussed.

MEDICAL DEFINITION OF NIPPLE CONFUSION

Two classifications of nipple confusion are recommended to distinguish the impact of artificial nipples during the newborn period from their influence after breast-feeding is well established. We propose that the term ''nipple confusion type A'' be used to describe a neonate's difficulty in exhibiting the correct oral configuration, latching technique, and suckling pattern necessary to extract milk from the breast after exposure to an artificial teat. Typically, this phenomenon occurs when an artificial nipple is introduced before the successful establishment of breast-feeding. It is especially likely to occur when sucking the artificial nipple results in more rapid flow of fluid than is available from the breast.

The term ''nipple confusion'' should not be applied to situations in which a newborn infant displays a primary inability to suckle the breast effectively, without prior exposure to an artificial teat such as a bottle nipple, pacifier, or adult finger. Rather, the term should describe only those instances in which an infant who may or may not yet have breast-fed successfully has been offered an artificial nipple and subsequently has difficulty breast-feeding effectively.

HYPOTHESES TO EXPLAIN NIPPLE CONFUSION

We propose four working hypotheses to explain the phenomenon of nipple confusion.

(1) A neonate may have limited ability to adapt to various oral configurations. When a newborn infant who has been breast-fed is given an artificial teat to suck, such as a pacifier, bottle nipple, or adult finger, this stimulus may intercept the physiologic action of normal breast-feeding, and the infant may readjust to a sucking pattern that compresses and controls the teat. In addition, if a higher volume and faster flow of fluid is obtained by bottle feeding than by breast-feeding, the infant may adapt his or her oral configuration to control the increased fluid flow.

(2) A form of ''imprinting'' may occur in the immediate postpartum period. If the first feeding after birth is given by bottle, the artificial nipple may be imprinted in the infant and make subsequent attempts at breast-feeding more difficult.

(3) Newborn infants may be vulnerable to nipple confusion because of the relatively low volume of colostrum available with breast-feeding in the first few days of life. Before full lactogenesis, the amount of colostrum available

Table I. Maternal lactation risk factors predisposing to nipple confusion

Variability in nipples
Very large or small nipples
Flat, inverted, or excessively long nipples
Abnormal breasts
Hypoplastic or markedly asymmetric breasts
Previous breast surgery that has severed milk ducts
Delayed or absent lactogenesis
Low milk supply
Maternal illness (hypertension, HELLP, diabetes mellitus, infection, anemia)
Maternal-infant separation
Previous history of insufficient lactation or inadequate weight gain in previous breast-fed infant
Difficulty learning proper breast-feeding technique

HELLP, Hemolysis, elevated liver enzymes, and low platelet count.

Table II. Infant lactation risk factors predisposing to nipple confusion

Prematurity, ≤37 wk
Apgar <5 at 1 min or <7 at 5 min
Birthweight <6 lb (2700 gm)
Small for gestational age or intrauterine growth retardation
Large for gestational age
Infant of diabetic mother
Hypoglycemia
Multiple births
Medical illness (oxygen requirement, cardiac defect, infection)
Neonatal hyperbilirubinemia, especially requiring phototherapy
Neuromotor/developmental problems (Down syndrome, hypotonia, dysfunctional sucking)
Oral anatomic problems (cleft lip/palate, micrognathia, ankyloglossia, high arched palate)
Difficulty latching on correctly or sustaining sucking

is small, and even after the true milk comes in, infants must nurse correctly to obtain generous quantities during breast-feeding. Measurements of milk intake by breast-fed newborn infants have documented intakes of about an ounce (30 ml) in the first 24 hours after birth.[13] Thus if a neonate is given the opportunity to feed from a 3- or 4-ounce (90 to 120 ml) bottle on the first day of life, at a time when only a minimum quantity of milk would be available during a single breast-feeding session, the infant might act accustomed to a more rapid flow of milk and act fretful during attempts at breast-feeding.

(4) Infants who have difficulty with their initial attempts at breast-feeding may be more prone to manifest nipple confusion. Not only is the poorly feeding infant more likely to receive supplemental bottle feedings, but an infant who has not learned to grasp and suckle the maternal nipple correctly is likely to perceive bottle feeding as easier and more rewarding than attempts at the breast.

POTENTIAL RISK FACTORS FOR NIPPLE CONFUSION

The vulnerability of individual infants to nipple confusion may be exacerbated by various risk factors that can jeopardize either correct nipple attachment or the extraction of milk during breast-feeding. Breast-fed infants who have difficulty obtaining milk will be more likely to prefer bottle feeding if given the opportunity. Examples of such predisposing factors are listed in Tables I and II.

Many of the proposed maternal risk factors relate to either improper infant grasp of the nipple, low milk production, or impaired milk flow. It stands to reason that breast-feeding would be facilitated for the infant of a mother with a protuberant nipple, generous colostrum/milk supply, and a free flow of milk. Conversely, the infant of a mother with poor nipple definition, minimal colostrum/milk production, or obstructed milk flow would be more susceptible to having bottle feedings interfere with the successful establishment of breast-feeding.

Some women have variations of nipple size or shape, developmental anomalies of the breast, or diagnostic or cosmetic breast surgery that impair nipple grasp, milk production, or milk emptying. Clinicians must reject the outdated concept that every breast is ideal for breast-feeding. Inspection of the breasts and nipples should readily identify women with anatomic risk factors. Illness, maternal-infant separation, previous breast-feeding failure, delayed or absent lactogenesis, and difficulty learning proper breast-feeding technique are other maternal factors that may place an infant at increased risk for nipple confusion.

Certain infant factors also are suggested to predispose neonates to nipple confusion. Whenever suckling effectiveness is decreased because of prematurity, intrauterine growth retardation, birth asphyxia, hyperbilirubinemia, neuromotor problems, respiratory distress, or other medical illness, infants are at increased risk for inadequate breast-feeding. Such neonates will be more vulnerable to nipple confusion if offered feedings by bottle. Some infants have medical indications for supplemental milk, such as hypoglycemia, excessive weight loss, or maternal-infant separation, which increase the likelihood that they will receive some bottle feedings. Any oral anatomic abnormality also can impair an infant's ability to breast-feed effectively, increasing the likelihood that supplemental milk will be required and making an infant more vulnerable to nipple confusion. Such problems include moderate to marked micrognathia, cleft lip or cleft palate, or ankyloglossia.

In addition to the maternal and infant risk factors cited, characteristic differences exist between the human nipple and artificial nipples that may contribute to nipple confusion. A particular infant's response to bottle feeding may be influenced by physical features (such as the texture, shape, and elasticity of the artificial nipple), sensory characteristics (such as odor, taste, and temperature of the artificial nipple), and the fluid flow rate.

CLINICAL RECOMMENDATIONS TO MINIMIZE THE OCCURRENCE OF NIPPLE CONFUSION TYPE A

On the basis of the proposed risk factors just outlined, it is possible to construct a profile of the infant who has difficulty learning to breast-feed, who has a medical indication for supplementation, or whose mother has flat or inverted nipples and a low volume of milk. This common scenario poses a familiar clinical dilemma—how best to provide the required supplement without jeopardizing breast-feeding. Does one use a traditional bottle and nipple unit or deliberately avoid bottle nipples by instituting cup, dropper, or spoon feedings? Although it is not known conclusively whether alternative methods of supplementing feedings improve an infant's chances of ultimately breast-feeding, it would seem prudent to avoid bottle feedings in vulnerable infants when possible. Many practitioners have acquired considerable experience with alternative feeding methods, which appear to be quite harmless. As long as numerous cases of breast-feeding failure are anecdotally linked with nipple confusion, further exploration of alternative feeding methods seem warranted.

A similar argument could be made against giving pacifiers to breast-fed infants until nursing is well established. Furthermore, avoiding use of artificial nipples with breast-fed newborn infants is an integral component of the World Health Organization/UNICEF Baby Friendly Hospital Initiative, a global campaign aimed at removing obstacles to breast-feeding that a woman may encounter in the hospital.[14, 15]

It should be emphasized that whenever a breast-fed newborn does not nurse effectively, rapid involution of maternal milk supply can result and further compound the feeding difficulty. Thus if maternal or infant risk factors are present that threaten the successful initiation of breast-feeding, it is advisable to prescribe a rental grade electric breast pump to empty the maternal breasts at regular intervals to establish and preserve a generous supply of milk. Nipple confusion is more likely to be overcome when a free flow of milk is readily available.

NIPPLE CONFUSION TYPE B

Some practitioners broaden the definition of nipple confusion to include situations in which an older infant who isproficient at breast-feeding refuses to drink from a bottle. We propose that this phenomenon, also known as "bottle refusal," be called nipple confusion type B to distinguish it from nipple confusion in a newborn infant who has never learned to breast-feed well. Bottle refusal or nipple confusion type B is a frustrating problem for a substantial number of breast-feeding women who want their infants to drink from a bottle because they wish to return to work, are ill, or elect to be separated from their infants for other reasons.

No baseline data exist to document the incidence of bottle refusal in breast-fed infants or the average duration required to accustom an exclusively breast-fed infant to periodic bottle feeding. However, in our practices we receive numerous inquiries from mothers who wish to return to work and are extremely distraught that their infants will not take a bottle. This common dilemma adds to the stress experienced by breast-feeding mothers in the workforce. Women anticipating returning to work may introduce bottle feedings prematurely in hopes of preventing subsequent bottle refusal. This practice, in turn, may undermine the successful initiation of breast-feeding.

Nipple confusion type B also can apply to subsequent breast-feeding difficulty or bottle feeding preference displayed by infants who previously nursed well until bottle feedings were introduced. We suspect that most of these cases are related to declining maternal milk volume associated with excessive supplementation and maternal-infant separation. Infants may lose interest in nursing when the milk volume is limited, preferring to consume ad lib quantities of milk by bottle.

RECOMMENDATIONS FOR FUTURE STUDIES

Currently, it is unclear whether the phenomena of nipple confusion type A and nipple confusion type B are separate or related problems. Further studies are necessary to confirm our hypotheses regarding the underlying mechanisms involved in nipple confusion and to address various unanswered questions regarding these entities.

We have designed a pilot study to investigate nipple confusion type B. This phenomenon is initially simpler to study because it involves healthy, older infants who are proficient at breast-feeding. We intend to examine different nipple-bottle systems to determine whether one system is more readily accepted by breast-fed infants or facilitates transfer between breast and bottle without undermining breast-feeding. Such a feeding system would be very useful in clinical practice because it would allow necessary supplementation without jeopardizing the continuation of breast-feeding.

After the completion of this pilot work, we plan to conduct further studies to investigate nipple confusion among breast-fed neonates who receive bottles before breast-feeding is well established. It is our hope that these studies will shed light on the cause of nipple confusion type A and nipple confusion type B, and further elucidate the risk factors associated with these problems.

REFERENCES

1. American Academy of Pediatrics Committee on Nutrition. The use of whole cow's milk in infancy. Pediatrics 1992;89: 1105-9.
2. Ryan AS, Rush D, Krieger FW, Lewandowski GE. Recent declines in breast-feeding in the United States, 1984 through 1989. Pediatrics 1991;88:719-27.
3. La Leche League International. The womanly art of breast-feeding, 35th anniversary ed. Franklin Park, Ill.: La Leche League International, 1991:331.
4. Mohrbacher N, Stock J. The breastfeeding answer book. Franklin Park, Ill.: La Leche League International, 1991:253.
5. Helliker K. Dying for milk. Wall Street Journal 1994 July 22:A1, A4.
6. Cronenwett L, Stukel T, Kearney M, et al. Single daily bottle use in the early weeks postpartum and breast-feeding outcome. Pediatrics 1992;90:760-6.
7. Walker M. Nipple confusion [Letter]. Pediatrics 1993;92:297.
8. Newman J. Nipple confusion. Pediatrics 1993;92:297-8.
9. Mulford C. Nipple confusion. Pediatrics 1993;92:298-9.
10. Heery L. Nipple confusion [Letter]. Pediatrics 1993;92:299.
11. Auerbach K. Nipple confusion. Pediatrics 1993;92:299-300.
12. Frederickson D. Nipple confusion. Pediatrics 1993;92:300-1.
13. Casey CE, Neifert MR, Seacat JM, Neville MC. Nutrient intake by breast-fed infants during the first five days after birth. Am J Dis Child 1986;140:933-6.
14. Kyenkya-Isabirye M. UNICEF launches the Baby-Friendly Hospital Initiative. MCN 1992;17:177-9.
15. Wolf H, Charrondiere R, Helsing E. First "baby-friendly" hospitals in Europe. Lancet 1993;341:440.

Imaging evaluation of breast-feeding and bottle-feeding systems

Arthur J. Nowak, DMD, Wilbur L. Smith, MD, and Allen Erenberg, MD

From the Departments of Pediatrics, Pediatric Dentistry, and Radiology, University of Iowa, Iowa City, and the Department of Pediatrics, University of Kansas Medical Center, Kansas City

Objective: **To compare infant sucking and swallowing patterns during feeding with a new artificial nipple and during breast-feeding.**
Methods: **Fifteen healthy, term infants were fed successfully for 1 week with use of the new tricut nipple; then each infant's oral cavity was examined during feeding by using real-time ultrasonography. Measurements of nipple length and compression were made, together with observations concerning the integrity of the seal formed by the infant's mouth around the nipple. These data were compared with similar data from previous studies of 16 breast-fed infants.**
Results: **Although no artificial feeding system exactly simulates breast-feeding, the new tricut nipple was sucked in a manner similar to the way the human nipple is sucked and delivered milk posteriorly to the foramen cecum region of the tongue, just as the breast does.**
Conclusion: **Although further studies are necessary to evaluate other characteristics of the new tricut nipple, the measurements from this investigation are useful additions to the ultrasound data these investigators have accumulated on various artificial feeding systems. These data may also prove helpful in determining the most appropriate nipples for infants with various feeding disorders. (J PEDIATR 1995;126:S130-4)**

Despite the advantages of breast-feeding, many women opt to bottle feed their infants occasionally or routinely. They may need to return to work, school, or other activities and may want to extend the duration of breast-feeding by having their infants bottle fed expressed milk in their absence. They may adopt bottle feeding because of perceived convenience of the method. All these mothers are soon faced with another decision: the selection of an appropriate artificial feeding system. Many artificial nipples are currently available, all with various claims as to their efficacy and similarity to the mother's breast. The validity of these claims must be evaluated objectively through techniques that examine an infant's interaction with the feeding system without jeopardizing his or her safety.

Supported in part by a grant from Johnson & Johnson Consumer Products, Inc., Skillman, N.J.

Reprint requests: Arthur J. Nowak, DMD, Department of Pediatric Dentistry DSB-S-204, University of Iowa Hospitals and Clinics, Iowa City, IA 52242.

0022-3476/95/$3.00 + 0 **9/0/64224**

Early studies of the mechanisms of sucking and swallowing in the late 1950s used cineradiology; unfortunately, this technique exposed infants to the risks of radiation.[1] During the past 10 years, our studies have used noninvasive ultrasonography to investigate normal movements of the tongue and mandible during sucking and swallowing[2] and to compare the shapes of artificial nipples and the human breast during sucking and swallowing.[3, 4] Ultrasound studies permit imaging in the normal feeding position for mother and infant, whether breast-feeding or bottle feeding.

This study compares measurements of length, compressibility, and other characteristics of a newly designed tricut nipple with measurements from a previous study[3] of the human nipple.

METHODS

Fifteen healthy term infants, 2 to 15 weeks of age (mean age of 7.2 weeks), with no congenital disorders were

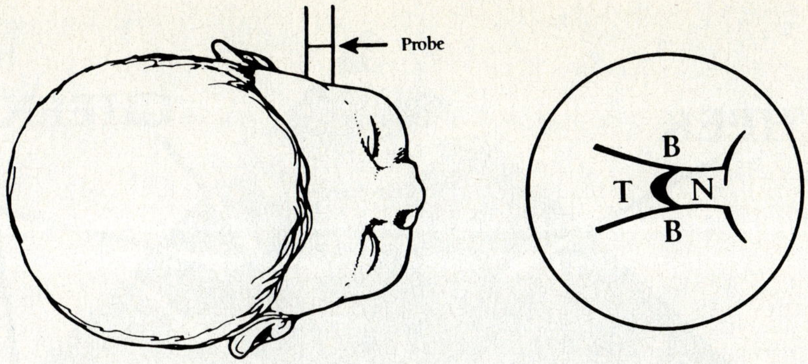

Fig. 1. Schemas of axial projection or transverse plane. *B*, Buccal surfaces; *N*, nipple; *T*, tongue.

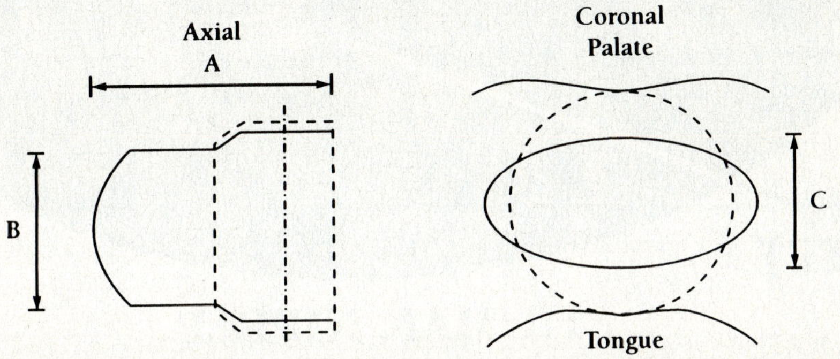

Fig. 2. Diagram of nipple deformation in axial and coronal projections. *Solid lines* indicate nipple at full suck; *dashed lines*, nipple at rest; *interrupted dashed lines*, plane in which coronal images were obtained. *A* measurement indicates elongation of nipple; *B* measurement indicates increase in width of nipple (lateral compression or axial compression); *C* measurement indicates decrease in height of nipple (flattening or coronal compression).

recruited from the University of Iowa Hospitals and Clinics' Department of Obstetrics and Gynecology, the Newborn Unit, and the Child Health Care Clinic of the Department of Pediatrics. Informed consent was obtained from the parents, and the protocol was approved by the Human Subjects Review Committee.

Parents were asked to use the new tricut nipple for bottle-feeding their infants and to return after approximately 1 week of successful feeding for ultrasonography of the infant's oral cavity during feeding. Axial and coronal projections were studied during active feeding (Fig. 1).

A high-resolution, real-time mechanical sector scanner with a 5 MHz transducer was used for ultrasound imaging. The studies were recorded on videotape, and the images were evaluated by step-frame analysis with use of a videotape editor. The changes in the dimensions of the artificial nipple during three active suck cycles were measured in each plane with a Helios Dial Caliper (Helios, Inc., Longmont, Colo.). The measurements were repeated by two of the investigators independently, and interexaminer and intraexaminer agreement was within 0.5 mm.

In the axial plane, the ratio of the length of the nipple at full suck to the length of the nipple at rest describes the percentage increase in length during sucking. The ratio of the axial width of the nipple at full suck to the width of the nipple at rest describes the percentage increase in lateral (side-to-side) compression. The coronal axis is used to measure the percentage increase in nipple flattening, determined by the ratio of the height of the nipple at maximum compression to the height of the nipple at rest (Figs. 1 and 2).

The results with the new artificial nipple were compared with similar data obtained from a previous study of 16 breast-fed infants[3] by using a Student *t* test (SAS Version 6; SAS Institute, Cary, N.C.).

RESULTS

Images obtained in the axial plane (with use of the horizontal transbuccal approach) during active suck on the new tricut nipple and the human nipple are shown in Fig. 3. Infants fed with the tricut nipple had sucking mechanisms similar to those of breast-fed infants. The infant's tongue-

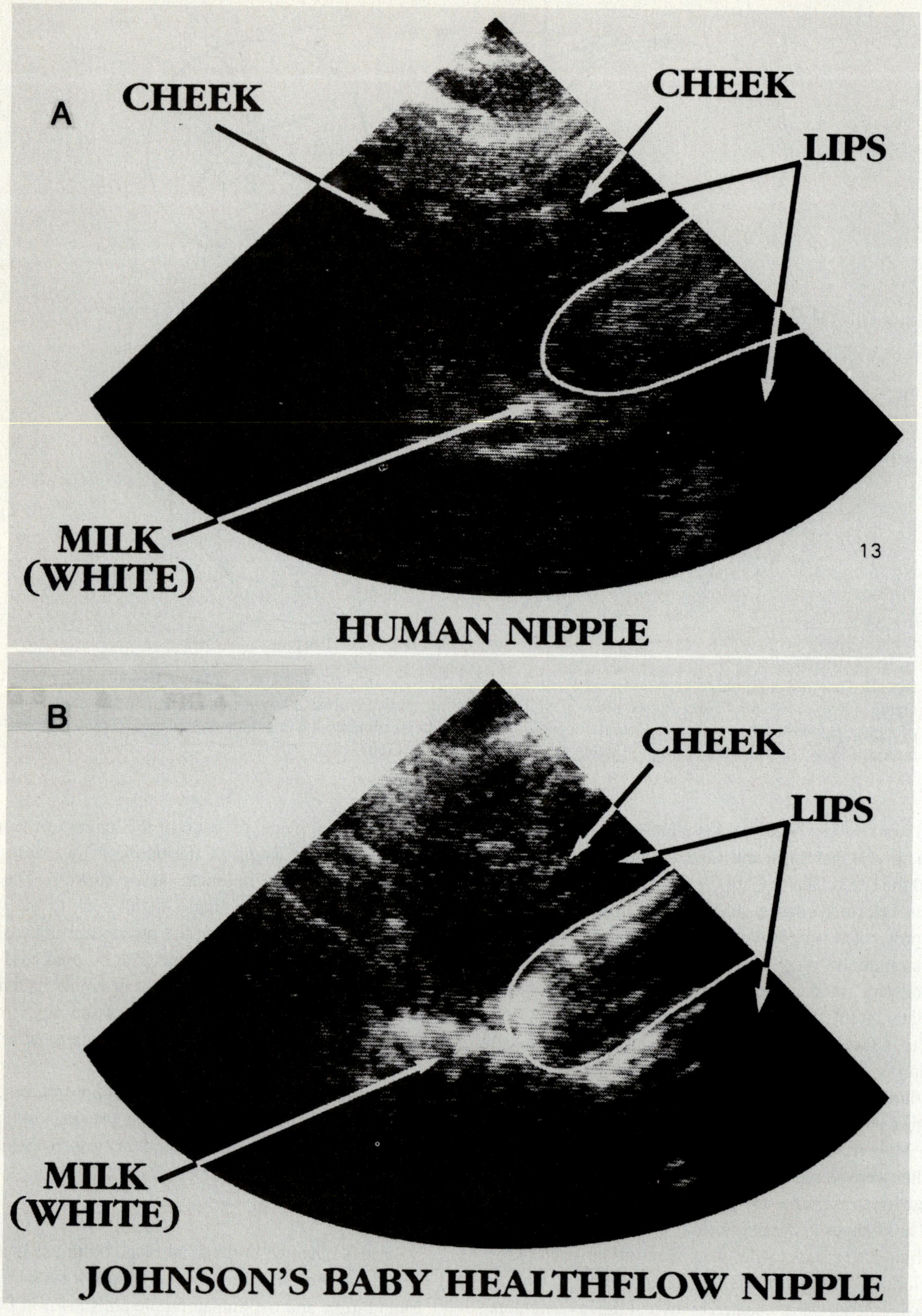

Fig. 3. Axial ultrasound study of human nipple (**A**) and a new artificial nipple (**B**) within oral cavity during feeding. Note elongation of human nipple versus artificial nipple. Infants' lips appear at *right* of image; light material beyond tip of nipple is milk.

Table I. Percent change in dimensions of tricut nipple during suck

Axial length		Axial compression		Coronal compression	
Mean	SD	Mean	SD	Mean	SD
122.2	6.4	78.5	12.8	69.0	11.1

Percentages calculated as (Dimension at Maximum Suck/Resting Dimension) × 100. Resting dimension is 100%.

Table II. Comparison between human breast and tricut nipple: Percent change in dimensions of nipples during suck

	Axial length		Axial compression		Coronal compression	
	Mean	SD	Mean	SD	Mean	SD
Breast	208.5	4.6	73.6	2.5	56.1	1.5
Tricut nipple	122.28	6.4	78.51	12.8	69.06	11.1
	$p = 0.0001$*		$p = 0.54$		$p = 0.0068$*	

*Significant at p ≤0.05, Student *t*-test (SAS Version 6).

jaw-hyoid axis was elevated, the infant pulled on the nipple and elongated it, and the milk was ejected in response to negative pressure after the infant's tongue elevated to meet the nipple, slightly after the nipple reached maximal elongation.

The new tricut nipple elongated during feeding to interact with the tongue; however, it was not as elastic as the human nipple. The tricut nipple reached a maximal lengthening ratio of 122.2% ± 6.4% (Table I).

In the axial plane, the tricut nipple was readily compressible and penetrated into the oral pharynx because of its manufactured length. The axial compression, but not the coronal compression, was nearly identical to that of the human nipple during active feeding (Table II).

Like other artificial nipples, the tricut nipple formed a tight seal when an infant's lips and cheeks were positioned around the nipple. An effective seal is critical if an infant is to generate adequate sucking pressure.[5] The dorsum of the tongue forms a groove to conduct milk backward, and the tongue elevates to compress the epiglottis and close the nasopharynx.

DISCUSSION

This study and others[2-4, 6, 7] have demonstrated that real-time ultrasonography can be useful for visualizing intraoral events during feeding. Changes in the dimensions of human and artificial nipples can be measured and compared on the basis of information generated by noninvasive ultrasonography.

When infant feeding is observed, the timing of images is critical. Nutritive suck occurs in bursts punctuated by pauses. Suck rates in term infants range from 40 to 100 per minute. Although the suck rate remains fairly constant, the pauses increase as an infant becomes satiated. Thus, sucking patterns and nipple management can vary widely throughout a feeding. In our studies, therefore, ultrasound examinations were confined to the first 2 minutes of active feeding.

Our results with the tricut nipple indicate that one of the principal differences between the human and the artificial nipple is elongation. In active feeding, the human nipple stretches to more than 200% of its resting length. This elasticity probably represents an advantage for the infant because the elongation enables the nipple to deliver milk to the foramen cecum region at the posterior of the tongue. Therefore, once the milk is ejected from the breast, swallowing is automatic or reflexive in nature.

Because the tricut nipple is designed to be longer in the axial plane, it stretches to 120% of its resting length. Even so, it delivers milk to the posterior of the tongue. Greater elasticity does not appear to be necessary, because the resting length of the tricut nipple is almost twice that of the human nipple.

As is true for the breast, milk expression from the tricut nipple occurs in response to the vacuum created by negative pressure caused by the rapid enlargement of the infant's oral cavity. Additional studies are necessary to evaluate other properties of the tricut nipple, such as milk-flow characteristics and the pressure generated by the infant during sucking.

In our experience, ultrasound imaging of an infant's oral cavity during feeding has been of value in diagnosing various feeding disorders. It is our hope that data on artificial nipples from studies such as this will be helpful in identifying artificial devices that are optimal for feeding infants with these disorders.

REFERENCES

1. Ardran GM, Kemp FH. A correlation between suckling pressure and the movements of the tongue. Acta Paediatr Scand 1959;48:261-72.
2. Smith WL, Erenberg A, Nowak A, Franken E. Physiology of sucking in the normal term infant using real-time US. Radiology 1985;156:379-81.
3. Smith WL, Erenberg A, Nowak A. Imaging evaluation of the human nipple during breast-feeding. Am J Dis Child 1988; 142:76-8.
4. Nowak A, Smith WL, Erenberg A. Imaging evaluation of artificial nipples during bottle-feeding. Arch Pediatr Adolesc Med 1994;148:40-2.
5. Matthew OP. Science of bottle feeding. J PEDIATR 1991; 119:511-9.
6. Weber F, Woolridge MW, Baum JD. An ultrasonographic study of the organisation of sucking and swallowing by newborn infants. Dev Med Child Neurol 1986;28:19-24.
7. Bu'Lock F, Woolridge MW, Baum JD. Development of co-ordination of sucking, swallowing and breathing: ultrasound study of term and preterm infants. Dev Med Child Neurol 1990;32:669-78.